Chronic Kidney Disease, Dialysis, and Transplantation

A Companion to Brenner and Rector's The Kidney

Chronic Kidney Disease, Dialysis, and Transplantation

A Companion to Brenner and Rector's The Kidney

Second Edition

Brian J.G. Pereira, M.D., M.B.A.
Professor of Medicine
Tufts University School of Medicine
President and Chief Executive Officer, NEHCF
Tufts-New England Medical Center
Boston, Massachusetts

Mohamed H. Sayegh, M.D., F.A.H.A
Director, Transplantation Research Center
Brigham and Women's Hospital
Associate Professor of Medicine
Harvard Medical School
Boston, Massachusetts

Peter G. Blake, M.B., F.R.C.P.C., F.R.C.P.I
Professor of Medicine
University of Western Ontario
Chair of Nephrology
London Health Sciences Center
London, Ontario, Canada

SECTION EDITORS

Vaidyanathapuram S. Balakrishnan, M.D., M.R.C.P.
Assistant Professor
Tufts University School of Medicine
Division of Nephrology, Department of Medicine
Tufts-New England Medical Center
Boston, Massachusetts

Bertrand L. Jaber, M.D.
Assistant Professor
Tufts University School of Medicine
Vice-Chairman, Department of Medicine
Caritas-St. Elizabeth's Medical Center
Boston, Massachusetts

Annamaria T. Kausz, M.D., M.S.
Assistant Professor of Medicine
Tufts-University School of Medicine
Division of Nephrology, Department of Medicine
Tufts-New England Medical Center
Boston, Massachusetts

Colm C. Magee, M.D., M.P.H.
Instructor in Medicine
Harvard Medical School
Staff Physician
Renal Division
Brigham and Women's Hospital
Boston, Massachusetts

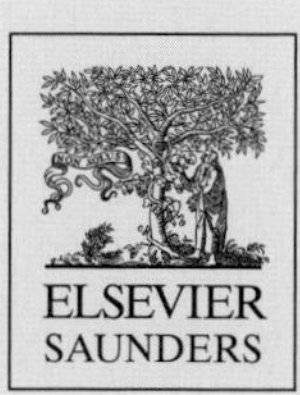

ELSEVIER
SAUNDERS
An Imprint of Elsevier

The Curtis Center
170 S Independence Mall W 300E
Philadelphia, Pennsylvania 19106

Chronic Kidney Disease, Dialysis, and Transplantation
A Companion to Brenner and Rector's The Kidney
Second Edition

ISBN: 1-4160-0158-1

NOTICE

Nephrology is an ever-changing field. Standard safety precautions must be followed, but as new research and clinical experience broaden our knowledge, changes in treatment and drug therapy may become necessary or appropriate. Readers are advised to check the most current product information provided by the manufacturer of each drug to be administered to verify the recommended dose, the method and duration of administration, and contraindications. It is the responsibility of the licensed prescriber, relying on experience and knowledge of the patient, to determine dosages and the best treatment for each individual patient. Neither the publisher nor the author assumes any liability for any injury and/or damage to persons or property arising from this publication.

Previous edition copyrighted 2000.

Library of Congress Cataloging-in-Publication Data

Chronic kidney disease, dialysis, and transplantation : a companion to Brenner and Rector's the kidney / [edited by Brian J.G. Pereira, Mohamed Sayegh, Peter Blake.–2nd ed.
p. ; cm.
Rev. ed. of: Dialysis and transplantation / [edited by] William F. Owen Jr., Brian J.G. Pereira, Mohamed H. Sayegh. 1st ed. c2000.
Includes bibliographical references and index.
ISBN 1-4160-0158-1
1. Hemodialysis. 2. Kidneys–Transplantation. I. Pereira, Brian J. G. II. Sayegh, Mohamed H. III. Blake, Peter Gerard, 1956- IV. Dialysis and transplantation. V. Brenner & Rector's the kidney.
[DNLM: 1. Renal Dialysis. 2. Kidney Failure, Chronic–therapy. 3. Kidney Transplantation. WJ 378 C55675 2005]
RC901.7.H45D5226 2005
616.6'1–dc22

2004051160

Acquisitions Editor: Susan Pioli
Developmental Editor: Alison Nastasi
Publishing Services Manager: Joan Sinclair
Project Manager: Cecelia Bayruns

Printed in China

Last digit is the print number: 9 8 7 6 5 4 3 2 1

To my wife, Sunita,
and children, Natasha and Nikhil,
for their constant support and understanding

To my mentors,
Drs. Kirpal Chugh, Nicolaos Madias,
and Andrew Levey
Brian J. G. Pereira

To my two brothers,
Dr. Sard H. Sayegh and Abdul Hafiz H. Sayegh,
for their continuous support of my career
through the years
Mohamed H. Sayegh

Thank you to Rose
for all her love and support
and to Matthew and Andrew
for keeping me grounded
Peter G. Blake

Contents

Contributors

Stuart Abramson, M.D., M.P.H.
Maine Nephrology Associates, Portland, Maine

Miriam J. Alter, Ph.D.
Associate Director for Epidemiologic Science, Division of Viral Hepatitis, Centers for Disease Control and Prevention, Atlanta, Georgia

Matthew J. Arduino, M.S., Dr.P.H.
Supervisory Research Microbiologist, Division of Healthcare Quality Promotion, Centers for Disease Control and Prevention, Atlanta, Georgia

George R. Aronoff, M.D., F.A.C.P.
Professor of Medicine and Pharmacology; Chief, Division of Nephrology, Department of Medicine, University of Louisville School of Medicine, Louisville, Kentucky

Vaidyanathapuram S. Balakrishnan, M.D., M.R.C.P.
Assistant Professor, Tufts University School of Medicine, Division of Nephrology, Department of Medicine, Tufts-New England Medical Center, Boston, Massachusetts

Joanne M. Bargman, M.D., F.R.C.P.C.
Professor of Medicine, University of Toronto; Staff Nephrologist, University Health Network, Toronto, Ontario, Canada

Peter G. Blake, M.B., F.R.C.P.C., F.R.C.P.I
Professor of Medicine,University of Western Ontario, Chair of Nephrology, London Health Sciences Center, London, Ontario, Canada

Joseph V. Bonventre, M.D., Ph.D.
Professor of Medicine, Harvard Medical School; Division Chief, Renal Section, Brigham and Women's Hospital, Boston, Massachusetts

Marilia Cascalho, M.D., Ph.D.
Director, Transplantation Biology, Departments of Surgery, Immunology and Pediatrics, Mayo Clinic, Rochester, Minnesota

Vimal Chadha, M.D.
Assistant Professor of Pediatrics, Virginia Commonwealth University Medical Center, Chair, Section of Pediatric Nephrology, Richmond, Virginia

Christopher T. Chan, M.D., F.R.C.P.C.
Medical Director-Home Hemodialysis, Division of Nephrology, Toronto General Hospital, University Health Network; Assistant Professor–Faculty of Medicine, University of Toronto, Toronto, Ontario, Canada

Anil Chandraker, M.D., C.H.B., M.R.C.P.
Transplant Research Center, Brigham and Women's Hospital, Boston, Massachusetts

Glenn M. Chertow, M.D., M.P.H.
Associate Professor, Division of Nephrology, Department of Medicine, University of California, San Francisco, School of Medicine, San Francisco, California

William R. Clark, M.D.
Clinical Assistant Professor of Medicine, Indiana University School of Medicine; Baxter Healthcare, Indianapolis, Indiana

Allan J. Collins, M.D., F.A.C.P.
Professor of Medicine, University of Minnesota, Minneapolis, Minnesota

Josef Coresh, M.D., Ph.D., M.H.S.
Professor, Departments of Epidemiology and Biostatistics, Johns Hopkins University School of Hygiene and Public Health; Professor, Department of Medicine, Johns Hopkins University School of Medicine, Baltimore, Maryland

Bryan M. Curtis, M.D., F.R.C.P.C.
Kidney Foundation of Canada Research Fellow, Division of Nephrology and Clinical Epidemiology Unit, Patient Research Centre, Health Sciences Centre, Memorial University of Newfoundland Faculty of Medicine, St. John's, Newfoundland, Canada

Gabriel M. Danovitch, M.D.
Professor of Medicine and Medical Director, Kidney Transplant Program, University of California, Los Angeles, David Geffen School of Medicine, Los Angeles, California

Simon J. Davies, M.D., F.R.C.P.
Professor, Institute of Science and Technology in Medicine, Keele University, Keele, England; Clinical Director, Department of Nephrology, University Hospital of North Staffordshire, Stoke-on-Trent, England

Francis L. Delmonico, M.D.
Professor of Surgery, Harvard Medical School; Director of Renal Transplantation, Massachusetts General Hospital, Boston, Massachusetts

Laura M. Dember, M.D.
Associate Professor of Medicine, Boston University School of Medicine; Director of Dialysis, Boston University Medical Center, Boston, Massachusetts

Thomas A. Depner, M.D.
Professor, Department of Internal Medicine, University of California, Davis, School of Medicine; Medical Director, University Dialysis Clinic, Sacramento, California

Rita De Smet, M.Sc., Ing.
Renal Division, Department of Internal Medicine, University Hospital Ghent, Ghent, Belgium

Bradley S. Dixon, M.D.
Associate Professor, Department of Internal Medicine, University of Iowa, Iowa City, Iowa

Jeremy S. Duffield, M.R.C.P., Ph. D.
Renal Fellow/NKRF Senior Fellow, Harvard Institutes of Medicine (BWH), Boston, Massachusetts

Nahel Elias, M.D.
Department of Surgery, Harvard Medical School; Massachusetts General Hospital, Boston, Massachusetts

Joseph A. Eustace, M.B., M.H.S., M.R.C.P.I.
Assistant Professor, Departments of Medicine and Epidemiology, Johns Hopkins University School of Medicine; Medical Director, Bond Street Dialysis Unit, Johns Hopkins University Hospital, Baltimore, Maryland

Martin S. Favero, Ph.D.
Director, Scientific and Clinical Affairs, Advanced Sterilization Products, Johnson & Johnson, Irvine, California

Steven Fishbane, M.D.
Associate Professor of Medicine, State University of New York (SUNY) at Stony Brook School of Medicine, Stony Brook, New York; Director of the Dialysis Network, Associate Chairman of Medicine, and Associate Director of Nephrology, Winthrop-University Hospital, Mineola, New York

Jay A. Fishman, M.D.
Director, Transplant Infectious Disease & Compromised Host Program, Massachusetts General Hospital; Associate Professor of Medicine, Harvard Medical School, Boston, Massachusetts

Dayong Gao, Professor
UK Alumni Professor of Mechanical Engineering, University of Kentucky, College of Engineering, Department of Mechanical Engineering, Lexington, Kentucky

John S. Gill, M.D., M.S.
Assistant Professor of Medicine, University Of British Columbia, St. Paul's Hospital, Vancouver, B.C., Canada; Adjunct Assistant Professor, Division of Nephrology, Department of Medicine, Tufts-New England Medical Center, Boston, Massachusetts

Griet Glorieux, M.Sc., Ph.D.
Renal Division, Department of Internal Medicine, University Hospital Ghent, Ghent, Belgium

Simin Goral, M.D.
Associate Professor of Medicine, Division of Nephrology, University of Pennsylvania Medical Center, Philadelphia, Pennsylvania

William E. Harmon, M.D.
Division of Nephrology, Department of Medicine, Harvard Medical School; Department of Nephrology, Children's Hospital, Boston, Massachusetts

Olof Heimbürger, M.D., Ph.D.
Division of Renal Medicine, Department of Clinical Science, Karolinska Instituet, and Senior Physician, Department of Renal Medicine, Karolinska University Hospital at Huddinge, Stockholm, Sweden

J. Harold Helderman, M.D.
Professor of Medicine, Microbiology, and Immunology; Chief, Renal Transplant Program; Medical Director, Vanderbilt Transplant Center, Vanderbilt University Medical Center, Nashville, Tennessee

Lee W. Henderson, M.D., F.A.C.P.
Renal Division, Baxter Healthcare Corporation, McGaw Park, Illinois

Jonathan Himmelfarb, M.D.
Clinical Professor of Medicine, University of Vermont College of Medicine, Burlington, Vermont; Director of Nephrology and Transplantation, Maine Medical Center, Portland, Maine

Michelle Hladunewich, M.D.
Assistant Professor of Medicine, University of Toronto Hospitals, Toronto, Ontario, Canada

Zhongping Huang, M.D.
Department of Mechanical Engineering, University of Kentucky, Lexington, Kentucky

Bertrand L. Jaber, M.D.
Assistant Professor, Tufts University School of Medicine; Vice-Chairman, Department of Medicine Caritas-St. Elizabeth's Medical Center, Boston, Massachusetts

Dicken S.C. Ko, M.D., F.R.C.S.(C.), F.A.C.S.
Assistant Professor of Surgery, Departments of Surgery and Urology, Harvard Medical School; Massachusetts General Hospital, Boston, Massachusetts

Holly Kramer, M.D., M.P.H.
Department of Preventive Medicine and Epidemiology, Loyola University Medical Center, Maywood, Illinois

Alan M. Krensky, M.D.
Stanford University, Stanford, California

Richard Lafayette, M.D.
Associate Professor of Medicine; Associate Chairman, Clinical Affairs, Department of Medicine, Stanford University School of Medicine; Clinical Chief, Division of Nephrology, Stanford University Medical Center, Stanford, California

Norbert Hendrik Lameire, M.D., Ph.D.
Professor of Medicine, Renal Division, Department of Internal Medicine, University Hospital Ghent, Ghent, Belgium

James P. Lash, M.D.
Associate Professor of Clinical Medicine; Program Director, Nephrology Fellowship, Section of Nephrology, Department of Medicine, University of Illinois at Chicago College of Medicine; University of Illinois at Chicago Medical Center, Chicago, Illinois

Adeera Levin, M.D., F.R.C.P.C.
Professor of Medicine, Division of Nephrology, University of British Columbia Faculty of Medicine; St. Paul's Hospital, Vancouver, British Columbia, Canada

John K. Leypoldt, Ph.D.
Research Professor of Medicine and Adjunct Professor of Bioengineering, Dialysis Program, University of Utah; Veterans Affairs Salt Lake City Health Care System, Salt Lake City, Utah

Philip Kam-Tao Li, M.D., F.R.C.P., F.A.C.P.
Chief of Nephrology and Consultant Physician, Department of Medicine & Therapeutics, Prince of Wales Hospital; Chinese University of Hong Kong, Hong Kong

Orfeas Liangos, M.D.
Clinical Research Fellow, Division of Nephrology, Tufts-New England Medical Center, Boston, Massachusetts

Colm C. Magee, M.D., M.P.H.
Instructor in Medicine, Harvard Medical School, Staff Physiscian Renal Division, Brigham and Women's Hospital, Boston, Massachusetts

Naveed Masani, M.D.
Attending Nephrologist, Winthrop-University Hospital, Mineola, New York

Tahsin Masud, M.D.
Assistant Professor of Medicine, Department of Medicine, Renal Division, Emory University School of Medicine, Atlanta, Georgia

Philip McFarlane, M.D., F.R.C.P.C.
Associate Professor of Medicine, University of Toronto Faculty of Medicine; Medical Director, Home Dialysis, Division of Nephrology, St. Michael's Hospital, Toronto, Ontario, Canada

Ravindra L. Mehta, M.B.B.S., M.D., F.A.C.P.
Professor of Clinical Medicine, Associate Chair for Clinical Affairs, Department of Medicine, Division of Nephrology, University of California, School of Medicine, San Diego, California

David C. Mendelssohn, M.D., F.R.C.P.C.
Associate Professor of Medicine, University of Toronto Faculty of Medicine, Toronto, Ontario, Canada; Head, Division of Nephrology, Medical Director of Dialysis, Humber River Regional Hospital, Weston, Ontario, Canada

William E. Mitch, M.D.
Edward Randall Distinguished Professor of Medicine; Department of Medicine, University of Texas Medical Branch at Galveston, Galveston, Texas

Sharon M. Moe, M.D.
Associate Professor of Medicine, Associate Dean for Research Support, Indiana University School of Medicine; Director of Nephrology, Wishard Memorial Hospital, Indianapolis, Indiana

Anupama Mohanram, M.D.
Renal Fellow, UT Southwestern Medical Center, Dallas, Texas

Donald A. Molony, M.D.
Professor of Medicine, Department of Internal Medicine, Division of Renal Diseases and Hypertension, University of Texas Houston Medical School, Houston, Texas

Bhamidipati V.R. Murthy, M.D., D.M.
Assistant Professor, Department of Internal Medicine, Division of Renal Diseases and Hypertension, University of Texas Houston Medical School, Houston, Texas

Nader Najafian, M.D.
Instructor of Medicine, Harvard Medical School; Renal Division, Brigham and Women's Hospital; Transplantation Research Center, Brigham and Women's Hospital and Children's Hospital, Boston, Massachusetts

Cynthia Nast, M.D.
Professor of Pathology, Department of Pathology, David Geffen School of Medicine at UCLA and Cedars Sinai Medical Center, Los Angeles, California

Gihad E. Nesrallah, M.D., F.R.C.P.C., F.A.C.P.
Staff Nephrologist, Division of Nephrology, Department of Internal Medicine, Humber River Regional Hospital, Toronto, Ontario, Canada

Daniel Norman, M.D.
Division of Pulmonary, Critical Care and Sleep Medicine, Beth Israel Deaconess Medical Center, Harvard Medical School, Boston, Massachusetts

Brenda M. Ogle, Ph.D.
Director, Transplantation Biology, Departments of Surgery, Immunology and Pediatrics, Mayo Clinic, Rochester, Minnesota

Yvonne M. O'Meara, M.D.
Department of Nephrology, Mater Hospital, Dublin, Ireland

Dimitrios G. Oreopoulos, M.D., Ph.D., F.R.C.P.C., F.A.C.P.
Professor of Medicine, Toronto Western Hospital, Toronto, Ontario, Canada

Brian J.G. Pereira, M.D., M.B.A.
Professor of Medicine, Tufts University School of Medicine, President and Chief Executive Officer, NEHCF, Tufts-New England Medical Center, Boston, Massachusetts

Phuong-Chi T. Pham, M.D.
Associate Professor of Medicine, Division of Nephrology, Department of Medicine, David Geffen School of Medicine at UCLA and Olive View–UCLA Medical Center, Sylmar, California

Phuong-Thu T. Pham, M.D.
Assistant Professor of Medicine, Nephrology Division, Kidney and Pancreas Transplantation, Department of Medicine, University of California, Los Angeles, David Geffen School of Medicine, Los Angeles, California

Andreas Pierratos, M.D., F.R.C.P.C.
Associate Professor of Medicine, University of Toronto Faculty of Medicine, Toronto, Ontario, Canada; Humber River Regional Hospital, Weston, Ontario, Canada

Jeffrey L. Platt, M.D.
Director, Transplantation Biology, Departments of Surgery, Immunology and Pediatrics, Mayo Clinic, Rochester, Minnesota

Sarah Prichard, M.D., F.R.C.P.C.
Professor of Medicine, Division of Nephrology, Department of Medicine, McGill University Faculty of Medicine, Montreal, Quebec, Canada

Emilio Ramos, M.D.
University of Maryland School of Medicine, Division of Nephrology, Baltimore, Maryland

Madhumathi Rao, M.D., F.R.C.P. (U.K.)
Instructor of Medicine, Division of Nephrology, Department of Medicine, Turfts University School of Medicine; Tufts-New England Medical Center, Boston, Massachusetts

Denise Sadlier, M.B., M.R.C.P.I.
Department of Medicine and Therapeutics, Mater Misericordiae University Hospital, Conway Institute of Biomolecular and Biomedical Research, University College Dublin; Dublin Molecular Medicine Centre, Dublin, Ireland

Mark J. Sarnak, MD
Associate Director, Research Training Program, and Assistant Professor, Division of Nephrology, Department of Medicine, Tufts University School of Medicine; Tufts-New England Medical Center, Boston, Massachusetts

Robert C. Stanton, M.D.
Assistant Professor in Medicine, Harvard Medical School; Chief, Nephrology Section, Joslin Diabetes Center, Boston, Massachusetts

Rita Suri, M.D., F.R.C.P.C.
Staff Nephrologist, London Health Sciences Centre and Assistant Professor of Medicine, University of Western Ontario, London, Canada

Cheuk-Chun Szeto, M.D., M.R.C.P.
Department of Medicine & Therapeutics, Prince of Wales Hospital, Shatin, Hong Kong

Geoffrey S. Teehan, M.D., M.S.
Division of Nephrology, Department of Medicine, Tufts-New England Medical Center, Boston, Massachusetts

Elias D. Thodis, M.D.
Assistant Professor of Nephrology, Demokritus University of Thrace, Alexandroupolis, Greece

Robert Thomas, MD
Division of Pulmonary, Critical Care and Sleep Medicine, Beth Israel Deaconess Medical Center, Harvard Medical School, Boston, Massachusetts

Jerome Tokars, M.D., M.P.H.
Medical Epidemiologist, Division of Healthcare Quality Promotion, Centers for Disease Control and Prevention, Atlanta, Georgia

Robert D. Toto, M.D.
Professor of Medicine; Director, Patient-Oriented Research in Nephrology, University of Texas Southwestern Medical Center, Dallas, Texas

Kathryn Tuohy, M.D.
Division of General Internal Medicine, Brown Medical School; Rhode Island Hospital, Providence, Rhode Island

Raymond Camille Vanholder, M.D., Ph.D.
Professor of Medicine, Renal Division, Department of Internal Medicine, University Hospital Ghent, Ghent, Belgium

Vassilis Vargemezis, M.D.
Department of Renal Medicine, Democritus University of Thrace, University Hospital, Alexandroupolis, Greece

Flavio Vincenti, M.D.
Professor of Clinical Medicine, Kidney Transplant Service, Department of Medicine, University of California, San Francisco, School of Medicine, San Francisco, California

Bradley A. Warady, M.D.
Professor of Pediatrics, University of Missouri-Kansas City School of Medicine; Associate Chair of Pediatrics, Chief, Section of Pediatric Nephrology; Director, Dialysis and Transplantation; The Children's Mercy Hospital, Kansas City, Missouri

Daniel E. Weiner, M.D., M.S.
Division of Nephrology, Department of Medicine, Tufts-New England Medical Center, Boston, Massachusetts

Mark E. Williams, M.D., F.A.C.P.
Associate Clinical Professor in Medicine, Harvard Medical School; Nephrology Section, Joslin Diabetes Center, Boston, Massachusetts

Jane Y. Yeun, M.D.
Associate Professor, Director, Nephrology Fellowship Program, University of California Davis Health Center, Department of Medicine, Sacramento, California; Staff Nephrologist, Sacramento Veterans Administration Medical Center, Department of Medicine, Mather, California

Preface

For the past two decades, *The Kidney,* by Drs. Barry M. Brenner and Floyd Rector, has been the central resource for authoritative and current information in the field of nephrology. However, the continuing expansion in the understanding of the pathophysiology and management of kidney diseases, dialysis, and transplantation and rapid advances in technology led to the need for more focused accompaniments to *The Kidney.* Consequently, a series of companion textbooks emerged; the first edition of our textbook, *Dialysis and Transplantation,* was the second in this series. The intent of our initial venture was to provide readers with a seamless flow of information regarding the management of the patient with end-stage renal disease (ESRD), including hemodialysis, peritoneal dialysis, and transplantation. In pursuit of this goal, we sought to provide an overview of the principles of management of the patient with ESRD as well as a more focused examination of the physiologic principles and clinical application of the different modes of kidney replacement therapy.

Since the release of the first edition of our textbook, there have been tremendous advances in the field of kidney disease. The publication of the National Kidney Foundation Kidney Disease Outcomes Quality Initiative (NKF KDOQI) guidelines has led to a new nomenclature and staging of patients with chronic kidney disease (CKD) and has focused the nephrology community on the magnitude of the problem. Since most of the comorbidity and complications of CKD begin early in the course of the disease, we have chosen to expand the scope of this textbook to include the entire spectrum of CKD, including the period prior to dialysis or transplantation. Hence the new title, *Chronic Kidney Disease, Dialysis, and Transplantation.* We undertook this revision with the understanding that the treatment of patients with ESRD is complex, and the field is rapidly changing. The past few years have witnessed new frontiers in the understanding of the pathophysiology, prevalence, and possible interventions with respect to cardiovascular disease, other comorbidity, and complications of CKD. Likewise, there has been considerable progress in the study of the physiologic basis of dialysis and its complications and the immunologic basis of allograft tolerance and rejection. Advances in pharmaceutical technology and biotechnology have brought new and effective therapies into clinical use, and the results of several pivotal clinical trials have challenged established concepts in patient management. Finally, the continuing efforts of professional societies to improve the quality of patient care have resulted in the development of new evidence-based clinical practice guidelines and clinical performance measures. These developments have mandated a new look at the management of the patient with CKD. Consequently, we invited distinguished scientists and educators in the field of kidney disease to provide an in-depth review—from the laboratory to the clinic. Each author was challenged to discuss the fundamental concepts behind the management of the patient with ESRD, to provide a comprehensive critique of clinical trials, and to present rational recommendations for clinical treatment.

Our strategy was to cover the most clinically relevant issues in dialysis and transplantation and to classify them under the broad sections of CKD, complications of CKD, hemodialysis, peritoneal dialysis, transplantation, acute renal failure, and economic issues. Each section was overseen by a section editor. Each chapter is self-contained and provides the reader with a thorough review of the subject along with a complete list of key references. Diagnostic and treatment algorithms have been used whenever possible. With an eye on the future, our contributors were encouraged to identify major unanswered questions, to suggest future clinical trials, and to highlight promising experimental strategies. We have applied a strong editorial policy to ensure that chapters remain balanced and that they conform to these principles. The editorial team has changed; Dr William Owen has departed and Dr. Peter G. Blake has joined us. In addition, we have had the privilege of working with an extraordinary team of section editors, Drs. Bertrand L. Jaber, V. S. Balakrishnan, Annamaria T. Kausz, and Colm Magee, who have brought additional rigor and vitality to the process

In summary, we endeavored to significantly revise the first edition of out textbook, *Dialysis and Transplantation,* and substantially expanded the scope in this edition, *Chronic Kidney Disease, Dialysis, and Transplantation.* Readers are encouraged to refer to *The Kidney* or other companions in this series for a detailed discussion of other issues in nephrology. We intend to maintain this textbook as a work in progress and to update it periodically as the relentless advances in the field mandate. During the coming years, we welcome comments, critiques, and suggestions from our readers as we strive to deliver a comprehensive and contemporary textbook on dialysis and transplantation.

Brian J.G. Pereira
Mohamed H. Sayegh
Peter G. Blake
EDITORS

Chronic Kidney Disease, Dialysis, and Transplantation

A Companion to Brenner and Rector's The Kidney

SECTION A

Chronic Kidney Disease

Chapter 1

Chronic Kidney Disease: Definition and Epidemiology

Joseph A. Eustace, M.B., M.H.S., M.R.C.P.I. •
Josef Coresh, M.D., Ph.D.

The developed world is suffering from an epidemic of kidney disease, the full spectrum of which is only beginning to be understood. Figure 1–1 illustrates the "pyramid" of chronic kidney disease (CKD), including estimates of the number of individuals at each stage in the United States. Kidney failure is the most visible aspect of this spectrum, but it represents only a minority of the total population affected by kidney disease. In the United States the age, race, and gender adjusted incidence of kidney failure requiring maintenance renal replacement therapy (that is, who have end-stage renal disease, ESRD) has increased over threefold in the last two decades, to a current rate of 334 persons per million population (pmp).[1] Although the annual rate of increase in the incidence rate has slowed to less than 1% for the last 2 years, given the expected demographic trends in the general population, by 2030 there are projected to be 2.2 million Americans who will require maintenance dialysis or kidney transplantation.[1] Similar trends, though of lesser magnitude, have been reported worldwide. In different national registries the rate of increase in incidence has uniformly been highest in the elderly. The U.S. race and gender adjusted incidence rates in subjects older than 75 years is 100-fold higher than those of individuals younger than 20 years, while globally the burden of kidney disease is disproportionately borne by the socially disadvantaged and by racial minorities.[1]

In addition to those patients with ESRD, at least 8.0 million Americans were estimated to have moderately or severely decreased kidney function, CKD stages III–IV.[2] The extent to which changes in the prevalence of CKD parallel the increase in ESRD over the last decade is unknown. The presence of CKD is clinically important, not only because such patients are at increased risk of progressing to kidney failure, but also because CKD is independently associated with complications that are likely to directly contribute to poor health-related outcomes, the most important of which is increased cardiovascular disease morbidity and mortality. As a result, a person over age 65 with severe CKD is several times more likely to die than to progress to requiring dialysis.[1] Increasing evidence suggests that some of the increased mortality risk is the result of CKD and that some of this attributable risk is amenable to intervention.

In recognition of the current health crisis associated with kidney failure, with its ever increasing prevalence, morbidity, mortality, and great cost ($20 billion for the U.S. ESRD program in 2000), the most recent U.S. Public Health strategy, "Healthy People, 2010," has for the first time devoted a separate chapter to CKD. Unfortunately, despite the evident importance of CKD we have very limited data on its epidemiology within the general population. Renal failure registry data is unlikely to be representative of the broader spectrum of CKD, while clinical reports, by necessity, emphasize forms of kidney disease that more readily come to clinical attention. The epidemiology of CKD is, therefore, incompletely described and much of the available data is not generalizable. What is known is that there is a wide degree of variability both within and between countries in the occurrence, clinical characteristics, and outcomes of patients with kidney failure and that there has been substantial changes in these parameters over time.

DEFINITION OF CHRONIC KIDNEY DISEASE

Terminology

Investigation of the epidemiology of CKD has to date been hampered by the lack of a uniform terminology. Traditionally, a wide and confusing combination of expressions, in English, Latin, and ancient Greek, have been used interchangeably to describe a persistent decrement in kidney function.[3] To help introduce a uniform terminology the National Kidney Foundation (NKF) in its Kidney Disease Outcomes Quality Initiative (KDOQI) has recently proposed a formal definition for CKD (Table 1–1).[2] This definition provides a necessary and essential foundation to help standardize current medical

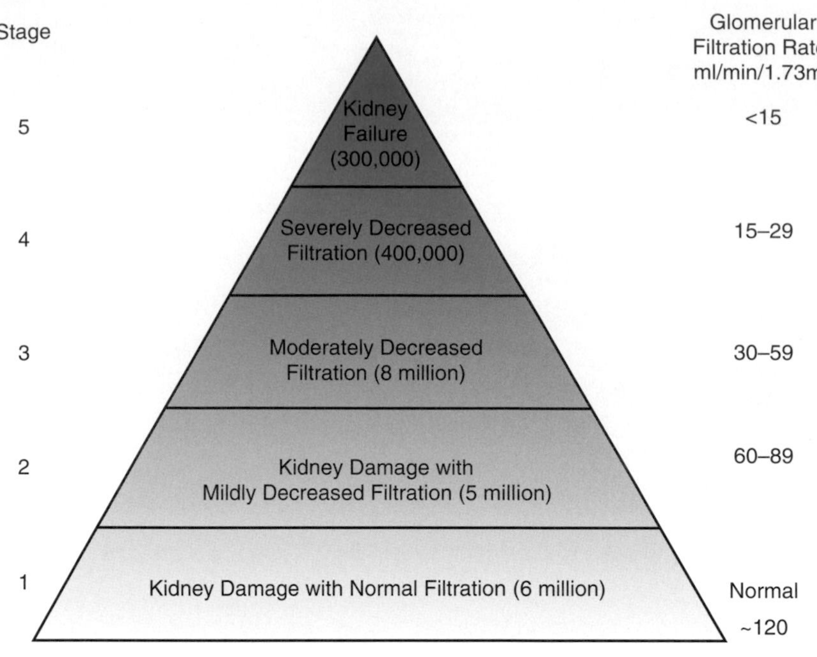

Figure 1-1 The spectrum of chronic kidney disease in the United States. *From USRDS (1988), includes approximately 230,000 patients treated by dialysis, and assuming 70,000 additional patients not on dialysis. Other estimates are from NHANES III (1988–1994): 15,600 individuals representing a U.S. population of 177 million age greater than age 20. Percentages total to greater than 100% because NHANES III may not have included dialysis patients. GFR estimated from serum creatinine using MDRD Study equation based on age, gender, race, and calibration for serum creatinine. For Stages 1 and 2, CKD is based on the persistence of positive spot albumin-to-creatinine ratio greater than or equal to 17 mg/g in men or greater than or equal to 25 mg/g in women. Persistence of microalbuminuria estimates are based on a subsample (54% of those with GFR>90, N= 102; 73% of those with GFR 60–90, N= 44).

Table 1-1 Definition of Chronic Kidney Disease

1. Kidney damage for ≥3 months, as defined by structural or functional abnormalities of the kidney, with or without decreased GFR, manifest by *either*:
   - Pathological abnormalities; or
   - Markers of kidney damage, including abnormalities in the composition of the blood or urine, or abnormalities in imaging tests
2. GFR <60 mL/min/1.73 m^2 for ≥3 months, with or without kidney damage

(From the National Kidney Foundation KD: Clinical Practice Guidelines for Chronic Kidney Disease: Evaluation, Classification, and Stratification. Am J Kidney Dis 2002; 39 (suppl 1): S1-S266. Copyright 2002, with permission from the National Kidney Foundation.)

Table 1-2 Stages of Chronic Kidney Disease

Stage	Description	GFR (mL/min/1.73 m^2)
1	Kidney damage with normal or ↑ GFR	≥90
2	Kidney damage with mild ↓ GFR	60–89
3	Moderate ↓ GFR	30–59
4	Severe ↓ GFR	15–29
5	Kidney failure	<15 (or dialysis)

Chronic kidney disease is defined as either kidney damage or GFR <60 mL/min/1.73 m^2 for ≥3 months. Kidney damage is defined as pathologic abnormalities or markers of damage, including abnormalities in blood or urine tests or imaging studies. (From the National Kidney Foundation KD: Clinical Practice Guidelines for Chronic Kidney Disease: Evaluation, Classification, and Stratification. Am J Kidney Dis 2002; 39 (suppl 1): S1-S266. Copyright 2002, with permission from the National Kidney Foundation.)

communication as well as to help make such communication more readily intelligible to the patient. It further serves to help identify and focus formal research in areas where it has traditionally been lacking, to facilitate appropriate population-based screening, and to encourage the timely prevention and treatment of kidney disease, as well as support formal quality improvement initiatives.

The NKF guidelines support the uniform use of the expression "chronic kidney disease" (CKD) to represent the entire spectrum of disease that occurs following the initiation of kidney damage. The severity of the resulting syndrome is denoted by a staging scheme that extends from occult kidney damage, with well-preserved function (stage I) down to the level of kidney failure requiring renal replacement therapy (stage V) (Table 1–2). As the English word *kidney* lacks a ready adjectival form, in this chapter we will continue to use the expression "renal" in this setting. We use the term *azotemia* to mean the overall toxicity state that accumulates with kidney dysfunction, without any implication at the overall severity of this state, and *uremia* to refer to the constellation of frequently subjective complications that develop with advanced azotemia and which necessitate the initiation of renal replacement therapy. Because the expression "end-stage renal disease" (ESRD) is widely used in regulatory and administrative circles, and it is codified in U.S. law, the KDOQI guidelines continue to use this expression to represent those subjects receiving or eligible for renal replacement therapy either by some form of dialysis or by transplantation.

NKF Definition of Chronic Kidney Disease

CKD is defined as *the presence of objective kidney damage and/or the presence of a glomerular filtration rate of 60 mL/min/1.73 m² body surface area, or less, for at least 3 months, irrespective of the underlying etiology of the kidney damage* (Table 1–1). Evidence of kidney damage may be either structural or functional in nature and may derive from renal histology or from the results of appropriate urine, blood, or renal imaging studies. The commonest and most readily available marker of kidney damage resulting in glomerular dysfunction is the presence of proteinuria. Similarly, the presence of abnormal sediment on urine microscopy or the demonstration of multiple cysts on renal imaging in a patient with a family history of polycystic kidney disease would meet the requirement for objective kidney damage. Because the relationship of hypertension to kidney disease is complex and varied, hypertension by itself is not included in the above definition; instead the presence or absence of hypertension is noted separately in conjunction with the presence or absence and the severity of CKD (Table 1–3).

In accordance with the KDOQI definition, a documented GFR of below 60 mL/min/1.73 m² fulfills the definition of CKD without requiring any additional evidence of underlying kidney damage. This cutoff in GFR was selected because it represents over a 50% reduction in kidney function as compared to the level for young healthy adults, and it is supported by accumulating evidence demonstrating the presence of complications as the glomerular filtration rate falls below 60 mL/min/1.73 m².[2] Patients with a GFR between 60 and 89, without evident kidney disease, are not defined as having CKD but are instead referred to as having a decreased GFR, either with or without the associated presence of high blood pressure (Table 1–3). This approach avoids potentially misclassifying the renal function in otherwise healthy elderly patients with a decreased glomerular filtration rate as a consequence of aging without any other evidence of kidney damage, while at the same time recognizing the increased risk of such patients for actually developing CKD as a consequence of their lower baseline GFR.

Change in Glomerular Filtration Rate with Age

The glomerular filtration rate is known to vary substantially with age, as well as with pregnancy,[4] dietary protein intake,[5] and certain medications, such as angiotensin converting enzyme inhibitors. Glomerular filtration rate increases during early infancy, reaching normal adult levels at approximately age 2 years. The glomerular filtration rate subsequently declines with increasing age. Although the changes in early infancy are clearly physiologic, the nature and consequences of the decrement that occurs with old age are not fully understood. In a cross-sectional study mean (sd) extrapolated GFR among 72 healthy adults males, as measured by iothalamate clearance, varied from 128 mL/min/1.73m² at ages 20 to 29 to 58 mL/min/1.73m² for 80 to 89 years old.[2] More recently a similar relationship was described in a study of 159 subjects, whose GFR was measured using urinary insulin clearance (Figure 1–2).[6]

Autopsy studies have shown a decrease in kidney weight and volume that occurs between the 5th and 9th decades of life. This is predominantly the result of a loss of renal mass from the outer cortex.[7] This results from a decrease in cortical capillary mass with resulting glomerular tuft collapse and eventual hyalinization of the tuft.[6] This capillary loss leads to a decrease in the total glomerular filtration surface area, thereby leading to a reduced glomerular ultrafiltration capacity, as measured by the glomerular ultrafiltration coefficient (K_f) and, consequently, reduced renal plasma flow.[8] Histologically, these changes are represented by the presence

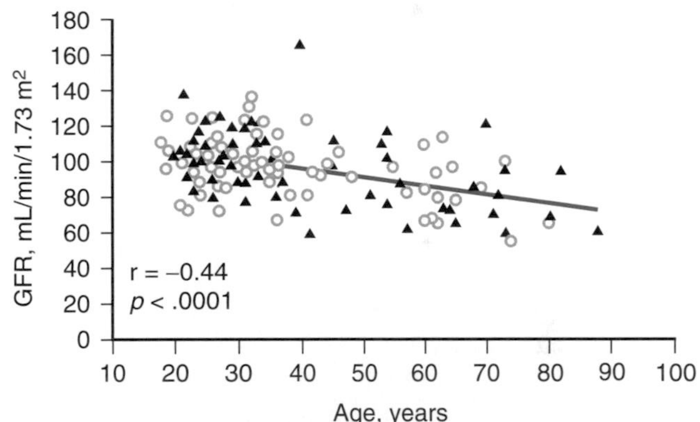

Figure 1–2 Glomerular filtration rate plotted as a function of age, in women *(circles)* and men *(triangles)*. (From Hoang K, Tan J, Derby G, et al: Determinants of glomerular hypofiltration in aging humans. Kidney Int 2003; 64:1417–1424.)

Table 1–3 Definition and Stage of Chronic Kidney Disease

GFR (mL/min/1.73 m²)	With Kidney Damage*		Without Kidney Damage*	
	With HBP†	Without HBP†	With HBP†	Without HBP†
≥90	1	1	"High blood pressure"	"Normal"
60–89	2	2	"High blood pressure with ↓ GFR"	"↓ GFR"‡
30–59	3	3	3	3
15–29	4	4	4	4
<15 (or dialysis)	5	5	5	5

Shaded area represents chronic kidney disease; numbers designate stage of chronic kidney disease.
*Kidney damage is defined as pathologic abnormalities or markers of damage, including abnormalities in blood or urine tests or imaging studies.
†High blood pressure is defined as ≥140/90 in adults and >90th percentile for height and gender in children.
‡May be normal in infants and in the elderly.

of glomerulosclerosis, the prevalence of which increases in a linear fashion after the 5th decade of life,[9,10] reaching 10% to 40% of glomeruli in patients older than 60 years.[9,11] In the cortex, glomerulosclerosis is eventually accompanied by obliteration of arteriolar supply and subsequent absorption of the obsolescent glomeruli. As a consequence, there is an absolute reduction in the number of glomeruli with age. The mean number of glomeruli, estimated by a stereological technique, was 560×10^3 in subjects older than 55 years as compared to 695×10^3 for subjects younger than 55 years ($p < .001$).[12] Whether these age-related changes represent a true physiologic effect or are instead the result of occult pathology is unknown; however, this issue has developed considerable importance with the increasing use of elderly living transplant donors and of extended criteria allografts of cadaveric origin.

Glomerular Filtration Rate and Gender

GFR levels have frequently been reported to be lower in any given age group in women as compared with men, the average difference after adjustment for body surface area being approximately 8%.[2] Women also develop treated ESRD at a lower rate than men, and female animals often show protection against progressive kidney disease compared to male animals.[13] GFR is known to increase substantially during and immediately following pregnancy, reaching 140% to 165% of nonpregnant levels by the second trimester.[4] This elevation persists until approximately gestational week 36, and thereafter starts to decrease but may not return to the previous baseline until several weeks postpartum.[14] As a consequence, the accurate diagnosis of CKD is particularly challenging during pregnancy.

SEVERITY OF CHRONIC KIDNEY DISEASE STAGE

Diagnostic Schema

Traditionally CKD has been classified using a variety of different schema that are based on clinical-pathologic features; these include:

1. The degree of proteinuria/albuminuria (normal, microalbuminuria, subnephrotic, nephrotic).
2. The rate of progression, which we arbitrarily define as stable (GFR: <1.0 mL/min/1.73 m²/year), slow progression (GFR: 1.0-3.9 mL/min/1.73 m²/year), fast progression (GFR: 4+ mL/min/1.73 m²/year), or rapidly progressive (progressing to kidney failure within several weeks or months of clinical onset).
3. The underlying diagnostic category (e.g., vascular, glomerular, tubulointerstitial) or specific diagnosis (e.g., diabetic glomerulosclerosis).
4. The presumed pathogenic mechanisms (e.g., autoimmune, lysosomal storage disease, allergic).
5. The basis of specific tests (e.g., ANCA positive vasculitis).

The utility of the above schema varies in different clinical circumstances. They all focus on the underlying primary cause of the kidney dysfunction and, as such, are typically used by nephrologists primarily in a diagnostic context and to help determine disease specific management and prognosis.

Rationale for a Severity Staging System in CKD

The diagnostic schema ignore the fact that as patients pass through the continuum of progressive kidney damage, there are predictable complications, such as the development of anemia and an elevated parathyroid hormone level, and predictable management issues, such as dialysis access preparation and pre-ESRD vaccination, which are common to progressive kidney disease in general, regardless of the specific underlying etiology. Increasing evidence documents the development of prognostically important complications that are associated with the degree of kidney dysfunction and that begin long before the occurrence of terminal kidney failure.[2] Traditionally, the clinical recognition and management of these complications, which often don't impact kidney disease progression itself, has not been systematic. Failure to focus on these issues has resulted in patients initiating dialysis with multiple inadequately controlled, CKD-related complications.[15] While the level of awareness for these complications has greatly increased over the last decade, there has traditionally been no standardized framework upon which to base relevant clinical practice. The NKF KDOQI staging system for CKD was developed in part to help address this need. This staging system may in some way be considered as representative of the "azotemic burden" that results from a given degree of kidney damage and the associated complications that may typically be expected to occur given the severity or "stage" of an individual's CKD. The staging system is based on the glomerular filtration rate, using this as the best single measure representative of global kidney function. Although the division of what is a continuum of change into specified categories is by nature arbitrary, from a practical standpoint, this simplification facilitates the recognition and management of CKD, which may otherwise be neglected if the primary focus is aimed exclusively at the underlying etiology and cause-specific management.

NKF Stage of Chronic Kidney Disease

CKD is divided into five stages, with the higher stage being associated with worse kidney function. Stage I represents subjects who do not have a clear filtration deficit and is defined as a normal or elevated kidney function (GFR > 90 mL/min/1.73 m²) in association with evidence of kidney damage; this latter is defined broadly but is most often represented by the presence of persistent albuminuria. Stage II is a mild reduction in kidney function (GFR 60–89 mL/min/1.73 m²) that occurs in association with kidney damage. CKD stages III and IV correspond to moderately and severely decreased kidney function (GFR of 30–59 and 15–29 mL/min/1.73 m², respectively). This large a decrement in kidney function is classified as CKD regardless of the presence of additional evidence of kidney damage. Stage V represents kidney failure, defined by either a GFR of below 15 or the need for dialysis therapy (Table 1–2). This staging system focuses on the severity of kidney dysfunction rather than on diagnostic considerations; as such, this complements and in no way replaces traditional classification schemes based on etiology. It is important to recognize the distinction between chronic stage of kidney disease and markers of etiology and progression of kidney disease. As shown in Table 1–4, CKD stage is an excellent measurement of severity

Table 1–4 Importance of CKD Stage, Type of Kidney Disease and Level of Proteinuria in Determining Outcomes in CKD

Outcome	Importance for Different Outcomes		
	CKD Stage	Type of Kidney Disease (Diagnosis)[†]	Proteinuria
Concurrent complications[*]	+++	+	+
Prognosis (next 10 years)			
Risk of CVD or mortality	+++	+	++
Risk of kidney failure	+++	++	+
Rate of decline in GFR	+	+++	+++

[*] Concurrent complications include hypertension, anemia, malnutrition, bone disease, neuropathy and decreased quality of life.
[†] For example, diabetic kidney disease, glomerular diseases, vascular diseases (such as hypertensive nephrosclerosis), tubulointerstitial diseases (including disease due to obstruction, infection, stones, and drug toxicity or allergy), and cystic disease (including polycystic kidney disease).

and a predictor of the risk of comorbidity and complications. However, the underlying diagnosis and the presence of proteinuria are better predictors of the rate of decline in GFR.

Chronic Kidney Disease and Transplantation

In keeping with the NKF definition, nearly all patients who undergo kidney transplantation continue to be defined as having CKD, the stage of which is determined by the level of allograft function. Only those patients with an allograft function of less than 15 mL/min/1.73 m^2 would be classified as having kidney failure (CKD stage V). The majority of allografts would be expected to result in CKD stages II to IV, which appears appropriate given the azotemic burden associated with failing allograft function and the often suboptimal management of the associated complications.[16] It is unknown whether the occurrence of complications is the same regardless of whether the residual GFR arises from a single functional kidney (as with a failing allograft) or from two kidneys.

CKD EPIDEMIOLOGY: DATA SOURCES

ESRD Registries

The available evidence suggests that throughout the 1980s and 1990s there was a sustained global increase in the number of new (incident) and established (prevalent) patients with treated kidney failure. The most reliable data demonstrating this increase comes from ESRD registries, such as the United States Renal Data System (USRDS), which tracks most patients in the United States who are treated with either maintenance dialysis or transplantation. Data from Western Europe is collated by the European Renal Association/ European Dialysis and Transplant Association (ERA/EDTA) registry based on several national and regional registries. These European registries track renal replacement therapy from the first day of treatment and are voluntary, however, on validation studies they have shown patient registration levels in excess of 95%. Registries of kidney failure treatment are also available in other countries, including Japan and Australia/New Zealand. However, although the NKF definition of CKD stage V includes all patients with a GFR of below 15 mL/min/1.73 m^2, the available data from renal replacement registries only include those who have progressed to the need for requiring dialysis, who are offered and accept renal replacement therapy at that time, and, in the case of the USRDS, for some analyses those who have been on a stable modality for at least 60 days; ESRD registry data therefore is not representative of even the entire spectrum of patients with CKD stage V.

In view of the above-mentioned limitations particular caution is required in comparing ESRD registry data from different regions and countries. Sources of variation may result from true differences in the incidence of CKD (either biologic or environmental in origin), differences in the rate of progression of the renal injury, differences in patient survival with CKD (in part due to differential competing mortality rates), and differences in the recognition, referral, and acceptance (by either the dialysis program or by the patient) for renal replacement therapy, as well as administrative differences in the registration and classification of patients within the individual dialysis registry.

CKD Stages I to IV

Unfortunately, data on the epidemiology of the earlier stages of CKD within the general population are still limited. It is likely that only a minority of patients with CKD actually progress to treatment by renal replacement therapy and so end up being identified in the ESRD registries; instead the majority of subjects die with CKD. In addition, some patients may maintain stable, though reduced, GFR and suffer complications of CKD without ever progressing to renal failure. As a result, ESRD trends provide only limited insights into the total morbidity and mortality associated with CKD. Several factors hinder the ready description and investigation of the epidemiology of early stages of CKD. As early CKD is typically clinically silent, both patients and physicians often fail to recognize its occurrence.[17] The symptoms that do occur are usually nonspecific and are typically not appreciated until late in the natural history of the condition. Complications of CKD are often attributed to preexisting comorbid disease or to old age rather than to kidney disease. Part of this failure to detect CKD relates to the widespread use of unadjusted serum creatinine as a screening test for the measurement of kidney function, despite the fact that in many cases of substantial kidney disease, especially in elderly subjects, the serum creatinine fails to rise above the population-derived reference range. Further compounding this has been a long-standing mistaken clinical tendency to interpret modest elevations in serum creatinine as representing only a minor clinically insignificant degree of kidney damage, and so systematically underestimate the severity of CKD even when its presence is recognized. Due to the lack of formal screening programs and inadequate recognition of CKD, most hospital and clinic based series of CKD are by necessity limited to diseases that do come to clinical attention, either as a result of the rapid rate of progression, advanced kidney disease or the development of associated features such as a frank nephrotic syndrome. As a consequence such case series are unlikely to be representative of the true burden of CKD, especially nonproteinuric forms. The most generalizable data come from population surveys for prevalence of CKD and its complications. Progression data require prospective follow-up, but the relatively slow progression of CKD requires a large sample size and long duration of follow-up. Administrative data on Medicare patients with diagnosed CKD as well as data from health care organizations are often less detailed but provide a powerful source for following large groups of individuals.

U.S. Prevalence Estimates

The Third National Health and Nutritional Examination Survey (NHANES III) has provided a valuable source of data to estimate the prevalence of CKD and associated complications in the United States.[2] Between 1988 and 1994, this program used a complex multistage sampling scheme to quantitate the state of health and health related behaviors, with inferences that are applicable to the general noninstitutionalized U.S. population. Subgroups at the extremes of age, as well as racial minorities, were over-sampled to provide more reliable estimates within these populations among surveyed adults. A serum creatinine level was measured on 16,589 study participants, thus allowing estimation of their GFR, calculation of the point prevalence of CKD, and examination on a cross-sectional basis of the various complications associated with different stages of kidney disease. Calibration of the serum creatinine assay to the laboratory where the MDRD equation was developed allows for a reliable estimate of GFR.[18] Additional data will be available from the continuation of NHANES, the next wave of which will provide data from 1999 to 2000. Valuable population-based data are available from other large cross-sectional surveys in the United States and internationally, although they don't use national probability samples, thus limiting their generalizability.

KIDNEY FAILURE (CKD STAGE V)

Incidence of Renal Replacement Therapy for ESRD in the United States

Relatively precise data regarding the use of renal replacement therapy to treat end-stage renal disease within the United States are available from the annual data report of the U.S. Renal Data System (USRDS), which tracks data on the vast majority of subjects within the United States who have a functioning renal allograft or are treated with maintenance dialysis. Throughout the 1980s and 1990s the incidence of ESRD treated by renal replacement therapy in the United States increased exponentially; the incidence rate (adjusted for age, race, and gender) in calendar years 1981, 1991, and 2001 increased from 91 per million population (pmp) to 223 pmp and to 334 pmp, respectively. However, in the 2 most recent years for which data are available, the adjusted incidence rate, although still increasing, has started to slow; the increases in the adjusted incidence rate for years 2000 and 2001 were both approximately 1% (Figure 1–3). The actual number of incident U.S. patients in 2001 was 93,327 patients, up from 91,449 patients the previous year.

Gender

The race and age adjusted incidence of ESRD is significantly higher in males (404 per million population) than in females (280 per million population), and the gender specific incidence rate has similarly tended to increase at a faster rate for males.

Age

The incidence of ESRD varies dramatically with age; the 2001 race and gender adjusted rates per million for those over age 75 is 100 times higher than for those less than age 20

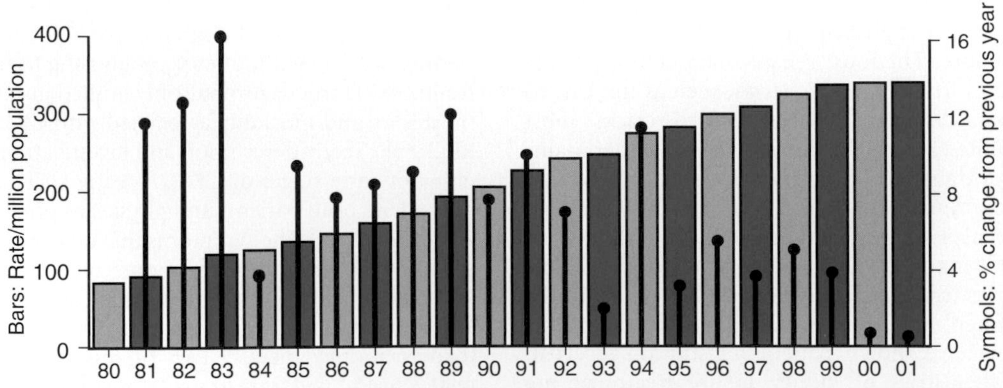

Figure 1–3 Age, race, and gender adjusted incidence of end-stage renal disease within the United States *(bars)*, and annual percent change relative to the previous year. (From U.S. Renal Data System: USRDS 2003 Annual Data Report: Atlas of end-stage renal disease in the United States. Bethesda, MD, National Institutes of Health, 2003, pp 1–560.)

(Figure 1–4). The rate of increase in incidence has also been much higher in the older categories; over the last decade the adjusted incidence rates for those age 75 and above has almost doubled (from 782 pmp to 1542), the adjusted rate among those age 65 to 74 increased by almost 50% (from 938 pmp to 1402 pmp), with only a slightly lower rate of increase (45%) among those age 45 to 64 (from 432 pmp to 625 pmp). The rate of increase for those younger than 45 years has been much lower; the incidence rate among those age 20 to 44 increased by 15% (from 104 pmp to 120 pmp), while the increase among those younger than 20 years was only 7% (from 14 pmp to 15 pmp). The increase in the oldest age category as compared with the 65- to 74-year-olds is likely to be a consequence of both increased intake into the ESRD program of very old subjects as well as the increased incidence of ESRD arising from diseases that increase in frequency with aging. The trends seen in the 45- to 65-year-old category are possibly more representative of changes in actual incidence of ESRD because they are potentially less influenced by secular trends in accepting patients for renal replacement therapy. It is very likely that the great increase in ESRD incidence within the United States is not simply the result of increased acceptance of subjects into treatment programs but also represents a substantial increase in the number of subjects at risk for ESRD, although this effect has not been adequately quantified.

Race

Although Caucasians have the lowest absolute age and gender adjusted incidence rate of treated ESRD, the rate of increase in incidence over the decade from 1991 to 2001 has been greatest in Caucasians (56%) and Asians (54%) as compared to African-Americans (40%) and Native Americans (20%). The reasons for these differentials are likely to be complex and cannot be explained purely by the better longevity of Caucasians as the results persist following adjustment for age. Some of these may be related to differences in access to or quality of health care delivery or trends in diabetes incidence and care.

Geographic Variation

Although the incidence of ESRD is high throughout the United States, there is nevertheless substantial geographic variation across states (Figure 1–5). In 2001 the state specific incidence rates varied by 2.7-fold despite adjusting for the age, race, gender, and population of the state; the adjusted rate was lowest for Montana at 143 per million population and highest for West Virginia at 387 per million population. Some of this variability is likely to relate to differences in geographic availability of renal replacement therapy as well as clinical practice patterns.

Modality

According to USRDS data, in 2001, 86,289 patients were initially treated with hemodialysis, 6991 patients initiated peritoneal dialysis, and 2412 underwent preemptive renal transplantation without prior dialysis. Between 1997 and 2001, the incidence rates of hemodialysis increased 3.3% per year, incidence rates for preemptive transplantation increased 8.9% per year, and in contrast the rate for peritoneal dialysis decreased by 4% per year. Of those treated with peritoneal dialysis, approximately half were treated with a cycler, a proportion that has steadily increased over time.

Incidence of Renal Replacement Therapy for ESRD in Europe

Similar to the U.S. experience, there has been a dramatic increase in the incidence of patients treated with renal replacement therapy throughout much of Europe; whether

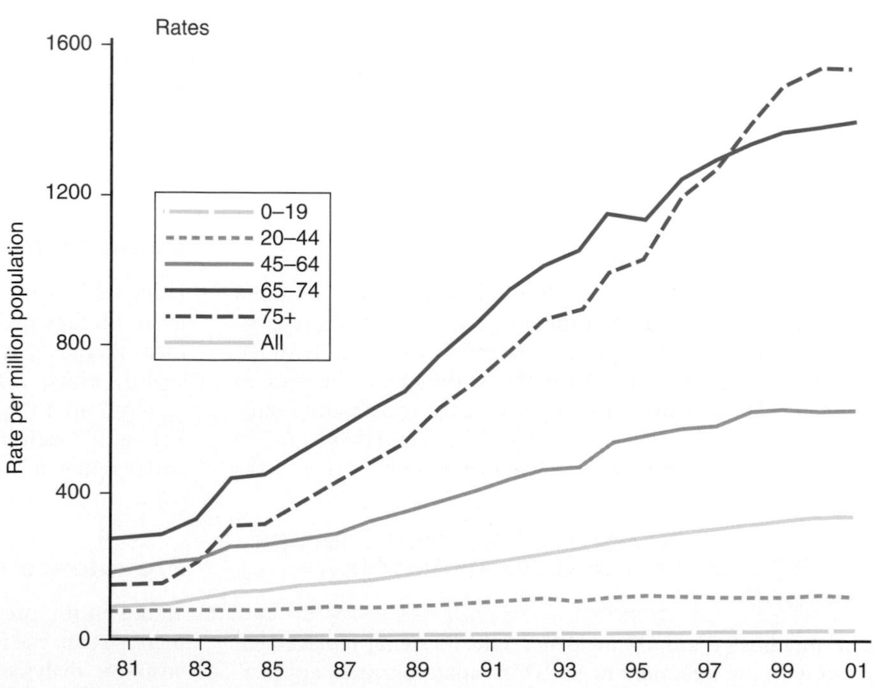

Figure 1–4 Race and gender adjusted incidence rate of end-stage renal disease by age category. (From U.S. Renal Data System: USRDS 2003 Annual Data Report: Atlas of end-stage renal disease in the United States. Bethesda, MD, National Institutes of Health, 2003, pp 1–560.)

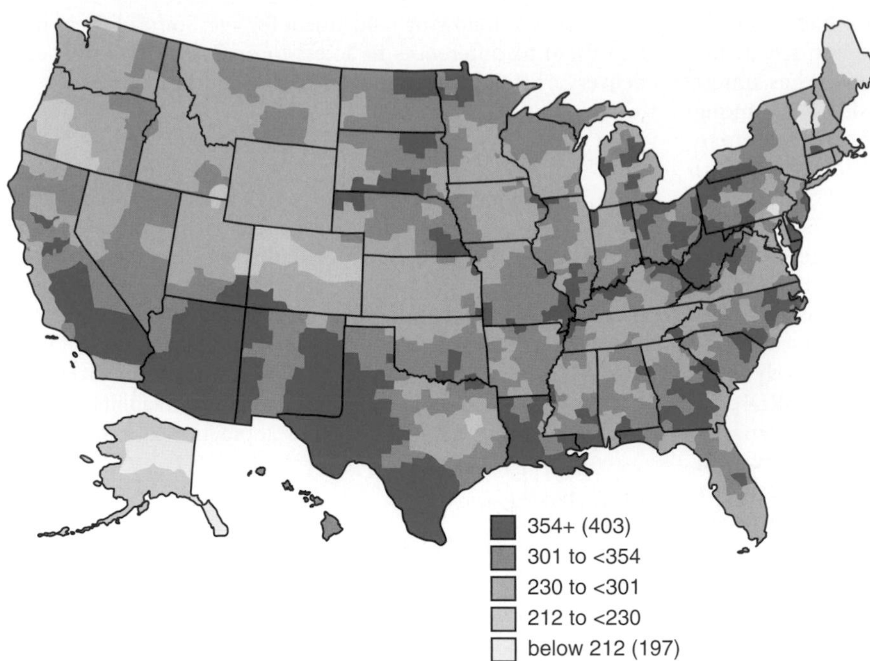

Figure 1–5 Geographic variation in age, race, and gender adjusted incidence rates for ESRD, per million population. (From U.S. Renal Data System: USRDS 2003 Annual Data Report: Atlas of end-stage renal disease in the United States. Bethesda, MD, National Institutes of Health, 2003, pp 1–560.)

this trend is also starting to slow in Europe is unclear. Stengel and colleagues[19] reported the change in incidence rates between 1990 and 1999 in nine Western European national ESRD registries (Austria, Belgium, Denmark, Finland, Greece, The Netherlands, Norway, Spain, UK [Scotland]). The age and gender adjusted incidence rates were calculated over this time period by Poisson regression using the mid-year census population estimates to calculate the population at risk. Analysis shows that the age and gender adjusted incidence rate increased 47% from 79.4 per million population (pmp) for 1990 to 1991 up to 117.1 pmp from 1998 to 1999. Thus the age and gender adjusted incidence rate in Europe remains about one-third that of the United States. The incidence rate of renal replacement therapy in Western Europe increased in an approximately linear fashion, at an overall mean rate of 4.8% per year (range between countries: 2.1% – 6.4%). In the United States incidence rates increased faster for men than for women, with overall increases of 5.2% versus 4% per year, respectively. Adjusted incidence rates were relatively stable for patients less than 45 years old but increased by 2.2% per year in the 45- to 64-year-old age group (from 135.3 to 203.1 pmp); by 7.0% in the 65- to 74-year-old age group (from 290.9 to 490.1 pmp), and over threefold (from 140.9 to 540.4 pmp) in those over age 75. Although the trend in adjusted incidence in all of the constituent registries was toward a significant increase, there was substantial variation between countries, especially for older patients; the rate of increase in incidence for patients above 75 years over the decade examined increased by a factor of 2.1 in The Netherlands, 6.6 in Scotland, 9.3 in Denmark, and 30.6 in Finland.

Incidence of Renal Replacement Therapy for ESRD in Asia and Australia/New Zealand

The unadjusted annual incidence rate for renal replacement therapy in the treatment of ESRD in Japan increased approximately threefold from 81.3 pmp in 1982 up to 252 pmp in 2001. Despite the relatively homogenous Japanese population and uniform health care, as in the United States there are substantial variations in ESRD incidence rates across regions; the incidence and rate of increase varied from 140 pmp and 9.1 pmp per year up to 179 pmp and 12 pmp per year across different regions.[20] The unadjusted incidence rate in Taiwan (331 pmp) is similar to that in the United States, and it has increased at almost double the U.S. rate (15%) over the last 4 years.

The unadjusted incidence rates in Australia and New Zealand are considerably less than that described above with unadjusted incidence rates of 92 and 107 pmp, respectively. As in other countries, there has been a substantial, in the Australian case twofold, increase in the annual incidence rate. As seen elsewhere the increase in overall incidence has largely been the result of an increase among those over age 65, with rates being relatively steady for those younger than 65, while racial minorities and people of native descent, such as Australian Aboriginals or New Zealand Maori Islanders, bear a disproportionate degree of the overall burden of ESRD.[21]

Cumulative Lifetime Risk of ESRD

Using a Markoff model, it has been estimated that the cumulative lifetime risk for requiring maintenance renal replacement therapy was approximately 1 in 40 for Caucasian males, slightly under 1 in 50 for Caucasian females, and approximately 1 in 13 for African-Americans of either gender.[22] By age 56, the estimated cumulative risk of ESRD in black men and women already exceeds the lifetime risk among their white American counterparts.

Prevalence of Stage V CKD

Trends in the prevalence of ESRD have shown an even larger increase than the incidence trends discussed above because survival on dialysis has improved over time. As reported by

USRDS, the age, race, and gender adjusted point prevalence count, as of December 31, 2001, was 405,081 persons, equivalent to an adjusted prevalence rate of 1392 per million population. This rate is 1.7-fold higher than in 1991 and 5.6-fold higher than in 1981. Currently, approximately 60% of the ESRD population is Caucasian, 31% is African-American, 4.1% is Asian, and 1.5% is Native-American, revealing a substantial overrepresentation of racial minorities in the burden of ESRD. Although the highest incidence of ESRD is seen in patients older than 74 years, the highest prevalence occurs in the 65- to 74-year-old group (4791 pmp) as compared to 4098 pmp for those greater than age 74 and 2905 pmp for 45 to 64 year olds. This difference results from differential incidence rates as well as differential survival rates on dialysis. Because of the age structure of the general population, the largest number of ESRD patients is between the ages of 45 and 64 years (41% of ESRD patients). The adjusted prevalence for 20 to 44 year olds was 813 and for those less than 20 years old it was 78 pmp. As in the incidence statistics, the prevalence is higher for males than for females, with adjusted prevalence rates of 1670 and 1163 pmp, respectively. Of the prevalence U.S. ESRD population, currently 65% of patients are treated with hemodialysis, 28% by renal transplant, and 7% by peritoneal dialysis, the latter being evenly split between noncycler and cycler-based techniques. More recent data suggest that the proportion of patients treated by a cycler-based therapy is even higher than this.

Although the prevalence rate of ESRD in the United States is extremely high, it is not unique. In 2001 the total Japanese prevalence count of ESRD was 209,036, equivalent to an unadjusted rate of 1642 pmp, a rate that exceeds the unadjusted prevalence rate for the United States. The 2001 unadjusted prevalence rate for Taiwan, 1423 pmp, was similar to the U.S. rate. The point prevalence as of December 31, 2000, in Australia was 334 pmp and in New Zealand it was 247 pmp. In Western Europe Luxemburg and Germany have the highest prevalence rates, while in central Europe the Czech Republic has the highest rate (Figure 1–6). Some of these lower observed rates correspond to lower availability of treatment. Thus the rates are likely to represent an underestimate of the true burden of disease.

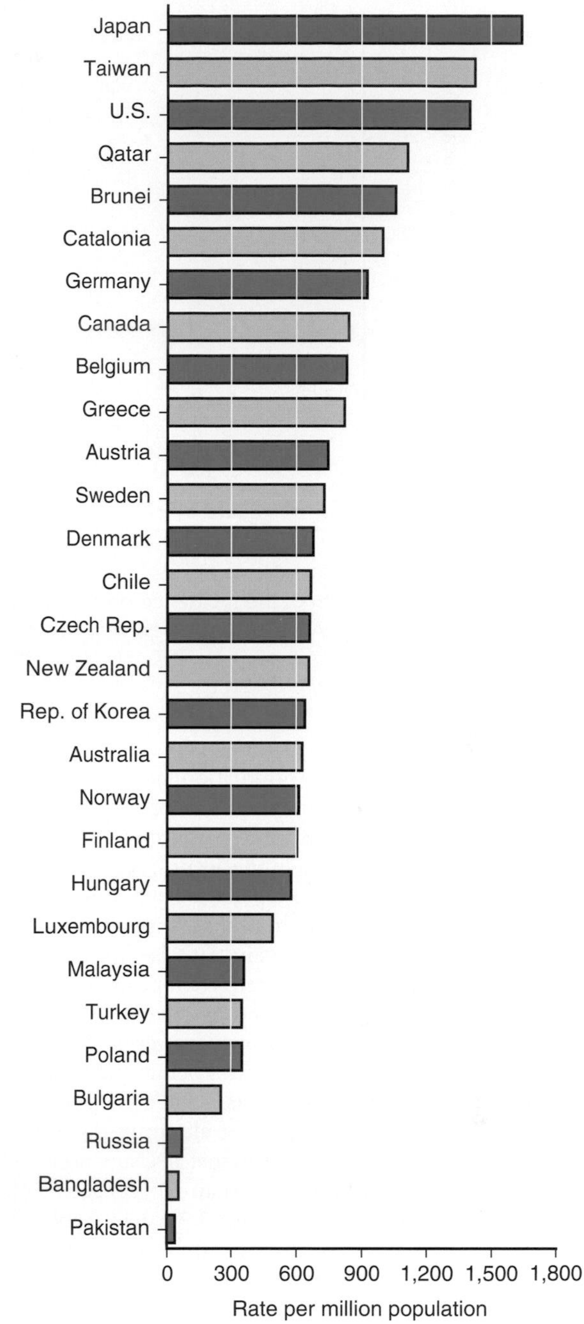

Figure 1–6 International comparison of the unadjusted prevalence of ESRD. (From U.S. Renal Data System: USRDS 2003 Annual Data Report: Atlas of end-stage renal disease in the United States. Bethesda, MD, National Institutes of Health, 2003, pp 1–560.)

Projected U.S. Prevalence Rates

Adjusting for the expected change in population demographics and growth, it is estimated that by the year 2030 the number of patients with ESRD in the United States is likely to increase to 2.24 million subjects, with half of the subjects being over age 65 and the majority of them being non-Caucasian (Figure 1–7).

CKD STAGES I TO IV

Prevalence data are available from national probability samples and large screening efforts. Earlier reports focused on urine dipstick and serum creatinine. Later reports focus on estimating GFR and application of the CKD staging system.

Prevalence of Kidney Damage: Albuminuria and/or Hematuria

The precise prevalence of kidney damage in the general population is unknown. From an epidemiologic perspective, the best studied marker of kidney damage has been albuminuria. Other potential markers of kidney damage such as urinary sediment and renal imaging have not been studied as systematically.[2,23]

U.S. Prevalence

Data from the NHANES III Survey revealed that at the time the study was conducted (1988–1994) approximately 11.7% of

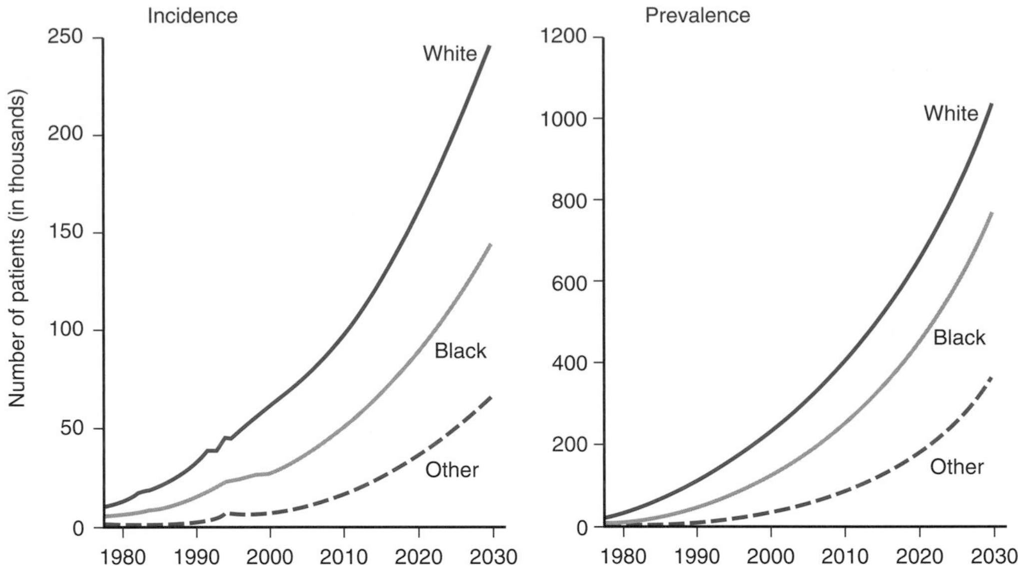

Figure 1–7 Projected growth of the incidence and prevalence ESRD population, by race. (From U.S. Renal Data System: USRDS 2003 Annual Data Report: Atlas of end-stage renal disease in the United States. Bethesda, MD, National Institutes of Health, 2003, pp 1–560.)

the noninstitutionalized U.S. population had an abnormal urinary albumin to creatinine ratio.[24] This equates to approximately 20.2 million adults with microalbuminuria. In a subsample from this study that underwent repeated testing, clinical macroalbuminuria always persisted, while only 61% of those with microalbuminuria had a positive result on the repeated test. Whether this reflects initial false positive results or alternatively the presence of intermittent proteinuria and if the latter, the significance of this finding relative to the risk of progressive kidney disease is unknown; however, it is notable that even the presence of albuminuria below the traditional definition of microalbuminuria is associated with increased cardiovascular risk.[25] The presence of albuminuria varies by age and the presence or absence of diabetes. Using nongender specific cutoffs, among adults older than 70 years 26.6% had microalbuminuria (<30 mg/day) and 3.7% had frank albuminuria (>300 mg/day); in those aged 60 to 69, the prevalence was 16.2% and 2%; and in those aged 40 to 59 years it was 9.1% and 1%, respectively. As expected, the prevalence was higher in diabetics; in diabetics over age 70 the prevalence of microalbuminuria was 43.2% and of frank albuminuria it was 8.4%, in nondiabetics it was 24.2% and 3.0%, respectively.[24] It is noteworthy that when gender-specific cutoffs are used, which attempt to estimate the spot albumin-to-creatinine ratio which would correspond to 30 and 300 mg/day of albumin excretion, the cutoffs are lower (17 and 255 mg/g for men and 35 and 350 mg/g for women) and the prevalence estimates are somewhat higher.[26] However, the current consensus is in favor of using nongender-specific cutoffs to maintain simplicity and consistency with American Diabetic Association guidelines.[27,28]

Cardia Study

In a study of 2582 healthy black and white young adults enrolled in the Cardia Study, using the average of the albumin to creatinine ratios obtained at 10 and 15 years of follow-up, the prevalence of microalbuminuria was 6.4% and of macroalbuminuria it was 0.7%. Levels tended to be higher in African-Americans than in Caucasians and in males compared to females, and for those with impaired baseline fasting glucose levels.[29]

AusDiab Kidney Study

The population prevalence of kidney damage in Australia has been estimated in the AusDiab Kidney Study[30]; 11,247 noninstitutionalized Australians, aged 25 years or older, were randomly surveyed using a stratified clustered selection method, and examined for indicators of CKD including the presence of proteinuria, dipstick hematuria, or an estimated creatinine clearance below 60 mL/min using the Cockcroft-Gault equation. The study sample comprised 92.9% Caucasians and 5.5% Asians. Overall, 2.4% of participants were found to have a urinary protein to creatinine ratio of 200 mg/g or higher (approximately 250 mg/day). The prevalence was similar in men and women and increased eightfold with age, from 0.8% for 25 to 44 year olds to 6.6% in the 65 and older group. Almost half a percent (0.4%) of subjects had proteinuria in excess of approximately 1 g/day. The prevalence of dipstick positive hematuria of "+1" or greater was approximately 1 in 20 (4.6%) and was more common in women than in men, especially in younger age groups. Over 1 in 10 participants (11.2%) had a Cockcroft Gault creatinine clearance of less than 60 mL/min/1.73 m^2; the risk of reduced renal function was higher in women than in men and increased significantly with age, from 0.01% in the 25- to 44-year-old group to 54.8% for those 65 years and older; 6.4% of the population had all three findings of hematuria, proteinuria, and reduced renal function. Of the patients with proteinuria, in approximately half (46.8%) it was an isolated finding, in a third (34.8%) it was associated with a creatinine clearance of less than 60 mL/min/1.73 m^2 and in an eighth (12%) it was associated with hematuria. Of those with hematuria 1 in 8 (12.1%) had a reduced GFR, 1 in 20 (5.7%) had proteinuria and 1 in 50 (2.1%) had both. Most (87%) patients with a GFR of less than 60 mL/min/1.73 m^2 had neither proteinuria nor hematuria, 7% had proteinuria, and 5% had hematuria, while 1% had both. These results show that reduced GFR is related to but by no means synonymous with either hematuria or proteinuria in the general population.

Okinawa Screen Study

In 1983 107,192 Japanese on the island of Okinawa underwent a population-based kidney disease screening program. Similar to the findings in the AusDiab study the prevalence of hematuria increased linearly over a ninefold range with age in men, from 0.9% at ages 18 to 29, to 8.2% in those 80 years and older; hematuria was more common in women, especially at younger ages (7.3% at 18–29 years and 15.3% at age 80 and older). The prevalence of proteinuria, defined as +1 or greater proteinuria by dipstick, was high in both men (4% for 18–29 year olds, 6% for those over 80) and women (3% and 7%, respectively). The prevalence of proteinuria and hematuria combined was less than 2% in all age groups for both genders.[31]

Prevalence of Elevated Serum Creatinine

The majority of studies have defined the presence of CKD in terms of an elevated serum creatinine. This approach has several important limitations. Because there is no universal standard for the calibration of the serum creatinine assay, serum creatinine results may differ substantially between different laboratories.[18,32] Furthermore, as the serum creatinine level is dependent on both the daily creatinine production rate as well as its excretion rate, individuals with lower muscle mass and thus lower creatinine generation rates will have a lower serum creatinine at any given level of kidney function. Thus an elderly individual may have a serum creatinine within the population reference range despite substantially reduced kidney function, while, in general, women will have lower levels of kidney function as compared to men at a given serum creatinine level.[18] These limitations are demonstrated in a cross-sectional study of 2781 unselected outpatients in British Columbia who had serum creatinine measurements arranged by their community physician.[33] Subjects had a mean (standard deviation) age of 57[18] years and were defined as having hypercreatininemia if their serum creatinine was greater than 1.5 mg/dL (130 Umol/L) and an abnormal creatinine clearance if their Cockcroft Gault estimated creatinine clearance of below 50 mL/min. Of the population examined 6.5% had abnormal serum creatinine, whereas an additional 13.9% of the population had an estimated creatinine clearance below 50 despite having a serum creatinine that was within the assay reference range. The proportion of subjects with an abnormal Cockcroft Gault, despite creatinine within the normal range, increased from 0.8% for those aged 40 to 49, to 1.6% for those aged 50 to 59, to 12.6% for those aged 60 to 69, and to 47.3% for those aged greater than 70 years. Given the above limitations, studies based on serum creatinine assessments alone often underestimate the true prevalence of CKD.

NHANES III

An early analysis of NHANES III data reported the prevalences of serum creatinine at or above 1.5, 1.7, and 2.0 mg/dL to be 5%, 1.9%, and 0.6% for men, and 1.6%, 0.7%, and 0.3% for women.[34] Applying these percentages to the 1990 U.S. Census population results in the estimates of 6.2, 2.5, and 0.8 millions of Americans having serum creatinine levels at or above these cutoffs, respectively.

Reykjavik Study

A much lower prevalence of CKD has been reported in Iceland, a country where the prevalence of end-stage renal disease (approximately 55 per million population) is much lower than in the United States. This study examined the initial prevalence of an elevated serum creatinine above 1.7 mg/dL (150 Umol/L) and the subsequent renal outcome among 18,912 people who were living in Reykjavik, Iceland, as of 1967.[35] The estimated GFR at the time of study entry was between 30 to 35 mL/min/1.73 m^2, confirming that the above creatinine cutoff was representative of patients with CKD stage IV. The overall survey response rate was approximately 70%, with participation being lower in older age groups; the response rate among 75- to 79-year-olds was 53%. At baseline, 45 patients were found to have confirmed elevations in serum creatinine; of these the elevations were transient in three individuals, 39% of the subjects had proteinuria, 12% had diabetes, and 67% had hypertension. The crude prevalence of creatinine above 1.7 mg/dL was 0.22%, which was substantially higher for men (0.28%) than among women (0.15%). Some of this gender-related effect is likely to have resulted from the use of a gender independent cutoff for creatinine despite the typically greater muscle mass and consequent creatinine generation rate in men as compared to women. The prevalence of elevated serum creatinine increased with age. Over a median follow-up of 7.5 years, 27% of subjects maintained a relatively stable function with a yearly decline in estimated GFR of less than 1 mL/min/1.73 m^2, while two-thirds had progressively decreasing kidney function. These historic prevalence estimates from Iceland are therefore considerably less than those identified more recently within the United States in NHANES III, even when using results specific to non-Hispanic whites in the latter study. However, the degree to which these differences relate to methodologic differences in the design and conduct of the studies, to secular trends, or to true biologic effects or variation in clinical practice is unknown. Of note, in sharp contrast to the current U.S. experience, in the Reykjavik study only 1 person out of almost 19,000 subjects had kidney damage attributed to diabetes.

Prevalence of CKD in a Southwestern U.S. Health Maintenance Organization

The prevalence of elevated serum creatinine in the Southwestern United States has been reported from 199,065 enrollees in a health maintenance organization, using gender-specific creatinine cutoffs (serum creatinine of >1.2 mg/dL for women and >1.4 mg/dL for men). At least one gender-specific elevation in serum creatinine level was found in 7.1% of subjects and a sustained elevation, on at least two occasions at least 90 days apart, was found in 1.7%. Applying these proportions to the 1990 census data, they estimated a prevalence of 9.1 million Americans in 1990 who would have at least one elevated serum creatinine and 4.2 million Americans with at least two elevated creatinines.[36]

Framingham Study

The prevalence of hypercreatininemia has also been reported from the Framingham cohort. A creatinine cutoff of 1.36 mg/dL (120 Umol/L) for men and 1.54 mg/dL (136 Umol/L) for females were derived from the 97.5 percentile of the serum creatinine distribution in a subgroup of 3241 study subjects, with a mean (sd) age of 47 (13.7) years and who were free of known renal, cardiovascular, and hypertensive disease or diabetes. Eight percent of women and 8.9% of men had elevated serum creatinine levels above these levels.[37]

Okinawa Screening Study

In the Okinawa Screening Study, 1.1% of women and 3.1% of men had serum creatinine levels above 1.4 mg/dL (124 Umol/L) and 1.5 mg/dL (133 Umol/L), respectively. However, this assay was only performed on 14,607 members of the original cohort who were discovered on initial screening to have either an abnormal urinalysis or an elevated blood pressure.[31]

Prevalence of CKD Stages

The initial NKF Guidelines for CKD apply the CKD definition and stages to NHANES III data to obtain overall U.S. population-based prevalence estimates, and subsequent publications detail the methods and the prevalence in high- and low-risk subgroups.[18,30,38] This approach, which relies on an estimated GFR derived from the calibrated serum creatinine assay overcomes most of the limitations of using serum creatinine levels alone. This analysis estimates that during 1988 to 1994 approximately 8 million Americans had glomerular filtration rates of below 60 mL/min/1.73 m^2 and 19 million had CKD stages I to V. Table 1–5 shows the absolute number of subjects and the proportion of the general noninstitutionalized U.S. population with the different stages of CKD. The AusDiab study used the presence of either proteinuria or hematuria on a dipstick, rather than persistent microalbuminuria, as markers of kidney damage, which resulted in low estimates of CKD stages I and II of 0.9% and 2%.[30] In contrast, the prevalence of CKD stage III was 10.9%, higher than the 4.3% estimate in the United States. However, the numbers are not directly comparable because different equations and serum creatinine methods were used. The prevalence of CKD stage IV was 0.3%, similar to the U.S. estimate of 0.4% at this lower GFR range, where creatinine calibration has a smaller impact. The prevalence of stage V in AusDiab was 0.003% but individuals on dialysis may be less likely to participate in population surveys. Therefore, the prevalence of stage V in the K/DOQI report is based on USRDS data, rather than NHANES data.

ETIOLOGY OF KIDNEY DISEASE

A detailed review of the epidemiology, natural history, and management of the specific conditions that give rise to kidney disease is beyond the scope of this chapter, but we review below some of the salient epidemiologic aspects of the more notable conditions. Information on population-based epidemiology of many of these conditions is extremely limited, most notably by the lack of any widespread or uniform registry of CKD patients. Registries do exist for ESRD, which track the attributed etiology of kidney failure, however, by definition these registries only include patients who progress to and are accepted for renal replacement therapy, and as such they reflect the most progressive forms of diseases causing CKD. The distribution of etiologies in the ESRD registries is similarly influenced by the natural history of the underlying condition, the efficacy of available treatment and practice patterns regarding disease recognition and management, as well as by potential referral and selection biases. Furthermore, in many cases recognition of CKD is often delayed until late in the disease course, when the patient has already developed advanced kidney damage, making it difficult to accurately establish the underlying cause and rendering the attributed diagnosis essentially a matter of speculation. The attributed etiology of kidney failure in the USRDS registry is collected on a regulatory form, completion of which may default in whole or in part to administrative or clinical support staff, while alternatively the physician certifying the patient as starting ESRD is often not the same physician who managed the patient's CKD, and thus even the physician may have incomplete knowledge of the pre-ESRD diagnostic workup.

Table 1–5 Prevalence of GFR Category: NHANES III 1988–1994, U.S. Adults (Age =20)

Stages and Prevalence of Chronic Kidney Disease (Age ≥ 20)				
		GFR	**Prevalence***	
Stage	**Description**	**(mL/min/1.73 m^2)**	**N (1000s)**	**%**
1	Kidney damage with normal or ↑ GFR	≥90	5,900	3.3
2	Kidney damage with mild ↓ GFR	60–89	5,300	3.0
3	Moderate ↓ GFR	30–59	7,600	4.3
4	Severe ↓ GFR	15–29	400	0.2
5	Kidney failure	<15 (or dialysis)	300	0.1

*Data for Stages 1–4 from NHANES III (1988–1994)[1]. Population of 177 million adults age ≥20 years. Data for Stage 5 from USRDS (1998)[2] include approximately 230,000 patients treated by dialysis, and assume 70,000 additional patients not on dialysis. GFR estimated from serum creatinine using MDRD Study equation based on age, gender, race and calibration for serum creatinine. For Stages 1 and 2, kidney damage estimated by spot albumin-to-creatinine ratio >17 mg/g in men or >25 mg/g in women on two measurements. (Copyright 2002, with permission from the National Kidney Foundation.)

Alternatively, clinical studies reporting the etiology of kidney disease are typically based on case series or biopsy series conducted in a single hospital or unit, often a tertiary referral center, and as such are heavily influenced by referral and selection biases, while in most cases the catchment area and population at risk can only be roughly approximated.

Diabetes

There has been a dramatic and global increase in the incidence and prevalence of diabetes over the last 2 decades. Distinguishing the relative contribution of type I versus type II diabetes to the incidence of kidney failure is difficult because many ESRD databases do not reliably make this distinction and, in addition, the diagnostic criteria have changed over time. However, the natural history of diabetic glomerulosclerosis appears to be similar for both type I and type II diabetes, if subjects are matched for an equal duration of diabetes. In clinical practice the duration of type II diabetes prior to clinical diagnosis is less predictable.

Nephropathy from Type I Diabetes

The incidence of type I diabetes has progressively increased over last several decades,[39] despite that the incidence of renal disease in type I diabetics appears to have either declined,[40] or at least been held steady.[41] The prime determinants of the rate of progression appears to be the degree of hypertensive and glycemic control.[42] In a cohort of 1075 subjects diagnosed with type I diabetes in Allegheny County, Pennsylvania, the cumulative incidence of ESRD was 11.3% at 25 years of diabetes, with an unadjusted incidence rate of 521/100,000 person years (95% CI: 424–629). The 20-year cumulative incidence rate for ESRD significantly declined in consecutive cohorts with regard to year of diagnosis from 9.1% for 1965 to 1969, 4.7% for 1970 to 1974 and 3.6% for 1975 to 1979.[43]

Nephropathy from Type II Diabetes

There has proportionately been a far greater increase over the last 2 decades in the incidence of type II diabetic nephropathy. This has paralleled the increased prevalence of type II diabetes, which itself has been associated with increased rates of obesity and sedentary lifestyles.[44] The increase in type II diabetic renal disease has occurred despite the proven benefit of secondary prevention with tight glycemic and antihypertensive control,[45,46] as well as potential primary preventative measures with lifestyle modification and pharmacotherapy.[47, 48] The implementation of these preventative strategies remains markedly suboptimal. In one survey the prevalence of diabetes in the United States increased by over a third, from 4.9% in 1990 to 6.5% in 1998, while the percentage of subjects with a BMI greater than 30 kg/m^2 increased from 11.1% to 18%.[49] In a prospective study of 155,774 patients in the Netherlands followed between 1998 to 2000, the age and gender adjusted prevalence rates of type II diabetes increased from 2.2% to 2.7%, and patients over 70 years of age accounted for over half of these subjects.[50]

In keeping with this dramatic increase in the prevalence of type II diabetes over the last 2 decades and the underutilization of preventative management strategies, there has been a dramatic increase in ESRD rates attributed to diabetic kidney disease. This increase has been one of epidemic proportion, and it has substantially contributed to the overall increased rates of ESRD. In the United States the age, race, and gender adjusted incidence rate of ESRD attributed to diabetes has doubled over the last decade, to a current adjusted rate of 148 pmp in 2001. The adjusted incidence rate peaks in the 65- to 74-year-old age group and is almost threefold higher in African-Americans than in Caucasians. Comparing data from NHANES III with NHANES II, between 1978 and 1991 the self reported prevalence of diabetes among 30 to 74 year olds increased 59%, and this increase was estimated to be responsible for 28% of the increase in incidence of ESRD over this period.[51] These trends are likely to have been further accentuated over the last decade. Similar trends, though of a lower magnitude, have been reported in Europe, though with substantial variability between countries, the 1999 age and gender adjusted incidence rate being 10.2 pmp in Norway and 39.3 pmp in Austria. That the incidence of diabetic kidney disease plays a major role in explaining the variability in ESRD rates was shown in Austria, where the age adjusted overall incidence rate of ESRD in the Tyrol region is 97.9 pmp/year (95% CI, 86.9–109.1), as compared to 120.9 pmp/year (95% CI, 116.9–124.5) for the rest of the country. On examining the cause-specific ESRD rates, most of these differences between regions are explained by differences in the rates of diabetic nephropathy and vascular nephropathy; the distribution of other etiologies for renal failure being similar. These differences are not obviously explained by differential rates of selection for dialysis or by available access to renal replacement programs in the Tyrol as compared to the rest of Austria. However, compared to the rest of Austria, the population in Tyrol has lower average body mass indices, a higher percentage who take regular physical exercise, and a lower overall rate of diabetes.[52]

Hypertension/Ischemic Kidney Disease

Hypertension is the second most common attributed etiology of ESRD in the United States, and from 1990 to 2001 the adjusted incidence rate of ESRD attributed to hypertension increased by almost 50%, although in the last 3 years this rate of increase appears to be slowing. The 2001 age, gender, and race adjusted incidence rate was 89 per million U.S. population. The reported incidence increases with age, while the age and gender adjusted incidence rate is over three times higher in African-Americans than in Caucasians. In Europe the incidence of ESRD attributed to hypertensive renovascular disease has also increased, though this increase has been predominantly limited to subjects over age 65. Its incidence varies widely between countries, with an adjusted rate of 5.8 pmp in Finland and 21 pmp in Norway.

The accuracy with which hypertension is attributed as the cause of ESRD has been widely questioned. Indeed, even whether nonmalignant hypertension can cause de novo kidney disease at all, especially in Caucasians, is controversial.[53] In contrast, there is abundant evidence that hypertension, especially systolic hypertension, is a powerful promoter of kidney damage, which may exacerbate the renal injury and rate of renal decline that occurs from a given disease.[54] There is also clear evidence that hypertension predates an increased risk of ESRD.[55–57] In addition, control of blood pressure clearly decreases the risk of CKD progression. A causal relationship between hypertension and CKD is difficult to establish because hypertension is a frequent consequence of CKD and thus is likely to be present in a large proportion of subjects with CKD regardless of their initial etiology. This is especially problematic given the large proportion of CKD patients who present with advanced CKD at the time of nephrology referral. In addition, the clinical definition of hypertensive kidney failure has been relatively loose and has not typically required demonstration of supportive evidence in the form of hypertensive damage at other nonrenal vascular beds.

Some of the recent increased incidence in ESRD is likely to have resulted from decreasing competing mortality rates as a consequence of improved stroke and/or myocardial infarction survival, with such survivors subsequently developing kidney disease as a renal manifestation of their diffuse atherosclerosis. However, in an analysis comparing the potential effect of stroke and heart attack survival on the incidence of ESRD between 1978 and 1991, the effect was relatively modest, and improved survival following stroke and/or myocardial infarction explained only 4.8% of the increase in incidence of ESRD over the examined period. Nevertheless it remains intuitive, if unproven, that a decrease in competing mortality, in the continued presence of diffuse atherosclerosis, is likely to increase the prevalence of ischemic renal vascular disease and to have contributed to the observed increase in ESRD attributed to hypertension. In addition, the aggressive management of large vessel atherosclerosis, with repeated endovascular cannulation for diagnostic or therapeutic purposes, is likely to predispose to cholesterol embolization with resultant renal injury. In a study of 1786 consecutive Japanese patients 40 years of age and older undergoing left heart catheterization, the incidence of definite cholesterol emboli was 0.66% and that of possible cholesterol emboli was an additional 0.73%.[58] In addition, radiologic contrast agents cause acute kidney damage and may contribute to an increased risk of ESRD.[59]

Glomerulonephritis

With the exception of some rare diseases such as Goodpasture's disease and ANCA associated pauci-immune vasculitis, most forms of glomerulonephritis cannot be readily diagnosed by serologic tests alone; therefore, the accuracy with which the occurrence of different forms of glomerulonephritis are estimated will vary directly with the timing and frequency with which kidney biopsies are performed. The increased utilization and demonstrated safety of percutaneous kidney biopsy, especially with the assistance of real-time sonographic guidance, had led to increased rates of biopsy and diagnosis of patients with less overt forms of glomerulonephritis and increasing recognition of the spectrum of findings associated with glomerulonephritis. However, kidney biopsy rates vary widely; for example, they are reported to be several times higher in Australia than in Italy.[60, 61] Similarly, in response to a questionnaire, 21% of nephrologists from Australia and New Zealand said they would perform a kidney biopsy in a patient with less than 1 gm of proteinuria/day, as compared to 14% of nephrologists from Europe and 0% from the United States.[62] Patients with isolated hematuria are more likely to undergo renal biopsy in many areas of Asia than in either the United States or Europe.[63] Given this great degree of variability, it is almost impossible to make comparisons either over time or between different sites. Given the high frequency of patients who present late to nephrology clinics, who may have established CKD and resulting small kidneys and thus do not, undergo kidney biopsy, the true incidence of the various forms of glomerulonephritis remains uncertain. In distinction to the overall spectrum of glomerulonephritis, those patients who develop frank nephrotic syndrome typically do present for medical evaluation and often are biopsied if they do not have long-standing diabetes. Changes in the identified etiology of the nephrotic syndrome therefore are more likely to be revealing of true changes in prevalence over time and less influenced by referral practices. Mindful of these limitations, it is interesting to note that in Europe the incidence of glomerulonephritis reported by the Danish National Kidney Biopsy Registry has remained relatively constant over the time period from 1985 to 1997; the incidence of biopsy proven glomerulonephritis overall was 39.2 cases per million population per year, the incidence peaked in the 60- to 70-year-old group, which was over twice that for patients in the 20- to 40-year-old group.[64] A similar estimate of the incidence of glomerulonephritis comes from Italy, where the rate was calculated as being 47 cases per million population per year.[65]

IgA Nephropathy

IgA nephropathy is the most common overall primary form of glomerulonephritis found on kidney biopsy worldwide. It is uncommon in children, rare in African-Americans, and may on occasion be familial. It is a particularly common diagnosis among Asians and is responsible for almost 50% of biopsy-proven glomerulonephritis from Japan.[66] The overall prevalence of IgA nephropathy varies substantially, in part related to varying practice patterns with regard to biopsy of patients with nonnephrotic proteinuria or isolated hematuria. Thus, the prevalence is substantially higher in Japan where there is routine screening of patients for proteinuria than, for example, in Canada or in the United States, where in the absence of formal screening program patients typically present later in their disease course. In comparing outcomes between different countries, it is important to note that countries with screening programs are more likely to identify patients with mild disease—and thus a potentially better prognosis—as well as demonstrate a substantial lead time bias effect on kidney survival. In a study from Singapore examining the frequency of glomerulonephritis over the last two decades, IgA nephropathy remained the single most common form of glomerulonephritis, representing 56% of biopsies. However, over time, there has been a decrease in the frequency of IgA nephropathy and an increase in the frequency of minimal change disease, which is now the most common underlying diagnosis found in patients with nephrotic syndrome in that country.[67]

FSGS and Membranous

Traditionally, membranous nephropathy has been the most common primary cause of adult nephrotic syndrome in both the United States and Europe. Over the last 20 years, however, there has been a significant increase in the frequency of idiopathic Focal Segmental Glomerulosclerosis (FSGS), which has now become the most common cause of idiopathic nephrotic syndrome among adults in the United States. This increased frequency is especially evident in African-Americans but is also present in Caucasians. The frequency of FSGS among patients undergoing biopsy for nephrotic range proteinuria increased from 29% between 1975 and 1985 to 38% between 1985 and 1994.[68] Barisoni and colleagues[69] noted that the frequency of all forms of FSGS diagnosed by kidney biopsy increased sevenfold between 1974 and 1993, while Haas and colleagues[70] confirmed a similar increase in the Midwestern United States. The frequency of idiopathic FSGS increased from 4% to 12% over a 20-year period; during this time frame, the proportion of patients with membranous glomerulopathy, approximately 9%, did not change, whereas the proportion with minimal change nephropathy declined. In the study, the proportion of patients presenting with frank nephrotic syndrome and the racial characterization of the population remained relatively constant over the study period, arguing against changes in the demographic makeup of the population or changes in kidney biopsy rates as being the primary cause for the observed increased incidence of FSGS. The incidence of FSGS is four times higher in African-Americans than in Caucasians.[68] In an analysis of the changing incidence of glomerulonephritis as the cause of ESRD, Braden and colleagues[71] confirmed FSGS to be the most common cause among black subjects and its increasing incidence among white subjects, among whom it has replaced membranous nephropathy as the most common cause of nephrotic syndrome. There has similarly been an increased incidence of FSGS in Hispanic patients, among whom this is noted to be the second most common cause of primary glomerulonephritis after IgA nephropathy. FSGS is also common in areas of the Middle East, present in 41% of kidney biopsies for nephrotic syndrome in Saudi Arabia; intermediate frequencies are described in Europe (6%–15%); and the lowest frequencies are described in Asia (2%–11%).[63]

HIV-Associated Nephropathy and Collapsing Glomerulopathy

The incidence of secondary FSGS due to HIVAN (HIV associated nephropathy) initially mirrored the prevalence of the HIV epidemic among African-Americans. More recently, these rates have leveled off, presumably due to the more widespread use of effective, highly active antiretroviral therapy. While the histologic appearance of HIVAN has typically shown collapsing features, an idiopathic form of this histologic finding had not been described prior to 20 years ago but is now increasingly recognized, especially in HIV negative African-American patients. This entity has more than doubled in frequency, from 11% of all cases of idiopathic FSGS between 1979 and 1985 to 24% between 1990 and 1993.[69] The pathogenesis with this variant of FSGS and the reason for this increased frequency over time remains unclear, but it has been speculated that it may be the result of an infectious agent, for example parvovirus B19 infection,[72] or an interaction of environmental factors such as the increased frequency of obesity in genetically predisposed individuals.

Vasculitides

Comparison of the occurrence of vasculitis is particularly susceptible to selection and referral biases, with the majority of the limited number of reports coming from single tertiary referral centers with relatively small and often poorly defined source populations. Different diagnostic criteria, for example, the 1990 American College of Rheumatology vasculitis criteria, as compared to the Chapel Hill Consensus Conference definitions, further complicates the examination of trends over time. Furthermore, the introduction in the mid-1980s of relatively specific antineutrophil cytoplasmic antibodies (ANCA) associated with Wegener's granulomatosis, microscopic polyangiitis, and Churg-Strauss syndrome have allowed for more ready identification of cases, especially those with atypical features.

An examination of the incidence of systemic vasculitis from two regional referral centers, one in Norfolk, England, and the other in Lugo, Spain, using Chapel Hill consensus conference definitions, found similar overall incidence of primary systemic vasculitis in the two regions. The incidence in Norfolk was 18.9 cases per million population (pmp) while in Spain it was 18.3 pmp. The incidence of Wegener's granulomatosis in Norfolk (10.6 pmp) was greater than in Spain (4.9 pmp). This has been interpreted as being in keeping with anecdotal trend for higher incidence of Wegener's granulomatosis at northern latitudes, a similar predisposition having been proposed for giant cell arteritis. In both the English and the Spanish centers, there was a marked increase in the incidence with advancing age, with peak incidence at ages 65 to 74 (52.9 pmp).[73]

A study from northern Norway over a 15-year period, based on hospital discharge records from all 11 hospitals in the region as well as from two renal pathology services, and using American College of Rheumatology 1990 criteria, found an incidence per million population for Wegener's granulomatosis of 5.2 (95% confidence interval (CI) 2.7–9.0) between 1984 and 1988, which had risen to 12.0 (95% CI 8.0–17.3) between 1994 and 1998. The respective point prevalence increased from 30.4 pmp (95% CI 16.6–51.0) to 95.1 pmp (95% CI 96.1–129.0). The incidence was higher in men than in women, with again a peak incidence in the 65- to 74-year-old group. However, it is impossible to determine how much of that increased incidence over time relates to improved diagnosis secondary to the widespread introduction of ANCA testing.

The incidence of vasculitis has been estimated based on all hospital and outpatient unit records as well as pathology and immunology results within a five million population, living within two large mixed rural and urban areas of north and south Germany. Over a 2-year period (1998–1999), 473 individuals were diagnosed as having incident primary systemic vasculitis. The unadjusted incidence rates in north Germany for all primary systemic vasculitides were 54 cases pmp/year in 1998 and 48 pmp/year in 1999, compared to rates in the south of 48 pmp in 1998 and 41 pmp in 1999. The incidence rates for ANCA associated vasculitis were 11 and 9.5 pmp in 1998 and 1999, respectively, in the north and 9 and 7 pmp in the south. Overall, Wegener's granulomatosis was the most frequent type of ANCA associated vasculitis diagnosed. There was no significant difference in the type of vasculitis identified between northern and southern Germany, or between urban or rural areas.

Tubulointerstitial Kidney Disease

The diagnosis of chronic tubulointerstitial kidney disease is especially difficult to make because it is often clinically silent: Patients usually lack substantial proteinuria and have a bland urinary sediment. Primary tubulointerstitial disease may occur as a consequence of allergic reaction, toxic exposures, or more rarely due to autoimmune mechanisms. The incidence of chronic interstitial nephritis is unknown. The increased use of exotic herbal preparation for a variety of purported reasons, including slimming regimens, has resulted in the increased recognition of an aggressive form of tubulointerstitial disease, referred to as Chinese herb nephropathy, characterized by minimal glomerular findings and a rapid, often irreversible decline in renal function.[74] Balkan nephropathy has been a long recognized form of severe tubulointerstitial disease; endemic to the Balkans, its etiology is unknown but is believed to result from an environmental exposure, the leading candidate being contamination of cereals or pork products by Ochratoxin A.

The association between analgesic use and renal failure remains complex and controversial and raises a variety of issues that demonstrate the potential limitations of observational epidemiology, especially retrospective studies.[75–77] While the nephrotoxic consequences of some agents such as phenacetin is well established, the association between currently used analgesics, such as nonsteroidal anti-inflammatory preparations or the Cox-2 inhibitors,[75] with long-term kidney dysfunction has been demonstrated in several studies but remains unproven. Lead has long been recognized as a potential nephrotoxin and cause of interstitial kidney disease, though the population-related renal consequences of lead exposure have been poorly defined. In a recent analysis based on NHANES III data, higher lead levels in the general population were associated with higher prevalence of CKD.[78] The highest population quartile of lead exposure as compared to the lowest quartile was associated with a 2.6 (95% CI: 1.5–4.5) higher odds of CKD, suggesting the possibility that prolonged exposure to even low environmental lead levels may contribute to kidney damage.

PATIENT OUTCOMES

Treatment with renal replacement therapy continues to be complicated by extremely high morbidity and mortality, though these have slowly improved over time. The 1-year, all modality (transplantation and dialysis) survival rate, adjusted for age, race, gender, and ESRD etiology increased from 73.8% in 1980 to 79.8% in 2000; the 5-year survival rate increased from 31.2% to 38.8%, respectively. Examining dialysis specific survival rates, 1-year survival improved between 1980 and 2000 from 74.8% to 79.2% and the 5-year survival rate increased from 29.5% to 34.4%. This improvement has occurred despite a marked increase in the degree of comorbidity among incident patients during this time. Among prevalent dialysis patients the overall age, race, and gender adjusted mortality rates fell by approximately 10% over the last decade. However, this improvement is the result of a decrease in mortality for patients who have been treated with dialysis for less than 3 years; the mortality rate for those dialyzed for 3 or more years has steadily increased (Figure 1–8).[79] The latter increase may reflect sicker patients surviving the first years on dialysis. The decline in prevalent mortality rates since 1980 has been less impressive for African-Americans, a 12.3% reduction, as compared to 13.5% for Caucasians, 18.2% for Native-Americans, and 29% for Asians.

The comparison of survival among transplant recipients as compared to dialysis treated patients is inherently biased because it does not take into account the selection bias that results from the screening of potential transplant candidates and the exclusion of high-risk subjects. A fairer comparison is to examine outcomes between transplant recipients and those individuals who are successfully wait-listed but who continue on dialysis while waiting for a transplant. This analysis continues to show approximately threefold lower mortality for transplanted as compared to wait-listed subjects.[80]

ESRD Hospitalization rates

Hospital admission rates have remained relatively constant within the dialysis population over the last decade in the United States.[1] Hospitalization rates are highest for patients with primary diagnosis of diabetes (2.4 admissions per patient year in 2001) and lowest for glomerulonephritis (1.7 admission per patient year, in 2001). Hospitalization days per patient year have steadily decreased over the last decade, by 19% for those with a primary diagnosis of glomerulonephritis and 21% for those with a primary diagnosis of

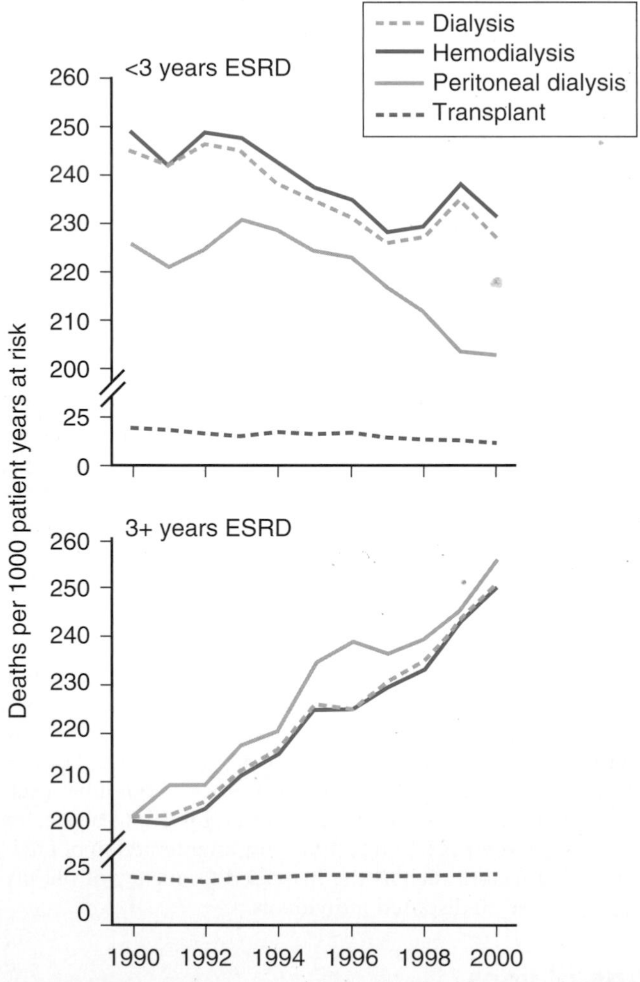

Figure 1–8 Prevalence mortality rates by duration of ESRD and modality. (From U.S. Renal Data System: USRDS 2003 Annual Data Report: Atlas of end-stage renal disease in the United States. Bethesda, MD, National Institutes of Health, 2003, pp 1–560. Copyright 2002, with permission from the National Kidney Foundation.)

diabetes (to 10 and 18 days a year, respectively, in 2001). Similar trends have been seen in the transplant population (1.26 and 0.76 hospitalizations for a total of 10 and 5 days a year in 2001 for ESRD attributed to diabetes and glomerulonephritis, respectively).

Outcomes in CKD Stages I to IV

Data from population-based studies and clinical populations are increasingly showing the gradual increase in kidney related complications at lower levels of GFR. These relationships are discussed in detail in subsequent chapters. Cross-sectional analyses indicate that many complications are noticeably more common at a GFR below 60 mL/min/1.73 m^2.[2] In addition, prospective data showing a higher risk of cardiovascular disease and mortality at lower kidney function are increasing.[81]

Expected Remaining Years of Life

The limitations of our current strategies for managing CKD are clearly evident in the limited expected remaining years of life for patients treated with dialysis, which are only one-third to one-sixth that of the age matched general U.S. population. The lowest ratios are found for white females. Thus, for a white 45-year-old on maintenance dialysis, the remaining years of life are 6.3 for a male and 6.0 years for a female, as compared to the general population remaining years of life of 32.4 and 36.6 years, respectively. The equivalent figures for an African-American male and female are 7.7 and 7.3 years of life on dialysis, as compared to 27.8 and 33 years in the general population.[1]

SUMMARY

The epidemiology of CKD is becoming better understood. In addition to the epidemic increase of treated kidney failure, the large burden of earlier stages of CKD is now better appreciated. A standardized definition and staging system complements the exiting etiologic classification of disease and focuses on complications common to all types of CKD. Management of CKD complications are important to prevent not only further CKD progression but also the associated morbidity and mortality that precede the onset of kidney failure and often result in mortality prior to initiation of dialysis. Improved understanding of the epidemiology (distribution and determinants) of CKD will be important in devising and tracking the implementation of strategies for improved diagnosis and treatment of all stages of CKD.

References

1. U.S. Renal Data System: USRDS 2003 Annual Data Report: Atlas of end-stage renal disease in the United States. Bethesda, MD, National Institutes of Health, 2003, pp 1–560.
2. National Kidney Foundation KD: Clinical practice guidelines for chronic kidney disease: Evaluation, classification and stratification. Am J Kidney Dis 2002; 39(suppl 1):S1–S266.
3. Hsu C, Chertow G: Chronic renal confusion: Insufficiency, failure, dysfunction, or disease. Am J Kidney Dis 2000; 36(2):415–418.
4. Sturgiss S, Dunlop W, Davison J: Renal haemodynamics and tubular function in human pregnancy. Clin Obstet Gynaecol 1994; 8:209–234.
5. Lew S, Bosch J: Effect of diet on creatinine clearance and excretion in young and elderly healthy subjects and in patients with renal disease. J Am Soc Nephrol 1991; 2(4):856–865.
6. Hoang K, Tan J, Derby G, et al: Determinants of glomerular hypofiltration in aging humans. Kidney Int 2003; 64:1417–1424.
7. Lindeman R: Overview: Renal physiology and pathophysiology of aging. Am J Kidney Dis 1990; 16:275–282.
8. McManus J, Lupton C: Ischemic obsolescence of renal glomeruli. Lab Invest 1960; 9:413–434.
9. Kasiske B: Relationship between vascular disease and age-associated changes in the human kidney. Kidney Int 1987; 31:1153–1159.
10. Muruve N, Steinbecker K, Luger A: Are wedge biopsies of cadaveric kidneys obtained at procurement reliable? Transplantation 2000; 69:2384–2388.
11. Kappel B, Olsen S: Cortical interstitial tissue and sclerosed glomeruli in the normal human kidney, related to age and sex. Virchows Arch A Pathol Anat Histol 1980; 387:271–277.
12. Nyengaard J, Bendtsen T: Glomerular number and size in relation to age, kidney weight, and body surface in normal man. Anat Rec 1992; 232:194–201.
13. Sandberg K, Ji H: Sex and the renin angiotensin system: Implications for gender differences in the progression of kidney disease. Adv Ren Replace Ther 2003; 10(1):15–23.
14. Davison J, Dunlop W, Ezimokhai M: 24-hour creatinine clearance during the third trimester of normal pregnancy. Br J Obstet Gynaecol 1980; 87:106–109.
15. Obrador G, Pereira B, Kausz A: Chronic kidney disease in the United States: An underrecognized problem. Semin Nephrol 2002; 22(6):441–448.
16. Gill J, Abichandani R, Khan S, et al: Opportunities to improve the care of patients with kidney transplant failure. Kidney Int 2002; 61(6):2193–2200.
17. McClellan W, Knight D, Karp H, Brown W: Early detection and treatment of renal disease in hospitalized diabetic and hypertensive patients: Important differences between practice and published guidelines. Am J Kidney Dis 1997; 29(3):368–375.
18. Coresh J, Astor B, McQuillan G, et al: Calibration and random variation of the serum creatinine assay as critical elements of using equations to estimate glomerular filtration rate. American Journal of Kidney Diseases 2002; 39(5):920–929.
19. Stengel B, Billon S, van Dijk PCW, et al: Trends in the incidence of renal replacement therapy for end-stage renal disease in Europe, 1990–1999. Nephrol Dial Transplant 2003; 18(9):1824–1833.
20. Usami T, Sato R, Yoshida A, Kimura G: Regional variation in end-stage renal disease. Opin Nephrol Hypertens 2002; 11:343–346.
21. McDonald S, Graeme R, Kerr P, Collins J: ESRD in Australia and New Zealand at the end of millennium: A report from the ANZ-DATA registry. Am J Kidney Dis 2004; 40:1122–1131.
22. Kiberd B, Clase C: Cumulative risk for developing end-stage renal disease in the U.S. population. J Am Soc Nephrol 2002; 13:1635–1644.
23. Paivansolo M, Huttunen K, Suramo I: Ultrasonographic findings in renal parenchymal diseases. Scand J Urol Nephrol 1985; 19:119–123.
24. Jones C, Francis M, Eberhardt M, et al: Microalbuminuria in the U.S. population: Third National Health and Nutrition Examination Survey. Am J Kidney Dis 2002; 39(3):445–459.
25. Gerstein HC, Mann JFE, Yi Q, et al: Albuminuria and risk of cardiovascular events, death, and heart failure in diabetic and non-diabetic individuals. JAMA 2001; 286(4):421–426.
26. Mattix HJ, Hsu Cy, Shaykevich S, Curhan G: Use of the albumin/creatinine ratio to detect microalbuminuria: Implications of sex and race. J Am Soc Nephrol 2002; 13(4):1034–1039.
27. Molitch ME, DeFronzo RA, Franz MJ, et al: Nephropathy in diabetes. Diabetes Care 2004; 27(suppl 1):S79–S83.

28. Keane W, Eknoyan G: Proteinuria, albuminuria, risk, assessment, detection, elimination (PARADE): A position paper of the National Kidney Foundation. Am J Kidney Dis 1999; 33(5):1004–1010.
29. Stehman-Breen CO, Gillen D, Steffes M, et al: Racial differences in early-onset renal disease among young adults: The Coronary Artery Risk Development in Young Adults (CARDIA) Study. J Am Soc Nephrol 2003; 14(9):2352–2357.
30. Chadban SJ, Briganti EM, Kerr PG, et al: Prevalence of kidney damage in Australian adults: The AusDiab Kidney Study. J Am Soc Nephrol 2003; 14(7 suppl 2):S131–S138.
31. Iseki K: The Okinawa screening program. J Am Soc Nephrol 2003; 14(7 suppl 2):S127–S130.
32. Ross J, Miller W, Myers G, Praestgaard J: The accuracy of laboratory measurements in clinical chemistry: A study of 11 routine chemistry analytes in the College of American Pathologists chemistry survey with fresh frozen serum, definitive methods, and reference methods. Arch Pathol Lab Med 1998; 122:587–608.
33. Duncan L, Heathcote J, Djurdjev O, Levin A: Screening for renal disease using serum creatinine: Who are we missing? Nephrol Dial Transplant 2001; 16:1042–1046.
34. Jones C, McQuillan G, Kusek J, et al: Serum creatinine levels in the U.S. population: Third National Health and Nutrition Examination Survey. Am J Kidney Dis 1998; 32(6):992–999.
35. Magnason R, Indridason O, Sigvaldason H, et al: Prevalence and progression of CRF in Iceland: A population-based study. Am J Kidney Dis 2002; 40(5):955–963.
36. Nissenson A, Pereira B, Collins A, Steinberg E: Prevalence and characteristics of individuals with chronic kidney disease in a large health maintenance organization. Am J Kidney Dis 2001; 37(6):1177–1183.
37. Culleton B, Larson M, Evans JC, et al: Prevalence and correlates of elevated serum creatinine levels. Arch Intern Med 1999; 159:1785–1790.
38. Coresh J, Astor B, Greene T, et al: Prevalence of chronic kidney disease and decreased kidney function in the adult U.S. population: Third National Health and Nutrition Examination Survey. Am J Kidney Dis 2003; 41(1):1–12.
39. Onkamo P, Vaananen S, Karvonen M, et al: Worldwide increase in incidence of type I diabetes: The analysis of the data on published incidence trends. Diabetologia 1999; 42:1395–1403.
40. Harvey J, Rizvi K, Craney L, et al: Population-based survey and analysis of trends in the prevalence of diabetic nephropathy in type I diabetes. Diabetic Med 2001; 18:998–1002.
41. Rossing P, Hougaard P, Parving H: Risk factors for development of incipient and overt diabetic nephropathy in type I diabetic patients. A 10-year prospective observational study. Diabetes Care 2002; 25:859–864.
42. Bojestig M, Arnqvist H, Hermansson G, et al: Declining incidence of nephropathy in insulin-dependent diabetes mellitus. N Engl J Med 1994; 330:15–18.
43. Nishimura R, Dorman J, Bosnyak Z, et al: Incidence of ESRD and survival after renal replacement therapy in patients with type I diabetes: A report from the Allegheny County Registry. Am J Kidney Dis 2003; 42(1):117–124.
44. Hu F, Manson J, Stampfer M, et al: Diet, lifestyle, and the risk of type II diabetes mellitus in women. N Engl J Med 2001; 345:790–797.
45. UK Prospective Diabetes Study Group. Efficacy of atenolol and captopril in reducing risk of macrovascular and microvascular complications in type II diabetes: UKPDS 39. BMJ 1998; 317(7160):713–720.
46. Stratton IM, Adler AI, Neil HA, et al: Association of glycaemia with macrovascular and microvascular complications of type II diabetes (UKPDS 35): Prospective observational study. BMJ 2000; 321(7258):405–412.
47. Diabetes Prevention Program Research Group. Reduction in the incidence of type II diabetes with lifestyle intervention or metformin. N Engl J Med 2002; 346(6):393–403.
48. Tuomilehto J, Lindstrom J, Eriksson JG, et al: Prevention of type II diabetes mellitus by changes in lifestyle among subjects with impaired glucose tolerance. N Engl J Med 2001; 344(18): 1343–1350.
49. Mokdad AH, Ford ES, Bowman BA, et al: Diabetes trends in the U.S.: 1990–1998. Diabetes Care 2000; 23(9):1278–1283.
50. Ubink-Veltmaat L, Bilo H, Groenier K, et al: Prevalence, incidence and mortality of type II diabetes mellitus revisited: A prospective population-based study in the Netherlands (ZODIAC-1). Eur J Epidemiol 2003; 18(8):793–800.
51. Muntner P, Coresh J, Powe N, Klag M: The contribution of increased diabetes prevalence and improved myocardial infarction and stroke survival to the increase in treated end-stage renal disease. J Am Soc Nephrol 2003; 14:1568–1577.
52. Wimmer F, Oberaigner W, Kramar R, Mayer G: Regional variability in the incidence of end-stage renal disease: An epidemiological approach. Nephrol Dial Transplant 2003; 18(8):1562–1567.
53. Hsu C: Does non-malignant hypertension cause renal insufficiency? Evidence-based perspective. Curr Opin Nephrol Hypertens 2002; 11:267–272.
54. Young J, Klag M, Muntner P, et al: Blood pressure and decline in kidney function: Findings from the Systolic Hypertension in the Elderly Program (SHEP). J Am Soc Nephrol 2002; 13(11): 2776–2782.
55. Haroun M, Jaar B, Hoffman S, et al: Risk factors for chronic kidney disease: A prospective study of 23,534 men and women in Washington County, Maryland. J Am Soc Nephrol 2003; 14:2934–2941.
56. Klag MJ, Whelton PK, Randall BL, et al: Blood pressure and end-stage renal disease in men. N Engl J Med 1996; 334(1):13–18.
57. Perry HM Jr, Miller JP, Fornoff JR, et al: Early predictors of 15-year end-stage renal disease in hypertensive patients. Hypertension 1995; 25(4):587–594.
58. Fukumoto Y, Tsutsui H, Tsuchihashi M, et al: The incidence and risk factors of cholesterol embolization syndrome, a complication of cardiac catheterization: A prospective study. J Am Coll Cardiol 2003; 42(2):211–216.
59. Muntner P, Coresh J, Klag M, et al: Exposure to radiologic contrast media and an increased risk of treated end-stage renal disease. Am J Med Sci 2003; 326:353–359.
60. Briganti EM, Dowling J, Finlay M, et al: The incidence of biopsy-proven glomerulonephritis in Australia. Nephrol Dial Transplant 2001; 16(7):1364–1367.
61. Schena FP: Survey of the Italian Registry of Renal Biopsies. Frequency of the renal diseases for 7 consecutive years. The Italian Group of Renal Immunopathology. Nephrol Dial Transplant 1997; 12(3):418–426.
62. Fuiano G, Mazza G, Comi N, et al: Current indications for renal biopsy: A questionnaire-based survey. Am J Kidney Dis 2000; 35(3):448–457.
63. Kitiyakara C, Kopp J, Eggers P: Trends in the epidemiology of focal segmental glomerulosclerosis. Semin Nephrol 2003; 23:172–182.
64. Heaf J, Lokkegaard H, Larsen S: The epidemiology and prognosis of glomerulonephritis in Denmark 1985–1997. Nephrol Dial Transplant 1999; 14(8):1889–1897.
65. Stratta P, Segoloni G, Canavese C, et al: Incidence of biopsy-proven primary glomerulonephritis in an Italian province. Am J Kidney Dis 1996; 27(5):631–639.
66. Anonymous. Nationwide and long-term survey of primary glomerulonephritis in Japan as observed in 1,850 biopsied cases. Nephron 1999; 82(3):205–213.
67. Woo K, Chiang G, Pall A, et al: The changing pattern of glomerulonephritis in Singapore over the past two decades. Clin Nephrol 1999; 52:96–102.
68. Korbet S, Genchi R, Borok R, Schwartz M: The racial prevalence of glomerular lesions in nephrotic adults. Am J Kidney Dis 1996; 27(5):647–651.

69. Valeri A, Barisoni L, Appel G, et al: Idiopathic collapsing focal segmental glomerulosclerosis: A clinicopathological study. Kidney Int 1996; 50:1734–1746.
70. Haas M, Meehan S, Karrison T, Spargo B: Changing etiologies of unexplained adult nephrotic syndrome: A comparison of renal biopsy findings from 1976–1979 and 1995–1997. Am J Kidney Dis 1997; 30(5):621–631.
71. Braden G, Mulhern J, O'Shea M, et al: Changing incidence of glomerular diseases in adults. Am J Kidney Dis 2000; 35(5):878–883.
72. Tanawattanacharoen S, Falk R, Jennette J, Kopp J: Parvovirus B19 DNA in kidney tissue of patients with focal segmental glomerulosclerosis. Am J Kidney Dis 2000; 35:1166–1174.
73. Watts R, Gonzalez-Gay M, Lane S, et al: Geoepidemiology of systemic vasculitis: Comparison of the incidence in two regions of Europe. Ann Rheum Dis 2001; 60:170–172.
74. Chang C, Wang Y, Yang A, Chiang S: Rapidly progressive interstitial renal fibrosis associated with Chinese herbal medications. Am J Nephrol 2001; 21:441–448.
75. Galli G, Panzetta G: Do non-steroidal anti-inflammatory drugs and COX-2 selective inhibitors have different renal effects. J Nephrol 2002; 15:480–488.
76. Henrich W, Agodoa L, Barrett B, et al: Analgesics and the kidney: Summary and recommendations to the Scientific Advisory Board of the National Kidney Foundation from an ad hoc committee of the National Kidney Foundation. Am J Kidney Dis 1996; 27:162–165.
77. Klag MJ, Whelton PK, Perneger T: Analgesics and chronic renal disease. Curr Opin Nephrol Hypertens 1996; 5:236–241.
78. Muntner P, He J, Vupputuri S, et al: Blood lead and chronic kidney disease in the general United States population: Results from NHANES III. Kidney Int 2003; 63(3):1044–1050.
79. National Institutes of Health NIDDK. USRDS 2002 Annual Data Report: Atlas of end-stage renal disease in the United States. Bethesda, MD, National Institutes of Health, 2003, 16–28.
80. Meier-Kriesche H, Ojo AO, Port FK, et al: Survival improvement among patients with end-stage renal disease: Trends over time for transplant recipients and wait-listed patients. J Am Soc Nephrol 2001; 12(6):1293–1296.
81. Coresh J, Astor B, Sarnak M: Evidence for increased cardiovascular disease risk in patients with chronic kidney disease. Curr Opin Nephrol Hypertens 2004; 13:73–81.

Measurement of Kidney Function

Anupama Mohanram, M.D. • Robert D. Toto, M.D.

The accurate measurement of kidney function is essential for the evaluation and management of kidney disease. This is especially important because early kidney disease is silent. Furthermore, staging by level of kidney function facilitates determination of not only kidney disease but also associated risks, such as cardiovascular disease, bone disease, and anemia. By measuring kidney function over time, one can monitor the course of kidney disease and the effects of therapies directed at slowing the progression of kidney disease. The National Kidney Foundation (NKF) recommends estimation of glomerular filtration rate (GFR) for staging the severity of chronic kidney disease (CKD), as shown in Table 2–1.[1]

GLOMERULAR FILTRATION RATE

Glomerular filtration rate is a standard measure of kidney function; it is the clearance by filtration of a marker from plasma by the kidneys and represents renal excretory function. Level of GFR correlates with structural kidney damage; however, in certain disease processes GFR may be normal or even elevated in the presence of significant kidney disease. Consequently, a normal GFR alone does not exclude kidney disease. GFR should be used in conjunction with other clinical parameters for diagnosis and management.

There is a great deal of variability in GFR for normal subjects,[2] and factors such as exercise and protein intake can influence GFR. Normal ranges for GFR are age and gender dependent. Table 2–2 demonstrates the mean GFR from the Third National Health and Nutrition Survey by age[3] and levels of kidney function in the Scandinavian population by age and gender. GFR is generally higher among men compared to women: mean adult values for GFR are 130 mL/min/1.73 m^2 for men and 120 mL/min/1.73 m^2 for women. Kidney function is expected to decline with advancing age, and the rate of decline of creatinine clearance, estimated from 24-hour urine collections, increases with advancing age.[4] Despite these factors, GFR is very useful for following kidney function over time for a given individual.

There are a variety of methods for estimating or measuring GFR, ranging from prediction equations based on serum creatinine (SCr) to complicated repeated measures of urine and serum samples, and each method has its own advantages and disadvantages.

Clearance Methods

Renal Clearance

The basic formula for measuring renal clearance of any substance is the product of the urine concentration of marker and the urine flow rate in mL/min divided by the plasma concentration of marker. For optimal GFR measurement, a marker is given via continuous infusion in order to achieve and maintain a stable plasma level of the marker. The marker may be given intravenously or subcutaneously and is followed by repeated collections of urine samples approximately every 30 to 45 minutes (Figure 2–1). The plasma concentration of the marker is usually measured at the midpoint of the urine collection period or as the log mean of two measures taken before and after each urine collection period. Urine is optimally collected with a properly positioned bladder catheter. However, in most instances bladder catheters are not employed to measure renal clearance; consequently, errors in measurement may occur due to incomplete bladder emptying, particularly in diabetics and children.

Plasma Clearance

The advantage of plasma clearance methods is that urine collection is not required. To measure plasma clearance, the marker may be given as a continuous injection or as a single bolus injection. If the marker is given as a continuous injection, plasma concentration is determined at steady-state. When the marker's distribution space and the marker's plasma level are constant, the rate of infusion and the rate of elimination will be the same. However, steady-state may not be achieved for 3 to 24 hours, which may limit use of this test. The basic formula for plasma clearance for a continuous infusion is the infusion rate of marker in mL/min divided by the plasma concentration of marker in mg/dL.

When a marker is given as a single injection, plasma clearance can be modeled as a two-compartment model (Figure 2–2) or as a single-compartment model (Figure 2–3) in order to measure GFR. The two-compartment model requires multiple measures of plasma concentration of marker over time. These measured concentrations of marker over time are then modeled as two phases of plasma clearance. Phase one is a slow elimination phase and represents movement of the marker from the intravascular space to the extravascular space. Phase two is the rapid elimination phase and represents plasma clearance of the marker, which is assumed to be the same as the renal clearance of the marker. This assumption is incorrect for some markers, such as Chromium ethylenediamine tetra-acetic acid (^{51}Cr-EDTA). Extra-renal clearance of such markers leads to overestimation of glomerular filtration rate by up to 10%.

For most markers, the two-compartment model accounts for all plasma clearance of marker. Two lines are determined in order to calculate GFR by the two-compartment model. The first line is a best fit regression of the terminal elimination phase (depicted by slope k_1 and intercept A in Figure 2–2). The second line is the best fit of the difference between actual

Table 2–1 Stages of Chronic Kidney Disease

Stage of CKD	Description	Glomerular Filtration Rate (mL/min/1.73 m²)
1	Kidney damage (such as proteinuria) with normal or increased GFR	>90
2	Kidney damage with mildly decreased GFR	60–89
3	Moderately decreased GFR	30–59
4	Severely decreased GFR	15–29
5	Kidney failure	<15 or dialysis

Staging for chronic kidney disease based on glomerular filtration rate as defined by the National Kidney Foundation. (From Eknoyan G, Levin NW: K/DOQI clinical practice guidelines for chronic kidney disease: Evaluation, classification, and stratification. Am J Kidney Dis 2002; 39[2]:S14-S266.)

values and values calculated from the line fitted to the terminal elimination phase (depicted by slope k_2 and intercept B in Figure 2–2). Glomerular filtration rate (two-compartment method) is calculated as follows:

$$\text{GFR} = [\text{Marker}] \times k_1 \times k_2 / (Ak_2 + Bk_1)$$

where [Marker] is the amount of marker given.

One can also determine GFR for a one-compartment model based on these regression analyses. Glomerular filtration rate (one-compartment method) is calculated as follows[5–7]:

$$\text{GFR} = [\text{Marker}] \times k_1 / A$$

Figure 2–3 shows a single-compartment model after a single injection. When plasma clearance is modeled as a single compartment, the area below the dotted line is used as the area under the curve (AUC) and corresponds to the rapid elimination phase. This model assumes total excretion of the marker. Because the slow elimination phase is not included, the AUC by the one-compartment method is slightly lower than the actual AUC, leading to overestimation of plasma clearance.[8]

MARKERS FOR MEASURING GLOMERULAR FILTRATION RATE

An ideal marker should be freely filtered, not protein bound, eliminated solely by the kidney and not metabolized, reabsorbed, or secreted by the renal tubules. One should be able to measure the marker by a reproducible and accessible laboratory assay without interference from other compounds. In addition, an ideal marker is one that is safe, readily available, and inexpensive. Less ideal markers may impart radiation exposure, require intravenous access for infusions, and require multiple sampling of blood and/or urine, via bladder catheterization. Although there is no ideal marker, inulin has been considered the gold standard. The major markers are discussed in this section and summarized in Table 2–3.

Exogenous Clearance Markers

Inulin

Inulin is the gold standard among markers because it allows for the most accurate measure of glomerular filtration rate. However, it is not practical for clinical use because it is expensive, in short supply, and it must be given intravenously.[9] It remains useful as a research tool given its accuracy.

Inulin (MW 5200 daltons [Da]) is an inert plant-derived fructose polymer. It does not bind to plasma proteins, is freely filtered and excreted by the kidney, and it is not reabsorbed or secreted by the tubule. There is no extra-renal metabolism of inulin. It can be measured in urine and plasma with the caveat that high glucose levels can interfere with the anthrone assay used to measure inulin.

There are several methods for measuring clearance with inulin; one such method is explained here. The patient begins the day by drinking water (10–15 mL/kg) after an overnight fast and is encouraged to continue drinking water in order to attain a urine flow rate of 4 mL/min. An intravenous loading dose of inulin is administered prior to beginning an inulin infusion in order to achieve steady-state (typically 45–60 minutes). After inulin is given, urine is collected every 30 minutes by bladder catheterization in order to avoid variability in measurement. Plasma inulin levels are also measured. Clearance is then calculated from an average of 3 to 5 measures based on the steady-state assumption that when the volume of distribution stabilizes, then infusion is equal to elimination.

This technique is considered cumbersome for clinical practice because it requires intravenous access for a constant infusion, oral water loading and need for bladder catheterization, and a prolonged time (more than 6 hours) to complete the procedure. Another caveat is that if the patient does not keep up with water loading, inulin elimination is decreased. Given these difficulties, newer techniques use an inulin bolus and no infusion. Bolus dosing without infusion results in lower levels of inulin that can now be measured by high pressure liquid chromatography. Inulin clearance with continuous intravenous infusion remains the gold standard for estimating GFR; however, due to the inconveniences mentioned, other markers have been used as described below.

Iothalamate

Iothalamate is convenient to administer both in clinical as well as in research settings. The radioiodinated form has advantages compared to using inulin since the radioiodinated iothalamate, ^{125}I-iothalamate, can be administered as a single subcutaneous injection for renal clearance measurement, making it an attractive method for estimating GFR.

Sodium iothalamate (MW 614 Da) is a derivative of triidobenzoic acid. It is a high osmolar ionic radiocontrast agent that is slightly protein bound.[10] Clearance measurements using sodium iothalamate are reasonably accurate, but overestimate inulin clearance by about 7% because of a constant rate of proximal tubular secretion. It can be given subcutaneously as the ^{125}I-nuclide and is relatively convenient for clinical management as well as for research purposes. A small amount undergoes extra-renal metabolism via the liver, biliary tract, and small intestine, which is more pronounced for patients with advanced CKD.[11] However, the nuclide is very expensive, requires special handling and

Table 2–2 Glomerular Filtration Rate, Plasma Creatinine, and Creatinine Excretion in Adults by Increasing Age

	NHANES Population[2]	Scandinavian Population[40]					
	Males and Females	Males			Females		
Age (yr)	Average GFR (mL/min/1.73m^2)	Serum creatinine (mg/dL ± SD)	Urinary creatinine (mg/kg/24 hr ± SD)	$C_{creatinine}$ (mL/1.73m^2)	Serum creatinine (mg/dL ± SD)	Urinary creatinine (mg/kg/24 hr ± SD)	$C_{creatinine}$ (mL/1.73m^2)
20–29	116	0.99 ± 0.16	23.8 ± 2.3	110	0.89 ± 0.17	19.7 ± 3.9	95
30–39	107	1.14 ± 0.22	21.9 ± 1.5	97	0.91 ± 0.17	20.4 ± 3.9	103
40–49	99	1.10 ± 0.20	19.7 ± 3.2	88	1.00 ± 0.24	17.6 ± 3.9	81
50–59	93	1.16 ± 0.17	19.3 ± 2.9	81	0.99 ± 0.26	14.9 ± 3.6	74
60–69	85	1.15 ± 0.14	16.9 ± 2.9	72	0.97 ± 0.17	12.9 ± 2.6	63
70–79	75	1.03 ± 0.22	14.2 ± 3.0	64	1.02 ± 0.23	11.8 ± 2.2	54
80–89		1.06 ± 0.25	11.7 ± 4.0	47	1.05 ± 0.22	10.7 ± 2.5	46
90–99		1.20 ± 0.16	9.4 ± 3.2	34	0.91 ± 0.12	8.4 ± 1.4	39

Second column shows population mean GFR from the Third National Health and Nutrition Survey (NHANES III), calculated by the Modification of Diet in Renal Disease formula. The remainder of this table shows creatinine concentrations and clearance by age and gender for a Scandinavian population of hospitalized patients with normal serum creatinine. Note that for these patients with normal creatinine, with advancing age, the trend is for decrease in urinary creatinine and decrease in measured creatinine clearance. Also note that overall, women tend to have lower urinary creatinine and clearance than men. (From Coresh J, Astor BC, Greene T, et al: Prevalence of chronic kidney disease and decreased kidney function in the adult U.S. population: Third National Health and Nutrition Examination Survey. Am J Kidney Dis 2003; 41[1]:1-12; and Kampmann J, Siersbaek-Nielsen K, Kristensen M, Hansen JM: Rapid evaluation of creatinine clearance. Acta Med Scand 1974; 196(6):517-520. Used with permission.)

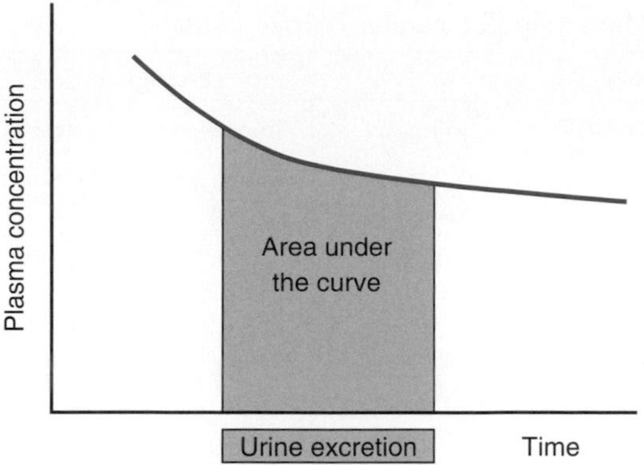

Figure 2–1 Renal clearance. This cartoon shows plasma concentration of a marker versus time. To calculate renal clearance of a marker, divide the amount of the marker that is excreted in the urine by the area under the curve (AUC): Clearance = [Urine excretion]/AUC. (Adapted from Horio M, Orita Y, Fukunaga M: Assessment of renal function. *In* Johnson RJ, Feehally J [eds]: Comprehensive Clinical Nephrology. London, Mosby, 2000, pp 3.1–3.6.)

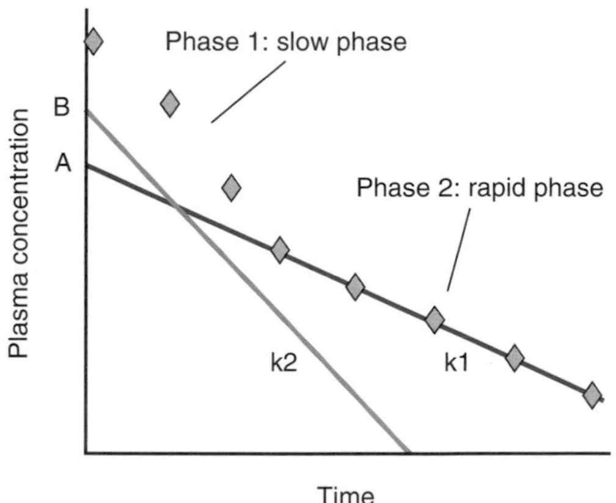

Figure 2–2 Plasma clearance curve after single injection—two-compartment model. In this cartoon, diamonds depict measured plasma concentration over time for a marker. Phase 1, the slow elimination phase, represents movement of the marker from the intravascular space to the extravascular space. Phase 2, the rapid elimination phase, represents renal elimination of the marker. The two-compartment model accounts for all plasma clearance of marker. The first line (slope k_1 and intercept A) is the best fit of the terminal elimination phase, the rapid phase, by least squares method. The second line (slope k_2 and intercept B) shows the best fit of the difference between actual values and values calculated from the line fitted to the terminal elimination phase. Glomerular filtration rate (two-compartment method) is calculated as follows: GFR = $[\text{Marker}]k_1\ k_2/(Ak_2 + Bk_1)$, where [Marker] is the amount of marker given.
Glomerular filtration rate (one-compartment method) is calculated as follows: GFR = $[\text{Marker}]k_1/A$. (Adapted from Silkensen JR, Kasiske BL: Laboratory assessment of kidney disease: Clearance, urinalysis, and kidney biopsy. *In* Brenner BM [ed]: The Kidney. Philadelphia, WB Saunders, 2004, pp 1107-1137.)

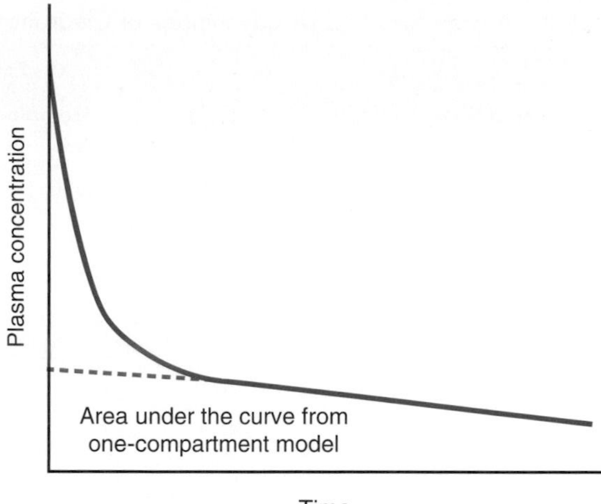

Figure 2–3 Plasma clearance after single injection—single-compartment model. When plasma clearance is modeled as a single compartment, the area below dotted line is used as the AUC and corresponds to the rapid elimination phase, as shown here. This model assumes total excretion of the marker. Because the slow elimination phase is not included, the AUC by the one-compartment method is slightly lower than the actual AUC, leading to overestimation of plasma clearance. (Adapted from Horio M, Orita Y, Fukunaga M: Assessment of renal function. *In* Johnson RJ, Feehally J [eds]: Comprehensive Clinical Nephrology. London, Mosby, 2000, pp 3.1–3.6.)

documentation, exposes the patient to radiation, and therefore cannot be made widely available to practice or research environments.

Although the amount of radiation used for GFR studies is lower than the amount used for radiologic procedures, these markers are concentrated in the urinary system, and exposure is a safety concern.[12] Furthermore, there is some risk of thyroid uptake, but this can be prevented with pretreatment of oral iodine (Lugol's solution). Radiation exposure is an even greater concern in pregnant women and in children. Alternative markers should be considered in patients who are allergic to iodinated compounds or contrast media. We recommend use of creatinine or cystatin C or, if possible, inulin to measure GFR in those at risk for allergic reaction to iodinated compounds, although there is some evidence that pretreatment with corticosteroids and antihistamines may reduce this risk.[13]

Continuous I.V. infusion and subcutaneous methods are available for cold iothalamate.[14–16] The cost of cold iothalamate is low, making this marker an attractive alternative to radionuclide management. Subcutaneous injection of cold iothalamate can be employed to measure GFR but requires access to high performance liquid chromatography (HPLC) or capillary electrophoresis to measure accurately low blood and urine levels of the marker. Whether using cold or hot iothalamate, GFR is overestimated when compared to inulin.[17]

Table 2–3 Advantages and Disadvantages of Clearance Markers for Measuring Glomerular Filtration Rate

	Exogenous					Endogenous	
Markers and Characteristics	**Inulin**	**Iothalamate Hot**	**Iothalamate Cold**	**51Cr-EDTA**	**Iohexol**	**Creatinine**	**Cystatin C**
Trade Name	**NA**	**Glofil**	**Conray**	**Codigo**	**Omnipaque**	**NA**	**NA**
Size (daltons)	5200	614	614	292	821	113	13000
Safe	Y	R, I*	I	R*	I	Y	Y
Expensive marker	Y	Y	N	N	N	N	N
Freely filtered	Y	Y	Y	Y	Y	Y	Y
Protein bound	N	L	L	L	L	N	N
Renal tubular metabolism	N	Y	Y	Y	Y	Y	Y
Extra-renal metabolism	N	Y	Y	Y	Y	Y	N
Commonly used for patient care	N	N	N	N*	N	Y	N
Intravenous administration	Y	Y	Y	Y	Y	NA	NA
Subcutaneous administration	N	Y	Y	Y	N	NA	NA
Plasma clearance method	N	Y	Y	Y	Y	N	N
Renal clearance method	Y	Y	Y	N	N	Y	Y
May require advanced method for assay	Y	N	Y	N	Y	N	Y
Colorimetric assay	Y†	N	N	N	N	N	N
HPLC	Y	N	Y	N	Y	N	Y
Capillary electrophoresis	N	N	Y	N	N	N	N
X-ray fluoroscopy	N	N	N	N	Y	N	Y
Latex immunoassay	N	N	N	N	N	N	Y
Assay Interference	Y†	N	N	N	Y‡	Y§	N
GFR compared to inulin	NA	O	O	Ur, Op	S	O	S

This table shows the major advantages and disadvantages of the clearance markers for GFR discussed in the text.
HPLC, high performance liquid chromatography; *Y*, yes; *N*, no; *NA*, not applicable; *L*, little (<10%); *I*, iodinated compound; *R*, radioactive; *S*, similar; *Ur*, underestimates by renal clearance method; *Up*, overestimates by plasma clearance method; *O*, overestimates;
*May need to preadminister Lugol's solution.
† Anthrone method: high glucose concentration can interfere, leading to false positive; alternate enzymatic assay less available than anthrone assay.
‡ Jaffe method: high glucose, fructose, pyruvate, acetoacetate, uric acid, ascorbic acid, plasma proteins, bilirubin and cephalosporins can interfere; enzymatic method: high glucose, ethamsylate and metamizol can interfere.
§ Lacks FDA approval.

Chromium Ethylenediamine Tetra-Acetic Acid (^{51}Cr-EDTA)

Plasma clearance of ^{51}Cr-EDTA has been studied extensively and is widely used in Europe to measure GFR. It is an impractical method for routine estimation of renal function because it is time-consuming; however, it is frequently employed for clinical studies. Because it is a radio-labeled marker, it exposes the patient to radiation and its associated risks. Also, this agent is not approved by the Food and Drug Administration, thus limiting its application in the United States.

^{51}Cr-EDTA (MW 292 Da) is freely filtered and not metabolized by the renal tubule. It is slightly protein bound,[18] and 10% may be subject to extra-renal metabolism.[19–21] Early studies demonstrated good agreement between renal clearance of inulin and plasma clearance of a single injection of ^{51}Cr-EDTA.[22,23] More recent studies have shown that renal clearance of ^{51}Cr-EDTA underestimates inulin clearance, and that plasma clearance of ^{51}Cr-EDTA overestimates it.[9] It should be noted that plasma clearance and not renal clearance is the preferred method for estimating GFR with Cr-EDTA. Despite the slight overestimate of GFR by plasma clearance, the precision of this technique is superior to that of most other markers. A single sampling of ^{51}Cr-EDTA is preferred because the single-sample method is associated with fewer errors compared to two samples.[24]

Iohexol

Iohexol is popular in Europe and Australia.[25,26] Clearance of iohexol can be calculated after 3 hours with a single measurement for patients with normal renal function. The linear model is similar to that of inulin,[27] and iohexol clearance is an accurate marker of GFR[28] not affected by level of renal function or gender.[29] However, iohexol is generally not available in clinical practice because it is time-consuming and requires access to advanced assay methods.

Iohexol (MW 821 Da) is a low osmolar nonionic radiocontrast agent. Iohexol is usually given intravenously and can be measured by X-ray fluorescence, chemical detection of iodine, or HPLC.[27] HPLC is more precise and more accurate.[30] A single measurement has been shown to be adequate for patients with GFR ranging from 4 to 139 mL/min/1.73m^2.[28,31] Iohexol has been studied in diabetics and is a reasonable marker for GFR in this population.[25] In a pediatric population, Iohexol was superior to several methods of estimating GFR, including serum creatinine-based equations and serum cystatin C.[32] In patients with gynecologic cancer, iohexol was equivalent to ^{51}Cr-EDTA and superior to creatinine for measuring GFR.[33]

Endogenous Clearance Markers

Serum Creatinine and Blood Urea Nitrogen

The two most commonly employed endogenous markers of kidney function are serum creatinine and blood urea nitrogen (BUN). A major advantage of endogenous markers of renal function is their safety, unlike potential contrast allergy or radiation exposure with certain other methods. However, there are numerous limitations to these markers.

Serum creatinine (MW 113 Da) is commonly used to assess kidney function, and it is incorporated into a variety of equations to estimate GFR. Serum creatinine is not protein-bound and is freely filtered. The production of serum creatinine depends on muscle mass, which is influenced by age, weight, and gender.[34] Serum creatinine is also influenced by diet and kidney filtration and secretion, which can result in a variation on a daily basis.[35] Creatinine is secreted in the proximal tubule, and its secretion can be inhibited by medications such as cimetidine, probenecid, and trimethoprim.[36] It is this tubular secretion that contributes to overestimation of GFR with serum creatinine. Because serum creatinine is not linearly related to GFR, its measurement alone is not recommended to assess kidney function accurately (i.e., GFR).

Blood urea (MW 60 Da) is a function of urea production, renal excretion, and breakdown by gut bacteria. Urea production depends on protein intake and breakdown, which, in turn, depends on diet, liver function, and kidney function. Urea is reabsorbed in the tubules. Other factors that influence BUN are diuretic use and sodium depletion.[37,38] Other issues to consider are reduced production of BUN and creatinine in the setting of liver disease and reduced muscle mass in the elderly or chronically ill; both patient types might still have chronic kidney disease despite normal appearing BUN and/or creatinine. Both examples illustrate that reliance on level of BUN or creatinine alone or together for estimation of kidney function may be misleading. The consequences include both misdiagnosis of kidney disease and potential harm from overdosing medications that are dependent upon renal excretion.

Creatinine Clearance: 24-Hour Urine Collection

Obtaining a 24-hour urine collection is a common method for measuring creatinine clearance. Typically, urine collection is started in the morning, following the first void, and continues all day and overnight, and ends with collection of the first void the following morning.[39] There may be errors in timing and collecting urine, both in the inpatient and outpatient setting. Properly collected urines can yield reasonably accurate estimates, but the method remains imprecise. This method lacks precision as a predictor of GFR.[34] Creatinine clearance overestimates GFR due to tubular secretion of creatinine. Fractional overestimation of GFR increases with more advanced CKD. Table 2–2 shows serum creatinine, 24-hour urine creatinine, and creatinine clearance for a series of hospitalized Scandinavian patients with serum creatinine in the normal range, categorized by age group and gender.[40] Note that men tend to have higher urinary creatinine and clearance compared to women, and with advancing age, urinary creatinine decreases as does clearance. These findings are likely a reflection of differences in body composition, that is, muscle mass. The accuracy and precision of creatinine clearance are highly dependent on patient compliance with urine collection procedures. That is, under-collection or over-collection of the sample markedly influences both accuracy and precision. In fact, the precision of serum creatinine based estimates of GFR are better than 24-hour urine creatinine clearance.[39]

Tubular secretion contributes to overestimation of GFR with serum creatinine; blockade of tubular secretion with cimetidine (1200 mg/day) improves accuracy of creatinine clearance such that it approaches inulin clearance.[34] However, this method requires careful timing of both cimetidine dosing and creatinine measurement.[36] Furthermore, with more advanced stages of CKD, there is more extra-renal breakdown of creatinine in the small bowel, leading to further imprecision of the assessment of kidney function, using urine collection methods.[9]

Creatinine clearance tends to overestimate GFR, whereas urea clearance tends to underestimate GFR. Taking advantage of this fact, the average of the creatinine clearance and urea clearance has been shown to correlate more closely with actual GFR in individuals with chronic kidney disease.[41,42]

Given the problems with 24-hour urine collection for estimation of creatinine clearance or GFR, the National Kidney Foundation has recommended estimating GFR or creatinine clearance from regression equations based on serum creatinine (see later text).

Creatinine Clearance During Water Loading

Creatinine clearance can also be measured during acute water loading. The protocol is similar to that used for renal clearance of inulin or iothalamate, except that endogenous creatinine in blood and urine is the marker for estimating GFR. This method is inexpensive because the creatinine assay is widely available, reproducible, and not costly. However, like other renal clearance techniques, it is time-consuming. It can be done concomitantly with iothalamate or inulin methods.[43]

Serum Cystatin C

Serum cystatin C (cysC) is an endogenous protein that was first proposed as a marker for GFR in 1985.[44] CysC (MW 13 kilodaltons [kD]) is a positively charged cysteine proteinase inhibitor that has a pH of 9.0. It is filtered freely and completely reabsorbed and catabolized in the proximal tubule, resulting in its complete elimination.[45] Even though it is a safe marker, factors limiting its current use include reduced access and higher cost of laboratory methods for measuring cysC as compared to SCr, which may make it a less attractive alternative for clinical use.

CysC shows great promise as a novel marker for GFR because it does not have the same limitations as serum creatinine. CysC is produced constitutively at a constant rate in all nucleated cells, and, unlike creatinine, several studies have shown that it is not affected by muscle mass, gender, or diet. Furthermore, CysC is not altered by inflammatory states. Past the age of 50 years, and again past the age of 70 years, patients have an increase in serum cysC due to age-related decrease in GFR.[46,47] Another advantage of CysC is that it may be useful for detecting renal impairment in advance of elevation of serum creatinine.

The methodology for measuring cysC has improved. The initial method for detecting cysC was a radioimmunoassay, followed by fluorescent and enzymatic immunoassays. Newer studies are based on latex immunoassay, by particle-enhanced turbidimetric immunoassay (PETIA), and by particle-enhanced nephelometric immunoassay (PENIA). The newer studies have improved precision and speed compared to older studies. The nephelometric assay has improved precision compared to other techniques, and cysC values are similar for men and women as well as for African-Americans and whites.[48]

Although some studies have shown that cysC is superior to serum creatinine for assessing kidney function or estimating GFR, others have shown equivalence of the two markers. Some studies evaluated correlation between 1/cysC and a standard marker, whereas other studies evaluated the receiver operating characteristic (ROC) for cysC versus serum creatinine. Some of the studies that did not show a difference between the two did show a trend for superiority of cysC. Reasons for non-superiority of cysC may have been due to type II error secondary to small sample size,[49] the chosen reference standards for GFR, use of earlier methods of measuring cysC, and the use of different units for GFR (not including body surface area). Because of these points, a meta-analysis of studies comparing cysC and creatinine correlation coefficients (54 studies) and ROC (11 studies) was conducted,[50] which demonstrated that cysC was significantly better for both of these parameters (Table 2–4). This study also showed that nephelometric assays exhibited significantly higher correlation coefficients than other methods for measuring cysC.

Although prior studies have shown that cysC is related to GFR without the limitations of serum creatinine (it is unrelated to age, body mass, gender), a more recent cross-sectional study suggests otherwise. In this study of 8058 individuals (mostly Caucasian), factors that were related to cysC were determined through multivariate linear regression, after adjusting for creatinine clearance. The factors independently associated with higher cysC levels were older age, male gender, height, weight, current cigarette smoking, and higher serum C-reactive protein.[51] This study also found that although cysC was a better predictor of creatinine clearance by 24-hour urine, it was not a better predictor than serum creatinine when factors such as age, weight, and gender were also considered. This study demonstrates that further studies of cysC are needed and in more heterogeneous populations. Whether cysC is better than serum creatinine at detecting smaller and earlier changes in GFR remains controversial.[48]

Pediatric populations may benefit from GFR estimation using cysC, because cysC after the age of 1 year is comparable to adults. The assay for serum creatinine is less accurate because children have lower serum creatinine due to their lower muscle mass. In a review of five pediatric studies evaluating different parameters, two showed that cysC was significantly superior to serum creatinine, whereas the other three showed equivalence. Few children below the age of 4 were included in these studies, and it is hypothesized that this group would benefit the most from the use of cysC versus serum creatinine.[48]

Patients with cirrhosis of the liver also tend to have lower serum creatinine and lower muscle mass as well as increased tubular secretion of creatinine, making serum creatinine a problematic marker for GFR. In a study of 44 cirrhotics without evidence of renal disease (normal urinalysis and no proteinuria), patients with more advanced liver disease by Child-Pugh criteria had higher levels of cysC. There was correlation between 1/serum creatinine and 1/cysC. Only cysC correlated with GFR,

Table 2–4 Results of Meta-Analysis of Cystatin C Studies

Comparison	Parameter		N		N	p
		1/Cystatin C		**1/Serum Creatinine**		
Correlation coefficient	Mean r (95%CI)	0.816 (0.804, 0.826)	3703	0.742 (0.726, 0.758)	3101	<.001
		Cystatin C		**Serum Creatinine**		
ROC-plot AUC	Mean (95%CI)	0.926 (0.892, 0.960)	997	0.837 (0.796, 0.878)	997	<.001
		Nephelometric Assay		**Other Assays**		
Correlation coefficient	Mean r (95%CI)	0.846 (0.832–0.859)	1698	0.784 (95%CI, 0.766–0.801)	1953	<.001

This table shows three different comparisons related to studies of cystatin C. The first comparison shows correlation coefficients for the inverse of cystatin C (versus a variety of markers as reference standards, including serum creatinine) and the inverse of serum creatinine. The second comparison is between the receiver operating characteristic curves (ROC) that plot sensitivity by 1-specificity, measured as area under the curve (AUC) for cystatin C (versus reference standard such as inulin or other exogenous marker, and not serum creatinine) and for serum creatinine. The third comparison shows correlation coefficients for the nephelometric assay for cystatin C versus all other assays for cystatin C. There were too few studies in this meta-analysis to compare ROC plots of AUC for assays. (From Dharnidharka VR, Kwon C, Stevens G: Serum cystatin C is superior to serum creatinine as a marker of kidney function: A meta-analysis. Am J Kidney Dis 2002; 40[2]:221-226.)

and cysC had a higher sensitivity for detecting reduced GFR.[52] Further studies of cysC are needed in this population.

More studies are needed to determine the utility of cysC as a marker in chemotherapy patients. One study showed decreased GFR by cysC, however, a second methodology was not used for comparison.[53] Theoretically, certain malignancies may have elevated levels of cysC from cell death or tumor burden. One study has shown that tumor burden does not affect cysC levels.[54]

There have been numerous studies of cysC in the transplant population ranging from detecting the return of renal function in the immediate post-transplant period[55] to detecting graft failure. Although some studies have shown superiority of cysC, the results have been mixed, and most studies do not include a comparative gold standard. Several studies suggest that cysC underestimates GFR by 10% to 25% in renal transplant patients.[56,57] Elevated cysC levels could be due to assay interference by immunosuppressive drugs, backleak of cysC due to renal damage, increased protein binding, or increased cell turnover. The potential interaction between steroids and cysC has not been determined. Studies of asthmatic patients[58] and renal transplant patients treated with steroids have shown that treatment with steroids increases cysC,[59] whereas a study of patients with nephrotic syndrome treated with steroids did not show increased cysC.[60] On the other hand, cyclosporine has been shown to decrease cysC.[58]

Further studies are needed to evaluate the utility of using cysC as a marker for GFR in specific populations such as children, kidney transplant recipients, chemotherapy patients, and cirrhotics. It is certainly reasonable to follow patients over time with GFR determined by serum creatinine, given the higher cost of the cysC assay. However, in order to detect early disease, prior studies have shown that cysC is superior to serum creatinine as an endogenous marker for GFR.

FORMULAS FOR ESTIMATING GLOMERULAR FILTRATION RATE

In clinical practice and in research environments it is often impractical or impossible to truly measure GFR. Consequently, several mathematic models based on serum creatinine have been developed in order to estimate glomerular filtration rate. For this reason, various methods utilizing serum markers of renal function have been developed to provide indirect estimates of GFR without the inconvenience of time commitment and repeated collections of blood and urine. Two of the most commonly used equations are the Cockcroft-Gault equation and the Modification of Diet in Renal Disease (MDRD) equation. These two equations are recommended by the clinical practice guidelines in the National Kidney Foundation Kidney Disease Outcomes Quality Initiative Clinical Practice Guidelines for Chronic Kidney Disease for estimating GFR in adults.[1]

Cockcroft-Gault Equation

The Cockcroft-Gault equation was developed to estimate creatinine clearance and is subject to the same limitations as creatinine.[61]

$$\text{Creatinine clearance (mL/min)} = \frac{(140-\text{age}) \times \text{Body weight (kg)}}{72 \times \text{serum creatinine (mg/dL)}}$$

For females, multiply by 0.85.

This formula has been evaluated in different patient populations (e.g., diabetics, critically ill patients) and has been shown to be accurate and more precise than creatinine clearance by 24-hour urine, especially between 20 to 100 mL/min.[34] An online calculator for GFR estimated by the Cockcroft-Gault equation is available through the NKF Web site: *http://www.kidney.org/professionals/kdoqi/gfr_page.cfm*, but this calculation is easily done on paper or with a standard hand-held calculator.

Modification of Diet in Renal Disease (MDRD) Equation

Levey and colleagues[62] developed a prediction equation for estimated GFR (eGFR) based on serum creatinine and demographic and serum variables obtained for the Modification of Diet in Renal Disease (MDRD) study. In the MDRD study, 1628 mostly nondiabetic patients had GFR measured by ^{125}I-iothalamate and estimates based on creatinine clearance and prediction equations. Serum creatinine and other measures at baseline were used to develop the final MDRD study prediction equation by a stepwise regression analysis that included independent predictors of GFR. The formula was developed initially in data from a subset of patients and then tested in the remainder of MDRD subjects. Figure 2–4 depicts the relationship between GFR predicted by MDRD and GFR measured by ^{125}I-iothalamate. Figure 2–5 shows the improved fit of MDRD versus other equations, compared to GFR.

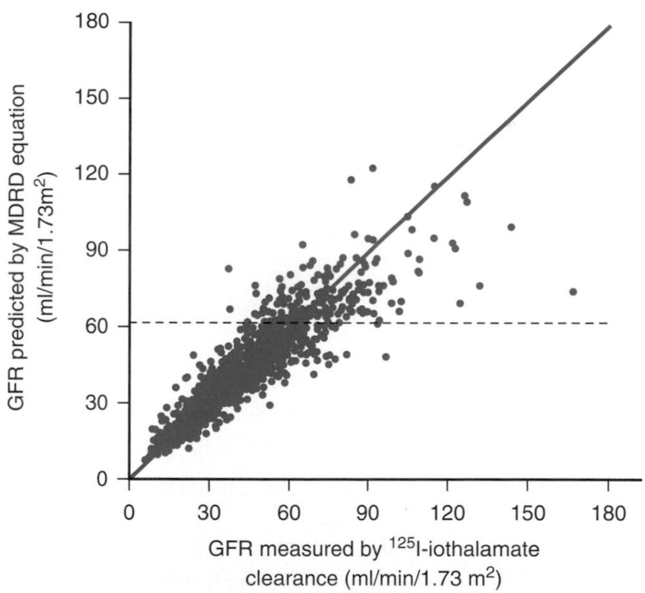

Figure 2–4 Relationship between GFR predicted by MDRD equation and GFR measured by 125-I-iothalamate.[62] This graph shows the relationship between GFR as predicted by one of the MDRD equations (calculated from demographic and serum variables, no urine variables) and GFR as measured by inulin clearance. Each point shows the relationship at baseline in the study. The solid line is the line of identity.[62] There is a strong correlation between predicted and mean GFR. However, as seen here, there is considerable variability. For a predicted GFR of 60 mL/min/1.73 m^2, the measured GFR ranges from 40 to 95 mL/min/1.73 m^2, as shown by the dashed line.

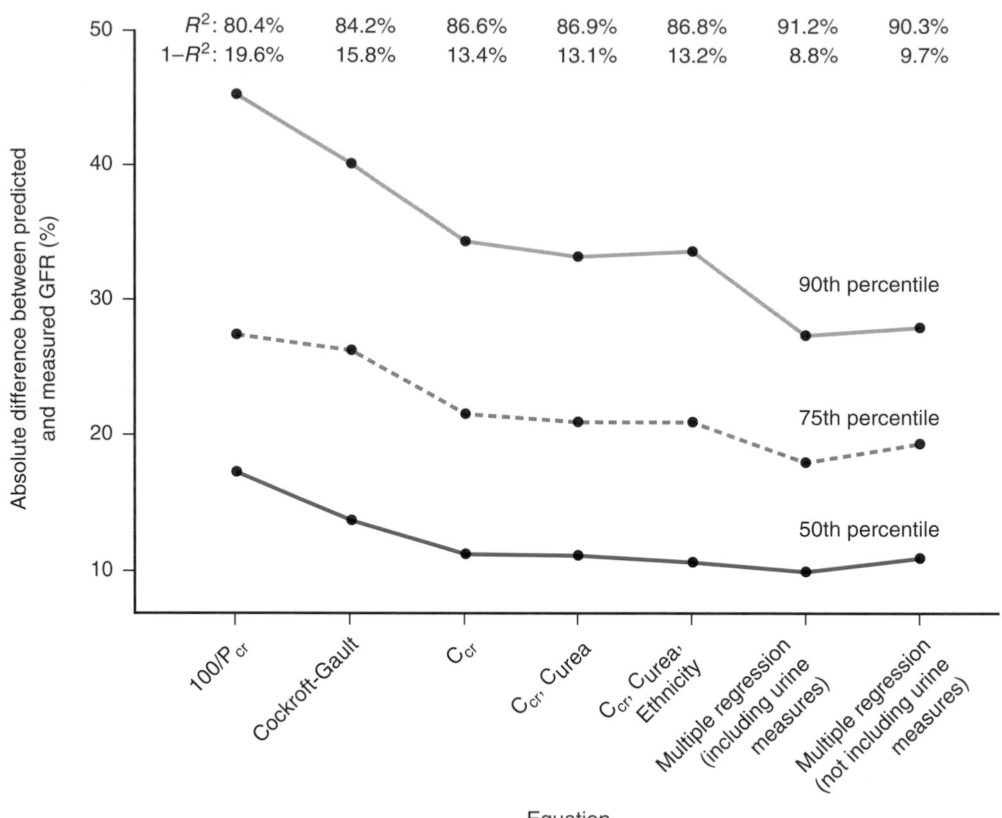

Figure 2–5 MDRD predicted and measured GFR by different prediction equations.[62] The R^2 values show percentage of variance of the log of GFR accounted for in the MDRD validation sample (n= 558) by equations derived from the training sample (n= 1070). The values of 1 to R^2 indicate the percentage of variance in log GFR that is unexplained by each equation. Note that this value is decreased by 50% from $100/P_{cr}$ to the multiple regression models. Although the multiple regression model that includes urine measurements has the closest values to measured GFR, this model does not add much to the multiple regression model that does not include urine measurements. C_{cr}, creatinine clearance; C_{urea}, urea clearance; P_{cr}, serum creatinine concentration.

The four variable MDRD equation includes age, race, gender, and serum creatinine,[62] as shown here:

$$\text{GFR (mL/min/1.73 m}^2) = 186 \times (\text{serum creatinine}^{(-1.154)}) \times (\text{age}^{(-0.203)})$$

For females, multiply by 0.742.
For African-Americans, multiply by 1.21.

This formula is not one that can be calculated easily by hand at the bedside like the Cockcroft-Gault equation. Rather, a calculator or personal digital assistant may be used at the bedside to determine GFR from the MDRD equation. An estimated GFR calculator for adults based on MDRD is available at the NKF Web site: *http://www.kidney.org/professionals/kdoqi/gfr_page.cfm.*

The MDRD formula is not without limitations, however. It has not been validated in specific populations such as children, the elderly, diabetics, and patients with liver disease. Only 12% of MDRD enrollees were African-American.[62] This equation, like others, is modeled after a steady-state model. Therefore, these equations should not be applied to patients with changing kidney function. Given the impact of dietary intake on creatinine, a fasting creatinine is preferred. The MDRD equation can overestimate and underestimate true GFR. Most importantly, the MDRD equation has not been validated in a prospective study directly comparing it to a renal clearance marker. In the African-American Study of Kidney Disease and Hypertension (AASK) study ad hoc analysis, overall estimated GFR (MDRD equation) and measured GFR (iothalamate clearance) provided similar results in terms of the outcome of rate of decline in GFR. However, there were subtle differences in some of the other GFR based outcomes. These findings suggest that additional prospective studies are needed to provide further validation of the MDRD equation.[63] At this time, the MDRD equation is widely used to estimate glomerular filtration rate and to stage chronic kidney disease. In the future, better estimation equations using serum creatinine and other factors known to influence kidney function should be developed. This is an important priority of ongoing research in this field.

Children

The Schwartz and Counahan-Barratt formulas are the two most convenient and practical formulas for estimating GFR in children.[64] The Counahan-Barratt formula is as follows[65]:

$$\text{GFR (mL/min/1.73 m}^2\text{)} = 0.43 \times \text{Height (cm)} \div \text{serum creatinine (mg/dL)}$$

The Schwartz formula estimates creatinine clearance as follows[66-68]:

$$\text{GFR (mL/min/1.73 m}^2\text{)} = 0.55 \times \text{Height (cm)} \div \text{serum creatinine (mg/dL)}$$

For children younger than 1 year of age, the constant is 0.45, and for adolescent boys, the constant is 0.7. Pediatric GFR calculators are available at the NKF Web site: *http://www.kidney.org/professionals/kdoqi/gfr_page.cfm.*

CONCLUSION

GFR is the preferred method for assessing kidney function and staging CKD for the purpose of diagnosis, prognosis, and management. There are several methods for measuring and estimating GFR. Each method has particular strengths, weaknesses, and limitations. Inulin clearance remains the gold standard. For clinical purposes, creatinine and cysC are good markers for measuring GFR. For clinical management, serum creatinine-based estimates of GFR, including the Cockcroft-Gault and MDRD equations, are the preferred methods. For research purposes, inulin and iothalamate clearances are accurate, reliable, and reproducible measures of GFR. Although cysC appears to be a promising new endogenous marker for measuring GFR, further studies are needed.

ACKNOWLEDGMENTS

This manuscript was supported by NIH grants numbers 1 F32-DK62687-01 and 5-K-24 02818-02.

References

1. Eknoyan G, Levin NW: K/DOQI clinical practice guidelines for chronic kidney disease: Evaluation, classification, and stratification. Am J Kidney Dis 2002; 39(2):S14-S266.
2. Wesson LG: Renal function. *In* Wesson LG (ed): Physiology of The Human Kidney. New York, Grune & Stratton, 1969.
3. Coresh J, Astor BC, Greene T, et al: Prevalence of chronic kidney disease and decreased kidney function in the adult U.S. population: Third National Health and Nutrition Examination Survey. Am J Kidney Dis 2003; 41(1):1-12.
4. Lindeman RD, Tobin JD, Shock NW: Association between blood pressure and the rate of decline in renal function with age. Kidney Int 1984; 26(6):861-868.
5. Silkensen JR, Kasiske BL: Laboratory assessment of kidney disease: Clearance, urinalysis, and kidney biopsy. *In* Brenner BM (ed): The Kidney. Philadelphia, WB Saunders, 2004, pp 1107-1137.
6. Bianchi C, Donadio C, Tramonti G: Noninvasive methods for the measurement of total renal function (Review, 48 refs). Nephron 1981; 28(2):53-57.
7. Farmer CD, Tauxe WN, Maher FT, Hunt JC: Measurement of renal function with radioiodinated diatrizoate and omicron-iodohippurate. Am J Clin Pathol 1967; 47(1):9-16.
8. Horio M, Orita Y, Fukunaga M: Assessment of renal function. *In* Johnson RJ, Feehally J (eds): Comprehensive Clinical Nephrology. London, Mosby, 2000, pp 3.1–3.6.
9. Levey AS: Measurement of renal function in chronic renal disease (Review, 129 refs). Kidney Int 1990; 38(1):167-184.
10. Riep RJ, Nelp WB: Mechanism of excretion of radioiodinated sodium iothalamate. Radiology 1969; 93(4):807-811.
11. Nissen D(ed): Mosby's Drug Consult. St. Louis, MO, Mosby, 2004.
12. Smith T, Veall N, Altman DG: Dosimetry of renal radiopharmaceuticals: The importance of bladder radioactivity and a simple aid for its estimation. Br J Radiol 1981; 54(647):961-965.
13. Lasser EC, Berry CC, Talner LB, et al: Pretreatment with corticosteroids to alleviate reactions to intravenous contrast material. N Engl J Med 1987; 317(14):845-849.
14. Isaka Y, Fujiwara Y, Yamamoto S, et al: Modified plasma clearance technique using nonradioactive iothalamate for measuring GFR. Kidney Int 1992; 42(4):1006-1011.
15. Gaspari F, Mosconi L, Vigano G, et al: Measurement of GFR with a single intravenous injection of nonradioactive iothalamate. Kidney Int 1992; 41(4):1081-1084.
16. Wilson DM, Bergert JH, Larson TS, Liedtke RR: GFR determined by nonradiolabeled iothalamate using capillary electrophoresis. Am J Kidney Dis 1997; 30(5):646-652.
17. Perrone RD, Steinman TI, Beck GJ, et al: Utility of radioisotopic filtration markers in chronic renal insufficiency: Simultaneous comparison of 125I-iothalamate, 169Yb-DTPA, 99mTc-DTPA, and inulin. The Modification of Diet in Renal Disease Study (See comment). Am J Kidney Dis 1990; 16(3):224-235.
18. Babiker MM: Binding of [51Cr]ethylene diamine tetra acetate to proteins of human plasma. J Physiol (Lond) 1986; 374:117-122.
19. Moore AE, Park-Holohan SJ, Blake GM, Fogelman I: Conventional measurements of GFR using 51Cr-EDTA overestimate true renal clearance by 10 percent (See comment). Eur J Nucl Med Mol Imaging 2003; 30(1):4-8.
20. Rehling M, Moller ML, Thamdrup B, et al: Simultaneous measurement of renal clearance and plasma clearance of 99mTc-labelled diethylenetriaminepenta-acetate, 51Cr-labelled ethylenediaminetetra-acetate and inulin in man. Clin Sci (Colch) 1984; 66(5):613-619.
21. Mortensen JB, Rodbro P: Comparison between total and renal plasma clearance of [51Cr] EDTA. Scand J Clin Lab Invest 1976; 36(3):247-249.
22. Brochner-Mortensen J, Giese J, Rossing N: Renal inulin clearance versus total plasma clearance of 51Cr-EDTA. Scand J Clin Lab Invest 1969; 23(4):301-305.
23. Hagstam KE, Nordenfelt I, Svensson L, Svensson SE: Comparison of different methods for determination of glomerular filtration rate in renal disease. Scand J Clin Lab Invest 1974; 34(1):31-36.
24. De Sadeleer C, Piepsz A, Ham HR: Influence of errors in sampling time and in activity measurement on the single sample clearance determination. Nucl Med Commun 2001; 22(4):429-432.
25. Houlihan C, Jenkins M, Osicka T, et al: A comparison of the plasma disappearance of iohexol and 99mTc-DTPA for the measurement of glomerular filtration rate (GFR) in diabetes. Aust N Z J Med 1999; 29(5):693-700.
26. Frennby B, Sterner G: Contrast media as markers of GFR. Eur Radiol 2002; 12(2):475-484.
27. Nilsson-Ehle P: Iohexol clearance for the determination of glomerular filtration rate: 15 years' experience in clinical practice. The electronic journal of the International Federation of Clinical Chemistry 13(2):1-5.
28. Rydstrom M, Tengstrom B, Cederquist I, Ahlmen J: Measurement of glomerular filtration rate by single-injection, single-sample techniques, using 51Cr-EDTA or iohexol. Scand J Urol Nephrol 1995; 29(2):135-139.
29. Gaspari F, Perico N, Matalone M, et al: Precision of plasma clearance of iohexol for estimation of GFR in patients with renal disease. J Am Soc Nephrol 1998; 9(2):310-313.

30. Rocco MV, Buckalew VM Jr, Moore LC, Shihabi ZK: Capillary electrophoresis for the determination of glomerular filtration rate using nonradioactive iohexol. Am J Kidney Dis 1996; 28(2): 173-177.
31. Brandstrom E, Grzegorczyk A, Jacobsson L, et al: GFR measurement with iohexol and 51Cr-EDTA. A comparison of the two favoured GFR markers in Europe. Nephrol Dial Transplant 1998; 13(5):1176-1182.
32. Hjorth L, Wiebe T, Karpman D: Correct evaluation of renal glomerular filtration rate requires clearance assays. Pediatr Nephrol 2002; 17(10):847-851.
33. Lundqvist S, Edbom G, Groth S, et al: Iohexol clearance for renal function measurement in gynaecologic cancer patients. Acta Radiol 1996; 37(4):582-586.
34. Toto RD: Conventional measurement of renal function utilizing serum creatinine, creatinine clearance, inulin and para-aminohippuric acid clearance (Review, 21 refs). Curr Opin Nephrol Hypertens 1995; 4(6):505-509.
35. Mayersohn M, Conrad KA, Achari R: The influence of a cooked meat meal on creatinine plasma concentration and creatinine clearance. Br J Clin Pharmacol 1983; 15(2):227-230.
36. van Acker BA, Koomen GC, Koopman MG, et al: Creatinine clearance during cimetidine administration for measurement of glomerular filtration rate (See comment). Lancet 1992; 340 (8831):1326-1329.
37. Kamm DE, Wu L, Kuchmy BL: Contribution of the urea appearance rate to diuretic-induced azotemia in the rat. Kidney Int 1987; 32(1):47-56.
38. Dal Canton A, Fuiano G, Conte G, et al: Mechanism of increased plasma urea after diuretic therapy in uraemic patients. Clin Sci (Colch) 1985; 68(3):255-261.
39. Toto RD, Kirk KA, Coresh J, et al: Evaluation of serum creatinine for estimating glomerular filtration rate in African Americans with hypertensive nephrosclerosis: Results from the African-American Study of Kidney Disease and Hypertension (AASK) Pilot Study. J Am Soc Nephrol 1997; 8(2):279-287.
40. Kampmann J, Siersbaek-Nielsen K, Kristensen M, Hansen JM: Rapid evaluation of creatinine clearance. Acta Med Scand 1974; 196(6):517-520.
41. Lavender S, Hilton PJ, Jones NF: The measurement of glomerular filtration-rate in renal disease. Lancet 1969; 2(7632):1216-1218.
42. Lubowitz H, Slatopolsky E, Shankel S, et al: Glomerular filtration rate. Determination in patients with chronic renal disease. JAMA 1967; 199(4):252-256.
43. Coresh J, Toto RD, Kirk KA, et al: Creatinine clearance as a measure of GFR in screenees for the African-American Study of Kidney Disease and Hypertension pilot study. Am J Kidney Dis 1998; 32(1):32-42.
44. Grubb A, Simonsen O, Sturfelt G, et al: Serum concentration of cystatin C, factor D and beta 2-microglobulin as a measure of glomerular filtration rate. Acta Med Scand 1985; 218(5):499-503.
45. Grubb AO: Cystatin C: Properties and use as diagnostic marker (Review, 183 refs). Adv Clin Chem 2000; 35:63-99.
46. Finney H, Newman DJ, Price CP: Adult reference ranges for serum cystatin C, creatinine and predicted creatinine clearance. Ann Clin Biochem 2000; 37(Pt 1):49-59.
47. Finney H, Bates CJ, Price CP: Plasma cystatin C determinations in a healthy elderly population. Arch Gerontol Geriatr 1999; 29(1):75-94.
48. Laterza OF, Price CP, Scott MG: Cystatin C: An improved estimator of glomerular filtration rate? [See comment; Review; 69 refs]. Clin Chem 2002; 48(5):699-707.
49. Coll E, Botey A, Alvarez L, et al: Serum cystatin C as a new marker for noninvasive estimation of glomerular filtration rate and as a marker for early renal impairment (See comment). Am J Kidney Dis 2000; 36(1):29-34.
50. Dharnidharka VR, Kwon C, Stevens G: Serum cystatin C is superior to serum creatinine as a marker of kidney function: A meta-analysis. Am J Kidney Dis 2002; 40(2):221-226.
51. Knight EL, Verhave JC, Spiegelman D, et al: Factors influencing serum cystatin C levels other than renal function and the impact on renal function measurement. Kidney Int 2004; 65:1416-1421.
52. Woitas RP, Stoffel-Wagner B, Flommersfeld S, et al: Correlation of serum concentrations of cystatin C and creatinine to inulin clearance in liver cirrhosis. Clin Chem 2000; 46(5):712-715.
53. Stabuc B, Vrhovec L, Stabuc-Silih M, Cizej TE: Improved prediction of decreased creatinine clearance by serum cystatin C: Use in cancer patients before and during chemotherapy. Clin Chem 2000; 46(2):193-197.
54. Finney H, Williams AH, Price CP: Serum cystatin C in patients with myeloma. Clin Chim Acta 2001; 309(1):1-6.
55. Christensson A, Ekberg J, Grubb A, et al: Serum cystatin C is a more sensitive and more accurate marker of glomerular filtration rate than enzymatic measurements of creatinine in renal transplantation. Nephron Physiol 2003; 94(2):19-27.
56. Le Bricon T, Thervet E, Froissart M, et al: Plasma cystatin C is superior to 24-h creatinine clearance and plasma creatinine for estimation of glomerular filtration rate 3 months after kidney transplantation (Comment). Clin Chem 2000; 46(8 Pt 1):1206-1207.
57. Bokenkamp A, Domanetzki M, Zinck R, et al: Cystatin C serum concentrations underestimate glomerular filtration rate in renal transplant recipients (See comment). Clin Chem 1999; 45(10): 1866-1868.
58. Cimerman N, Brguljan PM, Krasovec M, et al: Serum cystatin C, a potent inhibitor of cysteine proteinases, is elevated in asthmatic patients. Clin Chim Acta 2000; 300(1-2):83-95.
59. Risch L, Herklotz R, Blumberg A, Huber AR: Effects of glucocorticoid immunosuppression on serum cystatin C concentrations in renal transplant patients. Clin Chem 2001; 47(11):2055-2059.
60. Bokenkamp A, van Wijk JA, Lentze MJ, Stoffel-Wagner B: Effect of corticosteroid therapy on serum cystatin C and beta2-microglobulin concentrations. Clin Chem 2002; 48(7):1123-1126.
61. Cockcroft DW, Gault MH: Prediction of creatinine clearance from serum creatinine. Nephron 1976; 16:31-41.
62. Levey AS, Bosch JP, Lewis JB, et al: A more accurate method to estimate glomerular filtration rate from serum creatinine: A new prediction equation. Ann Intern Med 1999; 130(6):461-470.
63. Lewis J, Greene T, Appel L, et al: A Comparison of Iothalamate-GFR and Serum Creatinine-Based Outcomes: Acceleration in the Rate of GFR Decline in the African American Study of Kidney Disease and Hypertension (AASK) (in press).
64. Hogg RJ, Furth S, Lemley KV, et al: National Kidney Foundation's Kidney Disease Outcomes Quality Initiative clinical practice guidelines for chronic kidney disease in children and adolescents: Evaluation, classification, and stratification. Pediatrics 2003; 111 (6 Pt 1):1416-1421.
65. Counahan R, Chantler C, Ghazali S, et al: Estimation of glomerular filtration rate from plasma creatinine concentration in children. Arch Dis Child 1976; 51(11):875-878.
66. Schwartz GJ, Gauthier B: A simple estimate of glomerular filtration rate in adolescent boys. J Pediatr 1985; 106(3):522-526.
67. Schwartz GJ, Feld LG, Langford DJ: A simple estimate of glomerular filtration rate in full-term infants during the first year of life. J Pediatr 1984; 104(6):849-854.
68. Schwartz GJ, Haycock GB, Edelmann CM Jr, Spitzer A: A simple estimate of glomerular filtration rate in children derived from body length and plasma creatinine. Pediatrics 1976; 58(2): 259-263.

Chapter 3

Diabetic Kidney Disease

Mark E. Williams, M.D., F.A.C.P. • Robert C. Stanton, M.D.

According to the annual health report from the U.S. Department of Health and Human Services, the epidemic of diabetes mellitus in the United States continues to get worse. The percentage of Americans diagnosed with diabetes increased 27% between 1997 and 2000, and the percentage of Americans diagnosed with diabetes in 2002 rose to 6.5%, up from 5.1% in 1997.[1] The number of Americans diagnosed with diabetes mellitus has increased 61% over the last decade and will more than double by 2010. The incidence of diabetic nephropathy has more than doubled in the past decade,[2] due largely to increasing prevalence of type II diabetes.[3] Diabetic nephropathy now accounts for nearly 45% of new cases of end-stage renal disease (ESRD) in the United States,[4,5] with hypertension and glomerulonephritis being the second and third most common causes, respectively. The percentage of new cases of ESRD due to diabetes has been rising steadily for 25 years and is expected to continue to rise, largely contributing to the expected doubling of the number of patients with ESRD in the United States. This is considered to be due to the epidemic of type II diabetes that is occurring in the United States and throughout the world. Between 1992 and 2001, the size of the Medicare chronic kidney disease (CKD) population increased by 53%[5] (Figure 3–1). Results from the NHANES III study, published in 2002, documented that one third of diabetics demonstrated either microalbuminuria (MA) or macroalbuminuria.[6]

Proteinuria and progressive loss of kidney function are the clinical hallmarks of diabetic CKD. In the natural history of the disease.[7] Proteinuria is preceded by stages of excessive glomerular filtration and of microalbuminuria, which signals an increased risk of progression to overt nephropathy. A progressive increase in proteinuria subsequently leads to a variable decline in renal function. Proteinuria signifies evidence of glomerular damage and may be viewed as a measure of the severity of diabetic glomerulopathy. Early clinical reports noted nephrotic syndrome in 87% of type I and 70% of type II diabetic patients, and end-stage renal failure in up to 75% of diabetic patients within 15 years of developing proteinuria.[4] Factors that cause progression of kidney disease continue to be actively investigated and include glomerular hypertension and hypertrophy, activation of coagulation pathways, biochemical damage from hyperglycemia, and lipid deposition.

Two decades of progress in retarding the progression of renal disease were recently reviewed.[8] Until the mid-1970s, it was generally accepted that no treatment could slow the progression of diabetic nephropathy.[9] There is current agreement that the course of diabetic nephropathy can be impacted when interventions are implemented at the earliest possible time.[10] Current challenges in the management of the diabetic patient at risk for chronic kidney disease include nephropathy screening, early interventions to delay progression, and modification of disease comorbidities[11] (Figure 3–2). Later in the course, priorities become prevention of complications of uremia and preparation for renal replacement therapy. Diabetes is a chronic illness and diabetes care is complex.[4] This chapter reports on the complexity of diabetic nephropathy, its clinical hallmarks, proteinuria and loss of kidney function, and its primary therapy, renin-angiotensin blockade. It details the current approaches to management and describes potential new treatment strategies under current investigation.[12]

EPIDEMIOLOGY AND GENETICS

It is generally accepted that 25% to 40% of patients with either type I or type II diabetes will develop diabetic nephropathy.[13–16] There are certain subgroups that have a higher incidence and prevalence of diabetic nephropathy. Young and colleagues[17] showed that in the United States, African-Americans, Hispanics, Asians, and Native Americans all have a higher likelihood of developing diabetic nephropathy as compared to Caucasians, even when correcting for socioeconomic status, age, and gender. There may even be gender differences within racial groups. Crook and colleagues[18] reported a twofold increase in ESRD in African-American women as compared to African-American men.

The typical initial manifestation of diabetic nephropathy is detection of urinary albumin above normal levels (microalbuminuria, 30–300 mg/24 hr). It had been thought that microalbuminuria was present in 100% of the cases of diabetic nephropathy, but recent studies show that the initial pattern of expression is changing, with patients presenting with increased creatinine and normoalbuminuria.[14] This changing pattern might be due to changes in therapy, as over the past 10 years there has been increasing recognition of the importance of achieving tight control of blood sugar[19] and of maintaining ever lower targets for optimal blood pressure.[20] Importantly, not all patients who develop microalbuminuria will progress.[14] Caramori and colleagues[14,21,22] reviewed this a few years ago, noting that the prior estimate that 80% or more of patients with microalbuminuria will progress to proteinuria, and ever worsening renal function is contradicted by a number of studies, suggesting that only 30% to 40% will progress. This is still a highly significant number of patients and, as discussed later, comprise an ever growing proportion of the ESRD population.[23] Cases of diabetic nephropathy are typically not seen before 5 years of diabetes in type I patients, and the incidence then rises over the ensuing 10 years. This suggests that a relatively long exposure to the pathophysiologic processes associated with diabetic complications is required to cause kidney damage. In contrast, patients with type II diabetes might have diabetic nephropathy at the time of diagnosis, but true duration of diabetes in type II patients

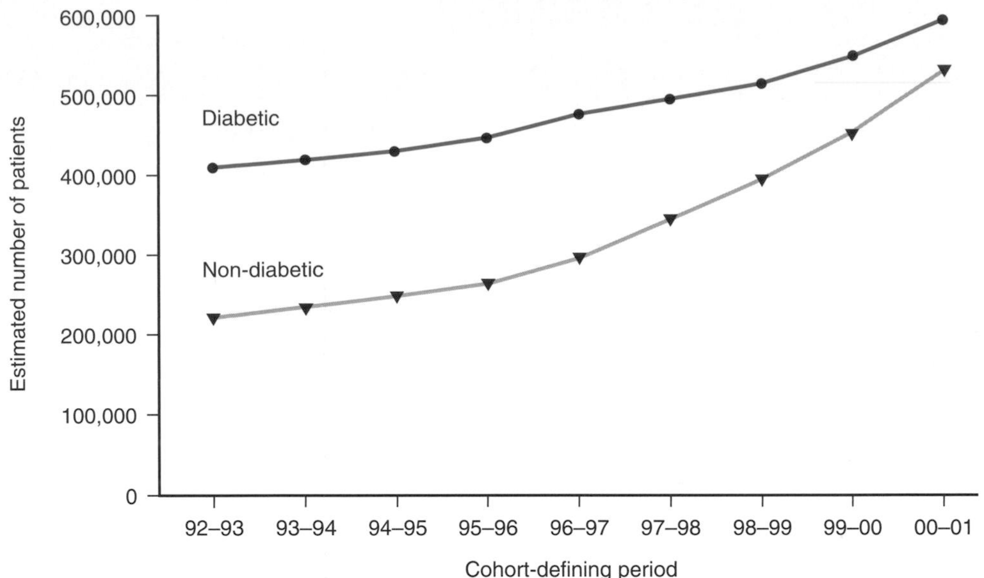

Figure 3–1 Trends in the size of the Medicare chronic kidney disease population, by diabetic status, from 1992 to 2001. Estimated from patients enrolled in any 2 consecutive calendar years. (From U.S. Renal Data System: USRDS 2003 annual data report. Bethesda, MD, National Institutes of Health, National Institute of Diabetes and Digestive and Kidney Diseases, 2003.)

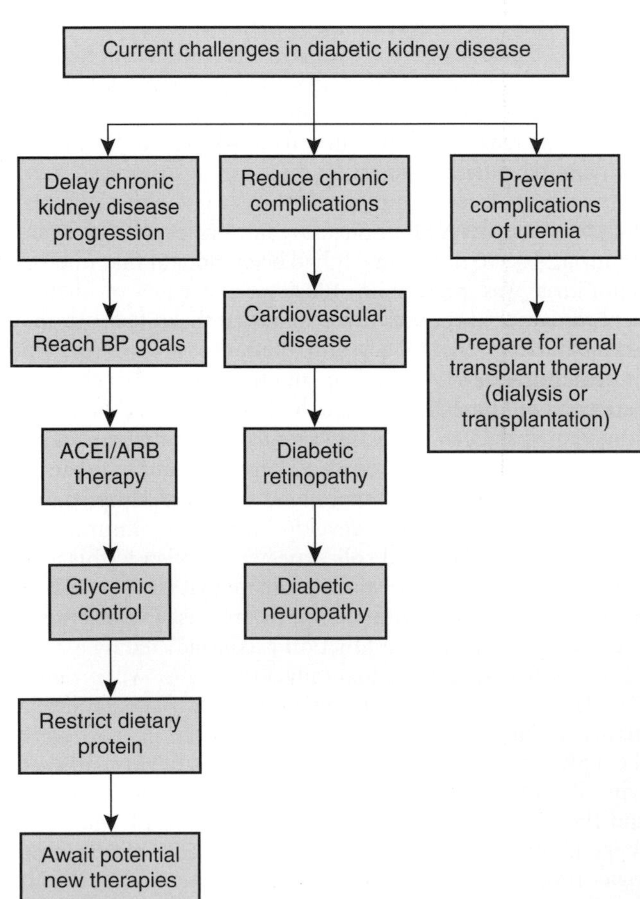

Figure 3–2 Current challenges in management of diabetic kidney disease.

is unknown in most cases. There may also be changing patterns of the incidence and prevalence of diabetic nephropathy. Bojestig and colleagues[15] reported that patients who developed diabetes between 1961 and 1965 had a cumulative incidence for diabetic nephropathy of 28%, whereas those who developed diabetes between 1971 and 1975 had a cumulative incidence of only 5.8%. Hovind and colleagues[24] recently reported similar findings for diabetic nephropathy and diabetic retinopathy. Although no specific reasons are given for these changes, one might surmise that improved blood sugar and blood pressure control might play a significant role.

In addition to treatment effects, there may be a genetic predisposition to develop diabetic nephropathy. Genetic determinants and their impact on the initiation and progression of diabetic nephropathy continue to be actively investigated.[25] Several observational studies have suggested that the ACE genotype may influence progression of diabetic nephropathy. The D allele of the insertion (I)/deletion (D) polymorphism of the ACE gene (ACE/ID) is strongly associated with progressive loss of kidney function.[26] In a recent study of type I diabetic nephropathy patients, the D allele of the ACE ID polymorphism was associated with accelerated progression of nephropathy.[27] Analysis of the clinical course of 168 proteinuric type II patients for 10 years revealed that almost all patients with the DD genotype progressed to end-stage renal disease (ESRD) within 10 years.[28] ACE gene polymorphism is associated with increased progression even during ACE inhibitor therapy[29]; however, a recent report showed protection from progression of diabetic nephropathy in type I patients with ACE II and DD genotypes treated with losartan.[30]

Although there are suggestive studies for a genetic association, no definitive answer is forthcoming. For example, a report from the Pittsburgh epidemiology of diabetes complications study[31] evaluated the relationship of genetic associations with apolipoprotein E, ACE I/D, and lipoprotein lipase *Hind*III polymorphisms with overt diabetic nephropathy (defined as >200 μg/min, which is equivalent to >300 mg/24 hours of albumin excretion in the urine). Only in specific subgroups were there positive predictive values for these genes. In fact, insulin resistance, hypertension, and lipid abnormalities were much stronger predictors. However, there is strong evidence that specific genes are involved in the development and progression of diabetic nephropathy.

A national effort to address the genetics of kidney disease in diabetes has been launched as a joint endeavor of the Juvenile Diabetes Research Foundation, the Centers for Disease Control and Prevention, the George Washington University, and the Joslin Diabetes Center. The Genetics of Kidneys in Diabetes (GoKinD) Study was initiated in order to develop a repository of DNA and clinical information on patients with type I diabetes and diabetic nephropathy (see http://www.gokind.org). "The fundamental aim of GoKinD is to provide a resource to facilitate investigator-initiated research into the genetic basis of diabetic nephropathy. Decisions regarding the genes and chromosomal regions to be studied will be made by individual investigators and subject to a competitive review process." The goal is to recruit 2200 patients with type I diabetes in order to identify genes that may play a role in the development of the diabetic nephropathy. The specific aims of the study are to evaluate genes from: (1) Case trios: 600 type I diabetic patients with diabetes duration at least 10 years and clinically diagnosed diabetic nephropathy together with their parents; (2) Cases: 500 type I diabetic patients with diabetes duration at least 10 years and clinically diagnosed diabetic nephropathy for whom parents are not available; (3) Control trios: 500 type I diabetic patients with normoalbuminuria and diabetes duration at least 15 years together with their parents; and (4) Controls: 500 type I diabetic patients with normoalbuminuria and diabetes duration at least 15 years for whom parents are not available. Recruitment ended on June 30, 2004. This database will hopefully provide researchers with the necessary information in order to identify genes involved in the pathogenesis of diabetic nephropathy.

NATURAL HISTORY

The earliest known manifestation of diabetic nephropathy is the presence of microalbuminuria. Protein excretion in the urine is normally less than 100 to 200 mg/24 hours, and urinary albumin excretion is normally less than 30 mg/24 hours. Excretion of more than 30 mg/24 hours (microalbuminuria) is abnormal but may be transient due to such circumstances as exercise, pregnancy, and medications. If persistent, it may reflect the presence of kidney damage. Many studies have shown that the presence of microalbuminuria is a very significant risk factor for progression of kidney disease and for the development and progression of cardiovascular disease.[32–35] Indeed, the Seventh Report of the Joint National Committee on Prevention, Detection, Evaluation, and Treatment of High Blood Pressure (JNC VII) hypertension treatment guidelines from the National Institutes of Health (NIH) lists the presence of microalbuminuria (the range is >30 mg/24 hr) as a major risk factor for cardiovascular disease.[36] Persistent microalbuminuria in a diabetic patient generally signifies the presence of diabetic nephropathy; as noted earlier, between 30% to 40% and up to 80% of patients with microalbuminuria will progress to overt proteinuria.[14] Although albumin excretion rate is currently considered the principal predictor for progression of diabetic nephropathy, this is not applicable to individuals presenting with increased creatinine and normoalbuminuria and may not be applicable even to patients with microalbuminuria in the era of tighter glycemic and blood pressure control and wide spread use of angiotensin converting enzyme inhibition. A recent study by Perkins and colleagues[37] showed that in type I diabetic patients, there was as much as a 50% chance for regression of microalbuminuria to normal levels, which was correlated with blood pressure and lipid control but not the use of angiotensin converting enzyme inhibitors.

Both type I and II diabetic patients with microalbuminuria are at risk for progression to overt nephropathy. Without specific treatment, up to 80% of patients with type I DM and 25% to 40% of patients with type II DM with sustained MA will eventually develop overt nephropathy.[34] A recent prospective study in Italy indicated that 4% of type II diabetic patients with MA progressed to overt nephropathy every year.[39]

First observed in diabetic patients over a century ago, clinical proteinuria was described in a pathologic report of diabetic glomerulosclerosis by Kimmelstiel and Wilson[40] in 1936. The natural sequence of proteinuria followed by loss of kidney function was not described until decades later. The natural history of diabetic nephropathy, including changes in glomerular filtration and proteinuria and stages of preventive treatment, is shown in Figure 3–3. The average time to proteinuria from the diagnosis of diabetes in type I patients is 19 years; the interval is shorter but variable in type II patients. Several definitions of persistent proteinuria in diabetes are now in use (Table 3–1), and they refer to albuminuria as well as to increased total urinary protein excretion.[41] Yearly increases in protein excretion average about 20% but with wide standard deviations. Untreated, up to 75% of proteinuric type I and type II patients may become nephritic.[42] Progressive loss of kidney function occurs over several years without intervention in type I patients. The overall sequence is similar in type II patients[4,43] (Figure 3–4), but the exact onset of diabetes may be uncertain, pathology not related to or atypical for diabetic nephropathy may exist, and the decline in function may be more variable. In its most advanced stages, diabetic glomerular proteinuria becomes less selective, with a significant leak of large proteins, such as albumin and IgG, and with tubular proteinuria.

Although all ESRD patients have significantly greater morbidity and mortality compared to the general population, patients who also have diabetes have an even greater likelihood of concurrent conditions, such as peripheral vascular disease, neuropathy, and progressive cardiovascular disease. These conditions may greatly affect lifestyle and shorten life spans.

Cardiovascular disease frequently confounds the natural history of diabetic kidney disease, and, as recently reviewed, the renin-angiotensin system (RAS) appears to have an important role in the pathophysiology of both diabetic renal and cardiovascular disease. It is, thus, not surprising that kidney disease is an independent risk factor for cardiovascular disease.[45] Microalbuminuria, even without elevated serum creatinine, has been shown to be associated with an increased risk of cardiovascular events, including stroke, myocardial infarction, and mortality[46,47] in both diabetic and nondiabetic individuals.

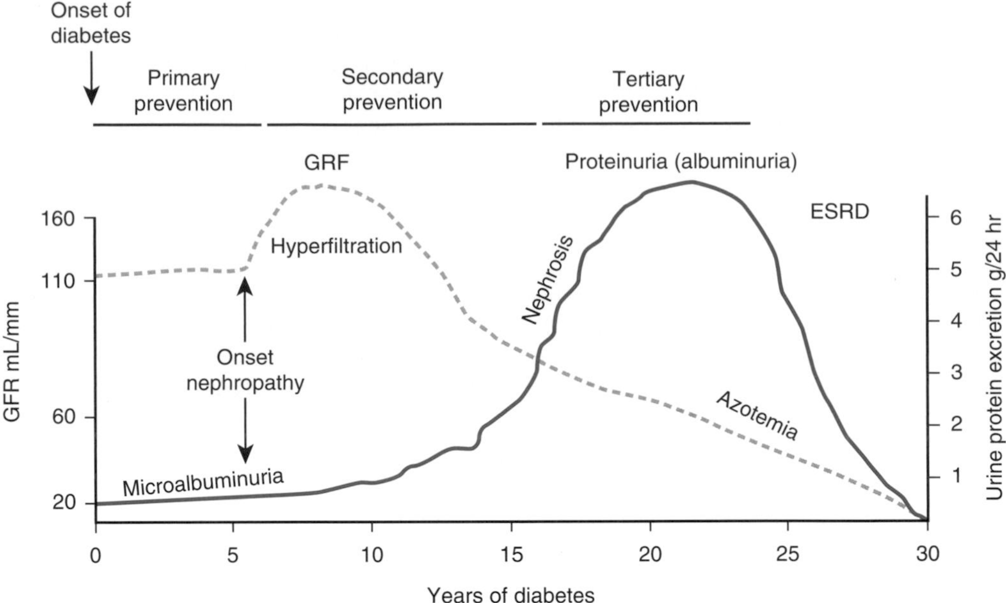

Figure 3–3 The natural history of diabetic kidney disease. Changes in glomerular filtration rate (GFR) and microalbuminuria/proteinuria are shown. Progressive loss of kidney function occurs over years, without successful intervention. Following the onset of diabetes in susceptible individuals, treatment of diabetic nephropathy may be primary (reduce the development of microalbuminuria), secondary (prevent the transition to overt nephropathy), or tertiary (slow the progression of established nephropathy to ESRD).

Table 3–1 Definitions of Abnormalities in Urinary Albumin and Protein Excretion

	Laboratory Test	MA	Albuminuria or Proteinuria
Urine albumin	Spot albumin/ creatinine ratio	17–250 mcg albumin/mg creatinine (males) 25–355 mcg albumin/mg creatinine (females)	> 250 mcg albumin/mg creatinine (males) > 355 mcg albumin/mg creatinine (females)
	24-hour collection	30–300 mg/24 hr	> 300 mg/24 hr
Urine total protein	Spot protein/creatinine ratio	?	> 0.20 mg protein/mg creatinine
	24-hour collection	?	> 300 mg/24 hr

Given the similarities between the renal and systemic vasculature, elevated urinary albumin excretion is felt to reflect damage to both the glomerulus and blood vessels. Clinically, MA is associated with a variety of cardiovascular risk factors, including hypertension, insulin resistance, atherogenic dyslipidemia, and obesity. The Framingham Heart Study first demonstrated that relevance of proteinuria to cardiovascular prognosis.[48] A recent study of type II diabetes confirmed the higher mortality associated with proteinuria.[49] Over a 5-year period, there was a fivefold excess risk for cardiovascular mortality for nephropathic patients (37%) compared to patients without nephropathy (8%), which was independent of other risk factors, including creatinine, age, and glycemic control. The risk of cardiovascular disease associated with diabetic kidney disease was also demonstrated in a recent observational study of 3608 patients enrolled in a multivessel coronary artery disease registry.[50] Among patients without diabetes, mortality at 7 years was 12% among patients without chronic kidney disease and 39% among patients with chronic kidney disease (serum creatinine >1.5 mg/dL) (Figure 3–5). Among diabetic patients without chronic kidney disease, mortality was only slightly higher than for nondiabetic patients with kidney disease. However, when both diabetes and chronic kidney disease were present, the mortality risk was additive (70%) during the 7-year observation period.[50]

Given this information, efforts to reduce cardiovascular risk are as equally, if not more, imperative as efforts to reduce progression of kidney disease?fortunately, there is a large overlap in the recommended interventions. For diabetic nephropathy, treatment may be primary (reduce the development of MA), secondary (prevent the transition to overt nephropathy), or tertiary (slow the progression of established nephropathy to ESRD)[51] (Figure 3–3).

MECHANISM

Diabetic proteinuria reflects glomerular damage and increased glomerular permeability to macromolecules, although the exact molecular mechanisms are still being defined. In general, protein permeability across the filtration barrier is affected by the hemodynamic pressure gradient across the glomerular basement membrane and separate factors involving the filtration barrier itself, including the pore size and extent of anion

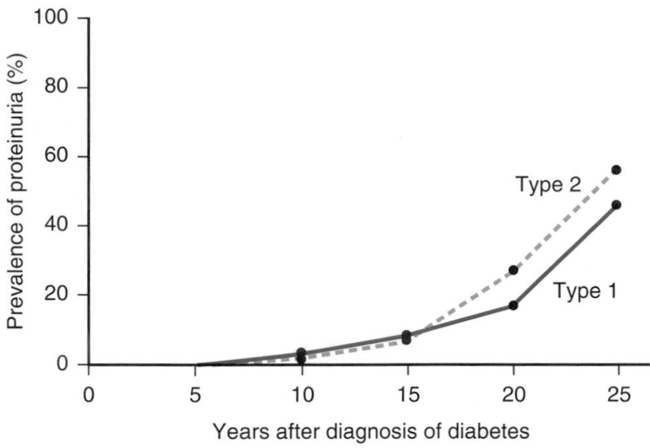

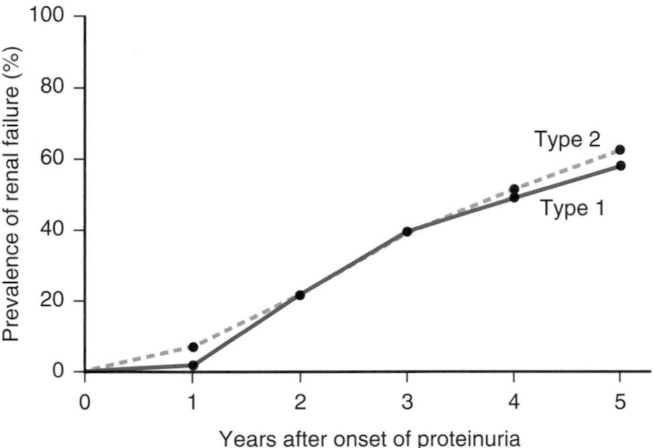

Figure 3–4 Proteinuria and progression to end-stage renal disease in diabetic nephropathy in type I and type II diabetic patients. Similar rates of proteinuria and time of progression from onset of proteinuria to kidney failure may occur in both types of diabetes. (From Ritz E, Orth SO: Nephropathy in patients with type 2 diabetes mellitus. N Engl J Med 1999; 341:1127-1133.)

charges. In diabetic nephropathy, both hemodynamic and intrinsic basement membrane factors contribute to proteinuria.[2] For example, angiotensin II combines hemodynamic actions such as induction of systemic vasoconstriction, increased glomerular arteriolar resistance, and increase in glomerular capillary pressure, with nonhemodynamic actions such as increased glomerular capillary permeability, reduction in filtration surface area, enhancement of extracellular matrix proteins, and stimulation of renal proliferation and fibrogenic chemokines, including monocyte chemoattractant protein-1 and transforming growth factor-B. The role of these factors in chronic kidney disease progression was recently reviewed.[52]

Although some pathologic changes characteristic of diabetic glomerulosclerosis, such as increased basement membrane width and mesangial expansion (Figures 3–6*A* and *B*), are known to precede the development of diabetic proteinuria, other changes such as mesangial and interstitial expansion correlate with the degree of albuminuria. The structural basis for the protein passage resides either in the glomerular basement membrane or in the nearby epithelial cell layer. Two adjacent molecular filters are felt to control glomerular permselectivity: the basement membrane itself and the slit diaphragm (Figure 3–6*C*). The glomerular basement membrane in humans is a complex tripartite structure of endothelial cells with fenestrations, dense basement membrane fibrils, and the outer visceral podocyte cells. The slit diaphragm arises between the interdigitating foot processes of the podocytes.

Glomerular hypertension, favorable in the short term, creates detrimental long-term nonhemodynamic consequences. According to a dominant theory of diabetic nephropathy based on animal models, glomerular hemodynamic forces lead to upregulation of fibrotic and inflammatory processes, resulting in structural damage.[53] The progression from normoalbuminuria to overt proteinuria in diabetes correlated in one study with a reduction in size and charge selectivity of the filtration barrier[54] and in other studies with a reduction in slit-pore density. More recent investigation has emphasized the role of extracellular matrix proteins[55] and glomerular podocyte injury and loss, and increased foot process width, which are prominent ultrastructural abnormalities in nephropathy in type I and type II diabetes.[56–58] Several mechanisms of podocyte loss have been speculated, including modulation of nephrin expression,[59] a transmembrane protein

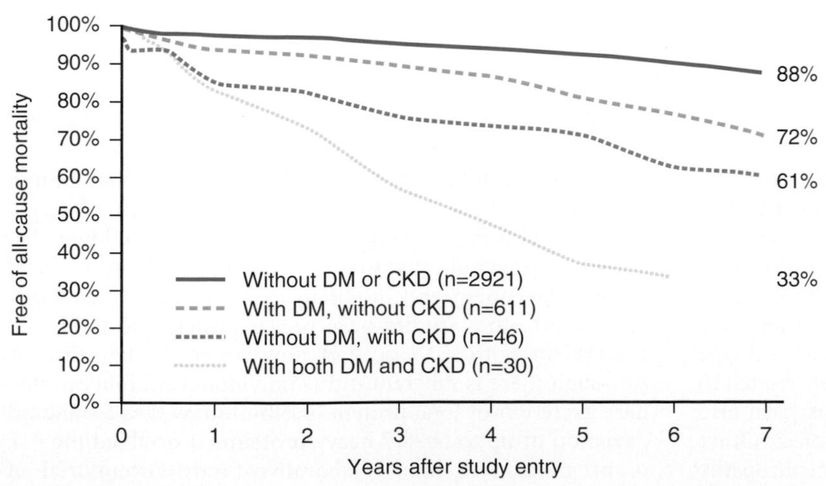

Figure 3–5 Survival curves (all-cause mortality) for cohorts of patients defined by chronic kidney disease and diabetes mellitus. (From Szczech LA, et al: Outcomes of patients with chronic renal insufficiency in the Bypass Angioplasty Revascularization Investigation. Circulation 2002; 105:2253-2258.)

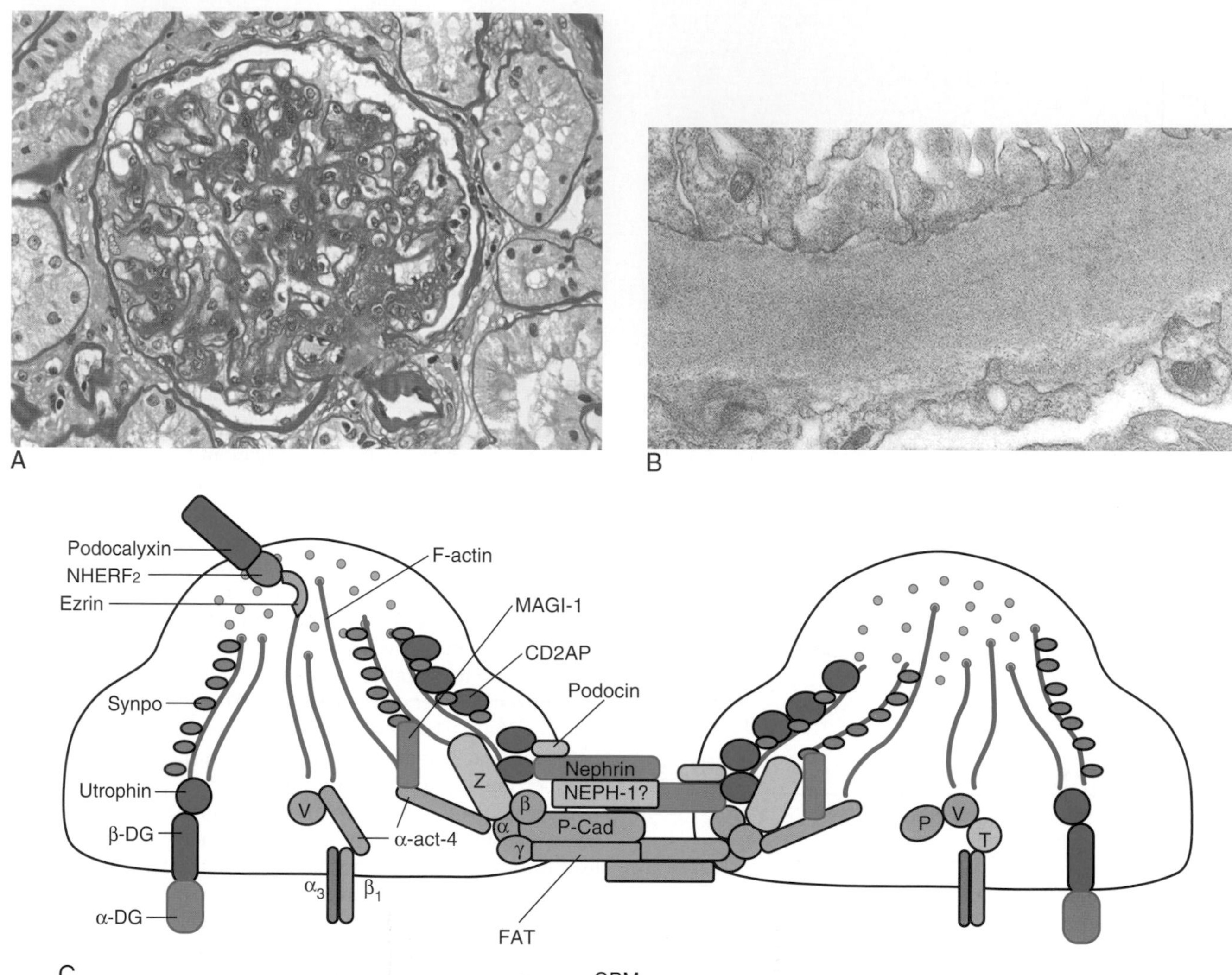

Figure 3–6 ***A,*** Pathologic changes of advanced diabetic nephropathy. PAS stain shows a diffusely expanded mesangial matrix with some associated proliferation. Peripheral capillary loop basement membranes are thickened. A hyaline deposit is present in the adjacent arteriole (original magnification 40X). ***B,*** Electron microscopy showing homogeneously increased glomerular basement membrane, with relative preservation of podocyte foot process and unremarkable endothelial cytoplasm (original magnification 6610X). ***C,*** The barrier to proteinuria. Schematic drawing of the visceral glomerular epithelial cells (podocytes) lining the outer aspect of the glomerular basement membrane. Foot processes are connected by the slit diaphragm with nephrin, podocin, and other proteins. Proposed mechanisms of diabetic proteinuria include structural changes to the basement membrane, hemodynamic injury to podocytes, decreased number of podocytes, damaged slit diaphragm components, and reduced expression of nephrin. (Reprinted with permission from Mundel P, Shankland S: Podocyte biology and response to injury. J Am Soc Nephrol 2002; 13:3005-3015.)

gene product localized to the area of and integral to the formation of the zipper-like slit diaphragm filtration structure between foot processes. There appear to be decreased protein levels of nephrin and podocin, despite an increase in their glomerular mRNA levels in several acquired human diseases, including diabetic nephropathy.[60] Some human data suggest a downregulation of nephrin expression in both type I and type II diabetic nephropathy,[61,62] which may be inversely related to the amount of proteinuria.[63] Podocin mutations have also been described in a variety of proteinuric conditions.[64] Other postulated factors in the pathogenesis of diabetic nephropathy factors include inflammation[65] and defective tubular albumin retrieval.[66]

A variety of experimental models and human kidney diseases have now indicated that proteinuria should be accepted as an independent and modifiable risk factor for renal disease,[67] and other studies have linked proteinuria to risk of ESRD,[68] in both diabetic and nondiabetic kidney disease. Although there is inherent intra-individual variability in urinary excretion of total protein or albumin, with a a standard deviation of up to 50%,[69] heavy proteinuria doubled the risk of progression in the Collaborative Study Group trial of

Captopril in type I diabetes[70] and may contribute to mortality risk.[71] Of two more recent well-known studies in type II patients, the IDNT (Irbesartan Diabetic Nephropathy Trial)[72] and RENAAL (Reducton of Endpoints in Non-insulin-dependent Diabetes Mellitus with the Angiotensin II Antagonist Losartan),[73] proteinuria was a prospective outcome measure only in the latter. Although no relationship of baseline proteinuria to renal outcomes was included in the original report, subsequent analysis reported proteinuria to be the most important predictor of ESRD.[74,75] For the IDNT, unpublished data revealed an increased risk of progression when baseline proteinuria equaled 3 to 4 g/24 hr.[76]

Although there is no proof of concept from clinical interventional trials that specific titration against the level of proteinuria improves the efficacy of renoprotective therapy, many consider the ultimate goal of proteinuria remission (<1 g/day) to be valid.[8] Targeting proteinuria reduction in patients with established diabetic nephropathy in order to accomplish slowing of renal progression is generally accomplished with agents that reduce both blood pressure and proteinuria. Data are very limited on therapies that might reduce proteinuria through other primary mechanisms, without correcting hypertension.

Diabetic nephropathy is an ideal disease model for testing the use of proteinuria as a surrogate end point.[77] Because early intervention is critical in diabetic nephropathy, a surrogate marker would be valuable.[78] However, disadvantages include the intraindividual variability in proteinuria, uncertainty regarding meaningful reduction in proteinuria, and the dearth of drugs with specific antiproteinuric effects. The relationship of proteinuria to the course of diabetic nephropathy is complex, and strict interpretation of available data does not readily lead to a specific goal for proteinuria reduction.

TREATMENT

Detection of Nephropathy

The presence of microalbuminuria in diabetic patients is considered indicative of nephropathy. Since it cannot be predicted who is going to develop nephropathy, widespread screening is recommended:

1. All diabetic patients should be tested yearly by examining urine for albumin starting immediately for patients with type II diabetes and after 3 to 5 years for patients with type I diabetes. Although 24-hour urine collections are ideal, the albumin/creatinine (a/c) ratio in a spot urine sample has been shown to accurately reflect the 24-hour urine collection,[38] thus is currently the recommended test for both screening and monitoring.
2. Considering the importance of early, aggressive treatment, tight control of blood sugar and blood pressure, and use of either ACE inhibitors or angiotensin receptor blockers should be undertaken in all patients with persistent microalbuminuria.

BLOOD SUGAR CONTROL

Many studies have demonstrated the critical importance in tight control of blood sugar in order to prevent the development or slow the progression of diabetic nephropathy.[79–82] The importance of tight control was definitively shown for patients with type I diabetes in the Diabetes Complications and Control Trial (DCCT).[79] In the initial study, 1441 patients with type I diabetes mellitus were studied for a mean of 6.5 years. One group received conventional treatment (mean glycosylated hemoglobin [Hgb A1c] 9.1), and another was treated intensively (Hgb A1c 7.2). With intensive therapy, there was a 39% reduction in microalbuminuria and 54% reduction in progression from microalbuminuria to overt proteinuria (defined as >300 mg/24 hours), compared to conventional therapy. Critical follow-up studies have continued to show the benefit of tight control of blood glucose in patients with type I diabetes. At the end of the DCCT, the patients in the conventional-therapy group were offered intensive therapy, and the care of all patients was transferred to their own physicians. Nephropathy was evaluated on the basis of urine specimens obtained from 1302 patients during the 3rd or 4th year after the end of the original DCCT study, approximately half from each treatment group. The median Hgb A1c values of the conventional-therapy group were 8.2%, and the intensive-therapy group's were 7.9%. Nevertheless, new cases of microalbuminuria were detected in 11% of 573 patients in the former conventional-therapy group, compared with 5% of 601 patients in the former intensive-therapy group, representing a 53% odds reduction. This longer follow-up demonstrates the importance of early aggressive management of blood sugar. It is quite common for blood glucose control to worsen over years of diabetes mellitus therapy, likely related to a combination of decreasing effectiveness of insulin due to multiple factors (e.g., changing metabolic requirements, resistance to effects of injected insulin), difficulty in maintaining the strict intensive regimen, age of the patient, genetic factors, and other as yet unanticipated factors. But even with worsening in the Hgb A1c, there were still benefits from keeping the blood sugar as tightly controlled as possible. The DCCT study organization recently reported on an 8-year follow-up study[83] (EDIC). As in the 4-year follow-up study, there was a narrowing of the difference between the Hgb A1c values of the original intensive therapy group (Hgb A1c 8.0%) and the conventional therapy group (Hgb A1c 8.2%), yet there was still a 57% risk reduction for the development of microalbuminuria in the original intensive therapy group as compared to the conventional therapy group. The risk reduction for progression to overt proteinuria from microalbuminuria was a remarkable 84% for intensive therapy compared to conventional therapy.

Patients with type II diabetes also benefit from tight control of blood sugar, as demonstrated in the United Kingdom Prospective Diabetes Study (UKPDS).[82] In this very large study of 3867 individuals with type II diabetes, the conventional therapy group averaged a Hgb A1c of 7.9%, whereas the intensively treated group had a Hgb A1c 7.0%. Intensive treatment was associated with a 33% risk reduction for developing microalbuminuria, and a 42% risk reduction for progression of microalbuminuria to proteinuria over 15 years. In addition, the risk reduction for doubling of serum creatinine was 67%. These results from both the DCCT and the UKPDS strongly support early and aggressive management of blood sugar as a highly effective approach for slowing the development and progression of diabetic kidney disease. The American Diabetes Association's official position is that the blood sugar treatment goal for all patients with diabetes should be a Hgb A1c of less than 7% in order to reduce the risk of diabetic nephropathy.[84]

HYPERTENSION

In the United States alone, at least 11 million diabetic patients (or 60% of all diabetics) are afflicted with hypertension. It has been emphasized that the risks of elevated blood pressures are greater for the diabetic than for the nondiabetic population.[85] Both systolic and diastolic hypertension accelerate the progression of microvascular complications such as nephropathy[10,86] as well as cardiovascular complications of diabetes, and even high normal blood pressure levels place patients in a high-risk category.[87] However, the majority of diagnosed hypertensives are inadequately controlled.[88] Overall, the prevalence of hypertension in the diabetic population is at least double that in the nondiabetic population (Table 3–2). The causes are complex and likely multifactorial (Figure 3–7).

Although hypertension is a typical manifestation of kidney disease, for 2 decades it has also been recognized as an early abnormality of nephropathy,[89] and hypertension may also be associated with the insulin resistance syndrome. In addition to genetics, several other factors contribute to hypertension in diabetic patients.[90] Intensive insulin treatment with near normal glycemia reduces the incidence of hypertension, an effect shown by the DCCT to be sustained for years after intensive treatment has stopped.[83] In general, hypertension in both type I and type II diabetes is characterized by expanded plasma volume, increased peripheral vascular resistance, and suppressed plasma renin activity. Systolic hypertension has been attributed to loss of elastic compliance in atherosclerotic large vessels.[10] In patients with type I diabetes, a rise in systemic blood pressure may precede the presence of kidney impairment, becoming manifest about the time the patient develops MA or even prior to a rise in urinary albumin excretion.[91] Microalbuminuria and its progression to overt nephropathy are associated with further increases in blood pressure.[92] In type II diabetes, overt hypertension or more subtle circadian blood pressure abnormalities are frequently present prior to proteinuria, so many patients with microalbuminuria are hypertensive.[93] In fact, hypertension is present at the time of diagnosis of type II diabetes in about one-third of patients.[10]

An association between the level of blood pressure and the clinical hallmarks of diabetic nephropathy, that is, degree of albuminuria[94] and chronic kidney disease progression, has been known for many years. In the last 2 decades, both observational and interventional studies have revealed that hypertension

Table 3–2 Prevalence of Hypertension in Diabetes Mellitus

Diabetes Type	Stage	Prevalence
1	No proteinuria	44%
	Proteinuria	67%
	Elevated serum creatinine	92%
2	No proteinuria	70%
	Proteinuria	83%
	Elevated serum creatinine	100%

(From Ritz E, et al: Hypertension and vascular disease as complications of diabetes. *In* Laragh JH, Brenner BM [eds]: Hypertension: Pathophysiology, Diagnosis, and Management. New York, Raven Press, 1990.)

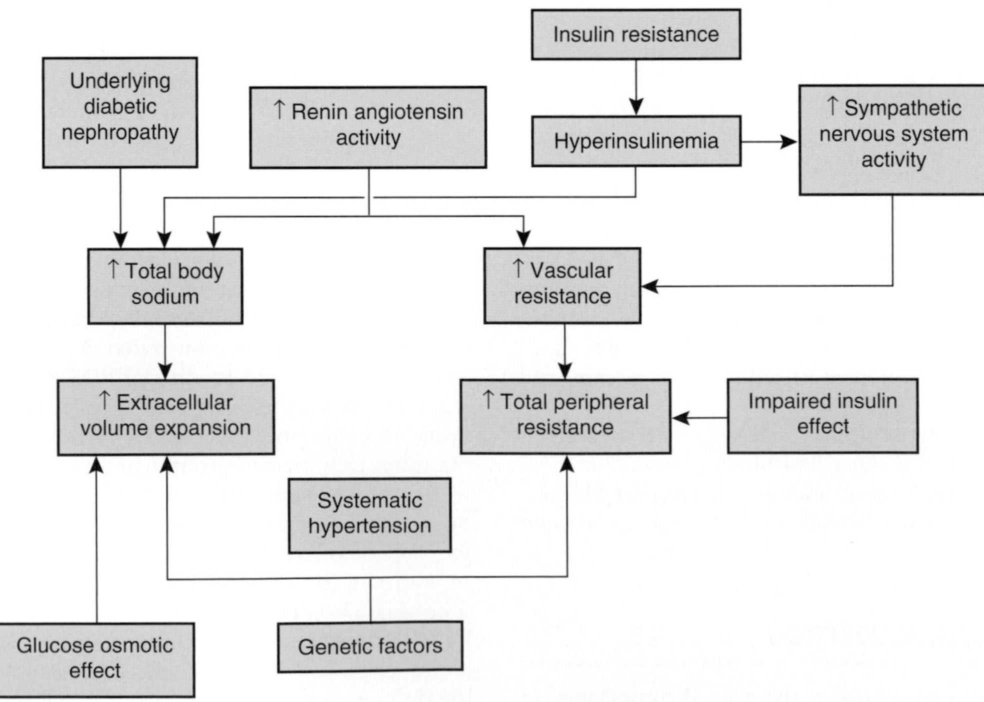

Figure 3–7 Mechanism of hypertension in diabetic kidney disease.

accelerates loss of renal function in both type I and type II patients.[95] In a recent study, each 10 mmHg increase in blood pressure was associated with about 1 cc/minute greater loss in glomerular filtration rate per year.[96] Although both systolic and diastolic blood pressures are associated with albuminuria in diabetes,[97] baseline systolic blood pressure was recently shown to be a stronger predictor of nephropathy than diastolic pressure in the RENAAL study of type II diabetics.[98]

Reports initially establishing the benefit of aggressive blood pressure control on slowing the decline in glomerular filtration rate did not emphasize that rising proteinuria was reversed and then reduced to less than 50% of the pretreatment value[99] (Figure 3–8). This and similarly important early studies showing that effective blood pressure control reduces proteinuria and slows renal progression have been corroborated.[53,100] For both primary and secondary prevention of chronic kidney disease progression in diabetic patients, clinical trials and meta-analyses have now demonstrated the beneficial effects of normalizing blood pressure.[101] More recently, the effect of intensive blood pressure control on the course of type I diabetic nephropathy was evaluated in patients who had participated in the Collaborative Study Group Captopril Study.[102] In this study using ramipril in combination with other agents, with an average 6 mmHg difference in mean arterial pressure over 24 months, proteinuria decreased by 50% in the intensive blood pressure group (MAP ≤92 mmHg) and increased by about 50% in the less intensive group (MAP 100–197 mmHg). Rates of decline in renal function during the intervention did not differ. Aggressive blood pressure treatment also induced remission of proteinuria and slowed decline of renal function in a prospective trial of 300 type I diabetics, with a mean arterial pressure of 100 mmHg achieved predominantly with ACEI.[103] The relevance of intensive blood pressure control (mean BP 128/75 mmHg) versus conventional control (mean BP 137/81 mmHg) to nephropathy progression in type II diabetic patients was evaluated by Schrier and colleagues.[104] Fewer intensively treated patients developed microalbuminuria or progressed to overt albuminuria. Growing evidence suggests that significant proteinuria is associated with cardiovascular disease in patients with diabetes, so proteinuria reduction may add to the cardiovascular risk reduction associated with hypertension control. Effective antihypertensive management is considered one of the most important interventions for delaying progression of diabetic nephropathy, almost regardless of the class of agent used. When antihypertensive therapy is initiated, an initial drop in kidney function may typically occur.[105] Reductions in pressure are associated with lowering of glomerular capillary pressure and diminished proteinuria.[106]

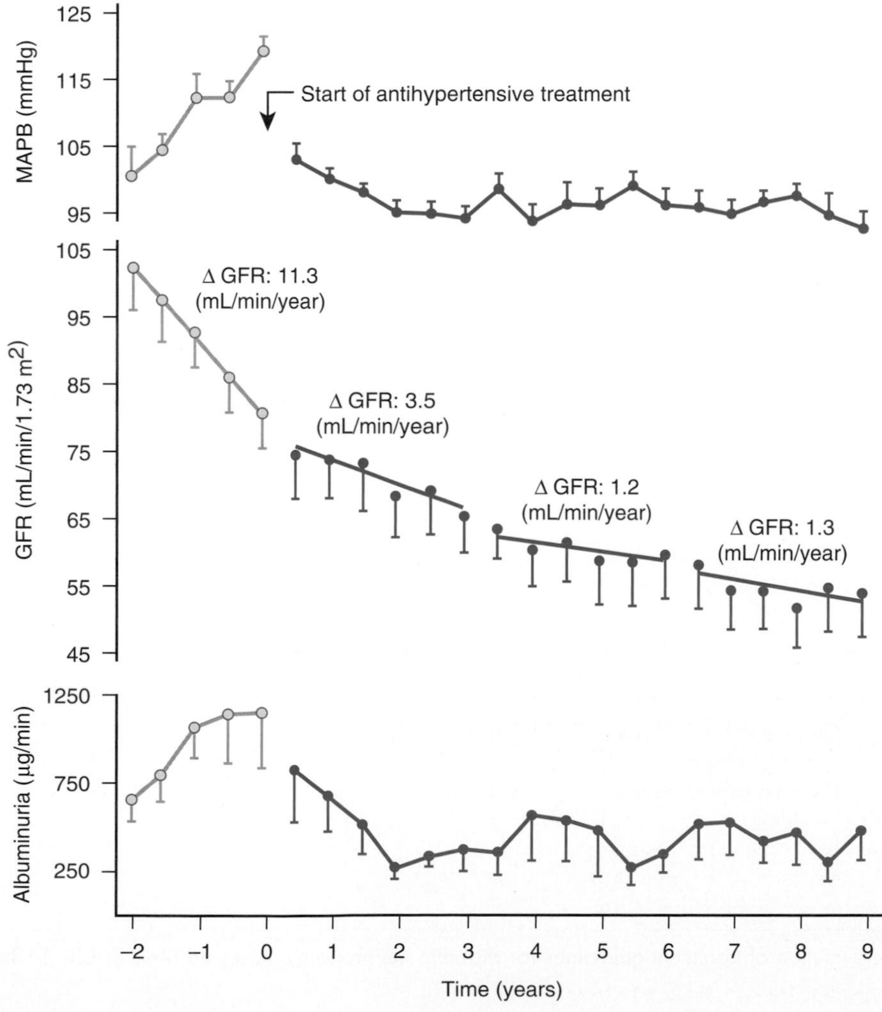

Figure 3–8 Early report by Parving and colleagues on the benefit of antihypertensive treatment on kidney function in diabetic nephropathy. With a fall in average blood pressures in nine patients from 143/96 mmHg to 129/84 mmHg, albuminuria was reduced by 50%. (From Parving H-H, et al: Effective an antihypertensive treatment postpones renal insufficiency in diabetic nephropathy. Br Med J 1987; 294:1443-1447.)

Based on available evidence that blood pressure readings above 125/75 mmHg increased the risk of ESRD in diabetic patients, a consensus statement from the National Kidney Foundation (NKF) published in 2000 advised treatment goals of less than that.[107] Since then, several expert panels, including the NKF and the American Diabetes Association (ADA), have adopted blood pressure targets of less than 130/80 mmHg as optimal for renal and cardiovascular protection in the diabetic patient with nephropathy[88,108–110] (Table 3–3). The National Kidney Foundation is currently working on new Blood Pressure Guidelines, which should be released in 2004 or 2005. A combination regimen of three or more drugs may be required. Clinical trial data suggest that mean arterial pressures of 92 mmHg or lower (corresponding to a blood pressure of about 130/70 mmHg) achieve greater preservation of renal function. Targets for high levels of isolated systolic hypertension (<180 mmHg) are less certain; systolic pressure should be lowered gradually, as tolerated.[109]

The optimal level of blood pressure decrease to achieve cardiovascular risk reduction is unclear[111] but may be answered in 2008 by the Action to Control Cardiovascular Risk in Diabetes (ACCORD) trial. Although data to evaluate the risks associated with low ranges of systolic blood pressure in diabetic kidney disease are not sufficient, pressures less than 100 to 110 mmHg should be avoided. Paradoxically, the fear of reducing systemic pressures too far may have contributed to failure to achieve lower blood pressure goals. Nonetheless, three large studies, the systolic hypertension in the Elderly Program (SHEP),[112] the Hypertension Optimal Treatment trial (HOT),[113] and the United Kingdom Prospective Diabetes Study (UKPDS)[114] have supported the notion that aggressive blood pressure lowering may not be harmful.

Several studies have underlined the challenge of achieving blood targets even in the clinical trial setting.[115] In the RENAAL study, for example, while systolic blood pressure was a stronger predictor of renal outcomes than diastolic pressure, less than half of patients achieved blood pressure goals during the treatment phase.[98] Hypertension may require selections from several different classes of drugs, and there are special considerations in the choice of antihypertensive treatment for the hypertensive diabetic (Table 3–4). Recent clinical trials have confirmed the poor response of diabetic nephropathy to

Table 3–3 Recent Blood Pressure Management Guidelines Issued by the Joint National Committee on Prevention, Detection, Evaluation, and Treatment of High Blood Pressure (JNC), the World Health Organization-International Society of Hypertension (WHO-ISH), the National Kidney Foundation (NKF), and the American Diabetes Association (ADA)

Year	Source	Patient Population	Target BP	Notes
1997	Sixth report of the Joint National Committee for Prevention, Detection, Evaluation, and Treatment of High Blood Pressure (JNC – VI)	Chronic kidney disease or diabetes mellitus	<130/<85	If diabetes or kidney disease
1999	World Health Organization/ International Society for Hypertension (WHO/ISH)		<130/<85	
2000	National Kidney Foundation special report	Chronic kidney disease	<130/<80	<125/<75 for proteinuria > 1 g/day and renal insufficiency
2000	American Diabetes Association	Chronic kidney disease or diabetes mellitus	<130/<85	For isolated systolic hypertension and systolic blood pressure >180 mmHg, lower BP in stages
2003	Seventh report of the Joint National Committee for Prevention, Detection, Evaluation, and Treatment of High Blood Pressure (JNC – 7)	Chronic kidney disease or diabetes mellitus	<130/<80	For diabetes or chronic kidney disease (gfr < 60 mL/min/1.73m^2 albumiuria)
2003	American Diabetes Association	Chronic kidney disease or diabetes mellitus	<130/<80	
2004	National Kidney Foundation K/DOQI Clinical Practice Guidelines on hypertension and antihypertensive agents in CKD	Diabetic kidney disease	<130/<80	

(Modified with permission from Bakris GL: The evolution of treatment guidelines for diabetic nephropathy. Postgrad Med 2003; 113: 35-50.)

treatment. An analysis of the NHANES III database indicated that only 11% of diabetic nephropathy patients being treated for hypertension achieved blood pressure goals of less than 130/85.[116] Furthermore, over a third of patients in ARB clinical trials with type II diabetic nephropathy progressed to primary renal end points.[72,73] In a recent trial implementing a stepped-care approach treatment algorithm, centered on maximal doses of ACEI or ARBs, only one third of patients reached target blood pressures of less than 130/80.[90] Target systolic blood pressure levels were even more difficult to control. A recent report of hypertensive military veterans indicated that, for patients with diabetes and renal disease, blood pressure control continues to fall short of guideline-recommended levels.[117] Combination therapy with agents that are tolerated and do not exacerbate existing metabolic problems are desirable.[118] Diuretics should be included in the antihypertensive regimen.

RENIN-ANGIOTENSIN BLOCKADE

By the late 1980s, basic research studies identifying the importance of elevations of glomerular plasma flow, glomerular capillary pressures, and single-nephron glomerular hyperfiltration in experimental diabetes had led to the recognition that angiotensin converting enzyme inhibition could modify the glomerular hyperfiltration and prevent the glomerular damage characteristic of the diabetic rat model.[119] The fact that other antihypertensive agents lacked these beneficial effects supported the key notion that intraglomerular hypertension was itself deleterious, and that ACEI had intrarenal effects independent of their antihypertensive properties. Several subsequent clinical trials in a spectrum of progressive renal diseases have demonstrated the benefit of ACEI in delaying progression of disease.[120] These observations were most significantly validated in type I diabetic kidney disease in the Collaborative Study Group trial with captopril, published in 1993,[121] comparing the ACEI with placebo in patients with creatinine of less than 2.5 mg/dL and urinary protein excretion of 500 mg/day or greater. Captopril slowed the progression of kidney disease by 50% and proved to reduce urinary protein excretion, despite comparable median blood pressures in the two groups. Median 24-hour urinary protein excretion was decreased by the 3-month visit in the captopril-treated group, and the reduction of almost 30% persisted throughout the study.[122] In large, randomized, controlled trials of type I diabetics, ACEI diminish proteinuria and slow the progression of diabetic nephropathy[11,101] in patients with microalbuminuria and overt proteinuria. Other randomized, controlled trials have suggested that reduction in proteinuria is associated with slowing of renal progression in patients with overt nephropathy. ACEI reduce the level of proteinuria more than equivalent antihypertensive doses of other classes of agents (Figure 3–9),[123] although the proteinuria advantage is lost as the systemic blood pressure declines.[43,106] A small subset of patients treated in a clinical trial setting appear to achieve proteinuria remission, and renal decline becomes nonprogressive.[124]

Analogous studies in patients with type II diabetic nephropathy have been less demonstrative of benefit. In contrast to type I patients, renal protection in type II diabetic

Table 3–4 Special Considerations in the Selection of Antihypertensive Medications for the Diabetic Patient

Drug Class	Special Considerations
Diuretic	Edema common in diabetic nephropathy; thiazides not effective in renal insufficiency.
Angiotensin-converting enzyme (ACE) inhibitor	Treatment of choice; Reduce proteinuria and protect from progression; Risk of hyperkalemia; Risk of worsening renal function; No adverse effects on glucose or lipid levels; Avoid in renal failure.
Angiotensin receptor blocker	Alternative to ACE inhibitor May use in combination with ACE inhibitor;
Calcium-channel blocker	Variable effects on diabetic nephropathy.
β-Blocker	No long-term data on diabetic nephropathy; Increased risk of hypoglycemia; May mask warning signs of hypoglycemia; Use if history of myocardial infarction or tachycardia.
α-Blockers	Never shown to reduce disease progression; Neutral effect on proteinuria; Orthostatic hypotension; Neutral on lipids and glucose intolerance; Recent concern about congestive heart failure.

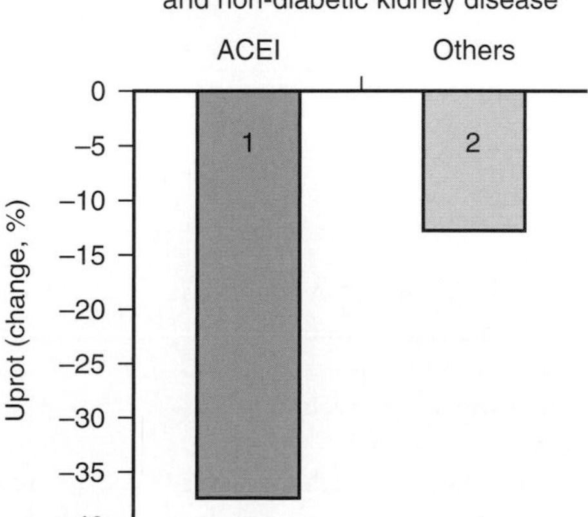

Figure 3–9 Effects of blood pressure-lowering agents in diabetic kidney disease. Shown are mean results for proteinuria obtained in studies that compared the effects of an ACEI with another antihypertensive agent. (From Gansevoort, Sluiter WJ, Bemmelder MH, et al: Nephrol Dial Transplant 1995; 10: 1963-1974.)

nephropathy compared against other antihypertensive agents has been less consistently demonstrated,[101] and results remain inconclusive,[125–127] possibly because of small sample sizes and use of surrogate outcomes. The clinical benefit to reduce proteinuria appears to be less significant in type II nephropathy.[128] Long-term protection was best shown in a 7-year study comparing the effects of enalapril and placebo in 94 type II normotensive patients with microalbuminuria.[125] A 5-year study period comparing the ACEI with placebo was followed by 2 additional years, during which all patients could choose enalapril or placebo. Initial ACEI therapy resulted in stable kidney function and albuminuria and reduced the risk of nephropathy by 42%; albuminuria worsened in the placebo group. Enalapril-treated patients who subsequently declined treatment noted a rise in albuminuria, whereas the placebo-treated patients who chose ACEI therapy had a reduction in albuminuria. A recent meta-analysis of ACEI in type II diabetic nephropathy indicated that ACEI produce significant reductions in proteinuria, although the effect is heterogeneous.[129] Overall, ACEI may provide similar results in type II as in type I diabetic nephropathy.

Relevant ACEI drug actions (Table 3–5) may include systemic and intrarenal hemodynamic effects, improvements in the filtration barrier, blockade of increased intrarenally-generated angiotension II,[130,131] reduced interstitial expansion,[132] tissue fibrosis[133] and extracellular expansion, attenuation of diabetes-associated reduction in nephrin expression,[59,61] and restoration of tubular albumin reabsorption.[134] Systemically, increasing attention is being given to the role of tissue-based RAS and the utility of blockade on other end-organ damage due to diabetes, primarily cardiovascular. ACEI slow the rise in creatinine and reduce the level of proteinuria more than equivalent doses of other classes of antihypertensive agents do, although event rates in clinical trial comparisons are similar when mean systemic pressure is less than 95 mmHg.[92] Extrarenal advantages of ACEI include lack of effects on lipid or glucoses levels and more effective regression of cardiac ventricular hypertrophy.

Angiotensin II receptor blockers have effects in experimental models of diabetic kidney disease to reduce proteinuria, glomerular hypertrophy, and glomerulosclerosis, similar to ACEI. ARBs share these effects with ACEI (Table 3–5) and provide a superior safety profile, including less risk of cough, angioedema, and significant hyperkalemia. Over recent years, data from clinical trials have demonstrated the beneficial effects of controlling blood pressure in secondary prevention of progression of chronic kidney disease in type II patients.[101] Published studies have included the RENAAL (Reduction of Endpoints in Non-insulin dependent diabetes mellitus with the Angiotensin II Antagonist Losartan)[73] and IDNT (Irbesartan Diabetic Nephropathy Trial).[72,135–137] In the RENAAL study, losartan was compared to conventional antihypertensive therapy in 1513 type II diabetic patients with diabetic nephropathy. Fewer ARB-treated patients reached the primary composite end point of doubling of serum creatinine, end-stage renal disease, or death (Table 3–6), and more achieved reduction in proteinuria. No improvement in all-cause mortality or cardiovascular morbidity and mortality occurred, although the rate of first hospitalizations for heart failure was reduced in the losartan group. A post-hoc analysis indicated that proteinuria, which was reduced by losartan, was the single most powerful predictor of ESRD in the study patients.[74] In the IDNT trial, the ARB irbesartan was compared with the calcium channel blocker amlodipine and placebo in 1715 type II diabetic patients with hypertension and nephropathy. Risk reduction for the primary composite end point was reduced by irbesartan compared with either amlodipine or placebo. Two subsequent evaluations of projected survival and health care cost-effectiveness of irbesartan in type II diabetes and nephropathy, based on treatment-specific probabilities derived from the IDNT, have indicated that the ARB improved survival, delayed onset of ESRD by over 1 year, and was the least costly treatment, compared to amlodip-

Table 3–5 Comparison of Clinical Effects of Angiotensin-Converting-Enzyme Inhibitors (ACEI) and Angiotensin II (Type I) Receptor Blockers (ARBs)

Effect	ACE Inhibitors	ARBs
Biologic effects		
Inhibit ACE and angiotensin-II synthesis	Yes	No
Blockade of angiotensin receptor	No	Yes
Increased plasma renin levels	Yes	Yes
Affects angiotensin-II formed by alternate pathways	No	Yes
Increased bradykinin levels	Yes	No
Side effects		
Cough, urticaria, angioedema	Yes	Less likely
Hyperkalemia	Yes	Milder
Deterioration of renal function	Potential	Potential
Contraindication in pregnancy	Yes	Yes
Approved indications		
Treatment of hypertension	Yes	Yes
Treatment of diabetic nephropathy	Yes (captopril)	Yes

Table 3–6 Results of Clinical Trials of Angiotensin Receptor Blockers in Type II Diabetic Kidney Disease

End Point	IDNT (Irbesartan)	RENAAL (Losartan)
Doubling of creatinine, ESRD, or death	20%	16%
Doubling of creatinine	33%	25%
ESRD	23%	28%
Overall death rate	NS	NS
Cardiovascular end points	NS	NS
First CHF hospitalization	23%	32%
Reduction in proteinuria	33%	35%

IDNT, irbesartan diabetic nephropathy trial; *RENAAL,* reduction of endpoints in NIDDM with the angiotensin II antagonist losartan. (See text.) Shown are percent risk reductions for study end points, and the percent reduction in proteinuria in the treatment group. (Data from Lewis EJ, Hunsicker LG, Clarke WR, et al: Renoprotective effect of the angiotensin-receptor antagonist ibesartan in patients with nephropathy due to type 2 diabetes. N Engl J Med 2001; 345:845–860; and Brenner BM, Cooper ME, De Zeeuw D, et al: Effects of Losartan on renal and cardiovascular outcomes in patients with type 2 diabetes and nephropathy. N Engl J Med 2001; 345:861–869.)

ine and control.[138,139] In both the RENAAL and IDNT studies, results were achieved in the absence of strict blood pressure control. In RENAAL, the target blood pressures (taken prior to the medication dose) of 140/90 during treatment was reached in only 47% of losartan and 40% of placebo patients.[45] In addition, examination of RENAAL and IDNT data has indicated that 43.5% of patients taking losartan and 32.6% taking irbesartan still reached a primary end point in the studies. Results of the RENAAL and IDNT studies have led to regulatory drug approval for ARBs in initial therapy for hypertensive type II diabetic patients with proteinuric renal disease. Economic evaluation of the IDNT has demonstrated the cost-effectiveness of the ARB compared to amlodipine or placebo.[137,138]

The previous review indicates that both ACEI and ARBs have demonstrated favorable effects on the progression of diabetic kidney disease.[108,140] Practice guidelines developed by the American Diabetes Association, the Joint National Commission (JNC), and the National Kidney Foundation support the uses of both ACEI and ARBs in initial therapy regimens for diabetic patients. Other studies, primarily in nondiabetic patients, have indicated that the nephroprotective effects of ARBs are similar to ACEI in reducing proteinuria. The time course of reduction in blood pressure and lowering of proteinuria are concordant.[141] ACEI may be preferred in both type I and type II patients with proteinuria, but ARBs may be substituted in patients intolerant of ACEI.

ARBs and ACEI interrupt the renin-angiotensin system through different mechanisms and could be synergistic in providing a higher degree of RAS blockade and renoprotection.[142,143] Theoretic advantages of combination therapy include blockade by the ARB of chymase-generated angiotensin II, lack of effect of the ARB on inhibition of kinin degradation and on aldosterone suppression, and improved receptor blockade by the ARB when AII production has been diminished.[144,145] More recent data suggest that combination therapy with angiotensin receptor antagonists and ACEI at standard clinical doses is superior to maximal recommended doses of ACEI with regard to lowering blood pressure levels, with ACEI/ARB combinations leading to greater reductions in blood pressure than either class used alone.[140] Limited data also suggest that combination therapy is also significantly more effective in reducing levels of proteinuria.[144] In type I patients, dual blockade with benazepril and valsartan compared to monotherapy with each in an identical dose was compared to placebo over 8-week treatment periods. Although benazepril and valsartan were equally effective in reducing blood pressure and albuminuria, dual blockade produced an additive reduction in albuminuria of 43%, and a modest further reduction in systolic and diastolic blood pressure.[96] Combination therapy was well-tolerated, consistent with previous trials, alleviating concerns that combination therapy might lead to more serious hyperkalemia.[143] The CALM study evaluated responses in type II diabetic patients with microalbuminuria. Reductions in albumin excretion were 50% with combination therapy, 39% with lisinopril, and 24% with candesartan.[146] A similar blinded short-term study in type II patients demonstrated similar reductions in albuminuria and blood pressure with dual blockade compared with maximal doses of candesartan and an ACEI.[147] An ACEI and ARB in maximal standard doses were effective as combined therapy in a recent nondiabetic trial, with a safety profile no different than the ACEI alone.[148] These recent clinical trials supporting combination therapy in the treatment of type I diabetic patients were recently reviewed[149] However, a clinical trial using an AT1 antagonist added to a usual maximal dose of the ACEI lisinopril did not show superior benefit to the ACEI alone, including many patients with diabetic nephropathy.[150] Further trials may be needed before combination therapy can be considered standard therapy.[151]

Several studies have attempted to identify ways to maximize the antiproteinuric effects of RAS blockade by increasing dosages of agents used to maximum tolerated nonhypotensive doses. In a study of nondiabetic proteinuria patients, the ACEI ramipril titrated up to 20 mg/day reduced proteinuria by 29% compared to baseline, about three times that of comventional dosages in a comparable study.[152] However, another ACEI study showed no impact of supramaximal doses over maximal antihypertensive doses.[153]

Because cardiovascular disease is a leading cause of mortality in diabetes, particularly in type II patients, and proteinuria is a powerful predictor of cardiovascular morbidity and mortality, cardioprotection is an important challenge in the management of patients with diabetic nephropathy. Several randomized studies of ACEI in diabetic patients with hypertension have demonstrated reductions in cardiovascular events, including Heart Outcomes Prevention Evaluation (HOPE) and microHope,[154] Captopril Prevention Project (CAPP),[155] and Fosinopril versus Amlodipine Cardiovascular Events Trial (FACET).[156] However, a recent meta-analysis of the effects of ACEI in diabetics and nondiabetics with chronic kidney disease did not reveal decreased mortality in patients with overt proteinuria treated with ACEI.[120] In the Collaborative Study Group Captopril Study, the 50% reduction in risk for the combined end points of death, dialysis, and transplantation included eight deaths in the captopril group and four deaths in the control group. The benefit of angiotensin receptor antagonists in reducing cardiovascular end points has been less consistent. Both the IDNT[111] and RENAAL studies showed no significant differences in cardiovascular outcomes with ARB therapy, except for similar reductions in hospitalizations for congestive heart failure. However, each trial was designed to evaluate renal, not cardiovascular, outcomes. The recent Losartan Intervention For Endpoint Reduction in Hypertension (LIFE) study showed more promise, with the ARB losartan more effective than conventional therapy in reducing cardiovascular morbidity and mortality in mostly type II diabetic patients with hypertension and left ventricular hypertrophy. However, there are no human data that prove cardioprotection independent of blood pressure when ARBs are given for renoprotection.[157] In addition, there have been no trials directly comparing ACEI and ARBs in cardioprotection in patients with diabetic nephropathy. The recent Optimal Therapy in Myocardial Infarction with the Angiotensin II Antagonist Losartan (OPTIMAAL) study comparing losartan and captopril in over 5000 patients with myocardial infarction reported a slightly higher cardiovascular death rate with the ARB.[158] Taking into account the results of these trials, some controversy remains regarding the selection of ACEI or ARB for cardiorenal protection in type II patients with diabetic nephropathy.[159]

NOVEL THERAPIES

Based on experimental models of diabetic kidney disease, advanced glycation end products (AGEs) have been postulated to play a role in human diabetic nephropathy.[160–162] Biologically active AGEs, formed from complex nonenzymatic glycosylation reactions of proteins, lipids, and nucleotides, can result in cross-linking between proteins, post-AGE receptor tissue effects, and altered cellular functions.[163] Several different AGE compounds have been identified in diabetic glomerulopathy lesions.[164] Toxic potential of AGEs has been described for mesangial cells, where overproduction of collagen, oxidative stress, and upregulation of insulin-like growth factor, transforming growth factor, and extracellular matrix components occur, and for tubular cells, where AGE binding may lead to tubulointerstitial fibrosis.

Pharmacologic inhibitors of AGE formation, including pimagedine[165] and pyridoxamine,[166] have been in development for several years and recently reached clinical development. Pimagedine inhibits AGE formation by binding irreversibly to reactive intermediates of early glycated products.[167,168] A major phase III clinical trial of pimagedine in type I diabetic nephropathy has recently been published.[169] In a randomized, double-blind, placebo-controlled multicenter study design, patients with established diabetic nephropathy were followed for a median of 2.5 years. Almost all were also on ACEI or ARB therapy. Both doses of the AGE inhibitor produced a statistical reduction in urinary protein excretion compared to placebo. In a subset with over 2 g of proteinuria per 24 hours, doubling of serum creatinine was less likely. In addition to a transient flu-like illness and anemia, pimagedine also produced unexpected toxicity in the form of ANCA positivity and a small number of cases of glomerulonephritis. A newer AGE inhibitor, pyridoxamine, is related to the natural compound, pyridoxine (vitamin B6), and appears to act at a later stage of the AGE biosynthetic pathway by inhibiting post-Amadori activity.[170] A recent phase II study of proteinuric type I and II diabetic patients with serum creatinine levels less than 2 mg/dL demonstrated that the agent was safe and well-tolerated.[171] Preliminary efficacy analysis indicated a reduction in urinary protein excretion and blunted rise in serum creatinine over 6 months. Other AGE inhibitors are also currently being evaluated.[172]

There are other new approaches to the treatment of diabetic nephropathy. These are based on an ever-growing mechanistic understanding of the causes of diabetic nephropathy where specific pathogenic roles for protein kinase C,[173] oxidative stress,[174] and transforming growth factor β have been well-established in animal models of diabetes.

Protein kinase C (PKC) is comprised of a family of serine/threonine kinases that have been shown to play important roles in a number of physiologic and pathophysiologic intracellular processes.[175] Research by King,[174] Whiteside,[176,177] and others has established that activation of PKCβ and PKCδ likely play important pathophysiologic roles in the development of diabetic nephropathy. A highly specific inhibitor (LY333531) directed against PKCβ has been shown to be very effective in preventing the development of diabetic retinopathy and in slowing the development of diabetic nephropathy in animals.[178] In 1996, Ishii and colleagues[179] reported in Science that LY333531 prevented the typical increase in glomerular filtration rate seen in diabetic rats and reduced albuminuria by 60%. In 1996, Koya and colleagues[179] studied the effect of oral PKCβ inhibition on mesangial cells from diabetic rats. They found that glucose-induced increases in arachidonic acid release, prostaglandin E 2 production, and inhibition of Na-K ATPase activities in the cultured mesangial cells were completely prevented by the addition of LY333531. They also found that PKCβ inhibition prevented the increased mRNA expression of transforming growth factor β1 and reduced expression of extracellular matrix components such as fibronectin and type IV collagen in the glomeruli of diabetic rats in parallel with inhibition of glomerular PKC activity. A detailed review of LY333531 and its potential may be found in a recent review by Tuttle and Anderson.[180] Similar but even more promising results for PKCβ inhibition have been found for the prevention of diabetic retinopathy. A worldwide trial of the PKCβ inhibitor is currently underway for retinopathy. Nephropathy trials are to be started in the near future.

Much research has shown that increased oxidative stress is likely a critical factor in the development of diabetic nephropathy.[173] Because of this a variety of trials of antioxidants in people and animals have been done. The animal studies strongly suggest that the addition of antioxidants can significantly slow development of diabetic nephropathy.[173] For example, work by Koya and colleagues[181] has shown that heme oxygenase 1 mRNA expression, which was increased 16-fold in glomeruli of diabetic rats, had virtually no increase in animals treated with the antioxidants vitmamin E or probucol. Other studies in animals have shown beneficial effects for other antioxidants such as alpha lipoic acid and taurine. Some studies in small numbers of patients suggest that antioxidants may be of benefit.[182, 183] Currently, there are a number of studies aimed at determining whether antioxidants such as vitamin E have a therapeutic role in the treatment of diabetic nephropathy. But to date the human studies have been disappointing. It is possible that the currently available antioxidants are not effective as used. There are likely many reasons for this. For example, it is possible that the antioxidant tissue levels are increased adequately with current approaches. It is also possible that a better understanding of the mechanisms responsible for the increased oxidative stress will lead to the development of more targeted approaches to controlling levels of reactive oxygen species. For example, recent work suggests that mitochondria are a major source of reactive oxygen species[184] and that deficiencies in intracellular antioxidants both may play major roles in the development of increased oxidative stress.[185,186] Thus, therapies specifically targeted at mitigating the effects of mitochondrial oxidant production[187] and increasing specific intracellular antioxidants might provide powerful new treatments for diabetic nephropathy.

Another potential mechanism that holds much promise for therapy is inhibition of transforming growth factor β (TGFβ). Diabetic nephropathy is associated with glomerulosclerosis and tubulointerstitial fibrosis. TGFβ is a protein that is prosclerotic and has been strongly implicated in the pathogenesis of diabetic nephropathy. Ziyadeh and colleagues[188,189] have done many studies showing that high glucose upregulates TGFβ and that specific monoclonal neutralizing antibodies and antisense oligonucleotides prevent the accumulation of mesangial matrix proteins in diabetic animals. Furthermore, long-term TGFβ inhibition in *db/db* mice prevented mesangial matrix expansion and preserved creatinine clearance.[190] Interestingly, there was no change in albuminuria. Because of this promising results, studies are being done to determine whether inhibition of

TGFβ will help to treat progression of diabetic nephropathy in humans. Pirfenidone inhibits the actions of TGFβ and has been used to treat pulmonary fibrosis.[191] Shumar and colleagues[192] are now using pirfenidone in an NIH sponsored clinical trial to determine whether it can prevent worsening of diabetic nephropathy.

At this time there is no clear approach to complete prevention or cure for diabetic nephropathy. An intriguing, although drastic, possible approach to treating diabetic kidney disease is pancreas transplantation. Fioretto and colleagues[193] studied patients up to 10 years post-pancreas transplants and showed by renal biopsy that there was a clear regression of disease that was not evident 5 years post-transplant. Clearly, this approach cannot be widely used because the risks of immunosuppression and the relative lack of pancreases make this approach useful only in a select number of patients. Of interest are islet cell transplants that should work as effectively as pancreas transplants and, hopefully, be safer to do.

ACKNOWLEDGMENTS

The authors wish to thank Kristy Frain for assistance in preparation of the manuscript and to acknowledge Dr. Isaac Stillman for his expert contribution of kidney pathology material.

References

1. U.S. Department of Health and Human Services. Health United States, 2003. *www.cdc.gov/nchs*
2. Caramori ML, Mauer M: Diabetes and nephropathy. Curr Opin Nephrol Hypertens 2003; 12:273–282.
3. Harvey JN: Trends in the prevalence of diabetic nephropathy in type 1 and type 2 diabetes. Curr Opin Nephrol Hypertens 2003; 12:317–322.
4. American Diabetes Association. Diabetic Nephropathy. Diabetes Care 2002; 25:S85-S89.
5. U.S. Renal Data System: USRDS 2003 annual data report. Bethesda, MD, National Institutes of Health, National Institute of Diabetes and Digestive and Kidney Diseases, April 2003.
6. Garg AX, Kiberd BA, Clark WF, et al: Albuminuria and renal insufficiency prevalence guides population screening: Results from the NHANES III. Kidney Intern 2002; 61:2165–2175.
7. Klein R, Kelin BEK, Moss SE: The incidence of gross proteinuria in people with insulin-dependent diabetes mellitus. Arch Int Med 1991; 151:1344–1348.
8. Brenner BM: Retarding the progression of renal disease. Nephrology forum. Kidney Intern 2003; 64:370–378.
9. Christensen CK, Mogensen CE: Effect of antihypertensive treatment on progression of incipient diabetic nephropathy. Hypertension 1985; 7:109–113.
10. American Diabetes Association. Diabetic nephropathy. Diabetes Care 2003; 26(S1): S94–S98.
11. Mohanram A, Toto RD: Outcome studies in diabetic nephropathy. Semin Nephrol 2003; 23:255–271.
12. Locatelli F, Canaud B, Eckardt KU, et al: The importance of diabetic nephropathy in current nephrological practice. Nephrol Dial Transplant 2003; 18:1716–1725.
13. Parving HH, Hovind P: Microalbuminuria in type 1 and type 2 diabetes mellitus: Evidence with angiotensin converting enzyme inhibitors and angiotensin II receptor blockers for treating early and preventing clinical nephropathy. Curr Hypertens Rep 2002; 4(5):387–393.
14. Caramori LM, Fioretto P, Mauer M: The need for early predictors of diabetic nephropathy risk: Is albumin excretion rate sufficient? Diabetes 2000; 49:1399–1408.
15. Bojestig M, Arnqvist HJ, Hermansson G, et al: Declining incidence of nephropathy in insulin-dependent diabetes mellitus. N Engl J Med 1994; 330:15–18.
16. Rossing P, Rossing K, Jacobsen P, Parving HH: Unchanged incidence of diabetic nephropathy in IDDM patients. Diabetes 1995; 44:739–743.
17. Young BA, Maynard C, Boyko EJ: Racial differences in diabetic nephropathy, cardiovascular disease, and mortality in a national population of veterans. Diabetes Care 2003; 26(8):2392–2399.
18. Crook ED, Wofford P, Oliver B: Advanced diabetic nephropathy disproportionately affects African-American females: Cross-sectional analysis and determinants of renal survival in an academic renal clinic. Ethnicity & Disease 2003; 13(1):28–33.
19. Writing Team for Diabetes Control and Complications Trial. Sustained effect of intensive treatment of type 1 diabetes mellitus on development and progression of diabetic nephropathy: The Epidemiology of diabetes interventions and complications study. JAMA 2003; 290:2159–2167.
20. Newton C, Raskin P: Blood pressure control: Effects on diabetic nephropathy progression: How low does blood pressure have to be? Curr Diabetes Rep 2002; 2:530–538.
21. Forsblom CM, Groop P-H, Ekstrand A, Groop LC: Predictive value of microalbuminuria in patients with insulin dependent diabetes of long duration. BMJ 1992; 305:1051–1053.
22. Rudberg S, Persson B, Dahlquist G: Increased glomerular filtration rate as a predictor of diabetic nephropathy: An 8-year prospective study. Kidney Int 1992; 41:822–828.
23. USRDS Web site, http://www.usrds.org
24. Hovind P, Tarnow L, Rossing K, et al: Decreasing incidence of severe diabetic microangiopathy in type 1 diabetes. Diabetes Care 2003; 26:1258–1264.
25. Merta M, Reiterova J, Rysava R, et al: Genetics of diabetic nephropathy. Nephrol Dial Transplant 2003; 18:24–25.
26. Cambien F, Poirier O, Lecerf L, et al: Deletion polymorphism in the gene for angiotensin-converting enzyme is a potent risk factor for myocardial infarction. Nature 1992; 359:641–644.
27. Jacobsen P, Tarnow L, Carstensen B, et al: Genetic variation in the renin-angiotensin system and progression of diabetic nephropathy. J Am Soc Nephrol 2003; 14:2843–2850.
28. Yoshida H, Kuriyama S, Atsumi Y, et al: Angiotensin I converting enzyme gene polymorphism in non-insulin dependent diabetes mellitus. Kidney Int 1996; 50:657–664.
29. Penno G, Chaturvedi N, Talmud P, et al: Effect of angiotensin converting enzyme (ACE) gene polymorphism on progression of renal disease and the influence of ACE inhibition in IDDM patients: Findings from the EUCLID randomized controlled trial. Diabetes 1998; 47:1507–1511.
30. Andersen S, Tarnow L, Cambien F, et al: Long-term renoprotective effects of losartan in diabetic nephropathy. Diabetes Care 2003; 26:1501–1506.
31. Orchard TJ, Chang YF, Ferrell RE, et al: Nephropathy in type 1 diabetes: A manifestation of insulin resistance and multiple genetic susceptibilities? Further evidence from the Pittsburgh Epidemiology of Diabetes Complication Study. Kidney Int 2002; 62(3):963–970.
32. Parving H-H, Oxenboll B, Svendsen PA, et al: Early detection of patients at risk of developing diabetic nephropathy: A longitudinal study of urinary albumin excretion. Acta Endocrinol 1982; 100:550–555.
33. Viberti GC, Hill RD, Jarrett RJ, et al: Microalbuminuria as a predictor of clinical nephropathy in insulin-dependent diabetes mellitus. Lancet 1982; 1:1430–1432.
34. Mogensen CE, Christensen CK: Predicting diabetic nephropathy in insulin-dependent patients. N Engl J Med 1984; 311:89–93.
35. Mogensen CE: Microalbuminuria as a predictor of clinical diabetic nephropathy. Kidney Int 1987; 31:673–689.

36. Chobanian AV, Bakris GL, Black HR, et al: National Heart, Lung, and Blood Institute Joint National Committee on Prevention, Detection, Evaluation, and Treatment of High Blood Pressure. National High Blood Pressure Education Program Coordinating Committee. The Seventh Report of the Joint National Committee on Prevention, Detection, Evaluation, and Treatment of High Blood Pressure: The JNC 7 report. JAMA 2003; 289: 2560–2572.
37. Perkins BA, Ficociello LH, Silva KH, et al: Regression of microalbuminuria in type 1 diabetes. N Engl J Med 2003; 348:2285–2293.
38. Bakker AJ: Detection of microalbuminuria: Receiver operating characteristic curve analysis favors albumin-to-creatinine ratio over albumin concentration. Diabetes Care 1999; 22:307–313.
39. Bruno G, Merletti F, Biggeri A, et al: Progression to overt nephropathy in type 2 diabetes: The Casale Monferrato study. Diabetes Care 2003; 26:2150–2155.
40. Kimmelstiel P, Wilson C: Intercapillary lesions in glomeruli of kidney. Am J Path 1936; 12:83–98.
41. Eknoyan G, Hostettler T, Bakris GL, et al: Proteinuria and other markers of chronic kidney disease: A position statement of the National Kidney Foundation (NKF) and the National Institute of Diabetes and Digestive Kidney Diseases (NIDDK). Am J Kidney Dis 2003; 42:617–622.
42. Goldstein DA, Massry SG: Diabetic nephropathy. Clinical course and effect of hemodialysis. Nephron 1978; 20:286–296.
43. Ritz E, Orth SO: Nephropathy in patients with type 2 diabetes mellitus. N Engl J Med 1999; 341:1127–1133.
44. Volpe M, Savoia C, De Paolis P, et al: The renin-angiotensin system as a risk factor and therapeutic target for cardiovascular and renal disease. J Am Soc Nephrol 2002; 13:S173–S178.
45. Bakris GL: NephSAP: Nephrology Self-Assessment Program. J Am Soc Nephrol 2003:2–6.
46. Ritz E: Albuminuria and vascular damage: The vicious twins. N Engl J Med 2003; 348:2349-2352.
47. Gerstein HC, Mann JFE, Yi Q, et al: Albuminuria and risk of cardiovascular events, death, and heart failure in diabetic and nondiabetic individuals. JAMA 2001; 286:421–426.
48. Segura J, Campo C, Ruilope LM: Proteinuria: An underappreciated risk factor in cardiovascular disease. Curr Cardiol Rep 2002; 4:458–462.
49. Jude EB, Anderson SG, Cruickshank JK, et al: Natural history and prognostic factors of diabetic nephropathy in type 2 diabetes. Quarterly J Med 2002; 95:371–377.
50. Szczech LA, Best PJ, Crowley E, et al: Bypass Angioplasty Revascularization Investigation (BARI) Investigators. Outcomes of patients with chronic renal insufficiency in the bypass angioplasty revascularization investigation. Circulation 2002; 105:2253–2258.
51. Parving H-H: Diabetic nephropathy: Prevention and treatment. Kidney Int 2001; 60:2041–2055.
52. Klahr S, Morrissey J: Progression of chronic renal disease. Am J Kidney Dis 2003; 41:S3–S7.
53. Hostetter TH: Mechanisms of diabetic nephropathy. Am J Kidney Dis 1994; 23:188–192.
54. Myers BD, Winetz JA, Chui F, et al: Mechanisms of proteinuria in diabetic nephropathy: A study of glomerular barrier function. Kidney Int 1982; 21:633–641.
55. Lee SH, Bae JS, Park SH, et al: Expression of TGF-beta-induced matrix protein beta Ig-h3 is upregulated in the diabetic rat kidney and human proximal tubular epithelial cells treated with high glucose. Kidney Int 2003; 64:1012 –1021.
56. Pagtalunan ME, Miller PL, Jumping-Eagle S, et al: Podocyte loss and progressive glomerular injury in type II diabetes. J Clin Invest 1997; 99:342-348.
57. Steffes MW, Schmidt D, McCrery R, et al: International Diabetic Nephropathy Study Group. Glomerular cell number in normal subjects and in type 1 diabetic patients. Kidney Int 2001; 59:2104–2113.
58. Vestra MD, Masiero A, Roiater AM, et al: Is podocyte injury relevant in diabetic nephropathy? Diabetes 2003; 52:1013–1035.
59. Kelly DJ, Aaltonen P, Cox AJ, et al: Expression of the slit-diagram protein, nephrin, in experimental diabetic nephropathy: Differing effects of anti-proteinuric therapies. Nephrol Dial Transplant 2002; 17:1327–1332.
60. Koop K, Eikmans M, Baelde HJ, et al: Expression of podocyte-associated molecules in acquired human kidney diseases. J Am Soc Nephrol 2003; 14:2063–2071.
61. Doublier S, Salvidio G, Lupia E, et al: Nephrin expression is reduced in human diabetic nephropathy. Diabetes 2003; 52: 1023–1030.
62. Cooper ME, Mundel P, Noner G: Role of nephrin in renal disease including diabetic nephropathy. Semin Nephrol 2002; 22: 393–398.
63. Langham RG, Kelly DJ, Cox AJ, et al: Proteinuria and the expression of the podocyte slit diaphragm protein, nephrin, in diabetic nephropathy: Effects of angiotensin converting enzyme inhibition. Diabetologia 2002; 45:1572–1576.
64. Caridi G, Bertelli R, Di Duca M, et al: Broadening the spectrum of diseases related to podocin mutations. J Am Soc Nephrol 2003; 14:1278–1286.
65. Navarro JF, Mora C, Maca M, et al: Inflammatory parameters are independently associated with urinary albumin in type 2 diabetes mellitus. Am J Kidney Dis 2003; 42:53–61.17.
66. Russo LM, Bakris GL, Comper WD: Renal handling of albumin: A critical review of basic concepts and perspective. Am J Kidney Dis 2002; 39:899–919.
67. Keane WF, Eknoyan G: Proteinuria, Albuminuria, Risk, Assessment, Detection, Elimination PARADE: A position paper of the National Kidney Foundation. Am J Kidney Dis 1999; 33:1004–1010.
68. Locatelli F, Del Vecchio L, D'Amico M, et al: Is the agent or the blood pressure level that matters for renal protection in chronic nephropathies? J Am Soc Nephrol 2002; 13:S196–S201.
69. Parving H-H, Smidt UV, Friisberg B, et al: A prospective study of glomerular filtration rate and arterial blood pressure in insulin-dependent diabetes with diabetic nephropathy. Diabetologia 1981; 20:457–461.
70. Breyer JA, Bain RP, Evans JK, et al: Predictors of the progression of renal insufficiency in patients with insulin-dependent diabetes and overt nephropathy. Kidney Int 1996; 50:1651–1658.
71. Watkins PJU, Blainey JD, Brewer DB, et al: The natural history of diabetic renal disease. Quart J Med 1972; XLI:437–456.
72. Lewis EJ, Hunsicker LG, Clarke WR, et al: Renoprotective effect of the angiotensin-receptor antagonist irbesartan in patients with nephropathy due to type 2 diabetes. N Engl J Med 2001; 345:851–860.
73. Brenner BM, Cooper ME, De Zeeuw D, et al: Effects of Losartan on renal and cardiovascular outcomes in patients with type 2 diabetes and nephropathy. N Engl J Med 2001; 345:861–869.
74. Keane WF, Brenner BM, Zeeuw D, et al: The risk of developing end-stage renal disease in patients with type 2 diabetes and nephropathy: The RENAAL Study. Kidney Int 2003; 63: 1499–1507.
75. Keane WF, Lyle PA: Recent advances in management of type 2 diabetes and nephropathy: Lessons from the RENAAL study. Am J Kidney Dis 2003; 41(3 suppl 1): S22–S25.
76. Weir MR: Diabetes and hypertension: How low should you go and with which drugs? Am J Hypertens 2001; 14:17s–26s.
77. Hostetter TH: Prevention of end-stage renal disease due to type 2 diabetes. N Engl J Med 2001; 345:910–911.
78. Campbell RC, Ruggenenti P, Remuzzi G: Halting the progression of chronic nephropathy. J Am Soc Nephrol 2002; 13: S190–S195.
79. The Diabetes Control and Complications Trial Research Group. The effect of intensive treatment of diabetes on the development and progression of long-term complications in insulin-dependent diabetes mellitus. N Engl J Med 1993; 329:977–986.

80. The Diabetes Control and Complications Trial Research Group. Retinopathy and nephropathy in patients with type 1 diabetes four years after an intensive trial with insulin. N Engl J Med 2000; 342:381–389.
81. Ohkubo Y, Kishikawa H, Araki E, et al: Intensive insulin therapy prevents the progression of diabetic microvascular complications in Japanese patients with non-insulin-dependent diabetes mellitus: A randomized prospective 6-year study. Diabetes Res Clin Pract 1995; 28:103.
82. Intensive blood-glucose control with sulphonylureas or insulin compared with conventional treatment and risk of complications in patients with type 2 diabetes (UKPDS 33). UK Prospective Diabetes Study Group. Lancet 1998; 352:837–853.
83. Writing Team for Diabetes Control and Complications Trial. Sustained effect of intensive treatment of type 1 diabetes mellitus on development and progression of diabetic nephropathy: The Epidemiology of diabetes interventions and complications study. JAMA 2003; 290:2159–2167.
84. American Diabetes Association. Diabetic nephropathy. Diabetes Care 2003; 26(S1):S94–S98.
85. Kaplan NM: Critique of recommendations from working group on hypertension in diabetes. Am J Kidney Dis 1989; 13:38–40.
86. Jandeleit-Dahm K, Cooper ME: Hypertension and diabetes. Curr Opin Nephrol Hypertens 2002; 11:221–228.
87. Bakris GL: The evolution of treatment guidelines for diabetic nephropathy. Postgrad Med 2003; 113:35–50.
88. WHO, ISH Writing Group: 2003 World Health Organization (WHO)/International Society of Hypertension (ISH) statement on management of hypertension. J Hypertens 2003; 21: 1983–1992.
89. Mogensen CE: Long-term antihypertensive treatment inhibiting progression of diabetic nephropathy. Br Med J 1982; 285: 685–688.
90. Tomlinson JW, Owen KR, MRCP, et al: Treating hypertension in diabetic nephropathy. Diabetes Care 2003; 26:1802–1805.
91. Thomas W, Shen Y, Molitch ME, et al: Rise in albuminuria and blood pressure in patients who progressed to diabetic nephropathy in the diabetes control and complications trial. J Am Soc Nephrol 2001; 12:333–340.
92. Ismail N, Becker B, Strzelczyk P, et al: Renal disease and hypertension in non-insulin-dependent diabetes mellitus. Kidney Int 1999; 55:1–28.
93. Remuzzi G, Schieppati A, Ruggenenti P: Nephropathy in patients with type 2 diabetes. N Engl J Med 2002; 346:1145–1151.
94. Jarrett RJ: Hypertension in diabetic patients and differences between insulin-dependent diabetes mellitus and non-insulin-dependent diabetes mellitus. Am J Kidney Dis 1989; 13:14–16.
95. Adamczak M, Zeier M, Dikow R, et al: Kidney and hypertension. Kidney Int Suppl 2002; 80:62–67.
96. Jacobsen P, Andersen S, Jensen BR, et al: Additive effect if ACE inhibition and angiotensin II receptor blockade in type 1 diabetic patients with diabetic nephropathy. J Am Soc Nephrol 2003; 14: 992–999.
97. Savage S, Nagel NJ, Estacio RO, et al: Clinical factors associated with urinary albumin excretion in type II diabetes. Am J Kidney Dis 1995; 25:836–844.
98. Bakris GL, Weir MR, Shanifar S, et al: Effects of blood pressure level on progression of diabetic nephropathy. Results from the RENAAL study. Arch Intern Med 2003; 163:1555–1565.
99. Parving H-H, Andersen AR, Smidt UM, et al: Effect of antihypertensive treatment on kidney function in diabetic nephropathy. Br Med J 1987; 294:1443–1447.
100. Lasaridis AN, Sarafidis PA: Diabetic nephropathy and antihypertensive treatment: What are the lessons from clinical trials? Am J Hypertens 2003; 16:689–697.
101. Brenner BM, Zagrobelny J: Clinical renoprotection trials involving angiotensin II-receptor antagonists and angiotensin-converting enzyme inhibitors. Kidney Int 2003; 83:S77–S85.
102. Lewis JB, Berl T, Bain RO, et al: Effect of intensive blood pressure control on the course of type 1 diabetic nephropathy. Am J Kidney Dis 1999; 34:809–817.
103. Hovind P, Rossing P, Tarnow L, et al: Remission and regression in the nephropathy of type 1 diabetes when blood pressure is controlled aggressively. Kidney Int 2001; 60:277–283.
104. Schrier RW, Estacio RO, Esler A, et al: Effects of aggressive blood pressure control in normotensive type 2 diabetic patients on albuminuria, retinopathy, and strokes. Kidney Int 2001; 61:1086–1097.
105. Hansen HO, Rossing P, Tarnow L, et al: Increased glomerular filtration rate after withdrawal of long-term antihypertensive treatment in diabetic nephropathy. Kidney Int 1995; 47: 1726–1731.
106. Weidmann P, Boehlen LM, deCourten M: Effects of different antihypertensive drugs on human diabetic proteinuria. Nephrol Dial Transplant 1993; 8:582–584.
107. Bakris GL, Williams M, Dworkin L, et al: Preserving renal function in adults with hypertension and diabetes: A consensus approach. Am J Kidney Dis 2000; 26:646–661.
108. Chabanian AV, Bakris GL, Black HR, et al: National High Blood Pressure Education Program Coordinating Committee. The Seventh Report of the Joint National Committee on Prevention, Detection, Evaluation and Treatment of High Blood Pressure: The JNC7 Report. JAMA 2003; 289:2560–2572.
109. American Diabetes Association. Treatment of hypertension in adults with diabetes. Diabetes Care 2003; 26:S80–S82.
110. Kidney Disease Outcome Quality Initiatives. K/DOQI clinical practice guidelines for chronic kidney disease: Evaluation, classification, and stratification. Am J Kidney Dis 2002; 39:S1–S231.
111. Berl T, Hunsicker LG, Lewis JB, et al: Cardiovascular outcomes in the Irbesartan Diabetic Nephropathy Trial of patients with type 2 diabetes and overt nephropathy. Ann Intern Med 2003; 138:542–549.
112. Perry HM Jr, Davis BR, Price TR, et al: Effect of treating isolated systolic hypertension on the risk of developing various types and subtypes of stroke: The systolic hypertension in the elderly program (SHEP). JAMA 2000; 284:465–471.
113. Hansson L, Zanchetti A, Carruthers SG, et al: Effects of intensive blood-pressure lowering and low-dose aspirin in patients with hypertension: Principal results of the Hypertension Optimal Treatment (HOT) randomized trial. Lancet 1998; 351: 1755–1762.
114. Adler AI, Stratton IM, Neil HA, et al: Association of systolic blood pressure with macrovascular and microvascular complications of type 2 diabetes *UKPDS 36: Prospective observational study. BMJ 2000; 321:412–419.
115. Boero R, Prodi E, Elia F, et al: How well are hypertension and albuminuria treated in type II diabetic patients? J Hum Hypertens 2003; 17:413–418.
116. Garg J, Bakris GL: Treatment of hypertension in patients with renal disease. Cardiovasc Drugs Ther 2002; 16:503-510.
117. Borzecki AM, Wong AT, Hickey EC, et al: Hypertension Control Arch Intern Med 2003; 163:2705–2711.
118. Kurihama S, Tomonari H, Tokudome G, et al: Anti-proteinuric effects of combined antihypertensive therapies in patients with overt type 2 diabetic nephropathy. Hypertens Res 2002; 25: 849–855.
119. Zatz R, Dunn BR, Meyer TW, et al: Prevention of diabetic glomerulopathy by pharmacological amelioration of glomerular capillary hypertension. J Clin Invest 1986; 77:1993–2001.
120. Kshirsagar AB, Joy MS, Hogan S, et al: Effect of ACE inhibitors in diabetic and nondiabetic chronic renal disease: A systematic overview of randomized placebo-controlled trials. Am J Kidney Dis 2000; 35:695–707.
121. Lewis EJ, Hunsicker LG, Bain RP, et al: The effect of angiotensin-converting enzyme inhibition on diabetic nephropathy. N Engl J Med 1993; 329:1456–1462.

122. Lewis EJ: Captropril in type I diabetic nephropathy. *In* Black HR (ed): Clinical Trials in Hypertension. New York, Marcel Dekker, 2001, p 451–468.
123. Gansevoort RT, Sluiter WJ, Bemmelder MH, et al: Antiproteinuric effect of blood-pressure-lowering agents: A meta-analysis of comparative trials. Nephrol Dial Transplant 1995; 10:1963–1974.
124. Hebert LA, Bain RP, Verme D, et al: Remission of nephrotic-range proteinuria in type 1 diabetes. Kidney Int 1994; 46:1688–1693.
125. Ravid M, Lang R, Rachmani R, et al: Long-term renoprotective effect of angiotensin-converting enzyme inhibition in non-insulin-dependent diabetes mellitus: A 7-year follow-up study. Arch Intern Med 1996; 156:286–289.
126. Lebovitz HE, Wiegmann TB, Cnan A, et al: Renal protective effects of enalapril in hypertensive NIDDM: Role of baseline albuminuria. Kidney Int Suppl 1994; 45:S150–S155.
127. Bakris GL, Copley JB, Vicknair N, et al: Calcium channel blockers versus other antihypertensive therapies on progression of NIDDM associated nephropathy. Kidney Int 1996; 50: 1641–1650.
128. Ruggenenti P, Perna A, Benei R, et al: In chronic nephropathies prolonged ACE inhibition can induce remission: Dynamics of time-dependent changes in GFR. J Am Soc Nephrol 1999; 10:997–1006.
129. Hamilton RA, Kane MP, Demers J: Angiotensin-converting enzyme inhibitors and type 2 diabetic nephropathy: A meta-analysis. Pharmacotherapy 2003; 23:909–915.
130. Carey RM, Siragy HM: The intrarenal renin-angiotensin system and diabetic nephropathy. Trends Endocrinol Metab 2003; 14:247–281.
131. Gilbert RE, Cooper ME: The tubulointerstitium in progressive diabetic kidney disease: More than an aftermath of glomerular injury? Kidney Int 1999; 56:1627–1637.
132. Cordonnier DJ, Pinel N, Barro C, et al: Expansion of cortical interstitium is limited by converting enzyme inhibition in type 2 diabetic patients with glomerulosclerosis. J Am Soc Nephrol 1999; 10:1253–1263.
133. Amann B, Tinzmann R, Angelkort B: ACE inhibitors improve diabetic nephropathy through suppression of renal MCP-1. Diabetes Care 2003; 26:2421–2425.
134. Tojo A, Onozato ML, Kurihara H, et al: Angiotensin II blockade restores albumin reabsorption in the proximal tubules of diabetic rats. Hypertens Res 2003; 26:413–419.
135. Ruilope LM, Luno J: Angiotensin blockade I type 2 diabetic renal disease. Kidney Int 2002; 62(S82):S61–S63.
136. Parving H-H: Angiotensin II receptor blockade in the prevention of diabetic nephropathy. Am J Clin Proc 2002; 3:21–26.
137. Gilbert RE, Krum H, Wilkinson-Berka J, et al: The renin-angiotensin system and the long-term complications of diabetes: Pathophysiological and therapeutic considerations. Diabet Med 2003; 20:607–621.
138. Rodby RA, Chiou CF, Boprenstein J, et al: The cost-effectiveness of irbesartan in the treatment of hypertensive patients with type 2 diabetic nephropathy. Clin Ther 2003; 25:2102–2119.
139. Palmer AJ, Annemans L, Roze S, et al: An economic evaluation of irbesartan in the treatment of patients with type 2 diabetes, hypertension and nephropathy: Cost effectiveness of Irbesartan in diabetic nephropathy trial (IDNT) in the Belgian and French settings. Nephrol Dial Transplant 2003; 18:2059–2066.
140. Thurman JM, Schrier RW: Comparative effects of angiotensin-converting enzyme inhibitors and angiotensin receptor blockers on blood pressure and the kidney. Cardiosource 2003; 114:588–598.
141. Andersen S, Jacobsen P, Tarnow L, et al: Time course of the antiproteinuric and antihypertensive effect of losartan in diabetic nephropathy. Nephrol Dial Transplant 2003; 18:293–297.
142. Sowers JR, Haffner S: Treatment of cardiovascular and renal risk factors in the diabetic hypertensive. Hypertension 2002; 40:781–788.
143. Hilgers KF, Mann JF: ACE inhibitors versus AT1 receptor antagonists in patients with chronic renal disease. J Am Soc Nephrol 2002; 13:1100–1108.
144. Rosner MH, Okusa MD: Combination therapy with angiotensin-converting enzyme inhibitors and angiotensin receptor antagonists in the treatment of patients with type 2 diabetes mellitus. Arch Intern Med 2003; 163:1025–1029.
145. Herbert LA, Silmer WA, Falkenhain ME, et al: Renoprotection: One or many therapies? Kidney Int 2001; 59:1211–1226.
146. Mogensen CE, Neldham S, Tikkanen I, et al: Randomized controlled trial of dual blockade of renin-angiotensin systems in patients with hypertension, microalbuminuria, and non-insulin-dependent diabetes: The Candesartan and Lisinopril Microalbuminuria (CALM) study. The Calm Study Group. Br Med J 2000; 321:1440–1444.
147. Rossing K, Jacobsen P, Pietraszek L, et al: Renoprotective effects of adding angiotensin II receptor blocker to maximal recommended doses of ACE inhibitor in diabetic nephropathy: A randomized double blind crossover trial. Diabetes Care 2003; 26:2268–2274.
148. Nakao N, Yoshimura A, Morita H, et al: Combination treatment of angiotensin-II receptor blocker and angiotensin-converting-enzyme inhibitor in non-diabetic renal disease (COOPERATE): A randomized controlled trial. Lancet 2003; 361:117–124.
149. Sowers JR: Diabetic nephropathy and concomitant hypertension: A review of recent ADA recommendations. Am J Clin Proc 2002; 3:27–33.
150. Agarwal R: Add-on angiotensin receptor blockade with maximized ACE inhibition. Kidney Int 2001; 59:2282–2289.
151. Finnegan PM, Gleason BL: Combination ACE Inhibitors and Angiotensin II receptor blockers for hypertension. Ann Pharmacother 2003; 37:886–889.
152. Pisoni R, Ruggenenti P, Sangalli F, et al: Effect of high dose ramipril with or without indomethacin on glomerular selectivity. Kidney Int 2002; 62:1010–1019.
153. Haas M, Leko MZ, Erler C, et al: Antiproteinuric versus antihypertensive effects of high-dose ACE inhibitor therapy. Am J Kidney Dis 2002; 40:458–463.
154. Gerstein HC, Yusuf S, Mann JFE, et al: Heart Outcomes Prevention Evaluation Study Investigators. Effects of ramipril on cardiovascular and microvascular outcomes in people with diabetes mellitus: Results of the HOPE study and MICRO-HOPE substudy. Lancet 2000; 355:253–259.
155. Hansson L, Lindholm LH, Niskanen L, et al: Effect of angiotensin-converting enzyme inhibition compared with conventional therapy on cardiovascular morbidity and mortality in hypertension: The Captopril Prevention Project (CAPP) randomized trail. Lancet 1999; 353:611–615.
156. Tatti P, Pahor M, Byington RP, et al: Outcome results of the Fosinopril versus Amlodipine cardiovascular events trial (FACET) in patients with hypertension and NIDDM. Diabetes Care 1998; 21:597–603.
157. Opie LH, Parving H: Diabetic nephropathy. Circulation 2002; 106:643.
158. Dickstein K, Kjeknus J: OPTIMAAL Steering Committee of the OPTIMAAL Study Group. Effects of losartan and captopril on mortality and morbidity in high-risk patients after acute myocardial infarction: The OPTIMAAL randomized trial. Lancet 2002; 360:752–760.
159. Defarrari G, Ravera M, Deferrari L, et al: Renal and cardiovascular protection in type 2 diabetes mellitus: Angiotensin II receptor blockers. J Am Soc Nephrol 2002; 13:S224–S229.
160. Williams ME: New therapies for advanced glycation end product nephrotoxicity: Current challenges. Am J Kidney Dis 2003; 41:S42–S47.
161. Forbes JM, Cooper ME, Oldfield MD, et al: Role of advanced glycation end products in diabetic nephropathy. J Am Soc Nephrol 2003; 14:S54–S258.

162. Raj DSC, Choudhury D, Welbourne TC, et al: Advanced glycation end-products: A nephrologist's perspective. Am J Kidney Dis 2000; 35:365–380.
163. Brownlee M: Biochemistry and molecular cell biology of diabetic complications. Nature 2001; 414:813–820.
164. Horie K: Immunohistochemical colocalization of glycoxidation products and lipid peroxidation products in diabetic renal glomerular lesions. Implication for glycoxidative stress in the pathogenesis of diabetic nephropathy. J Clin Invest 1997; 100: 2995–2999.
165. Yousef S, Nguyen DJ, Soulis T, et al: Effects of diabetes and aminoguanidine therapy in renal advanced glycation end-product binding. Kidney Int 1999; 55:907–916.
166. Degenhardt TP, Alderson NL, Arrington DD, et al: Pyridoxamine inhibits early renal disease and dyslipidemia in the streptozotocin-diabetic rat. Kidney Int 2000; 61:939–950.
167. Abdel-Rahman E, Bolton WK: Pimagedine: A novel therapy for diabetic nephropathy. Expert Opin Invest Drugs 2002; 11: 565–574.
168. Thornalley PJ: Use of aminoguanidine (pimagedine) to prevent the formation of advanced glycation endproducts. Arch Biochem Biophys 2003; 419:31–40.
169. Bolton KW, Cattran DC, Williams ME, et al: Randomized trial of an inhibitor of formation of advanced glycation end products in diabetic nephropathy. Am J Nephrol 2004; 24:32–40.
170. Alderson NL, Chachich ME, Yousef NN, et al: The ACE inhibitor pyridoxamine inhibits lipemia and development of renal and vascular disease in Zucker obese rats. Kidney Int 2003; 63:2123–2133.
171. Williams ME, Bolton WK, Degenhardt TP, et al: A phase 2 clinical trial of pyridoxamine (Pyridorin) in type 1 and type 2 diabetic patients with overt nephropathy (PYR-206). J Am Soc Nephrol 2004; 14:7A.
172. Vasan S, Foiles P, Founds H: Therapeutic potential of breakers of advanced glycation end product-protein crosslinks. Arch Biochem Biophys 2003; 419:89–96.
173. Kuroki T, Isshiki K, King GL: Oxidative stress: The lead or supporting actor in the pathogenesis of diabetic complications. J Am Soc Nephrol 2003; 14(8 suppl 3):S216–S220.
174. Way KJ, Katai N, King GL: Protein kinase C and the development of diabetic vascular complications. Diabetic Med 2001; 18(12):945–959.
175. Koya D, King GL: Protein kinase C activation and the development of diabetic complications. Diabetes 1998; 47(6): 859–866.
176. Kapor-Drezgic J, Zhou X, Babazono T, et al: Effect of high glucose on mesangial cell protein kinase C-delta and -epsilon is polyol pathway-dependent. J Am Soc Nephrol 1999; 10(6): 1193–1203.
177. Glogowski EA, Tsiani E, Zhou X, et al: High glucose alters the response of mesangial cell protein kinase C isoforms to endothelin-1. Kidney Int 1999; 55(2):486–499.
178. Koya D, Haneda M, Nakagawa H, et al: Amelioration of accelerated diabetic mesangial expansion by treatment with a PKC beta inhibitor in diabetic db/db mice, a rodent model for type 2 diabetes. FASEB J 2000; 14(3):439–447.
179. Ishii H, Jirousek MR, Koya D, et al: Amelioration of vascular dysfunctions in diabetic rats by an oral PKC beta inhibitor. Science 1996; 272(5262):728–731.
180. Tuttle KR, Anderson PW: A novel potential therapy for diabetic nephropathy and vascular complications: Protein kinase C beta inhibition (Review, 79 refs). Am J Kidney Dis 2003; 42(3): 456–465.
181. Koya D, Hayashi K, Kitada M, et al: Effects of antioxidants in diabetes-induced oxidative stress in the glomeruli of diabetic rats. J Am Soc Nephrol 2003; 14(8 suppl 3):S250–S253.
182. Morcos M, Borcea V, Isermann B, et al: Effect of alpha-lipoic acid on the progression of endothelial cell damage and albuminuria in patients with diabetes mellitus: An exploratory study. Diabetes Research & Clinical Practice. 2001; 52(3): 175–183.
183. Hirnerova E, Krahulec B, Strbova L, et al: Effect of vitamin E therapy on progression of diabetic nephropathy. Vnitrni Lekarstvi 2003; 49(7):529–534.
184. Brownlee M: Biochemistry and molecular cell biology of diabetic complications. Nature 2001; 414:813–820.
185. Ceriello A, Morocutti A, Mercuri F, et al: Defective intracellular antioxidant enzyme production in type 1 diabetic patients with nephropathy. Diabetes 2000; 49(12):2170–2177.
186. Zhang Z, Apse K, Pang J, Stanton RC: High glucose inhibits glucose 6-phosphate dehydrogenase via cAMP in aortic endothelial cells. J Biol Chem 2000; 275:40042–40047.
187. Hammes HP, Du X, Edelstein D, et al: Benfotiamine blocks three major pathways of hyperglycemic damage and prevents experimental diabetic retinopathy. Nature Medicine 2003; 9(3):294–299.
188. Ziyadeh FN, Sharma K, Ericksen M, Wolf G: Stimulation of collagen gene expression and protein synthesis in murine mesangial cells by high glucose is mediated by autocrine activation of transforming growth factor-beta. J Clin Invest 1994; 93:536–542.
189. Han DC, Hoffman BB, Hong SW, et al: Therapy with antisense TGF-Beta 1 oligodeoxynucleotides reduces kidney weight and matrix mRNAs in diabetic mice. Am J Physiol 2000; 278:F628–F634.
190. Ziyadeh FN, Hoffman BB, Han DC, et al: Long-term prevention of renal insufficiency, excess matrix gene expression, and glomerular mesangial matrix expansion by treatment with monoclonal antitransforming growth factor-beta antibody in db/db diabetic mice. Proc Natl Acad Sci U S A 2000; 97:8015–8020.
191. Raghu G, Johnson WC, Lockhart D, Mageto Y: Treatment of idiopathic pulmonary fibrosis with a new antifibrotic agent, pirfenidone: Results of a prospective, open-label phase II study. Am J Respir Crit Care Med 1999; 159(4 Pt 1): 1061–1069.
192. McGowan T, Dunn SR, Sharma K: Treatment of db/db mice with pirfenidone leads to improved histology and serum creatinine. J Am Soc Nephrol 2000; 11:A2814.
193. Fioretto P, Steffes MW, Sutherland DE, et al: Reversal of lesions of diabetic nephropathy after pancreas transplantation. N Engl J Med 1998; 339(2):69–75.

Nondiabetic Kidney Disease

James P. Lash, M.D. • Holly Kramer, M.D., M.P.H.

The term *nondiabetic kidney disease* encompasses a wide array of diseases, including glomerular diseases other than diabetes, vascular diseases other than renal artery disease, tubulointerstitial diseases, and cystic disease.[1] Grouping together such a diverse group of disorders has obvious limitations, and the use of the term "nondiabetic" is somewhat counterintuitive. However, the study of specific causes of kidney disease is limited by the relative rarity of individual diseases and makes it necessary to group together multiple etiologies of kidney disease. The term "nondiabetic kidney disease" is useful from the perspective of epidemiologic and clinical trials and in the clinical approach to patients with kidney disease. This chapter will review the epidemiology of nondiabetic kidney disease, screening strategies, risk factors for development and progression, clinical interventional trials, and treatment recommendations. This chapter will not focus on assessment of kidney function or treatment of cardiovascular disease (CVD), which are the topics of Chapters 3 and 5, respectively.

EPIDEMIOLOGY

In the United States we are facing an epidemic of kidney disease with the number of prevalent end-stage renal disease (ESRD) patients expected to double over the next decade.[2] This increase in the number of ESRD patients will have a substantial impact on health care systems, with costs projected to exceed 28 billion dollars annually.[2] The majority of end-stage kidney disease in the United States is attributable to nondiabetic kidney disease. From 1990 to 2000, nondiabetic kidney disease accounted for 98% of incident ESRD cases among individuals less than 20 years of age, 53% of individuals between 20 and 64 years of age, and 58% of those age 65 or older.[3] However, the percentage of kidney disease attributable to nondiabetic causes differs by race/ethnicity group (shown in Table 4–1). Among Native Americans and Hispanics, diabetic kidney disease accounts for greater than 60% of incident ESRD cases. Hypertension is the single most common cause of nondiabetic kidney disease in all race/ethnicity groups, accounting for approximately one third of all new ESRD cases among blacks in the United States and approximately one-fourth of new ESRD cases among whites and Asians.[3]

In 2002, the National Kidney Foundation (NKF) published the Kidney Disease Outcomes Quality Initiative (K/DOQI) Clinical Practice Guidelines for Chronic Kidney Disease (CKD).[4] These guidelines facilitate development of a clinical action plan to treat CKD. In these guidelines, CKD was defined as the presence of kidney damage or a glomerular filtration rate (GFR) less than 60 mL/min/1.73 m^2 body surface area for 3 months or greater. Kidney damage may be indicated by increased urine albumin excretion, histologic changes, or abnormalities in the urine sediment and/or imaging tests. CKD was divided into five stages depending on the estimated GFR (Table 4–2). The clinical action plan for stages I through III includes the treatment of comorbid conditions and interventions for the slowing of CKD progression. Preparation for renal replacement therapy should be initiated during stage IV, whereas stage V indicates need for renal replacement therapy once symptoms of uremia ensue.

Information on the epidemiology of CKD in the United States is mostly based on data from the Third National Health and Nutrition Examination Survey (NHANES III). This was a multistage complex probability sample of the total civilian noninstitutionalized population, 2 months of age or older, in the United States, which oversampled young children, older persons, non-Hispanic blacks, and Mexican-Americans. Data on health and nutrition, and blood and urine samples were collected from over 33,000 men, women, and children over a 6-year period (1988–1994). GFR was estimated from the serum creatinine using the modified Modification of Diet in Renal Disease (MDRD) GFR prediction formula,[5] and urine albumin excretion was assessed by measuring the albumin/creatinine ratios in the spot urine samples.

From these data, the number of U.S. adults with CKD was estimated to be 19 million, not including 0.3 million requiring renal replacement therapy, such as hemodialysis or kidney transplantation.[6] Among nondiabetic white and black U.S. adults, 13% have an estimated GFR less than 60 mL/min/1.73 m^2.[4] The prevalence of increased urine albumin excretion, defined as an albumin/creatinine ratio greater than 17 in men mg/g and greater than 25 mg/g in women among nondiabetic adults, ranges from 6.6% in 20- to 39-year-olds to 27.2% in adults age 70 years or greater.[4] Overall, approximately 3.9% of nondiabetic U.S. adults have CKD stages III to V (GFR < 60 mL/min/1.73 m^2), not including individuals requiring renal replacement therapy.[4] Information from NHANES III also suggests that a substantial proportion of type II diabetics with stages III to V CKD may not have diabetic nephropathy. Approximately one third of the estimated 1.1 million type II diabetics with GFR less than 60 mL/min/1.73 m^2 have no retinopathy, microalbuminuria, or macroalbuminuria.[7] In the absence of albuminuria and diabetic retinopathy, reduced GFR in these adults with type II diabetes is probably due to some other process such as aging, hypertension, or renal vascular disease. More studies are needed to confirm this hypothesis.

POPULATIONS AT RISK FOR NONDIABETIC CHRONIC KIDNEY DISEASE

Patients with systemic disorders associated with kidney disease, such as hypertension, autoimmune diseases, and recurrent kidney stones, are all at increased risk for CKD.[6]

Table 4–1 Percentage of Incident End-Stage Kidney Disease from 1990-2000 Due to Nondiabetic Kidney Disease by Race/Ethnicity

Nondiabetic Kidney Disease	Whites	Blacks	Asians	Native-Americans	Hispanics
Hypertension	24.0%	32.9%	23.5%	11.0%	16.5%
Glomerulonephritis/vasculitis	12.0%	10.4%	17.3%	10.4%	11.2%
Interstitial Nephritis	4.8%	2.0%	2.9%	1.8%	2.4%
Cystic disease/hereditary	3.8%	1.5%	2.2%	1.2%	2.5%
Cancers/tumors	2.4%	1.3%	0.8%	0.8%	1.0%
Miscellaneous	3.7%	4.7%	1.6%	1.7%	2.1%
Unknown	5.7%	5.1%	5.5%	3.9%	4.1%
Total	56.5%	57.95	53.8%	30.8%	39.8%

(Adapted from the U.S. Renal Data System, USRDS 2002 Annual Data Report: Atlas of End-Stage Renal Disease in the United States. Bethesda, MD, National Institutes of Health, National Institute of Diabetes and Digestive and Kidney Diseases, 2002.)

Table 4–2 Stages of Chronic Kidney Disease

Stage	Description	GFR (mL/min/1.73 m²)
1	Kidney damage with normal or ↑ GFR*	≥ 90
2	Kidney damage with mild ↓ GFR*	60–89
3	Moderate ↓ GFR	30–59
4	Severe ↓ GFR	15–29
5	Kidney failure	< 15 or dialysis

*Kidney damage defined as by increased urine albumin excretion (spot urine albumin/creatinine ratio > 17 in men and > 25 in women), abnormal urine sediment, imaging tests or histologic abnormalities. (Adapted from the National Kidney Foundation K/DOQI Clinical Practice Guidelines for Chronic Kidney Disease.)

Autoimmune disorders, such as systemic lupus erythematosus, are not uncommonly associated with glomerular diseases, which may go undetected unless the urine is screened for an abnormal sediment and proteinuria. Chronic infections, recurrent kidney stones, and abuse of anti-inflammatory drugs may all increase the risk of developing tubulointerstitial disease. Cystic diseases are usually associated with a strong family history but may occur spontaneously. Risk factors and clinical indicators for nondiabetic kidney disease are shown in Table 4–3.

Certain race/ethnicity groups and individuals with a family history of kidney disease are also considered to be at increased risk. Currently, over 1% of African-Americans have a serum creatinine greater than 2.0 mg/dL compared to only 0.3% of Caucasians.[8] In addition, the prevalence of increased urine albumin excretion is 30% higher among African-Americans and 20% higher among Mexican-Americans compared to whites after adjustment for blood pressure and presence of diabetes.[9] Other high-risk groups include American-Indians and Asians.[6] Because socioeconomic status, access to health care, and diet are all independent determinants of ESRD risk,[10,11] physicians should also consider screening patients with low income and education levels, especially if other susceptibility factors are present, such as hypertension or older age.

GENETICS OF NONDIABETIC KIDNEY DISEASE

Kidney disorders inherited in a Mendelian pattern are due to single-gene mutations and follow specific inheritance patterns (e.g., autosomal dominant, X-linked recessive, etc.). Approximately 8% of ESRD cases are attributed to Mendelian disorders, with polycystic kidney disease accounting for approximately half of these.[3] Examples of Mendelian kidney diseases and their associated genetic defects are shown in Table 4–4.

The majority of nondiabetic kidney diseases do not exhibit Mendelian inheritance patterns, but familial aggregation strongly suggests a polygenic effect. For example, the odds of having a first-degree relative with kidney failure was threefold higher among 612 patients with ESRD due to non-Mendelian kidney disease compared to the control group (patients' spouses).[12] Freedman and colleagues[13] examined family history data from 4365 dialysis patients, and 14% of Caucasian and 23% of African-American adults reported a first- or second-degree relative with ESRD. Family history of ESRD also varied by kidney disease etiology with 22% of patients with diabetes mellitus, 19% with hypertension, and 23% with glomerulonephritis reporting a family history of end-stage kidney disease.

The basis of racial differences implicating genetic etiology is more problematic due to lifestyle and environmental differences between populations. Marked race/ethnicity differences in kidney disease prevalence are most notable for hypertensive nephrosclerosis.[3] Although hypertension is more frequent in blacks compared to whites, the 20-fold higher risk of hypertensive kidney in these populations cannot be fully accounted by the increased prevalence of hypertension in this population. Although genetics potentially play a role, race/ethnicity differences in kidney disease prevalence could also be due to shared environmental exposures, such as socioeconomic status, access to health care and diet, which are all independent determinants of ESRD risk.[10,11,14] Most likely, non-Mendelian kidney diseases are influenced by multiple environmental factors and a varying number of genetic loci, which could interact with each other and with multiple environmental factors.

The human genome project has identified and catalogued over 1 million genetic variations such as variable number tandem repeats, insertion/deletion polymorphisms, and

Table 4–3 Risk Factors and Clinical Indicators of Nondiabetic Kidney Disease

Kidney Disease	Risk Factors	Clinical Indicators of Kidney Disease
Glomerular	Autoimmune diseases, systemic infections (e.g., endocarditis, visceral abscesses), drug exposures, cancers, family history of glomerular disease	Proteinuria (protein/creatinine ratio > 0.3 g/g or albumin/creatinine ratio > 30 mg/g), dysmorphic RBCs or RBC casts in urine
Vascular	Hypertension, family history of vascular diseases	Microalbuminuria
Tubulointerstitial	Infections, kidney stones, chronic obstruction, drugs (e.g., NSAIDS)	WBCs or WBC casts in urine, hydronephrosis
Cystic	Family history	Bilateral cysts

(Adapted from the National Kidney Foundation K/DOQI Clinical Practice Guidelines for Chronic Kidney Disease.)

Table 4–4 Examples of Mendelian Kidney Diseases and Associated Genetic Defects

Gene	Gene Product	Disease	Reference
NPHS2	Podocin	Autosomal recessive steroid resistant nephrotic syndrome	123
ACTN4	α-actinin-4	Autosomal dominant focal segmental glomerulosclerosis	124
NPHS1	Nephrin	Nephrotic syndrome of Finnish type	125
COL4A5	α-5 Chain Type IV Collagen	X-linked dominant Alport's syndrome	126
COL4A3	α-3 Chain Type IV Collagen	Autosomal dominant and autosomal recessive Alport's syndrome	127–130
GAL	α-Galactosidase A	X-linked Fabry's disease	131
PKD-1	Polycystin-1	Autosomal dominant polycystic kidney disease-1	132, 133
PKD-2	Polycystin-2	Autosomal dominant polycystic kidney disease-2	134, 135

single nucleotide polymorphisms, and over 600 studies have reported positive associations between a genetic variant and a common disease.[15] However, only 4% of 166 reported associations between a particular genetic variant and a common disease have been consistently replicated.[15] Some explanations for the lack of reproducibility are type I errors (significant findings due to chance alone), publication bias (negative findings are less likely to be published than positive findings), and population stratification (one subgroup has a higher frequency of disease and a particular genetic variant unrelated to disease compared to the other group leading to false a positive association).[15]

Such inconsistencies also apply to studies of genetic factors and kidney disease. For example, many studies have investigated the angiotensin converting enzyme (ACE) gene because ACE plays such an important role in renal physiologic processes and the development of kidney disease. The presence (insertion) or absence (deletion) of a 287 base pair Alu sequence [(I/D) polymorphism] within the ACE gene has been associated with both diabetic and nondiabetic kidney diseases in several studies, but almost every positive association has been countered by subsequent studies that failed to confirm the original findings.[16] Advances in molecular genetics show great promise in unraveling diseases with strong genetic effects, but it remains unclear how genetic epidemiology will impact the diagnosis and treatment of common polygenic disorders, including kidney disease.[17] Examples of potential candidate genes for risk of non-Mendelian kidney diseases are shown in Table 4–5.

SCREENING FOR NONDIABETIC KIDNEY DISEASE

Urinary Protein Excretion

Urine protein excretion in healthy men and women ranges from 30 to 200 mg/day. Tamm-Horsfall protein accounts for the majority of this protein, while approximately 10% to 30% is albumin, depending on the amount of protein excreted in the urine.[22] A positive dipstick test for proteinuria indicates urine protein excretion greater than 300 mg/L and should subsequently be quantified.

Previously, a timed urine collection has been considered the gold standard for quantifying protein excretion. However, due to diurnal variance in urinary protein excretion and difficulty in obtaining adequate and/or accurate timed urine collections, the NKF recommends the use of the protein/creatinine ratio measured in spot urine samples to quantitate urinary protein excretion.[4] If the GFR remains stable, then the excretion of creatinine will be fairly constant. Ginsberg and colleagues[23] compared spot urine protein/creatinine ratios to timed urine collections in 46 patients with kidney disease and stable kidney function and noted a high correlation ($(r = 0.97)$. Assuming that urinary protein excretion is constant, dividing the urine protein concentration by the urine creatinine concentration cancels out the time factor, and the calculated ratio reflects the cumulative protein excretion over a 24-hour period.[23] Because creatinine is a metabolic by-product of skeletal muscle creatine and phosphocreatine metabolism, its excretion is lower in subjects with lower muscle mass such as women or the elderly compared to individuals with higher muscle mass such as

Table 4–5 Potential Candidate Genes for Non-Mendelian Kidney Diseases

Gene	Gene Product Activities	References
Transforming growth factor-β (TGF-β1)	Modulates cellular growth, matrix degradation and production	136, 137
G Protein β-3 subunit (GBN3)	Mediate receptor-stimulated intracellular calcium mobilization	138–140
Endothelial nitric oxide synthase (NOS1)	Nitric oxide mediates vasorelaxation by activating soluble guanylate cyclase and suppresses vascular smooth muscle cell proliferation and platelet aggregation	141, 142
Aldosterone synthase (CYP11B2)	Catalyzes the production of aldosterone from its precursor	143–146
Endothelin-1 (EDN1)	Vasoconstrictor which also stimulates angiotensin II and aldosterone production	147–151
CD-2 associated protein (CD2AP)	Important for intracellular trafficking	152, 153

young men. Thus, protein/creatinine ratios may underestimate or overestimate protein excretion in individuals with high or low muscle mass, respectively.[23]

The spot urine protein/creatinine ratio is a simple test, which can be used to monitor protein excretion. As a general rule, a urine protein to creatinine ratio greater than 1000 mg/g indicates glomerular disease while nonglomerular disease such as tubulointerstitial and vascular diseases tend to have urine protein/creatinine ratios less than 1000 mg/g. Nevertheless, a protein/creatinine ratio greater than 200 mg/g warrants further evaluation.[1] However, determining level of albuminuria is a more sensitive screening tool for the presence of CKD.

Microalbuminuria

Albumin excretion rates greater than 30 mg/day (20–200 mcg/min) are considered abnormal, however, standard urine dipsticks cannot detect urinary albumin concentration less than 300 mg/L, leading to the term *microalbuminuria.* Microalbuminuria is a more sensitive marker of kidney disease than total protein excretion, thus, when "screening" adults for kidney disease, physicians should use either an albumin-specific dipstick to detect microalbuminuria or measure the albumin/creatinine ratio in a spot urine sample.[22]

According to the American Diabetes Association, the gold standard for measuring urine albumin excretion is a 24-hour urine collection.[24] However, a more convenient method to detect microalbuminuria is the albumin (mg)/creatinine (g) ratio (ACR) measured in a random urine specimen[4]; this may also actually be less prone to errors due to improper collection and variations in 24-hour protein excretion. Currently, the NKF recommends using a spot urine ACR obtained under standardized conditions (first voided, morning, mid-stream specimen) to detect microalbuminuria.[4] First void morning samples are recommended because upright posture,[25] exercise,[26,27] and smoking[28] may all increase urine albumin excretion.

The ACR threshold to define microalbuminuria remains controversial. The NKF K/DOQI Workgroup recommends an ACR cut-point greater or equal to 30 mg/g in both men and women.[6] Others advocate the use of sex-specific cut-points, which reflect sex differences in creatinine excretion to define microalbuminuria (≥17 mg/g in men and ≥25 mg/g in women).[9] The ACR values 17 to 250 mcg/mg in men and 25 to 355 mcg/mg in women corresponded to 30 to 300 mcg/min of urine albumin excretion measured in timed urine specimens, respectively, and were the 95th percentile ACR values among 218 nondiabetic healthy men and women, respectively.[29] Using a single ACR threshold to define microalbuminuria may thus underestimate microalbuminuria in subjects with higher muscle mass (men) and possibly in certain race/ethnicity groups.[9]

Increased urine albumin excretion should be confirmed in a subsequent urine sample within 3 months. The NHANES III repeated spot urine collections in a subsample of 1241 participants, including diabetics. Among those with microalbuminuria in the first urine specimen, only 63% had increased urine albumin excretion in the second urine specimen.[30] However, all individuals with macroalbuminuria (ACR > 250 mg/g in men and > 355 mg/g in women) in the first urine sample had increased urine albumin excretion in the second urine sample.[30] A positive and persistent urine albumin dipstick or increased albumin/creatinine ratio on at least two occasions over a 3-month period indicates the presence of CKD.[1]

Microalbuminuria and the Risk of Progression of Nondiabetic Kidney Disease

The presence of increased urine albumin excretion has been hypothesized to reflect increased glomerular pressure,[31,32] which could predict a faster rate of GFR decline over time.[33,34] A cross-sectional study of 7728 nondiabetic subjects noted an independent association between increased GFR and microalbuminuria, while overt proteinuria (> 300 mg/24 hr) was associated with a higher odds of decreased GFR compared to subjects without increased urine albumin excretion (< 15 mg/24 hours).[35] However, data from cross-sectional studies cannot determine the temporal relationship between changes in urine albumin excretion and GFR. One retrospective study of 141 hypertensives without end-organ damage reported that GFR loss was significantly higher in subjects with microalbuminuria compared to those without microalbuminuria with similar baseline GFR, after 7 years of follow-up (−12.1 ± 2.77 versus −7.1 ± 0.88 mL/min, $P < .05$).[36] However, the small number of subjects, and the different antihypertensive regimens in the subjects, with and without microalbuminuria, limits the interpretability of these results.

Among men and women with a history of cardiovascular disease enrolled in the Heart Outcomes and Prevention Evaluation (HOPE) study, nondiabetic subjects with baseline microalbuminuria were 19-fold more likely to develop overt proteinuria compared to nondiabetics without baseline microalbuminuria, after a median follow-up of 4.5 years (6.6% vs. 0.34%; $P < .001$),[37] an association which persisted after adjustment for age, sex, smoking, hypertension, increased cholesterol, obesity, and increased serum creatinine levels. Whether these findings would apply to nondiabetic populations without established vascular disease is not certain.

Microalbuminuria and the Risk of Cardiovascular Disease

Microalbuminuria is not only a marker of CKD, but it also serves to identify individuals who are at high risk for cardiovascular events. Increased urine albumin is associated with an increased risk for development of both macrovascular (coronary and peripheral arteries)[38–40] and microvascular (retina and glomeruli) disease.[41–44] Multiple cross-sectional studies have demonstrated an independent relationship between microalbuminuria and several cardiovascular risk factors, including cholesterol,[45] insulin resistance,[46] C-reactive protein,[47] and hypertension.[48,49] Individuals with microalbuminuria are also more likely to have subclinical cardiovascular disease such as increased thickness of the intima and media layers of the carotid artery[50] and increased left ventricular mass.[51,52] Aside from reflecting the presence of cardiovascular risk factors, microalbuminuria may be a more important independent predictor of future cardiovascular events than cholesterol or hypertension.[53–55] Among the nondiabetic HOPE study participants, the adjusted relative risk of a major cardiovascular event (myocardial infarction, stroke, or cardiovascular death) was 61% higher in subjects with microalbuminuria compared to those without microalbuminuria (95% Confidence Interval [CI] 1.36-1.90).[54] All-cause mortality was also increased in nondiabetic individuals with microalbuminuria (Relative Risk 2.00; 95% CI 1.65-2.41).[54] The association between microalbuminuria and increased risk of cardiovascular mortality has also been demonstrated in the general U.S. population[53] and in healthy adults living in Norway.[56]

Pathophysiologic Implications of Microalbuminuria

It has been hypothesized that increased urine albumin excretion reflects the presence of widespread vascular disease and endothelial dysfunction,[57] but data supporting this theory are somewhat limited. Endothelial damage leads to the release of von Willebrand factor (vWF), which is synthesized and stored in endothelial cells.[58] A few studies have noted an association between serum vWF levels and increased urine albumin excretion, but the results have been mixed.[59–61] In a small study of 64 healthy nondiabetics between the ages of 40 to 65 without microalbuminuria, increased levels of vWF at baseline (≥ 1.12 units/mL) were associated with significantly higher increases in urine albumin excretion after 4 years.[59] These findings, however, were not confirmed in subsequent larger cohort studies.[60,61]

Other indicators of endothelial function include cellular adhesion molecules such as intercellular adhesion molecule 1 (ICAM-1) and endothelial selectin (E-selectin). These proteins are synthesized and expressed by activated endothelial cells and mediate the adhesion and transendothelial migration of leukocytes.[62] Information with respect to the association between ICAM-1 and E-selectin and urine albumin excretion is currently limited. Among 191 type II diabetics followed for a mean of 9 years, baseline values of E-selectin greater than 79 mcg/L were associated with a twofold higher risk of developing microalbuminuria compared to levels less than 58 mcg/L (95% CI 1.24-3.32) after adjustment for demographic values and prior cardiovascular disease.[63] This study also noted that baseline C-reactive protein levels independently predicted the development of microalbuminuria. These results were similar to a study by Jager and colleagues,[60] where a 50% increase in baseline C-reactive protein levels increased the risk of developing microalbuminuria by 16% (95% CI 1.03-1.30) in both diabetic and nondiabetic subjects.[60]

Importance of Microalbuminuria Screening in Nondiabetics

The Seventh Report of the Joint National Committee (JNC 7) on Prevention, Detection, Evaluation, and Treatment of High Blood Pressure recommends checking a urinalysis and estimating GFR in all hypertensive patients prior to the initiation of therapy, but measurement of urine albumin excretion is considered optional.[64] However, without routine surveillance of urine albumin excretion, some hypertensive patients may not be adequately treated according to JNC VII guidelines, which recommend a BP goal less than 130/80 mmHg in the presence of CKD.

Several large trials have suggested that interventions in nondiabetic patients with microalbuminuria may improve clinical outcomes. Among the nondiabetic HOPE Study participants, treatment with ramipril decreased risk of cardiovascular events (myocardial infarction, stroke, or cardiovascular death) associated with presence of microalbuminuria by 50%.[54] Ramipril also decreased the risk for all-cause mortality in patients with microalbuminuria. The Losartan Intervention for Endpoint reduction (LIFE) Study, a randomized trial of losartan versus atenolol in nondiabetic patients with essential hypertension, measured the urine albumin/creatinine ratio and left ventricular hypertrophy by echocardiography at baseline and after 1 year of antihypertensive treatment. Left ventricular hypertrophy regressed with antihypertensive treatment, and echocardiographic changes were significantly associated with decreases of the urine albumin/creatinine ratio after controlling for changes in systolic blood pressure.[52]

Neither of these studies showed that the identification of microalbuminuria would change the overall clinical management of these patients, and some physicians doubt that routine testing of microalbuminuria will improve clinical outcomes in a general population.[65] However, the presence of microalbuminuria may indicate the presence of risk factors not routinely measured in primary care settings such as insulin resistance or left ventricular hypertrophy. Due to the important implications of persistent microalbuminuria, physicians may be more aggressive in treating patients with microalbuminuria. Finally, testing for microalbuminuria is not time-consuming, costly, or difficult for patients or physicians, and may provide valuable information on both kidney disease and cardiovascular risk.

OTHER STUDIES FOR ASSESSMENT OF NONDIABETIC KIDNEY DISEASE

Glomerular Filtration Rate (GFR)

The clearance of markers such as inulin and ^{125}I-iothalamate have been considered the gold standard for measuring GFR because they are not secreted or reabsorbed after being filtered by the kidney. However, administering these exogenous markers is very time-consuming and expensive and not practical for most clinical settings. In 1976 Cockroft and Gault developed a formula to estimate creatinine clearance, which incorporates age and body weight in order to account for age and sex differences in muscle mass.[18]

$$\frac{(140\text{-age in years}) \times (\text{body weight in kilograms}) \times (0.85 \text{ if female})}{\text{serum creatinine (mg/dL)} \times 72}$$

The Cockroft-Gault equation predicts creatinine clearance, which includes tubular excretion and intestinal catabolism in addition to GFR. Thus, creatinine clearance may overestimate GFR by as much as 16% to 25%.[19] Levey and colleagues[5] developed a newer prediction equation using demographic and laboratory data collected from subjects enrolled in the Modification of Diet in Renal Disease (MDRD) Study. The variables that jointly predicted GFR measured by the clearance of ^{125}I-iothalamate in a training sample (1070 randomly selected subjects) were determined using stepwise regression. These equations were then validated in the remaining 558 subjects.

$$\text{GFR} = 186 \times [\text{Plasma Creatinine}]^{-1.154} \times [\text{Age}]^{-0.203} \times [0.742 \text{ if female}] \times [1.210 \text{ if black}]$$

This prediction equation is easily implemented and does not require a timed urine collection, but the validity of this equation has yet to be tested in a group of patients with normal kidney function. A more detailed discussion of kidney function testing is provided in Chapter 2.

Urine Sediment

Urine sediments should be examined in all patients with CKD and in patients who are at high risk of developing kidney disease.[6] Ideally, the urine should be a first void morning specimen, because formed elements will more likely be seen in highly concentrated urine with a low urine pH. When examining the urine sediment, clinicians should carefully look for cellular elements such as red blood cells (RBCs), white blood cells (WBCs), or casts. Casts, formed in the renal tubules, are comprised of Tamm-Horsfall protein[20] and may also contain cells (RBCs, WBCs, renal tubule cells), cellular debris, crystals, and fat. These cellular elements may not be diagnostic of a specific disease process but may help narrow the diagnosis and determine the need for further work-up such as a kidney biopsy. Microscopic hematuria should be verified in subsequent urine samples in order to rule out transient hematuria due to exercise, menstruation, or trauma to the urethra from sexual activity.[21] If the RBCs appear dysmorphic, especially in the presence of decreased GFR and/or spot urine protein/creatinine ratio greater than 0.3, further evaluation, such as kidney biopsy may be warranted. Dysmorphic RBCs may originate from the glomeruli while RBCs of normal morphology, especially in the absence of proteinuria, may be shed from the lower urinary tract. The presence of RBC casts indicates a glomerular disease process such as IgA nephropathy, vasculitis, or anti-GBM disease. In contrast, the presence of dysmorphic RBCs by itself does not definitively rule in a glomerular lesion. For more information on urine sediment findings and associated kidney diseases, see Table 4–6.

Imaging Studies

Imaging studies are frequently used in the work-up of kidney disease, and these tests can provide valuable information for the physician evaluating a patient with CKD (Table 4–7). Ultrasound of the kidneys is inexpensive and easily performed with little discomfort to the patient and may reveal obstruction, asymmetry in size, increased echogenicity, or abnormalities in kidney size. Ultrasound may also provide a definitive diagnosis, such as multiple bilateral cysts in a patient with a family history of polycystic kidney disease, or bilateral hydronephrosis in a patient with known prostatic hypertrophy. In addition, the kidney ultrasound may determine whether further work-up is necessary. For example, if a patient presents with severely decreased GFR and is found to have small, scarred kidneys bilaterally, the physician may opt to not pursue further work-up because the disease is chronic and irreversible.

HYPERTENSION IN NONDIABETIC KIDNEY DISEASE

Hypertension Prevalence and Role as Risk Factor for Progression

The prevalence of hypertension (HTN) in nondiabetic kidney disease has been found to be high in clinical trials. The prevalence was 92% in the Angiotensin-Converting Enzyme-Inhibition in Progressive Renal Insufficiency (AIPRI) Study and 84%[66] in the Ramipril Efficacy in Nephropathy (REIN) Study.[67,68] Table 4–8 details the prevalence of HTN in the MDRD Study for types of nondiabetic kidney disease.[69] Observational studies and clinical trials have established that there is a strong relationship between uncontrolled HTN and risk for progressive kidney failure.[70–72] Furthermore, systolic blood pressure has been found to have a larger impact on the progression of kidney disease than diastolic blood pressure.[73–76] Despite the well established importance of HTN, there is ample evidence that HTN remains poorly controlled in this population.[4]

Clinical Interventional Studies

Table 4–9 provides an overview of the major trials conducted in patients with nondiabetic kidney disease. We will review in detail three of the largest studies and two important meta-analyses.

Angiotensin-Converting Enzyme-Inhibition in Progressive Renal Insufficiency (AIPRI)

The Angiotensin-Converting Enzyme-Inhibition in Progressive Renal Insufficiency (AIPRI) Study included 583 participants

Table 4–6 Urine Sediment

Finding	Normal	Pathologic	References
Cells			
RBCs	Up to 2-3/HPF; Transient microscopic hematuria may be noted with vigorous exercise	Dysmorphic RBCs may indicate glomerular disease, whereas RBCs with normal morphology may indicate a lower urinary tract lesion	21, 154, 155
WBCs	Up to 2-3/HPF	Infection or inflammation, pyelonephritis, interstitial nephritis	156, 157
Renal tubule		Large numbers indicate tubular damage	158–162
Transitional		Large numbers may indicate inflammation of bladder or ureters or be seen after bladder instrumentation	163, 164
Epithelial	Indicates contamination of urine		
Casts			
RBC	*	Indicates glomerular disease but may also be seen with renal infarction or pyelonephritis	21, 164, 165
WBC	*	Interstitial nephritis, pyelonephritis, renal infarction, glomerulonephritis	165
Waxy		Broad waxy casts may indicate advanced disease†	165
Granular casts	Small numbers may be seen with strenuous exercise	Large numbers, especially coarse brown (muddy) casts, suggestive of acute tubular necrosis	166–168
Hyaline	Exercise, dehydration, diuretic use, fever	Large wide hyaline casts may indicate advanced kidney disease†	166–169

*Always pathologic.
†Does not indicate a specific kidney disease.

Table 4–7 Abnormal Findings on Imaging Studies in Nondiabetic Kidney Disease

Imaging Study	Possible Diseases
Ultrasound	
Hydronephrosis	Obstruction
Asymmetry in size	Renal artery stenosis, unilateral obstruction
Scarring	Tubulointerstitial disease due to stones or infection
Small kidneys	Chronic kidney disease*
Large kidneys	Infiltrative disorders, tumors, HIV nephropathy, amyloidosis, growth hormone tumor
Increased echogenicity	Glomerular disease, tubulointerstitial diseases, cystic disease
CT scan without contrast	
Collecting system dilation	Ureteral or bladder outlet obstruction
Calculi	Kidney stone disease
CT scan with contrast	Kidney tumors, cysts
Helical CT scan with contrast	Renal artery stenosis
Magnetic resonance imaging	Tumors, renal vein thrombosis, cysts
Magnetic resonance angiography	Renal artery stenosis

*Does not indicate a specific kidney disease.
(Adapted from the National Kidney Foundation K/DOQI Clinical Practice Guidelines for Chronic Kidney Disease.)

with a variety of nondiabetic kidney diseases (glomerular disease, 33%; tubulointerstitial, 18%; hypertensive nephrosclerosis, 16%; diabetic nephropathy, 3%).[66] Participants were randomized to benazepril or placebo. The primary outcome was doubling of the serum creatinine or ESRD. After 3 years, the risk in the benazepril group for reaching the primary end point was 53%. The risk reduction was greatest for those with a glomerular disease and for those with a baseline protein excretion greater than 1 g/day.

Ramipril Efficacy in Nephropathy (REIN) Study

The Ramipril Efficacy in Nephropathy (REIN) Study included 352 patients with chronic nondiabetic nephropathies who

Table 4–8 Prevalence of HTN by Type of Nondiabetic Kidney Disease in MDRD Study

Type of Kidney Disease	Prevalence (%)
Glomerular diseases	85%
Vascular diseases	100%
Tubulointerstitial diseases	62%
PKD	87%

(Modified with permission from National Kidney Foundation. K/DOQI Clinical Practice Guidelines for Chronic Kidney Disease: Blood pressure management and use of antihypertensive agents in chronic kidney disease. Am J Kidney Dis 2004; 43:S1–S290.)

were randomized to receive ramipril or placebo. Prior to randomization, patients were stratified by level of proteinuria (stratum 1: proteinuria > 1 g/day and < 3 g/day; stratum 2: ≥ 3 g/day).[67,77] The primary end points were changed in iohexol measured GFR and time to ESRD. In stratum 2, the trial was terminated early because the ramipril group had a slower decline in GFR, a greater decrement in proteinuria, and improved renal survival as measured by the composite outcome of doubling of serum creatinine or ESRD (Figure 4–1). In stratum 1, the decline in GFR did not differ significantly between the ramipril and placebo groups. The relative risk for ESRD was 2.72 for the placebo group compared to the ramipril group. Baseline urinary protein excretion of greater than 1.5 gm was associated with a faster rate of GFR decline and for this subgroup, ramipril was associated with a slower decline in GFR (0.31 mL/min/month versus 0.40 mL/min/month) and decreased development of ESRD (18% vs. 52%).

African-American Study of Kidney Disease and Hypertension (AASK)

The African-American Study of Kidney Disease and Hypertension (AASK) was a randomized trial in patients with hypertensive nephrosclerosis.[78] In this trial, 1094 African-American participants were randomly assigned to a usual blood pressure goal or to a lower pressure goal and to initial treatment with one of three drugs (an ACE inhibitor, ramipril; a β-blocker, metoprolol; or a nondihydropyridine calcium channel blocker, amlodipine). The usual blood pressure goal was a mean arterial pressure (MAP) of 102 to 107 mmHg (corresponding to a BP of less than 140/90 mmHg) and the low blood pressure goal was a MAP of less than 92 mmHg (corresponding to a BP of less than 125/75 mmHg). The main outcome measures were rate of change in GFR slope and a composite outcome of reduction in GFR of 50% or more, ESRD, or death. The amlodipine arm was terminated early because an interim analysis found ramipril to be more beneficial than amlodipine.[79] There was no benefit in terms of slowing progression with lower BP (Figure 4–2*A*). However, a trend was seen favoring the lower blood pressure target in individuals with higher baseline proteinuria levels and an opposite trend in participants with little or no proteinuria. In the final analysis, there was no difference in GFR slope between the drug groups (Figure 4–2*B*). However, the ramipril group had a risk reduction in the clinical composite outcome of 22% compared to metoprolol and 38% compared to amlodipine (Table 4–10).

Meta-Analyses

The ACE Inhibition in Progressive Renal Disease (AIPRD) Study Group performed a patient-level meta-analysis of 1860 subjects with nondiabetic kidney disease enrolled in 11 randomized trials of ACE inhibitors to slow progression of kidney disease.[80] In these pooled studies, the mean duration of follow-up was 2.2 years. Individuals treated with ACE inhibitors had a greater decrease in systolic and diastolic blood pressure (Figure 4–3*A*). After adjusting for baseline characteristics and longitudinal changes in systolic blood pressure, ACE inhibitors were more effective in reducing proteinuria, reducing the risk for end-stage renal disease (relative risk, RR of 0.69) and in reducing the risk for the composite outcome of doubling of serum creatinine or ESRD (RR 0.70) (Figures 4–3*B*, *C*, and *D*).

In another analysis of the same database, this group of investigators also examined the relationship of levels of blood pressure and urine protein excretion with the progression of kidney disease.[76] These analyses demonstrated a strong, graded relationship between higher levels of systolic BP and urine protein excretion and the risk for kidney disease

Table 4–9 Summary of Clinical Interventional Trials of Nondiabetic Kidney Disease

Study or Author	N	Baseline GFR (mL/min/1.73 m^2) or Serum Creatinine	Baseline Proteinuria (mg/24 hr)	Intervention	Kidney Disease Progression	Methodologic Quality
ACE-versus placebo						
AIPRI	583	2.1 mg/dL	1800 mg	Benazepril	*	A
REIN	186	49 mL/min	1700 mg	Ramipril	*	B
REIN	166	40 mL/min	5600 mg	Ramipril	*	B
ACE versus other agents						
Hannedouche	100	2.9 mg/dL	No data	Enalapril	*	B
Chinotti	131	36 mL/min	506 mg	Lisinopril	*	A
AASK	1094	45 mL/min	600 mg	Ramipril	*	A
van Essen	103	51 mL/min	2500 mg	Enalapril	NS	A

*coding connotes that intervention fared better than comparison group.
NS, no statistical difference detected. (Modified with permission from National Kidney Foundation. K/DOQI Clinical Practice Guidelines for Chronic Kidney Disease: Blood pressure management and use of antihypertensive agents in chronic kidney disease. Am J Kidney Dis 2004; 43:S1–S290.)

Figure 4–1 Kidney Survival in Stratum 2 of the REIN Study S. (Used with permission from Randomized placebo-controlled trial of effect of ramipril on decline in glomerular filtration rate and risk of terminal renal failure in proteinuric, nondiabetic nephropathy. The GISEN Group [Gruppo Italiano di Studi Epidemiologici in Nefrologia]. Lancet 1997; 349[9069]:1857-1863.)

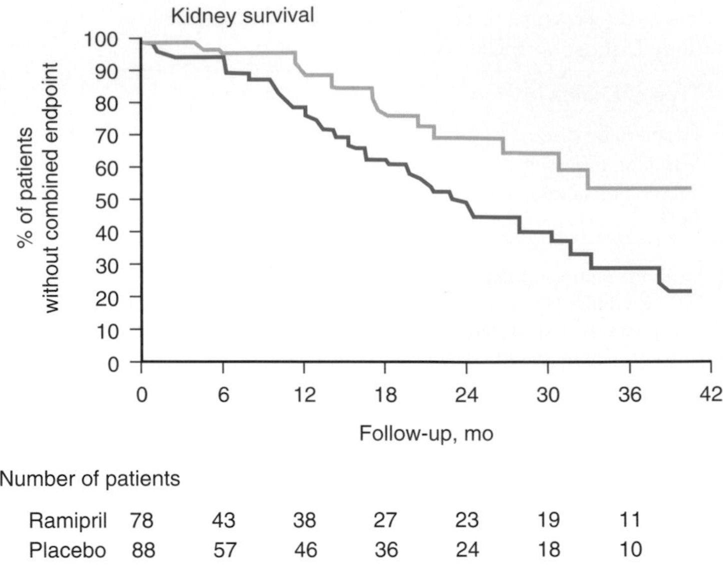

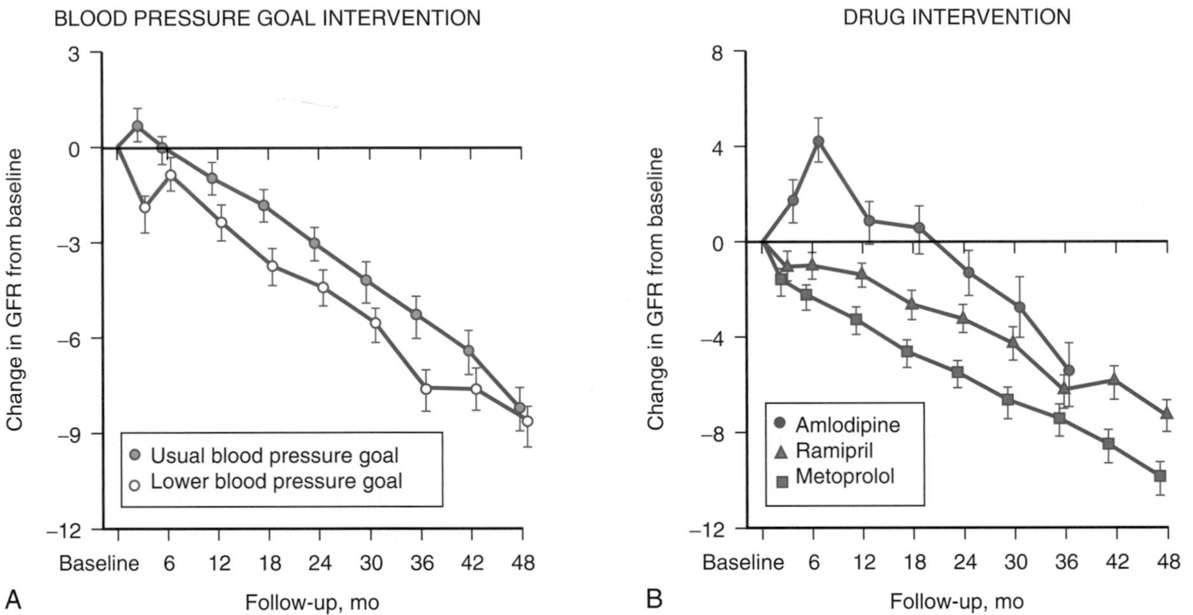

Figure 4–2 Mean change in glomerular filtration rate by randomized group in the AASK trial. ***A*** depicts BP goal intervention, and ***B*** depicts drug intervention. (Used with permission from Wright JT Jr, Bakris G, Greene T, et al: Effect of blood pressure lowering and antihypertensive drug class on progression of hypertensive kidney disease: Results from the AASK trial. JAMA 2002; 288[19]:2421-2431.)

progression. After adjusting for the level systolic blood pressure, diastolic blood pressure level was not found to be a risk factor for the progression of kidney disease. The lowest risk for kidney disease progression was seen in patients with a systolic BP of 110 to 129 and urine protein excretion of less than 2.0 g/day. Moreover, the relationship between the systolic BP and the risk for kidney disease progression was influenced by the level of proteinuria (Figure 4–4). In patients with more than 1.0 g/day of proteinuria, the risk for kidney disease progression increased significantly when systolic blood pressure was greater than 120 to 130 mmHg. However, in patients with less than 1.0 g/day of proteinuria, the risk for kidney disease progression was relatively constant over a range of systolic blood pressures between 110 to 159 mmHg. The study group also found that a systolic blood pressure of less than 110 was associated with a nearly fivefold increased risk of kidney disease progression among individuals with more than 1.0 g/day of proteinuria. In interpreting these results, it is important to recognize that the analyzed clinical trials were not primarily designed to evaluate the effect of lowering blood pressure and urinary protein excretion. In addition, the confidence intervals for the risk of kidney disease progression were wide. Nonetheless, the authors argue that the findings are strongly statistically significant and corroborate the results of other studies. As discussed in the accompanying editorial, the findings regarding the increased risk of lower levels of blood pressure need to be viewed with caution.[81] It is unclear whether this was the result of renal hypoperfusion or related to

Table 4–10 Analysis of Clinical Event Composite Outcomes in the AASK Trial

			Drug Intervention					
	Lower vs. Usual Blood Pressure Goal Intervention		Ramipril vs. Metoprolol		Metoprolol vs. Amlodipine		Ramipril vs. Amlodipine	
Outcomes	**% Risk Reduction (95% Confidence Interval)**	***P* Value**	**% Risk Reduction (95% Confidence Interval)**	***P* Value**	**% Risk Reduction (95% Confidence Interval)**	***P* Value**	**% Risk Reduction (95% Confidence Interval)**	***P* Value**
GFR event, ESRD, or death	2 (−22 to 21)	.85	22 (1 to 38)	.04	20 (−10 to 41)	.17	38 (14 to 56)	.004
GFR event or ESRD	−2 (−31 to 20)	.87	22 (−2 to 41)	.07	24 (−9 to 47)	.13	40 (14 to 59)	.006
ESRD or death	12 (−13 to 32)	.31	21 (−5 to 40)	.11	42 (17 to 60)	.003	49 (26 to 65)	<.001
ESRD alone	6 (−29 to 31)	.72	22 (−10 to 45)	.16	59 (36 to 74)	<.001	59 (36 to 74)	<.001

GFR, glomerular filtration rate; *ESRD*, end-stage renal disease. All risk reductions adjusted for prespecified covariates: baseline proteinuria, mean arterial pressure, sex, history of heart disease, and age. Risk difference for ESRD or death composite and ESRD alone also adjusted for baseline GFR. GFR event, ESRD, or death: main secondary composite clinical outcome with 340 events, including 179 declining GFR events and 84 additional participants with ESRD events; ESRD or death: composite end point with 251 events, including 171 ESRD events and 80 deaths; and ESRD alone: end point with 171 events and deaths censored in this analysis.

(Used with permission from Wright JT Jr, Bakris G, Greene T, et al: Effect of blood pressure lowering and antihypertensive drug class on progression of hypertensive kidney disease: Results from the AASK trial. JAMA 2002; 288[19]:2421-2431.)

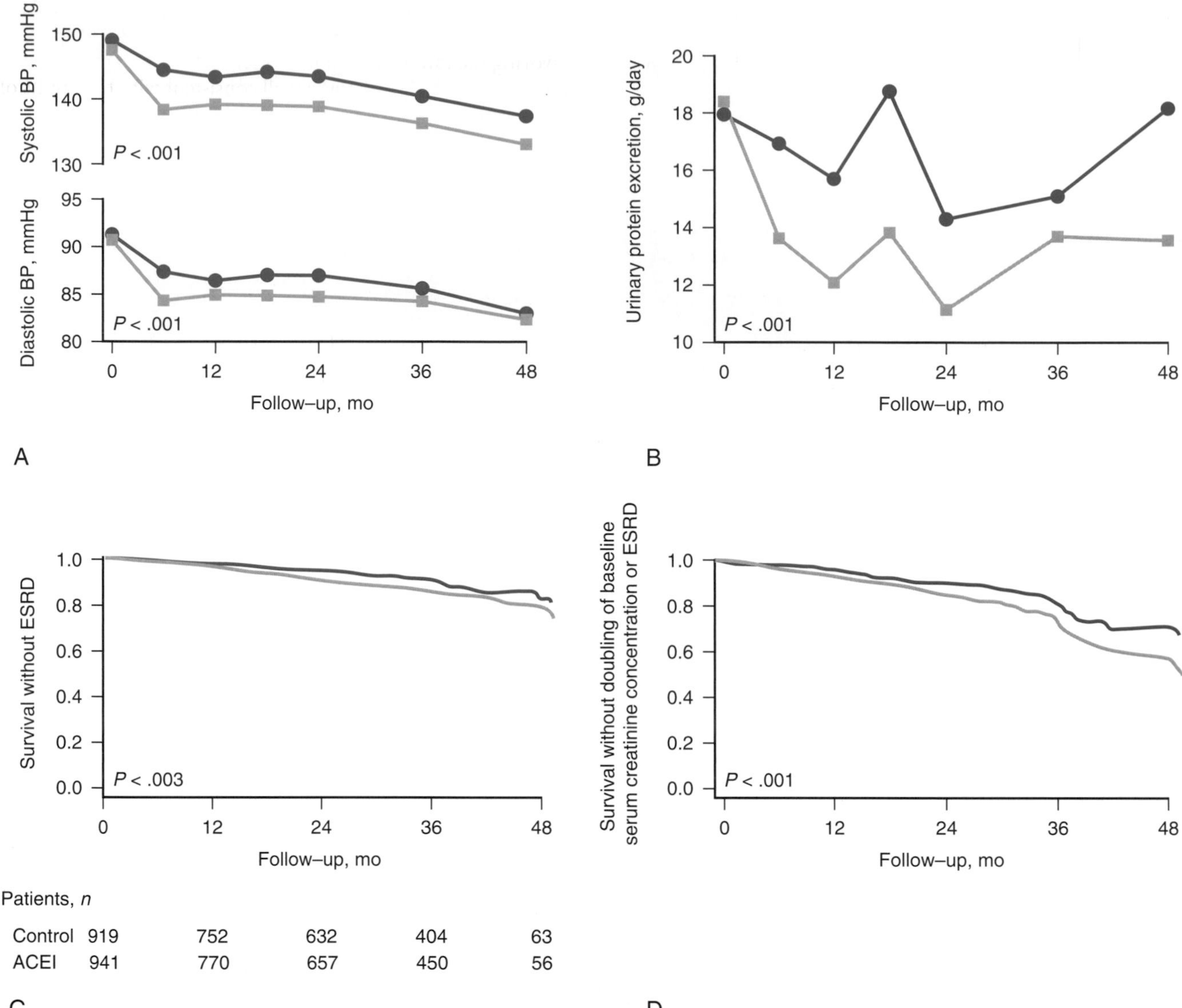

Figure 4–3 Blood pressure ***(A)***, urinary protein excretion ***(B)***, survival without end-stage renal disease (ESRD) ***(C)***, or the combined outcome of doubling baseline serum creatinine concentration or ESRD ***(D)*** during follow-up among patients taking ACEI (*dotted line*) and controls (*solid line*). (Used with permission from Jafar TH, Schmid CH, Landa M, et al: Angiotensin-converting enzyme inhibitors and progression of nondiabetic renal disease. A meta-analysis of patient-level data. Ann Intern Med 2001; 135[2]:73-87.)

independent factors, such as poor underlying health in the individuals with lower blood pressure.

Blood Pressure Goal

The Seventh Report of the Joint National Committee on Prevention, Detection, Evaluation, and Treatment of High Blood Pressure recommends a target blood pressure goal of less than 140/90 mmHg or less than 130/80 mmHg for patients with chronic kidney disease.[82] This blood pressure goal corresponds to the achieved systolic blood pressure in many of the clinical studies reviewed in Table 4–9, which provide strong evidence that this goal is beneficial for both CVD risk reduction and for slowing the progression of kidney disease. This blood pressure goal has been recommended by the K/DOQI Work Group on Blood Pressure Management and other published guidelines.[83] Two large clinical trials have examined the impact of a lower blood pressure goal on the progression of nondiabetic kidney disease. In the Modification of Diet in Renal Disease (MDRD) Study and the AASK trial, patients were randomized to a mean arterial pressure (MAP) goal of less than 92 mmHg (equivalent to a blood pressure less than 125/75 mmHg) or to a MAP goal of less than 107 mmHg (equivalent to a blood pressure less than 140/90 mmHg). The MDRD Study included predominantly nondiabetic kidney disease of various causes, and participants had a mean baseline proteinuria of 2.2 g/day.[84] By post hoc analysis, a beneficial effect of the lower BP goal was observed in patients with higher rates of urinary protein excretion (Figure 4–5). In the AASK Study, participants had a mean baseline proteinuria of about 0.6 g/day. As dis-

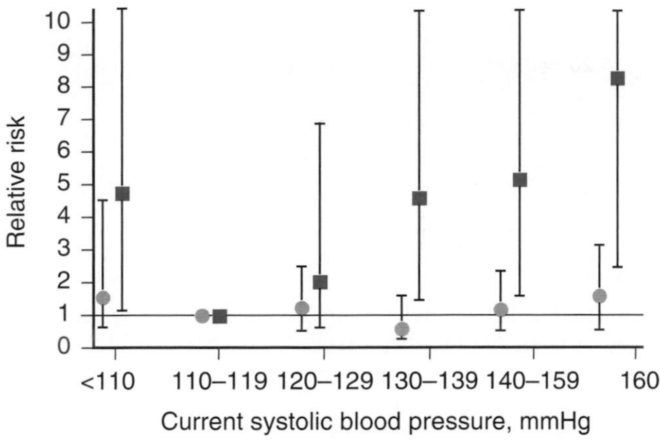

Figure 4–4 Meta-analysis: Relative risk for kidney disease progression based on current level of systolic blood pressure and current urine protein excretion. (Used with permission from Jafar T, Stark P, Schmid CH, et al: Progression of chronic kidney disease: The role of blood pressure control, proteinuria, and angiotensin-converting enzyme inhibition. A patient-level meta-analysis. Ann Intern Med 2003; 139[4]:244-252.)

cussed earlier, there was no significant beneficial effect of the lower BP goal (Figure 4–2).[78] Nonetheless, a trend was detected favoring the lower BP goal in participants with higher baseline proteinuria. These findings are all consistent with the results of the meta-analysis by Jafar and colleagues.[76]

Choice of Antihypertensive Agent

ACE Inhibitors

As summarized earlier, a number of large scale studies have demonstrated that ACE inhibitors reduce kidney end points in nondiabetic kidney disease. In the first meta-analysis by Jafar and colleagues,[80] the relative risk for kidney disease progression associated with ACE inhibitors was 0.67. Moreover, the beneficial effect was greater in patients with higher levels of proteinuria. Conversely, the strength of evidence favoring the use of ACE inhibitors was weaker for subclasses of nondiabetic kidney disease characterized by low levels of proteinuria (polycystic kidney disease and tubulointerstitial disease).

Number of Agents Required and Diuretics

Most patients with nondiabetic CKD will require multiple antihypertensive agents to achieve blood pressure control. In several large trials, at least two to three antihypertensive agents were required to achieve blood pressure control (Table 4–11).

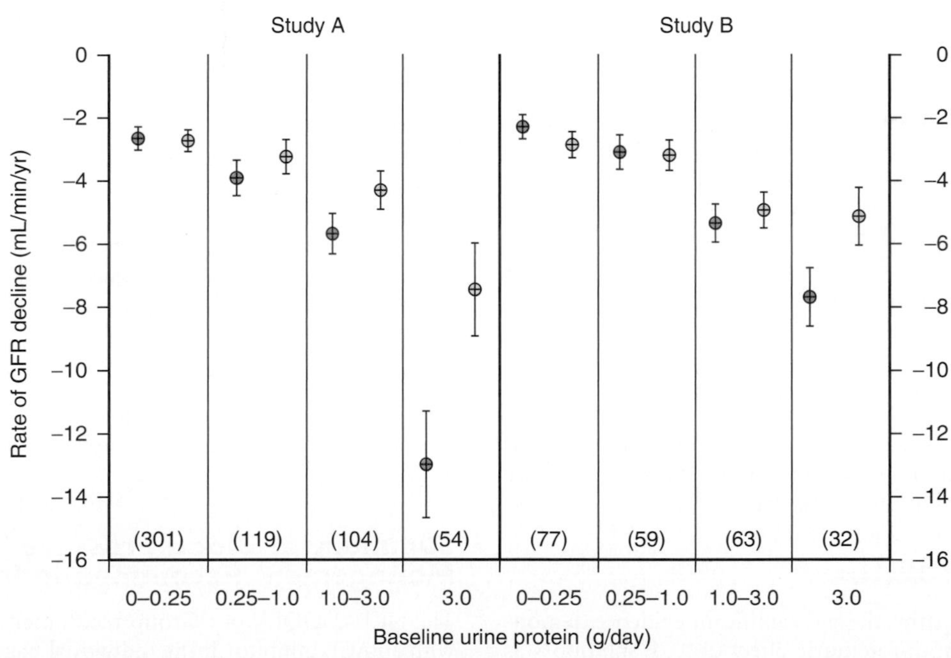

Figure 4–5 MDRD study: Effect of strict blood pressure control by baseline proteinuria. For Study A (baseline GFR 25-55 ml/min/1.73 m^2), estimated mean (±SE) rates of decline in GFR from baseline to 3 years, based on a 2-slope model are shown. For Study B (baseline GFR 13-24 ml/min/1.73 m^2), mean (±SE) rates of decline in GFR are estimated from the 1-slope informative censoring model. Closed circles designate the usual blood pressure group; open circles designate the low blood pressure group. The number in parentheses in each column is the total number of patients in both blood pressure groups who had a least one follow-up measurement. Greater baseline proteinuria is associated with a steeper mean GFR decline and with a greater benefit form the low blood pressure goal (P=.02 in Study A; P=.01 in Study B). (Used with permission from Klahr S, Levey AS, Beck GJ, et al: The effects of dietary protein restriction and blood-pressure control on the progression of chronic renal disease. Modification of Diet in Renal Disease Study Group. N Engl J Med 1994; 330[13]:877-884.)

Table 4–11 Summary of Number of Antihypertensive Agents to Reach Target Blood Pressure

Study, Year, Reference	Target BP	Achieved BP	Mean Number of Agens
AASK, 2002	<125/75	125/76	3.5
	<140/90	140/84	2.7
MDRD, 1997 (study A only)	<125/75	125/78	1.9
	<140/90	138/78	1.5
AIPRI, 1996	Diastolic = 90	135/84 (ACE inhibitor)	1.7
		144/89 (placebo)	2.1

(Modified with permission from National Kidney Foundation. K/DOQI Clinical Practice Guidelines for Chronic Kidney Disease: Blood pressure management and use of antihypertensive agents in chronic kidney disease. Am J Kidney Dis 2004; 43:S1–S290.)

Moreover, in most of the clinical studies, diuretics were prescribed in addition to ACE inhibitors.[78]

The ALLHAT study raised questions regarding the relative benefits of ACE inhibitors versus diuretics in CKD. A recent post-hoc analysis of the large subgroup of nondiabetics with estimated GFR less than 60 mL/min/1.73 m^2 demonstrated no beneficial effects of an ACE inhibitor (lisinopril) compared to a diuretic (chlorthalidone) on decline in GFR or onset of kidney failure over a 4-year interval.[85] However, evidence suggests that diuretics potentiate the effects of ACE inhibitors, which may partially explain the lack of beneficial effect seen in ACE inhibitors compared to diuretics.

Angiotensin Receptor Blockers (ARB) and Combined ACE Inhibitor/ARB Therapy

Though extensively studied in diabetic kidney disease, the impact of angiotensin receptor blockers (ARB) has not been well studied in nondiabetic kidney disease. Although it might be reasonable to assume that ARBs would also be of benefit in nondiabetic kidney disease, only limited evidence is available at this point. Combined ACE inhibitor and ARB therapy was studied in the COOPERATE study.[86] In this trial, 263 participants with nondiabetic kidney disease (65% had glomerular disease, 24% with IgA) were randomized to either ACE inhibitor (trandolapril), ARB (losartan), or ACE inhibitor and ARB combination (trandolapril and losartan). As demonstrated in Figure 4–6, combination therapy was more effective in reducing the progression of kidney disease than therapy with each agent alone. Though combination therapy may be a consideration for an individual proteinuric patient who is refractory to either agent alone, it is premature to recommend this approach for all patients with nondiabetic kidney disease until it is confirmed in other large trials.

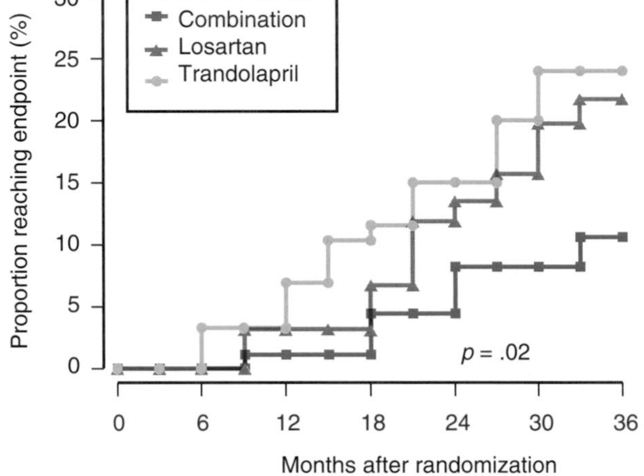

Number at risk

Losartan	89	88	84	79	65	59	47
Trandolapril	86	85	83	75	72	63	58
Combination	88	87	86	83	76	73	67

Figure 4–6 Proportion of patients reaching a kidney end point in the COOPERATE study. (Used with permission from Nakao N, Yoshimura A, Morita H, Kayono T, Ideura T et al: Combination treatment of angiotensin-II receptor blocker and angiotensin-converting-enzyme inhibitor in non-diabetic renal disease COOPERATE: A randomised controlled trial. Lancet 2003; 361[9352]:117-124.)

Calcium Channel Blockers

In diabetic nephropathy, there is significant evidence demonstrating a greater antiproteinuric effect of ACE inhibitors as compared to dihydropyridine calcium channel blockers (CCB). The AASK Study was the first large study to examine the impact of a dihydropyridine CCB on nondiabetic kidney disease. As described earlier, when compared with amlodipine, both ramipril and metoprolol reduced the risk of kidney failure and of kidney failure and death combined.[78,79] In addition, the rise in proteinuria was significantly higher in the amlodipine group than in the other two drug groups. For these reasons, the K/DOQI Work Group recommended that dihydropyridine CCBs should not be used in nondiabetic kidney disease in the absence of therapy with an ACE inhibitor or an ARB.

Summary of Blood Pressure Management Recommendations

The NKF-/DOQI Work Group recommended initial therapy with an ACE inhibitor if the individual has proteinuria, and a diuretic is preferred as the first line additional agent if one is required to achieve target blood pressure. A blood pressure goal of less than 130/80 is recommended by both K/DOQI and JNC 7.[4,64] As discussed earlier, for patients with higher levels of proteinuria, current evidence suggests that an even lower blood pressure goal may be beneficial.[76] Table 4–12 outlines the treatment approach recommended by the K/DOQI Work Group and emphasizes the importance of stratifying patients by level of proteinuria. As discussed later

Table 4–12 Target Blood Pressure and Antihypertensive Agents in Nondiabetic Kidney Disease

Clinical Assessment	Target Blood Pressure	Recommended Agents for CKD	Additional Agents to Reduce CVD Risk and Reach Target Blood Pressure
Blood pressure ≥130/80 mmHg and spot urine total protein-to-creatinine ratio ≥200 mg/g	<130/80 mmHg	ACE inhibitor	Diuretic preferred, then β-blocker or calcium channel blocker
Blood pressure <130/80 mmHg and spot urine total protein-to-creatinine ratio ≥200 mg/g	<130/80 mmHg	ACE inhibitor	Diuretic preferred, then β-blocker or calcium channel blocker
Blood pressure ≥130/80 mmHg and spot urine total protein-to-creatinine ratio <200 mg/g	<130/80 mmHg	None preferred	Diuretic preferred, then ACE inhibitor, ARB, β-blocker or calcium channel blocker

(Used with permission from National Kidney Foundation. K/DOQI Clinical Practice Guidelines for Chronic Kidney Disease: Blood pressure management and use of antihypertensive agents in chronic kidney disease. Am J Kidney Dis 2004; 43:S1–S290.)

in this chapter, other interventions of potential benefit include smoking cessation, low protein diet, and treatment of hyperlipidemia.

ROLE OF OTHER FACTORS IN THE PROGRESSION OF DIABETIC NEPHROPATHY

Dietary Protein Restriction

Although several large trials of dietary protein restriction for the slowing of CKD progression have been completed, the National Kidney Foundation K/DOQI guidelines state that currently available data are too inconclusive to support or not support dietary protein restriction to reduce GFR loss.[4] The Modification of Diet in Renal Disease (MDRD) Study, the largest randomized trial of dietary protein restriction in patients with CKD to date, did not determine definitively whether protein restriction retards CKD progression.[84] Diabetic patients requiring insulin were excluded from the study. Participants with moderately reduced GFR (25–55 mL/min/1.73 m^2) were randomized to either a low protein intake (0.58 gm/kg/day) or usual protein intake (1.3 gm/kg/day) and to a usual blood pressure control group (mean arterial pressure, 107 mmHg) or a low blood pressure control group (mean arterial pressure 92 mmHg). Patients with severely reduced GFR were randomized to low protein intake (0.58 gm/kg/day) and very low protein intake (0.28 gm/kg/day) supplemented with keto acid-amino supplements and a usual or low blood pressure control group. Mean follow-up was 2.2 years. After study completion, GFR decline was found to be 3.8 mL/min/year in patients with moderately decreased GFR and 4.0 mL/min/year among adults with severely decreased GFR. The total number of subjects needed for adequate power was based on a predicted GFR decline of 6 mL/min/year. Due to the slower GFR decline, fewer patients reached the end point (need for renal replacement therapy), and the study had less power overall than expected to determine whether protein restriction ameliorates GFR loss.[87] The risk of ESRD requiring renal replacement therapy or death was reduced by 35% in the low protein group compared to usual protein intake, but the 95% confidence intervals included 1. Risk of ESRD and/or death was similar between the low protein and the very low protein groups among patients with severely reduced GFR (Relative Risk 0.93; 95% CI 0.65, 1.3), but these patients had no usual protein intake arm.[88]

The possibility that GFR loss would not be constant was not incorporated into the original MDRD Study design.[88] GFR decline was actually 1.6 mL/min faster with protein restriction during the first 4 months compared to those assigned to the usual protein diet among patients with moderately reduced GFR. After the first 4 months, GFR decline was then noted to be 1.1 mL/min/year (28%) slower than the usual protein group, but the large increase in GFR decline during the first 4 months led to no overall significant difference between the two groups over the entire study period. However, the MDRD investigators contend that a 28% reduction in GFR decline may translate into clinically meaningful differences in the length of time a particular patient progresses to end-stage renal disease, even preventing older patients from ever reaching this end point. Patients with severely decreased GFR assigned to the very low protein intake group had a 19% slower rate of GFR decline but the difference was not statistically significant. Secondary analyses of the MDRD data have found that every 0.2 g/kg/day decrease in protein intake significantly reduces GFR decline by 30% among patients with severely reduced GFR.[88] No significant association was noted between protein intake and GFR decline among patients with moderately reduced GFR. It must be noted that this degree of protein restriction is difficult to maintain without close supervision by a dietitian and supplementation with essential amino acids, thus, it may be difficult to incorporate into usual clinical practice.

A meta-analysis of five studies (including the MDRD Study) pooled information from a total of 1413 patients with nondiabetic kidney disease to assess the efficacy of dietary protein restriction on CKD progression.[89] Low protein diets decreased the risk of ESRD or mortality by 33% (95% CI 0.50, 0.89). These results did not appear to be confounded by blood pressure because there were no significant differences in pooled mean arterial blood pressure between the low protein and usual protein diet groups. This decrease in risk of ESRD was similar to the risk reduction with low protein intake observed in the MDRD patients with moderately reduced GFR. Changes in GFR with protein restriction could not be determined with meta-analysis due to heterogeneity in assessing GFR among the different studies.

Although dietary protein restriction does appear to ameliorate the progression of kidney disease, the evidence is certainly not overwhelming. The decision to restrict dietary protein intake should incorporate the patient's ability to comply with the diet and maintain close follow-up with the physician and dietitian in order to avoid malnutrition. Moreover, patients should be advised on the current evidence and be involved in the decision-making process.

Smoking

Multiple studies have documented the strong association between smoking and mortality due to cardiovascular disease and cancers, including renal cell carcinoma.[90] Although all physicians are strongly encouraged to prescribe smoking cessation to their patients who continue to smoke, the importance of smoking cessation for the prevention of kidney disease has been poorly emphasized in the nephrology community despite increasing evidence of the adverse effects of smoking on kidney function.[91]

In nonsmokers, nicotine acutely increases renal vascular resistance and decreases GFR.[28] After a 48-hour abstinence from cigarettes, healthy volunteers were requested to smoke two cigarettes. During this 10-minute smoking period, GFR and renal plasma flow were assessed by measuring ^{111}In-diethylenetriamine penta-acetic acid (DTPA) and ^{131}I-hippurate clearances, respectively. GFR decreased by 15% from baseline values (115 ± 15.2 mL/min/1.73 m^2 to 97.3 ± 16.9 mL/min/1.73 m^2) while mean arterial pressure and renal vascular resistance increased. The investigators then repeated the study in seven occasional smokers with IgA nephropathy (serum creatinine ranged from 0.79 to 1.68 mg/dL). Although the increase in mean arterial pressure among the subjects with IgA nephropathy paralleled the mean arterial pressure increase in the healthy controls, no consistent decrease in GFR or increase in renal vascular resistance was noted. However, the urine albumin/creatinine ratio significantly increased in six to seven subjects with IgA nephropathy. No increase in urine albumin excretion was noted in the healthy volunteers with undetectable urine albumin concentrations at baseline, whereas the median urine albumin creatinine ratio among the subjects with IgA nephropathy was 55.5 mg/g.[28] A dose of nicotine gum revealed identical findings; thus, the renal hemodynamic changes with tobacco use were confirmed to be mediated by nicotine.

Halimi and colleagues[92] performed a similar study in 9 chronic smokers and 10 nonsmokers, but the chronic smokers refrained from smoking only 2 hours prior to the study. After chewing 4 mg of nicotine gum, both GFR and effective renal plasma flow decreased by 15% compared to baseline levels among the nonsmokers while no changes in GFR or effective renal plasma flow were noted in the smokers. The short tobacco abstinence period in the smoking group may explain the lack of changes in GFR and effective renal plasma flow.[92] Gambaro and colleagues[93] measured GFR and renal plasma flow in 30 healthy smokers and 24 age and sex matched healthy nonsmokers. There was no significant difference in GFR between the two groups, but renal plasma flow was significantly lower in the smokers compared to nonsmokers (199.2 mL/min/1.73 m^2 vs. 256.6; $P < .005$). In addition, endothelin-1 levels were measured in the two groups and were noted to be significantly higher in the smokers compared to nonsmokers (25.0 pmol/L vs. 21.6; $P < .001$).[93]

Smoking and CKD: Cross-Sectional Studies

Among 1567 nondiabetic men and women who participated in the Gubbio Population Study, smokers were almost twofold more likely to have microalbuminuria (urine albumin excretion 20 to 199 μg/min) compared to nonsmokers.[94] Similar results were noted in a study of 28,000 nondiabetic French adults recruited during routine medical checkups from nine social medical centers.[95] The AusDiab Kidney Study examined the association between smoking and markers of kidney function (estimated creatinine clearance and spot urine/protein ratios) in a nationally representative sample of over 11,000 Australian normotensive, nondiabetic adults.[96] Each 10-pack year smoking increase among current tobacco users was associated with a 3.2 mL/min/1.73 m^2 lower creatinine clearance compared to individuals who never smoked. The association between smoking and decreased creatinine clearance was stronger in men than in women, but this was probably due to the fact that men smoked substantially more cigarettes per day than women in this population. The number of cigarettes smoked per day was also associated with proteinuria as assessed by spot urine protein/creatinine ratios, but the results were not statistically significant.[96] A population based survey of 7476 nondiabetic residents of Groningen, the Netherlands, also observed a twofold higher prevalence of microalbuminuria among current smokers compared to never-smokers.[97]

Smoking and CKD: Prospective Studies

The consistent and strong link between smoking and markers of kidney disease observed in cross-sectional studies has, for the most part, been supported by several investigations using large cohorts. For example, the PREVEND (Prevention of Renal and Vascular End Stage Disease) Study, a population-based survey of residents of Groningen, the Netherlands, noted an independent association between current smoking status and risk of developing microalbuminuria or a decreased GFR (2 standard deviations less than the mean GFR among healthy nondiabetic subjects without microalbuminuria).[97] Current smokers were almost twofold more likely to develop microalbuminuria and 58% more likely to develop decreased GFR compared to nonsmokers. In addition, a dose response was noted: The higher the number of cigarettes smoked per day, the higher the risk of microalbuminuria or decreased GFR. The HOPE study noted a 20% higher risk of the development of new proteinuria (microalbuminuria or dipstick positive proteinuria) among current smokers compared to never-smokers.[37] However, approximately half of the

HOPE study participants were diabetic and all were considered high risk for cardiovascular events. When the investigators stratified the HOPE study participants by presence of diabetes mellitus, the association between smoking and development of new proteinuria in nondiabetics was no longer statistically significant.[37] Several smaller studies have also reported that smoking accelerates the progression of kidney disease associated with primary glomerulopathies such as lupus nephritis[98] and polycystic kidney disease.[99]

Why Does Smoking Increase the Risk for Chronic Kidney Disease in Nondiabetics?

It is well established that chronic smoking increases blood pressure levels by stimulation of the sympathetic system leading to increased levels of circulating catecholamines, endothelin-1 and subsequent activation of the renin-angiotensin system. The hypertension induced by chronic exposure to nicotine may lead to arteriole damage in multiple organs, including the kidney.[100–102] Orth[103] proposed a mechanistic pathway whereby nicotine exposure leads to activation of the renin-angiotensin system and subsequent kidney damage (Figure 4–7). Cigarette smoke also contains carbon monoxide, which may by itself activate the renin angiotensin system or lead to kidney damage due to chronic hypoxia in the tubulointerstitium.[104] Kidney damage may also be mediated by increased thrombogenesis from cigarette smoke[105,106] leading to glomerular intracapillary thrombosis and subsequent endothelial damage.

Cardiovascular mortality is over 10-fold higher in dialysis patients compared to the general population,[107] and CKD is an independent predictor of cardiovascular events and mortality.[53,54,108,109] Therefore, all individuals with kidney disease or those who are at high risk for the development of kidney disease should strongly be advised on the advantages of smoking cessation and encouraged to quit.

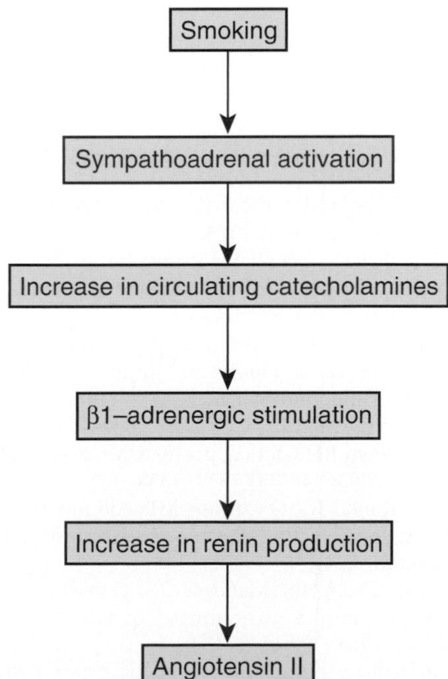

Figure 4–7 Sequence of smoking-induced activation of the renin-angiotensin system: A proposed mechanism of smoking-induced renal damage. (Reproduced with permission from Orth SR: Smoking and the kidney. J Am Soc Nephrol 2002; 13[6]:1663-1672.)

Lipid Abnormalities

Lipid abnormalities are more common in patients with CKD compared to the general population,[109] and lipid laden (foamy) macrophages and lipid deposits may be noted histologically in a variety of glomerulopathies.[110] In light of these findings, many investigators have hypothesized that lipid abnormalities participate in the development and progression of kidney disease. Oxygen radicals formed by mesangial and tubular cells in the presence of angiotensin II oxidize lipoproteins. These oxidized lipoproteins stimulate cytokine production and inflammatory cell migration leading to subsequent cell death and glomerulosclerosis.[111,112] Research supporting this theory include the acceleration of glomerulosclerosis in animal models with lipid rich diets,[113–115] and the decrease in albuminuria and glomerulosclerosis with lipid lowering treatment after 5/6 nephrectomy in rats.[116]

Clinical studies, however, have not demonstrated a consistent association between lipid abnormalities and the development of nondiabetic kidney disease. Using data from the Atherosclerotic Risk in Communities Study, a cohort of middle-aged adults recruited from four U.S. communities, investigators examined the association between baseline lipid levels and changes in serum creatinine after 3 years of follow-up.[117] Several types of lipid abnormalities were included, such as total cholesterol, triglycerides, HDL, LDL, Lp(a), apolipoprotein A, and apolipoprotein B. Patients taking lipid-lowering agents at baseline and those with an elevated baseline creatinine (≥ 2.0 mg/dL in men and ≥ 1.8 mg/dL in women) were excluded from the analyses. After adjustment for blood pressure, age, sex, and race, only baseline serum levels of HDL and triglycerides remained significant predictors of a ≥ 0.4 mg/dL creatinine increase from baseline. However, insulin resistance confounded this association because no significant association between HDL and triglycerides and serum creatinine changes was noted after adjustment for serum insulin levels.

Similar results were also observed in the Helsinki Heart Study, a 5-year randomized trial of gemfibrozil versus placebo in middle-aged healthy men with hyperlipidemia.[118] Enrollment criteria included absence of cardiovascular disease and normal serum creatinine, and patients with dipstick positive proteinuria were excluded from the analyses. Baseline serum triglycerides and HDL levels did not predict changes in serum creatinine over the 5-year period. However, the ratio of LDL/HDL was associated with a significantly higher change in serum creatinine among hypertensives and was noted in both treatment groups. In normotensive patients, changes in serum creatinine did not differ by level of the LDL/HDL ratio, regardless of the treatment group.[118] The null findings in these studies may have been due to the relatively short follow-up period.

Cohort studies with adequate follow-up to examine changes in kidney function include the Physicians Health Study. This study examined whether baseline lipid levels predicted an increased serum creatinine (≥ 1.5 mg/dL) after a 14-year follow-up period in over 4000 initially healthy men.[119]

After adjustment for multiple covariates, a baseline total cholesterol level greater than or equal to 240 mg/dL increased the risk of an elevated serum creatinine by 77%, while HDL levels less than 40 mg/dL increased the risk by over twofold. Hsu and colleagues[120] reported similar results in nondiabetic ambulatory patients followed at a university teaching hospital. Baseline serum cholesterol greater than 350 mg/dL increased the risk of developing CKD (GFR < 60 mL/min/1.73 m^2) by fourfold after a mean of 5 years compared to adults with baseline serum cholesterol less than 250 mg/dL.

Few studies have examined whether lipid abnormalities accelerate the progression of GFR loss in patients with established nondiabetic kidney disease. In 44 adult nondiabetic patients with CKD (mean GFR 40 mL/min/1.73 m^2), plasma concentrations of triglyceride rich apolipoprotein Bc particles were reported to be highly and significantly correlated with rate of GFR loss (r=0.43).[121] However, this study did not determine whether apolipoprotein Bc concentrations independently predicted progression of kidney disease. The Modification of Diet in Renal Disease Study, which included 840 patients with chronic kidney disease of different causes, noted an independent association between GFR decline and baseline HDL levels, but the association was limited to patients with baseline GFR levels greater than 25 mL/min/1.73 m^2.[122] Overall, the cumulative evidence suggests that lipid abnormalities influence the progression of GFR loss in patients with established kidney disease and may also increase the risk of developing CKD in healthy men.

AREAS FOR FUTURE RESEARCH

There are numerous areas for future research in nondiabetic kidney disease. Some important potential areas include: studying the potential protective effects of ARBs and other classes of antihypertensive agents, either alone or in combination with ACE inhibitors. In addition, more work is needed to better determine the optimal levels of blood pressure control for different levels of proteinuria of nondiabetic CKD. The impact of smoking cessation and treatment of hyperlipidemia also remains to be explored. Although this chapter has not focused on CVD in nondiabetics, interventional studies are needed to investigate interventions to reduce the toll of CVD in nondiabetic CKD. Finally, there is a need for the development of more precise diagnostic techniques for differentiating between types of nondiabetic CKD, as well as larger studies focusing on individual types of nondiabetic CKD. As discussed, the term "nondiabetic kidney disease" has obvious limitations because it encompasses such a broad array of disease. It is our hope that this term will one day be an anachronism, once we have reached a better understanding of the pathophysiology and treatment of individual causes of kidney disease.

References

1. Levey AS: Clinical practice. Nondiabetic kidney disease. N Engl J Med 2002; 347(19):1505–1511.
2. Xue JL, Ma JZ, Louis TA, Collins AJ: Forecast of the number of patients with end-stage renal disease in the United States to the year 2010. J Am Soc Nephrol 2001; 12(12):2753–2758.
3. US Renal Data System. USRDS 2002 annual data report: Atlas of end-stage renal disease in the United States. Bethesda, MD, National Institutes of Health, National Institute of Diabetes and Digestive Disease and Kidney Disease, 2002.
4. National Kidney Foundation. K/DOQI clinical practice guidelines for chronic kidney disease: Evaluation, classification, and stratification. Am J Kidney Dis 2002; 39:S46–S103.
5. Levey AS, Bosch JP, Breyer Lewis J, et al: A more accurate method to estimate glomerular filtration rate from serum creatinine. Ann Intern Med 1999; 139:461–470.
6. Levey AS, Coresh J, Balk E, et al: National Kidney Foundation practice guidelines for chronic kidney disease: Evaluation, classification, and stratification. Ann Intern Med 2003; 139(2): 137–147.
7. Kramer HJ, Nguyen QD, Curhan G, Hsu CY: Renal insufficiency in the absence of albuminuria and retinopathy among adults with type 2 diabetes mellitus. JAMA 2003; 289(24):3273–3277.
8. Jones CA, McQuillan GM, Kusek JW, et al: Serum creatinine levels in the US population: Third National Health and Nutrition Examination Survey 8. 6. Am J Kidney Dis 1998; 32(6):992-999.
9. Mattix HJ, Hsu C, Curhan GC: Use of the albumin/creatinine ratio to detect microalbuminuria: Implications of sex and race. J Am Soc Nephrol 2002; 13:1034–1039.
10. Reddan DN, Szczech LA, Klassen PS, Owen W Jr: Racial inequity in America's ESRD program. Semin Dial 2000; 13:399–403.
11. Byrne C, Nedelman J, Luke RG: Race, socioeconomic status, and the development of end-stage renal disease. Am J Kidney Dis 1994; 23:16–22.
12. O'Dea DF, Murphy SW, Hefferton D, Parfrey PS: Higher risk for renal failure in first-degree relatives of white patients with end-stage renal disease: a population-based study. Am J Kidney Dis 1998; 32(5):794–801.
13. Freedman BI, Soucie JM, McClellan WM: Family history of end-stage renal disease among incident dialysis patients. J Am Soc Nephrol 1997; 8(12):1942–1945.
14. Adrogue HJ, Wesson DE: Role of dietary factors in the hypertension of African Americans. Semin Nephrol 1996; 16(2):94–101.
15. Hirschhorn JN, Lohmueller K, Byrne E, Hirschhorn K: A comprehensive review of genetic association studies. Genet Med 2002; 4(2):45–61.
16. Taal MW: Angiotensin-converting enzyme gene polymorphisms in renal disease: clinically relevant? Curr Opin Nephrol Hypertens 2000; 9(6):651–657.
17. Cooper RS, Psaty BM: Genomics and medicine: Distraction, incremental progress, or the dawn of a new age? Ann Intern Med 2003; 138(7):576–580.
18. Cockroft DW, Gault MH: Prediction of creatinine clearance from serum creatinine. Nephron 1976; 16:31–41.
19. Rolin HI, Hall PM, Wei R: Inaccuracy of estimated creatinine clearance for prediction of iothalamate glomerular filtration rate. Am J Kidney Dis 1984; 4:48–54.
20. Rutecki GJ, Goldsmith C, Schreiner GE: Characterization of proteins in urinary casts. Fluorescent-antibody identification of Tamm-Horsfall mucoprotein in matrix and serum proteins in granules. N Engl J Med 1971; 284(19):1049–1052.
21. Cohen RA, Brown RS: Clinical practice. Microscopic hematuria. N Engl J Med 2003; 348(23):2330–2338.
22. Shihabi ZK, Konen JC, O'Connor ML: Albuminuria vs urinary total protein for detecting chronic renal disorders. Clin Chem 1991; 37(5):621–624.
23. Ginsberg JM, Chang BS, Matarese RA, Garella S: Use of single voided urine samples to estimate quantitative proteinuria. N Engl J Med 1983; 309:1543–1546.
24. American Diabetes Association. Diabetic nephropathy: Clinical practice recommendations 2001. Diabetes Care 2001; 24(suppl 1):S69–S72.
25. Rowe DJ, Bagga H, Betts PB: Normal variations in rate of albumin excretion and albumin to creatinine ratios in overnight and daytime urine collections in non-diabetic children. Br Med J (Clin Res Ed) 1985; 291(6497):693–694.

26. Kramer BK, Kernz M, Ress KM, et al: Influence of strenuous exercise on albumin excretion. Clin Chem 1988; 34(12): 2516–2518.
27. Poortmans JR: Postexercise proteinuria in humans. Facts and mechanisms. JAMA 1985; 253(2):236–240.
28. Ritz E, Benck U, Franek E, et al: Effects of smoking on renal hemodynamics in healthy volunteers and in patients with glomerular disease. J Am Soc Nephrol 1998; 9(10):1798–1804.
29. Warram JH, Gearin G, Laffel L, Krolewski AS: Effect of duration of type I diabetes on the prevalence of stages of diabetic nephropathy defined by urinary albumin/creatinine ratio. J Am Soc Nephrol 1996; 7:930–937.
30. Coresh J, Astor BC, Greene T, et al: Prevalence of chronic kidney disease and decreased kidney function in the adult US population: Third National Health and Nutrition Examination Survey. 2. Am J Kidney Dis 2003; 41(1):1–12.
31. Bianchi S, Bigazi R, Campese VM: Microalbuminuria in essential hypertension: Significance, pathophysiology, and therapeutic implications. Am J Kidney Dis 1999; 6:973–995.
32. Lowenstein J, Beranbaum ER, Chasis H, DS. B.[AU: Is this last name correct?]: Intrarenal pressure and exaggerated natriuresis in essential hypertension. Clinical Science 1970; 38:359–374.
33. Simons JL, Provoost AP, Anderson S, et al: Modulation of glomerular hypertension defines susceptibility to progressive glomerular injury. Kidney Int 1994; 46(2):396–404.
34. Neuringer JR, Brenner BM: Hemodynamic theory of progressive renal disease: A 10-year update in brief review. Am J Kidney Dis 1993; 22(1):98–104.
35. Pinto-Sietsma SJ, Janssen WM, Hillege HL, et al: Urinary albumin excretion is associated with renal functional abnormalities in a nondiabetic population. Kidney Int 2000; 11:1882–1888.
36. Bigazzi R, Bianchi S, Baldari D, VM C: Microalbuminuria predicts cardiovascular events and renal insufficiency in patients with essential hypertension predicts. J Hypertens 1998; 16: 1325–1333.
37. Mann JF, Gerstein HC, Yi QL, et al: Development of renal disease in people at high cardiovascular risk: Results of the HOPE randomized study. J Am Soc Nephrol 2003; 14(3):641–647.
38. Cerasola G, Cottone S, D'Ignoto G, et al: Micro-albuminuria as a predictor of cardiovascular damage in essential hypertension. J Htn 1989; 7:S332–S333.
39. Stehouwer CD, Nauta JJ, Zeldenrust GC, et al: Urinary albumin excretion, cardiovascular disease, and endothelial dysfunction in non-insulin-dependent diabetes mellitus. Lancet 1992; 340: 319–323.
40. Yudkin JS, Forrest RD, Jackson CA: Microalbuminuria as predictor of vascular disease in non-diabetic subjects. Lancet 1988; 2:530–533.
41. Mogensen CE: Systemic blood pressure and glomerular leakage with particular reference to diabetes and hypertension. J Intern Med 1995; 235:297–316.
42. Parving HH, Oxenboll B, Svendsen PA: Early detection of patients at risk of developing diabetic nephropathy: A prospective study of urinary albumin excretion. Acta Endocrinol 1982; 100:550.
43. Klein R, Klein BE, Moss SE: The Wisconsin epidemiological study of diabetic retinopathy: A review. Diabetes Metab Rev 1989; 5(7):559–570.
44. Kofoed-Enevoldsen A, Jensen T, Borch-Johnsen K, Deckert T: Incidence of retinopathy in type 1 (insulin-dependent) diabetes: Association with clinical nephropathy. J Diabet Complications 1987; 3:96–99.
45. Campese VM, Bianchi S, Bigazzi R: Association between hyperlipidemia and microalbuminuria in essential hypertension. Kidney Int 1999; 56:S10–S13.
46. Bianchi S, Bigazzi R, Quinones Galvan A, et al: Insulin resistance in microalbuminuric hypertension. Sites and mechanisms. Hypertension 1995; 26(5):789–795.
47. Festa A, D'agostino R, Howard G, et al: Inflammation and microalbuminuria in nondiabetic and type 2 diabetic subjects: The Insulin Resistance Atherosclerosis Study. Kidney Int 2000; 58:1703–1710.
48. Martinez MA, Moreno A, de Carcer AA, et al: Frequency and determinants of microalbuminuria in mild hypertension: A primary-care based study. J Htn 2001; 19:319–326.
49. Giaconi S, Levanti C, Fommei E, et al: Microalbuminuria and casual and ambulatory blood pressure monitoring in normotensives and in patients with borderline and mild essential hypertension. Am J Hypertens 1989; 2(4):259–261.
50. Bigazzi R, Bianchi S, Nenci R, et al: Increased thickness of the carotid artery in patients with essential hypertension and microalbuminuria. J Hum Htn 1995; 9:827–833.
51. Wachtell K, Palmieri V, Olsen MH, et al: Urine albumin/creatinine ratio and echocardiographic left ventricular structure and function in hypertensive patients with electrocardiographic left ventricular hypertrophy. Am Heart J 2002; 143:319–326.
52. Olsen MH, Wachtell K, Borch-Johnsen K, et al: A blood pressure independent association between glomerular albumin leakage and electrocardiographic left ventricular hypertrophy. The LIFE Study. Losartan Intervention For Endpoint reduction. J Hum Hypertens 2002; 16(8):591–595.
53. Munter P, He J, Hamm L, et al: Renal insufficiency and subsequent death resulting from cardiovascular disease in the United States. J Am Soc Nephrol 2002; 13:745–753.
54. Gerstein HC, Mann JF, Yi Q, et al: Albuminuria and risk of cardiovascular events, death and heart failure in diabetic and nondiabetic individuals. JAMA 2001; 286:421–426.
55. Ljungman S, Wikstrand J, Hartford M, Berglund G: Urinary albumin excretion?a predictor of risk of cardiovascular disease. A prospective 10-year follow-up of middle aged nondiabetic normal and hypertensive men. Am J Htn 1996; 9:770–778.
56. Romundstad S, Holmen J, Kvenild K, et al: Microalbuminuria and all-cause mortality in 2089 apparently healthy individuals: A 4.4-year follow-up study. The Nord-Trondelag Health Study (HUNT), Norway. Am J Kidney Dis 2003; 42(3):466–473.
57. Deckert T, Feldt-Rasmussen B, Borch-Johnsen K, et al: Albuminuria reflects widespread vascular damage. The steno hypothesis. Diabetologia 1989; 32(4):219–226.
58. Lip G, Blann A: von Willebrand factor: A marker of endothelial dysfunction in vascular disorders? Cardiovasc Research 1997; 34:255–265.
59. Clausen P, Feldt-Rasmussen B, Jensen G, Jensen JS: Endothelial haemostatic factors are associated with progression of urinary albumin excretion in clinically healthy subjects: A 4-year prospective study. Clin Sci (Lond) 1999; 97(1):37–43.
60. Jager A, van Hinsbergh VW, Kostense PJ, et al: C-reactive protein and soluble vascular cell adhesion molecule-1 are associated with elevated urinary albumin excretion but do not explain its link with cardiovascular risk. Arterioscler Thromb Vasc Biol 2002; 22(4):593–598.
61. Yokoyama H, Jensen JS, Myrup B, et al: Raised serum sialic acid concentration precedes onset of microalbuminuria in IDDM. A 10-year follow-up study. Diabetes Care 1996; 19(5): 435–440.
62. Hartwell DW, Wagner DD: New discoveries with mice mutant in endothelial and platelet selectins. Thromb Haemost 1999; 82(2):850–857.
63. Stehouwer CD, Gall MA, Twisk JW, et al: Increased urinary albumin excretion, endothelial dysfunction, and chronic low-grade inflammation in type 2 diabetes: Progressive, interrelated, and independently associated with risk of death. Diabetes 2002; 51(4):1157–1165.
64. Chobanian AV, Bakris GL, Black HR, et al: The Seventh Report of the Joint National Committee on Prevention, Detection, Evaluation, and Treatment of High Blood Pressure: The JNC 7 report. JAMA 2003; 289(19):2560–2572.

65. Donnelly R, Rea R: Microalbuminuria: How informative and reliable are individual measurements? J Htn 2003; 21: 1229–1233.
66. Maschio G, Alberti D, Locatelli F, et al: Angiotensin-converting enzyme inhibitors and kidney protection: The AIPRI trial. The ACE Inhibition in Progressive Renal Insufficiency (AIPRI) Study Group. J Cardiovasc Pharmacol 1999; 33(suppl 1): S16–S20.
67. Randomised placebo-controlled trial of effect of ramipril on decline in glomerular filtration rate and risk of terminal renal failure in proteinuric, non-diabetic nephropathy. The GISEN Group (Gruppo Italiano di Studi Epidemiologici in Nefrologia)67. 1. Lancet 1997; 349(9069):1857–1863.[
68. Ruggenenti P, Perna A, Gherardi G, et al: Renoprotective properties of ACE-inhibition in non-diabetic nephropathies with non-nephrotic proteinuria68. 1. Lancet 1999; 354(9176): 359–364.
69. Buckalew VM Jr, Berg RL, Wang SR, et al: Prevalence of hypertension in 1795 subjects with chronic renal disease: The modification of diet in renal disease study baseline cohort. Modification of Diet in Renal Disease Study Group69. 1. Am J Kidney Dis 1996; 28(6):811–821.
70. Brazy PC, Stead WW, Fitzwilliam JF: Progression of renal insufficiency: Role of blood pressure. Kidney Int 1989; 35(2):670–674.
71. Shulman NB, Ford CE, Hall WD, et al: Prognostic value of serum creatinine and effect of treatment of hypertension on renal function. Results from the hypertension detection and follow-up program. The Hypertension Detection and Follow-up Program Cooperative Group71. 3. Hypertension 1989; 13(5 suppl): I80–I93.
72. Walker WG, Neaton JD, Cutler JA, et al: Renal function change in hypertensive members of the Multiple Risk Factor Intervention Trial. Racial and treatment effects. The MRFIT Research Group72. 1. JAMA 1992; 268(21):3085–3091.
73. Klag M, Whelton P, Randall B, et al: Blood pressure and end-stage renal disease in men. N Engl J Med 1996; 334:13–18.
74. Klag MJ, Whelton PK, Randall BL, et al: End-stage renal disease in African-American and white men. 16-year MRFIT findings74. 2. JAMA 1997; 277(16):1293–1298.
75. Young JH, Klag MJ, Muntner P, et al: Blood pressure and decline in kidney function: Findings from the Systolic Hypertension in the Elderly Program (SHEP)75. 1. J Am Soc Nephrol 2002; 13(11):2776–2782.
76. Jafar T, Stark P, Schmid CH, et al: Progression of chronic kidney disease: The role of blood pressure control, proteinuria, and angiotensin-converting enzyme inhibition. A patient-level meta-analysis. Ann Intern Med 2003; 139(4):244–252.
77. Ruggenenti P, Perna A, Gherardi G, et al: Renoprotective properties of ACE-inhibition in non-diabetic nephropathies with non-nephrotic proteinuria. Lancet 1999; 354(9176):359–364.
78. Wright JT Jr, Bakris G, Greene T, et al: Effect of blood pressure lowering and antihypertensive drug class on progression of hypertensive kidney disease: Results from the AASK trial. JAMA 2002; 288(19):2421–2431.
79. Agodoa LY, Appel L, Bakris GL, et al: Effect of ramipril vs amlodipine on renal outcomes in hypertensive nephrosclerosis: A randomized controlled trial. JAMA 2001; 285(21):2719–2728.
80. Jafar TH, Schmid CH, Landa M, et al: Angiotensin-converting enzyme inhibitors and progression of nondiabetic renal disease. A meta-analysis of patient-level data. Ann Intern Med 2001; 135(2):73–87.
81. Mulrow C, Townsend R: Guiding lights for antihypertensive treatment in patients with nondiabetic chronic renal disease: Proteinuria and blood pressure levels? Ann Intern Med 139(4):296–298.
82. Chobanian AV, Bakris GL, Black HR, et al: The Seventh Report of the Joint National Committee on Prevention, Detection, Evaluation, and Treatment of High Blood Pressure: The JNC 7 report82. 1. JAMA 2003; 289(19):2560–2572.
83. National Kidney Foundation. K/DOQI Clinical Practice Guidelines for Chronic Kidney Disease: Blood Pressure Management and Use of Antihypertensive Agents in chronic kidney disease. Am J Kidney Dis 2004; 43:S1–S290.
84. Klahr S, Levey AS, Beck GJ, et al: The effects of dietary protein restriction and blood-pressure control on the progression of chronic renal disease. Modification of Diet in Renal Disease Study Group84. 2. N Engl J Med 1994; 330(13):877–884.
85. Rahman M, Cutler J, Davis B, et al: ALLHAT Collaborative Research Group. Renal outcomes in hypertensive patients with impaired renal function. Am J Kidney Dis 2003; 41:A6.
86. Nakao N, Yoshimura A, Morita H, et al: Combination treatment of angiotensin-II receptor blocker and angiotensin-converting-enzyme inhibitor in non-diabetic renal disease (COOPERATE): A randomised controlled trial. Lancet 2003; 361(9352):117–124.
87. Levey AS, Greene T, Beck GJ, et al: Dietary protein restriction and the progression of chronic renal disease: What have all of the results of the MDRD study shown? Modification of Diet in Renal Disease study group. J Am Soc Nephrol 1999; 10(11): 2426–2439.
88. Levey AS, Greene T, Beck GJ, et al: Dietary protein restriction and the progression of chronic renal disease: What have all of the results of the MDRD study shown? Modification of Diet in Renal Disease study group. J Am Soc Nephrol 1999; 10(11): 2426–2439.
89. Pedrini MT, Levey AS, Lau J, et al: The effect of dietary protein restriction on the progression of diabetic and nondiabetic renal diseases: A meta-analysis. Ann Intern Med 1996; 124(7):627–632.
90. McGinnis JM, Foege WH: Actual causes of death in the United States. JAMA 1993; 270(18):2207–2212.
91. Orth SR, Ritz E, Schrier RW: The renal risks of smoking. Kidney Int 1997; 51(6):1669-1677.
92. Halimi JM, Philippon C, Mimran A: Contrasting renal effects of nicotine in smokers and non-smokers. Nephrol Dial Transplant 1998; 13(4):940–944.
93. Gambaro G, Verlato F, Budakovic A, et al: Renal impairment in chronic cigarette smokers. J Am Soc Nephrol 1998; 9(4): 562–567.
94. Cirillo M, Senigalliesi L, Laurenzi M, et al: Microalbuminuria in nondiabetic adults: Relation of blood pressure, body mass index, plasma cholesterol levels, and smoking: The Gubbio Population Study. Arch Intern Med 1998; 158(17):1933–1939.
95. Halimi JM, Giraudeau B, Vol S, et al: Effects of current smoking and smoking discontinuation on renal function and proteinuria in the general population. Kidney Int 2000; 58(3):1285–1292.
96. Briganti EM, Branley P, Chadban SJ, et al: Smoking is associated with renal impairment and proteinuria in the normal population: The AusDiab kidney study. Am J Kidney Dis 2002:40.
97. Pinto-Sietsma SJ, Mulder J, Janssen W, et al: Smoking is related to albuminuria and abnormal renal function in non-diabetic persons. Ann Intern Med 2000; 133:585–591.
98. Ward MM, Studenski S: Clinical prognostic factors in lupus nephritis. The importance of hypertension and smoking. Arch Intern Med 1992; 152:2082–2088.
99. Chapman AB, Johnson AM, Gabow PA, Schrier RW: Overt proteinuria and microalbuminuria in autosomal dominant polycystic kidney disease. J Am Soc Nephrol 1994; 5(6):1349–1354.
100. Auerbach O, Hammond EC, Garfinkel L: Thickening of walls of arterioles and small arteries in relation to age and smoking habits. N Engl J Med 1968; 278:980–984.
101. Black HR, Zeevi GR, Silten RM, Walker Smith GJ: Effect of heavy cigarette smoking on renal and myocardial arterioles. Nephron 1983; 34(3):173–179.
102. Lhotta K, Rumpelt HJ, Konig P, et al: Cigarette smoking and vascular pathology in renal biopsies. Kidney Int 2002; 61(2): 648–654.

103. Orth SR: Smoking and the kidney. J Am Soc Nephrol 2002; 13(6):1663–1672.
104. Fine LG, Bandyopadhay D, Norman JT: Is there a common mechanism for the progression of different types of renal diseases other than proteinuria? Towards the unifying theme of chronic hypoxia. Kidney Int Suppl 2000; 75:22–26.
105. Hioki H, Aoki N, Kawano K, et al: Acute effects of cigarette smoking on platelet-dependent thrombin generation. Eur Heart J 2001; 22(1):56–61.
106. Newby DE, Wright RA, Labinjoh C, et al: Endothelial dysfunction, impaired endogenous fibrinolysis, and cigarette smoking: A mechanism for arterial thrombosis and myocardial infarction. Circulation 1999; 99(11):1411–1415.
107. Parfrey PS, Foley RN: The clinical epidemiology of cardiac disease in chronic renal failure. J Am Soc Nephrol 1999; 10(7): 1606–1615.
108. Mann J, Gerstein HC, Pogue J, et al: Renal insufficiency as a predictor of cardiovascular outcomes and the impact of ramipril: The HOPE randomized trial. Ann Intern Med 2001; 134:629–636.
109. Culleton BF, Larson MG, Wilson PW, et al: Cardiovascular disease and mortality in a community-based cohort with mild renal insufficiency. Kidney Int 1999; 56(6):2214–2219.
110. Keane WF, Kasiske BL, O'Donnell MP: Lipids and progressive glomerulosclerosis. A model analogous to atherosclerosis. Am J Nephrol 1988; 8(4):261–271.
111. Wanner C, Greiber S, Kramer-Guth A, et al: Lipids and progression of renal disease: Role of modified low density lipoprotein and lipoprotein(a). Kidney Int Suppl 1997; 63:102–106.
112. Keane WF: The role of lipids in renal disease: Future challenges. Kidney Int Suppl 2000; 75:27–31.
113. French SW, Yamanaka W, Ostwald R: Dietary induced glomerulosclerosis in the guinea pig. Arch Pathol 1967; 83(2):204–210.
114. Kasiske BL, O'Donnell MP, Schmitz PG, et al: Renal injury of diet-induced hypercholesterolemia in rats. Kidney Int 1990; 37(3):880–891.
115. Wellmann KF, Volk BW: Renal changes in experimental hypercholesterolemia in normal and in subdiabetic rabbits. I. Short term studies. Lab Invest 1970; 22(1):36–49.
116. Kasiske BL, O'Donnell MP, Garvis WJ, Keane WF: Pharmacologic treatment of hyperlipidemia reduces glomerular injury in rat 5/6 nephrectomy model of chronic renal failure. Circ Res 1988; 62(2):367–374.
117. Muntner P, Coresh J, Smith JC, et al: Plasma lipids and risk of developing renal dysfunction: The atherosclerosis risk in communities study. Kidney Int 2000; 58(1):293–301.
118. Manttari M, Tiula E, Alikoski T, Manninen V: Effects of hypertension and dyslipidemia on the decline in renal function. Hypertension 1995; 26(4):670–675.
119. Schaeffner ES, Kurth T, Curhan GC, et al: Cholesterol and the risk of renal dysfunction in apparently healthy men. J Am Soc Nephrol 2003; 14(8):2084–2091.
120. Hsu CY, Bates DW, Kuperman GJ, Curhan GC: Diabetes, hemoglobin A(1c), cholesterol, and the risk of moderate chronic renal insufficiency in an ambulatory population. Am J Kidney Dis 2000; 36:272–281.
121. Samuelsson O, Attman PO, Knight-Gibson C, et al: Complex apolipoprotein B-containing lipoprotein particles are associated with a higher rate of progression of human chronic renal insufficiency. J Am Soc Nephrol 1998; 9(8):1482–1488.
122. Hunsicker LG, Adler S, Caggiula A, et al: Predictors of the progression of renal disease in the Modification of Diet in Renal Disease Study. Kidney Int 1997; 51(6):1908–1919.
123. Boute N, Gribouval O, Roselli S, et al: NPHS2, encoding the glomerular protein podocin, is mutated in autosomal recessive steroid-resistant nephrotic syndrome. Nat Genet 2000; 24(4): 349–354.
124. Kaplan JM, Kim SH, North KN, et al: Mutations in ACTN4, encoding alpha-actinin-4, cause familial focal segmental glomerulosclerosis. Nat Genet 2000; 24(3):251–256.
125. Kestila M, Lenkkeri U, Mannikko M, et al: Positionally cloned gene for a novel glomerular protein—nephrin—is mutated in congenital nephrotic syndrome. Mol Cell 1998; 1(4):575–582.
126. Barker DF, Pruchno CJ, Jiang X, et al: A mutation causing Alport syndrome with tardive hearing loss is common in the western United States. Am J Hum Genet 1996; 58(6):1157–1165.
127. Knebelmann B, Forestier L, Drouot L, et al: Splice-mediated insertion of an Alu sequence in the COL4A3 mRNA causing autosomal recessive Alport syndrome. Hum Mol Genet 1995; 4(4):675–679.
128. Mochizuki T, Lemmink HH, Mariyama M, et al: Identification of mutations in the alpha 3(IV) and alpha 4(IV) collagen genes in autosomal recessive Alport syndrome. Nat Genet 1994; 8(1): 77–81.
129. Jefferson JA, Lemmink HH, Hughes AE, et al: Autosomal dominant Alport syndrome linked to the type IV collage alpha 3 and alpha 4 genes (COL4A3 and COL4A4). Nephrol Dial Transplant 1997; 12(8):1595–1599.
130. van der Loop FT, Heidet L, Timmer ED, et al: Autosomal dominant Alport syndrome caused by a COL4A3 splice site mutation. Kidney Int 2000; 58(5):1870–1875.
131. Eng CM, Desnick RJ: Molecular basis of Fabry disease: Mutations and polymorphisms in the human alpha-galactosidase A gene. Hum Mutat 1994; 3(2):103–111.
132. Reeders ST, Breuning MH, Davies KE, et al: A highly polymorphic DNA marker linked to adult polycystic kidney disease on chromosome 16. Nature 1985; 317(6037):542-544.
133. The polycystic kidney disease 1 gene encodes a 14 kb transcript and lies within a duplicated region on chromosome 16. The European Polycystic Kidney Disease Consortium. Cell 1994; 77(6):881–894.
134. Kimberling WJ, Kumar S, Gabow PA, et al: Autosomal dominant polycystic kidney disease: Localization of the second gene to chromosome 4q13-q23. Genomics 1993; 18(3):467–472.
135. Peters DJ, Spruit L, Saris JJ, et al: Chromosome 4 localization of a second gene for autosomal dominant polycystic kidney disease. Nat Genet 1993; 5(4):359–362.
136. Suthanthiran M, Li B, Song JO, et al: Transforming growth factor-beta 1 hyperexpression in African-American hypertensives: A novel mediator of hypertension and/or target organ damage. Proc Natl Acad Sci U S A 2000; 97(7):3479–3484.
137. Suthanthiran M, Khanna A, Cukran D, et al:Transforming growth factor-beta 1 hyperexpression in African American end-stage renal disease patients. Kidney Int 1998; 53(3):639–644.
138. Dong Y, Zhu H, Sagnella GA, et al: Association between the C825T polymorphism of the G protein beta3-subunit gene and hypertension in blacks. Hypertension 1999; 34(6):1193–1196.
139. Siffert W, Rosskopf D, Moritz A, et al: Enhanced G protein activation in immortalized lymphoblasts from patients with essential hypertension. J Clin Invest 1995; 96(2):759–766.
140. Siffert W: Molecular genetics of G proteins and atherosclerosis risk. Basic Res Cardiol 2001; 96(6):606–611.
141. Taddei S, Virdis A, Mattei P, et al: Defective L-arginine-nitric oxide pathway in offspring of essential hypertensive patients. Circulation 1996; 94(6):1298–1303.
142. Tsukada T, Yokoyama K, Arai T, et al: Evidence of association of the ecNOS gene polymorphism with plasma NO metabolite levels in humans. Biochem Biophys Res Commun 1998; 245(1):190–193.
143. Quan ZY, Walser M, Hill GS: Adrenalectomy ameliorates ablative nephropathy in the rat independently of corticosterone maintenance level. Kidney Int 1992; 41(2):326–333.
144. Davies E, Holloway CD, Ingram MC, et al: Aldosterone excretion rate and blood pressure in essential hypertension are related to polymorphic differences in the aldosterone synthase gene CYP11B2. Hypertension 1999; 33(2):703–707.
145. Greene EL, Kren S, Hostetter TH: Role of aldosterone in the remnant kidney model in the rat. J Clin Invest 1996; 98(4): 1063–1068.

146. Delles C, Erdmann J, Jacobi J, et al: Aldosterone synthase (CYP11B2) -344 C/T polymorphism is associated with left ventricular structure in human arterial hypertension. J Am Coll Cardiol 2001; 37(3):878–884.
147. Rabelink TJ, Kaasjager KA, Boer P, et al: Effects of endothelin-1 on renal function in humans: Implications for physiology and pathophysiology. Kidney Int 1994; 46(2):376–381.
148. Hocher B, Thone-Reineke C, Rohmeiss P, et al: Endothelin-1 transgenic mice develop glomerulosclerosis, interstitial fibrosis, and renal cysts but not hypertension. J Clin Invest 1997; 99(6): 1380–1389.
149. Treiber FA, Barbeau P, Harshfield G, et al: Endothelin-1 gene Lys198Asn polymorphism and blood pressure reactivity. Hypertension 2003; 42(4):494–499.
150. Barden AE, Herbison CE, Beilin LJ, et al: Association between the endothelin-1 gene Lys198Asn polymorphism blood pressure and plasma endothelin-1 levels in normal and pre-eclamptic pregnancy. J Hypertens 2001; 19(10):1775–1782.
151. Tiret L, Poirier O, Hallet V, et al: The Lys198Asn polymorphism in the endothelin-1 gene is associated with blood pressure in overweight people. Hypertension 1999; 33(5):1169–1174.
152. Lehtonen S, Zhao F, Lehtonen E: CD2-associated protein directly interacts with the actin cytoskeleton. Am J Physiol Renal Physiol 2002; 283(4):734–743.
153. Kim JM, Wu H, Green G, et al: CD2-associated protein haploinsufficiency is linked to glomerular disease susceptibility. Science 2003; 300(5623):1298–1300.
154. Larcom RC, Carter GH: Erythrocyes in urinary sediment: Identification and normal limits. J Lab Clin Med 1948; 33: 875–880.
155. Fairley KF, Birch DF: Hematuria: A simple method for identifying glomerular bleeding. Kidney Int 1982; 21(1):105–108.
156. Monte-Verde D, Nosanchuk JS: The sensitivity and specificity of nitrite testing for bacteriuria. Lab Med 1981; 12:755.
157. Kesson AM, Talbott JM, Gyory AZ: Microscopic examination of urine. Lancet 1978; 2:809–812.
158. Prescott LF: The normal urinary excretion rates of renal tubular cells, leucocytes and red blood cells. Clin Sci (Lond) 1966; 31:425.
159. Racusen LC, Fivush BA, Li YL, et al: Dissociation of tubular cell detachment and tubular cell death in clinical and experimental "acute tubular necrosis". Lab Invest 1991; 64(4): 546–556.
160. Mandal AK: Transmission electron microscopy of urinary sediment in renal disease. Semin Nephrol 1986; 6(4):346–370.
161. Mandal AK, Mize GN, Birnbaum DB: Transmission electron microscopy of urinary sediment in aminoglycoside nephrotoxicity. Ren Fail 1987; 10(2):63–81.
162. Segasothy M, Fairley KF, Birch DF, Kincaid-Smith P: Immunoperoxidase identification of nucleated cells in urine in glomerular and acute tubular disorders. Clin Nephrol 1989; 31(6):281–291.
163. Schumann GB: Epithelial cells observed in urine. Urine sediment examination. Baltimore, MD, Williams & Wilkins, 1980, pp 60–87.
164. McBride LJ: Microscopic examination of urine sediment. Textbook of Urinalysis and Body Fluids. Philadelphia, PA, Lippincott, 1998.
165. Schumann GB: Renal casts. Urine Sediment Examination. Baltimore, MD, Williams & Wilkins, 1980, pp 89–110.
166. Foster GS: Excessive physical exertion and its effect on the kidneys. JAMA 1939; 112:891–895.
167. Schrier RW, Hano J, Keller HI, et al: Renal, metabolic, and circulatory responses to heat and exercise. Studies in military recruits during summer training, with implications for acute renal failure. Ann Intern Med 1970; 73(2):213–223.
168. Behrman RA: Urinary findings before and after a marathon race. N Engl J Med 1941; 225:801.
169. Imhof PR, Hushak J, Schumann G, et al: Excretion of urinary casts after the administration of diuretics. Br Med J 1972; 2(807):199–202.

Chapter 5

The Role of the Chronic Kidney Disease Clinic

Bryan M. Curtis, M.D., F.R.C.P.C. • Adeera Levin, M.D., F.R.C.P.C.

The purpose of this chapter is to outline the structure and function of a clinic-based approach for the comprehensive care of patients with chronic kidney disease (CKD Care) and describe some of the potential utilities of such a clinic. The described structure and function may serve as a template for the future development of such clinics. To ensure a context for such a clinic we also review the evidence and rationale supporting this concept. Unlike the paradigm for diabetes, or more recently for heart failure, the role of a clinic facilitating the care of patients with CKD has not been as clearly defined. Thus, data to support the concept and implementation are relatively scant, much being drawn from logical arguments as well as from experience with other chronic diseases.

This chapter will describe CKD as an important health problem, key goals of care, and the evidence on which these are founded. It will also describe the principles of chronic disease management and a model of integrated multidisciplinary team-based care structured on these goals. To complete the chapter, we will review ongoing and future clinical trials to ensure that the reader is prepared for upcoming publications.

Kidney Disease Is an Important Health Care Concern

The burden of disease and the growing population of patients with end-stage renal disease (ESRD) remain exceedingly high. In the United States a diagnosis of ESRD may impart more lost life years than prostate or colorectal cancer.[1] As of 2001 in the United States, there were over 290,000 patients on dialysis and over 15,000 patients with kidney transplants.[2] Population studies such as the NHANES III cross-sectional survey of 29,000 persons revealed that 3% of people over age 17 had elevated creatinine.[3] It is estimated that by 2030, the number of patients with ESRD may reach 2.24 million.[2] Furthermore, the direct cost of caring for a patient on dialysis can cost over $50,000 (U.S.) annually.[4,5]

Kidney Disease Is Largely Due to Chronic Diseases

In North America CKD is largely due to diabetes and hypertension,[2] both relatively easy to identify and treat with evidence-based interventions. The NHANES III survey, for example, showed that an elevated creatinine was more common in people with hypertension.[3] Furthermore, clinical trials and prospective cohort studies have identified risk factors associated with accelerated loss of kidney function. In patients with CKD secondary to diabetic, glomerular and hypertensive/vascular diseases, the strongest predictors of more rapid progression are hypertension, especially systolic,[6–14] and the degree and/or persistence of proteinuria.[15–18]

Historically, the focus of CKD care was to coordinate placement of vascular access, to attend to uremic symptoms and complications, and to provide dialysis. However, the focus has changed; not only is it increasingly recognized that the majority of patients with CKD do not progress to ESRD due to varying rates of progression[11,17] and competing risks for death,[19] but also conditions associated with CKD itself, such as anemia and malnutrition, impart significant morbidity. Moreover, there is now a greater appreciation of the epidemiology of the disease, which has led clinicians to understand that the major competing risk for dialysis therapy was death from cardiovascular disease (CVD). Evidence has accumulated regarding the need for more proactive care and institution of strategies to delay progression. Thus, the focus of CKD care has broadened to include CVD risk reduction, in addition to or concomitant with, reducing the progression of kidney decline.[20] As our understanding has grown of the pathophysiology of kidney disease, and CVD within the CKD population, it has become clearer that the treatment and care options are increasingly complex. In addition, it was logical that identification and intervention in the population with earlier stages of CKD would provide the greatest opportunity to reduce morbidity and mortality.

Goals of Therapy

The goals of therapy (Figure 5–1) are to (1) delay progression of CKD, (2) delay/treat known CVD comorbidities, (3) manage uremic complications (such as anemia, mineral metabolism, nutrition, blood pressure), (4) ensure modality choice and timely placement of access or transplant workup, and (5) initiate timely kidney replacement therapy, including preemptive transplantation where feasible. Each of these goals requires education of patients and caregivers, as well as communication between them, and comanagement by different caregivers within medicine, including allied health professionals. With the one aim to maintain health, it is essential that the structure of the clinic reflect all goals and the demand for communication and investigation, to ensure success.

Staging and Terminology for CKD and Impact on Need for Coordinated Care

In 2002 the National Kidney Foundation sponsored Kidney Disease Outcomes Quality Initiative (K/DOQI) published guidelines targeting earlier evaluation and intervention in patients with CKD.[21] Using evidence-based review, the cornerstone of the working group was the establishment of five

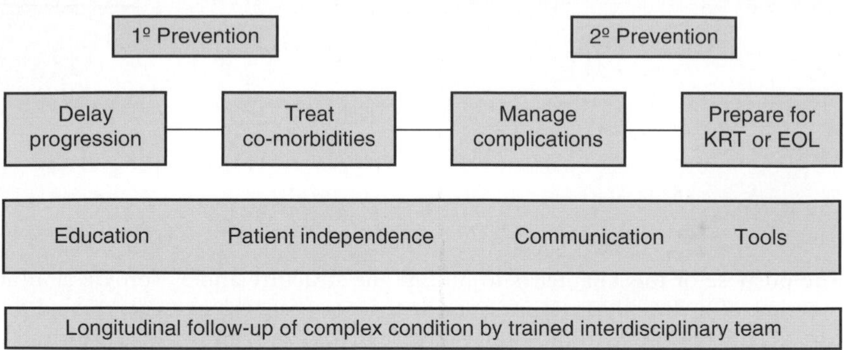

Figure 5–1 Care Goals and Elements of CKD Programs. *EOL*, End of life. *KRT*, Kidney replacement therapy.

Table 5–1 Five Stages of Chronic Kidney Disease

Stage	GFR (ml/min/1.73 m²)	Description
1	>90	Kidney Damage With Normal or ↑ GFR
2	60-89	Kidney Damage With Mild ↓ GFR
3	30-59	Moderate ↓ GFR
4	15-29	Severe ↓ GFR
5	< 15 or (or dialysis)	Kidney Failure

Adapted from Am J Kidney Dis. 2002 Feb;39(2 Suppl 2):S1-246.

stages of kidney disease (Table 5–1). Importantly, the classification system focused on estimated glomerular filtration rate (GFR) rather then serum creatinine levels alone, because use of serum creatinine alone may lead to overestimation or underestimation of kidney function in those with low (i.e., elderly, women) or high (i.e., muscular males, blacks) muscle mass, respectively. The new system based the classification not only on severity of kidney function decline, but also on the presence of conditions associated with the kidney disease, such as proteinuria and hypertension. In attempting to clarify the historic terms, which are confusing and sometimes misleading (pre-dialysis, progressive renal disease, progressive renal insufficiency), this new definition and classification system is an important tool, which aids in the understanding of CKD and will help standardize its definition. A universal language or terminology will facilitate knowledge acquisition by the medical community, patients, and public bodies and improve research clarity and applicability.

The estimates of populations with CKD that were generated from the new classification system, and the NHANES population database, have helped identify the large burden of CKD that potentially exists in the community. The focus on earlier identification will result in increased referrals for diagnosis, care, and follow-up that will overwhelm current nephrology resources, thus the need to create the appropriately structured care delivery systems described herein and to educate other health care providers in CKD care.

Referral

Late referral to nephrology has been recognized as a problem for many years, because it is associated with increased cost.[22–25] Published recommendations emphasize timely referral to maximize potential gains from involvement of specialized nephrology teams.[26] The appropriate time of referral to a nephrologist is debatable for many reasons, including: (1) other physicians should be capable to manage earlier stages of CKD, (2) estimated high numbers of patients overwhelm current nephrology resources, and (3) many patients with early stages of CKD may not progress. Nonetheless, a minimum recommendation would be for referral at GFR levels of less than 60 mL/min/1.73m^2 if the primary caregiver cannot identify the cause of the disease or requires help in the management of disease. All patients with GFR less than 30 mL/min/1.73m^2 should be seen by a nephrology team in order to ensure adequate psychologic and clinical preparation for kidney replacement therapy,[26,27] unless the patient is of an age or has a condition that leads them to not consider chronic dialysis. The new CKD staging system focused on GFR estimation should reduce some of the problems of late referral due to misinterpretation of serum creatinine values.

OVERVIEW OF CKD CLINIC

Philosophic Basis

Clinics for the care of CKD should be based on the fundamental principle of ensuring the delivery of longitudinal, complex care to a large diverse group of individuals. This requires that the structure of the clinic and services offered optimize communication within and between individuals, including the patient and other physicians and medical teams.

Role of Multidisciplinary Clinics

The importance of early referral to nephrologists is not disputed,[26] because identification of the myriad of abnormalities and plans for their treatment is best achieved in consultation with a specialist. However, the ability of nephrologists "alone" to attend to the multiple and complex aspects of care in this patient group is debated.[28] A multicenter cohort of patients starting dialysis demonstrated that even those patients known to nephrologists for greater than 3 months have suboptimal care. In this study, one third did not have permanent access ready for dialysis initiation, mean hemoglobin was 94 g/L, and mean albumin was below 34 g/L.[29] In another multicenter study of patients with CKD followed by nephrologists, the majority of patients had blood pressure over recommended targets, and only 50% were taking angiotensin converting enzyme (ACE) inhibitors. Furthermore, despite a history of significant heart disease and 66% prevalence of dyslipidemia, only 22% of at-risk patients were on lipid lowering medications. Abnormalities of calcium, phosphate, and parathyroid hormone levels were also demonstrated with only 15% of patients receiving therapy.[30] While there are undoubtedly patient and compliance factors that explain why patients with CKD under the care of nephrologists do not have optimal care, it is also probable that patients were not provided the appropriate elements of care. It is important to note, however, that it was these studies and others that contributed to the recognition of the importance of CKD care and lack of attention to it.

Given the multiplicity of goals of CKD care, the complexity of treatment options, and educational needs, it is clear that a team of individuals will be required. Treatment targets, such as blood pressure, may be reached by involving expert nurses, pharmacists, or other members of the team in conjunction with the physician.[31] Thus, a team approach with well-defined roles, responsibilities, and objectives appears to be both logical and practical. Improved patient care and outcomes due to a multidisciplinary team clinic have been demonstrated in disciplines such as diabetology,[32,33] cardiology,[34–36] rheumatology,[37–39] and oncology.[40] Similarly, compared to standard care by a nephrologist alone, there is evidence of benefit of a multidisciplinary care (MDC) team approach in the care of patients with CKD.[41–43] It appears that outcomes can be improved with protocol-based blood work, clinic visits, and education. This requires involvement of a patient educator, dietitian, social worker, and physician.

There has been only one randomized, controlled trial of case management in CKD, published by Harris and associates,[44] and it did not show a benefit to case management in CKD. However, the intervention in that study was limited to written suggestions made to primary care physicians and the assigned clinic patients did not receive any specific treatment for anemia, mineral metabolism, or for preparation for dialysis/transplant. Failure to show a benefit in the Harris study may well have been due to the failure of individual primary care physicians (PCP) to implement the recommendations from the clinic. Given that PCPs are inundated with protocols and guidelines for the management of numerous chronic conditions, it is unrealistic to expect them to be able to fully attend to the many complex issues of advancing CKD.

Structure and Definition of Multidisciplinary Clinics

These definitions help to clarify the definition of a multidisciplinary team as intended by the authors. It allows the readers to determine what type of resources they currently have available and may help in the interpretation of clinical studies so that similar types of clinics can be compared. Clinic structures can be categorized as follows with respect to multidisciplinary teams:

Formal Multidisciplinary Team

Nurses, nurse educators, dietitians, social workers, and physicians allied in a formal relationship, who interact with the patient and each other defines a multidisciplinary team. Although it is recognized that there are a number of different configurations due to funding and local health care system issues, for the purpose of definition, this team is readily identifiable as dedicated (part time or full time) to CKD care, and may or may not have team rounds or meetings to discuss patient care.

Informal Multidisciplinary Resources

Nurses, social workers, dietitians, and physicians associated with the kidney team to whom patients are referred may constitute informal resources. In such a schema, patient access is dependent of individual patient needs, and the group of individuals may or may not interact as a team or be necessarily dedicated to the longitudinal follow-up of patients. Each team member is able to interact with the patient on a regular basis as necessary, but no coordination with other team members is inherent to its structure.

No Multidisciplinary Team

Nurses, social workers, and dietitians may or may not be available to the patient. There is no team structure or function.

KEY GOALS OF CKD CARE

The following section describes the key goals of comprehensive CKD care, citing evidentiary basis as appropriate for the described strategies, including diagnosis, education, delay of progression, identification and treatment of comorbidities associated with CKD, and of complications of CKD. As well, the institution of primary prevention strategies, including vaccination programs and the preparation of patients for renal replacement therapy as appropriate, will be discussed. The goals described are comprehensive and complex, thus the need for a protocolized structured delivery system, such as a formal clinic.

Diagnosis

The first goal of the nephrology clinic medical staff should be to attempt to establish or confirm a diagnosis and to determine the rate of progression of kidney disease.

The nephrologist should ensure that appropriate tests have been undertaken to establish a diagnosis. Kidney biopsy or imaging may be helpful,[26] especially to rule out any potentially treatable or reversible etiologies such as rapidly progressive glomerulonephritis or obstruction. In early visits, reversible causes of kidney disease should be sought, even if a chronic etiology is suspected, especially if there has been a rapid decline in kidney function. In addition to diagnostic tests, review of current medications to ensure the absence of nephrotoxic medications is prudent. Further workup includes a review of family history and medications, and a search for systemic disease, including diabetes, vascular disease, connective tissue disorders, infections, and malignancy. Several contributory factors may coexist. The extent of comorbidities, especially the commonly associated vascular diseases[45] should be continually assessed. Although established kidney disease may progress even if the original cause is removed,[46] similar interventions that can slow loss of kidney function may prevent cardiovascular complications. Potentially harmful interventions, such as iodinated intravenous contrast dye, must be reviewed with the patient so that educated decisions may be made regarding their use.

Education

Patient education and awareness are an integral component of the clinic. Education is important from a decision-making perspective as well as to alleviate fear and psychologic suffering. Educated patients are more likely to take an active part in their care, with better outcomes noted in other chronic diseases.[47–49] Ideally, involvement of family members or other support network individuals should be encouraged. The clinic environment can provide a set of resources as well as sessions related to patient education. Minimal education should include the following, presented at the appropriate stages of CKD:

- Explanation of normal kidney function, blood pressure, and laboratory test results and their significance.
- Explanation of specific disease conditions, symptoms, and complications of CKD.
- Dietary teaching and diabetes education, if appropriate.
- Ensuring that patient understanding of medications is adequate.
- Discussions about vein preservation (blood taking and blood pressure).
- Erythropoietin hormone therapy teaching, including: importance of anemia and its treatment; ensure patient understanding of dose changes; warning of the side effects of iron therapy; self-administration or local administration by PCP or community nurse; and provision of educational materials to PCP.
- Discussion of choices for treating ESRD, including conservative therapy, hemodialysis, peritoneal dialysis, and transplant.
- The education effort can be augmented with pamphlets or video materials. Using the principles of adult learning, regular reinforcement of the key messages should be incorporated into the education program.

Delay of Progression

The cornerstone of CKD care is to delay progression of kidney disease and, thereby, reduce complications related to kidney failure. The evidence is relatively consistent in citing that interruption of the renin-angiotensin system (RAS) is a key component to delaying progression. Control of hypertension and reduction of proteinuria are important consequences of RAS interruption and are described more fully later.

Hypertension Treatment

Blood pressure goals should be based on the average of two or more seated readings on each of two or more office visits.[50] There is substantial evidence to support the optimal and target blood pressure of less than 130/80 mmHg in patients with established kidney disease, as suggested in the guidelines of the Seventh Joint National Committee for Prevention, Detection, Evaluation and Treatment of High Blood Pressure.[11,50–53] The goals are to reduce the rate of decline of kidney function[56] and decrease cardiovascular events and mortality. The recommended target blood pressure for patients with proteinuria greater than 1 g/day is less than 125/75.[53] This is based on evidence of slower progression of kidney failure at this level of blood pressure in a large randomized trial, which showed the greatest gain in those with the most proteinuria.[11–12] Patients with kidney disease often need between three and four different medications in addition to lifestyle modification in order to achieve this goal.[55] ACE inhibitors, angiotensin receptor blockers, β-blockers, calcium channel blockers, and diuretics are key drug classes for achieving blood pressure control.[11, 57–59]

Proteinuria Reduction

Patients with CKD and persistent proteinuria of greater than 3 g/day may progress to requiring dialysis or transplant within 2 years.[6, 60, 61] A number of large, randomized, controlled trials demonstrated the efficacy of ACE inhibitors in slowing progression of kidney disease, reducing proteinuria, and also in regressing left ventricular hypertrophy.[62–68] As some of these trials were placebo-controlled, it is difficult to be sure that the benefit was drug specific and not just due to blood pressure lowering. Nevertheless, follow-up studies suggest that long-term ACE inhibition, as a component of a blood pressure therapy, can be associated with stabilization and even improvement of kidney function.[68] Prophylactic use can also be justified in type II diabetics, because ACE inhibition preserved kidney function for over 6 years in normotensive type II diabetics without microalbuminuria.[69] More recently, the use of angiotensin receptor blockers (ARB) have been shown to reduce the time to doubling of serum creatinine, reduction of proteinuria, and time to dialysis.[57,58,70] All of these recent studies have been performed in diabetics. Mann and associates[71] have demonstrated the utility of ace inhibitor use in patients with established CVD, diabetes plus one risk factor, and kidney disease, in a subanalysis of HOPE. More recently, a trial demonstrated that dual blockade of the renin-angiotensin system with both an angiotensin-converting enzyme inhibitor and an angiotensin-II receptor blocker (vs. monotherapy and placebo) may offer additional renal and cardiovascular protection in type I diabetic patients with diabetic nephropathy.[70]

Management of Comorbidity: Secondary Prevention

Cardiovascular Disease

CKD is a risk factor for vascular events and death.[72,73] Creatinine values as low as 130 to 150 μmol/L confer a threefold risk of death within 8 years.[72] Cardiovascular death is 25 times as common as death due to kidney failure in type II diabetics with microalbuminuria.[74] The prevalence of cardiomyopathy, symptomatic heart failure, and symptomatic ischemic heart disease is very high at dialysis initiation.[75] This suggests that the later stages of CKD are a state of high cardiac risk.

Reversible cardiac risk factors, identified in these earlier stages, persist following entry to dialysis. Left ventricular hypertrophy (LVH) occurs in the CKD population, and its prevalence is inversely related to the level of declining kidney function.[76] Anemia and hypertension are also risk factors for progressive LV growth.[76] In kidney transplant recipients, a model of CKD, hypertension is a risk factor for LV growth, de novo heart failure, and de novo ischemic heart disease.[77,78] Anemia predisposes to de novo heart failure, as does hypoalbuminemia.[78] In addition, dyslipidemia and smoking are risk factors for ischemic heart disease.[79,80]

The National Kidney Foundation convened a task force in 1997 to specifically examine the epidemic of CVD in chronic kidney disease.[81] With a focus on decreasing death rates via strategies for prevention of disease, the task force considered whether strategies learned from the general population are applicable to patients with CKD. Recognized traditional risk factors identified in the general population include diabetes, hypertension, smoking, family history of coronary disease, male gender, older age, high low-density lipoprotein cholesterol, low high-density lipoprotein cholesterol, physical inactivity, menopause, and psychologic stress (Table 5–2).

As CKD progresses, additional risk factors related to chronic uremia also emerge. Excess cardiac risk may also be due to hemodynamic and metabolic perturbations, including fluid overload, anemia, malnutrition, hypoalbuminemia, inflammation, dyslipidemia, prothrombotic factors, hyperhomocysteinemia, increased oxidative stress, divalent ion abnormalities, vascular calcification, and hyperparathyroidism.[82,83]

Patients with kidney failure therefore require assessment and therapy for vascular disease and associated risk factors. It should be noted that many risk factors for CVD are also associated with the risk of progression of chronic kidney failure.[84] Thus, risk factor reduction strategies used to prevent CVD in the general population can be applied to patients with CKD and may slow the progression of kidney disease as well.[84] It remains unclear whether a raised serum creatinine is a marker for more severe hypertension, diabetes mellitus, and vascular disease, which causes death, or a marker for some intrinsic property of kidney disease, which accelerates CVD. However, some factors more peculiar to kidney disease (anemia, hypoalbuminemia, dyslipidemia) induce cardiac risk and may be amenable to intervention.

Table 5–2 Risk Factors for Cardiovascular Disease*

Traditional	Uremic
Diabetes	Hemodynamic overload
Hypertension	Anemia
History of smoking	Malnutrition
Family history of coronary disease	Hypoalbuminemia
Male gender	Inflammation
Older age	Prothrombotic factors
Dyslipidemia	Hyperhomocysteinemia
Proteinuria	Increased oxidative stress
Physical inactivity	Divalent ion abnormalities
Menopause	Vascular calcification
Psychological stress	Hyperparathyroidism

→ **Progression of CKD**

*As CKD progresses there is a parallel evolution of risk factors from taonal to those characteristic of chronic uremia.

Anemia

It has become increasingly evident that anemia is an important predictor of morbidity and mortality in the dialysis population.[85–87] It is associated with ischemic heart disease, left ventricular hypertrophy, and impaired quality of life.[85,87,88] Correction of anemia in CKD improves physical function, energy, cognitive function, and sexual function.[85,89–92]

Treatment of anemia with erythropoietin is effective. Studies are currently underway to determine whether early initiation of therapy among individuals with earlier stages of CKD is effective in preventing CVD, decreasing progression of kidney disease, or improving QOL.[87,93,94] There is evidence to suggest that iron supplementation in early kidney disease is important to maintain erythropoiesis, and that erythropoietin therapy is needed to maintain hemoglobin levels. Specific targets for hemoglobin levels have not yet been determined, though levels between 110 and 125 g/L are the current recommended guidelines.[85,95,96]

Mineral Metabolism

There is evidence to support the efficacy of calcium and/or vitamin D supplementation for treatment of hyperparathyroidism.[97–100] At the current time, recommendations regarding target values for patients with earlier stages of CKD have been extrapolated from those for patients with ESRD. We propose an approach that attempts to prevent hyperparathyroidism and its associated long-term complications. Phosphate reduction using dietary restriction, and inexpensive phosphate binders/calcium supplementation in those who have evidence of elevated intact parathyroid hormone (iPTH), and low normal calcium levels is reasonable. Vitamin D analogues are useful for those in whom PTH remains elevated despite calcium supplementation and phosphate restriction. Physiologic release of hormones is pulsatile and, thus, intermittent oral vitamin D therapy is recommended. Unfortunately, evidence for the effectiveness of therapeutic strategies and for specific target levels of each of the variables mentioned above is not available for earlier stages of CKD. Adherence to the principle of prevention, combined with early identification of calcium, phosphate, and PTH abnormalities at early stages of CKD, should lead to minimizing hyperplasia of the parathyroid glands and the attendant metabolic derangements. Future studies will need to address long-term targets and therapeutic strategies.

Nutrition

Malnutrition is common in patients with later stages of CKD. There is a strong association between decreased albumin and worse nutritional status, and adverse outcomes.[89,101–103] Even small decreases in albumin are associated with increased mortality. Unfortunately, albumin is a late index of malnutrition and is a negative acute phase reactant. Acidosis is also a contributor to protein breakdown and mineral metabolism aberrations. Thus, assessment of nutritional status generally requires the expertise of a dietitian.

Low protein diets have been extensively studied as a means to slow the progression of kidney disease, with mixed results. Meta-analyses and a large, randomized trial suggest that the impact may be slight.[11,104–106] Optimal dietary protein intake is not clear,[104] and there is a potential for protein malnutrition. Appropriate nutritional counseling to avoid malnutrition, acidosis, and phosphate excess is important. There are extensive guidelines for assessment of nutritional status and dietary management proposed by the National Kidney Foundation.[107] Ensuring adherence to a prescribed diet is difficult and requires frequent, continuous input from dietitians. This becomes especially important as the patient approaches ESRD, since worsening malnutrition may become the principal indication to initiate dialysis.

Management of Comorbidity: Primary Prevention

Primary prevention strategies are also important in the management of patients with CKD and may sometimes be overlooked due to the time-intensive management of conditions associated with uremia. Vaccinations, use of aspirin and lipid lowering agents and other CVD primary prevention strategies, as well as diabetes control, smoking cessation, and lifestyle modification are important. This section briefly touches on these strategies in CKD patients.

Vaccinations

Hepatitis B infection remains a concern in dialysis populations, and current recommendations are to vaccinate if eligible. In addition, there are recommendations to vaccinate patients with CKD against pneumococcal infections and influenza, which are common sources of morbidity in patients with chronic illnesses. Vaccination programs have been less successful among CKD patients compared to the general population, both in terms of implementation and response to vaccine. Reasons for poor response include malnutrition, uremia, and generalized immunosuppressive state of patients with CKD. However, variations in vaccination dose and dosing schedule to increase response rates in dialysis patients have been tried with reasonable success, which could be implemented among patients at all stages of CKD. In general, patients with higher GFR levels are more likely to respond with seroconversion to hepatitis B[108] and other vaccines. This reinforces the need to identify CKD early and provide comprehensive care.

Aspirin

The use of low dose aspirin should be considered to reduce the risk of subsequent CVD in patients with coronary artery disease or in those who are at high risk of developing coronary disease,[81] which included most patients with CKD. Recommendations to use aspirin should take into consideration the individual patient's risks of bleeding or other complications of aspirin. If there are contraindications to aspirin use, the use of other antiplatelet agents could be considered.

Dyslipidemia

There are no trials showing that treating dyslipidemia slows the progression of kidney disease. Based on randomized trial evidence of cardiovascular protection, current guidelines recommend an aggressive approach to lipid abnormalities in diabetics and other high-risk patients, which would include those with CKD.[52,109] Thus, best practice would suggest following the guidelines of the National Cholesterol Education Program Adult Treatment Panel II for initial classification, treatment initiation, and target cholesterol levels for diet or drug therapy.[110] Finally, the Heart Protection Study suggested benefit in treating patients with coronary disease, other occlusive arterial disease, or diabetes largely irrespective of initial cholesterol concentrations.[111]

Diabetes Control

Optimal glycemic control in those patients with diabetes mellitus should be encouraged and facilitated with referral to a diabetes clinic if possible. Tight glucose control in both types I and II diabetes may prevent or stabilize the early stages of microvascular complications, including nephropathy.[112,113] The impact seems to be sustainable for years.[114] However, diabetic control has not been shown to slow progression of advanced diabetic nephropathy. Furthermore, as kidney function deteriorates, diabetes management will require modification.

Lifestyle Modification

Smoking cessation is recommended for many reasons, including the possibility that it may slow loss of kidney function.[115,116] Obesity, poor diet, and sedentary lifestyle contribute to diabetes, hypertension, and vascular disease. Current recommendations are thus to achieve and maintain an ideal body mass index and moderate level of physical activity for 30 minutes per day for most days of the week.[81]

Rehabilitation

Cost of kidney disease from loss of work and associated loss of QOL is substantial. Strategies to enable patients to remain working or return to work should be in place and may involve referral to work retraining programs or occupational therapists, if available.[43,117]

PREPARATION FOR KIDNEY REPLACEMENT THERAPY

Preparation for kidney replacement therapy should be based on a good basic knowledge of kidney function, ideally a long process that begins well before the imminent need for initiation exists. Modality selection is done collaboratively with the team and the patients, with an attempt to ensure that patients maintain independent care status and choose modalities that foster such independence. The appropriate timing of initiation of dialysis remains unclear, but it is certain that it must be individualized and must be based generally on a combination of low GFR, patient symptoms, and other factors. Close follow-up of patients at the later stages of CKD, with objective assessment of global functioning, permits appropriate timing of dialysis initiation.

Modality Selection and Access Placement

Modality selection is a decision for the informed patient. It is unknown whether peritoneal dialysis or hemodialysis imparts a survival advantage over the other, as neither randomized trials have been done nor is one feasible in the future. Transplantation is a medically and economically superior treatment[128] for kidney replacement therapy and is associated with higher quality of life. At any given time approximately 50% to 60% of patients receiving dialysis are eligible for transplantation, but estimates are not available for those with earlier stages of CKD. Not all patients are eligible for transplantation, such as those with severe underlying illness. Preemptive transplantation, that is, before the need for dialysis, is generally possible for only those with an available live donor. In the United States, approximately 30% of transplants are from living donors, and a fifth of these are unrelated to the recipient.

It is clear that for some people, contraindications to one of the modalities may exist; for example, extensive prior abdominal surgery may negate the possibility of peritoneal dialysis. Importantly, the patient's desire to undertake chronic dialysis must be closely explored, because there may be some with serious underlying illnesses who choose to not undertake renal replacement therapy.

The options for kidney replacement therapy need to be reviewed with the patient, and access should be planned appropriately, if needed. The reality of how long it takes to decide on modality, get access placed, and let access mature should be stressed to patients, as should the possibility that the first access may not work. A perspective on the relative amount of time required to prepare for each of the options, including transplantation, should be provided. It should also be stressed that the presence of a working access (such as a functioning fistula) does not mean the patient has to start dialysis any earlier. A functioning, albeit unused, access only ensures that additional procedures such as placement of a temporary catheter, might be avoided.

Lack of preparation for dialysis increases morbidity and cost.[118–120] Cost and morbidity implications of temporary catheter access are extensive. They include the cost of catheters, insertion fees, radiology tests, and costs associated with complications such as infection and thrombosis, as well as the pain, discomfort, and time of the patient.

Planning for kidney replacement therapy should begin at least 6 months in advance of anticipated start. According to most published guidelines,[95] access should be created at GFR at approximately 20 to 25 mL/min in those who are anticipated to progress and who do not have a reasonable chance for a preemptive transplant. Reasons for lack of access at dialysis start may include patient factors such as denial of inevitable dialysis, being too sick to undergo permanent access procedures, or late decision to undertake chronic dialysis. However, this may also reflect the CKD team's inability to predict dialysis start, lack of resources, or poor planning. Late recognition of CKD and late referral to nephrology contribute to the problem.

In consultation with the patients and the clinic team, optimal timing around education, decision making, and access creation should be undertaken.

Timely Initiation

When to initiate dialysis is a complex decision that involves the consideration of many variables. There are some easily identified absolute indications for initiation,[121] however, debate exists with respect to "timely" dialysis when these indicators are not so apparent. Indeed, since the 1970s Bonomini[102, 122–125] has argued for initiation of dialysis before clinically significant markers of uremia appear. His studies suggested a positive association between residual kidney function at dialysis initiation and clinical outcomes. Unfortunately, lead-time bias, patient selection, or referral bias may favor outcomes in the population of patients starting "timely" dialysis. Further complicating the issue is the lack of a tool to define where a patient is on the time line of CKD, for both planning and comparison of study results. To date, there is no solid evidence regarding how "early" dialysis should be started for optimizing patient outcomes.

Presently, two main indices for initiating dialysis for the treatment of kidney failure following progression of CKD are: (1) low GFR and (2) symptoms or signs of uremia, or evidence of malnutrition.[95] Despite the lack of firm evidence, the National Kidney Foundation guidelines, first published in 1997 and updated in 2000, recommend that patients should begin dialysis when the GFR falls below 10.5 mL/min/1.73m^2 (approximates a Kt/V_{urea} of 2.0), unless edema-free body weight is stable or increased, the normalized protein nitrogen appearance nPNArate is greater than or equal to 0.8 gm/kg/day, and there are no clinical signs or symptoms of uremia.[126] More recently, the Canadian Society of Nephrology has recommended that dialysis should be initiated when the GFR is less than 12 mL/min if evidence of uremia or malnutrition (nPNA $<$ 0.8 g/kg/day, or clinical evidence of malnutrition) exists. Despite these and other guidelines, when to initiate dialysis remains debatable. Overall, the key factor is to avoid commencing dialysis when the patient is so ill that education opportunities and the chances for maintaining independence are impaired.

Hemodialysis

The goal is a nontraumatic start to hemodialysis care, and the CKD clinic staff should ensure the appropriate commencement of dialysis, including ensuring that patients have appropriate vascular access and are oriented to the hemodialysis unit. Schedules should be coordinated with appropriate team members in the hemodialysis unit, family members, and other medical professionals. The CKD clinic should send initial dialysis orders and transfer summaries to the hemodialysis unit.

Peritoneal Dialysis

Patients should be oriented to the peritoneal dialysis unit and staff. The role of the CKD clinic in organizing peritoneal dialysis catheter placement will vary from center to center. However, the timing, placement, and preliminary education should be done in concert with the peritoneal dialysis team. As in hemodialysis, specific orders and transfer summaries should be sent to the peritoneal dialysis unit and the training/initiating schedule coordinated with appropriate team members, family members, and other health professionals.

Transplant

As part of the educational process early in the course of CKD, the concepts of transplantation and living donation should be explored with patients and families. The CKD clinic working closely with the transplant assessment team can help determine eligibility for a transplant. Furthermore, a CKD clinic can facilitate preemptive transplantation, which is generally only possible if the patient with CKD has an available live donor.

Conservative Care

Not all patients will desire or benefit from kidney replacement therapy; longer-term education, longer follow-up time, and an established relationship with CKD team members will facilitate making this choice. In these cases, the CKD clinic staff may be the first to be aware of the wishes of the patients and families, and other caregivers should be informed of these decisions. Once such a decision is made, end-of-life wishes should be formalized, in particular extent of resuscitation attempts, with appropriate consent and documentation. Resources to ensure appropriate supportive care short of dialysis should be mobilized, because much can be done to maintain a patient who chooses to not undertake chronic dialysis. The patient should have referral for home care and for palliative care when appropriate. Patients may benefit from remaining in the care of the CKD team as plans of care may require revision or the patient may change his mind.

CLINIC LOGISTICS

Services

The CKD clinic would presumably exist within a health care system and society where the common goal is the health of the patients. Comprehensive care delivered in only one location is presumed to be beneficial. The frequency with which any individual patient accesses care is determined by the specific circumstances of the medical system, the other physicians involved in patient care, additional comorbid conditions, as well as the specific stage of disease. The clinic should provide a wide range of services for patients with kidney disease, and their physicians, with the overall goals of:

1. Ensuring patient and family understanding of kidney disease.
2. Ensuring understanding of health care system/hospital and outpatient systems and services available to kidney patients.
3. Identifying potential issues related to long-term patient management.
4. Facilitating longitudinal and parallel care of patients with CKD.

Key Components of the Clinic

The clinic should ideally be an outpatient facility providing easy access to all facilities and personnel in one location. This permits familiarity with team members and access to ancillary services as needed. If also located in proximity to the hospital or dialysis center, it provides familiarity with the respective hospital services and locations. Non-English patients should have interpreters provided and booked for entire duration of the clinic visit. It helps if interpreters are able to return with specific patients to facilitate continuity. An information package should be available and given out at the first visit, including an introduction to how the clinic works and various educational materials, including goals and expectations. Patients and families should also have an introduction to team members and explanation of roles and responsibilities. Finally, the clinic should facilitate peer support for patients with CKD.

In addition to ongoing assessment of patient by the team through regular clinic visits, weekly multidisciplinary rounds should be organized to facilitate communication and develop or adjust plan of care. This will allow for comprehensive follow-up by nurses, clerical staff, and others and facilitate:

- Bookings for tests (US, CT, etc.) and referrals to other specialists
- Medication changes/tolerance, etc.
- Reminders for appointments/blood work.
- Follow-up of test results.
- Liaison with laboratories and pharmacies.
- Liaison with GP and other consultants, including palliative care team (in hospital or community).
- Patients should receive education about kidney or kidney/pancreas transplant and screening for potential donors and referrals as appropriate.

Individual Roles

In order for any team to function, definition and clarification of roles of the individuals involved are important. Below are listed key roles and responsibilities for each of the key staff deemed important in the delivery of CKD care. The specifics may vary depending on local issues, but the principal roles need to be clearly defined.

Nurse

The CKD nurses function as case managers and facilitate care of patients, directly and through physician and team member liaison. Nursing support should be available 5 days a week by telephone or in person to triage medical concerns, answer questions, provide education or emotional support and referral to other team members or community resources. This should allow for ongoing collaboration and reevaluation with the patient, and facilitate changes in care plan with input from team members. A regular review of symptoms, medications, and monitoring of lab work results should occur, again responding to critical values by notifying physician, patient, and dietitian as necessary. The nurse should be able to liaise with family physicians, consultants, and other chronic disease clinics (e.g., diabetes, health heart, heart function clinic).

Nurses should be able to implement protocols such as hepatitis screening and vaccination program or peri-angiogram protocols. Similarly, they should be able to arrange treatment and procedures such as I.V. iron and transfusions or arrange referral for dialysis access and follow-up care. If patients progress to kidney failure, then the nurse should ensure coordination of initiation of dialysis or referral for transplantation and transfer of relevant data to dialysis or transplant facility. Finally, they should coordinate services in remote settings for the convenience of patients.

Dietitian

Patients should receive individualized diet education and counseling regarding CKD, diabetes, and heart disease, from a dietitian knowledgeable about the nutritional abnormalities of CKD. The dietitian should review diet history, habits and nutritional health, and advise patient about food choices and meal ideas. There should be a periodic dietary review, including blood work, to help reach goals and to avoid malnutrition.

Social Worker

Social workers may provide assistance with emotional and practical concerns of patients and their families, and assess emotional needs or potential issues that may arise, such as acceptance of kidney failure and end-of-life issues. The social worker should have a mechanism to liaise with psychiatry as needed. They also advocate on patient's behalf to ensure maximum allowable benefit from available resources such as home support, financial assistance, employment/retraining, and housing, and may need to assist the patient with insurance issues, including referral to institutional financial counselors.

Pharmacist

If possible, pharmacy services should be available for initial medication review and follow-up. They may advise about medication costs, pill burden, and possible interactions. They may also provide education and support as needed.

Clerical or Administrative Support

Clinics should have a dedicated unit coordinator/clerical support worker. Their main role is to ensure that data and patient charts are maintained accurately. A paper/electronic chart should be established with complete information available and maintained with ongoing follow-up data. This will include data such as labs, medications, and comorbidities. The coordinator is an essential component of the team as the organization of booking and coordinating appointments with other clinics, consultants, diagnostics, and community resources and follow-up is essential. Additionally, they are integral for information and chart transfer to programs within the kidney programs such as dialysis or transplant clinic. They may also triage patient concerns with the team and have appointment reminders for patients. Finally, they should identify interpreter requests and book interpreters as needed.

CKD Clinic Role in Longitudinal Care: Different Stages of CKD

Given the current estimates of the CKD population (between 10 and 20 million in the United States), it is unlikely that the optimal resources described in this chapter are available to all patients with CKD. It is still debated whether a nephrologist must see all patients with early CKD, as it is not clear who will and will not progress. Although there is consensus that nephrologists and teams need to see the patients at least 6 months, and ideally 12 months, prior to dialysis start for access, there remains skepticism regarding the utility of nephrology input prior to that time.

Although much has been learned about care of patients close to initiating dialysis, it is not known how to optimally care for patients in early CKD (frequency of visits, frequency of blood work, when to initiate "early" drug therapy, etc.). It seems reasonable that a "phased" approach is applicable. As outlined, the focus of the clinic must be adjustable from early disease detection and risk factor modification to preparing for kidney replacement therapy. Key at all phases would be communication and education between patients, medical caregivers, and allied health teams (Figure 5–2).

One end of the spectrum is an early referral (stage I or II) and a broad plan outlined to another caregiver about goals of treatment for that caregiver to follow. Patients could be familiarized with the clinic and kidney disease at this initial period and then referred back to the clinic if the kidney function deteriorates, for further education and refinement of management plan. Both the patient and the other caregiver are informed that the clinic is available when needed for either informal consultation or formal evaluation. The other end of the spectrum is for the clinic to assume most of the care, if not all, surrounding issues pertaining to kidney disease and other issues such as diabetes management. In between, the clinic could do a formal initial evaluation and then arrange follow-up once every year or so. To date there are no studies that have systematically evaluated the impact of different methods of care at earlier stages of CKD, though a number of trials are being planned.

CKD Clinic Role in Parallel Care: Integrating with Other Caregivers

An important issue in dealing with individual patients who are obtaining care in parallel locations (i.e., family physicians, diabetic services, and CKD clinic) is communication. The clinic should be viewed as a resource to both patients and parallel caregivers such as family and other physicians, and as such, could integrate care with other caregivers. For example, other caregivers could call to seek advice regarding safety of medications, and the clinic can serve as a facility to follow the patients during acute events (e.g., increased creatinine around diarrhea and temporarily holding the ace inhibitor). It is vital for such a clinic to communicate information about patient status, medications, plans, and so forth, not only to the patient but to all other caregivers involved (family physicians, diabetes clinics, hospital charts).

When inpatients are accessing different care systems due to the complex nature of their disease or due to practical issues such as locale, it is not so clear how to determine the responsibility of each of the individual medical practitioners. Should the CKD clinic assume the ace inhibitor is being managed by the heart failure clinic? Or does the CKD clinic assume the diabetes clinic is managing the blood sugar control or counseling about smoking cessation? At what point in the stage of CKD does the CKD clinic take a more active role? These are not questions that will be answered in clinical trials, so practical solutions to the issue of responsibility for care implementation will need to be developed. Again the key issue here is the communication between different physician group and medical teams and customization to individual patient and health care system particulars. There is an accumulating body of literature[47–49] that suggests involvement of the patient in all implementation plans, and knowledge of and active involvement in therapy targets and test results improve the ability of physicians to implement care strategies.

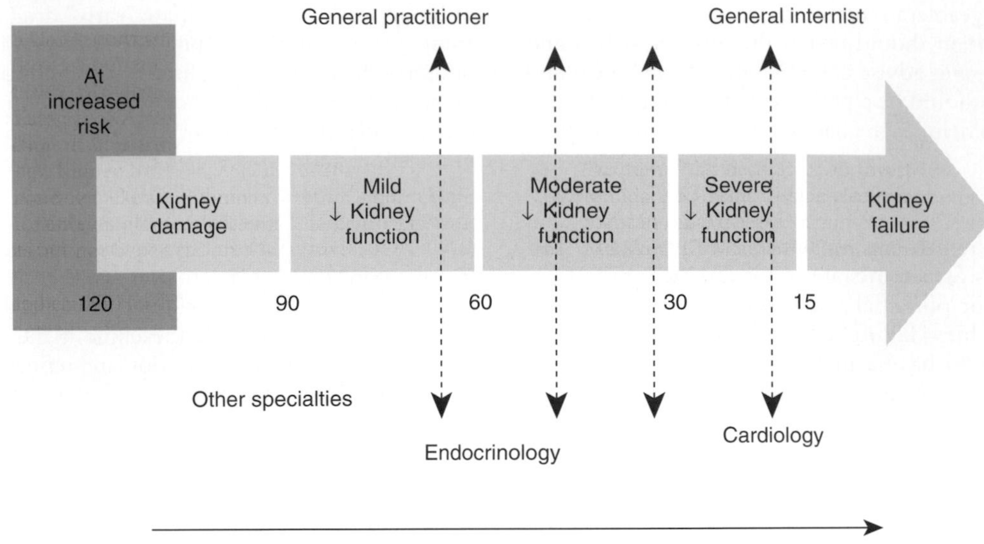

Figure 5–2 Integration of care over the progression of CKD (Longitudinal Care) and between other caregivers (Parallel Care).

Other Benefits of the CKD Clinic and Organized Protocolized Care

The key to the care of patients with chronic diseases is acknowledgment of the complexity of the condition(s) and the need for longitudinal follow-up by a well-trained team. As in oncology, rheumatology, and other areas of medicine, the care of CKD patients requires some adoption of protocols for investigation, therapy, and follow-up (Figure 5–3 and Table 5–3). In so doing, we will be able to develop sensible strategies based on data, and management of selected conditions will be uniformly undertaken. The systematic evaluation and management of patients with chronic diseases has been demonstrated to reduce resource utilization and to enhance patient compliance.

Table 5–3 Example of a Protocol for Follow-up/Blood Work Intervals*

Minimum follow-up/bloodwork intervals as a function of kidney function		
Creatinine Clearance (mL/min)	**Interval between visits/bloodwork**	
	Diabetics	**Non-diabetics**
31-60	3 months	3 months
15-30	2 months	3 months
10-14	1 month	2 months
<10	1 month	1 month

*Maximum intervals (or minimum frequency) between visits are given for stable patients. Shorter intervals may be necessary at discretion of physician or specialized nurse in less stable patients, or be specified in therapy titration algorithms (e.g., initiation of erythropoietin replacement therapy).

The additional advantages to the clinic models for the care of CKD include the ability to optimize all aspects of care by using individual team member's expertise more appropriately and to optimize follow-up and monitoring of large groups of patients in one area. Furthermore, a clinic-based approach would allow database development and evaluation of outcomes in large cohorts of patients, the ability to enroll patients in clinical trials, and importantly, the adoption of newer proven therapies may be easier in a clinic setting than in individual physician offices.

The clinic structure may also ensure that patients have access to appropriate current information and materials that may not be available in individual physician offices. Also, it will permit coordination of care plans and execution of those plans within any health system structure.

Barriers to care or implementation of strategies can be identified in a clinic setting. The costs and the number of medications required for CKD is becoming progressively daunting and leads to problems with compliance. These problems are more likely to be identified within a clinic setting, where social workers, pharmacists, and others may identify issues not identified by physicians. The importance of an asymptomatic condition can be reinforced in clinic settings where the patient–team interaction is far longer than the usual patient–doctor interaction.[41] Although there may be multiple problems and barriers that interfere with achieving the care goals in any one individual, the presence of an organized team approach is more likely to ensure the identification of those barriers in a timely manner.

FUTURE STUDIES

The CAN-CARE (Canadian Care Prior to Dialysis) Study is a prospective multicenter cohort study of incident patients with estimated GFR less than 50 mL/min referred to nephrol-

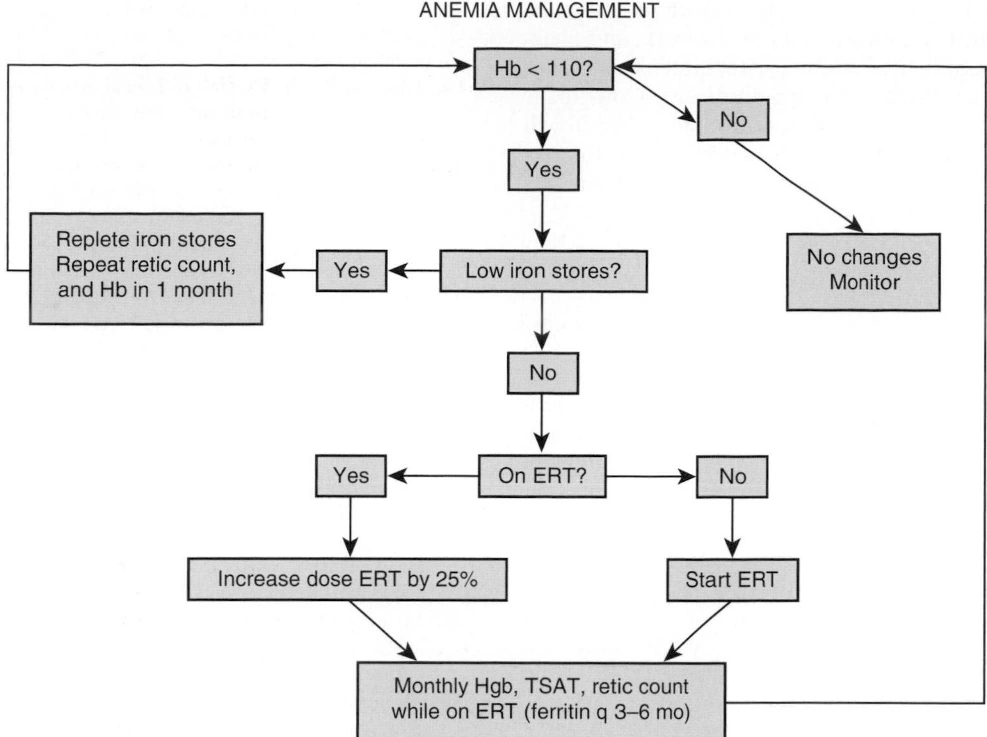

Figure 5–3 An example of a protocol for anemia management that may guide therapy by physician or specialized nurse. It assumes all secondary causes of anemia have been ruled out. *ERT,* erythropoietin replacement therapy (erythropoietin or darbopoieten); *Hb,* hemoglobin.

ogists across Canada. Enrollment began November 2000 with a planned follow-up of up to 4 years. The objectives are to describe: (1) the specific care ("elements") these patients receive over time, (2) the prevalence of cardio-renal risk factors at referral and at 12 and 24 months, and (3) the link between specific elements of care and outcomes/quality of life. The Study of Treatment for Renal Insufficiency: Data and Evaluation (STRIDE) registry will study data on prevalent CKD patients in nephrology practices in the United States.[128] The Chronic Renal Insufficiency Cohort (CRIC) Study will examine risk factors for progression of CKD and CVD among those patients. The main goal is to develop models identifying high-risk subgroups and, subsequently, increase application of preventive therapies.[129] The Kidney Early Evaluation Program (KEEP) was implemented to increase awareness of kidney disease among those at highest risk and, subsequently, to improve outcomes through early detection and referral for care. The KEEP 2.0 screening program identified persons with reduced kidney function and suboptimal care. The KEEP 3.0 will continue to identify individuals at high risk for kidney disease and will address educational needs by randomly assigning participants to one of several educational programs.[130]

The Can-Prevent trial is a proposed Canada-wide multicenter clinical trial to address the hypothesis that compared to usual care, a nurse supported by a nephrologist, running a multiple risk factor intervention and disease management clinic for people with moderate chronic kidney disease identified by laboratory based case-finding, will reduce or delay the onset of advanced kidney disease, cardiovascular events, and death. The study will also assess the effect on health care resource use, costs, and quality of life. Measurements of quality of life (QOL) in kidney patients have demonstrated worsening QOL as a function of anemia and need for dialysis. A systematic study of QOL prior to dialysis has not been undertaken, because there is a lack of organized access to this group of patients. Well designed studies are needed to better understand the impact of various therapeutic regimens on patient perceptions of health and wellness. Furthermore, the study will measure aspects of the professional care delivered (e.g., time spent, education provided) and assess the association of these with outcome. Interventions applied will include lowering blood pressure to target, maximal use of renin-angiotensin system interruption, treatment of dyslipidemia, prophylactic aspirin when indicated, treatment of renal anemia, disordered calcium/phosphate and parathyroid metabolism, use of β-blockers in heart failure and post myocardial infarction, control of diabetes, and smoking cessation.

CONCLUSION

Kidney disease involves the complex physical, mental, and social aspects of health mandating an understanding and rational utilization of available resources. Opportunities exist to improve early identification and follow-up of patients with CKD and to ensure better outcomes overall, regardless of whether patients ultimately require dialysis.

In order to focus on these complex aspects of care, the inclusion of medical, nursing, dietary, social work, and pharmacy staff in a coordinated system, with protocolized goals and systematic approaches to longitudinal follow-up is required. It is hoped that the information supplied herein will help develop templates and deliveries of care models for further evaluation, so that, ultimately, the outcomes of patients with CKD at all stages of disease are improved.

References

1. Kiberd BA, Clase CM: Cumulative risk for developing end-stage renal disease in the U.S. population. J Am Soc Nephrol 2002; 13:1635–1644.
2. U.S. Renal Data System. USRDS 2003 Annual Data Report: Atlas of end-stage renal disease in the United States. Bethesda, MD, National Institutes of Health, National Institute of Diabetes and Digestive and Kidney Diseases, 2003.
3. Coresh J, Wei GL, McQuillan G, et al: Prevalence of high blood pressure and elevated serum creatinine level in the United States: Findings from the Third National Health and Nutrition Examination Survey (1988–1994). Arch Intern Med 2001; 161:1207–1216.
4. Goeree R, Manalich J, Grootendorst P, et al: Cost analysis of dialysis treatments for end-stage renal disease (ESRD). Clin Invest Med 1995; 18(6):455–464.
5. Lee H, Manns B, Taub K, et al: Cost analysis of ongoing care of patients with end-stage renal disease: The impact of dialysis modality and dialysis access. Am J Kidney Dis 2002; 40(3):611–622.
6. Ruggenenti P, Gambara V, Perna A, et al: The nephropathy of non-insulin dependent diabetes: Predictors of outcome relative to diverse patterns of renal injury. J Am Soc Nephrol 1998; 9:2336–2343.
7. Biesenbach G, Janko O, Zazgornik J: Similar rate of progression in the predialysis phase in Type I and Type II diabetes mellitus. Nephrol Dial Transplant 1994; 9:1097–1110.
8. Perneger TV, Brancati FL, Whelton PK, Klag MJ: End-stage renal disease attributable to diabetes mellitus. Ann Intern Med 1994; 121:912–918.
9. Marcantoni C, Jafar TH, Oldrizzi L, et al: The role of systemic hypertension in the progression of nondiabetic renal disease. Kidney Int 2000; 75:S44–S48.
10. Perry HM, Miller JP, Fornoff JR, et al: Early predictors of 15-year end-stage renal disease in hypertensive patients. Hypertension 1995; 25(part 1):587–594.
11. Klahr S, Levey AS, Beck GJ, et al: Modification of Diet in Renal Disease Study Group: The effects of dietary protein restriction and blood pressure control on the progression of chronic renal disease. New Engl J Med 1994; 330:877–884.
12. Peterson JC, Adler S, Burkart IM, et al: Blood pressure control, proteinuria, and the progression of renal insufficiency. Kidney Int 1992; 42:452–458.
13. Oldrizzi L, Bright C, De Biase V, Maschio G: The place of hypertension among the risk factors for renal function in chronic renal failure. Am J Kidney Dis 1993; 21(suppl 2):119–123.
14. He J, Whelton PK: Elevated systolic blood pressure as a risk factor for cardiovascular and renal disease. J Hypertens 1999; 17(suppl 2):S7–S13.
15. Walser M: Progression of chronic renal failure in man. Kidney Int 1990; 37:1195–1210.
16. Nolin L, Courteau M: Management of IgA nephropathy: Evidence-based recommendations. Kidney Int 1999; 70: S56–S62.
17. Hunsicker LG, Adler S, Caggiula A, et al: Modification of Diet in Renal Disease Study Group: Predictors of the progression of renal disease in the Modification of Diet in Renal Disease Study. Kidney Int 1997; 51:1908–1919.
18. Keane WF: Proteinuria: Its clinical importance and role in progressive renal disease. Am J Kidney Dis 2000; 35(4 suppl 1):S97–S105.
19. Muntner P, Jiang H, Hamm L, et al: Renal insufficiency and subsequent death resulting from cardiovascular disease in the United States. J Am Soc Nephrol 2002; 13:745–753.
20. Culleton BF, Larson MG, Wilson PWF, et al: Cardiovascular disease and mortality in a community-based cohort with mild renal insufficiency. Kidney Int 1999; 56:2214–2219.
21. National Kidney Foundation: K/DOQI clinical practice guidelines for chronic kidney disease: Evaluation, classification, and stratification. Am J Kidney Dis 2002; 39(2 suppl 1):S1–S266.
22. Levin A: Consequences of late referral on patient outcomes. Nephrol Dial Transplant 2000; 15(suppl 3):8–13.
23. Stack AG: Impact of timing of nephrology referral and pre-ESRD care on mortality risk among new ESRD patients in the United States. Am J Kidney Dis 2003; 41(2):310–318.
24. Kinchen KS, Sadler J, Fink N, et al: The timing of specialist evaluation in chronic kidney disease and mortality. Ann Intern Med 2002; 137(6):479–486.
25. McLaughlin K, Manns B, Culleton B, et al: An economic evaluation of early versus late referral of patients with progressive renal insufficiency. Am J Kidney Dis 2001; 38(5):1122–1128.
26. Mendelssohn DC, Barrett BJ, Brownscombe LM, et al: Elevated levels of serum creatinine: Recommendations for management and referral. Can Med Assoc J 1999; 161(4):413–417.
27. McClellan WM, Knight DF, Karp H, Brown WW: Early detection and treatment of renal disease in hospitalized diabetic and hypertensive patients: Important differences between practice and published guidelines. Am J Kidney Dis 1997; 29(3):368–375.
28. Obrador G, Ruthazer R, Arora P, et al: Prevalence of and factors associated with suboptimal care before the initiation of dialysis in the United States. JASN 1999; 10:1793–1800.
29. Curtis BM, Barrett BJ, Jindal K, et al: Canadian survey of clinical status at dialysis initiation 1998–1999: A multicenter prospective survey. Clin Nephrol 2002; 58(4):282–288.
30. Levin A, Djurdjev O, Barrett B, et al: Cardiovascular disease in patients with chronic kidney disease: Getting to the heart of the matter. Am J Kidney Dis 2001; 38(6):1398–1407.
31. Balas EA, Weingarten S, Garb CT, et al: Improving preventive care by prompting physicians. Arch Intern Med 2000; 160:301–308.
32. Gaede P, Vedel P, Parving HH, Pedersen O: Intensified multifactorial intervention in patients with type II diabetes mellitus and microalbuminuria: The steno type II randomised study. Lancet 1999; 353:617–622.
33. Norris SL, Nichols PJ, Caspersen CJ, et al: The effectiveness of disease and case management for people with diabetes: A systematic review. Am J Prev Med 2002; 22:15–38.
34. Harris DE, Record NB, Gipson GW, Pearson TA: Lipid lowering in a multidisciplinary clinic compared with primary physician management. Am J Cardiol 1998; 81:929–933.
35. McAlister FA, Lawson FM, Teo KK, Armstrong PW: A systematic review of randomized trials of disease management programs in heart failure. Am J Med 2001; 110:378–384.
36. McDonald K, Ledwidge M, Cahill J, et al: Heart failure management: Multidisciplinary care has intrinsic benefit above the optimization of medical care. J Card Fail 2002; 8(3):142–148.
37. Vliet Vlieland TP, Breedveld FC, Hazes JM: The two-year follow-up of a randomized comparison of in-patient multidisciplinary team care and routine out-patient care for active rheumatoid arthritis. Br J Rheumatol 1997; 36(1):82–85.
38. Vliet Vlieland TP, Zwinderman AH, Vandenbroucke JP, et al: A randomized clinical trial of in-patient multidisciplinary treatment versus routine out-patient care in active rheumatoid arthritis. Br J Rheumatol 1996; 35(5):475–482.
39. Prier A, Berenbaum F, Karneff A, et al: Multidisciplinary day hospital treatment of rheumatoid arthritis patients. Evaluation after two years. Rev Rhum Engl Ed 1997; 64:7–9, 443–450.

40. Gabel M, Hilton NE, Nathanson SD: Multidisciplinary breast cancer clinics. Do they work? Cancer 1997; 79(12):2380–2384.
41. Levin A, Lewis M, Mortiboy P, et al: Multidisciplinary predialysis programs: Quantification and limitations of their impact on patient outcomes in two Canadian settings. Am J Kidney Dis 1997; 29(4):533–540.
42. Klang B, Bjorvell H, Berglund J, et al: Predialysis patient education: Effects on functioning and well-being in uremic patients. J Adv Nursing 1998; 28:36–44.
43. Rasgon SA, Chemleski BL, Ho S: Benefits of a multidisciplinary predialysis program in maintaining employment among patients on home dialysis. Adv Perit Dial 1996; 12:132–135.
44. Harris LE, Luft FC, Rudy DW, et al: Effects of multidisciplinary case management in patients with chronic renal insufficiency. Am J Med 1998; 105:546–548.
45. Sarnak MJ, Levey AS: Cardiovascular disease and chronic renal disease: A new paradigm. Am J Kidney Dis 2000; 35(4 suppl 1):S117–S131.
46. Klahr S, Schreiner G, Ichikawa I: The progression of renal disease. New Engl J Med 1988; 318:1657–1666.
47. Loveman E, Cave C, Green C, et al: The clinical and cost-effectiveness of patient education models for diabetes: A systematic review and economic evaluation. Health Technol Assess 2003; 7(22):iii, 1–190.
48. Latos D, Schatell D: The nephrologist's critical role in patient education. Adv Ren Replace Ther 2003; 10(2):146–149.
49. Wright SP, Walsh H, Ingley KM, et al: Uptake of self-management strategies in a heart failure management programme. Eur J Heart Fail 2003; 5(3):371–380.
50. Aram VC, George LB, Henry RB et al: The National High Blood Pressure Education Program Coordinating Committee: The Seventh Report of the Joint National Committee on Prevention, Detection, Evaluation, and Treatment of High Blood Pressure. JAMA 2003; 289:2560–2571.
51. Bakris GL, Williams M, Dworkin L, et al: Preserving renal function in adults with hypertension and diabetes: A consensus approach. National Kidney Foundation Hypertension and Diabetes Executive Committees Working Group. Am J Kidney Dis 2000; 36(3):646–661.
52. Meltzer S, Leiter L, Daneman D, et al: 1998 clinical practice guidelines for the management of diabetes in Canada. Can Med Assoc J 1998; 159(8 suppl):S1–S29.
53. 1999 Canadian recommendations for the management of hypertension. Can Med Assoc J 1999; 161(12 suppl):S13.
54. U.K. Prospective Diabetes Study (UKPDS) Group: Tight blood pressure control and risk of macrovascular and microvascular complications in type II diabetes: UKPDS 38. BMJ 1998; 317:703–713.
55. Hansson L, Zanchetti A, Carruthers SG, et al: Effects of intensive blood-pressure lowering and low dose aspirin in patients with hypertension: Principal results of the hypertension optimal treatment (HOT) randomised trial. Lancet 1998; 351:1755–1762.
56. Estacio RO, Gifford N, Jeffers BW, Schrier RW: Effect of blood pressure control on diabetic microvascular complications in patients with hypertension and type II diabetes. Diabetes Care 2000; 23(suppl 2):B54–B64.
57. Brenner BM, Cooper ME, deZeeuw D, et al: RENAAL Study Investigators: Effects of losartan on renal and cardiovascular outcomes in patients with type II diabetes and nephropathy. N Engl J Med 2001; 345:861–869.
58. Lewis EJ, Hunsicker LG, Clarke WR, et al: Renoprotective effect of the angiotensin receptor antagonist irbesartan in patients with nephropathy due to type II diabetes. N Engl J Med 2001; 345:851–860.
59. Keane WF, Brenner BM, De Zeeuw D, et al: The risk of developing end-stage renal disease in patients with type II diabetes and nephropathy: The RENAAL Study. Kidney Int 2003; 63(4):1499.
60. Locatelli F, Marcelli D, Comelli M, et al: Proteinuria and blood pressure as causal components of progression to end-stage renal failure. Nephrol Dial Transplant 1996; 11:461–467.
61. The GISEN Group: Randomised placebo-controlled trial of effect of ramipril on decline in glomerular filtration rate and risk of terminal renal failure in proteinuric, non-diabetic nephropathy. Lancet 1997; 349:1857–1863.
62. Lewis EJ, Hunsicker LG, Bain RP, Rohde RD: The effect of angiotensin-converting-enzyme inhibition on diabetic nephropathy. The Collaborative Study Group. N Engl J Med 1993; 329:1456–1461.
63. Ravid M, Savin H, Jutrin I, et al: Long-term stabilizing effect of angiotensin-converting enzyme inhibition on plasma creatinine and on proteinuria in normotensive type II diabetic patients. Ann Intern Med 1993; 118:577–581.
64. Philipp T, Anlauf M, Distler A, et al: HANE Trial Research Group: Randomised, double blind, multicentre comparison of hydrochlorothiazide, atenolol, nitrendipine, and enalapril in antihypertensive treatment: Results of the HANE study. BMJ 1997; 315:154–159.
65. Estacio RO, Jeffers BW, Hiatt WR, et al: The effect of nisoldipine as compared with enalapril on cardiovascular outcomes in patients with non-insulin-dependent diabetes and hypertension. N Engl J Med 1998; 338:645–651.
66. Ravid M, Lang R, Rachmani R, Lishner M: Long-term renoprotective effect of angiotensin-converting enzyme inhibition in non-insulin-dependent diabetes mellitus: A 7-year follow-up study. Arch Intern Med 1996; 156:286–289.
67. Giatras I, Lau J, Levey AS: Angiotensin-Converting-Enzyme Inhibition and Progressive Renal Disease Study Group: Effect of angiotensin-converting enzyme inhibitors on the progression of nondiabetic renal disease: A meta-analysis of randomized trials. Ann Intern Med 1997; 127:337–345.
68. Ruggenenti P, Perna A, Gherardi G, et al: gruppo Italiano di Studi in Nefrologia (GISEN): Renal function and requirement for dialysis in chronic nephropathy patients on long-term ramipril: REIN follow-up trial. Lancet 1998; 352: 1252–1256.
69. Ravid M, Brosh D, Levi Z, et al: Use of enalapril to attenuate decline in renal function in normotensive, normoalbuminuric patients with type II diabetes mellitus. Ann Intern Med 1998; 128:982–988.
70. Jacobsen P, Andersen S, Jensen BR, Parving HH: Additive effect of ACE inhibition and angiotensin II receptor blockade in type I diabetic patients with diabetic nephropathy. Am Soc Nephrol 2003; 14(4):992–999.
71. Mann JF, Gerstein HC, Pogue J, et al: Renal insufficiency as a predictor of cardiovascular outcomes and the impact of ramipril: The HOPE randomized trial. Ann Intern Med 2001; 134(8):629–636.
72. Shulman NB, Ford CE, Hall D, et al: Prognostic value of serum creatinine and effect of treatment of hypertension on renal function. Hypertension 1989; 13(suppl 1):I80–I93.
73. Kannel WB, Stampfer MJ, Castelli WP, Verter J: The prognostic significance of proteinuria: The Framingham study. Am Heart J 1984; 108(5):1347–1352.
74. Schmitz A, Vaeth M: Microalbuminuria: A major risk factor in non-insulin dependent diabetes. A 10-year follow-up study of 503 patients. Diabetes Med 1988; 5:126–134.
75. Curtis BM, Parfrey PS: How can the cardiac death rate be reduced in dialysis patients? Semin Dial 2002; 15(1):22–24.
76. Levin A, Singer J, Thompson CR, et al: Prevalent left ventricular hypertrophy in the predialysis population: Identifying opportunities for intervention. Am J Kidney Dis 1996; 27(3): 347–354.
77. Rigatto C, Foley RN, Kent GM, et al: Long-term changes in left ventricular hypertrophy after renal transplantation. Transplantation 2000; 27;70(4):570–575.

78. Rigatto C, Jeffrey J, Foley R, et al: Risk factors for de novo congestive heart failure in renal transplant recipients (Abstract, A3708). J Am Soc Nephrol 2000; 11:705A.
79. Rigatto C, Jeffrey J, Foley R, et al: Risk factors for de novo ischemic heart disease in renal transplant recipients (Abstract, A3709). J Am Soc Nephrol 2000; 11:705A.
80. Kasiske BL, Guijarro C, Massy ZA, et al: Cardiovascular disease after renal transplantation. J Am Soc Nephrol 1996; 7(1):158–165.
81. National Kidney Foundation Task Force on Cardiovascular Disease: Controlling the epidemic of cardiovascular disease in chronic renal disease. Am J Kidney Dis 1998; 32(suppl 3): S1–S199.
82. Foley RN, Parfrey PS, Sarnak MJ: Clinical epidemiology of cardiovascular disease in chronic renal disease. Am J Kidney Dis 1998; 32(suppl 3):112–119.
83. Parfrey PS (ed): Cardiac disease in chronic uremia: Uremia-related risk factors. Seminars in Dialysis 1999; 12:61–132.
84. Sarnak MJ, Levey AS: Cardiovascular disease and chronic renal disease: A new paradigm. Am J Kidney Dis 2000; 35(4 suppl 1):S117–S131.
85. Levin A: How should anaemia be managed in pre-dialysis patients? Nephrol Dial Transplant 1999; 14(suppl 2):66–74.
86. NKF–DOQI clinical practice guidelines for the treatment of anemia of chronic renal failure: National Kidney Foundation–Dialysis Outcomes Quality Initiative. Am J Kidney Dis 1997; 30(4 suppl 3):S192–S240.
87. Levin A, Thompson CR, Ethier J, et al: Left ventricular mass index increase in early renal disease: Impact of decline in hemoglobin. Am J Kidney Dis 1999; 34(1):125–134.
88. Harnett JD, Kent GM, Foley RN, Parfrey PS: Cardiac function and hematocrit level. Am J Kidney Dis 1995; 25(4 suppl 1):S3–S7.
89. Lowrie EG, Lew NL: Death risk in hemodialysis patients: The predictive value of commonly measured variables and an evaluation of death rate differences between facilities. Am J Kidney Dis 1990; 15(5):458–482.
90. Madore F, Lowrie EG, Brugnara C, et al: Anemia in hemodialysis patients: Variables affecting this outcome predictor. J Am Soc Nephrol 1997; 8(12):1921–1929.
91. Silverberg D, Blum M, Peer G, Iaina A: Anemia during the predialysis period: A key to cardiac damage in renal failure. Nephron 1998; 80(1):1–5.
92. Silberberg J, Racine N, Barre P, Sniderman AD: Regression of left ventricular hypertrophy in dialysis patients following correction of anemia with recombinant human erythropoietin. Can J Cardiol 1990; 6(1):1–4.
93. Collins AJ, Ma JZ, Xia A, Ebben J: Trends in anemia treatment with erythropoietin usage and patients' outcomes. Am J Kidney Dis 1998; 32(6 suppl 4):S133–141.
94. Levin A: Anaemia in the patient with renal insufficiency: Documenting the impact and reviewing treatment strategies. Nephrol Dial Transplant 1999; 14:2, 292–295.
95. Churchill DN (chairperson): 1999 Clinical Practice Guidelines of the Canadian Society of Nephrology for Treatment of Patients with Chronic Renal Failure. J Am Soc Nephrol 1999; 10(suppl 13).
96. Jacobs C, Horl WH, Macdougall IC, et al: European best practice guidelines 9–13: Anaemia management. Nephrol Dial Transplant 2000; 15(suppl 4):33–42.
97. Rostand G, Frueke TB: Parathyroid hormone, vitamin D and cardiovascular disease in chronic renal failure. Kidney Int 1999; 56(2):383–392.
98. Fournier A, Aparicio M: Recommendations for clinical practice concerning the prevention of renal osteodystrophy before extra-renal purification. Nephrologie 1998; 19:129–130.
99. Nordal KP, Dahl E, Halse J, et al: Long-term low-dose calcitriol treatment in predialysis chronic renal failure: Can it prevent hyperparathyroid bone disease? Nephrol Dial Transplant 1995; 10:203–206.
100. Combec C, Aparicio M: Phosphorus and protein restriction and parathyroid function in chronic renal failure. Kidney Int 1994; 46:1381–1386.
101. Hakim R, Levin N: Malnutrition in hemodialysis patients. Am J Kidney Dis 1993; 21:125–137.
102. Churchill DN: An evidence-based approach to earlier initiation of dialysis. Am J Kidney Dis 1997; 30(6):899–906.
103. Culp K, Flanigan M, Lowrie EG, et al: Modeling mortality risk in hemodialysis patients using laboratory values as time-dependent covariates. Am J Kidney Dis 1996; 28(5):741–746.
104. Kasiske BL, Lakatua JDA, Ma JZ, Louis TA: A meta-analysis of the effects of dietary protein restriction on the rate of decline in renal function. Am J Kidney Dis 1998; 31:954–961.
105. Fouque D, Wang P, Laville M, Boissel JP: Low protein diets delay end-stage renal disease in non-diabetic adults with chronic renal failure. Cochrane Database Syst Rev 2000; 2:CD001892.
106. Waugh NR, Robertson AM: Protein restriction for diabetic renal disease. Cochrane Database Syst Rev 2000; 2:CD002181.
107. Clinical Practice Guidelines for Nutrition in Chronic Renal Failure. Am J Kidney Dis 2000; 35(suppl 2):S56–S64.
108. Da Roza G, Loewen A, Djurdjev O, et al: Stage of chronic kidney disease predicts seroconversion after hepatitis B immunization: Earlier is better. Am J Kidney Dis 2003 (in press).
109. Frohlich J, Fodor G, McPherson R, et al: Rationale for and outline of the recommendations of the Working Group on Hypercholesterolemia and Other Dyslipidemias: Interim report. Dyslipidemia Working Group of Health Canada. Can J Cardiol 1998; 14(suppl A):17A–21A.
110. Summary of the second report of the National Cholesterol Educational Program (NCEP): Expert panel on detection evaluation and treatment of high blood cholesterol in adults. JAMA 1993; 269:3015–3023.
111. Heart Protection Study Collaborative Group: MRC/BHF Heart Protection Study of cholesterol lowering with simvastatin in 20,536 high-risk individuals: A randomised placebo-controlled trial. Lancet 2002; 360(9326):7–22.
112. The Diabetes Control and Complications Trial Research Group: The effect of intensive therapy of diabetes on the development and progression of long-term complications in insulin-dependent diabetes mellitus. New Engl J Med 1993; 329:977–986.
113. U.K. Prospective Diabetes Study (UKPDS) Group: Intensive blood-glucose control with sulphonylureas or insulin compared with conventional treatment and risk of complications in patients with type II diabetes (UKPDS 33). Lancet 1998; 352(9131):837–853.
114. The Diabetes Control and Complications Trial/Epidemiology of Diabetes Interventions and Complications Research Group: Retinopathy and nephropathy in patients with type I diabetes four years after a trial of intensive therapy. New Engl J Med 2000; 342:381–389.
115. Regalado M, Yang S, Wesson DE: Cigarette smoking is associated with augmented progression of renal insufficiency in severe essential hypertension. Am J Kidney Dis 2000; 35:687–694.
116. Orth SR, Stockmann A, Conradt C, et al: Smoking as a risk factor for end-stage renal failure in men with primary renal disease. Kidney Int 1998; 54:926–931.
117. Rasgon S, Schwankovsky L, James-Rogers A, et al: An intervention for employment maintenance among blue-collar workers with end-stage renal disease. Am J Kidney Dis 1993; 22:403–412.
118. Ifudu O, Dawood M, Homel P, Friedman EA: Excess morbidity in patients starting uremia therapy without prior care by a nephrologist. Am J Kidney Dis 1996; 28(6):841–845.
119. Jungers P, Zingraff J, Albouze G, et al: Late referral to maintenance dialysis: Detrimental consequences. Nephrol Dial Transplant 1993; 8:1089–1093.
120. Schmidt RJ, Domico JR, Sorkin MI, Hobbs G: Early referral and its impact on emergent first dialyses, health care costs, and outcome. Am J Kidney Dis 1998; 32(2):278–283.

121. Hakim RM, Lazarus JM: Initiation of dialysis (editorial). J Am Soc Nephrol 1995; 6(5):1319–1328.
122. Bonomini V, Vangelista A, Stefoni S: Early dialysis in renal substitute programs. Kidney Int 1978; 13:S112–S116.
123. Bonomini V: Early dialysis. Nephron 1979; 24:157–160.
124. Bonomini V, Baldrati L, Stefoni S: Comparative cost/benefit analysis in early and late dialysis. Nephron 1983; 33:1–4.
125. Bonomini V, Feletti C, Scolari MP, Stefoni S: Benefits of early initiation of dialysis. Kidney Int 1985; 28(suppl 17): S57–S59.
126. Laupacis A, Keown P, Pus N, et al: A study of the quality of life and cost-utility of renal transplantation. Kidney Int 1996; 50: 235–242.
127. Clinical Practice Guidelines for Hemodialysis Adequacy. Am J Kidney Dis 1997; 30(suppl 3):S15–S66.
128. Rao M, Kausz AT, Mitchell D, et al: The Study of Treatment for Renal Insufficiency: Data and Evaluation (STRIDE), a national registry of chronic kidney disease. Semin Dial 2002; 15(5):366–369.
129. Feldman HI, Appel LJ, Chertow GM, et al: Chronic Renal Insufficiency Cohort (CRIC) Study Investigators: The Chronic Renal Insufficiency Cohort (CRIC) Study: Design and methods. J Am Soc Nephrol 2003; 14(7 suppl 2):S148–S153.
130. Ohmit SE, Flack JM, Peters RM, et al: Longitudinal study of the National Kidney Foundation's (NKF) Kidney Early Evaluation Program (KEEP). J Am Soc Nephrol 2003; 14(7 suppl 2): S117–S121.

Complications of Chronic Kidney Disease

Chapter 6

Uremic Toxicity

Raymond Camille Vanholder, M.D., Ph.D. • Griet Glorieux, M.Sc., Ph.D. • Rita De Smet, M.Sc., Ing. • Norbert Hendrik Lameire, M.D., Ph.D.

The uremic syndrome is a complex of biologic and biochemical alterations that result in a host of failing organs and disturbing symptoms. It originates from the retention of solutes, that under normal conditions are cleared by the kidneys into the normal urine, although derangements of hormonal, metabolic, and enzymatic axes also play a role. The impact of retention is underscored by the clinical improvement resulting from dialysis and kidney transplantation.

The uremic syndrome is characterized by a deterioration of biochemical and physiologic functions (Table 6–1), in parallel with the progression of renal failure. This results in a variable number of symptoms, which mimic the picture of exogenous poisoning. Although the link between clinical deterioration and uremia has already been recognized decades ago, and although the number of new pathophysiologic elements provided in this area has risen exponentially over the last few years, our knowledge about the responsible factors remains incomplete.

In this chapter, the current knowledge about the uremic syndrome, its clinical and biochemical characteristics, and the factors playing a role in its development will be reviewed.

CLINICAL CHARACTERISTICS

Cardiovascular System

Cardiovascular anomalies occur almost invariably when renal function deteriorates[1]: hypertension, congestive heart failure, valvular stenosis or insufficiency and accelerated atheromatosis are among the most frequent epiphenomena.[2–4] Cardiovascular death is the most frequent cause of mortality in patients with end-stage renal disease.[5] A major point of concern in the uremic population is the accelerated development of atheromatosis, which starts already in the pre-dialytic phase.[6] Recently, atheromatosis has been classified as an inflammatory, rather than a degenerative disease.[7] Also in renal failure, inflammation and cardiovascular disease have been linked to each other.[8–10] Recently, a failure of the arterial vessel wall to relax,[11] resulting in systolic hypertension and diastolic hypotension, as well as an accelerated deposition of calcium in the vessel wall, even in young patients, has been described.[12] These events result in an inadequate coronary perfusion, since blood stream through the coronaries normally takes place during diastole.

Pericarditis has become rare with the advent of adequate dialysis strategies, except in patients who are referred too late and/or in patients with major access problems.

Cardiac hypertrophy and dilated cardiomyopathy are common findings in end-stage renal failure.[13] Myocardial dysfunction is related to an increase in myocardial cell calcium content.[14] Increased cytosolic Ca^{++} is also related to increased peripheral vascular resistance and hypertension.[15] Endothelium-dependent vasodilation is impaired in uremia.[16,17]

In spite of elevated circulating catecholamines, a diminished response of the cardiac α- and β-receptors has been reported,[18] which may be related to uremic autonomic neuropathy. Vasoconstrictive response during postural stress is lacking.[19] Moreover, the binding properties of catecholamines to vascular and myocardial adrenergic receptors may be altered.[20]

Apart from changes in systolic cardiac contractility, a decrease in diastolic compliance also plays a major pathophysiologic role.[21] This alteration is not necessarily related to previous hypertension. The basic mechanism is associated with an activation of interstitial cells and increased volume of interstitial cell nuclei and cytoplasm, whereby uremia increases myocardial interstitial ground substance.[21]

Although the importance of cardiovascular changes has been emphasized in end-stage renal failure,[22] uremia-induced atherogenic alterations probably start to take place much earlier, especially in patients with additional risk factors.[23]

Although many factors and retention solutes seem to be involved in cardiovascular disturbances of uremia, at present pro-inflammatory agents such as the cytokines,[8] oxidation products[24] and glycation products[25] are considered the main culprits. In view of its role in the general population,[26] also the role of homocysteine has been considered,[27] but its

Table 6–1 The Uremic Syndrome — Main Clinical Alterations

1) Cardiovascular system	– growth retardation
– atheromatosis	– hyperparathyroidism
– arteriosclerosis	– hypogonadism
– cardiomyopathy	– impotence, diminished libido
– decreased diastolic compliance	*6) Bone disease*
– hyper/hypotension	– adynamic bone disease
– pericarditis	– amyloidosis (β_2-microglobulin)
2) Nervous system	– defective calcitriol metabolism
– concentration disturbances	– osteitis fibrosa
– cramps	– osteomalacia
– dementia	– oseoporosis
– depression	*7) Skin*
– fatigue	– melanosis
– headache	– pruritus
– motor weakness	– uremic frost
– polyneuritis	*8) Gastro-intestinal system*
– reduced sociability	– anorexia
– restless legs	– dyspepsia
– sleep disorders	– gastro-intestinal ulcers
– stupor, coma	– hiccup
3) Hematological system / coagulation	– nausea, vomiting
– anemia	– pancreatitis
– bleeding	*9) Pulmonary system*
– hypercoagulability	– pleuritis
4) Immunological system	– pulmonary edema
– inadequate antibody formation	– sleep apnoea syndrome
– stimulation of inflammation (baseline)	*10) Miscellaneous*
– susceptibility to cancer	– hypothermia
– susceptibility to infection	– thirst
5) Endocrinology	– uremic foetor
– dyslipidemia	– weight loss
– glucose intolerance	

relevance remains difficult to prove in the uremic population.[28] Phosphate and an increased calcium-phosphate product are also considered to play a germane role[29] by provoking calcium deposition in the vessel wall. Also, hyperparathyroidism induces vascular calcification, essentially of the small and medium-sized vessels.[30] The guanidine asymmetric dimethyl arginine (ADMA) which is known to inhibit nitric oxide (NO) generation, has been related to vascular damage.[31]

Nervous System

During the progress of renal failure, uremic encephalopathy may develop alone or in combination with peripheral neuropathy.[32] The spectrum of central neuropathy is variable and ranges from minor mental disturbances to coma, but in the case of adequate dialysis, encephalopathy is exceptional today. Sleep disorders, on the other hand, are frequent, often in the context of the obstructive sleep apnea syndrome.[33] Brain stem-evoked potentials are disturbed, both in the pre-dialysis stage and after dialysis has been started.[34]

Also clinically overt peripheral polyneuropathy is exceptional today, although less pronounced variants that are only detectable by electromyography still persist, even in patients treated by acceptable dialysis, according to the current standards. Data regarding the responsible toxins are scarce; a substantial part of the presently available evidence points in the direction of the guanidines.[35] A recent comprehensive study disclosed an additional number of potential culprits, essentially small protein-bound compounds, such as spermine, spermidine and *p*-cresol.[36] Peripheral polyneuropathy might be improved by the application of large pore/high-flux membranes, which points to a role for larger "middle" molecules,[37] although this effect might as well be the result of the biocompatibility of these membranes.Vitamin and trace element deficiencies might additionally contribute to this problem.[38, 39]

HEMATOLOGY

Until the therapeutic applicability of recombinant erythropoietin, uremic anemia was one of the main components of the unsatisfactory quality of life of many renal failure patients. Anemia is mainly attributable to inappropriate erythropoietin production by the failing kidneys, but also defective body iron stores, resistance to iron, vitamin deficiencies, and increased blood losses might be at play, as well as erythrocyte fragility, in part related to hyperparathyroidism.[40]

The role of uremic retention solutes in the inhibition of erythropoiesis remains a matter of debate. The polyamines spermine and spermidine were suspected to inhibit hematopoiesis *in vitro*.[41,42] Segal and associates[46] suggested, however, that their inhibitory effect was aspecific,[43] and the above impact of polyamines on hematopoiesis was, to our knowledge, never confirmed. Other uremic retention solutes that have been incriminated are furancarboxylic acid (3-carboxy-4-methyl-5-propyl-2-furanpropionic acid [CMPF]),[44] parathyroid hormone,[45] and the inflammatory cytokines.

Insulin-like growth factor I (IGF-I) may modulate erythropoiesis by enhancing the effect of erythropoietin. A highly significant correlation was found in hemodialysis patients between IGF-I and hematocrit values.[47]

COAGULATION

Coagulation disturbances in uremia are reflected by an enhanced bleeding tendency, as well as by hypercoagulability. Other, nontoxic factors, such as the bioincompatibility of dialyzer membranes and circuits, are equally involved.

Uremic bleeding tendency is multifactorial. Platelet alterations (adherence, aggregation), anemia, hyperparathyroidism, and disturbances of prostaglandin production play a role.[48,49] The number of circulating thrombocytes remains unaltered in uremia, pointing to the role of functional changes in the induction of coagulation disturbances. Thrombocyte retention by glass beads,[50] aggregation response to adenosine diphosphate and collagen,[51] exposure of fibrinogen receptor,[51] cyclo-oxygenase activity,[52] and carbohydrate metabolism[53] are disturbed in renal failure.

Until a few years ago, no specific inhibitor of coagulation had been identified. More recently, nitric oxide (NO) was incriminated as a potential inducer of defective coagulation in at least a part of the uremic population.[54] In many uremic patients, however, NO-activity is inhibited,[55] which at least in theory should result in hypercoagulability.

In spite of the fact that a tendency for bleeding is found in most patients, isolated defects such as elevated amplitudes at thromboelastography[56] and increased von Willebrand factor activity,[57] point to hypercoagulability. Retention of altered fibrinogen fragments might modify coagulatory function and platelet response.[58]

IMMUNE STATUS

The susceptibility to infections, increased incidence of cancer, the burnout of immunologic disorders, and the presence of an inadequate antibody response, illustrate immune dysfunction in uremia. It is apparent at different levels: abnormalities of polymorphonuclear cell function (disturbances of locomotion and phagocytosis), changes in levels and quality of immunoglobulins, reticuloendothelial dysfunction, and disturbed cell-mediated immunity.[59,60] The number of circulating leukocytes remains unaltered, pointing to functional changes.

Bacterial infection remains one of the most prevalent clinical complications. A crucial role in the host-defense against bacterial infection is occupied by phagocytes.[61] Failure of phagocytes to ingest microparticles and to kill bacteria, points to a depression of their functional capacity.[59,60,62] The start of hemodialysis induces a further depression in polymorphonuclear functional response,[62,63] but an improvement is observed when patients remain on dialysis for longer periods.[64]

Cellular immunity primarily involves T-lymphocytes and their production of lymphokines. Granulocytes and macrophages interfere with each other as effector cells of this system. Many cellular functions such as T-cell growth factor activity, T-cell subset identification, metabolic responsiveness, lymphatic immune response and/or proliferation, and E-rosette forming capacity are disturbed. Raskova and associates[65] demonstrated that B-cell activation and immunoregulation, as well as helper T-cell functions, are quantitatively deficient. Lymphocyte response to stimulation is disturbed in cultured cells from dialyzed patients.[66] T-cell adhesion to extracellular matrix proteins is depressed in the presence of uremic sera.[67] Impaired proliferation of peripheral blood leukocytes and T-cell activation have been attributed to an accessory cell defect in the B7/CD28 pathway.[68] *In vitro* restoration of this B7/CD28 pathway reconstitutes leukocytic cellular function.

Many toxins have been claimed to suppress immune function: endorphins, phenols, indoles, parathyroid hormone, several peptidic structures, *p*-cresol, guanidino compounds, and advanced glycation end products, inhibit activated immune cell functional capacity.[25,59,69–74]

Other toxic factors might be involved, such as the disruption of protective skin barriers by vascular access, the bioincompatibility of dialyzers,[62] vitamin D deficiency or resistance,[75] infection-prone anatomic anomalies (e.g., polycystic kidney disease, vesicoureteral reflux, and cardiac valvular damage),[59] dysfunction of opsonins,[76] iron overload,[77] and anemia.[78]

In contrast to the ineffective response towards stimuli and infectious agents, the baseline uremic immune status is activated.[79,80] This results in a hyperoxidative condition and in an oxidative modification of molecules and structures.[24] This mechanism is most likely involved in atherogenesis and cardiovascular damage.[80]

ENDOCRINOLOGY

Carbohydrate Metabolism

Alterations of glucose-induced insulin secretion,[81] and target organ insensitivity to insulin,[82] are reflected by glucose intolerance,[83] which is not related to a decrease of insulin receptor binding or receptor kinase activity,[84] but to a decrease of glucose transport sites.[85,86] Remarkably, 1,25-dihydroxycholecalciferol corrects glucose-intolerance in hemodialysis patients.[87]

MacCaleb and associates[88] characterized and partially purified a peptide from uremic serum, which induces insulin resistance, although without exact identification. Dzúrik and associates[89–91] suggested hippuric acid, 5-hydroxyindoleacetic acid, and pseudouridine as potential inhibitors.

Glucagon levels are elevated because of inadequate renal metabolism.[92]

Thyroid Hormone

Levels of T3 and T4 may be depressed, in spite of a euthyroid appearance.[93] Both 3-carboxy-4-methyl-5-propyl-2-furanpropionic acid (CMPF) and indoxyl sulfate inhibit the deiodination of thyroxine by cultured hepatocytes.[94] The release of thyroid stimulating hormone (TSH) is suppressed, possibly by a dopamine-dependent mechanism.[95]

Growth Hormones

Baseline levels of growth hormone (GH) progressively increase during the progression of renal failure. Nevertheless, growth retardation is one of the onerous facets of pediatric nephrology. Contributing factors are the resistance to growth hormone,[96] malnutrition, acidosis, renal osteodystrophy, hyperparathyroidism, and inadequate gonadotropic hormone secretion.[97] Hepatic insulin-like growth factor-1 (IGF-1) expression is reduced in uremia, whereas the production of IGF-binding proteins is enhanced.[98] The administration of recombinant human GH and of IGF corrects the growth disturbances of uremic children[97,99] and improves protein utilization in stable hemodialyzed adults.[100,101] Use of this compound should, however, be avoided in critically ill patients, where protein turnover is accelerated.[102] Children with GH deficiency have higher plasma levels of soluble CD30, which is an index of Th2 lymphocyte activation.[103]

In uremic rats, the prevalence of growth hormone receptors in growth plates is decreased, and this defect is corrected by the administration of GH combined to IGF-I.[104]

Reproductive Hormones

Advanced renal failure results in reproductive abnormalities in both men and women. The cyclic peaks that are normally observed immediately before ovulation, do not occur in uremia,[105] pointing to a disregulation of the hypothalamic-pituitary-ovarian axis. Uremic men are often infertile and/or impotent. This is associated with an increase of plasma LH and FSH levels and a decrease of testosterone and results in compromised spermatogenesis. Prolactin levels are elevated, which induces galactorrhea and amenorrhea in women and impotence in men.[106] One of the epiphenomena of reduced gonadotropin pulsatility during pubertal maturation is growth retardation.[107]

BONE DISEASE

Uremic bone disease is a multifactorial problem, depending upon diverging mechanisms such as hyperparathyroidism, aluminum toxicity, vitamin D deficiency and resistance, intrinsic osteopenia, and amyloidosis.[108] Also, inflammatory elements might suppress bone formation.[109] Defective production of IGF-1 may play a role in deficient bone formation.[110] A low molecular weight inhibitor of cartilage sulfation, with negative influence on bone cell proliferation, has been detected in the plasma of dialysis patients.[111] Andress and associates[113–115] described an inhibitor of osteoblast mitogenesis with a molecular weight range between 750 and 900 dalton (D).[112] Several authors found evidence that uremic retention solutes reduce the molecular response to active vitamin D and its analogues.

Hyperparathyroidism as such is the result of relative hypocalcemia, hypovitaminosis D, and resistance to vitamin D.[116] Although it was accepted that hyperphosphatemia indirectly caused hyperparathyroidism, it was recently demonstrated that hyperphosphatemia also directly stimulated the response of the parathyroid gland.[117]

Therapeutic maneuvers to refrain parathyroid response, such as administration of oral calcium salts or vitamin D analogues, might as a counterbalance enhance calcium load and hence vascular calcification. The advent of noncalcium phosphate binders[118] and calcimimetics[119] might help to overcome this dysbalance.

Uremia-associated amyloidosis is a disease that mainly strikes the bone, tendons, and joints. $ß_2$-microglobulin is the main component of this amyloid.[120] Several modifications have been proposed to participate in amyloid formation: proteolysis of the N-terminus of $ß_2$-microglobulin,[121] deamination of Asn17,[122] and modification of $ß_2$-microglobulin by Advanced Glycation End Products (AGEs).[123] Other protein components of amyloid than $ß_2$-microglobulin, such as α_2-macroglobulin,[124] glycosaminoglycans,[125] and amyloid P components,[126] may also play a pathogenetic role. Furthermore, to explain the predilection of this disease for synovial and periarticular structures, a role for local predisposing factors should be postulated.[127]

Probably because of the recent adaptation in our therapeutic arsenal, the incidence of uremia-related amyloidosis has followed a pattern of decreasing frequency.[128]

PRURITUS

Several factors have been incriminated: increased serum vitamin A, hyperparathyroidism, high skin contents of divalent cations, mast cell proliferation with increased release of histamine, liver dysfunction, and/or abnormal cutaneous innervation.[129] Erythropoietin treatment may improve pruritic complaints.[130] Parathyroid hormone and phosphorus are the main responsible toxins.

PROGRESSION OF RENAL DISEASE

Motojima and associates[131] found compelling evidence that one or more ultrafiltrable uremic retention solutes were involved in the progression of glomerulosclerosis. Later studies by Niwa and associates[132,133] identified indoxyl sulfate as one of the responsible molecules. The administration of an oral sorbent alleviated the overload of indoxyl sulfate on remnant proximal tubular epithelial cells[134] and reduced the gene expression of Tissue Growth Factor-β1 (TGF-ß1) and of tissue inhibitor of metalloproteinase-1 (TIMP-1), which resulted in a delay of the progression of chronic renal failure. Sympathetic overactivity may also play a role in this progression.[135]

MALNUTRITION

A substantial number of end-stage renal disease (ESRD) and pre-ESRD patients suffer from malnutrition,[136] and a link between malnutrition, cardiovascular disease, and inflammation has been proposed.[8,9,80,136] Several pro-inflammatory compounds such as AGE, advanced oxidation end products (AOPP), and cytokines are accumulated in renal failure and might play a role in this process.[137] Leptin, a 16 kD suppressor of appetite, is retained in renal failure[138] and does so more in patients with a loss of body mass.[139]

Apart from inflammation, central and gastrointestinal mechanisms are involved in malnutrition. Brain serotonin hyperproduction, related to disturbances of tryptophan metabolism, has been related to uremic anorexia.[140] Gastric emptying disturbances are observed in a substantial fraction of the uremic population.[141,142] Also, acidosis provokes uremic catabolism,[143,144] by induction of proteolysis and resistance to growth hormones.

END-STAGE RENAL FAILURE

Until a few years ago, it was current practice to wait with the start of renal replacement until the creatinine clearance reached a level of 5 mL/min or less. Already more than a decade ago, some authors advocated the start of dialysis at an earlier stage (Ccrea 10–15 mL/min),[145] although well controlled studies proving the benefit of this approach were, to our knowledge, never published.

More recently, it became clear that the normalized clearance of low molecular weight molecules such as urea (Kt/V), which is a current marker of dialysis adequacy, is much lower in patients awaiting dialysis, than the values pursued once dialysis has been started.[146]

Studies still need to be undertaken to define the exact values of renal function at which dialysis should be initiated, although recent guidelines forward a cutoff value of weekly Kt/V of 2.0, a native creatinine clearance of 12 mL/min, or a GFR of 15 mL/min, in the presence of symptoms.[147–149] It should be noted that symptoms that are seemingly uremic, may be induced by nonuremic mechanisms such as the concomitant presence of hepatic failure, cerebrovascular disease or diabetes mellitus, disturbances of electrolyte and water homeostasis, and drug intoxication. An incorrect interpretation of these signs will result in the inappropriate start of renal replacement therapy. On the other hand, damaging side effects, such as vascular lesions and endothelial dysfunction, might occur early during progression,[150] so that even an earlier start than advocated at present might be desirable, if such an early start is not responsible for its own specific morbidity and mortality.[151]

Recent observational evidence points to a similar outcome of early and late start,[152] but it is practically impossible to avoid selection bias in this type of study.[153]

UREMIC SOLUTE RETENTION

General Classification of the Uremic Solutes

A gradual retention of a large number of organic metabolites of proteins, fatty acids, and carbohydrates characterizes the progression of renal failure, whereby partial metabolization and elimination by other than renal pathways may compensate for the loss of renal clearance. Some of the retained compounds are proven toxins. Toxicity is not a simple monofactorial process whereby only one or a few toxins affect many different metabolic processes at a time. Other retained substances are nontoxic but can be used as markers of retention.

A recent survey of the literature revealed the retention in uremia of at least 90 compounds, of which the concentration had been reported.[154] It is very likely that this is only the tip of the iceberg.

Under normal conditions, the glomerular filter clears molecules with a molecular weight up to ± 58,000 D. All of these substances are supposed to be retained in renal failure. An additional role should be attributed to changes in tubular secretion, reabsorption, and metabolic breakdown, which are all altered when renal mass decreases. The molecules metabolized by the kidneys may have a higher molecular weight (>58,000 D) than those cleared. Renal and nonrenal metabolization of solutes and nonrenal clearance may in their turn be inhibited following uremic retention.

Uremic retention products are arbitrarily subdivided according to their molecular weight.[155,156] Low molecular weight molecules are characterized by a molecular weight (MW) up to 500 D (e.g., urea [MW: 60], creatinine [MW: 113]). They can further be subdivided in protein bound and nonprotein bound molecules. Substances with a molecular weight range above 500 D are called middle molecules (e.g., parathyroid hormone [MW: 9,424], β_2-microglobulin [MW: 11,818]). Several clinical, metabolic, and/or biochemical disturbances such as food intake, apolipoprotein (apo) A-I secretion, osteoblast mitogenesis, cell growth, lymphocyte proliferation, and interleukin production are caused by uremic compounds that conform with the middle molecular weight range.[112,157–161] Several of the recently defined uremic compounds, for example, β_2-microglobulin (β_2-M), various peptides, some of the AGE, as well as PTH, conform with the definition of the middle molecules (MM) (see following).

Dialysis membranes with the capacity to remove MM (high-flux membranes) have been related to lower mortality,[162–166] as well as a slower loss of residual renal function,[167] less preponderant dyslipidemia,[168] improvement of polyneuropathy,[169] and a lower prevalence of the carpal tunnel syndrome.[170] However, these highly efficient membranes are often at the same time less complement activating than unmodified cellulose, in many studies their counterpart. Hence, the relative importance of the removal of MM versus biocompatibility related events is not always clear. Two studies, however, point to an independent benefit of large molecule removal. Leypoldt and associates[171] demonstrated that independent from urea removal, MM clearance correlated to patient survival. In a study applying nothing but synthetic membranes, large pore size was associated with a better survival.[172]

In the prospective randomized HEMO-study, however, no significant impact on mortality was found for high-flux dialyzers upon primary analysis, although there was a trend.[173] Upon secondary analysis a benefit was found for large pore membranes regarding cardiovascular events.[173] Patients who had been treated long-term on dialysis received an extra benefit.

Removal of larger molecules is more efficient when the high-flux membranes are used in a convective mode[174]; no data is available whether this affects mortality. Convective treatment modalities have a positive impact on the development of the carpal tunnel syndrome.[170] On line hemodiafiltration with large convective volumes results in a rise of erythrocyte counts and a decrease of erythropoietin needs.[175] Even if highly efficient dialysis is clinically superior, its cost effectiveness still needs to be demonstrated.

Small protein-bound compounds such as hippuric acid or *p*-cresol behave like MM during dialysis, due to their high protein binding. Their removal by classical hemodialysis systems, even with large pore membranes, remains disappointingly low,[176] which may be attributed to the complex distribution and intra-dialytic kinetics of these compounds. Therefore, alternative removal strategies than the classical ones should be considered, such as adsorption, changes in timeframes, use of protein-leaking membranes, and/or stimulation of metabolic pathways.

Peritoneal dialysate is a much richer source of protein bound compounds than hemodialysate,[177] since peritoneal pore size allows the transfer of substantial quantities of albumin together with its bound moieties, which is not the case for even the most open hemodialyzer membranes. Also, the continuous timeframe might enhance the removal of these compounds.[178]

Until recently, no data had confirmed a potential clinical impact of protein bound molecules. Recently, a correlation of free *p*-cresol with hospitalization rate and hospitalization for infection was confirmed.[179]

MAIN UREMIC RETENTION PRODUCTS

Several uremic retention solutes influence biologic functions. Other compounds have no proven direct toxicity but may be useful markers of uremic retention. A review of the most currently known uremic retention solutes with their molecular weight is given in Table 6–2. It should be acknowledged that anorganic compounds such as water and potassium exert toxicity as well. In what follows, we will concentrate on the organic retention compounds.

Table 6–2 Major Uremic Retention Solutes and their Molecular Weight (Daltons)

Compound	MW	Compound	MW
ADMA/SDMA	202	Adrenomedullin	5729
ANF	3080	Benzylalcohol	108
β-endorphin	3465	β-guanidinopropionic acid	131
β_2-microglobulin	11818	CGRP	3789
Cholecystokinin	3866	CIP	8500
Clara cell protein	15800	CML	188
CMPF	240	Complement factor D	23750
Creatine	131	Creatinine	113
Cystatin C	13300	Cytidine	234
DIP I	14400	DIP II	24000
3-Deoxyglucosone	162	Dimethylarginine	202
Endothelin	4283	γ-guanidinobutyric acid	145
Glomerulopressin	500	GIP I	28000
GIP II	25000	Guanidine	59
Guanidinoacetic acid	117	Guanidinosuccinic acid	175
Hippuric acid	179	Homoarginine	188
Homocysteine	135	Hyaluronic acid	25000
Hypoxanthine	136	Imidazolone	203
Indole-3-acetic acid	175	Indoxyl sulfate	251
Leptin	16000	Melatonin	126
Methylguanidine	73	Myoinositol	180
Neuropeptide Y	4272	Orotic acid	156
Orotidine	288	o-OH-hippuric acid	195
Oxalate	90	P-cresol	108
p-OH-hippuric acid	195	Parathyroid hormone	9225
Pentosidine	135	Phenylacetylglutamine	264
Phenol	94	Phosphate	96
Pseudouridine	244	Putrescine	88
Retinol binding protein	21200	Spermine	202
Spermidine	145	Thymine	126
Trichloromethane	119	Tryptophan	202
Urea	60	Uric acid	168
Uridine	244	Xanthine	152

The underlined compounds conform with the definition of MM (MW between 7500 and 12,000 Daltons, or above). *ADMA,* asymmetrical dimethylarginine; *SDMA,* symmetrical dimethylarginine; *ANF,* atrial natriuretic factor; *CGRP,* calcitonin gene related peptide; *CIP,* chemotaxis inhibiting protein; *CMPF,* 3-carboxy-4-methyl-5-propyl-2-furanpropionic acid; *CML,* carboxymethyllysine; *DIP I,* degranulation inhibiting protein I; *DIP II,* degranulation inhibiting protein II; *GIP I,* granulocyte inhibiting protein I; *GIP II,* granulocyte inhibiting protein II.

Advanced Glycation End Products (AGE)

As first described by Maillard,[180] glucose and other reducing sugars react nonenzymatically with free amino groups to form reversible Schiff base adducts (in days) and stable Amadori products (in weeks), which are then converted into AGE through chemical rearrangements and degradation reactions. Several AGE-compounds are peptide-linked degradation products[181] (MW 2000–6000 D), although the baseline AGE-products such as pentosidine, 2-(2-fuoryl)-4(5)-(2-furanyl)-1H-imidazole (FFI), imidazolone, 3-deoxyglucosone, pyrrole aldehyde, and N^{ε}–(carboxymethyl)lysine have a substantially lower MW (Table 6–2).

AGE are retained not only in renal failure but also in diabetes mellitus and aging,[182] where they are held responsible for tissular damage and functional disturbances. In the uremic population, the level of glucose-modified proteins is higher than in diabetics without renal failure,[183] and AGE-concentration does not depend on the glycemic status.[184,185] The production of AGE in ESRD has been related to oxidative and carbonyl stress, rather than to reactions with glucose.[186] Not all AGE-generation is oxidative, however. Imidazolone, a nonoxidative AGE, is found as well in serum and urine of uremic patients.[187]

Schiff base formation affects the interaction of the vitamin D receptor with responsive DNA-elements, such as osteocalcin, vitamin D-responsive elements (VDRE), or constructed VDRE in transfected cells.[188] AGE provoke monocyte activation,[189] as well as the induction of interleukin-6, tumor necrosis factor-α, and interferon-γ generation.[190] AGE-modified $ß_2$-M may play a role in the generation of dialysis-associated amyloidosis [123] (see later text). Serum pentosidine levels are higher in patients with dialysis-related amyloidosis, compared to their amyloid-free counterpart.[191] AGE can react with and chemically inactivate nitric oxide (NO),[192] a potent endothelium-derived vasodilator, anti-aggregant, and antiproliferative factor. Inversely, NO inhibits the formation of AGE.[193] AGE are also related to oxidative protein modification.[24] 3-Deoxyglucosone inactivates glutathione peroxidase, a key enzyme in the neutralization of hydrogen peroxide.[194] Transferrin and lysozyme, after contact with AGE-modified albumin, lose their immune-enhancing properties.[195] AGE accumulate in atheromatous plaque of the aortic wall of subjects with ESRD, where they may contribute to a more rapid progression of atherosclerosis.[191] There is, however, no observational study in uremia, linking AGE directly to atherogenesis.

Early glycation of proteins induces an increase of glucose uptake and accelerated apoptotic cell death of polymorphonuclears (PMNL).[25] Late glycation products increase PMNL chemotaxis.[25] Other recent data suggest that whereas AGE increase baseline leukocyte response, activated response to infectious stimuli is blunted.[74] This suggests a dual response, related at the clinical level to both atherogenesis and susceptibility to infection.[75]

Most of the biologic actions of AGE that have been registered up to now, have not, however, been obtained with AGE recovered from uremic or diabetic serum, but with AGE artificially prepared in the laboratorium.[75] In vivo collected uremic human serum albumin appeared to be only minimally AGE-modified.[196] It remains unclear which AGE exert toxicity in vivo, and what their real toxicity is.

Concentrations in ESRD patients might be attributed to increased uptake, production, and/or retention. During industrial food processing, cooking procedures and storage of foods, food proteins are modified by carbohydrates,[197–199] and those are absorbed via the gastrointestinal tract.[184] The healthy kidneys are responsible for not only glomerular filtration but also for tubular reabsorption and degradation of AGE.[200,201] Specific receptors for AGE have been identified (RAGE) and their expression is enhanced during uremia.[202] AGE binding to RAGE has been shown to stimulate mesothelial cell activity and results in overexpression of vascular cell adhesion molecule (VCAM-1), which activates human peritoneal cells and promotes local inflammation, implicating the development of tubular injury.[203]

In spite of continuous contact with glucose via the dialysate, CAPD patients do not have higher serum AGE levels than hemodialysis patients.[181] Nevertheless, protein glycation has been demonstrated in the peritoneal membrane.[204] The heat sterilization of glucose-containing peritoneal dialysate induces the formation of glucose degradation products (GDP), which are precursors of AGE.[205] GDP inhibit leukocyte response, and this effect is attenuated when heat sterilization is replaced by other procedures (e.g., filter sterilization).[206]

Removal of AGE is significantly more important with high-flux hemodialysis than with conventional dialysis with low-flux membranes.[207] Even then steady state serum levels still remain substantially above normal. Concentrations of AGE are subjected to a post-dialytic rebound[207] but are normalized by kidney transplantation. Nevertheless, albumin-bound pentosidine remains longer elevated after transplantation than free pentosidine,[208] whereas intratissular levels of AGE also remain elevated for a longer period than plasma levels.[209] In hemodialyzed ESRD patients, a decrease in AGE-apolipoprotein B is observed after 8 weeks of treatment with high-flux AN69 dialyzers, compared to low-flux polysulfone.[210] This effect could be attributed mainly to adsorption to the dialysis membrane and is paralleled by a decrease in total apolipoprotein B, pointing to a possible positive effect of AGE-removal on overall dyslipidemia. AGE show a marked heterogeneity in removal pattern, even during high-flux dialysis.[198,211] It is unclear which compounds could be representative by their removal pattern in a way that they could serve as a marker for the overall group of AGE.

Recently, Miyata and associates[212] demonstrated that two widely used families of antihypertensive agents, the angiotensin converting enzyme inhibitors, as well as the angiotensin II type I receptor antagonists, attenuated *in vitro* the production of AGE.

$ß_2$-Microglobulin ($ß_2$-M)

$ß_2$-M (MW approximately 12,000 D) is a component of the major histocompatibility antigen. Uremia-related amyloid is to a large extent composed of $ß_2$-M and is essentially found in the osteo-articular system and in the carpal tunnel, although deposition can be systemic as well.[213,214] Uremia-related amyloidosis becomes most often clinically apparent after several years of chronic renal failure and/or in the aged.[215] Recent data, however, show that amyloidosis develops earlier than previously suspected,[216,217] even in patients not yet submitted to dialysis.[218] According to the most recent studies, its prevalence tends to decrease.[219]

The exact pathophysiology of this disease remains largely unknown. In several studies, it was impossible to relate ß$_2$-M serum concentrations to the development of ß$_2$-M amyloidosis.[220–222]

AGE (see earlier text) and ß$_2$-M amyloidosis are closely connected. AGE-modified ß$_2$-M has been identified in amyloid of hemodialyzed patients.[223] At least three major AGE-modifications of ß$_2$-M have been recovered: pentosidine-ß$_2$-M,[184] carboxymethyllysine-ß$_2$-M,[186,223] and imidazolone-ß$_2$-M.[224] AGE-modified ß$_2$-M enhances monocytic migration and cytokine secretion,[225] suggesting that foci containing AGE-ß$_2$-M may initiate inflammatory response, leading to bone and joint destruction. AGE-ß$_2$-M was shown to delay monocyte apoptosis and to alter their phenotype.[226] Recent studies, however, suggest that macrophage infiltrates might be a secondary phenomenon.[227,228] Next to macrophages, fibroblasts seem to also play a key role in the pathogenesis of amyloidosis.[229]

Other modifications that have been proposed to participate in amyloid generation are proteolysis of the N-terminus of ß$_2$-M[121,230] and deamination of the Asn-17.[122,231] Some arguments, such as the lack of a higher clinical incidence of ß$_2$-M-amyloidosis in diabetic dialysis patients,[232] who generate large quantities of AGE in the presence of hyperglycemia, cast a doubt on the patho-physiologic role of AGE in amyloid formation. Possibly, the AGE-transformation plays a more important role in the inflammation surrounding ß$_2$-M-amyloid than in its generation.

Long-term hemodialysis with large pore membranes results in a progressive decrease of pre-dialysis ß$_2$-M concentrations; the levels remain, however, far above normal, even after intensive removal therapy.[233,234] Long-term dialysis with large-pore dialyzers results in a lower prevalence of dialysis-related amyloidosis and/or carpal tunnel syndrome.[162,170,235,236] Whether this benefit is attributable to a better removal of ß$_2$-M, to lower complement and leukocyte activating capacity, or to protection against the transfer of dialysate impurities into the bloodstream (e.g., lipopolysaccharides)[219] is not evident, because most of the dialyzers associated with a lower incidence of amyloidosis have all three abovementioned properties.

Because ß$_2$-M is only removed by dialyzers with a large pore size, its kinetic behavior might be representative for other large molecules. Behavior of ß$_2$-M during dialysis is, however, not necessarily representative for that of other MM. Discrepancies in behavior in the long run have been demonstrated in relation to other MM, such as complement factor D.[237]

Recently, several devices with strong adsorptive capacity for ß$_2$-M have been developed.[238,239]

The clinical expression of dialysis-related amyloidosis disappears after kidney transplantation, but the underlying pathologic processes such as bone cysts and tissular ß$_2$-M remain preserved.[240] Possibly, immunosuppressive therapy plays a role in the regression of the symptomatology.

ß$_2$-M-related compounds might also be involved in other aspects of the uremic syndrome. One of the peptides with granulocyte inhibitory effect described by Haag-Weber and associates[70] has partial homology with ß$_2$-M.

3-Carboxy-4-Methyl-5-Propyl-2-Furanpropionic Acid (CMPF)

One of the urofuranic acids, 3-Carboxy-4-methyl-5-propyl-2-furanpropionic acid (CMPF) is a lipophilic and strongly protein-bound uremic solute and one of the major inhibitors of the protein binding of drugs[241,242] and of bilirubin.[243] CMPF and bilirubin share the binding site for dicarboxylate molecules on human serum albumin.[244] CMPF is also a potent binding inhibitor for salicylic acid and phenole red (site I).[245] The renal clearance of CMPF is strongly reduced in renal failure,[246] which results in a marked rise of its serum concentration.[247] CMPF inhibits the renal uptake of para-amino hippuric acid (PAH) in rat kidney cortical slices[248] and causes a decrease in renal excretion of several drugs, of their metabolites, and of endogenously produced organic acids that are removed via the PAH pathway. *In vivo* CMPF clearance in the rat is inhibited by PAH and probenecid.[249] CMPF inhibits hepatic glutathione-S-transferase,[250] deiodination of T4 and T3 by cultured hepatocytes,[94] ADP-stimulated oxidation of NADH-linked substrates in isolated mitochondria,[251] and erythropoiesis.[252]

Costigan and associates[252–255] demonstrated a correlation between plasma concentration of CMPF and neurologic abnormalities and a negative correlation with blood hemoglobin.

CMPF levels are lower in CAPD than in hemodialysis. This might be attributed to the slower removal pattern and/or to the more important losses of the proteins that bind CMPF. Differences in residual renal function may also be involved in this effect, but this aspect has not yet been evaluated. The strong protein binding of CMPF[176] hampers its removal during hemodialysis, which is virtually nil.[176] Alternative removal strategies, such as adsorption or strategies that modify generation, should be considered.[256] Protein leaking hemodialysis induces a reduction of CMPF and is at the same time related to a rise in pre-dialysis hematocrit.[44]

Complement Factor D

Plasmatic concentrations of complement factor D increase in uremia, essentially because of alterations in renal removal.[257–259] Complement factor D exerts specific protease activity on its natural substrate, complement factor B, which results in an activation of the alternative complement pathway. This effect could in part be responsible for the baseline inflammatory status observed in chronic renal disease.[260] Furthermore, complement factor D was shown to adversely affect stimulated PMNL functions.[261] Some dialysis membranes remove complement factor D,[262] and this is at least in part attributed to adsorption.[257]

Creatinine

Creatinine belongs to the large group of guanidines (see later text). Because of the specific value of creatinine as a marker of renal function, this compound will be discussed separately.

The rise in serum creatinine during renal failure is not linearly related to the decrease in glomerular filtration rate (GFR), which may decrease by more than 50% without marked changes in serum creatinine. Changes become more prominent in the lower range of filtration. The determination of creatinine clearances as a parameter of renal function leads to an overestimation of true GFR, due to the secretion of creatinine in the renal tubular system. Unfortunately, the evolution of this tubular secretion does not parallel that of GFR. Some authors try to obtain a more accurate estimation of GFR by blocking the tubular secretion of creatinine, for example, by cimetidine.[263] Others calculate the mean of urea and creatinine clearance, although this approach remains a matter of debate.[264]

In spite of the extensive use of creatinine as a marker of uremic toxin retention, it has been held responsible for only a few uremic side effects, such as chloride channel blocking[265,266] and the reduction of the contractility of cultured myocardial cells,[267] however, at concentrations exceeding those encountered in ESRD. Injection of creatinine in uremic rats shortens their life span.[268] Creatinine is also a precursor of the toxic compound methylguanidine.[269,270] It interferes with some of the central neurologic functions.[266,271]

Serum creatinine concentration is not only the resultant of uremic retention but also of muscular breakdown; therefore, a high serum creatinine may be the consequence of high muscular mass, and hence an indicator of metabolic well-being. Morbidity and mortality in hemodialyzed patients are positively correlated with serum creatinine.[269]

Cytokines

In view of the strong associations between atherosclerosis, malnutrition, and inflammation,[272] it may be speculated that factors associated with malnutrition and inflammation may contribute to the excess prevalence of cardiovascular disease. The causes of inflammation in ESRD patients are probably multifactorial. All available evidence suggests that the pro-inflammatory cytokine system activity is elevated in ESRD patients.[273] It has been hypothesized that epoetin resistance is due to enhanced levels of immune activation because chronic inflammation can modify the process of erythropoiesis, which is probably mediated via pro-inflammatory cytokines.[274] The accumulation of TNF-α may contribute to the development of neurologic and hematologic complications in uremia; it has been suggested that TNF-α may, indeed, be considered a uremic toxin.[275] Several lines of evidence suggest that decreased renal clearance might play an important role.[276] However, as the half-life of various cytokines is short and local tissue cytokine inactivation may be the most important pathway of cytokine degradation, more research is needed to determine the relative importance of the kidney in cytokine clearance. Recently, the importance of the IL-10 genotype, which determines the production of the anti-inflammatory cytokine IL-10 on uremia- and dialysis-induced chronic inflammation, has been demonstrated.[277]

Glomerulopressin

Glomerulopressin is a low molecular weight (<500 D) hepatic hormone, which increases glomerular capillary pressure and enhances glomerular filtration rate.[278] Circulating levels are elevated in chronic renal failure.[279] Removal by dialysis is 75% of that of urea. Production is stimulated by dietary protein ingestion.[280] This hormone is possibly related to the progression of renal failure subsequent to high protein intake.

Guanidines

The group of the guanidines is composed by several structural metabolites of arginine. Among them are well known uremic retention solutes, such as creatinine and guanidine and newly detected moieties, such as asymmetric and symmetric dimethylarginine (ADMA and SDMA). Creatinine has been discussed separately.

Guanidine compound levels have been determined in serum, urine, cerebrospinal fluid, and brains of uremic patients.[281,282] Four compounds, creatinine, guanidine, guanidinosuccinic acid (GSA), and methylguanidine (MG) are highly increased.

Several of the guanidine compounds modify key biologic functions. GSA inhibits the production by 1α-hydroxylase of the active vitamin D metabolite, 1,25-$(OH)_2VitD_3$ (calcitriol)[283] and interferes with activation of ADP-induced platelet factor 3,[284] at concentrations currently found in hemodialyzed uremics.[285,286] A mixture of guanidine compounds suppresses the natural killer cell response to interleukin-2[73] and free radical production by neutrophils.[287] GSA, γ-guanidinobutyric acid, methylguanidine, homoarginine, and creatine induce seizures after systemic and/or cerebroventricular administration to animals.[265,266] GSA plays an important role in the hyperexcitability of the uremic brain.[35] Recent studies using the patch clamp technique suggest that GSA and MG might act as competitive antagonists at the transmission site of the γ-aminobutyric $acid_A$ ($GABA_A$) receptor.[271] GSA probably also acts as a selective agonist at the *N*-methyl-D-aspartate (NMDA) receptor.[288,289] GSA displays *in vivo* and *in vitro* neuroexcitatory effects that are mediated by ligand- and voltage-gated Ca^{2+} channels, suggesting an involvement of the guanidines in the central nervous complications of uremia.[36]

Arginine enhances NO-production. Some of the other guanidines, such as arginine-analogues, are strong inhibitors of NO-synthase. The inhibition of NO-synthesis results in saphenous[290] and mesenteric vasoconstriction,[291] hypertension,[292] ischemic glomerular injury,[293] immune dysfunction,[294] and neurologic changes.[295] NO-synthase is inhibited in chronic renal failure,[296] and the capacity of the NO-system to regulate hemodynamics is disturbed.[297] The strongest NO-synthase inhibitors are synthetic. ADMA is the most specific endogenous compound that inhibits NO-synthase. ADMA accumulates in the body during the development of renal failure,[298,299] related to decreased renal excretion but possibly also to suppressed enzymatic degradation by dimethylarginine dimethylaminohydrolase.[300] In addition, ADMA is produced in human endothelial cells.[301] The increase in SDMA is more pronounced, but this compound is biologically less active. In the brain, ADMA causes vasoconstriction and inhibition of acetylcholine-induced vasorelaxation.[302] Also in thoracic and radial vessels, ADMA induces contractions.[303] Recently, estrogen has been shown to alter the metabolism of ADMA, reducing the circulating concentration *in vivo*.[304] Methylguanidine, another endogenous guanidine, also shows a certain inhibitory activity on cytokine- and endotoxin-inducible NO-synthase, be it to a limited extent.[187]

In contradiction to the hypothesis of inhibition of NO-synthase in uremia, Noris and associates[54,305] described an enhanced NO-production in patients susceptible to uremic bleeding tendency. Possibly, this effect is limited to a subgroup of the uremic population. GSA might induce NO-production.

In the renal proximal convoluted tubule of rats with renal failure, the generation out of arginine of guanidinoacetic acid and creatine is depressed,[306] whereas the synthesis of GSA, guanidine, and methylguanidine is markedly increased, due to urea recycling.

Dialytic removal of guanidine compounds is subjected to a substantial variability.[286] Possibly, tissular distribution or protein binding play a role. In spite of a low MW, removal by hemodialysis of ADMA is only in the range of 20% to 30%.[299]

Hippuric Acid

Hippuric acid interferes with the transport of a variety of organic acids at the cortical tubular level,[307] the chorioid plexus of the brain, the ciliary body of the eye, the thyroid, the liver, and the erythrocytes.[308] Hippuric acid causes net fluid secretion in isolated proximal straight tubules of the rabbit.[309] Indirect data reported by MacNamara and associates[310] and by Gulyassy and associates,[311] and more direct studies on ultrafiltrate collected from dialyzed patients,[241,312] demonstrate an interference of hippuric acid with the protein binding of drugs. According to Dzúrik and associates,[313] hippurate interferes with glucose tolerance.

Hippuric acid is largely originated from the transformation of the quinic acid moiety of chlorogenic acid—the ester of caffeic acid—with quinic acid.[314] The intestinal flora may contribute to the generation of hippuric acid and hydroxyphenylpropionic acid.[315] The protein binding of hippuric acid tends to increase during dialysis.[316] Procentual dialytic removal is, however, close to that of urea,[176] possibly because protein binding is only moderate.

Homocysteine

Homocysteine (Hcy), a sulphur-containing amino acid, is produced by the demethylation of dietary methionine. Retention results in the cellular accumulation of S-adenosyl homocysteine (AdoHcy), an extremely toxic compound, which competes with S-adenosyl-methionine (AdoMet) and inhibits methyltransferase.[317] Moderate hyperhomocysteinemia, caused by a heterozygous deficiency of Hcy breakdown or by vitamin B_6, B_{12} or folate deficiency, is an independent risk factor for cardiovascular disease in the general population.[26,318] Reduced and oxidized forms of Hcy are present in the plasma, and total fasting levels are a reflection of intracellular metabolism and cellular excretion of Hcy.[27]

Hcy increases the proliferation of vascular smooth muscle cells, one of the most prominent hallmarks of atherosclerosis.[319] Moderate hyperhomocysteinemia may involve endothelial dysfunction and generate reactive oxygen species.[320] The administration of excess quantities of the Hcy precursor methionine to rats induces atherosclerosis-like alterations in the aorta.[321] Hcy also disrupts several anticoagulant functions in the vessel wall, which results in enhanced thrombogenicity.[322]

Patients with chronic renal failure have total serum Hcy levels twofold to fourfold above normal. The serum concentration depends not only on the degree of kidney failure, but also on nutritional intake (e.g., of methionine),[323] vitamin status (e.g., of folate),[324,325] genetic factors,[326–328] and decreased renal metabolization.[317] Almost all filtered Hcy is reabsorbed in the tubular system so that urinary excretion is minimal.[329] Detoxification by remethylation of homocysteine to methionine is inhibited in hemodialysis patients,[330,331] possibly due to folate resistance.[27]

Hyperhomocysteinemia is the most prevalent cardiovascular risk factor in ESRD[328,332] and is also present in kidney transplant recipients with cardiovascular disease.[333] In dialysis patients, there is a direct correlation between plasma homocysteine levels and the odds ratio for vascular complications.[332] Plasma homocysteine and cardiac mass correlate to each other.[334] In a study by Suliman and associates,[323] however, total plasma Hcy was lower in hemodialysis patients with cardiovascular disease than in those without. In this study, a correlation was found between total Hcy and serum albumin, pointing to a negative impact of malnutrition on Hcy concentrations. According to Shemin and associates,[335–337] hyperhomocysteinemia is also an independent risk factor for vascular access thrombosis. Such a relation was, however, not confirmed.

Hcy is partly bound to albumin, which hampers removal by hemodialysis. Hyperhomocysteinemia is more pronounced in hemodialysis patients than in PD.[325] In hemodialyzed patients, homocysteine levels correlate with plasma folate[324,325] and with the activity of enzymes that are at play in Hcy metabolism. Even with peritoneal dialysis, it is impossible to reduce total Hcy plasma levels to normal.[338] The application of amino acid containing PD fluids tends to increase the plasma homocysteine level.[339]

Dialysis with extremely leaky hemodialyzer membranes with large pore size (so-called super-flux membranes) results in a progressive decline of pre-dialysis plasma homocysteine concentrations.[340,341] This effect has at least in part been attributed to changes in homocysteine metabolism, induced by enhanced middle molecule removal through these highly efficient membranes.

Hcy levels can be reduced by folic acid, vitamin B_6, and vitamin B_{12}.[342,343] The population with ESRD might require high quantities of vitamins.[344] In pre-dialysis outpatients, folic acid (5 mg/day) causes a consistent decrease in Hcy levels.[345] Oral supplementation with high doses of folic acid (15 mg/day) and pyridoxine (200 mg/day) for 4 weeks in hemodialysis patients reduces Hcy but does not restore levels to normal.[346] Extremely high doses of 30 to 60 mg folic acid per day have no additional impact.[347] In ESRD patients, vitamin B_{12} alone reduces plasma Hcy levels, if it is administered to patients with low vitamin B_{12} plasma levels.[348] Patients on a high dose of vitamin B_{12} show a lower total Hcy than those on a high dose of folic acid.[349]

Possibly, the disappointing efficiency of folic acid might be related to an impairment of the metabolization of folic acid to 5-methyltetrahydrofolate (MTHF), which is the active compound in the remethylation pathway.[350] In an attempt to obviate such a deficiency, Bostom and associates[351] directly administered oral MTHF (17 mg/day) to hemodialyzed patients. No benefit was found, however. Touam and associates,[350] on the other hand, could reduce total Hcy to normal in approximately 80% of the studied population, by the administration of folinic acid, a precursor of MTHF. The folinic acid was administered IV (50 mg/week) and combined with pyridoxine (250 mg, three times weekly).[350] Therefore, it is not clear which element in this therapeutic strategy is responsible.[351] Since the supplementation with folate is inexpensive and relatively harmless, there is no formal objection against its therapeutic use.

Direct clinical proof of the benefit of a lower Hcy concentration in uremia is not available. Even when it was possible to decrease Hcy levels therapeutically, carotid artery stiffness was not altered,[28] but this finding might have been the consequence of too-late therapeutic intervention. Also, endothelial function was not improved, however.[352]

Hyaluronic acid

Hyaluronic acid concentration increases above normal in the large majority of patients with chronic renal failure.[353] The basic entity is a nonpolymerized molecule of 25 kD, but the compound may be present in a polymerized form as well. Concentrations correlate with β_2-microglobulin but not with creatinine. High values are found especially in patients with a bad clinical condition. In hemodialysis patients, hyaluronic acid correlates negatively with serum albumin[354] and is a strong independent predictor of long-term survival.[355–357]

Hyaluronic acid enhances the expression of the adhesion molecule VCAM-1[358,359] and of monocyte chemoattractant protein-1.[360] Hyaluronan stimulates cyclooxigenase type 2 (COX-2) and subsequent thromboxane A2 (TXA2) production in renal tubular cells and macrophages and therefore could play a role in inflammatory renal lesions.[361] Increased hyaluronan also promotes proliferation of rat interstitial fibroblasts, which could play a role in the pathogenesis of interstitial fibrosis.[362] These elements might be of relevance to the loss of residual renal function.

Indoles

Indoles are found in various plants and herbs and are produced by the intestinal flora. Several indolic metabolites are retained in uremia.[363] Indole itself is oxidized to indoxyl sulfate and various indigoid pigments by cytochrome P450.[364] CYP2E1, the major isoform of the isoenzyme P450, is responsible for the microsomal oxidation of indole to indoxyl.[365] Indoxyl sulfate, tryptophan, melatonin, and indole-3-acetic acid all are indoles. Indoxyl sulfate and melatonin are discussed under separate headings (see later text).

As a protein-bound compound, indole-3-acetic acid enhances drug toxicity by competition for protein binding and inhibition of tubular secretion.[241,366] Indole-3-acetic acid has been related to encephalopathy as well.[367] After oxidation, it becomes cytotoxic.[368]

Not all indoles show a similar kinetic behavior. Some of them do not even conform with the strict definition of uremic retention solutes, because their global concentration in ESRD is low rather than high (e.g., tryptophan),[369] but this decrease in concentration affects mainly the protein bound fraction, which is probably functionally inactive.[369] A relative increase of free plasma tryptophan has been described in uremia.[140] The decrease in plasma tryptophan is related to shifts in metabolic pathways that, at the same time, result in an increase of concentration of other related metabolites, such as quinolinic acid and kynurenine.[370] These compounds may exert neurotoxicity.[371] Central increases of free tryptophan have been related to anorexia.[140] This effect might be attributed to the generation of serotonin,[140] which also plays a role in thrombogenesis.[372]

The administration of AST-120, an oral adsorbent of uremic toxins, significantly reduced plasma indoxyl sulfate levels, increased tryptophan levels and improved the tryptophan plasma protein-binding ratio.[373] AST-120 improved partly the nutritional state, possibly by correcting the impaired metabolism of tryptophan.[373] Quinolinic acid is an endogenous excitotoxic agonist of NMDA-receptors[374] and an inhibitor of hepatic phosphoenolpyruvate carboxykinase and gluconeogenesis.[375] Quinolinic acid may also inhibit cardiac contractility[376] and may initiate lipid peroxidation in the brain.[377]

Indoxyl Sulfate

Indoxyl sulfate is metabolized by the liver from indole, which is produced by the intestinal flora as a metabolite of tryptophan. It enhances drug toxicity by competition with acidic drugs at the protein binding sites,[312,378] inhibits the active tubular secretion of these compounds,[366] and inhibits deiodination of thyroxin 4 by cultured hepatocytes.[94]

It is known that uremic retention solutes induce glomerular sclerosis.[131] The oral administration of indole or indoxyl sulfate to uremic rats causes a faster progression of glomerular sclerosis and of renal failure.[133] This effect is possibly mediated by the renal gene expression of transforming growth factor ß (TGFß), tissue inhibitor of metalloproteinase-1 (TIMP-1) and pro-α1 (type I) collagen.[134,379] Indoxyl sulfate as well as other protein bound solutes were shown to induce direct proximal tubular injury via organic anion transporter 1-mediated uptake.[380] In animals, progression of renal failure is refrained by adsorbent administration, together with a diminished expression of the abovementioned factors.[134] A similar attenuating effect is observed on the progression of diabetic nephropathy, based on the same mechanisms.[381,382]

Reduction of serum indoxyl sulfate concentration, by intraintestinal absorption of the precursor indole, reduces uremic itching.[383] AST-120 retards the development of acquired renal cystic disease and aortic calcification[384] and ameliorates tubulointerstitial injury by reducing the expression in the kidneys of ICAM-1, concopontin, TGF-β1 and clusterin in uninephrectomized rats.[382]

The oral administration of bifidobacterium longum, in gatro-resistant seamless capsules (Bifina) reduces serum levels of indoxyl sulfate in hemodialysis patients.[385]

Because of protein binding (approximately 100% in normal subjects and 90% in uremics), the intra-dialytic behavior of indoxyl sulfate diverges from that of other small compounds such as creatinine. If the percentage removal of creatinine during one hemodialysis session is approximately 50%, removal of indoxyl sulfate is only 0% to 20%.[252,386,387] Removal by CAPD is more effective.[252] High-flux hemodialysis does not enhance removal.[176] Alternative extracorporeal removal procedures such as hemoperfusion might be considered. Dialysis against albumin-containing dialysate removes albumin-bound uremic toxins such as indoxyl sulfate more efficiently than conventional dialysis and may be useful for reducing these compounds.[388]

Melatonin

The pineal hormone melatonin plays a role in the regulation of the hypothalamic-pituitary axis, sleep pattern, mood changes, cellular immunity, antibody response, and skin pigmentation, all of which are altered in end-stage renal disease. Melatonin inhibits the expression of lipopolysaccharide induced NO-synthase,[389] and acts as a free radical scavenger and an antioxidant,[390-393] although some authors attribute pro-oxidant activity to this compound.[394] Vaziri and associates[395] found no differences in early morning serum melatonin between healthy subjects and dialyzed uremic patients. In contrast, Viljoen and associates[396] demonstrated elevated melatonin levels in patients with CRF. Hemodialysis has no effect on the concentration of these compounds. The fluctuating concentration pattern, that normally occurs in healthy subjects, is absent in dialyzed uremics.[395]

Methylamines

Methylamine, dimethylamine, and trimethylamine are retained in uremia,[397,398] especially intracellularly.[397] The generation of methylamine increases after intake of fish, seafood, and vegetables (tomatoes, pears, peas).[399]

Maxfield and associates[400] demonstrated *in vitro* inhibition of fibroblast cellular function in the presence of methylamines. Increased deamination of methylamines might play a role in oxidative stress and atherogenesis.[398,401] Dimethylamine and trimethylamine inhibit human erythrocyte choline uptake.[402] Methylamine might play a role in central nervous disturbances.[399] At least at supraphysiologic concentrations, such as those occurring in normal renal medulla, methylamines counteract the biologic effects of urea.[403] This protective effect might be at play in uremia as well.[404] Trimethylamine oxide (TMA-O) protects myosin structures against urea-induced effects (2–8 mol/L).[405]

The gastrointestinal degradation of l-carnitine to trimethylamine and other compounds might limit the usefulness of long-term oral l-carnitine administration to hemodialysis patients.[406]

Myoinositol

An increased concentration of myoinositol has been found in uremic nervous tissue (cauda equina nerve), compared to tissue from nonuremic patients.[407] Sciatic nerve conduction velocity is decreased in rats after administration of myoinositol,[408] suggesting a possible role of this compound in peripheral neuropathy. Myoinositol also inhibits proliferation of Schwann cells, as estimated from their [^{3}H]-thymidine uptake.[409]

Myoinositol serves as a clinically relevant osmolyte in the cerebral nervous system[410] and inhibits red blood cell membrane ATPases at concentrations above 50 μmol/L, which corresponds to the high-normal physiologic range of concentration in uremic serum.[411]

Orthohydroxyhippuric and Parahydroxyhippuric Acid

In spite of its low molecular weight, orthohydroxyhippuric acid is characterized by a middle molecular intradialytic behavior because of its protein binding.[412,413] It interferes with the albumin binding of acidic drugs.[414] The urinary excretion of this glycine conjugate is increased in catabolic patients.[415] Possible precursors are compounds from the tyrosine-dopa-catecholamine pathway, and salicylate.[416] Use and abuse of salicylate and related compounds was a current cause of end-stage renal failure at the moment of the detection of orthohydroxyhippuric acid as a so-called uremic toxin. Therefore, the endogenous origin of orthohydroxyhippuric acid has always been a matter of debate.

Parahydroxyhippuric acid is a substance with a structural relationship to hippurate.[415] It is one of the uremic retention solutes that interfere with protein binding of organic acid drugs.[241] Recently, it was demonstrated to inhibit cellular CA^{++}-ATP-ase.[417] Parahydroxyhippuric acid and orthohydroxyhippuric acid together with other protein bound uremic solutes, were shown to cause tubular damage, albeit to a lesser extent than indoxyl sulfate or indoleacetic acid.[380]

Oxalate

In ESRD patients without primary hyperoxaluria, oxalate plasma levels are increased approximately 40-fold, compared to healthy controls.[418] Secondary oxalosis in ESRD patients without primary hyperoxaluria can be complicated by deposition of calcium oxalate in the myocardium, bone, articular surfaces, skin and blood vessels, especially if dialysis is inefficient, or in the presence of excessive intake of oxalate precursors (ascorbic acid, green leafy vegetables, rhubarb, tea, chocolate or beets[419]) or of inflammatory bowel disease.[420]

In rats with chronic renal failure, pyridoxine depletion resulted in increased urinary oxalate excretion and depressed renal function.[421] However, pyridoxine supplementation up to 300 mg/day for 1 month did not reduce plasma levels in CAPD patients.[422] Pyridoxine at 800 mg/day, on the other hand, caused a decrease in hemodialysis patients,[423] however, in combination with gastrointestinal intolerance.

Peritoneal clearance of oxalate is less than 10% of the normal renal clearance, which results in oxalate accumulation in CAPD patients.[422] Also in hemodialysis, oxalate levels are not restored to normal because removal does not match generation, and clearances are lower than those of urea.[325,424]

Oxidation Products

Oxidative capacity is increased in uremia[425-427] both before and after the start of dialysis, which points to a general uremic mechanism.[24] The Fenton reaction results in the generation of hydroxyl radicals, which react with proteins, causing structural modifications and irreparable damage.[428] Uremic patients also show an impaired antioxidant response, partly related to plasma glutathione deficiency.[429]

The concentrations of advanced oxidation protein products (AOPP) are increased in the plasma of uremic patients.[24,430] AOPP act in their turn as mediators of oxidative stress and monocyte respiratory burst.[24] Albumin seems to be one of the target proteins of these oxidative reactions.[24,431] Structural modification of albumin may alter its binding capacity for drugs and other solutes.[432] Modification of hemoglobin to glutathionylhemoglobin has been proposed as another marker of oxidative stress.[433]

Low-density lipoprotein (LDL) from uremic patients is more susceptible to oxidation than that from control subjects[434] (oxidized LDL [oxLDL]). This chemically modified LDL is more readily accumulated in macrophages, which results in the development of foam cells, an early event in atherogenesis. LDL autoantibodies against oxLDL have been demonstrated in ESRD, especially in hemodialyzed patients.[435] Oxidative modification of the protein moiety of LDL is a trigger of macrophage respiratory burst.[436,437] The LDL of chronic renal failure patients treated by hemodialysis and peritoneal dialysis is potentially more atherogenic, since it induces greater monocyte-endothelial adhesion.[438] The repeated use of vitamin E–coated hemodialyzers improves neutrophil function, oxidant stress and LDL concentrations, compared to uncoated cellulosic membranes.[439]

Malondialdehyde levels are increased in ESRD.[440] The capacity of malondialdehyde to form DNA adducts[441] may play a pathophysiologic role in carcinogenesis. Low-dose I.V. folinic acid given to dialysis patients reduced the levels of serum malondialdehyde and thus improved the cardiovascular risk profile.[442]

Several small molecular compounds might also be modified by oxidation. Organic chloramines are generated by the chemical binding of hypochlorite, a free radical produced by activated leukocytes, to retained organic compounds.[443] Chloramines increase endothelial permeability[444] and affect liver function and perfusion pressure.[445] They have a longer life span than genuine hypochlorite. In as far as binding occurs with liposoluble compounds, such as spermine or spermidine,[446] removal by hemodialysis will be hampered, whereas the capacity to penetrate cellular membranes and to cause toxic metabolic effects will be enhanced. Preliminary data with hemolipodialysis, a strategy that incorporates liposomes and antioxidants, suggest an attenuation of oxidation with this procedure.[447]

Parathyroid Hormone (PTH)

PTH, an MM with an MW of ± 9000 daltons (D), is generally recognized as a major uremic toxin, although its increased concentration during ESRD is merely attributable to enhanced glandular secretion, rather than to decreased removal by the kidneys. Excess PTH gives rise to an increase in intracellular calcium, which results in functional disturbances of virtually every organ system, including bone mineralization, pancreatic response to glucose, erythropoiesis, cardiovascular, and immune and liver function.[30,448-452] PTH is one of the few substances that has been causally linked to uremic neuropathy.[453] It also plays a role in fibroblast activation[448] and has been related to uremic pruritus.

Paradoxically, moderate hyperparathyroidism (intact PTH 60–200 ng/mL; normal range up to 60 ng/mL) has been demonstrated to improve the osseous response of uremic patients. If PTH remains in the lower range, patients may suffer from relative hypoparathyroidism, which results in aplastic bone, inadequate calcium handling, incapacity of the bone to buffer calcium,[454] and redistribution of body calcium stores leading to metastatic tissue calcification.[455] The current test methods for the determination of PTH-levels overestimate true concentrations, because they react as well with intact PTH as with functionally inactive fragments.[456] As a consequence, it has been suggested that to have a normal bone turnover, PTH-levels measured by classical methods should be two to three times above the upper normal limit.[451] At present, new test methods have been developed that estimate only intact PTH.[456,457]

The increased PTH concentration in uremia is the result of a number of compensatory homeostatic mechanisms. Hyperparathyroidism results from phosphate retention, decreased production of calcitriol (1,25 $[OH]_2$ vitamin D_3) and/or hypocalcemia. Remarkably enough, metabolic acidosis in rats reduces hyperparathyroidism, probably by enhancing phosphate excretion.[458] In HD patients, however, correction of metabolic acidosis reduced intact PTH levels in the presence of secondary hyperparathyroidism.[459] PTH-related peptide (PTHrP) enhances the secretion of PTH in response to hypocalcemia.[460]

Therapy with calcitriol alone or one of its analogues lowers serum PTH levels,[461] which not only suppresses PTH release, but also restores the secretory reserve of the parathyroid gland during hypocalcemia.[461] Uremia is, however, not only characterized by a depressed production of calcitriol, but also by resistance to this hormone; this resistance is induced by uremic biologic fluids, such as ultrafiltrate and chromatographic fractions of this ultrafiltrate.[113]

Downregulation of PTH-PTHrP receptor mRNA expression is observed in liver, kidney, and heart of rats with advanced chronic renal failure[462,463] and in bone from uremic patients.[464] Parathyroidectomy does not entirely prevent PTH/PTHrP receptor downregulation,[465] suggesting that this alteration depends on more than elevated PTH alone. Also, calcium receptors might show an abnormal function.[116]

Only dialysis membranes with a large pore size remove PTH.[466] Differences in concentration at the end of the dialysis session are, however, subtle[466] and presumably without clinical relevance. Increased removal will probably be compensated by enhanced endocrine production (trade-off). A more efficient way to correct parathyroid hormone hypersecretion is the correction of the plasma calcium, calcitriol, and phosphorus.[467] If these interventions remain ineffective, parathyroidectomy is the ultimate therapeutic resource. In the future, it might become possible to suppress the by-effects of hyperparathyroidism, such as hypercalcemia, by the administration of PTH antagonists. Serum calcium was, however, not lowered by the PTH antagonist BIM-44002, in a recent study in hypercalcemic hyperparathyroid patients.[468] Another pharmacologic option for the future are the calcimimetics.[469, 470] Apart from hypocalcemia, side effects are very rare.[471] A calcium-free phosphate binder (Renagel) is now commercially available with promising results.[472] Another calcium-free phosphate binder that became recently available is lanthanum carbonate. This compound is a trace element but it seems possible to administer it safely without its deposition in the bone. New vitamin D analogues that have less calcemic and phosphatemic effects are under development.[473] All these newly developed measures should help in combating hyperparathyroidism without increasing circulating calcium levels. In contrast, the traditional therapeutic options such as classical vitamin D analogues and calcium salts, easily induce hypercalcemia, hence increasing the risk for calcium deposition in the tissues and vascular damage.

Peptides

Peptides constitute a heterogeneous group of molecules. In general, peptides can be considered as typical MM • $ß_2$-M and PTH have been discussed previously.

Granulocyte inhibiting protein I (GIP I–28 kD), recovered from uremic sera or ultrafiltrate, suppresses the killing of invading bacteria by polymorphonuclear cells.[474] The compound has structural analogy with the variable part of kappa light chains. Free immunoglobulin light chains (25 kD) increase the number of viable neutrophils by inhibiting spontaneous apoptotic cell death.[71] Another peptide with granulocyte inhibitory effect (GIP II–9.5 kD) is partially homologous with $ß_2$-M and inhibits granulocyte glucose uptake and respiratory burst activity.[70] A degranulation inhibiting protein (DIP–24 kD), identical to angiogenin, was isolated from $ß_2$-M plasma ultrafiltrate of uremic patients.[475] The structure responsible for the inhibition of degranulation is different from the sites that are responsible for the angiogenic or ribonucleic activity of angiogenin. A structural variant of ubiquitin inhibits polymorphonuclear chemotaxis (chemotaxis inhibiting protein–CIP–8.5 kD).[476]

Atrial natriuretic peptide (ANP–3.1 kD) and endothelin (3.5 kD) are elevated in dialysis patients and may play a role in the regulation of blood pressure.[477] ANP levels correlate with left atrial size, fluid overload, and decreased systemic clearance.[478] ANP-fragments have been detected in uremia[479] and are removed by dialyzer membrane adsorption.[479] Endothelin causes peripheral insulin resistance, even at concentrations that induce no blood flow changes[480] and may play a role in uremic hypertension.[16,481,482] Progression of renal failure,[481] reduction of number of cardiac capillaries,[483] myocardial fibrosis,[484] as well as left ventricular dysfunction[485] are prevented by endothelin receptor blockade. Endothelin release is opposed by nitric oxide, especially in erythropoietin-treated uremic rats.[486,487]

The opioid peptides ß-endorphin (3.5 kD), methionine-enkephalin (0.6 kD) and ß-lipotropin (1.9 kD) are elevated in dialyzed patients,[488] although some studies do not confirm this rise in concentration.[489] Delta sleep-inducing peptide (0.9 kD) may modulate sleep-wakefulness.[490] Most toxic actions of this group of peptides remain speculative. ß-endorphins might downmodulate T-cell response.[491]

Neuropeptide Y (NPY–4.3 kD) is increased in uremia[492] and tends to increase further during hemodialysis.[493] It is a 36 amino acid peptide with renal vasoconstrictive activity.[494] Recently, plasma NPY was found to predict incident cardiovascular complications in end-stage renal disease.[495] NPY also acts as an orexigen.[496] Uremic patients with anorexia have lower neuropeptide Y levels.[140,496] The concentration of the anorexigen cholecystokinin (CCK) is increased in most patients with chronic renal failure.[496]

Adrenomedullin, a 52-amino acid and potent hypotensive peptide, is found at markedly increased concentrations in chronic renal failure patients[497] and activates inducible nitric oxide synthase.[498] Apart from enhancing the risk for hypotension under certain conditions, this factor may be involved in defensive mechanisms preventing or counterbalancing the damage to the cardiovascular system in chronic renal failure.

Cystatin C (13.3 kD), Clara cell protein (CC16) (15.8 kD), and retinol binding protein (RBP) (21.2 kD) are elevated in renal failure.[499] Cystatin C is an inhibitor proteinase and cathepsins.[500] CC16 is an α-microprotein, playing an immunosuppressive role in the airways.[501] Leptin, a 16 kD plasma protein that suppresses appetite[502] induces weight reduction in mice[503] and has been suggested to play a role in the decreased appetite of uremic patients.[504] Most,[138,505-507] but not all, ESRD-patients[508-510] have inappropriately high leptin levels. The rise in serum leptin is mostly attributed to decreased renal elimination[505,511-514] and is almost entirely limited to a rise in the free (non-protein-bound) concentration.[505] Increased leptin is associated with low protein intake and loss of lean tissue in chronic renal failure patients.[504] Recent data suggest an inverted correlation between leptin and indices of nutritional status, such as serum albumin or lean body mass,[515] and a direct correlation with C-reactive protein (CRP).[506] In a recent study in CAPD-patients, serum leptin showed a progressive rise only in those patients developing body weight loss over time.[139] The ratio of serum leptin to body fat mass is higher in hemodialysis patients than in controls[516] and correlates with subsequent body weight loss.[517] Dialysis patients with the highest leptin/fat mass ratio have low protein intakes and lower lean tissue mass.[504] Erythropoietin treatment results in a decline of leptinemia and an improvement of nutritional status.[518]

However, leptin levels are also elevated in obese people and are hence not necessarily related to reduced appetite. Body fat and serum leptin also correlate in uremia.[506] Female gender and obesity are important factors that affect serum leptin also in ESRD-patients.[519] Several authors found no correlation between leptinemia and markers of protein malnutrition.[507,520,521] The administration of cytokines, such as IL-1ß and TNF-α, has been shown to increase serum leptin levels.[522,523] However, Don and associates[524] suggest that in ESRD-patients, leptin may be depressed during inflammation and may actually act as a negative acute phase reactant. Therefore, the biochemical role of leptin in renal failure remains inadequately defined.

Phenylacetylglutamine

Phenylacetylglutamine is a metabolite of phenylalanine,[525] is found at increased concentrations in uremic plasma and ultrafiltrate,[526] and is removed during dialysis in parallel to urea and creatinine.[527] No biologic effects have been demonstrated, although several structural precursors and analogues inhibit tumor growth and induce differentiation.[528]

Phenols

Phenol depresses various functional parameters of enzymatic activity in polymorphonuclear leukocytes.[529] A depressive effect was demonstrated on the 3′:5′-cyclic monophosphate response of the neostriatum to dopamine.[530] This effect was abolished after conjugation of phenol to phenylglucuronide. These findings may be relevant to hepatic and uremic coma. Phenol prevents *in vitro* the inhibition of parathyroid cell proliferation induced by calcitriol.[531]

P-cresol, a phenolic volatile compound with a MW of only 108.1 D, is retained in renal failure,[532] induces LDH-leakage from rat liver slices,[533] blocks liver mitochondrial respiration,[534] and inactivates the transformation of dopamine to norepinephrine by ß-hydroxylase.[535] Several other functions, such as drug protein binding[310] and cell growth,[536] oxygen uptake,[537] and membrane permeability[538] are affected as well. *P*-cresol inhibits various metabolic processes related to the production by activated phagocytes of free radicals, which are involved in the destruction of invading bacteria.[72] Aluminum uptake by hepatocytes and the toxic effect of aluminum on these hepatocytes are increased in the presence of *p*-cresol.[539] A similar toxic effect was also observed on neuroblastoma and erythroleukemia cells.[539] *P*-cresol and phenol inhibit platelet-activating factor (PAF) synthesis by phagocytic leukocytes,[540] and *p*-cresol inhibits detoxification of arsenic by methylation.[541] It also alters neuronal cell function.[36] *P*-cresol is produced by the intestinal flora, as a result of the metabolism of tyrosine[542] but might be generated from environmental sources as well.[543] Prevention of the intestinal absorption of p-cresol by administration of oral sorbent decreases serum concentration in rats.[544] Changes of composition of intestinal flora might influence p-cresol generation.[545]

P-cresol is lipophilic and protein-bound, and its removal by hemodialysis is markedly less than that of urea and creatinine.[176,256] Daily hemodialysis results in lower pre-dialysis serum p-cresol levels compared to conventional alternate day dialysis.[546] In a hemodialysis setting, the removal of p-cresol and that of urea and creatinine are not correlated,[176] demonstrating that the latter markers are not representative for the intradialytic behavior of protein-bound p-cresol. P-cresol levels are markedly lower in PD, compared to hemodialysis.[547] Rises in free p-cresol during hemodialysis with heparin as an anticoagulant, appeared to be artifactual.[178] Hypoalbuminemia and a rise in total p-cresol are correlated to an increase of the free active fraction of p-cresol.[179] A correlation between free p-cresol and hospitalization rate was demonstrated.[179] Patients hospitalized for infection also had a higher free p-cresol.[179] In rats with normal renal function, the total clearance of p-cresol largely exceeded the renal clearance in contrast to creatinine, for which renal clearance equals total clearance.[548] The distribution volume of p-cresol is approximately four times larger than that of creatinine, and is not significantly affected by renal failure.[549] The intravenous administration of p-cresol results in the immediate metabolization of the compound into p-cresylglucuronide,[550] pointing to the role of metabolism in the removal of this compound.

Phosphate

High phosphate levels are associated with pruritus and hyperparathyroidism.[551] They affect PTH levels indirectly by decreasing Ca^{++} and calcitriol,[552] but also by direct stimulation of PTH secretion.[553,554] Phosphorus causes a decrease in the activity of spermine/spermidine N^1-acetyltransferase, the enzyme responsible for polyamine degradation,[555] and is also engaged in intestinal dysfunction and proliferation of the intestinal villi.[555] Low dietary phosphate prevents parathyroid hyperplasia in early uremia, whereas a high dietary phosphate enhances the production of tumor growth factor α (TGF-α), which functions as an autocrine signal to further stimulate growth.[556]

Hyperphosphatemia is not only a direct cause of hyperparathyroidism,[557] but also the result of the action of PTH on the bone. The administration of calcitriol in an attempt to control PTH produces hyperphosphatemia as well.[558]

The blood phosphorus concentration is the result of protein catabolism and protein intake as well as of the ingestion of other sources (e.g., Coca-Cola). Restriction of oral intake increases the risk of protein malnutrition,[551] which can be avoided by the administration of oral phosphate binders.[559] Until recently, these consisted mainly of aluminum or calcium salts. The effect of the latter, however, is often insufficient, especially in subjects with a high phosphorus intake. The presence of a high calcium-phosphate product results in tissular deposition of calcium. New phosphate binders such as lanthanum carbonate, sevelamer hydrochloride and trivalent iron-containing compounds offer the advantage that they contain no calcium, so that the risk of hypercalcemia is reduced.[560–563] Whether these compounds are more efficient phosphate binders is, however, less obvious. Sevelamer hydrochloride has a lipid lowering effect[564] and reduces cardiovascular calcification.[565] Lanthanum is a cationic trace element[563] and in this regard could impose similar problems as aluminum if absorbed into the body.

Phosphorus is a small water soluble molecule, but with a retention and removal pattern that hardly mimics that of any other molecule. Cellular clearance during hemodialysis is markedly lower than that of urea,[566] resulting in a substantial post-dialysis rebound.[567] Removal seems to be effective only during the initial phase of a hemodialysis session, after which transfer from the intracellular compartment becomes the rate-limiting step.[568] Alternative dialytic strategies such as daily dialysis,[569,570] slow prolonged dialysis sessions,[570] or hemodiafiltration[571] all might improve phosphate removal. The application of daily dialysis even results in a decreased intake of peroral phosphate binders.[569,570] The serum phosphate levels in nocturnal hemodialysis patients are better under control compared with daily hemodialysis or conventional hemodialysis patients,[572] although oral phosphate binders may still be required.[573] High-flux hemodialysis fails to produce higher phosphate removal.[574] Gotch and associates[575] describe a kinetic model of inorganic phosphorus mass balance in hemodialysis therapy to monitor the individual effects of diet, dialysis and binders, to optimize inorganic phosphorus mass balance, and to reduce phosphate accumulation in the tissues.

Currently, 60% of hemodialysis patients in the United States have serum phosphate levels higher than 5.5 mg/dL.[576] Such high phosphate levels are directly correlated to mortality,[29] which appears to be linked to a high Ca × P product and an enhanced tissular deposition of Ca-containing complexes, for example, in vessel walls.[29,577]

Phosphorus and uremic serum upregulate osteopontin expression in vascular smooth muscle cells,[578] which might explain, at least in part, the trend for vessel calcification in relation to hyperphosphatemia.

Polyamines

Spermine is a polycathionic polyamine, which inhibits erythropoiesis.[42] Other polyamines, such as spermidine, putrescine, and cadaverine, are also found at increased concentrations in renal failure and inhibit erythroid colony formation in a dose-dependent manner.[41] Polyamines have a high affinity for body proteins and cells. In uremic serum, the polyamines are conjugated to protein carriers, resulting in complexes with molecular weights from 1500 to 5000 D.[579] Polyamines might play a role in anorexia, vomiting, ataxia, seizures, hypothermia and immune deficiency.[580] The accumulation of putrescine may lead to oxidative stress causing cell death.[581] Putrescine inhibits *in vitro* cell growth and alters cytoplasmic, mitochondrial and nuclear membrane structures at high concentrations, where it causes irreversible cell degeneration at lower concentration.[160] Several polyamines interfere with the NMDA receptor,[582] and subsequently with channel conductance and Ca^{++} permeability of brain cells,[36] but spermine might induce neurotoxicity by other pathways as well.[583] Spermine reduces intracellular free calcium in permeabilized pancreatic islets[584] and inhibits NO-synthase.[585] Polyamines antagonize platelet aggregation.[586] Polyamine-related cytotoxicity is attributed to the generation of acrolein as a result of polyamine oxidation by amine oxidase.[587] Polyamine-protein conjugates have been shown to accumulate in uremia and, in vitro, these substances inhibit erythroid proliferation.[588] Oxidation of polyamines by amine oxidase results in cytotoxic compounds, with a potential role in brain damage.[589,590] Remarkably, a potent antiglycation effect of the polyamines spermine and spermidine at physiologic concentrations has been observed, comparable to the effect of aminoguanidine and carnosine.[591]

One of the problems with the polyamines is the relative impermeability of the cell membrane for these compounds, which will result in a multicompartmental behavior during dialysis.[41]

Pseudouridine

Pseudouridine accumulates in uremia in parallel to creatinine.[592] Dzúrik and associates[91] demonstrated inhibition of glucose utilization in isolated rat soleus muscle. Other pyrimidine derivatives, such as orotic acid, orotidine, uridine, and thymine also accumulate in uremic plasma; the concentrations of orotic acid and orotidine are further increased by allopurinol administration.[593]

Purines

Uric acid, xanthine, hypoxanthine, cytidine, and guanosine are the most important purines retained in uremia. The purines disturb calcitriol production and to a lesser extent also its metabolization.[594] Administration of purines to animals results in a net decrease of serum calcitriol and of the binding of vitamin D receptor to DNA-chromatin.[594] A decrease of uric acid in response to allopurinol administration results in a rise of plasma calcitriol levels.[595] Purines are involved in the resistance to calcitriol of immune competent cells,[115] by a reduction of the expression of the lipopolysaccharide receptor CD14 on the surface of monocytes. Xanthine and hypoxanthine have been implicated as modulators of neurotransmission and may be related to poor appetite and weight loss.[596] Both xanthine and hypoxanthine induce vasoconstriction, inhibit platelet induced vasorelaxation,[597] and disturb endothelial barriers.[598] Hypoxanthine also blocks detoxification by methylation of arsenic.[541] Uric acid acts as an antioxidant and hence reduces oxidative stress,[599, 600] although this effect is mainly limited to *in vitro* conditions.[430,599] In young children with chronic renal failure, cytidine is found in cerebrospinal fluid at concentrations that are at least 10 times above normal, and that are also higher than the corresponding concentrations in blood.[601] Based on indirect arguments, this finding has been related to delayed cognitive development.

In spite of a markedly diminished urinary secretion of uric acid in renal failure, the rise in plasma uric acid levels is only moderate because of net intestinal secretion.[602] Uric acid is a small water soluble compound that is removed by hemodialysis from the plasma in a similar way as urea,[387] but removal from the intracellular compartment is by far not as efficient.[603] Possibly, other uremic toxins play a role in the inhibition of this transfer. Dialytic removal of xanthine and hypoxanthine shows no correlation with that of urea and creatinine.[387] Microencapsulated genetically engineered E. Coli cells have been developed, which have the capacity to lower uric acid both *in vitro* and *in vivo.*[604]

Trace Elements

Sources of trace element accumulation are dialysate, food intake, drugs, and prosthetic materials. Retention is the consequence of insufficient renal elimination. Although alterations in concentration of trace elements modify a host of biologic functions, it has been difficult to demonstrate a link between trace element accumulation and uremic side effects.[39]

Aluminum accumulates as a result of its presence in dialysate, or of excessive intake of aluminum hydroxide as a phosphate binder. It provokes mental changes (aluminum encephalopathy) and osteomalacia as a result of the competition of aluminum with calcium at the bone matrix.[605] Aluminum intoxication has become less prevalent, since the implementation of more adequate water treatment systems.

Iron overload results in a baseline activation of leukocyte biologic activity,[606] which is related to chronic inflammation and possibly atherogenesis, and in a depressed response of the leukocytes upon activation,[606] linked to an increased susceptibility to infection. Fortunately, iron overload has become less frequent since the introduction of erythropoietin.

The concentration of other elements, such as copper, cadmium, mercury, chromium, strontium, and molybdene is also increased.[607-610] In recent studies, retention of arsenic has been evidenced in a substantial segment of the uremic population.[609,611] For some trace elements, such as zinc, bromine, selenium, rubidium and caesium, a decreased concentration has been reported.[609,612,613] Selenium deficiency might be related to atherogenesis.[614] Selenium supplementation not only prevents oxidative stress but renal structural energy as well.[615]

Trihalomethanes

Trihalomethanes are common contaminants of chlorinated tap water, which are found in dialysate if they are incompletely eliminated by water treatment systems. They are present at increased concentrations in the blood of hemodialyzed patients,[616] are potentially mutagenic, carcinogenic,[617-619] and a possible cause of spontaneous abortion.[620]

Urea

For the extensive number of toxicity studies to which urea has been submitted, the number in which a well defined adverse biochemical or physiologic impact has been reported at concentrations currently encountered in uremia is relatively low. Interestingly, in a classical study by Johnson and associates,[621] long lasting dialysis against dialysate containing high urea concentrations had no consistent impact on uremic clinical symptoms. More recently, two large controlled clinical studies, the ADEMEX and the HEMO-study, could not demonstrate an impact of enhanced urea removal on survival outcome.[173,622]

Lim and associates[623,624] have shown that urea inhibits NaK2Cl cotransport in human erythrocytes, as well as a number of cell volume sensitive transport pathways. A heat shock response is elicited by urea in human neuroblastoma cells, which might be a factor playing a role in uremic neurotoxicity. In a recent study by Moeslinger and associates,[625] urea was shown to induce macrophage proliferation by inhibition of inducible nitric oxide synthesis (iNOS). This inhibition of iNOS occurs at the posttranscriptional level.[626] Urea inhibits *in vitro* L-arginine transport and endothelial NO-synthase activity,[627] but *in vivo*, 7 days of urea administration to rats had no impact on renal cortical L-arginine concentration or on NO-synthase activity.[628] Urea increases the expression of the oxidative stress-responsive transcription factor, Gadd153/ CHOP.[629]

It has been suggested that *in vivo*, urea toxicity is counterbalanced by the methylamines, which are retained in parallel in renal failure.[404] A direct proof of this effect has, however, not yet been delivered. Trimethylamine oxide (TMA-O) protects myosin structures against urea-induced effects (2–8 mol/L).[405] Urea, when administered alone to bilaterally nephrectomized rats, shortens their life span.[268] This could possibly be attributed to an osmotic effect.

Urea is also the precursor of some of the guanidines, especially guanidinosuccinic acid (see earlier text), which by themselves induce direct biochemical alterations. As the uremic retention solute with the highest net concentration, urea may also be involved in dialysis disequilibrium, if the decrease in plasma concentration during dialysis occurs too rapidly. Urea may also be a source of generation of cyanate and isocyanic acid, and these might be at the origin of carbamoylation, resulting in structural and functional changes of amino acids and proteins.[630-634] Serum urea is the most consistent predictor of carbomylated hemoglobin in uremia.[631] Spontaneous dissociation of urea to isocyanate has been held responsible for the decreased affinity of oxygen for hemoglobin.[635]

Urea is unequivocally recognized as a marker of solute retention and removal in dialyzed patients. It is one of the few solutes that has been correlated convincingly with clinical outcome of hemodialysis.[636] However, it is not the peak concentration per se, but the low reduction ratios during dialysis together with the high ambient level (time average) that are related to increased mortality.[637] Therefore, dynamic urea kinetic parameters, reflecting dialytic removal (total clearance normalized for distribution volume–Kt/V) are more valuable indices of dialysis adequacy than static parameters (e.g., pre-dialysis urea concentrations). Standard Kt/V (stdKt/V) enables the quantitative comparison of dose with widely varying dialysis schedules.[638] High blood concentrations of urea do not necessarily relate to poor outcome if removal is sufficient, such as in continuous ambulatory peritoneal dialysis (CAPD) patients and/or in patients receiving high protein diet.[639] The reason for this apparent paradox is that urea concentration is not only influenced by dialytic removal but also by protein intake, which is actually a factor related to a good metabolic status.

One might question the validity and representativity of urea as a marker for the retention and the removal of other solutes. Biochemical systems are, at least in part, affected by compounds with a kinetic behavior that largely differs from that of urea (e.g., MM, protein bound solutes). Even if dialytic removal from the plasma is similar, as is the case for other small, water soluble, non-protein-bound compounds such as creatinine or uric acid,[387] the shift from intracellular to the plasma might occur at a different rate,[603] again resulting in divergent kinetics.

FACTORS INFLUENCING UREMIC SOLUTE CONCENTRATION (TABLE 6–3)

Removal Pattern

Conventional hemodialysis easily removes small water-soluble compounds, such as urea and creatinine, which are the most current markers of uremic retention and removal. Urea removal is linked to dialysis-related mortality.[640] Removal pattern of urea and creatinine is markedly different from that of many other uremic solutes with proven toxicity. MM are better removed by hemodialyzers containing membranes with larger pore size, and by convection (e.g., hemodiafiltration).[234] Also CAPD results in a relatively more efficient removal of MM, compared to conventional hemodialysis.

Table 6–3 Factors Influencing Solute Concentration in Dialyzed Patients

Solute-related factors
Compartmental distribution
Intracellular concentration
Resistance of cell membrane
Protein binding
Electrostatic charge
Steric configuration
Molecular weight
Hydrophilicity/lipophilicity
Patient-related factors
Distribution volume and body weight
Intake and generation
Solute
Metabolic precursors
Residual renal function
Access quality
Metabolic generation
Metabolic degradation
Absorption from the intestine
Haematocrit
Blood viscosity
Serum albumin concentration
Dialysis-related factors
Dialysis time
Interdialytic intervals
Blood flow
Mean blood flow
Blood flow pattern
Shear in dialyzer
Blood distribution
Dialysate flow
Dialysate distribution
Dialysate processing (single pass/batch)
Dialyzer surface
Dialyzer volume
Dialyzer membrane resistance
Dialyzer pore size
Dialyzer hydrophilicity/hydrophobicity
Adsorption
On the membrane
On other constituents of the circuit
Ultrafiltration rate
Intradialytic changes in efficacy
Changes with a direct impact on solute related factors
Blood pH
Heparinization
Free fatty acid concentration
Hemodynamic stability during dialysis

Protein bound molecules behave during dialysis like larger (middle) molecules. Nevertheless, their removal will insufficiently be influenced by an increase in pore size,[176] unless the carrier proteins (mainly albumin) are removed at the same time, but this enhances the risk of caloric malnutrition. Until recently, the current dialytic methods offer no satisfactory possibilities to remove protein-bound compounds, except for PD.[256]

In recent studies, however, super flux cellulose triacetate as well as so-called protein-leaking membranes were shown to enhance removal of protein-bound molecules,[340, 341] although it remains unclear whether this effect is the result of enhanced removal unto or through the membrane, or of improved metabolism. Likewise, super flux polysulphone dialysis could decrease pre-dialysis AGE-concentration.[641]

Adsorption

Adsorption on specifically designed devices may be a promising solution for the elimination of difficult to remove molecules, such as the protein bound compounds, and renewed interest has recently been gained for this concept.[642-644] Adsorption already occurs on most hemodialysis membranes, but surface is not sufficient to allow adequate removal. The most acceptable option is the development of chemical polymers that contain structures in which the targeted molecules perfectly fit. As most small water-soluble molecules are easily removed by diffusion, it is of greater interest to develop devices with high adsorptive surface area (> 200 m^2) for large and/or lipophilic molecules. The question arises whether the adsorptive capacity of such devices will be sufficient, especially if confronted with toxins with a multicompartmental distribution.

Sorbent techniques can be used to extract compounds from dialysate (e.g., hemadsorption,[645] hemolipodialysis,[646] from ultrafiltrate[647,648] in a regeneration procedure before the treated ultrafiltrate is returned to the blood stream, from plasma[649,650] if combined with plasma filtration, or directly from blood.[238,651-653]

Removal of protein bound compounds during hemodialysis might be increased by the addition of albumin to the dialysate,[388,654] which is efficient but expensive.

Alternative Time Frames

Even under optimal conditions, Kt/V_{urea} in PD-patients is low compared to the values obtained in hemodialysis-patients, but the clinical status of patients treated with both modalities is similar. This suggests that other compounds than urea, presumably with dissimilar physical characteristics, play a role in uremic toxicity, and/or that the slow toxin removal by PD and/or its capacity to remove protein-bound moieties, may have an additional beneficial impact.[177,655] Because removal is more gradual with continuous strategies, more compounds will be cleared, especially those with low clearance rates. Continuous hemodialysis strategies, slow, low efficiency dialysis applied over prolonged time periods, or daily dialysis might therefore result in more adequate toxin removal. While shifting patients from alternate day high-flux hemodialysis to daily overnight slow online hemodiafiltration, Raj and associates[656] were able to provoke an additional decline in pre-dialysis serum $ß_2$-microglobulin concentration.

Likewise, similar or lower phosphate plasma levels have been observed with daily hemodialysis, compared to classical alternate day hemodialysis, in spite of a lower intake of phosphate binders.[569,570] Several studies suggest an improvement of clinical status if patients are submitted to daily and/or slow prolonged hemodialysis.[569,657] This has been confirmed recently in a well-conducted controlled study.[491] AGE-levels were lower in patients treated by daily dialysis than if the same patients were submitted to an alternative day scheme, in spite of identical weekly dialysis time and similar Kt/V.[301] Similarly, the pre-dialysis concentration of several protein bound molceules was decreased significantly after 6 months of daily hemodialysis treatment.[546]

Intracellular Shifts and Removal

Uremic solutes accumulate not only in the plasma but also in the cell, where most of the biologic activity is exerted. Removal of intracellular compounds across the cell membrane may be delayed during dialysis, resulting in multicompartmental kinetics, as removal will largely be limited to the plasmatic compartment. Even small water soluble compounds, such as urea, which are not subjected to resistance during their passage through the cell membrane, may display a multicompartmental behavior,[658] due to sequestration of certain body compartments. One of the consequences is a rebound at the end of the dialysis session.[659] In rats, the protein-bound toxin *p*-cresol was shown to distribute over a volume that exceeded the rat's weight by a factor of two to three,[548] which might explain its difficult removal even with the most efficient dialysis strategies.[176]

NONDIALYTIC FACTORS

Nutritional and Environmental Effects

Most toxins or their precursors enter the body via the gastrointestinal route. The metabolic processes that are generated by the intestinal flora play a role in this process. Inhibition of intestinal absorption, and modifications in the composition of the intestinal flora could influence solute concentration.[544,660,661] A specific oral sorbent (AST120) decreases serum indoxyl sulfate and *p*-cresol in uremic rats.[133,544,662,663] A few potassium and phosphate binders are applied in the clinical setting today, but in general, the resources to decrease intestinal delivery of uremic solutes are insufficiently explored.

A number of toxins are produced from protein breakdown or from metabolization of amino acids. Therefore, protein restriction might reduce toxicity, were it not that protein malnutrition increases morbidity and mortality by itself.[637]

Several toxins or their precursors, such as AGEs, trace elements, conservation agents (e.g., benzylalcohol as a precursor of hippuric acid), or vitamin C (precursor of oxalate), are present in food; these compounds are not necessarily linked to protein intake, the classically accepted main source of uremic toxin generation. Other rarely considered sources are forensic contact with volatile precursors (e.g., toluene), that are inhaled or swallowed, the intake of herbal medicines, and psychedelic drugs, or contact with environmental noxes, leached from elements of the dialysis circuit or from the dialysate (e.g., glucose degradation products present in heat-sterilized glucose-containing PD-solutions).

Pharmacologic Interaction

One of the future aspects of the treatment of uremia will consist of influencing toxin metabolization by drugs or other compounds. Some elements are known already as of today. Allopurinol decreases uric acid.[664] Rhubarb tannins decrease the concentration of urea, creatinine, guanidino-succinic acid and methylguanidine in rats with renal failure.[665] Vitamin C increases urinary excretion of CMPF.[666] Homocysteine can be lowered in uremic patients by supplementation of folic acid, pyridoxine and/or vitamin B_{12}.[344,346,348,667,668] Pyridoxine also reduces oxalate levels.[423] Aminoguanidine has the presumed property to reduce AGE generation.[669] The *in vivo* effect of aminoguanidine is not entirely convincing, but other inhibitors of AGE formation, which might turn out to be more efficient, will become available in the future.[670]

In a recent study, Lesaffer and associates[549] demonstrated in uremic rats that not only renal but also nonrenal clearance was dramatically inhibited. Enhancing metabolic clearance, for example, by applying the principles as they are in vigor during artificial liver treatment, might be of help as well in the uremic population.

Most uremic patients receive several drugs, which can result in: (1) accumulation of the mother compound because of decreased renal clearance and/or decreased metabolization by the kidneys or other organs; (2) interference of drugs with protein binding and/or tubular secretion of uremic toxins; and (3) the generation of drug metabolites that are not excreted by the failing kidneys, and that exert toxic side effects on their own.

Residual Renal Function

The impact of residual renal function on uremic retention is substantial.[636] This relative contribution is even more important for larger molecules and molecules with multicompartmental behavior, which are removed less efficiently by the dialysis procedure. Therefore, the longer preservation of residual renal function with CAPD compared to conventional hemodialysis[671, 672] may have a substantial impact on toxicity. Also with high flux biocompatible membranes, residual renal function is preserved longer.[167, 673]

Uremic retention solutes have been held responsible for a faster deterioration of residual renal function.[131] At least one of these compounds, indoxyl sulfate, is removed more efficiently by CAPD.[133]

CONCLUSIONS

The uremic syndrome is the result of a complex set of biochemical and pathophysiologic disturbances, emanating in a state of generalized malaise and dysfunction. This condition is related to the retention of a host of compounds; many of them exert a negative impact on key functions of the body; those molecules have consequently been identified as uraemic toxins. Up to now, the toxic action of single solutes has repeatedly been studied, but the intermutual interference between compounds has rarely been considered. Although solute retention is one of the major pathophysiologic events, deficiencies are functionally important as well.

Removal and generation of many compounds with proven biologic or biochemical impact, especially toxins that are hydrophobic and/or not generated from protein breakdown, can hardly be predicted by the intradialytic behavior of urea, a current marker but a small water soluble compound generated from protein, with relatively little biologic impact.

Solute clearance eventually reaches a plateau as dialyzer blood flow and/or dialysate flow are increased; this plateau is reached much sooner for molecules with a higher molecular weight. As a result, clearance of MM stricto sensu is relatively blood and dialysate flow independent. Only an increase of dialysis time, dialyzer surface area, ultrafiltration rates and/or dialyzer pore size can enhance their removal.

Removal of solutes that behave like larger molecules due to their protein binding, multicompartmental distribution and/or lipophilicity, will be less affected by the use of high flux dialyzers and/or dialyzers with a larger pore size. To improve the clearances of these "new definition MM," it may be necessary to develop renal replacement systems with different characteristics, for example, specific adsorption systems and/or procedures that allow a slower exchange of solutes.

Earlier concepts of charcoal adsorption, eventually largely abandoned, should perhaps be reconsidered, especially for the removal of organic acids. More specific and/or more efficient adsorptive systems may be needed, however. As an alternative, adsorption of toxins or of their precursors may be pursued at the intestinal level. Another alternative to be considered is dialysis against recycled albumin-containing dialysate, to allow a better diffusion of protein bound toxic compounds.[388] Finally, a last alternative could be the use of protein permeable membranes, to remove larger molecules as well as protein bound substances.[340] Whether the amount of removal will be sufficient to reduce uremic toxicity, whether this removal will not enhance or induce protein malnutrition, and whether the cost of such procedures will outweigh the benefit remains a matter of debate. Even if solute removal is improved by alternative strategies, mass transfer may be limited if the compounds of interest are distributed over multiple compartments.

The next step is to pursue more specific removal. However, before this can be realized, we will need to know more about the toxic compounds responsible for these disturbances. Some progress has been made in this area during the last few years. What is still lacking is a structural approach, comparing a large panel of putative toxins, at well defined concentrations, and with well defined test methods. The subsequent step is then to launch controlled studies, whereby therapeutic strategies that remove the toxins that have been characterized, will be tested on their impact on morbidity and mortality.

We are convinced that our views on how to enhance uremic toxin removal need to be changed. Increasing pore size, alone or in combination with adaptations in dialyzer geometry, is certainly not the only solution, and might have come close to its maximal capacity.

References

1. Lazarus JM, Lowrie EG, Hampers CL, Merrill JP: Cardiovascular disease in uremic patients on hemodialysis. Kidney Int Suppl 1975; 167–175.
2. Lameire N, Vanholder RC, Van Loo A, et al: Cardiovascular diseases in peritoneal dialysis patients: The size of the problem. Kidney Int Suppl 1996; 56:S28–S36.
3. Parfrey PS, Harnett JD, Barre PE: The natural history of myocardial disease in dialysis patients. J Am Soc Nephrol 1991; 2:2–12.

4. Wray TM, Stone WJ: Uremic pericarditis: A prospective echocardiographic and clinical study. Clin Nephrol 1976; 6:295–302.
5. Foley RN, Parfrey PS: Cardiovascular disease and mortality in ESRD. J Nephrol 1998; 11:239–245.
6. Levin A, Thompson CR, Ethier J, et al: Left ventricular mass index increase in early renal disease: Impact of decline in hemoglobin. Am J Kidney Dis 1999; 34:125–134.
7. Ross R: Atherosclerosis: An inflammatory disease. N Engl J Med 1999; 340:115–126.
8. Stenvinkel P: Inflammatory and atherosclerotic interactions in the depleted uremic patient. Blood Purif 2001; 19:53–61.
9. Kaysen GA: The microinflammatory state in uremia: Causes and potential consequences. J Am Soc Nephrol 2001; 12:1549–1557.
10. Zoccali C, Benedetto FA, Mallamaci F, et al: Inflammation is associated with carotid atherosclerosis in dialysis patients. Creed Investigators. Cardiovascular Risk Extended Evaluation in Dialysis Patients. J Hypertens 2000; 18:1207–1213.
11. Guerin AP, London GM, Marchais SJ, Metivier F: Arterial stiffening and vascular calcifications in end-stage renal disease. Nephrol Dial Transplant 2000; 15:1014–1021.
12. Goodman WG, Goldin J, Kuizon BD, et al: Coronary-artery calcification in young adults with end-stage renal disease who are undergoing dialysis. N Engl J Med 2000; 342:1478–1483.
13. Parfrey PS, Harnett JD, Griffiths SM, et al: Congestive heart failure in dialysis patients. Arch Intern Med 1988; 148: 1519–1525.
14. Rostand SG, Sanders C, Kirk KA, et al: Myocardial calcification and cardiac dysfunction in chronic renal failure. Am J Med 1988; 85:651–657.
15. Lindner A, Kenny M, Meacham AJ: Effects of a circulating factor in patients with essential hypertension on intracellular free calcium in normal platelets. N Engl J Med 1987; 316:509–513.
16. Morris ST, McMurray JJ, Spiers A, Jardine AG: Impaired endothelial function in isolated human uremic resistance arteries. Kidney Int 2001; 60:1077–1082.
17. Morris ST, McMurray JJ, Rodger RS, Jardine AG: Impaired endothelium-dependent vasodilatation in uraemia. Nephrol Dial Transplant 2000; 15:1194–1200.
18. Rambausek M, Mann JF, Mall G, et al: Cardiac findings in experimental uremia. Contrib Nephrol 1986; 52:125–133.
19. Kong CH, Thompson FD: Hemodynamic responses to head-up tilt in uremic patients. Clin Nephrol 1990; 33:283–287.
20. Meggs LG, Ben Ari J, Gammon D, et al: Effect of chronic uremia on the cardiovascular alpha 1 receptor. Life Sci 1986; 39:169–179.
21. Mall G, Rambausek M, Neumeister A, et al: Myocardial interstitial fibrosis in experimental uremia: Implications for cardiac compliance. Kidney Int 1988; 33:804–811.
22. Foley RN, Parfrey PS, Sarnak MJ: Epidemiology of cardiovascular disease in chronic renal disease. J Am Soc Nephrol 1998; 9:S16–S23.
23. Hemmelgarn BR, Ghali WA, Quan H, et al: Poor long-term survival after coronary angiography in patients with renal insufficiency. Am J Kidney Dis 2001; 37:64–72.
24. Witko-Sarsat V, Friedlander M, Nguyen KT, et al: Advanced oxidation protein products as novel mediators of inflammation and monocyte activation in chronic renal failure. J Immunol 1998; 161:2524–2532.
25. Cohen G, Rudnicki M, Walter F, et al: Glucose-modified proteins modulate essential functions and apoptosis of polymorphonuclear leukocytes. J Am Soc Nephrol 2001; 12:1264– 1271.
26. Boushey CJ, Beresford SA, Omenn GS, Motulsky AG: A quantitative assessment of plasma homocysteine as a risk factor for vascular disease. Probable benefits of increasing folic acid intakes. JAMA 1995; 274:1049–1057.
27. Massy ZA: Importance of homocysteine, lipoprotein (a) and non-classical cardiovascular risk factors (fibrinogen and advanced glycation end-products) for atherogenesis in uraemic patients. Nephrol Dial Transplant 2000; 15(suppl 5):81–91.
28. van Guldener C, Lambert J, ter Wee PM, et al: Carotid artery stiffness in patients with end-stage renal disease: No effect of long-term homocysteine-lowering therapy. Clin Nephrol 2000; 53:33–41.
29. Block GA, Hulbert-Shearon TE, Levin NW, Port FK: Association of serum phosphorus and calcium × phosphate product with mortality risk in chronic hemodialysis patients: A national study. Am J Kidney Dis 1998; 31:607–617.
30. Rostand SG, Drueke TB: Parathyroid hormone, vitamin D, and cardiovascular disease in chronic renal failure. Kidney Int 1999; 56:383–392.
31. Zoccali C, Benedetto FA, Maas R, et al: Asymmetric dimethylarginine, C-reactive protein, and carotid intima-media thickness in end-stage renal disease. J Am Soc Nephrol 2002; 13: 490–496.
32. Fraser CL, Arieff AI: Nervous system complications in uremia. Ann Intern Med 1988; 109:143–153.
33. Kimmel PL, Miller G, Mendelson WB: Sleep apnea syndrome in chronic renal disease. Am J Med 1989; 86:308–314.
34. Gafter U, Shvili Y, Levi J, et al: Brainstem auditory evoked responses in chronic renal failure and the effect of hemodialysis. Nephron 1989; 53:2–5.
35. D'Hooge R, Pei YQ, Manil J, De Deyn PP: The uremic guanidino compound guanidinosuccinic acid induces behavioral convulsions and concomitant epileptiform electrocorticographic discharges in mice. Brain Res 1992; 598:316–320.
36. D'Hooge R, Van de Vijver G, Van Bogaert PP, et al: Involvement of voltage- and ligand-gated Ca2+ channels in the neuroexcitatory and synergistic effects of putative uremic neurotoxins. Kidney Int 2003; 63:1764–1775.
37. Robles NR, Murga L, Galvan S, et al: Hemodialysis with cuprophane or polysulfone: Effects on uremic polyneuropathy. Am J Kidney Dis 1993; 21:282–287.
38. Moriwaki K, Kanno Y, Nakamoto H, et al: Vitamin B6 deficiency in elderly patients on chronic peritoneal dialysis. Adv Perit Dial 2000; 16:308–312.
39. Vanholder R, Cornelis R, Dhondt A, Lameire N: The role of trace elements in uraemic toxicity. Nephrol Dial Transplant 2002; 17(suppl 2):2–8.
40. Bogin E, Massry SG, Levi J, et al: Effect of parathyroid hormone on osmotic fragility of human erythrocytes. J Clin Invest 1982; 69:1017–1025.
41. Kushner D, Beckman B, Nguyen L, et al: Polyamines in the anemia of end-stage renal disease. Kidney Int 1991; 39:725–732.
42. Radtke HW, Rege AB, LaMarche MB, et al: Identification of spermine as an inhibitor of erythropoiesis in patients with chronic renal failure. J Clin Invest 1981; 67:1623–1629.
43. Segal GM, Stueve T, Adamson JW: Spermine and spermidine are non-specific inhibitors of in vitro hematopoiesis. Kidney Int 1987; 31:72–76.
44. Niwa T, Asada H, Tsutsui S, Miyazaki T: Efficient removal of albumin-bound furancarboxylic acid by protein-leaking hemodialysis. Am J Nephrol 1995; 15:463–467.
45. Urena P, Eckardt KU, Sarfati E, et al: Serum erythropoietin and erythropoiesis in primary and secondary hyperparathyroidism: Effect of parathyroidectomy. Nephron 1991; 59:384–393.
46. Macdougall IC: Role of uremic toxins in exacerbating anemia in renal failure. Kidney Int Suppl 2001; 78:S67–S72.
47. Urena P, Bonnardeaux A, Eckardt KU, et al: Insulin-like growth factor I: A modulator of erythropoiesis in uraemic patients? Nephrol Dial Transplant 1992; 7:40–44.
48. Larsson SO: On coagulation and fibrinolysis in renal failure. Scand J Haematol Suppl 1971; 15:1–59.
49. Remuzzi G: Bleeding in renal failure. Lancet 1988; 1:1205–1208.
50. Remuzzi G, Livio M, Marchiaro G, et al: Bleeding in renal failure: Altered platelet function in chronic uraemia only partially corrected by haemodialysis. Nephron 1978; 22: 347–353.
51. Di Minno G, Cerbone A, Usberti M, et al: Platelet dysfunction in uremia. II. Correction by arachidonic acid of the impaired

exposure of fibrinogen receptors by adenosine diphosphate or collagen. J Lab Clin Med 1986; 108:246–252.
52. Remuzzi G, Benigni A, Dodesini P, et al: Reduced platelet thromboxane formation in uremia. Evidence for a functional cyclooxygenase defect. J Clin Invest 1983; 71:762–768.
53. Tison P, Cernacek P, Silvanova E, Dzurik R: Uremic "toxins" and blood platelet carbohydrate metabolism. Nephron 1981; 28: 192–195.
54. Noris M, Benigni A, Boccardo P, et al: Enhanced nitric oxide synthesis in uremia: Implications for platelet dysfunction and dialysis hypotension. Kidney Int 1993; 44:445–450.
55. Vaziri ND: Effect of chronic renal failure on nitric oxide metabolism. Am J Kidney Dis 2001; 38:S74–S79.
56. Holloway DS, Vagher JP, Caprini JA, et al: Thrombelastography of blood from subjects with chronic renal failure. Thromb Res 1987; 45:817–825.
57. Warrell RP Jr, Hultin MB, Coller BS: Increased factor VIII/von Willebrand factor antigen and von Willebrand factor activity in renal failure. Am J Med 1979; 66:226–228.
58. Kozek-Langenecker SA, Masaki T, Mohammad H, et al: Fibrinogen fragments and platelet dysfunction in uremia. Kidney Int 1999; 56:299–305.
59. Vanholder R, Ringoir S: Infectious morbidity and defects of phagocytic function in end-stage renal disease: A review (editorial). J Am Soc Nephrol 1993; 3:1541–1554.
60. Goldblum SE, Reed WP: Host defenses and immunologic alterations associated with chronic hemodialysis. Ann Intern Med 1980; 93:597–613.
61. Lewis SL, Van Epps DE: Neutrophil and monocyte alterations in chronic dialysis patients. Am J Kidney Dis 1987; 9:381–395.
62. Vanholder R, Ringoir S, Dhondt A, Hakim R: Phagocytosis in uremic and hemodialysis patients: A prospective and cross sectional study. Kidney Int 1991; 39:320–327.
63. Vanholder R, Ringoir S: Polymorphonuclear cell function and infection in dialysis. Kidney Int Suppl 1992; 38:S91–S95.
64. Vanholder R, Van Biesen W, Ringoir S: Contributing factors to the inhibition of phagocytosis in hemodialyzed patients. Kidney Int 1993; 44:208–214.
65. Raskova J, Ghobrial I, Czerwinski DK, et al: B-cell activation and immunoregulation in end-stage renal disease patients receiving hemodialysis. Arch Intern Med 1987; 147:89–93.
66. Ladefoged J, Langhoff E: Accessory cell functions in mononuclear cell cultures uremic patients. Kidney Int 1990; 37:126–130.
67. Hershkoviz R, Korzets Z, Rathaus M, et al: Inhibition by uraemic sera of CD4+ T-cell adhesion to extracellular matrix components. Nephrol Dial Transplant 1995; 10:2065–2069.
68. Girndt M, Kohler H, Schiedhelm-Weick E, et al: T cell activation defect in hemodialysis patients: Evidence for a role of the B7/CD28 pathway. Kidney Int 1993; 44:359–365.
69. Haag-Weber M, Horl WH: Dysfunction of polymorphonuclear leukocytes in uremia. Semin Nephrol 1996; 16:192–201.
70. Haag-Weber M, Mai B, Horl WH: Isolation of a granulocyte inhibitory protein from uraemic patients with homology of beta 2-microglobulin. Nephrol Dial Transplant 1994; 9:382–388.
71. Cohen G, Rudnicki M, Horl WH: Uremic toxins modulate the spontaneous apoptotic cell death and essential functions of neutrophils. Kidney Int 2001; 59(suppl 78):S48–S52.
72. Vanholder R, de Smet R, Waterloos MA, et al: Mechanisms of uremic inhibition of phagocyte reactive species production: Characterization of the role of p-cresol. Kidney Int 1995; 47:510–517.
73. Asaka M, Iida H, Izumino K, Sasayama S: Depressed natural killer cell activity in uremia. Evidence for immunosuppressive factor in uremic sera. Nephron 1988; 49:291–295.
74. Bernheim J, Rashid G, Gavrieli R, et al: In vitro effect of advanced glycation end-products on human polymorphonuclear superoxide production. Eur J Clin Invest 2001; 31: 1064–1069.
75. Glorieux G, Vanholder R, Lameire N: Advanced glycation and the immune system: Stimulation, inhibition or both? Eur J Clin Invest 2001; 31:1015–1018.
76. Schena FP, Pertosa G: Fibronectin and the kidney. Nephron 1988; 48:177–182.
77. Flament J, Goldman M, Waterlot Y, et al: Impairment of phagocyte oxidative metabolism in hemodialyzed patients with iron overload. Clin Nephrol 1986; 25:227–230.
78. Veys N, Vanholder R, Ringoir S: Correction of deficient phagocytosis during erythropoietin treatment in maintenance hemodialysis patients. Am J Kidney Dis 1992; 19:358–363.
79. Ikizler TA, Wingard RL, Harvell J, et al: Association of morbidity with markers of nutrition and inflammation in chronic hemodialysis patients: A prospective study. Kidney Int 1999; 55: 1945–1951.
80. Zimmermann J, Herrlinger S, Pruy A, et al: Inflammation enhances cardiovascular risk and mortality in hemodialysis patients. Kidney Int 1999; 55:648–658.
81. Fadda GZ, Akmal M, Premdas FH, et al: Insulin release from pancreatic islets: Effects of CRF and excess PTH. Kidney Int 1988; 33:1066–1072.
82. Mak RH, DeFronzo RA: Glucose and insulin metabolism in uremia. Nephron 1992; 61:377–382.
83. DeFronzo RA, Andres R, Edgar P, Walker WG: Carbohydrate metabolism in uremia: A review. Medicine 1973; 52:469–481.
84. Cecchin F, Ittoop O, Sinha MK, Caro JF: Insulin resistance in uremia: Insulin receptor kinase activity in liver and muscle from chronic uremic rats. Am J Physiol 1988; 254:E394-E401.
85. Schmitz O, Arnfred J, Orskov L, et al: Influence of hyperglycemia on glucose uptake and hepatic glucose production in non-dialyzed uremic patients. Clin Nephrol 1988; 30:27–34.
86. Jacobs DB, Hayes GR, Truglia JA, Lockwood DH: Alterations of glucose transporter systems in insulin-resistant uremic rats. Am J Physiol 1989; 257:E193-E197.
87. Mak RH: Intravenous 1,25 dihydroxycholecalciferol corrects glucose intolerance in hemodialysis patients. Kidney Int 1992; 41:1049–1054.
88. McCaleb ML, Izzo MS, Lockwood DH: Characterization and partial purification of a factor from uremic human serum that induces insulin resistance. J Clin Invest 1985; 75:391–396.
89. Spustova V, Dzurik R: Effect of hippurate on glucose utilization in rat kidney cortex slices. Ren Physiol Biochem 1991; 14:42–47.
90. Sebekova K, Spustova V, Dzurik R: Inhibition of glucose uptake by 5-hydroxyindoleacetic acid in the isolated rat soleus muscle. Int Urol Nephrol 1996; 28:123–131.
91. Dzurik R, Spustova V, Lajdova I: Inhibition of glucose utilization in isolated rat soleus muscle by pseudouridine: Implications for renal failure. Nephron 1993; 65:108–110.
92. Katz AI, Emmanouel DS: Metabolism of polypeptide hormones by the normal kidney and in uremia. Nephron 1978; 22: 69–80.
93. Kalk WJ, Morley JE, Gold CH, Meyers A: Thyroid function tests in patients on regular hemodialysis. Nephron 1980; 25:173–178.
94. Lim CF, Bernard BF, de Jong M, et al: A furan fatty acid and indoxyl sulfate are the putative inhibitors of thyroxine hepatocyte transport in uremia. J Clin Endocrinol Metab 1993; 76: 318–324.
95. Elias AN, Vaziri ND, Pandian MR, et al: Dopamine and TSH secretion in uremic male rats. Horm Res 1987; 27:102–108.
96. Schaefer F, Chen Y, Tsao T, et al: Impaired JAK-STAT signal transduction contributes to growth hormone resistance in chronic uremia. J Clin Invest 2001; 108:467–475.
97. Hanna JD, Krieg RJ Jr, Scheinman JI, Chan JC: Effects of uremia on growth in children. Semin Nephrol 1996; 16:230–241.
98. Tonshoff B, Powell DR, Zhao D, et al: Decreased hepatic insulin-like growth factor (IGF)-I and increased IGF binding protein–1 and –2 gene expression in experimental uremia. Endocrinology 1997; 138:938–946.

99. Lippe B, Fine RN, Koch VH, Sherman BM: Accelerated growth following treatment of children with chronic renal failure with recombinant human growth hormone (somatrem): A preliminary report. Acta Paediat Scand Suppl 1988; 343:127–131.
100. Ziegler TR, Lazarus JM, Young LS, et al: Effects of recombinant human growth hormone in adults receiving maintenance hemodialysis. J Am Soc Nephrol 1991; 2:1130–1135.
101. Mehls O, Haas S: Effects of recombinant human growth hormone in catabolic adults with chronic renal failure. Growth Horm IGF Res 2000; 10(suppl B):S31–S37.
102. Biolo G: Can we increase protein synthesis by anabolic factors? Am J Kidney Dis 2001; 37:S115–S118.
103. Barbano G, Cappa F, Prigione I, et al: Plasma levels of soluble CD30 are increased in children with chronic renal failure and with primary growth deficiency and decrease during treatment with recombination human growth hormone. Nephrol Dial Transplant 2001; 16:1807–1813.
104. Edmondson SR, Baker NL, Oh J, et al: Growth hormone receptor abundance in tibial growth plates of uremic rats: GH/IGF-I treatment. Kidney Int 2000; 58:62–70.
105. Krieg RJ, Tokieda K, Chan JC, Veldhuis JD: Impact of uremia on female reproductive cyclicity, ovulation, and luteinizing hormone in the rat. Kidney Int 2000; 58:569–574.
106. Biasioli S, Mazzali A, Foroni R, et al: Chronobiological variations of prolactin (PRL) in chronic renal failure (CRF). Clin Nephrol 1988; 30:86–92.
107. Schaefer F, Stanhope R, Scheil H, et al: Pulsatile gonadotropin secretion in pubertal children with chronic renal failure. Acta Endocrinol (Copenh) 1989; 120:14–19.
108. Ritz E, Matthias S, Seidel A, et al: Disturbed calcium metabolism in renal failure: Pathogenesis and therapeutic strategies. Kidney Int Suppl 1992; 38:S37–S42.
109. Gonzalez EA: The role of cytokines in skeletal remodelling: Possible consequences for renal osteodystrophy. Nephrol Dial Transplant 2000; 15:945–950.
110. Andress DL, Pandian MR, Endres DB, Kopp JB: Plasma insulin-like growth factors and bone formation in uremic hyperparathyroidism. Kidney Int 1989; 36:471–477.
111. Phillips LS, Fusco AC, Unterman TG, del Greco F: Somatomedin inhibitor in uremia. J Clin Endocrinol Metab 1984; 59:764–772.
112. Andress DL, Howard GA, Birnbaum RS: Identification of a low molecular weight inhibitor of osteoblast mitogenesis in uremic plasma. Kidney Int 1991; 39:942–945.
113. Patel SR, Ke HQ, Vanholder R, et al: Inhibition of calcitriol receptor binding to vitamin D response elements by uremic toxins. J Clin Invest 1995; 96:50–59.
114. Hsu CH, Patel SR, Young EW: Mechanism of decreased calcitriol degradation in renal failure. Am J Physiol 1992; 262:F192-F198.
115. Glorieux G, Hsu CH, de Smet R, et al: Inhibition of calcitriol-induced monocyte CD14 expression by uremic toxins: Role of purines. J Am Soc Nephrol 1998; 9:1826–1831.
116. Drueke TB: The pathogenesis of parathyroid gland hyperplasia in chronic renal failure. Kidney Int 1995; 48:259–272.
117. Estepa JC, Aguilera-Tejero E, Lopez I, et al: Effect of phosphate on parathyroid hormone secretion in vivo. J Bone Miner Res 1999; 14:1848–1854.
118. Amin N: The impact of improved phosphorus control: Use of sevelamer hydrochloride in patients with chronic renal failure. Nephrol Dial Transplant 2002; 17:340–345.
119. Urena P: Use of calcimimetics in uremic patients with secondary hyperparathyroidism: Review. Artif Organs 2003; 27: 759–764.
120. Gejyo F, Yamada T, Odani S, et al: A new form of amyloid protein associated with chronic hemodialysis was identified as beta 2-microglobulin. Biochem Biophys Res Commun 1985; 129: 701–706.
121. Linke RP, Hampl H, Lobeck H, et al: Lysine-specific cleavage of beta 2-microglobulin in amyloid deposits associated with hemodialysis. Kidney Int 1989; 36:675–681.
122. Odani H, Oyama R, Titani K, et al: Purification and complete amino acid sequence of novel beta 2-microglobulin. Biochem Biophys Res Commun 1990; 168:1223–1229.
123. Miyata T, Oda O, Inagi R, et al: Beta 2-Microglobulin modified with advanced glycation end products is a major component of hemodialysis-associated amyloidosis. J Clin Invest 1993; 92:1243–1252.
124. Argiles A, Mourad G, Gouin-Charnet A, Schmitt-Bernard CF: Antiproteases and cells in the pathogenesis of beta(2)-microglobulin amyloidosis: Role of alpha(2)-macroglobulin and macrophages. Nephron 2000; 86:1–11.
125. Snow AD, Willmer J, Kisilevsky R: Sulfated glycosaminoglycans: A common constituent of all amyloids? Lab Invest 1987; 56: 120–123.
126. Holck M, Husby G, Sletten K, Natvig JB: The amyloid P-component (protein AP): An integral part of the amyloid substance? Scand J Immunol 1979; 10:55–60.
127. Floege J, Ketteler M: Beta2-microglobulin-derived amyloidosis: An update. Kidney Int Suppl 2001; 78:S164–S171.
128. Ketteler M, Bongartz P, Westenfeld R, et al: Association of low fetuin-A (AHSG) concentrations in serum with cardiovascular mortality in patients on dialysis: A cross-sectional study. Lancet 2003; 361:827–833.
129. Ponticelli C, Bencini PL: Uremic pruritus: A review (editorial). Nephron 1992; 60:1–5.
130. De Marchi S, Cecchin E, Villalta D, et al: Relief of pruritus and decreases in plasma histamine concentrations during erythropoietin therapy in patients with uremia. N Engl J Med 1992; 326:969–974.
131. Motojima M, Nishijima F, Ikoma M, et al: Role for "uremic toxin" in the progressive loss of intact nephrons in chronic renal failure. Kidney Int 1991; 40:461–469.
132. Miyazaki T, Ise M, Hirata M, et al: Indoxyl sulfate stimulates renal synthesis of transforming growth factor-beta 1 and progression of renal failure. Kidney Int Suppl 1997; 63: S211–S214.
133. Niwa T, Ise M: Indoxyl sulfate, a circulating uremic toxin, stimulates the progression of glomerular sclerosis. J Lab Clin Med 1994; 124:96–104.
134. Miyazaki T, Aoyama I, Ise M, et al: An oral sorbent reduces overload of indoxyl sulphate and gene expression of TGF-beta1 in uraemic rat kidneys (in process citation). Nephrol Dial Transplant 2000; 15:1773–1781.
135. Rump LC, Amann K, Orth S, Ritz E: Sympathetic overactivity in renal disease: A window to understand progression and cardiovascular complications of uraemia? Nephrol Dial Transplant 2000; 15:1735–1738.
136. Caravaca F, Arrobas M, Pizarro JL, Sanchez-Casado E: Uraemic symptoms, nutritional status and renal function in pre-dialysis end-stage renal failure patients. Nephrol Dial Transplant 2001; 16:776–782.
137. Vanholder R, Argiles A, Baurmeister U, et al: Uremic toxicity: Present state of the art. Int J Artif Organs 2001; 24:695–725.
138. Fontan MP, Rodriguez-Carmona A, Cordido F, Garcia-Buela J: Hyperleptinemia in uremic patients undergoing conservative management, peritoneal dialysis, and hemodialysis: A comparative analysis. Am J Kidney Dis 1999; 34:824–831.
139. Stenvinkel P, Lindholm B, Lonnqvist F, et al: Increases in serum leptin levels during peritoneal dialysis are associated with inflammation and a decrease in lean body mass. J Am Soc Nephrol 2000; 11:1303–1309.
140. Aguilera A, Selgas R, Codoceo R, Bajo A: Uremic anorexia: A consequence of persistently high brain serotonin levels? The tryptophan/serotonin disorder hypothesis. Perit Dial Int 2000; 20:810–816.

141. van Vlem B, Schoonjans R, Vanholder R, et al: Delayed gastric emptying in dyspeptic chronic hemodialysis patients. Am J Kidney Dis 2000; 36:962–968.
142. De Schoenmakere G, Vanholder R, Rottey S, et al: Relationship between gastric emptying and clinical and biochemical factors in chronic haemodialysis patients. Nephrol Dial Transplant 2001; 16:1850–1855.
143. Lim VS, Kopple JD: Protein metabolism in patients with chronic renal failure: Role of uremia and dialysis. Kidney Int 2000; 58:1–10.
144. Mitch WE: Mechanisms accelerating muscle atrophy in catabolic diseases. Trans Am Clin Climatol Assoc 2000; 111:258–269.
145. Bonomini V, Feletti C, Stefoni S, Vangelista A: Early dialysis and renal transplantation. Nephron 1986; 44:267–271.
146. Tattersall J, Greenwood R, Farrington K: Urea kinetics and when to commence dialysis. Am J Nephrol 1995; 15:283–289.
147. NKF-DOQI clinical practice guidelines for peritoneal dialysis adequacy. National Kidney Foundation. Am J Kidney Dis 1997; 30:S67–S136.
148. Churchill DN, Blake PG, Jindal KK, et al: Clinical practice guidelines for initiation of dialysis. Canadian Society of Nephrology. J Am Soc Nephrol 1999; 10(suppl 13):S289–S291.
149. Section I. Measurement of renal function, when to refer and when to start dialysis. Nephrol Dial Transplant 2002; 17(suppl 7):7–15.
150. Thambyrajah J, Landray MJ, McGlynn FJ, et al: Abnormalities of endothelial function in patients with predialysis renal failure. Heart 2000; 83:205–209.
151. Burkart JM, Satko SG: Incremental initiation of dialysis: One center's experience over a two-year period. Perit Dial Int 2000; 20:418–422.
152. Korevaar JC, Jansen MA, Dekker FW, et al: When to initiate dialysis: Effect of proposed U.S. guidelines on survival. Lancet 2001; 358:1046–1050.
153. Lameire N, Biesen WV, Vanholder R: Initiation of dialysis: Is the problem solved by NECOSAD? Nephrol Dial Transplant 2002; 17:1550–1552.
154. Vanholder R, de Smet R, Glorieux G, et al: Review on uremic toxins: Classification, concentration, and interindividual variability. Kidney Int 2003; 63:1934–1943.
155. Vanholder R, de Smet R: Pathophysiologic effects of uremic retention solutes. J Am Soc Nephrol 1999; 10:1815–1823.
156. Vanholder R, de Smet R, Hsu C, et al: Uremic toxicity: The middle molecule hypothesis revisited. Semin Nephrol 1994; 14:205–218.
157. Anderstam B, Mamoun AH, Sodersten P, Bergstrom J: Middle-sized molecule fractions isolated from uremic ultrafiltrate and normal urine inhibit ingestive behavior in the rat. J Am Soc Nephrol 1996; 7:2453–2460.
158. Mamoun AH, Sodersten P, Anderstam B, Bergstrom J: Evidence of splanchnic-brain signaling in inhibition of ingestive behavior by middle molecules. J Am Soc Nephrol 1999; 10:309–314.
159. Kamanna VS, Kashyap ML, Pai R, et al: Uremic serum subfraction inhibits apolipoprotein A-I production by a human hepatoma cell line. J Am Soc Nephrol 1994; 5:193–200.
160. Stabellini G, Mariani G, Pezzetti F, Calastrini C: Direct inhibitory effect of uremic toxins and polyamines on proliferation of VERO culture cells. Exp Mol Pathol 1997; 64:147–155.
161. Severini G, Diana L, Di Giovannandrea R, Sagliaschi G: Influence of uremic middle molecules on in vitro stimulated lymphocytes and interleukin–2 production. ASAIO J 1996; 42: 64–67.
162. Koda Y, Nishi S, Miyazaki S, et al: Switch from conventional to high-flux membrane reduces the risk of carpal tunnel syndrome and mortality of hemodialysis patients. Kidney Int 1997; 52:1096–1101.
163. Hornberger JC, Chernew M, Petersen J, Garber AM: A multivariate analysis of mortality and hospital admissions with high-flux dialysis. J Am Soc Nephrol 1992; 3:1227–1237.
164. Hakim RM, Held PJ, Stannard DC, et al: Effect of the dialysis membrane on mortality of chronic hemodialysis patients. Kidney Int 1996; 50:566–570.
165. Chandran PK, Liggett R, Kirkpatrick B: Patient survival on PAN/AN69 membrane hemodialysis: A ten-year analysis. J Am Soc Nephrol 1993; 4:1199–1204.
166. Bloembergen WE, Hakim RM, Stannard DC, et al: Relationship of dialysis membrane and cause-specific mortality. Am J Kidney Dis 1999; 33:1–10.
167. Hartmann J, Fricke H, Schiffl H: Biocompatible membranes preserve residual renal function in patients undergoing regular hemodialysis. Am J Kidney Dis 1997; 30:366–373.
168. Blankestijn PJ, Vos PF, Rabelink TJ, et al: High-flux dialysis membranes improve lipid profile in chronic hemodialysis patients. J Am Soc Nephrol 1995; 5:1703–1708.
169. Malberti F, Surian M, Farina M, et al: Effect of hemodialysis and hemodiafiltration on uremic neuropathy. Blood Purif 1991; 9: 285–295.
170. Locatelli F, Marcelli D, Conte F, et al: Comparison of mortality in ESRD patients on convective and diffusive extracorporeal treatments. The Registro Lombardo Dialisi E Trapianto. Kidney Int 1999; 55:286–293.
171. Leypoldt JK, Cheung AK, Carroll CE, et al: Effect of dialysis membranes and middle molecule removal on chronic hemodialysis patient survival. Am J Kidney Dis 1999; 33:349–355.
172. Port FK, Wolfe RA, Hulbert-Shearon TE, et al: Mortality risk by hemodialyzer reuse practice and dialyzer membrane characteristics: Results from the USRDS Dialysis Morbidity and Mortality Study. Am J Kidney Dis 2001; 37:276–286.
173. Eknoyan G, Beck GJ, Cheung AK, et al: Effect of dialysis dose and membrane flux in maintenance hemodialysis. N Engl J Med 2002; 347:2010–2019.
174. Dellanna F, Wuepper A, Baldamus CA: Internal filtration: Advantage in haemodialysis? Nephrol Dial Transplant 1996; 11(suppl 2):83–86.
175. Maduell F, del Pozo C, Garcia H, et al: Change from conventional haemodiafiltration to on-line haemodiafiltration. Nephrol Dial Transplant 1999; 14:1202–1207.
176. Lesaffer G, de Smet R, Lameire N, et al: Intradialytic removal of protein-bound uraemic toxins: Role of solute characteristics and of dialyser membrane. Nephrol Dial Transplant 2000; 15:50–57.
177. Gulyassy PF: Can dialysis remove protein bound toxins that accumulate because of renal secretory failure? ASAIO J 1994; 40:92–94.
178. de Smet R, van Kaer J, Liebich H, et al: Heparin-induced release of protein-bound solutes during hemodialysis is an in vitro artifact. Clin Chem 2001; 47:901–909.
179. de Smet R, van Kaer J, van Vlem B, et al: Toxicity of free p-cresol: A prospective and cross-sectional analysis. Clin Chem 2003; 49:470–478.
180. Brownlee M, Cerami A, Vlassara H: Advanced glycosylation end products in tissue and the biochemical basis of diabetic complications. N Engl J Med 1988; 318:1315–1321.
181. Papanastasiou P, Grass L, Rodela H, et al: Immunological quantification of advanced glycosylation end-products in the serum of patients on hemodialysis or CAPD. Kidney Int 1994; 46:216–222.
182. Thorpe SR, Baynes JW: Role of the Maillard reaction in diabetes mellitus and diseases of aging. Drugs Aging 1996; 9:69–77.
183. Makita Z, Radoff S, Rayfield EJ, et al: Advanced glycosylation end products in patients with diabetic nephropathy. N Engl J Med 1991; 325:836–842.
184. Miyata T, Ueda Y, Shinzato T, et al: Accumulation of albumin-linked and free-form pentosidine in the circulation of uremic patients with end-stage renal failure: Renal implications in the pathophysiology of pentosidine. J Am Soc Nephrol 1996; 7:1198–1206.
185. Monnier VM, Sell DR, Nagaraj RH, et al: Maillard reaction-mediated molecular damage to extracellular matrix and other

tissue proteins in diabetes, aging, and uremia. Diabetes 1992; 41(suppl 2):36–41.

186. Miyata T, Wada Y, Cai Z, et al: Implication of an increased oxidative stress in the formation of advanced glycation end products in patients with end-stage renal failure. Kidney Int 1997; 51:1170–1181.

187. Franke S, Niwa T, Deuther-Conrad W, et al: Immunochemical detection of imidazolone in uremia and rheumatoid arthritis. Clin Chim Acta 2000; 300:29–41.

188. Patel SR, Koenig RJ, Hsu CH: Effect of Schiff base formation on the function of the calcitriol receptor. Kidney Int 1996; 50:1539–1545.

189. Friedlander MA, Witko-Sarsat V, Nguyen AT, et al: The advanced glycation end product pentosidine and monocyte activation in uremia. Clin Nephrol 1996; 45:379–382.

190. Imani F, Horii Y, Suthanthiran M, et al: Advanced glycosylation end product-specific receptors on human and rat T-lymphocytes mediate synthesis of interferon gamma: Role in tissue remodeling. J Exp Med 1993; 178:2165–2172.

191. Sakata S, Takahashi M, Kushida K, et al: The relationship between pentosidine and hemodialysis-related connective tissue disorders. Nephron 1998; 78:260–265.

192. Bucala R, Tracey KJ, Cerami A: Advanced glycosylation products quench nitric oxide and mediate defective endothelium-dependent vasodilatation in experimental diabetes. J Clin Invest 1991; 87:432–438.

193. Asahi K, Ichimori K, Nakazawa H, et al: Nitric oxide inhibits the formation of advanced glycation end products. Kidney Int 2000; 58:1780–1787.

194. Niwa T, Tsukushi S: 3-deoxyglucosone and AGEs in uremic complications: Inactivation of glutathione peroxidase by 3-deoxyglucosone. Kidney Int Suppl 2001; 78:S37–S41.

195. Li YM, Tan AX, Vlassara H: Antibacterial activity of lysozyme and lactoferrin is inhibited by binding of advanced glycation-modified proteins to a conserved motif (see comments). Nat Med 1995; 1:1057–1061.

196. Thornalley PJ, Argirova M, Ahmed N, et al: Mass spectrometric monitoring of albumin in uremia. Kidney Int 2000; 58:2228–2234.

197. Koschinsky T, He CJ, Mitsuhashi T, et al: Orally absorbed reactive glycation products (glycotoxins): An environmental risk factor in diabetic nephropathy. Proc Natl Acad Sci USA 1997; 94:6474–6479.

198. Henle T, Deppisch R, Beck W, et al: Advanced glycated end-products (AGE) during haemodialysis treatment: Discrepant results with different methodologies reflecting the heterogeneity of AGE compounds. Nephrol Dial Transplant 1999; 14: 1968–1975.

199. Friedman M: Prevention of adverse effects of food browning. Adv Exp Med Biol 1991; 289:171–215.

200. Miyata T, Ueda Y, Horie K, et al: Renal catabolism of advanced glycation end products: The fate of pentosidine. Kidney Int 1998; 53:416–422.

201. Gugliucci A, Bendayan M: Renal fate of circulating advanced glycated end products (AGE): Evidence for reabsorption and catabolism of AGE-peptides by renal proximal tubular cells. Diabetologia 1996; 39:149–160.

202. Abel M, Ritthaler U, Zhang Y, et al: Expression of receptors for advanced glycosylated end-products in renal disease. Nephrol Dial Transplant 1995; 10:1662–1667.

203. Boulanger E, Wautier MP, Wautier JL, et al: AGEs bind to mesothelial cells via RAGE and stimulate VCAM–1 expression. Kidney Int 2002; 61:148–156.

204. Lamb EJ, Cattell WR, Dawnay AB: In vitro formation of advanced glycation end products in peritoneal dialysis fluid. Kidney Int 1995; 47:1768–1774.

205. Linden T, Forsback G, Deppisch R, et al: 3-Deoxyglucosone, a promoter of advanced glycation end products in fluids for peritoneal dialysis. Perit Dial Int 1998; 18:290–293.

206. Wieslander AP, Kjellstrand PT, Rippe B: Heat sterilization of glucose-containing fluids for peritoneal dialysis: Biological consequences of chemical alterations. Perit Dial Int 1995; 15:S52–S59.

207. Makita Z, Bucala R, Rayfield EJ, et al: Reactive glycosylation end products in diabetic uraemia and treatment of renal failure. Lancet 1994; 343:1519–1522.

208. Miyata T, Ueda Y, Yoshida A, et al: Clearance of pentosidine, an advanced glycation end product, by different modalities of renal replacement therapy. Kidney Int 1997; 51:880–887.

209. Hricik DE, Wu YC, Schulak A, Friedlander MA: Disparate changes in plasma and tissue pentosidine levels after kidney and kidney-pancreas transplantation. Clin Transplant 1996; 10:568–573.

210. Fishbane S, Bucala R, Pereira BJ, et al: Reduction of plasma apolipoprotein-B by effective removal of circulating glycation derivatives in uremia. Kidney Int 1997; 52:1645–1650.

211. Jadoul M, Ueda Y, Yasuda Y, et al: Influence of hemodialysis membrane type on pentosidine plasma level, a marker of "carbonyl stress." Kidney Int 1999; 55:2487–2492.

212. Miyata T, van Ypersele de Strihou C, Ueda Y, et al: Angiotensin II receptor antagonists and angiotensin-converting enzyme inhibitors lower in vitro the formation of advanced glycation end products: Biochemical mechanisms. J Am Soc Nephrol 2002; 13:2478–2487.

213. Campistol JM, Sole M, Munoz-Gomez J, et al: Systemic involvement of dialysis-amyloidosis. Am J Nephrol 1990; 10:389–396.

214. Guz G, Ozdemir BH, Sezer S, et al: High frequency of amyloid lymphadenopathy in uremic patients. Ren Fail 2000; 22:613–621.

215. Kessler M, Netter P, Azoulay E, et al: Dialysis-associated arthropathy: A multicentre survey of 171 patients receiving haemodialysis for over 10 years. The Co-operative Group on Dialysis-associated Arthropathy. Br J Rheumatol 1992; 31:157–162.

216. Jadoul M, Garbar C, Vanholder R, et al: Prevalence of histological beta2-microglobulin amyloidosis in CAPD patients compared with hemodialysis patients. Kidney Int 1998; 54:956–959.

217. Jadoul M, Garbar C, Noel H, et al: Histological prevalence of beta 2-microglobulin amyloidosis in hemodialysis: A prospective post-mortem study. Kidney Int 1997; 51:1928–1932.

218. Moriniere P, Marie A, el Esper N, et al: Destructive spondyloarthropathy with beta 2-microglobulin amyloid deposits in a uremic patient before chronic hemodialysis. Nephron 1991; 59:654–657.

219. Schwalbe S, Holzhauer M, Schaeffer J, et al: Beta 2-microglobulin associated amyloidosis: A vanishing complication of long-term hemodialysis? Kidney Int 1997; 52:1077–1083.

220. Gejyo F, Homma N, Suzuki Y, Arakawa M: Serum levels of beta 2-microglobulin as a new form of amyloid protein in patients undergoing long-term hemodialysis. N Engl J Med 1986; 314: 585–586.

221. Walz G, Kunzendorf U, Schwarz A, et al: Elevated tissue polypeptide antigen as a risk factor for carpal tunnel syndrome in haemodialyzed patients. Nephron 1988; 50:83–84.

222. Hurst NP, van den BR, Disney A, et al: "Dialysis related arthropathy": A survey of 95 patients receiving chronic haemodialysis with special reference to beta 2 microglobulin related amyloidosis. Ann Rheum Dis 1989; 48:409–420.

223. Niwa T, Sato M, Katsuzaki T, et al: Amyloid beta 2-microglobulin is modified with N epsilon-(carboxymethyl)lysine in dialysis-related amyloidosis. Kidney Int 1996; 50:1303–1309.

224. Niwa T, Katsuzaki T, Miyazaki S, et al: Amyloid beta 2-microglobulin is modified with imidazolone, a novel advanced glycation end product, in dialysis-related amyloidosis. Kidney Int 1997; 51:187–194.

225. Miyata T, Inagi R, Iida Y, et al: Involvement of beta 2-microglobulin modified with advanced glycation end products in the pathogenesis of hemodialysis-associated amyloidosis. Induction of human monocyte chemotaxis and macrophage secretion of tumor necrosis factor-alpha and interleukin–1. J Clin Invest 1994; 93:521–528.

226. Hou FF, Miyata T, Boyce J, et al: Beta(2)-microglobulin modified with advanced glycation end products delays monocyte apoptosis. Kidney Int 2001; 59:990–1002.
227. Garcia-Garcia M, Argiles, Gouin-Charnet A, et al: Impaired lysosomal processing of beta2-microglobulin by infiltrating macrophages in dialysis amyloidosis. Kidney Int 1999; 55:899–906.
228. Garbar C, Jadoul M, Noel H, van Ypersele de Strihou C: Histological characteristics of sternoclavicular beta 2-microglobulin amyloidosis and clues for its histogenesis. Kidney Int 1999; 55:1983–1990.
229. Jaradat MI, Schnizlein-Bick CT, Singh GK, Moe SM: Beta(2)-microglobulin increases the expression of vascular cell adhesion molecule on human synovial fibroblasts. Kidney Int 2001; 59:1951–1959.
230. Linke RP, Hampl H, Bartel-Schwarze S, Eulitz M: Beta 2-microglobulin, different fragments and polymers thereof in synovial amyloid in long-term hemodialysis. Biol Chem Hoppe Seyler 1987; 368:137–144.
231. Ogawa H, Saito A, Oda O, et al: Detection of novel beta 2-microglobulin in the serum of hemodialysis patients and its amyloidogenic predisposition. Clin Nephrol 1988; 30: 158–163.
232. Lehnert H, Jacob C, Marzoll I, et al: Prevalence of dialysis-related amyloidosis in diabetic patients. Diabetes Amyloid Study Group. Nephrol Dial Transplant 1996; 11:2004–2007.
233. Canaud B, Assounga A, Kerr P, et al: Failure of a daily haemofiltration programme using a highly permeable membrane to return beta 2-microglobulin concentrations to normal in haemodialysis patients. Nephrol Dial Transplant 1992; 7:924–930.
234. Locatelli F, Mastrangelo F, Redaelli B, et al: Effects of different membranes and dialysis technologies on patient treatment tolerance and nutritional parameters. The Italian Cooperative Dialysis Study Group. Kidney Int 1996; 50:1293–1302.
235. Chanard J, Bindi P, Lavaud S, et al: Carpal tunnel syndrome and type of dialysis membrane. BMJ 1989; 298:867–868.
236. van Ypersele de Strihou C, Jadoul M, Malghem J, et al: Effect of dialysis membrane and patient's age on signs of dialysis-related amyloidosis. The Working Party on Dialysis Amyloidosis. Kidney Int 1991; 39:1012–1019.
237. Ward RA, Schmidt B, Hullin J, et al: A comparison of on-line hemodiafiltration and high-flux hemodialysis: A prospective clinical study. J Am Soc Nephrol 2000; 11:2344–2350.
238. Ronco C, Brendolan A, Winchester JF, et al: First clinical experience with an adjunctive hemoperfusion device designed specifically to remove beta(2)-microglobulin in hemodialysis. Blood Purif 2001; 19:260–263.
239. Ameer GA, Grovender EA, Ploegh H, et al: A novel immunoadsorption device for removing beta2-microglobulin from whole blood. Kidney Int 2001; 59:1544–1550.
240. Mourad G, Argiles A: Renal transplantation relieves the symptoms but does not reverse beta 2-microglobulin amyloidosis. J Am Soc Nephrol 1996; 7:798–804.
241. de Smet R, Vogeleere P, van Kaer J, et al: Study by means of high-performance liquid chromatography of solutes that decrease theophylline/protein binding in the serum of uremic patients. J Chromatogr A 1999; 847:141–153.
242. Takamura N, Maruyama T, Otagiri M: Effects of uremic toxins and fatty acids on serum protein binding of furosemide: Possible mechanism of the binding defect in uremia (see comments). Clin Chem 1997; 43:2274–2280.
243. Tsutsumi Y, Maruyama T, Takadate A, et al: Decreased bilirubin-binding capacity in uremic serum caused by an accumulation of furan dicarboxylic acid. Nephron 2000; 85:60–64.
244. Tsutsumi Y, Maruyama T, Takadate A, et al: Interaction between two dicarboxylate endogenous substances, bilirubin and an uremic toxin, 3-carboxy-4-methyl-5-propyl-2-furanpropanoic acid, on human serum albumin. Pharm Res 1999; 16:916–923.
245. Sarnatskaya VV, Lindup WE, Niwa T, et al: Effect of protein-bound uraemic toxins on the thermodynamic characteristics of human albumin. Biochem Pharmacol 2002; 63: 1287–1296.
246. Sato M, Koyama M, Miyazaki T, Niwa T: Reduced renal clearance of furancarboxylic acid, a major albumin-bound organic acid, in undialyzed uremic patients. Nephron 1996; 74: 419–421.
247. Sassa T, Matsuno H, Niwa M, et al: Measurement of furancarboxylic acid, a candidate for uremic toxin, in human serum, hair, and sweat, and analysis of pharmacological actions in vitro. *Arch Toxicol* 2000; 73:649–654.
248. Henderson SJ, Lindup WE: Renal organic acid transport: Uptake by rat kidney slices of a furan dicarboxylic acid which inhibits plasma protein binding of acidic ligands in uremia. J Pharmacol Exp Ther 1992; 263:54–60.
249. Costigan MG, Lindup WE: Plasma clearance in the rat of a furan dicarboxylic acid which accumulates in uremia. Kidney Int 1996; 49:634–638.
250. Mabuchi H, Nakahashi H: Inhibition of hepatic glutathione S-transferases by a major endogenous ligand substance present in uremic serum. Nephron 1988; 49:281–283.
251. Niwa T, Aiuchi T, Nakaya K, et al: Inhibition of mitochondrial respiration by furancarboxylic acid accumulated in uremic serum in its albumin-bound and non-dialyzable form. Clin Nephrol 1993; 39:92–96.
252. Niwa T, Yazawa T, Kodama T, et al: Efficient removal of albumin-bound furancarboxylic acid, an inhibitor of erythropoiesis, by continuous ambulatory peritoneal dialysis. Nephron 1990; 56:241–245.
253. Costigan MG, Callaghan CA, Lindup WE: Hypothesis: Is accumulation of a furan dicarboxylic acid (3-carboxy–4-methyl–5-propyl–2-furanpropanoic acid) related to the neurological abnormalities in patients with renal failure? Nephron 1996; 73:169–173.
254. Costigan MG, Yaqoob M, Lindup WE: Retention of an albumin-bound furan dicarboxylic acid in patients with chronic renal failure or after a kidney transplant. Nephrol Dial Transplant 1996; 11:803–807.
255. Niwa T: Organic acids and the uremic syndrome: Protein metabolite hypothesis in the progression of chronic renal failure. Semin Nephrol 1996; 16:167–182.
256. Vanholder R, de Smet R, Lameire N: Protein-bound uremic solutes: The forgotten toxins. Kidney Int Suppl 2001; 78:S266–S270.
257. Pascual M, Schifferli JA: Adsorption of complement factor D by polyacrylonitrile dialysis membranes. Kidney Int 1993; 43:903–911.
258. Pascual M, Steiger G, Estreicher J, et al: Metabolism of complement factor D in renal failure. Kidney Int 1988; 34:529–536.
259. Volanakis JE, Barnum SR, Giddens M, Galla JH: Renal filtration and catabolism of complement protein D. N Engl J Med 1985; 312:395–399.
260. Deppisch RM, Beck W, Goehl H, Ritz E: Complement components as uremic toxins and their potential role as mediators of microinflammation. Kidney Int Suppl 2001; 78:S271–S277.
261. Cohen G, Haag-Weber M, Horl WH: Immune dysfunction in uremia. Kidney Int Suppl 1997; 62:S79–S82.
262. Strobel WM, Gurke T, Schifferli JA: Lowering plasma levels of complement factor D with AN69 dialysis membranes. J Clin Apheresis 1999; 14:188–189.
263. Kemperman FA, Silberbusch J, Slaats EH, et al: Glomerular filtration rate estimation from plasma creatinine after inhibition of tubular secretion: Relevance of the creatinine assay. Nephrol Dial Transplant 1999; 14:1247–1251.
264. Petersen LJ, Petersen JR, Talleruphuus U, et al: Glomerular filtration rate estimated from the uptake phase of 99mTc-DTPA renography in chronic renal failure. Nephrol Dial Transplant 1999; 14:1673–1678.

265. De Deyn PP, Macdonald RL: Guanidino compounds that are increased in cerebrospinal fluid and brain of uremic patients inhibit GABA and glycine responses on mouse neurons in cell culture (see comments). Ann Neurol 1990; 28:627–633.
266. D'Hooge R, Pei YQ, Marescau B, De Deyn PP: Convulsive action and toxicity of uremic guanidino compounds: Behavioral assessment and relation to brain concentration in adult mice. J Neurol Sci 1992; 112:96–105.
267. Weisensee D, Low-Friedrich I, Riehle M, et al: In vitro approach to "uremic cardiomyopathy." Nephron 1993; 65:392–400.
268. Levine S, Saltzman A: Are urea and creatinine uremic toxins in the rat? Ren Fail 2001; 23:53–59.
269. Lowrie EG, Lew NL: Death risk in hemodialysis patients: The predictive value of commonly measured variables and an evaluation of death rate differences between facilities. Am J Kidney Dis 1990; 15:458–482.
270. Yokozawa T, Fujitsuka N, Oura H, et al: Purification of methylguanidine synthase from the rat kidney. Nephron 1993; 63:452–457.
271. D'Hooge R, De Deyn PP, Van de Vijver G, et al: Uraemic guanidino compounds inhibit gamma-aminobutyric acid-evoked whole cell currents in mouse spinal cord neurones. Neurosci Lett 1999; 265:83–86.
272. Stenvinkel P, Heimburger O, Paultre F, et al: Strong association between malnutrition, inflammation, and atherosclerosis in chronic renal failure. Kidney Int 1999; 55:1899–1911.
273. Kimmel PL, Phillips TM, Simmens SJ, et al: Immunologic function and survival in hemodialysis patients. Kidney Int 1998; 54:236–244.
274. Macdougall IC, Cooper AC: Erythropoietin resistance: The role of inflammation and pro-inflammatory cytokines. Nephrol Dial Transplant 2002; 17(suppl 11):39–43.
275. Espinoza M, Aguilera A, Auxiliadora BM, et al: Tumor necrosis factor alpha as a uremic toxin: Correlation with neuropathy, left ventricular hypertrophy, anemia, and hypertriglyceridemia in peritoneal dialysis patients. Adv Perit Dial 1999; 15:82–86.
276. Descamps-Latscha B, Herbelin A, Nguyen AT, et al: Balance between IL–1 beta, TNF-alpha, and their specific inhibitors in chronic renal failure and maintenance dialysis. Relationships with activation markers of T cells, B cells, and monocytes. J Immunol 1995; 154:882–892.
277. Girndt M, Sester U, Sester M, et al: The interleukin–10 promoter genotype determines clinical immune function in hemodialysis patients. Kidney Int 2001; 60:2385–2391.
278. del Castillo E, Fuenzalida R, Uranga J: Increased glomerular filtration rate and glomerulopressin activity in diabetic dogs. Horm Metab Res 1977; 9:46–53.
279. Zhou XJ, Vaziri ND, Kaupke CJ: Effects of chronic renal failure and hemodialysis on plasma glomerulopressin. Int J Artif Organs 1993; 16:180–184.
280. Alvestrand A, Bergstrom J: Glomerular hyperfiltration after protein ingestion, during glucagon infusion, and in insulin-dependent diabetes is induced by a liver hormone: Deficient production of this hormone in hepatic failure causes hepatorenal syndrome. Lancet 1984; 1:195–197.
281. De Deyn PP, Marescau B, D'Hooge R, et al: Guanidino compound levels in brain regions of non-dialyzed uremic patients. Neurochem Int 1995; 27:227–237.
282. De Deyn PP, Marescau B, Cuykens JJ, et al: Guanidino compounds in serum and cerebrospinal fluid of non-dialyzed patients with renal insufficiency. Clin Chim Acta 1987; 167:81–88.
283. Patel S, Hsu CH: Effect of polyamines, methylguanidine, and guanidinosuccinic acid on calcitriol synthesis. J Lab Clin Med 1990; 115:69–73.
284. Horowitz HI, Cohen BD, Martinez P, Papayoanou MF: Defective ADP-induced platelet factor 3 activation in uremia. Blood 1967; 30:331–340.
285. De Deyn P, Marescau B, Lornoy W, et al: Guanidino compounds in uraemic dialysed patients. Clin Chim Acta 1986; 157:143–150.
286. De Deyn P, Marescau B, Lornoy W, et al: Serum guanidino compound levels and the influence of a single hemodialysis in uremic patients undergoing maintenance hemodialysis. Nephron 1987; 45:291–295.
287. Hirayama A, Noronha-Dutra AA, Gordge MP, et al: Inhibition of neutrophil superoxide production by uremic concentrations of guanidino compounds. J Am Soc Nephrol 2000; 11:684–689.
288. D'Hooge R, Pei YQ, De Deyn PP: N-methyl-D-aspartate receptors contribute to guanidinosuccinate-induced convulsions in mice. Neurosci Lett 1993; 157:123–126.
289. De Deyn PP, D'Hooge R, Van Bogaert PP, Marescau B: Endogenous guanidino compounds as uremic neurotoxins. Kidney Int Suppl 2001; 78:S77–S83.
290. MacAllister RJ, Whitley GS, Vallance P: Effects of guanidino and uremic compounds on nitric oxide pathways. Kidney Int 1994; 45:737–742.
291. White R, Barefield D, Ram S, Work J: Peritoneal dialysis solutions reverse the hemodynamic effects of nitric oxide synthesis inhibitors (published erratum appears in Kidney Int 1997; 51(3):978.). Kidney Int 1995; 48:1986–1993.
292. Rees DD, Palmer RM, Moncada S: Role of endothelium-derived nitric oxide in the regulation of blood pressure. Proc Natl Acad Sci USA 1989; 86:3375–3378.
293. Baylis C, Mitruka B, Deng A: Chronic blockade of nitric oxide synthesis in the rat produces systemic hypertension and glomerular damage. J Clin Invest 1992; 90:278–281.
294. Liew FY, Millott S, Parkinson C, et al: Macrophage killing of Leishmania parasite in vivo is mediated by nitric oxide from L-arginine. J Immunol 1990; 144:4794–4797.
295. Johns RA, Moscicki JC, DiFazio CA: Nitric oxide synthase inhibitor dose-dependently and reversibly reduces the threshold for halothane anesthesia. A role for nitric oxide in mediating consciousness? Anesthesiology 1992; 77:779–784.
296. Mendes Ribeiro AC, Brunini TM, Ellory JC, Mann GE: Abnormalities in L-arginine transport and nitric oxide biosynthesis in chronic renal and heart failure. Cardiovasc Res 2001; 49:697–712.
297. Passauer J, Bussemaker E, Range U, et al: Evidence in vivo showing increase of baseline nitric oxide generation and impairment of endothelium-dependent vasodilation in normotensive patients on chronic hemodialysis. J Am Soc Nephrol 2000; 11:1726–1734.
298. Al Banchaabouchi M, Marescau B, Possemiers I, et al: NG, NG-dimethylarginine and NG, NG-dimethylarginine in renal insufficiency. Pflugers Arch 2000; 439:524–531.
299. MacAllister RJ, Rambausek MH, Vallance P, et al: Concentration of dimethyl-L-arginine in the plasma of patients with end-stage renal failure. Nephrol Dial Transplant 1996; 11:2449–2452.
300. Kielstein JT, Frolich JC, Haller H, Fliser D: ADMA (asymmetric dimethylarginine): An atherosclerotic disease mediating agent in patients with renal disease? Nephrol Dial Transplant 2001; 16:1742–1745.
301. Boger RH, Bode-Boger SM, Tsao PS, et al: An endogenous inhibitor of nitric oxide synthase regulates endothelial adhesiveness for monocytes. J Am Coll Cardiol 2000; 36: 2287–2295.
302. Faraci FM, Brian JE Jr, Heistad DD: Response of cerebral blood vessels to an endogenous inhibitor of nitric oxide synthase. Am J Physiol 1995; 269:H1522-H1527.
303. Segarra G, Medina P, Vila JM, et al: Contractile effects of arginine analogues on human internal thoracic and radial arteries. J Thorac Cardiovasc Surg 2000; 120:729–736.
304. Holden DP, Cartwright JE, Nussey SS, Whitley GS: Estrogen stimulates dimethylarginine dimethylaminohydrolase activity and the metabolism of asymmetric dimethylarginine. Circulation 2003; 108:1575–1580.

305. Noris M, Remuzzi G: Uremic bleeding: Closing the circle after 30 years of controversies? Blood 1999; 94:2569–2574.
306. Levillain O, Marescau B, De Deyn PP: Guanidino compound metabolism in rats subjected to 20% to 90% nephrectomy. Kidney Int 1995; 47:464–472.
307. Boumendil-Podevin EF, Podevin RA, Richet G: Uricosuric agents in uremic sera. Identification of indoxyl sulfata and hippuric acid. J Clin Invest 1975; 55:1142–1152.
308. Cathcart-Rake W, Porter R, Whittier F, et al: Effect of diet on serum accumulation and renal excretion of aryl acids and secretory activity in normal and uremic man. Am J Clin Nutr 1975; 28:1110–1115.
309. Porter RD, Cathcart-Rake WF, Wan SH, et al: Secretory activity and aryl acid content of serum, urine, and cerebrospinal fluid in normal and uremic man. J Lab Clin Med 1975; 85:723–731.
310. McNamara PJ, Lalka D, Gibaldi M: Endogenous accumulation products and serum protein binding in uremia. J Lab Clin Med 1981; 98:730–740.
311. Gulyassy PF, Bottini AT, Stanfel LA, et al: Isolation and chemical identification of inhibitors of plasma ligand binding. Kidney Int 1986; 30:391–398.
312. Vanholder R, Van Landschoot N, de Smet R, et al: Drug protein binding in chronic renal failure: Evaluation of nine drugs. Kidney Int 1988; 33:996–1004.
313. Dzurik R, Spustova V, Gerykova M: Pathogenesis and consequences of the alteration of glucose metabolism in renal insufficiency. Adv Exp Med Biol 1987; 223:105–109.
314. Gonthier MP, Verny MA, Besson C, et al: Chlorogenic acid bioavailability largely depends on its metabolism by the gut microflora in rats. J Nutr 2003; 133:1853–1859.
315. Williams RE, Eyton-Jones HW, Farnworth MJ, et al: Effect of intestinal microflora on the urinary metabolic profile of rats: A (1)H-nuclear magnetic resonance spectroscopy study. Xenobiotica 2002; 32:783–794.
316. Farrell PC, Gotch FA, Peters JH, et al: Binding of hippurate in normal plasma and in uremic plasma pre- and post-dialysis. Nephron 1978; 20:40–46.
317. Perna AF, Ingrosso D, De Santo NG, et al: Mechanism of erythrocyte accumulation of methylation inhibitor S-adenosylhomocysteine in uremia. Kidney Int 1995; 47:247–253.
318. Clarke R, Daly L, Robinson K, et al: Hyperhomocysteinemia: An independent risk factor for vascular disease (see comments). N Engl J Med 1991; 324:1149–1155.
319. Tsai JC, Perrella MA, Yoshizumi M, et al: Promotion of vascular smooth muscle cell growth by homocysteine: A link to atherosclerosis. Proc Natl Acad Sci USA 1994; 91:6369–6373.
320. Massy ZA, Ceballos I, Chadefaux-Vekemens B, et al: Homocyst(e)ine, oxidative stress, and endothelium function in uremic patients. Kidney Int Suppl 2001; 78:S243–S245.
321. Matthias D, Becker CH, Riezler R, Kindling PH: Homocysteine induced arteriosclerosis-like alterations of the aorta in normotensive and hypertensive rats following application of high doses of methionine. Atherosclerosis 1996; 122: 201–216.
322. Harpel PC, Zhang X, Borth W: Homocysteine and hemostasis: Pathogenic mechanisms predisposing to thrombosis. J Nutr 1996; 126:1285S–1289S.
323. Suliman ME, Qureshi AR, Barany P, et al: Hyperhomocysteinemia, nutritional status, and cardiovascular disease in hemodialysis patients. Kidney Int 2000; 57:1727–1735.
324. van Guldener C, Janssen MJ, De Meer K, et al: Effect of folic acid and betaine on fasting and postmethionine-loading plasma homocysteine and methionine levels in chronic haemodialysis patients. J Intern Med 1999; 245:175–183.
325. Moustapha A, Gupta A, Robinson K, et al: Prevalence and determinants of hyperhomocysteinemia in hemodialysis and peritoneal dialysis. Kidney Int 1999; 55:1470–1475.
326. Hultberg B, Andersson A, Sterner G: Plasma homocysteine in renal failure. Clin Nephrol 1993; 40:230–235.
327. Fodinger M, Mannhalter C, Wolfl G, et al: Mutation (677 C to T) in the methylenetetrahydrofolate reductase gene aggravates hyperhomocysteinemia in hemodialysis patients. Kidney Int 1997; 52:517–523.
328. Bostom AG, Shemin D, Lapane KL, et al: Hyperhomocysteinemia and traditional cardiovascular disease risk factors in end-stage renal disease patients on dialysis: A case-control study. Atherosclerosis 1995; 114:93–103.
329. Refsum H, Helland S, Ueland PM: Radioenzymic determination of homocysteine in plasma and urine. Clin Chem 1985; 31:624–628.
330. van Guldener C, Kulik W, Berger R, et al: Homocysteine and methionine metabolism in ESRD: A stable isotope study. Kidney Int 1999; 56:1064–1071.
331. McGregor DO, Dellow WJ, Lever M, et al: Dimethylglycine accumulates in uremia and predicts elevated plasma homocysteine concentrations. Kidney Int 2001; 59:2267–2272.
332. Robinson K, Gupta A, Dennis V, et al: Hyperhomocysteinemia confers an independent increased risk of atherosclerosis in end-stage renal disease and is closely linked to plasma folate and pyridoxine concentrations. Circulation 1996; 94:2743–2748.
333. Massy ZA, Chadefaux-Vekemans B, Chevalier A, et al: Hyperhomocysteinaemia: A significant risk factor for cardiovascular disease in renal transplant recipients. Nephrol Dial Transplant 1994; 9:1103–1108.
334. Blacher J, Demuth K, Guerin AP, et al: Association between plasma homocysteine concentrations and cardiac hypertrophy in end-stage renal disease. J Nephrol 1999; 12:248–255.
335. Shemin D, Lapane KL, Bausserman L, et al: Plasma total homocysteine and hemodialysis access thrombosis: A prospective study. J Am Soc Nephrol 1999; 10:1095–1099.
336. Sirrs S, Duncan L, Djurdjev O, et al: Homocyst(e)ine and vascular access complications in haemodialysis patients: Insights into a complex metabolic relationship. Nephrol Dial Transplant 1999; 14:738–743.
337. Manns BJ, Burgess ED, Parsons HG, et al: Hyperhomocysteinemia, anticardiolipin antibody status, and risk for vascular access thrombosis in hemodialysis patients. Kidney Int 1999; 55:315–320.
338. Vychytil A, Fodinger M, Papagiannopoulos M, et al: Peritoneal elimination of homocysteine moieties in continuous ambulatory peritoneal dialysis patients. Kidney Int 1999; 55:2054–2061.
339. Brulez HF, van Guldener C, Donker AJ, ter Wee PM: The impact of an amino acid-based peritoneal dialysis fluid on plasma total homocysteine levels, lipid profile and body fat mass. Nephrol Dial Transplant 1999; 14:154–159.
340. Van Tellingen A, Grooteman MP, Bartels PC, et al: Long-term reduction of plasma homocysteine levels by super-flux dialyzers in hemodialysis patients. Kidney Int 2001; 59:342–347.
341. Galli F, Benedetti S, Buoncristiani U, et al: The effect of PMMA-based protein-leaking dialyzers on plasma homocysteine levels. Kidney Int 2003; 64:748–755.
342. Ubbink JB, Vermaak WJ, van der MA, Becker PJ: Vitamin B–12, vitamin B–6, and folate nutritional status in men with hyperhomocysteinemia. Am J Clin Nutr 1993; 57:47–53.
343. Bostom AG, Gohh RY, Beaulieu AJ, et al: Treatment of hyperhomocysteinemia in renal transplant recipients. A randomized, placebo-controlled trial. Ann Intern Med 1997; 127:1089–1092.
344. Wilcken DE, Dudman NP, Tyrrell PA, Robertson MR: Folic acid lowers elevated plasma homocysteine in chronic renal insufficiency: Possible implications for prevention of vascular disease. Metabolism 1988; 37:697–701.
345. Jungers P, Joly D, Massy Z, et al: Sustained reduction of hyperhomocysteinaemia with folic acid supplementation in predialysis patients. Nephrol Dial Transplant 1999; 14:2903–2906.
346. Suliman ME, Divino Filho JC, Barany P, et al: Effects of high-dose folic acid and pyridoxine on plasma and erythrocyte sulfur

amino acids in hemodialysis patients. J Am Soc Nephrol 1999; 10:1287–1296.

347. Sunder-Plassmann G, Fodinger M, Buchmayer H, et al: Effect of high dose folic acid therapy on hyperhomocysteinemia in hemodialysis patients: Results of the Vienna multicenter study. J Am Soc Nephrol 2000; 11:1106–1116.
348. Dierkes J, Domrose U, Ambrosch A, et al: Supplementation with vitamin B12 decreases homocysteine and methylmalonic acid but also serum folate in patients with end-stage renal disease. Metabolism 1999; 48:631–635.
349. Hoffer LJ, Bank I, Hongsprabhas P, et al: A tale of two homocysteines and two hemodialysis units. Metabolism 2000; 49:215–219.
350. Touam M, Zingraff J, Jungers P, et al: Effective correction of hyperhomocysteinemia in hemodialysis patients by intravenous folinic acid and pyridoxine therapy. Kidney Int 1999; 56: 2292–2296.
351. Bostom AG, Shemin D, Bagley P, et al: Controlled comparison of L-5-methyltetrahydrofolate versus folic acid for the treatment of hyperhomocysteinemia in hemodialysis patients (published erratum appears in Circulation 2000; 102(5):598). Circulation 2000; 101:2829–2832.
352. Thambyrajah J, Landray MJ, McGlynn FJ, et al: Does folic acid decrease plasma homocysteine and improve endothelial function in patients with predialysis renal failure? Circulation 2000; 102:871–875.
353. Turney JH, Davison AM, Forbes MA, Cooper EH: Hyaluronic acid in end-stage renal failure treated by haemodialysis: Clinical correlates and implications. Nephrol Dial Transplant 1991; 6:566–570.
354. de Medina M, Ashby M, Diego J, et al: Factors that influence serum hyaluronan levels in hemodialysis patients. ASAIO J 1999; 45:428–430.
355. Lipkin GW, Forbes MA, Cooper EH, Turney JH: Hyaluronic acid metabolism and its clinical significance in patients treated by continuous ambulatory peritoneal dialysis. Nephrol Dial Transplant 1993; 8:357–360.
356. Woodrow G, Turney JH, Davison AM, Cooper EH: Serum hyaluronan concentrations predict survival in patients with chronic renal failure on maintenance haemodialysis. Nephrol Dial Transplant 1996; 11:98–100.
357. Stenvinkel P, Heimburger O, Wang T, et al: High serum hyaluronan indicates poor survival in renal replacement therapy. Am J Kidney Dis 1999; 34:1083–1088.
358. Schawalder A, Oertli B, Beck-Schimmer B, Wuthrich RP: Regulation of hyaluronan-stimulated VCAM–1 expression in murine renal tubular epithelial cells. Nephrol Dial Transplant 1999; 14:2130–2136.
359. Oertli B, Beck-Schimmer B, Fan X, Wuthrich RP: Mechanisms of hyaluronan-induced up-regulation of ICAM–1 and VCAM–1 expression by murine kidney tubular epithelial cells: Hyaluronan triggers cell adhesion molecule expression through a mechanism involving activation of nuclear factor-kappa B and activating protein–1. J Immunol 1998; 161: 3431–3437.
360. Beck-Schimmer B, Oertli B, Pasch T, Wuthrich RP: Hyaluronan induces monocyte chemoattractant protein–1 expression in renal tubular epithelial cells. J Am Soc Nephrol 1998; 9:2283–2290.
361. Sun LK, Beck-Schimmer B, Oertli B, Wuthrich RP: Hyaluronan-induced cyclooxygenase–2 expression promotes thromboxane A2 production by renal cells. Kidney Int 2001; 59:190–196.
362. Takeda M, Babazono T, Nitta K, Iwamoto Y: High glucose stimulates hyaluronan production by renal interstitial fibroblasts through the protein kinase C and transforming growth factor-beta cascade. Metabolism 2001; 50:789–794.
363. Ludwig GD, Senesky D, Bluemle LW Jr, Elkinton JR: Indoles in uraemia: Identification by countercurrent distribution and paper chromatography. Am J Clin Nutr 1968; 21:436–450.
364. Gillam EM, Notley LM, Cai H, et al: Oxidation of indole by cytochrome P450 enzymes. Biochemistry 2000; 39:13817–13824.
365. Banoglu E, Jha GG, King RS: Hepatic microsomal metabolism of indole to indoxyl, a precursor of indoxyl sulfate. Eur J Drug Metab Pharmacokinet 2001; 26:235–240.
366. Depner TA: Suppression of tubular anion transport by an inhibitor of serum protein binding in uremia. Kidney Int 1981; 20:511–518.
367. Greco AV, Mingrone G, Favuzzi A, et al: Subclinical hepatic encephalopathy: Role of tryptophan binding to albumin and the competition with indole–3-acetic acid. J Investig Med 2000; 48:274–280.
368. Folkes LK, Wardman P: Oxidative activation of indole–3-acetic acids to cytotoxic species: A potential new role for plant auxins in cancer therapy. Biochem Pharmacol 2001; 61:129–136.
369. Walser M, Hill SB: Free and protein-bound tryptophan in serum of untreated patients with chronic renal failure. Kidney Int 1993; 44:1366–1371.
370. Saito K, Fujigaki S, Heyes MP, et al: Mechanism of increases in L-kynurenine and quinolinic acid in renal insufficiency. Am J Physiol Renal Physiol 2000; 279:F565-F572.
371. Stone TW: Neuropharmacology of quinolinic and kynurenic acids. Pharmacol Rev 1993; 45:309–379.
372. Malyszko JS, Malyszko J, Pawlak K, et al: Importance of serotonergic mechanisms in the thrombotic complications in hemodialyzed patients treated with erythropoietin. Nephron 2000; 84:305–311.
373. Tsubakihara Y, Takabatake Y, Oka K, et al: Effects of the oral adsorbent AST–120 on tryptophan metabolism in uremic patients. Am J Kidney Dis 2003; 41:S38–S41.
374. Perkins MN, Stone TW: Pharmacology and regional variations of quinolinic acid-evoked excitations in the rat central nervous system. J Pharmacol Exp Ther 1983; 226:551–557.
375. McDaniel HG, Reddy WJ, Boshell BR: The mechanism of inhibition of phosphoenolpyruvate carboxylase by quinolinic acid. Biochim Biophys Acta 1972; 276:543–550.
376. Beskid M, Finkiewicz-Murawiejska L, Obminski Z, Wolska B: Quinolinic acid: A modulator of the heart calcium channel in the rat and a binder of calcium ions. Exp Pathol 1991; 41:110–114.
377. Rios C, Santamaria A: Quinolinic acid is a potent lipid peroxidant in rat brain homogenates. Neurochem Res 1991; 16:1139–1143.
378. Sakai T, Yamasaki K, Sako T, et al: Interaction mechanism between indoxyl sulfate, a typical uremic toxin bound to site II, and ligands bound to site I of human serum albumin. Pharm Res 2001; 18:520–524.
379. Aoyama I, Miyazaki T, Takayama F, et al: Oral adsorbent ameliorates renal TGF-beta 1 expression in hypercholesterolemic rats. Kidney Int Suppl 1999; 71:S193–S197.
380. Motojima M, Hosokawa A, Yamato H, et al: Uraemic toxins induce proximal tubular injury via organic anion transporter 1-mediated uptake. Br J Pharmacol 2002; 135:555–563.
381. Aoyama I, Shimokata K, Niwa T: Oral adsorbent AST–120 ameliorates interstitial fibrosis and transforming growth factor-beta(1) expression in spontaneously diabetic (OLETF) rats. Am J Nephrol 2000; 20:232–241.
382. Aoyama I, Niwa T: An oral adsorbent ameliorates renal overload of indoxyl sulfate and progression of renal failure in diabetic rats. Am J Kidney Dis 2001; 37:S7–S12.
383. Niwa T, Emoto Y, Maeda K, et al: Oral sorbent suppresses accumulation of albumin-bound indoxyl sulphate in serum of haemodialysis patients. Nephrol Dial Transplant 1991; 6:105–109.
384. Ishikawa I, Araya M, Hayama T, et al: Effect of oral adsorbent (AST–120) on renal function, acquired renal cysts and aortic calcification in rats with adriamycin nephropathy. Nephron 2002; 92:399–406.
385. Takayama F, Taki K, Niwa T: Bifidobacterium in gastro-resistant seamless capsule reduces serum levels of indoxyl sulfate in patients on hemodialysis. Am J Kidney Dis 2003; 41:S142–S145.

386. Niwa T, Takeda N, Tatematsu A, Maeda K: Accumulation of indoxyl sulfate, an inhibitor of drug-binding, in uremic serum as demonstrated by internal-surface reversed-phase liquid chromatography. Clin Chem 1988; 34:2264–2267.
387. Vanholder RC, De Smet RV, Ringoir SM: Assessment of urea and other uremic markers for quantification of dialysis efficacy. Clin Chem 1992; 38:1429–1436.
388. Abe T, Abe T, Ageta S, et al: A new method for removal of albumin-binding uremic toxins: Efficacy of an albumin-dialysate. Ther Apher 2001; 5:58–63.
389. Crespo E, Macias M, Pozo D, et al: Melatonin inhibits expression of the inducible NO-synthase II in liver and lung and prevents endotoxemia in lipopolysaccharide-induced multiple organ dysfunction syndrome in rats. FASEB J 1999; 13: 1537–1546.
390. Ha H, Yu MR, Kim KH: Melatonin and taurine reduce early glomerulopathy in diabetic rats. Free Radic Biol Med 1999; 26:944–950.
391. Beyer CE, Steketee JD, Saphier D: Antioxidant properties of melatonin: An emerging mystery (published erratum appears in Biochem Pharmacol 1999; 57(9):1077). Biochem Pharmacol 1998; 56:1265–1272.
392. Qi W, Reiter RJ, Tan DX, et al: Inhibitory effects of melatonin on ferric nitrilotriacetate-induced lipid peroxidation and oxidative DNA damage in the rat kidney. Toxicology 1999; 139:81–91.
393. Herrera J, Nava M, Romero F, Rodriguez-Iturbe B: Melatonin prevents oxidative stress resulting from iron and erythropoietin administration. Am J Kidney Dis 2001; 37:750–757.
394. Wolfler A, Caluba HC, Abuja PM, et al: Prooxidant activity of melatonin promotes fas-induced cell death in human leukemic Jurkat cells. FEBS Lett 2001; 502:127–131.
395. Vaziri ND, Oveisi F, Wierszbiezki M, et al: Serum melatonin and 6-sulfatoxymelatonin in end-stage renal disease: Effect of hemodialysis. Artif Organs 1993; 17:764–769.
396. Viljoen M, Steyn ME, van Rensburg BW, Reinach SG: Melatonin in chronic renal failure. Nephron 1992; 60:138–143.
397. Ihle BU, Cox RW, Dunn SR, Simenhoff ML: Determination of body burden of uremic toxins. Clin Nephrol 1984; 22:82–89.
398. Yu PH, Dyck RF: Impairment of methylamine clearance in uremic patients and its nephropathological implications. Clin Nephrol 1998; 49:299–302.
399. Mitchell SC, Zhang AQ: Methylamine in human urine. Clin Chim Acta 2001; 312:107–114.
400. Maxfield FR, Willingham MC, Davies PJ, Pastan I: Amines inhibit the clustering of alpha2-macroglobulin and EGF on the fibroblast cell surface. Nature 1979; 277:661–663.
401. Yu PH, Deng YL: Endogenous formaldehyde as a potential factor of vulnerability of atherosclerosis: Involvement of semicarbazide-sensitive amine oxidase-mediated methylamine turnover. Atherosclerosis 1998; 140:357–363.
402. Flanagan GJ, O'Kelly J, Rae C, et al: Human erythrocyte choline uptake in uraemia: The role of intracellular substrate and an investigation into the effects of haemodialysis. Clin Sci (Colch) 1996; 91:353–358.
403. Burg MB, Peters EM, Bohren KM, Gabbay KH: Factors affecting counteraction by methylamines of urea effects on aldose reductase. Proc Natl Acad Sci USA 1999; 96:6517–6522.
404. Lee JA, Lee HA, Sadler PJ: Uraemia: Is urea more important than we think? (See comments). Lancet 1991; 338:1438–1440.
405. Ortiz-Costa S, Sorenson MM, Sola-Penna M: Counteracting effects of urea and methylamines in function and structure of skeletal muscle myosin. Arch Biochem Biophys 2002; 408:272–278.
406. Evans A: Dialysis-related carnitine disorder and levocarnitine pharmacology. Am J Kidney Dis 2003; 41:S13–S26.
407. Niwa T, Asada H, Maeda K, et al: Profiling of organic acids and polyols in nerves of uraemic and non-uraemic patients. J Chromatogr 1986; 377:15–22.
408. Clements RS Jr, DeJesus PV Jr, Winegrad AI: Raised plasma-myoinositol levels in uraemia and experimental neuropathy. Lancet 1973; 1:1137–1141.
409. Niwa T, Sobue G, Maeda K, Mitsuma T: Myoinositol inhibits proliferation of cultured Schwann cells: Evidence for neurotoxicity of myoinositol. Nephrol Dial Transplant 1989; 4:662–666.
410. Fisher SK, Novak JE, Agranoff BW: Inositol and higher inositol phosphates in neural tissues: Homeostasis, metabolism and functional significance. J Neurochem 2002; 82:736–754.
411. Moeckel GW, Shadman R, Fogel JM, Sadrzadeh SM: Organic osmolytes betaine, sorbitol and inositol are potent inhibitors of erythrocyte membrane ATPases. Life Sci 2002; 71:2413–2424.
412. Asaba H: Accumulation and excretion of middle molecules. Clin Nephrol 1983; 19:116–123.
413. Zimmerman L, Bergstrom J, Jornvall H: A method for separation of middle molecules by high performance liquid chromatography: Application in studies of glucuronyl-o-hydroxyhippurate in normal and uremic subjects. Clin Nephrol 1986; 25:94–100.
414. Lichtenwalner DM, Suh B, Lichtenwalner MR: Isolation and chemical characterization of 2-hydroxybenzoylglycine as a drug binding inhibitor in uremia. J Clin Invest 1983; 71:1289–1296.
415. Altschule MD, Hegedus ZL: Orthohydroxyhippuric (salicyluric) acid: Its physiologic and clinical significance. Clin Pharmacol Ther 1974; 15:111–117.
416. Krivosikova Z, Spustova V, Dzurik R: A highly sensitive HPLC method for the simultaneous determination of acetylsalicylic, salicylic and salicyluric acids in biologic fluids: Pharmacokinetic, metabolic and monitoring implications. Methods Find Exp Clin Pharmacol 1996; 18:527–532.
417. Jankowski J, Tepel M, Stephan N, et al: Characterization of p-hydroxy-hippuric acid as an inhibitor of Ca2+-ATPase in end-stage renal failure. Kidney Int Suppl 2001; 78:S84–S88.
418. Marangella M, Vitale C, Petrarulo M, et al: Bony content of oxalate in patients with primary hyperoxaluria or oxalosis-unrelated renal failure. Kidney Int 1995; 48:182–187.
419. Abuelo JG, Schwartz ST, Reginato AJ: Cutaneous oxalosis after long-term hemodialysis. Arch Intern Med 1992; 152:1517–1520.
420. Marangella M, Vitale C, Petrarulo M, et al: Pathogenesis of severe hyperoxalaemia in Crohn's disease-related renal failure on maintenance haemodialysis: Successful management with pyridoxine. Nephrol Dial Transplant 1992; 7:960–964.
421. Wolfson M, Cohen AH, Kopple JD: Vitamin B-6 deficiency and renal function and structure in chronically uremic rats. Am J Clin Nutr 1991; 53:935–942.
422. Marangella M, Bagnis C, Bruno M, et al: Determinants of oxalate balance in patients on chronic peritoneal dialysis. Am J Kidney Dis 1993; 21:419–426.
423. Morgan SH, Maher ER, Purkiss P, et al: Oxalate metabolism in end-stage renal disease: The effect of ascorbic acid and pyridoxine. Nephrol Dial Transplant 1988; 3:28–32.
424. Marangella M, Petrarulo M, Mandolfo S, et al: Plasma profiles and dialysis kinetics of oxalate in patients receiving hemodialysis. Nephron 1992; 60:74–80.
425. McLeish KR, Klein JB, Lederer ED, et al: Azotemia, TNF alpha, and LPS prime the human neutrophil oxidative burst by distinct mechanisms. Kidney Int 1996; 50:407–416.
426. Ridker PM, Cushman M, Stampfer MJ, et al: Inflammation, aspirin, and the risk of cardiovascular disease in apparently healthy men (published erratum appears in N Engl J Med 1997; 337(5):356) (see comments). N Engl J Med 1997; 336:973–979.
427. Schwedler S, Schinzel R, Vaith P, Wanner C: Inflammation and advanced glycation end products in uremia: Simple coexistence, potentiation or causal relationship? Kidney Int Suppl 2001; 78:S32–S36.
428. Dean RT, Wolff SP, McElligott MA: Histidine and proline are important sites of free radical damage to proteins. Free Radic Res Commun 1989; 7:97–103.

429. Weinstein T, Chagnac A, Korzets A, et al: Haemolysis in haemodialysis patients: Evidence for impaired defence mechanisms against oxidative stress. Nephrol Dial Transplant 2000; 15: 883–887.
430. Nguyen-Khoa T, Massy ZA, Witko-Sarsat V, et al: Critical evaluation of plasma and LDL oxidant-trapping potential in hemodialysis patients. Kidney Int 1999; 56:747–753.
431. Himmelfarb J, McMonagle E: Albumin is the major plasma protein target of oxidant stress in uremia. Kidney Int 2001; 60:358–363.
432. Sarnatskaya VV, Ivanov AI, Nikolaev VG, et al: Structure and binding properties of serum albumin in uremic patients at different periods of hemodialysis. Artif Organs 1998; 22:107–115.
433. Takayama F, Tsutsui S, Horie M, et al: Glutathionyl hemoglobin in uremic patients undergoing hemodialysis and continuous ambulatory peritoneal dialysis. Kidney Int Suppl 2001; 78:S155–S158.
434. Maggi E, Bellazzi R, Falaschi F, et al: Enhanced LDL oxidation in uremic patients: An additional mechanism for accelerated atherosclerosis? Kidney Int 1994; 45:876–883.
435. Maggi E, Bellazzi R, Gazo A, et al: Autoantibodies against oxidatively-modified LDL in uremic patients undergoing dialysis. Kidney Int 1994; 46:869–876.
436. Drueke TB, Khoa TN, Massy ZA, et al: Role of oxidized low-density lipoprotein in the atherosclerosis of uremia. Kidney Int Suppl 2001; 78:S114–S119.
437. Nguyen-Khoa T, Massy ZA, Witko-Sarsat V, et al: Oxidized low-density lipoprotein induces macrophage respiratory burst via its protein moiety: A novel pathway in atherogenesis? Biochem Biophys Res Commun 1999; 263:804–809.
438. O'Byrne D, Devaraj S, Islam KN, et al: Low-density lipoprotein (LDL)-induced monocyte-endothelial cell adhesion, soluble cell adhesion molecules, and autoantibodies to oxidized-LDL in chronic renal failure patients on dialysis therapy. Metabolism 2001; 50:207–215.
439. Tsuruoka S, Kawaguchi A, Nishiki K, et al: Vitamin E-bonded hemodialyzer improves neutrophil function and oxidative stress in patients with end-stage renal failure. Am J Kidney Dis 2002; 39:127–133.
440. Daschner M, Lenhartz H, Botticher D, et al: Influence of dialysis on plasma lipid peroxidation products and antioxidant levels. Kidney Int 1996; 50:1268–1272.
441. Voitkun V, Zhitkovich A: Analysis of DNA-protein crosslinking activity of malondialdehyde in vitro. Mutat Res 1999; 424: 97–106.
442. Apeland T, Mansoor MA, Seljeflot I, et al: Homocysteine, malondialdehyde and endothelial markers in dialysis patients during low-dose folinic acid therapy. J Intern Med 2002; 252: 456–464.
443. Witko V, Nguyen AT, Descamps-Latscha B: Microtiter plate assay for phagocyte-derived taurine-chloramines. J Clin Lab Anal 1992; 6:47–53.
444. Tatsumi T, Fliss H: Hypochlorous acid and chloramines increase endothelial permeability: Possible involvement of cellular zinc. Am J Physiol 1994; 267:H1597-H1607.
445. Bilzer M, Lauterburg BH: Effects of hypochlorous acid and chloramines on vascular resistance, cell integrity, and biliary glutathione disulfide in the perfused rat liver: Modulation by glutathione. J Hepatol 1991; 13:84–89.
446. Thomas EL, Grisham MB, Jefferson MM: Myeloperoxidase-dependent effect of amines on functions of isolated neutrophils. J Clin Invest 1983; 72:441–454.
447. Wratten ML, Sereni L, Tetta C: Hemolipodialysis attenuates oxidative stress and removes hydrophobic toxins. Artif Organs 2000; 24:685–690.
448. Amann K, Ritz E, Wiest G, et al: A role of parathyroid hormone for the activation of cardiac fibroblasts in uremia. J Am Soc Nephrol 1994; 4:1814–1819.
449. Rao DS, Shih MS, Mohini R: Effect of serum parathyroid hormone and bone marrow fibrosis on the response to erythropoietin in uremia (see comments). N Engl J Med 1993; 328:171–175.
450. Massry SG, Smogorzewski M: Mechanisms through which parathyroid hormone mediates its deleterious effects on organ function in uremia. Semin Nephrol 1994; 14:219–231.
451. Torres A, Lorenzo V, Hernandez D, et al: Bone disease in predialysis, hemodialysis, and CAPD patients: Evidence of a better bone response to PTH. Kidney Int 1995; 47:1434–1442.
452. Bommer J, Strohbeck E, Goerich J, et al: Arteriosclerosis in dialysis patients. Int J Artif Organs 1996; 19:638–644.
453. Di Paolo B, Cappelli P, Spisni C, et al: New electrophysiological assessments for the early diagnosis of encephalopathy and peripheral neuropathy in chronic uraemia. Int J Tissue React 1982; 4:301–307.
454. Kurz P, Monier-Faugere MC, Bognar B, et al: Evidence for abnormal calcium homeostasis in patients with adynamic bone disease. Kidney Int 1994; 46:855–861.
455. Mawad HW, Sawaya BP, Sarin R, Malluche HH: Calcific uremic arteriolopathy in association with low turnover uremic bone disease. Clin Nephrol 1999; 52:160–166.
456. Slatopolsky E, Finch J, Clay P, et al: A novel mechanism for skeletal resistance in uremia. Kidney Int 2000; 58:753–761.
457. Gao P, Scheibel S, D'Amour P, et al: Development of a novel immunoradiometric assay exclusively for biologically active whole parathyroid hormone 1–84: Implications for improvement of accurate assessment of parathyroid function. J Bone Miner Res 2001; 16:605–614.
458. Jara A, Gonzalez S, Felsenfeld AJ, et al: Failure of high doses of calcitriol and hypercalcaemia to induce apoptosis in hyperplastic parathyroid glands of azotaemic rats. Nephrol Dial Transplant 2001; 16:506–512.
459. Movilli E, Zani R, Carli O, et al: Direct effect of the correction of acidosis on plasma parathyroid hormone concentrations, calcium and phosphate in hemodialysis patients: A prospective study. Nephron 2001; 87:257–262.
460. Lewin E, Almaden Y, Rodriguez M, Olgaard K: PTHrP enhances the secretory response of PTH to a hypocalcemic stimulus in rat parathyroid glands. Kidney Int 2000; 58:71–81.
461. Ramirez JA, Goodman WG, Belin TR, et al: Calcitriol therapy and calcium-regulated PTH secretion in patients with secondary hyperparathyroidism. Am J Physiol 1994; 267:E961-E967.
462. Urena P, Kubrusly M, Mannstadt M, et al: The renal PTH/PTHrP receptor is down-regulated in rats with chronic renal failure. Kidney Int 1994; 45:605–611.
463. Smogorzewski M, Tian J, Massry SG: Down-regulation of PTH-PTHrP receptor of heart in CRF: Role of [Ca2+]i. Kidney Int 1995; 47:1182–1186.
464. Picton ML, Moore PR, Mawer EB, et al: Down-regulation of human osteoblast PTH/PTHrP receptor mRNA in end-stage renal failure. Kidney Int 2000; 58:1440–1449.
465. Urena P, Mannstadt M, Hruby M, et al: Parathyroidectomy does not prevent the renal PTH/PTHrP receptor down-regulation in uremic rats. Kidney Int 1995; 47:1797–1805.
466. D'Amour P, Jobin J, Hamel L, L'Ecuyer N: iPTH values during hemodialysis: Role of ionized Ca, dialysis membranes and iPTH assays. Kidney Int 1990; 38:308–314.
467. Lau AH, Kuk JM, Franson KL: Phosphate-binding capacities of calcium and aluminum formulations. Int J Artif Organs 1998; 21:19–22.
468. Rosen HN, Lim M, Garber J, et al: The effect of PTH antagonist BIM–44002 on serum calcium and PTH levels in hypercalcemic hyperparathyroid patients. Calcif Tissue Int 1997; 61:455–459.
469. Fox J, Lowe SH, Petty BA, Nemeth EF: NPS R–568: A type II calcimimetic compound that acts on parathyroid cell calcium receptor of rats to reduce plasma levels of parathyroid hormone and calcium. J Pharmacol Exp Ther 1999; 290:473–479.
470. Goodman WG, Frazao JM, Goodkin DA, et al: A calcimimetic agent lowers plasma parathyroid hormone levels in patients with secondary hyperparathyroidism. Kidney Int 2000; 58: 436–445.

471. Olgaard K, Lewin E: Prevention of uremic bone disease using calcimimetic compounds. Annu Rev Med 2001; 52:203–220.
472. Inoue H, Kagoshima M, Kaibara K: Effects of anion exchange resin as phosphate binder on serum phosphate and iPTH levels in normal rats. Int J Artif Organs 2000; 23:243–249.
473. Martin KJ, Gonzalez EA, Gellens M, et al: 19-Nor-1-alpha-25-dihydroxyvitamin D2 (Paricalcitol) safely and effectively reduces the levels of intact parathyroid hormone in patients on hemodialysis. J Am Soc Nephrol 1998; 9:1427–1432.
474. Horl WH, Haag-Weber M, Georgopoulos A, Block LH: Physicochemical characterization of a polypeptide present in uremic serum that inhibits the biological activity of polymorphonuclear cells. Proc Natl Acad Sci USA 1990; 87:6353–6357.
475. Tschesche H, Kopp C, Horl WH, Hempelmann U: Inhibition of degranulation of polymorphonuclear leukocytes by angiogenin and its tryptic fragment. J Biol Chem 1994; 269:30274–30280.
476. Cohen G, Rudnicki M, Horl WH: Isolation of modified ubiquitin as a neutrophil chemotaxis inhibitor from uremic patients. J Am Soc Nephrol 1998; 9:451–456.
477. Lipkin GW, Dawnay AB, Harwood SM, et al: Enhanced natriuretic response to neutral endopeptidase inhibition in patients with moderate chronic renal failure. Kidney Int 1997; 52:792–801.
478. Paniagua R, Franco M, Rodriguez E, et al: Impaired atrial natriuretic factor systemic clearance contributes to its higher levels in uremia. J Am Soc Nephrol 1992; 2:1704–1708.
479. Franz M, Woloszczuk W, Horl WH: Adsorption of natriuretic factors in uremia. Semin Nephrol 2001; 21:298–302.
480. Ottosson-Seeberger A, Lundberg JM, Alvestrand A, Ahlborg G: Exogenous endothelin–1 causes peripheral insulin resistance in healthy humans. Acta Physiol Scand 1997; 161:211–220.
481. Brochu E, Lacasse S, Moreau C, et al: Endothelin ET(A) receptor blockade prevents the progression of renal failure and hypertension in uraemic rats. Nephrol Dial Transplant 1999; 14:1881–1888.
482. Brochu E, Lacasse S, Lariviere R, et al: Differential effects of endothelin–1 antagonists on erythropoietin-induced hypertension in renal failure. J Am Soc Nephrol 1999; 10: 1440–1446.
483. Amann K, Munter K, Wessels S, et al: Endothelin A receptor blockade prevents capillary/myocyte mismatch in the heart of uremic animals. J Am Soc Nephrol 2000; 11:1702–1711.
484. Nabokov AV, Amann K, Wessels S, et al: Endothelin receptor antagonists influence cardiovascular morphology in uremic rats. Kidney Int 1999; 55:512–519.
485. Wolf SC, Gaschler F, Brehm S, et al: Endothelin-receptor antagonists in uremic cardiomyopathy. J Cardiovasc Pharmacol 2000; 36:S348–S350.
486. Moreau C, Lariviere R, Kingma I, et al: Chronic nitric oxide inhibition aggravates hypertension in erythropoietin-treated renal failure rats. Clin Exp Hypertens 2000; 22:663–674.
487. Dumont Y, D'Amours M, Lebel M, Lariviere R: Supplementation with a low dose of L-arginine reduces blood pressure and endothelin–1 production in hypertensive uraemic rats. Nephrol Dial Transplant 2001; 16:746–754.
488. Hegbrant J, Thysell H, Ekman R: Elevated plasma levels of opioid peptides and delta sleep-inducing peptide but not of corticotropin-releasing hormone in patients receiving chronic hemodialysis. Blood Purif 1991; 9:188–194.
489. Letizia C, Mazzaferro S, De Ciocchis A, et al: Effects of haemodialysis session on plasma beta-endorphin, ACTH and cortisol in patients with end-stage renal disease. Scand J Urol Nephrol 1996; 30:399–402.
490. Skagerberg G, Bjartell A, Vallet PG, Charnay Y: Immunocytochemical demonstration of DSIP-like immunoreactivity in the hypothalamus of the rat. Peptides 1991; 12:1155–1159.
491. Amati L, Caradonna L, Magrone T, et al: In vitro effects of naloxone on T-lymphocyte-dependent antibacterial activity in hepatitis C virus (HCV) infected patients and in inflammatory bowel disease (IBD) patients. Immunopharmacol Immunotoxicol 2001; 23:1–11.
492. Bald M, Gerigk M, Rascher W: Elevated plasma concentrations of neuropeptide Y in children and adults with chronic and terminal renal failure. Am J Kidney Dis 1997; 30:23–27.
493. Hegbrant J, Thysell H, Ekman R: Circulating neuropeptide Y in plasma from uremic patients consists of multiple peptide fragments. Peptides 1995; 16:395–397.
494. Bischoff A, Avramidis P, Erdbrugger W, et al: Receptor subtypes Y1 and Y5 are involved in the renal effects of neuropeptide Y. Br J Pharmacol 1997; 120:1335–1343.
495. Zoccali C, Mallamaci F, Tripepi G, et al: Prospective study of neuropeptide Y as an adverse cardiovascular risk factor in end-stage renal disease. J Am Soc Nephrol 2003; 14:2611–2617.
496. Aguilera A, Codoceo R, Selgas R, et al: Anorexigen (TNF-alpha, cholecystokinin) and orexigen (neuropeptide Y) plasma levels in peritoneal dialysis (PD) patients: Their relationship with nutritional parameters. Nephrol Dial Transplant 1998; 13:1476–1483.
497. Ishimitsu T, Nishikimi T, Saito Y, et al: Plasma levels of adrenomedullin, a newly identified hypotensive peptide, in patients with hypertension and renal failure. J Clin Invest 1994; 94:2158–2161.
498. Ikeda U, Kanbe T, Shimada K: Adrenomedullin increases inducible nitric oxide synthase in rat vascular smooth muscle cells stimulated with interleukin–1. Hypertension 1996; 27: 1240–1244.
499. Kabanda A, Jadoul M, Pochet JM, et al: Determinants of the serum concentrations of low molecular weight proteins in patients on maintenance hemodialysis. Kidney Int 1994; 45:1689–1696.
500. Cimerman N, Prebanda MT, Turk B, et al: Interaction of cystatin C variants with papain and human cathepsins B, H and L. J Enzyme Inhib 1999; 14:167–174.
501. Peri A, Cordella-Miele E, Miele L, Mukherjee AB: Tissue-specific expression of the gene coding for human Clara cell 10-kD protein, a phospholipase A2-inhibitory protein. J Clin Invest 1993; 92:2099–2109.
502. Pelleymounter MA, Cullen MJ, Baker MB, et al: Effects of the obese gene product on body weight regulation in ob/ob mice (see comments). Science 1995; 269:540–543.
503. Halaas JL, Gajiwala KS, Maffei M, et al: Weight-reducing effects of the plasma protein encoded by the obese gene (see comments). Science 1995; 269:543–546.
504. Young GA, Woodrow G, Kendall S, et al: Increased plasma leptin/fat ratio in patients with chronic renal failure: A cause of malnutrition? Nephrol Dial Transplant 1997; 12: 2318–2323.
505. Sharma K, Considine RV, Michael B, et al: Plasma leptin is partly cleared by the kidney and is elevated in hemodialysis patients. Kidney Int 1997; 51:1980–1985.
506. Heimburger O, Lonnqvist F, Danielsson A, et al: Serum immunoreactive leptin concentration and its relation to the body fat content in chronic renal failure. J Am Soc Nephrol 1997; 8:1423–1430.
507. Merabet E, Dagogo-Jack S, Coyne DW, et al: Increased plasma leptin concentration in end-stage renal disease. J Clin Endocrinol Metab 1997; 82:847–850.
508. Stenvinkel P, Heimburger O, Lonnqvist F: Serum leptin concentrations correlate to plasma insulin concentrations independent of body fat content in chronic renal failure. Nephrol Dial Transplant 1997; 12:1321–1325.
509. Fouque D, Juillard L, Lasne Y, et al: Acute leptin regulation in end-stage renal failure: The role of growth hormone and IGF–1. Kidney Int 1998; 54:932–937.
510. Garibotto G, Russo R, Franceschini R, et al: Inter-organ leptin exchange in humans. Biochem Biophys Res Commun 1998; 247:504–509.
511. Nordfors L, Lonnqvist F, Heimburger O, et al: Low leptin gene expression and hyperleptinemia in chronic renal failure. Kidney Int 1998; 54:1267–1275.

512. Cumin F, Baum HP, Levens N: Leptin is cleared from the circulation primarily by the kidney. Int J Obes Relat Metab Disord 1996; 20:1120–1126.
513. Cumin F, Baum HP, de Gasparo M, Levens N: Removal of endogenous leptin from the circulation by the kidney. Int J Obes Relat Metab Disord 1997; 21:495–504.
514. Zeng J, Patterson BW, Klein S, et al: Whole body leptin kinetics and renal metabolism in vivo. *Am J Physiol* 1997; 273:E1102-E1106.
515. Johansen KL, Mulligan K, Tai V, Schambelan M: Leptin, body composition, and indices of malnutrition in patients on dialysis. J Am Soc Nephrol 1998; 9:1080–1084.
516. Nishikawa M, Takagi T, Yoshikawa N, et al: Measurement of serum leptin in patients with chronic renal failure on hemodialysis. Clin Nephrol 1999; 51:296–303.
517. Odamaki M, Furuya R, Yoneyama T, et al: Association of the serum leptin concentration with weight loss in chronic hemodialysis patients. Am J Kidney Dis 1999; 33:361–368.
518. Kokot F, Wiecek A, Mesjasz J, et al: Influence of long-term recombinant human erythropoietin (rHuEpo) therapy on plasma leptin and neuropeptide Y concentration in haemodialysed uraemic patients. Nephrol Dial Transplant 1998; 13:1200–1205.
519. Stenvinkel P, Lonnqvist F, Schalling M: Molecular studies of leptin: Implications for renal disease. Nephrol Dial Transplant 1999; 14:1103–1112.
520. Rodriguez-Carmona A, Perez FM, Cordido F, et al: Hyperleptinemia is not correlated with markers of protein malnutrition in chronic renal failure. A cross-sectional study in predialysis, peritoneal dialysis and hemodialysis patients. Nephron 2000; 86:274–280.
521. Dagogo-Jack S, Ovalle F, Landt M, et al: Hyperleptinemia in patients with end-stage renal disease undergoing continuous ambulatory peritoneal dialysis. Perit Dial Int 1998; 18:34–40.
522. Janik JE, Curti BD, Considine RV, et al: Interleukin 1 alpha increases serum leptin concentrations in humans. J Clin Endocrinol Metab 1997; 82:3084–3086.
523. Zumbach MS, Boehme MW, Wahl P, et al: Tumor necrosis factor increases serum leptin levels in humans. J Clin Endocrinol Metab 1997; 82:4080–4082.
524. Don BR, Rosales LM, Levine NW, et al: Leptin is a negative acute phase protein in chronic hemodialysis patients. Kidney Int 2001; 59:1114–1120.
525. Yang D, Beylot M, Agarwal KC, et al: Assay of the human liver citric acid cycle probe phenylacetylglutamine and of phenylacetate in plasma by gas chromatography-mass spectrometry. Anal Biochem 1993; 212:277–282.
526. Zimmerman L, Egestad B, Jornvall H, Bergstrom J: Identification and determination of phenylacetylglutamine, a major nitrogenous metabolite in plasma of uremic patients. Clin Nephrol 1989; 32:124–128.
527. Zimmerman L, Jornvall H, Bergstrom J: Phenylacetylglutamine and hippuric acid in uremic and healthy subjects. Nephron 1990; 55:265–271.
528. Copland JA, Hendry LB, Chu CK, et al: Inhibition of estrogen stimulated mitogenesis by 3-phenylacetylamino–2,6-piperidinedione and its para-hydroxy analog. J Steroid Biochem Mol Biol 1993; 46:451–462.
529. Wardle EN, Williams R: Polymorph leucocyte function in uraemia and jaundice. Acta Haematol 1980; 64:157–164.
530. Turner GA, Wardle EN: Effect of unconjugated and conjugated phenol and uraemia on the synthesis of adenosine 3′:5′-cyclic monophosphate in rat brain homogenates. Clin Sci Mol Med 1978; 55:271–275.
531. Canalejo A, Almaden Y, de Smet R, et al: Effects of uremic ultrafiltrate on the regulation of the parathyroid cell cycle by calcitriol. Kidney Int 2003; 63:732–737.
532. Niwa T: Phenol and p-cresol accumulated in uremic serum measured by HPLC with fluorescence detection. Clin Chem 1993; 39:108–111.
533. Thompson DC, Perera K, Fisher R, Brendel K: Cresol isomers: Comparison of toxic potency in rat liver slices. Toxicol Appl Pharmacol 1994; 125:51–58.
534. Kitagawa A: Effects of cresols (o-, m-, and p-isomers) on the bioenergetic system in isolated rat liver mitochondria. Drug Chem Toxicol 2001; 24:39–47.
535. Goodhart PJ, DeWolf WE Jr, Kruse LI: Mechanism-based inactivation of dopamine beta-hydroxylase by p-cresol and related alkylphenols. Biochemistry 1987; 26:2576–2583.
536. Yokoyama MT, Tabori C, Miller ER, Hogberg MG: The effects of antibiotics in the weanling pig diet on growth and the excretion of volatile phenolic and aromatic bacterial metabolites. Am J Clin Nutr 1982; 35:1417–1424.
537. Lascelles PT, Taylor WH: The effect upon tissue respiration in vitro of metabolites which accumulate in uraemic coma. Clin Sci 1966; 31:403–413.
538. Heipieper HJ, Keweloh H, Rehm HJ: Influence of phenols on growth and membrane permeability of free and immobilized Escherichia coli. Appl Environ Microbiol 1991; 57: 1213–1217.
539. Abreo K, Sella M, Gautreaux S, et al: P-cresol, a uremic compound, enhances the uptake of aluminum in hepatocytes. J Am Soc Nephrol 1997; 8:935–942.
540. Wratten ML, Tetta C, de Smet R, et al: Uremic ultrafiltrate inhibits platelet-activating factor synthesis. Blood Purif 1999; 17:134–141.
541. De Kimpe J, Cornelis R, Vanholder R: In vitro methylation of arsenite by rabbit liver cytosol: Effect of metal ions, metal chelating agents, methyltransferase inhibitors and uremic toxins. Drug Chem Toxicol 1999; 22:613–628.
542. de Smet R, Glorieux G, Hsu C, Vanholder R: P-cresol and uric acid: Two old uremic toxins revisited. Kidney Int Suppl 1997; 62:S8–S11.
543. Anderson IB, Mullen WH, Meeker JE, et al: Pennyroyal toxicity: Measurement of toxic metabolite levels in two cases and review of the literature (see comments). Ann Intern Med 1996; 124:726–734.
544. Niwa T, Ise M, Miyazaki T, Meada K: Suppressive effect of an oral sorbent on the accumulation of p-cresol in the serum of experimental uremic rats. Nephron 1993; 65:82–87.
545. Fujiwara S, Seto Y, Kimura A, Hashiba H: Establishment of orally-administered Lactobacillus gasseri SBT2055SR in the gastrointestinal tract of humans and its influence on intestinal microflora and metabolism. J Appl Microbiol 2001; 90:343–352.
546. Fagugli RM, de Smet R, Buoncristiani U, et al: Behavior of non-protein-bound and protein-bound uremic solutes during daily hemodialysis. Am J Kidney Dis 2002; 40:339–347.
547. Lameire N, Vanholder R, de Smet R: Uremic toxins and peritoneal dialysis. Kidney Int Suppl 2001; 78:S292–S297.
548. Lesaffer G, de Smet R, D'heuvaert T, et al: Kinetics of the protein-bound, lipophilic, uremic toxin p-cresol in healthy rats. Life Sci 2001; 69:2237–2248.
549. Lesaffer G, de Smet R, D'heuvaert T, et al: Comparative kinetics of the uremic toxin p-cresol versus creatinine in rats with and without renal failure. Kidney Int 2003; 64:1365–1373.
550. Lesaffer G, de Smet R, Belpaire FM, et al: Urinary excretion of the uraemic toxin p-cresol in the rat: Contribution of glucuronidation to its metabolization. Nephrol Dial Transplant 2003; 18:1299–1306.
551. Coburn JW, Salusky IB: Control of serum phosphorus in uremia (editorial). N Engl J Med 1989; 320:1140–1142.
552. Llach F: Secondary hyperparathyroidism in renal failure: The trade-off hypothesis revisited. Am J Kidney Dis 1995; 25: 663–679.

553. de Francisco AL, Cobo MA, Setien MA, et al: Effect of serum phosphate on parathyroid hormone secretion during hemodialysis. Kidney Int 1998; 54:2140–2145.
554. Combe C, Aparicio M: Phosphorus and protein restriction and parathyroid function in chronic renal failure. Kidney Int 1994; 46:1381–1386.
555. Imanishi Y, Koyama H, Inaba M, et al: Phosphorus intake regulates intestinal function and polyamine metabolism in uremia. Kidney Int 1996; 49:499–505.
556. Dusso AS, Pavlopoulos T, Naumovich L, et al: P21(WAF1) and transforming growth factor-alpha mediate dietary phosphate regulation of parathyroid cell growth. Kidney Int 2001; 59:855–865.
557. Almaden Y, Canalejo A, Hernandez A, et al: Direct effect of phosphorus on PTH secretion from whole rat parathyroid glands in vitro. J Bone Miner Res 1996; 11:970–976.
558. Rodriguez M, Felsenfeld AJ, Williams C, et al: The effect of long-term intravenous calcitriol administration on parathyroid function in hemodialysis patients. J Am Soc Nephrol 1991; 2: 1014–1020.
559. Schiller LR, Santa Ana CA, Sheikh MS, et al: Effect of the time of administration of calcium acetate on phosphorus binding (see comments). N Engl J Med 1989; 320:1110–1113.
560. Hergesell O, Ritz E: Phosphate binders on iron basis: A new perspective? Kidney Int Suppl 1999; 73:S42–S45.
561. Hsu CH: Are we mismanaging calcium and phosphate metabolism in renal failure? Am J Kidney Dis 1997; 29:641–649.
562. Bleyer AJ, Burke SK, Dillon M, et al: A comparison of the calcium-free phosphate binder sevelamer hydrochloride with calcium acetate in the treatment of hyperphosphatemia in hemodialysis patients (see comments). Am J Kidney Dis 1999; 33:694–701.
563. Hutchison AJ: Calcitriol, lanthanum carbonate, and other new phosphate binders in the management of renal osteodystrophy. Perit Dial Int 1999; 19(suppl 2):S408–S412.
564. Wilkes BM, Reiner D, Kern M, Burke S: Simultaneous lowering of serum phosphate and LDL-cholesterol by sevelamer hydrochloride (RenaGel) in dialysis patients. Clin Nephrol 1998; 50:381–386.
565. London GM: Cardiovascular calcifications in uremic patients: Clinical impact on cardiovascular function. J Am Soc Nephrol 2003; 14:S305–S309.
566. Kerr PG, Lo A, Chin M, Atkins RC: Dialyzer performance in the clinic: Comparison of six low-flux membranes. Artif Organs 1999; 23:817–821.
567. Haas T, Hillion D, Dongradi G: Phosphate kinetics in dialysis patients. Nephrol Dial Transplant 1991; 6(suppl 2): 108–113.
568. Pohlmeier R, Vienken J: Phosphate removal and hemodialysis conditions. Kidney Int Suppl 2001; 78:S190–S194.
569. Kooistra MP, Vos J, Koomans HA, Vos PF: Daily home haemodialysis in the Netherlands: Effects on metabolic control, haemodynamics, and quality of life. Nephrol Dial Transplant 1998; 13:2853–2860.
570. Mucsi I, Hercz G, Uldall R, et al: Control of serum phosphate without any phosphate binders in patients treated with nocturnal hemodialysis. Kidney Int 1998; 53:1399–1404.
571. Zehnder C, Gutzwiller JP, Renggli K: Hemodiafiltration: A new treatment option for hyperphosphatemia in hemodialysis patients. Clin Nephrol 1999; 52:152–159.
572. Lindsay RM, Alhejaili F, Nesrallah G, et al: Calcium and phosphate balance with quotidian hemodialysis. Am J Kidney Dis 2003; 42:24–29.
573. Lindsay RM, Kortas C: Hemeral (daily) hemodialysis. Adv Ren Replace Ther 2001; 8:236–249.
574. Gutzwiller JP, Schneditz D, Huber AR, et al: Increasing blood flow increases kt/V(urea) and potassium removal but fails to improve phosphate removal. Clin Nephrol 2003; 59: 130–136.
575. Gotch FA, Panlilio F, Sergeyeva O, et al: A kinetic model of inorganic phosphorus mass balance in hemodialysis therapy. Blood Purif 2003; 21:51–57.
576. Block GA, Port FK: Re-evaluation of risks associated with hyperphosphatemia and hyperparathyroidism in dialysis patients: Recommendations for a change in management. Am J Kidney Dis 2000; 35:1226–1237.
577. Amann K, Gross ML, London GM, Ritz E: Hyperphosphataemia: A silent killer of patients with renal failure? Nephrol Dial Transplant 1999; 14:2085–2087.
578. Chen NX, O'Neill KD, Duan D, Moe SM: Phosphorus and uremic serum up-regulate osteopontin expression in vascular smooth muscle cells. Kidney Int 2002; 62:1724–1731.
579. Stabellini G, Calastrini C, Scapoli L, et al: The effect of polyamines and dialysate fluid on extracellular matrix synthesis in VERO cell cultures. J Nephrol 2002; 15:539–546.
580. Campbell RA: Polyamines and uremia. Adv Exp Med Biol 1987; 223:47–54.
581. Erez O, Goldstaub D, Friedman J, Kahana C: Putrescine activates oxidative stress dependent apoptotic death in ornithine decarboxylase overproducing mouse myeloma cells. Exp Cell Res 2002; 281:148–156.
582. Rock DM, Macdonald RL: Spermine and related polyamines produce a voltage-dependent reduction of N-methyl-D-aspartate receptor single-channel conductance. Mol Pharmacol 1992; 42:157–164.
583. Segal JA, Skolnick P: Spermine-induced toxicity in cerebellar granule neurons is independent of its actions at NMDA receptors. J Neurochem 2000; 74:60–69.
584. Lenzen S, Rustenbeck I: Effects of IP3, spermine, and Mg2+ on regulation of Ca2+ transport by endoplasmic reticulum and mitochondria in permeabilized pancreatic islets. Diabetes 1991; 40:323–326.
585. Szabo C, Southan GJ, Wood E, et al: Inhibition by spermine of the induction of nitric oxide synthase in J774.2 macrophages: Requirement of a serum factor. Br J Pharmacol 1994; 112: 355–356.
586. de la Pena NC, Sosa-Melgarejo JA, Ramos RR, Mendez JD: Inhibition of platelet aggregation by putrescine, spermidine, and spermine in hypercholesterolemic rabbits. Arch Med Res 2000; 31:546–550.
587. Sharmin S, Sakata K, Kashiwagi K, et al: Polyamine cytotoxicity in the presence of bovine serum amine oxidase. Biochem Biophys Res Commun 2001; 282:228–235.
588. Galli F, Beninati S, Benedetti S, et al: Polymeric protein-polyamine conjugates: A new class of uremic toxins affecting erythropoiesis. Kidney Int Suppl 2001; 78:S73–S76.
589. Seiler N: Oxidation of polyamines and brain injury. Neurochem Res 2000; 25:471–490.
590. Kaasinen K, Koistinaho J, Alhonen L, Janne J: Overexpression of spermidine/spermine N-acetyltransferase in transgenic mice protects the animals from kainate-induced toxicity. Eur J Neurosci 2000; 12:540–548.
591. Gugliucci A, Menini T: The polyamines spermine and spermidine protect proteins from structural and functional damage by AGE precursors: A new role for old molecules? Life Sci 2003; 72:2603–2616.
592. Dzurik R, Lajdova I, Spustova V, Opatrny K Jr: Pseudouridine excretion in healthy subjects and its accumulation in renal failure. Nephron 1992; 61:64–67.
593. Daniewska-Michalska D, Motyl T, Gellert R, et al: Efficiency of hemodialysis of pyrimidine compounds in patients with chronic renal failure. Nephron 1993; 64:193–197.
594. Hsu CH, Patel SR, Young EW, Vanholder R: Effects of purine derivatives on calcitriol metabolism in rats. Am J Physiol 1991; 260:F596-F601.
595. Vanholder R, Patel S, Hsu CH: Effect of uric acid on plasma levels of 1,25(OH)2D in renal failure. J Am Soc Nephrol 1993; 4:1035–1038.

596. Simmonds HA, Cameron JS, Morris GS, et al: Purine metabolites in uraemia. Adv Exp Med Biol 1987; 223:73–80.
597. Yang BC, Khan S, Mehta JL: Blockade of platelet-mediated relaxation in rat aortic rings exposed to xanthine-xanthine oxidase. Am J Physiol 1994; 266:H2212-H2219.
598. Berman RS, Martin W: Arterial endothelial barrier dysfunction: Actions of homocysteine and the hypoxanthine-xanthine oxidase free radical generating system. Br J Pharmacol 1993; 108: 920–926.
599. Bergesio F, Monzani G, Ciuti R, et al: Total antioxidant capacity (TAC): Is it an effective method to evaluate the oxidative stress in uraemia? J Biolumin Chemilumin 1998; 13:315–319.
600. Meucci E, Littarru C, Deli G, et al: Antioxidant status and dialysis: Plasma and saliva antioxidant activity in patients with fluctuating urate levels. Free Radic Res 1998; 29:367–376.
601. Gerrits GP, Monnens LA, De Abreu RA, et al: Disturbances of cerebral purine and pyrimidine metabolism in young children with chronic renal failure. Nephron 1991; 58:310–314.
602. Vaziri ND, Freel RW, Hatch M: Effect of chronic experimental renal insufficiency on urate metabolism. J Am Soc Nephrol 1995; 6:1313–1317.
603. Langsdorf LJ, Zydney AL: Effect of uremia on the membrane transport characteristics of red blood cells. Blood 1993; 81:820–827.
604. Prakash S, Chang TM: In vitro and in vivo uric acid lowering by artificial cells containing microencapsulated genetically engineered E. coli DH5 cells. Int J Artif Organs 2000; 23:429–435.
605. Fernandez-Martin JL, Canteros A, Alles A, et al: Aluminum exposure in chronic renal failure in Iberoamerica at the end of the 1990s: Overview and perspectives. Am J Med Sci 2000; 320:96–99.
606. Patruta SI, Edlinger R, Sunder-Plassmann G, Horl WH: Neutrophil impairment associated with iron therapy in hemodialysis patients with functional iron deficiency. J Am Soc Nephrol 1998; 9:655–663.
607. Borguet F, Cornelis R, Delanghe J, et al: Study of the chromium binding in plasma of patients on continuous ambulatory peritoneal dialysis. Clin Chim Acta 1995; 238:71–84.
608. Wallaeys B, Cornelis R, Mees L, Lameire N: Trace elements in serum, packed cells, and dialysate of CAPD patients. Kidney Int 1986; 30:599–604.
609. Van Renterghem D, Cornelis R, Vanholder R: Behaviour of 12 trace elements in serum of uremic patients on hemodiafiltration. J Trace Elem Electrolytes Health Dis 1992; 6:169–174.
610. D'Haese PC, Couttenye MM, Lamberts LV, et al: Aluminum, iron, lead, cadmium, copper, zinc, chromium, magnesium, strontium, and calcium content in bone of end-stage renal failure patients. Clin Chem 1999; 45:1548–1556.
611. De Kimpe J, Cornelis R, Mees L, et al: More than tenfold increase of arsenic in serum and packed cells of chronic hemodialysis patients. Am J Nephrol 1993; 13:429–434.
612. Van Renterghem D, Cornelis R, Mees L, Vanholder R: The effect of adding Br or Zn supplements to the dialysate on the concentrations of Br and Zn in the blood of hemodialysed patients. J Trace Elem Electrolytes Health Dis 1992; 6:105–109.
613. Mahajan SK: Zinc metabolism in uremia. Int J Artif Organs 1988; 11:223–228.
614. Zima T, Tesar V, Mestek O, Nemecek K: Trace elements in end-stage renal disease. II. Clinical implication of trace elements. Blood Purif 1999; 17:187–198.
615. Reddi AS, Bollineni JS: Selenium-deficient diet induces renal oxidative stress and injury via TGF-beta1 in normal and diabetic rats. Kidney Int 2001; 59:1342–1353.
616. Cailleux A, Subra JF, Riberi P, Allain P: Uptake of trihalomethanes by patients during hemodialysis. Clin Chim Acta 1989; 181:75–80.
617. Landi S, Hanley NM, Warren SH, et al: Induction of genetic damage in human lymphocytes and mutations in Salmonella by trihalomethanes: Role of red blood cells and GSTT1-1 polymorphism. Mutagenesis 1999; 14:479–482.
618. Melnick RL, Kohn MC, Dunnick JK, Leininger JR: Regenerative hyperplasia is not required for liver tumor induction in female B6C3F1 mice exposed to trihalomethanes (see comments). Toxicol Appl Pharmacol 1998; 148:137–147.
619. Coffin JC, Ge R, Yang S, et al: Effect of trihalomethanes on cell proliferation and DNA methylation in female B6C3F1 mouse liver. Toxicol Sci 2000; 58:243–252.
620. Waller K, Swan SH, DeLorenze G, Hopkins B: Trihalomethanes in drinking water and spontaneous abortion (see comments). Epidemiology 1998; 9:134–140.
621. Johnson WJ, Hagge WW, Wagoner RD, et al: Effects of urea loading in patients with far-advanced renal failure. Mayo Clin Proc 1972; 47:21–29.
622. Paniagua R, Amato D, Vonesh E, et al: Effects of increased peritoneal clearances on mortality rates in peritoneal dialysis: ADEMEX, a prospective, randomized, controlled trial. J Am Soc Nephrol 2002; 13:1307–1320.
623. Lim J, Gasson C, Kaji DM: Urea inhibits NaK2Cl cotransport in human erythrocytes. J Clin Invest 1995; 96:2126–2132.
624. Maddock AL, Westenfelder C: Urea induces the heat shock response in human neuroblastoma cells. J Am Soc Nephrol 1996; 7:275–282.
625. Moeslinger T, Friedl R, Volf I, et al: Urea induces macrophage proliferation by inhibition of inducible nitric oxide synthesis (see comments). Kidney Int 1999; 56:581–588.
626. Prabhakar SS, Zeballos GA, Montoya-Zavala M, Leonard C: Urea inhibits inducible nitric oxide synthase in macrophage cell line. Am J Physiol 1997; 273:C1882-C1888.
627. Xiao S, Wagner L, Mahaney J, Baylis C: Uremic levels of urea inhibit L-arginine transport in cultured endothelial cells. Am J Physiol Renal Physiol 2001; 280:F989-F995.
628. Xiao S, Erdely A, Wagner L, Baylis C: Uremic levels of BUN do not cause nitric oxide deficiency in rats with normal renal function. Am J Physiol Renal Physiol 2001; 280:F996-F1000.
629. Zhang Z, Yang XY, Cohen DM: Urea-associated oxidative stress and Gadd153/CHOP induction. Am J Physiol 1999; 276: F786-F793.
630. Kraus LM, Kraus AP Jr: Carbamoylation of amino acids and proteins in uremia. Kidney Int Suppl 2001; 78:S102–S107.
631. Kairaitis LK, Yuill E, Harris DC: Determinants of haemoglobin carbamoylation in haemodialysis and peritoneal dialysis patients. Nephrol Dial Transplant 2000; 15:1431–1437.
632. Haley RJ, Ward DM: Nonenzymatically glucosylated serum proteins in patients with end-stage renal disease. Am J Kidney Dis 1986; 8:115–121.
633. Fluckiger R, Harmon W, Meier W, et al: Hemoglobin carbamoylation in uremia. N Engl J Med 1981; 304:823–827.
634. Kwan JT, Carr EC, Neal AD, et al: Carbamoylated haemoglobin, urea kinetic modelling and adequacy of dialysis in haemodialysis patients. Nephrol Dial Transplant 1991; 6:38–43.
635. Monti JP, Brunet PJ, Berland YF, et al: Opposite effects of urea on hemoglobin-oxygen affinity in anemia of chronic renal failure. Kidney Int 1995; 48:827–831.
636. Vanholder RC, Ringoir SM: Adequacy of dialysis: A critical analysis (editorial). Kidney Int 1992; 42:540–558.
637. Owen WF Jr, Lew NL, Liu Y, et al: The urea reduction ratio and serum albumin concentration as predictors of mortality in patients undergoing hemodialysis (see comments). N Engl J Med 1993; 329:1001–1006.
638. Depner TA: Daily hemodialysis efficiency: An analysis of solute kinetics. Adv Ren Replace Ther 2001; 8:227–235.
639. Blumenkrantz MJ, Kopple JD, Moran JK, Coburn JW: Metabolic balance studies and dietary protein requirements in patients undergoing continuous ambulatory peritoneal dialysis. Kidney Int 1982; 21:849–861.
640. Bloembergen WE, Stannard DC, Port FK, et al: Relationship of dose of hemodialysis and cause-specific mortality. Kidney Int 1996; 50:557–565.

641. Stein G, Franke S, Mahiout A, et al: Influence of dialysis modalities on serum AGE levels in end-stage renal disease patients. Nephrol Dial Transplant 2001; 16:999–1008.
642. Winchester JF, Ronco C, Brady JA, et al: Sorbent augmented dialysis: Minor addition or major advance in therapy? Blood Purif 2001; 19:255–259.
643. Botella J, Ghezzi PM, Sanz-Moreno C: Adsorption in hemodialysis. Kidney Int Suppl 2000; 76:S60–S65.
644. La Greca G, Brendolan A, Ghezzi PM, et al: The concept of sorbent in hemodialysis. Int J Artif Organs 1998; 21:303–308.
645. Steczko J, Bax KC, Ash SR: Effect of hemodiabsorption and sorbent-based pheresis on amino acid levels in hepatic failure. Int J Artif Organs 2000; 23:375–388.
646. Wratten ML, Navino C, Tetta C, Verzetti G: Haemolipodialysis. Blood Purif 1999; 17:127–133.
647. Marinez de Francisco AL, Ghezzi PM, Brendolan A, et al: Hemodiafiltration with online regeneration of the ultrafiltrate. Kidney Int Suppl 2000; 76:S66–S71.
648. de Francisco AL, Pinera C, Heras M, et al: Hemodiafiltration with on-line endogenous reinfusion. Blood Purif 2000; 18:231–236.
649. Falkenhagen D, Strobl W, Vogt G, et al: Fractionated plasma separation and adsorption system: A novel system for blood purification to remove albumin bound substances. Artif Organs 1999; 23:81–86.
650. Tetta C, Cavaillon JM, Schulze M, et al: Removal of cytokines and activated complement components in an experimental model of continuous plasma filtration coupled with sorbent adsorption. Nephrol Dial Transplant 1998; 13:1458–1464.
651. Gejyo F, Homma N, Hasegawa S, Arakawa M: A new therapeutic approach to dialysis amyloidosis: Intensive removal of beta 2-microglobulin with adsorbent column. Artif Organs 1993; 17:240–243.
652. Nakazawa R, Azuma N, Suzuki M, et al: A new treatment for dialysis-related amyloidosis with beta 2-microglobulin adsorbent column. Int J Artif Organs 1993; 16:823–829.
653. Ronco C, Ghezzi PM, Morris A, et al: Blood flow distribution in sorbent beds: Analysis of a new sorbent device for hemoperfusion. Int J Artif Organs 2000; 23:125–130.
654. Stange J, Ramlow W, Mitzner S, et al: Dialysis against a recycled albumin solution enables the removal of albumin-bound toxins. Artif Organs 1993; 17:809–813.
655. Gulyassy PF, Depner TA, Shearer GC: Comparison of binding by concentrated peritoneal dialysate and serum. ASAIO J 1993; 39:M569-M572.
656. Raj DS, Ouwendyk M, Francoeur R, Pierratos A: Beta(2)-microglobulin kinetics in nocturnal haemodialysis. Nephrol Dial Transplant 2000; 15:58–64.
657. Fagugli RM, Buoncristiani U, Ciao G: Anemia and blood pressure correction obtained by daily hemodialysis induce a reduction of left ventricular hypertrophy in dialysed patients (Letter). Int J Artif Organs 1998; 21:429–431.
658. Vanholder R, Burgelman M, de Smet R, et al: Two-pool versus single-pool models in the determination of urea kinetic parameters. Blood Purif 1996; 14:437–450.
659. Pedrini LA, Zereik S, Rasmy S: Causes, kinetics and clinical implications of post-hemodialysis urea rebound. Kidney Int 1988; 34:817–824.
660. Hida M, Aiba Y, Sawamura S, et al: Inhibition of the accumulation of uremic toxins in the blood and their precursors in the feces after oral administration of Lebenin, a lactic acid bacteria preparation, to uremic patients undergoing hemodialysis. Nephron 1996; 74:349–355.
661. Ling WH, Hanninen O: Shifting from a conventional diet to an uncooked vegan diet reversibly alters fecal hydrolytic activities in humans. J Nutr 1992; 122:924–930.
662. Niwa T, Yazawa T, Ise M, et al: Inhibitory effect of oral sorbent on accumulation of albumin-bound indoxyl sulfate in serum of experimental uremic rats. Nephron 1991; 57:84–88.
663. Niwa T, Miyazaki T, Hashimoto N, et al: Suppressed serum and urine levels of indoxyl sulfate by oral sorbent in experimental uremic rats. Am J Nephrol 1992; 12:201–206.
664. Boss GR, Seegmiller JE: Hyperuricemia and gout. Classification, complications and management. N Engl J Med 1979; 300:1459–1468.
665. Yokozawa T, Fujioka K, Oura H, et al: Effects of rhubarb tannins on uremic toxins. Nephron 1991; 58:155–160.
666. Shinzato T, Morita H, Maeda K: Metabolism and kinetics of propylurofuranic acid in end-stage renal failure. ASAIO J 1994; 40:94–96.
667. Bostom AG, Shemin D, Lapane KL, et al: High dose-B-vitamin treatment of hyperhomocysteinemia in dialysis patients. Kidney Int 1996; 49:147–152.
668. Ingrosso D, Cimmino A, Perna AF, et al: Folate treatment and unbalanced methylation and changes of allelic expression induced by hyperhomocysteinaemia in patients with uraemia. Lancet 2003; 361:1693–1699.
669. Raj DS, Choudhury D, Welbourne TC, Levi M: Advanced glycation end products: A nephrologist's perspective. Am J Kidney Dis 2000; 35:365–380.
670. Miyata T, Kurokawa K, van Ypersele de Strihou C: Advanced glycation and lipoxidation end products: Role of reactive carbonyl compounds generated during carbohydrate and lipid metabolism (In process citation). J Am Soc Nephrol 2000; 11:1744–1752.
671. Rottembourg J: Residual renal function and recovery of renal function in patients treated by CAPD. Kidney Int Suppl 1993; 40:S106–S110.
672. Lysaght MJ, Vonesh EF, Gotch F, et al: The influence of dialysis treatment modality on the decline of remaining renal function. ASAIO Trans 1991; 37:598–604.
673. McKane W, Chandna SM, Tattersall JE, et al: Identical decline of residual renal function in high-flux biocompatible hemodialysis and CAPD. Kidney Int 2002; 61:256–265.

Anemia in Chronic Kidney Disease

Steven Fishbane, M.D. • Naveed Masani, M.D.

Anemia is a frequent complication of chronic kidney disease (CKD). When cardiac output and blood oxygenation are constant, hemoglobin concentration is the variable that determines oxygen delivery to the body's tissues. The anemic patient suffers the consequences of reduced systemic oxygen delivery, with fatigue being the most pronounced symptom. The body's attempts to compensate for anemia lead to secondary pathology, such as left ventricular hypertrophy of the heart, with its attendant increase in risk for adverse outcomes. Patients with CKD are often exposed to years of anemia (if untreated) with important effects on quality of life and cardiac function.

The prevalence of anemia in CKD depends on both the severity of renal insufficiency (CKD stage) and the definition of anemia. In a study of patients seen in nephrology practices in Boston (Figure 7–1), hematocrit (Hct) less than 36% was found in 45% of patients with serum creatinine (SCr) less than 2 mg/dL; 50% with SCr 2.1 to 3 mg/dL; 58% with SCr 3.1 to 4 mg/dL; and 92% with SCr greater than 4 mg/dL.[1] In end-stage renal disease (ESRD, CKD Stage V) the prevalence, if untreated, increases to greater than 90%.[2]

Most patients with ESRD receive erythropoietin replacement treatment (rHuEPO); however, in earlier stages of CKD anemia may go unrecognized and rHuEPO treatment may be underutilized. In a recent analysis of Medicare beneficiaries who, as patients, started hemodialysis, 60% had Hct less than 30%, and only 15.6% had ever been treated with rHuEPO.[3] Similarly, Obrador and colleagues[4] found that among 155,051 patients new to dialysis between 1995 and 1997, only 23% had been treated with rHuEPO during their years with CKD. Moreover, of those patients with Hct less than 28%, only 20% had received rHuEPO treatment.[4]

PATHOGENESIS

The most common form of anemia in CKD is one of reduced erythrocyte production, with cells generally normal in size and shape.[4,5] Bone marrow studies fail to show the expected increase in erythropoiesis as compensation for anemia. In the past many believed that circulating uremic factors inhibited marrow erythropoiesis.[6–8] A preponderance of evidence now demonstrates that inadequate stimulation of erythropoiesis is the primary defect. The kidneys in CKD may continue to produce erythropoietin, but the quantity produced is insufficient to support normal oxygen delivery.[9,10] Eschbach and colleagues,[11] in seminal studies performed in sheep, clearly demonstrated the importance of erythropoietin deficiency as the primary cause of the anemia of CKD. In the years since rHuEPO replacement treatment was first used, the clinical effectiveness of rHuEPO has been the strongest confirmatory evidence for the primacy of erythropoietin deficiency.

Erythropoietin is a glycoprotein hormone, and its known receptor is a member of the cytokine receptor superfamily.[12] The hormone is produced in response to hypoxic conditions that cause reduced systemic oxygen delivery.[13,14] Hypoxia is sensed in erythropoietin-producing renal peritubular cells by the recently discovered hypoxia inducible factor-1.[15,16] This protein degrades rapidly when normal oxygen tension is present. In hypoxic conditions it is stabilized[17,18] and interacts with the oxygen-sensitive promoter of the erythropoietin gene, resulting in upregulated erythropoietin production.[19] In nonuremic subjects, plasma erythropoietin levels range from 0.01 to 0.03 U/mL. When hypoxia or anemia is present, levels may increase up to 100- to 1000-fold.[20]

Most of the body's erythropoietin production occurs in the kidney, and the primary site of action is in erythroid tissues of the bone marrow. Binding of erythropoietin to its receptor leads to a cascade of signal transduction events that work to stimulate erythrocyte production.[21–25] This occurs in intermediate-stage erythroid burst-forming units (BFU-E) and erythroid colony-forming units (CFU-E), where cell proliferation is stimulated and programmed cell death is reduced.[26] Serum hemoglobin levels increase, systemic oxygen delivery improves, and the stimulus for erythropoietin production decreases.

Although erythropoietin deficiency is the primary cause in over 90% of cases of anemia in CKD, other etiologic factors may be present. Indeed, the patient with CKD may suffer from any of the large number of causes of anemia for which people in the general population are at risk. This would include common causes of anemia, such as iron deficiency, folic acid or vitamin B12 deficiency, bleeding, hemolysis, and myelodysplastic syndromes. Of particular importance in patients with CKD is iron deficiency, a subject that will be discussed in great detail in subsequent sections.

Consequences of Anemia in Chronic Kidney Disease and the Effects of Treatment

Increased Risk of Mortality and Morbidity

It is biologically plausible that anemia could increase the risk of death in CKD. Anemia reduces oxygen delivery to tissues, which could adversely impact on organ function. For patients with chronic organ dysfunction, such as congestive heart failure or coronary artery disease, reduced oxygen supply could potentially increase the risk for ischemic adverse events. Furthermore, maladaptive compensations for anemia, such as left ventricular hypertrophy, might independently increase the risk for mortality. To date, however, no studies have rigorously proven that anemia in CKD causes an increase in mortality risk. Instead, a number of observational studies have successfully

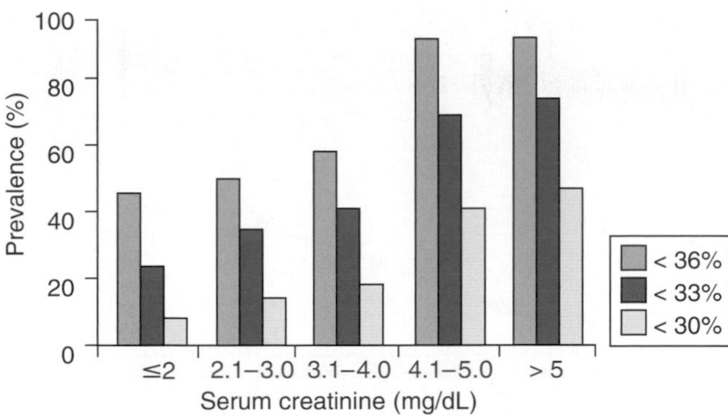

Figure 7–1 Prevalence of anemia in chronic kidney disease.(Adapted from Kazmi et al: AM J Kidney Dis 2001; 38[4]: 803–812.1)

associated anemia in CKD with an increased risk of death. Among a large cohort of patients with ESRD, Ma and colleagues[27] found the risk of death for patients with Hct less than 30% to be increased by 12% to 33%, compared to those patients with higher Hct values. Foley and colleagues[28] prospectively followed 432 ESRD patients and found that each 1 g/dL increase in Hgb was associated with a decrease in mortality risk of 14%. Similar observational findings were reported by Lowrie and Lew.[29] In a post hoc analysis of a large congestive heart failure study, Al-Ahmad and colleagues[30] found that anemia was an independent risk factor for mortality. Every 1% decrease in Hct was associated with a 3% increase in mortality risk. Despite sophisticated multivariate analyses, these studies cannot fully exclude the possibility that low Hct was simply a marker for sicker patients, and that anemia may not be causally linked to an increased mortality risk. Besarab and colleagues[31] reported the results of an interventional study that offered some potential to examine this issue from a different perspective. Patients with preexisting cardiac disease on hemodialysis were randomized to rHuEPO treatment targeted to a low or normal level of Hct. The study did not find anemia, or a lower Hct level, to result in greater mortality risk; in fact, there was a trend to greater mortality in the normal Hct group. Further research will be needed to fully elucidate the relationship of anemia and its treatment to death risk in CKD.

Hospitalization risk in relation to anemia in CKD has also been studied by observational analyses. Collins and colleagues[32] found the risk of hospitalization to be lower in hemodialysis patients with higher Hct values. In the Hct category of 36% to 39%, the risk was 16% to 22% lower than when the Hct was 33% to 36%. Similar findings in hemodialysis patients were reported by Churchill and colleagues.[33] Xue and colleagues[3] studied the pre-ESRD period and found that lower Hct values were associated with greater hospitalization risk. As for mortality, the studies cannot demonstrate that anemia is causally linked to greater risk.

Reduced Quality of Life

Fatigue is the cardinal symptom of anemia.[34] It is often associated with dyspnea and loss of stamina and may result in diminished overall quality of life (QOL). A good-sized body of evidence has accumulated demonstrating that partial or complete correction of anemia in CKD improves measures of QOL.[35–41] A recent systematic review analyzed 16 studies composed of 2253 patients with CKD. The baseline Hct averaged 24.4%, and the mean increase after treatment was 8.3%. Meta-analysis showed a consistent positive correlation between change in Hct and change in QOL measures ($P < .001$).[42] Moreno and colleagues[39] raised Hct from 30% to 38.4% in 156 selected hemodialysis patients. The functional status and quality of life improved significantly with increased Hct.[39] Painter and colleagues[41] found that normalization of Hct accompanied by exercise training led to a significant increase in exercise capacity, although not to normal levels.[41] In contrast, employment status does not seem to improve with anemia treatment.[43] In a recent study of 126 CKD patients with coexistent severe congestive heart failure, Silverberg and colleagues[44] treated with rHuEPO to raise mean hemoglobin levels to approximately 13.1 g/dL. Subjects' functional status, fatigue, and shortness of breath improved significantly, and hospitalization over the next year was reduced by 95% (Figure 7–2).[44]

Reduced Brain and Cognitive Function

Neurocognitive function in relation to CKD and anemia has been examined in several reported studies. Marsh and colleagues[45] studied 24 hemodialysis patients treated with rHuEPO to increase Hct from a mean of 23.7% to 36.5%. An electrophysiologic parameter was found to improve, as were most neuropsychological test results. Temple and colleagues[46] partially corrected anemia in 17 peritoneal dialysis patients and found that IQ results improved as did other measures of cognitive function. Pickett and colleagues[47] studied the effect of normalization of Hct in 20 hemodialysis patients and found improvement in various tests of brain function. These results are consistent with the finding in dogs that systemic oxygen consumption is optimized when Hct is in the normal range.[48,49] Benz and colleagues[50] normalized Hct in 10 hemodialysis patients and found that various measures of sleep function improved significantly.

	Before	After
Hemoglobin (g/dL)	10.3	13.1*
Serum creatinine (mg/dL)	2.4	2.3
NYHA class (1–4)	3.8	2.7*
Fatigue/SOB index	8.9	2.7*
Hospitalization	3.7	0.2*
Systolic BP (mm Hg)	132	131
Diastolic BP (mm Hg)	75	76

* p value < .05

Figure 7–2 Effect of epoietin treatment in congestive heart failure: 126 patients with chronic kidney disease and severe congestive heart failure treated with rHuEPO. (Adapted from Silverberg et al: Perit Dial Int 2001; 21[suppl 3]:S236-S240.)

Cardiac Complications

Left ventricular hypertrophy (LVH) and dilatation develop as compensation for anemia in CKD.[51–53] Levin and colleagues[53,54] found that left ventricular mass index (LVMI) correlated with hemoglobin concentration in pre-ESRD CKD patients. For each decrease of 1 g/dL in serum hemoglobin, LVH risk increased by 6%. Furthermore, they found that worsening of LVMI over a 1-year period correlated with lower hemoglobin levels.[53,54] Harnett and colleagues[55] found that 75% of patients who started dialysis in the United States had LVH present, and that anemia was an important risk factor for LVH.

The importance of the association between anemia and LVH cannot be understated. In nonuremic populations there is a significant and independent relationship between LVH and risk of death.[56,57] Among patients with kidney disease the same relationship holds true.[58] Given the high cardiovascular death rate of hemodialysis patients,[59] the great prevalence of LVH at the onset of hemodialysis,[55] the role of LVH in increasing death risk, and the importance of anemia in the pre-ESRD period as a predictor of LVH, a chain of logic can be constructed that links anemia in the CKD period with subsequent poor outcomes of hemodialysis patients. In fact, Levin and colleagues[53] found that the prevalence of LVH increased progressively with decreasing creatinine clearance levels (Figure 7–3). The causality relationship between anemia and LVH risk in CKD has not yet been sufficiently examined in interventional studies. In uncontrolled studies of partial anemia correction with rHuEPO, regression of LVH has been demonstrated in hemodialysis[60–62] and pre-ESRD CKD patients.[63,64] In one fair-sized randomized controlled trial, Foley and colleagues[65] randomized 146 hemodialysis patients with LVH or left ventricular dilatation to anemia correction to hemoglobin levels of 10.0 or 13.5 g/dL. No difference was found between the groups in subsequent changes in LVH. Therefore, no definitive conclusions can be reached as to whether anemia is causally linked to LVH in CKD. Further randomized controlled trials are in progress.

Ischemic heart disease is a frequent problem for patients with CKD. It is plausible that anemia could increase the risk of ischemia in patients with coronary obstructive disease by reducing coronary oxygen delivery. Conlon and colleagues,[66] in a randomized controlled study of 31 hemodialysis patients, found no reduction in silent ischemia episodes with treatment to a normal Hct level. In contrast, Wizemann and colleagues,[67] in an uncontrolled study of 81 hemodialysis patients, found that partial correction of anemia led to significant reductions in exercise-induced electrocardiograph changes. Hase et al[68] studied the effect of rHuEPO treatment in nine hemodialysis patients with coronary artery disease. Mean hemoglobin concentrations increased from 7.9 g/dL to 10.4 g/dL. Exercise duration improved by approximately 40%, and electrocardiographic ischemic changes were reduced. The effect of anemia or anemia treatment on cardiac mortality is discussed separately above.

Treatment with Recombinant Human Erythropoietin (rHuEPO)

Erythropoietin is a glycoprotein hormone synthesized and released primarily by peritubular type I interstitial cells located in the renal cortex. The native compound is composed of 166 amino acids, although in the circulating form there are only 165 amino acids. It is N-glycosylated at three amino acids and O-glycosylated at one, Ser126.[69] The gene for erythropoietin was cloned by Jacobs and colleagues[70] in 1985. Within 2 years clinical studies were published demonstrating the safety and efficacy of a recombinant form of the hormone.[71,72] The U.S. Food and Drug Administration approved rHuEPO for the treatment of anemia of kidney disease in 1989.

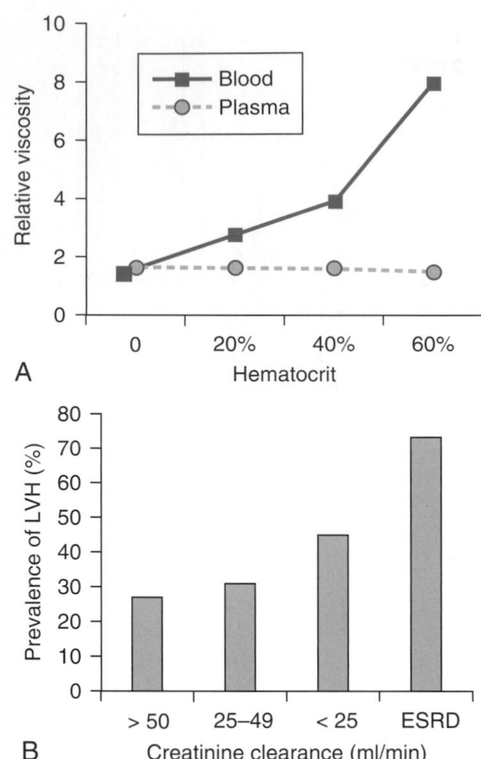

Figure 7–3 ***A,*** Relative viscosity as measured by viscometer. ***B,*** Prevalence of LVH increases as the creatinine clearance decreases. (Adapted from Levin A, Singer J, Thompson CR, et al: Prevalent left ventricular hypertrophy in the predialysis population: identifying opportunities for intervention. Am J Kidney Dis 1996; 27:347-354, and Foley RN, Parfrey PS, Morgan J, et al: Effect of hemoglobin levels in hemodialysis patients with asymptomatic cardiomyopathy. Kidney Int 2000; 58:1325-1335.

Recombinant human erythropoietin (rHuEPO or epoetin) is a generic term that encompasses all genetically produced forms of erythropoietin. The drugs are produced through recombination of the human erythropoietin gene with Chinese hamster ovary cells.[73,74] Four forms of the drug are currently available: epoetin-α, epoetin-β, epoetin-Ω, and darbepoetin-α. Epoetin-α, epoetin-β, and epoetin-Ω are indistinguishable from the native human hormone and are very similar in clinical characteristics. Darbepoetin-α has a modified carbohydrate content that yields a longer serum half-life.[75] The drug contains five N-linked carbohydrate chains as opposed to the three contained in standard epoetin. This results in improved serum half-life, despite decreased erythropoietin receptor affinity. Darbepoetin-α has approximately three times the half-life of standard epoetin-α, with an intravenous administration half-life of approximately 25 hours (compared to 8 hours for epoetin-α).[75,76] It is not clear whether the longer half-life allows for extended dosing intervals relative to other forms of rHuEPO.[77–81]

Dose, Route of Administration, Titration, and Monitoring

Because of easy access to the circulation and practicality, rHuEPO administration for patients on maintenance hemodialysis is typically via the intravenous route. The typical starting dose of epoetin-α is 120 to 180 U/kg, divided three times per week.[82] Darbepoetin-α may be started at a dose of 25 mcg once weekly. Since erythropoiesis takes time, and since newly made erythrocytes join a large pool of existing cells in circulation, there will usually not be an increase in serum hemoglobin for 2 to 4 weeks after the initiation of treatment. The rate of response varies between patients and is related to the dose chosen. In the initial clinical trials of epoetin-α, doses as high as 500 U/kg were used, resulting in an overly rapid increase of as much as 10 Hct points in 3 weeks.[71]

Certain factors may preclude epoetin from achieving its maximum efficacy, including reduced iron stores, presence of infection, lack of adequate dialysis, hyperparathyroidism, and chronic inflammation, which results in a reticuloendothelial blockade and impaired iron release.[83] Although controversial, it appears that angiotensin-converting enzyme inhibitors and angiotensin-II receptor blockers may also result in relative erythropoietin resistance and the need for higher doses.[84,85] When a patient's response to rHuEPO is inadequate, a careful search for factors that may lead to hyporesponsiveness should be undertaken. As discussed in subsequent sections, iron deficiency may be the most important of these factors.

During the initiation of rHuEPO treatment, hemoglobin and Hct levels should be checked every 1 to 2 weeks. The goal should be for Hct to increase by approximately 0.5 to 1.5 points per week. The target is to raise the Hct to a range of 33% to 36% (hemoglobin 11 to 12 g/dL).[82] Once the goals of therapy are reached, hemoglobin/hematocrit monitoring can be reduced to every 2 to 4 weeks. Because of the important link between iron supply and erythropoiesis, iron stores should be tested every month during the initiation of rHuEPO treatment and every 3 months thereafter.

The target hemoglobin concentration for CKD patients treated with rHuEPO has been the subject of some controversy.[86] Normal Hct values for adults are 36% to 46%, with the lower part of the range applying to women. Most interventional studies in CKD have evaluated the effect of rHuEPO treatment for raising Hct from levels below 30% to levels between 30% and 36%. The effects analyzed have generally been outcomes such as need for blood transfusion, Hct level achieved, or measures of quality of life or functional status. These studies have generally demonstrated good efficacy for rHuEPO treatment within these parameters and support the current Kidney Disease Outcomes Quality Initiative (K/DOQI™) target hemoglobin level (11 to 12 g/dL).[82] There has been only one published, well powered interventional study that has examined the effect of normalizing Hct. Besarab and colleagues[31] studied 1233 hemodialysis patients randomized to an Hct of approximately 30% or 42%. The primary finding was of no benefit and, in fact, suggested a trend toward a greater mortality risk in the higher Hct group. In a recent cost effectiveness analysis, Tonelli and colleagues[87] found no value to raising hemoglobin levels above 12 g/dL in hemodialysis patients. Similarly, a recent systematic literature review by Strippoli and colleagues[88] did not result in a benefit for higher Hct levels. Therefore, the current target hemoglobin level of 11 to 12 g/dL would seem to be quite adequate.

The route of administration for rHuEPO is usually intravenous for hemodialysis patients and subcutaneous for patients with earlier stages of CKD or for those on peritoneal dialysis. Convenience tends to be the main driver of the route selected. However, there is a difference in efficacy that has been consistently demonstrated in clinical trials.[89–91] In one study, Kaufman and colleagues[89] randomly assigned 208 hemodialysis patients to treatment with epoetin-α, either by intravenous or subcutaneous routes. The main result was a mean 32% reduction in epoetin dose requirements when the drug was administered by the subcutaneous route. McClellan and colleagues[90] studied administrative data on 7092 hemodialysis patients and found that the subcutaneous route yielded equivalent Hct outcomes with an approximate 14% reduction in dose requirement. It is likely that when rHuEPO is administered intravenously, the very high plasma levels of erythropoietin immediately after injection fully saturate erythropoietin receptors. Some drug may be metabolized before there is any interaction with receptors, essentially wasting the drug. Subcutaneous dosing results in a slower accumulation phase in plasma and less saturation of erythropoietin receptors.[82] However, despite the strong data and national guidelines supporting subcutaneous administration, most hemodialysis patients are still treated with intravenous rHuEPO. This is probably the result of patient and provider preference.

Potential Adverse Effects of Treatment

A variety of side effects may be seen with epoetin therapy, including hypertension, seizures, increased arteriovenous (AV) graft clotting, and the recently described phenomenon of pure red cell aplasia. Hypertension develops or worsens in approximately 25% to 35% of patients treated with rHuEPO.[92,93] This may be countered with additional antihypertensive therapy or with reduction of the dry weight of hemodialysis patients. Unless the extremely rare complication of hypertensive encephalopathy is encountered, rHuEPO therapy need not be discontinued.[93] Particular care must be taken with patients with progressive CKD, where hypertension is the major driver of disease progression. Worsening hypertensive control in these patients may outweigh any benefits derived from rHuEPO treatment. In a study of rats with CKD (renal ablation), Garcia and colleagues[94] found that rHuEPO treatment resulted in uncontrolled hypertension and faster disease progression. Hypertension should first be under good control before rHuEPO is initiated in patients with CKD. Blood pressure should be carefully monitored during all phases of treatment and, especially, after the rHuEPO dose is increased.

The etiology of the rHuEPO-induced hypertension is incompletely understood and is probably multifactorial. Factors implicated in the pathobiology include (1) an increase in blood viscosity, (2) improved cardiac output, (3) increased synthesis of endothelin-1 and an imbalance in vasoactive hormones and autacoids, (4) reduction in vasodilatation as compensation for anemia, and (5) improved vascular responsiveness to circulating catecholamines.[93, 95–97] Not one of these factors has yet been identified as the primary cause of hypertension. Interestingly, Caravaca and colleagues[98] found that hypertension risk was reduced by approximately 95% in patients who were taking antiplatelet drugs at the time of their rHuEPO treatment. The authors suggested that changes in platelet aggregability induced by rHuEPO might play an important role in the pathogenesis of the hypertension.

Blood viscosity increases as Hct rises. The relationship is nonlinear, with the rate of rise of viscosity increasing at high levels of Hct (Figure 7–3). Treatment with rHuEPO increases Hct and blood viscosity, and there has been a concern that either native vessel or graft thrombosis risk may be increased. Recently, Wun and colleagues[99] found venous thrombosis risk in cervical cancer patients treated with rHuEPO to be increased 10.3-fold compared to non-rHuEPO-treated patients. A trial study of Hct normalization in hemodialysis patients resulted in a trend toward a greater risk of myocardial infarction among patients randomized to the higher Hct group.[31] Churchill and colleagues[100] studied hemodialysis vascular access thrombosis and found that rHuEPO treatment was associated with increased risk in AV grafts but not in fistulas. In contrast, Besarab and colleagues[101] did not find an increased risk of vascular access clotting during rHuEPO treatment. In general, until the magnitude of risk for thrombosis is better understood, limiting target hemoglobin to 12 g/dL is probably reasonable.

The effects on native AV fistula stenosis have also been studied with respect to rHuEPO therapy. A 3-year, placebo-controlled, prospective study in hemodialysis patients evaluated the effects of rHuEPO treatment on the progression of native AV fistula stenoses. Treatment with rHuEPO was not found to accelerate the development of stenoses. Interestingly, the treatment group was found to have a statistically significant decrease in plasma values of platelet-derived growth factor and vascular cell adhesion molecule-1, signaling molecules that tend to favor neointimal proliferation.[102]

The development of pure red cell aplasia (PRCA) during rHuEPO therapy, secondary to the formation of anti-erythropoietin antibodies, was first reported in 2002.[103–105] The antibodies have a strong neutralizing capability, blocking erythropoiesis and erythroid colony formation from normal bone marrow. Over a 3-year period, 13 patients who were receiving epoetin-α for chronic kidney disease developed transfusion-dependent anemia anywhere from 3 to 67 months after initiation of treatment. After discontinuing rHuEPO, six patients regained erythropoietic activity after being treated with immunosuppressants or a renal allograft, while three remain transfusion-dependent more than 2 years later. Many other cases have now been reported in Europe and elsewhere, while the incidence in the United States appears to be extremely rare. One possible explanation for the recent development of PRCA is a difference in stabilizing agents used in rHuEPO production. The vast majority of reported cases occurred with only one type of epoetin-α formulation, Eprex (Johnson & Johnson). In 1998 the European formulation of this drug was changed at the request of regulatory agencies, with the replacement of human serum albumin (HSA), by polysorbate 80 and glycine. There was a clear temporal relationship between this formulation change and with the suddenly increased incidence of PRCA. In contrast, the incidence of PRCA has remained low with HSA-containing epoetin-α products. It may be that this formulation change was a major cause of the rapid increase in PRCA cases. There is little reason to believe that PRCA is an important problem with other forms of rHuEPO. Another interesting finding is that in all cases in which the route of administration could be determined, the drug was administered subcutaneously. It is possible that interaction of the drug with tissue proteins, without the stabilizing effect of HSA, may occasionally render the drug immunogenic. The incidence is not completely clear, but probably less than 1 in 10,000 patients is treated with Eprex.

Pure red cell aplasia should be considered when a patient who has previously responded to rHuEPO suddenly becomes unresponsive. Usual causes of hyporesponse, as described above, should be excluded. The diagnosis of PRCA is confirmed by analysis of bone marrow biopsy samples, with the demonstration of no erythroid precursors. Anti-erythropoietin antibodies can be demonstrated in serum by immunoprecipitation. Treatment with Eprex (or other rHuEPO) should be discontinued and no other rHuEPO treatment initiated. Immunosuppressive treatment (steroids, immunoglobulin, plasmapheresis, corticosteroids) may help to restore marrow erythropoietic function.

Iron Management in Chronic Kidney Disease

Introduction

Monitoring of iron status and treatment of iron deficiency are essential components of the treatment of anemia in CKD. It has long been recognized that insufficient iron storage diminishes the effectiveness of rHuEPO therapy.[106] Iron deficiency may occur at any stage of CKD but is particularly frequent among hemodialysis patients.[82] Although the exact incidence of iron deficiency in hemodialysis patients is not known, it occurs in the majority of patients.[107]

Pathobiology of Iron Deficiency in Chronic Kidney Disease

Iron balance in man reflects a homeostatic system in which dietary iron absorption is adjusted based on iron losses and storage. Dietary intake of iron is usually far in excess of actual need, therefore it is unusual for iron deficiency to develop on the basis of inadequate intake.[108,109] Rather, excess external loss of iron causes most cases of iron deficiency. In hemodialysis patients iron losses are common for several reasons. First, a certain amount of blood and iron are left behind in the dialysis lines and filter at the end of each treatment.[110] Iron is also lost as a result of frequent venipuncture for laboratory testing, surgical blood loss, gastrointestinal bleeding, and vascular access accidents.[111,112] The second reason for iron deficiency in hemodialysis patients is insufficient absorption of dietary iron resulting from the use of phosphate binders. This effect may be less profound with sevelamer than with calcium- and aluminum-containing binders.[113,114] If phosphate binders are not used, basal absorption of dietary iron may be unimpaired in hemodialysis patients.[115] The third reason for the high incidence of iron deficiency in hemodialysis patients is the accelerated demand for storage iron caused by rHuEPO therapy. Normal total body iron stores are 3000 to 4000 mg. A much smaller quantity of iron, 3 mg, is in circulation at any given moment.[108] During the intensified erythropoietic stimulus of rHuEPO treatment, this small amount of circulating iron may be rapidly exhausted, leading to iron deficient erythropoiesis, even if there is stainable iron in storage tissues.[116] For peritoneal dialysis patients and CKD patients not yet on dialysis, iron deficiency is probably a less frequent occurrence because there is less blood loss. However, there is little published data to critically assess the incidence of iron deficiency in these populations.

Monitoring and Diagnosis of Iron Deficiency in Chronic Kidney Disease

The K/DOQI™ anemia guidelines recommend that during the initiation of rHuEPO treatment, iron status should be tested every month in patients not receiving iron repletion.[82] Once rHuEPO dosing and iron maintenance have stabilized, the guidelines recommend monitoring every 3 months. Two tests, serum ferritin and transferrin saturation, have been widely used for the diagnosis of iron deficiency in CKD.

Serum ferritin is a marker for iron storage and believed to reflect iron deficiency in CKD patients when less than 100 ng/mL.[82] The diagnostic value of serum ferritin, however, is limited by its behavior as a potent acute phase reactant.[117] Clinical settings often arise in CKD where ferritin values may be high, even in the presence of iron deficiency, resulting in a test sensitivity of only 41% to 60% in hemodialysis patients.[118–120] Given the low sensitivity, a high or normal serum ferritin is not sufficient to exclude the possibility of iron deficiency. Serum ferritin should not be used by itself for the assessment of iron status in patients with CKD.

Transferrin saturation (TSAT) is a measure of the availability of circulating iron, calculated as TSAT = (serum iron/total iron binding capacity) × 100. K/DOQI™ guidelines recommend using a value of less than 20% as an indicator of iron deficiency in patients with CKD.[82] This test, although reasonably sensitive, has a specificity measured in hemodialysis patients of only 36% to 63%.[118–120] As a result, low values of transferrin saturation cannot reliably make the diagnosis of iron deficiency in this patient population, and results are often falsely positive. Because of transferrin saturation's poor specificity and serum ferritin's poor sensitivity, it is not surprising that concurrently measured specimens often paradoxically suggest iron deficiency by transferrin saturation and iron overload by serum ferritin (such discordant results are frequently due to the effects of inflammation).[121,122] Both tests are further limited by their great variability. Recently, the coefficient of variation for both tests was greater than 40%.[123]

The weakness in the predictive values of serum ferritin and transferrin saturation leads logically to the conclusion that the tests are most helpful when serum ferritin is less than 100 ng/mL (highly predictive of iron deficiency) or TSAT is greater than 20% (highly predictive of iron sufficiency). All other test results are too inaccurate to be used in isolation as a guide for iron management. Rather, the clinician must consider the patient's serum hemoglobin concentration and rHuEPO dose requirements as part of the overall context of iron treatment decisions.

Other tests have been used with varying success to improve the accuracy of the monitoring of iron status in CKD. The percentage of hypochromic red blood cells (PHR) appears to be a helpful test of iron status in patients on hemodialysis.[124] Tessitore and colleagues[125] found that it had the greatest utility of any test in the diagnosis of iron deficiency. When PHR was greater than 6%, the efficiency was 89.6%, indicating excellent discriminative ability.[125] The test has one important limitation, that is, it is affected by changes in erythrocyte size. When samples are stored or shipped, the cell size may be significantly altered.[126] In the United States, the majority of laboratory samples for hemodialysis are shipped to central locations. This may help explain PHR's inconsistent results in several studies[127,128] and may limit its practicality and usefulness.

Reticulocyte hemoglobin content (CHr) is a direct measure of iron status at the level of the final precursor to mature erythrocytes, the reticulocyte. Because it is a measure of content instead of concentration, it is unaffected by changes in cell volume. In addition, since reticulocytes circulate only for approximately 24 hours,[129] test results are a "snapshot," indicating very acute changes in iron status. Studies have generally found this test to be an accurate measure of iron status in hemodialysis patients.[125,127,128,130,131] In a preliminary analysis of 32 hemodialysis patients, CHr had a sensitivity of 100% and specificity of 80%, superior to the accuracy of serum ferritin, transferrin saturation, and percent hypochromic red blood cells.[128] In a more recent three-center study, 157 hemodialysis patients were randomized to iron treatment based on (1) CHr less than 29 pg or (2) serum ferritin less than 100 ng/mL or transferrin saturation less than 20%. When treatment was based on CHr the total cost of anemia care was significantly reduced, driven by greater than 50% reduction in IV-iron dosing. Furthermore, the variability of the test was far less than that for serum ferritin or transferrin saturation.[123] Generally, a CHr value of less than 29 to 33 pg indicates a need for more intensive iron treatment in patients with CKD.

Iron Treatment in Chronic Kidney Disease

K/DOQI™ anemia treatment guidelines recommend iron treatment in CKD when the serum ferritin is less than 100 ng/mL or the TSAT is less than 20%.[82] Iron replacement may be by oral or intravenous routes. Oral supplementation of iron offers the benefits of simplicity, low cost and safety, but efficacy may be limited. K/DOQI™ guidelines recommend that when oral iron is used in adults, 200 mg of elemental iron should be administered daily in two to three divided doses.[82] A variety of different oral iron drugs are available over the counter or by prescription. All of the agents may cause gastrointestinal side effects such as dyspepsia, constipation and bloating,[132] and there is little evidence to differentiate between them based on efficacy or tolerability.

The efficacy of oral iron in CKD has been rigorously studied only in the subset of patients on hemodialysis, and the results have been disappointing. Macdougall and colleagues[133] found that during the initiation of rHuEPO treatment that oral iron was no more effective than no iron treatment.[133] Similarly, Wingard and colleagues[134] treated 46 hemodialysis patients with oral iron for 6 months and found that most patients had Hct less than 30% and declining iron stores.[134] Markowitz and colleagues[135] studied 49 hemodialysis patients in a double-blinded, randomized controlled trial and found no difference in efficacy between oral iron polysaccharide and placebo.[135] Fudin and colleagues[136] studied 39 iron deficient subjects at the initiation of hemodialysis and found no difference in subsequent hemoglobin levels between oral iron and no iron treatment.[136] Taken together, these findings indicate that oral iron does not have demonstrable efficacy for iron replacement in hemodialysis patients. In contrast, among CKD patients not yet on dialysis and those on peritoneal dialysis, ongoing iron losses are far less than what hemodialysis patients experience. Accordingly, they have lesser needs for iron supplementation and may benefit from oral iron treatment. There are, however, few published data to support this assumption.

The reasons for the lack of efficacy of oral iron treatment in hemodialysis patients are multiple. First, compliance with oral iron therapy may be poor, although there are few published reports that cover this issue. Factors impacting on compliance with oral iron include gastrointestinal side effects,[132] the need to take the pills between meals, the obligatory intake of three pills per day with most supplements to attain adequate elemental iron intake,[137] and poor education of patients of the purpose and goals of iron therapy.

The effectiveness of oral iron in CKD patients may be enhanced through several practices: (1) The dose should provide at least 200 mg of elemental iron per day[82] (for ferrous sulfate, this would be approximately three 325 mg tablets per day), (2) the pills should be taken between meals and should be spaced at least 1 hour apart from ingestion of phosphate binders, and (3) since iron is absorbed proximally in the gastrointestinal tract, delayed-release iron supplements should probably be avoided.

Because of the poor efficacy of oral iron in hemodialysis patients, there has been a great increase in recent years in the use of intravenous iron in this and other stages of CKD. A large number of studies have consistently pointed to the excellent efficacy of intravenous iron in CKD.[133,136,138–144] Treatment results in the ability to consistently reach target hemoglobin levels and/or to achieve a significant reduction in rHuEPO dose requirements. Our group randomized hemodialysis patients to treatment with oral iron or intravenous iron dextran 200 mg per week. Despite having adequate iron test results at baseline, patients responded with higher Hct levels and a 46% reduction in mean rHuEPO dose.[138] As a result of the large body of evidence demonstrating the efficacy of intravenous iron treatment, both the European Best Practice Guidelines for the management of anemia and the K/DOQI™ place intravenous iron as a key facet of care for hemodialysis patients.[82,145] As discussed above, other CKD patients have lesser degrees of blood loss, and oral iron therapy may often suffice.

The primary goal of intravenous iron therapy is to optimally support erythropoiesis, allowing target hemoglobin levels to be reached. To achieve this goal, the amount of iron administered and the resulting levels of iron tests will vary for different patients. In general terms, the K/DOQI™ anemia guidelines recommend that serum ferritin be kept greater than 100 mg/dL and transferrin saturation be greater than 20%.[82] How high above these levels is optimal for supporting rHuEPO therapy is unclear. However, with repeated dosing of intravenous iron, iron storage may increase to potentially unsafe levels. At the present time, it is not known what levels of serum ferritin or transferrin saturation indicate such iron overload.[146] European and American practice guidelines recommend that intravenous iron not be administered if serum ferritin is greater than 800 to 1000 ng/mL.[82,145]

Intravenous iron supplementation in CKD can be delivered using different dosing strategies. For patients on hemodialysis, the ready availability of vascular access during the dialysis treatment leads to great flexibility in dosing. One of two approaches is generally used. The first anticipates ongoing iron losses by providing a regular weekly (or another interval) dose of iron. The quantity administered depends on the iron needs of the individual patient; for the most part 25 to 100 mg per week should be sufficient. Based on quarterly iron test results, the dose can be adjusted to achieve the desired level of iron storage and hemoglobin level. An alternative dosing strategy is to treat with no regular intravenous iron dose and, rather, to check iron tests every 3 months; if iron deficiency develops, the recommended strategy is to treat with a more intense, repletive course of iron. Typically, 1000 mg of iron will be dosed over the course of 10 consecutive hemodialysis treatments. Both of these treatment approaches are convenient and easy to monitor. There are few published data to establish the superiority of either approach.

Intravenous iron treatment is occasionally needed for patients treated with peritoneal dialysis or CKD not yet on dialysis. As opposed to hemodialysis, where vascular access is readily available, for these patients establishing access may be inconvenient. Therefore, the treatment approach seeks to use larger iron doses given with fewer repetitions. A typical approach is to administer 250 mg of iron over 1 to 2 hours, with repeated doses given for 1 to 3 weeks as needed.[147,148]

There are currently three forms of intravenous iron that are most frequently used in the United States and in Europe. Iron dextran is a simple complex in which a dense iron core is surrounded by a shell of glucose polymers that extend out radially from the iron center.[149] The complex binds iron tightly, releasing iron into the reticuloendothelial system, where iron is cleaved from the dextran component. Iron is released into the circulation where it associates with serum transferrin.[150] The drug has well-demonstrated efficacy, but its safety is less than desired because of the occasional occurrence of anaphylaxis.[151] This complication is believed to be a result of the dextran component, although the pathogenesis is incompletely understood. Some patients have been found to have preformed dextran antibodies,[152] and the anaphylaxis may not be associated with typical manifestations, such as IgE or immune complex mediation.[153] Indeed, there is some evidence for direct unstimulated release of mediators from mast cells.[153] The incidence of iron dextran-related anaphylaxis has been found to be from 0.6% to 0.7% of all patients treated.[154,155] A history of multiple previous drug allergies may identify patients at particular risk.[155] Because of the problem of anaphylaxis and the availability of nondextran containing a form of intravenous iron, iron dextran use should probably be limited to patients who have received the drug over a long period without problems occurring.

Sodium Ferric Gluconate Complex (SFGC) is a form of intravenous iron in which the iron core is surrounded by sucrose (20% of weight) and a gluconate function that is important for stability. The apparent molecular weight by gel chromatography is 350,000 ± 23,000 daltons (Da).[156] The drug has been used for several decades with excellent safety[151] and efficacy reported.[157] The risk for allergic and anaphylactic type reaction appears to be dramatically reduced compared to iron dextran. Michael and colleagues[158] reported on single dose exposure in a randomized, controlled double-blinded study of 2503 hemodialysis patients. There was only one immediate type of reaction found: a rate of 0.04%. This compares to a rate of 0.61% for iron dextran calculated from an accompanying meta-analysis.[158]

Iron sucrose is a polynuclear iron (III)-hydroxide complex composed of approximately 30% sucrose. The apparent molecular weight is 34,000 to 60,000 Da.[159] This drug, like SFGC, has been used for several decades with good reports of efficacy and safety.[160] Charytan and colleagues[160] administered iron sucrose 100 mg intravenously for 10 consecutive hemodialysis treatments and found a significant increase in Hgb and transferrin saturation and ferritin levels.[160] Van Wyck and colleagues[161] tested iron sucrose in 23 hemodialysis patients who were previously allergic to iron dextran. They found no severe reactions in 223 administered doses of iron sucrose. Silverberg and colleagues[162] treated 73 hemodialysis and peritoneal dialysis patients with intravenous iron sucrose 100 mg twice monthly and found significant increases in Hct and reductions in rHuEPO dose requirements of up to 75.7%.[162]

There is little published data directly comparing the efficacy and safety of sodium ferric gluconate to iron sucrose. One study by Kosch and colleagues[163] randomized 59 hemodialysis patients to intravenous treatment with either iron sucrose administered in a dose of 250 mg iron diluted in 100 mL normal saline given over 60 minutes once per month or ferric gluconate, 62.5 mg given once per week in a slow push injection (5 min). Serum ferritin, transferrin saturation, and hemoglobin rose significantly and similarly in both groups. There were no significant differences between the two drugs in efficacy or safety end points.[163]

Iron Treatment Safety

The main safety concern in the use of intravenous iron is risk for anaphylaxis. When iron sucrose or ferric gluconate is used instead of iron dextran, the risk, as discussed earlier, is greatly reduced. Large database reviews have suggested a slightly increased risk of death with repeated intravenous iron dosing.[164] Other safety concerns generally relate to iron's oxidizing potential or its ability to serve as a growth factor for microorganisms. The potential risk for iron overload, infection, oxidative tissue damage, and cardiovascular disease is discussed in Chapter 9.

Iron overload is best understood through familiarity with the disease state hemosiderosis and the related genetic disorder hemochromatosis. In these states, many years of excessive iron storage lead gradually to evidence of tissue damage, including restrictive cardiomyopathy, pancreatic damage, arthritis, and other pathologic changes.[165] It is unlikely that intravenous iron treatment would ever lead to such a state of iron overload unless monitoring of treatment was completely disregarded. Current recommendations of the K/DOQI™ anemia practice guidelines are that intravenous iron not be administered if serum ferritin is greater than 800 ng/mL or if transferrin saturation is greater than 50%.[82] In the era prior to the introduction of rHuEPO, Gokal and colleagues[166] and Ali and colleagues[167] found evidence of iron overload in multiple transfused hemodialysis patients, some of whom had been treated with intravenous iron as well. During the same era, various researchers associated elevated iron stores with an increased risk for adynamic bone disease,[168] hepatomegaly,[169] and cardiomyopathy.[170]

The risk of infection related to intravenous iron treatment extends from the observation that iron is a key growth factor for many microorganisms.[171] Bullen and colleagues[172,173] found that bacteria injected into animals did not cause infection unless iron was first injected. In fact, iron injection led to the development of overwhelming sepsis.[172,173] Others have found that desferrioxamine iron chelation may be associated with risk of severe infections (probably as a result of providing an iron supply to bacteria or fungi).[174] In addition, intravenous iron treatment has been associated with reduced white blood cell function.[175–177] These and other findings establish that it is at least plausible that iron treatment could promote infection.

The extent to which intravenous iron treatment actually promotes infection (if at all) is uncertain. Most attempts to evaluate the relationship between iron and potential infection risk have focused on iron storage as measured by serum ferritin. Indeed, several investigators found that higher levels of serum ferritin were associated with an increased risk of infection.[178–180] This methodology may be faulty, however, in that serum ferritin behaves as an intense acute phase reactant.[181] The relationship between serum ferritin and infection risk may not indicate causality. Rather, patients with increased infection risk or with early occult infection may have elevated serum ferritins on the basis of the acute phase response. The ability to more rigorously explore the relationship would require a greater understanding of infection risk factors and inflammatory markers to power more effective multivariate analyses. Of note, a large, prospective European multicenter study found no association between serum ferritin and risk for bacteremia.[182] The relationship of intravenous iron treatment itself to infection risk was studied by Jean and colleagues.[183] These investigators found that among patients with hemodialysis catheters in place, intravenous iron dosing was associated with a greater risk for bacteremia.[183] Similarly, Canziani and colleagues[184] studied 111 hemodialysis patients and found that higher doses of intravenous iron sucrose were associated with increased infection risk. In contrast to these studies, Hoen and colleagues[185] found no relationship between intravenous iron dosing and infection risk.

Parkkinen and colleagues[186] evaluated the relationship between intravenous iron treatment and infection risk in a novel manner. A small group of hemodialysis patients were injected with intravenous iron sucrose at a typical 100 mg dose. Half of the patients were found to have significant amounts of free iron in circulation at 3.5 hours after dosing. Plasma samples from all patients were incubated with *Staphylococcus epidermidis.* For patients with no free iron present, there was no growth of bacteria. Among patients with free iron present there was a significant linear relationship between the quantity of free iron and the degree of bacterial growth.[186] These findings suggest that free iron present after intravenous iron injection might predispose to bacterial growth. By extension, it would probably be reasonable to avoid intravenous iron treatment during episodes of bacteremia.

Iron is a powerful oxidizing substance, and the body has highly conserved mechanisms to prevent tissues from being directly exposed to iron. In storage pools, iron is tightly bound within the protective shells of ferritin and hemosiderin. In circulation, iron is protected by transferrin, and release of iron to tissues is a highly regulated receptor-mediated process.[187–188] After intravenous iron dosing, the drug should be taken up from circulation by the reticuloendothelial system with later release of iron into the circulation for carriage by transferrin.

Any direct and immediate release of iron after injection into the circulation could potentially overwhelm the ability of transferrin to bind the iron. Free, unprotected iron may then be present in circulation, with the potential to cause oxidative tissue damage and to induce the production of reactive oxygen species.

Early studies of intravenous iron and release of free iron may have used faulty methodology, including drug bound iron in the measurement of serum free iron.[189] More recent studies have used better analytic techniques to measure free iron. Parkkinen and colleagues[186] found that after injection of 100 mg of iron sucrose, transferrin saturation rose dramatically within 10 minutes, indicating immediate release of iron from the drug into the circulation. Free iron was detected in the circulation in 50% of patients at 3.5 hours after injection. Patients with lower levels of serum transferrin were much more likely to have free iron present. As discussed previously, the plasma of the patients with free iron present promoted growth of *S. epidermidis.*[186] Similarly, Kooistra and colleagues[190] and Rooyakkers and colleagues[191] found that injection of iron sucrose led to free iron in plasma of hemodialysis patients and normal volunteers, respectively. In the latter study, free iron release was associated with increased reactive oxygen species in plasma and reduced forearm blood flow.[191] Roob and colleagues[192] found that iron sucrose injection in hemodialysis patients led to free iron release and oxidation, which could be attenuated by pretreatment with vitamin E. Taken together, these and other studies indicate that intravenous iron injection does appear to be associated with some free iron appearance in plasma. The effect of the free iron on the health of patients and clinically important outcomes is not yet known. Recent studies have shown some evidence of protein oxidation and a possible association with accelerated atherosclerosis.[193,194] In another report, oxidized fibrinogen was found after intravenous ferric gluconate injection.[195] It is the opinion of the authors that all intravenous iron drugs have the potential for the release of at least small amounts of free iron after injection, with the potential for a resulting increase in oxidative stress. The ability of cellular antioxidant systems to cope with this stress has not yet been adequately studied.

The potential association of iron treatment with accelerated cardiovascular disease risk has been proposed based on iron's oxidative properties and the relationship between oxidation and atherosclerosis risk.[196] The link was first proposed by Sullivan[197] in 1981, with the suggestion that iron deficiency might protect against atherosclerotic disease. With the high prevalence of cardiac disease among patients with end-stage kidney disease[198] and frequent use of iron supplementation in this population, any relationship between the two may be clinically relevant. However, there are few reports addressing this subject specifically in patients with renal failure, so a potentially misleading approach was extrapolated from studies in other populations. In one such study, Salonen and colleagues[199] examined risk for myocardial infarction in 1931 middle-aged Finnish men. Serum ferritin greater than 200 ng/mL was found to be an independent risk factor for cardiac disease. In contrast, Magnusson and colleagues[200] studied over 2000 subjects and found no relationship between serum ferritin and cardiac risk. Similarly, other results from the literature have been mixed, with more negative than positive studies.[199-208] Indeed, a natural model to explore the relationship exists in the form of hereditary hemochromatosis. In patients with this disease and extensive iron overload, Miller and Hutchins[209] have found a rate of severe coronary artery disease of only 12%, compared to 39% of controls with normal iron stores. Given the complexity of this subject and its possible implications for therapy with iron and rHuEPO, further research in this area is clearly needed.

References

1. Kazmi WH, Kausz AT, Khan S, et al: Anemia: An early complication of chronic renal insufficiency. Am J Kidney Dis 2001; 38(4):803–812.
2. Eschbach JW, Adamson JW: Anemia of end-stage renal disease ESRD. Kidney Int 1985; 28:1–5.
3. Xue JL, St Peter WL, Ebben JP, et al: Anemia treatment in the pre-ESRD period and associated mortality in elderly patients. Am J Kidney Dis 2002; 40(6):1153–1161.
4. Obrador GT, Ruthazer R, Arora P, et al: Prevalence of and factors associated with suboptimal care before initiation of dialysis in the United States. J Am Soc Nephrol 1999;10(8): 1793–1800.
5. Loge JP, Lange RD, Moore CV: Characterization of the anemia associated with chronic renal insufficiency. Am J Med 1958; 24:4–18.
6. Radtke HW, Rege AB, Lamarche B, et al: Identification of spermine as an inhibitor of erythropoiesis in patients with chronic renal failure. J Clin Invest 1981; 67:1623–1629.
7. Massry SG: Is parathyroid hormone an uremic toxin? Nephron 1977; 19:125–130.
8. Fisher JW, Hatch FE, Roh BL, et al: Erythropoietin inhibitor in kidney extracts and plasma from anemic uremic human subjects. Blood 1968; 31(4):440–452.
9. Erslev AJ, Besarab A: The rate and control of baseline red cell production in hematologically stable patients with uremia. J Lab Clin Med 1995; 126:283–286.
10. Eschbach JW: The anemia of chronic renal failure: Pathophysiology and the effects of recombinant erythropoietin. Kidney Int 1989; 35:134–148.
11. Eschbach JW, Detter JC, Adamson JW: Physiologic studies in normal and uremic sheep. II. Changes in erythropoiesis and oxygen transport. Kidney Int 1980;18(6):732–745.
12. Noguchi CT, Bae KS, Chin K, et al: Cloning of the human erythropoietin receptor gene. Blood 1991; 78:2548–2556.
13. Ge RL, Witkowski S, Zhang Y, et al: Determinants of erythropoietin release in response to short-term hypobaric hypoxia. J Appl Physiol 2002; 92(6):2361–2367.
14. Levine BD: Intermittent hypoxic training: Fact and fancy. High Alt Med Biol 2002; 3:177–193.
15. Ema M, Taya S, Yokotani N, et al: A novel bHLH-PAS factor with close sequence similarity to hypoxia-inducible factor 1α regulates the VEGF expression and is potentially involved in lung and vascular development. Proc Natl Acad Sci USA 1997; 94:4273–4278.
16. Fisher JW: Erythropoietin: Physiology and pharmacology update. Exp Biol Med (Maywood). 2003; 228(1):1–14.
17. Ivan M, Kondo K, Yang H, et al: HIFα targeted for VHL-mediated destruction by proline hydroxylation: Implications for O_2 sensing. Science 2001; 292:464–468.
18. Epstein ACR, Gleadle JM, McNeill LA, et al: C. elegans EGL-9 and mammalian homologs define a family of dioxygenases that regulate HIF by propyl hydroxylation. Cell 2001; 107:43–54.
19. Gopfert T, Gess B, Eckardt KV, Kurtz A: Hypoxia signalling in the control of erythropoietin gene expression in rat hepatocytes. J Cell Physiol 1996; 168(2):354–361.
20. Graber SE, Krantz SB: Erythropoietin and the control of red cell production. Ann Rev Med 1978; 29:51–66.

21. Fisher JW: Erythropoietin: Physiology and pharmacology update. Exp Biol Med 2003; 228(1):1–14.
22. Neubauer H, Cumano A, Muller M, et al: Jak2 deficiency defines an essential developmental checkpoint in definitive hematopoiesis. Cell 1998; 93:397–409.
23. Carroll MP, Spivak JL, McMahon M, et al: Erythropoietin induces Raf-1 activation is required for erythropoietin-mediated proliferation. J Biol Chem 1991; 266:14964–14969.
24. Fujitani Y, Hibi M, Fukada Y, et al: An alternative pathway for STAT activation that is mediated by the direct interaction between Jak and Stat. Oncogene 1997; 14:751–761.
25. Nagata Y, Kiefer F, Watanabe T, Todokoro K: Activation of hematopoietic progenitor kinase-1 by erythropoietin. Blood 1999; 93:3347–3354.
26. Adamson JW: The relationship of erythropoietin and iron metabolism to red blood cell production in humans. Semin Oncol 1994; 21(2 Suppl 3):9–15.
27. Ma JZ, Ebben J, Xia H, Collins AJ: Hematocrit level and associated mortality in hemodialysis patients. J Am Soc Nephrol 1999; 10(3):610–619.
28. Foley RN, Parfrey PS, Harnett JD, et al: The impact of anemia on cardiomyopathy, morbidity, and mortality in end-stage renal disease. Am J Kidney Dis 1996; 28(1):53–61.
29. Lowrie EG, Lew N: Death risk in hemodialysis patients: The predictive value of commonly measured variables and an evaluation of death rate differences between facilities. Am J Kidney Dis 1990; 15(5):458–482.
30. Al-Ahmad A, Rand WM, Manjunath G, et al: Reduced kidney function and anemia as risk factors for mortality in patients with left ventricular dysfunction. J Am Coll Cardiol 2001; 38(4):955–962.
31. Besarab A, Bolton WK, Browne JK, et al: The effects of normal as compared with low hematocrit values in patients with cardiac disease who are receiving hemodialysis and epoetin. N Engl J Med 1998; 339(9):584–590.
32. Collins AJ, Li S, St Peter W, et al: Death, hospitalization, and economic associations among incident hemodialysis patients with hematocrit values of 36% to 39%. J Am Soc Nephrol 2001; 12(11):2465–2473.
33. Churchill DN, Taylor DW, Cook RJ, et al: Canadian hemodialysis morbidity study. Am J Kidney Dis 1992; 19(3):214–234.
34. Larsh SE: Anemia and symptoms. Ann Intern Med 1967; 66(1):234–235.
35. Canadian Erythropoietin Study Group. Association between recombinant human erythropoietin and quality of life and exercise capacity of patients receiving hemodialysis. Br Med J 1990; 300:573–578.
36. Laupacis A, Wong C, Churchill D: The use of generic and specific quality-of-life measures in hemodialysis patients treated with erythropoietin. The Canadian Erythropoietin Study Group. Control Clin Trial 1991; 12(suppl 4):68–179.
37. McMahon LP, Dawborn JK: Subjective quality of life assessment in hemodialysis patients at different levels of hemoglobin following use of recombinant human erythropoietin. Am J Nephrol 1992; 12:162–169.
38. Moreno F, Aracil FJ, Perez R, Valderrabano F: Controlled study on the improvement of quality of life in elderly hemodialysis patients after correcting end-stage renal disease-related anemia with erythropoietin. Am J Kidney Dis 1996; 27:548–556.
39. Moreno F, Sanz-Guajardo D, Lopez-Gomez JM, et al: Increasing the hematocrit has a beneficial effect on quality of life and is safe in selected hemodialysis patients. J Am Soc Nephrol 2000; 11:335–342.
40. McMahon LP, Mason K, Skinner SL, et al: Effects of haemoglobin normalization on quality of life and cardiovascular parameters in end-stage renal failure. Nephrol Dial Transplant 2000; 15:1425–1430.
41. Painter P, Moore G, Carlson L, et al: Effects of exercise training plus normalization of hematocrit on exercise capacity and health-related quality of life. Am J Kidney Dis 2002; 39(2):257–265.
42. Ross SD, Fahrbach K, Frame D, et al: The effect of anemia treatment on selected health-related quality-of-life domains: A systematic review. Clin Ther 2003; 25(6):1786–1805.
43. Wolcott DL, Marsh JT, La Rue A, et al: Recombinant human erythropoietin treatment may improve quality of life and cognitive function in chronic hemodialysis patients. Am J Kidney Dis 1989; 14(6):478–485.
44. Silverberg DS, Wexler D, Blum M, et al: Aggressive therapy of congestive heart failure and associated chronic renal failure with medications and correction of anemia stops or slows the progression of both diseases. Perit Dial Int 2001; 21(suppl 3):S236–S240.
45. Marsh JT, Brown WS, Wolcott D, et al: RHuEPO treatment improves brain and cognitive function of anemic dialysis patients. Kidney Int 1991; 39(1):155–163.
46. Temple RM, Deary IJ, Winney RJ: Recombinant erythropoietin improves cognitive function in patients maintained on chronic ambulatory peritoneal dialysis. Nephrol Dial Transplant 1995; 10(9):1733–1738.
47. Pickett JL, Theberge DC, Brown WS, et al: Normalizing hematocrit in dialysis patients improves brain function. Am J Kidney Dis 1999; 33(6):1122–1130.
48. Crowell JW, Frod RG, Lews VM: Oxygen transport in hemorrhagic shock as a function of the hematocrit ratio. Am J Physiol 1959; 196(5):1033–1038.
49. Jan KM, Chien S: Effect of hematocrit variations on coronary hemodynamics and oxygen utilization. Am J Physiol 1977; 233(1):106–113.
50. Benz RL, Pressman MR, Hovick ET, Peterson DD: A preliminary study of the effects of correction of anemia with recombinant human erythropoietin therapy on sleep, sleep disorders, and daytime sleepiness in hemodialysis patients (The SLEEPO study). Am J Kidney Dis 1999; 34(6):1089–1095.
51. Harnett JD, Kent GM, Barre PE, et al: Risk factors for the development of left ventricular hypertrophy in a prospective cohort of dialysis patients. J Am Soc Nephrol 1994; 4:1486–1490.
52. Parfrey PS, Foley RN, Harnett JD, et al: Outcome and risk factors for left ventricular disorders in chronic uremia. Nephrol Dial Transplant 1996; 11:1277–1285.
53. Levin A, Singer J, Thompson CR, et al: Prevalent left ventricular hypertrophy in the predialysis population: Identifying opportunities for intervention. Am J Kidney Dis 1996; 27: 347–354.
54. Levin A, Thompson CR, Ethier J, et al: Left ventricular mass index increase in early renal disease: Impact of decline in hemoglobin. Am J Kidney Dis 1999; 34(1):125–134.
55. Harnett JD, Kent GM, Foley RN, Parfrey PS: Cardiac function and hematocrit level. Am J Kidney Dis 1995; 25(4 Suppl 1):S3-S7.
56. Frohlich E: Left ventricular hypertrophy as a risk factor. Cardiol Clin 1986; 4:137–145.
57. Kannel WB, Abbott R: A prognostic comparison of asymptomatic left ventricular hypertrophy and unrecognized myocardial infarction: The Framingham Study. Am Heart J 1986; 111: 391–397.
58. Silberberg JS, Barre PE, Prichard SS, Sniderman AD: Impact of left ventricular hypertrophy on survival in end-stage renal disease. Kidney Int 1989; 36:286–290.
59. Devereaux PJ, Schunemann HJ, Ravindran N, et al: Comparison of mortality between private for-profit and private not-for-profit hemodialysis centers: A systematic review and meta-analysis. JAMA 2002; 288(19):2449–2457.
60. Silberberg J, Racine N, Barre P, Sniderman AD: Regression of left ventricular hypertrophy in dialysis patients following correction of anemia with recombinant human erythropoietin. Can J Cardiol 1990; 6:31–37.

61. Cannella G, La Canna G, Sandrini M, et al: Reversal of left hypertrophy following recombinant human erythropoietin treatment of anaemic dialysed uremic patients, Nephrol Dial Transplant 1991; 6:31–37.
62. Massimetti C, Pontillo D, Feriozzi S, et al: Impact of recombinant human erythropoietin treatment on left ventricular hypertrophy and cardiac function in dialysis patients. Blood Purif 1998; 16(6):317–324.
63. Portoles J, Torralbo A, Martin P, et al: Cardiovascular effects of recombinant human erythropoietin in predialysis patients. Am J Kidney Dis 1997; 29(4):541–548.
64. Hayashi T, Suzuki A, Shoji T, et al: Cardiovascular effect of normalizing the hematocrit level during erythropoietin therapy in predialysis patients with chronic renal failure. Am J Kidney Dis 2000; 35(2):250–256.
65. Foley RN, Parfrey PS, Morgan J, et al: Effect of hemoglobin levels in hemodialysis patients with asymptomatic cardiomyopathy. Kidney Int 2000; 58(3):1325–1335.
66. Conlon PJ, Kovalik E, Schumm D, et al: Normalization of hematocrit in hemodialysis patients does not affect silent ischemia. Ren Fail 2000; 22(2):205–211.
67. Wizemann V, Kaufmann J, Kramer W: Effect of erythropoietin on ischemia tolerance in anemic hemodialysis patients with confirmed coronary artery disease. Nephron 1992; 62(2): 161–165.
68. Hase H, Imamura Y, Nakamura R, et al: Effects of rHuEPO therapy on exercise capacity in hemodialysis patients with coronary artery disease. Jpn Circ J 1993; 57(2):131–137.
69. Williams DM, Zimmers TA, Pierce JH, et al: The expression and role of human erythropoietin receptor in erythroid and nonerythroid cells. Ann N Y Acad Sci 1994; 718:232–243.
70. Jacobs K, Shoemaker C, Rudersdorf R, et al: Isolation and characterization of genomic and cDNA clones of human erythropoietin. Nature 1985; 313(6005):806–810.
71. Eschbach JW, Egrie JC, Downing MR, et al: Correction of the anemia of end-stage renal disease with recombinant human erythropoietin. Results of a combined phase I and II clinical trial. N Engl J Med 1987; 316(2):73–78.
72. Akizawa T, Koshikawa S, Takaku F, et al: Clinical effect of recombinant human erythropoietin on anemia associated with chronic renal failure. A multi-institutional study in Japan. Int J Artif Organs 1988; 11(5):343–350.
73. Lin FK, Suggs S, Lin CH, et al: Cloning and expression of the human erythropoietin gene. Proc Natl Acad Sci 1985; 82: 7580–7584.
74. Egrie JC, Strickland TW, Lane J, et al: Characterization and biological effects of recombinant human erythropoietin. Immunobiology 1986; 72:213–224.
75. Nissenson A: Novel erythropoiesis stimulating protein for managing the anemia of chronic kidney disease. Am J Kidney Dis 2001; 38(6):1390–1397.
76. Macdougall IC, Gray SJ, Elston O, et al: Pharmacokinetics of novel erythropoiesis stimulating protein compared with epoetin α in dialysis patients. J Am Soc Nephrol 1999; 10(11):2392–2395.
77. Barnett AL, Cremieux PY: Dose conversion from epoetin-α to darbepoetin-α for patients with chronic kidney disease receiving hemodialysis. Pharmacotherapy 2003; 23(5):690–693.
78. Locatelli F, Olivares J, Walker R, et al: Novel erythropoiesis stimulating protein for treatment of anemia in chronic renal insufficiency. Kidney Int 2001; 60(2):741–747.
79. Nissenson A: Novel erythropoiesis stimulating protein for managing the anemia of chronic kidney disease. Am J Kidney Dis 2001; 38(6):1390–1397.
80. Nissenson A, Swan S, Lindberg JS, et al: Randomized, controlled trial of darbepoetin-α for the treatment of anemia in hemodialysis patients. Am J Kidney Dis 2002; 40(1):110–118.
81. Macdougall IC: An overview of the efficacy and safety of novel erythropoiesis stimulating protein (NESP). Nephrol Dial Transplant 2001; 16(suppl 3):14–21.
82. National Kidney Foundation. K/DOQI™ Clinical Practice Guidelines for Anemia of Chronic Kidney Disease, 2000. Am J Kidney Dis 2001; 37(suppl 1):S182-S238.
83. Ifudu O: Care of patients undergoing hemodialysis. N Engl J Med 1998; 339:1054–1062.
84. Albitar S, Genin R, Fen-Chong M, et al: High dose enalapril impairs the response to erythropoietin in hemodialysis patients. Nephrol Dial Transplant 1998; 13:1206.
85. Odabas AR, Cetinkaya R, Selcuk Y, et al: The effect of high dose losartan on erythropoietin resistance in patients undergoing hemodialysis. Paminerva Medica 2003; 45:59–62.
86. Minetti L: Erythropoietin treatment in renal anemia. How high should the target hematocrit be? J Nephrol 1997; 10(3): 117–119.
87. Tonelli M, Winkelmayer WC, Jindal KK, et al: The cost-effectiveness of maintaining higher hemoglobin targets with erythropoietin in hemodialysis patients. Kidney Int 2003; 64(1): 295–304.
88. Strippoli GF, Manno C, Schena FP, Craig JC: Haemoglobin and haematocrit targets for the anaemia of chronic renal disease. Cochrane Database Syst Rev 2003; (1):CD003967.
89. Kaufman JS, Reda DJ, Fye CL, et al: Subcutaneous compared with intravenous epoetin in patients receiving hemodialysis. Department of Veterans Affairs cooperative study group on erythropoietin in hemodialysis patients. N Engl J Med 1998; 339(9):578–583.
90. McClellan WM, Frankenfield DL, Wish JB, et al: End-Stage Renal Disease Core Indicators work group. Subcutaneous erythropoietin results in lower dose and equivalent hematocrit levels among adult hemodialysis patients: Results from the 1998 End-Stage Renal Disease Core Indicators Project. Am J Kidney Dis 2001; 37(5):E36.
91. Paganini EP, Eschbach JW, Lazarus JM, et al: Intravenous versus subcutaneous dosing of epoetin-α in hemodialysis patients. Am J Kidney Dis 1995; 26(2):331–340.
92. Nowicki M: Erythropoietin and hypertension. J Hum Hypertens 1995; 9(2):81–88.
93. Luft FC: Erythropoietin and arterial hypertension. Clin Nephrol 2000; 53(suppl 1):S61-S64.
94. Garcia DL, Anderson S, Rennke HG, Brenner BM: Anemia lessens and its prevention with recombinant human erythropoietin worsens glomerular injury and hypertension in rats with reduced renal mass. Proc Natl Acad Sci U S A 1988; 85(16):6142–6146.
95. Bode-Boger SM, Boger RH, Kuhn M, et al: Recombinant human erythropoietin enhances vasoconstrictor tone via endothelin-1 and constrictor prostanoids. Kidney Int 1996; 50:1255.
96. Vaziri ND: Mechanism of erythropoietin-induced hypertension. Am J Kidney Dis 1999; 33(5):821–828.
97. Jones MA, Kingswood JC, Dallyn PE, et al: Changes in diurnal blood pressure variation and red cell and plasma volumes in patients with renal failure who develop erythropoietin-induced hypertension. Clin Nephrol 1995; 44(3):193–200.
98. Caravaca F, Pizarro JL, Arrobas M, et al: Antiplatelet therapy and development of hypertension induced by recombinant human erythropoietin in uremic patients. Kidney Int 1994; 45(3):845–851.
99. Wun T, Law L, Harvey D, et al: Increased incidence of symptomatic venous thrombosis in patients with cervical carcinoma treated with concurrent chemotherapy, radiation, and erythropoietin. Cancer 2003; 98(7):1514–1520.
100. Churchill DN, Muirhead N, Goldstein M, et al: Probability of thrombosis of vascular access among hemodialysis patients treated with recombinant human erythropoietin. J Am Soc Nephrol 1994; 4(10):1809–1813.
101. Besarab A, Medina F, Musial E, et al: Recombinant human erythropoietin does not increase clotting in vascular accesses. ASAIO Trans 1990; 36(3):M749-M753.

102. De Marchi S, Cecchin E, Falleti E, et al: Long-term effects of erythropoietin therapy on fistula stenosis and plasma concentrations of PDGF and MCP-1 in hemodialysis patients. J Am Soc Nephrol 1997; 8:1147–1156.
103. Casadevall N, Nataf J, Viron B, et al: Pure red-cell aplasia and antierythropoietin antibodies in patients treated with recombinant erythropoietin. N Engl J Med 2002; 346(7):469–475.
104. Casadevall N: Antibodies against rHuEPO: Native and recombinant. Nephrol Dial Transplant 2002; 17(suppl 5):42–47.
105. Macdougall IC: An overview of the efficacy and safety of novel erythropoiesis stimulating protein (NESP). Nephrol Dial Transplant 2001; 16(Suppl):14–21.
106. Eschbach JW, Adamson JW: Guidelines for recombinant human erythropoietin therapy. Am J Kidney Dis 1989; 14(2 suppl 1): 2–8.
107. Macdougall IC: Meeting the challenges of a new millennium: Optimizing the use of recombinant human erythropoietin. Nephrol Dial Transplant 1998; 13(Suppl 2):23–27.
108. Brittenham GM: Disorders of iron metabolism: Iron deficiency and overload. *In* Hoffman R, Benz EJ Jr, Shattil SJ, et al (eds): Hematology Basic Principles and Practice, 2nd ed. New York, Churchill Livingstone, 1995.
109. Bridges KR, Seligman PA: Disorders of iron metabolism. *In* Handin RI, Lux SE, Stossel TP (eds): Blood: Principles and Practice of Hematology. Philadelphia, Lippincott, 1995, p.1433–1472.
110. Van Wyck DB: Iron management during recombinant human erythropoietin therapy. Am J Kidney Dis 1989; 14(2 suppl 1): 9–13.
111. Akmal M, Sawelson S, Karubian F, Gadallah M: The prevalence and significance of occult blood loss in patients with predialysis advanced chronic renal failure (CRF), or receiving dialytic therapy. Clin Nephrol 1994; 42(3):198–202.
112. Fishbane S, Maesaka JK: Iron management in end-stage renal disease. Am J Kidney Dis 1997; 29(3):319–333.
113. Pruchnicki MC, Coyle JD, Hoshaw-Woodard S, Bay WH: Effect of phosphate binders on supplemental iron absorption in healthy subjects. J Clin Pharmacol 2002; 42(10):1171–1176.
114. Cook JD, Dassenko SA, Whittaker P: Calcium supplementation: Effect on iron absorption. Am J Clin Nutr 1991; 53(1):106–111.
115. Skikne BS, Ahluwalia N, Fergusson B, et al: Effects of erythropoietin therapy on iron absorption in chronic renal failure. J Lab Clin Med 2000; 135(6):452–458.
116. Brugnara C, Colella GM, Cremins J, et al: Effects of subcutaneous recombinant human erythropoietin in normal subjects: Development of decreased reticulocyte hemoglobin content and iron-deficient erythropoiesis. J Lab Clin Med 1994; 123(5): 660–667.
117. Rogers JT, Bridges KR, Durmowicz GP, et al: Translational control during the acute phase response. Ferritin synthesis in response to interleukin-1. J Biol Chem 1990; 265(24):14572–14578.
118. Fishbane S, Kowalski EA, Imbriano LJ, Maesaka JK: The evaluation of iron status in hemodialysis patients. J Am Soc Nephrol 1996; 7:2654–2657.
119. Kalantar-Zadeh K, Hoffken B, Wunsch H, et al: Diagnosis of iron deficiency anemia in renal failure patients during the post-erythropoietin era. Am J Kidney Dis 1995; 26:292–299.
120. Low CL, Bailie GR, Eisele G: Sensitivity and specificity of transferrin saturation and serum ferritin as markers of iron status after intravenous iron dextran in hemodialysis patients. Ren Fail 1997; 19(6):781–788.
121. Rahmati MA, Craig RG, Homel P, et al: Serum markers of periodontal disease status and inflammation in hemodialysis patients. Am J Kidney Dis 2002; 40(5):983–989.
122. Owen WF, Lowrie EG: C-reactive protein as an outcome predictor for maintenance hemodialysis patients. Kidney Int 1998; 54(2):627–636.
123. Fishbane S, Shapiro W, Dutka P, et al: A randomized trial of iron deficiency testing strategies in hemodialysis patients. Kidney Int 2001; 60:2406–2411.
124. Macdougall IC: What is the most appropriate strategy to monitor functional iron deficiency in the dialysed patient on rHuEPO therapy? Merits of percentage hypochromic red cells as a marker of functional iron deficiency. Nephrol Dial Transplant 1998; 13:847–849.
125. Tessitore N, Solero GP, Lippi G, et al: The role of iron status markers in predicting response to intravenous iron in haemodialysis patients on maintenance erythropoietin. Nephrol Dial Transplant 2001; 16:1416–1423.
126. Olivieri O, de Franceschi L, de Gironcoli M, et al: Potassium loss and cellular dehydration of stored erythrocytes following incubation in autologous plasma: Role of the KCl cotransport system. Vox Sang 1993; 65:95–102.
127. Cullen P, Soffker J, Hopfl M, et al: Hypochromic red cells and reticulocyte haemoglobin content as markers of iron-deficient erythropoiesis in patients undergoing chronic haemodialysis. Nephrol Dial Transplant 1999; 14:659–665.
128. Fishbane S, Galgano C, Langley RC Jr, et al: Reticulocyte hemoglobin content in the evaluation of iron status of hemodialysis patients. Kidney Int 1997; 52:217–222.
129. Koepke JF, Koepke JA: Reticulocytes. Review. Clin Lab Haematol 1986; 8(3):169–179.
130. Bhandari S, Norfolk D, Brownjohn A, Turney J: Evaluation of RBC ferritin and reticulocyte measurements in monitoring response to intravenous iron therapy. Am J Kidney Dis 1997; 30:814–821.
131. Mittman N, Sreedhara R, Mushnick R, et al: Reticulocyte hemoglobin content predicts functional iron deficiency in hemodialysis patients receiving rHuEPO. Am J Kidney Dis 1997; 30(6):912–922.
132. Hallberg L, Ryttinger L, Solvell L: Side effects of oral iron therapy. A double-blind study of different iron compounds in tablet form. Acta Med Scand 1966; (Suppl)459:3–10.
133. Macdougall IC, Tucker B, Thompson J, et al: A randomized controlled study of iron supplementation in patients treated with erythropoietin. Kidney Int 1996; 50:1694–1699.
134. Wingard RL, Parker RA, Ismail N, Hakim RM: Efficacy of oral iron therapy in patients receiving recombinant human erythropoietin. Am J Kidney Dis 1995; 25:433–439.
135. Markowitz GS, Kahn GA, Feingold RE, et al: An evaluation of the effectiveness of oral iron therapy in hemodialysis patients receiving recombinant human erythropoietin. Clin Nephrol 1997; 48:34–40.
136. Fudin R, Jaichenko J, Shostak A, et al: Correction of uremic iron deficiency anemia in hemodialyzed patients: A prospective study. Nephron 1998; 79:299–305.
137. Eisen SA, Miller DK, Woodward RS, et al: The effect of prescribed daily dose frequency on patient medication compliance. Arch Intern Med 1990; 150:1881–1884.
138. Fishbane S, Frei GL, Maesaka J: Reduction in recombinant human erythropoietin doses by the use of chronic intravenous iron supplementation. Am J Kidney Dis 1995; 26:41–46.
139. Sunder-Plassmann G, Horl WH: Importance of iron supply for erythropoietin therapy. Nephrol Dial Transplant 1995; 10:2070–2076.
140. Taylor JE, Peat N, Porter C, Morgan AG: Regular low-dose intravenous iron therapy improves response to erythropoietin in haemodialysis patients. Nephrol Dial Transplant 1996; 11: 1079–1083.
141. Senger JM, Weiss RJ: Hematologic and erythropoietin responses to iron dextran in the hemodialysis environment. ANNA J 1996; 23(3):319–323.
142. Fishbane S, Lynn RI: The efficacy of iron dextran for the treatment of iron deficiency in hemodialysis patients. Clin Nephrol 1995; 44:238–240.

143. Besarab A, Amin N, Ahsan M, et al: Optimization of epoetin therapy with intravenous iron therapy in hemodialysis patients. J Am Soc Nephrol 2000; 11:530–538.
144. Ahsan N: Intravenous infusion of total dose iron is superior to oral iron in treatment of anemia in peritoneal dialysis patients: A single center comparative study. J Am Soc Nephrol 1998; 9(4): 664–668.
145. European Best Practice Guidelines for the management of anaemia in patients with chronic renal failure. Working party for European Best Practice Guidelines for the management of anaemia in patients with chronic renal failure. Nephrol Dial Transplant 1999; 14(Suppl 5):1–50.
146. Ali M, Rigolosi R, Fayemi AO, et al: Failure of serum ferritin levels to predict bone-marrow iron content after intravenous iron-dextran therapy. Lancet 1982; 1(8273):652–655.
147. Javier AM: Weekly administration of high-dose sodium ferric gluconate is safe and effective in peritoneal dialysis patients. Nephrol Nurs J 2002; 29(2):183–186.
148. Jain AK, Bastani B: Safety profile of a high dose ferric gluconate in patients with severe chronic renal insufficiency. J Nephrol 2002; 15(6):681–683.
149. Kumpf VJ, Holland EG: Parenteral iron dextran therapy. DICP 1990; 24(2):162–166.
150. Geisser P, Baer M, Schaub E: Structure/histotoxicity relationship of parenteral iron preparations. Arzneimittelforschung 1992; 42(12):1439–1452.
151. Faich G, Strobos J: Sodium ferric gluconate complex in sucrose: Safer intravenous iron therapy than iron dextrans. Am J Kidney Dis 1999; 33(3):464–470.
152. Fleming LW, Stewart WK, Parratt D: Dextran antibodies, complement conversion and circulating immune complexes after intravenous iron dextran therapy in dialyzed patients. Nephrol Dial Transplant 1992; 7(1):35–39.
153. Novey HS, Pahl M, Haydik I, Vaziri ND: Immunologic studies of anaphylaxis to iron dextran in patients on renal dialysis. Ann Allergy 1994; 72(3):224–228.
154. Hamstra RD, Block MH, Schocket AL: Intravenous iron dextran in clinical medicine. JAMA 1980; 243(17):1726–1731.
155. Fishbane S, Ungureanu VD, Maesaka JK, et al: The safety of intravenous iron dextran in hemodialysis patients. Am J Kidney Dis 1996; 28:529–534.
156. Ferrlecit Product Insert, Watson Pharmaceuticals, Morrisstown, NJ.
157. Fudin R, Jaichenko J, Shostak A, et al: Correction of uremic iron deficiency anemia in hemodialyzed patients: A prospective study. Nephron 1998; 79:299–305.
158. Michael B, Coyne DW, Fishbane S, et al: Sodium ferric gluconate complex in hemodialysis patients: Adverse reactions compared to placebo and iron dextran. Kidney Int 2002; 61: 1830–1839.
159. Package insert: Venofer™ iron sucrose injection, American Regent Labs, Shirley, New Hampshire.
160. Charytan C, Levin N, Al-Saloum M, et al: Efficacy and safety of iron sucrose for iron deficiency in patients with dialysis-associated anemia: North American clinical trial. Am J Kidney Dis 2001; 37(2):300–307.
161. Van Wyck DB, Cavallo G, Spinowitz BS, et al: Safety and efficacy of iron sucrose in patients sensitive to iron dextran: North American clinical trial. Am J Kidney Dis 2000; 36(1):88–97.
162. Silverberg DS, Blum M, Peer G, et al: Intravenous ferric saccharate as an iron supplement in dialysis patients. Nephron 1996; 72(3):413–417.
163. Kosch M, Bahner U, Bettger H, et al: A randomized, controlled parallel-group trial on efficacy and safety of iron sucrose (Venofer) vs. iron gluconate (Ferrlecit) in haemodialysis patients treated with rHuEPO. Nephrol Dial Transplant 2001; 16(6):1239–1244.
164. Feldman HI, Santanna J, Guo W, et al: Iron administration and clinical outcomes in hemodialysis patients. J Am Soc Nephrol 2002; 13(3):734–744.
165. Ajioka RS, Kushner JP: Clinical consequences of iron overload in hemochromatosis homozygotes. Blood 2003; 101(9): 3351–3353.
166. Gokal R, Millard PR, Weatherall DJ, et al: Iron metabolism in haemodialysis patients. A study of the management of iron therapy and overload. Q J Med 1979; 48(191):369–391.
167. Ali M, Fayemi AO, Rigolosi R, et al: Hemosiderosis in hemodialysis patients. An autopsy study of 50 cases. JAMA 1980; 244(4):343–345.
168. Van de Vyver FL, Visser WJ, D'Haese PC, De Broe ME: Iron overload and bone disease in chronic dialysis patients. Nephrol Dial Transplant 1990; 5(9):781–787.
169. Schafer AI, Cheron RG, Dluhy R, et al: Clinical consequences of acquired transfusional iron overload in adults. N Engl J Med 1981; 304(6):319–324.
170. Bregman H, Gelfand MC, Winchester JF, et al: Iron-overload-associated myopathy in patients on maintenance haemodialysis: A histocompatibility–linked disorder. Lancet 1980; 2(8200): 882–885.
171. Bullen JJ: Iron and infection. Eur J Clin Microbiol 1985; 4(6):537–539.
172. Rogers HJ, Bullen JJ, Cushnie GH: Iron compounds and resistance to infection. Further experiments with Clostridium welchii type A in vivo and in vitro. Immunology 1970; 19(4): 521–538.
173. Bullen JJ, Ward CG, Wallis SN: Virulence and the role of iron in pseudomonas aeruginosa infection. Infect Immun 1974; 10(3): 443–450.
174. Jones RL, Peterson CM, Grady RW, et al: Effects of iron chelators and iron overload on salmonella infection. Nature 1977; 267(5607):63–65.
175. Patruta SI, Edlinger R, Sunder-Plassmann G, Horl WH: Neutrophil impairment associated with iron therapy in hemodialysis patients with functional iron deficiency. J Am Soc Nephrol 1998; 9(4):655–663.
176. Deicher R, Ziai F, Cohen G, et al: High-dose parenteral iron sucrose depresses neutrophil intracellular killing capacity. Kidney Int 2003; 64(2):728–736.
177. Sengoelge G, Kletzmayr J, Ferrara I, et al: Impairment of transcendothelial leukocyte migration by iron complexes. J Am Soc Nephrol 2003; 14(10):2639–2644.
178. Kessler M, Hoen B, Mayeux D, et al: Bacteremia in patients on chronic hemodialysis. A multicenter prospective survey. Nephron 1993; 64:95–100.
179. Hoen B, Kessler M, Hestin D, Mayeux D: Risk factors for bacterial infections in chronic haemodialysis adult patients: A multicentre prospective survey. Nephrol Dial Transplant 1995; 10: 377–381.
180. Tielemans CL, Lenclud CM, Wens R, et al: Critical role of iron overload in the increased susceptibility of haemodialysis patients to bacterial infections. Beneficial effects of desferrioxamine. Nephrol Dial Transplant 1989; 4:883–887.
181. Rogers JT, Bridges KR, Durmowicz GP, et al: Translational control during the acute phase response. Ferritin synthesis in response to interleukin-1. J Biol Chem 1990; 265(24):14572–14578.
182. Hoen B, Paul-Dauphin A, Hestin D, Kessler M: EPIBACDIAL: A multicenter prospective study of risk factors for bacteremia in chronic hemodialysis patients. J Am Soc Nephrol 1998; 9:869–876.
183. Jean G, Charra B, Chazot C, et al: Risk factor analysis for long-term tunneled dialysis catheter-related bacteremias. Nephron 2002; 91:399–405.
184. Canziani ME, Yumiya ST, Rangel EB, et al: Risk of bacterial infection in patients under intravenous iron therapy: Dose versus length of treatment. Artif Organs 2001; 25(11):866–869.
185. Hoen B, Paul-Dauphin A, Kessler M: Intravenous iron administration does not significantly increase the risk of bacteremia in chronic hemodialysis patients. Clin Nephrol 2002; 57:457–461.

186. Parkkinen J, von Bonsdorff L, Peltonen S, et al: Catalytically active iron and bacterial growth in serum of haemodialysis patients after i.v. iron-saccharate administration. Nephrol Dial Transplant 2000; 15(11):1827–1834.
187. Aisen P: Transferrin, the transferrin receptor, and the uptake of iron by cells. Met Ions Biol Syst 1998; 35:585–631.
188. Griffiths WJ, Kelly AL, Cox TM: Inherited disorders of iron storage and transport. Mol Med Today 1999; 5(10):431–438.
189. Seligman PA, Schleicher RB: Comparison of methods used to measure serum iron in the presence of iron gluconate or iron dextran. Clin Chem 1999; 45(6 Pt 1):898–901.
190. Kooistra MP, Kersting S, Gosriwatana I, et al: Nontransferrin-bound iron in the plasma of haemodialysis patients after intravenous iron saccharate infusion. Eur J Clin Invest 2002; 32(suppl 1):36–41.
191. Rooyakkers TM, Stroes ES, Kooistra MP, et al: Ferric saccharate induces oxygen radical stress and endothelial dysfunction in vivo. Eur J Clin Invest 2002; 32(suppl 1):9–16.
192. Roob JM, Khoschsorur G, Tiran A, et al: Vitamin E attenuates oxidative stress induced by intravenous iron in patients on hemodialysis. J Am Soc Nephrol 2000; 11(3):539–549.
193. Tovbin D, Mazor D, Vorobiov M, et al: Induction of protein oxidation by intravenous iron in hemodialysis patients: Role of inflammation. Am J Kidney Dis 2002; 40(5):1005–1012.
194. Drueke T, Witko-Sarsat V, Massy Z, et al: Iron therapy, advanced oxidation protein products, and carotid artery intima-media thickness in end-stage renal disease. Circulation 2002; 106(17): 2212–2217.
195. Michelis R, Gery R, Sela S, et al: Carbonyl stress induced by intravenous iron during haemodialysis. Nephrol Dial Transplant 2003; 18(5):924–930.
196. Albertini R, Moratti R, De Luca G: Oxidation of low-density lipoprotein in atherosclerosis from basic biochemistry to clinical studies. Curr Mol Med 2002; 2(6):579–592.
197. Sullivan JL: Iron and the sex difference in heart disease risk. Lancet 1981; 1:1293–1294.
198. Parfrey PS, Foley RN: The clinical epidemiology of cardiac disease in chronic renal failure. J Am Soc Nephrol 1999; 10: 1606–1615.
199. Salonen JT, Nyyssonen K, Korpela H, et al: High stored iron levels are associated with excess risk of myocardial infarction in Eastern Finnish men. Circulation 1992; 86:803–811.
200. Magnusson MK, Sigfusson N, Sigvaldason H, et al: Low iron-binding capacity as a risk factor for myocardial infarction. Circulation 1994; 89:102–108.
201. Salonen JT, Nyyssonen K, Salonen R: Body iron stores and the risk of coronary heart disease. N Engl J Med 1994; 331:1159.
202. Klipstein-Grobusch K, Koster JF, Grobbee DE, et al: Serum ferritin and risk of myocardial infarction in the elderly: The Rotterdam study. Am J Clin Nutr 1999; 69:1231–1236.
203. Tuomainen TP, Punnonen K, Nyyssonen K, Salonen JT: Association between body iron stores and the risk of acute myocardial infarction in men. Circulation 1998; 97:1461– 1466.
204. Marniemi J, Jarvisalo J, Toikka T, et al: Blood vitamins, mineral elements and inflammation markers as risk factors of vascular and non-vascular disease mortality in an elderly population. Int J Epidemiol 1998; 27:799–807.
205. Kiechl S, Willeit J, Egger G, et al: Body iron stores and the risk of carotid atherosclerosis: Prospective results from the Bruneck study. Circulation 1997; 96:3300–3307.
206. Aronow WS, Ahn C: Three-year follow-up shows no association of serum ferritin levels with incidence of new coronary events in 577 persons aged > or = 62 years. Am J Cardiol 1996; 78: 678–679.
207. Manttari M, Manninen V, Huttunen JK, et al: Serum ferritin and ceruloplasmin as coronary risk factors. Eur Heart J 1994; 15:1599–1603.
208. Frey GH, Krider DW: Serum ferritin and myocardial infarct. W V Med J 1994; 90:13–15.
209. Miller M, Hutchins GM: Hemochromatosis, multiorgan hemosiderosis, and coronary artery disease. JAMA 1994; 272(3): 231–233.

Renal Osteodystrophy

Sharon M. Moe, M.D.

INTRODUCTION AND REVIEW OF MINERAL HOMEOSTASIS

In people with healthy kidneys, normal serum levels of phosphorus and calcium are maintained through the interaction of two hormones: parathyroid hormone (PTH) and $1,25(OH)_2D$ (calcitriol), the active metabolite of vitamin D3. These two hormones act on three primary target organs: bone, kidney, and intestine. The kidneys play a critical role in the regulation of normal serum calcium and phosphorus levels, and thus, derangements occur quickly in patients with chronic kidney disease (CKD). The result is abnormal serum concentrations of calcium and phosphorus and impaired bone remodeling, which together can lead to fractures and extraskeletal manifestations such as vascular calcification. These abnormalities are linked and are important causes of morbidity and mortality in patients on dialysis. There is a 2-fold to 87-fold increased risk of hip fracture in dialysis patients compared to age matched individuals in the general population at ages 80 and 40, respectively.[1–3] The mortality rate after a hip fracture in a dialysis patient is double that of the general population.[4] Similarly, dialysis patients have twofold to fivefold more coronary artery calcification than age matched non-dialysis patients with angiographically proven coronary artery disease.[5] Aorta, carotid, and peripheral artery vascular calcification is also common and is associated with increased mortality.[6] These processes may be linked, because epidemiology data in the general population[7–10] and in dialysis patients[5] have shown that as bone mineral content decreases, vascular calcification increases. In addition, recent evidence shows that vascular calcification is a cell mediated process that resembles osteogenesis[11–14] and is worsened by hyperphosphatemia.[15, 16] In turn, hyperphosphatemia is associated with increased mortality.[17, 18] Thus, abnormalities of bone strength, vascular calcification, and mineral metabolism are interrelated and associated with increased morbidity and mortality in CKD.

In the past, the term *renal osteodystrophy* was equated only with abnormalities of bone turnover, but a recent expert consensus panel convened by the National Kidney Foundation determined that renal osteodystrophy is a complex disorder of compromised bone strength in CKD patients.[19–21] Whereas *osteoporosis* is a term used to describe fragile bones prone to fracture in the general population assessed by dual x-ray absorptiometry (DEXA), *renal osteodystrophy* should be the principal term to describe fragile bones prone to fracture and other morbidities in CKD. Renal osteodystrophy is a function of bone turnover (assessed by bone biopsy), bone density (assessed by DEXA or quantitative-CT [qCT]) and bone architecture, but the principal determinant of bone fragility in CKD is abnormal bone turnover. While DEXA is useful in predicting fractures in the general population,[22] this has not been shown in CKD patients. DEXA can only detect the overall density but not how the bone is arranged, and the latter is determined principally by bone turnover. Thus, with the dramatic abnormalities in bone turnover in advanced CKD, the sensitivity and specificity of DEXA for predicting fractures is likely altered. Last, CKD patients have relative hypogonadism, or "renopause," and the impact of these abnormalities on bone fragility are unclear. Low bone mass that is common in dialysis and CKD patients[23–27] is one factor, of many, that lead to increased bone fragility. Thus, although DEXA is a diagnostic tool, and low DEXA is associated with increased mortality in a small study,[28] therapeutic decisions should not be based on these results alone and should be based on multiple factors. Furthermore, there is more data to support therapeutic interventions for abnormal bone turnover than there is for abnormal bone mass or architecture in CKD patients. Therefore, the remainder of this chapter will focus on abnormalities of bone turnover. To do so, a brief review of parathyroid hormone physiology and measurement, vitamin D metabolism, and bone histology are presented.

Parathyroid Hormone

The primary function of PTH is to maintain calcium homeostasis by (1) increasing bone mineral dissolution, thus releasing calcium and phosphorus; (2) increasing renal reabsorption of calcium and excretion of phosphorus; and (3) enhancing the gastrointestinal absorption of both calcium and phosphorus indirectly through its effects on the synthesis of $1,25(OH)_2D$. In healthy subjects, this increase in serum PTH level in response to hypocalcemia effectively restores serum calcium levels and maintains serum phosphorus levels. The kidneys are of key importance in this normal homeostatic response, and thus patients with CKD may not be able to appropriately correct abnormalities in serum ionized calcium.

PTH is cleaved to an 84 amino acid protein in the parathyroid gland, where it is stored with fragments in secretory granules for release. Once released, the circulating 1–84 amino acid protein has a half-life of 2 to 4 minutes. It is then cleaved into N-terminal, C-terminal, and mid-region fragments of PTH, which are metabolized in the liver and kidney.[29,30] PTH secretion occurs in response to hypocalcemia, hyperphosphatemia, and $1,25(OH)_2D$ deficiency. The extracellular concentration of ionized calcium is the most important determinant of minute-to-minute secretion of PTH from stored secretory granules in response to hypocalcemia. The secretion of PTH in response to low levels of ionized calcium is a sigmoidal relationship, frequently referred to as the calcium-PTH curve (Figure 8–1). The rapid response, within seconds, of changes in ionized calcium concentration has long been hypothesized to be due to a calcium sensing receptor. This calcium sensing receptor (CaR) has now been sequenced and cloned and is a member of the G-protein receptor superfamily, with a seven

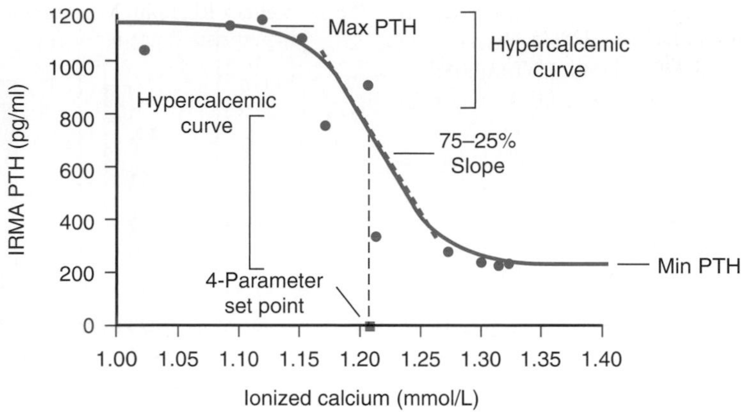

Figure 8–1 **The ionized calcium-PTH curve** as calculated from data obtained from an actual hemodialysis patient. Data is obtained during successive dialysis sessions against a low calcium dialysate (hypocalcemic) curve and high calcium dialysate (hypercalcemic) curve and fitted mathematically using the four-parameter model *(solid line)*. The maximal (max) PTH and minimal (min) PTH are indicated. The four-parameter set point *(solid square)* is the ionized calcium corresponding to a PTH midway between max and min PTH. The 75% to 25% non-normalized slope *(dashed line)* is also shown. (From Ouseph R, Leiser JD, Moe SM: Calcitriol and the parathyroid hormone-ionized calcium curve: A comparison of methodologic approaches. J Am Soc Nephrol 1996; 7:497–505, with permission.)

membrane-spanning domain.[31] Inactivating mutations have been associated with neonatal severe hyperparathyroidism and benign familial hypocalcuric hypercalcemia.[32] These patients have asymptomatic elevations of serum calcium in the presence of nonsuppressed PTH, representing a true shift to the right of this curve. Activating mutations have been found in patients with autosomal dominant hypocalcemia.[33] The CaR has also been localized to the thyroid C-cells and the kidney, predominantly in the thick ascending limb, where it controls renal excretion of calcium in response to changes in serum calcium.[34,35]

PTH secretion is also regulated by vitamin D. 1,25$(OH)_2$D decreases PTH synthesis by binding to the vitamin D response element on the PTH gene. 1,25$(OH)_2$D also regulates the expression of the vitamin D receptor itself and regulates parathyroid cell proliferation.[36] In addition, elevated serum phosphorus also regulates proliferation of parathyroid cells and stimulates PTH secretion.[37] The mechanism of this appears to be mediated via post-translational binding proteins[38, 39] and down regulation of the CaR.[40]

Early studies indicated that the calcium-PTH curve was shifted to the right in CKD creating an altered set point, defined as the calcium concentration that results in 50% maximal PTH secretion.[41, 42] The extrapolation of this data to clinical practice was that patients with renal failure required supra-physiologic serum levels of calcium to suppress PTH. However, several studies failed to confirm these findings.[43] Others show phosphorus to be a major regulator. In rats fed a high phosphorus diet, the mRNA and protein expression of the CaR is downregulated in PTH glands.[40] In parathyroid glands removed from patients with severe secondary hyperparathyroidism, there was altered sensitivity to calcium (a shift to the right of the curve) when glands were incubated in the presence of phosphorus.[44] An in vivo study in dialysis patients demonstrated that an infusion of phosphorus shifts the calcium-PTH curve to the right.[45] These studies indicate that phosphorus may regulate the CaR. Thus, it is possible that some of the earlier discrepancy in the literature regarding possible alterations of the set point in renal failure may have been due to differences in serum phosphorus levels in the various studies,[46] although methodologic differences can also explain some of this discrepancy.[43] This interrelationship of calcium, phosphorus, and calcitriol in regulating PTH synthesis is complex and nearly impossible to fully evaluate in humans, because changes in one leads to rapid changes in the other parameters. However, based on available literature, it appears that calcium is more important in stimulating PTH release, whereas calcitriol is more important in inhibiting PTH release. The presence of hyperphosphatemia impairs both of these homeostatic mechanisms.

PTH binds to the PTH receptor, which is a member of the G-protein linked seven membrane spanning receptor family.[47] PTH receptors are ubiquitously located in the body, although most abundantly in the kidney and bone. PTH induced signaling predominately affects mineral metabolism, however, there are many extraskeletal manifestations of PTH excess. These include encephalopathy, anemia, extraskeletal calcification, peripheral neuropathy, cardiac dysfunction, hyperlipidemia, and impotence.[48–51]

There has been a progression of increasingly sensitive assays developed to measure PTH over the past few years. The major difficulty in accurately measuring PTH is the presence of circulating fragments, particularly in the presence of CKD.[29, 30] Initial measurements of PTH using C-terminal assays were inaccurate in patients with renal disease due to impaired renal excretion of fragments, and thus retention, and measurement of these inactive fragments. The development of the N-terminal assay brought hope of a more accurate reflection of end-organ effects of PTH, but it also detected inactive metabolites. The development of a two-site antibody test (commonly called INTACT assay) offered hope for improved ability to only detect entire length (active) PTH molecules. In this assay, a capture antibody binds to the N-terminus and a second antibody binds to the C-terminus.[52] This intact assay is more discriminatory than N- or C-terminal assays in patients with renal failure,[53] however, its ability to discriminate between low and high bone turnover in dialysis patients as compared to bone histology is limited to very low levels (< 100–150 pg/mL) and very high levels (> 500 pg/mL).[54,55] Furthermore, racial differences exist. In one series, the mean intact PTH level was 460 ± 110 pg/mL in African-Americans with bone biopsy proven low turnover bone disease compared to 144 ± 43 pg/mL in Caucasians with the same degree of bone turnover.[56]

Recent data indicates that this intact assay also detects accumulation of C-terminal fragments, commonly referred to as "7–84," although the precise sequence is unknown.[57] In parathyroidectomized rats, the injection of a truly whole 1–84 amino acid PTH was able to induce bone resorption, whereas the 7–84 amino acid fragment was antagonistic.[58,59] Two new assays are now available that truly only detect the 1–84 amino acid full length molecule called whole PTH (CAP) assay (Scantabodies, Inc., San Diego, CA) or bio-active PTH (Nichols Institute, San Juan, CA). In dialysis patients, initial studies demonstrated that the measurement of the intact PTH led to results that were always greater than the whole (1–84 amino acid only) assay, regardless of whether the patients had low or high PTH levels.[58–60] While this new assay offers hope of better reproducibility across laboratories, its role in the diagnosis of underlying bone histology is controversial. An initial study demonstrated that the whole PTH was superior to the former intact assay and that a ratio of the 1–84 amino acid to 7–84 amino acid (active/antagonist) PTH levels less than one was predictive of underlying low turnover bone disease and more accurate than either assay alone.[61] However, two subsequent studies failed to confirm these findings and found no difference in the area under a receiver operating curve (ROC) with the traditional intact and 1–84 assays[62,63] (Figure 8–2). The patient characteristics, especially serum calcium levels, and vitamin D use were different in these three studies. This is important, as a recent study demonstrated that although both 1–84 and non-1–84 fragments are secreted from the PTH gland in response to serum calcium levels, the secretory responses are not proportional.[64] Thus, different serum levels of calcium will result in different ratios of fragments. The clinical use of these PTH assays for the diagnosis of renal osteodystrophy will be discussed later.

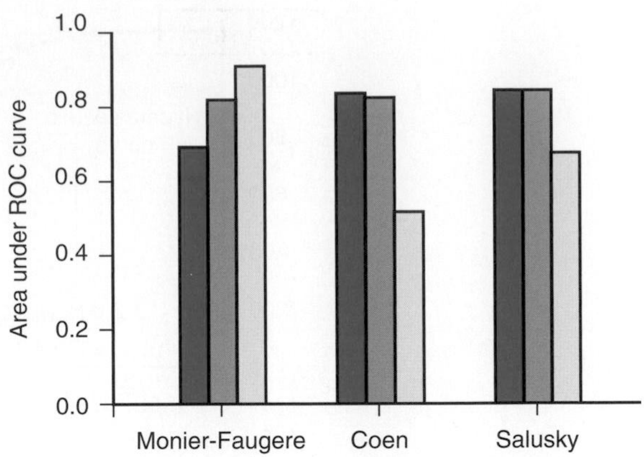

Figure 8–2 Value of PTH assays to determine the presence of low turnover bone disease by biopsy. This graph depicts the area under the receiver operating curves (ROC) for the intact PTH assay *(black bar)*, the 1–84 PTH assay *(light gray bar)*, and the ratio of the intact PTH assay result divided by the circulating C terminal fragments *(white bar)*. The circulating C terminal fragments are calculated as the difference of the intact PTH and the 1–84 PTH results. These ROC curves are from three separate studies with 51,[61] 35,[62] and 33[63] subjects, respectively. The data demonstrate that there are discrepancies in the diagnostic value of these assays among these three studies. (Reprinted with permission from Moe SM: Management of renal osteodystrophy in peritoneal dialysis patients. Perit Dial Int 2004; 24:209-216, with permission.)

Vitamin D

Although vitamin D_3 is metabolically inactive, it is metabolized in the liver to 25(OH)D, and then converted in the kidney via the 1-α-hydroxylase enzyme to $1,25(OH)_2D$, which has a number of important effects.[65] Its most important function is exerted on the small intestine, where it regulates the intestinal absorption of calcium, and, to a lesser degree, phosphorus.[66] Apart from its effect on calcium and phosphorus levels, $1,25(OH)_2D$ also directly suppresses PTH synthesis, as described above,[67] and may be important for normal bone turnover by enhancing formation of osteoclasts.[68] Elevated serum levels of PTH increases 1-α-hydroxylase activity in the kidney, thereby raising serum $1,25(OH)_2D$ levels. This results in a rise in serum calcium, and then $1,25(OH)_2D$ feeds back on the parathyroid gland, decreasing PTH secretion, thus completing the typical endocrine feedback loop. PTH does not directly inhibit its own synthesis, which is one reason why PTH levels increase in the presence of renal failure where $1,25(OH)_2D$ is no longer synthesized in sufficient amounts. The 1-α-hydroxylase enzyme in the kidney is also the site of regulation of $1,25(OH)_2D$ synthesis by numerous other factors, including low calcium, low phosphorus, estrogen, prolactin, growth hormone, and $1,25(OH)_2D$ itself.[69] Thus, there is $1,25(OH)_2D$ deficiency in essentially all patients with CKD, with an inability to respond appropriately to normal physiologic stimuli.

In addition, many dialysis patients are also deficient in the precursor vitamin D_3 due to inadequate dietary intake and lack of sunlight[70] (Figure 8–3). Cholesterol is synthesized to 7-dehydrocholesterol, which in turn is metabolized in the skin to vitamin D_3. This reaction is facilitated by ultraviolet light and, therefore, reduced in individuals with high skin melanin content and inhibited by sunscreen of SPF 8 or greater. In addition, there are dietary sources of vitamin D_2 and vitamin D_3. Once in the blood, vitamins D_2 and D_3 bind with vitamin D binding protein and are carried to the liver where they are hydroxylated to yield 25(OH)D, often called calcidiol. Thus, calcidiol levels in the blood are a direct assessment of nutritional (dietary) intake of vitamin D. Calcidiol is then converted in the kidney to $1,25(OH)_2D$ by the action of 1α-hydroxylase. This active metabolite is also degraded by another kidney enzyme, 24,25-hydroxylase, providing the primary metabolism of the active compound. However, this same 24,25 hydroxylase also hydroxylates 25(OH)D, yielding $24,25(OH)_2D$, which may have an important effect in bone.[71] However, the predominate effects of vitamin D in the body are exerted through the actions of $1,25(OH)_2D$ (calcitriol).

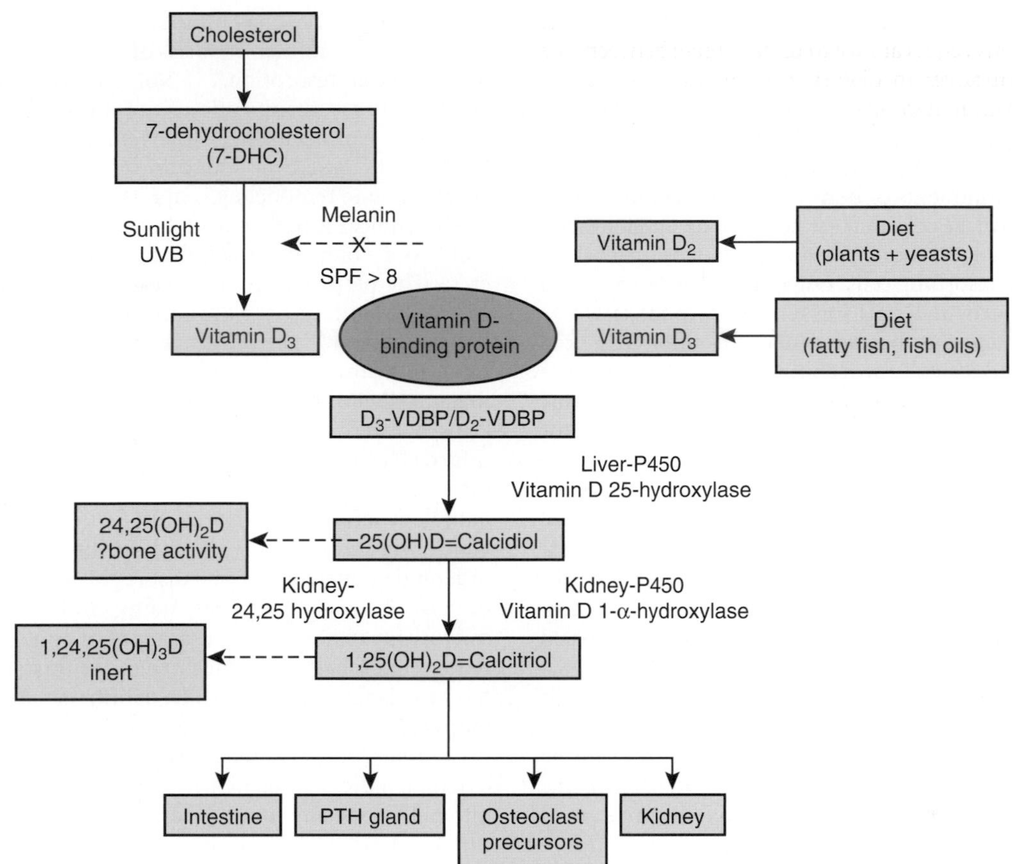

Figure 8–3 Overview of vitamin D metabolism. Vitamin D is obtained from dietary sources and is metabolized via ultraviolet light from 7-DHC in the skin (which is inhibited by sunscreen > SPF 8 and decreased with increased skin melanin content). Both sources of vitamin D_2 and vitamin D_3 bind to vitamin D binding protein (VDBP) and circulate to the liver. In the liver, vitamin D is hydroxylated to 25(OH)D, commonly referred to as calcidiol. Calcidiol is then further metabolized to calcitriol by the 1-α–hydroxylase enzyme at the level of the kidney. The active metabolite $1,25(OH)_2D$ (calcitriol) acts principally on the target organs of the intestine, parathyroid (PTH) gland, bone cell precursors, and the kidney. Calcitriol is metabolized to the inert $1,24,25(OH)_3D$ through the action of the 24,25-hydroxylase enzyme. Calcidiol is similarly hydroxylated to $24,25(OH)_2D$, which has unknown actions in humans but may be important in bone mineralization.

Hormone $1,25(OH)_2D$ mediates its cellular function via both genomic and nongenomic mechanisms. $1,25(OH)_2D$ circulates in the blood stream with vitamin D binding protein. The free form of $1,25(OH)_2D$ enters the target cell where it interacts with its nuclear vitamin D receptor (VDR). This complex then combines with the retinoic acid X receptor to form a heterodimer, which, in turn, interacts with the vitamin D response element (VDRE) on the target gene. The findings of VDRE on multiple genes and VDR in multiple organ systems point to the widespread systemic effects of vitamin D.[70,72,73] In particular, vitamin D is important in cell differentiation and proliferation, which has led to its therapeutic use in cancer and skin disorders.[70,74] In addition to these nongenomic effects, $1,25(OH)_2D$ facilitates the uptake of calcium by enhancing the production of the calcium transport protein calbindin (9kd in intestine and 28kd in kidney).[75,76] Lastly, $1,25(OH)_2D$ activates voltage dependent calcium channels, with increased intracellular calcium.[77] In order to target $1,25(OH)_2D$ to more specific cellular functions, the structure has been altered to produce several "designer" vitamin D analogues that are in clinical use today. The vitamin D analogues for use in renal failure are designed to maximize the effects on the PTH gland and minimize the effects on the intestine. Some of these vitamin D analogues may be less hypercalcemic and may be useful in patients with renal failure as described later.

Bone Biology

The majority of the total body stores of calcium and phosphorus are located in bone. Trabecular (cancellous) bone is located predominately in the epiphyses of the long bones, which is 15% to 25% calcified and serves a metabolic function with a relatively short turnover rate of 45Ca. In contrast, cortical (compact) bone is in the shafts of long bones and is 80% to 90% calcified. This bone serves primarily as a protective and mechanical function and has a calcium turnover rate of months. Bone consists principally (90%) of highly organized cross-linked fibers of type I collagen; the remainder consists of proteoglycans, and "non-collagen" proteins such as osteopontin, osteocalcin, osteonectin, and alkaline phosphatase. Hydroxyapatite ($Ca_{10}(PO_4)_6(OH)_2$) is the major bone salt.

The cellular components of bone are of utmost importance and consist of cartilage cells that are key to bone development, osteoblasts that are the bone forming cells, and osteoclasts that are the bone resorbing cells. Osteoblasts are derived from progenitor mesenchymal cells located in the bone marrow. They are then induced to become osteoprogenitor cells, then endosteol or periosteol progenitor cells, then mature osteoblasts. The control of this differentiation pathway is due to bone morphogenic proteins and the transcription factor Cbfa1 early and other hormones and cytokines later. Once bone formation is complete, osteoblasts may undergo apoptosis, or become quiescent cells trapped within the mineralized bone in the form of osteocytes.[78,79] The osteocytes are interconnected through a series of cannaliculi. Although these cells were previously thought to be of little importance, it is now clear that they serve to transmit the initial signaling involved with mechanical loading.[80]

Osteoclasts are derived from hematopoietic precursor cells that differentiate and are somehow "signaled" to arrive at a certain place in the bone. Once there, they fuse to form the multinucleated cells known as osteoclasts, which become highly polarized, reabsorbing bone through the release of degradative enzymes. They move along a resorption surface via changes in the cytoskeleton. PTH, cytokines, and $1,25(OH)_2D$ are all important in inducing the fusion of the committed osteoclast precursors. Once resorption is complete, estrogens, bisphosphonates, and cytokines can induce, and PTH can inhibit apoptosis.[78,81,82] Numerous hormones and cytokines have been evaluated, mostly in vitro, for their role in controlling osteoclast function.

The control of bone remodeling is highly complex but appears to occur in very distinct phases: (1) osteoclast resorption, (2) reversal, (3) pre-osteoblast migration and differentiation, (4) osteoblast matrix (osteoid or unmineralized bone) formation, (5) mineralization, and (6) quiescent stage. At any one time, less than 15% to 20% of the bone surface is undergoing remodeling, and this process in a single bone remodeling unit can take 3 to 6 months.[83] How a certain piece of bone is chosen to undergo a remodeling cycle and how the osteoclasts and osteoblasts signal each other are not completely clear.

Recently, the discovery of the osteoprotegerin (OPG) and RANK (receptor activator of nuclear-factor κB) system has shed new light on the control of osteoclast function and the long observed coupling of osteoblasts and osteoclasts. RANK is located on osteoclasts, and the RANK ligand (RANK-L) on osteoblasts. Osteoblasts also synthesize the protein OPG, which can bind to RANK-L on osteoblasts and inhibit the subsequent binding of RANK-L to RANK on osteoclasts, thus inhibiting bone resorption. Alternatively, if OPG production is decreased, the RANK-L can bind with RANK on osteoclasts and induce osteoclastic bone resorption. This fascinating control system is regulated by nearly every cytokine and hormone thought important in bone remodeling, including PTH, $1,25(OH)_2D$, estrogen, glucocorticoids, interleukins, prostaglandins, and members of the TGF-β superfamily of cytokines.[84–86] OPG has been successful in preventing bone resorption in animal models of osteoporosis and tumor induced bone resorption.[87,88] Not surprisingly, this system is being tested as a therapeutic agent for osteoporosis, and initial studies appear promising.[89] Interestingly, abnormalities in the OPG/RANK have been found in renal failure,[90] although the effect on bone remodeling is not yet clear.

The clinical assessment of bone remodeling is best done with a bone biopsy of the trabecular bone, usually at the iliac crest. The patient is given a tetracycline derivative approximately 1 month prior to the bone biopsy and a different tetracycline derivative 3 to 5 days prior to the biopsy. Tetracycline binds to hydroxyapatite and emits fluorescence, thereby serving as a label of the bone. A core of predominately trabecular bone is taken and embedded in a plastic material and sectioned. The use of this plastic material is why only some laboratories are equipped to process bone biopsies. Typical pathology labs normally decalcify tissue and paraffin embed, which will destroy the very architecture that is necessary to differentiate metabolic bone disorders. The sections can then be visualized with special stains and under fluorescent microscopy to determine the amount of bone between the two tetracycline labels, or that formed in the time interval between the two labels. This dynamic parameter assessed on bone biopsy is the basis for assessing bone turnover, which is key in discerning types of renal osteodystrophy. In addition to dynamic indices, bone biopsies can be analyzed by histomorphometry for many static parameters as well. The nomenclature for these assessments has been standardized.[91]

Clinically, bone biopsies are most useful for differentiating types of renal osteodystrophy, as well as other undiagnosed metabolic disorders. However, with the advent of several new markers of bone turnover, the use of bone biopsy has recently been reserved primarily for the diagnosis of renal osteodystrophy and for research purposes.[92,93] For renal osteodystrophy the most important parameters are osteoid (unmineralized bone) area as a percent of total bone area, and fibrosis. These two static parameters, together with the dynamic bone turnover assessed by bone formation rate or activation frequency can distinguish the various forms of renal osteodystrophy (Table 8–1).

THE SPECTRUM OF ABNORMAL BONE TURNOVER IN CKD

Bone turnover is tightly regulated by numerous hormones and cytokines, of which PTH is of key importance. In situations where PTH is elevated, bone turns over with excessive rapidity, replacing lamellar bone with structurally inferior woven bone. In addition, both osteoblastic bone formation and osteoclastic bone resorption are accelerated, and fibrosis eventually develops, a pathology referred to as osteitis fibrosa cystica. In contrast, low-turnover bone disease is usually observed in the presence of normal to low levels of PTH. In osteomalacia, aluminum is deposited at the mineralization front, blocking mineralization. This leads to an accumulation of osteoid, or unmineralized bone, and is the hallmark of osteomalacia. In adynamic, or aplastic, bone disease is characterized by normal amounts of osteoid, an absence of tissue fibrosis, decreased numbers of osteoblasts and osteoclasts, and low rates of bone formation.[92]

Table 8–1 Histologic Classification of Renal Osteodystrophy

Lesion	Area of Fibrosis (% of tissue area)	Area of Osteoid (% of total bone area)	Bone Formation Rate ($\mu m^2/mm^2$ tissue area/day)
Mild	<0.5	<15	>108
Osteitis fibrosa	>0.5	<15	X
Mixed	>0.5	>15	X
Osteomalacia	<0.5	>15	X
Adynamic	<0.5	<15	<108
Normal range	0	1–7	108–500

X is not a diagnostic criterion. (Adapted from Sherrard DJ, Hercz G, Pei Y, et al: The spectrum of bone disease in end-stage renal failure: An evolving disorder. Kidney Int 1993; 43:436–442.)

The prevalence of different forms of renal osteodystrophy has changed over the past decade. Whereas osteitis fibrosa cystica had previously been the predominant lesion, the prevalence of mixed uremic osteodystrophy and adynamic bone disease has recently increased. However, the overall percentage of patients with high bone formation compared to low bone formation has not changed dramatically over the last 20 to 30 years, but osteomalacia has been essentially replaced with adynamic bone disease[92,94–98] (Figure 8–4). In patients not yet on dialysis, the series of bone biopsies yield widely different results, depending on the level of GFR and the country in which the study was done[99–105] (Figure 8–5). However, it is clear from these data that histologic abnormalities of bone begin very early in the course of chronic kidney disease.

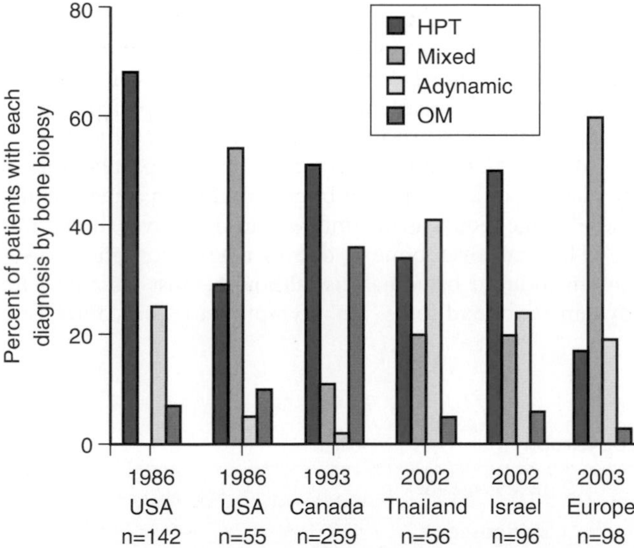

Figure 8–4 The spectrum of histologic types of renal osteodystrophy in patients with chronic kidney stage V. This graph represents the distribution of various pathologic forms of renal osteodystrophy in studies over the past 30 years. There is considerable variability on the number of patients with each histologic subtype in the studies, likely dependent on the geographic location and the criteria of inclusion into the research study. Data are from bone biopsy series done on patients undergoing dialysis in the United States,[94,95] Canada,[92] Thailand,[96] Israel[97] and Europe,[98] with the number of subjects in each study listed. *HPT*, hyperparathyroidism; *Mixed*, mixed uremic osteodystrophy; *Adynamic*, adynamic bone disease; *OM*, osteomalacia.

Diagnosis of Abnormal Bone Turnover

Studies evaluating the ability of the serum concentration of intact PTH to predict both low and high turnover bone disease have been disappointing. In general, the risk of high-turnover bone disease increases with the concentration of intact PTH.[54,55] However, the ability to reliably predict the presence of high-turnover bone disease is poor until intact PTH levels of 450 to 500 pg/mL are reached. Levels of intact PTH under 100 pg/mL are fairly reliable for the prediction of low-turnover bone disease,[54] but again, not perfect. Based primarily on these studies, the K/DOQI guidelines recommend a target intact PTH level of 150 to 300 pg/mL.[106] Unfortunately, these studies that correlate intact PTH with bone histology were done prior to the widespread use of vitamin D derivatives and may not be applicable in the current treatment environment. Thus, in general, levels of intact PTH below 100 to 150 pg/mL are indicative of low turnover bone, whereas levels of intact PTH greater than 450 to 500 pg/mL are indicative of high turnover bone on biopsy. Levels in between those two cutoff levels are not predictive of underlying bone histology, creating a clinical challenge for nephrologists. As described previously, the new whole or bioactive 1–84 amino acid PTH assay may offer improved diagnostic capabilities, but this remains to be proven.

Obviously, it is not practical to have all patients undergo a bone biopsy. Thus, we must use clinical judgment, PTH hormone levels, and various other bone markers. Initially, there was great hope for the new bone markers such as osteocalcin and bone specific alkaline phosphatase to be predictive of underlying bone histology. Unfortunately, these specialized tests offer little additive value to our usual measurement of calcium, phosphorus, PTH, and total alkaline phosphatase.[107] This is also true for patients not yet on dialysis, where a recent study in 84 subjects determined that measurement of intact PTH, bone alkaline phosphatase, total alkaline phosphatase, or osteocalcin had sensitivities of 72% to 83%, but specificity of 53% to 67% to discriminate adynamic bone from other types of renal osteodystrophy.[108] A new assay that measures circulating tartrate-resistant acid phosphatase 5b (TRACP) as

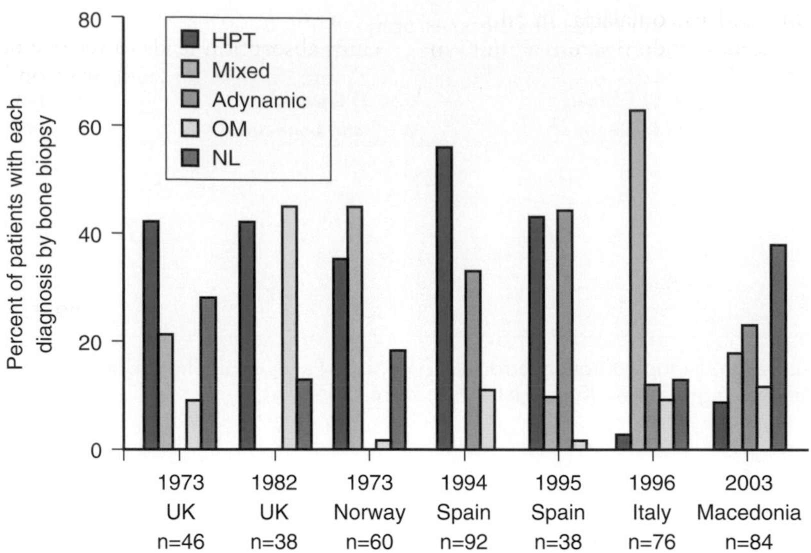

Figure 8–5 **The spectrum of histologic types of renal osteodystrophy in patients with chronic kidney disease stages III and IV**. This graph represents the distribution of various pathologic forms of renal osteodystrophy in studies over the past 30 years. There is considerable variability on the number of patients with each histologic subtype in the studies, likely dependent on the geographic location and the magnitude and cause of chronic kidney disease of the subjects. Data are from bone biopsy series done on patients with chronic kidney disease in the United Kingdom in 1973,[99] 1982,[100] Norway,[101] Spain in 1994[102] and 1995,[103] Italy in 1996,[104] and Macedonia in 2003,[105] with the number of subjects in each study listed. *HPT*, hyperparathyroidism; *Mixed*, mixed uremic osteodystrophy; *Adynamic*, adynamic bone disease; *OM*, osteomalacia; *NL*, normal.

a marker of osteoclast activity may be promising,[109] but more evaluation is necessary. Thus, in the absence of a perfect marker, we must look at multiple variables (Table 8–2).

In contrast to the hypophosphatemia and hypercalcemia observed in primary hyperparathyroidism, patients with secondary hyperparathyroidism tend to be hyperphosphatemic (which leads to increased PTH). The serum level of calcium is variable and depends on the overall calcium balance, type of phosphate binder, vitamin D therapy, and calcium dialysate concentration. However, in advanced cases of secondary hyperparathyroidism, patients are both hypercalcemic and hyperphosphatemic, in part because of the efflux from bone. It is also important to look at the trend of PTH values with time. Clearly, if the PTH concentration is above 300 pg/mL by intact assay *and* consistently rising, then the patient almost certainly has high-turnover bone. In contrast, patients with low-turnover bone are often hypercalcemic, in part because of the inability of low-turnover bone to buffer an acute calcium load.[110] Bone biopsy is the only way to definitively differentiate if low-turnover bone is due to adynamic bone or aluminum induced osteomalacia, although most patients with adynamic bone disease are asymptomatic in contrast to

Table 8–2 Features of High-Turnover and Low-Turnover Renal Osteodystrophy

	High Turnover	Low Turnover
PTH	Increased	Decreased
Alkaline phosphatase	Increased	Normal
Bone alkaline phosphatase	Increased	Normal or decreased
Osteocalcin	Increased	Normal
Calcium	Variable	Can be increased
Phosphorus	Increased	Normal or increased
DFO stimulation test	Normal	Normal (adynamic) Elevated delta (aluminum OM)
Skeletal radiographs	Resorption, sclerosis	Normal
Symptoms	Usually asymptomatic, unless very severe disease	Asymptomatic (adynamic) Symptomatic (aluminum OM)

DFO, deferoxamine; *OM*, osteomalacia (From Moe SM. Calcium, phosphorus, and vitamin D metabolism in renal disease and chronic renal failure. *In* Kopple JD, Massry SG [eds]: Nutritional Management of Renal Disease. Philadelphia, Lippincott Williams & Wilkins, 2004, pp 261–285.)

patients with aluminum induced osteomalacia. In addition, deferoxamine stimulation tests and random serum aluminum levels can occasionally be helpful, as discussed later.[111, 112]

HIGH-TURNOVER BONE DISEASE

Pathogenesis of Secondary Hyperparathyroidism

As detailed previously, the kidney plays an integral role in the maintenance of normal calcium and phosphorus homeostasis and bone health. As a result, severe abnormalities can occur in the presence of CKD (Figure 8–6). As CKD disease advances, the reduced mass of functioning renal tissue is unable to excrete the normal dietary intake of phosphorus. Early on, the serum level of phosphorus is maintained via stimulation of parathyroid hormone release, leading to the development of secondary hyperparathyroidism, the "trade-off" hypothesis.[113] Phosphorus retention further limits calcitriol production by inhibiting the activity of 1-α-hydroxylase, which converts 25(OH)-vitamin D into active $1,25(OH)_2D$ (calcitriol). The decreased $1,25(OH)_2D$ directly increases PTH release further and leads to decreased calcium and phosphorus absorption from the gastrointestinal tract. The impaired intestinal calcium absorption leads to relative decreases in serum ionized calcium, further augmenting secondary hyperparathyroidism. Over time, the parathyroid glands become less sensitive to the feedback suppression of calcium and calcitriol, causing continual secretion of PTH and secondary hyperparathyroidism.[114] Continual stimulation of PTH secretion has been shown to induce irreversible hyperplasia of the parathyroid glands in uremic rats[115] through a number of abnormalities of gene and growth factor expression.[36] The continued elevated levels of PTH lead to increased bone remodeling or high-turnover bone.

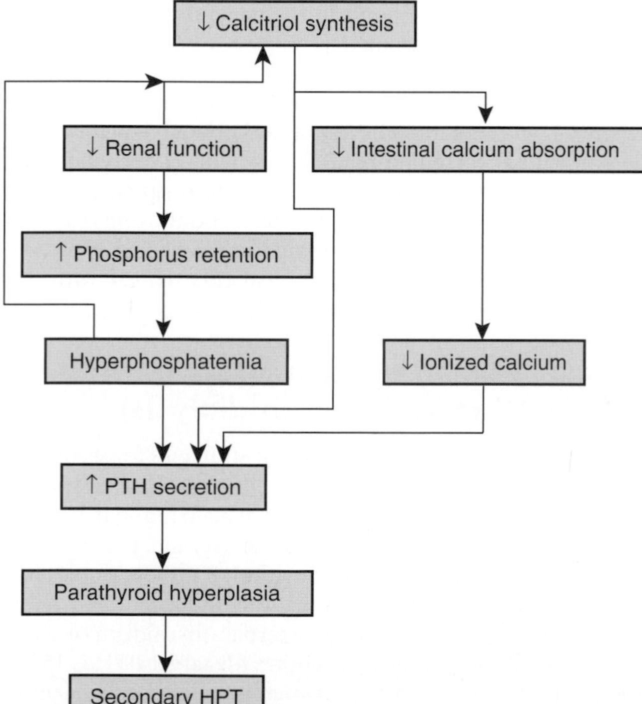

Figure 8–6 The pathogenesis of secondary hyperparathyroidism in chronic kidney disease. Excess parathyroid hormone secretion occurs in response to hypocalcemia, hyperphosphatemia, and decreased conversion of vitamin D to the active form, calcitriol. (Reprinted from Moe SM, Drueke TB: Management of secondary hyperparathyroidism: The importance and the challenge of controlling parathyroid hormone levels without elevating calcium, phosphorus, and calcium-phosphorus product. Am J Nephrol 2003; 23:369–379, with permission.)

As indicated in Figure 8–6, hyperphosphatemia has been shown to be one of the most important factors in the pathogenesis of secondary hyperparathyroidism. Although early studies suggested hyperphosphatemia induced decline in serum calcitriol (leading to low serum calcium), was the initial stimulus for enhanced PTH secretion,[116] more recent evidence suggests that elevated serum phosphorus levels promote PTH secretion directly, independent of changes in serum calcium or calcitriol. Phosphorus restriction in dogs with renal failure[117] and in patients with chronic renal failure[118] have been shown to decrease PTH secretion directly, independently of changes in serum calcium or calcitriol. In uremic rats, phosphorus directly stimulates parathyroid gland hyperplasia.[115] Moreover, high phosphorus levels have been shown to directly stimulate PTH secretion in intact rat parathyroid glands in vitro.[117,119] In addition, in the presence of increased phosphorus load, the PTH-calcium curve is probably shifted to the right, creating resistance at the level of the PTH gland.[46] Thus, there is now substantial evidence to support that phosphorus, calcium, and $1,25(OH)_2D$ all act directly, and independently, to regulate PTH secretion. Therefore, all three factors are targeted for the prevention and treatment of secondary hyperparathyroidism.

GENERAL TREATMENT STRATEGIES FOR SECONDARY HYPERPARATHYROIDISM

The National Kidney Foundation has recently published clinical practice guidelines (Kidney Disease Outcomes Quality Initiative (K/DOQI)[106] on the management of renal osteodystrophy in all stages of chronic kidney disease. A summarized version of these guidelines are in Tables 8–3 and 8–4 and will be subsequently discussed.

Chronic Kidney Disease (CKD) Stage III (GFR 30–60 mL/min) and Stage IV (GFR 15–30 mL/min)

The treatment of secondary hyperparathyroidism should begin early in the course of CKD. Serum phosphorus levels are normally maintained within a narrow range, typically 2.5 to 4.5 mg/dL (0.8–1.5 mmol/L). Approximately 1000 to 1800 mg of phosphorus is ingested daily in the average Western diet.[120,121] Of this amount, about 30% is excreted through the gastrointestinal tract, and 70% is excreted by the kidneys.[113] The dietary sources of phosphorus include all meats, dairy products, and many cereals and grains, thus making dietary restriction nearly impossible. The amount of phosphorus excreted by the kidneys is determined by the balance between

Table 8–3 Summary of K/DOQI Guidelines for Chronic Kidney Disease Stages III and IV

- Normalize serum phosphorus by diet and phosphorus binder therapy, 2.7–4.6 mg/dL; begin when *either* elevated serum phosphorus *or* elevated serum PTH.
- Treat nutritional vitamin D deficiency if serum 25-hydroxyvitamin D is <30 ng/mL.
- Treat elevated PTH with calcitriol or other "less hypercalcemic" vitamin D analogues to target of 35–70 (CKD III) or 70–110 (CKD IV) pg/mL by intact assay.
- Normalize serum calcium.

(From K/DOQI NKF: Clinical practice guidelines for bone metabolism and disease in chronic kidney disease. Am J Kidney Dis 2003; 42:S1–S201.)

Table 8–4 Summary of K/DOQI Guidelines for Chronic Kidney Disease Stage V

- Normalize serum phosphorus by diet and phosphorus binder therapy, 3.5–5.5 mg/dL; limit elemental calcium intake from binders to 1500 mg/day.
- Treat elevated PTH with calcitriol or other "less hypercalcemic" vitamin D analogues to target of 150–300 pg/mL by intact assay.
- Normalize serum calcium, ideally < 9.5 mg/dL, and always < 10.2 mg/dL; Ca X P < 55 mg^2/dL^2.

(From K/DOQI NKF: Clinical practice guidelines for bone metabolism and disease in chronic kidney disease. Am J Kidney Dis 2003; 42:S1–S201.)

ultrafiltration and reabsorption. As renal function declines, serum phosphorus levels are maintained through a compensatory decrease in the rate of renal tubular reabsorption of phosphorus, mediated in part by elevation in the serum PTH.[113] This adaptation allows for maintenance of normal serum phosphorus levels until the glomerular filtration rate (GFR) falls below 20 to 25 mL/min, at which point elevation in the serum PTH level cannot further increase phosphorus excretion, and hyperphosphatemia develops.[113,122,123] Thus, normal serum phosphorus levels are maintained well into advanced stages of renal failure but at the cost of worsening secondary hyperparathyroidism.

Based on animal data, the key to the successful treatment of secondary hyperparathyroidism is to prevent the development of hyperplasia, because once that stage is reached, regression is unlikely.[124] Thus, more aggressive and frequent monitoring of serum PTH is recommended by the K/DOQI guidelines, including assessment every 12 months in CKD stage III, and every 3 months in CKD stage IV.[106] Treatment should probably begin at levels of intact PTH of 70 to 110 pg/mL in order to prevent hyperparathyroidism.[106]

Thus, the mainstay of therapy at this level of GFR should be to control hyperparathyroidism by (1) dietary phosphate restriction and phosphate binders and (2) increase calcitriol by either giving calcidiol or active vitamin D sterols, such as calcitriol. In CKD stages III and IV, the K/DOQI guidelines recommend measuring 25(OH)D (calcidiol) levels if the PTH is elevated. If low, this vitamin D of nutritional origin can be replaced with ergocalciferol. This substrate should then be converted by the remaining renal mass to active calcitriol that will suppress PTH. Data in non-CKD patients who are calcidiol-deficient demonstrates that hyperparathyroidism can be corrected by repleting these levels with oral ergocalciferol.[125] However, this remains to be proven in CKD patients, and it is not clear just how much renal mass is required for conversion of 25(OH)D to $1,25(OH)_2D$. Nonetheless, studies have demonstrated that CKD patients commonly have low levels of 25(OH)D,[126,127] and in the general population deficiency is associated with hip fractures, low bone mineral density, immunologic defects, and possibly cancer.[70] If calcidiol levels are normal and PTH increased, treatment with active vitamin D sterols should be initiated. Although an early study demonstrated worsening renal failure with active vitamin D therapy,[128] other studies have failed to demonstrate this.[129,130] If vitamin D analogues are begun, close monitoring of serum calcium, phosphorus, and creatinine are indicated. However, there are no long-term studies of patients treated with this regimen.

Chronic Kidney Disease Stage V (GFR < 15 mL/min, or on dialysis)

For patients on dialysis, the treatment strategies for secondary hyperparathyroidism are threefold: (1) phosphate restriction and use of phosphate binders, (2) normalizing, but not elevating, serum calcium, and (3) use of vitamin D analogues. The current strategy is to monitor serum PTH levels quarterly, although more frequent monitoring is indicated, and reimbursed, in cases of more severe hyperparathyroidism or when therapy is adjusted. As detailed above, the target PTH is 150 to 300 pg/mL by the intact assay, which is roughly equivalent to 75 to 150 by the whole or bioactive "1–84" assays.

Control of Phosphorus

Successful clinical management of phosphorus consists of several core components: a low phosphorus diet, adequate dialysis, and safe and effective phosphate-binding therapy. The efficacy of each of these components depends on patient compliance, the key for improving phosphorus control.

Phosphorus is contained in almost all foods. Unfortunately, foods high in phosphorus are generally also high in protein.

National Kidney Foundation Dialysis Outcomes Quality Initiative (NKF/DOQI) dietary guidelines for patients on maintenance hemodialysis include a daily intake of 1.2 g of protein per kg body weight.[131] Protein requirements are even higher in patients receiving CAPD than in hemodialysis patients.[66,132] As a result, it is challenging to balance dietary phosphate restriction against the need for adequate protein intake, especially with malnutrition present in up to 50% of dialysis patients.[133] Indeed, most well nourished dialysis patients are in positive phosphorus balance. Roughly 60% to 70% of consumed phosphate is absorbed, so about 4000 to 5000 mg of phosphorus per week enters the extracellular fluid. Therefore, dietary phosphorus restriction alone, although an important component of effective phosphorus management, is not sufficient to control serum phosphorus levels in most dialysis patients.

With the limitations of dietary phosphorus restriction, dialysis plays an important role in removing excess phosphorus from the patient's blood, eliminating about 2700 to 3000 mg phosphorus per week.[134] However, a significant amount of the total body phosphorus is found in the intracellular compartment. Thus, the amount of phosphorus that can be removed during a single dialysis session is limited. Kinetic studies indicate that phosphorus is cleared more efficiently in the first half of a hemodialysis treatment, when serum levels are highest.[135] This correlation partly accounts for the rapid fall in serum phosphorus during the first 1 to 2 hours of treatment, followed by a plateau during which serum phosphorus levels remain between 1.9 and 3.4 mg/dL. The rate of phosphorus removal significantly decreases in the second half of treatment and is generally followed by a rebound in serum phosphorus levels in the first 3 to 4 hours following dialysis treatment.[136,137] Nocturnal hemodialysis and other slow continuous methods offer a hope for the future, as patients using these methods have normal or low phosphorus levels.[138]

Phosphate Binders

Because of the limitations associated with dietary phosphorus restriction and the phosphorus removal with dialysis, dietary phosphate binders are required in nearly all dialysis patients. Unfortunately, no binder is perfect and the best binder is one the patient will take consistently. Thus, a trial of multiple binder regimens is often required. The dose of phosphate binder should be titrated to dietary intake of phosphorus for both the initial starting dose and subsequent dose adjustments.

Aluminum hydroxide is extremely efficient as a phosphate binder and, consequently, was the primary phosphate binder used from the time of its introduction in 1941 until the mid-1980s. Subsequently, it has been recognized that aluminum is absorbed from the gastrointestinal tract and accumulation of even small amounts of aluminum in the body can cause toxic side effects, such as aluminum bone disease (osteomalacia), dementia, myopathy, and anemia.[66,139,140] It is now recognized that all dialysis patients receiving aluminum-containing binders are at risk for development of aluminum bone disease and other symptoms of aluminum intoxication, although diabetic patients[141] and children[142] are at particularly high risk. Thus, aluminum-containing binders should be administered only when all other resources to control phosphorus have been exhausted, and only for intervals of up to 4 weeks.[106]

Of the available calcium-containing binders, both calcium carbonate and calcium acetate have proven efficacy compared to placebo.[143,144] In addition, calcium containing phosphate binders have been shown to effectively lower phosphorus levels and to help prevent the development of secondary hyperparathyroidism.[66] Sensitive balance studies have demonstrated less calcium absorption from calcium acetate compared to calcium carbonate on a gram per gram basis.[145,146] However, studies have not consistently demonstrated that calcium acetate can lead to less hypercalcemic episodes.[147] Over the last 10 years, these two calcium containing phosphate binders have become the mainstay of therapy, with choice depending primarily on patient preference. Other calcium supplements that have been used as phosphate binders include calcium ketoamino acids,[148] calcium ketovaline,[149] and calcium citrate. However, calcium citrate should be avoided as citrate can increase intestinal absorption of aluminum.[150] The main side effects of calcium containing phosphate binders are constipation, inability to swallow the tablets due to their size, altered taste, and increased calcium load leading to positive calcium balance.

Serum calcium levels are normally tightly controlled within a narrow range, usually 8.5 to 10.5 mg/dL (2.1 to 2.6 mmol/L). However, the serum calcium level is a poor reflection of overall total body calcium, because serum levels are only 0.1% to 0.2% of extracellular calcium, which in turn is only 1% of total body calcium. The remainder is stored in bone. However, ionized calcium, generally 40% of total serum calcium levels is physiologically active and is maintained in the normal range by inducing increases in the secretion of parathyroid hormone (PTH). PTH acts to increase bone resorption, increase renal calcium reabsorption, and to increase the conversion of 25(OH)D to $1,25(OH)_2D$ in the kidney. The latter increases gastrointestinal calcium absorption. In individuals with normal homeostatic mechanisms, these interactions of PTH and vitamin D metabolites at target organs, including the kidney, maintain the serum ionized calcium level within the normal range to ensure proper cellular function and to ensure normal bone growth. In normal individuals, the net calcium balance (intake–output) varies with age. Children and young adults are usually in a slightly positive net calcium balance to enhance linear growth; beyond ages 25 to 35, when bones stop growing, the calcium balance tends to be neutral.[151] Normal individuals have protection against calcium overload by virtue of their ability to reduce intestinal absorption of calcium and to increase renal excretion of calcium in response to excessive calcium intake by actions of PTH and calcitriol. However, in CKD the ability to maintain normal homeostasis, including a normal serum ionized calcium level and appropriate calcium balance for age, is lost.

The K/DOQI guidelines recommend a limit on the daily ingestion of calcium in the form of calcium containing phosphate binders to be 1500 mg elemental calcium per day. This is assuming a 500 mg intake per day from diet, yielding 2000 mg per day.[106] This level is slightly below the Institute of Medicine's recommended maximum intake of calcium of 2500 mg per day for healthy adults.[152] In patients with CKD stage V, the primary intake of calcium is from calcium containing phosphate binders. Early metabolic studies demonstrated that approximately 18% to 20% of calcium is absorbed from the intestine.[153,154] Figure 8–7 shows net calcium intake per day for hemodialysis and peritoneal dialysis

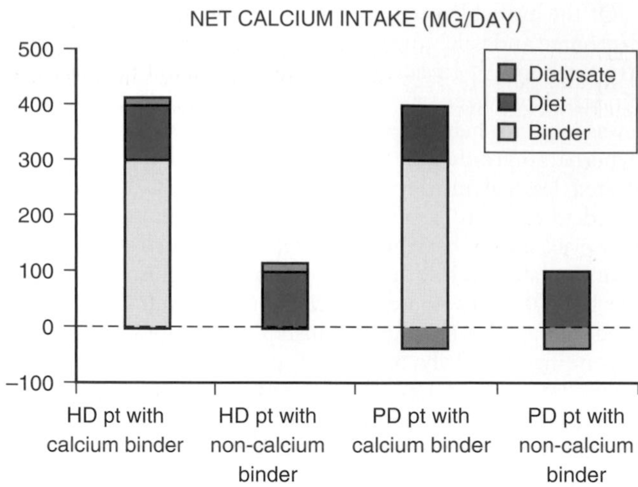

Figure 8-7 Calcium balance in hemodialysis and peritoneal dialysis in the presence and absence of calcium containing phosphate binders. Estimated net calcium intake per day in a prototype dialysis patient comes from three sources: dialysate (2.5 meq/L calcium concentration; *dark gray bars*), diet of 500 mg elemental calcium per day (*black bars*), and phosphate binder (*light gray bars*). The left two bars are from a patient undergoing hemodialysis on calcium containing phosphate binder containing 1500 mg elemental calcium (*first bar*) and on a noncalcium containing binder (*second bar*). The third and fourth bars are similar data in a prototype patient undergoing continuous ambulatory peritoneal dialysis of four exchanges per day. These data assume an absorption of 20% of ingested calcium from diet[132,154] and binder,[145] which would be 100 mg from a 500 mg calcium diet, and 300 mg from an intake of phosphate binders containing 1500 mg of elemental calcium. As depicted graphically, the main contribution to daily calcium intake is from calcium containing phosphate binders, whereas a relatively small amount of calcium is taken in from hemodialysis,[134] and a small efflux is observed in peritoneal dialysis, depending on the ultrafiltration.[155] These data represent calcium intake, and the calcium excretion will primarily be in the form of stool, sweat, and residual renal function and will vary from 150 to 300 mg/day.[154]

patients. If patients are taking 2000 mg per day in total calcium intake (1500 mg from binder and 500 mg from diet), and 20% is absorbed, then the net intake is 400 mg/day. On hemodialysis days, this figure is slightly greater because approximately 50 mg of calcium is infused with a 4-hour dialysis treatment, using 2.5 meq/L dialysate calcium concentration.[134] In peritoneal dialysis patients there is a slight efflux of calcium, using a 2.5 meq/L dialysate in four daily exchanges.[155] The excretion of calcium in stool and sweat ranges from 150 to 250 mg/day,[152] and if patients have residual urine output, the excretion rate may increase slightly. Thus, the patients will still be in positive calcium balance at this K/DOQI maximum when taking 1500 mg of calcium containing phosphate binders. In an anuric patient, this positive calcium load has only two "compartments" to go to: bone and extraskeletal locations. If the bone is normally remodeling the calcium should be deposited there, however, normal bone is not common in dialysis patients. If no calcium containing phosphate binder is taken, the patients will be in neutral, to slightly negative balance depending on stool and sweat output. It is important to emphasize three points: First, this 1500 mg maximum intake of elemental calcium from phosphate binders in the K/DOQI guidelines is based on opinion, because there are no recent formal metabolic balance studies. Second, in patients taking vitamin D, the intestinal absorption of calcium will be increased, and thus the amount of calcium in the form of binder should be decreased. Third, in patients with low-turnover bone disease, the bone cannot take up calcium,[110] and that is the rationale for the K/DQOI recommendation that calcium containing phosphate binders not be used in patients with intact PTH levels of less than 150 pg/mL.[106]

The noncalcemic, nonaluminum/metal phosphate binder, sevelamer, received FDA approval in 1998 in the United States. This binder is effective in controlling serum phosphorus[156,157] and leads to equivalent phosphate control but less hypercalcemia than does calcium acetate.[158,159] In addition, this phosphate binder can be used together with calcium containing phosphate binders and may allow the use of more vitamin D.[160] This phosphate binder is also unique in that it lowers total cholesterol levels, principally by lowering LDL levels.[158,160,161] Recently, this phosphate binder was compared to calcium containing phosphate binders (both calcium acetate and calcium carbonate) in a randomized, controlled year-long study. Subjects treated with both binders showed excellent and similar serum phosphorus and calcium × phosphorus products. However, sevelamer led to less hypercalcemia and less over-suppression of PTH. In addition, calcium containing phosphate binders (both calcium acetate and calcium carbonate), but not sevelamer, lead to progressive coronary artery and aorta calcification by electron beam CT.[159,162] Of note, the average elemental calcium content of subjects taking calcium acetate was 1.1 g/day, below the K/DOQI maximum, and yet calcification progressed. The reason for the attenuation of vascular calcification in subjects receiving sevelamer is not clear but may be reduced calcium load, fewer episodes of hypercalcemia, lower LDL cholesterol, or less over-suppression of PTH. The main side effects of sevelamer are gastrointestinal distress, such as bloating, flatulence, and occasional diarrhea. Unfortunately, sevelamer is much more expensive than the other phosphate binders and generally not affordable for patients in the United States without prescription drug coverage.

Lanthanum carbonate, a heavy metal, has been effective in animal studies[163] and in dialysis patients in a preliminary report[164] and a large clinical trial.[165] It is pending FDA approval. Much concern has been raised for the potential toxicity of lanthanum because a very small amount is absorbed from the gastrointestinal tract. However, 80% of lanthanum excretion is via biliary tract, and 20% is via urinary excretion, in contrast to 100% urinary excretion of another metal, aluminum. Thus, the intestinal absorption of lanthanum is less than that of aluminum, and the predominant route of excretion is biliary not urinary.[98,165] A study evaluating bone biopsies in dialysis patients at baseline and 1 year after lanthanum use did not demonstrate the development of osteomalacia in any patient, and, of interest, a considerable number of patients taking calcium containing phosphate binder developed adynamic bone disease.[98] The eventual approval of lanthanum will offer another noncalcemic binder to the list of options for our patients. The drug is also chewable and, thus, may be helpful in individuals who have difficulty swallowing pills.[165]

Other phosphate binders that are available include magnesium carbonate, usually in combination with calcium acetate. Magnesium carbonate is an effective phosphate binder. However, the dialysate magnesium concentration should be lowered in patients taking oral magnesium,[166] which is not practical given that most dialysis units utilize central delivery systems of standardized dialysis baths. Furthermore, no long-term studies have been done. This is of particular concern given that serum magnesium levels are a poor reflection of total body magnesium. Most recent on the horizon are ferric compounds,[167–169] which appear effective in limited studies. Finally, a mixed magnesium and iron compound also has preliminary efficacy *in vitro*.[170]

The breadth of choices of phosphate binders and the number of agents in development indicate that these medications continue to be the Achilles heel of dialysis patients with large numbers of pills required to control serum phosphorus and gastrointestinal side effects, leading to patient noncompliance. However, the physician and dietitian should be aggressive in finding a regimen agreeable to the patient. Frequent snacking without phosphate binders, and taking calcium based binders with oral iron supplements, which limit effectiveness, can also lead to hyperphosphatemia and can be easily adjusted. Last, some of the serum phosphorus derives from bone, such that patients with high bone turnover due to severe hyperparathyroidism may have hyperphosphatemia despite compliance with phosphate binders.

Therapy with Vitamin D Analogues

Berl and associates[171] first demonstrated that orally administered $1,25(OH)_2D$, but not vitamin D_3, suppressed PTH in patients with renal failure, confirming that hydroxylation of the sterol at the level of the kidney is required for its actions on PTH. The intravenous formulation was introduced in 1984 by Slatopolsky and associates,[41] who found excellent suppression of PTH in patients given high dose (4 mcg) intravenous calcitriol thrice weekly on hemodialysis. Andress[172] subsequently demonstrated improvement in bone histology with intravenous therapy. Unfortunately, this therapy, although quite effective, led to uniform elevations in serum calcium. We subsequently demonstrated that in patients with mild to moderate hyperparathyroidism, low doses (0.5 to 1 mcg) given intravenously thrice weekly was effective in suppressing PTH with time and led to only minimal rise in serum calcium levels.[173]

Based on these and many other studies, intravenous pulse calcitriol was felt to be the optimal therapy to allow greater bioavailability to the parathyroid gland and bypass some of the intestinal absorption of calcium and phosphorus. However, in Japan, where intravenous medications are not paid for as they are in the United States, oral pulse calcitriol proved equally efficacious to intravenous calcitriol.[174] Subsequent studies have also demonstrated that oral and intravenous calcitriol are equally efficacious with a similar incidence of hypercalcemia and hyperphosphatemia, at least in patients with mild to moderate secondary hyperparathyroidism.[175,176] This was followed by our study in peritoneal dialysis patients[177] and that of Hermann[178] in hemodialysis patients, demonstrating that daily and pulse therapy of calcitriol, when given in equivalent weekly doses, were also equally efficacious in suppressing PTH. Thus, these studies demonstrate that calcitriol is effective for the treatment of secondary hyperparathyroidism regardless of its route and frequency of administration. However, most of these studies treated only mild to moderate hyperparathyroidism. The vitamin D receptor (VDR) is down-regulated in the PTH glands in advanced hyperparathyroid disease, based on examination of tissue removed during parathyroidectomy.[179] In these patients, very high doses may indeed be required. In addition, none of these regimens completely remove the problematic side effect of increased intestinal calcium and phosphorus absorption, leading to the aggressive development of analogues with increased potency at the PTH gland compared to the intestine.

Two "less calcemic" analogues are commercially available in the United States: 19-nor-$1,25(OH)_2D_2$ (paricalcitol) and $1\text{-}\alpha(OH)D_2$(doxercalciferol) and others are available outside the United States.[180] All of these analogues appear effective in suppressing hyperparathyroidism in patients on dialysis.[129,181–186] Paricalcitol appears superior to calcitriol in terms of its hypercalcemic and hyperphosphatemic effects in comparison studies in rats[187] and possibly humans.[188] A recent secondary analysis of a trial comparing paricalcitol and calcitriol has recently been published. This study found that although there was no difference between these vitamin D preparations in the number of subjects who had a single episode of hypercalcemia, paricalcitol led to less sustained hypercalcemia.[189] There are no direct comparative trials of doxercalciferol to calcitriol. The lack of comparative trials makes blanket endorsement of preferential use of any of these analogues over calcitriol premature, and the K/DQOI guidelines found no evidence for superiority but did recommend that a trial of less calcemic analogues be utilized in patients prone to hypercalcemia because of the large base of anecdotal experience. Unfortunately, demonstrating this in a randomized, comparative trial is difficult, given that the concomitant use of different phosphate binders may alter serum calcium and phosphorus levels independent of the effects of the vitamin D analogues. Doxercalciferol is also available orally, and a direct comparison study of the oral and intravenous formulations indicate that the oral agent may lead to more hypercalcemia than the intravenous formulation.[129]

Interestingly, a recent study evaluating a large provider database found that patients treated exclusively with paricalcitol had a 16% reduction in mortality compared to patients treated exclusively with calcitriol.[190] This effect prevailed across many independent analyses of potential confounders, and there was no difference in serum calcium, phosphorus, and PTH in the two groups. However, it should be emphasized that these results need prospective confirmation. The two groups were slightly different at baseline, no phosphate binder data were available, and the rationale of the prescribing physician in choosing one vitamin D form over another cannot be assessed in such a retrospective review.[191] This also raises the possibility that nonskeletal effects of vitamin D on immune function and cell proliferation may be important and differ among analogues. It also raises the question: Do all dialysis patients need some vitamin D? Unfortunately, in the absence of functioning kidneys, the adverse effects of hypercalcemia may outweigh any improvement in immune function.[192]

Despite aggressive use of calcitriol and other vitamin D analogues, a significant number of patients remain refractory to therapy, either because of hyperphosphatemia and/or hypercalcemia leading to an elevated calcium × phosphorus product, or advanced hyperplasia of the parathyroid glands, rendering the secretion of PTH unsuppressible. In these patients surgical parathyroidectomy offers the only current solution to the ill effects of hyperparathyroidism. Katoh and associates[193] have suggested using PTH gland imaging to determine who will and will not respond to calcitriol therapy by detecting enlarged parathyroid glands, but this has not become widely accepted and requires a skilled ultrasonographer. The surgical technique utilized for parathyroidectomy is not as important as the skills of the surgeon. The patient who undergoes a parathyroidectomy gets immediate relief of musculoskeletal discomfort and a rapid fall in both serum calcium and phosphorus due to the "hungry bone" syndrome. The potential adverse effects of the surgery are primarily recurrent laryngeal nerve damage, in addition to the risk of anesthesia. There has been a tendency to avoid this procedure, but in my opinion, we probably underutilize it. Prior to the parathyroidectomy, a bone biopsy should be done to rule out coexistent aluminum bone disease in anyone with significant aluminum exposure. The problem is that the amount of "significant" exposure is unique for each patient leading some experts to argue that a biopsy should be done in all cases preoperatively.[194] However, patients given infrequent "rescue" therapy with aluminum for hyperphosphatemia do not require a bone biopsy.

Calcimimetics

New to the horizon are the calcimimetics, pharmaceutical agents that increase the sensitivity of the calcium sensing receptor in the parathyroid gland, leading to suppression of PTH release. The first generation agents were shown to be very effective in suppressing PTH in animal models of renal failure and improving bone histology.[195,196] The initial trial in humans was encouraging,[197] however, the agent had poor bioavailability and potential drug interactions. This led to the second generation agent, AMG073, or Cinacalcet (Amgen, Inc, Thousand Oaks, CA). In the initial studies, this agent proved quite effective in suppressing PTH but with some hypocalcemia.[198] The phase II trials had dramatic results: effective suppression of PTH and lowering of both calcium and phosphorus, leading to a reduction in the calcium × phosphorus product.[199] Phase III data confirm these results.[200] Preliminary composite data from all phase III studies in over 1100 patients around the world demonstrate that use of this agent can lead to suppression of PTH with a lowering of the calcium × phosphorus product,[201] allowing achievement of the current K/DOQI guidelines in many more patients than current regimens. The ability of calcimimetics to lower the calcium × phosphorus product clearly differentiates this agent from vitamin D compounds that uniformly raise the calcium × phosphorus product. Thus, calcimimetics will become an important therapeutic option for secondary hyperparathyroidism.

LOW-TURNOVER BONE DISEASE

Aluminum Induced Osteomalacia

As detailed earlier, low-turnover bone disease in dialysis patients is generally due to aluminum induced osteomalacia or adynamic bone. In aluminum induced osteomalacia, aluminum deposits at the mineralization front, leading to impaired mineralization and subsequent accumulation of unmineralized bone, or osteoid. The potential toxicity of aluminum was initially recognized by Alfrey and associates,[202,203] who identified a fatal neurologic syndrome in dialysis patients consisting of dyspraxia, seizures, and EEG abnormalities in association with high brain aluminum levels on autopsy. The source of aluminum in these severe cases was felt to be elevated concentrations in dialysate water. Subsequently, aluminum containing phosphate binders were also identified as a source.[204–206] The additional symptoms of fractures, myopathy, and microcytic anemia were described several years after the initial reports of the neurologic syndrome.[206,207] In the more recent (late 1980s) Toronto bone biopsy study, where unselected patients at three dialysis units underwent bone biopsies and noninvasive tests ($n = 259$), 69 patients had aluminum bone disease defined as greater than 25% surface aluminum staining. In this series, aluminum bone disease was the most common bone histologic disorder associated with proximal myopathy, pathologic fractures, unexplained bone pain, microcytic anemia, and hypercalcemia.[112] The ingestion of aluminum containing phosphate binders, sucralfate, and some over the counter antacids can also lead to aluminum accumulation.[208] Children, diabetics, and individuals taking citrate are at increased risk of developing the disease.[142,150,209]

The diagnosis of aluminum induced bone disease can be difficult, because aluminum toxicity is due to tissue burden not serum levels. Milliner and associates[111] first described the deferoxamine stimulation test where serum aluminum levels are induced to rise by administering the chelator deferoxamine. An increment in plasma aluminum concentration of 200 μg/L was the threshold for best specificity (93%) but poor sensitivity (43%). Pei and associates[112] later found that the specificity of the deferoxamine stimulation test improved in patients with low levels of intact PTH (< 200 pg/mL). However, the sensitivity of the test remains poor at 48% to 66%. Also, serum aluminum levels are not predictive with poor sensitivity and specificity in asymptomatic patients.[210] Thus, bone biopsy remains the gold standard. Treatment of aluminum bone disease is with deferoxamine, 1 g/week post hemodialysis or intraperitoneally. The duration of therapy must be individualized but is usually 6 months to 1 year. The treatment is quite beneficial, with a dramatic improvement in musculoskeletal symptoms[140] and bone histology[211] in nearly all patients. Unfortunately, the treatment is not without adverse effects, including hearing loss, retinal damage, and infection with mucormycosis. The latter is nearly always fatal.[212] However, these adverse effects were much more common when patients were treated with deferoxamine at each dialysis treatment, as opposed to the current standard therapy of once weekly administration. Fortunately, this disease is now uncommon, at least in the United States, where aluminum containing phosphate binders are rarely utilized.

Adynamic Bone Disease

In adynamic bone disease, there is a paucity of cells with resultant low bone turnover. In addition, in contrast to osteomalacia, in adynamic bone there is no increase in osteoid or unmineralized bone. The lack of bone cell activity led to the initial description of the disease as "aplastic" bone disease. Early studies felt the disease was still due to aluminum, but it was later identified in the absence of positive staining for aluminun.[153,213] The disease is increasing in prevalence, and is particularly common in peritoneal dialysis patients.[92,214] The etiology of adynamic bone disease is unknown but risk factors include age, over-suppression of PTH with vitamin D and calcium containing phosphate binders, diabetes, peritoneal dialysis, and possibly calcium overload.[92,110,215,216] In addition, there is evidence for altered osteoblast response to PTH due to downregulation of the PTH receptor in renal failure,[217] which further contributes to the paucity of cells observed in adynamic bone disease. Circulating fragments of PTH (so called 7–84 amino acid fragments) may also be antagonists to PTH,[58,59] resulting in an effective resistance to 1–84 amino acid at the level of bone. There is also abnormal regulation of cell differentiation in the presence of renal failure, which may explain, in part, the relative paucity of cells in adynamic bone, although this remains to be proven.

Various risk factors have been identified: diabetes, peritoneal dialysis, older age, high calcium dialysate, and Caucasian race.[102,215,216,218,219] In addition, some of the low PTH is secondary to over-suppression with calcitriol[220] or with calcium load, as changing to a low calcium dialysate[221] or sevelamer, a non-calcium containing phosphate binder,[222] can increase the PTH. Patients with adynamic bone disease are often asymptomatic, however, they are at increased risk of hypercalcemia due to the inability of bone to buffer an acute calcium load.[110] Symptoms can usually help differentiate aluminum induced bone disease, which is often symptomatic, from adynamic bone disease, which is nearly always asymptomatic. The lack of cells in adynamic bone disease may impair the ability of bone to repair microfractures and predispose to clinical fractures. Indeed, low levels of PTH have been identified as risk factors for fracture,[4,223] which are particularly common in patients with end-stage renal disease.[3,4] However, these studies did not examine bone histology. Clearly, longitudinal studies of patients with biopsy proven adynamic bone disease are needed.

EXTRASKELETAL CALCIFICATION OR: WHAT IS THE OPTIMAL SERUM PHOSPHORUS, CALCIUM, AND CALCIUM × PHOSPHORUS PRODUCT?

In the past, a calcium × phosphorus product of 70 mg^2/dL^2 was considered the threshold above which calcitriol should not be given. This was felt to be the level above which metastatic calcification occurred. Unfortunately, this level of 70 was based on theoretical, in vitro data and extrapolations from case reports.[224–226] In addition, this number originated when the process of extraskeletal calcification was felt to be purely due to physiochemical interactions and supersaturation of sera with calcium and phosphorus. However, there is now clear evidence that vascular calcification is not purely a physiochemical process. In arteries from patients with atherosclerotic and medial calcification, *ex vivo* and *in vitro* data support that vascular smooth muscle cells can produce bone matrix proteins and mineralize similar to osteoblasts.[227–231] We have also demonstrated the presence of these "bone" matrix proteins in calcification of the arterioles of skin (calciphylaxis/calcific uremic arteriolopathy) and in medial and intimal calcification in the inferior epigastric artery of dialysis patients.[16,232,233] Thus, vascular calcification is clearly a cell mediated process. *In vitro* work has demonstrated that vascular smooth muscle cells can mineralize in the presence of elevated phosphorus concentrations,[15] similar to the mechanisms for phosphorus induced bone mineralization. The in vitro concentrations required to induce mineralization in vascular smooth muscle cells are well within the range of serum phosphorus observed in the majority of dialysis patients. In addition, uremic sera, even without elevated phosphorus concentrations, can induce vascular calcification in vitro to a greater extent and faster than normal sera.[234] Thus, uremia and altered mineral metabolism may lead to, or accelerate, vascular calcification.

Epidemiologic studies have demonstrated that the serum phosphorus and the calcium × phosphorus product are associated with poor outcomes. Lowrie and associates[17] found that serum phosphorus levels greater than 7.0 mg/dL were associated with increased mortality, and Block[18] found that serum phosphorus levels greater than 6.5 mg/dL were associated with increased mortality. The latter study also demonstrated that a calcium × phosphorus product greater than 73 mg^2/dL^2 was associated with increased mortality, principally due to the effects of phosphorus.[18] These studies were from data sets from over 10 years ago, during the widespread use of aluminum containing phosphate binders, and prior to aggressive use of vitamin D metabolites for the treatment of secondary hyperparathyroidism. However, the association of elevated serum phosphorus and mortality was recently confirmed by Block and associates,[235] who found an 88% higher relative risk of death for hemodialysis patients with serum phosphorus levels greater than 9 mg/dL, compared to patients with phosphorus levels in the reference range of 5 to 6 mg/dL. He also found that the relative risk of death correlated directly to serum calcium levels, rising 47% as the calcium level rises from 9 to 9.5 mg/dL to greater than 11 mg/dL.[235] Elevated serum phosphorus is also associated with poor outcomes in European studies.[236] A recent cohort study also demonstrated that management of calcium-phosphorus metabolism (defined as measuring PTH, or prescribing vitamin D or phosphate binders) prior to beginning dialysis was independently associated with a 35% decrease likelihood of death in the first year of dialysis.[237] These studies provide the rationale for the K/DOQI targets (Tables 8–3 and 8–4).[106] Furthermore, a preliminary report demonstrated that achievement of these K/DOQI target values for PTH and the calcium × phosphorus led to reduced mortality.[238]

The leading cause of mortality in dialysis patients is cardiovascular disease, and there is growing evidence for an adverse effect of mineral metabolism on the vascular system. Vascular calcification has become easier to document with the advances in imaging in the recent decade, including electron beam CT,[5] spiral CT,[11] and duplex ultrasonography.[239] These techniques are thought to be more reproducible than the older method of observing progression of vascular calcification on plain radiographs. Electron beam CT and spiral CT allows rapid imaging of the heart in diastole, such that calcification in the coronary arteries can be easily distinguished and quantified. Braun and associates[5] found in 1996 that hemodialysis patients had markedly increased coronary artery calcification compared to age and sex matched nonrenal failure individuals with angiographically proven coronary artery disease. Furthermore, valvular calcification was present in 50% of patients, and the coronary artery calcification increased in all 57 patients over the course of 1 to 2 years. Goodman and associates[240] found that this calcification also affected children and young adults on dialysis. They demonstrated that the patients with increased coronary artery calcification were on dialysis for a longer period of time, had an elevated calcium × phosphorus product, increased intake of calcium containing phosphate binder, a trend toward higher phosphorus levels, and no difference in the serum calcium levels. Kimura and associates[241] found an elevated calcium × phosphorus product greater than or equal to 60 mg^2/dL^2 on more than 25% of measurements correlated with severity of aortic calcification by abdominal CT. Marchais and associates[242] found that patients with hyperphosphatemia greater than 6.2 mg/dL had higher diastolic and mean blood pressure and increased cardiac index caused by increased stroke index and heart rate. They also found increased carotid artery tensile stress in the patients who were hyperphosphatemic.[242] This same group subsequently found that increased arterial calcification was associated with increased intake of calcium containing phosphate binders[243] and mortality.[6] In vascular calcification of the small arterioles of the skin (calciphylaxis or calcific uremic arteriolopathy), we found elevated phosphorus and calcium × phosphorus product to be a risk factor in a case control study.[16] This was confirmed by Mazhar and associates,[244] who found that the risk of calcific uremic arteriolopathy increased 3.51-fold for each mg/dL increase in serum phosphorus levels. Last, elevated serum phosphorus, calcium, calcium × phosphorus product, and PTH were all greater in peritoneal dialysis patients with valvular calcification,[245,246] and the presence of valvular calcification was predictive of all cause and cardiovascular mortality.[246] These data are supported by that of Rubel and associates,[247] demonstrating a serum phosphorus level of greater than or equal to 5.0 mg/dL (1.62 mmol/L) was independently associated with having undergone a cardiac valve replacement procedure. Thus, elevated serum phosphorus, and calcium × phosphorus product, is associated with accelerated vascular and valvular calcification, and in vitro data support a direct role of phosphorus and other uremic toxins in this process.[15,232,248,249] In summary, there is mounting evidence that disturbances of mineral metabolism in renal failure contributes to the excessive cardiovascular disease observed in dialysis patients. Thus, we need to strive for lower values in our patients,[250] which are reflected in the target goals for the new bone and mineral KDOQI: serum phosphorus levels at 3.5 to 5.5 mg/dL. Calcium × phosphorus produce below 55 mg^2/dL^2 and serum PTH levels near 150 to 200 pg/mL.[106]

Post Renal Transplant Bone Disease

Ideally, all of these complications of calcium and phosphorus imbalance and renal osteodystrophy would be improved with renal transplantation. Unfortunately, in many cases, renal transplantation returns individuals to chronic kidney disease (as opposed to normal renal function), and thus transplant patients still suffer from renal osteodystrophy. There are limited studies evaluating bone histology in recipients of renal transplants. There appears to be a persistent mineralization defect.[251] In some studies bone turnover normalized,[251] but in others, there is low turnover with histology consistent with adynamic bone disease.[252] Aluminum staining resolves in the majority of patients. However, longitudinal studies are lacking. There does appear to be a consistent decrease in bone mineral content by densitometry, although more recent studies[253–255] have not found the dramatic decrease initially described,[251] perhaps due to the current practice of reducing steroid dose more rapidly. There is an increased risk of fracture, although this risk is less than that observed with other solid organ transplants.[256–260] The combination of a kidney-pancreas transplant increases fracture risk above that associated with renal transplant alone.[261]

The use of corticosteroids is the major determinant of low bone mineral content, as these agents impair calcium absorption from the gastrointestinal tract and inhibit bone cell recruitment and function.[255,262] The diagnosis of corticosteroid induced osteoporosis is best done with dual x-ray absorptiometry (DEXA) of the hips and spine for assessment of changes in trabecular bone. Osteoporosis, regardless of its etiology, is defined by the World Health Organization as a t-score less than 2.5 standard deviations from the norm, which is a young adult mean. The rationale for use of this comparison group is that it is measuring current bone mass to peak bone mass, which is obtained near ages 30 to 35. Furthermore, this value is the threshold below which there is increased fracture risk in postmenopausal women.[22] This threshold value was recently confirmed for nonrenal transplant corticosteroid induced osteoporosis.[263] However, as indicated earlier in this chapter, abnormal bone turnover may alter the predictive value of DEXA in patients with CKD and, thus, preexisting bone turnover likely affects the assessment and outcomes of bone disease in transplant recipients.

The treatment for corticosteroid induced osteoporosis is similar to that for other forms of osteoporosis: antiresorptive agents (osteoclast inhibitors), such as bisphosphonates, calcitonin, and estrogen in deficient women. There is substantial evidence from controlled trials in nontransplant corticosteroid induced osteoporosis that these agents, particularly bisphosphonates, are effective in preventing steroid induced osteoporosis.[264–266] However, there are limited data on treatments with bisphosphonates in renal transplantation recipients, and early uncontrolled data supported the use of bisphosphonates.[254,267] Recently, there have been several studies supporting the use of bisphosphonates postrenal transplant. In randomized, controlled trials, intravenous pamidronate[268,269] and zoledronic acid[270] were associated with improved bone mineral density in renal transplant recipients. In a few patients, bone biopsies demonstrated reduced activation frequency but increased trabecular thickness.[269, 270] Thus, although there is concern about potential long-term consequences, the data to date support the use of antiresorptive therapies to prevent corticosteroid induced osteoporosis. This last point deserves further emphasis: They are only effective in *preventing* bone loss and must be administered during the large dose of steroids given in the first 6 months posttransplant. Furthermore, in a long-term (4 years) follow-up study of 17 male renal transplant recipients, two doses of intravenous pamidronate, given at the time of transplant and 1 month later, continued to show protective effects of bone mineral density 4 years later.[268] This conservative approach of short-term, limited administration of bisphosphonates is recommended given the current practice to quickly decrease steroid dose and limited data on potential long-term adverse effects of bisphosphonates on bone histology.

CONCLUSION

Multiple abnormalities of bone and mineral metabolism are observed in patients with chronic kidney disease. Our understanding of the cellular biology of parathyroid hormone and vitamin D in the last decade have led to new therapies that allow more aggressive treatment of renal osteodystrophy with less toxicity. This latter point is particularly important with the strong data associating abnormal mineral metabolism with cardiovascular disease, the leading cause of death in dialysis patients. Although significant progress has been made in our understanding of these disease states, there is much more knowledge to be gained.

ACKNOWLEDGMENTS

This chapter is dedicated to John and Michelle Moe for their unending support and patience. The author would like to thank Michelle Murray for her expert administrative support in the preparation of this chapter.

References

1. Stehman-Breen CO, Sherrard DJ, Alem AM, et al: Risk factors for hip fracture among patients with end-stage renal disease. Kidney Int 2000; 58:2200–2205.
2. Ball AM, Gillen DL, Sherrard D, et al: Risk of hip fracture among dialysis and renal transplant recipients. JAMA 2002; 288:3014–3018.
3. Alem AM, Sherrard DJ, Gillen DL, et al: Increased risk of hip fracture among patients with end-stage renal disease. Kidney Int 2000; 58:396–399.
4. Coco M, Rush H: Increased incidence of hip fractures in dialysis patients with low serum parathyroid hormone. Am J Kidney Dis 2000; 36:1115–1121.
5. Braun J, Oldendorf M, Moshage W, et al: Electron beam computed tomography in the evaluation of cardiac calcification in chronic dialysis patients. Am J Kidney Dis 1996; 27: 394–401.
6. London GM, Guerin AP, Marchais SJ, et al: Arterial media calcification in end-stage renal disease: Impact on all-cause and cardiovascular mortality. Nephrol Dial Transplant 2003; 18: 1731–1740.
7. Boukhris R, Becker KL: Calcification of the aorta and osteoporosis. A roentgenographic study. JAMA 1972; 219:1307– 1311.
8. Banks LM, Lees B, MacSweeney JE, Stevenson JC: Effect of degenerative spinal and aortic calcification on bone density measurements in post-menopausal women: Links between osteoporosis and cardiovascular disease? European J Clin Invest 1994; 24:813–817.
9. Kiel DP, Hannan MT, Cupple LA, et al: Low bone mineral density (BMD) is associated with coronary artery calcification. JBMR 2000; 15:S160.
10. Hak AE, Pols HA, van Hemert AM, et al: Progression of aortic calcification is associated with metacarpal bone loss during menopause: A population-based longitudinal study. Arteriosclerosis, Thrombosis & Vascular Biology 2000; 20: 1926–1931.
11. Moe SM, Duan D, Doehle DP, et al: Uremia induces the osteoblast differentiation factor Cbfa1 in human blood vessels. Kidney Int 2003; 63:1003-1011.
12. Parhami F, Basseri B, Hwang J, et al: High-density lipoprotein regulates calcification of vascular cells. Circ Res 2002; 91:570–576.
13. Chen NX, O'Neill KD, Duan D, Moe SM: Phosphorus and uremic serum up-regulate osteopontin expression in vascular smooth muscle cells. Kidney Int 2002; 62:1724–1731.
14. Reslerova M, Moe SM: Vascular calcification in dialysis patients: Pathogenesis and consequences. Am J Kidney Dis 2003; 41:S96–S99.
15. Jono S, McKee MD, Murry CE, et al: Phosphate regulation of vascular smooth muscle cell calcification. Circ Res 2000; 87:E10–E17.
16. Ahmed S, O'Neill KD, Hood AF, et al: Calciphylaxis is associated with hyperphosphatemia and increased osteopontin expression by vascular smooth muscle cells. Am J Kidney Dis 2001; 37:1267–1276.
17. Lowrie EG, Lew NL: Death risk in hemodialysis patients: The predictive value of commonly measured variables and an evaluation of death rate differences between facilities. Am J Kidney Dis 1990; 15:458–482.
18. Block GA, Hulbert-Shearon TE, Levin NW, Port FK: Association of serum phosphorus and calcium x phosphate product with mortality risk in chronic hemodialysis patients: A national study. Am J Kidney Dis 1998; 31:607–617.
19. Delling G, Amling M: Biomechanical stability of the skeleton: It is not only bone mass, but also bone structure that counts. Nephrol Dial Transplant 1995; 10:601–606.
20. Moe S, Drueke T: Controversies in mineral metabolism in chronic kidney disease: A bridge to improving healthcare outcomes and quality of life in patients with CKD. Am J Kidney Dis 2004; 43:S52-S57.
21. Cunningham J, Sprague SM Cannata-Andia J, et al: Osteoporosis in chronic kidney disease. Am J Kidney Dis 2004; 43: S66-S71.
22. Hui SL, Slemenda CW, Johnston CC Jr: Age and bone mass as predictors of fracture in a prospective study. J Clin Invest 1988; 81:1804–1809.
23. Stehman-Breen CO, Gillen D, Gipson D: Prescription of hormone replacement therapy in postmenopausal women with renal failure. Kidney Int 1999; 56:2243–2247.
24. Baszko-Blaszyk D, Grzegorzewska AE, Horst-Sikorska W, Sowinski J: Bone mass in chronic renal insufficiency patients treated with continuous ambulatory peritoneal dialysis. Adv Perit Dial 2001; 17:109–113.
25. Fontaine MA, Albert A, Dubois B, et al: Fracture and bone mineral density in hemodialysis patients. Clin Nephrol 2000; 54:218–226.
26. Stehman-Breen C: Bone mineral density measurements in dialysis patients. Semin Dial 2001; 14:228–229.
27. Urena P, Bernard-Poenaru O, Ostertag A, et al: Bone mineral density, biochemical markers and skeletal fractures in haemodialysis patients. Nephrol Dial Transplant 2003; 18:2325– 2331.
28. Taal MW, Roe S, Masud T, et al: Total hip bone mass predicts survival in chronic hemodialysis patients. Kidney Int 2003; 63:1116–1120.
29. Martin KJ, Hruska KA, Lewis J, et al: The renal handling of parathyroid hormone. Role of peritubular uptake and glomerular filtration. J Clin Invest 1977; 60:808–814.
30. Segre GV, Perkins AS, Witters LA, Potts J Jr: Metabolism of parathyroid hormone by isolated rat Kupffer cells and hepatocytes. J Clin Invest 1981; 67:449–457.

31. Brown EM, Gamba G, Riccardi D, et al: Cloning and characterization of an extracellular Ca(2+)-sensing receptor from bovine parathyroid. Nature 1993; 366:575–580.
32. Pollak MR, Brown EM, Chou YH, et al: Mutations in the human Ca(2+)-sensing receptor gene cause familial hypocalciuric hypercalcemia and neonatal severe hyperparathyroidism. Cell 1993; 75:1297–1303.
33. Pollak MR, Brown EM, Estep HL, et al: Autosomal dominant hypocalcaemia caused by a Ca(2+)-sensing receptor gene mutation. Nat Genet 1994; 8:303–307.
34. Hebert SC: Extracellular calcium-sensing receptor: Implications for calcium and magnesium handling in the kidney. Kidney Int 1996; 50:2129–2139.
35. Brown EM, Pollak M, Hebert SC: Sensing of extracellular Ca2+ by parathyroid and kidney cells: Cloning and characterization of an extracellular Ca(2+)-sensing receptor. Am J Kidney Dis 1995; 25:506–513.
36. Drueke TB: Cell biology of parathyroid gland hyperplasia in chronic renal failure. J Am Soc Nephrol 2000; 11:1141–1152.
37. Naveh-Many T, Rahamimov R, Livni N, Silver J: Parathyroid cell proliferation in normal and chronic renal failure rats. The effects of calcium, phosphate, and vitamin D. J Clin Invest 1995; 96:1786–1793.
38. Moallem E, Kilav R, Silver J, Naveh-Many T: RNA-protein binding and post-transcriptional regulation of parathyroid hormone gene expression by calcium and phosphate. J Biol Chem 1998; 273:5253–5259.
39. Yalcindag C, Silver J, Naveh-Many T: Mechanism of increased parathyroid hormone mRNA in experimental uremia: Roles of protein RNA binding and RNA degradation. J Am Soc Nephrol 1999; 10:2562–2568.
40. Brown AJ, Ritter CS, Finch JL, Slatopolsky EA: Decreased calcium-sensing receptor expression in hyperplastic parathyroid glands of uremic rats: Role of dietary phosphate. Kidney Int 1999; 55:1284–1292.
41. Slatopolsky E, Weerts C, Thielan J, et al: Marked suppression of secondary hyperparathyroidism by intravenous administration of 1,25-dihydroxy-cholecalciferol in uremic patients. J Clin Invest 1984; 74:2136–2143.
42. Delmez JA, Tindira C, Grooms P, et al: Parathyroid hormone suppression by intravenous 1,25-dihydroxy-vitamin D. A role for increased sensitivity to calcium. J Clin Invest 1989; 83: 1349–1355.
43. Ouseph R, Leiser JD, Moe SM: Calcitriol and the parathyroid hormone-ionized calcium curve: A comparison of methodologic approaches. J Am Soc Nephrol 1996; 7:497–505.
44. Almaden Y, Hernandez A, Torregrosa V, et al: High phosphate level directly stimulates parathyroid hormone secretion and synthesis by human parathyroid tissue in vitro. J Am Soc Nephrol 1998; 9:1845–1852.
45. de Francisco AL, Cobo MA, Setien MA, et al: Effect of serum phosphate on parathyroid hormone secretion during hemodialysis. Kidney Int 1998; 54:2140–2145.
46. Felsenfeld AJ, Rodriguez M: Phosphorus, regulation of plasma calcium, and secondary hyperparathyroidism: A hypothesis to integrate a historical and modern perspective. J Am Soc Nephrol 1999; 10:878–890.
47. Juppner H, Abou-Samra AB, Freeman M, et al: A G protein-linked receptor for parathyroid hormone and parathyroid hormone-related peptide. Science 1991; 254:1024–1026.
48. Massry SG: Neurotoxicity of parathyroid hormone in uremia. Kidney Int Suppl 1985; 17:S5–S11.
49. Slatopolsky E, Martin K, Hruska K: Parathyroid hormone metabolism and its potential as a uremic toxin. Am J Physiol 1980; 239:F1–F12.
50. Potts JT Jr: Non-traditional actions of parathyroid hormone: An overview. Miner Electrolyte Metab 1995; 21:9–12.
51. Feinfeld D: The role of parathyroid hormone as a uremic toxin: Current concepts. Semin Dial 1992; 5:48–53.
52. Endres DB, Villanueva R, Sharp CF Jr, Singer FR: Measurement of parathyroid hormone. Endocrinol Metab Clin North Am 1989; 18:611–629.
53. Cohen-Solal ME, Sebert JL, Boudailliez B: Comparison of intact, midregion, and carboxy-terminal assays of parathyroid hormone for the diagnosis of bone disease in hemodialyzed patients. J Clin Endocrinol Metab 1991; 73:516–524.
54. Wang M, Hercz G, Sherrard DJ, et al: Relationship between intact 1–84 parathyroid hormone and bone histomorphometric parameters in dialysis patients without aluminum toxicity. Am J Kidney Dis 1995; 26:836–844.
55. Qi Q, Monier-Faugere MC, Geng Z, Malluche HH: Predictive value of serum parathyroid hormone levels for bone turnover in patients on chronic maintenance dialysis. Am J Kidney Dis 1995; 26:622–631.
56. Sawaya BP, Butros R, Naqvi S, et al: Differences in bone turnover and intact PTH levels between African American and Caucasian patients with end-stage renal disease. Kidney Int 2003; 64:737–742.
57. Gao P, Scheibel S, D'Amour P, et al: Development of a novel immunoradiometric assay exclusively for biologically active whole parathyroid hormone 1–84: Implications for improvement of accurate assessment of parathyroid function. J Bone Miner Res 2001; 16:605–614.
58. Slatopolsky E, Finch J, Clay P, et al: A novel mechanism for skeletal resistance in uremia. Kidney Int 2000; 58:753–761.
59. Malluche HH, Mawad H, Trueba D, Monier-Faugere MC: Parathyroid hormone assays: Evolution and revolutions in the care of dialysis patients. Clin Nephrol 2003; 59:313–318.
60. John MR, Goodman WG, Gao P, et al: A novel immunoradiometric assay detects full-length human PTH but not amino-terminally truncated fragments: Implications for PTH measurements in renal failure. J Clin Endocrinol Metab 1999; 84:4287–4290.
61. Monier-Faugere MC, Geng Z, Mawad H, et al: Improved assessment of bone turnover by the PTH-(1–84)/large C-PTH fragments ratio in ESRD patients. Kidney Int 2001; 60:1460–1468.
62. Coen G, Bonucci E, Ballanti P, et al: PTH 1–84 and PTH "7–84" in the noninvasive diagnosis of renal bone disease. Am J Kidney Dis 2002; 40:348–354.
63. Salusky IB, Goodman WG, Kuizon BD, et al: Similar predictive value of bone turnover using first- and second-generation immunometric PTH assays in pediatric patients treated with peritoneal dialysis. Kidney Int 2003; 63:1801–1808.
64. Santamaria R, Almaden Y, Felsenfeld A, et al: Dynamics of PTH secretion in hemodialysis patients as determined by the intact and whole PTH assays. Kidney Int 2003; 64:1867– 1873.
65. Brickman AS, Coburn JW, Massry SG, Norman AW: 1,25 Dihydroxyvitamin D3 in normal man and patients with renal failure. Ann Intern Med 1974; 80:161–168.
66. Delmez JA, Slatopolsky E: Hyperphosphatemia: Its consequences and treatment in patients with chronic renal disease. Am J Kidney Dis 1992; 19:303–317.
67. Silver J, Naveh-Many T, Mayer H, et al: Regulation by vitamin D metabolites of parathyroid hormone gene transcription in vivo in the rat. J Clin Invest 1986; 78:1296–1301.
68. Roodman GD, Ibbotson KJ, MacDonald BR, et al: 1,25-Dihydroxyvitamin D3 causes formation of multinucleated cells with several osteoclast characteristics in cultures of primate marrow. Proc Natl Acad Sci U S A 1985; 82: 8213–8217.
69. Holick MF, Krane SM, Potts JT Jr: Calcium, Phosphorus, and Bone Metabolism: Calcium-Regulating Hormones. New York, McGraw-Hill, 1994.
70. Holick MF: Vitamin D: Photobiology, Metabolism, Mechanism of Action, and Clinical Applications, 4th ed. Philadelphia, Lippincott Williams & Wilkins, 1999.

71. Gal-Moscovici A, Rubinger D, Popovtzer MM: 24,25-Dihydroxyvitamin D3 in combination with 1,25-dihydroxy vitamin D3 ameliorates renal osteodystrophy in rats with chronic renal failure. Clin Nephrol 2000; 53:362–371.
72. Milde P, Merke J, Ritz E, et al: Immunohistochemical detection of 1,25-dihydroxyvitamin D3 receptors and estrogen receptors by monoclonal antibodies: Comparison of four immunoperoxidase methods. J Histochem Cytochem 1989; 37:1609–1617.
73. Berger U, Wilson P, McClelland RA, et al: Immunocytochemical detection of 1,25-dihydroxyvitamin D receptors in normal human tissues. J Clin Endocrinol Metab 1988; 67:607– 613.
74. Rice JS, Haverty T: Vitamin D and immune function in uremia. Semin Cell Biol 1990; 3:237–239.
75. Reichel H, Koeffler HP, Norman AW: The role of the vitamin D endocrine system in health and disease (see comments). N Engl J Med 1989; 320:980–991.
76. Levitan IB: It is calmodulin after all! Mediator of the calcium modulation of multiple ion channels. Neuron 1999; 22:645–648.
77. Hoenderop JG, van der Kemp AW, Hartog A, et al: Molecular identification of the apical Ca2+ channel in 1, 25-dihydroxyvitamin D3-responsive epithelia. J Biol Chem 1999; 274:8375–8378.
78. Teitelbaum SL: Bone resorption by osteoclasts. Science 2000; 289:1504–1508.
79. Rodan GA, Martin TJ: Role of osteoblasts in hormonal control of bone resorption: A hypothesis. Calcif Tissue Int 1981; 33: 349–351.
80. Turner CH, Chandran A, Pidaparti RM: The anisotropy of osteonal bone and its ultrastructural implications. Bone 1995; 17:85–89.
81. Bonn D: Crumbling bones yield to molecular biology. Lancet 1999; 353:1596.
82. Blair HC: How the osteoclast degrades bone. Bioessays 1998; 20:837–846.
83. Parfitt AM: Targeted and nontargeted bone remodeling: Relationship to basic multicellular unit origination and progression. Bone 2002; 30:5–7.
84. Hofbauer LC, Khosla S, Dunstan CR, et al: The roles of osteoprotegerin and osteoprotegerin ligand in the paracrine regulation of bone resorption. J Bone Miner Res 2000; 15:2–12.
85. Lories RJ, Luyten FP: Osteoprotegerin and osteoprotegerin-ligand balance: A new paradigm in bone metabolism providing new therapeutic targets. Clin Rheumatol 2001; 20:3–9.
86. Sasaki N, Kusano E, et al: Glucocorticoid decreases circulating osteoprotegerin (OPG): Possible mechanism for glucocorticoid induced osteoporosis. Nephrol Dial Transplant 2001; 16:479–482.
87. Simonet WS, Lacey DL, Dunstan CR, et al: Osteoprotegerin: A novel secreted protein involved in the regulation of bone density. Cell 1997; 89:309–319.
88. Akatsu T, Murakami T, Ono K, et al: Osteoclastogenesis inhibitory factor exhibits hypocalcemic effects in normal mice and in hypercalcemic nude mice carrying tumors associated with humoral hypercalcemia of malignancy. Bone 1998; 23: 495–498.
89. Bekker PJ, Holloway D, Nakanishi A, et al: The effect of a single dose of osteoprotegerin in postmenopausal women. J Bone Miner Res 2001; 16:348–360.
90. Kazama JJ, Shigematsu T, Tsuda E, et al: Increased circulating osteoprotegerin/osteoclastogenesis inhibitory factor (OPG/OCIF) in patients with chronic renal failure. Am J Kidney Dis 2002; 39:525–537.
91. Parfitt AM, Drezner MK, Glorieux FH, et al: Bone histomorphometry: Standardization of nomenclature, symbols, and units. Report of the ASBMR Histomorphometry Nomenclature Committee. J Bone Miner Res 1987; 2:595–610.
92. Sherrard DJ, Hercz G, Pei Y, et al: The spectrum of bone disease in end-stage renal failure: An evolving disorder. Kidney Int 1993; 43:436–442.
93. Sprague SM: The role of the bone biopsy in the diagnosis of renal osteodystrophy. Semin Dial 2000; 13:152–155.
94. Llach F, Felsenfeld AJ, Coleman MD, et al: The natural course of dialysis osteomalacia. Kidney Int Suppl 1986; 18:S74–S79.
95. Faugere MC, Malluche HH: Stainable aluminum and not aluminum content reflects bone histology in dialyzed patients. Kidney Int 1986; 30:717–722.
96. Changsirikulchai S, Domrongkitchaiporn S, Sirikulchayanonta V, et al: Renal osteodystrophy in Ramathibodi Hospital: Histomorphometry and clinical correlation. J Med Assoc Thai 2000; 83:1223–1232.
97. Gal-Moscovici A, Popovtzer MM: Parathyroid hormone-independent osteoclastic resorptive bone disease: A new variant of adynamic bone disease in haemodialysis patients. Nephrol Dial Transplant 2002; 17:620–624.
98. D'Haese PC, Spasovski GB, Sikole A, et al: A multicenter study on the effects of lanthanum carbonate (fosrenol) and calcium carbonate on renal bone disease in dialysis patients. Kidney Int Suppl 2003:S73–S78.
99. Ingham JP, Stewart JH, Posen S: Quantitative skeletal histology in untreated end-stage renal failure. Br Med J 1973; 2: 745–748.
100. Eastwood JB: Quantitative bone histology in 38 patients with advanced renal failure. J Clin Pathol 1982; 35:125–134.
101. Dahl E, Nordal KP, Attramadal A, et al: Renal osteodystrophy in predialysis patients without stainable bone aluminum. A cross-sectional bone-histomorphometric study. Acta Med Scand 1988; 224:157–164.
102. Hernandez D, Concepcion MT, Lorenzo V, et al: Adynamic bone disease with negative aluminum staining in predialysis patients: Prevalence and evolution after maintenance dialysis. Nephrol Dial Transplant 1994; 9:517–523.
103. Torres A, Lorenzo V, Hernandez D, et al: Bone disease in predialysis, hemodialysis, and CAPD patients: Evidence of a better bone response to PTH. Kidney Int 1995; 47:1434–1442.
104. Coen G, Mazzaferro S, Ballanti P, et al: Renal bone disease in 76 patients with varying degrees of predialysis chronic renal failure: A cross-sectional study. Nephrol Dial Transplant 1996; 11:813–819.
105. Spasovski GB, Bervoets AR, Behets GJ, et al: Spectrum of renal bone disease in end-stage renal failure patients not yet on dialysis. Nephrol Dial Transplant 2003; 18:1159–1166.
106. K/DOQI NKF: Clinical practice guidelines for bone metabolism and disease in chronic kidney disease. Am J Kidney Dis 2003; 42:S1–S201.
107. Urena P, De Vernejoul MC: Circulating biochemical markers of bone remodeling in uremic patients. Kidney Int 1999; 55: 2141–2156.
108. Bervoets AR, Spasovski GB, Behets GJ, et al: Useful biochemical markers for diagnosing renal osteodystrophy in predialysis end-stage renal failure patients. Am J Kidney Dis 2003; 41:997–1007.
109. Chu P, Chao TY, Lin YF, et al: Correlation between histomorphometric parameters of bone resorption and serum type 5b tartrate-resistant acid phosphatase in uremic patients on maintenance hemodialysis. Am J Kidney Dis 2003; 41: 1052–1059.
110. Kurz P, Monier-Faugere MC, Bognar B, et al: Evidence for abnormal calcium homeostasis in patients with adynamic bone disease. Kidney Int 1994; 46:855–861.
111. Milliner DS, Nebeker HG, Ott SM, et al: Use of the deferoxamine infusion test in the diagnosis of aluminum-related osteodystrophy. Ann Intern Med 1984; 101:775–779.
112. Pei Y, Hercz G, Greenwood C, et al: Non-invasive prediction of aluminum bone disease in hemo- and peritoneal dialysis patients. Kidney Int 1992; 41:1374–1382.
113. Slatopolsky E, Bricker NS: The role of phosphorus restriction in the prevention of secondary hyperparathyroidism in chronic renal disease. Kidney Int 1973; 4:141–145.

114. Feinfeld DA, Sherwood LM: Parathyroid hormone and 1,25(OH)2D3 in chronic renal failure. Kidney Int 1988; 33: 1049–1058.
115. Slatopolsky E, Finch J, Denda M, et al: Phosphorus restriction prevents parathyroid gland growth. High phosphorus directly stimulates PTH secretion in vitro. J Clin Invest 1996; 97: 2534–2540.
116. Portale AA, Halloran BP, Morris RC Jr: Physiologic regulation of the serum concentration of 1,25-dihydroxyvitamin D by phosphorus in normal men. J Clin Invest 1989; 83:1494–1499.
117. Lopez-Hilker S, Dusso AS, Rapp NS, et al: Phosphorus restriction reverses hyperparathyroidism in uremia independent of changes in calcium and calcitriol. Am J Physiol 1990; 259: F432–F437.
118. Combe C, Aparicio M: Phosphorus and protein restriction and parathyroid function in chronic renal failure. Kidney Int 1994; 46:1381–1386.
119. Silver J, Moallem E, Kilav R, et al: New insights into the regulation of parathyroid hormone synthesis and secretion in chronic renal failure. Nephrol Dial Transplant 1996; 11(suppl 3):2–5.
120. Nordin BE: Absorption of Calcium, Phosphorus and Magnesium. New York, Churchill Livingstone, 1976.
121. Delmez JA: Avoiding renal osteodystrophy in peritoneal dialysis patients. Semin Dial 1995; 8:373–377.
122. Slatopolsky E, Robson AM, Elkan I, Bricker NS: Control of phosphate excretion in uremic man. J Clin Invest 1968; 47: 1865–1874.
123. Brenner BM: Disturbances of Renal Function. New York, McGraw-Hill, 1994.
124. Slatopolsky E, Brown A, Dusso A: Role of phosphorus in the pathogenesis of secondary hyperparathyroidism. Am J Kidney Dis 2001; 37:S54–S57.
125. Malabanan A, Veronikis IE, Holick MF: Redefining vitamin D insufficiency. Lancet 1998; 351:805–806.
126. Koenig KG, Lindberg JS, Zerwekh JE, et al: Free and total 1,25-dihydroxyvitamin D levels in subjects with renal disease. Kidney Int 1992; 41:161–165.
127. Ishimura E, Nishizawa Y, Inaba M, et al: Serum levels of 1, 25-dihydroxyvitamin D, 24,25-dihydroxyvitamin D, and 25-hydroxyvitamin D in nondialyzed patients with chronic renal failure. Kidney Int 1999; 55:1019–1027.
128. Christiansen C, Rodbro P, Christensen MS, et al: Deterioration of renal function during treatment of chronic renal failure with 1,25-dihydroxycholecalciferol. Lancet 1978; 2:700–703.
129. Maung HM, Elangovan L, Frazao JM, et al: Efficacy and side effects of intermittent intravenous and oral doxercalciferol (1alpha-hydroxyvitamin D[2]) in dialysis patients with secondary hyperparathyroidism: A sequential comparison. Am J Kidney Dis 2001; 37:532–543.
130. Baker LR, Abrams L, Roe CJ, et al: 1,25(OH)2D3 administration in moderate renal failure: A prospective double-blind trial. Kidney Int 1989; 35:661–669.
131. Kopple JD: National Kidney Foundation K/DOQI clinical practice guidelines for nutrition in chronic renal failure. Am J Kidney Dis 2001; 37:S66–S70.
132. Blumenkrantz MJ, Kopple JD, Moran JK, Coburn JW: Metabolic balance studies and dietary protein requirements in patients undergoing continuous ambulatory peritoneal dialysis. Kidney Int 1982; 21:849–861.
133. Pastan S, Bailey J: Dialysis therapy. N Engl J Med 1998; 338:1428–1437.
134. Hou SH, Zhao J, Ellman CF, et al: Calcium and phosphorus fluxes during hemodialysis with low calcium dialysate. Am J Kidney Dis 1991; 18:217–224.
135. Zucchelli P, Santoro A: Inorganic phosphate removal during different dialytic procedures. Int J Artif Organs 1987; 10:173–178.
136. Haas T, Hillion D, Dongradi G: Phosphate kinetics in dialysis patients. Nephrol Dial Transplant 1991; 6:108–113.
137. Winchester JF, Rotellar C, Goggins M, et al: Calcium and phosphate balance in dialysis patients. Kidney Int Suppl 1993; 41:S174–S178.
138. Mucsi I, Hercz G, Uldall R, et al: Control of serum phosphate without any phosphate binders in patients treated with nocturnal hemodialysis. Kidney Int 1998; 53:1399–1404.
139. Kates DM: Control of hyperphosphatemia in renal failure: Role of aluminum. Semin Dial 1996; 9:310–315.
140. Nebeker HG, Coburn JW: Aluminum and renal osteodystrophy. Annu Rev Med 1986; 37:79–95.
141. Andress DL: Aluminum bone disease in chronic renal failure. Semin Dial 1990; 3:27–32.
142. Andreoli SP, Bergstein JM, Sherrard DJ: Aluminum intoxication from aluminum-containing phosphate binders in children with azotemia not undergoing dialysis. N Engl J Med 1984; 310:1079–1084.
143. Slatopolsky E, Weerts C, Lopez-Hilker S, et al: Calcium carbonate as a phosphate binder in patients with chronic renal failure undergoing dialysis. N Engl J Med 1986; 315:157–161.
144. Emmett M, Sirmon MD, Kirkpatrick WG, et al: Calcium acetate control of serum phosphorus in hemodialysis patients. Am J Kidney Dis 1991; 17:544–550.
145. Sheikh MS, Maguire JA, Emmett M, et al: Reduction of dietary phosphorus absorption by phosphorus binders. A theoretical, in vitro, and in vivo study. J Clin Invest 1989; 83:66–73.
146. Mai ML, Emmett M, Sheikh MS, et al: Calcium acetate, an effective phosphorus binder in patients with renal failure. Kidney Int 1989; 36:690–695.
147. d'Almeida Filho EJ, da Cruz EA, Hoette M, et al: Calcium acetate versus calcium carbonate in the control of hyperphosphatemia in hemodialysis patients. Sao Paulo Med J 2000; 118:179–184.
148. Macia M, Coronel F, Navarro JF, et al: Calcium salts of ketoamino acids, a phosphate binder alternative for patients on CAPD. Clin Nephrol 1997; 48:181–184.
149. Schaefer K, von Herrath D, Erley CM, Asmus G: Calcium ketovaline as new therapy for uremic hyperphosphatemia. Miner Electrolyte Metab 1990; 16:362–364.
150. Nolan CR, Califano JR, Butzin CA: Influence of calcium acetate or calcium citrate on intestinal aluminum absorption. Kidney Int 1990; 38:937–941.
151. Heaney R, Skillman T: Secretion and excretion of calcium by the human gastrointestinal tract. J Lab Clin Med 1964; 64:29–41.
152. Institute of Medicine: Dietary References Intakes: Calcium, Phosphorus, Magnesium, Vitamin D, and Fluoride. Washington D. C., National Academy Press, 1997.
153. Coburn JW, Hartenbower DL, Massry SG: Intestinal absorption of calcium and the effect of renal insufficiency. Kidney Int 1973; 4:96–104.
154. Coburn JW, Koppel MH, Brickman AS, Massry SG: Study of intestinal absorption of calcium in patients with renal failure. Kidney Int 1973; 3:264–272.
155. Bender FH, Bernardini J, Piraino B: Calcium mass transfer with dialysate containing 1.25 and 1.75 mmol/L calcium in peritoneal dialysis patients. Am J Kidney Dis 1992; 20: 367–371.
156. Chertow GM, Burke SK, Lazarus JM, et al: Poly[allylamine hydrochloride] (RenaGel): A noncalcemic phosphate binder for the treatment of hyperphosphatemia in chronic renal failure. Am J Kidney Dis 1997; 29:66–71.
157. Slatopolsky EA, Burke SK, Dillon MA: RenaGel, a nonabsorbed calcium- and aluminum-free phosphate binder, lowers serum phosphorus and parathyroid hormone. The RenaGel Study Group. Kidney Int 1999; 55:299–307.
158. Bleyer AJ, Burke SK, Dillon M, et al: A comparison of the calcium-free phosphate binder sevelamer hydrochloride with calcium acetate in the treatment of hyperphosphatemia in hemodialysis patients. Am J Kidney Dis 1999; 33:694–701.

159. Chertow GM, Burke SK, Raggi P: Sevelamer attenuates the progression of coronary and aortic calcification in hemodialysis patients. Kidney Int 2002; 62:245–252.
160. Chertow GM, Dillon M, Burke SK, et al: A randomized trial of sevelamer hydrochloride (RenaGel) with and without supplemental calcium. Strategies for the control of hyperphosphatemia and hyperparathyroidism in hemodialysis patients. Clin Nephrol 1999; 51:18–26.
161. Burke SK, Dillon MA, Hemken DE, et al: Meta-analysis of the effect of sevelamer on phosphorus, calcium, PTH, and serum lipids in dialysis patients. Adv Ren Replace Ther 2003; 10: 133–145.
162. Chertow GM, Raggi P, McCarthy JT, et al: The effects of sevelamer and calcium acetate on proxies of atherosclerotic and arteriosclerotic vascular disease in hemodialysis patients. Am J Nephrol 2003; 23:307–314.
163. Graff L, Burnel D: A possible non-aluminum oral phosphate binder? A comparative study on dietary phosphorus absorption. Res Commun Mol Pathol Pharmacol 1995; 89: 373–388.
164. Dewberry K, Fox J, Stewart J, et al: Lanthanum carbonate: A novel non-calcium containing phosphate binder. J Am Soc Neph 1997; 8:A2610.
165. Joy MS, Finn WF: Randomized, double-blind, placebo-controlled, dose-titration, phase III study assessing the efficacy and tolerability of lanthanum carbonate: A new phosphate binder for the treatment of hyperphosphatemia. Am J Kidney Dis 2003; 42:96–107.
166. Delmez JA, Kelber J, Norword KY, et al: Magnesium carbonate as a phosphorus binder: A prospective, controlled, crossover study. Kidney Int 1996; 49:163–167.
167. Hsu CH, Patel SR, Young EW: New phosphate binding agents: Ferric compounds. J Am Soc Nephrol 1999; 10:1274–1280.
168. Hergesell O, Ritz E: Stabilized polynuclear iron hydroxide is an efficient oral phosphate binder in uraemic patients. Nephrol Dial Transplant 1999; 14:863–867.
169. Chang JM, Hwang SJ, Tsai JC, et al: Effect of ferric polymaltose complex as a phosphate binder in haemodialysis patients (Letter). Nephrol Dial Transplant 1999; 14:1045–1047.
170. Zhu H, Webb M, Buckley J, Roberts NB: Different Mg to Fe ratios in the mixed metal MgFe hydroxy-carbonate compounds and the effect on phosphate binding compared with established phosphate binders. J Pharm Sci 2002; 91:53–66.
171. Berl T, Berns AS, Hufer WE, et al: 1,25 Dihydroxycholecalciferol effects in chronic dialysis. A double-blind controlled study. Ann Intern Med 1978; 88:774–780.
172. Andress DL, Norris KC, Coburn JW, et al: Intravenous calcitriol in the treatment of refractory osteitis fibrosa of chronic renal failure (see comments). N Engl J Med 1989; 321:274–279.
173. Sprague SM, Moe SM: Safety and efficacy of long-term treatment of secondary hyperparathyroidism by low-dose intravenous calcitriol. Am J Kidney Dis 1992; 19:532–539.
174. Tsukamoto Y, Nomura M, Takahashi Y, et al: The "oral 1,25-dihydroxyvitamin D3 pulse therapy" in hemodialysis patients with severe secondary hyperparathyroidism. Nephron 1991; 57:23–28.
175. Quarles LD, Yohay DA, Carroll BA, et al: Prospective trial of pulse oral versus intravenous calcitriol treatment of hyperparathyroidism in ESRD. Kidney Int 1994; 45:1710–1721.
176. Levine BS, Song M: Pharmacokinetics and efficacy of pulse oral versus intravenous calcitriol in hemodialysis patients. J Am Soc Nephrol 1996; 7:488–496.
177. Moe SM, Kraus MA, Gassensmith CM, et al: Safety and efficacy of pulse and daily calcitriol in patients on CAPD: A randomized trial. Nephrol Dial Transplant 1998; 13:1234–1241.
178. Herrmann P, Ritz E, Schmidt-Gayk H, et al: Comparison of intermittent and continuous oral administration of calcitriol in dialysis patients: A randomized prospective trial. Nephron 1994; 67:48–53.
179. Drueke TB: Parathyroid gland hyperplasia in uremia. Kidney Int 2001; 59:1182–1183.
180. Brown AJ, Dusso AS, Slatopolsky E: Vitamin D analogues for secondary hyperparathyroidism. Nephrol Dial Transplant 2002; 17(suppl 10):10–19.
181. Martin KJ, Gonzalez EA, Gellens M, et al: 19-Nor-1-alpha-25-dihydroxyvitamin D2 (Paricalcitol) safely and effectively reduces the levels of intact parathyroid hormone in patients on hemodialysis. J Am Soc Nephrol 1998; 9:1427–1432.
182. Frazao JM, Chesney RW, Coburn JW: Intermittent oral 1-alpha-hydroxyvitamin D2 is effective and safe for the suppression of secondary hyperparathyroidism in haemodialysis patients. 1alphaD2 Study Group. Nephrol Dial Transplant 1998; 13(suppl 3):68–72.
183. Frazao JM, Elangovan L, Maung HM, et al: Intermittent doxercalciferol (1alpha-hydroxyvitamin D[2]) therapy for secondary hyperparathyroidism. Am J Kidney Dis 2000; 36:550–561.
184. Tan AU Jr, Levine BS, Mazess RB, et al: Effective suppression of parathyroid hormone by 1 alpha-hydroxy-vitamin D2 in hemodialysis patients with moderate to severe secondary hyperparathyroidism. Kidney Int 1997; 51:317–323.
185. Akiba T, Marumo F, Owada A, et al: Controlled trial of falecalcitriol versus alfacalcidol in suppression of parathyroid hormone in hemodialysis patients with secondary hyperparathyroidism. Am J Kidney Dis 1998; 32:238–246.
186. Yasuda M, Akiba T, Nihei H: Multicenter clinical trial of 22-oxa-1,25-dihydroxyvitamin D3 for chronic dialysis patients. Am J Kidney Dis 2003; 41:S108–S111.
187. Slatopolsky E, Finch J, Ritter C, et al: A new analog of calcitriol, 19-nor-1,25-(OH)2D2, suppresses parathyroid hormone secretion in uremic rats in the absence of hypercalcemia. Am J Kidney Dis 1995; 26:852–860.
188. Coyne DW, Grieff M, Ahya SN, et al: Differential effects of acute administration of 19-Nor-1,25-dihydroxy-vitamin D2 and 1,25-dihydroxy-vitamin D3 on serum calcium and phosphorus in hemodialysis patients. Am J Kidney Dis 2002; 40: 1283–1288.
189. Sprague SM, Llach F, Amdahl M, et al: Paricalcitol versus calcitriol in the treatment of secondary hyperparathyroidism. Kidney Int 2003; 63:1483–1490.
190. Teng M, Wolf M, Lowrie E, et al: Survival of patients undergoing hemodialysis with paricalcitol or calcitriol therapy. N Engl J Med 2003; 349:446–456.
191. Drueke TB, McCarron DA: Paricalcitol as compared with calcitriol in patients undergoing hemodialysis. N Engl J Med 2003; 349:496–499.
192. Moe SM, Zekonis M, Harezlak J, et al: A placebo-controlled trial to evaluate immunomodulatory effects of paricalcitol. Am J Kidney Dis 2001; 38:792–802.
193. Katoh N, Nakayama M, Shigematsu T, et al: Presence of sonographically detectable parathyroid glands can predict resistance to oral pulsed-dose calcitriol treatment of secondary hyperparathyroidism. Am J Kidney Dis 2000; 35:465–468.
194. Malluche H: Renal bone disease 1982 to 1994: Continued need for bone biopsies. Mediguide to Nephrology 1995; 3:1–8.
195. Wada M, Nagano N, Furuya Y, et al: Calcimimetic NPS R-568 prevents parathyroid hyperplasia in rats with severe secondary hyperparathyroidism. Kidney Int 2000; 57:50–58.
196. Chin J, Miller SC, Wada M, et al: Activation of the calcium receptor by a calcimimetic compound halts the progression of secondary hyperparathyroidism in uremic rats. J Am Soc Nephrol 2000; 11:903–911.
197. Antonsen JE, Sherrard DJ, Andress DL: A calcimimetic agent acutely suppresses parathyroid hormone levels in patients with chronic renal failure. Rapid communication. Kidney Int 1998; 53:223–227.
198. Goodman WG, Frazao JM, Goodkin DA, et al: A calcimimetic agent lowers plasma parathyroid hormone levels in patients

with secondary hyperparathyroidism. Kidney Int 2000; 58: 436–445.
199. Lindberg JS, Moe SM, Goodman WG, et al: The calcimimetic AMG 073 reduces parathyroid hormone and calcium x phosphorus in secondary hyperparathyroidism. Kidney Int 2003; 63: 248–254.
200. Block GA, Martin KJ, de Francisco AL, et al: Cinacalcet for secondary hyperparathyroidism in patients receiving hemodialysis. N Engl J Med 2004; 350:1516–1525.
201. Moe SM, Coburn JW, Quarles LD, et al: Achievement of proposed NKF-K/DOQI bone metabolism and disease targets: Treatment with cinacalcet HCL in dialysis patients with uncontrolled secondary hyperparathyroidism (HPT). J Am Soc Nephrol 2003; 14:48A.
202. Alfrey AC, Mishell JM, Burks J, et al: Syndrome of dyspraxia and multifocal seizures associated with chronic hemodialysis. Transactions ASAIO J 1972; 18:257–261.
203. Alfrey AC, LeGendre GR, Kaehny WD: The dialysis encephalopathy syndrome. Possible aluminum intoxication. N Engl J Med 1976; 294:184–188.
204. Platts MM, Anastassiades E: Dialysis encephalopathy: Precipitating factors and improvement in prognosis. Clin Nephrol 1981; 15:223–228.
205. Platts MM, Goode GC, Hislop JS: Composition of the domestic water supply and the incidence of fractures and encephalopathy in patients on home dialysis. Br Med J 1977; 2:657–660.
206. Alfrey AC: Aluminum intoxication (editorial). N Engl J Med 1984; 310:1113–1115.
207. Parkinson IS, Ward MK, Feest TG, et al: Fracturing dialysis osteodystrophy and dialysis encephalopathy. An epidemiological survey. Lancet 1979; 1:406–409.
208. Burgess E, Muruve D, Audette R: Aluminum absorption and excretion following sucralfate therapy in chronic renal insufficiency. Am J Med 1992; 92:471–475.
209. Andress DL, Kopp JB, Maloney NA, et al: Early deposition of aluminum in bone in diabetic patients on hemodialysis. N Engl J Med 1987; 316:292–296.
210. Kausz AT, Antonsen JE, Hercz G, et al: Screening plasma aluminum levels in relation to aluminum bone disease among asymptomatic dialysis patients. Am J Kidney Dis 1999; 34: 688–693.
211. Andress DL, Nebeker HG, Ott SM, et al: Bone histologic response to deferoxamine in aluminum-related bone disease. Kidney Int 1987; 31:1344–1350.
212. Boelaert JR, Fenves AZ, Coburn JW: Deferoxamine therapy and mucormycosis in dialysis patients: Report of an international registry. Am J Kidney Dis 1991; 18:660–667.
213. Moriniere P, Cohen-Solal M, Belbrik S, et al: Disappearance of aluminic bone disease in a long term asymptomatic dialysis population restricting A1(OH)3 intake: Emergence of an idiopathic adynamic bone disease not related to aluminum. Nephron 1989; 53:93–101.
214. Hutchison AJ, Whitehouse RW, Freemont AJ, et al: Histological, radiological, and biochemical features of the adynamic bone lesion in continuous ambulatory peritoneal dialysis patients. Am J Nephrol 1994; 14:19–29.
215. Malluche HH, Monier-Faugere MC: Risk of adynamic bone disease in dialyzed patients. Kidney Int Suppl 1992; 38:S62–S67.
216. Couttenye MM, D'Haese PC, Deng JT, et al: High prevalence of adynamic bone disease diagnosed by biochemical markers in a wide sample of the European CAPD population. Nephrol Dial Transplant 1997; 12:2144–2150.
217. Picton ML, Moore PR, Mawer EB, et al: Down-regulation of human osteoblast PTH/PTHrP receptor mRNA in end-stage renal failure. Kidney Int 2000; 58:1440–1449.
218. Couttenye MM, D'Haese PC, Van Hoof VO, et al: Low serum levels of alkaline phosphatase of bone origin: A good marker of adynamic bone disease in haemodialysis patients. Nephrol Dial Transplant 1996; 11:1065–1072.
219. Gupta A, Kallenbach LR, Zasuwa G, Divine GW: Race is a major determinant of secondary hyperparathyroidism in uremic patients. J Am Soc Nephrol 2000; 11:330–334.
220. Goodman WG, Ramirez JA, Belin TR, et al: Development of adynamic bone in patients with secondary hyperparathyroidism after intermittent calcitriol therapy. Kidney Int 1994; 46:1160–1166.
221. Montenegro J, Saracho R, Gonzalez O, et al: Reversibility of parathyroid gland suppression in CAPD patients with low i-PTH levels. Clin Nephrol 1997; 48:359–363.
222. Moe SM, Peterson JM, Murphy CL, et al: Sevelamer HCL improves parathyroid hormone (PTH) and bone function in peritoneal dialysis (PD) patients with probable low turnover bone disease. Am J Kidney Dis 2001; 37:A25.
223. Atsumi K, Kushida K, Yamazaki K, et al: Risk factors for vertebral fractures in renal osteodystrophy. Am J Kidney Dis 1999; 33:287–293.
224. Shear M, Kramer B: Composition of bone. III. Physicochemical mechanism. J Biol Chem 1928; 79:125–145.
225. Nordin B: Primary and secondary hyperparathyroidism. Adv Intern Med 1957; 9:81–105.
226. Parfitt AM: Soft-tissue calcification in uremia. Arch Intern Med 1969; 124:544–556.
227. Bostrom K, Watson KE, Horn S, et al: Bone morphogenetic protein expression in human atherosclerotic lesions. J Clin Invest 1993; 91:1800–1809.
228. Fitzpatrick LA, Severson A, Edwards WD, Ingram RT: Diffuse calcification in human coronary arteries. Association of osteopontin with atherosclerosis. J Clin Invest 1994; 94:1597– 1604.
229. Shanahan CM, Cary NR, Metcalfe JC, Weissberg PL: High expression of genes for calcification-regulating proteins in human atherosclerotic plaques. J Clin Invest 1994; 93:2393–2402.
230. Shanahan CM, Cary NR, Salisbury JR, et al: Medial localization of mineralization-regulating proteins in association with Monckeberg's sclerosis: Evidence for smooth muscle cell-mediated vascular calcification. Circulation 1999; 100:2168–2176.
231. Proudfoot D, Shanahan CM, Weissberg PL: Vascular calcification: New insights into an old problem (editorial; comment). J Pathol 1998; 185:1–3.
232. Moe SM, Duan D, Doehle BP, et al: Uremia induces the osteoblast differentiation factor Cbfa1 in human blood vessels. Kidney Int 2003; 63:1003–1011.
233. Moe SM, Chen NX: Calciphylaxis and vascular calcification: A continuum of extra-skeletal osteogenesis. Pediatr Nephrol 2003; 18:969–975.
234. Chen N, Moe S: Vascular calcification in chronic kidney disease. Semin Nephrol 2004; 24:61–68.
235. Block GA, Klassen PS, Lazarus JM, et al. Excess mortality associated with disorders of mineral metabolism in hemodialysis. J Am Soc Nephrol (in press).
236. Ansell BM, Feest T, Taylor H: Serum phosphate and dialysis mortality in 1998: A multi-centre study from the UK. Nephrol Dial Transplant 2000:A182.
237. Winkelmayer WC, Levin R, Avorn J: The nephrologist's role in the management of calcium-phosphorus metabolism in patients with chronic kidney disease. Kidney Int 2003; 63:1836–1842.
238. Block GA, Klassen P, Danese M, et al: Association between proposed NKF-K/DOQI bone metabolism and disease guidelines and mortality risk in hemodialysis patients. J Am Soc Nephrol 2003; 14:474A.
239. London GM, Marchais SJ, Guerin AP, et al: Arterial structure and function in end-stage renal disease. Nephrol Dial Transplant 2002; 17:1713–1724.
240. Goodman WG, Goldin J, Kuizon BD, et al: Coronary-artery calcification in young adults with end-stage renal disease who are undergoing dialysis. N Engl J Med 2000; 342:1478–1483.
241. Kimura K, Saika Y, Otani H, et al: Factors associated with calcification of the abdominal aorta in hemodialysis patients. Kidney Int Suppl 1999; 71:S238–S241.

242. Marchais SJ, Metivier F, Guerin AP, London GM: Association of hyperphosphataemia with haemodynamic disturbances in end-stage renal disease. Nephrol Dial Transplant 1999; 14:2178–2183.
243. Guerin AP, London GM, Marchais SJ, Metivier F: Arterial stiffening and vascular calcifications in end-stage renal disease. Nephrol Dial Transplant 2000; 15:1014–1021.
244. Mazhar AR, Johnson RJ, Gillen D, et al: Risk factors and mortality associated with calciphylaxis in end-stage renal disease. Kidney Int 2001; 60:324–332.
245. Wang AY, Woo J, Wang M, et al: Association of inflammation and malnutrition with cardiac valve calcification in continuous ambulatory peritoneal dialysis patients. J Am Soc Nephrol 2001; 12:1927–1936.
246. Wang AY, Wang M, Woo J, et al: Cardiac valve calcification as an important predictor for all-cause mortality and cardiovascular mortality in long-term peritoneal dialysis patients: A prospective study. J Am Soc Nephrol 2003; 14:159–168.
247. Rubel JR, Milford EL: The relationship between serum calcium and phosphate levels and cardiac valvular procedures in the hemodialysis population. Am J Kidney Dis 2003; 41:411–421.
248. Giachelli CM: Vascular calcification: In vitro evidence for the role of inorganic phosphate. J Am Soc Nephrol 2003; 14: S300–S304.
249. Chen N, Moe S: Vascular calcification in chronic kidney disease. Semin Nephrol 2004; 24:61–68.
250. Block GA, Port FK: Re-evaluation of risks associated with hyperphosphatemia and hyperparathyroidism in dialysis patients: Recommendations for a change in management. Am J Kidney Dis 2000; 35:1226–1237.
251. Julian BA, Laskow DA, Dubovsky J, et al: Rapid loss of vertebral mineral density after renal transplantation. N Engl J Med 1991; 325:544–550.
252. Monier-Faugere MC, Mawad H, Qi Q, et al: High prevalence of low bone turnover and occurrence of osteomalacia after kidney transplantation. J Am Soc Nephrol 2000; 11:1093–1099.
253. Kosch M, Hausberg M, Link T, et al: Measurement of skeletal status after renal transplantation by quantitative ultrasound. Clin Nephrol 2000; 54:15–21.
254. Fan SL, Almond MK, Ball E, et al: Pamidronate therapy as prevention of bone loss following renal transplantation1 (see comments). Kidney Int 2000; 57:684–690.
255. Lindberg JS, Moe SM: Osteoporosis in end-stage renal disease. Semin Nephrol 1999; 19:115–122.
256. Grotz WH, Mundinger FA, Gugel B, et al: Bone mineral density after kidney transplantation. A cross-sectional study in 190 graft recipients up to 20 years after transplantation. Transplantation 1995; 59:982–986.
257. Grotz WH, Mundinger FA, Gugel B, et al: Bone fracture and osteodensitometry with dual energy X-ray absorptiometry in kidney transplant recipients. Transplantation 1994; 58: 912–915.
258. Epstein S, Shane E, Bilezikian JP: Organ transplantation and osteoporosis. Curr Opin Rheumatol 1995; 7:255–261.
259. Rodino MA, Shane E: Osteoporosis after organ transplantation. Am J Med 1998; 104:459–469.
260. Shane E, Rivas M, McMahon DJ, et al: Bone loss and turnover after cardiac transplantation. J Clin Endocrinol Metab 1997; 82:1497–1506.
261. Ramsey-Goldman R, Dunn JE, Dunlop DD, et al: Increased risk of fracture in patients receiving solid organ transplants. J Bone Miner Res 1999; 14:456–463.
262. Moe SM: The treatment of steroid-induced bone loss in transplantation. Curr Opin Nephrol Hypertens 1997; 6:544–549.
263. Selby PL, Halsey JP, Adams KR, et al: Corticosteroids do not alter the threshold for vertebral fracture. J Bone Miner Res 2000; 15:952–956.
264. Eastell R, Reid DM, Compston J, et al: A UK Consensus Group on management of glucocorticoid-induced osteoporosis: An update. J Intern Med 1998; 244:271–292.
265. Adachi JD, Bensen WG, Bell MJ, et al: Salmon calcitonin nasal spray in the prevention of corticosteroid-induced osteoporosis. Br J Rheumatol 1997; 36:255–259.
266. Adachi JD, Bensen WG, Brown J, et al: Intermittent etidronate therapy to prevent corticosteroid-induced osteoporosis (see comments). N Engl J Med 1997; 337:382–387.
267. Geng Z, Monier-Faugere MC, Bauss F, Malluche HH: Short-term administration of the bisphosphonate ibandronate increases bone volume and prevents hyperparathyroid bone changes in mild experimental renal failure. Clin Nephrol 2000; 54:45–53.
268. Fan SL, Kumar S, Cunningham J: Long-term effects on bone mineral density of pamidronate given at the time of renal transplantation. Kidney Int 2003; 63:2275–2279.
269. Coco M, Glicklich D, Faugere MC, et al: Prevention of bone loss in renal transplant recipients: A prospective, randomized trial of intravenous pamidronate. J Am Soc Nephrol 2003; 14: 2669–2676.
270. Haas M, Leko-Mohr Z, Roschger P, et al: Zoledronic acid to prevent bone loss in the first 6 months after renal transplantation. Kidney Int 2003; 63:1130–1136.
271. Moe SM: Calcium, phosphorus, and vitamin D metabolism in renal disease and chronic renal failure. *In* Kopple JD, Massry SG (eds): Nutritional Management of Renal Disease. Philadelphia, Lippincott Williams & Wilkins, 2004, pp 261–285.
272. Moe SM: Management of renal osteodystrophy in peritoneal dialysis patients. Perit Dial Int (in press).
273. Moe SM, Drueke TB: Management of secondary hyperparathyroidism: The importance and the challenge of controlling parathyroid hormone levels without elevating calcium, phosphorus, and calcium-phosphorus product. Am J Nephrol 2003; 23:369–379.

Cardiovascular Disease in Patients with Chronic Kidney Disease

Daniel E. Weiner, M.D., M.S. • Mark J. Sarnak, M.D.

Cardiovascular disease is the leading cause of morbidity and mortality in patients with chronic kidney disease (CKD). This increased risk of cardiovascular disease may begin during the earlier stages of CKD before the onset of kidney failure. Notably, patients with CKD have a very high prevalence of cardiovascular disease risk factors such as diabetes and hypertension, but they are also exposed to other nontraditional, uremia-related cardiovascular disease risk factors. Much of the burden of cardiovascular disease in CKD may be due to atherosclerosis, but it is apparent that patients with cardiovascular disease also have a high prevalence of arteriosclerosis and disorders of left ventricular (LV) structure and function.

In this chapter, we discuss the epidemiology and pathophysiology of cardiovascular disease in patients with CKD, with a focus on dialysis patients and nontransplant recipients with stages 1 through 4 CKD. We also discuss the different manifestations of cardiovascular disease in kidney disease and review diagnostic and therapeutic options.

EPIDEMIOLOGY

Dialysis

Among dialysis patients, cardiovascular disease (CVD) is the leading cause of mortality, accounting for nearly 45% of deaths; approximately 20% of cardiac deaths are attributed directly to acute myocardial infarction (AMI).[1] This high burden of CVD mortality is well illustrated by comparing CVD mortality in the dialysis population to the general population; at all ages in both men and women, mortality due to CVD is 10 to 30 times higher in dialysis patients (Figure 9–1).[2]

In theory, the high CVD mortality rate in dialysis patients may be due to both a high prevalence of CVD and a high case fatality rate. In fact, both are true. Based on data obtained from medical evidence forms, at the time of initiation of kidney replacement therapy nearly 40% of patients have known coronary disease, over 40% have congestive heart failure, approximately 20% have peripheral vascular disease, and over 10% have had strokes or transient ischemic attacks.[3] The prevalence of CVD at initiation of dialysis is even higher if claims data are used instead of the Medical Evidence Form.

Dialysis patients with CVD also have a very high case fatality rate. Herzog and associates,[4] retrospectively studied outcomes of 34,189 dialysis patients and noted a 60% 1-year mortality and 90% 5-year mortality rate following AMI.

Stages 1 to 4 CKD

CVD Morbidity and Mortality

The high prevalence of CVD in incident dialysis patients suggests that CVD develops prior to the onset of kidney failure. Several studies have shown that manifestations of CVD may be seen relatively early in CKD. For example, in a cross-sectional study of 175 patients, 27% of patients with creatinine clearance above 50 mL/min had LVH, while 31% of patients with creatinine clearance between 25 and 49 mL/min and 45% of patients with creatinine clearance below 25 mL/min had LVH.[5] This contrasts with a prevalence of LVH of less than 20% in patients of similar age in the general population.[6]

Similarly, patients with CKD have a higher prevalence of coronary artery disease, heart failure, and CVD risk factors than those without CVD and suffer from CVD events at higher rates.[7–10] For example, among patients with reduced kidney function in the Cardiovascular Health Study (CHS), comprised entirely of subjects aged 65 years and older, 26% had coronary artery disease, 8% had heart failure, and 55% had hypertension at baseline. This is compared with subjects in the same study without CKD, where 13%, 3%, and 36% had coronary artery disease, heart failure, and hypertension at baseline, respectively. Notably, subjects with CKD had a rate of CVD events of 102 per 1000 patient years, while those without CKD had an event rate of 44 per 1000 patient years.[11] Similar findings were noted in the Atherosclerosis Risk in Communities (ARIC) Study, a community-based cohort of individuals aged 45 to 64 years. In ARIC, subjects with CKD had a baseline prevalence of coronary artery disease, cerebrovascular disease, and diabetes of 11%, 10%, and 24%, respectively, and the rate of CVD events was 26 per 1000 patient years. In comparison, subjects without CKD had a baseline prevalence of coronary artery disease, cerebrovascular disease and diabetes of 4.1%, 4.4%, and 13% respectively, and the rate of CVD events was 9 per 1000 patient years.[12]

CKD as an Independent Risk Factor for CVD

Several studies have demonstrated that in patients with CVD or at high risk for CVD, the presence of CKD is an independent risk factor for future CVD outcomes. For example, in the Studies of Left Ventricular Dysfunction (SOLVD) trial examining subjects with left ventricular ejection fraction below 40%, subjects with CKD had a 40% increased risk of mortality and a 50% to 70% increased risk of death due to heart failure.[13] Similarly, in the Heart Outcomes and Prevention Evaluation (HOPE) Trial, patients with CKD had a 40% increased risk of the composite outcome of myocardial infarction, CVD death,

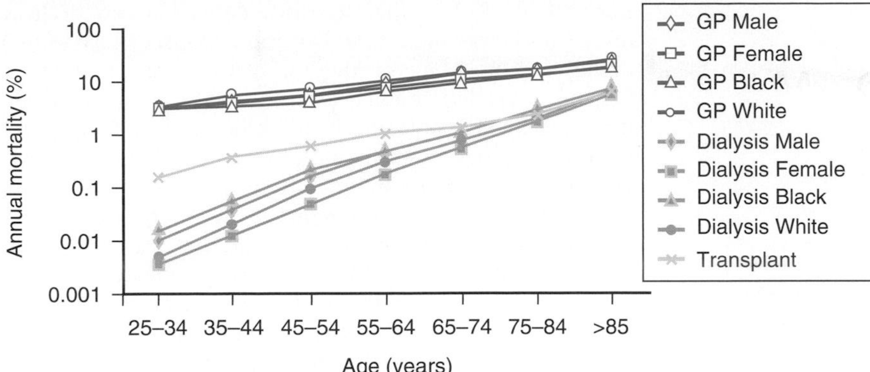

Figure 9–1 Cardiovascular mortality in the general population and dialysis population stratified by sex and race. (Data from Foley RN, Parfrey PS, Sarnak MJ: Clinical epidemiology of cardiovascular disease in chronic renal disease. Am J Kidney Dis 1998; 32[5 suppl 3]:S112–S119.)

and stroke.[14] These results have also been seen in subjects following myocardial infarction.[8–12]

In community studies, the independent effect of kidney function has been less conclusive. For example, analyses of the Framingham Heart Study cohort and the National Health and Nutrition Examination Survey I (NHANES I) did not demonstrate that CKD was an independent risk factor for CVD outcomes.[15,16] In contrast, in ARIC and CHS, CKD was an independent risk factor for CVD outcomes; however, the impact of CKD was diminished after adjusting for traditional CVD risk factors (Figure 9–2).

There are several reasons why CKD may be an independent risk factor for CVD outcomes. These include, but are not limited to, residual confounding from traditional risk factors and insufficient adjustment for nontraditional risk factors. Additionally, CKD may be a marker of the severity of either diagnosed or undiagnosed vascular disease. Furthermore, patients with CKD may not receive sufficient therapy for their disease, including medications such as aspirin, β-blockers and angiotensin converting enzyme inhibitors, as well as diagnostic and therapeutic procedures.

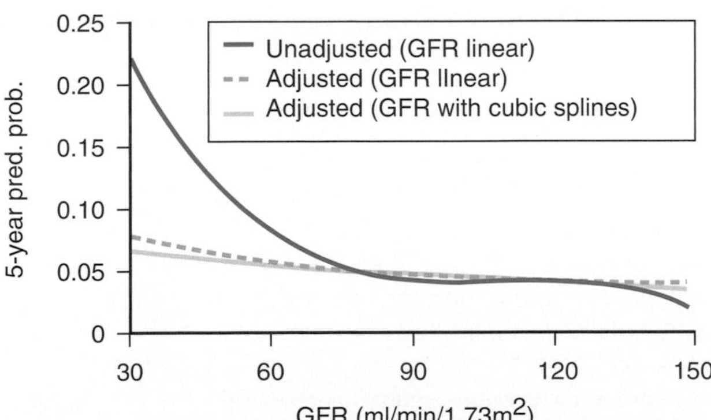

Figure 9–2 Smoothed 5-year predicted probability of developing atherosclerotic cardiovascular disease (ASCVD) by level of GFR in the ARIC Study. The linear model includes GFR as a continuous variable in a Cox regression while the cubic spline model includes a cubic transition between linear segments with five knots. (From Manjunath G, Tighiouart H, Ibrahim H, et al: Level of kidney function as a risk factor for atherosclerotic cardiovascular outcomes in the community. J Am Coll Cardiol 2003; 41[1]:47–55.)

Proteinuria as an Independent Risk Factor for CVD

Proteinuria, manifest as either microalbuminuria or macroalbuminuria, is associated with a higher prevalence of surrogates of CVD, including left ventricular hypertrophy in patients with hypertension[17] and arterial intima-media thickening in patients with diabetes.[18] Proteinuria detected by a urine dipstick examination was an independent risk factor for CVD outcomes in the Framingham cohort.[19,20] Other studies have confirmed this finding in diabetic and hypertensive patients.[21,22]

Several recent studies have expanded on the importance of microalbuminuria as a CVD risk factor. Secondary evaluation of the HOPE Trial data as well as evaluations of population-based cohorts in Norway and the Netherlands expanded on prior evaluations of proteinuria to show that microalbuminuria, even in very low quantities, may independently predict CVD outcomes (Figure 9–3).[23–25]

There are several reasons why microalbuminuria may be an independent risk factor for CVD outcomes. Microalbuminuria may represent kidney disease itself, with an associated risk of subsequent CKD progression and development of macroalbuminuria. Microalbuminuria may also represent the kidney manifestation of systemic endothelial disease burden, or may be associated with systemic inflammatory markers and abnormalities in the coagulation and fibrinolytic systems.[26]

RISK FACTORS

Much of the increased burden of CVD in CKD is due to increased prevalence of both traditional and nontraditional risk CVD factors. Traditional risk factors are factors identified in the Framingham Heart Study as conferring increased risk of cardiovascular disease in the general population. Traditional risk factors include older age, diabetes and hypertension, all of which are highly prevalent in patients with CKD. Nontraditional risk factors are defined as those factors that increase in prevalence as kidney function declines and that have been hypothesized to be CVD risk factors in this population (Table 9–1).

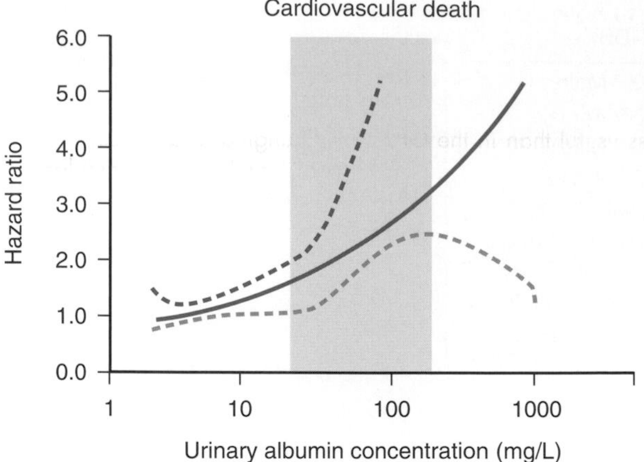

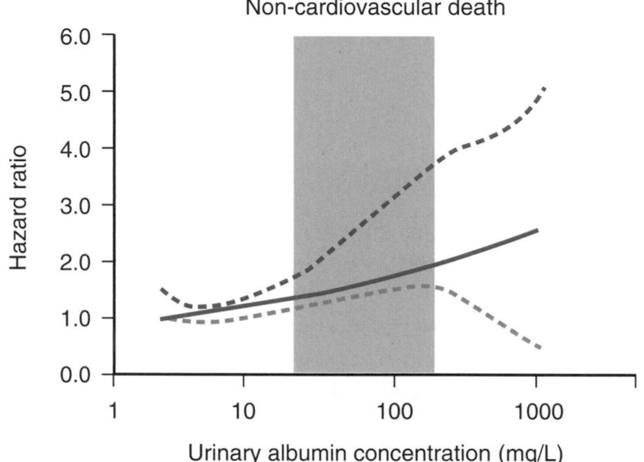

Figure 9–3 Microalbuminuria. Adjusted effect of urinary albumin concentration (UAC) on the hazard of cardiovascular and noncardiovascular death. Shaded areas represent the upper and lower limit of current definition of microalbuminuria (20 to 200 mg/L). (From Hillege HL, Fidler V, Diercks GF, et al: Urinary albumin excretion predicts cardiovascular and noncardiovascular mortality in general population. Circulation 2002; 106[14]:1777–1782.)

Most CVD risk factors lead to atherosclerosis, arteriosclerosis, cardiomyopathy, or any combination of these three conditions (Table 9–2). Atherosclerosis, defined as an occlusive disease of the vasculature, and arteriosclerosis, defined as non-occlusive remodeling of the vasculature, may manifest as ischemic heart disease and heart failure (HF). Some risk factors, including dyslipidemia and hyperhomocysteinemia, primarily predispose to development and progression of atherosclerosis, while others, including volume overload and elevated calcium-phosphorus product, may predispose to arteriosclerosis. Still other risk factors, including anemia and the presence of arteriovenous fistulae, may predispose to cardiac remodeling and left ventricular hypertrophy. Essential to the understanding of CVD in CKD is an understanding of the interplay of these various risk factors in patients with kidney disease.

Traditional Cardiovascular Disease Risk Factors

Blood Pressure in Dialysis Patients

Hypertension is both a cause as well as a result of kidney disease. About 70% to 80% of patients with stages 1 through 4 CKD have hypertension, and the prevalence of hypertension increases as glomerular filtration rate (GFR) declines, such that over 80% to 90% of patients starting dialysis are hypertensive (Figure 9–4).[27, 28]

"U"-shaped relationship

The relationship between hypertension and CVD outcomes in the dialysis patient is complex, with increased adverse CVD events and mortality at both markedly elevated post-dialysis systolic blood pressures (>180 mmHg) as well as lower blood pressures (<110 mmHg) (Figure 9–5).[29,30] Reflecting perhaps increased arterial stiffness, pulse pressure, and when evaluated in conjunction with systolic blood pressure, may more accurately predict CVD outcomes than systolic blood pressure alone.[31]

Hypertension

It is important to note that high blood pressure has been associated with CVD outcomes in dialysis patients. For example, hyper-

Table 9–1 Traditional and Nontraditional Cardiovascular Risk Factors in Chronic Kidney Disease

Traditional Risk Factors	Nontraditional Factors
Older age	Albuminuria
Male gender	Homocysteine
Hypertension	Lipoprotein (a) and apo (a) isoforms
Higher LDL cholesterol	Lipoprotein remnants
Lower HDL cholesterol	Anemia
Diabetes	Abnormal calcium/phosphate metabolism
Smoking	Extracellular fluid volume overload
Physical inactivity	Electrolyte imbalance
Menopause	Oxidative stress
Family history of cardiovascular disease	Inflammation (C-reactive protein)
Left ventricular hypertrophy	Malnutrition
	Thrombogenic factors
	Sleep disturbances
	Altered nitric oxide/endothelin balance

(Reproduced and modified with permission from Sarnak MJ, Levey AS: Cardiovascular disease and chronic renal disease: A new paradigm. Am J Kidney Dis 2000; 35[4 suppl 1]:S117–S131.)

Table 9–2 Spectrum of CVD in CKD: Differences from the General Population

Types of CVD	Pathology	Surrogates	Clinical Presentations of CVD
Arterial Vascular Disease	Atherosclerosis	Inducible ischemia, carotid IMT, EBCT (may be less useful than in the GP for atherosclerosis because of medial rather than intimal calcification), ischemia by EKG	IHD (myocardial infarction, angina, sudden cardiac death), cerebrovascular disease, PVD, HF
	Arteriosclerosis: Dilated and noncompliant large vessels	Aortic pulse wave velocity, calcification of the aorta, LVH (indirectly), increased pulse pressure	IHD, HF
Cardiomyopathy	Concentric LVH as well as LV dilatation with proportional hypertrophy	LVH, systolic dysfunction, and diastolic dysfunction by echocardiogram. LVH by EKG	HF, hypotension, IHD

IMT, intima-media thickness; *EBCT*, electron beam computed tomography; *IHD*, ischemic heart disease; *CAD*, coronary disease; *HF*, heart failure; *GP*, general population; *LVH*, left ventricular hypertrophy; *LVMI*, left ventricular mass index; *PVD*, peripheral vascular disease; *EKG*, electrocardiogram; *CVD*, cardiovascular disease; *CKD*, chronic kidney disease. (Reproduced with permission of Sarnak MJ, Levey AS, Schoolwerth AC, et al: Kidney disease as a risk factor for development of cardiovascular disease: A statement from the American Heart Association Councils on Kidney in Cardiovascular Disease, High Blood Pressure Research, Clinical Cardiology, and Epidemiology and Prevention. Circulation 2003; 108(17):2154–2169.)

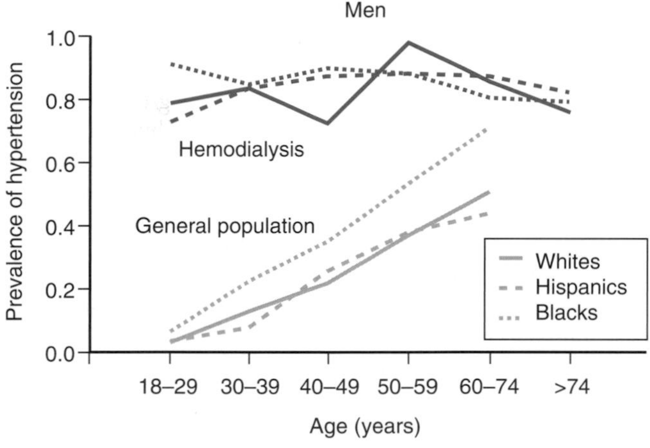

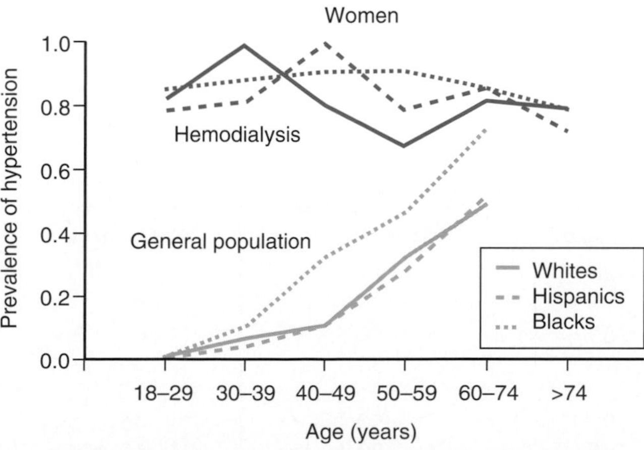

Figure 9–4 The prevalence of hypertension in chronic dialysis patients as compared to the general population. (Reprinted with permission from Agarwal R, Nissenson AR, Batlle D, et al: Prevalence, treatment, and control of hypertension in chronic hemodialysis patients in the United States. Am J Med 2003; 115[4]:291–297.)

tension is an independent risk factor for ischemic heart disease, LVH, heart failure,[32] and cerebral hemorrhage.[33] Hypertension is likely under-treated in dialysis patients[34,35]; unfortunately, there are no large trials to date that examine blood pressure goals and medication regimens in dialysis patients.

Low blood pressure

There are two potential reasons that low blood pressure may be associated with adverse outcomes in dialysis patients. First, hypotension may be associated with other comorbid conditions, including heart failure and cardiomyopathy. Second, low blood pressure may predispose dialysis patients to experiencing intradialytic hypotension, which itself may lead to ischemic events.

Intradialytic hypotension is a relatively common occurrence during hemodialysis and may also be an independent

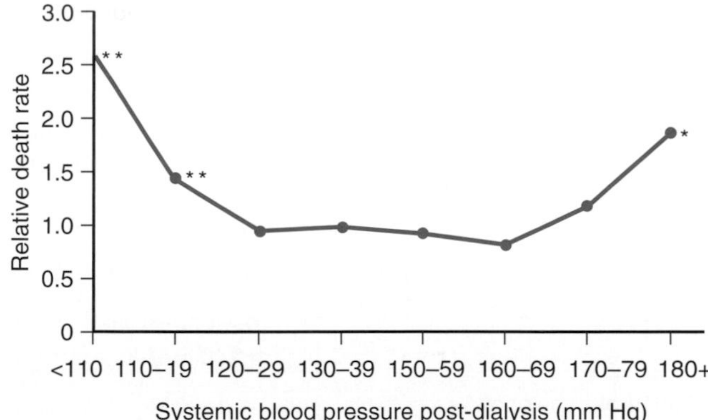

Figure 9–5 Systolic blood pressure post-dialysis (SBP; time-varying) and CVD mortality in hemodialysis patients 1992 to 1996. The "U" curve relationship between SBP post-dialysis and mortality is: SBP < 110 mmHg, RR = 2.62; SBP 110 to 119 mmHg, RR = 1.48; SBP ≥ 180 mmHg, RR = 1.86. $P < .01$ for SBP < 110 mmHg and $p < .05$ for SBP between 110–119 and > 180 mmHg versus the reference group. (Reproduced with permission from Zager PG, Nikolic J, Brown RH, et al: "U" curve association of blood pressure and mortality in hemodialysis patients. Medical Directors of Dialysis Clinic, Inc., Kidney Int 1998; 54[2]:561–569.)

risk factor for CVD outcomes, perhaps representing either the inability of the heart or blood vessels to appropriately respond to reduced blood pressure or, alternatively, heart failure itself in the absence of overt volume overload. Hypotension, particularly in the presence of reduced preload from ultrafiltration, may represent the inability of a noncompliant left ventricle to compensate for decreased left ventricular filling pressures.

Stages 3 to 4 CKD

Blood pressure in stages 3 to 4 CKD has been investigated in more detail than in dialysis patients, although the focus of most studies has been on retarding progression of kidney disease rather than assessing CVD outcomes. In this section, we will discuss the prevalence of hypertension in CKD, its association with CVD, and therapeutic recommendations.

Prevalence

Hypertension is highly prevalent in patients with CKD. In a Canadian evaluation of patients with creatinine clearance below 75 mL/min, 80% had hypertension (defined as blood pressure greater than 140/90 mm Hg or use of anti-hypertensive medications),[36] while the prevalence of hypertension was 70% in the NHANES III population with CKD.[37] Hypertension was more commonly seen with CKD due to glomerular disease than tubulointerstitial disease.[38]

Progression of CKD

Elevated systolic blood pressure is an independent risk factor for CVD outcomes in both diabetic[39,40] and nondiabetic patients.[41] A secondary analysis of the MDRD study showed a 35% increased risk of hospitalization for CVD for each 10-point increase in systolic blood pressure, and this increased risk remained significant even after adjusting for other traditional risk factors.[42] Increased risk of progression of kidney disease is also associated with poor blood pressure control, with the lowest risk of kidney disease progression seen in treated hypertensive patients who achieved systolic blood pressure reduction to 110 and 119 mmHg, primarily in patients with proteinuria.[43]

Therapy

Angiotensin converting enzyme (ACE) inhibitors and angiotensin receptor blockers (ARBs) are the preferred anti-hypertensive medications in patients with CKD. Several studies have shown a reduction in progression of CKD using these medications, particularly in patients with proteinuria.[23,43–48] Notably, in a subgroup analysis of patients with CKD in the HOPE study, ACE inhibitors were beneficial for reducing CVD events in patients with either preexisting vascular disease or diabetes combined with an additional cardiovascular risk factor.[14] Based on this evidence, the National Kidney Foundation (NKF) has published practice guidelines that recommend a target blood pressure of 130/80 mmHg in all CKD patients.[48a]

Dyslipidemia

Patients with earlier stages of CKD frequently have diabetes and hypertension. In the United States, this metabolic syndrome is frequently accompanied by dyslipidemia and, in particular, elevated LDL cholesterol. Additionally, nephrotic-range proteinuria can also exacerbate hyperlipidemia and hypertriglyceridemia. In the absence of severe proteinuria, as CKD progresses levels of LDL cholesterol may normalize reflecting progressive malnutrition.[49] HDL cholesterol is often low, while triglycerides are generally moderately elevated. Other abnormalities include increased levels of lipoprotein(a), a higher proportion of atherogenic, oxidized LDL-C and abnormal concentrations of apolipoproteins that comprise the major lipoproteins (Table 9–3).

Despite these changes, approximately 50% of prevalent hemodialysis patients have LDL cholesterol over 100 mg/dL and non-HDL cholesterol levels over 130 mg/dL.[50] In peritoneal dialysis (PD) patients, the prevalence of hyperlipidemia is approximately 70%, although PD patients have a somewhat more atherogenic lipid panel than their HD counterparts, with increased LDL-C, apolipoprotein B, oxidized LDL-C, triglycerides, and Lp(a) and decreased HDL-C. Therefore, despite the fact that total cholesterol levels are often relatively normal, significant dyslipidemia is highly prevalent in the CKD population.

In hemodialysis patients, the relationship between cholesterol levels and coronary heart disease mortality is more complex than in the general population. A review of observational studies of dialysis patients found a "reverse epidemiology" between cholesterol levels and risk of death.[20] Contrary to what has been observed in the general population, low cholesterol levels were associated with a higher death rate in dialysis

Table 9–3 Lipid Abnormalities by Target Population (approximate percentage)

	Total Cholesterol > 240 mg/dL	LDL Cholesterol > 130 mg/dL	HDL Cholesterol < 35 mg/dL	Triglycerides > 200 mg/dL
General Population*	20	40	15	15
CKD Stages 1–4†				
with Nephrotic Syndrome‡	90	85	50	60
without Nephrotic Syndrome‡	30	10	35	40
CKD Stage 5†				
Hemodialysis	20	30	50	45
Peritoneal Dialysis	25	45	20	50

Reproduced and modified with permission from Kasiske.[168]
*Data from National Health and Nutrition Examination Survey (NHANES) III and the Framingham Offspring Study.[169,170]
†Data extracted from multiple observational studies.[168]
‡Nephrotic proteinuria was defined as > 3 g of total protein excretion in 24 hours

patients. For example, in an analysis of data from more than 12,000 hemodialysis patients, patients with low total cholesterol levels (<100 mg/dL) had a more than fourfold increase in risk of death compared with patients whose cholesterol levels were between 200 and 250 mg/dL.[51] In one study, hypocholesterolemia was associated with low serum albumin and elevated levels of C-reactive protein (CRP), possibly implicating hypocholesterolemia as a surrogate for malnutrition and inflammation. In that same study, although hypocholesterolemia was more closely associated with all-cause mortality, hyperlipidemia was also a strong predictor of cardiovascular death.[52] Similar findings were noted in a recent evaluation of the CHOICE study, an incident cohort of dialysis patients, where, after taking inflammation and malnutrition into account, higher levels of total serum cholesterol were associated with adverse CVD outcomes and mortality.[53]

Although the results of currently ongoing randomized, controlled trials are necessary to examine whether lipid-lowering treatment is beneficial in patients with CKD, the National Kidney Foundation (NKF) has recently published guidelines as part of their Kidney/Dialysis Outcomes Quality Initiative (K/DOQI) for the treatment of dyslipidemia in CKD. These recommendations stress that all patients with CKD, even in the absence of known CVD, be considered to be at the highest risk for CVD outcomes. Lipid levels should be treated to the lowest levels recommended for the general population (namely LDL-C < 100 mg/dL and non-HDL-C < 130 mg/dL) (Table 9–4).[54]

Diabetes Mellitus

Diabetes accounts for over 40% of the dialysis population in the United States and is increasingly the cause of kidney failure in other countries.[1]

Dialysis

The presence of diabetes in dialysis patients is an independent risk factor for ischemic heart disease, heart failure, and all-cause mortality.[55,56] Diabetic dialysis patients also have worse long-term outcomes following coronary interventions than nondiabetic patients with CKD.[57,58]

However, there is suggestive evidence that the management of diabetes in the dialysis unit has been suboptimal as marked by lower than expected rates of hemoglobin A1C assessment and yearly eye examinations.[59] Unlike in the general population, there have been no studies in the dialysis population of the relationship between strict glycemic control and CVD outcomes. The net benefit of rigid diabetes control may be smaller in the dialysis population because microvascular and macrovascular complications already exist and because of a potentially increased risk of hypoglycemia; however, hyperglycemia may still worsen retinopathy, hasten the loss of residual kidney function, cause or worsen peripheral neuropathy, and increase the risk of infection.

Stages 1 to 4 CKD

Diabetes mellitus is the most common cause of stages 1 to 4 CKD, with microalbuminuria as the first clinical manifestation of diabetic nephropathy. In the general population, diabetes is a powerful risk factor for cardiovascular outcomes.[60] The same holds true for patients with CKD.[61]

Left Ventricular Hypertrophy and Cardiomyopathy

LVH is highly prevalent in both stages 3 and 4 CKD and dialysis patients and represents a physiologic adaptation to a long-term increase in myocardial work requirements.

Pathogenesis

LVH may be thought of as resulting from either pressure or volume overload. Pressure overload results from increased cardiac afterload, often due to hypertension, aortic stenosis, and reduced arterial compliance from arteriosclerosis.[62,63] Some evidence suggests that increased vascular calcification in dialysis patients may also contribute to this phenomenon.[63] Volume overload may be related to anemia, developing when the heart attempts to compensate for decreased peripheral oxygen delivery.[64,65] Other causes of volume overload include increased extracellular volume seen in dialysis patients[66,67] and the presence of arteriovenous fistulae.

Most LVH is initially concentric, representing a uniform increase in wall thickness secondary to pressure overload from hypertension or aortic stenosis. The concentric thickening of the wall of the left ventricle allows for generation of greater intraventricular pressure, effectively overcoming increased afterload. Volume overload may result in eccentric hypertrophy secondary to the addition of new sarcomeres in series. Eccentric hypertrophy is defined by an increased LV diameter with a proportional increase in LV wall thickness. As this process progresses, capillary density decreases and subendocardial perfusion is reduced. Myocardial fibrosis may ensue and, with sustained maladaptive forces, myocyte death occurs. The end point of this cycle is often dilated cardiomyopathy with eventual reduction in systolic function (Figure 9–6).[68]

Although LVH was identified early on the Framingham population as a CVD risk factor, LVH in dialysis results from the confluence of at least one major traditional risk factor (hypertension)

Table 9–4 Treatment Recommendations for Dyslipidemia in Dialysis Patients

Dyslipidemia	Treatment Goal	Initial Regimen	Increased Regimen	Alternative Regimen
TG ≥ 500 mg/dL	TG < 500 mg/dL	TLC	TLC + Fibrate or Niacin	Fibrate or Niacin
LDL 100–129 mg/dL	LDL < 100 mg/dL	TLC	TLC + low dose statin	Bile acid seq or Niacin
LDL ≥ 130 mg/dL	LDL < 100 mg/dL	TLC + low dose statin	TLC + max. dose statin	Bile acid seq or Niacin
TG ≥ 200 mg/dL and non-HDL ≥ 130 mg/dL	Non-HDL < 130 mg/dL	TLC + low dose statin	TLC + max. dose statin	Fibrate or Niacin

TLC, therapeutic lifestyle changes; *TG*, triglycerides; *HDL*, high-density lipoprotein cholesterol; *LDL*, low-density lipoprotein cholesterol. (Adapted with permission from National Kidney Foundation, Kidney Disease Outcomes Quality Initiative. Am J Kidney Dis 2003; 41 [4 suppl 3]:S40.)

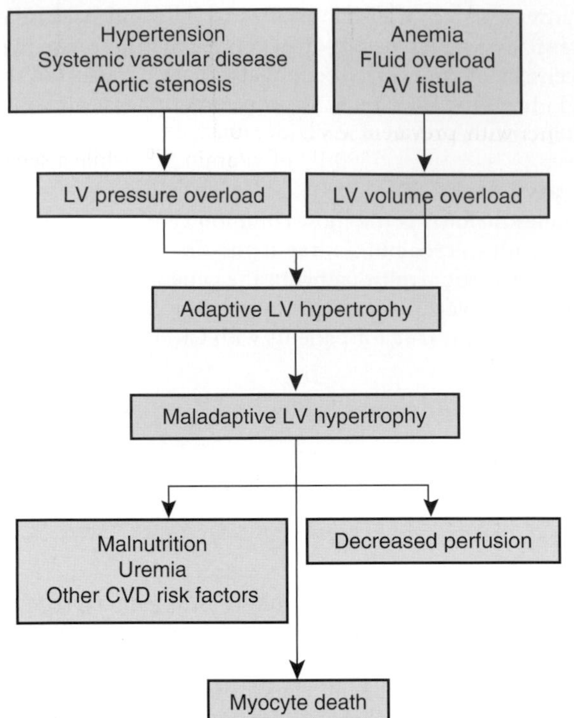

Figure 9–6 Progression of cardiac dysfunction in kidney disease patients. (Adapted from Parfrey PS, Foley RN: The clinical epidemiology of cardiac disease in chronic renal disease. J Am Soc Nephrol 1995; 10:1606-1615.

and several nontraditional risk factors (anemia, chronic volume overload, uremia, and possibly hyperparathyroidism).

Epidemiology

Studies have shown a prevalence of LVH of 20% to 50% in the pre-dialysis population, with LVH being more common at lower levels of kidney function, decreased hemoglobin, and increased systolic blood pressure. Among incident dialysis patients, as many as 70% may have LVH present by echocardiography,[5] while, among prevalent dialysis patients, LVH is present in 50% to 75% of patients when assessed by echocardiography.[69,70]

As in the general population, LVH is an independent risk factor for adverse CVD outcomes in dialysis patients.[71,72] Notably, both concentric LVH and dilated cardiomyopathy are independently associated with increased incidence of adverse CVD outcomes and all-cause mortality.[68]

Therapy

Given the complexity of the development of LVH, it presents a challenging target for therapy. Potentially modifiable risk factors include anemia, hypertension, extracellular volume overload, abnormal calcium and phosphorus metabolism, and arteriovenous fistulae. With attention to these risk factors prior to dialysis, LVH and its eventual cardiovascular sequelae may potentially be prevented.

Some data from small studies have suggested that with modification of risk factors, including anemia and systolic blood pressure as well as strict management of volume, regression of LVH can be induced in dialysis patients.[67,73–75] However, one recent study found that only a subset of patients treated with ACE inhibitor therapy had regression of LV mass; those who did not respond tended to have higher levels of C-reactive protein (CRP), perhaps implicating inflammation as a confounding factor in development of LVH.[76] Additionally, two randomized trials, one in dialysis patients and one in patients with stages 3 to 4 CKD, did not demonstrate any regression of LVH or decrease in LV mass with higher levels of hemoglobin.[77,78] The latter study is difficult to interpret given that diastolic blood pressure rose in the higher hemoglobin arm, follow-up was only 2 years, and the difference in achieved hemoglobin levels between the two groups was small. While future research in this field may reveal important genetic associations governing the renin-angiotensin-aldosterone system, therapy at this time is likely best directed at modifying the multiple risk factors for LVH in order to prevent its development, particularly in the pre-dialysis CKD population.

Other Traditional Risk Factors

Other traditional risk factors include advanced age, male sex, and smoking. Smoking represents an opportunity for intervention. Although there have been few studies examining specific effects of smoking in dialysis patients, a recent evaluation of U.S. Renal Data System (USRDS) data showed that smoking was a strong, independent risk factor for incident heart failure, incident peripheral vascular disease, and all-cause mortality. Importantly, dialysis patients who were former smokers were more similar to nonsmokers than current smokers in risk, demonstrating the potential benefit of smoking cessation efforts in dialysis patients.[79]

Nontraditional Risk Factors

Homocysteine

Homocysteine (Hcy), a metabolite of the essential amino acid methionine, has been implicated in the general population as a risk factor for myocardial infarction and stroke.[80,81] Hyperhomocysteinemia is much more common in dialysis patients than in the general population (Table 9–5). Normal plasma levels of Hcy range from 5 to 12 µmol/L, whereas dialysis patients have mean homocysteine levels of 24 µmol/L. Hcy levels increase proportionally as kidney function declines, with as many as 80% of dialysis patients classified as having hyperhomocysteinemia.[82] Much of this elevation is secondary to defective kidney clearance of homocysteine.[83]

Some but not all studies have demonstrated that hyperhomocysteinemia is an independent risk factor for CVD mortality in dialysis patients,[84] although the relationship is only modest.[85] However, it is important to note that Hcy levels are

Table 9–5 Comparison of Homocysteine Levels in Different Populations

Population	Mean HCY, µM (range: 10–90 percentile)
Stage 5 CKD	24 (19–39)
Kidney Transplant	15 (9–25)
CKD	15 (9–25)
General Population*	9 (6–12)

*In the age of folate supplementation.
(From Friedman et al. J Am Soc Nephrol 2001; 12:2181–2189.)

also correlated with nutritional status, and, in subjects who are nutritionally bereft, low levels of serum homocysteine are associated with adverse outcomes.[86]

Deficiencies of folate, vitamin B_{12}, and vitamin B_6 have all been linked to increased Hcy in the general population,[87] and therapy with these vitamins may both normalize Hcy levels and reduce CVD recurrence.[88,89] In the earlier stages of CKD, treatment with supraphysiologic doses of folic acid and B vitamins may also normalize Hcy levels; however, Hcy levels in dialysis patients are often somewhat resistant to folate and B vitamin administration, such that high dose supplementation may result in improvement but not normalization of homocysteine levels.[90] Extremely high flux dialyzers and daily nocturnal dialysis may also decrease lower homocysteine levels.[91,92] While trials are ongoing, to date there are no randomized, controlled trial data demonstrating the impact of Hcy-lowering therapy on CVD outcomes in dialysis patients.

Oxidant Stress and Inflammation

Oxidant stress has recently been proposed as a unifying concept linking both traditional and other nontraditional risk factors in CKD.[93] Whether or not this is the case, the hypothesis of oxidant stress is certainly illustrative of the multifactorial nature of CVD risk in CKD.

Oxidant stress may be defined as an imbalance between oxidants and antioxidants (oxidant defenses) that leads to tissue damage.[94] Most oxidation occurs in the mitochondria, although phagocytes also produce reactive oxygen (ROS) species in a "respiratory burst" designed to defend the body against infection. These ROS include hydrogen peroxide and superoxide anion, both of which function as precursors for generation of more powerful oxidants. These ROS eventually can oxidize lipids, proteins, carbohydrates, and nucleic acids, which can then be measured as markers of oxidant burden. This system is balanced by a series of antioxidant defenses, some of which work by enzymatically catalyzing reduction of oxidant species (e.g., superoxide dismutase, catalase) while others work nonenzymatically by scavenging for oxidants (e.g., glutathione, vitamin C).[95]

Numerous factors in the CKD patient population increase oxidant stress. These include inflammation, malnutrition (by reducing antioxidant defenses), uremic toxins, and potentially the dialysis procedure itself. Patients with CKD not only have higher levels of oxidant stress, but they also have decreased defenses, particularly plasma protein-associated free thiols such as glutathione.[93] This "double-hit" makes dialysis patients particularly vulnerable to sequelae of oxidant stress.

Several studies have been published that show a strong, independent association between inflammation and the risk of adverse CVD outcomes in dialysis patients.[69, 96, 97] Adverse CVD outcomes may be exacerbated by the role of oxidant stress in the development of anemia and malnutrition.[95] The dual presence of inflammation and oxidant stress may also increase the amount of atherogenic oxidized LDL, contributing to atherosclerotic disease.

At this time, specific treatment strategies for oxidant stress and inflammation in CKD have not been adopted. In the general population, therapy with statins and antioxidants has been investigated. Statins are associated with a greater beneficial effect on CVD events and mortality than would be expected by changes in the lipid profile alone. This may be due to a pleiotropic anti-inflammatory effect associated with statins,[98,99] which has also been appreciated in dialysis patients.[100]

Numerous studies have investigated the use of antioxidants for cardiovascular protection in the general population. The most notable demonstrated no benefit of vitamin E supplementation.[101] However, in dialysis patients, a study of 200 patients with prevalent CVD demonstrated a benefit associated with daily use of 800 IU of vitamin E[102] while a separate study showed a benefit with use of 600 mg of *N*-acetylcysteine twice daily.[103] Other investigations have used vitamin E–coated dialyzers and noted a decrease in oxidant stress.[104,105]

Other Nontraditional Risk Factors

Other nontraditional risk factors for CVD include anemia, derangements in calcium and phosphate metabolism, lipoprotein abnormalities, and sleep abnormalities. Some of these issues are discussed at length elsewhere in this text.

The contribution of anemia to increased CVD risk may be secondary to compensatory LVH as well as reflect high levels of inflammation and oxidant stress. Current research is also focusing on the effects of hyperphosphatemia and elevated calcium-phosphate product on arterial remodeling, as well as the effect of hyperparathyroidism on cardiomyopathy. Electron beam computed tomography has revealed extensive coronary artery calcification in dialysis patients and, in cross-sectional studies, this is associated with clinical CVD.[106] However, it remains to be determined whether reduction of serum phosphorus levels and calcium-phosphate product as well as treatment of hyperparathyroidism decreases CVD events. Other nontraditional risk factors include sleep abnormalities that are highly prevalent in dialysis patients and associated with coronary artery disease.[107] Nocturnal hypoxemia predicts CVD events[108] and may also represent a potentially modifiable risk factor.

ISCHEMIC HEART DISEASE

Epidemiology

Ischemic heart disease (IHD) is common in patients with stages 3 to 4 CKD and in dialysis patients. As discussed earlier, in patients aged 45 to 64 years with CKD, the rate of atherosclerotic events was approximately three times higher than the rate seen in patients with normal kidney function,[12] whereas, in the elderly, CVD event rates were approximately double those observed in the general population.[11]

In dialysis patients, rates are also high. A recent analysis of the USRDS Dialysis Morbidity and Mortality Study (DMMS) Wave 2 showed that the incidence of hospitalizations for acute coronary syndromes was 29 per 1000 person years and the incidence of AMI was 19 per 1000 person years.[109] Outcomes for patients with AMI are abysmal with 50% 1-year mortality and an 80% 3-year mortality.[109]

Pathophysiology

Atherosclerosis

Atherosclerosis is a disease of the arterial intima characterized by the presence of plaques and occlusive lesions. The development of atherosclerosis in patients with CKD is multifactorial and begins before kidney failure. Surrogates of atherosclerosis include both intima-media thickness of the carotid wall that is detectable by ultrasound[110,111] and inducible myocardial ischemia that is detectible by coronary stress tests (Table 9–2).[112] Electron beam computed tomography has emerged as a sensitive method to detect vascular calcification that correlates with atherosclerosis and predicts development of coronary artery disease in the general population.[113] However, it may not be an ideal method to detect atherosclerosis in CKD because it is unable to distinguish between intimal calcifications of atherosclerosis and medial calcification that is common in CKD.[114]

Arteriosclerosis

Arteriosclerosis is characterized by diffuse dilatation and hypertrophy of large arteries with loss of arterial elasticity. In CKD, this occurs in response to both atherogenic factors causing direct vascular injury as well as changes in the hemodynamic burden. Classically, in response to increased blood pressure, tensile stress is maintained by compensatory increase in arterial wall thickness. This pressure overload, discussed earlier in relation to LVH, manifests similarly in the arteries with arterial wall hypertrophy and increased arterial wall to lumen ratio. Concurrently, flow/volume overload manifests with proportional lumen and wall expansion. Overall, in dialysis patients, arteries undergo remodeling characterized by lumen dilatation as well as wall hypertrophy. This is often present at the onset of dialysis, implying development during the course of CKD.[115]

The manifestations of arteriosclerosis in CKD patients include LVH and changes in the blood pressure profile. Specifically, with loss of arterial elasticity, increased systolic blood pressure with or without a decrease in diastolic blood pressure is common. This results in an increased pulse pressure, which itself is an independent risk factor for mortality in dialysis patients.[116,117] The effects of arteriosclerosis are clinically significant and include LVH-related increased myocardial oxygen demand and altered coronary perfusion with subsequent subendocardial ischemia.[115]

Clinical Manifestations

Atherosclerosis and arteriosclerosis manifest with IHD (angina pectoris, myocardial infarctions, and sudden cardiac death), heart failure, and other vascular disease manifestations, including cerebrovascular disease and peripheral vascular disease (Table 9–2). As has been presented above, arteriosclerosis with or without atherosclerosis can cause cardiac remodeling, in particular LVH. Cardiac remodeling can in turn exacerbate arteriosclerosis and atherosclerosis in a vicious circle that results in ischemia, heart failure, and other sequelae of vascular disease.

Ischemic heart disease may be present without significant atherosclerosis. In one study, up to 50% of nondiabetic dialysis patients with symptoms of myocardial ischemia did not have significant large caliber coronary artery disease.[118] The authors hypothesized that the patients may have ischemia secondary to the combined effects of volume overload and LVH causing increased myocardial oxygen demand and small vessel coronary disease, and anemia causing decreased oxygen supply. Notably, this study was conducted in the era prior to erythropoietin use when severe anemia was more prevalent.

Diagnosis

Although IHD is extremely common in CKD, routine screening is not currently recommended in CKD patients in the absence of clinical manifestations of CVD. Available diagnostic tool are similar to those used in the general population and include resting echocardiography for evaluation of cardiac structure and function; exercise and pharmacologic stress testing for detection of perfusion defects; laboratory tests for assessment of both acute ischemia and chronic cardiac risk; and cardiac catheterization for description and possible repair of coronary anatomy.

Echocardiography

Echocardiography is a safe, accurate, and readily available tool for assessment of cardiac structure and function. However, assessment of left ventricular mass may be confounded by volume status and timing of dialysis, potentially leading to inaccuracies.[119–121]

Stress testing

Evaluation of IHD in dialysis patients is dependent on exercise capacity of the patient. Because many dialysis patients are unable to achieve adequate exercise levels for valid stress tests, pharmacologic stress tests are frequently used in this population; both pharmacologic thallium and echocardiographic evaluations are acceptable.[104] One reason for the infrequent use of stress testing not accompanied by an imaging modality is the high prevalence of baseline electrocardiogram abnormalities in the CKD population, making interpretation of changes difficult without accompanying thallium or echocardiographic images.

Angiography

Coronary angiography remains the gold standard for diagnosing flow-limiting lesions that may cause ischemia. Overall, angiography is relatively safe in the CKD population. However, nephrotoxicity secondary to contrast dye remains a major concern, particularly in patients with stages 3 and 4 CKD, as well as in stage 5 CKD patients with residual kidney function. Prevention and treatment of contrast nephropathy is beyond the scope of this chapter. One major advantage to angiography is the opportunity for revascularization concurrent with diagnosis.

Cardiac markers

Some evidence exists that elevated levels of cardiac troponin I may be most specific and sensitive for AMI in CKD,[122] but conclusive evidence is lacking as most studies evaluating this issue have excluded dialysis patients. When markers are initially equivocal, diagnosis of AMI in dialysis patients may be best accomplished by following the trend of levels of troponin I and/or creatine kinase-MB, as a sequential rise and fall in levels of these markers are consistent with acute cardiac damage.[123]

Several cardiac markers may be useful for CVD risk stratification. One study has shown that even minimal elevations in troponin T predicted all-cause mortality in dialysis patients, whereas another study showed that levels of troponin T above 0.10 ng/mL predicted coronary artery disease outcomes.[69,124] Troponin T may be a marker of chronic subendocardial ischemia and may correlate with LVH and other CVD risk factors. The prognostic utility of troponin I is probably more limited in this population.[124,125]

Treatment

Treatment of IHD should not be dependent on kidney function. Numerous studies have shown that dialysis patients with coronary artery disease benefit from appropriate interventions, including coronary artery bypass grafting (CABG) and angioplasty with stenting. As with most procedures, those done on an emergent basis are associated with worse outcomes. Although several studies have compared CABG with percutaneous transluminal coronary angioplasty (PTCA) with or without stent placement, none have been randomized trials. Results of observational studies are difficult to interpret given the inherent biases associated with patient selection for coronary interventions. The largest of these trials in dialysis utilized the USRDS database and noted better long-term survival for CABG and better short-term survival for PTCA.[58] Meanwhile, an investigation of admissions over an 8-year period of patients with stages 3 to 5 CKD for treatment of AMI revealed significantly improved survival in adjusted analysis for those treated with PTCA versus CABG. In this study, patients receiving either PTCA or CABG did better than those managed only medically.[126]

Chronic therapy for IHD involves management of both traditional and nontraditional risk factors described earlier. Although there are few trials of pharmacologic therapy for LVH, diabetes management and therapy of dyslipidemia in CKD, the management of hypertension has been more extensively investigated.

In studies of both diabetic and nondiabetic patients, ACE inhibitors have been shown to retard progression of kidney disease.[44,46] This has been most marked in patients with proteinuria. Additionally, in a subset of the HOPE trial examining patients with stage 3 to 4 CKD and at least one other CVD risk factor, ACE inhibitor therapy safely and effectively reduced cardiovascular outcomes.[14] ARBs have also been shown to reduce the progression of kidney disease but have not been evaluated sufficiently as CVD protective factors in CKD.[45,122,127] Therefore, whenever tolerated, ACE inhibitors remain a good option for prevention of CVD in patients with CKD.

In observational studies, β-blockers, ACE inhibitors, and also aspirin have all been shown to confer benefit in patients with stages 3 to 5 CKD and IHD.[8,9,128–130] Importantly, all of these studies demonstrated that patients with CKD were underprescribed these therapies, despite the apparent benefits.

There is a relatively small body of evidence focusing on the impact of treating nontraditional risk factors as part of a therapeutic regimen for patients with CKD and IHD. In particular, several studies have investigated treatment of anemia in CVD. In a large trial of dialysis patients with either HF or IHD, normalization of hematocrit with recombinant human erythropoietin resulted in a trend toward increased adverse events in the normal hematocrit arm.[131] Current trials are therefore evaluating whether treatment of anemia in the earlier stages of CKD may decrease CVD outcomes. With regard to other nontraditional risk factors, there are few trial data with clinical outcomes. As mentioned earlier, only with regard to oxidant stress have there been randomized trials showing a reduction in clinical events.[102,103]

HEART FAILURE

Despite the lack of a universally accepted definition, heart failure (HF) is generally characterized by volume overload, pulmonary edema, and dyspnea. Heart failure may occur as a result of left ventricular systolic dysfunction or diastolic dysfunction in which the left ventricle has a normal ejection fraction but impaired filling. Diastolic dysfunction is often associated with left ventricular hypertrophy and systemic hypertension. Systolic dysfunction often results from ischemic disease or hypertensive cardiomyopathy.

Diagnosis

Although the diagnosis of HF is clinical, echocardiography is invaluable for diagnosing both systolic and diastolic dysfunction. Several novel blood tests, including atrial natriuretic peptide and, in particular, brain natriuretic peptide, may correlate with cardiac function and predict future CVD events; these have not yet gained wide clinical use in patients with CKD.[132–134]

Treatment

Initial therapy of HF differs by stages of CKD, as loop diuretics remain a mainstay of therapy in pre-dialysis patients, whereas acute fluid overload in dialysis patients is treated with ultrafiltration. Chronic therapy for HF has not been adequately studied so most recommendations are either extrapolated from the general population or are based on smaller trials.

ACE inhibitors are of known benefit in the general population for treatment of HF with systolic dysfunction. In stages 3 and 4 CKD as well as in dialysis patients there is no reason to suspect that ACE inhibitors would not have a similar benefit. Although there are no large, randomized, controlled trials in CKD, some observational studies do suggest a benefit of ACE inhibitors independent of their blood pressure lowering effects in dialysis patients.[135] In the general population, ARBs remain a second line therapy to ACE inhibitors for HF, and this can likely be extrapolated to patients with CKD.

β-Blockers, another mainstay of HF therapy in the general population, are also beneficial in patients with CKD. A recent randomized trial in dialysis patients demonstrated that carvedilol reduced mortality in patients with left ventricular dysfunction.[129]

Cardiac glycosides are frequently used in HF in the general population where it has been shown that they improve morbidity but not mortality.[136] Although there are no specific studies of digoxin in CKD, this medication should be utilized judiciously with careful attention to dosage and drug levels, and, in dialysis patients, dialysate potassium concentration.

PERICARDIAL DISEASE

Epidemiology

Pericardial disease in CKD is generally associated with stage 5 CKD. It most commonly manifests as acute uremic or dialysis-associated pericarditis although chronic constrictive pericarditis may also be seen. Most estimates of the clinical incidence of pericardial disease in dialysis patients are less than 20%.[137]

Uremic pericarditis describes patients who develop clinical manifestations of pericarditis prior to or within 8 weeks of initiation of kidney replacement therapy. With the advent of modern dialysis, uremic pericarditis is exceedingly rare but remains an indication for and responds extremely well to initiation of dialysis.[138]

Dialysis-associated pericarditis by definition occurs after a patient is stabilized on dialysis. The precise etiology is unknown but may be related to inadequate dialysis and volume overload, although heparin use has been implicated.

Clinical Manifestations and Diagnosis

Pericarditis may be accompanied by nonspecific symptoms including chest pain, fever, chills, malaise, dyspnea, and cough. Physical examination may reveal a pericardial friction rub. When hemodynamically significant, pericardial disease accompanied by an effusion may be characterized by hypotension, particularly during the hemodialysis procedure.[139] Although other expected signs of pericardial effusion may be present, dialysis-related pericarditis often does not manifest with the classical electrocardiogram finding of diffuse ST segment elevation because there may only be minimal inflammation of the epicardium.[140] Echocardiography is helpful to confirm pericarditis in dialysis patients; however, effusions may be absent in patients who have adhesive, noneffusive pericarditis.

Treatment

Small, asymptomatic pericardial effusions are fairly common in dialysis patients and require no acute intervention, whereas larger effusions present a risk for tamponade. Intensification of hemodialysis is the mainstay of therapy but is only effective approximately 50% of the time.[138] Traditionally, heparin has been avoided during dialysis out of concern for hemorrhagic tamponade. Adjuvant medical therapies, including oral and parenteral glucocorticoids and nonsteroidal anti-inflammatory medications, have generally not been effective. For patients with hemodynamic instability, treatment consists of emergent drainage of the pericardial effusion. This is generally accomplished by pericardiocentesis or pericardiotomy with or without pericardiostomy for the instillation of long-acting, nonabsorbable glucocorticoids.[141]

VALVULAR DISEASE

Endocarditis

Epidemiology

Although unusual in the nonhemodialysis CKD population, infective endocarditis is a relatively common complication of hemodialysis when compared to rates in the general population.[142] This likely reflects several factors, including the relatively high incidence of bacteremia, common use of dialysis catheters, and the high prevalence of preexisting valvular abnormalities. Patients using catheters for hemodialysis access, more so than patients with AV grafts and fistulae, are prone to infection with subsequent hematogenous spread of bacteria to valves.[143–145] The vast majority of endocarditis in hemodialysis patients is secondary to gram-positive organisms, with *Staphylococcus aureus* predominating.[146–148]

Clinical Manifestations and Diagnosis

Dialysis patients with endocarditis usually have fever, murmurs, leukocytosis, and septic emboli may also be common. The mitral valve is the most commonly affected, followed by the aortic valve.[146–148] Diagnosis is chiefly dependent on positive blood cultures and clinical suspicion. Transthoracic and/or transesophageal echocardiography may be critical to making the diagnosis.

Treatment

Treatment of endocarditis begins with appropriate antibiotic therapy. Surgical intervention may also be appropriate, and indications for surgery are the same as in the general population: progressive valvular destruction, progressive heart failure, recurrent systemic emboli, and failure to respond to appropriate antibiotic therapy.

Even with therapy, survival is often poor, with case series showing 30% mortality during the initial hospitalization and 1-year mortality over 50%.[146–149] Factors associated with mortality include hypoalbuminemia, involvement of multiple valves, and severe valvular insufficiency. In one study, 30-day survival among patients who had surgery was 80% while it was only 47% among those managed medically.[147] In another small study, 50% (3/6) of patients who underwent surgery were alive at 1 year.[146] Although these studies are observational and not designed to compare surgical versus medical therapy, an important inference to be made is that hemodialysis patients with endocarditis should be considered surgical candidates if they have indications.

Prevention is, however, the best treatment for endocarditis in dialysis patients. Prevention is accomplished by complete treatment of known hematogenous infections and avoidance of access infection by use of sterile techniques and early placement and use of noncatheter-based dialysis access.

Mitral Annular Calcification

Mitral annular calcification may occur in 30% to 50% of patients on dialysis and is also common in patients during the earlier stages of CKD.[150, 151] It is recognized on echocardiography as a uniform echodense rigid band located near the base of the posterior mitral leaflet and may progressively involve the posterior leaflet. The pathogenesis of mitral calcification may be linked to altered calcium and phosphate metabolism.[151,152] Serious complications can include conduction abnormalities,[153] as well as embolic phenomena, mitral valve disease, and an increased risk of endocarditis.

Aortic Calcification and Stenosis

Epidemiology

Aortic valve calcification is the most common valvular abnormality in dialysis patients, occurring in 28% to 55% of patients. This prevalence is similar to that seen in the general population; however, dialysis patients experience aortic valve calcification 10 to 20 years earlier than the general population.[154] Age is the most significant risk factor for aortic valve calcification,[153] although elevated parathyroid hormone levels, elevated calcium and/or phosphorus levels, and dialysis vintage also appear to play a role.[155] Aortic valve calcification may itself pose a CVD risk beyond the increased risk of endocarditis; one study of elderly non-dialysis patients showed an independent association between aortic valve calcification and CVD outcomes.[156]

The most significant hazard associated with aortic valve calcification is the potential for development of progressive immobilization of the aortic leaflets, eventually restricting flow. Aortic stenosis exists when the valve leaflets thicken to the extent that commissural fusion can no longer occur and a pressure gradient develops across the aortic valve. In one study of dialysis patients, the estimated incidence of symptomatic aortic stenosis was 3.3% per year.[155] Progression of aortic valve disease to aortic stenosis in dialysis patients appears more rapid than that in the general population.[157] Very little evidence exists in the non-dialysis CKD population as to the prevalence and progression of valvular abnormalities.

Clinical Manifestations of Aortic Stenosis

Angina, heart failure, and syncope are the cardinal symptoms of critical aortic stenosis. Clinical evidence of aortic stenosis may be more readily evident in dialysis patients as they may have more frequent episodes of intradialytic hypotension, particularly as ultrafiltration can rapidly reduce preload. Frequent monitoring with echocardiography is important as dialysis patients may have very rapid progression of aortic valve disease.[154]

Treatment

Treatment of aortic stenosis is multifaceted, encompassing prevention of progression, prevention of endocarditis, and eventual repair of the valve. Management of calcium and phosphorus abnormalities are likely important in preventing worsening of aortic stenosis, although this has not been proven. Management of hypertension may also be important.

Valve replacement is the therapy of choice for critical aortic stenosis, and the timing of surgery is dependent on individual patient characteristics. Surgery should be performed before left ventricular contractility becomes diminished. There currently is no consensus for a benefit of either prosthetic versus bioprosthetic valves in dialysis patients.[158] The mortality rate for valve replacement is, however, much higher than in the general population (17% operative mortality for aortic valve replacement in dialysis patients, 23% for mitral valve replacement, 25% for aortic valve replacement and CABG, and 37% for mitral valve replacement and CABG).[159] However, in most cases the prognosis is worse if clinically indicated surgery is not performed or if emergent rather than elective surgery is performed.[150]

ARRHYTHMIAS AND SUDDEN CARDIAC DEATH IN CKD

Patients with CKD are at high risk for arrhythmia due to a high prevalence of LVH, HF, IHD, atrial enlargement, and valvular abnormalities. Hemodialysis patients are also exposed to rapid shifts in ions, including potassium, calcium, hydrogen, and magnesium.

Atrial Fibrillation

Both atrial and ventricular arrhythmias are common in dialysis patients. Mirroring the general population, atrial fibrillation is the most common of these arrhythmias, with an incidence of over 10%.[160] In the USRDS DMMS Wave 2 cohort, 123 out of 3374 patients (3.6%) were hospitalized with a primary diagnosis of atrial fibrillation (12.5 hospitalizations per 1000 person years).[161]

The major complications of atrial fibrillation include loss of the "atrial kick" and cardiac synchronicity leading to diminished cardiac function and occurrence of thromboembolic phenomena. Very little data exist as to how common thromboembolism is in dialysis patients with atrial fibrillation, although one small observational study showed a 1-year incidence of nearly 35%.[160] Optimal management involves rate control with or without restoration of sinus rhythm, although patients with symptoms may benefit from a return to sinus rhythm.[162–164] β-Blockers and calcium channel blockers are useful for rate control, whereas amiodarone is useful for both slowing the rate as well as for chemical cardioversion. Anticoagulation with warfarin has not been prospectively studied in dialysis patients, although analysis of the DMMS Wave 2 database showed a survival benefit for patients who were on warfarin at the time of hospitalization for atrial fibrillation.[161] At this time, the benefits and risks of anticoagulation in dialysis patients should be considered on an individual patient basis.

Ventricular Arrhythmias and Sudden Death

Ventricular arrhythmias and ectopy are also common in CKD. There are currently no data indicating that cardiac management of patients prone to arrhythmia should be any different than in the general population.

Identified arrhythmias and cardiac arrest of unknown cause account for 60% of cardiac deaths in dialysis patients.[165] During the first year of dialysis, the rate of cardiac arrest is 93 events per 1000 patient years; this nearly doubles by dialysis year 4 such that 43% of dialysis patients have had cardiac arrest by this time. Thirty-day survival after cardiac arrest is only 32% and 1-year survival 15%.

Potential strategies to reduce the risk of fatal cardiac arrhythmias include careful attention to fluid and electrolyte shifts. Other potential interventions may include routine use of β-blockers, although this has not been investigated. Finally, studies of the appropriate use of implantable defibrillators in dialysis patients are needed.

References

1. U.S. Renal Data System. USRDS 2000 Annual Data Report. Bethesda, MD, National Institutes of Health, National Institute of Diabetes and Digestive and Kidney Diseases, 2000.
2. Foley RN, Parfrey PS, Sarnak MJ: Epidemiology of cardiovascular disease in chronic renal disease. J Am Soc Nephrol 1998; 9(12 suppl):S16–S23.
3. U.S. Renal Data System. USRDS 2001 Annual Data Report. Bethesda, MD, National Institutes of Health, National Institute of Diabetes and Digestive and Kidney Diseases, 2001.
4. Herzog CA, Ma JZ, Collins AJ: Poor long-term survival after acute myocardial infarction among patients on long-term dialysis. N Engl J Med 1998; 339(12):799–805.
5. Levin A, Singer J, Thompson CR, et al: Prevalent left ventricular hypertrophy in the predialysis population: Identifying opportunities for intervention. Am J Kidney Dis 1996; 27(3):347–354.
6. Levy D, Garrison RJ, Savage DD, et al: Prognostic implications of echocardiographically determined left ventricular mass in the Framingham Heart Study. N Engl J Med 1990; 322(22): 1561–1566.
7. Shlipak MG, Simon JA, Grady D, et al: Renal insufficiency and cardiovascular events in postmenopausal women with coronary heart disease. J Am Coll Cardiol 2001; 38(3):705–711.

8. Shlipak MG, Heidenreich PA, Noguchi H, et al: Association of renal insufficiency with treatment and outcomes after myocardial infarction in elderly patients. Ann Intern Med 2002; 137(7):555–562.
9. Wright RS, Reeder GS, Herzog CA, et al: Acute myocardial infarction and renal dysfunction: A high-risk combination. Ann Intern Med 2002; 137(7):563–570.
10. Henry RM, Kostense PJ, Bos G, et al: Mild renal insufficiency is associated with increased cardiovascular mortality: The Hoorn Study. Kidney Int 2002; 62(4):1402–1407.
11. Manjunath G, Tighiouart H, Coresh J, et al: Level of kidney function as a risk factor for cardiovascular outcomes in the elderly. Kidney Int 2003; 63(3):1121–1129.
12. Manjunath G, Tighiouart H, Ibrahim H, et al: Level of kidney function as a risk factor for atherosclerotic cardiovascular outcomes in the community. J Am Coll Cardiol 2003; 41(1):47–55.
13. Dries DL, Exner DV, Domanski MJ, et al: The prognostic implications of renal insufficiency in asymptomatic and symptomatic patients with left ventricular systolic dysfunction. J Am Coll Cardiol 2000; 35(3):681–689.
14. Mann JF, Gerstein HC, Pogue J, et al: Renal insufficiency as a predictor of cardiovascular outcomes and the impact of ramipril: The HOPE randomized trial. Ann Intern Med 2001; 134(8):629–636.
15. Garg AX, Clark WF, Haynes RB, House AA: Moderate renal insufficiency and the risk of cardiovascular mortality: Results from the NHANES I. Kidney Int 2002; 61(4):1486–1494.
16. Culleton BF, Larson MG, Wilson PW, et al: Cardiovascular disease and mortality in a community-based cohort with mild renal insufficiency. Kidney Int 1999; 56(6):2214–2219.
17. Wachtell K, Olsen MH, Dahlof B, et al: Microalbuminuria in hypertensive patients with electrocardiographic left ventricular hypertrophy: The LIFE study. J Hypertens 2002; 20(3):405–412.
18. The Diabetes Control and Complications Trial Research Group: The effect of intensive treatment of diabetes on the development and progression of long-term complications in insulin-dependent diabetes mellitus. N Engl J Med 1993; 329(14): 977–986.
19. Culleton BF, Larson MG, Parfrey PS, et al: Proteinuria as a risk factor for cardiovascular disease and mortality in older people: A prospective study. Am J Med 2000; 109(1):1–8.
20. Kannel WB, Stampfer MJ, Castelli WP, Verter J: The prognostic significance of proteinuria: The Framingham study. Am Heart J 1984; 108(5):1347–1352.
21. Mogensen CE: Microalbuminuria predicts clinical proteinuria and early mortality in maturity-onset diabetes. N Engl J Med 1984; 310(6):356–360.
22. Bigazzi R, Bianchi S, Baldari D, Campese VM: Microalbuminuria predicts cardiovascular events and renal insufficiency in patients with essential hypertension. J Hypertens 1998; 16(9):1325–1333.
23. Gerstein HC, Mann JF, Yi Q, et al: Albuminuria and risk of cardiovascular events, death, and heart failure in diabetic and nondiabetic individuals. JAMA 2001; 286(4):421–426.
24. Romundstad S, Holmen J, Kvenild K, et al: Microalbuminuria and all-cause mortality in 2,089 apparently healthy individuals: A 4.4-year follow-up study. The Nord-Trondelag Health Study (HUNT), Norway. Am J Kidney Dis 2003; 42(3):466–473.
25. Hillege HL, Fidler V, Diercks GF, et al: Urinary albumin excretion predicts cardiovascular and noncardiovascular mortality in general population. Circulation 2002; 106(14):1777–1782.
26. Weiner DE, Sarnak MJ: Microalbuminuria: A marker of cardiovascular risk. Am J Kidney Dis 2003; 42(3):596–598.
27. Longenecker JC, Coresh J, Powe NR, et al: Traditional cardiovascular disease risk factors in dialysis patients compared with the general population: The CHOICE Study. J Am Soc Nephrol 2002; 13(7):1918–1927.
28. Uhlig K, Levey AS, Sarnak MJ: Traditional cardiac risk factors in individuals with chronic kidney disease. Semin Dial 2003; 16(2):118–127.
29. Port FK, Hulbert-Shearon TE, Wolfe RA, et al: Predialysis blood pressure and mortality risk in a national sample of maintenance hemodialysis patients. Am J Kidney Dis 1999; 33(3):507–517.
30. Zager PG, Nikolic J, Brown RH, et al: "U" curve association of blood pressure and mortality in hemodialysis patients. Medical Directors of Dialysis Clinic, Inc., Kidney Int 1998; 54(2):561–569.
31. Foley RN, Herzog CA, Collins AJ: Blood pressure and long-term mortality in United States hemodialysis patients: USRDS Waves 3 and 4 Study. Kidney Int 2002; 62(5):1784–1790.
32. Foley RN, Parfrey PS, Harnett JD, et al: Impact of hypertension on cardiomyopathy, morbidity and mortality in end-stage renal disease. Kidney Int 1996; 49(5):1379–1385.
33. Kawamura M, Fijimoto S, Hisanaga S, et al: Incidence, outcome, and risk factors of cerebrovascular events in patients undergoing maintenance hemodialysis. Am J Kidney Dis 1998; 31(6):991–996.
34. Agarwal R: Systolic hypertension in hemodialysis patients. Semin Dial 2003; 16(3):208–213.
35. Agarwal R, Nissenson AR, Batlle D, et al: Prevalence, treatment, and control of hypertension in chronic hemodialysis patients in the United States. Am J Med 2003; 115(4):291–297.
36. Tonelli M, Bohm C, Pandeya S, et al: Cardiac risk factors and the use of cardioprotective medications in patients with chronic renal insufficiency. Am J Kidney Dis 2001; 37(3):484–489.
37. Coresh J, Wei GL, McQuillan G, et al: Prevalence of high blood pressure and elevated serum creatinine level in the United States: Findings from the third National Health and Nutrition Examination Survey (1988–1994). Arch Intern Med 2001; 161(9):1207–1216.
38. Buckalew VM Jr, Berg RL, Wang SR, et al: Prevalence of hypertension in 1,795 subjects with chronic renal disease: The modification of diet in renal disease study baseline cohort. Modification of Diet in Renal Disease Study Group. Am J Kidney Dis 1996; 28(6):811–821.
39. Adler AI, Stratton IM, Neil HA, et al: Association of systolic blood pressure with macrovascular and microvascular complications of type II diabetes (UKPDS 36): Prospective observational study. BMJ 2000; 321(7258):412–419.
40. Davis TM, Millns H, Stratton IM, et al: Risk factors for stroke in type II diabetes mellitus: United Kingdom Prospective Diabetes Study (UKPDS) 29. Arch Intern Med 1999; 159(10): 1097–1103.
41. Jungers P, Massy ZA, Khoa TN, et al: Incidence and risk factors of atherosclerotic cardiovascular accidents in predialysis chronic renal failure patients: A prospective study. Nephrol Dial Transplant 1997; 12(12):2597–2602.
42. Lazarus JM, Bourgoignie JJ, Buckalew VM, et al: Achievement and safety of a low blood pressure goal in chronic renal disease. The Modification of Diet in Renal Disease Study Group. Hypertension 1997; 29(2):641–650.
43. Jafar TH, Stark PC, Schmid CH, et al: Progression of chronic kidney disease: The role of blood pressure control, proteinuria, and angiotensin-converting enzyme inhibition: A patient-level meta-analysis. Ann Intern Med 2003; 139(4):244–252.
44. Lewis EJ, Hunsicker LG, Bain RP, Rohde RD: The effect of angiotensin-converting-enzyme inhibition on diabetic nephropathy. The Collaborative Study Group. N Engl J Med 1993; 329(20): 1456–1462.
45. Lewis EJ, Hunsicker LG, Clarke WR, et al: Renoprotective effect of the angiotensin-receptor antagonist irbesartan in patients with nephropathy due to type II diabetes. N Engl J Med 2001; 345(12):851–860.
46. Jafar TH, Schmid CH, Landa M, et al: Angiotensin-converting enzyme inhibitors and progression of nondiabetic renal disease. A meta-analysis of patient-level data. Ann Intern Med 2001; 135(2):73–87.
47. Giatras I, Lau J, Levey AS: Effect of angiotensin-converting enzyme inhibitors on the progression of nondiabetic renal disease: A meta-analysis of randomized trials. Angiotensin-

Converting-Enzyme Inhibition and Progressive Renal Disease Study Group. Ann Intern Med 1997; 127(5):337–345.

48. Brenner BM, Cooper ME, de Zeeuw D, et al: Effects of losartan on renal and cardiovascular outcomes in patients with type II diabetes and nephropathy. N Engl J Med 2001; 345(12): 861–869.

48a. National Kidney Foundation. K/DOQI Practice Guidelines on Hypertension and Antihypertensive Agents in Chronic Kidney Disease. Am J Kidney Dis 2004; 43(suppl):S1-S290.

49. Attman PO, Samuelsson O, Alaupovic P: Lipoprotein metabolism and renal failure. Am J Kidney Dis 1993; 21(6):573–592.

50. National Kidney Foundation. K/DOQI Clinical Practice Guidelines for Managing Dyslipidemias in Chronic Kidney Disease. Am J Kidney Dis 2003; 41(suppl 3):S1–S92.

51. Lowrie EG, Lew NL: Death risk in hemodialysis patients: The predictive value of commonly measured variables and an evaluation of death rate differences between facilities. Am J Kidney Dis 1990; 15(5):458–482.

52. Iseki K, Yamazato M, Tozawa M, Takishita S: Hypocholesterolemia is a significant predictor of death in a cohort of chronic hemodialysis patients. Kidney Int 2002; 61(5): 1887–1893.

53. Liu Y, Coresh J, Eustace JA, et al: Association between cholesterol level and mortality in dialysis patients: Role of inflammation and malnutrition. JAMA 2004; 291(4):451–459.

54. National Kidney Foundation. K/DOQI Clinical Practice Guidelines for Managing Dyslipidemias in Chronic Kidney Disease. Am J Kidney Dis 2003; 41(suppl 3):S1–S92.

55. Cheung AK, Sarnak MJ, Yan G, et al: Atherosclerotic cardiovascular disease risks in chronic hemodialysis patients. Kidney Int 2000; 58(1):353–362.

56. Harnett JD, Foley RN, Kent GM, et al: Congestive heart failure in dialysis patients: Prevalence, incidence, prognosis and risk factors. Kidney Int 1995; 47(3):884–890.

57. Le Feuvre C, Borentain M, Beygui F, et al: Comparison of short- and long-term outcomes of coronary angioplasty in patients with and without diabetes mellitus and with and without hemodialysis. Am J Cardiol 2003; 92(6):721–725.

58. Herzog CA, Ma JZ, Collins AJ: Comparative survival of dialysis patients in the United States after coronary angioplasty, coronary artery stenting, and coronary artery bypass surgery and impact of diabetes. Circulation 2002; 106(17):2207–2211.

59. U.S. Renal Data System. USRDS 2000 Annual Data Report. Bethesda, MD, National Institutes of Health, National Institute of Diabetes and Digestive and Kidney Diseases, 1998.

60. Wilson PW, Castelli WP, Kannel WB: Coronary risk prediction in adults (the Framingham Heart Study). Am J Cardiol 1987; 59(14):91G–94G.

61. Weiner DE, Tighiouart H, Amin MG, et al: Chronic kidney disease as a risk factor for cardiovascular disease and all-cause mortality: A pooled analysis of community based studies. J Am Soc Nephrol 2004; 15(5):1307–1315.

62. Blacher J, Pannier B, Guerin AP, et al: Carotid arterial stiffness as a predictor of cardiovascular and all-cause mortality in end-stage renal disease. Hypertension 1998; 32(3):570–574.

63. Guerin AP, London GM, Marchais SJ, Metivier F: Arterial stiffening and vascular calcifications in end-stage renal disease. Nephrol Dial Transplant 2000; 15(7):1014–1021.

64. McMahon LP, Mason K, Skinner SL, et al: Effects of haemoglobin normalization on quality of life and cardiovascular parameters in end-stage renal failure. Nephrol Dial Transplant 2000; 15(9):1425–1430.

65. Levin A, Thompson CR, Ethier J, et al: Left ventricular mass index increase in early renal disease: Impact of decline in hemoglobin. Am J Kidney Dis 1999; 34(1):125–134.

66. Kong CH, Farrington K: Determinants of left ventricular hypertrophy and its progression in high-flux haemodialysis. Blood Purif 2003; 21(2):163–169.

67. Ozkahya M, Toz H, Qzerkan F, et al: Impact of volume control on left ventricular hypertrophy in dialysis patients. J Nephrol 2002; 15(6):655–660.

68. Middleton RJ, Parfrey PS, Foley RN: Left ventricular hypertrophy in the renal patient. J Am Soc Nephrol 2001; 12(5): 1079–1084.

69. deFilippi C WS, Rosanio S, Tiblier E, et al: Cardiac troponin T and C-reactive protein for predicting prognosis, coronary atherosclerosis, and cardiomyopathy in patients undergoing long-term hemodialysis. JAMA 2003; 290(3):353–359.

70. Foley RN, Parfrey PS, Harnett JD, et al: Clinical and echocardiographic disease in patients starting end-stage renal disease therapy. Kidney Int 1995; 47(1):186–192.

71. Zoccali C, Benedetto FA, Mallamaci F, et al: Prognostic impact of the indexation of left ventricular mass in patients undergoing dialysis. J Am Soc Nephrol 2001; 12(12):2768–2774.

72. Parfrey PS, Foley RN, Harnett JD, et al: Outcome and risk factors for left ventricular disorders in chronic uraemia. Nephrol Dial Transplant 1996; 11(7):1277–1285.

73. Paoletti E, Cassottana P, Bellino D, et al: Left ventricular geometry and adverse cardiovascular events in chronic hemodialysis patients on prolonged therapy with ACE inhibitors. Am J Kidney Dis 2002; 40(4):728–736.

74. Unger P, Wissing KM, de Pauw L, et al: Reduction of left ventricular diameter and mass after surgical arteriovenous fistula closure in renal transplant recipients. Transplantation 2002; 74(1):73–79.

75. Chan CT, Floras JS, Miller JA, et al: Regression of left ventricular hypertrophy after conversion to nocturnal hemodialysis. Kidney Int 2002; 61(6):2235–2239.

76. London GM, Marchais SJ, Guerin AP, et al: Inflammation, arteriosclerosis, and cardiovascular therapy in hemodialysis patients. Kidney Int Suppl 2003; 84:S88–S93.

77. Foley RN, Parfrey PS, Morgan J, et al: Effect of hemoglobin levels in hemodialysis patients with asymptomatic cardiomyopathy. Kidney Int 2000; 58(3):1325–1335.

78. Roger SD, McMahon LP, Clarkson A, et al: Effects of early and late intervention with epoetin alpha on left ventricular mass among patients with chronic kidney disease (stage III or IV): Results of a randomized clinical trial. J Am Soc Nephrol 2004; 15(1):148–156.

79. Foley RN, Herzog CA, Collins AJ: Smoking and cardiovascular outcomes in dialysis patients: The United States Renal Data System Wave 2 Study. Kidney Int 2003; 63(4):1462–1467.

80. Bostom AG, Silbershatz H, Rosenberg IH, et al: Nonfasting plasma total homocysteine levels and all-cause and cardiovascular disease mortality in elderly Framingham men and women. Arch Intern Med 1999; 159(10):1077–1080.

81. Bostom AG, Rosenberg IH, Silbershatz H, et al: Nonfasting plasma total homocysteine levels and stroke incidence in elderly persons: The Framingham Study. Ann Intern Med 1999; 131(5): 352–355.

82. Bostom AG, Lathrop L: Hyperhomocysteinemia in end-stage renal disease: Prevalence, etiology, and potential relationship to arteriosclerotic outcomes. Kidney Int 1997; 52(1):10–20.

83. Friedman AN, Bostom AG, Selhub J, et al: The kidney and homocysteine metabolism. J Am Soc Nephrol 2001; 12(10):2181–2189.

84. Mallamaci F, Zoccali C, Tripepi G, et al: Hyperhomocysteinemia predicts cardiovascular outcomes in hemodialysis patients. Kidney Int 2002; 61(2):609–614.

85. Clarke R, Lewington S, Landray M: Homocysteine, renal function, and risk of cardiovascular disease. Kidney Int Suppl 2003; 84:S131–S133.

86. Suliman ME, Qureshi AR, Barany P, et al: Hyperhomocysteinemia, nutritional status, and cardiovascular disease in hemodialysis patients. Kidney Int 2000; 57(4):1727–1735.

87. Selhub J, Jacques PF, Wilson PW, et al: Vitamin status and intake as primary determinants of homocysteinemia in an elderly population. JAMA 1993; 270(22):2693–2698.

88. Schnyder G, Roffi M, Pin R, et al: Decreased rate of coronary restenosis after lowering of plasma homocysteine levels. N Engl J Med 2001; 345(22):1593–1600.

89. Vermeulen EG, Stehouwer CD, Twisk JW, et al: Effect of homocysteine-lowering treatment with folic acid plus vitamin B6 on progression of subclinical atherosclerosis: A randomised, placebo-controlled trial. Lancet 2000; 355(9203):517–522.
90. Shemin D, Bostom AG, Selhub J: Treatment of hyperhomocysteinemia in end-stage renal disease. Am J Kidney Dis 2001; 38 (4 suppl 1):S91–S94.
91. Van Tellingen A, Grooteman MP, Bartels PC, et al: Long-term reduction of plasma homocysteine levels by super-flux dialyzers in hemodialysis patients. Kidney Int 2001; 59(1):342–347.
92. Friedman AN, Bostom AG, Levey AS, et al: Plasma total homocysteine levels among patients undergoing nocturnal versus standard hemodialysis. J Am Soc Nephrol 2002; 13(1): 265–268.
93. Himmelfarb J, Stenvinkel P, Ikizler TA, Hakim RM: The elephant in uremia: Oxidant stress as a unifying concept of cardiovascular disease in uremia. Kidney Int 2002; 62(5): 1524–1538.
94. Sies H: Oxidative stress: Oxidants and antioxidants. Exp Physiol 1997; 82(2):291–295.
95. Locatelli F, Canaud B, Eckardt KU, et al: Oxidative stress in end-stage renal disease: An emerging threat to patient outcome. Nephrol Dial Transplant 2003; 18(7):1272–1280.
96. Qureshi AR, Alvestrand A, Divino-Filho JC, et al: Inflammation, malnutrition, and cardiac disease as predictors of mortality in hemodialysis patients. J Am Soc Nephrol 2002; 13(suppl 1): S28–S36.
97. Spittle MA, Hoenich NA, Handelman GJ, et al: Oxidative stress and inflammation in hemodialysis patients. Am J Kidney Dis 2001; 38(6):1408–1413.
98. Sakai M, Kobori S, Matsumura T, et al: HMG-CoA reductase inhibitors suppress macrophage growth induced by oxidized low density lipoprotein. Atherosclerosis 1997; 133(1):51–59.
99. Kinlay S, Schwartz GG, Olsson AG, et al: High-dose atorvastatin enhances the decline in inflammatory markers in patients with acute coronary syndromes in the MIRACL study. Circulation 2003; 108(13):1560–1566.
100. Chang JW, Yang WS, Min WK, et al: Effects of simvastatin on high-sensitivity C-reactive protein and serum albumin in hemodialysis patients. Am J Kidney Dis 2002; 39(6):1213–1217.
101. Yusuf S, Dagenais G, Pogue J, et al: Vitamin E supplementation and cardiovascular events in high-risk patients. The Heart Outcomes Prevention Evaluation Study Investigators. N Engl J Med 2000; 342(3):154–160.
102. Boaz M, Smetana S, Weinstein T, et al: Secondary prevention with antioxidants of cardiovascular disease in end stage renal disease (SPACE): Randomised placebo-controlled trial. Lancet 2000; 356(9237):1213–1218.
103. Tepel M, van der Giet M, Statz M, et al: The antioxidant acetylcysteine reduces cardiovascular events in patients with end-stage renal failure: A randomized, controlled trial. Circulation 2003; 107(7):992–995.
104. Tsuruoka S, Kawaguchi A, Nishiki K, et al: Vitamin E-bonded hemodialyzer improves neutrophil function and oxidative stress in patients with end-stage renal failure. Am J Kidney Dis 2002; 39(1):127–133.
105. Miyazaki H, Matsuoka H, Itabe H, et al: Hemodialysis impairs endothelial function via oxidative stress: Effects of vitamin E-coated dialyzer. Circulation 2000; 101(9):1002–1006.
106. Raggi P, Boulay A, Chasan-Taber S, et al: Cardiac calcification in adult hemodialysis patients. A link between end-stage renal disease and cardiovascular disease? J Am Coll Cardiol 2002; 39(4): 695–701.
107. Unruh ML, Hartunian MG, Chapman MM, Jaber BL: Sleep quality and clinical correlates in patients on maintenance dialysis. Clin Nephrol 2003; 59(4):280–288.
108. Zoccali C, Mallamaci F, Tripepi G: Nocturnal hypoxemia predicts incident cardiovascular complications in dialysis patients. J Am Soc Nephrol 2002; 13(3):729–733.
109. Trespalacios FC, Taylor AJ, Agodoa LY, Abbott KC: Incident acute coronary syndromes in chronic dialysis patients in the United States. Kidney Int 2002; 62(5):1799–1805.
110. Shoji T, Emoto M, Tabata T, et al: Advanced atherosclerosis in predialysis patients with chronic renal failure. Kidney Int 2002; 61(6):2187–2192.
111. Nishizawa Y, Shoji T, Maekawa K, et al: Intima-media thickness of carotid artery predicts cardiovascular mortality in hemodialysis patients. Am J Kidney Dis 2003; 41(3 suppl 1):S76–S79.
112. Rabbat CG, Treleaven DJ, Russell JD, et al: Prognostic value of myocardial perfusion studies in patients with end-stage renal disease assessed for kidney or kidney-pancreas transplantation: A meta-analysis. J Am Soc Nephrol 2003; 14(2):431–439.
113. O'Rourke RA, Brundage BH, Froelicher VF, et al: American College of Cardiology/American Heart Association Expert Consensus document on electron-beam computed tomography for the diagnosis and prognosis of coronary artery disease. Circulation 2000; 102(1):126–140.
114. Qunibi WY, Nolan CA, Ayus JC: Cardiovascular calcification in patients with end-stage renal disease: A century-old phenomenon. Kidney Int Suppl 2002; 82:73–80.
115. London GM, Marchais SJ, Guerin AP, et al: Arterial structure and function in end-stage renal disease. Nephrol Dial Transplant 2002; 17(10):1713–1724.
116. Klassen PS, Lowrie EG, Reddan DN, et al: Association between pulse pressure and mortality in patients undergoing maintenance hemodialysis. JAMA 2002; 287(12):1548–1555.
117. Tozawa M, Iseki K, Iseki C, Takishita S: Pulse pressure and risk of total mortality and cardiovascular events in patients on chronic hemodialysis. Kidney Int 2002; 61(2):717–726.
118. Rostand SG, Kirk KA, Rutsky EA: Dialysis-associated ischemic heart disease: Insights from coronary angiography. Kidney Int 1984; 25(4):653–659.
119. Stewart GA, Foster J, Cowan M, et al: Echocardiography overestimates left ventricular mass in hemodialysis patients relative to magnetic resonance imaging. Kidney Int 1999; 56(6): 2248–2253.
120. Martin LC, Barretti P, Cornejo IV, et al: Influence of fluid volume variations on the calculated value of the left ventricular mass measured by echocardiogram in patients submitted to hemodialysis. Ren Fail 2003; 25(1):43–53.
121. Prisant LM, Kleinman DJ, Carr AA, et al: Assessment of echocardiographic left ventricular mass before and after acute volume depletion. Am J Hypertens 1994; 7(5):425–428.
122. Martin GS, Becker BN, Schulman G: Cardiac troponin-I accurately predicts myocardial injury in renal failure. Nephrol Dial Transplant 1998; 13(7):1709–1712.
123. Freda BJ, Tang WH, Van Lente F, et al: Cardiac troponins in renal insufficiency: Review and clinical implications. J Am Coll Cardiol 2002; 40(12):2065–2071.
124. Iliou MC, Fumeron C, Benoit MO, et al: Prognostic value of cardiac markers in ESRD: Chronic Hemodialysis and New Cardiac Markers Evaluation (CHANCE) study. Am J Kidney Dis 2003; 42(3):513–523.
125. Khan IA, Wattanasuwan N, Mehta NJ, et al: Prognostic value of serum cardiac troponin I in ambulatory patients with chronic renal failure undergoing long-term hemodialysis: A two-year outcome analysis. J Am Coll Cardiol 2001; 38(4): 991–998.
126. Keeley EC, Kadakia R, Soman S, et al: Analysis of long-term survival after revascularization in patients with chronic kidney disease presenting with acute coronary syndromes. Am J Cardiol 2003; 92(5):509–514.
127. Berl T, Hunsicker LG, Lewis JB, et al: Cardiovascular outcomes in the Irbesartan Diabetic Nephropathy Trial of patients with type II diabetes and overt nephropathy. Ann Intern Med 2003; 138(7):542–549.
128. Gottlieb SS, McCarter RJ, Vogel RA: Effect of beta-blockade on mortality among high-risk and low-risk patients after myocardial infarction. N Engl J Med 1998; 339(8):489–497.
129. Cice G, Ferrara L, D'Andrea A, et al: Carvedilol increases two-year survival in dialysis patients with dilated cardiomyopathy: A prospective, placebo-controlled trial. J Am Coll Cardiol 2003; 41(9):1438–1444.

130. Berger AK, Duval S, Krumholz HM: Aspirin, beta-blocker, and angiotensin-converting enzyme inhibitor therapy in patients with end-stage renal disease and an acute myocardial infarction. J Am Coll Cardiol 2003; 42(2):201–208.
131. Besarab A, Bolton WK, Browne JK, et al: The effects of normal as compared with low hematocrit values in patients with cardiac disease who are receiving hemodialysis and epoetin. N Engl J Med 1998; 339(9):584–590.
132. Naganuma T, Sugimura K, Wada S, et al: The prognostic role of brain natriuretic peptides in hemodialysis patients. Am J Nephrol 2002; 22(5/6):437–444.
133. Nakatani T, Naganuma T, Masuda C, et al: The prognostic role of atrial natriuretic peptides in hemodialysis patients. Blood Purif 2003; 21(6):395–400.
134. Zoccali C, Mallamaci F, Benedetto FA, et al: Cardiac natriuretic peptides are related to left ventricular mass and function and predict mortality in dialysis patients. J Am Soc Nephrol 2001; 12(7):1508–1515.
135. Efrati S, Zaidenstein R, Dishy V, et al: ACE inhibitors and survival of hemodialysis patients. Am J Kidney Dis 2002; 40(5):1023–1029.
136. The Digitalis Investigation Group: The effect of digoxin on mortality and morbidity in patients with heart failure. N Engl J Med 1997; 336(8):525–533.
137. Alpert MA, Ravenscraft MD: Pericardial involvement in end-stage renal disease. Am J Med Sci 2003; 325(4):228–236.
138. Rutsky EA, Rostand SG: Treatment of uremic pericarditis and pericardial effusion. Am J Kidney Dis 1987; 10(1):2–8.
139. Rostand SG, Rutsky EA: Pericarditis in end-stage renal disease. Cardiol Clin 1990; 8(4):701–707.
140. Gunukula SR, Spodick DH: Pericardial disease in renal patients. Semin Nephrol 2001; 21(1):52–56.
141. Buselmeier TJ, Davin TD, Simmons RL, et al: Treatment of intractable uremic pericardial effusion. Avoidance of pericardiectomy with local steroid instillation. JAMA 1978; 240(13): 1358–1359.
142. Abbott KC, Agodoa LY: Hospitalizations for bacterial endocarditis after initiation of chronic dialysis in the United States. Nephron 2002; 91(2):203–209.
143. Marr KA, Sexton DJ, Conlon PJ, et al: Catheter-related bacteremia and outcome of attempted catheter salvage in patients undergoing hemodialysis. Ann Intern Med 1997; 127(4): 275–280.
144. Little MA, O'Riordan A, Lucey B, et al: A prospective study of complications associated with cuffed, tunnelled haemodialysis catheters. Nephrol Dial Transplant 2001; 16(11):2194–2200.
145. Stevenson KB, Hannah EL, Lowder CA, et al: Epidemiology of hemodialysis vascular access infections from longitudinal infection surveillance data: Predicting the impact of NKF-DOQI clinical practice guidelines for vascular access. Am J Kidney Dis 2002; 39(3):549–555.
146. McCarthy JT, Steckelberg JM: Infective endocarditis in patients receiving long-term hemodialysis. Mayo Clin Proc 2000; 75(10): 1008–1014.
147. Doulton T, Sabharwal N, Cairns HS, et al: Infective endocarditis in dialysis patients: New challenges and old. Kidney Int 2003; 64(2):720–727.
148. Robinson DL, Fowler VG, Sexton DJ, et al: Bacterial endocarditis in hemodialysis patients. Am J Kidney Dis 1997; 30(4): 521–524.
149. Maraj S, Jacobs LE, Kung SC, et al: Epidemiology and outcome of infective endocarditis in hemodialysis patients. Am J Med Sci 2002; 324(5):254–260.
150. Umana E, Ahmed W, Alpert MA: Valvular and perivalvular abnormalities in end-stage renal disease. Am J Med Sci 2003; 325(4):237–242.
151. Maher ER, Young G, Smyth-Walsh B, et al: Aortic and mitral valve calcification in patients with end-stage renal disease. Lancet 1987; 2(8564):875–877.
152. Forman MB, Virmani R, Robertson RM, Stone WJ: Mitral annular calcification in chronic renal failure. Chest 1984; 85(3): 367–371.
153. Ribeiro S, Ramos A, Brandao A, et al: Cardiac valve calcification in haemodialysis patients: Role of calcium-phosphate metabolism. Nephrol Dial Transplant 1998; 13(8):2037–2040.
154. London GM, Pannier B, Marchais SJ, Guerin AP: Calcification of the aortic valve in the dialyzed patient. J Am Soc Nephrol 2000; 11(4):778–783.
155. Urena P, Malergue MC, Goldfarb B, et al: Evolutive aortic stenosis in hemodialysis patients: Analysis of risk factors. Nephrologie 1999; 20(4):217–225.
156. Otto CM, Lind BK, Kitzman DW, et al: Association of aortic-valve sclerosis with cardiovascular mortality and morbidity in the elderly. N Engl J Med 1999; 341(3):142–147.
157. Perkovic V, Hunt D, Griffin SV, et al: Accelerated progression of calcific aortic stenosis in dialysis patients. Nephron Clin Pract 2003; 94(2):C40-C45.
158. Herzog CA, Ma JZ, Collins AJ: Long-term survival of dialysis patients in the United States with prosthetic heart valves: Should ACC/AHA practice guidelines on valve selection be modified? Circulation 2002; 105(11):1336–1341.
159. Edwards FH, Peterson ED, Coombs LP, et al: Prediction of operative mortality after valve replacement surgery. J Am Coll Cardiol 2001; 37(3):885–892.
160. Vazquez E, Sanchez-Perales C, Borrego F, et al: Influence of atrial fibrillation on the morbido-mortality of patients on hemodialysis. Am Heart J 2000; 140(6):886–890.
161. Abbott KC, Trespalacios FC, Taylor AJ, Agodoa LY: Atrial fibrillation in chronic dialysis patients in the United States: Risk factors for hospitalization and mortality. BMC Nephrol 2003; 4(1):1.
162. Van Gelder IC, Hagens VE, Bosker HA, et al: A comparison of rate control and rhythm control in patients with recurrent persistent atrial fibrillation. N Engl J Med 2002; 347(23): 1834–1840.
163. Hagens VE, Ranchor AV, Van Sonderen E, et al: Effect of rate or rhythm control on quality of life in persistent atrial fibrillation. Results from the Rate Control Versus Electrical Cardioversion (RACE) study. J Am Coll Cardiol 2004; 43(2): 241–247.
164. Carlsson J, Miketic S, Windeler J, et al: Randomized trial of rate-control versus rhythm-control in persistent atrial fibrillation: The Strategies of Treatment of Atrial Fibrillation (STAF) study. J Am Coll Cardiol 2003; 41(10):1690–1696.
165. Herzog CA: Cardiac arrest in dialysis patients: Approaches to alter an abysmal outcome. Kidney Int Suppl 2003; 84: S197–S200.
166. Sarnak MJ, Levey AS: Cardiovascular disease and chronic renal disease: A new paradigm. Am J Kidney Dis 2000; 35(4 suppl 1):S117–S131.
167. Sarnak MJ, Levey AS, Schoolwerth AC, et al: Kidney disease as a risk factor for development of cardiovascular disease: A statement from the American Heart Association Councils on Kidney in Cardiovascular Disease, High Blood Pressure Research, Clinical Cardiology, and Epidemiology and Prevention. Circulation 2003; 108(17):2154–2169.
168. Kasiske BL: Hyperlipidemia in patients with chronic renal disease. Am J Kidney Dis 1998; 32(5 suppl 3):S142–S156.
169. Report of the National Cholesterol Education Program Expert Panel on Detection, Evaluation, and Treatment of High Blood Cholesterol in Adults. The Expert Panel. Arch Intern Med 1988; 148(1):36–69.
170. Schaefer EJ, Lamon-Fava S, Cohn SD, et al: Effects of age, gender, and menopausal status on plasma low density lipoprotein cholesterol and apolipoprotein B levels in the Framingham Offspring Study. J Lipid Res 1994; 35(5):779–792.

Management of the Diabetic End-Stage Renal Disease (ESRD) Patient: Dialysis and Transplantation

Kathryn Tuohy, M.D. • Mark E. Williams, M.D., F.A.C.P.

In 2001, the prevalence of adults in the United States diagnosed with diabetes was 7.9% (16.7 million Americans) while 35% of diabetics are estimated to remain undiagnosed. This represents an increase of 61% since 1990 (prevalence 4.9%) in the number of Americans diagnosed with diabetes, which is thought to be largely due to a concurrent increase in obesity and a sedentary lifestyle. African-Americans had the highest rate of diagnosed diabetes among all races, and adults with less than a high-school education were highest among levels of education. Of Americans over age 60, 15% had a diagnosis of diabetes.[1] The prevalent number of people with insulin-dependent (type I), and non–insulin-dependent (type II) diabetes has increased for three decades as a result of both improved survival and the aging of the population, as well as the increased prevalence of obesity. Approximately one million new cases of diabetes are diagnosed each year in patients over age 20 in the United States. Recent data estimate the lifetime risk of developing diabetes for individuals born in 2000 in the United States is approximately 35%.[2] Type I diabetes accounts for 5% to 10%, and type II diabetes accounts for 90% to 95% of all diagnosed cases of diabetes.[3] About 90% of diabetic patients older than 20 years have non–insulin-dependent diabetes. A recent report states that 30% of new cases of diabetes diagnosed in North Americans in the second decade of life are also type II.[4]

Diabetic patients are three times more likely than nondiabetic patients to be hospitalized. Adult patients with complications are the most frequently hospitalized.[5] Diabetic patients may account for up to 10% of bed days for nonobstetric, nonpsychiatric admissions,[6] and their average length of stay is longer than that of nondiabetic patients.[7] Health care costs directly attributable to diabetes care were estimated to be $91.8 billion in 2002. This does not include an additional estimated $40.2 billion in indirect costs (disability, work loss, premature mortality).[3]

Risk of death in patients with diabetes is twice that of patients without diabetes, and diabetes is the sixth leading cause of death in the United States.[3] Three quarters of deaths from type I diabetes are associated with renal failure. Despite modest advances in slowing its progression[8] and ongoing research into its primary prevention, diabetic nephropathy accounts for a larger proportion than ever of cases of end-stage renal disease (ESRD) in the United States (Figure 10–1). Projections indicate that by 2006 the incident number of patients with diabetes as the primary diagnosis for ESRD will equal all other causes, and by 2017 the prevalence will also be equal.[9] Notably, however, the growth in incident rates of ESRD due to diabetes has slowed in recent years, with the largest growth rates of diabetes as the primary cause of ESRD occurring in the Eastern, Southern, and Gulf Coast states. Also, although diabetes continues to be the most common cause of ESRD across all racial groups, it accounts for far higher rates among blacks, Hispanics, and Native Americans than in whites.[10]

Primary risk reduction was achieved with intensive insulin therapy in the Diabetes Care and Complications Trial (DCCT),[11] resulting in both a delay in onset and a decrease in complications of diabetic nephropathy. Improvements in patients at risk of developing ESRD have included the use of angiotensin-converting enzyme (ACE) inhibitors[12] and angiotensin receptor blockers (ARBs),[13] tight blood pressure control,[14] and improved glycemic control.[15,16] Between 1991 and 2001, hospital admission rates fell slightly for diabetic patients on dialysis and fell 13% for diabetic patients with a transplanted kidney. Also, diabetic patient survival has improved 17.3% on hemodialysis and 28% on peritoneal dialysis for the period of 1992 to 1996 as compared to 1987 to 1991.[9] In both diabetics and nondiabetics initiating dialysis, a higher glomerular filtration rate (GFR) predicts a higher likelihood of hospitalization, possibly reflecting a greater presence of comorbidities among patients who are pushed to start dialysis earlier.[10] The epidemic of diabetic ESRD appears to result from an increased prevalence of non–insulin-dependent diabetic patients, longer survival of all diabetic patients, and greater acceptance of ESRD treatment.[17]

Summary statistics from the 2002 U.S. Renal Data System (USRDS) report indicated that 110,041 diabetic patients were on dialysis and 21,132 had undergone transplantation by year's end of 2000, which is 34.6% of the 378,862 ESRD patients receiving Medicare benefits.[10] About 41,500 diabetic patients (44% of all new patients) initiated treatment that year. Approximately half were 65 years or older; less than 1% was younger than 20 years. Diabetic patients with ESRD now have a mean age of 64 years,[10] and about two-thirds have type II disease.[18] They make up the majority of diabetic patients on dialysis in some centers. Misclassification of the type of diabetes is common, however. For example, when clinical criteria (age, need for insulin, absence of ketoacidosis, body mass) are used, up to one-third may be misclassified as having type I disease, using C-peptide values as the gold standard. As a result, patients with type II diabetes may be underrepresented.[19]

Diabetic ESRD reflects the demographics of diabetes itself.[20] About 70% of diabetic patients with ESRD are white, and 30% are black.[21] Whereas the proportion of ESRD cases attributed to diabetes is higher in blacks,[10] type I diabetes is the predominant cause of ESRD in whites, and type II diabetes is the predominant cause in blacks. The prevalence of diabetes in the ESRD population in 1-year survivors on dialysis regardless of the primary cause of ESRD is quite high in the United States; 80% of Native Americans, 73% of Hispanics, 61% of Asians, 59% of blacks, and 58% of whites have diabetes at 1-year survival on dialysis.[10]

In this chapter, renal replacement options for the uremic diabetic patient are compared (Table 10–1). In the United States, diabetic patients are more likely than others to be managed on chronic hemodialysis and less likely to have a functioning transplant (Figure 10–2). For all ESRD modalities, diabetic patients are considerably costlier to treat than are nondiabetic patients. Compared with an average cost in 2000 of $67,600 annually for all patients, diabetic patients cost about $3500 more per year. The annual cost in 2000 for a diabetic patient on hemodialysis (HD) was about $72,000, which was $6500 more than that for a nondiabetic. The annual cost for a diabetic patient on peritoneal dialysis (PD) was about $61,000, which was $9200 more than that for a nondiabetic. During the last 10 years, the percentage of dialysis patients covered solely by Medicare has decreased.[10] In 2001, Medicare expenditures accounted for 63% of the total ESRD care costs, and patients with diabetes consumed the greatest amount of resources (Figure 10–3).[9]

Diabetic patients with ESRD are also at greatest risk for complications. Eighty-five percent have comorbid conditions. After 1-year of survival on dialysis, 38% of diabetics have some cardiovascular morbidity, compared with 30% of nondiabetics.[10] Whereas all uremic diabetic patients suffer from two chronic diseases, patients with type II diabetes are generally older and have more advanced coronary disease but

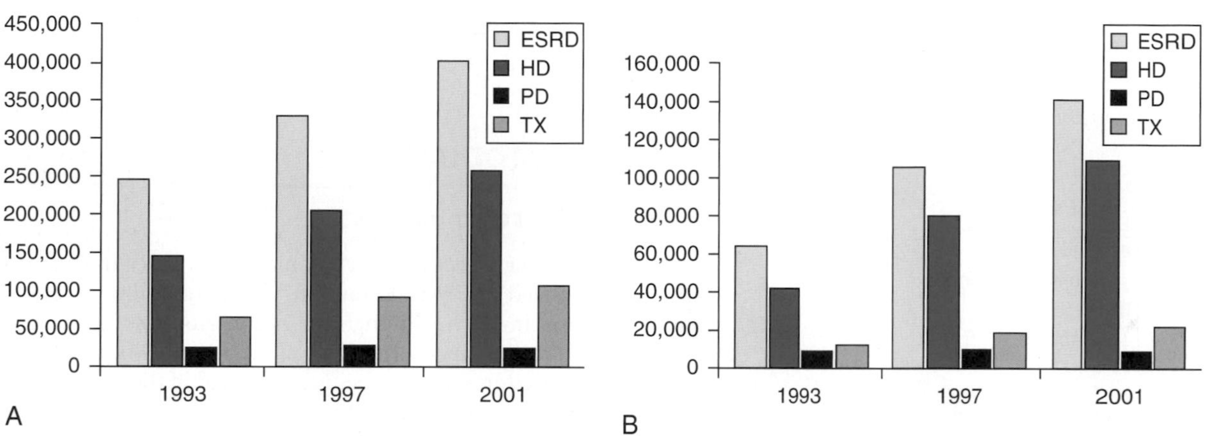

Figure 10–1 Point prevalence counts of patients with end-stage renal disease (ESRD) who were receiving Medicare benefits and who were alive on December 31, by treatment modality and year, 1993–2001. ***A,*** total ESRD population; ***B,*** diabetic ESRD population. (*ESRD,* all treatment modalities; *HD,* hemodialysis; *TX,* transplantation; *PD,* peritoneal dialysis.) A steady increase in total number of patients treated, and in the number treated with HD and TX, is shown, while the number of patients treated with PD has remained relatively stable. Diabetic ESRD continues to increase at a higher rate than other primary causes of renal failure. (Modified from U.S. Renal Data System: USRDS 2003 Annual Data Report. Bethesda, MD, National Institutes of Health, National Institute of Diabetes and Digestive and Kidney Diseases, 2003.)

Table 10–1 Renal Replacement Options for Uremic Diabetic Patients

	Hemodialysis	Peritoneal Dialysis	Transplantation
Advantages	Efficient Closer medical surveillance Ease of EPO administration Less protein loss IDPN available	Better tolerated Easy access Cardiovascular tolerance Intraperitoneal insulin Heparin use not necessary Potassium control Less hypoglycemia Less hypertension IDPN available	Superior survival Improved quality of life Improved nutrition Better rehabilitation Stable retinopathy Cost savings
Disadvantages	Vascular access necessary Inconvenient Cardiac stress Hypotension Hyperkalemia Hypoglycemia	Peritonitis Must be trainable Time commitment Technical failure Withdrawal Orthostatic hypotension More gastrointestinal complaints	Immunosuppression Poor glycemic control No improvement in cardiovascular mortality Fractures Infections

EPO, erythropoietin; *IDPN,* intradialytic parenteral nutrition.

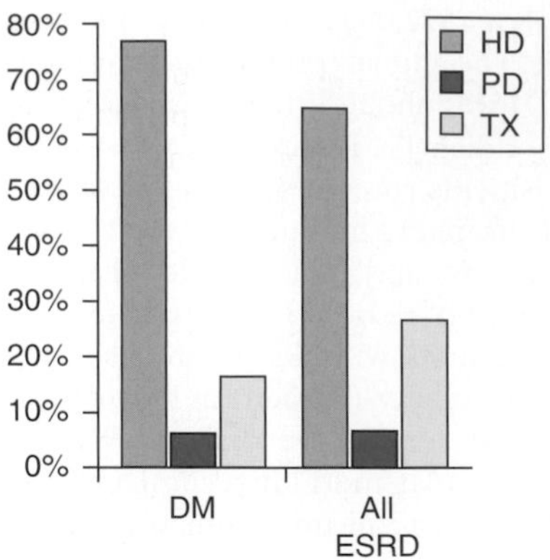

Figure 10–2 Treatment modalities for prevalent patients with end-stage renal disease who received Medicare benefits, according to diabetic status, 2000. *TX*, transplant; *PD*, peritoneal dialysis; HD, hemodialysis. (Modified from U.S. Renal Data System: USRDS 2003 Annual Data Report. Bethesda, MD, National Institutes of Health, National Institute of Diabetes and Digestive and Kidney Diseases, 2003.)

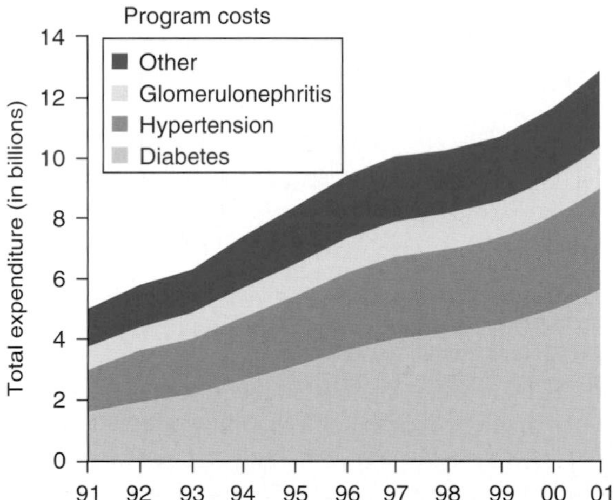

Figure 10–3 Costs in billions of dollars for prevalent patients receiving Medicare benefits by primary diagnosis. Diabetics consume the largest portion of Medicare expenditures reflecting the fact that they make up the greatest proportion of patients at the greatest per capita cost. (From U.S. Renal Data System: USRDS 2003 Annual Data Report. Bethesda, MD, National Institutes of Health, National Institute of Diabetes and Digestive and Kidney Diseases, 2003.)

better preserved vision than patients with type I disease. Detailed recommendations are available on the standards of medical care for diabetes.[22] Only a multidisciplinary team, including a nephrologist, vascular surgeon, cardiologist, ophthalmologist, podiatrist, nutrition expert, and transplantation specialist, can provide these patients with optimal management as renal failure progresses to ESRD. New complexities then emerge in the management strategy: insulin requirements decrease, retinopathy progresses, hypertension[23] and fluid retention worsen, and gastroparesis becomes refractory to medication. When ESRD is reached, complications are severe in half of patients, one third are blind, half have gastroparesis, and one in six have had a myocardial infarction. Other uremic problems are worsened by diabetes, such as nausea, vomiting, impotence, neuropathy, and vascular disease.

Although the optimal time to initiate dialysis has not been determined, dialysis should be initiated earlier in uremic diabetic patients to avoid life-threatening events[24] and accelerated retinopathy. Diabetic patients may have lower serum creatinine levels than nondiabetic patients but similar renal function by other parameters.[25] However, diabetics have higher GFRs at the time of initiation of dialysis than the overall population. This likely reflects a higher degree of comorbidity in diabetics necessitating earlier initiation of renal replacement therapy. A higher degree of comorbidity in patients initiating dialysis with a higher GFR is evidenced by the fact that the higher the GFR at the initiation of dialysis, the greater the probability of hospitalization and death.[10] Subsequent treatment goals include preserving vascular access, controlling hyperglycemia, preventing cardiac mortality, maintaining vision, avoiding limb amputation, and preventing malnutrition (Table 10–2).

HEMODIALYSIS

Vascular Access

Medicare spending for vascular access procedures during 2000 totaled nearly $200 million, almost doubling from $104 million in 1991. Although the number of vascular access procedures has increased fourfold between 1991 and 2000, these procedures are now being performed in the outpatient instead of the inpatient setting, resulting in a significant decrease in cost per procedure. Since 1991, arteriovenous fistula, synthetic graft, and catheter insertion costs have dropped 60%, 50%, and 50%, respectively, while the cost of vascular access complications have dropped almost 200%. The number of vascular access hospitalizations has declined 25% between 1991 and 2000, whereas the overall rates of hospitalizations for patients with ESRD has remained nearly the same, due to increased rates of hospitalization for circulatory and respiratory problems.[10] Suboptimal access has always been a problem in the total management of uremic diabetic patients and should be termed the *diabetic access syndrome*. Diabetic patients have the highest rate of access-related complications,[26–28] and access dysfunction is their most common problem. Less than half of diabetic patients have a permanent access placed or attempted before developing ESRD. Creating and preserving vascular access is one of the basic goals in management of the uremic diabetic patient.[29]

The diabetic access syndrome begins long before ESRD develops. As with nondiabetic patients, only about one-third of diabetic patients have been told to preserve their forearm vein for a permanent access.[30] The arterial inflow is usually inadequate because of atherosclerosis, and outflow veins are often scarred by phlebotomy or indwelling catheters.[31] Arteriovenous fistulas as initial permanent access have a higher primary failure rate in diabetic patients; 30% to 40% fail to develop and are never used.[32] A recent study reported an 85% greater likelihood of primary failure and a relative risk of 2.38% for ultimate failure of a native fistula in diabetics.[33] Alternative vessels may also be unsuitable for native fistulas. Distal arm vessels, the preferred site, may be fragile because of medial calcification. Because upper extremity fistulas are less

Table 10–2 Problem Evaluation in Diabetic Patients with End-Stage Renal Disease

Problem	Evaluation
Vascular access	Preservation of vasculature and early assessment for native fistula
Glycemic control	Hemoglobin A_{1c}, home glucose monitoring
Angina, myocardial infarction	Exercise treadmill test, P-thallium, echocardiography, catheterization
Visual impairment	Ophthalmic evaluation
Foot ulcers	Podiatric evaluation
Peripheral vascular disease, limb amputation	Doppler flow studies
Gastroparesis	Gastric-emptying study
Neuropathic problems	Electromyogram, neurology consultation
Malnutrition	Serum albumin level, dietary counseling, physical examination

prone to infection and vascular steal is less critical, an alternative is the brachiocephalic fistula.[34] Proximal radial artery to antebrachial vein may serve as a good alternative site even in diabetics.[35] Routine use of preoperative vein mapping is thought to enhance the efficacy of native fistulas.[36] Nonetheless, a minority of newly treated diabetic patients with ESRD has a satisfactory native vessel in place at initiation of dialysis. Other modes of hemoaccess, such as long-term catheters, upper extremity grafts, lower extremity grafts, or even conversion to peritoneal dialysis, may be needed.

Diabetic patients, especially older patients, are more likely to require temporary catheters or "permanent" tunneled venous catheters. Cuffed, dual-lumen tunneled venous catheters may provide long-term permanent access. In one center, catheter failure was a result of thrombosis or inadequate flow in about one third of patients and of infection in about one fourth of patients, most of whom had diabetes. The 6-month catheter survival rate was 53%. The major limiting factors in long-term catheter survival are infection and thrombosis.[37] Diabetes is an independent predictor of cuffed dialysis catheter failure.[38]

The risk of catheter-related infection is increased in diabetic patients, and *Staphylococcus aureus* nasal carriage may be more prevalent.[39] Infection may result from a break in sterile technique or poor exit site care, or rarely from injection of illicit drugs by the patient. Most cases of *S. aureus* bacteremia in hospitalized patients are associated with infections transmitted through venous catheters.[40] Infections are more common with temporary rather than cuffed hemodialysis catheters and are least common with arteriovenous fistulas or synthetic grafts.[41] Standard therapy of dialysis catheter-related bacteremia historically has been catheter removal and administration of systemic antibiotics, followed by placement of a new catheter at an alternate site. To avoid loss of potential future access sites, the standard of care is evolving toward guidewire catheter exchange at the same venous site, with a course of antibiotics, as long as there is no evidence of an overt subcutaneous tunnel infection,[42] or sepsis,[43] including staphylococcal, gram-negative, and yeast infections.

The risk of catheter-related thrombosis is also increased. Some data support the use of low-dose warfarin anticoagulation for permanent central venous catheters.[44] Catheter obstruction may require a venous stripping procedure or may be overcome by the intravenous administration of a thrombolytic agent, such as recombinant tissue plasminogen activator.[45,46] The danger of iatrogenic bleeding, such as retinal hemorrhage, is increased in patients with diabetes. Alternatively, a fibrin stripping procedure in interventional radiology may be helpful in restoring function in a poorly functioning catheter.[47]

Diabetic patients have been more likely to require a synthetic graft as primary access. In a 1996 report, diabetic patients were two to three times more likely to receive a graft than a fistula and were twice as likely to require a graft as nondiabetic patients.[48] However, recent data show that there is little difference in the rates of use of fistulas in diabetics versus nondiabetics, with fistulas being used in about 28% of new patient initiating hemodialysis in 2000. Overall graft use has decreased 15%, fistula use has increased 10%, and catheter use has increased 25% in the hemodialysis population, with increasing access salvage with angioplasty, stent, and surgical revision. It is not clear whether these patterns also hold true for the diabetic dialysis population specifically.[9] Polytetrafluoroethylene has become the material most frequently chosen but remains inferior to the arteriovenous fistula even when study groups are comparable in age, diabetic status, cardiovascular status, smoking status, and degree of hypertension.[49,50] Grafts have slightly better outcomes during the first 6 months than fistulas, but fistulas subsequently perform better. Uncontrolled studies show a mean patency duration of less than 2 years, about two-thirds the duration of fistulas. Compared with nondiabetic patients, hemodialysis graft survival is decreased in diabetic patients, and complications occur earlier.[28,51]

The most common complications of grafts are thrombosis, infection, and distal ischemia. The rates of thrombosis of synthetic grafts are high in dialysis patients in general, but the risks of thrombosis in hemodialysis patients with diabetes appear greater. According to 1997 USRDS data, of patients in need of a procedure to restore permanent access, those with diabetes were more likely to have surgical declotting and less likely to have angioplasty with thrombolysis.[30] Neointimal hyperplasia, the response to vascular injury associated with spontaneous vascular thrombosis,[52] occurs earlier and more extensively in the diabetic population.[53] Synthetic grafts activate platelets, and patients whose platelets aggregate more readily (such as those with diabetes) are at risk of graft thrombosis. Other diabetic factors that might worsen the process of vascular injury are unclear. Diabetic vasculopathy is an endothelial dysfunction characterized by basement membrane thickening and endothelial cell proliferation.[54] Arterial angioplasty procedures result in intimal hyperplasia, with smooth muscle cell proliferation and a matrix of connective tissue elements.[55] Diabetic patients are at increased risk of re-stenosis after coronary angioplasty.[56] The addition of intraluminal stent placement has decreased the risk of coronary artery re-stenosis,[57,58] however, it is not clear whether this is true in diabetics. Most cases of venous stenosis underlying graft thromboses occur at or near the venous anastomosis.[59] The hyperplastic response histologically includes collagen and proteoglycan. New techniques including drug-eluting stents are showing promise in decreasing in-stent coronary re-stenosis.[60]

Graft infection rates are increased fourfold compared with fistulas (see later).

Patients with diabetes are also more likely to develop arterial steal complications,[61] with ischemic pain or gangrene in the operated limb. Compromised vessels and microcirculation lead to necrosis and painful digital ulcerations. Tapered grafts do not appear to lower the risk of ischemia and, in fact, may reduce graft patency. Less common than overt steal, but also disabling, is ischemic monomelic neuropathy,[62] in which ischemia insufficient to produce finger ulcerations nonetheless causes severe nerve injury. In cases of arterial steal, noninvasive vascular studies, nerve conduction studies, and arteriography may be required. Lower extremity femoral artery–to–saphenous vein grafts are placed only as a last resort. Their patency rate is about 50% at 2 years.[63]

Many factors contribute to the low rate in the use of arteriovenous fistulas and to inferior access outcomes in diabetic patients. In addition to the factors described previously, they include late presentation or referral to the nephrologist[64] (as when suitability for dialysis is uncertain), indecision about the preferred dialysis modality, and rapid terminal loss of renal function. Aggressive diuresis for volume overload and contrast nephropathy commonly result in the latter.

Improving long-term access patency begins with increasing the number of native fistulas. More initial brachial fistula placements may be necessary.[65] Although diabetic patients are more likely to be viewed as poor candidates for a fistula, initial surgical evaluation should occur early enough to permit long maturation times of 4 months or more.[66] Surgical revisions, such as ligation of runoff vessels or bypass to improve arterial flow, may be required. The role of antiplatelet therapy in preventing dialysis graft thrombosis has not been proven, although it is used routinely for stroke, myocardial infarction, and maintenance of arterial graft patency.[67] Dipyridamole, whose action on platelets complements aspirin, has no added benefit in peripheral vascular disease. However, one prospective nonrandomized dialysis study showed that dipyridamole was beneficial in preventing thrombosis in newly placed grafts, whereas aspirin was not.[68] Diabetic patients were not separately analyzed in this study. A recent retrospective analysis suggested improved primary graft patency with the use of calcium channel blockers, improved secondary graft patency with aspirin, improved secondary fistula patency with angiotensin converting enzyme (ACE) inhibitors, and worse primary graft patency in patients receiving warfarin therapy.[69] Aspirin in routine doses appears to be safe in patients with diabetes, with no increased risk of vitreous or preretinal hemorrhage.[70] Because of increased platelet turnover in diabetic patients, at least 325 mg may be required.[71] Warfarin, in low doses, has been found to be ineffective in prolonging graft survival and was associated with increase in bleeding complications.[72] Although thrombolysis (tissue plasminogen activator with or without mechanical thrombolysis) has been effective in salvaging both fistulas and grafts,[73,74] no separate analysis of thrombolysis in diabetic patients has been done. One study found that recombinant erythropoietin use was associated with a mean increase in hematocrit from 23% to 34% and a 10% improvement in graft patency without increased risk of venous thrombosis.[75] Prospective monitoring of access flow rates in the dialysis unit on a routine basis is considered a reasonable way to monitor for impending access failure as well as response to therapy.[76]

Glycemic Control

Maintenance of glycemic control is a priority in diabetic patients with ESRD. An analysis of the DCCT concluded that, for eligible patients, intensive diabetes therapy results in improved quality and length of life.[77] Another clinical study of type I and type II diabetes further supported the DCCT recommendations to slow the progression of nephropathy.[78] Goals for glycemic control recently published by the American Diabetes Association are: (1) preprandial plasma glucose, 90 to 130 mg/dL, (2) 1 to 2 hours postprandial plasma glucose less than 180 mg/dL, and (3) hemoglobin A_{1C} less than 7.0%. In patients who are meeting preprandial targets, but not hemoglobin A_{1C} targets, reducing postprandial plasma glucose may improve A_{1C} values.[22] Among the necessary tasks of the nephrologist as primary care provider of the uremic diabetic patient is achieving glycemic control.[79] This can retard complications of microvascular disease, prevent catabolism, minimize infection, and limit hyperkalemia.[80] It may also be associated with shorter hospitalizations, improved gastroparesis and orthostatic hypotension, decreased incidence of heart failure and myocardial infarction, and higher serum albumin levels.[81]

The signs and symptoms of hyperglycemia are modified in dialyzed patients. Consequences of hyperglycemia in hemodialyzed patients are listed in Table 10–3. Excessive thirst owing to hyperglycemia results in excessive interdialytic weight gain. Interdialytic weight gain correlated inversely with glycemic control in one study.[82] Pulmonary edema and hypertension may also occur. Severe hyperosmolality may result in hyperkalemia.[83] Ketoacidosis is less common. Shifts in serum osmolality secondary to marked variation in blood glucose levels have been implicated in the development of central pontine myelinolysis. The demyelinating disorder occurred in a diabetic hemodialysis patient without significant changes in the serum sodium concentration.[84] Anorexia, nausea, vomiting, weakness, worsened gastroparesis, and altered mental status may also occur. The risk of infection may increase as a conse-

Table 10–3 Consequences of Hyperglycemia

Thirst, excessive fluid intake, weight gain between dialysis, hypertension
Pulmonary edema
Severe hyperkalemia
Diabetic ketoacidosis
Shifts in serum osmolality
Anorexia, nausea, vomiting, weakness
Increased risk of infection

quence of hyperglycemia. Because osmotic diuresis does not occur, volume depletion is not to be expected (unlike in patients with good renal function), and excessive volume replacement is contraindicated. Sustained severe hyperglycemia may produce only nonspecific symptoms.[85] In more modest forms of diabetes, hyperglycemia[86] may be latent but still potentially important as a contributor to complications.

Insulin dosing and glucoregulation are more complex in dialyzed diabetic patients.[87] In renal failure, reduced insulin degradation prolongs the duration of exogenous insulin, leading to decreased insulin requirements, particularly when insulin sensitivity is improved by dialysis. Hemodialysis improves glucose tolerance.[87] Smaller insulin doses suffice, and oral agents or even insulin may be discontinued in some patients. Metformin should be avoided in ESRD, but rosiglitazone and pioglitazone are hepatically cleared and can be used without dose adjustment. Glimepiride and glyburide should be used with caution in patients with ESRD. Glipizide is metabolized by the liver and is generally considered the sulfonylurea of choice in ESRD. Although repaglinide should not be used in ESRD, nateglinide can be used. Acarbose is also contraindicated in ESRD.[88] If caloric intake improves and weight increases on dialysis, insulin needs may increase.

Although dosing must be individualized, most patients do best with twice-daily dosing of intermediate (for basal requirements) and regular (for meal coverage) insulin. Long acting insulin (ultralente, glargine) should be used with caution in ESRD. Total daily doses are modest. The relative proportions of the insulin vary. Malnourished patients may do well with once-daily dosing. For simplicity, other patients may prefer a fixed 70:30 ratio of insulin. Some selected patients are willing to intensify their therapy with multiple injections. Of note, one report described proximal calciphylaxis in four cases of ESRD diabetes and suggested that sites of insulin injection led to the ischemic tissue necrosis.[89]

Home and dialysis unit glucose monitoring should be done frequently. Measurement of glycohemoglobin, which best reflects glycemic control over the previous 6- to 10-week period, has not been well standardized in uremic patients. A falsely high value of chromatographically measured glycosylated hemoglobin in uremia may result from an increase in carbamylated hemoglobin.[90] Affinity chromatography and immunoassays avoid analytic interference. Hemoglobin A_{1C} is the major component of glycohemoglobin and when measured by immunoassay accurately reflects glycemic control in a range of 6% to 7%. However, a hemoglobin A_{1C} greater than 7.5% may overestimate hyperglycemia in the diabetic uremic patient.[91] Another index of glycemic control, serum fructosamine, which is not affected by urea, has not gained acceptance.[92] A preprandial blood glucose of less than 130 mg/dL and a postprandial blood glucose of less than 180 mg/dL are suitable goals if undue risks of hypoglycemia can be avoided. The hemoglobin A_{1C} level should be checked monthly. A value of 7% or less reflects good glycemic control. A decrease of 1% results in 40% decrease in rates of subsequent microvascular complications (nephropathy, retinopathy, and neuropathy).[3]

Hyperglycemia is increasingly recognized as the major causative factor in irreversible tissue damage, leading to diabetic complications. A growing body of evidence has linked late diabetic complications to the accumulation of products of glucose-protein interactions.[93] Glucose normally reacts nonenzymatically with free amino groups of proteins to form a heterogeneous group of advanced glycation end products (AGEs) with cross-linking properties. AGEs appear to be degraded in the body and effectively cleared by the kidneys.[94] Buildup of AGEs is enhanced in ESRD,[95] and it is even more dramatic in diabetics with ESRD and may correlate with late complications.[96] Increased AGEs buildup in diabetic animal models has been documented in vascular, nerve, and kidney tissues. Multiple adverse consequences leading to tissue damage have been described.

Evidence suggests that AGE damage can be compounded in chronic renal failure because of renal retention of AGE-breakdown products and other glycated proteins. In fact, increased plasma and tissue AGEs occur in ESRD unrelated to hyperglycemia. For example, β_2-microglobulin isolated from amyloid deposits in patients with dialysis-related amyloidosis has been demonstrated to be modified by AGEs.[97] Advanced glycation in uremia has also been linked to oxidation processes and the availability of precursor molecules unrelated to hyperglycemia.[98]

AGEs are inefficiently cleared by conventional hemodialysis or peritoneal dialysis,[99] although high-flux dialysis or hemofiltration[100] may be more efficient.[101] Several different strategies for decreasing AGE levels have potential benefit including daily hemodialysis,[102] dietary AGE restriction,[103] ACE inhibitors and ARBs,[104] and compounds known to block AGE formation and AGE cross-linking activity in hemodialysis patients, such as aminoguanidine (pimagedine)[105] and a study drug, OBP-9195.[106] In fact, one study found that aminoguanidine therapy resulted not only in a decrease in AGEs, but also in a decrease in the overexpression of transforming growth factor-β and platelet derived growth factor-β (profibrotic cytokines) in renal tissue, suggesting a potential benefit in the pathogenesis of diabetic nephropathy.[107] Additional problems in managing AGE toxicity include establishing a standardized method of measurement of AGE levels and devising combination therapies.[108]

Hypoglycemia is a potentially serious complication in diabetic ESRD patients.[109] Severe episodes cause significant morbidity (including new retinal hemorrhages), or even mortality, and make tight glycemic control unfeasible. Dialyzed patients may refuse their morning insulin because blood sugar levels commonly decrease during treatment (despite the dialysate dextrose level of 200 mg/dL) as a result of glucose removal by dialysis[110] and a transient improvement in insulin sensitivity. Predisposing factors to hypoglycemia include: (1) decreased insulin clearance and gluconeogenesis by failed kidneys, (2) poor substrate for gluconeogenesis with decreased intake and absorption of food, and (3) impaired counter-regulatory responses. Hypoglycemic episodes may occur with exercise (such as seasonal walking or snow shoveling) or nocturnally. Malnourished diabetic patients with decreased glycogen stores are at highest risk. Important precipitating factors include alcohol (used uncommonly by diabetics), nonselective β-blockers (due to multiple effects), and sulfonylureas. The latter may cause hypoglycemic coma or severe brain damage. Risk is increased with chlorpropamide, tolazamide, and acetohexamide. Glipizide is the preferred oral agent because active metabolites accumulate with glyburide.

Diverse symptoms caused by hypoglycemia are predominantly neuroglycopenic and include headache, nausea, vomiting, confusion, drowsiness, lethargy, tremors, seizure, and unconsciousness; angina,[111] silent myocardial infarction, and elevated systemic blood pressure may also occur. Patients commonly are unaware of their hypoglycemia. Postdialysis hypoglycemia may place patients who drive home from their treatments at risk of having a motor vehicle accident. When hypoglycemia occurs with increasing frequency, the accuracy of insulin given at home should be verified, glucometer accuracy tested, insulin injection sites inspected for hypertrophy or lipoatrophy, and gastroparesis evaluated. Treatment of hypoglycemia should include glucose concentrate or tablets, honey or similar foods, and intravenous dextrose. High potassium containing juices such as orange juice and grapefruit juice should be avoided. Cranberry juice is a good alternative. The blood glucose level should be retested in 30 minutes.

Ischemic Heart Disease

Ischemic heart disease complicates the management of dialyzed diabetic patients and poses a major threat to survival. Diabetes itself is an independent risk factor for coronary artery disease,[112] which is found to some degree in nearly all diabetic patients older than 45 years.[113] The risk for development of coronary artery disease is dramatically increased in patients with type I diabetes and nephropathy.[114,115] Proteinuria predicts cardiovascular events in patients with type II disease as well, even after adjusting for other cardiovascular risk factors.[116] Adults with diabetes are two to four times more likely to have ischemic heart disease than nondiabetics, and heart disease is the leading cause of diabetes-related deaths.[3] ESRD carries a high cardiovascular mortality rate in all patients. In a study of more than 400 ESRD patients followed from the start of ESRD therapy, diabetes independently predicted cardiac death over a mean follow up of 41 months.[117] Recent USRDS data show that approximately 50% of ESRD patients with diabetes (whether or not it was the primary diagnosis) have atherosclerotic heart disease, compared to only 32% of nondiabetic ESRD patients. Cardiovascular event rates, including myocardial infarction, heart failure, cardiac arrest, and coronary revascularization, were highest among ESRD patients with primary diabetic nephropathy, intermediate among patients with a secondary diagnosis of diabetes, and lowest among nondiabetics. Event rates also increased with time after diagnosis of ESRD.[10]

Management must address individual coronary risk factors.[118] Age, hypercholesterolemia, hypertension, smoking, high hemoglobin A_{1C} levels, low high-density lipoprotein (HDL) cholesterol, duration of diabetes, obesity (mostly in type II diabetes), and hereditary factors are among those identified in diabetic patients with nephropathy. In addition, nontraditional risk factors should be considered, such as hyperhomocysteinemia, inflammation, calcium phosphate product, oxidant stress, and endothelial dysfunction.[119] In patients with non–insulin-dependent diabetes, population-based studies support a linear association of glycemic control with the risk of coronary heart disease,[120] perhaps related to the effects of hyperglycemia on endothelial lesions, smooth muscle proliferation, platelets, or advanced glycation end-products. Data also suggest that diabetes itself is an even greater risk factor in young patients, both white and black.[121] Plaque progression may also be related to vessel wall effects of AGEs[122] and cellular oxidative stress.[98,123] Diabetic patients have impaired platelet and fibrinolytic function.[124] Hyperlipidemia is an important atherogenic risk factor in dialysis patients, who are known to have elevated very-low-density lipoprotein (VLDL) and triglyceride levels and decreased HDL levels. Hypercholesterolemia and hypertriglyceridemia are common in diabetic patients before initiation of dialysis. Recent data indicate that improvement in the lipid panel in diabetics leads to a decreased risk of cardiovascular complications by up to 20% to 50%.[3] With ESRD, high cholesterol levels tend to remit, whereas triglyceride levels worsen. In addition, the apolipoprotein B/apolipoprotein A-1 ratio is an atherogenic index of uremia that is more elevated in dialyzed diabetic patients.[125] Lipoprotein A, or Lp(A), a recently emphasized risk factor, is also elevated in dialyzed patients.[126] Data suggest that hypertension increases coronary risk more in diabetic than in nondiabetic patients.[127]

Finally, limited data support an inverse relation of the dose of dialysis and coronary risk in diabetic patients.[128] A study of cause-specific ESRD mortality in the USRDS Case Mix Adequacy Study reported a relation between low dialysis dose and coronary artery disease mortality. The correlation appeared to be of even greater magnitude in diabetic patients.[129] More recently, the trend relating higher urea reduction ratios (URRs) to lower mortality (cardiac and other) showed a peak at a URR of 75% above which risk of death increased; this trend was not significantly different when comparing diabetics to nondiabetics.[10] This may reflect poor nutritional status and low initial blood urea nitrogen resulting in a high URR and is not likely to indicate that more dialysis is detrimental.

Clinical strategies to improve cardiac outcomes must improve coronary prevention and treatment (see later). The efficacy of coronary preventive measures in diabetic patients with ESRD is unclear. Dietary modification should include restricted cholesterol, saturated fats, and excess carbohydrates.[130] Caloric restriction is also necessary in obese patients. Tobacco use should be strongly discouraged.[131] All diabetic patients with ESRD are candidates for aggressive management of dyslipidemia. In cases in which cholesterol abnormalities predominate, 3-hydroxy-3-methylglutaryl-coenzyme A (HMG-CoA) reductase inhibitors can be used, with ongoing monitoring of liver function tests and muscle enzymes.[132] The new cholesterol lowering agent, ezetimibe, which inhibits cholesterol absorption, can be used in renal failure without dose adjustment. Hypertriglyceridemia can also be treated with gemfibrozil in reduced dose.

Earlier studies have shown some increase in cardiovascular death with diastolic blood pressure less than 85 mmHg in patients with ischemic cardiovascular disease,[133] however, the recent "Seventh Report of the Joint National Committee on Prevention, Detection, Evaluation, and Treatment of High Blood Pressure" (JNC 7) recommendations suggest that the target blood pressure in patients with hypertension and coexisting diabetes or kidney disease should be less than 130/80 mmHg, which is associated with a decreased incidence of cardiovascular events. Most patients with hypertension and diabetes or kidney disease will require two to three antihypertensive agents to reach target blood pressure.[134] Choices of antihypertensive agents will be discussed later. Control of hyperglycemia and abstention from alcohol and smoking are indicated. Exercise should be promoted. Dialysis adequacy should be maintained.

Because of risks of coronary vascular calcification, hyperphosphatemia should be corrected with phosphate binders, and excessive calcium intake in the form of phosphate binders should be avoided. Sevelamer is a non-calcium containing phosphate binder, which may be used instead of or in conjunction with calcium containing binders and may have an added beneficial effect on lipid profiles.[135] Hyperhomocysteinemia is now a recognized risk factor in atherosclerosis and is common in dialysis patients. Folate therapy has been shown to decrease homocysteine in dialysis patients.[136] Intensified dialysis treatment regimens may also aid in normalizing homocysteine levels in dialysis patients.[137] The effect this will have on long-term cardiovascular outcomes is not yet known. With the implication of oxidative stress (which is induced by hyperglycemia[98] and more prevalent among dialysis patients[138]) in accelerated atherosclerotic disease, the role of antioxidant therapy has also been proposed in diabetics with cardiovascular disease.[98] Because the risk of developing coronary artery disease is high in these patients, aggressive diagnostic testing for coronary artery disease is appropriate.

There is insufficient literature on the outcome of percutaneous transluminal coronary angioplasty in uremic diabetic patients. Although studies to date have shown survival in dialysis patients requiring coronary revascularization to be better with coronary artery bypass surgery than with percutaneous transluminal coronary angioplasty,[139–141] most comparisons do not evaluate the influence of coronary stenting. One prestent report suggested success rates of less than 60%, with high acute complication rates in dialysis patients undergoing angioplasty, and identified abnormal carbohydrate metabolism as a factor contributing to poor short- and long-term outcomes in dialyzed angioplasty patients.[139] A later report did compare bypass surgery, angioplasty, and angioplasty with stenting and found that stenting offered no advantage and that stenting outcomes are worse in diabetic dialysis patients than in nondiabetics.[142] Another recent report examined stenting procedures in dialysis patients compared to patients without renal disease and found that despite comparable angiographic results, re-stenosis and need for repeat procedures were twice as likely in the dialysis patients. However, most of the dialysis patients did not develop re-stenosis during follow-up, suggesting there is some role for stenting in managing dialysis patients.[143] Diabetes is independently associated with an increased rate of coronary re-stenosis[144] and of subsequent progression of coronary disease. Outcomes are better in diabetics with coronary artery disease after bypass surgery than after angioplasty even with stenting.[145,146]

Bypass surgery is the preferred method of revascularization in diabetic dialysis patients who are surgical candidates. Reports suggest increased perioperative morbidity, such as wound complications, but little or no increase in perioperative mortality after bypass surgery in diabetic versus nondiabetic patients.[147–149] The risk of complications, such as sternal wound infections, osteomyelitis, and wound dehiscence, may be increased.[149,150] For dialysis patients in general, the perioperative mortality rate ranges from slightly higher to double that of patients with normal renal function, but is still less than 10% on average.[139–140,151–154] Symptomatic relief and improved functional status can be achieved. In an outcome study of 84 ESRD patients, including about 30% with diabetes, subsequent cardiovascular events were greater after balloon angioplasty than after bypass surgery.[139] In another study of dialysis patients undergoing revascularization, diabetics had increased risk of cardiac death after angioplasty with or without stenting as compared to bypass surgery.[142] Most series have not analyzed diabetics separately.

In diagnosing acute myocardial infarction, cardiac troponin T levels are being increasingly used because of high specificity for acute coronary syndrome and a universal measuring technique. However, cardiac troponin T levels are difficult to interpret in the setting of end-stage renal disease as it is cleared by the kidney and often elevated in dialysis patients. Elevated cardiac troponin T levels are felt, however, to be associated with cardiovascular risk factors, ischemic heart disease, and left ventricular hypertrophy[155] and to be a marker for poor short-term prognosis[156] in asymptomatic dialysis patients.

Peripheral Vascular Disease

Occlusive peripheral vascular disease is discussed in greater detail under Transplantation. In the dialyzed diabetic patient, it may lead not only to extremity amputations but also, rarely, to necrosis of penile tissue, requiring penectomy.[157]

Hypertension

In the new JNC 7 recommendations, goal blood pressure in patients with diabetes or chronic kidney disease is less than 130/80 mmHg.[134] Nearly 75% of adults with diabetes have blood pressure above the target of 130/80 mmHg or are on antihypertensive therapy.[3] Almost all patients with diabetic nephropathy are hypertensive.[125] Hypertension affects more than 90% of diabetic patients with ESRD, in whom it is associated with both microvascular and macrovascular complications. In type I diabetics, hypertension is often the result of underlying nephropathy and usually becomes apparent with the development of microalbuminuria.[17] Hypertension then accentuates the nephropathy. In type II diabetics, hypertension is often present at the time of diagnosis of diabetes as part of the metabolic syndrome.[17] The causes of hypertension in diabetes include increased total body sodium (renal hypertension), heightened vascular reactivity to angiotensin and catecholamines, and a genetic predisposition. Mechanisms of hypertension in chronic kidney disease include extracellular fluid volume expansion, stimulation of renin-angiotensin-aldosterone system, increased sympathetic activity, alteration in endothelial-derived factors such as nitric oxide, erythropoietin administration, hyperparathyroidism with hypercalcemia, calcified arterial tree, and renal vascular disease.[159] Reduction in blood pressure slows progression to diabetic renal failure.[12,23]

In one report of hypertensive type II diabetics, a decrease in the systolic blood pressure of 10 mmHg resulted in a 12% decreased risk of macrovascular and microvascular diabetic complications, and the lowest risk was achieved with a systolic blood pressure below 120 mmHg. No threshold level below which the risk of complications was increased was observed.[160] Blood pressure control in diabetics is reported to decrease coronary artery disease and stroke by 33% to 50% and microvascular diabetic complications (nephropathy, retinopathy, and neuropathy) by 33%.[3] The management of hypertension in diabetic patients who have uremia is complicated by the presence of renal disease and renal replacement therapy. Blood pressure control is more difficult to achieve. The conventional blood pressure goal of 130/80 mmHg is frequently unrealistic in dialysis patients. In some reports, low pre- and post-dialysis systolic blood pressures (< 110 mmHg) in diabetic and nondiabetic dialysis patients have been associated with higher cardiovascular mortality.[161,162] Target blood pressure in the diabetic dialysis patient needs to be individualized.

One report found that 62% of dialysis patients have uncontrolled hypertension, defined as blood pressure greater than 160/90 mmHg.[163] Usually two or more medications are necessary to achieve blood pressure values of less than 130/80 mmHg.[164] Factors that should be considered when hypertension is uncontrolled include high interdialytic weight gain, holding medications pre-dialysis,[164] noncompliance with dialysis regimen (skipping or shortening treatments),[165] and inadequate fluid removal during dialysis. Although different methods to accurately determine a patient's "dry weight" have been proposed, including plasma atrial natriuretic peptide levels,[166,167] a standard does not exist and the clinician must make his or her best judgment. Other important factors that may contribute to inadequate blood pressure control are poor drug absorption (in the presence of gastroparesis) and dialyzability (atenolol, methyldopa, captopril).

Correction of hypertension in dialyzed diabetic patients by ultrafiltration is likely to be hampered by paradoxical reflex systolic hypertension, orthostatic hypotension, and the ongoing need for antihypertensive medication. Some reports suggest that longer[168] or more frequent[169] hemodialysis may be more effective in achieving ideal dry weight than short (3–4 hr) hemodialysis treatments three times per week. Interdialytic fluid gains and salt intake should be moderated and physical activity increased. Excessive alcohol intake should be avoided.[22] Hypertension in obese patients may respond to weight reduction. While on dialysis, severe hypertension, related in some cases paradoxically to ultrafiltration, may force the use of short-acting nifedipine or captopril.[170]

Antihypertensives in atherosclerotic patients with ESRD should include β-blockers[171] and calcium channel blockers.[172,173] Although there has been question of increased cardiovascular morbidity such as myocardial infarction in hypertensive patients on calcium channel blockers,[174] specifically in diabetics,[175,176] this risk has been refuted in subsequent studies,[173,177,178] even in the subset of hypertensive diabetics.[177,178] ACE inhibitors have been shown to promote regression of left ventricular hypertrophy[179] and to decrease cardiovascular mortality[180] in hypertensive dialysis patients, and to decrease cardiovascular morbidity and mortality as well as progression of nephropathy in patients with diabetes.[181] ARBs are effective and well-tolerated without dose adjustment in dialysis patients.[182] They prevent progression of diabetic nephropathy in patients with type II diabetes[183,184] and appear to offer some advantage in cardiovascular morbidity and mortality when compared to atenolol in hypertensive diabetic patients.[185] Although α-blockers may improve insulin sensitivity in type II diabetics with hypertension,[186] a recent study showed an increased risk of heart failure with α-blockers as compared to diuretics, ACE inhibitors, and calcium channel blockers and so should be used as a second or third line agent.[187] They may be preferentially added to a regimen in older men with obstructive symptoms of prostatic hypertrophy. A once weekly clonidine patch may be useful in patients who are noncompliant with medications.

In choosing a blood pressure medication regimen, side effects must also be considered. Beta-blockers may worsen hyperglycemia[188] and may also mask symptoms of hypoglycemia. Hypoglycemia has also been reported with ACE inhibitors, resulting from increased insulin sensitivity.[189] Orthostatic hypotension occurring with supine hypertension in patients with type I diabetes is worsened by α-blockers and vasodilators. Hyperlipidemia may be an adverse effect of β-blockers as well as of diuretics. Erectile dysfunction may be worsened by β-blockers and methyldopa. ACE inhibitors and angiotensin receptor blockers (ARBs) may be underused because of fear of hyperkalemia, although hyperkalemia seems to be less pronounced with ARBs.[190]

Overtreatment of hypertension in uremic patients at risk of coronary ischemia may be dangerous. Diabetic patients are at particular risk because intradialytic hypotension is more common in diabetics. Depressed counter-regulatory reflexes in response to hypovolemia are the major factor.[191] During tilt testing, blood pressure decreases further in diabetic patients because of a smaller rise in total peripheral resistance and an absent catecholamine response. Previously hypertensive patients may later develop sustained hypotension as autonomic neuropathy worsens and cardiac performance deteriorates. With drops in blood pressure, the hemodialysis access itself may be threatened because of low flow and risk of thrombosis.

Dialysis hypotension may respond to increased treatment time, increased target weight, limit in interdialytic weight gain, withholding of antihypertensive medications, sodium modeling to promote vascular refilling, and erythropoietin to correct coexisting anemia.[192] Symptomatic episodes require placement in Trendelenburg's posture, infusion of normal saline, cessation of negative dialysis pressure, reduction in blood flow to the dialyzer, cooling of dialysate, and administration of ephedrine or midodrine.[193] Possible underlying causes, such as coronary ischemia, sepsis, and pericardial tamponade, should be considered.

Retinopathy

Diabetes is the leading cause of blindness in adults aged 20 to 74 years, causing 12,000 to 24,000 new cases per year,[3] and is the most common cause of blindness in uremic patients. Ophthalmologic screening programs can prevent vision loss and are cost-effective.[194] The ocular complications in type I and type II diabetes are similar.[195] Progression of retinopathy is a major problem for dialyzed diabetic patients, whose sight is necessary for functional independence and rehabilitation. Type I diabetics rarely develop signs of retinopathy within the first 3 to 5 years of diagnosis of diabetes, but nearly all have evidence of retinopathy by 20 years after diagnosis, while 20% of type II diabetics have signs of retinopathy at the time of diagnosis of diabetes.[196] Almost all patients with type I diabetes have background or proliferative retinopathy when starting dialysis. Three-fourths have visual disturbances, and half have significant visual loss.[197] Up to one-third of type I and one-fifth of type II diabetic patients are blind at the initiation of dialysis.[198] The presence of albuminuria in type I diabetics[199] and in Hispanic type II diabetics[200] predicts the presence of diabetic retinopathy independent of glycemic control and duration of diabetes.

With current technology, dialysis does not appear to exacerbate vision loss.[201] Heparin administration, abrupt changes in glycemic control, and fluctuating blood pressure are factors that could potentially worsen retinopathy.[196] Heparin may worsen vitreous hemorrhage. Macular edema, on the other hand, may disappear with hemodialysis in the absence of proliferative retinopathy, leading to improvement in visual acuity.

The visual prognosis for uremic diabetic patients has improved because of collaboration among the nephrologist, the diabetologist, and the ophthalmologist. Therapy is primarily preventative and does not restore vision, therefore early intervention is mandatory to preserve sight. The stage of retinopathy determines the ophthalmologic treatment.[202] For macular edema, the most common cause of visual impairment in diabetes, focal photocoagulation therapy is beneficial[203] and should be combined with control of hypertension,[204] avoidance of fluid overload, and improved blood glucose control.[205,206] Diet, exercise, and smoking cessation should also be encouraged.[207] Visual acuity may be improved by resolution of macular edema after correction of anemia by erythropoietin.[208] Raising the red blood cell mass by treatment with erythropoietin may also improve retinal hard exudates.[209]

Patients with proliferative retinopathy are treated with panretinal photocoagulation to lessen the risk of extensive vitreous hemorrhage. Even florid diabetic retinopathy, which carries a high risk of blindness, can be improved with extensive full subconfluent panretinal photocoagulation.[210] For persistent vitreous hemorrhage, vitrectomy is indicated. Lens replacement and retinal reattachment may also preserve sight. Follow-up should be at 3- to 12-month intervals, depending on the severity of the retinopathy. With aggressive eye management, dialyzed patients can achieve a visual prognosis similar to those who undergo transplantation.[211]

Foot Care

Foot complications occur in one-quarter of diabetic patients with ESRD[212] and were twice as common as in those without ESRD in one study.[213] Notably, more than 60% of nontraumatic lower extremity amputations in the United States are in diabetic patients, and there were approximately 82,000 lower extremity amputations per year in diabetic patients between 1997 and 1999.[3] Amputations of the lower extremities are a major source of morbidity for dialyzed diabetic patients, occurring 10 times more frequently than in the general diabetic population,[213] but many are preventable.[214,215] Approximately 84% of amputations are preceded by foot ulcers, which are not less likely to heal in patients with diabetic nephropathy than in diabetics with normal renal function.[214] A reduction in amputation rates requires that both the patient and the ESRD specialist be educated about the need for prophylactic foot care and lifelong surveillance. The podiatrist and vascular surgeon must also be included on the dialysis team.

Risk factors leading to lower extremity amputation include sensory neuropathy, impaired circulation, and foot deformities. Patients with diabetes for more than 10 years, poor glycemic control, cardiovascular complications, retinopathy, or nephropathy are also at increased risk. Patients at particular risk (elderly patients, immobilized patients, and those with poor vision, foot deformity, or history of foot ulcer) should be identified and educated regarding foot care, including the absence of pain as a foot ulcer symptom, wearing protective footwear at all times, and avoiding exposure of neuropathic feet to heating pads.[216]

Extremities should be examined for absent pulses, poor hair growth, atrophic skin changes, and cool temperature. The feet should be visually inspected daily for foot ulcers, ingrown nails, and calluses. Minor skin disease such as dryness and tinea pedis should be identified and treated before evolving into a more serious problem.[216] In the hospitalized bed-confined patient, the heels must be given particular attention. Toe gangrene with painful petechiae suggests cholesterol microemboli.[217] Foot inspection at home depends on adequate vision or the presence of a sighted partner. A mirror may be necessary to inspect the bottoms of the feet. Hemodialysis treatments provide an opportunity for the dialysis unit team to inspect the patient's feet.

Foot ulcers should be aggressively debrided and protected from weight bearing. Underlying vascular insufficiency may cause impaired healing. In fact, in patients who underwent toe or forefoot amputation, success of revascularization, and not diabetes or presence of ESRD, predicted healing without need for more extensive (below or above the knee) amputation.[218]

Regular exercise should be encouraged to maintain circulation, unless an active or healing ulcer is present. Because even minor sores may progress unnoticed into major infections, foot discomfort should be taken seriously. Deep cultures, prompt ulcer debridement, cessation of weight bearing, broad-spectrum antibiotics, and noninvasive Doppler studies should be ordered promptly. Foot deformities may need correction. Cellulitis should be treated before extremity revascularization. Smoking should be discouraged. Hyperbaric oxygen therapy[219] and human skin equivalent[220] may also be beneficial in aiding wound healing of ischemic or neuropathic ulcers, respectively. Diabetic patients with lower limb disability make poor psychosocial adjustments to illness and should be psychologically prepared for a long period of convalescence.[221]

Infection

Because of factors such as altered host immunity due to uremic toxins, breakdown of protective barriers, affinity of bacteria for foreign materials, carriage of infective organisms, and malnutrition, the incidence of infection in uremic patients is high, with both common and opportunistic pathogens.[222] Therefore, a high index of suspicion for infection is appropriate. Bacteremia and death from infection are more common in dialyzed patients,[223] and infection is the second leading cause of death among ESRD patients.[224] Rates of hospitalization for infection are more than five times higher in diabetic dialysis patients compared to diabetic Medicare patients without chronic kidney disease.[10] Although overall rates of hospital admission in the ESRD population have remained fairly constant, admissions for infection have increased 12% to 21% in the ESRD population and 30% specifically in the hemodialysis population between 1991 and 2001.[9] This seems largely due to increased rates of vascular access infections, which have increased 87%, and pulmonary infections, which have increased 24% between 1991 and 2001 in hemodialysis patients.[9] Hospitalization rates for sepsis have also increased 69% in hemodialysis patients between 1991 and 1999.[9] Mortality from sepsis is 50-fold higher in dialysis patients than in the general population in both diabetics and nondiabetics.[225]

Indwelling dialysis catheters are more likely to be a nidus for infection than native or synthetic arteriovenous shunts,[224] and grafts are more likely to become infected than fistulas. Mortality due to access infections is greatest with catheters, less common with grafts, and least with fistulas.[226] The most common organism is *S. aureus*. More serious complications, such as infective endocarditis,[227] septic pulmonary emboli, osteomyelitis, meningitis, or visceral abscesses may occur in otherwise nonthreatening access infections. Catheter salvage with guidewire exchange does not appear to increase the risk of complications of catheter-related bacteremia.[228]

High nasal carriage of *S. aureus* in dialyzed patients may account for higher rates of self-infection than are seen in nondialyzed patients.[229] Nasal mupirocin can safely eradicate carriage of *S. aureus* and may lead to a reduction in bacteremia.[230] Prophylactic topical Polysporin™ Triple antibiotic ointment applied to catheter exit sites may also reduce the rate of infection and improve survival in hemodialysis patients.[231]

Illicit drug abuse appears to be uncommon in the diabetic dialysis population, occurring in less than 5% in one study.[232] Use of cocaine, however, was associated with increased bacterial infection rates that included cellulitis, sepsis, and abscesses, often virulent. Dialysis access infections were common. Although no cocaine user tested positive for human immunodeficiency virus, more than half tested positive for hepatitis B antibody. Morbidity was evidenced by a fivefold higher hospitalization cost in the illicit drug abuse population.

Bacteremia should be suspected in febrile patients on hemodialysis, and the access promptly inspected. Blood cultures should be obtained. Empiric vancomycin and gentamicin should be administered if the access appears responsible. Antibiotic coverage should be narrowed once culture and sensitivity results are available, and treatment should be continued to complete a 3-week course. Follow-up should include careful evaluation for metastatic complications (blood cultures, chest radiograph, echocardiogram). Exploration of the graft may be required; up to half of infected grafts can be salvaged, with exploration and careful resection of the infected portion. Partly revised grafts may continue to be used with caution. Infected tunneled catheters may be changed over a wire under sterile conditions in patients without signs of sepsis. If there is evidence of associated tunnel infection, the catheter may be changed over a guidewire with the creation of a new tunnel.[233]

Hyperkalemia

Significant hyperkalemia occurs in about 10% of chronically dialyzed patients, but it is more common in diabetic patients, in part, because of insulin deficiency or resistance. Hyperkalemia is worsened by severe hyperglycemia.[234] Even severe cases may be asymptomatic. Late cardiac manifestations may occur, including a prolonged PR interval and a sine wave pattern leading to cardiac standstill.[235] The management should take into account preexisting cardiac problems and concomitant medications that might cause bradyarrhythmias. Glucose need not accompany intravenous insulin in the acute treatment of hyperkalemia in the presence of hyperglycemia. Hyperkalemia may be worsened by severe constipation in patients with diabetic enteropathy.

Gastroparesis

Gastroparesis affects more than one third of diabetic patients with chronic renal failure and is more common in type I than in type II diabetes. Symptoms include nausea, vomiting, abdominal discomfort, and bloating.[236] Symptoms of reflux esophagitis may also occur. Upper gastrointestinal bleeding is less common. Variable fluid and food intake result in hypoglycemia or hyperglycemia and in variable weight gains or losses. Gastroparesis has been associated with poor survival, protein malnutrition, poor glycemic control, orthostatic hypotension, and a high frequency of other diabetic complications.

In symptomatic patients, gastric emptying studies, or magnetic resonance imaging with radiopaque markers (combined with upper endoscopy to exclude other causes[237]), along with improvement with prokinetic agents, confirm the diagnosis. Treatment includes six small meals per day, gastric motility stimulants, and avoidance of high fiber foods and medications that may slow gastric emptying. The prokinetic agent metoclopramide[238] has a variety of extrapyramidal side effects and may cause parkinsonism. These symptoms improve promptly with discontinuation of the drug. Cisapride also reduces gastric retention,[239] but it has been taken off the market because of serious drug interactions and cardiac dysrhythmias.[240] It can now only be obtained directly from the manufacturer in cases with documented need and low risk of complications (no prolonged QTc interval on ECG and no concurrent use of medications known to have a high incidence of interaction, such as macrolides, antifungals, and phenothiazines). Erythromycin is added in refractory cases, which may respond dramatically.[241] Early studies show that gastric pacing might improve symptoms of gastroparesis.[242] Enteral nutrition via jejunostomy tube or even parenteral nutrition may be necessary when severe episodes are prolonged.

Diabetic diarrhea due to enteropathy, although less common, also contributes to malnutrition, hypoglycemia, and weight loss. Uncontrolled diarrhea may interrupt dialysis treatments and sleep. A combination of factors seem to be responsible for diarrhea, including abnormal small bowel motility, bacterial overgrowth, and anorectal dysfunction.[243] Bowel motility disorders may respond to loperamide hydrochloride or diphenoxylate with atropine. Clonidine may be helpful in refractory cases.[244] A few case reports have shown some improvement in diarrheal symptoms with octreotide.[245] Severe cases involving bacterial overgrowth require broad-spectrum or rotating courses of antibiotics. Fat malabsorption or the less common protein-losing enteropathy should be excluded.

NUTRITION

Malnutrition is common among dialysis patients, with estimated rates of severe malnutrition affecting 20% to 36% of dialysis patients in one recent study based on multiple nutritional parameters including lean body mass, normalized protein catabolic rate, albumin and pre-albumin,[246] and up to 47% of hemodialysis patients based on lean body mass.[247] Likelihood of malnutrition increases with the duration on dialysis.[248] Malnutrition is well-recognized as a predictor of increased mortality in dialysis patients, with hypoalbuminemia, although it is a late marker of protein malnutrition due to its long half-life and the large hepatic synthetic capability, being a key predictor of death in patients with ESRD.[249] Because of the high prevalence of malnutrition among dialysis patients and its association with increased mortality, frequent assessment of a patient's nutritional status with early intervention, if malnutrition is present, is important.

There is a growing consensus that nutritional status should be evaluated by a panel of measures rather than by any one single measure.[250] Recent National Kidney Foundation K/DOQI™ guidelines suggest monthly screening for albumin less than 4.0 g/dL and protein catabolic rate less than 0.8 g/kg/day to identify malnutrition.[251] Also, low blood urea nitrogen, creatinine, and cholesterol as well as declining anthropometric measurements and dry weight may suggest worsening nutritional status. Anthropometric norms in dialysis patients have been established in one study.[252] These guidelines are directed toward the general dialysis population but should be followed in the diabetic dialysis population as well.

Although protein-energy malnutrition has achieved growing recognition as an important source of mortality risk in ESRD patients,[253] its true incidence in dialyzed diabetic patients is not known. Data suggest that diabetic patients with ESRD have a poor overall nutritional status,[254] more cachexia, and slightly lower serum albumin levels.[249] Diabetic patients also have lower serum creatinine levels, probably reflecting a poor nutritional status that partly accounts for their decreased dialysis survival. One study showed that the increased mortality rates in diabetic patients with ESRD was related partly, in a logistic regression analysis, to reductions in serum creatinine and albumin levels.[255] Recent USRDS data show an 8% to 9% increased risk of hospitalization for nondiabetic and diabetic dialysis patients with a body mass index (BMI) less than 20 kg/m^2 as compared to those with a BMI of 20 to 24 kg/m^2. The risk of hospitalization continues to decline in diabetics up to a BMI of 30 kg/m^2 or more.[9]

Protein malnutrition starts before initiation of dialysis,[256] and some recommendations are evolving toward initiating maintenance dialysis for deteriorating nutritional status.[251] Multiple causes contribute to hypoalbuminemia during ESRD, including (1) reduced rate of synthesis due to inadequate protein and caloric intake due to the anorexia of uremia, (2) increased catabolism associated with infection and the dialysis treatment itself, (3) external losses in the dialysate, (4) distribution within the body,[257,258] and (5) acidosis.[259] Bioincompatible membranes can induce an inflammatory response that contributes to decreased serum albumin.[260,261] Reuse of high-flux dialysis membranes processed with bleach seems to increase protein losses with successive uses.[262] The causes more important to diabetic patients are the synergistic effects of poor protein-calorie intake due to gastroparesis[263,264] and enteropathy, catabolic stress and intercurrent illnesses, decreased albumin synthesis due to inadequate insulin anabolic effects, and psychosocial factors. Albumin homeostasis may be abnormal in diabetic patients through a specific mechanism, since insulin is necessary for basal rates of albumin synthesis. Reduced albumin synthesis may result, in hypoinsulinemic patients, from a decrease in albumin transcription. A slight increase in the prevalence of hypoalbuminemia in dialyzed diabetic patients has been reported in some studies,[249,265] although it was not confirmed in the ESRD Core Indicator Project,[266] which surveyed only about 5% of in-center adult hemodialysis patients in the United States.

Treatment of malnutrition is multifactorial. Adequate dialysis should be achieved.[267,268] Adequate insulin dosing and glycemic control may improve protein balance. Factors that cause anorexia and increased protein catabolism should be eliminated. The dietary prescription should include greater than 1.2 g/kg/day of protein, 35 kcal/kg/day,[249] 35% fat with an increase in polyunsaturated fat, and 55% carbohydrate with a special effort to limit simple sugars and concentrated sweets. Oral dietary supplements given at hemodialysis to insure compliance resulted in increased serum albumin in a recent study.[269] Compliance with supplements is critical to the beneficial effect, and so in patients who do not like preparations specifically for kidney failure, nonspecific nutritional supplements may be preferred, if the higher intake of potassium and sodium is tolerated. Overnight enteral tube feeding may be beneficial in patients with severe anorexia unable to increase oral intake.[270] Intradialytic parenteral nutrition or total parenteral nutrition are other alternatives.[270] A retrospective analysis demonstrating an association between intradialytic parenteral nutrition and improved survival in malnourished chronic hemodialysis patients included more than one third diabetics in both the control and parenteral nutrition groups.[271] Of note, mortality in patients with nearly normal serum albumin levels (> 3.5 g/dL) who received intradialytic parenteral nutrition was increased. Another analysis examined intradialytic parenteral nutrition in chronic dialysis patients, including over 40% diabetics in both the treatment and control groups, and found a slight increased survival among treated diabetic patients over the 9-month treatment interval, with an increase in serum albumin among the survivors.[272] Newer forms of nutritional therapy being investigated include appetite stimulants like megestrol acetate,[270] growth factors like anabolic steroids (nandrolone)[273] and recombinant growth hormone,[274] oral essential amino acid supplements,[275] and carnitine supplementation.[276] None of these interventions have been specifically evaluated in dialyzed diabetic patients.

Nutritional prescriptions advocated for nondiabetic patients on dialysis also apply in general to diabetic patients. Management begins with early recognition of protein malnutrition and reversal of dietary protein restriction when dialysis commences. There should be monthly nutritional counseling by the dialysis dietician on nutritional needs, and the social worker can assist in solving reimbursement problems for those unable to afford a special diet or supplement. Serum glucose levels, hemoglobin A_{1C} values, lipid levels, and obesity management should be evaluated. Nutritional plans need to take into consideration individual, personal and cultural preferences and lifestyle.[22]

SURVIVAL

A steady improvement of survival of diabetics on hemodialysis occurred through the 1980s as a result of more effective control of hypertension and hyperglycemia. Survival has continued to improve throughout the 1990s, despite the overall aging of the diabetic population with ESRD. The survival for diabetics on hemodialysis has improved by 17.3% when the 1987 to 1991 incident cohort to the 1992 to 1996 incident cohort are compared.[9] In every study, however, morbidity and mortality remain significantly higher in diabetics than in nondiabetic patients. The inferior prognosis of diabetic patients on dialysis is due largely to ongoing progression of comorbid conditions. In addition, for elderly blacks and Hispanics with ESRD due to diabetes, inadequate medical care after the initial diagnosis of diabetes may contribute to worse outcomes.[277]

The overall mortality risk is increased about 1.2 to 1.6 times in diabetic patients with ESRD compared with nondiabetic patients with ESRD, depending on their underlying cause. The 1-, 2-, 5-, and 10-year patient survival estimates for diabetic and nondiabetic patients on dialysis in the United States are shown in Figure 10–4. Limited data show increased, very early (< 90 days) mortality for diabetics on dialysis; short-term survival may be even lower than expected, because Medicare reporting does not begin until the fourth month after initiation of dialysis.[278] Diabetic survival is mildly reduced at 1 year but falls off more significantly with increasing vintage on hemodialysis. While hospital admission rates have fallen slightly over the past decade for dialysis patients in the United States, hospital admission rates for diabetic patients continue to exceed those for nondiabetic patients.[9] Higher mortality rates for diabetic patients on dialysis extend throughout the world.[279]

Most of the excess mortality in diabetic hemodialysis patients is due to associated cardiovascular disease, which is greater in diabetic patients than in nondiabetic patients (Figure 10–5). Deaths resulting from cerebrovascular disease and sepsis are about 1.5-fold more common among diabetic than nondiabetic hemodialysis patients.[280] All causes of death occur more commonly in diabetic than in nondiabetic dialysis patients, except for malignancy, which may affect more nondiabetics.[9]

A growing number of studies have reported predictors of survival in ESRD diabetic patients. As in nondiabetic patients, survival is affected by comorbidity. As for all ESRD patients, the number of preexisting comorbid conditions at the start of dialysis has increased,[9,281] and the number is greater than for nondiabetic patients. Diabetic patients with higher estimated glomerular filtration rates have higher mortality rates, possibly reflecting higher comorbidity, necessitating earlier initiation of hemodialysis.[10] Increasing age is associated with increasing mortality risk for all patients on dialysis.[10] While females have a higher risk of mortality among the nondiabetic population, gender does not affect mortality risk in the diabetic population.[10] Although the USRDS does not include classification of diabetes type in its survival analysis, it has reported poorer survival rates in diabetic white Americans than in diabetic black Americans, Native-Americans, or Asian-Americans, suggesting a survival disadvantage for patients with type I diabetes.[9,282]

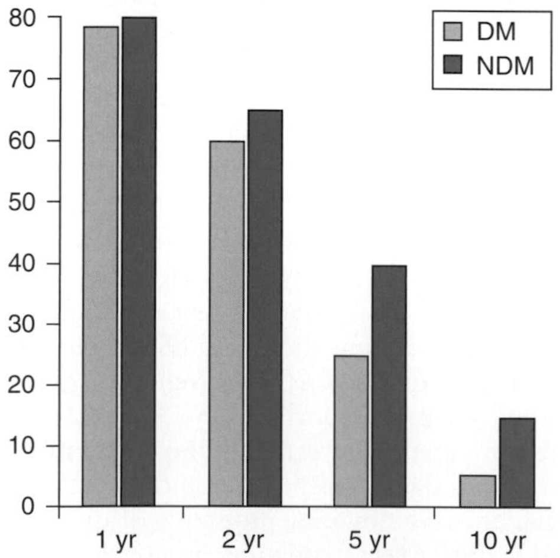

Figure 10–4 First, second, fifth, and tenth year patient survival estimates for diabetics and nondiabetics receiving dialysis, adjusted for age, gender, and race. Incident cohorts from 2001, 1999, 1996, and 1991, followed through 2001. (From U.S. Renal Data System: USRDS 2003 Annual Data Report. Bethesda, MD, National Institutes of Health, National Institute of Diabetes and Digestive and Kidney Diseases, 2003.)

White diabetic patients also have shorter dialysis survival times than diabetic Mexican-Americans.

Protein malnutrition, as indicated by a low serum albumin level, is a strong predictor of mortality, and similarly the BMI is associated with mortality with the highest risk at a BMI less than 20 kg/m^2 and the lowest risk at a BMI greater than 30 kg/m^2.[10] Low serum creatinine as a marker of diminished lean body mass has also been used as a marker of malnutrition and increased mortality.[283] Diabetic status itself becomes a weaker risk factor after nutritional baseline biochemical parameters are taken into account.[284]

Adequacy of dialysis also appears to influence survival. A number of studies describing a relationship between increasing dialysis delivery and lower all-cause mortality have included diabetic patients.[285] One study suggesting that diabetic patients receive lower doses of in-center dialysis than nondiabetic patients[286] is of concern because of data indicating a stronger influence of dialysis dose on diabetic patients than on nondiabetic patients.[287,288] Although an increasing URR or Kt/V as a marker for dialysis delivery has been associated with improved survival, patients with numbers in the top 10% to 20% for these parameters (URR > 75% and Kt/V > 1.6) have been found to have an increase in mortality, which is most likely reflecting protein-calorie malnutrition, which falsely elevates these parameters.[289] Recent USRDS data showed that in diabetics, increasing URRs are associated with decreasing mortality up to a URR of 70%, while the same is true up to a URR of 75% in nondiabetics.[10] The recent hemodialysis (HEMO) study prospectively examined more than 1800 dialysis patients, of whom nearly half were diabetics, and compared standard dose dialysis (Kt/V, 1.16; URR, 66%) to high dose dialysis (Kt/V, 1.53; URR, 75%). Hemodialysis patients did not experience a mortality benefit from a dose of dialysis greater than currently recommended in the United States.[290] Diabetic patients have equivalent 2-year survival on hemodialysis and peritoneal dialysis as long as adequacy is achieved.[291]

In addition to dialysis or transplantation, the other option in the management of uremic diabetic patients is withdrawal and death. Mortality by withdrawal from dialysis for diabetic patients is 1.3 times more common than in other diagnosis groups.[9] Reasons for withdrawal are similar for diabetic and nondiabetic patients.

PERITONEAL DIALYSIS

Although many advocate the use of peritoneal dialysis in uremic diabetic patients,[292, 293] it is the prevalent treatment option for less than 10% of diabetic adults in the United States.[9] The proportion of diabetic ESRD patients on peritoneal dialysis has declined over the past decade from about 11% in 1993 to 6% in 2001 (see Figure 10–1). Peritoneal dialysis is utilized more commonly among patients less than 20 years old (13.2% of ESRD patients) and less commonly among those aged 75 and over (4.3% of ESRD patients).[10] Its frequency as an ESRD treatment modality appears to be similar to that for nondiabetics. Almost half of the new patients begun on peritoneal dialysis are diabetic.[10] Increasing numbers of these patients are using *continuous cycling peritoneal dialysis* (CCPD). Of all diabetic patients initiating peritoneal dialysis in 2000, 25% began with continuous cycling and, of all prevalent diabetics on peritoneal dialysis in 2000, nearly half were using continuous cycling.[10]

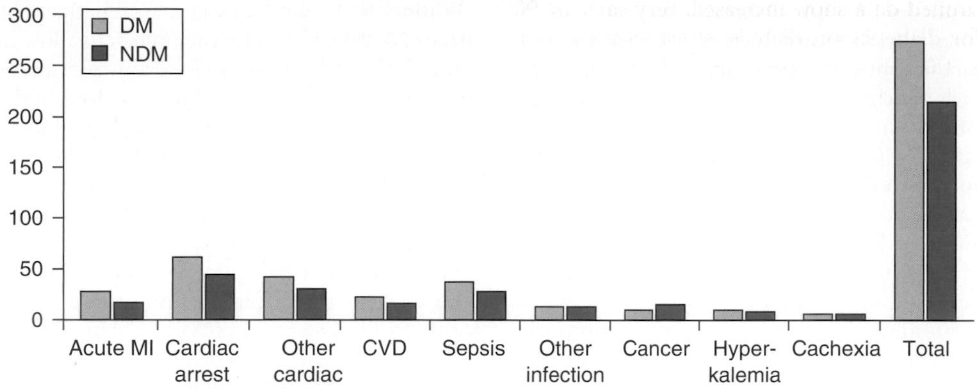

Figure 10–5 Death rates per 1000 patient years for patients on dialysis who received medicare benefits according to cause of ESRD (diabetes vs. all others), 1996–1998. *CVD*, cerebrovascular disease; *MI*, myocardial infarction. Combined cardiac causes were the most common recorded cause of death. Causes not shown include withdrawal from dialysis, acquired immunodeficiency syndrome, and hemorrhage. (From U.S. Renal Data System: USRDS 2000 Annual Data Report. Bethesda, MD, National Institutes of Health, National Institute of Diabetes and Digestive and Kidney Diseases, 2000.)

Peritoneal dialysis offers many advantages (see Table 10–1): (1) avoidance of vascular access problems, (2) a brief time to use after catheter placement, (3) better glycemic control through the use of intraperitoneal insulin, (4) milder fluid and electrolyte shifts, (5) avoidance of heparin, (6) lower vascular stress, (7) less antihypertensive therapy, and (8) better preservation of renal function.[294-296] Patients may also prefer it for psychosocial reasons, including lifestyle advantages, such as ease of travel and performance at home. CCPD may be preferred over *continuous ambulatory peritoneal dialysis* (CAPD) because it allows more flexibility for patients who continue to work, as the long dwell occurs during the daytime hours.[297] The disadvantages of peritoneal dialysis include risk of peritonitis, high rates of technical failure due to poor visual acuity and manual dexterity,[298] patient burnout, abdominal complaints, orthostatic hypotension, and in some cases, inadequate dialysis when residual renal function is lost (see Table 10–1).

Data to support the advantage of peritoneal dialysis in dialyzed diabetic patients are limited,[292,293] with some data suggesting that mortality for diabetics on dialysis is greater with peritoneal dialysis as compared to hemodialysis.[299] Most studies, however, once correcting for comorbidity, have not found a significant survival difference between hemodialysis and peritoneal dialysis in diabetic patients.[300,301] In the absence of hyperglycemia or advanced peritoneal microvascular disease, peritoneal transport and ultrafiltration, in most cases, are similar to those in nondiabetic patients. Hyperglycemic diabetic patients may have enhanced peritoneal transport by peritoneal equilibration tests, perhaps related to increased capillary permeability. Approximately 75% of patients remain on peritoneal dialysis after 3 years.[302]

Insulin and Glucose

An understanding of insulin and glucose physiology is essential to the care of diabetic patients on peritoneal dialysis. Glucose absorbed continuously from the dialysate may constitute one-quarter of daily caloric intake,[303] leading to poor glycemic control, hyperlipidemia, and weight gain. Adverse lipid effects include an increase in triglyceride and in plasma very low density lipoprotein levels. Glycemic control is a desirable therapeutic goal (see Box 10–1) that is associated with better outcomes and slower progression of diabetic complications, including less disabling gastroparesis and better patient and technique survival.[304] Peritoneal ultrafiltration is reduced even in the presence of moderate hyperglycemia.[305]

Intraperitoneal insulin administration may eliminate the need for injections, provides more consistent insulin absorption, lowers peripheral insulin levels, lessens the risk of hypoglycemia, and provides constant basal insulin dosing. Because it is absorbed (mainly by diffusion) into the portal venous system, detectable insulin blood levels occur within 15 minutes and peak at about 90 minutes. Fifty percent is absorbed by 8 hours of dwell time.[306] A high first-pass elimination of insulin occurs in the liver.[307] Some intraperitoneal insulin reaches the systemic circulation directly. Intraperitoneal insulin does not affect solute clearances, ultrafiltration rates, or absorption of glucose.[308]

The major benefit of intraperitoneal insulin is improved glycemic control.[309] In one report, the hemoglobin A_{1C} levels improved from 8.4% to 6.1% when diabetic peritoneal dialysis patients were switched from subcutaneous insulin to intraperitoneal insulin.[308] Initial concerns about higher peritonitis rates have waned, and the risk of peritonitis appears to be increased only minimally, if at all, with intraperitoneal insulin use.[302,306,308] In a comparison of subcutaneous and intraperitoneal administration of insulin, peritoneal insulin resulted in improved glycemic control, although it was associated with higher total cholesterol, low-density lipoprotein, and triglyceride levels, and 33% lower high-density lipoprotein levels, possibly because of a direct effect of insulin on the liver.[310] Although significant clinical benefit has not been proven in clinical trials, intraperitoneal insulin is preferred in most patients on CAPD. Use of intraperitoneal insulin in patients on automated cyclers is more complex, because it leaves less time for insulin absorption and does not provide daytime insulin, necessitating a daytime subcutaneous insulin injection.[311]

Icodextrin, a high molecular weight glucose polymer, is now available as an alternate osmotic agent to dextrose in peritoneal dialysis fluid. Its absorption from the peritoneal cavity is slow compared to dextrose, resulting in a longer and more effective ultrafiltration,[312] with less of an absorbed glucose load.[313] Patients with impaired ultrafiltration, such as diabetics, seem to derive the most benefit, obviating exposure to high dextrose-containing solutions, which are typically relied upon to promote ultrafiltration.[314] Limited data demonstrate decreased formation of advanced glycation end-products (AGEs) with icodextrin as compared to dextrose based dialysate fluid.[315,316] Accumulation of AGEs bound to receptors in the peritoneal membrane may stimulate fibrosis and ultrafiltration failure.[317] Hypoglycemia has been reported in diabetic patients using icodextrin dialysate, resulting from falsely high glucose values with some glucose monitoring assays, prompting inappropriately high dosing of insulin.[318,319] Other adverse effects of this fluid that have limited its use include sterile peritonitis, which can result in technique failure,[320,321] and cutaneous hypersensitivity reactions.[322] However, icodextrin has been more effective than dextrose in decreasing edema weight, especially during the long dwell of the day[312,323] and is also effective in preserving ultrafiltration during episodes of peritonitis.[324] Furthermore, early data suggest an improvement in quality of life in peritoneal dialysis patients using icodextrin solution versus dextrose solution.[325] The role of this costly therapy in diabetic patients on peritoneal dialysis remains to be determined.

Uremic patients are at risk for hypoglycemia because of impaired insulin degradation, improved insulin sensitivity, and poor nutrition. In uremic diabetic patients, excessive insulin or oral hypoglycemic agents may also contribute. Severe sequelae of hypoglycemia, including convulsions and brain damage, are known to occur. However, patients on CAPD using intraperitoneal insulin experience less variability in serum glucose levels, and hypoglycemic reactions are fewer and milder than with hemodialysis[326] or with subcutaneous insulin.[308,327] When severe hypoglycemic reactions occur in a diabetic patient on hemodialysis, peritoneal dialysis with intraperitoneal insulin may be preferable.

As with subcutaneous insulin, glycemic control during intraperitoneal insulin use is assessed by self-monitoring of blood glucose levels, office fasting blood sugars, and glycated hemoglobin values. Blood glucose levels should be checked at home two to four times daily, including before meals and at bedtime. Treatment objectives include preprandial blood sugars of less than 130 mg/dL and postprandial blood sugars of less than 180 mg/dL, with avoidance of hypoglycemia. Hemoglobin A_{1C} levels above 7.5% may be falsely elevated because of uremia, but hemoglobin A_{1C} goals should be measured regularly, preferably with an immunoassay to avoid analytic interference, and a goal of less than 7% should be sought.[91] Diabetes education using a calendar diary is essential.

When adding insulin into the bag of dialysate, limited insulin ultimately reaches the portal system (due to adherence to the plastic bag and tubing and dilution in the dialysate), so that the average dose is often two to three times the previous subcutaneous dose. Doses in type I diabetics may be substantially lower than in type II diabetics.[328] Doses, however, vary greatly and must be individualized.

To determine the initial intraperitoneal insulin dose for CAPD (Table 10–4), add up the total number of units of all types of insulin given subcutaneously and divide this evenly among four 2-liter bags, giving it all as regular insulin. Supplemental insulin is required to account for the dextrose in each exchange. For 1.5% dextrose solution, add 2 units, for 2.5% dextrose solution, add 4 units, and for 4.25% dextrose solution, add 6 units. Daytime exchanges should be timed to occur 20 minutes before each meal, to allow insulin absorption and dietary hyperglycemia to coincide. Blood glucose should be monitored fasting to adjust the dose in the overnight dwell and at 1 hour postprandial to adjust each daytime dwell as indicated in Table 10–4.[328] As metabolic control improves on CAPD, decreased insulin requirements may result.

In patients on cycling peritoneal dialysis, comparable glycemic control can be achieved. Because of higher ultrafiltration and reduced glucose absorption during the frequent short-dwell cycles, total insulin can be reduced to about 85% of that administered on CAPD.[329] Up to half the total dose can be given in the daytime dwell. Additional subcutaneous injections during the day may be required to help metabolize carbohydrate absorbed with meals.[328] Alternatively, cycling patients can be treated with twice-daily or more frequent subcutaneous dosing. Cycling patients who switch temporarily to CAPD should beware of the risk of hypoglycemia during the longer exchanges, which permit greater insulin absorption.

In patients with rapid peritoneal transport rates (as determined by the peritoneal equilibration test),[305] higher blood sugars reduce ultrafiltration and may also require more insulin. During infection, injuries, or emotional stress, extra insulin should be given, using "sick-day" rules, to prevent ketoacidosis. During episodes of peritonitis, insulin requirements vary widely: they are commonly increased but in some cases are reduced because of hypoglycemia. The insulin dose may also need to be adjusted for variable food intake or physical activity. The insulin dose should be reduced for exchanges prior to a procedure that requires fasting.

Peritonitis

Between 1991 and 2001, rates of hospitalization among peritoneal dialysis patients for peritonitis fell 47%,[9] presumably resulting from improved preventive techniques among peritoneal dialysis patients.[330,331] However, peritonitis remains one of the most common causes of hospital admission in peritoneal dialysis patients, accounting for about 15% of admissions in one recent study.[332] Peritonitis is the main cause of technique failure resulting in transfer to hemodialysis.[302,333] Demographic data in the past have associated diabetes with an increased risk of peritonitis.[334] In one registry, diabetes was an independent predictor of peritonitis,[335] and additional studies have reported worse complications of peritonitis in diabetic patients, including higher mortality rates.[302,336] Although theoretically more prone to peritonitis, diabetic patients in fact have an incidence of peritonitis similar to that of nondiabetic patients,[10,337] recently reported as 105 events per 1000 patient years at risk.[10] Another recent study reported that diabetes was not associated with worse outcomes in nearly 400 episodes of peritonitis.[338] Other data show an increased risk of tunnel infections without more frequent peritonitis.[339] Diabetics have significantly higher rates of hospital admission for peritoneal dialysis catheter complications than nondiabetics.[10] The duration of infection and the frequency of need for catheter removal appear similar in nondiabetic and diabetic patients. Organisms causing peritonitis are similar in these two populations on peritoneal dialysis.[340] Blind diabetic patients may have increased peritonitis rates and more severe disease. Overall, infections other than peritonitis more frequently cause death in diabetic patients on peritoneal dialysis.[341]

Table 10–4 Intraperitoneal Insulin Dosing in Peritoneal Dialysis

- Start CAPD with four daily exchanges each 2 L.
- Add up total subcutaneous insulin dose in units. Add one-fourth of the total as regular insulin to each bag of dialysate.
- For 1.5% dextrose, add 2 units regular insulin per bag.
  For 2.5% dextrose, add 4 units regular insulin per bag.
  For 4.25% dextrose, add 6 units regular insulin per bag.
- Perform each exchange 20 minutes before breakfast, lunch and dinner, and at 11 PM before bed.
- Check fasting and 1 hour postprandial blood sugars.
- Adjust insulin dose based on blood sugar as follows:

Fasting Glucose (mg/dL)	1 h Postprandial Glucose (mg/dL)	Insulin Adjustment (units)
	<40	−6
<40	40-80	−4
40-80	80-120	−2
80-180	120-180	0
180-240	180-240	+2
240-400	240-300	+4
>400	>300	variable

- For patients on CCPD, reduce the total daily insulin dose to 85%.
- Give up to half of this dose in the daytime dwell; use the remainder in cycled exchanges.
- Beware of the risk of hypoglycemia when the patient converts from CCPD to CAPD status.

CAPD, continuous ambulatory peritoneal dialysis; *CCPD*, continuous cyclic peritoneal dialysis. (From Tzamaloukas AH, Friedman EA: Diabetes. *In* Daugirdas JT, Blake PG, Ing TS [eds]: Handbook of Dialysis, 3rd ed. Lippincott, Williams & Wilkins, 2001, p 453.)

Chronic carriers of *S. aureus*, with or without diabetes, are at higher risk of exit-site infections and of tunnel infections.[342-344] Furthermore, carriers have a higher rate of *Staphylococcal peritonitis*. In one study, three fourths of diabetic patients on peritoneal dialysis were nasal carriers of *S. aureus* (twice the rate of nondiabetic patients).[342] In another report, diabetics tended to have higher rates of nasal carriage than exit site colonization with *S. aureus*, and nasal carriage was more important prognostically than positive exit-site culture in determining risk of *S. aureus* catheter-related infection. Diabetics were at significantly higher risk of *S. aureus* catheter infection than nondiabetics in this study.[345]

Eradication of the staphylococcal carrier state seems to reduce the risk of peritonitis and catheter loss.[346] In a large study population, of whom 30% were diabetic patients, mupirocin 2% ointment applied daily to the exit site was as effective as oral rifampin in preventing catheter-related *S. aureus* infection.[343] A recent review concluded that with either oral rifampin or mupirocin ointment, there was strong evidence that prophylaxis reduced the rate of exit-site infections, while the evidence for decreased rates of tunnel infections and peritonitis was weaker.[347] Although *S. aureus* catheter infections and peritonitis may be serious, the role of prophylaxis for all diabetic patients undergoing CAPD remains to be determined.[348] There is a growing consensus that at least those diabetic patients who are carriers of *S. aureus* should receive antibiotic prophylaxis.[345]

Initial treatment of peritonitis in diabetic patients should be similar to that in nondiabetic patients[343] and should follow the recent recommendations of the International Society for Peritoneal Dialysis.[349] In patients with residual urine output of greater than 100 mL/day, empiric therapy should consist of a first generation cephalosporin, such as cefazolin, and the third generation cephalosporin, ceftazidime, which can be mixed in the same bag for one exchange per day.[349] Because of the recent increase in vancomycin-resistant enterococci,[350] empiric use of vancomycin is now discouraged. Empiric use of cefazolin once daily intraperitoneally appears to be as effective in treatment of peritonitis as vancomycin.[351] Aminoglycoside exposure accelerates loss of residual renal function in peritoneal dialysis patients[352] and is therefore avoided in patients with urine output greater than 100 mL/day.

Fungal peritonitis is an uncommon but severe complication of peritoneal dialysis and may be caused by a growing list of fungal agents. *Candida albicans* is by far the most common.[353] Catheter removal is necessary in most cases of fungal or mycobacterial infections. Diabetes does not appear to predispose to fungal peritonitis.[340,353] However, diabetes was a risk factor for non-*Candida albicans* peritonitis in a recent, very small series of peritoneal dialysis patients.[354]

Gastroparesis

Diabetic gastroparesis is twice as common (70% vs. 37%) in type I than in type II diabetics.[355] Symptomatic gastroparesis may be aggravated by peritoneal dialysis and is an important cause of hospitalization.[356] Gastric emptying is delayed when the peritoneal cavity is full, even in nondiabetic peritoneal dialysis patients.[357] Gastric emptying is significantly slower with dextrose dialysate than with icodextrin dialysate, suggesting that impaired gastric emptying in peritoneal dialysis is not merely reflecting the effect of increased intraabdominal pressure due to the volume of dialysate.[358] Radionuclide gastric emptying results may not correlate with symptoms. A few small studies have reported delayed gastric emptying in approximately 50% of all CAPD patients even without symptoms.[359] Patients refractory to oral metoclopramide on CAPD may respond to intraperitoneal erythromycin, 100 mg/2 L dialysate, with exchanges 30 minutes before meals.[356] Improvement in the radionuclide gastric emptying study with treatment using prokinetic agents resulted in a significant increase in serum albumin levels reflecting improved nutritional status.[360]

Retinopathy

Although vision is less likely to deteriorate in diabetic patients who have undergone renal transplantation, loss of vision is independent of dialysis modality, having similar progression in patients on peritoneal dialysis and hemodialysis.[201,339] Blind patients have decreased technique survival rates.[361] Newer techniques are being developed to allow visually-impaired ESRD patients to perform peritoneal dialysis independently at home without increased risk of peritonitis.[362]

MALNUTRITION

Some reports show that serum albumin is only weakly correlated with other markers of nutritional status such as BMI, percent lean body mass, and a normalized protein equivalent of nitrogen appearance in peritoneal dialysis patients.[363,364] Whereas hypoalbuminemia predicts risk of mortality in the hemodialysis population, its validity is less established in diabetic patients on peritoneal dialysis.[365,366] A low serum albumin level was the variable most closely associated with death risk in a large national survey that included an analysis of peritoneal dialysis patients, 40% of whom were diabetic.[367] A recent report also proposed low prealbumin as a marker of malnutrition and decreased survival in peritoneal dialysis patients.[368] The 40% prevalence rate of protein-calorie malnutrition in patients on CAPD is greater than that in patients on hemodialysis,[369,370] and almost 10% of these patients have moderate to severe malnutrition. Protein malnutrition may be associated with a twofold increase in cachexia-related deaths in diabetic patients on peritoneal dialysis, compared with nondiabetic patients.[371] In one recent study, diabetic patients on peritoneal dialysis had a tendency toward lower serum albumin concentrations, and hypoalbuminemia was a marker of morbidity, especially related to an increased risk of hospitalization.[365]

Hypoproteinemia may be worse in diabetic than nondiabetic patients on peritoneal dialysis. Protein losses in the dialysate (5 to 15 g/day, two thirds of it albumin)[372] and inadequate protein intake are principal causes.[373] Diabetic patients may have greater peritoneal protein permeability than nondiabetic patients on CAPD.[374,375] The greatest protein losses occur during longer dwells, such as overnight, or during bouts of peritonitis. Ongoing urinary protein losses contribute in some patients. Better dialysis adequacy is associated with higher serum albumin.[376] Greater residual renal function has also been associated with higher dietary protein intake.[377] Malnutrition may be worsened by increased gastroparesis.[360] Markers of inflammation such as C-reactive protein correlate with a low serum albumin, suggesting that an acute phase response during peritoneal dialysis may also contribute to hypoalbuminemia.[378]

Because CAPD patients are able to increase nitrogen synthesis and become protein anabolic in response to increased dietary protein intake, a minimum daily protein intake of 1.2 g/kg is recommended.[369] Other measures available to improve the nutritional status of CAPD patients (including early initiation of dialysis, more intensive dialysis, nutritional counseling, and intraperitoneal amino acid solutions)[369] have not been specifically tested in diabetic patients. Nutritional supplementation with amino acid-containing dialysis solutions has been effective in inducing protein anabolism[379] and increasing serum albumin, prealbumin, and transferrin concentrations,[380] but has been associated with increased serum urea concentrations and metabolic acidosis.[381] A new peritoneal dialysis solution containing both glucose and amino acids has been shown to increase serum amino acid levels to normal without increasing urea, suggesting improved amino acid utilization for protein synthesis without increased urea.[382] Because inadequate dialysis is a risk factor for severe malnutrition in patients on peritoneal dialysis, an increase in the amount of dialysis delivered may be necessary when residual renal function is lost.[267,383] Transfer to continuous cycling peritoneal dialysis may result in improved caloric intake and diminished protein losses relative to CAPD.

SURVIVAL

Patient survival rates for diabetics on peritoneal dialysis have improved 28% from the cohort of patients on peritoneal dialysis between 1987 and 1991 to the cohort of patients on peritoneal dialysis between 1992 and 1996.[9] However, it remains true that uremic diabetic patients have lower survival rates than nondiabetic patients regardless of treatment modality[9,384,385] (Table 10–5). Differences in mortality rates of diabetic patients on peritoneal dialysis versus hemodialysis have generally been small.[386] According to the USRDS, mortality rates of diabetic patients with ESRD who were treated with peritoneal dialysis were slightly higher than those of patients undergoing hemodialysis.[9] A recent prospective analysis compared mortality in all ESRD patients on hemodialysis versus peritoneal dialysis and found that there was no significant difference in mortality during the first 2 years of therapy; however, after the first 2 years, patients on hemodialysis had a survival advantage.[387] Among patients older than age 65 beginning renal replacement therapy, the mortality over the first year on dialysis was higher for peritoneal dialysis patients than for hemodialysis patients, and this difference was more pronounced among diabetics.[388] A report from Europe looking specifically at type II patients found greater mortality in those on peritoneal dialysis than in those on hemodialysis over 14 months of follow-up.[389] Another recent report found that both diabetic and nondiabetic patients with underlying coronary artery disease had poorer survival on peritoneal dialysis than on hemodialysis.[390] Other studies that have shown a survival advantage for peritoneal dialysis over hemodialysis have attributed this to physician selection of healthier patients for peritoneal dialysis.[391,392] In addition, dia-

Table 10–5 Peritoneal Dialysis Outcomes in Diabetic Patients

- Inferior survival compared with that for nondiabetic patients on peritoneal dialysis (PD)
- Slightly inferior overall survival compared with that for diabetic patients on hemodialysis
- Better survival for young patients receiving PD
- Older diabetic patients (>60 yr) do better with hemodialysis
- Survival rates for patients with type I diabetes are better than those for patients with type II diabetes who are on PD
- Poor technique survival in patients with type II diabetes
- Causes of death similar to diabetic patients receiving hemodialysis

betes was a death risk predictor in a survey that included more than 1500 peritoneal dialysis patients.[367]

Recent data show 2-year survival for patients on peritoneal dialysis at 78%, with technique survival at 2 years of 62%.[393] Increased age, poor nutritional status, and presence of diabetes were predictors of decreased survival.[393] Previous data showed 1-, 2-, and 3-year survival rates for type I diabetic patients on CAPD of 92%, 75%, and 50%, respectively.[394] Survival rates have been better for type I than for type II diabetes at both 1-year (92% vs. 74%) and 2-year (65% vs. 23% vintage on CAPD.[395] Two recent reports demonstrated better early (1 year) survival with worse longer term (>1 year) survival for type II as compared to type I diabetics on peritoneal dialysis.[396,397] Survival rates at 1, 3, and 5 years for type I versus type II diabetics on CAPD were 89% versus 100%, 71% versus 69%, and 58% versus 39%, respectively. Both groups of diabetics had worse survival than nondiabetics, despite sufficient and comparable dialysis adequacies.[396] Long-term survival on peritoneal dialysis is better for type I than for type II diabetics.[398] Ten-year survival of patients started on peritoneal dialysis was 50% for type I diabetics and 11% for type II diabetics, including patients who had changed modality to hemodialysis or been transplanted.[399] In a review of age-adjusted CAPD outcomes at one facility in the United States over 10 years, the median survival in type I diabetes (21 months) did not statistically differ from rates from other major causes of ESRD, whereas type II patient survival was significantly worse (11 months).[400]

Compared to hemodialysis, peritoneal dialysis led to better survival for young patients (< 45 years old), whereas older patients (> 60 years old) with type II disease did better on hemodialysis.[395] Other data support an effect of age on outcomes in patients on CAPD.[339, 401] One report attributed all of the increased mortality in type I diabetics to comorbid cardiovascular disease and in type II diabetics to comorbid cardiovascular disease and increased age.[397] In an analysis of the Case Mix Severity Special Study of the USRDS, which included Medicare patients starting dialysis during 1986 to 1987, higher overall adjusted mortality for CAPD relative to hemodialysis was found among diabetic patients. Increased CAPD mortality was particularly evident in elderly patients with type II disease. In fact, the analysis revealed that younger patients on CAPD may have a lower mortality risk than those on hemodialysis, particularly because of fewer comorbid conditions. The best survival in peritoneal dialysis is achieved in younger patients who are initially free of cardiac disease and are nonsmokers. No similar relative mortality risk was found for nondiabetic patients selected for peritoneal or hemodialysis in the Case Mix Study.[402] Diabetic patients treated with peritoneal dialysis had higher hospitalization rates than those treated with hemodialysis, except for younger patients less than age 40.[9, 403]

Additional factors have been shown to influence outcomes in diabetic patients on peritoneal dialysis. Early referral to a nephrologist prior to initiation of peritoneal dialysis was associated with better survival in type II diabetics.[404] Survival was better in patients with greater residual renal function, although this was not specifically shown in diabetics.[405] A high peritoneal transport rate has been associated with poorer survival, although it seems to be a marker for diabetes, which is the most important risk factor for mortality in peritoneal dialysis patients, so that a high transport rate may not impose any independent risk for mortality.[406,407] In type II diabetics, better glycemic control prior to initiation of peritoneal dialysis (defined as hemoglobin A_{1C} <10% for at least 6 months prior to starting dialysis) was associated with better survival.[408] Independent predictors of mortality in peritoneal dialysis patients in the CANUSA study included increased age, insulin-dependent diabetes, cardiovascular disease, low albumin, poor nutritional status by global assessment, and lean body mass.[409] Another recent report identified independent predictors of mortality as increased age, diabetes, low albumin, elevated diastolic blood pressure, and increased lipoprotein(a) levels.[410]

Peritoneal dialysis technique survival, defined as remaining on this modality without either death or transfer to hemodialysis, may also be inferior in diabetic patients.[395, 411] Some studies[412] have also shown more frequent technique failure in diabetic patients when defined only as transfer to hemodialysis. However, subsequent reports have found similar technique survival for diabetics and nondiabetics on peritoneal dialysis,[385,413] although technique survival on peritoneal dialysis is worse than on hemodialysis.[385] Technique failure resulting from increased membrane permeability, loss of ultrafiltration, and fibrosis of the peritoneal membrane are hastened by accumulation of AGEs because of high glucose-containing peritoneal dialysis solutions in both diabetic and nondiabetic patients.[385] Few studies have compared technique survival in type I versus type II diabetes. CAPD technique survival rates (defined as removal from peritoneal dialysis or death) in type I diabetics were 75% at 1 year and 60% at 2 years, which were better than for type II diabetics. Type II diabetes is the main risk factor for poor technique survival, which is only 35% at 2 years and 18% at 3 years.[400] Technique survival did not differ between patients with type I and type II diabetes in the recent CANUSA study.[414] For technique survival in that analysis, death was censored.

The causes of mortality in patients on peritoneal dialysis are similar to those associated with hemodialysis. Nearly half of the deaths are cardiovascular. Death from acute myocardial infarction in patients on peritoneal dialysis, for example, is more than twice as common in diabetic patients than in nondiabetic patients. Diabetic patients on peritoneal dialysis also die nearly two times as often from cardiac arrest, septicemia, cerebrovascular disease, and hyperkalemia than do nondiabetic patients on peritoneal dialysis.[9] In addition, their hospital admission rates and lengths of stay are higher than those of nondiabetic patients.[9] Diabetic patients on peritoneal dialysis require less antihypertensive therapy,[415] have more gastroparesis, and may have an increased risk of lower extremity amputation. Experience with long-term survival is limited, but it is more likely with young age, absence of coronary disease, and good blood pressure control.[361]

TRANSPLANTATION

Although improved care of uremic diabetic patients has resulted in a growing population of diabetic transplant recipients,[416] diabetic transplant candidates remain disadvantaged. Diabetics are less likely to be wait-listed before the start of ESRD therapy, [417] and the percent of ESRD diabetics on the waiting list, compared to all causes, is lower.[418] Nonetheless, a large portion of the patients on the national deceased donor waiting list have diabetes.[419] Although the incidence of ESRD has continued to increase for diabetics and for all patients in the United States, however, the transplant rates have not kept pace, decreasing in 2000 to 3.7/100 patient years on dialysis for diabetics compared to 6.6/100 patient years for all ESRD patients (Figure 10–6). Diabetics comprise 44% of all incident ESRD patients but only 17% of those transplanted. The annual incidence rate decreased by 4.6% between 1996 and 2000. Diabetics comprise about 20% of recipients from both deceased and living donors. Of the incident ESRD population of diabetic patients, 13% received a kidney transplant in 2000.

Nonetheless, relatively low mortality rates have led to continued growth (annual change + 6%) in the number of prevalent diabetic transplant recipients. The number of diabetic recipients in the United States increased from 15,608 to 21,132, of a total of 103,809 recipients in year 2000. With improved short-term success rates, diabetic transplant recipients overwhelm the resources of the transplant center[420] and receive long-term follow-up care by community-based nephrologists.[421] Across the United States, point prevalence in ESRD networks varied somewhat, between 16.5% and 27.2%.[9] Most recipients have type I diabetes. By comparison, in few other countries do diabetic patients account for greater than 10% of the total renal transplant population.[416] Following transplantation, diabetic recipients are roughly one and one-half times more likely to have a hospital admission, with hospitalized days annually increased to 8.1 compared to 5.3 for all recipients. In addition to transplant care, management must address all the potential complications of diabetes. In advance of surgery, the candidate should have been evaluated for factors that could negatively affect transplantation outcomes (see Table 10–2). Postoperative management may be made difficult by the concurrent problems of glycemic control, gastroparesis, impaired wound healing, hypertension, malnutrition, and urinary retention. Insulin therapy, either intravenous or subcutaneous, should continue in the recovery room. Postoperative hyperkalemia is common, especially when graft function is delayed, and may require extra insulin or even acute dialysis.[422] Sodium polystyrene sulfonate, especially in sorbitol, should be avoided initially because of the risk of intestinal necrosis.[423] Given experimental evidence that sorbitol is toxic to bowel mucosa, administration with another vehicle may be indicated.[424,425]

Postoperative conversion to oral medications and fluids may be delayed because of gastric atony and bowel dysfunction. The promotility agent metoclopramide may increase cyclosporine levels, and erythromycin, also used for gastroparesis, may precipitate frank cyclosporine[426] or tacrolimus[427] toxicity by decreasing drug hepatic metabolism. Wound complications are more common in patients with diabetes. Because of slower neo-ureterocystotomy healing and coexisting bladder atony, an indwelling catheter should remain in place longer than for the nondiabetic recipient. Despite near doubling of insulin doses on average, glycemic control remains suboptimum in many patients.

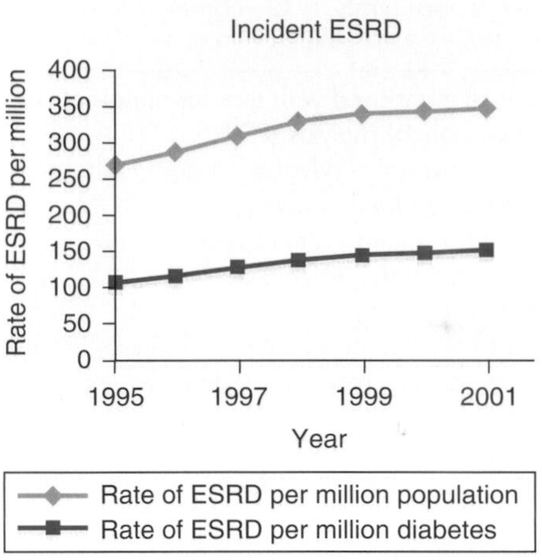

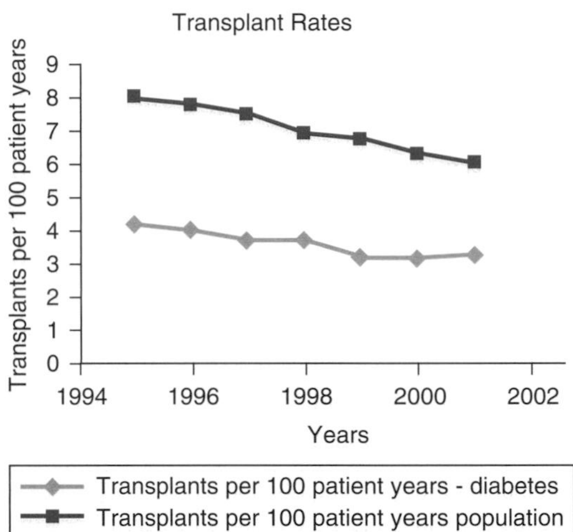

Figure 10–6 Incidence of ESRD and rate of transplantation (per 100 dialysis patient years), 1995 – 2001. Rates adjusted for age, gender, and race. Population estimates obtained from U.S. census data. (From U.S. Renal Data System: USRDS 2003 Annual Data Report: Atlas of End-Stage Renal Disease in the United States. Bethesda, MD, National Institutes of Health, National Institute of Diabetes and Digestive and Kidney Diseases, 2003.)

Ischemic Heart Disease

Although cardiovascular event rates are markedly higher in dialysis patients,[3] cardiovascular disease (coronary artery disease, peripheral vascular disease, and cerebrovascular disease) has emerged as the leading cause of death in kidney transplant recipients.[428,429] Transplantation is associated with atherogenesis accelerated by the combined effects of preexisting vascular disease and post-transplant factors. This premature development of atherosclerosis is multifactorial[430] because of traditional cardiovascular risk factors (including diabetes) and to factors uniquely related to chronic kidney disease, dialysis, and transplantation.[431,432]

The cumulative incidence of coronary artery disease over 15 years of transplantation is about 25%.[433] Cardiovascular disease accounts for about half of all deaths in ESRD patients and 17% to 50% of deaths among renal transplant recipients. The prevalence of all cardiovascular types at the time of transplantation was 12.9% in one study.[434] By the time of initiation of chronic dialysis treatment, 25% of patients have a history of ischemic heart disease.[435] Cardiovascular mortality rates in patients undergoing dialysis are nearly 15-fold higher than the normal population.[436] In the USRDS, cardiac mortality is high, with overall in-hospital mortality rates with myocardial infarction of 26%.[437] Diabetes is more prevalent in patients with documented cardiovascular events pre-transplant.[438] Diabetic patients manifest the highest cardiovascular morbity and mortality rates of any group of ESRD patients.[439] Overall mortality rates are two times higher when ESRD is secondary to diabetes mellitus, and the risk of death from cardiovascular disease is over two times higher,[440] with ischemic heart disease (IHD) accounting for most. With glomerulonephritis as a reference level for patients who died with functioning grafts, the relative risk by multivariate Cox proportional hazard regression was 1.93.[441] The risk of death in diabetic transplant recipients ages 55 to 64 years is 20 times that of the general population.[439]

The relationship between ischemic heart disease and markers of risk in transplant recipients has been studied to define high risk patients and the roles of individualized risk factor intervention.[433] Some risk factors for post-transplant cardiovascular disease are the same as for the general population, including gender, age, obesity, and a sedentary lifestyle.[442] Classic cardiovascular risk factors including hypertension, diabetes, smoking, and anemia, account for a large part but not for all of the excessive prevalence of IHD in the ESRD population.[438,443] Additional accepted factors altered by the uremic state include disordered lipid metabolism, secondary hyperparathyroidism, and hyperhomocyteinemia[444]; inflammation, oxidative stress, endothelial dysfunction, and apoptosis-related abnormalities in the vessel wall are under evaluation.[445] Among these, hypertension, hyperlipidemia, hyperhomocysteinemia, and hyperglycemia are modifiable by current treatments.

New IHD events continue to accrue many years after transplantation.[443] Following transplantation, significant risk factors for IHD include age, male gender, hyperlipidemia, delayed graft function, acute rejection, obesity, and diabetes.[446] Women are particularly vulnerable to the cardiovascular consequences of diabetes.[447] The roles of other potential factors such as hypercoagulability are currently being evaluated.[430] At early stages of diabetic nephropathy, coronary risk factors begin to aggregate, including lipids, growth factors,[448] and coagulation factors. In addition, cardiovascular disease in diabetic patients with nephropathy clusters in families, supporting an additional genetic mechanism of risk factor aggregation.[449] The mortality risk from cardiovascular causes in proteinuric type I diabetic patients is higher than in nonproteinuric diabetics.[450-452] Immunosuppressive therapy, particularly corticosteroids, may further aggravate risk factors for atherosclerotic vascular disease in transplant recipients.[439] Recently, decreased renal function has emerged as an additional risk factor for acute coronary syndromes in transplant recipients.[453] Many transplanted diabetic patients have mild to moderate renal insufficiency.[436] A recent study reported that higher rates of heart disease requiring hospitalization were associated with stage III chronic kidney disease, 1 to 3 years after transplantation. The association persisted after correction for other known cardiovascular risk factors.[454]

The high rates of serious and fatal IHD in diabetic transplant recipients underscores the need for a systematic approach that begins long before the development of ESRD. Clinical practice guidelines have recommended that screening tests in general should be based on the individual's risk estimate for IHD.[455] Increased graft and patient survival can be achieved using screening strategies to assign risk stratification and exclude those with significant coronary artery disease.[456] However, the most ESRD diabetic patients with severe coronary artery disease do not have tyical anginal symptoms,[457] although the presence of even asymptomatic coronary disease places ESRD diabetic patients at high risk for subsequent myocardial infarction.[458] Even in asymptomatic diabetic recipients, coronary stenosis over 50% is present in over half.[459]

Because of the high incidence of coronary ischemia and because they are more likely to have coronary ischemia that is unrecognized, screening of diabetic kidney transplant candidates undergo more cardiac screening tests than nondiabetics.[460] All symptomatic diabetic patients and high-risk type I patients require angiography; in all others, diabetes is a coronary risk factor, which will require noninvasive evaluation.[456] For preoperative screening alone, for example, diabetic candidates may have high risk for surgery based on standard criteria.[461] For those otherwise at low risk, the presence of diabetes still requires noninvasive cardiac testing. While most transplant centers use noninvasive cardiac tests to screen diabetic candidates,[462] no single cardiac screening test is superior. Uremic diabetic patients are commonly unable to perform adequately on exercise testing, and accuracy of radionuclide imaging in detecting coronary disease is suboptimal.[463] For example, thallium stress testing has low predictive value because of its high incidence of false-positive results, up to 50% in one study.[464] However, the addition of an imaging modality can increase the sensitivity and specificity of noninvasive testing.[465] Dipyridamole thallium imaging supplemented by echocardiography may be superior.[465] Electron beam computed tomography is of uncertain value at this time.

While therapeutic nihilism continues to affect cardiovascular management in ESRD patients,[464] pre-transplant patients with positive screening tests or with symptomatic coronary disease should undergo coronary angiography (Figure 10–7). One study utilized clinical criteria to define a group of type I patients at low risk of cardiac mortality (age $<$ 45 years, diabetic for $<$ 25 years, nonsmoker, normal electrocardiogram[466]), in whom coronary angiography can be avoided. However, no follow-up verification of low-risk status after transplantation has been reported. In patients with symptoms and significant ($>$ 70%) coronary stenosis, coronary bypass or

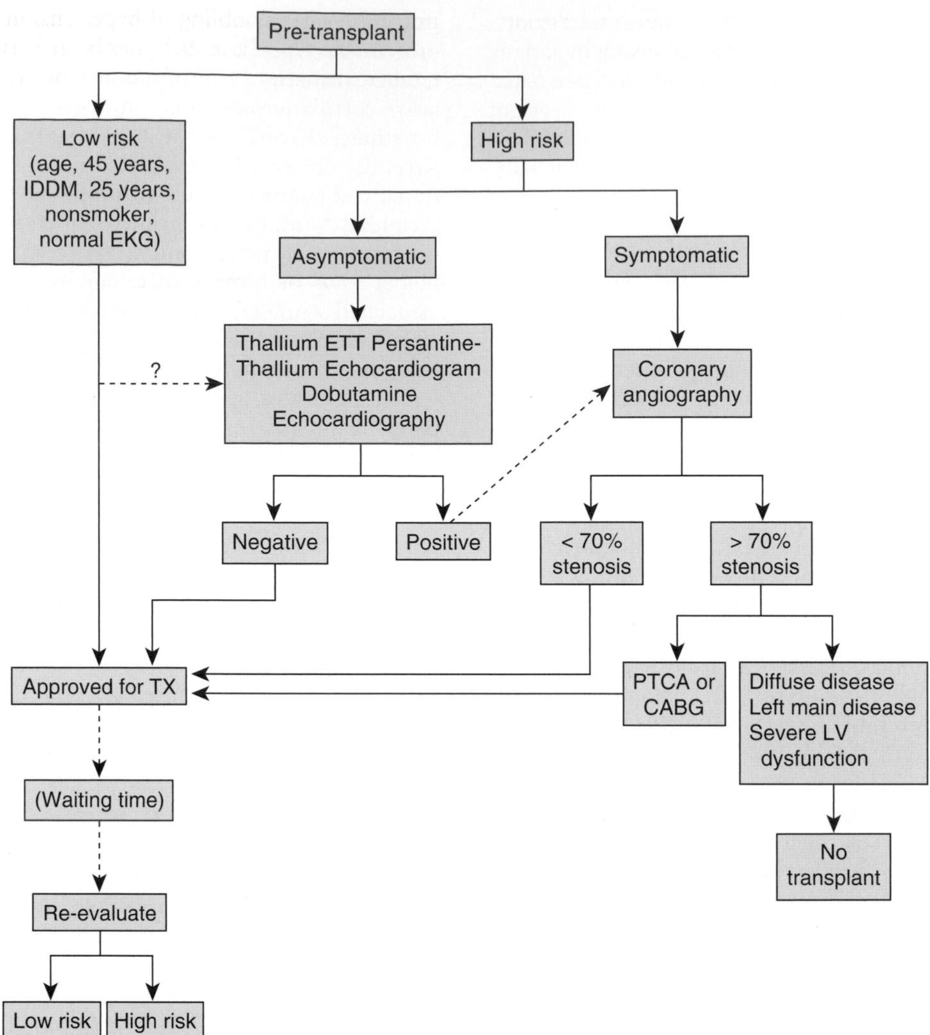

Figure 10–7 Algorithm for screening diabetic transplant candidates for coronary artery disease. (*CABG*, coronary artery bypass graft; *EKG*, electrocardiogram; *ETT*, exercise treadmill test; *LV*, left ventricular; *PTCA*, percutaneous transluminal coronary angioplasty; *TX*, transplantation. Data suggest that noninvasive evaluation or coronary angiography are necessary except for some in low-risk category. (Modified from Williams ME: Management of the diabetic transplant recipient. Kidney Int 1995; 48: 1660. Used with permission of Kidney International.)

angioplasty should be performed, although in the absence of stenting, the latter has a high rate of re-stenosis.[467] In a randomized series, a high rate of cardiovascular events was reported in diabetic patients with chronic renal failure and silent coronary disease that was treated medically (i.e., aspirin, calcium channel blockers), as compared with angioplasty or bypass surgery.[468] No similar studies involving lipid-lowering medical management has been done.

Patients with positive screening tests can nonetheless undergo transplantation if appropriate revascularization is performed. Myocardial revascularization surgery using cardiopulmonary bypass can be performed acceptable morbidity and mortality rates in transplant recipients in general.[469,470] Revascularization of advanced disease in symptom-free patients should probably depend on its location and severity. Patients with severe three-vessel disease or left main coronary disease causing severe left ventricular dysfunction may need to be excluded from transplantation. Further emphasis on risk factor management is needed to reduce cardiovascular mortality in the diabetic transplant recipient.[471]

Dyslipidemia

The prevalence of dyslipidemias in patients with chronic kidney disease is high, and only a minority of dialysis patients have normal lipid levels. Dyslipidemias are present in the majority of transplant recipients and are characterized by high total and LDL-cholesterol. Triglycerides are often increased, and, in some, HDL is low. Diabetes contributes synergistically to these unfavorable alterations in lipid profiles.[472] Transplant recipients may also have other nonclassical lioprotein abnormalities. The association of elevated lipid levels and cardiovascular disease or survival of diabetic transplant recipients, however, may be less obvious than in the general population.[473,474] Lipid values are persistently elevated in the first post-transplant year and may decrease partially thereafter.[475] The hyperlipidemic effect of steroids, which varies widely among patients, may result from stimulation of hepatic very low density lipoprotein synthesis, leading to increased plasma triglycerides and an increase in total serum cholesterol. Cyclosporine has also been implicated as a causative factor in some studies, although the effect is not well-understood. There is no evidence that tacrolimus or mycophenolate mofetil worsen lipoprotein metabolism. Hyperlipidemia is a significant side effect of sirolimus treatment, leading to remarkable increases in mean total cholesterol (50%), LDL-cholesterol (50%), and triglyceride levels (95%) in one study.[476] Specific data on diabetic recipients are not available.

No consensus exists on the ideal management of dyslipidemia in transplant recipients,[477] and adequate trials in the diabetic recipient have not been performed.[478] Lipid reduction strategies should include improved glycemic control,[479] appropriate exercise, and a lipid-lowering diet. However, dietary modifications, especially control of total caloric intake, may be safe but are generally unsuccessful.[480] Immunosuppressive options in high-risk patients generally include withdrawing prednisone, replacing cyclosporine, and avoiding use of sirolimus.[481] Concomitant cyclosporine may increase systemic exposure of all HMG-coA reductase inhibitors, but may be used safely in reduced doses.[482] Statins do not induce increased blood levels of cyclosporine. A recent single-center retrospective analysis showing improved survival in recipients treated with statins included 21% diabetics in the statin-treated population and 22% in the untreated population.[483]

Bile acid sequestrants may worsen high triglyceride levels, may cause gastrointestinal side effects in transplant recipients, and may further impair cyclosporine absorption in diabetic recipients. Nicotinic acid can lower low-density lipoprotein and increase high-density lipoprotein levels in transplant recipients, but may worsen insulin resistance and glycemic control. Fish oil supplements, an alternative best suited for high triglyceride levels, have not been tested in diabetic patients.

Peripheral Vascular Disease

In addition to coronary artery disease, diabetes mellitus leads to peripheral vascular disease with increased limb amputations.[484] Although less lethal than coronary disease, occlusive peripheral vascular disease also limits the success of renal transplants,[485] resulting in 20 times the increase in minor and major amputation rates in diabetic recipients. Pre-transplant large vessel disease is three times more common in diabetic recipients,[486] and vascular disease detected before transplantation doubles the risk of new disease afterward.[487] Pre-transplant coronary disease is associated with increased risk of peripheral vascular complications afterward and a sevenfold increase in risk of amputations.[452] Vascular calcification is an independent predictor of mortality in diabetic patients.[488] Smoking has a strong negative effect on amputation rates.[489] Many amputations are performed in younger recipients. Diagnostic studies show that abnormal toe/brachial pressures and pulse value recordings can be used to assess resting hemodynamics and peripheral vascular disease after renal transplantation.[490]

Hypertension

The etiology of post-transplant hypertension in the diabetic recipient is multifactorial.[491] While the prevalence of hypertension varies with the time after transplantation and the immunosuppressive regimen, it is likely that recipient factors such as pre-transplant hypertension and diabetes are contributors.[492] A near doubling of hypertension rates over time, to 80% to 90% of recipients,[493] has been attributed to the use of calcineurin inhibitors. Cyclosporine-treated patients are somewhat more likely to have hypertension (89%) than those receiving tacrolimus (78%).[494] The prevalence of hypertension in diabetes mellitus is about twice that of nondiabetics. Hypertension is present in most diabetics awaiting a transplant[495,496] and persisting post-transplantation. It is possible but not proven that diabetic recipients have more pronounced hypertension as a result of calcineurin inhibitors. The incidence of transplant renal artery stenosis does not appear to be increased.

Hypertension contributes to the high incidence of cardiovascular disease, mortality, and late allograft failure.[491] Even minor elevations of systolic and diastolic pressure may impact on graft survival. However, despite the growing number of diabetic transplant recipients, the impact of post-transplant hypertension has not been studied.

Numerous hypertension guidelines do not directly address the issue of post-transplant hypertension, including in the diabetic recipient.[497] Hypertension treatment goals have not been specified[498] but are based on those for the general population. Recent European practice guidelines mandated goals of less than 125/75 mmHg in proteinuric transplant recipients.[492] Pharmacologic therapy is usually necessary, and most conventional therapies have been demonstrated to be safe and effective in the general transplant population. The most commonly used therapeutic options such as calcium channel blockers and angiotensin converting enzyme inhibitors are equally effective in reducing blood pressure. Proteinuria in the transplant recipient is an indication for ACEI rather than for calcium channel blockers. ACEI slows progression of renal disease in diabetic nephropathy,[12] and retards experimental chronic allograft rejection.[499] Angiotensin receptor blockers are potentially and similarly useful.[500] However, a recent study showing the safety and efficacy in post-transplant patients included only a minority of diabetic recipients.[501] ACEI and ARBs have gained wider acceptance in the diabetic recipient and, when used cautiously, are probably effective[502,503] and may be renoprotective. Hyperkalemia and anemia may complicate their use.[504] Treatment failures of post-transplant hypertension may be common.[505] Twenty-four hour ambulatory blood pressure measurements may become a valuable clinical tool in assessing treatment efficacy. Blood pressure control may be improved when type I patients undergo combined kidney and pancreas transplantation.

Urologic Complications

Arising mainly from technical difficulties during the surgery,[506] urologic complications in general have decreased in renal transplant recipients. They remain almost twice as common in diabetic transplant recipients.[507] Diabetic bladder dysfunction and urinary retention commonly occur. Pre-transplant urologic evaluation, such as voiding cystourethrogram are performed in some centers but are not routinely indicated in the absence of voiding symptoms or urinary tract infections.[508] Two common urologic complications, postoperative urinary leaks and obstruction, have a technical basis not related to diabetes. Urinary fistulas are less common but occur more frequently in diabetic recipients. Urinary retention is managed with bladder retraining, cessation of anticholinergic drugs, and the use of parasympathetic medications. Emphysematous cystitis may be a sequela to neurogenic bladder or bladder outlet obstruction but responds to early diagnosis and treatment.[509] Long-term graft survival is not affected by surgically corrected urologic complications.[510]

Infectious Disease

Infectious complications after kidney transplantation remain a significant cause of morbidity and mortality for the diabetic recipient. Diabetes mellitus has been shown to be a predisposing factor for post-transplant surgical wound infections,[511] bowel perforations, urinary tract infections, including pyelonephritis,[509] and hospitalizations for sepsis.[512] In a large review of data from the USRDS, patients with ESRD renal transplantation resulting from diabetes was associated with a higher risk of sepsis due to gram-negative rods and to urinary tract infections.[512] Diabetic recipients are also prone to opportunistic infections. Persistent colonization or low-grade infection with *Candida* species is relatively common and can lead to emphysematous cystitis and pyelonephritis, papillary necrosis, renal or perinephric abscesses, and *Candida fasciitis*.[513] Colonization should respond to amphotericin bladder irrigation or oral fluconazole. Upper urinary tract infection requires intravenous amphotericin. Aggressive management is necessary to eradicate torulopsis species infection. Diabetes is the most common associated disease for tuberculosis in kidney transplant patients.[514] While mucormycosis is a rare fungal opportunistic infection, it is frequently associated with diabetes,[515] where it causes pulmonary,[516] cutaneous, or disseminated disease. Aggressive treatment with liposomal amphotericin and surgical resection of all infected tissue is required.[517]

Diabetic Retinopathy

As a consequence of the duration of diabetes and the presence of end-stage renal disease, advanced diabetic retinopathy is present in a high proportion of diabetic transplant recipients. Half of recipients are visually impaired, and visual acuity commonly deteriorates in the year preceding transplantation.[518] Whereas the incidence of sight-threatening complications in nondiabetic survivors of renal transplantation is low,[519] preservation of vision in the diabetic may require laser photocoagulation and vitrectomy. Retinopathy can stabilize in the majority of diabetic patients. Posterior subcapsular cataract formation with extended steroid use imposes significant additional impairment of visual acuity[520] and may account for later vision loss in many patients.[521] Ophthalmologic examination should occur every 6 months.

Fractures

Despite improved treatments of bone and mineral metabolism in end-stage renal disease, increased bone fracture rates in diabetic patients after kidney transplantation have been confirmed in recent studies.[522,523] One or more fractures occurred in about 20% of consecutive kidney recipients over about 4 decades in a cross-sectional study at a single center, with a mean follow-up of 6.5 years.[524] Kidney failure due to diabetes doubled the risk of fractures. The risk for foot or ankle fractures is increased almost fourfold in patients with type I diabetes. Diabetic patients have increased risk of hospitalization because of fractures and decreased survival.[525] In the nontransplant population without renal disease, some studies have suggested an increased risk for fractures with diabetes[526] related to peripheral neuropathy, propensity to falling episodes, and bone fragility, attributed to low bone mass and decreased bone turnover and cortical osteopenia.[527] Evidence has suggested that fewer fractures and increased bone density occur in type II diabetic patients, but osteopenia places type I patients at risk for fractures. Further risk factors for bone osteopenia in pre-transplant renal failure have been widely studied and include secondary hyperparathyroidism, metabolic acidosis, and risk of low turnover bone disease. When measured by dual-photon absorptiometry, bone density is lower in dialyzed diabetic patients than in nondiabetic patients.[528] Low bone turnover (aplastic) states,[529] associated with about half of cases in one study from a decade ago[530] with increased aluminum accumulation on bone surfaces, have emerged as the most common disorder in diabetic patients with end-stage renal disease.[531] Risk of later fractures is correlated with the duration of kidney failure pre-transplant.[524] The major factor implicated in accelerated bone loss following kidney transplantation is use of glucocorticoids, which reduce intestinal calcium absorption, increase resorption of bone, increase renal calcium excretion, enhance sensitivity to parathyroid hormone, and suppress gonadal hormones.[532] Post-transplant bone loss is predominantly the result of steroid-induced decrease in bone formation. Cyclosporine produces increased bone turnover and severe osteopenia in rats,[533] but its specific effects on bone in humans, particularly when used with steroids, is unresolved.[534] Transplantation in the cyclosporine era, which has been accompanied by lower steroid doses, has increased the risk of foot and ankle fractures.[524]

Because of the high fracture risk, diabetic transplant recipients are suitable for fracture prevention. Few randomized controlled trials have examined preventative states to reduce fractures among kidney transplant recipients in general. High levels of bone loss in the initial 6 months are associated with higher steroid doses. Diminished bone mass in diabetic recipients should be managed by steroid reduction, calcium (1–1.5 g/day), vitamin D supplementation, and exercises to prevent disuse osteodystrophy. In postmenopausal women, estrogen therapy is indicated. Calcitonin attenuates cyclosporine-induced bone loss.[535] Bisphosphonates have been shown, in prospective, randomized, controlled trials to delay post-transplant bone loss,[536-538] but have not been evaluated in diabetic recipients.

Post-Transplant Diabetes Mellitus

As transplant management has increasingly emphasized control of post-transplant complications, post-transplant diabetes mellitus (PTDM) has received additional attention recently as a relatively common and potentially preventable cause of adverse transplant outcomes and cost of care. Also termed new onset diabetes mellitus (NODM), it has recently been recognized as an independent predictor of graft failure and mortality that may impact on immunosuppressive drug selection.

Unlike diabetes mellitus itself, the definition of PTDM has not reached a consensus. Criteria vary from the accepted definition of diabetes (fasting plasma glucose 126 mg/dL, to 2-hr post-prandial 200 mg/dL in a standard oral glucose tolerance test, to consistent blood glucose levels over 140 mg/dL, to hyperglycemia with clinical symptoms of diabetes, to the requirement for insulin) in patients with no previous diagnosis of diabetes. The rates of detection vary with the definition of the condition used. The incidence is affected by the diabetogenic effects of prednisone, cyclosporine, and tacrolimus. While far less than some historical data show an incidence of up to 46% in patients treated with corticosteroids and azothiaprine,[539] more recent data indicate an incidence on cyclosporine/steroid and tacrolimus/steroid regimens of up to 20%, but more typically 5% to 10%. Concern about an increased risk associated with the use of tacrolimus (even with decreased steroid use) has been confirmed in some but not all studies ranging from 10% to 20%. Most cases occur within the first few months post-transplantation, but a recent large survey of Medicare beneficiaries who received their first kidney transplant between 1996 and 2000 revealed an incidence that increased from 16% to 24% in the interval from 12 to 36 months post-transplant (Figure 10–8).[540]

Although risk factors associated with PTDM among surveys do vary, consistent risk factors unrelated to immunosuppression include age, body mass index, African-American and Hispanic ethnicities, family history of diabetes, and hepatitis C.[540] Most studies have not shown a relationship to the cause of ESRD. Corticosteroids provoke glucose intolerance and diabetes by increasing insulin resistance and may also attenuate insulin secretion from the pancreatic β-cells.[541] The mechanisms for the diabetogenic effect of cyclosporine and tacrolimus are less defined but may involve the same combination of worsening insulin resistance and impaired insulin release. While PTDM might be expected to carry the same prognosis as diabetes itself, recent data have confirmed the risk of graft failure (1.63%), death-censored graft failure (1.46%), and mortality associated with it.[540] Despite the association between PTDM and tacrolimus, the drug was actually associated with improved graft survival in the same study. Management guidelines have recently been published[542] and focus attention on closer monitoring, more intensive glycemic control, including use of insulin, and individualization of the immunosuppressive regimen in patients difficult to control, including cessation of steroids in some cases, and conversion from tacrolimus to cyclosporine.[543] No controlled studies are available. Added Medicare costs are $21,500 per newly diabetic patient following renal transplantation.[544]

Recurrent/De Novo Diabetic Nephropathy

Diabetes mellitus remains the most common cause of end-stage renal disease in transplanted patients and may even be underdiagnosed in patients on the renal transplant waiting list.[545] Small series and large registries of transplanted patients indicate that 5% to 10% of allografts are affected by recurrent disease,[546] on average 36 months post-transplantation, that the half-life of allografts with recurrence is diminished, and rate of graft loss variably increased, ranging from a few up to over 50%.[547,548] Recurrence of diabetic nephropathy is an important problem in kidney recipients. Several series have indicated that recurrent diabetic histologic changes of mesangial expansion, glomerular basement membrane thickening, and arteriolar lesions can be found in nearly all transplanted diabetic patients after a few years.[549-551] Nodular glomerulosclerosis is less common and may occur in fewer than 20% of diabetic recipients even as late as 13 years after the procedure.[552,553] However, it remains difficult to accurately determine the incidence of recurrent diabetic nephropathy. Data are generally limited to allograft biopsy series done for clinical indications. Particularly in diabetic patients, renal biopsies to confirm their primary diagnosis are infrequently done. Histologic features may be mixed with those of rejection or drug nephrotoxicity. Some cases may be due to de novo rather than recurrent diabetic nephropathy.

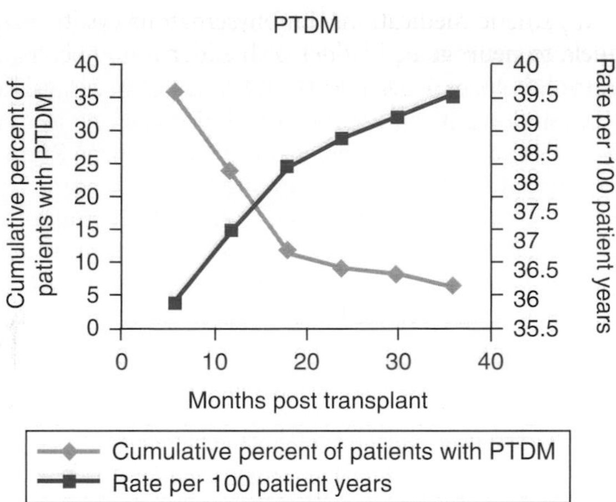

Figure 10–8 Incidence of new onset, post-transplant diabetes mellitus *(PTDM)* after kidney transplantation in adults. Incidence estimated from Cox proportional hazards model; adjusted for multiple covariates. (From U.S. Renal Data System: USRDS 2003 Annual Data Report: Atlas of End-Stage Renal Disease in the United States. Bethesda, MD, National Institutes of Health, National Institute of Diabetes and Digestive and Kidney Diseases, 2003.)

Clinical diagnosis of recurrent disease may develop sooner than previously reported but appears to still occur later than other diseases, between 42 and 118 months in a recent series.[554] As in nondiabetic recipients, the half-life of renal allografts with recurrent disease is diminished compared to those without recurrent disease, and allograft survival is reduced. However, the time course to recurrent diabetic renal failure is slow, with fewer than 10% of recipients with recurrence having graft loss after 13 years in one study.[555] Overall, graft loss attributed to recurrent disease in the UNOS registry data was 2%.[556] Additional combined registry data from two transplant centers indicated that 50% of patients with recurrent diabetic nephropathy lost their allografts.[557] With an increasing incidence of post-transplant diabetes mellitus, de novo diabetic transplant nephropathy is now being recognized. A recent study reported that de novo disease was as prevalent as recurrent diabetic nephropathy and had a similar time of occurrence.[558]

Clinical risk factors that predict de novo or recurrent allograft diabetic nephropathy remain uncertain. Known risk factors do not appear to distinguish those with recurrence from those without, except for a loose relation to glycemic control in some studies.[559] The role of angiotensin converting enzyme inhibitor/receptor blocker therapy in preventing histologic or clinical recurrence or de novo disease has not been evaluated. Progression of recurrent early diabetic lesions can be delayed by successful pancreas-after-kidney transplantation.[560] Recurrent diabetic nephropathy can be prevented after combined pancreas and kidney transplantation.[561] Long-term randomized studies will be required to further assess the impact of recurrent and de novo diabetic nephropathy and available treatments on allograft and patient survival.

SURVIVAL

The survival benefit of kidney transplant recipients varies with the original cause of ESRD. The increased number of prevalent diabetic transplant recipients (including high risk patients) in the United States reflects prevention of early graft loss[562] and improvement in short-term outcomes.[563] Although recent survival studies have analyzed outcomes in cadaveric or living donor kidney transplants versus kidney-pancreas recipients, data continue to confirm the survival advantage of kidney transplantation over dialysis for diabetic patients,[564] even those who qualify for a transplant.[565] Diabetic recipients have shared in the good outcomes of kidney tranplantation during the past two decades but have also benefited from better perioperative management, a reduction in steroid immunosuppression, and improved cardiovascular screening. Annual death rates for diabetic recipients of cadaveric transplants were half those for diabetics on the waiting list, and about one fourth those for all diabetic patients on dialysis in the United States in one study.[418] Long-term survival of diabetic transplant recipients exceeds that of diabetic patients on chronic dialysis,[566] even when selection bias is eliminated. The 30-day mortality rates are only slightly higher in diabetic than in other recipients.[567] Standard analysis shows patient survival curves that approximate those for nondiabetic patients (Figure 10–9). However, death rates post-transplantation are consistently highest among recipients with diabetic kidney disease, who have the poorest 5-year patient survival following transplantation from deceased donors (68% vs. 80% overall) or living donors (81% vs. 90% overall).[568] Annual death rates for diabetic recipients remain one and one-half times the overall death rates and have not significantly improved over the past 8 years.[569] Diabetes is an important determinant of death with a functioning transplant.

Although the increased number of diabetic transplant recipients (including high-risk patients) in the United States reflects improvements in short-term success rates as a result of prevention of early graft loss, diabetic ESRD patients are also more likely to receive a repeat transplant than those with other ESRD diagnoses.[570] For those type I diabetics wait-listed and previously transplanted, the survival advantage occurs earlier and is twice as great as for nondiabetic ESRD patients. Type II patients are less likely to be relisted.

Graft survival rates are shown in Figure 10–10. When graft loss due to recipient death is censored out, long-term graft survival in the diabetic recipient approaches that in nondiabetic patients. The leading overall causes of graft loss are allograft rejection and cardiovascular death. For example, late (5-year) graft loss is due to death in two thirds of diabetic recipients, twice the number in nondiabetics.[571] For older type II diabetic ESRD patients, the prognosis is worse whether renal replacement is dialysis or transplantation, although elderly patients who lack vascular complications may benefit from transplantation.[572] Risk factors for graft survival for deceased donors and living donor transplants are shown in Table 10–6.

REHABILITATION

A consequence of ESRD for the diabetic patients is deterioration of their psychologic and physical status. Many ESRD patients describe their physical condition prior to transplantation as poor[573] and lack abilities for even self-care at home. Rehabilitation of the dialyzed diabetic patient is marginally successful because of severe vision loss, limb amputation, stroke, and cardiac disability. For the diabetic transplant recipient, the goal of transplantation is improvement in well-being rather than cure of the underlying condition. Compared with dialysis, recipients of successful transplants are better rehabilitated, although diabetic recipients remain more impaired than nondiabetic recipients.[574] This is partly because of the inferior pre-transplantation health status of patients with diabetes. Most diabetic recipients experience a benefit in their general health[575] and may be spontaneously more active post-transplantation, but only one third are able to work.[576] Nondiabetic kidney transplant recipients are

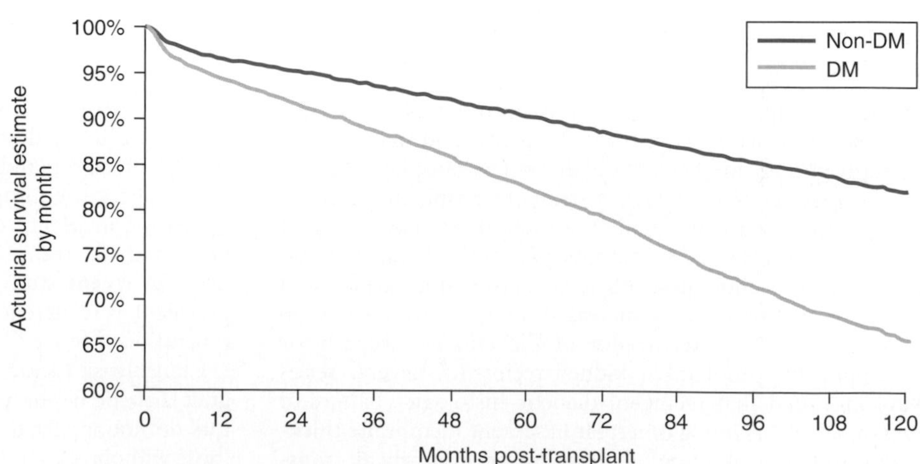

Figure 10–9 Actuarial patient survival estimate by month for 116,811 recipients of first kidney transplants between 1990 and 2001, followed until 12/31/2001 for a death event. Diabetes mellitus vs. nondiabetic primary cause of renal failure. (From U.S. Renal Data System: USRDS 2003 Annual Data Report: Atlas of End-Stage Renal Disease in the United States. Bethesda, MD, National Institutes of Health, National Institute of Diabetes and Digestive and Kidney Diseases, 2003.)

twice as likely as diabetics to return to full-time work. Vocational rehabilitation facilitates employment and plays an important role in determining quality of life.[577] Although nondiabetic transplant patients commonly report physical and psychologic quality of life status as similar to healthy controls,[578] the perceived health status is lower among diabetic recipients.[579] Exercise training may improve levels of physical functioning, such as muscle strength and exercise capacity.[580] When compared with patients continued on dialysis, the improvement in health status provided by a successful transplant for the diabetic recipient may actually exceed that of nondiabetic recipients.

SOCIOECONOMICS

Management of ESRD patients costs the Medicare system billions of dollars annually, and ESRD payment costs are growing more rapidly than general Medicare expenditures. ESRD accounts for an increasing percentage of Medicare programs, mostly due to the growing population of patients.[9] Direct expenditures for health care in diabetic patients are also billions of dollars in the United States. In diabetics, management of chronic complications accounts for one third of expenditures, and the annual management costs are about two times those for people without diabetes.[581] Management costs increase as diabetes complications progress. Dialysis increases the cost of diabetes care 11-fold.[582] Patients with diabetes continue to consume the greatest amount of ESRD resources and have the most pronounced growth in health services to Medicare.[9] Current data for the USRDS indicate that although the cost of transplantation in diabetic patients still exceeds that in nondiabetic patients, it is still the least expensive treatment of ESRD, when compared with dialysis[3] and costs fewer dollars per life-year saved.[583] Annualized dialysis costs, which are relatively stable over time, average 19% higher for diabetic patients than for the entire dialysis population.[584] The economic costs of transplantation to diabetic recipients is initially a little increased over that for nondiabetic patients, but annualized average costs rise to between one third and two thirds higher, largely because of increased hospitalization rates.[3] The Medicare costs of transplantation for diabetics compared to nondiabetics are particularly increased for recipients over age 65. Hospitalization constitutes a significant portion of resource utilization by kidney transplant recipients,[585] and in-patient transplant-related expenditures are 25% higher for diabetic recipients. However, overall annual cost savings, when compared with dialysis, were greater for diabetic than for nondiabetic patients by more than $1300, in one study.[586] The cost benefits of re-transplantation are not as significant.[587]

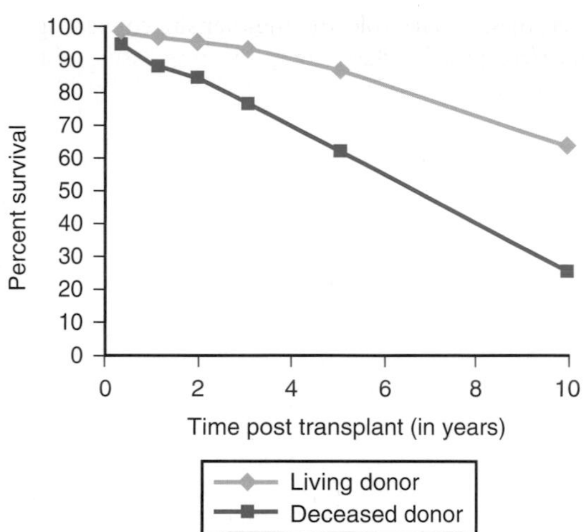

Figure 10–10 1994–2000 combined adjusted (Cox proportional hazards) deceased donor and living donor graft survival (months) for patients with ESRD due to diabetes. Probabilities are adjusted for age and race. (From U.S. Renal Data System: USRDS 2002 Annual Data Report: Atlas of End-Stage Renal Disease in the United States. Bethesda, MD, National Institutes of Health, National Institutes of Diabetes and Digestive and Kidney Diseases, 2002.)

Table 10–6 Risk Factors for Graft Survival for Deceased Donor Transplants and Living Donor Transplants

Primary Cause of ESRD	Percent of Patients	Hazard Ratio for All-Cause Graft Failure	Hazard Ratio for Death-Censored Graft Failure	Hazard Ratio for Death with Functioning Graft
Deceased donor transplants				
Diabetes	22.1	1.26	0.90	2.02
Hypertension	19.6	1.13	1.05	1.35
Glomerulitis	23.3	1.00	1.00	1.00
Cystic kidney disease	9.2	0.78	0.80	0.82
Other	25.8	1.01	0.87	1.36
Graft survival				
Diabetes	20.2	1.15	0.73	2.37
Hypertension	12.3	1.08	0.99	1.49
Glomerulitis	28.0	1.00	1.00	1.00
Cystic kidney disease	7.5	0.74	0.61	1.16
Other	34.1	0.88	0.74	1.40

Cox proportional hazards models modeling all-cause graft failure, death-censored graft failure, and death, 1995-2001 combined. Reference risk of 1.00 arbitrarily assigned to one category for each characteristic. (From U.S. Renal Data System: USRDS 2003 Annual Data Report: Atlas of End-Stage Renal Disease in the United States. Bethesda, MD, National Institutes of Health, National Institute of Diabetes and Digestive and Kidney Diseases, 2003.)

References

1. Mokdad AH, Ford ES, Bowman B, et al: Prevalence of obesity, diabetes, and obesity-related health risk factors, 2001. JAMA 2003; 289:76–79.
2. Narayan KMV, Boyle JP, Thompson TJ, et al: Lifetime risk for diabetes mellitus in the United States. JAMA 2003; 290: 1884–1890.
3. National Institute of Diabetes and Digestive and Kidney Diseases. National Diabetes Statistics fact sheet: General information and national estimates on diabetes in the United States, 2000. Bethesda, MD, U.S. Department of Health and Human Services, National Institutes of Health, 2002.
4. Rosenbloom AL, Joe JR, Young RS, et al: Emerging epidemic of type II diabetes in youth. Diabetes Care 1999; 22:345–354.
5. Harris MI: Medical care for patients with diabetes: Epidemiologic aspects. Ann Intern Med 1996; 124:117–122.
6. Currie CJ, Williams DR, Peters JR: Patterns of in and outpatient activity for diabetes: A district survey. Diabetes Med 1996; 13:273–280.
7. Aubert RE, Geiss LS, Ballard DJ, et al: Diabetes-related hospitalization and hospital utilization. *In* Harris MI, Cowie CC, Stern MP, et al (eds): Diabetes in America, 2nd ed. Bethesda, MD, National Institutes of Health, NIH Publ. No. 95–1468, 1995, p 571.
8. Breyer JA: Therapeutic intervention for nephropathy in type I diabetes mellitus. Semin Nephrol 1997; 17:114–123.
9. U.S. Renal Data System: USRDS 2003 annual data report. Bethesda, MD, National Institutes of Health, National Institute of Diabetes and Digestive and Kidney Diseases, April 2003.
10. U.S. Renal Data System: USRDS 2002 annual data report. Bethesda, MD, National Institutes of Health, National Institute of Diabetes and Digestive and Kidney Diseases, April 2002.
11. Diabetes Control and Complications Trial Research Group: The effects of intensive treatment of diabetes on the development and progression of long-term complications of insulin-dependent diabetes mellitus. N Engl J Med 1993; 329:977–986.
12. Lewis EJ, Hunsicker LG, Bain RP, et al: The effect of angiotensin-converting-enzyme inhibition on diabetic nephropathy. N Engl J Med 1993; 329:1456–1462.
13. Brenner BM, Cooper ME, de Zeeuw D, et al: Effects of losartan on renal and cardiovascular outcomes in patients with type II diabetes and nephropathy. N Engl J Med 2001; 345:861–869.
14. Adler AI, Stratton IM, Neil HA, et al: Association of systolic blood pressure with macrovascular and microvascular complications of type II diabetes (UKPDS): Prospective observational study. BMJ 2000; 321:412–419.
15. Molitch ME: The relationship between glucose control and the development of diabetic nephropathy in type I diabetes. Semin Nephrol 1997; 17:101–113.
16. Krolewski M, Eggers PW, Warram JH: Magnitude of end-stage renal disease in IDDM: A 35 year follow-up study. Kidney Int 1996; 50:2041–2046.
17. Position statement: Diabetic nephropathy. Diabetes Care 2003; 26:S94–S98.
18. U.S. Renal Data System: USRDS 1996 annual data report. Bethesda, MD, National Institutes of Health, National Institute of Diabetes and Digestive and Kidney Diseases, April 1996.
19. Benhamou PY, Marwah T, Balducci F, et al: Classification of diabetes in patients with end-stage renal disease. Clin Nephrol 1992; 38:239–244.
20. Friedman EA: Renal syndromes in diabetes. Endocrinol Metab Clin North Am 1996; 25:293–324.
21. Owen WF: Racial differences in incidence, outcome, and quality of life for African Americans on hemodialysis. Blood Purif 1996; 14:278–285.
22. Position statement: Standards of medical care for patients with diabetes mellitus. Diabetes Care 2003; 26:S33–S50.
23. Arauz-Pacheco C, Raskin P: Hypertension in diabetes mellitus. Endocrinol Metab Clin North Am 1996; 25:401–423.
24. Hakim RM, Lazarus JM: Initiation of dialysis. J Am Soc Nephrol 1995; 6:1319–1328.
25. Tattersall J, Greenwood R, Farrington K: Urea kinetics and when to commence dialysis. Am J Nephrol 1995; 15:283–289.
26. Feldman HI, Held PJ, Hutchinson JT, et al: Hemodialysis vascular access morbidity in the United States. Kidney Int 1993; 43:1091–1096.
27. U.S. Renal Data System: USRDS 1995 annual data report. Bethesda, MD, National Institutes of Health, National Institute of Diabetes and Digestive and Kidney Diseases, April 1995.
28. Windus DW, Jendrisak MD, Delmez JA: Prosthetic fistula survival and complications in hemodialysis patients: Effects of diabetes and age. Am J Kidney Dis 1992; 19:448–452.
29. Windus DW: The effect of comorbid conditions on hemodialysis patency. Adv Ren Replace Ther 1994; 1:148–154.
30. U.S. Renal Data System: USRDS 1997 annual data report. Bethesda, MD, National Institutes of Health, National Institute of Diabetes and Digestive and Kidney Diseases, April 1997.
31. Kaufman JL: The decline of the autogenous hemodialysis access site. Semin Dial 1995; 8:59–66.
32. Ravani P, Marcelli D, Malberti F: Vascular access surgery managed by renal physicians: The choice of native arteriovenous fistulas for hemodialysis. Am J Kidney Dis 2002; 40:1264–1276.
33. Rocco MV, Bleyer AJ, Burkart JM: Utilization of inpatient and outpatient resources for management of hemodialysis access complications. Am J Kidney Dis 1996; 28:250–256.
34. Bruns SD, Jennings WC: Proximal radial artery as inflow site for native arteriovenous fistula. J Am Col Surgeons 2003; 197:58–63.
35. Dalman RL, Harris EJ, Victor BJ, et al: Transition to all autogenous hemodialysis access: The role of preoperative vein mapping. Ann Vasc Surg 2002; 16:624–630.
36. Bender MHM, Bruyninckx CMA, Gerlog PGG: The brachiocephalic elbow fistula: A useful alternative angioaccess for permanent hemodialysis. J Vasc Surg 1994; 20:808–813.
37. Shaffer D, Madras PN, Williams ME, et al: Use of Dacron cuffed silicone catheters as long-term hemodialysis access. ASAIO J 1992; 38:55–58.
38. Little MA, O'Riordan A, Lucey B, et al: A prospective study of complications associated with cuffed, tunneled hemodialysis catheters. Nephrol Dial Transplant 2001; 16:2194–2200.
39. Breen JD, Karchmer AW: *Staphylococcal aureus* infections in diabetic patients. Infect Dis Clin North Am 1995; 9:11–24.
40. Gold HS, Karchmer AW: Catheter-associated *Staphylococcus aureus* bacteremia. Hosp Practice September 15, 1996, p 133–137.
41. Stevenson KB, Adcox MJ, Mallea MC, et al: Standardized surveillance of hemodialysis vascular access infections: 18-month experience at an outpatient, multifacility hemodialysis center. Infect Control Hosp Epidem 2000; 21:200–203.
42. Shaffer D: Catheter-related sepsis complicating long-term, tunneled central venous dialysis catheters: Management by guidewire exchange. Am J Kidney Dis 1995; 25:593–596.
43. Saad TF: Bacteremia associated with tunneled, cuffed hemodialysis catheters. Am J Kidney Dis 1999; 34:1114–1124.
44. Uldall R, Besley ME, Thomas A, et al: Maintaining the patency of double-lumen silastic jugular catheters for haemodialysis. Int J Artif Organs 1993;16:37–40.
45. Hilleman DE, Dunlay RW, Packard KA: Reteplase for dysfunctional hemodialysis catheter clearance. Pharmacother 2003; 23:137–141.
46. Daeihagh P, Jordan J, Chen R, et al: Efficacy of tissue plasminogen activator administration on patency of hemodialysis access catheters. Am J Kidney Dis 2000; 36:75–79.
47. Angle JF, Shilling AT, Schenk WG, et al: Utility of percutaneous intervention in the management of tunneled hemodialysis catheters. Cardiovasc Intervent Radiol 2003; 26:9–18.

48. Hirth RA, Turenne MN, Woods JD, et al: Predictors of type of vascular access in hemodialysis patients. JAMA 1996; 276: 1303–1308.
49. Turenne MN, Strawderman RL, Woods JD, et al: Vascular access survival in hemodialysis patients. Kidney Int 1996; 48:504.
50. Woods JD, Turenne MN, Strawderman RL, et al: Vascular access survival among incident hemodialysis patients in the United States. Am J Kidney Dis 1997; 30:50–57.
51. Goldwasser P, Ayram MM, Collier JT, et al: Correlates of vascular access occlusion in hemodialysis. Am J Kidney Dis 1994; 24:785–794.
52. Sukatme VP: Vascular access stenosis: Prospects for prevention and therapy. Kidney Int 1996; 49:1161–1174.
53. Taber TE, Maikranz PS, Haag BW, et al: Maintenance of adequate hemodialysis access. ASAIO J 1995; 41:842–846.
54. Davies MG, Hagen PO: The vascular endothelium: A new horizon. Ann Surg 1993; 218:593–609.
55. Swedberg SH, Brown BG, Sigley R, et al: Intimal fibromuscular hyperplasia at the venous anastomosis of PTFE grafts in hemodialysis patients. Circulation 1989; 80:1726–1736.
56. Carrozza JP, Kuntz RE, Fishman RF, et al: Restenosis after arterial injury caused by coronary stenting in patients with diabetes mellitus. Ann Intern Med 1993; 118:344–349.
57. Serruys PW, de Jaegere P, Kiemeneij F, et al: A comparison of balloon-expandable-stent implantation with balloon angioplasty in patients with coronary artery disease. Benestent study group. N Engl J Med 1994; 331:489–495.
58. Fischman DL, Leon MB, Baim DS, et al: A randomized comparison of coronary-stent placement and balloon angioplasty in the treatment of coronary artery disease. Stent restenosis study investigators. N Engl J Med 1994; 331:496–501.
59. Kanterman RY, Vesely TM, Pilgram TK, et al: Dialysis access grafts: Anatomic location of venous stenosis and results of angioplasty. Radiology 1995; 195:135–139.
60. Sousa JE, Costa MA, Abizaid AC, et al: Sustained suppression of neointimal proliferation by sirolimus-eluting stents: One-year angiographic an intravascular ultrasound follow-up. Circ 2001; 104:2007–2011.
61. Redfern AB, Zimmerman NB: Neurologic and ischemic complications of upper extremity vascular access for dialysis. J Hand Surg 1995; 20:199–204.
62. Hye RJ, Wolf YG: Ischemic monomelic neuropathy: An underrecognized complication of hemodialysis access. Ann Vasc Surg 1994; 8:578–582.
63. Taylor SM, Eaves GL, Weatherford DA, et al: Results and complications of arteriovenous access dialysis grafts in the lower extremity: A five-year review. Am Surg 1996; 62:188–191.
64. Ratcliffe PJ, Phillips RE, Oliver DO: Late referral for maintenance dialysis. Br Med J 1984; 288:441–443.
65. Sands JJ, Miranda CL: Increasing AV fistulas for hemodialysis access. Kidney Int 1996; 48:501.
66. National Kidney Foundation–Dialysis Outcome Quality Initiative Work Group: Patient evaluation prior to access placement: Timing of access placement. Am J Kidney Dis 1997; 30(suppl 3):S160.
67. Welch HJ, O'Donnell TF: Role of thrombolytic, antiplatelet, antithrombotic and other drugs in the management of failed arterial grafts. Semin Vasc Surg 1994; 7:201–209.
68. Sreedhara R, Himmelfarb J, Lazarus JM, et al: Anti-platelet therapy in graft thrombosis: Results of a prospective, randomized, double-blind study. Kidney Int 1994; 45:1477–1483.
69. Saran R, Dykstra DM, Wolfe RA, et al: Association between vascular access failure and the use of specific drugs: The Dialysis Outcomes and Practice Patterns Study (DOPPS). Am J Kidney Dis 2002; 40:1255–1263.
70. Chew EY, Klein ML, Murphy RP, et al: Effects of aspirin on vitreous/preretinal hemorrhage in patients with diabetes mellitus. Arch Ophthalmol 1995; 113:52–55.
71. Yudkin JS: Which diabetic patients should be taking aspirin? Br Med J 1995; 311:641–642.
72. Crowther MA, Clase CM, Margetts PJ, et al: Low-intensity warfarin is ineffective for the prevention of PTFE graft failure in patients on hemodialysis: A randomized controlled trial. J Am Soc Nephrol 2002; 13:2331–2337.
73. Schon D, Mishler R: Salvage of occluded autologous arteriovenous fistula. Am J Kidney Dis 2000; 36:804–810.
74. Cooper SG: Pulse-spray thrombolysis of thrombosed hemodialysis grafts with tissue plasminogen activator. Am J Roentgenol 2003; 180:1063–1066.
75. Martino MA, Vogel KM, O'Brien SP, et al: Erythropoietin therapy improves graft patency with no increased incidence of thrombosis or thrombophlebitis. J Am Col Surgeon 1998; 187: 616–619.
76. Schwab SJ, Oliver MJ, Suhocki, et al: Hemodialysis arteriovenous access: Detection of stenosis and response to treatment by vascular access blood flow. Kidney Int 2001; 59:358–362.
77. The Diabetes Control and Complications Trial Research Group: Lifetime benefits and costs of intensive therapy as practiced in the Diabetes Control and Complications Trial. JAMA 1996; 276:1409–1415.
78. Hillman R, Regan J, Rosen H: Effect of intensive treatment of diabetes on the risk of death or renal failure in NIDDM and IDDM. Diabetes Care 1997; 20:258–264.
79. Williams ME: Insulin management of a diabetic patient on hemodialysis. Semin Dialysis 1992; 5:69–77.
80. Gray H, O'Rahilly S: Toward improved glycemic control in diabetes: What's on the horizon? Arch Intern Med 1995; 155:1137–1142.
81. Tzamaloukas AH, Yuan ZY, Murata GH, et al: Clinical association of glycemic control in diabetics on CAPD. Adv Perit Dial 1993; 9:291–294.
82. Ifudu O, Dulin AL, Friedman EA: Interdialytic weight gain correlates with glycosylated hemoglobin in diabetic hemodialysis patients. Am J Kidney Dis 1994; 23:686–691.
83. Montoliu J, Revert L: Lethal hyperkalemia associated with severe hyperglycemia in diabetic patients with renal failure. Am J Kidney Dis 1985; 5:47–48.
84. Esforzado N, Poch E, Cases A, et al: Central pontine myelinolysis secondary to frequent and rapid shifts in plasma glucose in a diabetic haemodialysis patient. Nephrol Dial Transplant 1993; 8:644–646.
85. Al-Kudsi RR, Daugirdas JT, Ing JS, et al: Extreme hyperglycemia in dialysis patients. Clin Nephrol 1982; 17:228–231.
86. Williams ME: What are the clinically important consequences of ESRD-associated endocrine dysfunction? Semin Dial 1997; 10:11–21.
87. Mujais SK, Fadda G: Carbohydrate metabolism in end-stage renal disease. Semin Dial 1989; 2:46–52.
88. Charpentier G, Riveline JP, Varroud-Vial M: Management of drugs affecting blood glucose in diabetic patients with renal failure. Diabet Metabol 2000; 26(S4):73–85.
89. Ruggian JC, Maesaka JK, Fishbane S: Proximal calciphylaxis in four insulin-requiring diabetic hemodialysis patients. Am J Kidney Dis 1996; 28:409–414.
90. Smith WG, Holden M, Benton M, et al: Glycosylated and carbamylated haemoglobin in uremia. Nephrol Dial Transplant 1989; 4:96–100.
91. Joy MS, Cefalu WT, Hogan SL, et al: Long-term glycemic control measurements in diabetic patients receiving hemodialysis. Am J Kidney Dis 2002; 39:297–307.
92. Shoji T, Tabata T, Nishizawa Y, et al: Clinical availability of serum fructosamine measurement in diabetic patients with uremia. Nephron 1989; 51:338–343.
93. Vlassara H: Recent progress on the biologic and clinical significance of advanced glycosylation end products. J Lab Clin Med 1994; 124:19.

94. Vlassara H: Protein glycation in the kidney: Role of diabetes and aging. Kidney Int 1996; 49:1795–1804.
95. Weiss MF, Erhard P, Kader-Attia FA, et al: Mechanisms for the formation of glycoxidation products in end-stage renal disease. Kidney Int 2000; 57:2571–2585.
96. Dolhofer-Bliesener R, Lechner B, Gerbitz KD: Possible significance of advanced glycation end-products in serum in end-stage renal disease and in late complications of diabetes. Eur J Clin Chem Clin Biochem 1996; 34:355–361.
97. Niwa T, Katsuzaki T, Momoi T, et al: Modification of beta 2m with advanced glycation end-products as observed in dialysis-related amyloidosis by 3-DG accumulating in uremic serum. Kidney Int 1996; 49:861–867.
98. Miyata T, Wada Y, Cai Z, et al: Implication of an increased oxidative stress in the formation of advanced glycation end-products in patients with end-stage renal failure. Kidney Int 1997; 51:1170–1181.
99. Korbet SM, Makita Z, Firanek CA: Advanced glycosylation end-products in continuous ambulatory peritoneal dialysis patients. Am J Kidney Dis 1993; 22:588–591.
100. Odetti P, Cosso L, Pronzato MA: Plasma advanced glycosylation end-products in maintenance haemodialysis patients. Nephrol Dial Transplant 1995; 10:2110–2113.
101. Vlassara H: Serum advanced glycosylation end-products: A new class of uremic toxins? Blood Purif 1994; 12:54–59.
102. Floridi A, Antolini F, Galli F, et al: Daily haemodialysis improves indices of protein glycation. Nephrol Dial Transplant 2002; 17:871–878.
103. Uribarri J, Peppa M, Cai W, et al: Restriction of dietary glycotoxins reduces excessive advanced glycation end products in renal failure patients. J Am Soc Nephrol 2003; 14:728–731.
104. Miyata T, van Ypersele de Strihou C, Ueda Y, et al: Angiotensin II receptor antagonists and angiotensin-converting enzyme inhibitors lower in vitro the formation of advanced glycation end products: Biochemical mechanisms. J Am Soc Nephrol 2002; 13:2478–2487.
105. Abdel-Rahman E, Bolton WK: Pimagedine: A novel therapy for diabetic nephropathy. Expert Opin Investigat Drugs 2002; 11:565–574.
106. Nakamura S, Tachikawa T, Tobita K, et al: An inhibitor of advanced glycation end product formation reduces N epsilon-(carboxymethyl) lysine accumulation in glomeruli of diabetic rats. Am J Kidney Dis 2003; 41:S68–S71.
107. Kelly DJ, Gilbert RE, Cox AJ, et al: Aminoguanidine ameliorates overexpression of prosclerotic growth factors and collagen deposition in experimental diabetic nephropathy. J Am Soc Nephrol 2001; 12:2098–2107.
108. Williams ME: New therapies for advanced glycation end product nephrotoxicity: current challenges. Am J Kidney Dis 2003; 41:S42–S47.
109. Rodriguez VO, Arem R, Adrogue HJ: Hypoglycemia in dialysis patients. Semin Dial 1995; 8:95–99.
110. Rosborough DC, VanStone JC: Dialysate glucose. Semin Dial 1993; 6:260–266.
111. Duh E, Feinglos M: Hypoglycemia-induced angina pectoris in a patient with diabetes mellitus. Ann Intern Med 1994; 121: 945–946.
112. Raman M, Nesto RW: Heart disease in diabetes mellitus. Endocrinol Metab Clin North Am 1996; 25:425–438.
113. Nesto R, Zarich S, Jacoby R, et al: Heart disease in diabetes. *In* Kahn C, Weir G (eds): Joslin's Diabetes Mellitus. Philadelphia, Lea & Febiger, 1994.
114. Manske CL: Coronary artery disease in diabetic patients with nephropathy. Am J Hypertens 1993; 6:367S–374S.
115. Krolewski AS, Kosinski EJ, Warram JH, et al: Magnitude and determinants of coronary artery disease in juvenile-onset, insulin-dependent diabetes mellitus. Am J Cardiol 1987; 59:750–755.
116. Miettinen H, Haffner SM, Lehto S, et al: Proteinuria predicts stroke and other atherosclerotic vascular disease events in non-diabetic and non-insulin-dependent diabetic subjects. Stroke 1996; 27:2033–2039.
117. Foley RN, Parfrey PS, Harnett JD, et al: Clinical and echocardiographic disease in patients starting end-stage renal disease therapy. Kidney Int 1995; 47:186–192.
118. Ma KW, Greene EL, Raij L: Cardiovascular risk factors in chronic renal failure and hemodialysis populations. Am J Kidney Dis 1992; 19:505–513.
119. Prichard S: Risk factors for coronary artery disease in patients with renal failure. Am J Med Science 2003; 325:209–213.
120. Laakso M: Glycemic control and the risk for coronary heart disease in patients with non-insulin dependent diabetes mellitus. Ann Intern Med 1996; 124:127–130.
121. DeStefano F, Newman J: Comparison of coronary heart disease mortality risk between black and white people with diabetes. Ethn Dis 1993; 3:145–151.
122. Williams ME: Dam (AGE) in diabetic ESRD: Role of advanced glycosylation. Semin Dial 1996; 9:1–10.
123. Schleicher ED, Wagner E, Nerlich AG: Increased accumulation of the glycoxidation product N(ε)-(carboxymethyl) lysine in human tissues in diabetes and aging. J Clin Invest 1997; 99:457–468.
124. Davi G, Catalano I, Averna M, et al: Thromboxane biosynthesis and platelet function in type II diabetes mellitus. N Engl J Med 1990; 322:1769–1774.
125. Sakurai T, Oka T, Hasegawa H, et al: Comparison of lipids, apoprotein and associated activities between diabetic and nondiabetic end-stage renal disease. Nephron 1992; 61: 409–414.
126. Hirata K, Kikuchi S, Saku K, et al: Apolipoprotein (A) phenotypes and serum lipoprotein (A) levels in maintenance hemodialysis patients with/without diabetes mellitus. Kidney Int 1993; 44:1062–1070.
127. Ritz E, Strump FC, Katz F, et al: Hypertension and cardiovascular risk factors in hemodialyzed diabetic patients. Hypertension 1985; 7(suppl 2):118–124.
128. Collins A, Keshaviah P, Ma J, et al: Elderly dialysis patients have a lower risk of cardiac, infectious, and all deaths with a $Kt/V \geq 1.2$ for nondiabetic and $Kt/V \geq 1.4$ for diabetic patients. ASAIO J 1993; 22:79.
129. Bloembergen WE, Stannard DC, Port FK, et al: Relationship of dose of hemodialysis and cause-specific mortality. Kidney Int 1996; 50:557–565.
130. Avram MA, Blaustein DA: Causes, risks and therapy of hyperlipidemia in chronic dialysis patients. Semin Dial 1997; 10:267–274.
131. Biesenbach G, Zazgornik J: Influence of smoking on the survival rate of diabetic patients requiring hemodialysis. Diabetes Care 1996; 19:625–628.
132. Bertolini S, Bon GB, Campbell LM, et al: Efficacy and safety of atorvastatin compared to pravastatin in patients with hypercholesterolemia. Atherosclerosis 1997; 130:191–197.
133. Rosansky S: Treatment of hypertension in renal failure patients: When do we overtreat? When do we undertreat? Blood Purif 1996; 14:315–320.
134. Chobanian AV, Bakris GI, Black HR, et al: The seventh report of the joint national committee on prevention, detection, evaluation, and treatment of high blood pressure: The JNC 7 report. JAMA 2003; 289:2560–2572.
135. Cannata-Andia JB, Rodriguex-Garcia M: Hyperphosphatemia as a cardiovascular risk factor: How to manage the problem. Nephrol Dial Transplant 2002; 17(supp 11):16–19.
136. Billion S, Tribout B, Cadet E, et al: Hyperhomocysteinemia, folate and vitamin B12 in unsupplemented hemodialysis patients: Effect of oral therapy with folic acid and vitamin B12. Nephrol Dial Transplant 2002; 17:455–461.

137. Massy ZA: Potential strategies to normalize the levels of homocysteine in chronic renal failure patients. Kidney Int 2003; 84:S134–S136.
138. Chiarello PG, Vannucchi MT, Vannucchi H: Hyperhomocysteinemia and oxidative stress during dialysis treatment. Renal Failure 2003; 25:203–213.
139. Rinehart AL, Herzog CA, Collins AJ, et al: A comparison of coronary angioplasty and coronary artery bypass grafting outcomes in chronic dialysis patients. Am J Kidney Dis 1995; 25:281–290.
140. Herzog CA, Ma JZ, Collins AJ: Long-term outcomes of dialysis patients in the United States with coronary revascularization procedures. Kidney Int 1999; 56:324–332.
141. Szczech LA, Reddan DN, Owen WF, et al: Differential survival after coronary revascularization procedures among patients with renal insufficiency. Kidney Int 2001; 60:292–299.
142. Herzog CA, Ma JZ, Collins AJ: Comparative survival of dialysis patients in the United States after coronary angioplasty, coronary artery stenting, and coronary artery bypass surgery and impact of diabetes. Circulation 2002; 106:2207–2211.
143. Azar RR, Prpic R, Ho KK, et al: Impact of end-stage renal disease on clinical and angiographic outcomes after coronary stenting. Am J Cardiol 2000; 86:485–489.
144. Aronson D, Bloomgarden Z, Rayfield EJ: Potential mechanisms promoting restenosis in diabetic patients. J Am Coll Cardiol 1996; 27:528–535.
145. Comparison of coronary bypass surgery with angioplasty in patients with multivessel disease. The bypass angioplasty revascularization investigation (BARI) Investigators. N Engl J Med 1996; 335:217–225.
146. Abizaid A, Costa MA, Centemero M, et al: Clinical and economic impact of diabetes mellitus on percutaneous and surgical treatment of multivessel coronary disease in patients: Insights from the arterial revascularization therapy study (ARTS) trial. Circulation 2001; 104:533–538.
147. Owen CH, Cummings RG, Sell TL, et al: Coronary artery bypass grafting in patients with dialysis-dependent renal failure. Ann Thorac Surg 1994; 58:1729–1733.
148. Fietsam R, Bassett J, Glover JL: Complications of coronary artery surgery in diabetic patients. Am Surg 1991; 57: 551–557.
149. Maher M, Singh HP, Dias JS: Coronary artery bypass surgery in the diabetic patient. Ir J Med Sci 1995; 164:136–138.
150. Johnson WD, Pedraza PM, Kayser KL: Coronary artery surgery in diabetics: 261 Consecutive patients followed four to seven years. Am Heart J 1982; 104:823–827.
151. Batiuk TD, Kurtz SB, Oh JK, et al: Coronary artery bypass operation in dialysis patients. Mayo Clin Proc 1991; 66:45–53.
152. Zamora JL, Burdine JT, Karlberg H, et al: Cardiac surgery in patients with end-stage renal disease. Ann Thorac Surg 1986; 42:113–117.
153. Marshall WG Jr, Rossi NP, Meng RL, et al: Coronary artery bypass grafting in dialysis patients. Ann Thorac Surg 1986; 42(suppl 6):S12–S15.
154. Koyanagi T, Nishida H, Kitamura M, et al: Comparison of clinical outcomes of coronary artery bypass grafting and percutaneous transluminal coronary angioplasty in renal dialysis patients. Ann Thorac Surg 1996; 61:1793–1796.
155. Iliou MC, Fumeron C, Benoit MO, et al: Factors associated with increased serum levels of cardiac troponins T and I in chronic hemodialysis patients: Chronic hemodialysis and new cardiac markers evaluation (CHANCE) study. Nephrol Dial Transplant 2001; 16:1452–1458.
156. Aviles RJ, Askari AT, Lindahl B, et al: Troponin T levels in patients with acute coronary syndromes, with or without renal dysfunction. N Engl J Med 2002; 346:2047–2052.
157. Bali I, Abdu AF, Gloster ES, et al: Penectomy in diabetic patients undergoing maintenance dialysis. Am J Nephrol 1995; 15: 152–156.
158. Ritz E: Hypertension in diabetic nephropathy: Prevention and treatment. Am Heart J 1993; 125:1514–1519.
159. National Kidney Foundation. K/DOQI™ Clinical practice guidelines for chronic kidney disease: Evaluation, classification, and stratification. Am J Kidney Dis 2002; 39:S1–S246.
160. Adler AI, Stratton IM, Neil HA, et al: Association of systolic blood pressure with macrovascular and microvascular complications of type II diabetes (UKPDS 36): A prospective observational study. BMJ 2000; 321:412–419.
161. Zager PG, Nikolic J, Brown RH, et al: "U" curve association of blood pressure and mortality in hemodialysis patients. Kidney Int 1998; 54:561–569.
162. Port FK, Hubert-Shearon TE, Wolfe RA, et al: Predialysis blood pressure and mortality risk in a national sample of maintenance hemodialysis patients. Am J Kidney Dis 1999; 33: 507–517.
163. Rahman M, Dixit A, Donley V, et al: Factors associated with inadequate blood pressure control in hypertensive hemodialysis patients. Am J Kidney Dis 1999; 33:498–506.
164. Bakris GL, Williams M, Dworkin L, et al: Preserving renal function in adults with hypertension and diabetes: A consensus approach. National Kidney Foundation, Hypertension and Diabetes Executive Committees Working Group. Am J Kidney Dis 2000; 36:646–661.
165. Rahman M, Fu P, Sehgal AR, et al: Interdialytic weight gain, compliance with dialysis regimen and age are independent predictors of blood pressure in hemodialysis patients. Am J Kidney Dis 2000; 35:257–265.
166. Fishbane S, Natke E, Maesaka JK: Role of volume overload in dialysis-refractory hypertension. Am J Kidney Dis 1996; 28:257–261.
167. Jaeger JQ, Mehta RL: Assessment of dry weight in hemodialysis: An overview. J Am Soc Nephrol 1999; 10:392–403.
168. Katzarski KS, Charra B, Luik AJ, et al: Fluid state and blood pressure control in patients treated with long and short hemodialysis. Nephrol Dial Transplant 1999; 14:369–375.
169. Fagugli RM, Buoncristiani U, Ciao G, et al: Blood pressure reduction in hypertensive patients on daily hemodialysis. J Am Soc Nephrol 1998; 9:233A.
170. Wu SG, Lin SL, Shiao WY, et al: Comparison of sublingual captopril, nifedipine, and prazosin in hypertensive emergencies during hemodialysis. Nephron 1993; 65:284–287.
171. Braunwald E, Antman EM, Beasley JW, et al: ACC/AHA 2002 guidelines update for the management of patients with unstable angina and non-ST segment elevation myocardial infarction. J AM Coll Cardiol 2002; 40:1366–1374.
172. Caldwell BV: Treating hypertension in the diabetic patient: Therapeutic goals and the role of calcium channel blockers. Clin Ther 1993; 15:618–636.
173. Kestenbaum B, Gillen DL, Sherrard DJ, et al: Calcium channel blocker use and mortality among patients with end-stage renal disease. Kidney Int 2002; 61:2157–2164.
174. Psaty BM, Heckbert SR, Koepsell TD, et al: The risk of myocardial infarction associated with antihypertensive drug therapies. JAMA 1995; 274:620–625.
175. Estacio RO, Jeffers BW, Hiatt WR, et al: The effect of nisoldipine as compared with enalapril on cardiovascular outcomes in patients with non-insulin dependent diabetes and hypertension. N Engl J Med 1998; 338:645–652.
176. Tatti P, Pahor M, Byington RP, et al: Outcome results of the fosinopril versus amlodipine cardiovascular events randomized trial (FACET) in patients with hypertension and NIDDM. Diabetes Care 1998; 21:597–603.
177. DeLeeuw PW, Birkenhager WH: The effects of calcium channel blockers on cardiovascular outcomes: A review of randomized controlled trials. Blood Pressure 2002; 11:71–78.
178. Tuomilehto J, Rastenyte D, Birkenhager WH, et al: Effects of calcium channel blockade in older patients with diabetes and systolic hypertension. N Engl J Med 1999; 340:677–684.

179. Cannella G, Paoletti E, Delfino R, et al: Prolonged therapy with ACE inhibitors induces a regression of left ventricular hypertrophy of dialyzed uremic patients independently from hypotensive effects. Am J Kidney Dis 1997; 30:659–664.
180. Efrati S, Zaidenstein R, Dishy V, et al: ACE inhibitors and survival of hemodialysis patients. Am J Kidney Dis 2002; 40:1023–1029.
181. Heart Outcomes Prevention Study Investigators: Effects of ramipril on cardiovascular and microvascular outcomes in people with diabetes mellitus: Results of the HOPE study and MICRO-HOPE substudy. Lancet 2000; 355:253–259.
182. Toto R, Shultz P, Raij L, et al: Efficacy and tolerability of losartan in hypertensive patients with renal impairment. Hypertension 1998; 31:684–691.
183. Lewis EJ, Hunsicker LG, Clarke WR, et al: Renoprotective effect of the angiotensin-receptor antagonist irbesartan in patients with nephropathy due to type II diabetes. N Engl J Med 2001; 345:851–860.
184. Brenner BM, Cooper ME, deZeeuw D, et al: Effects of losartan on renal and cardiovascular outcomes in patients with type II diabetes and nephropathy. N Engl J Med 2001; 345: 861–869.
185. Lindholm LH, Ibsen H, Dahlof B, et al: Cardiovascular morbidity and mortality in patients with diabetes in the losartan intervention for endpoint reduction in hypertension study (LIFE): A randomized trial against atenolol. Lancet 2002; 359:1004–1010.
186. Giordano M, Matsuda M, Sanders L, et al: Effects of angiotensin-converting enzyme inhibitors, Ca2+ channel antagonists, and alpha-adrenergic blockers on glucose and lipid metabolism in NIDDM patients with hypertension. Diabetes 1995; 44: 665–671.
187. Davis BR, Cutler JA, Furberg CD, et al: Relationship of antihypertensive treatment regimens and change in blood pressures to risk for heart failure in hypertensive patients randomly assigned to doxazosin or chlorthalidone: Further analysis from the antihypertensive and lipid-lowering treatment to prevent heart attack trial. Ann Intern Med 2002; 137:313–320.
188. Gress TW, Nieto FJ, Shahar E, et al: Hypertension and antihypertensive therapy as risk factors for type II diabetes mellitus. Atherosclerosis risk in communities study. N Engl J Med 2000; 342:905–912.
189. Shorr RI, Ray WA, Daugherty JR, et al: Antihypertensives and the risk of serious hypoglycemia in older persons using insulin or sulfonylureas. JAMA 1997; 278:40–43.
190. Bakris GL, Siomos M, Richardson D, et al: ACE inhibition or angiotensin receptor blockade: impact on potassium in renal failure. VAL-K study group. Kidney Int 2000; 58:2084–2092.
191. Ribeiro AB: Abnormalities of systemic blood pressure in diabetes mellitus. Kidney Int 1992; 42:1470–1483.
192. National Kidney Foundation, Dialysis Outcome Quality Initiative Work Group: NKF-K/DOQI™ clinical practice guidelines for the treatment of anemia of chronic renal failure. Am J Kidney Dis 1997; 30(suppl 3):5192–5240.
193. Blowey DL, Balfe JW, Gupta I, et al: Midodrine efficacy and pharmacokinetics in a patient with recurrent intradialytic hypotension. Am J Kidney Dis 1996; 28:132–136.
194. Javitt JC, Aiello LP: Cost-effectiveness of detecting and treating diabetic retinopathy. Ann Intern Med 1996; 124:164–169.
195. Aiello LP, Cavallerano J, Bursell SE: Diabetic eye disease. Endocrinol Metab Clin North Am 1996; 25:271–291.
196. Position statement: Diabetic retinopathy. Diabetes Care 2003; 26:S99–S102.
197. Watanabe Y, Yuzawa Y, Mizumoto D, et al: Long-term follow up study of 268 diabetic patients undergoing haemodialysis, with special attention to visual acuity and heterogeneity. Nephrol Dial Transplant 1993; 8:725–734.
198. Whitley KY, Shapiro FL: Hemodialysis for end-stage diabetic nephropathy. *In* Friedman EA, L'Esperance FA (eds): Diabetic Renal-Retinal Syndrome, 3rd vol. Orlando, Grune & Stratton, 1986, p 349.
199. Gilbert RE, Tsalamandris C, Allen TJ, et al: Early nephropathy predicts vision-threatening retinal disease in patients with type I diabetes mellitus. J Am Soc Nephrol 1998; 9:85–89.
200. Estacio RO, McFarling E, Biggerstaff S, et al: Overt albuminuria predicts diabetic retinopathy in Hispanics with NIDDM. Am J Kidney Dis 1998; 31:947–953.
201. Diaz-Buxo JA, Burgess WP: Visual function in diabetic patients undergoing dialysis: Comparison of peritoneal and hemodialysis. Int J Artif Organs 1984; 7:257–262.
202. Berman DH, Garcia CA: Diabetic retinopathy: A review. Semin Dial 1989; 2:226–230.
203. Early Treatment Diabetic Retinopathy Study Research Group: Early photocoagulation for diabetic retinopathy: ET-DRS report no. 9. Ophthalmology 1991; 98:766–785.
204. UK Prospective Diabetes Study Group: Tight blood pressure control and the risk of macrovascular and microvascular complications in type II diabetes (UKPDS 38). BMJ 1998; 317:703–713.
205. Diabetes Control and Complications Trial Research Group: The effect of intensive treatment of diabetes on the development and progression of long-term complications in insulin-dependent diabetes mellitus. N Engl J Med 1993; 329:977–986.
206. UK Prospective Diabetes Study Group: Intensive blood-glucose control with sulfonylureas or insulin compared with conventional treatment and risk of complications in patients with type II diabetes (UKPDS 33). Lancet 1998; 352:837–853.
207. Gaede P, Vedel P, Larsen N, et al: Multifactorial intervention and cardiovascular disease in patients with type II diabetes. N Engl J Med 2003; 348:383–393.
208. Friedman EA, Brown CD, Berman DH: Erythropoietin in diabetic macular edema and renal insufficiency. Am J Kidney Dis 1995; 26:202–208.
209. Berman DH, Friedman EA: Partial absorption of hard exudates in patients with diabetic end-stage renal disease and severe anemia after treatment with erythropoietin. Retina 1994; 14:1–5.
210. Favard C, Guyot-Angenton C, Assouline M, et al: Full panretinal photocoagulation and early vitrectomy improve prognosis of florid diabetic retinopathy. Ophthalmology 1996; 103:561–574.
211. Berman DH, Friedman EA, Lundin AP: Aggressive ophthalmological management in diabetic end-stage renal disease: A study of 31 consecutively referred patients. Am J Nephrol 1992; 12:344–350.
212. Levin ME: Foot lesions in patients with diabetes mellitus. Endocrinol Metab Clin North Am 1996; 25:447–462.
213. Hill MN, Feldman HI, Hilton SC, et al: Risk of foot complications in long-term diabetic patients with and without ESRD: A preliminary study. ANNA J 1996; 23:381–386.
214. Deery HG Jr, Sangeorzan JA: Saving the diabetic foot with special reference to the patient with chronic renal failure. Infect Dis Clinics N Am 2001; 15:953–981.
215. Shaw JE, Boulton AJ, Gokal R: Management of foot problems in diabetes. Perit Dial Int 1996; 16(suppl 1):S279–S282.
216. Position statement: Preventive foot care in people with diabetes. Diabetes Care 2003; 26:S78–S79.
217. Levin ME: The diabetic foot: A primer for nephrologists. Semin Dial 1991; 4:258–263.
218. Yeager RA, Moneta GL, Edwards JM, et al: Predictors of outcome of forefoot surgery for ulceration and gangrene. Am J Surgery 1998; 175:388–390.
219. Faglia E, Favales F, Aldeghi A, et al: Adjunctive systemic hyperbaric oxygen therapy in treatment of severe prevalently ischemic diabetic foot ulcer. Diabetes Care 1996; 19:1338–1343.
220. Veves A, Falanga V, Armstrong DG, et al: Graftskin, a human skin equivalent, is effective in the management of noninfected neuropathic diabetic foot ulcers: A prospective randomized multicenter clinical trial. Diabetes Care 2001; 24:290–295.

221. Carrington AL, Mandsley SK, Morley M, et al: Psychological status of diabetic people with or without lower limb disability. Diabetes Res Clin Pract 1996; 32:19–25.
222. Vanholder R, VanBiesen W: Incidence of infectious morbidity and mortality in dialysis patients. Blood Purification 2002; 20:477–480.
223. U.S. Renal Data System: USRDS 1991 annual data report. Bethesda, MD, National Institutes of Health, National Institute of Diabetes and Digestive and Kidney Diseases, April 1991.
224. Sarnak MJ, Jaber BL: Mortality caused by sepsis in patients with end-stage renal disease compared with the general population. Kidney Int 2000; 58:1758–1764.
225. Fan PY, Schwab SJ: Vascular access: Concepts for the 1990s. J AM Soc Nephrol 1992; 3:1–11.
226. Pastan S, Soucie JM, McClellan WM: Vascular access and increased risk of death among hemodialysis patients. Kidney Int 2002; 62:620–626.
227. Mohamed M, Habte-Gabr E, Mueller W: Infected arteriovenous hemodialysis graft presenting as left and right infective endocarditis. Am J Nephrol 1995; 15:521–523.
228. Marr KA, Sexton DJ, Conlon PJ, et al: Catheter-related bacteremia and outcome of attempted catheter salvage in patients undergoing hemodialysis. Ann Intern Med 1997; 127:275–280.
229. Yu VL, Goetz A, Wagener M, et al: *Staphylococcus aureus* nasal carriage and infection in patients on hemodialysis: Efficacy of antibiotic prophylaxis. N Engl J Med 1986; 315:91–96.
230. Bommer J, Vergetis W, Hingst V: Elimination of cutaneous and mucosal Staph aureus by mupirocin nasal ointment—a randomized placebo controlled study. Kidney Int 1990; 37:289.
231. Lok CE, Stanley KE, Hux JE, et al: Hemodialysis infection prevention with polysporin ointment. J Am Soc Nephrol 2003; 14:169–179.
232. D'Elia JA, Weinrauch LA, Paine DF, et al: Increased infection rate in diabetic dialysis patients exposed to cocaine. Am J Kidney Dis 1991; 18:349–352.
233. Beathard GA: Management of bacteremia associated with tunneled-cuffed hemodialysis catheters. J Am Soc Nephrol 1999; 10:1045–1049.
234. Goldfarb S, Cox M, Singer I, et al: Acute hyperkalemia induced by hyperglycemia: Hormonal mechanisms. Ann Intern Med 1976; 84:426–432.
235. Williams ME: Hyperkalemia. Crit Care Clin 1991; 7:155–174.
236. Eisenberg B, Murata GH, Tzamaloukas AH, et al: Gastroparesis in diabetics on chronic dialysis: Clinical and laboratory associations and predictive features. Nephron 1995; 70:296–300.
237. Lehmann R, Borovicka J, Kunz P, et al: Evaluation of delayed gastric emptying in diabetic patients with autonomic neuropathy by a new magnetic resonance imaging technique and radio-opaque markers. Diabetes Care 1996; 19:1075–1082.
238. Snape WJ, Battle WM, Schwartz SS, et al: Metaclopramide to treat gastroparesis due to diabetes mellitus: A double-blind, controlled trial. Ann Intern Med 1982; 96:444–446.
239. Kawagishi T, Nishizawa Y, Okuno Y: Effect of cisapride on gastric emptying of indigestible solids and plasma motilin concentration in diabetic autonomic neuropathy. Am J Gastroenterol 1993; 88:933–938.
240. Wysowski DK, Bacsanyl J: Cisapride and fatal arrhythmia. N Engl J Med 1996; 335:290–291.
241. Fraser RJ, Mittal RK: Erythromycin: The mechanism of its prokinetic action in the treatment of gastroparesis. Gastroenterol 1994; 107:1904–1905.
242. McCallum RW, Chen JD, Lin Z, et al: Gastric pacing improves emptying and symptoms in patients with gastroparesis. Gastroenterol 1998; 114:456–461.
243. Valdovinos MA, Camilleri M, Zimmerman BR: Chronic diarrhea in diabetes mellitus: Mechanisms and an approach to diagnosis and treatment. Mayo Clin Proc 1993; 68:691–702.
244. Fedorak RN, Field M, Chang EB: Treatment of diabetic diarrhea with clonidine. Ann Intern Med 1985; 102:197–199.
245. von der Ohe MR: Diarrhoea in patients with diabetes mellitus. Eur J Gastroenterol Hepatol 1995; 7:730–736.
246. Aparicio M, Cano N, Chauveau P, et al: Nutritional status of hemodialysis patients: A French national cooperative study. French Study Group for Nutrition in Dialysis. Nephrol Dial Transplant 1999; 14:1679–1686.
247. Keshaviah PR, Nolph KD, Moore HL, et al: Lean body mass estimation by creatinine kinetics. J Am Soc Nephrol 1994; 4:1475–1485.
248. Chertow GM, Johansen KL, Lew N, et al: Vintage, nutritional status, and survival in hemodialysis patients. Kidney Int 2000; 57:1176–1181.
249. Owen WF, Lew NL, Liu Y, et al: The urea reduction ratio and serum albumen concentrations as predictors of mortality in patients undergoing hemodialysis. N Engl J Med 1993; 329:1001–1006.
250. Kopple JD: National kidney foundation K/DOQI™ clinical practice guidelines for nutrition in chronic renal failure. AM J Kidney Dis 2001; 37:S66–S70.
251. Dialysis Outcomes Quality Initiative Guidelines. Clinical practice guidelines for nutrition in chronic renal failure. I. Adult guidelines. A. Maintenance dialysis. Am J Kidney Dis 2000; 35:S1–S140.
252. Nelson EE, Hong CD, Pesce AL, et al: Anthropometric norms for the dialysis population. Am J Kidney Dis 1990; 16:32–37.
253. Lowrie EG, Lew NL: Death risk in hemodialysis patients: The predictive value of commonly measured variables and an evaluation of death rate differences between facilities. Am J Kidney Dis 1990; 15:458–482.
254. Miller DG, Levine S, Bistrian B, et al: Diagnosis of protein calorie malnutrition in diabetic patients on hemodialysis and peritoneal dialysis. Nephron 1983; 33:127–132.
255. Lowrie EG, Lew NL, Huang WH: Race and diabetes as death risk predictors in hemodialysis patients. Kidney Int 1992; 42(S38):S22–S31.
256. Kopple JD, Chumlea WC, Gassman JJ, et al: The Modification of Diet in Renal Disease study group: Relationship between GFR and nutritional status—results from the MDRD study (Abstract). J Am Soc Nephrol 1994; 5:335.
257. Kaysen GA, Rathore V, Shearer GC, et al: Mechanisms of hypoalbuminemia in hemodialysis patients. Kidney Int 1995; 48:510–516.
258. Bergstrom J: Why are dialysis patients malnourished? Am J Kidney Dis 1995; 26:229–241.
259. Pickering WP, Price SR, Bircher G, et al: Nutrition in CAPD: Serum bicarbonate and the ubiquitin-proteasome system in muscle. Kidney Int 2002; 61:1286–1292.
260. Tayeb JS, Provenzano R, El-Ghoroury M, et al: Effect of biocompatibility of hemodialysis membranes on serum albumen levels. Am J Kidney Dis 2000; 35:606–610.
261. Hakim RM, Wingard RL, Ikizler TA, et al: Effects of biocompatibility on nutritional status in chronic hemodialysis patients. J Am Soc Nephrol 1994; 25:451.
262. Kaplan AA, Halley SE, Lapkin RA, et al: Dialysate protein losses with bleach processed polysulphone dialyzers. Kidney Int 1995; 47:573–578.
263. DeSchoenmakere G, Vanholder R, Rottey S, et al: Relationship between gastric emptying and clinical and biochemical factors in chronic hemodialysis patients. Nephrol Dial Transplant 2001; 16:1850–1855.
264. Ross EA, Koo LC: Improved nutrition after the detection and treatment of occult gastroparesis in nondiabetic dialysis patients. Am J Kidney Dis 1998; 31:62–66.
265. Folsom AR, Ma J, Eckfeldt JH, et al: Low serum albumin: Association with diabetes mellitus and other cardiovascular risk factors. Ann Epidemiol 1995; 5:186–191.

266. End-Stage Renal Disease Core Indicators Project: 1996 Annual Report. Baltimore, Department of Health and Human Services, 1997.
267. Ikizler TA, Wingard RL, Hakim RM: Interventions to treat malnutrition in dialysis patients: The role of the dose of dialysis, intradialytic parenteral nutrition, and growth hormone. Am J Kidney Dis 1995; 26:256–265.
268. Lindsay RM, Spanner E, Heizlenheim RP, et al: Which comes first, Kt/V or PCR—chicken or the egg? Kidney Int 1992; 38:S32–S36.
269. Caglar K, Fedje L, Dimmitt R, et al: Therapeutic effects of oral nutritional supplementation during hemodialysis. Kidney Int 2002; 62:1054–1059.
270. Kopple JD: Therapeutic approaches to malnutrition in chronic dialysis patients: The different modalities of nutritional support. Am J Kidney Dis 1999; 33:180–185.
271. Chertow GM, Ling J, Lew N, et al: The association of intradialytic parenteral nutrition administration with survival in hemodialysis patients. Am J Kidney Dis 1994; 24:912–920.
272. Capelli JP, Kushner H, Camiscioli TC, et al: Effect of intradialytic parenteral nutrition on mortality rates in end-stage renal disease care. Am J Kidney Dis 1994; 23:808–816.
273. Johansen KL, Mulligan K, Schambelan M: Anabolic effects of nandrolone decanoate in patients receiving dialysis: A randomized controlled trial. JAMA 1999; 281:1275–1281.
274. Johannsson G, Bengtsson BA, Ahlmen J: Double-blind, placebo-controlled study of growth hormone treatment in elderly patients undergoing chronic hemodialysis: Anabolic effect and functional improvement. Am J Kidney Dis 1999; 33: 709–717.
275. Eustace JA, Coresh J, Kutchey C, et al: Randomized double-blind trial of oral essential amino acids for dialysis-associated hypoalbuminemia. Kidney Int 2000; 57:2527–2538.
276. Bellinghieri G, Santoro D, Calvani M: Carnitine and hemodialysis. Am J Kidney Dis 2003; 41:S116–S122.
277. Friedman EA: How can care of the diabetic ESRD patients be improved? Semin Dial 1991; 4:13–17.
278. Blau A, Ben-David A, Eliahou HE: High short-term mortality of diabetic patients entering dialysis. Israel J Med Sci 1994; 30:528–530.
279. Cordonnier D, Bayle F, Benhamou PY, et al: Future trends of management of renal failure in diabetics. Kidney Int 1993; 41:S8–S13.
280. U.S. Renal Data System: USRDS 2000 annual data report. Bethesda, MD, National Institutes of Health, National Institute of Diabetes and Digestive and Kidney Diseases, April 2000.
281. Collins AJ, Hanson G, Umen A, et al: Changing risk factor demographics in end-stage renal disease patients entering hemodialysis and the impact of long-term mortality. Am J Kidney Dis 1990; 15:422–432.
282. Medina RA, Pugh JA, Monterrosa A, et al: Minority advantage in diabetic end-stage renal disease survival on hemodialysis: Due to different proportions of diabetic type? Am J Kidney Dis 1996; 28:226–234.
283. Keshaviah PR, Nolph KD, Moore HL, et al: Lean body mass estimation by creatinine kinetics. J Am Soc Nephrol 1994; 4: 1475–1485.
284. Lowrie EG, Lew NL, Huang WH: Race and diabetes as death risk predictors in hemodialysis patients. Kidney Int 1992; 38:S22–S31.
285. Bloembergen WE, Stannard DC, Port FK, et al: Relationship of dose of hemodialysis and cause-specific mortality. Kidney Int 1996; 50:557–565.
286. Cheigh J, Raghavan J, Sullivan J, et al: Is insufficient dialysis a cause for high morbidity in diabetic patients (Abstract). J Am Soc Nephrol 1991; 2:317.
287. Held PJ, Port FK, Wolfe RA, et al: The dose of hemodialysis and patient mortality. Kidney Int 1996; 50:550–556.
288. Collins AJ, Ma JZ, Umen A, et al: Urea index and other predictors of hemodialysis patient survival. Am J Kidney Dis 1994; 23:272–282.
289. Chertow GM, Owen WF, Lazarus JM, et al: Exploring the J-shaped curve between urea reduction ratio and mortality. Kidney Int 1999; 56:1872–1878.
290. Eknoyan G, Beck GJ, Cheung AK, et al: Effect of dialysis dose and membrane flux in maintenance hemodialysis. N Engl J Med 2002; 347:2010–2019.
291. Keshaviah P, Collins AJ, Ma JZ, et al: Survival comparison between hemodialysis and peritoneal dialysis based on matched doses of delivered therapy. J Am Soc Nephrol 2002; 13:S48–S52.
292. Wolfe RA, Port FK, Hawthorne VM, et al: A comparison of survival among dialytic therapies of choice: In-center hemodialysis versus continuous ambulatory peritoneal dialysis at home. Am J Kidney Dis 1990; 15:433–440.
293. Nelson CB, Port FK, Wolfe RA, et al: Comparison of continuous ambulatory peritoneal dialysis and hemodialysis patient survival with evaluation of trends during the 1980s. J Am Soc Nephrol 1992; 3:1147–1155.
294. Johnston JR: Maintaining diabetic patients on long-term peritoneal dialysis. Semin Dial 1995; 8:390–396.
295. Moist LM, Port FK, Orzol SM, et al: Predictors of loss of residual renal function among new dialysis patients. J Am Soc Nephrol 2000; 11:556-564.
296. Jansen MA, Hart AA, Korevaar JC, et al: Predictors of the rate of decline of residual renal function in incident dialysis patients. Kidney Int 2002; 62:1046-1053.
297. Bro S, Bjorner JB, Tofte-Jensen P, et al: A prospective, randomized multicenter study comparing APD and CAPD treatment. Perit Dial Int 1999; 19:526-533.
298. Khanna R: Dialysis considerations for diabetic patients. Kidney Int 1993; 40:S58-S64.
299. Bloembergen WE, Port FK, Mauger EA, et al: A comparison of mortality between patients treated with hemodialysis and peritoneal dialysis. J Am Soc Nephrol 1995; 6:177-183.
300. Passadakis P, Thodis E, Vargemezis, et al: Long-term survival with peritoneal dialysis in ESRD due to diabetes. Clin Nephrol 2001; 56:257-270.
301. Passadakis P, Oreopoulos D: Peritoneal dialysis in diabetic patients. Adv Ren Repl Ther 2001; 8:22-41.
302. Woodrow G, Turney JH, Brownjohn AM: Technique failure in peritoneal dialysis and its impact on patient survival. Periton Dial Int 1997; 17:360-364.
303. Grodstein GP, Blumenkrantz MJ, Kopple JD, et al: Glucose absorption during continuous ambulatory peritoneal dialysis. Kidney Int 1981; 19:564-567.
304. Tzamaloukas AH, Yuan ZY, Murata GH, et al: Clinical associations of glycemic control in diabetics on CAPD. Adv Perit Dial 1993; 9:291-294.
305. Lamb EJ, Worrall J, Buhler R, et al: Effect of diabetes and peritonitis on the peritoneal equilibration test. Kidney Int 1995; 47:1760-1767.
306. Mactier RA, Khanna R: Intraperitoneal insulin in diabetic CAPD patients. Int J Artif Organs 1988; 11:9-12.
307. Wideroe TE, Dahl KJ, Smeby LC, et al: Pharmacokinetics of transperitoneal insulin transport. Nephron 1996; 74:283-290.
308. Quellhorst E: Insulin therapy during peritoneal dialysis: pros and cons of various forms of administration. J Am Soc Nephrol 2002; 13:S92-S96.
309. Khanna R: Peritoneal dialysis in diabetic end-stage renal disease. *In* Gokal R, Nolph KD (eds): The Textbook of Peritoneal Dialysis. Dordrecht, the Netherlands, Kluwer Academic Publishers, 1994, p 639.
310. Nevalainen P, Lahtela JT, Mustonen J, et al: The influence of peritoneal dialysis and the use of subcutaneous and intraperitoneal insulin on glucose metabolism and serum lipids in type I diabetic patients. Nephrol Dial Transplant 1997; 12:145-150.

311. Zimmerman SW, Sollinger H, Wakeen M, et al: Renal replacement therapy in diabetic nephropathy. Adv Ren Replace Ther 1994; 1:66–74.
312. Wolfson M, Piraino B, Hamburger RJ, et al: A randomized controlled trial to evaluate the efficacy and safety of icodextrin in peritoneal dialysis. Am J kidney Dis 2002; 40:1055-1065.
313. Frampton JE, Plosker GL: Icodextrin: A review of its use in peritoneal dialysis. Drugs 2003; 63:2079-2105.
314. Johnson DW, Agar J, Collins J, et al: Recommendations for the use of icodextrin in peritoneal dialysis patients. Nephrol 2003; 8:1-7.
315. Dawnay AB, Millar DJ: Glycation and advanced glycation end-product formation with icodextrin and dextrose. Perit Dial Int 1997; 17:9-10.
316. Posthuma N, ter Wee PM, Niessen H, et al: Amadori albumin and advanced glycation end-product formation in peritoneal dialysis using icodextrin. Perit Dial Int 2001; 21:43-51.
317. De Vriese AS, Flyvbjerg A, Mortier S, et al: Inhibition of the interaction of AGE-RAGE prevents hyperglycemia-induced fibrosis of the peritoneal membrane. J Am Soc Nephrol 2003; 14:2109-2118.
318. Oyibo SO, Pritchard GM, McLay L, et al: Blood glucose overestimation in diabetic patients on continuous ambulatory peritoneal dialysis for end-stage renal disease. Diabet Med 2002; 19:693-696.
319. Riley SG, Chess J, Donovan KL, et al: Spurious hyperglycaemia and icodextrin in peritoneal dialysis fluid. BMJ 2003; 327: 608-609.
320. Boer WH, Vos PF, Fiernen MW: Culture negative peritonitis associated with the use of icodextrin-containing dialysate in twelve patients treated with peritoneal dialysis. Perit Dial Int 2003; 23:33-38.
321. Basile C, De Padova F, Montanaro A, et al: The impact of relapsing sterile icodextrin-associated peritonitis on peritoneal dialysis outcome. J Nephrol 2003; 16:384-386.
322. Valance A, Lebrun-Vignes B, Descamps V, et al: Icodextrin cutaneous hypersensitivity: report of 3 psoriaform cases. Arch Dermatol 2001; 137:309-310.
323. Davies SJ, Woodrow G, Donovan K, et al: Icodextrin improves the fluid status of peritoneal dialysis patients: Results of a double-blind randomized controlled trial. J Am Soc Nephrol 2003; 14:2338-2344.
324. Posthuma N, ter Weel PM, Donker AJ, et al: Icodextrin use in CCPD patients during peritonitis: Ultrafiltration and serum disaccharide concentrations. Nephrol Dial Transplant 1998; 13:2341-2344.
325. Guo A, Wolfson M, Holt R: Early quality of life benefits of icodextrin in peritoneal dialysis. Kidney Int 2002; 62:S72-S79.
326. Tzamaloukas AH, Murata GH, Eisenberg B, et al: Hypoglycemia in diabetics on dialysis with poor glycemic control: Hemodialysis versus continuous ambulatory peritoneal dialysis. Int J Artif Organs 1992; 15:390-392.
327. Oskarsson PR, Lins PE, Backman L, et al: Continuous intraperitoneal insulin infusion partly restores the glucagons responses to hypoglycaemia in type I diabetic patients. Diabetes Metab 2000; 26:118-124.
328. Tzamaloukas AH, Friedman EA: Diabetes. *In* Daugirdas JT, Blake PG, Ing TS (eds): Handbook of Dialysis, 3rd ed. Philadelphia, Lippincott, Williams & Wilkins, 2001, p 453-465.
329. Aujla NS, Pirano B, Sorkin M: An intraperitoneal insulin regimen for diabetics on continuous cyclic peritoneal dialysis. Trans Am Soc Artif Intern Organs 1990; 36:119-121.
330. Voinescu CG, Khanna R: Peritonitis in peritoneal dialysis. Int J Artif Organs 2002; 25:249-260.
331. Grutzmacher P, Tsobanelis T, Bruns M, et al: Decrease in peritonitis rate by integrated disconnect system in patients on continuous ambulatory peritoneal dialtsis. Perit Dial Int 1993; 13:S326-S328.
332. Fried L, Abidi S, Bernardini J, et al: Hospitalization in peritoneal dialysis patients. Am J Kidney Dis 1999; 33:927-933.
333. Keane WF, Alexander SR, Bailie GR: Peritoneal dialysis–related peritonitis treatment recommendations: 1996 update. Perit Dial Int 1996; 16:557-573.
334. Port FK, Held PJ, Nolph KD, et al: Risk of peritonitis and technique failure by CAPD connection technique: A national study. Kidney Int 1992; 42:967-974.
335. Lindblad AS, Novak JW, Nolph KD: The USA Continuous Ambulatory Peritoneal Dialysis Registry: Characteristics of participants and selected outcome measures. *In* Nolph KD (ed): Peritoneal Dialysis. Dordrecht, the Netherlands, Kluwer Academic Publishers, 1989.
336. Traeneus A, Heimburger O, Lindholm B: Peritonitis in CAPD: Diagnostic findings, therapeutic outcome, and complications. Perit Dial Int 1989; 9:179-190.
337. Tzamaloukas AH, Murata GH, Lewis SL: Severity and complications of continuous ambulatory peritoneal dialysis peritonitis in diabetic and nondiabetic patients. Perit Dial Int 1993; 13(suppl 2):S236-S238.
338. Krishnan M, Thodis E, Ikonomopoulos D, et al: Predictors of outcome following bacterial peritonitis in peritoneal dialysis. Perit Dial Int 2002; 22:573-581.
339. Tzamaloukas AH, Yuan ZY, Balaskas E, et al: CAPD in end-stage patients with renal disease due to diabetes mellitus: An update. Adv Perit Dial 1992; 8:185-191.
340. Viglino G, Cancarini GC, Catizone L, et al: Italian Cooperative Peritoneal Dialysis Study Group: Ten years' experience of CAPD in diabetics: Comparison of results with nondiabetics. Nephrol Dial Transplant 1994; 9:1443-1448.
341. Bloembergen WE, Port FK: Epidemiologic perspective on infections in chronic dialysis patients. Adv Ren Replace Ther 1996; 3:201-207.
342. Luzar MA, Coles GA, Faller B, et al: *Staphylococcus aureus* nasal carriage and infection in patients on continuous ambulatory peritoneal dialysis. N Engl J Med 1990; 322:505-509.
343. Kraus ES, Spector DA: Characteristics and sequelae of peritonitis in diabetics and nondiabetics receiving chronic intermittent peritoneal dialysis. Medicine 1983; 62:52-57.
344. Sewell CM, Clarridge J, Lacke C, et al: Staphylococcal nasal carriage and subsequent infection in peritoneal dialysis patients. JAMA 1982; 248:1493-1495.
345. Vychytil A, Lorenz M, Schneider B, et al: New strategies to prevent Staphylococcus aureus infections in peritoneal dialysis patients. J Am Soc Nephrol 1998; 9:669-676.
346. Thodis E, Passadakis P, Vargemezis V, et al: Prevention of catheter related infections in patients on CAPD. Int J Artif Organs 2001; 24:671-682.
347. Ritzau J, Hoffman RM, Tzamaloukas AH: Effect of preventing Staphylococcus aureus carriage on rates of peritoneal catheter-related staphylococcal infections. Perit Dial Int 2001; 21: 471-479.
348. Bernardini J, Piraino B, Holley J, et al: A randomized trial of *Staphylococcus aureus* prophylaxis in peritoneal dialysis patients: Mupirocin calcium ointment 2% applied to the exit site versus cyclic oral rifampin. Am J Kidney Dis 1996; 27: 695-700.
349. Keane WF, Bailie GR, Boeschoten E, et al: Adult peritoneal dialysis-related peritonitis treatment recommendations: 2000 update. Perit Dial Int 2000; 20:396-411.
350. Boyle JF, Soumakis SA, Rendo A, et al: Epidemiologic analysis and genotypic characterization of a nosocomial outbreak of vancomycin-resistent enterococci. J Clin Microbiol 1993; 31:1280-1285.
351. Goldberg L, Clemenger M, Azadial B, et al: Initial treatment of peritoneal dialysis peritonitis without vancomycin with a once-daily cefazolin-based regimen. Am J Kidney Dis 2001; 37:49-55.

352. Shemin D, Maaz D, St Pierre D, et al: Effect of aminoglycoside use on residual renal function in peritoneal dialysis patients. Am J Kidney Dis 1999; 34:14-20.
353. Michel C, Courdavault L, al Khayat R, et al: Fungal peritonitis in patients on peritoneal dialysis. Am J Nephrol 1994; 14: 113-120.
354. Kleinpeter MA, Butt AA: Non Candida albicans fungal peritonitis in continuous ambulatory peritoneal dialysis patients. Adv Perit Dial 2001; 17:176-179.
355. Eisenberg B, Murata GH, Tzamaloukas AH, et al: Gastroparesis in diabetics on chronic dialysis: clinical and laboratory associations and predictive features. Nephron 1995; 70:296-300.
356. Gallar P, Oliet A, Vigil A, et al: Gastroparesis: An important cause of hospitalization in continuous ambulatory peritoneal dialysis patients, and the role of erythromycin. Perit Dial Int 1993; 13(suppl 2):S183-S186.
357. Schoonjans R, Van Vlem B, Vandamme W, et al: Gastric emptying of solids in cirrhotic and peritoneal dialysis patients: Influence of peritoneal volume load. Eur J Gastroenterol Hepatol 2002; 14:395-398.
358. Van V, Schoonjans RS, Struijk DG, et al: Influence of dialysate on gastric emptying time in peritoneal dialysis patients. Perit Dial Int 2002; 22:32-38.
359. Bird NJ, Streather CP, O'Doherty MJ, et al: Gastric emptying in patients with chronic renal failure on continuous ambulatory peritoneal dialysis. Nephrol Dial Transplant 1994; 9:287-290.
360. Ross EA, Koo LC: Improved nutrition after the detection and treatment of occult gastroparesis in nondiabetic dialysis patients. Am J Kidney Dis 1998; 31:62-66.
361. Balaskas EV, Yuan ZY, Gupta A, et al: Long-term continuous ambulatory peritoneal dialysis in diabetics. Clin Nephrol 1994; 42:54-62.
362. Bentley ML: Keep it simple! A touch technique peritoneal dialysis procedure for the blind and visually impaired. CAANT J 2001; 11:32-34.
363. Flanigan MJ, Rocco MV, Prowant B, et al: Clinical performance measures: The changing status of peritoneal dialysis. Kidney Int 2001; 60:2377-2384.
364. Flanigan MJ, Frankenfield DL, Prowant BF, et al: Nutritional markers during peritoneal dialysis: Data from the 1998 Peritoneal Dialysis Core Indicators Study. Perit Dial Int 2001; 21:345-354.
365. Spiegel DM, Anderson M, Campbell U, et al: Serum albumin: A marker for morbidity in peritoneal dialysis patients. Am J Kidney Dis 1993; 21:26-30.
366. Rocco MV, Jordan JR, Burkart JM: The efficacy number as a predictor of morbidity and mortality in peritoneal dialysis patients. J Am Soc Nephrol 1993; 4:1184-1191.
367. Lowrie EG, Huang WH, Lew NL: Death risk predictors among peritoneal dialysis and hemodialysis patients: A preliminary comparison. Am J Kidney Dis 1995; 26:220-228.
368. Mittman N, Avram MN, Oo KK, et al: Serum prealbumin predicts survival in hemodialysis and peritoneal dialysis: 10 years of prospective observation. Am J Kidney Dis 2001; 38: 1358-1364.
369. Wolfson M: Nutritional management of the continuous ambulatory peritoneal dialysis patient. Am J Kidney Dis 1996; 27: 744-749.
370. Young GA, Kopple JD, Lindholm B, et al: Nutritional assessment of continuous ambulatory peritoneal dialysis patients: An international study. Am J Kidney Dis 1991; 17:462-471.
371. Avram MM, Goldwasser P, Erroa M, et al: Predictors of survival in continuous ambulatory peritoneal dialysis patients: The importance of prealbumin and other nutritional and metabolic markers. Am J Kidney Dis 1994; 23:91-98.
372. Dulaney JT, Hatch FE: Peritoneal dialysis and loss of proteins: A review. Kidney Int 1984; 26:253-262.
373. Kopple JD, Blumenkrantz MJ: Nutritional requirements for patients undergoing continuous ambulatory peritoneal dialysis. Kidney Int 1983; 24(suppl 16):S295-S302.
374. Krediet RT, Zuyderhoudt FMJ, Boeschoten EW, et al: Peritoneal permeability to proteins in diabetic and nondiabetic continuous ambulatory peritoneal dialysis patients. Nephron 1986; 42:133-140.
375. Nakamoto H, Imai H, Kawanishi H, et al: Effects of diabetes on peritoneal function assessed by personal dialysis capacity test in patients undergoing CAPD. Am J Kidney Dis 2002; 40: 1045-1054.
376. Jager KJ, Merkus MP, Huisman RM, et al: Nutritional status over time in hemodialysis and peritoneal dialysis. J Am Soc Nephrol 2001; 12:1272-1279.
377. Wang AY, Sea MM, Ip R, et al: Independent effects of residual renal function and dialysis adequacy on actual dietary protein, calorie, and other nutrient intake in patients on continuous ambulatory peritoneal dialysis. J Am Soc Nephrol 2001; 12: 2450-2457.
378. Yeun JY, Kaysen GA: Acute phase proteins and peritoneal dialysate albumin loss are the main determinants of serum albumin in peritoneal dialysis patients. Am J Kidney Dis 1997; 30:923-927.
379. Wolfson M, Jones M: Intraperitoneal nutrition. Am J Kidney Dis 1999; 33:203-204.
380. Jones M, Hagen T, Boyle CA, et al: Treatment of malnutrition with 1% amino acid peritoneal dialysis solution: Results of a multicenter outpatient study. Am J Kidney Dis 1998; 32:761-769.
381. Bruno M, Bagnis C, Marangella M, et al: CAPD with an amino acid dialysis solution: A long-term, cross-over study. Kidney Int 1989; 35:1189-1194.
382. Canepa A, Carrea A, Menoni S, et al: Acute effects of simultaneous intraperitoneal infusion of glucose and amino acids. Kidney Int 2001; 59:1967-1973.
383. Jones MR: Preventing malnutrition in the long-term peritoneal dialysis patient. Semin Dial 1995; 8:347-352.
384. Markell MS, Friedman EA: Care of the diabetic patient with end-stage renal disease. Semin Nephrol 1990; 10:274-286.
385. Lee HB, Chung SH, Chu WS, et al: Peritoneal dialysis in diabetic patients. Am J Kidney Dis 2001; 38:S200-S203.
386. Passadakis P, Oreopoulos D: Peritoneal dialysis in diabetic patients. Adv Ren Repl Ther 2001; 8:22-41.
387. Foley RN, Parfrey PS, Harnett JD, et al: Mode of dialysis therapy and mortality in end-stage renal disease. J Am Soc Nephrol 1998; 9:267-276.
388. Winkelmayer WC, Glynn RJ, Mittleman MA, et al: Comparing mortality of elderly patients on hemodialysis versus peritoneal dialysis: A propensity score approach. J Am Soc Nephrol 2002; 13:2353-2362.
389. Vigneau C, Trolliet P, Labeeuw M, et al: Which method of dialysis for the type II diabetic? Nephrologie 2000; 21:173-178.
390. Ganesh SK, Hulbert-Shearon T, Port FK, et al: Mortality differences by dialysis modality among incident ESRD patients with and without coronary artery disease. J Am Soc Nephrol 2003; 14:415-424.
391. Miskulin DC, Meyer KB, Athienites NV, et al: Comorbidity and other factors associated with modality selection in incident dialysis patients: The Choice study. Choices for healthy outcomes in caring for end-stage renal disease. Am J Kidney Dis 2002; 39:324-336.
392. Heaf JG, Lokkegaard H, Madsen M: Initial survival advantage of peritoneal dialysis relative to haemodialysis. Nephrol Dial Transplant 2002; 17:112-117.
393. Brown EA, Davies SJ, Rutherford P, et al: Survival of functionally anuric patients on automated peritoneal dialysis: The European APD outcomes study. J Am Soc Nephrol 2003; 14: 2948-2957.

394. Kemperman FA, VanLeusen R, VanLiebergen, et al: Continuous ambulatory peritoneal dialysis (CAPD) in patients with diabetic nephropathy. Neth J Med 1991; 38:236-245.
395. Zimmerman SW, Oxton LL, Bidwell D, et al: Long-term outcome of diabetic patients receiving peritoneal dialysis. Perit Dial Int 1996; 15:63-68.
396. Olszowska A, Pietrzak B, Wankowicz Z: Survival of patients with diabetic nephropathy on continuous ambulatory peritoneal dialysis. Own experiences. Pol Arch Med Wewn 2001; 106:1041-1048.
397. Miguel A, Garcia-Ramon R, Perez-Contreras J, et al: Comorbidity and mortality in peritoneal dialysis: a comparative study of type I and II diabetes versus nondiabetic patients. Peritoneal dialysis and diabetes. Nephron 2002; 90:290-296.
398. Abdel-Rahman EM, Wakeen M, Zimmerman SW: Characteristics of long-term peritoneal dialysis survivors: 18 years experience in one center. Perit Dial Int 1997; 17:151-156.
399. Auinger M: CAPD (continuous ambulatory peritoneal dialysis) in diabetic nephropathy: Overview and general practice in the Lainz Hospital since 1982. Acta Med Austriaca 1999; 26: 154-158.
400. Rubin J, Hsuh K: Continuous ambulatory peritoneal dialysis: Ten years at one facility. Am J Kidney Disease 1991; 17:165-169.
401. Lindblad AS, Novak JW, Nolph KD: Continuous ambulatory peritoneal dialysis in the USA: Final report of the National CAPD Registry 1981–1988. Dordrecht, the Netherlands, Kluwer Academic Publishers, 1989.
402. Held PJ, Port FK, Turenne MN, et al: Continuous ambulatory peritoneal dialysis and hemodialysis: Comparison of patient mortality with adjustment for comorbid conditions. Kidney Int 1994; 45:1163-1169.
403. Habach G, Bloembergen WE, Mauger EA, et al: Hospitalization among United States dialysis patients: Hemodialysis versus peritoneal dialysis. J Am Soc Nephrol 1995; 5:1940-1948.
404. Wu MS, Lin CL, Chang CT, et al: Improvement in clinical outcomes by early nephrology referral in type II diabetics on maintenance peritoneal dialysis. Perit Dial Int 2003; 23:39-45.
405. Rocco MV, Frankenfield DL, Prowant B, et al: Risk factors for early mortality in U.S. peritoneal dialysis patients: Impact of residual renal function. Perit Dial Int 2002; 22:371-379.
406. Cueto-Manzano AM, Correa-Rotter R: Is high peritoneal transport rate an independent risk factor for CAPD mortality? Kidney Int 2000; 57:314-320.
407. Park HC, Kang SW, Choi KH, et al: Clinical outcomes in continuous ambulatory peritoneal dialysis patients is not influenced by high peritoneal transport status. Perit Dial Int 2001; 21:S80-S85.
408. Wu MS, Yu CC, Wu CH, et al: Pre-dialysis glycemic control is an independent predictor of mortality in type II diabetic patients on continuous ambulatory peritoneal dialysis. Perit Dial Int 1999; 19:S179-S183.
409. Canada-USA (CANUSA) Peritoneal Dialysis Study Group: Adequacy of dialysis and nutrition in continuous peritoneal dialysis: Association with clinical outcomes. J Am Soc Nephrol 1996; 7:198-207.
410. Iliescu EA, Marcovina SM, Morton AR, et al: Apolipoprotein(a) phenotype and lipoprotein(a) level predict peritoneal patient mortality. Perit Dial Int 2002; 22:492-499.
411. Serkes KD, Blagg CR, Nolph KD, et al: Comparison of patient and technique survival in continuous ambulatory peritoneal dialysis (CAPD) and hemodialysis: A multicenter study. Perit Dial Int 1990; 10:15-19.
412. Viglino G, Cancarini C, Catizone L, et al: Ten years experience of CAPD in diabetics: Comparison of results with nondiabetics. Nephrol Dial Transplant 1994; 9:1443-1448.
413. Huisman RM, Nieuwenhuizen MG, Th de Charro F: Patient-related and center-related factors influencing technique survival of peritoneal dialysis in the Netherlands. Nephrol Dial Transplant 2002; 17:1655-1660.
414. Churchill DN, Thorpe KE, Teehan BP: CANUSA Peritoneal Dialysis Study Group: Treatment of diabetics with end-stage renal disease: Lessons from the Canada-USA (CANUSA) Study of Peritoneal Dialysis. Semin Dial 1997; 10:215-219.
415. Amair P, Khanna R, Leibel B, et al: Continuous ambulatory peritoneal dialysis in diabetics with end-stage renal disease. N Eng J Med 1982; 306:625-630.
416. Williams ME: Management of the diabetic transplant recipient. Kidney Int 1995; 48:1660-1672.
417. Wolfe RA, Ashby VB, Milford EL, Bloembergen WE: Differences in access to cadaveric renal transplantation in the United States. Am J Kidney Dis 2002; 36:1025-1033.
418. Wolfe RA, Ashby VB, Milford EL, et al: Comparison of mortality in all patients on dialysis, patients on dialysis awaiting transplantation, and recipients of a first cadaveric transplant. N Engl J Med 1999; 341:1725-1731
419. UNOS Bulletin 1997; 2:4-5.
420. Howard AD: Long-term management of the renal transplant recipient: Optimizing the relationship between the transplant center and the community nephrologist. Am J Kidney Dis 2001; 38:S51-S57.
421. Cohen D, Galbraith C: General health management and long-term care of the renal transplant recipient. Am J Kidney Dis 2001; 38:S10-S24.
422. Adu D, Michael J, Turney J, et al: Hyperkalemia in cyclosporin-treated renal allograft recipients. Lancet 1983; 2:370-373.
423. Lillemoe KD, Romolo JL, Hamilton ST, et al: Intestinal necrosis due to sodium polystyrene (Kayexalate) in sorbitol enemas: Clinical and experimental support for the hypothesis. Surgery 1987; 101:267-271.
424. Roy-Chaurhury P, Meisels IS, Freedman S, et al: Combined gastric and ileocecal toxicity (serpiginous ulcers) after oral Kayexalate in sorbital therapy. Am J Kidney Dis 1997; 30: 120-126.
425. Rashid A, Hamilton SR: Necrosis of the gastrointestinal tract in uremic patients as a resuslt of sodium polystyrene sulfonate (Kayexalate) in sorbitol: An underrecognized condition. Am J Surg Pathol 1997; 21:60-65.
426. Freeman D, Grant D, Carruthers S: The cyclosporine-erythromycin interaction: Impaired first pass metabolism in the pig. Br J Pharmacol 1991; 103:1709-1715.
427. Moreno M, Latorre A, Manzanares C, et al: Clinical management of tacrolimus drug interactions in renal transplant patients. Transplant Proc 1999; 31:2252-2253.
428. Aakhus S, Dahl K, Wideroe TE: Cardiovascular morbidity and risk factors in renal transplant patients. Nephrol Dial Transplan 1999; 14:348-354.
429. Djamali D, Nalinee P, Pirsch JD: Outcomes in kidney transplantation. Sem In Nephrol 2003; 23:306-316.
430. Pascual M, Theruvath T, Tatsuo K, et al: Strategies to improve long-term outcomes after renal transplantation. N Eng J Med 2003; 346:580-582.
431. Ganesh SK, Hulbert-Shearon T, Port FK, et al: Differences by dialysis modality among incident patients with and without coronary artery disease. J Am Soc Nephr 2003; 14:415-424.
432. Prichard S: Risk factors for coronary artery disease in patients with renal failure. Am J Med Science 2003; 325:209-231.
433. Kasiske BL: Ischemic heart disease after renal transplantation. Kidney Int 2002; 61:356-359.
434. Kasiske BL: Risk factors for accelerated atherosclerosis in renal transplant recipients. Am Journal of Med 1988; 84:985-992.
435. Foley RN, Parfrey PS, Sarnak MJ: Epidemiology of cardiovascular disease in chronic renal disease. J Am Soc Nephr 1998; 9: S16-S23.
436. Best PJ, Holmes DR: Chronic kidney disease as a cardiovascular risk factor. Am Heart J 2003; 145:383-386.

437. Herzog CA, Logar CM, Beddhu S: Diagnosis and therapy of coronary artery disease in renal failure, end-stage renal disease, and renal transplant populations. N Eng J Med 1999; 325: 214-227.
438. Rice M, Martin J, Hathaway D, et al: Prevalence of cardiovascular risk factors before kidney transplantation. Prog Transplant 2002; 12:299-304.
439. Deminy EM: Cardiovascular disease after renal transplantation. Kidney Int 2002; 61:S78-S84.
440. Lindholm A, Albrechtsen D, Frodin L, et al: Ischemic heart disease: Major cause of death and graft loss after renal transplantation in Scandinavia. Transplant 1995; 60:451-457.
441. Ojo AO, Hanson JA, Wolfe RA, et al: Long-term survival in renal transplant recipients with graft function. Kidney Int 2000; 57:307-313.
442. Kasiske BL: Ischemic heart disease after renal transplantation. Kidney Int 2002; 61:356-369.
443. Kasiske BL: Cardiovascular disease after renal transplantation. Sem Nephrol 2000; 20:176-187.
444. Zoccali C, Mallamaci F, Tripepi G: Traditional and emerging cardiovascular risk factors in end-stage renal disease. Kidney Int 2003; S85:S105-S110.
445. Troyanov S, Hebert M, Masse M, et al: Soluble FAS: A novel predictor of atherosclerosis in dialysis patients. Am J Kidney Dis 2003; 41:1043-1051.
446. Hariharan S: Case 4: Cardiovascular risk in renal transplantation. Transplant 2003; 75:1610-1614.
447. Kannel WB: Metabolic risk factors for coronary heart disease in women: Perspective from the Framingham study. Am Heart J 1987; 114:413-417.
448. Lamberton RP, Goodman AD, Kassoff A, et al: Von Willebrand factors (VIII R: Ag), fibronectin, and insulin-like growth factors I and II in diabetic retinopathy and nephropathy. Diabetes 1984; 33:125-129.
449. Earle K, Walker J, Hill C, et al: Familial clustering of cardiovascular disease in patients with insulin-dependent diabetes and nephropathy. N Engl J Med 1992; 326:673-679.
450. Borch-Johnsen K, Kreiner S: Proteinuria: Value as predictor of cardiovascular mortality in insulin-dependent diabetes mellitus. Br Med J 1978; 294:1651-1656.
451. Friedman EA: Renal syndromes in diabetes. Endocrinol Metab Clin North Am 1996; 25:293-303.
452. Manske CL: Coronary artery disease in diabetic patients with nephropathy. Am J Hypertens 1993; 6:3675-3680.
453. Meir-Kriesche HU, Valiga R, Kaplan B: Decreased renal function is a strong risk factor for cardiovascular death after renal transplantation. Transplant 2003; 75:1291-1295.
454. Abbot KC, Bucci JR, Cruess D, et al: Graft loss and acute coronary syndromes after renal transplantation in the United States. J Am Soc Nephrol 2002; 13:2560-2569.
455. Rabbat CG, Treleaven DJ, Russell JD, et al: Prognostic value of myocardial perfusion studies in patients with end-stage renal disease assessed for kidney or kidney-pancreas transplantation: A meta-analysis. J Am Soc Nephr 2003; 14:431-439.
456. Ghods AJ, Ossareh S: Detection and treatment of coronary artery disease in renal transplantation candidates. Transpl Proc 2002; 34:2415-2417.
457. Braun WE, Phillips DF, Vidt DG: Coronary artery disease in diabetics with end-stage renal failure. Transplant Proc 1984; 16:603-608.
458. Bennett WM, Kloster F, Rosch J: Natural history of asymptomatic coronary arteriographic lesions in diabetic patieints with end-stage renal disease. Am J Med 1978; 65:779-784.
459. Manske CL, Wilson RF, Wang Y, et al: Atherosclerotic vascular complications in diabetic transplant candidates. Am J Kidney Dis 1997; 29:601-609.
460. Ramos EL, Kasiske BL, Alexander SR, et al: The evaluation of candidates for renal transplantation. Transplant 1994; 57: 490-498.
461. Kasiske BL, Vazquez MA, Harmon WE, et al: Recommendations for the outpatient surveillance of renal transplant recipients. J Am Soc Nephr 2000; 11:S1-S86.
462. Vandenberg BF, Rossen JD, Grover-McKay M, et al: Evaluation of diabetic patients for renal and pancreas transplantation. Transplant 1996; 62:1230-1235.
463. Holley JL, Fenton RA, Arthur RS: Thallium stress testing does not predict cardiovascular risk in diabetic patients with end-stage renal disease undergoing cadaveric renal transplantation. Am J Med 1991; 90:563-567.
464. Logar CM, Herzog CA, Beddhu S: Diagnosis and therapy of coronary artery disease in renal failure, end-stage renal disease, and renal transplant populations. Am J Med Sci 2003; 25: 214-227.
465. Weinrauch LA, D'Elia JA, Monaco AP, et al: Preoperative evaluation for diabetic renal transplantation: Impact of clinical, laboratory, and echocardiographic parameters on patient and allograft survival. Am J Med 1992; 93:19-25.
466. Manske L, Thomas W, Wang Y, et al: Screening diabetic transplant candidates for coronary artery disease: Identification of a low risk subgroup. Kidney Int 1993; 44:617-621.
467. Carrozza JP, Kuntz RE, Fishman RF, et al: Restenosis after arterial injury caused by coronary stenting in patients with diabetes mellitus. Ann Intern Med 1993; 118:344-351.
468. Manske CL, Wang Y, Rector T, et al: Coronary revascularization in insulin-dependent diabetic patients with chronic renal failure. Lancet 1992; 340:998-1002.
469. Reddy SV, Chen AC, Johnson HK, et al: Cardiac surgery after renal transplantation. Am J Surg 2002; 68:154-158.
470. Ozdemir FN, Yakupoglu A, Sezgin H, et al: Myocardial revascularization in renal transplant patients. Transplant Proc 2002; 34:2124-2125.
471. Rigatto C: Clinical epidemiology of cardiac disease in renal transplant recipients. Sem Dial 2003; 16:106-110.
472. Gonzalez AI, Schreier L, Elbert A, et al: Lipoprotein alternations in hemodialysis: Differences between diabetic and nondiabetic patients. Metabolism 2003; 52:116-121.
473. Cosio FG, Pesavento TE, Pelletier RP, et al: Patient survival after renal transplantation III: The effects of statins. Am J Kidney Dis 2002; 40:638-643.
474. Kasiske BL: Risk factors for accelerated atherosclerosis in renal transplant recipients. Am J Med 1998; 84:985-992.
475. Chueh SC, Kahan BD: Dyslipidemia in renal transplant recipients treated with a sirolimus and cyclosporine-based immunosuppressive regimen: Incidence, risk factors, progression and prognosis. Transplant 2003; 76:375-382.
476. Morrisett JD, Abdel-Fattah G, Hoogeveen R, et al: Effects of sirolimus on plasma lipids, lipoprotein levels, and fatty acid metabolism in renal transplant patients. Journ Lipid Res 2002; 43:1170-1180.
477. Pirch JD, D'Alessandro AM, Sollinger HW, et al: Hyperlipidemia and transplantation: Etiologic factors and therapy. J Am Soc Nephrol 1992; 2:238-244.
478. Kiberd BA, West KA: Targeting cardiovascular risk in renal transplantation. Transplant Proc 2001; 33:1117-1118.
479. Bastani B, Robinson S, Heisler T, et al: Post-transplant hyperlipidemia: Risk factors and response to dietary modification and gemfibrozil therapy. Clin Transplant 1995; 9:340-346.
480. Arnadottir M, Berg AL: Treatment of hyperlipidemia in renal transplant recipients. Transplant 1997; 63:339-345.
481. Kidney Disease Outcomes Quality Initiative (K/DOQI) Group. K/DOQI clinical practice guidelines for management of dyslipidemias in patients with kidney diesase. Am J Kidney Dis 2003; 1: S1-S910.

482. Asberg A: Interactions between cyclosporin and lipid-lowering drugs: Implications for organ transplant recipients. Drugs 2003; 63:367-378.
483. Cosio FG, Pesavento TE, Pelletier RP, et al: Patient survival after renal transplantation III: The effects of statins. Am J Kidney Dis 2002; 40:638-643.
484. Attinger CE, Ducic I, Neville RF, Abbruzzese MR: The relative roles of aggressive wound care versus revascularization in salvage of the threatened lower extremity in the renal failure diabetic patient. Plast Reconstr Surg 2002; 109:1281-1290.
485. Boucek P, Saudek F, Pokorna E, et al: Kidney transplantation in type II diabetic patients: A comparison with matched nondiabetic subjects. Nephr Dial Transplant 2002; 17:1678-1683.
486. Rao KV, Andersen RC: The impact of diabetes on vascular complications following cadaver renal transplantation. Transplant 1987; 43:193-199.
487. Lemmers MJ, Barry JM: Major role for arterial disease in morbidity and mortality after kidney transplantation in diabetic recipients. Diab Care 1991; 14:295-300.
488. Chen NX, Moe SM: Arterial calcification in diabetes. Curr Diab Res 2003; 3:28-32.
489. Kalker AJ, Pirsch JD, Deisey D, et al: Foot problems in the diabetic transplant recipient. Clin Transplant 1996; 10:503-510.
490. Makisalo H, Lepantalo M, Halme L, et al: Peripheral arterial disease as a predictor of outcome after renal transplantation. Transplant Intern 1998; 11:S140-S143.
491. Zhang R, Leslie B, Boudreaux JP, et al: Hypertension after kidney transplantation: Impact, pathogenesis and therapy. Am J Med Sci 2003; 325:202-208.
492. EBPG Expert Group on Renal Transplantation: European best practice guidelines for renal transplantation. Section IV: Long-term management of the transplant recipient. IV.5.2. Cardiovascular risks. Arterial hypertension. Nephrol Dial Transplant 2002; 17: 25-26.
493. Schwenger V, Zeier M, Ritz E: Hypertension after renal transplantation. Ann Transplant 2001; 6:25-30.
494. Ducloux D, Motte G, Kribs M, et al: Hypertension in renal transplantation: Donor and recipient risk factors. Clin Nephr 2002; 57:409-413.
495. Klein R, Klein BE, Lee KE, et al: The incidence of hypertension in insulin-dependent diabetes. Arch Intern Med 1996; 156: 622-628.
496. Ribiero AB: Abnormlities of systemic blood pressure in diabetes mellitus. Kidney Int 1992; 42:1470-1476.
497. Midtvedt K, Hartmann A: Hypertension after kidney transplantation: Are treatment guidelines emerging? Nephrol Dial Transplant 2002; 17:1166-1169.
498. Klassan DK: How aggressively should blood pressure be treated in renal transplant recipients? Curr Hypertens Rep 2000; 2: 473-477.
499. Benediktsson H,Chea R, Davidoff A, et al: Antihypertensive drug treatment in chronic renal allograft rejection in the rat: Effect on structure and function. Transplant 1996; 62: 1634-1642.
500. Del Castillo D, Campistol JM, Guirado I, et al: Efficacy and safety of losartan in the treatment of hypertension in renal transplant recipients. Kidney Int 1998; 68:S135-S139.
501. Stigant CE, Cohen J, Vivera M, et al: ACE inhibitors and angiotensin II antagonists in renal transplantation: An analysis of safety and efficacy. Am J Kidney Dis 2000; 35:58-63.
502. Mourad G, Ribstein J, Mimran A: Converting-enzyme inhibitor versus calaclium antagonist in cyclosporine-treated renal transplants. Kidney Int 1993; 43:419-426.
503. Leese GP, Vora JP: The management of hypertension in diabetes: With special reference to diabetic kidney disease. Diabetic Med 1996; 13:401-409.
504. Vlahakos D, Canzanello VJ, Madaio M, et al: Enalapril-associated anemia in renal transplant recipients treated for hypertension. Am J Kidney Dis 1991; 17:199-206.
505. Loghan-Adham M: Medication noncompliance in patients with chronic disease: Issues in dialysis and renal transplantation. Am J Manag Care 2003; 9:155-171.
506. Makisalo H, Eklund B, Salmela K, et al: Urological complications after 2084 consecutive kidney transplantations. Transpl Proc 1997; 29:152-153.
507. Elkhammas EA, Henry ML, Barone GW, et al: Urologic complications in diabetic recipients of combined kidney/pancreas grafts versus kidney grafts alone. Transplant Proc 1992; 24: 813-818.
508. Yang CC, Rohr MC, Assimos DG: Pretransplant urologic evaluation. Urology 1994; 43:169-173.
509. Alkalin E, Hyde C, Schmitt G, et al: Emphysematous cystitis and pyelitis in a diabetic renal transplant recipient. Transplant 1996; 62:1024-1027.
510. van Roijen JH, Kirkels WJ, Zieste, et al: Long-term graft survival after urological complications of 695 kidney transplantations. J Urol 2001; 165:1884-1887.
511. Humar A, Ramcharan T, Denny R, et al: Are complications after kidney transplant more common with modern immunosuppression? Transplant 2001; 72:1920-1923.
512. Abbot KC, Oliver JD, Hypolite I, et al: Hospitalizations for bacterial septicemia after renal transplantation in the United States. Am J Neph 2001; 21:120-127.
513. Wai PH, Ewing CA, Johnson LB, et al: Candida fasciitis following renal transplantation. Transplant 2001; 15:477-479.
514. Vachharajani T, Abreo K, Phadke A, et al: Diagnosis and treatment of tuberculosis in hemodialysis and renal transplant patients. Am J Nephr 2001; 20:273-277.
515. Demirag A, Elkhammas EA, Henry ML, et al: Pulmonary Rhizopus infection in a diabetic renal transplant recipient. Clin Transpl 2001; 14:8-10.
516. Satif S, Saffarian N, Bellovich K, et al: Pulmonary mucormycosis in diabetic renal allograft recipients. Am J Kidney Dis 1997; 29:461-464.
517. Jimenez C, Lumbreras C, Aguado JM, et al: Successful treatment of mucor infection after liver or pancreas-kidney transplantation. Transplant 2002; 73:476-480.
518. Khauli RB, Novick AC, Steinmuller DR, et al: Comparison of renal transplantation and dialysis in rehabilitation of diabetic end-stage renal disease patients. Urology 1986; 6:521-527.
519. Jayamanne DG, Porter R: Ocular morbidity following renal transplantation. Nephrol Dial Transplant 1998; 13:2070-2073.
520. Pai RP, Mitchell P, Chow VC, et al: Post transplant cataract: Lessons from kidney-pancreas transplantation. Transplant 2002; 69:1108-1114.
521. Ramsay RC, Knobloch WH, Barbosa JJ, et al: The visual status of diabetic patients after renal translantation. Am J Ophthalmol 1979; 87:305-311.
522. Nisbeth U, Lindh E, Ljunghall S, et al: Increased fracture rate in diabetes mellitus and females after renal transplantation. Transplant 1999; 67:1218-1222.
523. Nisbeth U, Lindh E, Liunghall S, et al: Fracture frequency after kidney transplantation. Transplant Proc 1994; 26:1764-1766.
524. O'Shaughnessy EA, Dahl DC, Smith CL, et al: Risk factors for fractures in kidney transplantation. Transplant 2002; 74: 362-366.
525. Abbot KC, Oglesby RJ, Hypolite IO, et al: Hospitalizations for fractures after renal transplantation in the United States. Ann Epidemiol 2001; 11:450-457.
526. VanDaele P, Stolk RP, Burger H, et al: Bone density in non-insulin dependent diabetes mellitus. Ann Intern Med 1995; 122:409-414.

527. Chiu MY, Sprague SM, Bruce DS, et al: Analysis of fracture prevalence in kidney-pancreas allograft recipients. J Am Soc Nephrol 1998; 9:677-683.
528. Nishitani H, Miki T, Morii H, et al: Decreased bone mineral density in diabetic patients on hemodialysis. Contrib Nephrol 1991; 90:223-230.
529. Gallar P, Oliet A, Vigil A, et al: Aplastic osteodystrophy without aluminum: The role of "suppressed" parathyroid function. Kidney Int 1993; 44:860-866.
530. Andress DL, Kopp JB, Maloney NA, et al: Early deposition of aluminum in bone in diabetic patients on hemodialysis. N Engl J Med 1989; 316:292-299.
531. Pei Y, Hercz G, Greenwood C, et al: Renal osteodystrophy in diabetic patients. Kidney Int 1993; 44:159-166.
532. Lukert BP, Raisz LG: Glucocorticoid-induced osteoporosis: Pathogenesis and management (Comments). Ann Intern Med 1990; 112:352.
533. Movsowitz C, Epstein S, Fallon M, et al: Cyclosporin-A in vivo produces severe osteopenia in the rat: Effect of dose and duration of administration. Endo 1988; 123:2571-2576.
534. Durieux S, Mercadal L, Orcel P, et al: Bone mineral density and fracture prevalence in long-term kidney graft recipients. Transplant 2002; 74:496-500.
535. Stein B, Takizawa M, Katz I, et al: Salmon calcitonin prevents cyclosporin-A-induced high turnover bone loss. Endo 1991; 129:92-99.
536. Jeal W, Barradell LB, McTavish D: Alendronate: A review of its pharmacological properties and therapeutic efficacy in postmenopausal osteoporosis. Drugs 1997; 53:415-420.
537. Haas M, Leko-Mohr Z, Roschger P, et al: Zoledronic acid to prevent bone loss in the first 6 months after renal transplantation. Kidney Int 2003; 63:1130-1136.
538. Cruz DN, Brickel HM, Wysolmerski JJ, et al: Treatment of osteoporosis and osteopenia in long-term renal transplant patients with alendronate. Am J Transplant 2002; 2:62-67.
539. First MR, Gerber DA, Hariharan S, et al: Posttransplant diabetes mellitus in kidney allograft recipients: Incidence, risk factors, and management. Transplant 2002; 73:379-386.
540. Kasiske BL, Snyder JJ, Gilbertson D, Matas AJ: Diabetes mellitus after kidney transplantation in the United States. Am J Transplant 2003; 3:178-185.
541. Hjelmesaeth J, Hartmann A, Kofstad J, Matas AJ: Glucose intolerance after transplantation depends upon prednisolone dose and recipient age. Transplant 1997; 64:979-983.
542. Davidson J, Wilkinson A, Dantal J, et al: New-onset diabetes after transplantation: 2003 International consensus guidelines. Transplant 2003; 75:S3–S24.
543. Moore R, Bocher A, Carter J, et al: Post-Transplant Diabetes Mellitus Advisory Board: Diabetes mellitus in transplantation: 2002 consensus guidelines. Transplant Proc 2003; 4:1265-1270.
544. Woodward RS, Schnitzler MA, Baty J, et al: Incidence and cost of new onset diabetes mellitus among U.S. wait-listed transplanted renal allograft recipients. Am J Transplant 2003; 3: 590-595.
545. Hergesell O, Zeier M: Underdiagnosis of diabetes mellitus in chronic dialysis patients on the renal transplant waiting list. Transplant Proc 2003; 35:1287-1289.
546. Hariharan S, Peddi VR, Savin VJ, et al: Recurrent and de novo renal diseases after renal transplantation: A report from the renal allograft disease registry. Am J Kidney Dis 1998; 31: 928-931.
547. Rao VK: Posttransplant medical complications. Surg Clin North Am 1998; 78:113-132.
548. Denton MD, Singh AK: Recurrent and de novo glomerulonephritis in the renal allograft. Sem Nephrol 2000; 20: 164-175.
549. Basadonna G, Matas AJ, Najarian JS, et al: Transplantation in diabetic patients: The University of Minnesota experience. Kidney Int 1992; 42:S193-S198.
550. Mauer SM, Barbosa J, Vernier RL, et al: Development of diabetic vascular lesions in normal kidneys transplanted into patients with diabetes mellitus. N Engl J Med 1976; 295:916-923.
551. Mauer SM, Steffes MW, Connett J, et al: The development of lesions in the glomerular basement membrane and mesangium after transplantation of normal kidneys transplanted into patients with diabetes mellitus. Diabetes 1983; 32:948-956.
552. Hariharan S, Smit RD, Viero R, et al: Diabetic nephropathy after renal transplantation. Clinical and pathological features. Transplant 1996; 62:632-638.
553. Mauer SM, Goetz FC, McHugh LE, et al: Long-term study of normal kidneys transplanted into patients with type I diabetes. Diabetes 1989; 38:516-522.
554. Hariharan S, Peddi VR, Savin VJ, et al: Recurrent and de novo renal diseases after renal transplantation: A report from the renal allograft disease registry. Am J Kidney Dis 1998; 31: 928-931.
555. Najarian JS, Kaufman DB, Fryd DS, et al: Survival into the second decade following kidney transplantation in type I diabetic patients. Transplant Proc 1989; 21:2012-2017.
556. Cecka JM, Terasacki PI, Cecka JM (eds): The UNOS Scientific Renal Transplant Registry in Clinical Transplantations, 1992. Los Angeles, CA, UCLA Tissue Typing Laboratory, 1993, pp 1-18.
557. EBPG Expert Group on Renal Transplantation. European best practice guidelines for renal transplantation. Section IV: Long-term management of the transplant recipient. IV.2.6. Chronic graft dysfunction. Late recurrence of other diseases. Nephr Dial Transplant 2002; 17:18-19.
558. Bhalla V, Nast CC, Stollenwerk N, et al: Recurrent and de novo diabetic nephropathy in renal allografts. Transplant 2003; 75:66-71.
559. Molitch ME: The relationship between glucose control and the development of diabetic nephropathy in type I diabetes. Semin Nephrol 1997; 17:101-112.
560. Bilous RW, Mauer SM, Sutherland DER, et al: The effects of pancreas transplantation on the glomerular structure of renal allografts in patients with insulin dependent diabetes. N Engl J Med 1989; 321:80-86.
561. Bohman SO, Tyden G, Wilezek, et al: Prevention of kidney graft diabetic nephropathy by pancreas transplantation in man. Diabetes 1985; 34:306-312.
562. Sutherland DER, Marrow CE, Fryd DS, et al: Improved patient and primary renal allograft survival in uremic diabetic recipients. Transplant 1982; 34:319-329.
563. Sutherland DER, Gores PF, Farney AC, et al: Evolution of kidney, pancreas, and islet transplantation for patients with diabetes at the University of Minnesota. Am J Surg 1993; 166:456-463.
564. Nishimura R, Dorman JS, Boynyak Z, et al: Incidence of ESRD and survival after renal replacement therapy in patients with type I diabetes: A report from the Allegheny county registry. Am J Kidney Dis 2003; 42:117-124.
565. Brunkhorst R, Lufft V, Dannenberg B, et al: Improved survival in patients with type I diabetes mellitus after renal transplantation compared with hemodialysis: A case-control study. Transplant 2003; 76:115-119.
566. Ojo AO, Hanson JA, Wolfe RA, et al: Long-term survival in renal transplant recipients with graft function. Kidney Int 2000; 57:307-313.
567. Port FK, Wolfe RA, Mauger EA, et al: Comparison of survival probabilities for dialysis patients versus cadaveric renal transplantation recipients. JAMA 1993; 270:1339-1345.

568. Gaston RS, Alveranga DY, Becker BN, et al: SRTR Report on the state of transplantation: Kidney and pancreas transplantation. Am J Transplant 2003; 3(Suppl 4):64-77.
569. OPTN/SRTR. 2002 Annual Report: The U.S. Organ Procurement and Transplantation Network and the Scientific Registry of Transplant Recipients. Transplant Data, 1992-2001.
570. Ojo AO, Wolfe RA, Agodoa LY, et al: Prognosis after primary renal transplant failure and the beneficial effects of repeat transplantation. Transplant 1998; 66:1651-1659.
571. Shaffer D, Simpson MA, Madras P, et al: Kidney transplantation in diabetic patients using cyclosporin. Arch Surg 1995; 130: 283-290.
572. Hirschl MM, Heinz G, Sunder-Plassmann G, et al: Renal replacement therapy in type II diabetic patients: 10 years' experience. Am J Kidney Dis 1992; 20:264-270.
573. Ostrowski M, Wesolowski T, Makar D, et al: Changes in patient's quality of life after renal transplantation. Transplant Proc 2002; 32:1371-1374.
574. Lim EC, Terasaki PI: Outcome of renal transplantation in different primary diseases. Clin Transplant 1991; 7:293-299.
575. Porter GA: Rehabilitation for end-stage renal disease patients: Reflections on a new treatment paradigm. Semin Dial 1994; 5:313-319.
576. Nielens H, Lejeune TM, Lalaoui A, et al: Increase of physical activity level after successful renal transplantation: A 5-year follow-up study. Nephr Dial Transplant 2003; 16:134-140.
577. Wlodarczyk Z, Badylak E, Glyda M, et al: Vocational rehabilitation following kidney transplantation. Ann Transplant 1999; 4:40-42.
578. Reimer J, Franke GH, Lutkes P, et al: Quality of life in patients before and after kidney transplantation. Psychother Psychosom Med Psychol 2002; 52:16-23.
579. Manninen DL, Evans RW: A longitudinal assessment of the health status of diabetic and nondiabetic renal transplant recipients. Clin Transp 1988; 4:203-210.
580. Painter P: Exercise after renal transplantation. Adv Ren Replace Ther 1999; 6:159-164.
581. Simpson SH, Corabian P, Jacobs P, et al: The cost of major comorbidity in people with diabetes mellitus. Can Medical Assoc 2003; 168:1661-1667.
582. Brandle M, Zhou H, Smith BR, et al: The direct medical cost of type II diabetes. Diab Care 2003; 26:2300-2304.
583. Winkelmayer WC, Weinstein MC, Mittleman MA, et al: Health economic evaluations: The special case of end-stage renal disease treatment. Med Decis Making 2002; 22:417-430.
584. Health Care Financing Research Report on End Stage Renal Disease. Department of Health and Human Services, Health Care Financing Administration Bureau of Data Management and Strategy, Baltimore, MD, 1991.
585. Khan S, Tighiouart H, Kalra A: Resources utilization among kidney transplant recipients. Kidney Int 2003; 64:657-664.
586. Smith DG, Harlan LC, Hawthorne VM: The charges for ESRD treatment of diabetes. J Clin Epidemiol 1989; 42:111-116.
587. Evans RW: A cost-outcome analysis of retransplantation: The need for accountability. Transplant Rev 1993; 7:163-170.

Nutrition in End-Stage Renal Disease

Tahsin Masud, M.D. • William E. Mitch, M.D.

There is abundant evidence that patients with chronic renal failure (CRF), including those treated by peritoneal or hemodialysis, have decreased body weight and subnormal values of serum proteins.[1–3] The mechanisms for these abnormalities are complex and have not been fully identified, but assigning these abnormalities to malnutrition is misleading, since it suggests that the abnormalities can be overcome simply by supplying more food or altering the composition of the diet. Although the focus of our discussion is geared toward nutrition in end-stage renal disease (ESRD) patients, issues also affecting patients with advanced CRF or acute renal failure (ARF) will be highlighted. We begin with a fundamental question: Why does ESRD state mimic malnutrition? Topics to address are: (1) the etiology of protein-calorie malnutrition (PCM) in renal disease, (2) methods for assessing nutritional status, (3) the strategy for successful nutritional intervention, and (4) recommendations for various nutrients intake for maintenance hemodialysis (MHD) or chronic peritoneal dialysis (CPD) patients. Important questions concerning low-protein diet will be addressed: (1) Does therapy with low-protein diets slow the progression of renal disease? (2) Are low-protein diets safe? and (3) Does delaying dialysis, using low-protein diets, affect patient outcome? Finally, the role of nutritional supplements in ESRD patients, including intradialytic parenteral nutrition (IDPN) will be discussed.

WHY DOES END-STAGE RENAL DISEASE MIMIC MALNUTRITION?

Studies of experimental uremia and investigations of patients with kidney failure have suggested several mechanisms that may account for the abnormalities mistakenly assigned to malnutrition (Figure 11–1).

Hypoalbuminemia

Approximately 63% of patients beginning ESRD therapy were found to have subnormal serum albumin levels (< 3.2 g/dL by bromocresol purple and < 3.5 g/dL by bromocresol green).[1] A low serum albumin level is clinically important because it is the strongest independent predictor of total and cardiovascular mortality in ESRD patients.[2,3] Much has been made of a low serum albumin being an index of malnutrition, yet there are several other causes for a dialysis patient to have a low serum albumin and loss of protein stores.[4] The serum albumin concentration is influenced by age, fluid overload, capillary leakage, and evidence of inflammation, in addition to dietary protein stores.[5,6] Regarding its clinical relevance, there is a strong association among atherosclerosis, a low serum albumin and a high C-reactive protein (CRP) level in pre-dialysis patients.[7] In dialysis patients, albumin generation and serum albumin levels are negatively correlated with markers of inflammation, including CRP, fibrinogen, and interleukin-6.[8,14] These findings suggest that inflammation, mediated by pro-inflammatory cytokines, decrease serum albumin levels but also cause loss of lean body mass plus the development of cardiovascular disease in kidney disease patients. The decline in protein stores, in this case, is linked to increased protein breakdown initiated by responses to inflammation rather than to an abnormal diet (as would be the case in malnutrition).[9] The reason for emphasizing this distinction is the persuasive evidence indicating that serum albumin increases when dietary protein of patients with renal insufficiency is restricted.[10,11] What is required in such patients is a strategy for attenuating inflammation followed by observation of changes in serum albumin. In summary, a normal or low serum albumin concentration may not accurately reflect total albumin content and should not be used as the sole indicator of protein stores.

Inflammation

Inflammation is ascribed as another cause of the problems attributed to malnutrition. Contact of blood with "foreign" surfaces, like the hemodialyzer membrane or peritoneal dialysate, activates several humoral and cellular pathways, with higher levels of CRP and other pro-inflammatory cytokines.[12–14]

Although cross-sectional studies suggest that dialysis patients have high circulating concentrations of cytokines, neither the source of inflammation nor the mechanism that increases the concentrations of these cytokines has been identified. Moreover, circulating concentrations of CRP and other cytokines are also elevated in elderly patients and in patients with congestive heart failure or diabetes.[15–17] These data, in addition to the observation that patients with chronic renal insufficiency who are pre-dialysis also have elevated concentrations of pro-inflammatory cytokines, indicate that the mechanism driving high circulating CRP concentration and inflammation includes other factors in addition to exposure of the patient's blood to dialysis membranes.[13,18,19]

The common thread in models of inflammatory conditions that cause loss of muscle mass is activation of protein breakdown, as has been demonstrated repeatedly in models of sepsis and inflammatory conditions. The administration of TNF-α (and other cytokines) to rodents can stimulate protein degradation in muscle, but it is difficult to assign this response to the action of a single cytokine.[20] To date, cytokine-activated mechanisms that lead to accelerated muscle proteolysis by the ubiquitin-proteasome system have not been identified fully, but, as with acidosis, the catabolic

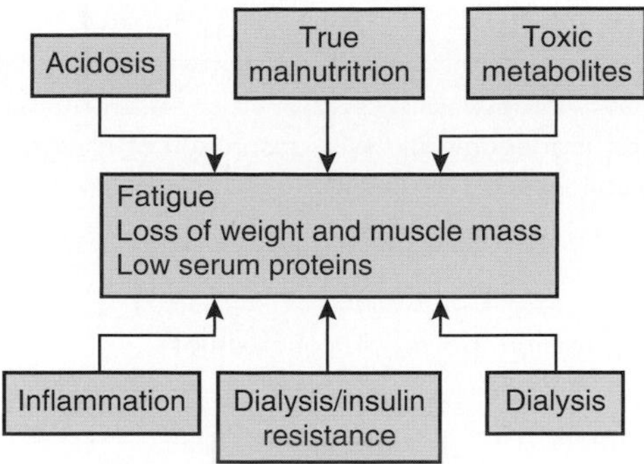

Figure 11–1 An inadequate diet or "true malnutrition" rarely leads to the fatigue, loss of lean body mass, and low serum proteins associated with loss of kidney function. More commonly, these problems are the result of catabolic mechanisms stimulated by renal insufficiency.

responses depend on the action of glucocorticoids.[21–24] In brief, both the mechanism causing the high concentrations of acute phase reactant proteins and the response of serum albumin to the removal of inflammatory stimuli need elucidation.

Metabolic Acidosis

Metabolic acidosis is common in kidney failure and acts to stimulate the irreversible destruction of essential, branched-chain amino acids. In addition, it accelerates the degradation of protein, especially muscle protein.[21,25] The increased breakdown of muscle protein is a result of activation of the ubiquitin-proteasome proteolytic system, the major system that degrades the bulk of protein in all cells, including muscle cells.[26,27] Recently, we obtained evidence that correcting acidosis in patients treated by chronic ambulatory peritoneal dialysis suppresses the ubiquitin-proteasome system and leads to gain of body weight.[28] There is also evidence that acidosis contributes to the low level of serum albumin in dialysis patients.[29,30] Acidosis in kidney failure, therefore, could contribute substantially to the abnormalities presumed to be caused by malnutrition.

Insulin Resistance

Another cause of the constellation of problems lumped under the diagnosis of malnutrition is resistance to the anabolic action of insulin. Experimentally, acute diabetes mellitus causes rapid loss of body weight and muscle mass due to activation of the ubiquitin-proteasome proteolytic system in muscle.[31] These catabolic responses are rapidly reversed by insulin but are independent of the acidosis of acute diabetes.[32] However, as in acidosis, sepsis, and even starvation, activation of accelerated muscle proteolysis by this system requires glucocorticoids.[33,34] Since diabetes is a common cause of ESRD and kidney failure causes resistance to the hypoglycemic action of insulin, it is likely that diabetes or insulin resistance plays a role in the abnormalities attributed to malnutrition.[35] It is tempting to speculate that the protein catabolism that occurs when patients are dialyzed against a glucose-free bath is related to a reduced stimulation of insulin release.[36]

Another potential cause of ESRD-associated abnormalities in weight, muscle mass, and serum proteins is the combination of accumulated wasted products and metabolic abnormalities caused by the loss of kidney function. Again, this mechanism is not directly linked to an inadequate diet and, in fact, an excess of protein-rich foods should only increase the accumulation of waste products like phosphates, acid, and nitrogen-containing products.[37] To date, there has been no cause-and-effect association found between the accumulation of nitrogen-containing waste products and a specific syndrome, despite intriguing investigations about links between unidentified "middle molecules" and depressed appetite.[38] Overall, evidence supporting this mechanism as a cause of the problems attributed to malnutrition is substantially weaker than for other mechanisms. Finally, Ikizler and colleagues[39] measured whole-body and muscle protein turnover in stable patients dialyzed with modern dialysis membranes. They found that whole-body degradation of protein, including muscle protein, was stimulated during hemodialysis. Because the catabolic response persisted after completion of the dialysis procedure, the authors concluded that the dialysis somehow induced the breakdown of protein.

PROTEIN-CALORIE MALNUTRITION IN RENAL FAILURE

The diagnosis of protein-calorie malnutrition (PCM) in dialysis patients is confounded by the lack of uniform criteria for its diagnosis and the difficulties in separating abnormal nutritional parameters caused by inflammation or complications of uremia. In cross-sectional and longitudinal surveys, the reported prevalence of PCM in dialysis patients varies from 25% to 75%.[40–47] Some ESRD patients have true protein-calorie malnutrition, a condition caused by inadequate nutrient intake, increased catabolism, or increased body requirement of nutrients[2,3] (Table 11–1). As noted, there are other reasons for the loss of protein mass.

Inadequate Protein and Calorie Intake

Anorectic pre-dialysis uremic patients regain appetite after beginning dialysis. It suggests that uremic toxins causing anorexia have been removed by dialysis.[48] Inadequate dialysis, therefore, may result in accumulation of uremic toxins that suppress appetite and cause malnutrition. Several studies in hemodialysis or chronic peritoneal dialysis (CPD) patients report a strong correlation between the dose of dialysis for small molecule removal (Kt/V_{urea}) and protein intake.[49–51] However, even patients with adequate dialysis often have anorexia. Anorexia may be caused by altered taste buds sensation or through complex interaction of various appetite modulators, with serotonin as a central cause of anorexia.[52] Catecholamine and serotonin pathways appear to be involved in the hypothalamic regulation of satiety center and high brain serotonin level, and a lower serotonin/dopamine ratio in the brain will cause anorexia. High plasma levels of anorectics, including tryptophan (a precursor of serotonin), cholecystokinin, leptin, pancreatic polypeptide, cytokines (TNF-α and IL-1), and deficiencies of nitric oxide and neuropeptide Y will each increase intracerebral serotonin.[52]

Table 11–1 Causes of Protein-Calorie Malnutrition in ESRD

Condition	Mechanisms
Inadequate protein or calorie intake	Anorexia: Uremic toxins, inadequate dialysis, absorption of glucose from dialysate, medications Diabetic gastropathy Dental status Volume overload Psychosocial factors: Depression, poverty, alcohol/drugs
Increase catabolic response	Low energy intake Acidosis Insulin resistance Inflammation, infection, sepsis Glucocorticoids
Increase requirement for protein and energy	Loss of nutrients during peritoneal and hemodialysis Increase in resting energy expenditure

Increased Catabolic Response

The maintenance of nitrogen balance in ESRD patients depends on an adequate energy intake.[49,53] Metabolic studies and K/DOQI™ guidelines recommend minimum energy intake of 35 kcal/kg/day,[54] but cross-sectional studies have shown that hemodialysis patients ingest far fewer calories.[55,56] Thus, inadequate energy intake could be an important factor contributing to impaired protein metabolism. Stimulation of protein breakdown by metabolic acidosis, inflammation, insulin resistance, and glucocorticoids have already been discussed.

Increased Requirement for Protein and Energy

Each dialysis session can result in removal of amino acids (about 10 to 12 g), some peptides, and smaller amounts of protein (< 1 to 3 g).[57–60] Significant losses of protein and amino acids have been documented across high-flux membranes that are treated with bleach and formaldehyde.[59,61] In general, the protein losses from reprocessed dialyzers are trivial until the number of reuses exceeds 10.[61] Protein losses in CPD patients are even higher, averaging about 5 to 15 g/day. During episodes of peritonitis, losses may be considerably higher.[62] Much of these losses consist of albumin. There are also immunoglobulins, peptides, and amino acids.[63] Amino acid losses average about 3 g/day.[64] Loss of protein and amino acid is too small to account fully for the increased protein requirements of dialysis patients, but the changes in plasma amino acid concentrations suggest these patients catabolize 25 to 30 g of body protein to compensate for these losses.[63]

Uremic complications can promote protein catabolism to increase dietary protein requirements.[65] The disorders favoring catabolism include resistance to insulin, growth hormone, and insulin-like growth factor-1 and both hyperglucagonemia and hyperparathyroidism.[65] Recent reports suggest that the resting energy expenditure (REE), as measured by indirect calorimetry in patients, is significantly higher in ESRD patients compared to CRF patients not on dialysis.[66,67] Earlier reports concluded that REE in dialysis patients is similar to that of healthy controls and pre-dialysis CRF patients.[68,69] The difference could be the more recent use of more accurate chamber indirect calorimeter. Increased energy requirements could contribute to the development of malnutrition.

ASSESSMENT OF NUTRITIONAL STATUS IN RENAL DISEASES

Since loss of lean body mass is a common problem for patients with ESRD, it is important to use longitudinal assessments of nutritional status to recognize substrate deficiencies early. No single assessment has been defined to evaluate variables that affect nutritional status, so a number of indices are needed to define the nutritional status of patients (Table 11–2).

There must be a medical history for the type of renal disease, comorbid conditions, plus a physical examination. The dietary history should include the amount and patterns of nutrient intake, and a dietitian should obtain information about socioeconomic circumstances that could interfere with a necessary diet. The energy level, appetite, physical activity, medications, and the use of dietary and herbal supplements, alcohol, and illicit drugs must also be documented.[70]

The most common methods for estimating intake in patients with renal disease are dietary recalls, dietary diaries, and determination of protein equivalent of nitrogen appearance. The dietary recall (usually obtained for previous 24 hours) is a simple, rapid method of obtaining a crude assessment of dietary intake.[54] Dietary diaries are written reports of foods consumed during a specified length of time (from 3 to 7 days). This method is not only a more reliable estimate of an individual's intake on average than on a single day, but it is also the only practical way to estimate energy intake. The validity and reliability of dietary interviews and diaries depend on the patient's ability to provide accurate data and the ability of the dietitian to conduct detailed and probing interviews.[54]

Protein Equivalent of Total Nitrogen Appearance (PNA)

Biochemical methods for estimating protein intake are based on the concept that ingested proteins plus the products arising from endogenous protein are metabolized to several

Table 11–2 Categories of Nutritional Assessment in Renal Patient

Clinical
Medical history
Physical examination
Psychosocial history
Dietary history
Diet history
Appetite assessment
Food habits and patterns
Fluid intake/balance: Interdialytic fluid gains
Dietary nutrient intake
Food intake records and dietary recall
Normalized protein equivalent of total nitrogen appearance (nPNA)
Biochemical measurements (pre-dialysis stablized)
Serum albumin, *serum prealbumin, serum transferrin*
Serum bicarbonate, serum potassium, serum glucose
Serum creatinine, urea nitrogen, calcium and phosphorus
Serum cholesterol
Kt/V or URR
Body composition
Anthropometric measurements
Creatinine kinetics
Bio-electrical impedance
Dual energy x-ray absorptiometery (DEXA)
Near infra-red interactance
Total body nitrogen, total body potassium
Subjective global assessment (SGA)
Categories shown in italics are not routinely recommended.

nitrogenous products (e.g., urea, amino acids, or creatinine). In the steady state (neither catabolism nor anabolism), the nitrogenous products that are removed from the body by urine, dialysate, stool, skin, and blood (total nitrogen appearance) are equal to the protein intake (6.25 g protein produces 1 g nitrogen).[71] There is a strong correlation between urea appearance rate (which can be easily calculated from urea dialysate and urine concentration) and total nitrogen appearance, so protein nitrogen appearance can be estimated from the urea appearance rate calculated as the urea accumulated in the body and how much is excreted.

Urea kinetics, calculated from the blood urea nitrogen (BUN), the properties of the dialyzer and the duration of dialysis treatment, is used to calculate protein nitrogen appearance in hemodialysis patients. There are formulas based on a three-BUN or two-BUN measurement.[72,73] The three-BUN method measures pre- and post-dialysis BUN of a single hemodialysis session plus the subsequent pre-dialysis BUN value.[72] The two-BUN method calculates PNA from a single dialysis session, using a computer iteration scheme eliminating need for a third BUN.[73] The two-BUN method is routinely incorporated into formal urea kinetic modeling because fewer BUN measurements are needed and the amount of dietary protein between the dialysis sessions does not influence the measurement. An error involving any of the variables for kinetic modeling will extend to the dietary protein estimates.[74] Graphical nomograms have been developed to estimate dietary protein from a pre-dialysis and post-dialysis BUN samples.[75]

The calculation of protein intake for CPD patient is simpler; it requires only the urea nitrogen excretion in urine and dialysate. Numerous equations proposed for calculating dietary protein were originally developed for chronic ambulatory dialysis patients but also applied to automated peritoneal dialysis patients.[76,77] Protein nitrogen appearance is usually normalized (nPNA) to some function of body weight (e.g., edema-free body weight or body weight derived from the urea distribution space [$V_{urea}/0.58$]).[54]

There are important limitations in interpreting urea kinetically derived estimates of dietary protein intake. First, in catabolic states (acidosis, infection, etc.), endogenous protein breakdown can increase urea appearance so protein nitrogen appearance will exceed protein intake estimates. Conversely, when a patient becomes anabolic protein nitrogen appearance will underestimate actual protein intake. Second, day-to-day variations in protein intake are reflected rapidly by the protein nitrogen appearance, so single measurement may not tell us about average protein intake over 1 month. Third, protein nitrogen appearance does accurately estimate intake at extremes of protein intake. This is a result of increased nitrogen losses through unmeasured pathways of excretion at higher protein intake and greater endogenous protein catabolism at lower protein intake.[78] Finally, normalizing protein nitrogen appearance to body weight can be misleading in obese, malnourished, or edematous patients. Therefore, K/DOQI™ guidelines for individuals who are less than 90% or greater than 115% of standard body weight, recommend using the adjusted edema-free body weight.[54]

In summary, protein nitrogen appearance reflects approximate protein intake in a stable dialysis patient. However, it should not be used as the sole means of assessing nutritional status, and one must be familiar with potential errors in its calculation and its limitations in interpreting dietary protein intake.

Biochemical Values and Nutritional Assessment

Serum Albumin, Prealbumin, and Transferrin

These proteins are biochemical markers often used to assess visceral protein stores, to monitor the adequacy of responses to a nutritional intervention, and to identify patients who are at risk for complications or are responding poorly to medical/surgical treatment. Besides the limitations of serum albumin as a marker of malnutrition (see previous), prealbumin has a short half-life (2 to 3 days) and is more sensitive to acute changes in protein status. Prealbumin is a retinol-binding protein that circulates in a 1:1 molar ratio to transport the alcohol form of vitamin A. The serum prealbumin level is a powerful predictor of survival in dialysis patients[79] and correlates directly with markers of visceral (albumin and cholesterol), somatic protein stores (creatinine), and recent protein intake.[80] Unfortunately, serum prealbumin is limited by many of the same factors as serum albumin; it is a negative acute-phase reactant. This retinol-binding protein is excreted and metabolized by the kidney in renal failure so it accumulates.[81] There is insufficient evidence to conclude that prealbumin as an indicator of nutritional status is more sensitive or accurate compared to serum albumin.[54]

Serum transferrin also has a short half-life (about 8 vs. 20 days for albumin), but as an indicator of malnutrition, the serum transferrin concentration is frequently reduced in renal failure independently of malnutrition, perhaps due to fluctuation in iron stores.[82] Serum transferrin increases in iron deficiency, in pregnancy, and in the early phases of acute hepatitis; it decreases with certain chronic infections, liver diseases, cancer, or iron loading. Finally, its concentration, like that of albumin, varies with hydration.

In summary, no single serum protein measurement is ideal for detecting malnutrition early, but repeatedly low values generally indicate that there is some degree of protein malnutrition.

Serum Bicarbonate

Dietary protein intake in dialysis patient is an important determinant of acid-base status since metabolism of amino acids, particularly cysteine and methionine, generates protons. Pre-dialysis or stable serum bicarbonate values below 22 mmol/L are indicative of metabolic acidosis in an ESRD patient. Metabolic acidosis affects nutrition by stimulating protein catabolism, and correction of acidosis decreases whole body protein degradation in dialysis patients.[83] Because of the inaccuracies in serum bicarbonate measurements, the reports that acidosis is not associated with malnutrition should be ignored.[84,85] For example, correction of metabolic acidosis in CPD patients improved the nutritional status and reduced hospitalization rates.[86] Oral bicarbonate supplements given to acidotic CPD patients resulted in improved nutritional status judged by subjective global assessment.[87] We recommend that pre-dialysis patients or dialysis patients should have stabilized serum bicarbonate levels above 22 mmol/L.

Serum Potassium

Low serum potassium levels in dialysis patients should raise the suspicion of a poor nutritional intake. Associated with a low serum albumin, low serum phosphorus and magnesium values are commonly found in severely malnourished nursing-home ESRD patients and those maintained on parenteral nutrition.[88] Increasing the dialysis dose may lead to significant hypokalemia in a large proportion of CPD patients, even when achieving DOQI targets.[89]

Serum Creatinine

In dialysis patients, the serum creatinine level is proportional to muscle mass and dietary meat intake.[90,91] The serum creatinine concentration was higher and predicted long-term survival (10–15 years on MHD and 10 years on CPD) compared to values in average-survival (< 5 years) ESRD patients.[92] A direct relationship has been reported between serum creatinine and albumin and prealbumin concentrations.[93,94] Individuals with low pre-dialysis or stabilized serum creatinine values (< 10 mg/dL) should be evaluated for protein-energy malnutrition and wasting of skeletal muscle.[54]

Serum Cholesterol

The serum cholesterol is another marker of increased risk of mortality in ESRD patient.[92,95–97] Surprisingly, it is an independent predictor of mortality in hemodialysis patients who have low-normal nonfasting values of serum cholesterol (< 150–180 mg/dL) compared to those with higher cholesterol levels.[95–98] The same relationship was not observed in CPD patients.[3,95,96] The pre-dialysis or stabilized serum cholesterol concentration is too insensitive to be used for assessment of nutritional status in ESRD patient.

Other biochemical measurements (serum glucose, calcium, and phosphorus) are not useful to assess nutritional status but are of immense importance for diet planning and overall nutritional management of individual dialysis patient.

Assessment of Body Composition

Methods to assess adipose stores and lean body mass range from simple techniques like anthropometrics and creatinine kinetics to utilization of sophisticated technology.

Anthropometry consists of a series of noninvasive, inexpensive, and easy to perform indices including body weight, percent of usual weight, skeletal frame size, body mass index, body fat, and fat-free mass.[54] A decline in anthropometric measurements can detect a loss of lean body mass during long-term evaluations. Unfortunately, very little data are available on how closely subnormal anthropometric values correlate with an adverse clinical outcome. Cross-sectional studies do show a strong linkage between large body size and reduced risk of mortality in hemodialysis patients.[99–101]

The anthropometrics measurement in "healthy" males (including diabetics) and most women on hemodialysis were similar to those of normal adults cited in the National Health and Nutrition Examination Survey (NHANES II) data.[102] However, women with diabetes or African-American diabetics over age 55 had lower triceps skin-fold thickness. There were no differences in anthropometric measurements between hemodialysis and peritoneal dialysis patients. The anthropometrics assessment of patients enrolled in Hemodialysis (HEMO) study revealed that the patients were, on average, lighter with less adipose and muscle tissue in comparison to healthy persons of same ages from NHANES II.[103] Importantly, the HEMO study patients may not be representative of the general ESRD population because patients with serum albumin less than 2.8 mg/dL or those with body weight greater than 85 kg were excluded from the enrollment.[104]

The reliability of anthropometric measurements depends heavily on the skill of the observer, the sites examined (e.g., the circumference of the dominant or nondominant arm when assessing muscle mass), and the degree of hydration. In hemodialysis patients, it is recommended that measures be completed after a treatment, using the arm without the dialysis access. Loss of fat from subcutaneous tissues occurs proportionately, so repeated measures from a selected group of sites in an individual patient can provide reliable information on trends of adipose stores.

Creatinine index is another simple method for estimating fat-free body mass in an ESRD patient.[105,106] There are several limitations of this method. First, rate of creatinine appearance is affected by dietary meat and residual renal function.[54] Second, there is mathematical coupling between weekly creatinine clearance and lean body mass in CPD patients, because both are calculated from the same 24-hour urine and dialysate collection.[107] Finally, the creatinine-based calculation of lean body mass in CPD patients was found to be highly variable compared to lean body mass based on total body potassium.[108]

Other methods of measuring body composition include bioelectrical impedance, dual-energy X-ray absorptiometry (DEXA), neutron activation, near infra-red interactance, magnetic resonance imaging, and computed tomography (Table 11–3). Each has advantages and disadvantages in ESRD patients.

SUBJECTIVE GLOBAL ASSESSMENT (SGA)

A clinical approach of assessing protein-calorie malnutrition that has recently become popular is subjective global assessment (SGA).[70] SGA is based on evaluating subjective and objective patient information, including medical history and physical examination, gastrointestinal symptoms, bodyweight patterns, and patient functional capacity, plus the presence of comorbid conditions that could affect nutritional requirements. The patient is assigned to one of the three nutritional status groups: (1) well nourished, (2) mild-moderately malnourished, or (3) severely malnourished. The SGA method has been used to assess the nutritional status of pre-dialysis[109] and CPD or hemodialysis patients.[110–112] Not all reports agree that SGA has sufficient accuracy for detecting protein-calorie malnutrition. Cooper and colleagues[113] compared SGA with total body nitrogen (neutron activation or "gold standard" marker) for nutritional status. SGA was found to be of limited value in determining malnutrition in patients with ESRD, predicting only 20% to 50% of patients who had evidence of significant nutritional compromise. The SGA did not sufficiently discriminate between mild to moderate and severe degrees of malnutrition.[113] Limitations of the SGA include a heavy reliance on subjective judgment, and SGA may not identify functional impairment due to malnutrition; it also does not identify the type or amount of nutritional support to provide repletion.[114]

In summary, no single parameters have been defined to evaluate the variables that affect the nutritional status of dialysis patient. Consequently, a complete nutritional evaluation is recommended, using all the categories in Table 11–2. A renal dietitian can perform the evaluation at the initiation of dialysis and should monitor post dialysis weights and biochemical parameters monthly. The comprehensive nutritional assessment is repeated every 6 months or more frequently in patients at high risk for malnutrition (e.g., the elderly, those with complicating diseases, etc.).

MANAGEMENT OF NUTRITIONAL ISSUES IN CRF AND ESRD

The goals of dietary therapy for patients with chronic renal failure are: (1) to diminish the accumulation of nitrogenous wastes and limit the metabolic disturbances characteristic of uremia, (2) to prevent malnutrition, and (3) to slow the progression of renal failure.

Protein-restricted diets improve uremic symptoms because they reduce the levels of uremic toxins, most of which result from the metabolism of protein. A low-protein diet also ameliorates specific complications of CRF, including metabolic acidosis, renal osteodystrophy, hyperkalemia, and hypertension, because a diet that is restricted in protein is invariably restricted in the quantities of sulfates, phosphates, potassium, and sodium eaten each day. Those considerations explain why dietary protein restriction has been used for decades to treat chronically uremic patients. Fundamental questions regarding use of low-protein diets in CRF patients are:

- Do they change the progression of renal failure?
- Do low-protein diets cause malnutrition?
- Does delaying the start of renal replacement therapy affect patient outcomes?

LOW-PROTEIN DIETS AND PROGRESSION OF CHRONIC RENAL FAILURE

A number of studies have examined the influence of dietary protein restriction on the progression of renal disease, but

Table 11–3 Assessment of Body Composition in Patients with Renal Disease

Test	Measure	Advantages	Disadvantages	Reference
Bioelectric impedance (BIA)	Total body water, Fat mass, Fat-free mass	Easy and practical in clinical setting	Results influenced by state of hydration	202
		Small coefficient of variation	Technique not validated in amputees	203,204
Dual-energy X-ray absorptiometry (DEXA)	Fat mass, Fat-free mass, bone mineral mass density	Independent of fluid status Small coefficient of variation	Expensive, require large set-up	205,206
Neutron activation	Total body potassium Total body nitrogen	High precision and reliability Independent of fluid status	Expensive, require large set-up	207,208
Near infra-red interactance	Body fat, fat-free mass	Independent of fluid status Validated for longitudinal assessment	Not compared to BIA or DEXA in dialysis patients	209

many of these reports suffer from problems in design, differences in measurement of efficacy, a limited sample size, and the type of diet and degree of compliance with the diet.[115] The randomized, controlled trials that have enrolled only insulin-dependent diabetes patients have shown improved preservation of kidney function in patients assigned to a low-protein diet when compared to patients eating unrestricted amounts of dietary protein.[116–119] The number of diabetic patients studied in these trials was generally small and the duration of follow-up was short. To examine this question in a larger number of patients, meta-analyses have been done in order to combine results from several studies. The results published by Fouque, Pedrini and colleagues[120–122] indicate a significant benefit from low-protein diets in preserving the renal function of diabetic patients.

Trials enrolling nondiabetic and non–insulin-dependant diabetic CRF patients in a randomized fashion have not consistently demonstrated that dietary protein restriction slows progression at least when analyzed according to the diet prescribed. The results of these trials are summarized in Table 11–3. The largest trial in this group was the Modification of Diet in Renal Disease, or MDRD, a study designed to test the effects of dietary protein restriction and different levels of blood pressure control on the progression of renal insufficiency (loss of GFR) in 840 patients.[123] In Study A, patients with GFRs of 25 to 55 mL/min/1.73 m^2 were randomly assigned to a usual protein diet (1.3 g/kg/day) or a low-protein diet (0.58 g/kg/day). In Study B, patients with GFRs of 13 to 24 mL/min/1.73 m^2 were randomly assigned to the same low-protein diet or to a very low-protein diet (0.28 g/kg/day) plus a mixture of ketoacids (to supply essential amino acid requirements). There was no control group eating an unrestricted diet in this group of patients with more advanced renal insufficiency. GFR was measured every 4 months as the renal clearance of $[I^{125}]$-iothalamate and the patients were followed for an average of 2.2 years; the results extrapolated to 3 years for all patients. There was no significant difference in the loss of GFR between the two diet groups in either Study A or in Study B, although there was a trend toward a slower decline in GFR in patients assigned to the lower protein diets.

Do the MDRD study results provide the last word on the influence of low-protein diets in preserving kidney function? Because there are shortcomings of the MDRD study, we do not believe these results demonstrate there is no slowing of the loss of renal function in patients eating a low-protein diet. First, the hypothesis being tested was that eating a protein-restricted diet will slow the loss of residual renal function, but the conclusions of the initial MDRD report[123] were based on the diet assignment, rather than achieved intake (Table 11–3). In fact, when the MDRD study results were analyzed according to compliance with the low-protein diets, there was significant slowing of the loss of GFR and a delay until patients

Table 11–3 Randomized Controlled Trials of Effect of Protein-Restricted Diets on the Progression of Renal Failure

Reference	No. of patients	Mean follow-up (months)	Prescribed protein for randomized groups (g/kg/day)	Actual protein intake (g/kg/day)	Outcome of trial
Jungers et al[210]	14	9	0.6 vs 0.4 plus KA	0.7 vs 0.4 plus KA	Time to dialysis longer and mean slope of $1/S_{cr}$ lower in KA group
Bergstörm et al[211]	16	12-24	Unrestricted vs 0.4 plus EAA	0.86 vs 0.65	Slope of $1/S_{cr}$ and drop in CrCl were similar
Ihle et al[212]	64	18	Unrestricted vs 0.4	>0.75 vs 0.4	Significantly less decrease in GFR and progression to end-stage in low protein group
Rosman et al[213]	239	48	Unrestricted vs 0.4-0.6	No data available	Renal survival better in low protein group after 2 years but no difference after 4 years
Locatelli et al[214]	456	24	1.0 vs 0.6	0.9 vs 0.78	No difference in renal survival
William et al[215]	95	19	>0.8 vs 0.6	1.0-1.14 vs 0.69	Rate of fall of CrCl and $1/S_{cr}$ similar
Klahr et al[123] Study A	585	26	1.3 vs 0.58	1.1 vs 0.77	The intention-to-treat analysis revealed no difference in GFR decline, when analysed by degree of compliance low protein group has significant slowing in GFR
Klahr et al[123] Study B	255	26	0.58 vs 0.28 plus KA	0.73 vs 0.48	No difference in slowing of GFR, on secondary analysis lower protein intake caused slower mean decline in GFR but no independent effect of KA
D Amico et al[216]	128	27	1.0 vs 0.6	1.1 vs 0.8	Low protein group had significant lower risk of progression

CrCl, creatinine clearance; *EAA*, essential amino acids; *GFR*, glomerular filtration rate; *KA*, ketoacids; S_{cr}, serum creatinine.

required dialysis.[124] Second, the criteria for entering the MDRD study did not include a requirement that patients were, in fact, losing renal function; approximately 15% of the Study A control group had no evidence of progressive loss of GFR, and this would increase the number of patients required to demonstrate a benefit from the dietary manipulations. Another factor that would increase the number of patients to be studied to detect a benefit was the finding that the overall rate of loss of renal function was slower than predicted. In this respect, it is interesting that meta-analyses utilizing results from several studies[120,121] led to the conclusion that dietary restriction was beneficial in preserving residual renal function. Third, there was a disproportionate number of patients (~20%) with polycystic kidney disease, and these patients had no benefit from the dietary restriction or from treating hypertension. Including these patients in the study might have obscured a benefit of the dietary manipulation. Fourth, patients in the MDRD study were given angiotensin-converting enzyme inhibitor therapy in a random fashion. Considering the beneficial effects of these drugs on progressive renal insufficiency,[125] their inclusion would make it more difficult to detect a benefit from the low-protein diet on preserving residual kidney function. Finally, the MDRD study lasted an average of only 2.2 years. This is important because the patients in Study A had an initial rapid loss of GFR just after institution of the low-protein diet, followed by a slower loss of GFR. If this slowing had persisted, it is possible that statistically significant slowing of progression may have been detected in a longer-term study. For example, in other large trials (e.g., the examination of the influence of strict control of hyperglycemia, the DCCT Trial), no benefit was apparent until 4 years of therapy.[126] Likewise, slowing of the loss of renal function in patients with IgA nephropathy during treatment with a fish oil supplement was not apparent until 3 years had passed.[127]

Do Low-Protein Diets Cause Malnutrition?

The finding that dialysis patients often have low levels of serum proteins and evidence of malnutrition has led some to suggest that low-protein diets should be used cautiously or avoided in pre-dialysis patients and that dialysis should be initiated early.[128,129] It is true that if CRF patients are not properly instructed and supervised, there may well be a spontaneous decrease in protein intake and deterioration of some nutritional indices. Another worrisome report is the association between hypoalbuminemia and increased mortality in hemodialysis patients,[130] but hypoalbuminemia in these patients can be linked as much to evidence of inflammation as it is to dietary inadequacy.[8,14,131] In fact, CRF patients treated with low-protein diets were found to have an increase in serum protein concentrations at the initiation of dietary therapy.[132,133] A low-protein diet is also associated with improved survival of CRF patients who subsequently began dialysis.[134] Finally, there is abundant evidence that with proper implementation, a low-protein diet yields neutral nitrogen balance and maintenance of normal serum proteins and anthropometric indices during long-term therapy.[135–137] Once on dialysis, patients treated with supplemented very low-protein diet (SVLPD) rapidly increase their protein intake and gain in lean body mass.[138] Follow-up for 5 years after initiation of renal replacement therapy (MHD and renal transplant), these patients revealed low mortality, correlating to age but not to nutritional parameters at the end of SVLPD therapy.[133]

Does Delaying the Start of Renal Replacement Therapy Affect Patient Outcomes?

NFK K/DOQI™ guidelines for peritoneal dialysis adequacy suggest that chronic dialysis should be initiated at a weekly renal Kt/V_{urea} of 2.0, which approximates a creatinine clearance of 9 to 14 mL/min/1.73 m^2 or glomerular filtration rate (arithmetic mean of the urea and creatinine clearances) of 10.5 mL/min/1.73 m^2. Unless patient has stable or increased edema-free body weight, sound nutritional status and complete absence of clinical symptoms or signs are attributable to uremia.[139] This recommendation was not evidence-based but an opinion relying on flawed or weak arguments.

The rationale given for this suggestion is that optimizing urea clearance once patients are on dialysis is a goal, so why accept much lower levels of urea clearance during the pre-dialysis phase of patient management? There is also concern that CRF patients spontaneously reduce their protein intake as renal function worsens,[128,140,141] and a low serum albumin and low residual renal function at the initiation of dialysis is associated with poor outcomes.[141,142] However, the K/DOQI™ work group did not consider the following facts. First, they assumed equivalence between the solute clearance from residual renal function and peritoneal dialysate. This is not supported by a re-analysis of results from the CANUSA study; the association between total clearance and patient survival was only accounted for by residual renal function not by peritoneal clearance.[143] The differential impact of residual renal clearance and peritoneal clearance on survival was confirmed by the prospective Netherlands Cooperative Adequacy of Dialysis Study of CAPD patients.[144] Second, there is abundant evidence that protein malnutrition is common in dialysis patients,[42–47] suggesting that dialysis therapy could itself be a contributing factor to malnutrition.[39] Finally, those studies reporting negative impact of a low residual renal function on survival at the start of dialysis therapy are flawed by failure to take account of lead-time bias. Lead-time bias refers to the effect whereby measuring survival from the start of dialysis increases apparent survival of those started with more residual renal function, that is, earlier in the course of the disease, than those who start dialysis with less residual renal function.[145] When CRF patients were followed from an estimated creatinine clearance (eC_{cr}) of 20 mL/min, and divided into early and late start groups by the median eC_{cr} (8.3 mL/min) for all patients at the initiation of dialysis, there was no benefit of survival from earlier initiation of dialysis.[146] A Cox proportional hazards model demonstrated a significant inverse relationship between eC_{Cr} at start of dialysis and survival (hazard ratio, 1.1; $P = .02$), that is, patients who started dialysis with a lower eC_{Cr} tended to survive longer.[146] More recently, Beddhu and colleagues[147] examined data from the dialysis Morbidity Mortality Study Wave II to evaluate if beginning dialysis at higher levels of creatinine clearance or GFR (estimated from the MDRD formula) would improve mortality. They found that initiation of dialysis was associated with an increase in mortality for each 5 mL/min increase in GFR. The authors concluded that there is insufficient evidence to advocate early initiation of dialysis.

In summary, there is no substantial evidence that survival improves with early initiation of dialysis in ESRD and that it is associated with a better health-related quality of life.[148]

The results of clinical trials evaluating effect of low-protein diets on the progression of CRF to date have not settled whether such diets will be effective in slowing the loss of residual renal function in a large proportion of patients. When properly applied, these diets do not lead to malnutrition, even in patients with advanced renal insufficiency.[10,11,136–138] For these reasons, we recommend instituting a low-protein diet in all patients who have symptoms attributable to uremia or for patients who exhibit progressive renal insufficiency, despite the proper management of known risk factors for progression such as control of blood pressure, use of drugs blocking angiotensin II responses to minimize proteinuria, hyperglycemia, and so forth. This will require education of the patient and interaction with a skilled dietitian who monitors intake of protein and calories and periodic assessment of the nutritional status of the patient.

DIETARY PROTEIN PRESCRIPTION FOR PRE-ESRD PATIENTS

Based on previous findings, we support the K/DOQI™ recommendations that patients with advanced renal disease (GFR < 25 mL/min), with or without symptoms attributable to uremia or with uncontrolled progressive renal insufficiency, be treated with a well-planned low-protein diet providing 0.6 g protein/kg/day[54] (Table 11–4). For individuals who will not accept such a diet or who are unable to maintain adequate protein-energy intake with such a diet, an intake can be increased up to 0.75 g protein/kg/day. Further increments in protein intake will not only generate more urea but it will also contribute to metabolic acidosis and renal osteodystrophy through hyperphosphatemia. At least 50% of the protein intake for all these patients should be of high biologic value. The diet should be designed by a nutritionist with an interest in the implementation of diets for CRF patients in order to take advantage of a patient's food preferences and to ensure an adequate intake of calories and vitamins, and so forth.

NUTRITIONAL MANAGEMENT OF DIALYSIS PATIENT

Nutritional management in ESRD patients is primarily directed toward prevention and correction of protein-calorie malnutrition. Management should include dietary counseling, adequate dialysis, avoidance of acidemia, and aggressive medical therapy and nutritional support during acute catabolic illnesses.[149,150] Correctly performed nutritional assessment should point out whether the problem is a result of low nutrient intake, poor assimilation, or increased catabolism. The single most decisive factor influencing protein-calorie nutritional status is probably their intake.[150]

DIETARY PROTEIN PRESCRIPTION FOR DIALYSIS PATIENTS

Hemodialysis patients have increased protein and amino acids losses into dialysate (see previous), as well as increased catabolism from the chronic inflammatory state of uremia, acidemia, or the dialysis procedure itself (e.g., exposure to hemodialyzer membranes, tubing, and catheters).[12–14,39] Measurement of nitrogen balance (NB) is the "gold standard" by which

Table 11–4 Recommended Nutrient Intake in Chronic Renal Failure and Dialysis Patients

	Chronic renal failure and renal transplant	End stage renal disease
Protein* (g/kg of ideal body weight)	GFR (mL/min/1.73 m²) >50 No restriction recommended 25-50 0.6 to 0.75 controlled <25 0.6 For early transplant recipient† For nephrotic patient‡	MHD 1.2 CPD 1.2 to 1.3 Revise goals to 1.0 to 1.1 if serum phosphorus difficult to control
Energy (kcal/kg of ideal body weight)	< 60 yrs old ≥35 > 60 yrs old 30 to 35	< 60 yrs old ≥35 > 60 yrs old 30 to 35
Carbohydrates	35% of non-protein calories	35% of non-protein calories
Fat	Polyunsaturated to saturated ratio of 2:1	Polyunsaturated to saturated ratio of 2:1
Phosphorus (mg)	800-1000 No restriction in transplant recipient if serum phosphorus is normal	800-1000 Individualized
Potassium	Individualized	
Sodium and water	As tolerated, to maintain body weight and blood pressure	As tolerated, to maintain body weight and blood pressure

* At least 50% of proteins should be of high biological value.
† Protein intake of 1.3 to 1.5 g/kg/day while on high doses of steroids.
‡ For nephrotic patients, 0.8 g of protein/kg and add 1 g of protein/g of proteinuria.
CPD, chronic peritoneal dialysis; *MHD*, maintenance hemodialysis.

dietary protein requirements are assessed. There have been only a small number of NB studies performed in hemodialysis patients, and most have shortcomings.[151–154] A small number of patients, short periods of observation, patients that were not always in a steady-state, inclusion of acidotic patients, and reliance on dietary histories for measuring nitrogen intake instead of duplicate diet analysis are some of the weaknesses of NB studies in MHD patients.[65] NB measurements reported in CPD patients suffer from similar limitations. Notwithstanding these limitations, the NB studies suggest that the average protein intake necessary to maintain nitrogen balance in hemodialysis patients is about 1.0 to 1.1 g protein/kg/day and 1.05 to 1.1 g protein/kg/day in CPD patients. The K/DOQI™ work group recommended adding 25% to the average protein intake to obtain safe protein intake (Table 11–4). Some experts believe this is too much protein, especially in anuric peritoneal dialysis patients, and likely to lead to hyperphosphatemia.[155]

ENERGY REQUIREMENTS

Few studies have examined the calorie requirements of CRF patients. In pre-dialysis patients, nitrogen balance with a low-protein diet improves when calorie intake rises; the recommended amount is 30 to 35 kcal/kg/day.[159] The same amount is recommended for dialysis patients. It is important to monitor calorie intake since a diet containing too few calories will compromise the patient's ability to achieve nitrogen balance and lead to loss of muscle mass. Unfortunately, there is no simple method of estimating calorie intake so the clinician must rely on repeated measurements of weight and muscle mass plus input from the dietitian.[159]

Dietary Phosphorus

An elevated serum phosphorus or calcium-phosphorus product, and secondary hyperparathyroidism not only causes renal osteodystrophy in dialysis patient but would also result in vascular and visceral calcification, contributing to the increased risk of cardiovascular deaths in ESRD patients.[156] With these concerns in mind, experts recommend that target serum levels should be 9.2 to 9.6 mg/dL for calcium, 2.5 to 5.7 mg/dL for phosphorus, less than 55 mg^2/dL^2 for serum calcium-phosphorus product, and 200 pg/mL for intact PTH.[157,158] Restriction of dietary phosphorus remains the cornerstone of therapy to prevent hyperparathyroidism and the complications of renal osteodystrophy. The recommended phosphorus allowance for a dialysis patient is 800 to 1000 mg/day and similar or a lower intake should be prescribed for pre-dialysis CRF patients.[158,159] Note that even a slightly elevated serum phosphorus level will stimulate parathyroid hormone production so it is important to initiate dietary phosphorus restriction early in the course of renal failure and, if this strategy is insufficient, an oral phosphate-binder will be needed. For patients who have a high serum calcium-phosphorus product, the initial choice should be a noncalcium containing phosphorus binder. If necessary, aluminum hydroxide should be used for only brief periods (especially in dialysis patients) to reduce the risk of aluminum toxicity. When serum calcium is low, calcium based phosphate binders (carbonate or acetate) should be preferred, because they are effective and cheap. For maximum efficacy, the binder should be taken with food.

Dietary Calcium

The tendency for the calcium intake of CRF patients to be inadequate can be aggravated by decreased intestinal calcium absorption linked to vitamin D deficiency. For this reason and because an excess of phosphates in intestinal secretions will bind calcium, the CRF patient requires an intake of 1.5 g calcium/day.[159] Since dairy products (an excellent source of calcium) are invariably restricted to achieve an adequate phosphorus restriction, eating this much calcium can be difficult. Calcium can be given as a phosphate binder, but calcium carbonate requires a more acidic gastric milieu to be effective; calcium acetate is effective even with gastric atrophy. For hemodialysis patients, pulse doses of vitamin D appear to be beneficial in suppressing parathyroid hormone production. Before beginning vitamin D therapy, serum phosphorus and calcium must be within the normal range in order to prevent hypercalcemia and calciphylaxis. Again, dietary education is critical since dietary indiscretion even by patients who are compliant with phosphate binders, leads to a rise in the calcium-phosphorus product, increasing the likelihood of spontaneous precipitation of calcium and phosphorus throughout the body.

Sodium

Control of blood pressure should be a part of any strategy directed at slowing the progression of CRF.[160] It is easy to achieve a recommended 2-g sodium diet when dietary protein is restricted, and it will potentiate the efficacy of antihypertensive medicines.[161] Moreover, in edematous states, it is difficult, if not impossible, to achieve a net loss of sodium (and hence, extracellular volume) with diuretics, unless dietary sodium is restricted. In dialysis patients, dietary sodium restriction is mandatory to minimize the interdialytic weight gain. Without such therapy, blood pressure is difficult to control and there are more intradialytic problems, including hypotensive episodes and cramps. Patients should be urged to monitor their weight as weight gain invariably signifies fluid retention from dietary indiscretion.

Trace Elements and Vitamin Requirements

In uremia there are significant alterations in the blood and tissue concentrations of trace elements and vitamins. These derangements are due to a decrease in glomerular filtration, impaired tubular function and protein binding of micronutrients. In addition, an inadequate diet or altered gastrointestinal absorption in patients with advanced uremia may limit the absorption of trace elements and vitamins. Dialysis can remove micronutrients, depending on their water solubility, membrane permeability and the gradient between the concentration of an element in serum and its concentration in the dialysate. Inadequate removal may lead accumulation and toxicity (e.g., vitamin A), and water-soluble vitamins can be lost during dialysis. The water-soluble vitamin requirements for dialysis patients are not different from healthy adults. Pharmacologic doses of folic acid are recommended for lowering plasma homocysteine levels, but whether this decreases cardiovascular risk in renal patients is yet to be established.[162] Vitamin C intake above 100 mg/day can lead to tissue deposition of oxalate crystals and hastening renal insufficiency and increasing the risk of myocardial infarction, shunt failure, and muscle weakness in dialysis patients. Vitamin A and retinol-binding protein plasma levels are increased in renal patients, so vitamin A containing multivitamin preparations for kidney disease patients should be avoided. There is no evidence that vitamin E reduces risk of cardiovascular events and routine supplementation is not recommended.[163] Patients with kidney disease eating an inadequate diet should take a multivitamin preparation that is formulated specifically for renal patients. For dialysis patients, deficiencies of water-soluble vitamins are common due to vitamin losses in the dialysate, poor oral intake and/or altered metabolism.

In summary, the daily requirements for most trace elements and vitamins in renal patients are quite similar to those of healthy adults (Table 11–5).[164]

NUTRITIONAL CARE OF PATIENTS WITH ACUTE RENAL FAILURE (ARF)

ARF, in association with multiple organ failure, has a very high in-hospital mortality rate averaging 40% to 65%.[165–167] In most cases death is due to underlying illnesses such as sepsis, cardiac failure, or hemorrhage rather than electrolyte disturbances or uremia. Evidence of protein losses is quite prevalent in ARF patients for multiple reasons. The main causes are coexisting catabolic illnesses, dialysis related amino acids and protein losses, reduced nutritional intake and preexisting malnutrition. The predominant feature of hypercatabolism is an increase in skeletal muscle protein breakdown, and the released amino acids are not effectively used for protein synthesis.[168–169] Hepatic uptake of amino acids from the circulation, gluconeogenesis, ureagenesis, and secretion of acute phase proteins are stimulated. Insulin resistance is the major stimulus for decreased protein synthesis and proteolysis. In animal models of uncomplicated ARF, increased muscle protein catabolism and decreased protein synthesis have been documented.[170,171] It is not clear whether increased catabolism is due to uremia or to the associated catabolic illnesses. There is little evidence in humans, that uncomplicated ARF patients have an abnormal nutritional status.[168]

Multiple studies have evaluated the effects of aggressive nutritional supplementation in attempts to reverse malnutrition and improve the prognosis of ARF patients.[172–175] However, the complexity of the disease process has precluded obtaining meaningful and clear-cut results from these clinical studies. Unfortunately, parenteral nutrition in ARF can have significant negative consequences such as fluid overload, mineral and electrolyte disturbances, acid-base disorders, hyperlipidemia, adverse effect of central venous catheter placement and infection, and need for more aggressive dialysis.[168]

Patients with ARF should be closely monitored for changes in nutritional status, and adequate protein and calories are needed. In non-catabolic patients and during the polyuric phase of ARF, a protein intake of 1 g/kg/day is required to achieve a positive nitrogen balance.[176] Larger amounts of dietary proteins will augment the accumulation of unexcreted waste products and prolong the uremic syndrome. A high-protein intake may also stimulate the need for dialysis,

Table 11–5 Comparison of the RDAs for Micronutrients in Healthy Subjects and the Measured Intake by Hemodialysis Patients, with Recommended Intake as the Percent of RDA for ESRD Patients

Micronutrient	RDA in healthy population	Observed intake in HD patients*	Recommended supplement as % of RDA
Zinc	8 mg in women 11 mg in men	N/A	None
Selenium	55 μg	N/A	None
Copper	900 μg	N/A	None
Thiamin	1.1 mg in women 1.2 in men	0.78-2.36 mg	100
Riboflavin	1.1 mg in women 1.3 mg in men	0.69-2.29 mg	100
Folic acid†	400 μg	71-378 μg	200-1000
Vitamin B_6	1.3 mg	0.64-2.14 mg	100
Vitamin B_{12}	2.4 μg	1.2-7.5 μg	100
Vitamin C	75 mg for women 90 mg for men	14-125 mg	120
Vitamin A	700 μg for women 900 μg for men	285-1385 μg	None
Vitamin E‡	15 mg	N/A	None

* Intake from Rocco MV and Makoff R. Seminars in Dialysis 1997; 10:272-277.
† Expressed as dietary folate equivalent.
‡ Represent α-tocopherol from only.
ESRD, end-stage renal disease; *HD*, hemodialysis; *RDA*, recommended dietary allowance.

which can by itself, stimulate protein degradation.[39] The extent of protein catabolism can be estimated from the urea nitrogen appearance and change in urea nitrogen pool.[168] For critically ill ARF patients on continuous renal replacement therapy (CRRT) amino acid/protein intake of 1.4 g/kg/day is recommended; a higher intake was ineffective in further ameliorating nitrogen balance.[169,177] Use of CRRT in catabolic ARF patients allows better fluid control, but the procedure presents additional nutritional challenges. Loss of amino acids and peptides can reach 6 to 15 g/day, depending upon the filtrate volume and/or dialysate flow, activation of inflammatory reaction through blood-membrane contact, loss of micronutrients such as water-soluble vitamins, and electrolyte derangements.[178,179] Hypophosphatemia and hypomagnesemia can develop in critically ill ARF patients who are receiving parenteral nutrition with restricted phosphate and magnesium content, especially if insulin is present. When regional citrate is used for anticoagulation, bicarbonate and/or lactate concentrations must be reduced to avoid inducing metabolic alkalosis. Moreover, serum ionized calcium should be monitored to prevent extreme derangements in serum calcium levels. The energy requirement in uncomplicated ARF is not different from healthy subject, about 25 to 30 kcal/kg/day. Even in hypercatabolic conditions, such as sepsis or multiple organ failure, energy intake should not exceed 35 kcal/kg/day.[169]

In summary, ARF occurring with critical illnesses induces net protein catabolism, primarily through enhanced proteolysis. Studies that have examined aggressive parenteral nutrition therapy in ARF have not provided conclusive evidence of enhanced survival or recovery of renal function with the therapy. Use of CRRT in critically ill ARF patient allows for liberalization of parenteral nutrition support by easier fluid management, though the procedure can increase catabolism and will require monitoring of electrolyte and acid-base status.

NUTRITIONAL ISSUES IN RENAL TRANSPLANT PATIENTS

A successful renal transplant into a patient with ESRD restores near-normal renal function and is expected to correct the nutritional abnormalities arising from uremia. The renal transplant recipient typically experiences a marked improvement of appetite leading to weight gain. Nevertheless, these patients face many nutritional challenges that demand close dietary monitoring. The commonly prescribed immunosuppressives (corticosteroids, calcineurin inhibitors, and sirolimus) are known to induce metabolic side effects such as protein hypercatabolism, hyperlipidemia, glucose intolerance, hyperkalemia, hypophosphatemia, hypomagnesemia, and obesity. The nutritional status after transplant is also determined by preexisting medical conditions such as protein losses, renal osteodystrophy, hyperlipidemia, and cardiovascular disease. Moreover, these patients suffer from declining renal function due to recurrent acute or chronic rejection, varying degree of proteinuria, hypertension, and poorly controlled diabetes. In early stages of the post renal transplant period the nutritional challenge is to counter the metabolic effects of protein hypercatabolism, hyperlipidemia, and hyperglycemia. For the stable transplant recipient, the nutritional status should be optimized, including weight gain, obesity, and lipid control. With a failing graft, nutritional management is similar to CRF pre-dialysis patients.

Dietary Protein and Calorie Prescription for Renal Transplant Patients

Early post-transplantation, there is a marked increase in amino acid and protein catabolism due to the use of large doses of steroids plus surgery related stresses. Patients with preexisting malnutrition are at risk for poor wound healing and susceptibility to infection. Based on these concerns, a dietary protein intake of 1.3 g/kg body weight/day is recommended for the early post renal transplant.[180] However, these recommendations are based on only a few nitrogen balance studies.[181] The optimum dietary protein intake for transplant patients on maintenance immunosuppressive therapy is not well-established. Transplant recipients have been shown to maintain neutral nitrogen balance on low-protein intake of 0.6 g/kg/day as long as their energy intake was maintained at least 28 kcal/kg/day.[182] Recently, results of a 12-year follow-up on renal function of transplant recipients consuming protein intake of 0.8 g/kg/day compared to those taking higher protein intake of 1.4 g/kg/day was reported.[183] Those with the lower protein intake maintained unchanged renal function, whereas patients with the higher protein intake lost more than 40% of excretory efficiency. Based on limited available data, it is reasonable to recommend protein intake of 0.8 g/kg/day along with minimal energy intake of 30 to 35 kcal/kg/day for stable renal transplant patient. Those patients with progressive graft failure should have a more stringent protein intake of 0.6 g/kg/day, because there is evidence that a low-protein diet is also associated with a reduction in proteinuria and decreased activity of renin-angiotensin system.[184] During an acute rejection episode requiring treatment with high doses of corticosteroids, protein catabolism increased, yielding high blood urea nitrogen levels. Protein restriction in such patients can lead to severe negative nitrogen balance, so increasing protein intake to 1.2 g/kg/day is appropriate.

Obesity, defined as body mass index (BMI) of more than 30 kg/m^2 or more than 130% ideal body weight, is present in 12% to 40% of recipients within 1 year after renal transplant.[185,186] Obesity is associated with decreased graft survival and increased prevalence of cardiovascular disease after transplantation.[185,187,188] For stable transplant recipients who require weight reduction, a caloric intake of 25 kcal/kg/day along with appropriate dietary and lifestyle measures, including an exercise program, should be recommended. Weight reduction diets in obese, hyperlipidemic transplant recipients cause a modest reduction in cholesterol levels, although "statin" drugs are usually required.[189] The American Heart Association's "one-step" diet is a reasonable initial approach for hyperlipidemic renal transplant patients. This diet, consisting of less than 300 mg of cholesterol per day (with a goal of less than 250 mg/day), 30% total calories as fat, 50% as carbohydrate, and 20% as protein, is easily attainable and is familiar to renal dietitians.[180]

Dietary Phosphorus and Calcium After Renal Transplantation

Hypercalcemia and low normal serum phosphorus levels can be observed after a successful kidney transplant. These biochemical changes are due to persistent hyperparathyroidism, improved PTH sensitivity and increased 1-hydroxylation of vitamin D.[190,191] The parathyroid-induced increase in renal tubular phosphate leak lowers serum phosphorus levels. A phosphaturic action of steroids must also be considered; an increase in serum phosphorus levels after reduction of steroid doses has been reported.[192]

The major improvement over a patient's pre-transplant renal diet is the liberalization of dietary phosphorus. Nevertheless, oral supplements of phosphates are required for periods of up to 1 year after renal transplant. In the absence of hypercalcemia, calcium intake should be around 1000 to 1500 mg/day by diet and supplements.

In summary, a successful renal transplant allows greater dietary freedom and resultant weight gain. Immunosuppressive medications contribute to the protein hypercatabolism, hyperlipidemia, hyperglycemia, and propensity toward weight gain. Protein requirements are high during the early phase, similar to the requirements of healthy adults. With failing graft function, protein restrictions are reinstituted. Further, maintenance of optimal body weight along with changes in lifestyle measures, including an exercise program, should be part of the nutritional management in all renal transplant recipients.

NUTRITIONAL SUPPORT IN DIALYSIS

Despite an aggressive nutritional approach, some ESRD patients have a steady decline in their nutritional status. Unfortunately, dietary counseling is not always successful to maintain an adequate protein and calorie intake.[193] In these circumstances other forms of nutritional intervention have been considered, including oral supplements and enteral or parenteral feeding. There are many commercially available oral nutrient supplements (Nepro®, Magnacal®, Suplena®, etc.) designed specially for renal patients. Use of oral nutritional supplements by malnourished hemodialysis patients have resulted in improvement of serum albumin and prealbumin levels,[193] an increase in protein catabolic rate,[194] and decreased risk of hospitalization.[195] All of these studies were nonrandomized and included a small, selected group of patients that were followed for 3 to 6 months. Two important limitations to long-term use of oral supplements are: (1) A substantial proportion of patients appear to tire of the supplement and will stop taking them, and (2) Medicare does not reimburse for oral supplements, which, when taken on a daily basis, are expensive.[193]

Enteral feeding through nasogastric or gastric tube is usually prescribed for sick dialysis patients, who are incapacitated by neurologic disorders or debilitating illnesses precluding self or assisted oral feeding. There are no data on the efficacy of this nutritional strategy for the prevention or treatment of malnutrition in adult dialysis patients. Tube feeding has been used successfully for many years to provide nutritional support for infants and children treated by dialysis.[193,196]

Intradialytic parenteral nutrition (IDPN) is the provision of nutrients by infusion into the blood stream during the hemodialysis procedure. The benefit may be an improvement in body weight (primarily excess fluid gain), serum markers of nutrition, and a decrease in mortality rates.[197,198] Foulks[199] reviewed all published literature on IDPN use in MHD patients, utilizing an evidence-based approach, and concluded that the data supporting the use of IDPN are weak and a clear recommendation cannot be made. Recently, Pupim and colleagues[200] examined the influence of IDPN on the protein catabolism caused by dialysis. They found that intravenous nutrition increased protein synthesis and decreased protein degradation but only during the dialysis. After dialysis and IDPN, protein degradation increased again. Thus, the influence of IDPN remains controversial. Moreover, this treatment is expensive and its use is severely restricted with Medicare-imposed strict criteria for reimbursement. A National Kidney Foundation position paper on IDPN use gives explicit guidelines for the use of IDPN.[201]

References

1. U.S. Renal Data Systems: Excerpts from the USRDS 2002 Annual DataReport: Atlas of End-Stage Renal Disease in the United States. Am J Kidney Dis 2003 (suppl 2); 41:S1-S260.
2. Lowrie EG, Lew NL. Death risk in hemodialysis patients: the predictive value of commonly measured variables and evaluation of death rate differences between facilities. Am J Kidney Dis 1990; 15:458.
3. Avram MM, Goldwasser P, Errora M, et al. Predictors of survival in continuous ambulatory peritoneal dialysis patients: the importance of prealbumin and other nutritional and metabolic parameters. Am J Kidney Dis 1994; 23:91.
4. Mitch WE. Malnutrition: a frequent misdiagnosis for hemodialysis patients. J. Clin. Invest 2002; 110:437.
5. Bergstorm J and Lindholm B. What are the causes and consequences of the chronic inflammatory state in chronic dialysis patients? Seminars in Dialysis 2000; 13:163-164.
6. Kaysen GA. Biological basis of hypo-albuminemia in ESRD. J. Am. Soc. Nephrol 1998; 9:2368-2376.
7. Stenvinkle P, Heimburger O, Paultre F, et al. Strong association between malnutrition, inflammation, and atherosclerosis in chronic renal failure. Kidney Int 1999; 55:1899.
8. Bologa RM, Levine DM, Parker TS, et al. Interleukin-6 predicts hypoalbuminemia, hypocholesrolemia, and mortality in hemodialysis patients. Am J Kidney Dis 1998; 32:107-114.
9. Kaysen GA, Dubin JA, Muller HG, Mitch WE, et al. Levels of alpha1 acid glycoprotein and ceruloplasmin predict future albumin levels in hemodialysis patients. Kidney Int 2001; 60:2360.
10. Walser M, Hill S. Can renal replacement be deferred by a supplemented very low protein diet? J Am Soc Nephrol 1999; 10:110.
11. Aparicio M, Chauveau P, De Precigout V, et al. Nutrition and outcome on renal replacement therapy of patients with chronic renal failure treated by a supplemented very low protein diet. J Am Soc Nephrol 2000; 11:708.
12. Qureshi AR, Alverstand A, Danielsson A, et al. Factors predicting malnutrition in hemodialysis patients: a cross-sectional study. Kidney Int 1998; 53:773-782.
13. Pereira BJ, Shapiro L, King AJ, et al. Plasma levels of IL-1 beta, TNF alpha and their specific inhibitors in undialyzed chronic renal failure, CAPD and hemodialysis patients. Kidney Int 1994; 45:890-896.
14. Caglar K, Peng Y, Pupim L. et al. Inflammatory signals associated with hemodialysis. Kidney Int 2002; 62:1408-16.
15. Yeh S-S, Schuster MW. Geriatric cachexia: the role of cytokines. Am J Clin Nutr 1999; 70:183-197.

16. McMurray J, Abdullah I, Dargie H, et al. Increased concentration of tumor necrosis factor in cachetic patients with severe chronic heart failure. Br Heart J 1991; 66:356-358.
17. Tan KB, Chow WS, Tam SC, et al. Atrovastatin lowers C-reactive protein and improves endothelium-dependent vasodilatation in type 2 diabetes mellitus. J Clin Endocrinol Metab 2002; 87: 563-568.
18. Pereira BJ, Shapiro L, King AJ, et al. Plasma levels of IL-1 beta, TNF alpha and their specific inhibitors in undialyzed chronic renal failure, CAPD and hemodialysis patients. Kidney Int. 1994;45:890-6.
19. Hakim RM, Breillatt J, Lazarus JM, et al. Complement activation and hypersensitivity reactions to dialysis membranes. N Engl J Med 1984; 311:878-882.
20. Goodman MN. Tumor necrosis factor induces skeletal muscle protein breakdown in rats. Am. J. Physiol 1991; 260:E727-E730.
21. May RC, Bailey JL, Mitch WE, Masud T,et al. Glucocorticoids and acidosis stimulate protein and amino acid catabolism in vivo. Kidney Int 1996; 49:679-683.
22. Tiao G. et al.1996. Energy-ubiquitin–dependent muscle proteolysis during sepsis in rats is regulated by glucocorticoids. J. Clin. Invest. 97:339-348.
23. Du J, Mitch WE, Wang X, and Price SR. Glucocorticoids induce proteasome C3 subunit expression in L6 muscle cells by opposing the suppression of its transcription by NF-kB. J. Biol. Chem 200; 275:19661-19666.
24. Mitch WE, and Price SR. Transcription factors and muscle cachexia: have we defined a therapeutic target? Lancet 2001; 357:734-735.
25. Hara Y, May RC, Kelly RA, and Mitch WE. Acidosis, not azotemia, stimulates branched-chain amino acid catabolism in uremic rats. Kidney Int 1987; 32:808-814.
26. Bailey JL, Wang X, England BK, et al. The acidosis of chronic renal failure activates muscle proteolysis in rats by augmenting transcription of genes encoding proteins of the ATP-dependent, ubiquitin-proteasome pathway. J. Clin. Invest 1996; 97:1447-1453.
27. Mitch WE, and Goldberg AL. Mechanisms of muscle wasting: the role of the ubiquitin-proteasome system. N. Engl. J. Med 1996; 335:1897-1905.
28. Pickering WP, Price SR, Bircher G, et al. Nutrition in CAPD: serum bicarbonate and the ubiquitin-proteasome system in muscle. Kidney Int 2002; 61:1286-1292.
29. Ballmer PE, McNurlan MA, Hulter HN, et al. Chronic metabolic acidosis decreases albumin synthesis and induces negative nitrogen balance in humans. J. Clin. Invest 1995; 95:39-45.
30. Movilli E, Zani R, Carli,et O, al.1998. Correction of metabolic acidosis increases serum albumin concentration and decreases kinetically evaluated protein intake in hemodialysis patients: a prospective study. Nephrol. Dial. Transplant 1998; 13:1719-1722.
31. Price SR, Bailey J, Wang X, et al. Muscle wasting in insulinopenic rats results from activation of the ATP-dependent, ubiquitin-proteasome pathway by a mechanism including gene transcription. J. Clin. Invest 1996; 98:1703-1708.
32. Mitch WE, Bailey J, Wang X, et al. Evaluation of signals activating ubiquitin-proteasome proteolysis in a model of muscle wasting. Am. J. Physiol 1999; 276:C1132-C1138.
33. Tiao G, Fagan J, Roegner V, et al. Energy-ubiquitin–dependent muscle proteolysis during sepsis in rats is regulated by glucocorticoids. J. Clin. Invest 1996; 97:339-348.
34. Wing SS., and Goldberg AL. Glucocorticoids activate the ATP-ubiquitin–dependent proteolytic system in skeletal muscle during fasting. Am. J. Physiol 1993; 264:E668-E676.
35. DeFronzo RA, Tobin JD, Rowe JW, et al. Glucose intolerance in uremia. J Clin Invest. 1978; 62:425-430.
36. Guiterrez A, Bergstrom J, alvestrand A. Hemodialysis-associated protein catabolism with and without glucose in the dialysis fluid. Kidney Int 1994; 46:814-822.
37. Hakim RM and Lazarus JM. Biochemical parameters in chronic renal failure. Am. J. Kidney Dis 1988; 9:238-247.
38. Anderstam B, Mamoun AH, Bergstrom J, et al. Middle-sized molecule fractions isolated from uremic ultrafiltrate and normal urine inhibit ingestive behavior in the rat. J. Am. Soc. Nephrol 1996; 7:2453-2460.
39. Ikizler TA, Pupim L, Brouillette JR, et al. Hemodialysis stimulates muscle and whole body protein loss and alters substrate oxidation. Am. J. Physiol 2002; 282:E107-E116.
40. Thunberg BJ, Swamy AP, Cestero RVM. Cross-sectional and longitudinal nutritional measurements in maintenance hemodialysis patients. Am J Clin Nutr 1981; 34:2005-2012.
41. Schoenfeld PY, Henry RR, Laird NM, et al. Assessment of nutritional status of the National Cooperative Dialysis Study population. Kidney Int 1983; 23 (suppl 13):80-88.
42. Marckmann P. Nutritional status of patients on hemodialysis and peritoneal dialysis. Clin Nephrol 1998; 29:75-78.
43. Enia G, Sicuso C, Alati G, et al. Subjective global assessment of nutrition in dialysis patients. Nephrol Dial Transplant 1993; 8:1094-1098.
44. Cianciaruso B, Brunori G, Kopple JD, et al. Cross-sectional comparison of malnutrition in continuous ambulatory peritoneal dialysis and hemodialysis patients. Am J Kidney Dis 1995; 26:475-86.
45. Tai TW, Chan AM, Cochran CC, et al. Renal dietitians' perspective: identification, prevalence, and intervention for malnutrition in dialysis patients in Texas. J Ren Nutr 1998; 8:188-98.
46. Mancini A, Grandaliano G, Magarelli P, et al. Nutritional status in hemodialysis patients and bioimpedance vector analysis. J Ren Nutr 2003; 3:199-204.
47. Rocco MV, Paranandi L, Burrowes JD, et al. Nutritional status in the HEMO Study cohort at baseline. Hemodialysis. Am J Kidney Dis 2002; 39:245-56.
48. Bergstörm J. Why are the dialysis patients malnourished? Am J Kidney Dis 1995; 26:229-241.
49. Bergstörm J, Fürst P, Alvestrand A, et al. Protein and energy intake, nitrogen balance and nitrogen losses in patients treated with continous ambulatory peritoneal dialysis. Kidney Int 1993; 44:1048-1057.
50. Lindsay RM, Spanner E. A hypothesis: the protein catabolic rate is dependent upon the type and amount of treatment in dialyzed uremic patients. Am J Kidney Dis 1989; 13:382-389.
51. Goodship THJ, Passlick-Deetjen J, Ward MK, et al.Adequacy of dialysis and nutritional status in CAPD. Nephrol Dial Transplant 1993; 8:1366-1371.
52. Aguilera A, Selgas R, Codoceo R, Bajo A. Uremic Anorexia: A consequence of persistently high brain serotonin levels? The Tryptophan/Serotonin disorder hypothesis. Perit Dial Int 2000; 20:810-816.
53. Slomowitz LA, Monteon FJ, Grosvenor M, et al. Effects of energy intake on nutritional status in maintenance hemodialysis patients. Kidney Int 1989; 35:704:711.
54. National Kidney Foundation: K/DOQI clinical practice guidelines for nutrition in chronic renal failure. Am J Kidney Dis 2000; 6 (suppl 2):S1-S140.
55. Lorenzo V, deBonis E, Rufino M, et al. Caloric rather than protein deficiency predominates in stable chronic hemodialysis patients. Nephrol Dial Transplant 1995; 10:1885-1889.
56. Burrows JD, Larive B, Cockram DB, et al. Effects of dietary intake, appetite, and eating habits on dialysis and non-dialysis days in hemodialysis patients: Cross-sectional results from HEMO study. J Renal Nutr 2003; 13:191-198.
57. Chazot C, Shahmir E, Matias B, et al. Dialytic nutrition: Provision of amino acids in dialysate during hemodialysis. Kidney Int 1997; 52:1663-1670.
58. Wolfson M, Jones MR, Kopple JD. Amino acid losses during hemodialysis with infusion of amino acids and glucose. Kidney Int 1986; 21:500-506.

59. Ikizler TA, Flakoll PJ, Parker RA, Hakim RM. Amino acid and albumin losses during hemodialysis. Kidney Int 1994; 46:830-837.
60. Kopple JD, Swendseid ME, Shinaberger JH, Umezawa CY: The free and bound amino acids removed by hemodialysis. ASAIO Trans 1973 ;19:309-313.
61. Kaplan AA, Halley SE, Lapkin RA, et al. Dialysate protein losses with processed polysulphone dialysers. Kidney Int 1995; 47:573-578.
62. Blumenkrantz MJ, Gahl GM, Kopple JD, Kamdar AV, Jones MR, Kessel M, Coburn JW: Protein losses during peritoneal dialysis. Kidney Int 1981; 19:593-602.
63. Ikizler TA, Hakim RM. Nutrition in end-satge renal disese. Kidney Int 1996; 50:343-357.
64. Kopple JD, Blumenkrantz MJ, Jones MR, et al. Plasma amino acid levels and amino acid losses during continuous ambulatory peritoneal dialysis. Am J Clin Nutr 1982; 36:395-402.
65. Kopple JD. The National Kidney Foundation K/DOQI clinical guidelines for dietary protein intake for chronic dialysis patients. Am J Kidney Dis 2001; 38(Suppl 4):S68-S73.
66. Neyra R, Chen KY, Sun M, et al. Increased resting energy expenditure in patients with end-stage renal disease. J Parenter Enteral Nutr 2003; 27:36-42.
67. Ikizler TA, Wingard RL, Sun M, et al. Increased energy expenditure in hemodialysis patients. J Am Soc Nephrol. 1996; 7:2646-53.
68. Kopple JD. Dietary protein and energy requirements in ESRD patients. Am J Kidney Dis 1998; 32(6 Suppl 4):S97-104.
69. Monteon FJ, Laidlaw SA, Shaib JK, et al. Energy expenditure in patients with chronic renal failure. Kidney Int 1986; 30:741-747.
70. Umeakunne K. Approaches to successful nutrition intervention in renal disease. In Mitch WE, Klahr S (eds)Handbook of Nutrition and Kidney, 4th Ed. Philadelphia: Lippincott Williams and Wilkins, 2002:292-325.
71. Vychytil A, Horl WH. Nutrition and peritoneal dialysis. In Mitch WE, Klahr S (eds)Handbook of Nutrition and Kidney, 4th Ed. Philadelphia: Lippincott Williams and Wilkins, 2002:233-271.
72. Depner TA. Quantification of dialysis. Urea modeling: the basics. Semin Dial 1991; 4:179-184.
73. Depner TA, Cheer A. Modeling urea kinetics with two vs. three BUN measurements. A critical comparison. J ASAIO Trans 1989; 35:499-502.
74. National Kidney Foundation. K/DOQI clinical practice guidelines for hemodialysis adequacy. Am J Kidney Dis 2000; 37:S15-S26.
75. Depner TA, Daugirdas JT. Equations for normalized protein catabolic rate based on two-point modeling of hemodialysis urea kinetics. J Am Soc Nephrol 1996; 7:780-785.
76. Bergstorm J, Heimburger O, Lindholm B. Calculation of the protein equivalent of total nitrogen appearance and total nitrogen appearance in chronic renal failure and CAPD patients. Which formula should be used? Perit Dial Int 1998; 18: 467-473.
77. Randerson DH, Chapman GV, FarrellPC. Amino acids and dietary status in CAPD patients, in Atkins RC, Thomson NM, Farrell PC (eds). Peritoneal Dialysis. Edinburough, UK, Churchill Livingstone 1981; pp 179-191.
78. Panzetta G, Tessitore N, Faccini G, et al. The protein catabolic rate as a measure of protein intake in dialysis patients: Usefulness and limits. Nephrol Dial Transplant 1990; 5(suppl 1): S125-S127.
79. Mittman N, Avram MM, Oo KK, et al. Serum prealbimin predicts survival in hemodialysis and peritoneal dialysis: 10 Years of propective observation. Am J Kidney Dis 2001; 38;1358-1364.
80. Neyra NR, Hakim RM, Shyr Y, et al. J Renal Nutr 2000; 10:184-190.
81. Cano N, Di Costanzo-Dufetel J, Calaf R, et al. Prealbumin-retinal-binding-protein-retinol complex in hemodialysis patients. Am J Clin Nutr 1988; 47:664-667.
82. Kopple JD, Swendseid ME. Protein and amino acid metabolism in uremic patients undergoing maintenance hemodialysis. Kidney Int Suppl 1975;2:S64-72.
83. Graham KA, Reaich D, Channon SM, et al. Correction of acidosis in hemodialysis decreases whole-body protein degradation. J Am Soc Nephrol. 1997; 8:632-637.
84. Uribarri J. Moderate metaboic acidosis and its effects on nutritional parameters in hemodialysis patients. Clin Nephrol 1997; 48:238-240.
85. Kirschbaum BB, Spurious Metabolic Acidosis in hemodialysis patients. Am J Kidney Dis 2000; 35:1068-1071.
86. Stein A, Moorhouse J, Iles-Smith H, et al. Role of an improvement in acid-base stats and nutrition in CAPD patietns. Kidney Int 1997; 52:1089-1095.
87. Szeto CC, Wong TY, Chow KM, et al. Oral sodium bicarbonate for the treatment of metabolic acidosis in peritoneal dialysis patients: a randomized placebo-control trial. J Am Soc Nephrol. 2003;14:2119-26.
88. Duerksen DR, Papineau N. Electrolyte abnormalities in patients with chronic renal failure receiving parenteral nutrition. J Parenter Enteral Nutr 1998; 22:102-4.
89. Newman LN, Weiss MF, Berger J, et al. The law of unintended consequences in action: increase in incidence of hypokalemia with improved adequacy of dialysis. Adv Perit Dial. 2000;16:134-7.
90. Blumenkrantz MJ, Kopple JD, Gutman RA, et al. Methods for assessing nutritional status of patients with renal failure. Am J Clin Nutr 1980; 33:1567-1585.
91. Borovnicar DJ, Wong KC, Kerr PG, et al. Total body protein status assessed by different estimates of fat-free mass in adult peritonea dialysis patients. Eur J Clin Nutr 1996; 50:607-616.
92. Avram MM, Bonomini LV, Sreedhara R, et al. Predictive value of nutritional markers (albumin, creatinine, cholesterol, and hematocrit) for patients on dialysis for up to 30 years. Am J Kidney Dis. 1996; 28:910-7.
93. Hans DS, Lee SW, Kang SW, et al. Factors affecting low values of serum albumin in CAPD patients. Adv Perit Dial 1996; 12:288-292.
94. Goldwasser P, Kaldas AI, Barth RH. Rise in serum albumin and creatinine in the first half year on hemodialysis. Kidney Int. 1999; 56:2260-8.
95. Lowrie EG, Haung WH, Lew NL. Death risk predictors among peritoneal and hemodialysis patients. A preliminary comparison. Am J Kidney Dis 1995; 26:220-228.
96. Avram MM, Mittman N, Bonomini L, et al. Markers for survival in dialysis.: A seven-year prospective study. Am J Kidney Dis 1995; 26:209-219.
97. Iseki K, Miyasato F, Tokuyama K, et al. Low diastolic blood pressure, hypoalbuminemia, and risk of death in a cohort of chronic hemodialysis patients. Kidney Int 1997; 51:1212-1217.
98. Piccoli GB, Quarello F, Salomone M, et al. Are serum albumin and cholesterol reliable outcome markers in elderly dialysis patients? Nephrol Dial Transplant 1995; 10(suppl 6):S72-S75.
99. Port FK, Ashby VB, Dhingra RK, et al. Dialysis dose and body mass index are strongly associated with survival in hemodialysis patients. J Am Soc Nephrol. 2002;13:1061-6.
100. Leavey SF, McCullough K, Hecking E, et al. Body mass index and mortality in 'healthier' as compared with 'sicker' haemodialysis patients: results from the Dialysis Outcomes and Practice Patterns Study (DOPPS). Nephrol Dial Transplant. 2001; 16:2386-94.
101. Wolfe RA, Ashby VB, Daugirdas JT, et al. Body size, dose of hemodialysis, and mortality. Am J Kidney Dis. 2000; 35:80-8.
102. Nelson EE, Hong CD, Pesce AL, et el. Anthropometric norms for the dialysis patient population. Am J Kidney Dis 1990; 16:32-37.
103. Chumlea WC, Dwyer J, Bergen C, et al. Nutritional status assessed from anthropometric measures in the HEMO study. J Renal Nutr 2003; 13:31-38.

104. Allon M, Depner TA, Radeva M, et al. Impact of dialysis dose and membrane on infection-related hospitalization and death: results of the HEMO Study. J Am Soc Nephrol. 2003; 14:1863-70.
105. Keshaviah P. Lean body mass estimation by creatinine kinetics. J Am Soc Nephrol 1994; 4:1475-1485.
106. Bhatla B, Moore H, Emerson P, et al. Lean body mass estimation by creatinine kinetics, bioimpedence, dual energy x-ray absorptiometry in patients on continuous ambulatory peritoneal dialysis. ASAIO J 1995; 41:M442-M446.
107. Szeto CC, Kong J, Wu AKL, et al. The role of lean body mass as a nutritional index in chinese peritoneal dialysis patients-comparison of creatinine kinetics method and anthrpometric method. Perit Dial Int 2000; 20:708-714.
108. Johansson AC, Attmen PO. Haraldsson B. Creatinine generation rate and lean body mass: a critical analysis in peritoneal dialysis patients. Kidney Int 1997; 51:855-859.
109. Heimburger O, Qureshi AR, Blaner WS, et al. Hand-grip muscle strength, lean body mass, and plasma proteins as markers of nutritional status in patients with chronic renal failure close to start of dialysis therapy. Am J Kidney Dis 2000; 36:1213-1225.
110. Young GA, Kopple JD, Lindholm B, et al: Nutritional assessment of continuous ambulatory peritoneal dialysis patients: An international study. Am J Kidney Dis 1991; 17:462-471.
111. Enia G, Sicuso C, Alati G, Zoccali C. Subjective global assessment of nutrition in dialysis patients. Nephrol Dial Transplant 1993; 8:1094-1098.
112. McCusker FX, Teehan BP, Thorpe KE, et al. How much peritoneal dialysis is required for the maintenance of a good nutritional state? Canada-USA (CANUSA) Peritoneal Dialysis Study Group. Kidney Int 1996; 50 (suppl56):S56-S61.
113. Cooper BA, Bartlett LH, Aslani A, et al. Validity of subjective global assessment as a nutritional marker in end-stage renal disease. Am J Kidney Dis. 2002; 40:126-32.
114. Goldstein-Fuchs DJ. Assesment of nutritional status in renal diseases. In Mitch WE, Klahr S (eds)Handbook of Nutrition and Kidney, 4th Ed. Philadelphia: Lippincott Williams and Wilkins, 2002:233-271.
115. Maroni BJ, Mitch WE. Role of nutrition in prevention of the progression of renal disease. Ann Rev Nutr 1997; 17:435-455.
116. Brouhard BH, LaGrone L. Effect of dietary protein restriction on functional renal reserve in diabetic nephropathy. Am J Med 1990; 89:427-431.
117. Zeller KR, Whittaker E, Sullivan L, Raskin P, Jacobson HR. Effect of restricting dietary protein on the progression of renal failure in patients with insulin-dependent diabetes mellitus. N Engl J Med 1991; 324:78-83.
118. Dullaart RP, Beusekamp BJ, Meijer S, van Doormaal JJ, Sluiter WJ. Long-term effects of protein-restricted diet on albuminuria and renal function in IDDM patients without clinical nephropathy and hypertension. Diabetes Care 1993; 16:483-492.
119. Raal FJ, Kalk WJ, Lawson M, Esser JD, Buys R, Fourie L et al. Effect of moderate dietary protein restriction on the progression of overt diabetic nephropathy: A 6-mo prospective study. Am J Clin Nutr 1994; 60:579-585.
120. Fouque D, Laville M, Boissel JP, Chifflet R, Labeeuw M, Zech PY. Controlled low protein diets in chronic renal insufficiency: meta-analysis. Br Med J 1992; 304:216-220.
121. Pedrini MT, Levey AS, Lau J, Chalmers TC, Wang PH. The effect of dietary protein restriction on the progression of diabetic and nondiabetic renal diseases: A meta-analysis. Ann Intern Med 1996; 124:627-632.
122. Fouque D, Wang P, Laville M, Boissel JP. Low protein diets delay end-stage renal disease in non diabetic adults with chronic renal failure. Nephrol Dial Transpl 2000; 15:1986-1992.
123. Klahr S, Levey AS, Beck GJ, Caggiula AW, Hunsicker LJ, Kusek JW et al. The effects of dietary protein restriction and blood-pressure control on the progression of chronic renal failure. N Engl J Med 1994; 330:878-884.
124. Levey AS, Adler S, Caggiula AW, England BK, Greene T, Hunsicker LG et al. Effects of dietary protein restriction on the progression of advanced renal disease in the Modification of Diet in Renal Disease Study. Am J Kid Dis 1996; 27:652-663.
125. Taal MW, Brenner BM. Renoprotective benefits of RAS inhibition: From ACEI to antiotensin II antagonists. Kidney Int 2000; 57:1803-1817.
126. DCCT Research Group. Effect of intensive therapy on the development and progression of diabetic nephropathy in the Diabetes Control and Complications Trial. Kidney Int 1995; 47:1703-1720.
127. Donadio JV, Bergstralh EJ, Offord KP, Spencer DC, Holley KE. A controlled trial of fish oil in IgA nephropathy. N Engl J Med 1994; 331:1194-1199.
128. Ikizler TA, Greene JH, Wingard RL, et al. Spontaneous dietary protein intake during progression of chronic renal failure. J Am Soc Nephrol 1995; 6:1386 1391.
129. Hakim RM & Lazarus JM: Initiation of dialysis. J Am Soc Nephrol 1995; 6:1319 1320.
130. Lowrie EG & Lew NL: Death risk in hemodialysis patients: The predictive value of commonly measured variables and an evaluation of the death rate differences among facilities. Am J Kidney Dis. 1990; 15:458 482.
131. Kaysen GA: Biological basis of hypoalbuminemia in ESRD. J Am Soc Nephrol 1998; 9:2368-2376.
132. Walser M: Does prolonged protein restriction preceding dialysis lead to protein malnutrition at the onset of dialysis? Kidney Int 1993; 44:1139-1144.
133. Aparicio M, Chauveau P, Precigout VD, et al. Nutrition and outcome on renal replacement therapy of patients with chronic renal failure treated by a supplemented very low protein diet. J Am Soc Nephrol 2000; 11:708-716.
134. Coresh J, Walser M, Hill S: Survival on dialysis among chronic renal failure patients treated with a supplemented low-protein diet before dialysis. J Am Soc Nephrol 1995; 6:1379-1385.
135. Masud T, Young VR, Chapman T, Maroni BJ: Adaptive responses to very low protein diets: The first comparison of ketoacids to essential amino acids. Kidney Int 45:1182-1192.
136. Tom K, Young VR, Chapman T, Masud T, Akpele L, Maroni BJ: Long-term adaptive responses to dietary protein restriction in chronic renal failure. Am J Physiol 1995; 268:E668-E677.
137. Bernhard J, Beaufrere B, Laville M, Fouque D. Adaptive response to a low-protein diet in predialysis chronic renal failure patients. J Am Soc Nephrol. 2001; 12:1249-54.
138. Vendrely B, Chauveau P, Barthe N, et al. Nutrition in hemodialysis patients previously on a supplemented very low protein diet. Kidney Int 2003; 63:1491-1498.
139. National Kidney Foundation. K/DOQI Clinical Practice Guidelines For Peritoneal Dialysis Adequacy. Am J Kidney Dis 2000; 37:S65-S136.
140. Pollock CA. Protein intake in renal disease. J Am Soc Nephrol 1997; 8:777-783.
141. Churchill DN, Taylor DW, Keshaviah PR, et al. Adequacy of dialysis and nutrition in continuous peritoneal dialysis: Association with clinical outcomes. J Am Soc Nephrol 1996; 7:198-207.
142. Bonmini V, Feletti C, Scolari MP, et al. Benefits of early initiation of dialysis. Kidney Int 1985; 28 (Suppl 17):S57-S59.
143. Bergman JM, thorpe KE, Churchill DN. Relative contribution of residual renal function and peritoneal clearance to adequacy of dialysis: a reanalysis of the CANUSA study. J Am Soc Nephrol 2001; 12:2158-2162.
144. Termorshuizen F, Korevaar JC, Dekker FW, et al. The relative importance of residual renal function compared with peritoneal clearance for patient survival and quality of life: An analysis of the netherlands cooperative study on the adequacy of dialysis (Necosad)-2. Am J Kidney Dis. 2003; 41: 1293-1302.

145. Korevaar JC, Jansen M, Dekker FW, et al. When to initiate dialysis: effect of proposed US guidelines on survival. Lancet 2001; 358:1046-1050.
146. Traynor JP, Simpson K, Geddes C, et al. Early Initiation of Dialysis Fails to Prolong Survival in Patients with End-Stage Renal Failure. J Am Soc Nephrol 2002; 13:2125-2132.
147. Beddhu S, Samove MH, Roberts MS, Stoddard GL, Ramkinmar N, Pappas LM, Cheung AK. Impact of timing of initiation of dialysis on mortality. J Am Soc Nephrol 2003; 14:2305-2312.
148. Korevaar JC, Jansen MAM, Dekker FW, et al. Evaluation of DOQI guidelines: early start of dialysis treatment is not associated with better health-related quality of life. Am J Kidney Dis. 2002; 39:108-15.
149. Mitch WE. Mechanisms causing loss of lean body mass in kidney disease. Am J Clin Nutr 1998; 67:359-365.
150. Kopple JD. Therapeutic approaches to malnutrition in chronic dialysis patients: The different modalities of nutritional support. Am J Kidney Dis. 1999; 33:180-185.
151. Ginn H, Frost A, Lacy W: Nitrogen balance in hemodialysis patients. Amer J Clin Nutr 1968; 21:385-393.
152. Borah M, Schoenfeld PY, Gotch FA, et al. Nitrogen balance in intermittent hemodialysis therapy. Kidney Int 1978; 14:491-500.
153. Ikizler TA, Greene JH, Yenicesu M, Schulman G, Wingard RL, Hakim RM: Nitrogen balance in hospitalized chronic hemodialysis patients. Kidney Int 1996; 50(suppl 57):S53-S56.
154. Rao M, Sharma M, Juneja R, et al. Calculated nitrogen balance in hemodialysis patients: Influence of protein intake. Kidney Int 2000; 58:336-345.
155. Uribarri J. DOQI guidelines for nutrition in long-term peritoneal dialysis patient: A dissenting view. Am J Kidney Dis 2001; 37:1313-1318.
156. Ganesh SK, Stack AG, Levin NW, et al. Association of elevated serum PO_4, CA X PO_4 product, and parathyroid hormone with cardiac mortality risk in chronic hemodialysis patients. J Am Soc Nephrol 2001; 12:2131-2138.
157. Block GA, Port FK. Re-evaluation of risks associated with hyperphosphatemia and hyperparathyroidism in dialysis patients: Recommendations for a change in management. Am J Kidney Dis 2000; 35:1226-1237.
158. National Kidney Foundation. K/DOQI guidelines for Bone Metabolism and Diseases in Chronic Kidne Disease. Am J Kidney 2003; 42(suppl3):S62-S83.
159. Maroni BJ. Requirements for protein, calories, and fat in the predialysis patient. In: Mitch WE, Klahr S, editors. Handbook of Nutrition and the Kidney. 3nd ed, p 144-165. Philadelphia, Lippincott-Raven., 1998.
160. Klahr S, Levey AS, Beck GJ, Caggiula AW, Hunsicker LJ, Kusek JW, et al. The effects of dietary protein restriction and blood-pressure control on the progression of chronic renal failure. N Engl J Med 1994; 330:878-884.
161. Mitch WE, Wilcox CS. Disorders of body fluids, sodium and potassium in chronic renal failure. Am J Med 1982; 72:536-550.
162. Westhuzen J. Folate supplementation in the dialysis patient-fragmantary evidence and tentative recommendations. Nephron Dial Transplant 1998, 13:2748-2750.
163. Yousuf S, Dagenais G, Pogue et el. Vitamin E supplementation and cardiovascular events in high-risk patients. The Heart Oucome Prevention Evaluation Study Inveestigators. N Engl J Med 2000, 342:154-160.
164. Masud T. Trace elements and vitamins in renal disease. In: Mitch WE, Klahr S (eds). Handbook of Nutrition and the Kidney. 4th ed,. Philadelphia, Lippincott Williams and Wilkins 2002; 233-252.
165. Chertow GM, Christiansen CL, Cleary PD, etal. Prognostic stratification in critically ill patients whith acute renal failure requiring dialysis. Arch Intern Med 1995; 155: 1505-1511.
166. Brivet FG, Kleinknecht DJ, Loirat P, et al. and The French Study Group on Acute Renal Failure Acute renal failure in intensive care units. Causes, outcome and prognostic factors of hospital mortality; a prospective, multicenter study. Crit Care Med 1996; 24: 192-198
167. Tonelli M, Manns B, Feller-Kopman D. Acute renal failure in the intensive care unit: a systematic review of the impact of dialytic modality on mortality and renal recovery. Am J Kidney Dis. 2002; 40:875-885.
168. Sponsel H, Conger JD. Is parenteral nutrition therapy of value in acute renal failure? Am J Kidney Dis 1995; 25:96-102.
169. Druml W. Nutritional management of acute renal failure. Am J Kidney Dis. 2001; 37(Suppl 2):S89-S94.
170. Mitch WE. Amino acid release from the hindquarter and urea appearance in acute uremia. Am J Physiol 1981; 241:E415-E419.
171. Salusky I, Flugel-Link R, Jones M, et al. Effect of acute uremia on protein degradation and amino acid release in the rat hemicorpus. Kidney Int 1983; 24(Suppl 16):S43-S47.
172. Abel R, Beck C, Abbot W, et al. Improved survival from acute renal failure after treatment with intravenous essential a-amino acids and glucose. N Engl J Med 1973; 288:695-699.
173. Baek S, Makaboli G, Bryan-Brown C, et al. The influence of parenteral nutrition on the course of acute renal failure. Surg Gynecol Obstet 1975; 141:405-408.
174. Pelosi G, Proitti R, Arcangeli A, et al. Total parenteral infusate, an approach to its optimal composition in post trauma acute renal failure. Resuscitation 1981; 9:45-51.
175. Fienstein EI, Blumenbrantz M, Healy M, et al. Clinical and metabolic responses to parenteral nutroition in acute renal failure. Medicine 1981; 60:124-137.
176. Druml W. Nutritional support in acute renal failure. In Mitch WE, Klahr S (eds)Handbook of Nutrition and Kidney, 4th Ed. Philadelphia: Lippincott Williams and Wilkins, 2002:273-291.
177. Macias WL, Alaka KJ, Murphy MH, et al. Impact of nutritional regimen on protein catabolism and nitrogn balance in patients with acute renal failure. J Parenter Enteral Nutr 1996; 20:56-62.
178. Davies SP, Reaveley DA, Brown EA, Kox WJ. Amino acid clearances and daily losses in patients with acute renal failure treated by continuous arteriovenous hemodialysis. Crit Care Med 1991; 19:1510-1515.
179. Davenport A, Roberts NB. Amino acid losses during continuous high-flux hemofiltration in the critically ill patient. Crit Care Med 1989, 17:1010-1015.
180. Bertolatus JA. Nutritional requirements of renal transplant patients. In Mitch WE, Klahr S (eds)Handbook of Nutrition and Kidney, 4th Ed. Philadelphia: Lippincott Williams and Wilkins, 2002:273-291.
181. Whittier FC, Evans DH, Dutton S. Nutrition in renal transplantation. Am J Kidney Dis 1985; 6:405-411.
182. Windus DW, Lacson S, Delmez JA. The short-term effects of a low-protein diet in stable renal transplant recipients. Am J Kidney Dis. 1991; 17:693-9.
183. Bernardi A, Biasia F, Pati T, et al. Long-term protein intake control in kidney transplant recipients: effect in kidney graft function and in nutritional status. Am J Kidney Dis. 2003, 41 (3 Suppl 1):S146-52.
184. Salahudeen AK, Hostetter TH, Raatz SK, et al. Effects of dietary protein in patients with chronic renal transplant rejection. Kidney Int. 1992; 41:183-90.
185. Johnson DW, Isbel NM, Brown AM, et al. The effect of obesity on renal transplant outcomes. Transplantation 2002; 74:675-81.
186. Baum CL, Thielke K, Westin E, et al. Predictors of weight gain and cardiovascular risk in a cohort of racially diverse kidney transplant recipients. Nutrition 2002;18:139-46.
187. EBPG Expert Group on Renal Transplantation. European best practice guidelines for renal transplantation. Section IV: Long-term management of the transplant recipient. IV.5.7.

Cardiovascular risks. Obesity and weight gain. Nephrol Dial Transplant 2002;17(Suppl 4):29-30.

188. Meier-Kriesche HU, Arndorfer JA, et al. The impact of body mass index on renal transplant outcomes: a significant independent risk factor for graft failure and patient death. Transplantation 2002; 73:70-4.

189. Moore RA, Callahan MF, Cody M, et al. The effect of the American Heart Association step one diet on hyperlipidemia following renal transplantation. Transplantation 1990;49:60-2.

190. Caravaca F, Fernandez MA, Ruiz-Calero R, et al. Effects of oral phosphorus supplementation on mineral metabolism of renal transplant recipients. Nephrol Dial Transplant 1998; 13:2605-11.

191. Reinhardt W, Bartelworth H, Jockenhovel F, et al. Sequential changes of biochemical bone parameters after kidney transplantation. Nephrol Dial Transplant 1998;13:436-42.

192. Higgins RM, Richardson AJ, Endre ZH, et al. Hypophosphatemia after renal transplantation: relationship to immunosuppressive drug therapy and effects on muscle detected by 31P nuclear magnetic resonance spectroscopy. Nephrol Dial Transplant 1990; 5:62-68.

193. Caglar K, Fedje L, Dimmitt R, Hakim RM, et al. Therapeutic effects of oral nutritional supplementation during hemodialysis. Kidney Int. 2002; 62:1054-1059.

194. Pate MG, Kitchen S, Miligan PJ. The effect of dietary supplements on the nPCR in stable hemodialysis patient. J Renal Nutr. 2000; 10:69-75.

195. Stieber AL, Handu DJ, Cataline Dr, et al. The impact of nutrition intervention on a reliable morbidity and mortality indicator: the hemodialysis-prognostic nutrition index. J Renal Nutr. 2003; 13:186-190.

196. Kuizon BD, Nelson PA, Salusky IB. Tube feeding in children with end-stage renal disease. Miner Electrolyte Metab 1997; 23: 306-310.

197. Cherry N, Shalansky K. Efficacy of intradialytic parenteral nutrition in malnourished hemodialysis patients. Am J Health Sys Pharm. 2002; 15:1736-1741.

198. Capelli JP, Kushner H, Camiscioli TC, et al. Effect of intradialytic parenteral nutrition on mortality rates in end-stage renal disease care. Am J Kidney Dis. 1994 ; 23:808-16.

199. Foulks C. An evidence-based evaluation of intradialytic parenteral nutrition. Am J Kidney Dis 1999; 33:186-192.

200. Pupim LB, Flakoll PJ, Brouillette JR, et al. Intradialytic parenteral nutrition improves protein and energy homeostasis in chronic hemodialysis patients. J Clin Invest 2002;110:483-92.

201. Kopple JD, Foulks CJ, Piraino B, et al. Proposed Health Care Financing Administration guidelines for reimbursement of enteral and parenteral nutrition. Am J Kidney Dis. 1995; 26:995-997.

202. Lukaski HC. Validation of body composition assessment techniques in the dialysis population. ASAIO J. 1997;43(3): 251-5.

203. Dumler F, Kilates C. Body composition analysis by bioelectrical impedance in chronic maintenance dialysis patients: comparisons to the National Health and Nutrition Examination Survey III. J Ren Nutr. 2003;13:166-72.

204. Dumler F, Kilates C. Use of bioelectrical impedance techniques for monitoring nutritional status in patients on maintenance dialysis. J Ren Nutr. 2000; 10:116-24.

205. Stenver DI, Gotfredsen A, Hilsted J, et al. Body composition in hemodialysis patients measured by dual-energy X-ray absorptiometry. Am J Nephrol. 1995; 15:105-10.

206. Konings CJ, Kooman JP, Schonck M, et al. Influence of fluid status on techniques used to assess body composition in peritoneal dialysis patients. Perit Dial Int. 2003; 23:184-90.

207. Stall S, DeVita MV, Ginsberg NS, et al. Body composition assessed by neutron activation analysis in dialysis patients. Ann N Y Acad Sci. 2000; 904:558-63.

208. Cooper BA, Aslani A, Ryan M, et al. Comparing different methods of assessing body composition in end-stage renal failure. Kidney Int. 2000; 58:408-16.

209. Kamyar Kalantar-Zadeh, Gladys Block, et al. Near infra-red interactance for longitudinal assessment of nutrition in dialysis patients. J Ren Nutr 2001; 11:23-31.

210. Junger P, Chauveau P, Ployard F et al: Comparison of ketoacids and low protein diet on advanced chronic renal failure progression. Kidney Int 1987; 32(suppl 22):S67-S71.

211. Bergstörm J, Alvestrand A, Bucht H et al: Stockholm clinical study on progression of chronic renal failure_An interim report. Kidney Int 1989; 36(suppl 27):S110-S114.

212. Ihle BU, Becker GJ, Whitworth JA et al: The effect of protein restriction on the progression of renal insufficiency. N Engl J Med 1989; 321:1773-1777.

213. Rosman JB, Langer K, Brandl M et al: Protein-restricted diets in chronic renal failure: A four year follow-up shows limited indications. Kidney Int 1989; 27;S96-S102.

214. Locatelli F, Alberti D, Graziani G et al: Propective randomized, multicentre trial of effect of protein restriction on progression of chronic renal insufficiency. North Italian Cooperative Study Group. Lancet 1991; 337:1299-1304.

215. Williams PS, Stevens ME, Fass G et al: Failure of dietary protein and phosphate restriction to retard the rate of progression of chronic renal failure: A prospective, randomized, controlled trial. Q J Med 1991; 81:837-855.

216. D'Amico G, Gentile MG, Fellin G et al: Effect of dietary protein restriction on the progression of renal failure: A prospective randomized trial. Nephrol Dial Transplant 1994; 9:1590-1594.

Inflammation in Chronic Kidney Disease

Madhumathi Rao, M.D., F.R.C.P. (U.K.) • Vaidyanathapuram S. Balakrishnan, M.D., M.R.C.P.

The last two decades have seen a rapid evolution in our understanding of the mechanisms underlying the various consequences of the uremic state. Our perception has advanced to include not only the uremic milieu and uremic toxins, but an inflammatory micro-environment that impacts a wide variety of organ systems and physiologic pathways. The "interleukin hypothesis" was proposed in 1983, incriminating interleukin-1 (IL-1) produced during dialysis as the cause of hypotension, fever, and other acute phase responses observed in patients on dialysis.[1] This ushered in an era of study of the role of cytokines as orchestrators of not only acute intradialytic complications, but of the acute phase response and the chronic inflammatory state that exists in patients with chronic kidney disease.

CYTOKINES AND THE ACUTE PHASE RESPONSE

The early observations of endogenous pyrogen (Interleukin-2 [IL-2]), the fever-causing molecule produced by inflammatory cells,[2] and of macrophage migration inhibiting substances produced by lymphocytes upon exposure to antigen,[3,4] led to an awareness of a complex network of cytokines regulating a wide variety of inflammatory and immune responses. Cytokines are polypeptides with a molecular weight of 10 to 45 kDa, with autocrine and paracrine actions. They are highly potent, active at picomolar and femtomolar concentrations, and are synthesized and secreted in response to cellular injury, mainly by—although not restricted to—mononuclear cells, including monocyte-macrophage cell populations and lymphocytes and neutrophils. Cytokines fall into five broad classes according to their salient biologic properties (Table 12–1).[5] Among these categories, the pro- and anti-inflammatory cytokines may be considered the most significant in mediating chronic inflammation in disease states.

The acute phase response is the systemic response to tissue injury and has an important adaptive and defensive role. A more narrow characterization that has emerged in recent years refers to the changes in concentration of a number of plasma proteins, mediated by cytokines produced in response to tissue injury. By definition, the plasma concentration of these acute-phase reactants (APRs) increases (positive APRs) or decreases (negative APRs) by at least 25% during acute inflammation.[6] The most striking increases are seen in levels of C-reactive protein (CRP) and serum amyloid A (SAA), with a 1000-fold or greater rise within a few days of a stimulus. In contrast, some plasma proteins, such as albumin and transferrin, consistently demonstrate a reduction in plasma concentration and therefore represent the "negative" APRs. Although most APRs are synthesized by hepatocytes, some are produced by other cell types, including monocytes, endothelial cells, fibroblasts, and adipocytes.

The acute phase response, including elevated levels of CRP, reflects the generation of pro-inflammatory cytokines. These include interleukin-6 (IL-6), interleukin-1β (IL-1β), tumor necrosis factor-α (TNF-α), to a lesser extent, interferon-χ, transforming growth factor-β1 (TGF-β1), and possibly interleukin-8 (IL-8). Cytokines operate both as a cascade and as a network, regulating the production of other cytokines and their receptors. The expression of genes for APRs is regulated mainly at the transcriptional level, but post-transcriptional and post-translational mechanisms also participate.[7,8]

The acute phase response is physiologically transient, but chronic inflammatory states are characterized by ongoing tissue injury that provides the repetitive stimuli for cytokine release and persistence of the acute phase response. This is true of the classic inflammatory arthritides, such as rheumatoid arthritis, other collagen vascular diseases, inflammatory bowel disease, chronic infections, and some cancers; a growing body of evidence now places chronic kidney disease (CKD) and end-stage renal disease (ESRD) in the same context. This persistent state of systemic inflammation that represents a sustained activation of the innate immune response presents with systemic manifestations, such as fever, anorexia, fatigue, and lethargy, that characterize many chronic inflammatory illnesses, including CKD. In addition, inflammation associated cytokines mediate the pathogenesis of the anemia of chronic disease and cachexia. Notably, over the last two decades research has established atherosclerosis as an inflammatory process, a concept that takes on additional significance with the observation that cardiovascular disease (CVD) is the most frequent cause of death in patients with CKD of any degree of severity. Cytokine production is also believed to play a role in the bone disease and immune dysfunction seen among uremic patients.

THE CHRONIC INFLAMMATORY STATE IN PATIENTS WITH CHRONIC KIDNEY DISEASE—THE EVOLUTION OF A CONCEPT

Mononuclear cell activation and cytokine production are well-known consequences of blood-dialyzer interactions. The interleukin hypothesis and subsequent research signified that release of pro-inflammatory cytokines was a critical mediator of acute intra-dialytic manifestations in hemodialysis patients. The extent of mononuclear cell activation is dependent on the dialyzer material used and is considered an

Table 12–1 Cytokine Classification

Class of Cytokine	Prototypical Members
Pro-inflammatory cytokines	IL-1, IL-6, TNF-α
Anti-inflammatory cytokines	IL-10
Lymphocyte growth and differentiation factors	IL-2, IL-4, IFN-χ
Hematopoietic colony-stimulating factors	G-CSF, GM-CSF, M-CSF
Mesenchymal cell growth factors	TGF-β1

index of biocompatibility. However, the recognition that the chronic morbidity of renal failure may be a function of a chronic inflammatory process, likely stemmed from the observation that a low serum albumin was one of the most powerful associates of mortality. This observation, borne by several large cross-sectional studies in dialysis patients in the late 1980s, identified hypoalbuminemia as both a marker of the malnourished state and an independent predictor of mortality.[9, 10] Originally attributed to protein-calorie malnutrition and uremic toxicity, it became increasingly clear that a simple deficiency of dietary protein intake, or underdialysis, was insufficient to explain the decline in serum albumin seen in dialysis patients. In addition, interventions such as intradialytic parenteral nutrition have failed to uniformly correct hypoalbuminemia.[11]

Thus, the notion that nonnutritional factors, including inflammation, may be a major cause of hypoalbuminemia was strengthened, and studies in chronic hemodialysis patients noted a high prevalence and coexistence of markers of malnutrition and chronic inflammation. In over 1000 randomly selected dialysis patients, Owen and Lowrie[12] found that the serum concentration of CRP exceeded the upper reference range value (<0.8 mg/dL) in approximately 35% of patients, and a prevalence of 46% was noted by Zimmermann[13] in 288 stable hemodialysis patients. Stenvinkel[14] studied 109 patients with pre-ESRD, and those with malnutrition as judged by a subjective global assessment (SGA) score 2 or greater had significantly higher levels of CRP and fibrinogen. While protein malnutrition can decrease albumin synthesis, this may also occur as part of the acute phase response. Although synthesis of APRs, even after an appropriate inflammatory stimulus, is impeded in protein malnutrition, cytokine release is unimpeded; hence, the inflammatory state is characterized by elevated APRs and pro-inflammatory cytokines in association with hypoalbuminemia.[15] Using this principle, Kaysen and colleagues[16] measured albumin synthesis, fractional catabolic rate, and the distribution of albumin in the vascular and extravascular compartments from the turnover of I-125 human albumin in two groups of hemodialysis patients with serum albumin less than 3.5 g/dL and greater than 4.0 g/dL. Albumin synthesis was significantly reduced in the low-albumin group, and there was a significant negative correlation between serum albumin and both CRP and SAA. Further credence of the impact of inflammation was lent by studies that showed a link between elevated levels of CRP and mortality in patients with CKD. Indeed, Yeun and colleagues[17] showed that inclusion of CRP in a regression model for mortality eliminated serum albumin as a predictor of risk.

Causes of the Inflammatory State in Patients with Chronic Kidney Disease/End-Stage Renal Disease

End-Stage Renal Disease

The causes of the inflammatory state are easier to appreciate in patients with ESRD. Recurrent blood-dialyzer membrane interactions and exposure to dialysis tubing trigger an ongoing inflammatory response, especially with bioincompatible membranes.[18,19] Direct contact of peripheral blood mononuclear cells (PBMC) with dialysis membrane and generation of active complement fragments (C3a, C5a, C5b-9) during hemodialysis play an important role in cytokine induction. Betz and colleagues[20] demonstrated that cuprophan membranes stimulate IL-1 expression in monocytes in the absence of complement. On the other hand, cellulosic membranes can activate through the alternative pathway, the complement cascade, and can generate active fragments able to stimulate cytokine gene expression and secretion by monocytes.

Bacterial contaminants, including lipopolysaccharide (LPS) fragments from poor quality of dialysis water and back-filtration or back-diffusion of contaminants, are another important trigger; indeed, the biologic activities of endotoxin are largely mediated by the cytokines TNF-α, IL-1, IL-6, and IFN-χ, and released from immune cells in response to endotoxin stimulation. Pertosa and colleagues[21] demonstrated that the basal release of TNF-α and IL-6 during hemodialysis was independent of the biocompatibility features of the membrane used but was considerably influenced by the endotoxin content of the dialysate. The contact with the dialysis membrane as well as the interactions with complement fractions, although able to induce a selective cytokine gene transcription in monocytes, does not always automatically stimulate the translation of the specific proteins; LPS or IL-1 is required as a second hit to induce a translational signal.[22]

Finally, the presence of foreign material in vascular accesses, such as polytetrafluoroethylene (PTFE) grafts, or intravenous catheters and their propensity to harbor chronic or recurrent latent infection are additional reasons for the inflammatory state in dialysis patients.[23]

Patients undergoing peritoneal dialysis have their unique set of factors that may enhance chronic inflammation, including episodes of overt or latent peritonitis or PD-catheter related infections and the constant exposure to PD solution, which may include bioincompatible substances or endotoxin.[24]

Chronic Kidney Disease

There is evidence that reduction in renal function per se may play a role in the genesis of inflammation in patients with CKD who are not yet on dialysis, through several mechanisms. Decreased clearance of pro-inflammatory cytokines may enhance overall inflammatory responses. The serum half-lives of pro-inflammatory cytokines, TNF-α and IL-1, are greater in animals without than with renal function.[25] In humans, declining renal function may also affect the levels of additional inflammatory molecules; serum CRP and IL-6 levels are inversely correlated with creatinine clearance.[26] In addition, with renal failure, other molecules that accumulate may provoke an inflammatory response. Advanced glycosylated end products (AGE), for example, clearly initiate inflammation in patients with renal failure.[27]

Volume overload and vascular congestion in patients with renal insufficiency may result in altered permeability of the gastrointestinal tract with accumulation of gut endotoxins that stimulate monocytes toward increased release of pro-inflammatory cytokines.[28] Other comorbid conditions in renal patients may be independently associated with an acute phase response and mechanisms that enhance the development of inflammation. Systemic autoimmune conditions and unrecognized persistent infections may all be contributors to inflammation among patients with decreased renal function.[29]

Oxidative Stress

Oxidative stress results from an imbalance between reactive oxygen species production and antioxidant defense mechanisms. Neutrophils obtained from patients with varying degrees of decline in GFR (creatinine clearance 6 to 35 mL/min/1.73 m^2) appear to exist in a primed state and show enhanced oxidative burst response upon stimulation by formyl peptides.[30] Factors that lead to neutrophil priming may be retained uremic toxins in pre-dialysis patients and LPS contamination of the dialysate in ESRD.[31] Dialyzer membrane bioincompatibility results in leukocyte activation and production of reactive oxygen species.[32] Pro-inflammatory cytokines, produced in response to either contact with membrane or endotoxin, contribute to this primed state.[33] Antioxidant defenses are also impaired in uremic patients who show diminished levels of reduced glutathione, selenium and vitamin E; hemodialysis contributes further to diffusive losses of hydrophilic vitamins such as ascorbic acid.[34] Data are beginning to emerge linking inflammation and oxidative stress in dialysis patients. Positive correlations between elevated CRP levels and plasma thiobarbituric acid reactive substances (TBARS) and plasma F_2 isoprostane levels, both measures of lipid peroxidation, and a negative correlation with plasma α-tocopherol levels have been shown.[35,36] These observations are consistent with the hypothesis that markers of inflammation and oxidant stress in dialysis patients are associated, and inflammation is associated with a depletion of antioxidants.

CYTOKINES AND THEIR REGULATORY NETWORKS

Classically, the immune system has been divided into innate and adaptive components. The former comprises the nonspecific resistance to pathogens, and the latter is characterized by antigen specificity and immunologic memory. The mammalian innate immune system consists of plasma proteins (such as complement), cells (such as neutrophils, macrophages, and natural killer cells), and physical barriers. The innate immune system recognizes and responds to a restricted set of highly conserved structures common to different pathogens. These pathogen-associated molecular patterns (PAMPs) include, among others, LPS, peptidoglycan, bacterial DNA, lipotechoic acid, mannans, and glucans. A family of receptors called "toll" receptors appear to initiate the innate immune response. At least 10 mammalian toll receptors have been identified, of which toll-like receptor–4 (TLR-4) is important in LPS recognition and responsiveness. TLR-4 defective mice show endotoxin hyporesponsiveness as well as an increased susceptibility to infection by gram-negative organisms. Recognition results in the release of inflammatory cytokines (IL-6, TNF-α, IL-1β) that mediate the biologic activities of LPS, and in concert with costimulatory molecules, initiate the adaptive immune response. Thus, cytokines produced in response to cellular injury are one of the major classes of compounds in this scheme that initiate and mediate inflammatory responses for both the innate and adaptive immune systems. They activate neutrophil chemotaxis and phagocytosis and modulate mononuclear cell function in T-cell immune regulation.[37,38]

Both IL-1 and TNF-α sequentially induce the production of IL-6, feedback upon each other, and initiate other cascades. Several of the metabolic effects of IL-1 and TNF-α are thought to be mediated by IL-6, which also appears to be the major mediator of the acute phase response in ESRD patients.[39,40] IL-10 provides a physiologic mechanism to limit the inflammatory response after its initiation and effector functions for defense have been accomplished. After a latency of 8 to 12 hours, the initial secretion of IL-6 and TNF-α is followed by IL-10 production by stimulated monocytes. TNF-α of itself up-regulates IL-10 production, and IL-10 downregulates and inhibits production of TNF-α, IL-1 β, and IL-6, providing an efficient autocrine feedback mechanism for controlling the very redundant pro-inflammatory cytokine production by monocytes. The precise mechanisms by which IL-10 mediates these inhibitory effects have not been determined; however, both transcriptional and post-transcriptional mechanisms have been proposed.[41–44]

Several inhibitors of cytokines have been characterized. The same cells that synthesize IL-1, TNF-α, and IL-6 also produce specific inhibitors: IL-1 receptor antagonist (IL-1 Ra), soluble TNF receptors (sTNFR), and soluble IL-6 receptors (sIL-6R). These inhibitors antagonize the biologic functions of their specific cytokine and extend their circulating half-lives. Whereas IL-1Ra acts as a competitive inhibitor of IL-1 binding to its type-I and type-II receptors, without agonist activity, sTNFR's and sIL-6R's are the extracellular ligand binding domains of their cell surface receptors that are shed upon stimulation and bind directly to the cytokine.[5,45]

Cytokine Dysregulation in Chronic Kidney Disease/End-Stage Renal Disease

Several studies have demonstrated elevated circulating levels of pro-inflammatory cytokines in patients on HD, although others have not corroborated this observation.[40,46] The reasons for variability among these studies could relate to different methodologic and biologic factors that affect the measurement of cytokines in HD patients.[47] Moreover, plasma levels of cytokines do not necessarily reflect cytokine synthesis in HD patients or inflammatory states. Measurement of cytokine synthesis by peripheral blood mononuclear cells (PBMC) probably offers a consistent method of assessing cytokine production in dialysis patients. Transcriptional activation of interleukin-1 (IL-1) in PBMC has been observed following a single passage through an unsubstituted cellulose dialyzer.[48] Consequently, PBMC isolated from patients on chronic HD demonstrate increased spontaneous IL-1 synthesis on incubation, despite the absence of exogenous stimuli. In contrast, in mononuclear cells isolated from healthy subjects, neither IL-1 protein nor mRNA for IL-1 is demonstrated by using Northern hybridization, and these cells fail to show evidence of IL-1 synthesis even after incubation for 24 hours.[49] Furthermore, PBMC from HD patients are "primed" to produce increased levels of IL-1 and TNF upon *in vitro* stimulation.[50–52] When stimulated with endotoxin, these cells synthesize as much as fivefold more IL-1 as compared to mononuclear cells from healthy subjects.[53] Similar results have been reported for the synthesis of TNF and IL-6.[54,55] Girndt and colleagues[56] used the cytoflow technique, a single-cell detection of cytokine production to measure the activation state of circulating monocytes. This technique revealed that only 15% to 20% of circulating monocytes were capable of cytokine production in healthy individuals, even after stimulation by endotoxin. In contrast, some 50% of circulating monocytes in HD patients were primed for cytokine production.

It has been proposed that counter-regulatory mechanisms may be insufficient to limit the heightened state of inflammation in patients with ESRD. The inflammation-limiting effect of IL-10 is functional in HD patients, although higher levels of the cytokine are needed to downregulate the overproduction of pro-inflammatory cytokines. Unlike TNF-α and IL-6, where higher levels are derived from a higher number of cytokine producing cells, IL-10 secretion is mainly enhanced by a higher level of secretion per single cell.[56] A transcriptional defect has been observed in IL-10 synthesis and may partly explain why the required elevation of IL-10 production appears to be limited in a significant proportion of ESRD patients.[57] There is evidence that monocytes differentiate into populations that mutually exclusively express either IL-6 or IL-10, and this may further contribute to the cytokine imbalance seen in ESRD.[56]

Cytokine-specific inhibitory proteins such as IL-1Ra and sTNFR are also elevated in HD patients. The molar ratios of plasma IL-1Ra:IL-1β range from 3:1 to 4:1 and the molar ratios of plasma sTNFR:TNF range from 13:1 to 38:1. Exposure to cuprophan membranes increases the peripheral blood mononuclear cell (PBMC) content of IL-1Ra, and the production of IL-1Ra upon endotoxin-stimulation by several-fold higher compared to undialyzed patients with CRF, CAPD patients, or healthy controls. However, in vivo studies have shown that a 1000-fold excess of IL-1Ra is required to block the hemodynamic effects of IL-1. Therefore, it appears unlikely that the levels of IL-1Ra and sTNFR observed in patients on HD are sufficient to block the systemic effects of IL-1 and TNF produced during dialysis. Therefore, such elevated plasma levels of inhibitory proteins are more likely to be "footprints" of IL-1 and TNF, respectively, or markers of monocyte activation produced during dialysis.[58] Indeed, elevated levels of IL-1 Ra have been shown to correlate with adverse cardiovascular events in HD patients.[59]

Genetic Factors

Circulating cytokine levels vary considerably among ESRD patients, and one may speculate that genetic factors, such as polymorphisms in genes encoding pro-inflammatory cytokines, may be involved in determining the individual inflammatory reaction in response to a given insult. Polymorphisms are the existence of two or more alleles at significant frequencies in a population, that may take the form of insertions/ deletions (I/D), minisatellites and microsatellites (dinucleotide, trinucleotide, and tetranucleotide repeats), and single nucleotide polymorphisms (SNPs). In this respect, a number of different cytokine polymorphisms might be of interest, serving as markers of susceptibility to or severity of disease.

In humans, the interleukin gene cluster on chromosome 2q12-14 contains the loci for IL-1α, IL-1β, their receptors, and IL-1Ra.[60] Specifically, for IL-1α, a genetic association exists between a promoter polymorphism and juvenile rheumatoid arthritis and early-onset Alzheimer's disease.[61,62] A second IL-1α variation within intron 6, a 46 bp tandem repeat (VNTR), also influences gene expression.[63] In addition, IL-1α and IL-1β genotypes are significantly associated with the severity of periodontal disease, whereas an IL-1Ra polymorphism contributes to the susceptibility to severe sepsis.[64,65] Several variants of IL-1β and IL-1Ra have been associated with chronic renal failure and diabetic nephropathy in Caucasians and African-Americans.[66–68] Berger and colleagues[69] recently reported that IL-1 gene polymorphisms are highly related to both plasma levels of CRP and fibrinogen in patients referred for angiography.

The human TNF-α gene maps to chromosome 6 (p21.1-21.3) within the human leucocyte antigen complex.[70] There are a number of different polymorphisms in the promoter region of TNF-α and also at least one in the coding region. The polymorphism at position -308 in the promoter region consisting of a G (-308G) in the common (wild-type) allele and an A (-308A) in the uncommon allele, modifies gene expression.[71] The TNF-α -308A allele has a prevalence of approximately 30% in the general white population.[72] *In vitro* studies show that the presence of this allelic variant displays increased gene transcription as compared with the wild-type allele and is associated with increased secretion of TNF-α from macrophages *in vitro* and elevated TNF-α blood levels in vivo. The TNF-α -308A allele has also been associated with adverse outcome in a variety of infectious and inflammatory diseases, including cerebral malaria, meningococcal disease, the sepsis syndrome, and celiac disease.[72–75] The TNF-α promoter gene is in linkage disequilibrium with several HLA alleles that may also be involved with the control of TNF-α secretion or that may be independent risk factors for the development of meningococcal disease or other forms of sepsis.[76]

Several SNPs have been identified within the IL-6 promoter region, the best studied being the -174G/C SNP. The C/C genotype has been related to higher levels of plasma IL-6, particularly after stresses such as surgical procedures.[77,78] In the general population, the C-allele has been associated with higher levels of CRP and has been linked to hypertension, coronary heart disease, and left ventricular hypertrophy.[79]

There is a large interindividual variation in IL-10 response to inflammation, at least 70% of which may be explained by genetic factors.[80] Indeed, the SNPs identified in the promoter region of the IL-10 gene are related to IL-10 expression and have been linked to the risk of both SLE[81] and inflammatory bowel disease.[82] Moreover, Girndt and colleagues[84] have recently shown that the IL-10-1082 SNP was associated with an increased risk of cardiovascular events[83] and immune dysfunction, characterized by poor rates of seroconversion after hepatitis-B vaccine in hemodialysis patients.

The human TGF-β1 gene is sited on chromosome 19 (q13.1-13.3) and at least seven polymorphic sites have been described, including three each in the promoter and coding regions.[85] Grainger and colleagues[86] demonstrated that the concentration of total TGF-β1(active + acid activable latent) in plasma was predominantly under genetic control with a heritability estimate of 54%. The presence of the C-509T promoter region polymorphism explained 8.2% of the additive genetic variance of total TGF-β1 concentration. In a study of lung transplant recipients, Awad and colleagues[87] showed that stimulated lymphocytes from patients homozygous for the G allele at the +915 position of the signal sequence (codon 25) produced higher levels of TGF-β1 compared to heterozygous patients (G/C). In a study of heart transplant recipients, Aziz and colleagues[88] showed that the codon 25 G/G genotype was associated with plasma levels about one and a half times higher than the G/C genotype. TGF-β appears to have a protective role in atherogenesis, and low plasma levels have been associated with clinical disease.[89] In a recent study of hemodialysis patients from Italy, serum levels of TGF-β1 were lower in patients with atherosclerotic disease, although there was no demonstrable relationship to TGF-β1 genotypes.[90] The ECTIM study showed an association between the G/C genotype at codon 25 and the risk of myocardial infarction.[85] Yokota and colleagues[91] showed that male subjects with the T allele at the +869 position of the signal peptide sequence region (genotypes T/C or T/T at codon 10), had a threefold higher risk of MI, and lower TGF-β1 levels, compared to males with the C/C genotype. Several other studies have been negative for an association between coronary disease and coding or promoter region polymorphisms in population groups without CKD.[92,93]

The innate immune system is the first line of defense against bacterial lipopolysaccharide (LPS). Two polymorphisms of the human TLR-4 gene, Asp299Gly and Thr399Ile, have been recently characterized.[94] These are associated with impaired bacterial endotoxin-induced signaling and the capacity to elicit inflammation. TLR-4 receptor mutations have been associated with an increased risk of gram-negative infections and gram-negative shock.[95] TLR-4 expression has been noted to be up-regulated in both human and murine atherosclerotic lesions.[96] These observations suggest that defects in TLR-4 signaling may exert opposing effects in the pathogenesis of gram-negative infections and atherosclerotic disease. This is especially significant in the context of microbial disease with organisms such as *Chlamydia pneumoniae* and *Helicobacter pylori* being implicated in the pathogenesis of atherosclerotic disease. Kiechl and colleagues[97] recently described an association between the Asp299Gly TLR-4 polymorphism (diminishing the inflammatory response to gram-negative pathogens) and a decreased risk of atherosclerosis in nonrenal patients.

Myeloperoxidase (MPO), another component of the defense system, is a hemoprotein expressed in polymorphonuclear leukocytes and monocytes that catalyzes the production of hypochlorous acid, enhancing the antimicrobial activity. MPO has recently been linked to several diseases, such as atherosclerosis and Alzheimer's disease.[98] A highly functional SNP that affects the transcription of MPO is located in the promoter region (463G/A)[99] and may be of interest due to a recent description of an association between this SNP and the presence of coronary artery disease.[100]

Another polymorphism that might contribute to different inflammatory responses is the C825T polymorphism in the GNB3 gene, encoding the ubiquitously expressed β3-subunit of the G proteins, which is involved in immune cell function in humans. In a preliminary prospective study including 228 HD patients, higher CRP levels and higher mortality were seen in T homozygotes, suggesting that the C825T polymorphism might influence mortality rate in HD patients.[101]

Consequences of the Inflammatory State in Patients with Chronic Kidney Disease/End-Stage Renal Disease

Hypoalbuminemia and Malnutrition

The reasons for malnutrition in dialysis patients are multifactorial and include disturbances in protein and energy metabolism, hormonal derangements, poor intake due to anorexia, and nausea and vomiting related to the uremic toxicity. Associated comorbidity (diabetes mellitus, diffuse vascular disease) and complications (pericarditis, infection, congestive heart failure) can also contribute to malnutrition. Thus poor nutrient intake, protein, and amino-acid losses during dialysis and catabolic stresses summarize the main mechanisms underlying dialysis-related malnutrition. The inflammatory response and cytokines mediate many of these mechanisms.[46,102,103]

TNF-α and IL-1 directly suppress appetite. Animal studies suggest that direct effects of these cytokines on the hypothalamic satiety center explain this anorectic effect. IL-6 and TNF-α induce muscle breakdown in rats and lead to a wasting illness similar to prolonged starvation and are known mediators of cancer cachexia.[104,105] These cytokines have both antianabolic and catabolic actions on muscle, upregulating ubiquitin-proteasome-mediated proteolysis and freeing amino acids for the synthesis of defensive proteins such as the APRs, ferritin, and CRP.[106,107] An established metabolic effect of chronic inflammation is cytokine-mediated hypermetabolism. Increased resting energy expenditure (REE) is observed in most of the chronic inflammatory states, again placing dialysis patients at increased risk for negative energy balance.[108] Chronic inflammation also produces insulin resistance and disrupts the growth hormone and insulin-like growth factor I axis, leading to decreased anabolism and increased leptin concentrations, which may induce anorexia due to its central effects.[109]

In the dialysis population, the most consistent relationships have been demonstrated between IL-6 and indices of malnutrition. Since both IL-1 and TNF-α sequentially induce the production of IL-6, some of their metabolic effects are thought to be mediated by IL-6. It is also notable that whereas most other cytokines function via paracrine/autocrine mechanisms, the major effects of IL-6 are a consequence of its concentration in the circulation and can take place at sites distinct from its site of secretion. IL-6 downregulates albumin synthesis, and the relationship between elevated levels of IL-6 and hypoalbuminemia has been noted by several investigators.[39] Kaizu and colleagues[110] reported that hemodialyzed patients with high plasma IL-6 concentration had lower serum albumin levels and greater weight loss over a 3-year period than patients with low plasma IL-6. Moreover the circulating IL-6 concentration was inversely correlated with serum albumin, cholinesterase, and mid-arm muscle area. In a more recent study these investigators showed a significant inverse association between IL-6 and measures of muscle wasting, using the creatinine generation rate from a creatinine kinetic model and thigh muscle area measured by computed tomography.[111] Bologa and colleagues[112] showed that in addition to the inverse correlation with serum albumin, higher levels of circulating TNF-α and IL-6 were also associated with lower levels of serum cholesterol. IL-6 remained the strongest predictor of mortality in this cohort, even after adjustment for potential confounders such as older age, hypoalbuminemia, and lower body mass index (BMI). While serum cholesterol was not a significant predictor of mortality, nonsurvivors were noted to have significantly lower levels of serum cholesterol. The link between elevated levels of circulating IL-6 and mortality has also been noted in patients with normal renal function and in the elderly.[113,114] Pecoits-Filho and colleagues[115] showed a strong predictive value of elevated IL-6 levels for poor outcome in an incident dialysis population that was starting either HD or PD.[115]

The Malnutrition-Inflammation-Atherosclerosis (MIA) Syndrome

Cardiovascular causes account for almost 50% of the reported causes of dialysis patient deaths in all age groups.[116,117] Considering that most dialysis patients die of atherosclerotic cardiovascular diseases, it is significant that hypoalbuminemia and other nutritional indicators are strong risk factors for early death. Several recent epidemiologic studies have demonstrated that inflammation per se may play an important role in the development of atherosclerosis and death from ischemic heart disease and cerebrovascular disease.[118] A series of recent publications mirror these associations between cardiovascular risk and a host of inflammatory biomarkers, including cytokines, cell adhesion molecules, and downstream players, such as CRP and SAA, in patients both with and without renal disease.[119] Experimental evidence suggests an important role of IL-6 in the atherosclerotic process. Injection of recombinant IL-6 exacerbates early atherosclerosis in ApoE-deficient mice, and increased IL-6 expression is found within the fibrous plaques of atherosclerotic lesions.[120,121] IL-6 is also an independent predictor of the progression of carotid atherosclerosis in patients on dialysis treatment,[122] and baseline levels of plasma IL-6 appear to predict patient survival similar to the reported associations for albumin and CRP.[112,115] Thus, the chronic inflammatory state contributes to malnutrition and atherosclerotic cardiovascular disease, both of which are strong predictors of mortality in dialysis patients. Foley and colleagues[123] found that among hemodialysis patients, a 1.0 g/dL fall in mean serum albumin was independently associated with the development of de novo and recurrent cardiac failure, de novo and recurrent ischemic heart disease, cardiac mortality, and overall mortality, the magnitude of increased risk ranging from 2.2 to 5.6.

There is thus considerable evidence for strong interactions between CVD, malnutrition, and a chronic inflammatory state, and nutritional and inflammatory markers are closely linked to CVD in CKD patients. Stenvinkel and colleagues[14] have therefore suggested the existence of a syndrome consisting of malnutrition, inflammation, and atherosclerosis (MIA syndrome) in patients with CKD. Elevated levels of pro-inflammatory cytokines could be the link between the high prevalence of inflammation, malnutrition, and CVD in patients with CKD. The MIA syndrome has also been invoked to explain the "reverse epidemiology" or "risk-factor paradox" seen in dialysis patients.[124] PEM and inflammation change many nutritional measures in the same direction. In contrast to the general population, where markers of overnutrition are associated with increased risk of CVD, markers of undernutrition such as low body mass index (BMI), reduced serum cholesterol, or creatinine concentration correlate with increased morbidity and mortality, including a higher risk of cardiovascular events and death, in dialysis patients. A similar reversal is also apparent for the relationship between plasma total homocysteine (tHcy) and cardiovascular risk. Homocysteine may induce vascular damage and promote atherogenesis by inducing platelet activation, oxidative stress, endothelial dysfunction, and hypercoagulability.[125] Although in the general population there is strong evidence that a mildly elevated plasma tHcy is an independent and graded risk factor for atherosclerosis,[126,127] in patients with ESRD, findings have been inconsistent, with some studies showing paradoxically lower levels in association with CVD.[128] Several studies have shown that tHcy levels are lower in malnourished ESRD patients as a direct consequence of PEM. Moreover, albumin is an important binding site for tHcy, and there is a direct relationship between serum albumin levels and tHcy. Thus, the presence of the MIA syndrome would be expected to confound the relationship between plasma tHcy and vascular disease.

Cardiovascular Disease

Atherosclerosis as an inflammatory lesion

In contrast to the traditional view that atherosclerosis is an acellular lesion composed of lipid deposits, recent understanding of the biology of atherosclerosis reveals the atheromatous lesion to be a site of active inflammation. Cytokines play differential roles in the pathogenesis and evolution of the lesion with pro- and anti-atherogenic effects influencing plaque characteristics and clinical outcomes. The classical pro-inflammatory cytokines, IL-1, TNF-α, and IL-6, typically mediate pro-atherogenic processes, whereas IL-10, an anti-inflammatory cytokine is considered anti-atherogenic, although this may be an oversimplification. Pro-atherogenic mechanisms include local effects on endothelial cells, VSMCs and monocytes, as well as various metabolic and coagulant mechanisms. IFN-χ and TGF-β1, mediate either pro- or anti-atherogenic effects depending on the stage of evolution of the lesion. The balance between pro- and anti-atherogenic cytokines probably depends, in part, upon the balance between the T_H1 and T_H2 lymphocyte subpopulations within the atherosclerotic plaque.[129]

The earliest stages of atherogenesis are associated with an enhanced expression of pro-inflammatory cytokines. Several pathologic processes that cause endothelial injury, including modified LDL, free radicals, hemodynamic stress, hypertension, or infectious microorganisms, stimulate cytokine release. Cytokines alter endothelial function, enhancing the expression of leukocyte adhesion molecules and chemokines. A strong positive correlation has been demonstrated between IL-6 levels and soluble intercellular adhesion molecule –1 (ICAM-1). Moreover, they interact with platelets and coagulation and fibrinolytic systems that are activated following endothelial injury. Monocyte and T-cell recruitment and migration of vascular smooth muscle cells (VSMCs) into the sub-intimal region are promoted, leading to the formation of foam cells and, eventually, the "fatty streak," which is the first macroscopic manifestation of atherosclerosis. Foam cells represent a rich source of cytokines, chemokines, growth factors, colony stimulating factors and proteolytic enzymes. IL-1, TNF-α, and IFN-χ, in turn, increase the expression of CD40 and CD40-ligand (CD40L), cell-associated members of the TNF-TNF receptor family. Subsequent ligand binding of CD40 by CD40L augments the surface expression of E- or P-selectin, ICAM-1, and vascular cell adhesion molecule –1 (VCAM-1) on cells found in plaques. These findings highlight the role of the foam cell in the plaque microenvironment and the potential autoregulatory, positive feedback loops that determine the chronic nature of atherosclerotic inflammation.[129]

Further plaque advancement depends upon the subintimal microenvironment. Replication and activation of both VSMCs and mononuclear phagocytes promote plaque growth and fibrous cap formation. Plaques composed of a lipid-rich core with numerous inflammatory cells, in particular, macrophages, are termed "vulnerable" because they are more prone to rupture. Pro-inflammatory cytokines, TNF-α and IL-1, stimulate the expression of matrix metallo-proteinases (MMPs) that degrade extracellular matrix (ECM). This weakens the fibrous cap that overlies the lipid core of the plaque and renders it more prone to rupture by hemodynamic stresses. The direct contact of blood coagulation mechanisms to tissue factor triggers thrombosis. When the prevailing fibrinolytic mechanisms outweigh the procoagulant pathways, a limited mural thrombus rather than a sustained and occlusive blood clot develops. Healing takes place with resorption of the mural thrombus and the elaboration of growth factors, such as platelet derived growth factor (PDGF) from platelets and TGF-β1 from VSMCs, macrophages, and activated platelets. TGF-β1 is the most potent stimulus known for interstitial collagen synthesis by VSMCs and appears to exert an important plaque stabilizing effect. A stable plaque has a thick fibrous cap, a smaller lipid pool, fewer inflammatory cells and a dense ECM, and is less prone to disruption.[129] Apart from increasing ECM synthesis, TGF-β1 increases the expression of tissue inhibitors of MMPs, TIMPs,[130] and interacts with the fibrinolytic cascade. Plasmin is the most important physiologic activator of TGF-β1, which, in turn, upregulates the expression of plasminogen activator inhibitor-1 (PAI-1).[131–133]

Inflammation and Other Cardiovascular Disease

Congestive heart failure is common among ESRD patients, and over 50% of such patients have evidence of PEM and hypoalbuminemia.[134] In its most serious form, cardiac cachexia is defined as the loss of more than 10% of lean body mass.[135] Plasma levels of TNF-α, IL-1, and IL-6 have been reported to be elevated in cardiac failure, presumably triggered by factors such as low tissue perfusion, hypoxia, hepatic congestion, and bowel wall edema.[136,137] Inflammatory cytokines are, in part, responsible for anorexia, increased muscle proteolysis, and increased resting energy expenditure. They also have a depressant action on the myocardium, thus inducing myocardial dysfunction. Stenvinkel and colleagues[138] evaluated cardiac troponin T (cTnT), a highly sensitive and specific marker of myocardial damage in ESRD patients starting dialysis and an independent predictor of mortality. They demonstrated positive correlations between cTnT and IL-6, and CRP, respectively, suggesting an association between inflammation and cTnT levels. Cardiac calcification of either coronary vessels or valves has been previously considered a passive degenerative process, but more recent studies have indicated the involvement of active inflammation. A recent study in a peritoneal dialysis cohort showed a significant relationship between cardiac valve calcification and elevated CRP, hypoalbuminemia and malnutrition assessed by SGA, even after adjustment for serum PTH and Ca-P metabolism.[139] Another study in peritoneal dialysis patients showed that the presence of coronary artery calcification measured by the Agatston score showed higher levels of IL-6, TNF-α, and CRP, although these associations did not retain significance on multivariate adjustment.[140]

Triggers for Inflammation

The traditional lipid-centric view contributed tremendously to progress in understanding the pathophysiology of atherosclerosis. The current model links inflammation to the role of lipids and dyslipidemia. Oxidative modification of low-density lipoprotein (LDL) yields biologically active compounds that induce the expression of adhesion molecules, chemokines, and pro-inflammatory cytokines.[141] Pro-inflammatory cytokines such as IL-1 and TNF-α inhibit the activity of lipolytic enzymes (lipoprotein lipase, hepatic triglyceride lipase, lecithin-cholesterol acyltransferase) that are responsible for the catabolism of triglyceride-rich apo-B containing lipoproteins and HDL.[142,143] Indeed, given that plasma levels and synthesis of these cytokines are elevated in dialysis patients, it follows that the uremic lipoprotein profile resembles the abnormalities seen in patients with acute infection, severe trauma, and myocardial infarction. The protective effect of HDL stems partly from its role in reverse cholesterol transport and in the transport of significant antioxidant enzymes (platelet activating factor acetyl hydroxylase and paraoxonase).[141] However, in the presence of inflammation, SAA associates with HDL, displacing apoA-I and redirecting HDL cholesterol from the liver to the macrophage for use in tissue repair, or even converting it to a nonfunctional or pro-inflammatory particle.[144] Lipoprotein (a) (Lp[a]) is another APR; IL-6 responsive elements have been identified in the 5′ flanking regulatory region of the apo(a) gene on chromosome 6.[145] Concentrations of Lp(a) increase during the acute phase response,[146] depending upon the size of the apo(a) isoform, which is inherited as an autosomal codominant trait.[147] Lp(a) is an LDL-like particle in which an apolipoprotein(a) (apo[a]) moiety is linked via a disulfide bond to apoB-100.[148] There is extensive homology between Lp(a) and plasminogen.[149] Lp(a) binds avidly to endothelial cells, macrophages, fibroblasts, and platelets, as well as the subendothelial matrix, where it may promote proliferation of VSMCs and chemotaxis of human monocytes.[150,151] By virtue of its structural homology to plasminogen, it competes for binding to plasminogen receptors and inhibits fibrinolysis at sites of tissue injury. It may also induce production of PAI-1 and inhibit secretion of tissue plasminogen activator (TPA).[152,153] Lp(a) also has the ability to deliver significant quantities of cholesterol to sites of vascular injury, 40% of its mass being represented by cholesterol. It is thus a highly atherothrombotic lipoprotein, triggering inflammatory, antifibrinolytic, and lipid mediated pathways in vascular injury. A recent meta-analysis of 27 prospective studies with a mean follow-up of 10 years showed that individuals with Lp(a) concentrations in the top tertile, had a risk ratio for coronary heart disease 1.6 times (95% CI: 1.4 to 1.8) that of individuals with Lp(a) concentrations in the bottom tertile. Adjustment for conventional risk factors did not diminish this association.[154]

Infectious agents, such as *Chlamydia pneumoniae, Helicobacter pylori,* herpes simplex virus, and cytomegalovirus, have been implicated in various epidemiologic studies as etiologic for atherosclerosis, of which the associations with *C. pneumoniae* have been the strongest.[155] The organism has been demonstrated within atherosclerotic lesions by immunostaining or PCR[156,157] and may potentially mediate both local effects and stimulate the production of IL-6 and the acute phase response.[122]

Other factors that may trigger inflammatory signals involved in atherogenesis include advanced glycosylated end products (AGE) that occur as a result of sustained hyperglycemia. AGE-modified proteins can augment the production of cytokines and other inflammatory pathways in endothelial cells.[158] Adipose tissue is an important source of pro-inflammatory cytokines, such as TNF-α and IL-6, and thus potentiates atherogenesis independent of its relationship to the metabolic syndrome and insulin resistance.[159]

C-Reactive Protein

CRP is the prototypical APR produced by the liver in response to various pro-inflammatory cytokines, namely IL-6, IL-1, and TNF-α. IL-6 binding elements are present in the promoter region of the CRP gene in hepatocytes.[160] Human CRP is a pentameric protein encoded by a gene on chromosome 1. It acts as an opsonin for bacteria, parasites, and immune complexes and can activate the classical pathway of complement. In addition, it binds to and effects the clearance of nuclear material from necrotic tissue and therefore provides a protective mechanism against the initiation of nuclear-antigen specific autoimmunity.[7]

Data from the Physician's Health Study first called attention to the importance of CRP as a marker of risk of MI in, apparently, healthy individuals.[118] In a recently reported meta-analysis of 14 prospective long-term studies of CRP and the risk of nonfatal myocardial infarction or death from coronary heart disease, the combined adjusted risk ratio was 1.9 (95% CI 1.5–2.3) among individuals in the top tertile of baseline CRP concentrations.[161] CRP also predicts recurrent events and mortality in patients with coronary, cerebrovascular, and peripheral vascular disease.[162] CRP has emerged as a remarkably robust marker of cardiovascular risk and meets the criteria required for clinical utility as a surrogate for cytokine stimulation. It is relatively stable from day to day in a given individual, with a plasma half-life of 19 hours and relatively constant fractional clearance rates in both healthy individuals and diseased states. It has a standardized and reproducible assay and adds to estimates of risk already provided by established markers.[163] The recent guidelines of the American Heart Association (AHA) address the potential role of CRP in cardiovascular risk assessment.[164]

There is evidence that CRP may be more than a marker of disease, playing a direct role in the pathogenesis of atherosclerosis. The protein is markedly upregulated in atheromatous plaques, the majority of foam cells beneath the endothelium showing positive staining for CRP. It promotes LDL cholesterol uptake by macrophages, binding to LDL and VLDL in a calcium-dependent fashion. It may induce the expression of intercellular adhesion molecules by endothelial cells and the production of tissue factor, an activator of the coagulation pathway, by monocytes. Indeed, it has been suggested that high CRP concentrations and the extent of its deposition in the atherosclerotic plaque may be associated with plaque vulnerability and occurrence of acute thrombotic events.[162,163]

Patients with CKD and ESRD show elevated CRP levels in keeping with the underlying chronic inflammatory state.[9,13] There is a close correlation between changes in plasma levels of IL-6 and levels of CRP.[115,165] The inverse relation with serum albumin levels among ESRD patients has already been discussed. Bergstrom and colleagues[166] were the first to show that elevated CRP was a strong predictor of mortality in HD patients, and later studies have supported this observation. Zimmermann[13] showed that all-cause mortality was 4.6-fold, and cardiovascular mortality was 5.5-fold higher among patients in the highest quartile of CRP compared to the lowest quartile. Yeun[17] also identified CRP levels as the most powerful predictor of all-cause and cardiovascular mortality. Similarly, Iseki and colleagues[167] showed a poorer survival among patients with an elevated CRP compared to those with normal levels. Mirroring the observations in the general population, hemodialysis patients with elevated serum CRP and serum amyloid A levels were shown to have significantly higher serum levels of Lp(a) and fibrinogen, and both were predictors of CVD and death.[13] The Cardiovascular Risk Extended Evaluation in Dialysis (CREED) study showed that CRP was an independent predictor of the number of atherosclerotic plaques in the carotid arteries of a chronic HD cohort.[168] Among patients with CKD, Stenvinkel[14] showed strong associations between inflammation (high CRP) and increased carotid intima media area and presence of carotid plaques. In a recent secondary analysis of the Modification of Diet in Renal Disease (MDRD) data, Menon and colleagues[169] showed that among patients with CKD and glomerular filtration rate (GFR) less than 60 mL/min/1.73m^2, CRP was inversely related to serum albumin, and patients with a high CRP level had a 1.73-fold increase in the odds of CVD.

Anemia and Unresponsiveness to Erythropoietin

Erythropoiesis is regulated by cytokines, and chronic inflammatory conditions characterized by high circulating cytokine levels often manifest anemia that is hyporesponsive to erythropoietin (EPO).[170] A significant proportion of dialysis patients show EPO resistance even after known causes such as iron deficiency, hyperparathyroidism, or aluminum overload have been excluded,[171] and altered cytokine production may be responsible for suppressing bone marrow erythropoiesis, EPO production, or impairing iron utilization. Serum ferritin is an APR and patients with refractory anemia due to inflammation characteristically have paradoxically elevated levels of ferritin. IL-1 and TNF-α inhibit EPO production *in vitro*; the inhibitory effect on erythroid colony formation in bone marrow cultured with uremic serum was reversed by the addition of specific anti-TNF-α antibodies.[172] Goicoechea[173] and, more recently, Kalantar-Zadeh[174] have shown in patients undergoing chronic HD, a significant and direct correlation between EPO dose and peripheral blood mononuclear cell (PBMC) associated TNF-α and IL-6 production and serum IL-6 levels, respectively.

Bone Disease

Cytokines such as IL-6 appear to play a role in regulating osteoblast/osteoclast interactions. Il-6 is produced by osteoblasts in response to parathyroid hormone (PTH) and may induce osteoclastogenesis and bone resorption. Indeed, some of the effects of calcitriol in bone may be mediated by IL-6. IL-1 and TNF-α also appear to exert osteoclastic effects. In addition, IL-1 upregulates the expression of the extracellular calcium-sensing receptor mRNA, inhibiting PTH secretion *in vitro*.[175]

IL-1, IL-6, and TNF-α stimulate β-2 microglobulin (β-2MG) release by leukocyte and endothelial cells.[176] They play an important role in the pathogenesis of amyloid bone disease in patients dialyzed with cellulosic membranes where complement activation and cytokine release culminates in enhanced β-2MG generation.[177,178]

Immune Dysfunction

Uremic patients on dialysis demonstrate an increased susceptibility to infections, which account for up to 15% of the mortality in this population.[117] Dysfunction of phagocytic cells related to blood-dialyzer interactions with bioincompatible cellulosic membranes, complement activation, and altered cytokine production are some of the nonspecific defects in host defenses. The immune system in HD patients is characterized by deficient effector function towards bacterial and viral infections. Other manifestations of this cellular immune defect include extended survival of skin allografts, marked decrease in delayed type hypersensitivity responses to cutaneous antigens, and reduced seroconversion after vaccination.[179] Part of the underlying defect is an impaired costimulatory signaling of antigen presenting cells towards T-lymphocytes.[180] Girndt and colleagues[181] showed in dialysis patients, a correlation between inflammatory activation, measured as the *in vitro* production of IL-6 and TNF-α by PBMC upon stimulation with LPS, and immunodeficiency, measured as nonresponsiveness to hepatitis B vaccination. The higher production of pro-inflammatory cytokines appeared to correlate with impairment of immune function and a higher production of IL-10, an anti-inflammatory cytokine, with good immune function. An intact counter-regulatory effect of IL-10 for reducing monokine synthesis thus appears to be necessary for immunocompetence. Indeed, Kimmel and colleagues[40] showed that elevations in pro-inflammatory cytokines such as IL-1 and TNF-α were independently associated with mortality, and circulating levels of IL-2 and IL-12, cytokines critical for T-cell growth and function, and T-cell number and function, were independently associated with survival. Related observations emerged from analyses of over 20,000 chronic dialysis patients in the Fresenius Medical Care data system. Total lymphocyte count was associated, albeit weakly with proxies for body protein content (albumin, creatinine) and inversely with death risk. Total neutrophil count, a crude marker of systemic inflammation, on the other hand, was inversely associated with proxies for body protein content and directly with death risk.[182] These findings underscore the intricate relationships between malnutrition, immune function, and clinical outcomes in ESRD patients with chronic inflammation as a unifying pathophysiology.

Metabolic Effects

TNF-α and IL-6 induce insulin resistance, and both cytokines cause dyslipidemia. Both TNF-α and IL-6 appear to be closely related to the control of body composition.[183,184] TNF-α is over-expressed in the adipose and muscle tissues in obese compared to lean subjects. IL-6 is also expressed in adipose tissue, and IL-6 deficient mice develop obesity.[185] TNF-α blocks the action of insulin in cell culture as well as in experimental animals.[186] The elevated levels of inflammatory cytokines such as TNF-α, IL-1β, and IL-6 are believed to mediate, in large part, the hyperglycemia with insulin resistance and profound negative nitrogen balance in the sepsis syndrome.[187] In a sample of patients from a population survey, serum IL-6 concentrations were higher in subjects with impaired glucose tolerance and type II diabetes than in the control subjects.[188] The dyslipidemic effects associated with the acute phase response that have been discussed earlier in this review, include elevation of circulating concentrations of Lp(a) and triglycerides, conversion of HDL into a proatherogenic form, and oxidation of LDL.

Inflammation as a Therapeutic Target

At the patient level, several questions remain and might be of clinical significance, such as the temporal patterns of the development of the inflammatory state and the identification of subsets of patients at greater risk for developing the inflammatory state and its consequences. A suggested approach to the management of the inflammatory aspects of the uremic state is schematized in Figure 12–1. At the current state of knowledge, we do not have a robust evidence base to propose specific strategies to counter inflammatory processes. However, within the framework of existing clinical guidelines there exists considerable potential to modify clinical outcomes.

Anti-inflammatory or anti-cytokine strategies (anti-TNF-α antibodies, soluble TNF-α receptors, and IL-1Ra) have been found to be extremely effective in limiting the inflammatory consequences of certain diseases, such as rheumatoid arthritis.[189] In the context of the patient with CKD, however, such therapies would be limited by the fact that there is no single target in the inflammatory response; the inflammatory state is already established in response to multiple factors and consists of the activation of multiple mediators. It can be argued that interventions should be directed to block the inflammation inducing stimuli upstream, such as the use of ultrapure water for dialysate, biocompatible membranes, and correction of acidosis. Clearance of larger molecules by dialytic or adsorbent therapies are potential avenues for the removal of β2-MG, leptin, or other proteins that potentiate the inflammatory response. Preliminary studies with an adsorbent column (BetaSorb) have shown that in addition to very efficient β2-MG clearance, there was a marked decrease in the ability of uremic serum to stimulate TNF-α production from a monocytic cell line.[190]

Observations from recent clinical trials have shown that HMG-CoA reductase inhibitors and ACE inhibitors appear to have anti-inflammatory effects beyond their lipid-lowering actions and antihypertensive actions, respectively.[191–193]

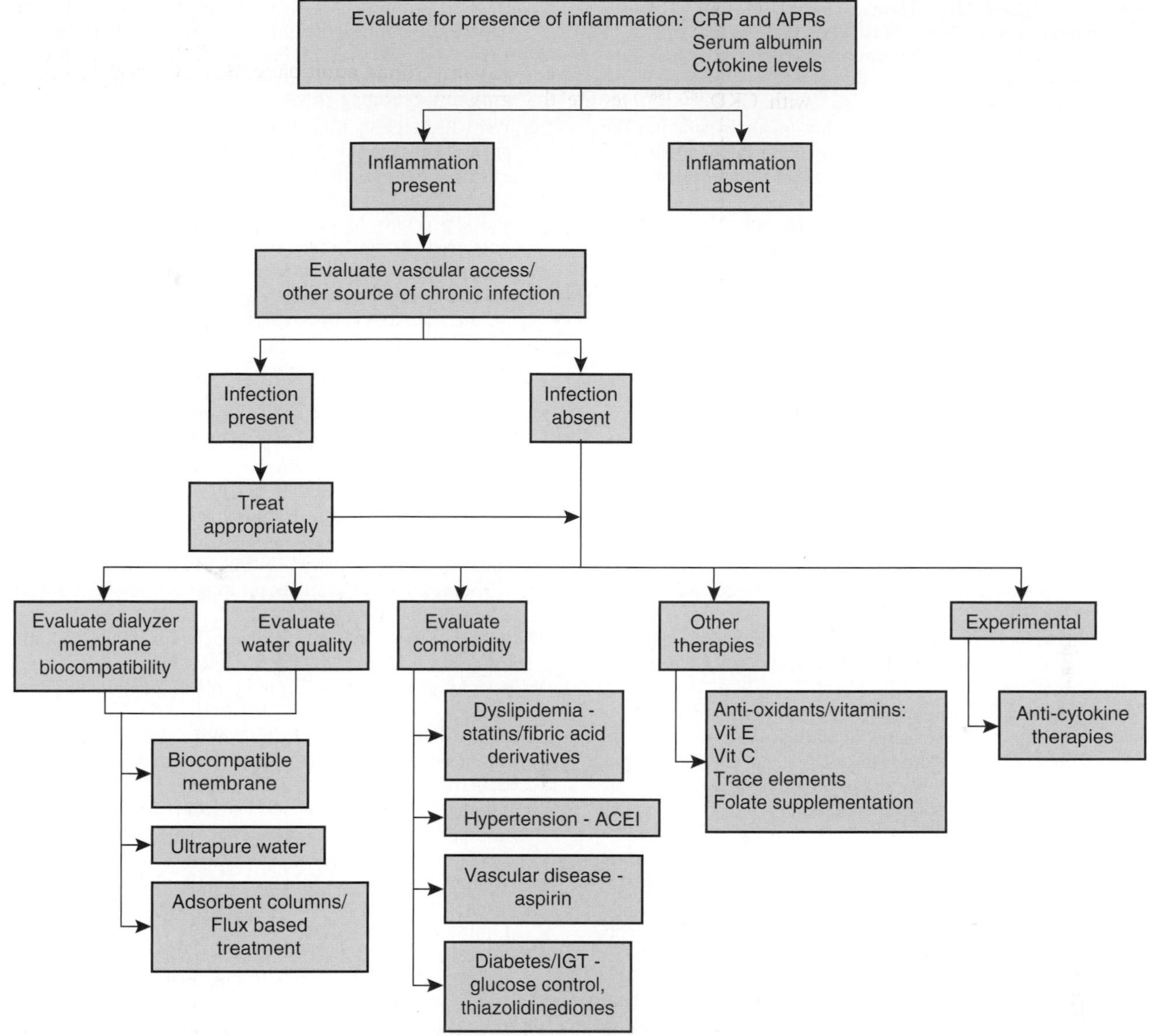

Figure 12–1 Management of inflammatory aspects of the uremic state in the patient with chronic kidney disease.

Aspirin is now known to reduce cardiovascular risk in direct relation to baseline levels of CRP.[118] The antioxidant and anti-inflammatory effects of vitamin E have been explored in several studies, such as the SPACE trial with benefit on cardiovascular end points.[194] The other group of drugs that may have beneficial effects on plaque biology, apart from their primary therapeutic indications include the fibric acid derivatives and thiazolidinediones that activate peroxisome proliferation activating receptor isoforms α and χ, respectively.[195] Thus, although there is some evidence that therapeutic avenues targeting chronic low grade inflammation might mitigate the cardiovascular consequences, malnutrition, and increased mortality among patients with kidney disease with evidence of systemic inflammation, prospective studies are required to evaluate these novel strategies and to define optimal therapeutic approaches.

References

1. Henderson LW, Koch KM, Dinarello CA, Shaldon S: Hemodialysis hypotension: The interleukin-1 hypothesis. Blood Purif 1983; 1:3-8.
2. Dinarello CA, Cannon BD, Wolff SM: New concepts on the pathogenesis of fever. Rev Infect Dis 1988; 10:168-189.
3. David JR: Delayed hypersensitivity *in vitro*: Its mediation by cell-free substances formed by lymphoid cell-antigen interactions. Proc Natl Acad Sci U S A 1966; 56:72-77.
4. Bloom BR, Bennett B: Mechanism of a reaction *in vitro* associated with delayed-type hypersensitivity. Science 1966; 153: 80-82.
5. Pereira BJ, Dinarello CA: Production of cytokines and cytokine inhibitory proteins in patients on dialysis. Nephrol Dial Transplant 1994; 9:60-71.
6. Morley JJ, Kushner I: Serum C-reactive protein levels in disease. Ann N Y Acad Sci 1982; 389:406-418.

7. Panichi V, Migliori M, De Pietro S, et al: Plasma C-reactive protein in hemodialysis. Blood Purif 1999; 17:142-148.
8. Gabay C, Kushner I: Mechanisms of disease: Acute-phase proteins and other systemic responses to inflammation. N Engl J Med 1999; 340:448-454.
9. Lowrie EG, Lew NL: Death risk in hemodialysis patients: The predictive value of commonly measured variables and an evaluation of death rate differences between facilities. Am J Kidney Dis 1990; 15:458-482.
10. Owen WF, Lew NL, Liu Y, et al: The urea reduction ratio and serum albumin concentration as predictors of mortality in patients undergoing hemodialysis. N Engl J Med 1993; 329:1001-1006.
11. Foulks C: An evidence based evaluation of intra-dialytic parenteral nutrition. Am J Kidney Dis 1999; 33:186-192.
12. Owen WF, Lowrie EG: C-reactive protein as an outcome predictor for maintenance hemodialysis patients. Kidney Int 1998; 54:627-636.
13. Zimmerman J, Herrlinger S, Pruy A, et al: Inflammation enhances cardiovascular risk and mortality in hemodialysis patients. Kidney Int 1999; 55:648-658.
14. Stenvinkel P, Heimburger O, Paultre F, et al: Strong association between malnutrition, inflammation, and atherosclerosis in chronic renal failure. Kidney Int 1999; 55:1899-1911.
15. Kaysen G: Hypoalbuminemia in dialysis patients. Semin Dial 1996; 9:249-256.
16. Kaysen GA, Stevenson FT, Depner TA: Determinants of albumin concentration in hemodialysis patients. Am J Kidney Dis 1997; 29:658-668.
17. Yeun JY, Levine RA, Mantadilok V, Kaysen GA: C-reactive protein predicts all-cause and cardiovascular mortality in hemodialysis patients. Am J Kidney Dis 2000; 35:469-476.
18. Schindler R, Boenisch O, Fischer C, Frei U: Effect of the hemodialysis membrane on the inflammatory reaction in vivo. Clin Nephrol 2000; 53:452.
19. Memoli B, Minutolo R, Bisesti V, et al: Collaborative Study Group on SMC Membrane: Changes of serum albumin and C-reactive protein are related to changes of interleukin-6 release by peripheral blood mononuclear cells in hemodialysis patients treated with different membranes. Am J Kidney Dis 2002; 39:266.
20. Betz M, Haensch GM, Rauterberg EW, et al: Cuprammonium membranes stimulate interleukin 1 release and arachidonic acid metabolism in monocytes in the absence of complement. Kidney Int 1988; 34:67-73.
21. Pertosa G, Gesualdo L, Bottalico D, Schena FP: Endotoxins modulate chronically tumour necrosis factor alpha and interleukin 6 release by uraemic monocytes. Nephrol Dial Transplant 1995; 10:328-333.
22. Schindler R, Gelfand J, Dinarello C: Recombinant C5a stimulates transcription rather than translation of IL-1 and TNF: Priming of mononuclear cells with recombinant C5a enhances cytokine synthesis induced by LPS, IL-1 or PMA. Blood 1990; 76:1631-1635.
23. Ayus JC, Sheikh-Hamad D: Silent infection in clotted hemodialysis access grafts. J Am Soc Nephrol 1998; 9:1314.
24. Yeun JY, Kaysen GA: Acute phase proteins and peritoneal dialysate albumin losses are the main determinants of serum albumin in peritoneal dialysis patients. Am J Kidney Dis 1997; 30:923.
25. Bemelmans MH, Gouma DJ, Buurman WA: Influence of nephrectomy on tumor necrosis factor clearance in a murine model. J Immunol 1993; 150:2007.
26. Panichi V, Migliori M, De Pietro S, et al: C-reactive protein in patients with renal diseases. Ren Fail 2001; 23:551.
27. Friedman EA: Advanced glycation end products in diabetic nephropathy. Nephrol Dial Transplant 1999; 14(suppl 3):1.
28. Hasper D, Hummel M, Kleber FX, et al: Systemic inflammation in patients with heart failure. Eur Heart J 1998; 19:761.
29. Keane WF, Collins AJ: Influence of comorbidity on mortality and morbidity in patients treated with hemodialysis. Am J Kidney Dis 1994; 24:1010.
30. Ward R, McLeish K: Polymorphonuclear leukocyte oxidative burst is enhanced in patients with chronic renal insufficiency. J Am Soc Nephrol 1995; 5:1697-1702.
31. McLeish KR, Klein JB, Lederer ED, et al: Azotemia, TNF-alpha, and LPS prime the human neutrophil oxidative burst by distinct mechanisms. Kidney Int 1996; 50:407-416.
32. Himmelfarb J, Lazarus J, Hakim R: Reactive oxygen species production by monocytes and polymorphonuclear leukocytes during dialysis. Am J Kidney Dis 1991; 17:271-276.
33. Ward R: Phagocytic cell function as an index of biocompatibility. Nephrol Dial Transplant 1994; 9(suppl 2):46-56.
34. Morena M, Cristol JP, Canaud B: Why hemodialysis patients are in a prooxidant state? What could be done to correct the pro/antioxidant imbalance. Blood Purif 2000; 18:191-199.
35. Nguyen-Khoa T, Massy ZA, Pascal De Bandt J, et al: Oxidative stress and hemodialysis: Role of inflammation and duration of dialysis treatment. Nephrol Dial Transplant 2001; 16: 335-340.
36. Handelman GJ, Walter MF, Adhikarla R, et al: Elevated plasma F2-isoprostanes in patients on long term dialysis. Kidney Int 2001; 51:1960-1966.
37. Rabb H: The T-cell as a bridge between innate and adaptive immunity. Kidney Int 2002; 61:1935-1946.
38. Aderem A: Role of toll-like receptors in inflammatory response in macrophages. Crit Care Med 2001; 29:S16-S18.
39. Pecoits-Filho R, Lindholm B, Axelsson J, Stenvinkel P: Update on interleukin-6 and its role in chronic renal failure. Nephrol Dial Transplant 2003; 18:1042-1045.
40. Kimmel PL, Phillips TM, Simmens SJ, et al: Immunologic function and survival in hemodialysis patients. Kidney Int 1998; 54:236-244.
41. Wang P, Wu P, Siegel MI, et al: IL-10 inhibits transcription of cytokine genes in human peripheral blood mononuclear cells. J Immunol 1994; 153:811-816.
42. Fiorentino DF, Zlotnik A, Mosmann TR, et al: IL-10 inhibits cytokine production by activated macrophages. J Immunol 1991; 147:3815-3822.
43. Donnelly RP, Freeman SL, Hayes MP: Inhibition of IL-10 expression by IFN-γ upregulates transcription of TNF-α in human monocytes. J Immunol 1995; 155:1420-1427.
44. De Waal Malefyt F, Abrams J, Bennett B, et al: Interleukin 10 (IL-10) inhibits cytokine synthesis by human monocytes: An autoregulatory role of IL-10 produced by monocytes. J Exp Med 1991; 174:1209-1220.
45. Hurst SM, Wilkinson TS, McLoughlin RM, et al: IL-6 and its soluble receptor orchestrate a temporal switch in the pattern of leukocyte recruitment seen during acute inflammation. Immunity 2001; 14:705-714.
46. Kaysen G: C-reactive protein: A story half told. Semin Dial 2000; 13:143-146.
47. Pereira BJ, Shapiro L, King AJ, et al: Plasma levels of IL-1 beta, TNF alpha and their specific inhibitors in undialyzed chronic renal failure, CAPD and hemodialysis patients. Kidney Int 1994; 45:890-896.
48. Schindler R, Linnenweber S, Shulze M, et al: Gene expression of interleukin-1β during hemodialysis. Kidney Int 1993; 43: 712-721.
49. Endres S, Cannon JG, Ghorbani R, et al: *In vitro* production of IL-1beta, IL-1alpha, TNF, and IL-2 in healthy subjects: Distribution, effect of cyclooxygenase inhibition and evidence of independent gene regulation. Eur J Immunol 1989; 19:2327-2333.

50. Lonnemann G, Bingel M, Koch KM, et al: Plasma interleukin-1 activity in humans undergoing hemodialysis with regenerated cellulosic membranes. Lymphokine Res 1987; 6:63-70.
51. Lonnemann G, Van Der Meer JW, Cannon JG, et al: Induction of tumor necrosis factor during extracorporeal blood purification. N Engl J Med 1987; 317:963-964.
52. Luger A, Kovarik J, Stummvoll HK, et al: Blood-membrane interaction in hemodialysis leads to increased cytokine production. Kidney Int 1987; 32:84-88.
53. Lonnemann G, Haubitz M, Schindler R: Hemodialysis-associated induction of cytokines. Blood Purif 1990; 8:214-222.
54. Memoli B, Libetta C, Rampino T, et al: Hemodialysis related induction of interleukin-6 production by peripheral blood mononuclear cells. Kidney Int 1992; 42:320-326.
55. Ryan J, Beynon H, Rees AJ, Cassidy MJ: Evaluation of the *in vitro* production of tumour necrosis factor by monocytes in dialysis patients. Blood Purif 1991; 9:142-147.
56. Girndt M, Sester U, Kaul H, Köhler H: Production of proinflammatory and regulatory monokines in hemodialysis patients shown at a single-cell level. J Am Soc Nephrol 1998; 9: 1689-1696.
57. Perianayagam M, Jaber B, Guo D, et al: Defective interleukin-10 synthesis by peripheral blood mononuclear cells among hemodialysis patients. Blood Purif 2002; 20:543-550.
58. Pereira BJ: Cytokine production in patients on dialysis (Review). Blood Purif 1995; 13:135-146.
59. Balakrishnan VS, Schmid CH, Jaber BL, et al: Interleukin-1 receptor antagonist synthesis by peripheral blood mononuclear cells: A novel predictor of morbidity among hemodialysis patients. J Am Soc Nephrol 2000; 11:2114-2121.
60. Manzoli A, Andreotti F, Varlotta C, et al: Allelic polymorphism of the interleukin-1 receptor antagonist gene in patients with acute or stable presentation of ischemic heart disease. Cardiologia 1999; 44:825-830.
61. Grimaldi LM, Casadei VM, Ferri C, et al: Association of early-onset Alzheimer's disease with an interleukin-1alpha gene polymorphism. Ann Neurol 2000; 47:361-365.
62. McDowell TL, Symons JA, Ploski R, et al: A genetic association between juvenile rheumatoid arthritis and a novel interleukin-1 alpha polymorphism. Arthritis Rheum 1995; 38:221-228.
63. Bailly S, Israel N, Fay M, et al: An intronic polymorphic repeat sequence modulates interleukin-1 alpha gene regulation. Mol Immunol 1996; 33:999-1006.
64. Kornman KS, Crane A, Wang HY, et al: The interleukin-1 genotype as a severity factor in adult periodontal disease. J Clin Periodontol 1997; 24(1):72-77.
65. Fang XM, Schroeder S, Hoeft A, Stuber F: Comparison of two polymorphisms of the interleukin-1 gene family: Interleukin-1 receptor antagonist polymorphism contributes to susceptibility to severe sepsis. Crit Care Med 1999; 27:1330-1334.
66. Loughrey BV, Maxwell AP, Fogarty DG, et al: An interleukin-1β allele, which correlates with a high secretor phenotype, is associated with diabetic nephropathy. Cytokine 1998; 10:984-988.
67. Freedman BI, Yu H, Spray BJ, et al: Genetic linkage analysis of growth factor loci and end-stage renal disease in African Americans. Kidney Int 1997; 51:819-825.
68. Blakemore AI, Cox A, Gonzalez AM, et al: Interleukin-1 receptor antagonist allele (IL1RN*2) associated with nephropathy in diabetes mellitus. Hum Genet 1996; 97:369-374.
69. Berger P, McConnell J, Nunn M, et al: C-reactive protein levels are influenced by common IL-1 gene variations. Cytokine 2002; 17:171-174.
70. Azzawi M, Hasleton P: Tumour necrosis factor alpha and the cardiovascular system: Its role in cardiac allograft rejection and heart disease. Cardiovasc Res 1999; 43:850-859.
71. Wilson AG, Symons JA, McDowell TL, et al: Effects of a polymorphism in the human tumor necrosis factor (alpha) promoter on transcriptional activation. Proc Natl Acad Sci U S A 1997; 94:3195-3199.
72. Mira JP, Cariou A, Grall F, et al: Association of TNF2, a TNF-alpha promoter polymorphism, with septic shock susceptibility and mortality: A multicenter study. JAMA 1999; 282: 561-568.
73. McManus R, Wilson AG, Mansfield J, et al: TNF2, a polymorphism of the tumour necrosis-alpha gene promoter, is a component of the celiac disease major histocompatibility complex haplotype. Eur J Immunol 1996; 26:2113-2118.
74. Nadel S, Newport MJ, Booy R, Levin M: Variation in the tumor necrosis factor-a promoter region may be associated with death from meningococcal disease. J Infect Dis 1996; 174:878-880.
75. McGuire W, Hill AV, Allsopp CE, et al: Variation in the TNF-alpha promoter region associated with susceptibility to cerebral malaria. Nature 1994; 371(6497):508-510.
76. Webb GC, Chaplin DD: Genetic variability at the human tumor necrosis factor loci. J Immunol 1990; 145:1278-1285.
77. Fishman D, Faulds G, Jeffery R, et al: The effect of novel polymorphisms in the interleukin-6 (IL-6) gene on IL-6 transcription and plasma IL-6 levels, and an association with systemic-onset juvenile chronic arthritis. J Clin Invest 1998; 102:1369-1376.
78. Brull DJ, Montgomery HE, Sanders J, et al: Interleukin-6 gene -174g/c and -572g/c promoter polymorphisms are strong predictors of plasma interleukin-6 levels after coronary artery bypass surgery. Arterioscler Thromb Vasc Biol 2001; 21: 1458-1463.
79. Humphries SE, Luong LA, Ogg MS, et al: The interleukin-6 174 G/C polymorphism is associated with risk of coronary heart disease and systolic blood pressure in healthy men. Eur Heart J 2001; 22:2219-2220.
80. Westendorp RG, Langermans JA, Huizinga TW, et al: Genetic influence on cytokine production and fatal meningococcal disease. Lancet 1997; 349:170-173.
81. Lazarus M, Hajeer AH, Turner D, et al: Genetic variation in the interleukin-10 gene promoter and systemic lupus erythematosus. J Rheumatol 1997; 24:2314-2317.
82. Tagore A, Gonsalkorale W, Pravica V, et al: Interleukin-10 (IL-10) genotypes in inflammatory bowel disease. Tissue Antigens 1999; 54:386-390.
83. Girndt M, Kaul H, Sester U, et al: Anti-inflammatory interleukin-10 genotype protects dialysis patients from cardiovascular events. Kidney Int 2002; 62:949-955.
84. Girndt M, Sester U, Sester M, et al: The interleukin-10 promoter genotype determines clinical immune function in hemodialysis patients. Kidney Int 2001; 60:2385-2391.
85. Cambien F, Ricard S, Troesch A, et al: Polymorphisms of the transforming growth factor-beta 1 gene in relation to myocardial infarction and blood pressure. The Etude Cas-Temoin de l'Infarctus du Myocarde (ECTIM) Study. Hypertension 1996; 28:881-887.
86. Grainger DJ, Heathcote K, Chiano M, et al: Genetic control of the circulating concentration of transforming growth factor type-β1. Hum Mol Genet 1999; 8:93-97.
87. Awad MR, El-Gamel A, Hasleton P, et al: Genotypic variation in the transforming growth factor-beta1 gene: Association with transforming growth factor-beta1 production, fibrotic lung disease, and graft fibrosis after lung transplantation. Transplantation 1998; 66:1014-1020.
88. Aziz TM, Burgess M, Hasleton PS, et al: Transforming growth factor beta: Association with arteriosclerosis and left ventricular dysfunction after heart transplantation. Transplant Proc 2001; 33:2334-2336.
89. Grainger DJ, Kemp PR, Metcalfe JC, et al: The serum concentration of active transforming growth factor-beta is severely depressed in advanced atherosclerosis. Nat Med 1995; 1:74-79.

90. Stefoni S, Cianciolo G, Donati G, et al: Low TGF-beta1 serum levels are a risk factor for atherosclerosis disease in ESRD patients. Kidney Int 2002; 61:324-335.
91. Yokota M, Ichihara S, Lin TL, et al: Association of a T29–C polymorphism of the transforming growth factor-beta1 gene with genetic susceptibility to myocardial infarction in Japanese. Circulation 2000; 101:2783-2787.
92. Syrris P, Carter ND, Metcalfe JC, et al: Transforming growth factor-beta1 gene polymorphisms and coronary artery disease. Clin Sci (Lond) 1998; 95:659-667.
93. Wang XL, Sim AS, Wilcken DE: A common polymorphism of the transforming growth factor-beta1 gene and coronary artery disease. Clin Sci (Lond) 1998; 95:745-746.
94. Arbour N, Lorenz E, Schutte B, et al: TLR4 mutations are associated with endotoxin hyporesponsiveness in humans. Nat Genet 2000; 25:187-191.
95. Butler B, Poltorak A: Sepsis and the evolution of the innate immune response. Crit Care Med 2001; 29(suppl):S2-S7.
96. Xu XH, Shah PK, Faure E, et al: Toll-like receptor 4 is expresed by macrophages in murine and human lipid-rich atherosclerotic plaques and upregulated by oxidized LDL. Circulation 2001; 104:3103-3108.
97. Kiechl S, Lorenz E, Reindl M, et al: Toll-like receptor 4 polymorphisms and atherogenesis. N Engl J Med 2002; 347: 185-192.
98. Hoy A, Leininger-Muller B, Kutter D, et al: Growing significance of myeloperoxidase in non-infectious disease. Clin Chem Lab Med 2002; 40:2-8.
99. Piedrafita FJ, Molander RB, Vansant G, et al: An Alu element in the myeloperoxidase promoter contains a composite SP1-thyroid hormone-retinoic acid response element. J Biol Chem 1996; 271:14412-14420.
100. Pecoits-Filho R, Stenvinkel P, Marchlewska A, et al: A functional variant of the myeloperoxidase gene is associated with cardiovascular disease in end stage renal disease patients. Kidney Int 2003; 84:S172-S176.
101. Zimmermann J, Wohrmann S, Passlick-Deetjen J, et al: G-protein beta-3 subunit 825 T-allele is associated with increased mortality in hemodialysis patients. J Am Soc Nephrol 2000:A1597.
102. Bergstrom J, Lindholm B: Malnutrition, cardiac disease and mortality: An integrated point of view. Am J Kidney Dis 1998; 32:834-841.
103. Stenvinkel P, Heimburger O, Lindholm B, et al: Are there two types of malnutrition in chronic renal failure? Evidence for relationships between malnutrition, inflammation and atherosclerosis (MIA syndrome). Nephrol Dial Transplant 2000; 15: 953-960.
104. Dinarello CA, Roubenoff RA: Mechanisms of the loss of lean body mass in patients on chronic dialysis. Blood Purif 1996; 14:388-394.
105. Flores EA, Bistrian BR, Pomposelli JJ, et al: Infusion of tumor necrosis factor/cachectin promotes muscle catabolism in the rat. A synergistic effect with interleukin 1. J Clin Invest 1989; 83:1614-1622.
106. Yeun JY, Kaysen G: Factors influencing serum albumin in dialysis patients. Am J Kidney Dis 1998; 32(suppl 4):S118-S125.
107. Lowrie E: Conceptual model for a core pathobiology of uremia with special reference to anemia, malnourishment, and mortality among dialysis patients. Semin Dial 1997; 10:115-129.
108. Roubenoff R, Roubenoff RA, Cannon JG, et al: Rheumatoid cachexia-cytokine driven hypermetabolism accompanying reduced body cell mass in chronic inflammation. J Clin Invest 1994; 93:2379-2386.
109. Ikizler T: What are the causes and consequences of the chronic inflammatory state in patients on chronic dialysis. Semin Dial 2000; 13:169-171.
110. Kaizu Y, Kimura M, Yoneyama T, et al: Interleukin-6 may mediate malnutrition in chronic hemodialysis patients. Am J Kidney Dis 1998; 31:93-100.
111. Kaizu Y, Ohkawa S, Odamaki M, et al: Association between inflammatory mediators and muscle mass in long-term hemodialysis patients. Am J Kidney Dis 2003; 42:295-302.
112. Bologa RM, Levine DM, Parker TS, et al: Interleukin-6 predicts hypoalbuminemia, hypocholesterolemia, and mortality in hemodialysis patients. Am J Kidney Dis 1998; 32:107-114.
113. Harris TB, Ferrucci L, Tracy RP, et al: Association of elevated interleukin-6 and C-reactive protein levels with mortality in the elderly. Am J Med 1999; 106(5):506-512.
114. Ridker PM, Rifai N, Stampfer MJ, Hennekens CH: Plasma concentrations of interleukin-6 and the risk of future myocardial infarction among apparently healthy men. Circulation 2000; 101:1767-1772.
115. Pecoits-Filho R, Barany P, Lindholm B, et al: Interleukin-6 is an independent predictor of mortality in patients starting dialysis treatment. Nephrol Dial Transplant 2002; 17: 1684-1688.
116. Foley R, Parfrey P, Sarnak M: Clinical epidemiology of cardiovascular disease in chronic renal failure. Am J Kidney Dis 1998; 32:S112-S119.
117. USRDS 2000 Annual Data Report: Atlas of end-stage renal disease in the United States. Bethesda, MD, National Institutes of Health, National Institute of Diabetes and Digestive and Kidney Diseases, 2000.
118. Ridker PM, Cushman M, Stampfer MJ, et al: Inflammation, aspirin, and the risk of cardiovascular disease in apparently healthy men. N Engl J Med 1997; 336:973-979.
119. Blake GJ, Ridker PM: Inflammatory bio-markers and cardiovascular risk prediction. J Intern Med 2002; 252:283-294.
120. Huber SA, Sakkinen P, Conze D, et al: Interleukin-6 exacerbates early atherosclerosis in mice. Arterioscler Thromb Vasc Biol 1999; 19:2364-2367.
121. Elhage R, Clamens S, Besnard S, et al: Involvement of interleukin-6 in atherosclerosis but not in the prevention of fatty streak formation by 17-beta-estradiol, in apolipoprotein deficient mice. Atherosclerosis 2001; 156:315-320.
122. Stenvinkel P, Heimburger O, Jogestrand T: Elevated interleukin-6 predicts progressive carotid artery atherosclerosis in dialysis patients: Association with chlamydia pneumonia seropositivity. Am J Kidney Dis 2002; 39:274-282.
123. Foley RN, Parfrey O, Harnett JD, et al: Hypoalbuminemia, cardiac mortality and morbidity in end stage renal disease. J Am Soc Nephrol 1996; 7:728-736.
124. Kalantar-Zadeh K, Block G, Humphreys MH, Kopple J: Reverse epidemiology of cardiovascular risk factors in maintenance dialysis patients. Kidney Int 2003; 63:793-808.
125. Lentz S: Homocysteine and vascular dysfunction. Life Sci 1997; 61:1205-1215.
126. Boushey CJ, Beresford SAA, Omenn GS, Motulsky AG: Quantitative assessment of plasma homocysteine as a risk factor for vascular disease. JAMA 1995; 274:1049-1057.
127. Clarke R, Daly L, Robinson K, et al: Hyperhomocysteinemia: An independent risk factor for vascular disease. N Engl J Med 1991; 324:1149-1155.
128. Suliman ME, Stenvinkel P, Barany P, et al: Hyperhomocysteinemia and its relationship to cardiovascular disease in ESRD: Influence of hypoalbuminemia, malnutrition, inflammation and diabetes mellitus. Am J Kidney Dis 2003; 41(suppl 1):S89-S95.
129. Young JL, Libby P, Schonbeck U: Cytokines in the pathogenesis of atherosclerosis. Thromb Haemost 2002; 88:554-567.
130. Li YY, McTiernan CF, Feldman AM: Interplay of matrix metalloproteinases, tissue inhibitors of metalloproteinases and their regulators in cardiac matrix remodeling. Cardiovasc Res 2000; 46:214-224.

131. Grainger DJ, Kirschenlohr H, Metcalfe JC, et al: Proliferation of human smooth muscle cells promoted by lipoprotein(a). Science 1993; 260:1655-1658.
132. Dennler S, Itoh S, Vivien D, et al: Direct binding of Smad3 and Smad4 to critical TGF beta-inducible elements in the promoter of human plasminogen activator inhibitor-type 1 gene. EMBO J 1998; 17:3091-3100.
133. Lyons RM, Gentry LE, Purchio AF, Moses HL: Mechanism of activation of latent recombinant transforming growth factor beta 1 by plasmin. J Cell Biol 1990; 110:1361-1367.
134. Carr JG, Stevenson LW, Walden JA, Heber D: Prevalence and hemodynamic correlates of malnutrition in severe congestive heart failure secondary to ischemic or idiopathic dilated cardiomyopathy. Am J Cardiol 1989; 63:709-713.
135. Freeman LM, Roubenoff RA: The nutritional implications of cardiac cachexia. Nutr Rev 1994; 52:340-347.
136. Munger MA, Johnson B, Amber IJ, et al: Circulating concentrations of proinflammatory cytokines in mild or moderate heart failure secondary to ischemic or idiopathic dilated cardiomyopathy. Am J Cardiol 1996; 77:723-727.
137. Levine B, Kalman J, Mayer L, et al: Elevated circulating levels of tumor necrosis factor in severe chronic heart failure. N Engl J Med 1990; 323:236-241.
138. Lowbeer C, Stenvinkel P, Pecoits-Filho R, et al: Elevated cardiac troponin T in predialysis patients is associated with inflammation and predicts mortality. J Intern Med 2003; 253:153-160.
139. Wang AY, Woo J, Wang M, et al: Association of inflammation and malnutrition with cardiac valve calcification in continuous ambulatory peritoneal dialysis patients. J Am Soc Nephrol 2001; 12:1927-1936.
140. Stompor T, Pasowicz M, Sullowicz W, et al: An association between coronary artery calcification score, lipid profile, and selected markers of chronic inflammation in ESRD patients treated with peritoneal dialysis. Am J Kidney Dis 2003; 41: 203-211.
141. Libby P, Ridker PM, Maseri A: Inflammation and atherosclerosis. Circulation 2002; 105:1135-1143.
142. Querfeld U, Ong JM, Prehn J, et al: Effects of cytokines on the production of lipoprotein lipase in cultured human macrophages. J Lipid Res 1990; 31:1379-1386.
143. Grunfeld C, Gulli R, Moser AH, et al: Effect of tumor necrosis factor administration in vivo on lipoprotein lipase activity in various tissues of the rat. J Lipid Res 1989; 30:579-585.
144. Navab M, Berliner JA, Watson AD, et al: The Yin and Yang of oxidation in the development of the fatty streak. A review based on the 1994 George Lyman Duff Memorial Lecture. Arterioscler Thromb Vasc Biol 1996; 16:831-842.
145. Wade DP, Clarke JG, Lindahl GE, et al: Genetic influences on lipoprotein(a) concentration. Biochem Soc Trans 1993; 21:499-502.
146. Kario K, Matsuo T, Kobayashi H, et al: High lipoprotein (a) levels in chronic hemodialysis patients are closely related to the acute phase reaction. Thromb Haemost 1995; 74:1020-1024.
147. Dieplinger H, Lackner C, Kronenberg F, et al: Elevated plasma concentrations of lipoprotein(a) in patients with end-stage renal disease are not related to the size polymorphism of apolipoprotein(a). J Clin Invest 1993; 91:397-401.
148. Milionis HJ, Winder AF, Mikhailidis DP: Lipoprotein (a) and stroke. J Clin Pathol 2000; 53:487-496.
149. Loscalzo J: Lipoprotein(a). A unique risk factor for atherothrombotic disease. Arteriosclerosis 1990; 10(5):672-679.
150. Poon M, Zhang X, Dunsky KG, et al: Apolipoprotein(a) induces monocyte chemotactic activity in human vascular endothelial cells. Circulation 1997; 96:2514-2519.
151. Grainger DJ, Kemp PR, Liu AC, et al: Activation of transforming growth factor-beta is inhibited in transgenic apolipoprotein(a) mice. Nature 1994; 370:460-462.
152. Levin EG, Miles LA, Fless GM, et al: Lipoproteins inhibit the secretion of tissue plasminogen activator from human endothelial cells. Arterioscler Thromb 1994; 14:438-442.
153. Li XN, Grenett HE, Benza RL, et al: Genotype-specific transcriptional regulation of PAI-1 expression by hypertriglyceridemic VLDL and Lp(a) in cultured human endothelial cells. Arterioscler Thromb Vasc Biol 1997; 17:3215-3223.
154. Danesh J, Collins R, Peto R: Lipoprotein(a) and coronary heart disease. Meta-analysis of prospective studies. Circulation 2000; 102:1082-1085.
155. Kalayoglu M, Libby P, Byrne GI: Chlamydia pneumoniae as an emerging risk factor in cardiovascular disease. JAMA 2002; 288:2724.
156. Ericson K, Saldeen TG, Lindquist O, et al: Relationship of Chlamydia pneumoniae infection to severity of human coronary atherosclerosis. Circulation 2000; 101:2568.
157. Kuo C, Shor A, Campbell LA, et al: Demonstration of Chlamydia pneumoniae in atherosclerotic lesions of coronary arteries. J Infect Dis 1993; 167:841.
158. Lopes-Virella MF, Virella G: The role of immune and inflammatory processes in the development of macrovascular disease in diabetes. Front Biosci 2003; 8:S750-S768.
159. Yudkin JS, Stehouwer CD, Emeis JJ, Coppack SW: C-reactive protein in healthy subjects: Associations with obesity, insulin resistance, and endothelial dysfunction: A potential role for cytokines originating from adipose tissue? Arterioscler Thromb Vasc Biol 1999; 19:972-978.
160. Weinhold B, Ruther U: Interleukin-6-dependent and -independent regulation of the human C-reactive protein gene. Biochem J 1997; 327:425-429.
161. Danesh J, Whincup P, Walker M, et al: Low grade inflammation and coronary heart disease: Prospective study and updated meta-analyses. BMJ 2000; 321:199-204.
162. Hackam DG, Anand SS: Emerging risk factors for atherosclerotic vascular disease: A critical review of the evidence. JAMA 2003; 290:932-940.
163. Arici M, Walls J: End-stage renal disease, atherosclerosis, and cardiovascular mortality: Is C-reactive protein the missing link? Kidney Int 2001; 59:407-414.
164. Shishehbor MH, Bhatt DL, Topol EJ: Using C-reactive protein to assess cardiovascular disease risk. Cleve Clin J Med 2003; 70:634-640.
165. Bergstrom J, Lindholm B: What are the causes and consequences of the chronic inflammatory state in chronic dialysis patients? Semin Dial 2000; 13:163-164.
166. Bergstrom J, et al: (Abstract). J Am Soc Nephrol 1995; 6:573.
167. Iseki K, Tozawa M, Yoshi S, Fukiyama K: Serum C-reactive protein (CRP) and risk of death in chronic dialysis patients. Nephrol Dial Transplant 1999; 14:1956-1960.
168. CREED (Cardiovascular Risk Extended Evaluation in Dialysis Patients) investigators: C-reactive protein and atherosclerosis in dialysis patients. Nephrol Dial Transplant 1998; 13: 2710-2711.
169. Menon V, Wang X, Greene T, et al: Relationship between C-reactive protein, albumin, and cardiovascular disease in patients with chronic kidney disease. Am J Kidney Dis 2003; 42:44-52.
170. Jongen-Lavrencic M, Peeters HR, Wognum A, et al: Elevated levels of inflammatory cytokines in bone marrow of patients with rheumatoid arthritis and anemia of chronic disease. J Rheumatol 1997; 24:1504-1509.
171. Tarng DC, Huang TP, Chen TW, Yang WC: Erythropoietin hyporesponsiveness: From iron deficiency to iron overload. Kidney Int Suppl 1999; 69(suppl):S107-S118.
172. Allen DA, Breen C, Yaqoob MM, Macdougall IC: Inhibition of CFU-E colony formation in uremic patients with inflammatory disease: Role of IFN-gamma and TNF-alpha. J Investig Med 1999; 47:204-211.

173. Goicoechea M, Martin J, de Sequera P, et al: Role of cytokines in the response to erythropoietin in hemodialysis patients. Kidney Int 1998; 54:1337-1343.
174. Kalantar-Zadeh K, McAllister CJ, Lehn RS, et al: Effect of malnutrition-inflammation complex syndrome on EPO hyporesponsiveness in maintenance hemodialysis patients. Am J Kidney Dis 2003; 42:761-773.
175. Pertosa G, Grandaliano G, Gesualdo L, Schena FP: Clinical relevance of cytokine production in hemodialysis. Kidney Int Suppl 2000; 76(suppl):S104-S111.
176. Zaoui PM, Stone WJ, Hakim RM: Effects of dialysis membranes on beta 2-microglobulin production and cellular expression. Kidney Int 1990; 38:962-968.
177. Miyata T, Inagi R, Iida Y, et al: Involvement of beta 2-microglobulin modified with advanced glycation end products in the pathogenesis of hemodialysis-associated amyloidosis. Induction of human monocyte chemotaxis and macrophage secretion of tumor necrosis factor-alpha and interleukin-1. J Clin Invest 1994; 93:521-528.
178. Ferreira A, Urena P, Ang KS, et al: Relationship between serum beta 2-microglobulin, bone histology, and dialysis membranes in uraemic patients. Nephrol Dial Transplant 1995; 10:1701-1707.
179. Cohen G, Haag-Weber M, Horl W: Immune dysfunction in uremia. Kidney Int 1997; 52:S79-S82.
180. Girndt M, Sester M, Sester U, et al: Molecular aspects of T- and B-cell function in uremia. Kidney Int Suppl 2001; 78: S206-S211.
181. Girndt M, Kohler H, Schiedhelm-Weick E, et al: Production of interleukin-6, tumor necrosis factor alpha and interleukin-10 *in vitro* correlates with the clinical immune defect in chronic hemodialysis patients. Kidney Int 1995; 47:559-565.
182. Lowrie E: Chronic inflammation and clinical outcome in adult hemodialysis patients. Kidney Int Suppl 2002; 61(suppl 80): S94-S98.
183. Zoccali C, Mallamaci F, Tripepi G: Adipose tissue as a source of inflammatory cytokines in health and disease: Focus on end-stage renal disease. Kidney Int Suppl 2003; suppl 84:S65-S68.
184. Feingold KR, Grunfeld C: Role of cytokines in inducing hyperlipidemia. Diabetes 1992; 41(suppl 2):97-101.
185. Wallenius V, Wallenius K, Ahren B, et al: Interleukin-6-deficient mice develop mature-onset obesity. Nat Med 2002; 8:75-79.
186. Hotamisligil GS, Arner P, Caro JF, et al: Increased adipose tissue expression of tumor necrosis factor-alpha in human obesity and insulin resistance. J Clin Invest 1995; 95:2409-2415.
187. Michie H: Metabolism of sepsis and multiple organ failure. World J Surg 1996; 20:460-464.
188. Muller S, Martin S, Koenig W, et al: Impaired glucose tolerance is associated with increased serum concentrations of interleukin-6 and co-regulated acute-phase proteins but not TNF-alpha or its receptors. Diabetologia 2002; 45:805-812.
189. Goldbach-Mansky R, Lipsky P: New concepts in the treatment of rheumatoid arthritis. Annu Rev Med 2003; 54:197-216.
190. Morena MD, Guo D, Balakrishnan VS, et al: Effect of a novel adsorbent on cytokine responsiveness to uremic plasma. Kidney Int 2003; 63:1150-1154.
191. Ridker PM, Rifai N, Pfeffer MA, et al: Long-term effects of pravastatin on plasma concentration of C-reactive protein. The Cholesterol and Recurrent Events (CARE) Investigators. Circulation 1999; 100:230-235.
192. Albert MA, Danielson E, Rifai N, et al: PRINCE Investigators. Effect of statin therapy on C-reactive protein levels: The pravastatin inflammation/CRP evaluation (PRINCE): A randomized trial and cohort study. JAMA 2001; 286:64-70.
193. Libby P: Current concepts of the pathogenesis of the acute coronary syndromes. Circulation 2001; 104:365-372.
194. Boaz M, Smetana S, Weinstein T, et al: Secondary prevention with antioxidants of cardiovascular disease in endstage renal disease (SPACE): Randomised placebo-controlled trial. Lancet 2000; 356:1213-1218.
195. Libby P, Aikawa M: Stabilization of atherosclerotic plaques: New mechanisms and clinical targets. Nat Med 2002; 8: 1257-1262.

Chapter 13

Sleep Disorders in Chronic Kidney Disease and Transplantation

Daniel Norman, M.D. • Robert Thomas, M.D.

OVERVIEW

Sleep and Sleep-Breathing: A Primer for the Nephrologist

The human sleep-wake cycle is primarily generated through interactions of the circadian system and a sleep homeostat. These two separate but interacting oscillatory processes mediate much of sleep or wake propensity at any given point in time. Sleep debt increases during wakefulness and dissipates during sleep. At the same time, the suprachiasmatic nucleus of the hypothalamus generates a wake or arousal signal that increases in strength throughout the biologic day, peaking in the evening hours at approximately 2200 hours, to keep us awake despite an increasing sleep debt in the evening hours. The strength of this signal then declines during the biologic night to reach a minimum at approximately 0600 hours, which coincides with the nadir of body temperature to help keep us asleep as we "pay off" our sleep debt into the early morning. In the absence of this circadian arousal signal, sleep-wake consolidation is lost, and the monophasic sleep-wake cycle is replaced by a polyphasic sleep-wake cycle.

Many protective mechanisms are compromised during sleep. The upper airway, a dynamic structure that serves functions in speech, swallowing, and respiration, is particularly vulnerable during sleep. Most patients with obstructive sleep-disordered breathing (SDB) have an anatomic predisposition (a smaller airway that is longer and laterally compressed) to airway collapse. However, during wakefulness, protective mechanisms maintain an open airway by increasing the activity of tongue and pharyngeal dilator muscles. These protective mechanisms can fail during sleep, with subsequent collapse of the pharyngeal airway behind the palate, tongue, or both. Control mechanisms are also important, because for any given anatomic abnormality, there is a wide spectrum of clinical disease. Disordered breathing events occur only during sleep, even in patients with the most severe obstructive disease. Instability of respiratory control can lead to periodic breathing with variable respiratory effort, and complete or partial obstruction can occur at the nadir of the ventilatory cycle. As a result, instability of respiratory control may contribute, in some individuals, to the development of obstructive disease. Such interactions of anatomy and control may be most important in populations with a high prevalence of mixed disease, including chronic renal failure and congestive heart failure.

Upper airway narrowing during sleep fluctuates continuously within a population and across nights within an individual. Predominantly obstructive and nonobstructive disease (central apneas; periodic breathing, including Cheyne-Stokes, hypoventilation) each has characteristic appearances on sleep studies. A polysomnogram, otherwise known as a sleep study, typically records information on sleep timing, staging, respiratory effort, air flow, muscle tone, oxyhemoglobin saturation, and limb movements. Apneas are complete or nearly complete cessations of airflow, and hypopneas are events of lesser severity. Study interpretation will typically include indices of the frequency of breathing disturbances during sleep, such as a respiratory disturbance index (RDI), an apnea-hypopnea index (AHI), or an oxygen desaturation index (ODI) (often the number of 4% desaturations per hour of sleep). There is still much uncertainty regarding the physiologically appropriate method of scoring abnormal breathing during sleep and phenotyping of the scored abnormality. When associated with desaturations and clinical symptoms, a count of 5 or more events per hour of sleep is considered a reasonable threshold to treat; when scoring regardless of desaturations, counts of close to 20 are at the upper end of normal. However, counts do not clearly reflect severity of individual events, because they do not necessarily reflect the duration, impact on sleep, and degree of autonomic activation at arousal from each event. The criteria used to score these events are especially relevant, because methods used in the older literature may not be comparable with the most recent. It is important to recognize that virtually all studies on sleep-breathing in the renal failure population used the less-sensitive thermal air sensors (thermistors) rather than the more sensitive nasal cannula-pressure transducer technique. This tends to underestimate diagnostic severity and overestimate therapeutic efficacy. In the absence of symptoms, the application of scoring results is even more problematic, but a count greater than 15 respiratory events that have oxygen desaturation per hour of sleep may be a reasonable threshold to recommend treatment in healthy and asymptomatic individuals.

Sleep in Renal Disease

Sleep disorders are very common in the setting of renal disease. Questionnaire-based studies have reported a prevalence of sleep disorders in 43% to 86% of patients with end-stage renal disease (ESRD) (vs. 12% of healthy controls).[1–4] Sleep symptoms become more frequent with the introduction of hemodialysis (HD),[3] are similar in prevalence among patients on hemodialysis or peritoneal dialysis,[1,5] and increase with the duration of dialysis therapy.[4] Sleep-related complaints are also more common with advanced age, male gender,[6] and increased caffeine intake.[1,6] Among HD patients, reports of daytime sleepiness are more common in those on the morning versus afternoon or evening dialysis shifts, and morning-shift patients also report the fewest hours of nightly sleep.[4]

Hemodialysis may result in the production of sleepiness-inducing cytokines,[7] and napping during the dialysis sessions is a very common occurrence.

Common sleep disorders in patients with renal disease include insomnia, circadian rhythm disturbances, obstructive and central sleep apnea, restless legs syndrome (RLS), and periodic limb movement disorder (PLMD). Sleep apnea is estimated to be 10 times more prevalent in patients with ESRD than in the general population.[8] In a study of an unselected series of patients with ESRD, 70% reported symptoms of excessive daytime somnolence and 31% demonstrated evidence of sleep disordered breathing (AHI = 5 events/hr).[9] Parker and colleagues[10] studied stable hemodialysis patients, excluding subjects if interview revealed symptoms of sleep apnea, RLS or PLMD, and then found that of the 46 "asymptomatic" participants, 33% displayed abnormal levels (defined by mean sleep latency < 8 min) of objective sleepiness by multiple sleep latency test (MSLT), 50% had evidence of sleep apnea (defined by a respiratory disturbance index of > 5 events/hr), and 50% had evidence of PLMD (PLM index > 5 events/hr).

Consequences of Abnormal Sleep in Renal Failure

Earlier data had to be extrapolated from work with the non-ESRD population, but there is now a body of research on the effects of sleep disorders directly related to patients with ESRD. A recent study by Bliwise and colleagues[11] reported that median survival among morning-shift HD patients is double that of afternoon-shift patients, and others have demonstrated that individuals undergoing morning HD have the fewest hours of nightly sleep[4] and are sleepier than those dialyzed at other times of the day.[2] PLMD predicts increased mortality risk among hemodialysis patients,[12] and after adjusting for age, sex, and number of years on dialysis, the presence of restless legs syndrome was associated with an astounding 80% greater risk of mortality over 2.5 years of follow-up in one surveyed series of hemodialysis patients.[13]

Cardiovascular Consequences

Obstructive sleep apnea is now accepted as an independent risk factor for the development of hypertension, arrhythmias, congestive heart failure, and stroke.[14] Given its high prevalence in this population, it is likely to play a significant role in cardiovascular morbidity in patients with renal disease.[15] Data from the Sleep Heart Health Study demonstrated clear associations between sleep apnea and the development of hypertension.[16] Episodic hypoxia causes surges in blood pressure, heart rate, and sympathetic activity in patients with sleep apnea and is associated with a loss of the normal "dip" in blood pressure seen in normal individuals during the night.[17] Patients with chronic renal failure show a similar blunting of the normal blood pressure decline at night,[18] and this blunting tends to become more severe in pre-dialysis patients as renal failure worsens.[19,20] A lack of normal blood pressure decline at night is a known predictor of end-organ damage in hypertensive patients,[21] a phenomenon to which SDB likely contributes. When patients who lack normal nocturnal decline in blood pressure are studied by polysomnography, many are found to have unrecognized sleep apnea.[22] Episodic hypoxia causes progressive increases in blood pressure in animal studies, mediated in part through rennin-angiotensin system activation, via increased renal sympathetic nerve activity.[23] A prospective study by Covic and colleagues,[21] using ambulatory blood pressure monitoring, demonstrated that lack of normal nocturnal blood pressure decline is surprisingly common among patients with ESRD (67% were nondippers), and that only the consistent nondippers in this cohort developed left ventricular dilation and hypertrophy by echocardiography over a 12-month period of follow-up. Another study demonstrated that lack of nocturnal decline in blood pressure in hemodialysis patients was associated with nocturnal hypoxemia, and that greater degrees of nocturnal hypoxemia were associated with greater left ventricular wall thickness and greater incidence of concentric hypertrophy.[25] In a study over 32 months of 50 uremic patients on dialysis without pre-existing pulmonary disease, nocturnal hypoxemia was a significant predictor of the incidence of cardiovascular events: each 1% decrease in average nocturnal oxyhemoglobin saturation associated with a 33% increase in risk of fatal and non-fatal cardiovascular events.[26] Thus, there is ample evidence that the nocturnal hypoxemia and sympathetic activation associated with SDB are physiologically detrimental to the ESRD patient.

Renal Consequences

The pathophysiologic changes associated with SDB, especially the intermittent, severe hypertensive surges, can also damage the kidneys. Compared with daytime blood pressure-matched controls who have a more normal decline in nocturnal blood pressure, nondippers have a faster rate of decline in renal function due to hypertensive nephrosclerosis.[27] Nocturnal hypertension also relates to the rate of decline in renal function in patients with IgA nephropathy.[19] Subnormal nocturnal blood pressure decline has also been linked to degree of urine albumin excretion within the normoalbuminuric range in patients with type I diabetes[28] and correlated with urine albumin excretion in microalbuminuric and normoalbuminuric patients with type II diabetes mellitus.[5] Microalbuminuria, in turn, is a strong predictor of total mortality and cardiovascular mortality and morbidity in this patient population.[29] Cross-sectional studies of type I diabetic patients with microalbuminuria have shown that the nocturnal blood pressure often fails to fall normally during sleep. A recent prospective study demonstrated that the increase in systolic blood pressure during sleep preceded the development of microalbuminuria and was thought to perhaps play a causative role in its development.[30] Among patients with obstructive sleep apnea syndrome, proteinuria correlates with both apnea hypopnea score and time spent with oxyhemoglobin saturation less than 90%.[31] Sklar and colleagues[32–34] demonstrated that 64% of obese apnea subjects had proteinuria (> 46 mcg/min), versus 14% of obese non-apnea subjects, and that apnea patients demonstrate reversibility of proteinuria following treatment of sleep apnea. Glomerular hyperfiltration is decreased by positive airway pressure treatment.[34] Other studies, however, suggest a lesser role for sleep apnea in the development of clinically significant proteinuria, but they do show links between arousal index and urine protein/creatinine ratio.[35] Natriuresis and diuresis decrease by approximately 50% in patients with severe sleep apnea with effective nasal continuous positive airway pressure (CPAP) therapy.[36]

Sleep apnea is also cited as a potential contributor to poor compliance with dialysis.[37] A questionnaire study demonstrated that 20% of the hemodialysis patients had prematurely discontinued dialysis at least once in the past. Self-reported premature discontinuation rates correlated significantly with self-reported sleep problems, sleep onset latency, diminished total sleep time, symptoms of restless legs, and transferrin saturation (which is indirectly linked to RLS).[13]

Sleep Disordered Breathing in the Post-Transplant Population

Perfect blood pressure control is an important goal after renal transplantation. Although there are reports of dramatic improvement in sleep disordered breathing in some patients following kidney transplantation,[38] (see later text) residual sleep apnea can compromise this goal and not be obvious by daytime office blood pressure measurements. The prevalence of significant SDB in unselected post-transplant patients is not known, but preliminary evidence suggests that "cure" cannot be taken for granted.[39] Does SDB-related sympathetic activation exacerbate that induced by cyclosporine and tacrolimus? Clearly, more research is needed in this area.

Metabolic and Infectious Consequences

Sleep deprivation in animal studies results in impairment of host defenses and invasion of bacteria into normally sterile body tissues, with bacterial overgrowth in the intestine and invasion in mesenteric lymph nodes apparent by day 5.[40] In humans, sleep deprivation increases C-reactive protein levels, an independent marker of adverse cardiovascular outcome.[41] Treatment of sleep apnea with CPAP results in diminution of the elevated levels of C-reactive protein and interleukin-6 found in patients with sleep apnea.[42] Severe SDB is associated with the "metabolic syndrome," and intermittent hypoxia models of sleep apnea worsen insulin resistance in animal[43] and human[44] studies, and improvements in insulin resistance in patients with sleep apnea have been shown following CPAP therapy.[45] Could the consequences of severely fragmented sleep amplify some of the metabolic abnormalities, especially increased inflammatory markers and cytokine activation, so commonly seen in ESRD? The metabolic consequences of sleep disorders, particularly sleep-disordered breathing is becoming increasingly recognized. These include insulin resistance, endothelial dysfunction, lipid peroxidation, and cytokine dysregulation.[46–49] Specific research on metabolic changes before and after therapy of sleep apnea in patients with ESRD may be forthcoming.

Quality of Life Consequences

Post-dialysis fatigue is reported in greater than half of patients on hemodialysis.[50] CAPD patients with sleep apnea (respiratory event index > 20/hr) score higher on the depression and anxiety scales of the Minnesota Multiphasic Personality Inventory II tests than those without sleep apnea.[38] Multivariate analyses of a cohort of adult hemodialysis patients revealed that sleep disturbances were linked to levels of pain, depression, and physical functioning.[51] The periodic leg movements (PLM) index correlates to Health & Functioning and Family subsets of quality of life indices in HD patients.[52] The percentage of ESRD patients with a professional activity is significantly higher (63%) for those with ODI less than 15 than those with ODI greater than 15 (21%).[53] A study of 46 HD patients by PSG, MSLT, and questionnaires revealed that 30% have abnormal levels of daytime somnolence, 32% have a mean sleep latency less than 8 minutes, and 13% have a mean sleep latency less than 5 minutes, demonstrating objective measures of severe daytime somnolence.[52] In these studies, MSLT score correlated with quality of life measures, but total recorded sleep time and Epworth Sleepiness Score did not, demonstrating the difficulty in identifying those with the greatest potential degree of impact from sleep disturbances.[52]

Medication use for symptom relief is common. Of those with RLS, 50% report taking a sedative, and frequency of sedative use correlates with severity of RLS.[2] Regular use of hypnotics or minor tranquilizers is reported by 39% of the HD population, with greater frequency of use among females than males.[4] The short- and long-term effects of increased sedative use among this population are largely unknown.

SPECIFIC DISORDERS: ETIOLOGY, DIAGNOSIS, AND MANAGEMENT

Sleep-Disordered Breathing

Prevalence

Polysomnographic studies have revealed sleep apnea prevalence rates of between 50% and 70% among patients with ESRD.[54] This is significantly greater than the prevalence in the general population, which in wide-scale studies ranges from 2% to 8%.[55,56] The prevalence of sleep apnea in ESRD does not seem to relate to the modality of therapy (HD vs. PD) and is often mixed (central and obstructive) in etiology.[54] Pfister and colleagues[53] studied 38 patients with ESRD by overnight ambulatory oximetry, revealing that 47% of ESRD patients (vs. 3% of healthy controls) have an ODI greater than 15. Of those ESRD patients who reported on questionnaire "excessively loud snoring," 88% had an ODI greater than 15, versus 13% of those without. ODI greater than 15 was found in 77% of those who were overweight, and those who had a systolic blood pressure greater than 140. Wadha and colleagues'[57] study of 30 randomly selected ESRD patients (half on HD, half on PD), demonstrated 53% to 60% had sleep apnea (RDI > 5 events/ hr), with the majority of events being obstructive. Similarly, Kimmel and colleagues[58] found that 9 of the 16 ESRD patients with symptomatic sleep apnea studied by overnight polysomnogram had primarily obstructive physiology, whereas in the remaining 7, greater than half of the respiratory events were of the central type. In other series, however, such as Pressman and colleagues'[59] study of eight ESRD patients referred to polysomnography for sleep complaints, central and mixed sleep apnea were more common than obstructive disease.

Mechanisms

There have been a large number of hypotheses proposed to explain the high prevalence of sleep apnea in patients with renal disease. Certainly, part of the explanation stems from the presence of confounders (age, diabetes, tobacco use, and obesity) common to patients with renal disease that are known risk factors for sleep apnea. Many other contributors to the increased prevalence of sleep apnea in renal disease have been proposed, however, including: (1) anemia, (2) ineffective clearance of endogenous substances/opioids that destabilize breathing, (3) diminished upper airway muscle tone from uremic neuropathy, (4) respiratory control instability due to uremic toxin effects on the central nervous system, (5) airway narrowing secondary to volume overload, (6) osmotic disequilibrium from hemodialysis, and (7) chronic metabolic acidosis/compensatory respiratory alkalosis, with an altered pCO_2 threshold (which may increase propensity for central sleep apnea).[38,58,60,61] Many of these proposed mechanisms, however, need further investigation and may be contradicted by other studies that demonstrate no correlation between some of these factors (i.e., degree of azotemia, bicarbonate concentration, or hematocrit) and severity of sleep apnea.[59] The use of testosterone in some patients to stimulate erythropoiesis has been proposed as another potential link between ESRD and sleep apnea but is not supported, because respiratory event indices are not associated with serum testosterone levels and do not change 2 months after discontinuation of testosterone supplements.[62]

Effects of Treatment in End-Stage Renal Disease

Fein and colleagues[63] described complete reversal of sleep apnea in one patient with uremia after the initiation of dialysis. However, adequacy of dialysis, as evaluated by Kt/V, correlates neither with the presence of sleep complaints on questionnaire nor with the number of respiratory events per hour on polysomnography in patients on HD or CAPD.[64] Kimmel and colleagues[58] found no correlation between carbon dioxide tension or plasma hydrogen ion concentration and number of disordered breathing events in a series of 13 ESRD or chronic renal insufficiency (CRI) patients who had both arterial blood gas analysis and polysomnography. Mendelson and colleagues'[65] polysomnographic study of 11 HD patients both on the day before and on the day of dialysis did not show a decrease in number of respiratory events on the nights following dialysis (132 events to 138 events per night on pre- and post-dialysis nights, respectively) or in level of oxyhemoglobin desaturation, but the study did show a smaller percentage of disordered breathing time comprised of central events on nights following dialysis versus nondialysis nights. When Kimmel and colleagues[58] compared hemodialysis patients with patients within "weeks to months" of initiating dialysis (mean serum creatinine and creatinine clearances of 6.8 mg/dL and 9.8 mL/min, respectively), no significant differences were found in the number of disordered breathing events or level of oxyhemoglobin desaturation between the two groups. Interestingly, two patients with chronic renal insufficiency were restudied by polysomnography after initiation of hemodialysis. One, who had clinically significant sleep apnea (defined as >30 total respiratory events on overnight study), continued to have sleep apnea but fewer events on the repeat study (numbers were not published). The other patient with CRI studied twice did not meet criteria (he had 5 total nocturnal respiratory events only) on the initial study but did meet criteria (>30 events overnight) for clinically significant sleep apnea on repeat study 18 months after the initiation of hemodialysis.[58] Although these results seem to refute a causative role for uremia in the development of sleep apnea, it is possible that the adequacy of dialysis achieved among patients involved in these studies was not sufficient to demonstrate a change in apnea frequency or severity.

Hanly and colleagues[66] studied 14 patients with ESRD by polysomnography during conventional, 4 hours at a time, thrice-weekly hemodialysis, and then again after switch to 8-hour nightly hemodialysis. Mean AHI was 25/hr on conventional hemodialysis, and dropped to 8/hr on nocturnal hemodialysis, and stayed lower at 13/hr 2 days after nocturnal hemodialysis was discontinued. Among the subset of 7 of the 14 patients having clinically significant sleep apnea, defined as AHI greater than 15 events per hour, transition to nocturnal hemodialysis was associated with an even more dramatic drop in AHI (from greater than 40/hr, to 9/hr on nocturnal hemodialysis, and to 19/hr 2 days after its discontinuation).[66] The changes described in transition to nocturnal hemodialysis were accompanied not only by a fall in serum creatinine concentration, but also by elevations in serum bicarbonate concentration and transcutaneous pCO_2.[66] The better treatment of metabolic acidosis and resultant movement of pCO_2 away from the apneic threshold may be partly responsible for the decline in AHI, by limiting central sleep apnea and periodic breathing (both thought to be linked to pCO_2) that, in turn, affect upper airway stability and may predispose to obstructive events.[66] The type of dialysate buffer used in hemodialysis may also have an impact on the type and severity of sleep apnea observed, as Jean and colleagues[67] demonstrated that in 10 HD patients studied polysomnographically after 6 HD sessions with either an acetate or bicarbonate buffer, and then again after six sessions with the other, the total number of respiratory events (from 114 to 64), particularly central apneas (from 33 to 3) and hypopneas (from 114 to 64), declined on the night following bicarbonate buffer HD. This change occurred despite no significant difference in arterial pH, pCO_2, and bicarbonate levels after dialysis with each of the two buffers, and was speculated to represent possible alteration of chemical ventilatory control by acetate buffers.[67]

In a study of 11 patients on peritoneal dialysis with polysomnography on two subsequent nights, one with and without PD fluid in the abdominal cavity, 6 were found to have clinically significant sleep apnea, and, although the total number of respiratory events, the distribution of these events between REM and NREM sleep, and the mean percentage of total disordered breathing time comprised of obstructive events did not change between the two nights, the degree of desaturation and wake after sleep time increased, and total sleep time decreased on nights with dialysate instilled versus empty nights.[68] The apneic patients had a significantly lower waking PaO_2 with dialysate instilled compared to empty nights, suggesting that they may have poor ability to compensate for the fluid load in the abdomen that could, in part, predispose them to sleep disordered breathing or greater oxyhemoglobin desaturation.[68]

Transplantation

Several case reports demonstrate significant improvements—and at times, resolution—of central and obstructive sleep apnea in dialysis patients after renal transplant.[38] Some of these cases have been quite spectacular, with patients with pre-transplant AHIs greater than 50 per hour manifesting post-transplant AHIs less than 10 per hour, accompanied by resolution of snoring, daytime somnolence, and nocturnal dyspnea.[39] Another striking example is a case report of a patient with severe sleep apnea, with pre-transplant polysomnography demonstrating an ODI of 133 per hour, and mean- and nadir-oxyhemoglobin saturations of 85% and 52%, respectively, who spent almost half of his total sleep time prior to transplantation with oxyhemoglobin saturations less than 80%. By the time of discharge from hospital following cadaveric kidney transplantation, this patient reported complete resolution of sleep-related symptoms, and on follow-up study, showed an ODI of 6 per hour and mean- and nadir-oxyhemoglobin saturations of 94% and 80%, respectively, demonstrating spectacular improvement in what had been primarily (88%) obstructive sleep-disordered breathing shortly after transplantation.[69] An ongoing study of the effects of transplantation on sleep-disordered breathing has been less impressive (Bertrand Jaber, M.D., personal communication), and resolution should not be taken for granted.

Standard Therapy

Nasal positive airway pressure (PAP) remains the optimal treatment for most patients with sleep apnea. Single night titration of nasal CPAP resulted in improvement in subjective sleep quality, number of awakenings and morning alertness, and objective measures, including reduction in stage I sleep, elevation of oxyhemoglobin saturation nadir (from mean of 79.5% pre-CPAP to 90% with titration), and a drop in apnea/hypopnea index (from mean 64/hr pre-treatment, to 6/hr during titration).[59] Given the known association of ESRD and mixed physiology disease, the failure rate and the need for bilevel ventilation could be expected to be high, but systematic large treatment trials have not been published. Weight reduction, avoidance of supine posture during sleep, maximizing nasal patency, avoidance of alcohol or other sedatives, are often-cited adjuncts in the treatment of sleep apnea but do not substitute for PAP therapy. Dental devices and surgical options also exist but have variable success rates and are less often used. A diet with high concentrations of branched-chain amino acids may improve central sleep apnea in chronic renal failure patients but appears to worsen obstructive disease and warrants further study.[70]

Restless Legs Syndrome and Periodic Limb Movement Disorder

Prevalence

Walker and colleagues'[2] questionnaire-based study of unselected patients in a hemodialysis unit indicates a prevalence of RLS in the HD population of 57%. Among these patients, 48% report severe symptoms, an equal proportion believe that RLS causes delays in their sleep onset, and a full 74% report excessive daytime somnolence.[2] Though RLS severity does not seem to correlate with serum creatinine levels, HD patients with RLS tend to have higher pre-dialysis urea and creatinine concentrations.[2] Restless legs symptoms have been associated with nocturnal awakening, sleep-onset latency, diminished total sleep time, pruritis, and the use of medications as sleep aids.[13] Periodic limb movements of sleep is a disorder that is characterized by rhythmic movements (usually the lower) of extremities during sleep that is often seen in patients with restless legs syndrome but may exist independently as well. PLM by sleep study in CAPD population is more common in those with higher intact PTH levels,[38] suggesting a possible contributor may be altered calcium homeostasis. Although it was previously thought to be a prevalent cause of sleep disruption, many in the sleep field now question the significance of PLMD role in sleep disturbance, because limb movements may be just a marker for arousals related to respiratory effort.[71] The presence of "significant" PLM (>25/hr) on PSG in CAPD patients is not predicted by sleep complaints, and is in fact less common in those who report leg twitching at night than those who do not.[38] Pressman and colleagues'[59] study of ESRD patients with symptomatic sleep apnea demonstrated a trend toward decline in PLMS with arousal during single night of CPAP titration study. The presence of PLMs by sleep study is related to mortality, with patients with ESRD who have a PLM index greater than 80 per hour and a median survival of 6 months.[12] In one study, PLM index actually appeared to be a better predictor of mortality in this population than more traditional indicators, including serum albumin concentration, hematocrit level, and urea reduction ratio.[53]

Mechanisms

Despite similar polysomnographic measures of sleep macroarchitecture (total sleep time, sleep efficiency, sleep latency, time spent awake, time spent in various sleep stages), uremic patients with RLS have significantly higher PLM indices during sleep and wakefulness and poorer subjective sleep quality compared to nonuremic patients with RLS symptoms of similar severity, indicating that uremia itself may (perhaps through increased excitability) contribute to greater impact of RLS on sleep.[72] Iron deficiency and abnormal iron transport mechanisms to the central nervous system are thought to be involved in the etiology of many cases of RLS and PLMD and are likely to play some role in the high prevalence of these disorders in patients with ESRD.[73] Magnetic resonance imaging utilizing special sequences can quantify iron in the basal ganglia but remains a research tool. Serum ferritin levels less than 50 mcg per liter are often used as an indirect marker and may indicate a prospect for improvement with iron replacement therapy.[73] Other potential contributors in patients with ESRD include uremic peripheral neuropathy[73] and spinal cord pathology, because spinal cord flexor withdrawal reflex excitability during sleep is increased in idiopathic RLS associated with renal failure.[74]

Effects of Treatment in End-Stage Renal Disease

Roger and colleagues[75] demonstrated that of the 55 ESRD patients studied, 40% had RLS and that treatment with erythropoietin in the affected group did result in a substantial improvement in symptoms. In addition, there have been some case reports of resolution of restless leg syndrome in a number of patients with ESRD after kidney transplantation,[76,77] but in a substantial proportion of these patients, RLS may gradually reappear.[77]

Standard Therapy

Guidelines for therapy of RLS in patients with renal disease are now available. Intravenous iron was an original treatment for RLS, and appropriate repletion of iron stores is still very important in this patient group.[73] In the hemodialysis population, correction of anemia through iron supplementation (including intravenous) and recombinant human EPO results in significant reduction of PLMS, arousing PLMS, and improves daytime alertness.[78] Levodopa/carbidopa is effective for the treatment of RLS in this poplulation,[79] but although it lowers PLMS indices, there is conflicting data on whether it causes subjective improvement in sleep quality.[80,81] There is now a clear preference for the newer dopamine agonists, such as pramipexole, pergolide, cabergoline, and ropinirole over levodopa/carbidopa as first-line therapy, because levodopa/carbidopa is associated with greater risk for augmentation of symptoms over time. (Augmentation refers to development of increased symptoms that start earlier in circadian time that temporarily respond to an increased dose.) The newer dopamine agonists, though generally well tolerated, are still not ideal. Pergolide therapy results in subjective improvement in restless legs symptoms, quality of sleep, and lowers PLMS indices, but it does not necessarily result in less interrupted sleep by polysomnography.[82,83] Pramipexole has few side effects, reduces severity of restless legs symptoms, and significantly lessens PLM while awake and PLM of sleep,[84] but does not significantly change sleep latency, sleep efficiency, or total hours of sleep time by pretreatment and posttreatment polysomnography.[84] Opioids are effective but are usually reserved for patients who fail dopamine agonist therapy.[85,86] Clonazepam, despite its widespread use in RLS, has extremely limited data supporting its efficacy[87,88]; thus it and other benzodiazepines are also considered second-line therapies.[89] Gabapentin may be an effective option for restless legs syndrome in hemodialysis patients who do not respond to other therapies, but needs further study.[73,90] Table 13–1 lists medications used for the treatment of RLS/PLMS, along with information on dosing and common side effects. Clinical trials are ongoing with several newer antiepileptics, such as levetiracetam (Keppra), so further choices may be available.

Insomnia and Circadian Rhythm Abnormalities

Insomnia is a rather nonspecific complaint from the pathophysiologic standpoint (difficulty initiating and maintaining sleep, poor subjective sleep quality, nocturnal awakenings), but 45% of hemodialysis patients reported it, and rates increase with age, morning hemodialysis, greater than 12 months duration of dialysis, and serum PTH levels.[91] Polysomnographic studies of stable HD patients not on sedatives, who report no symptoms of RLS or sleep apnea, reveal diminished total sleep times and sleep efficiency compared to age-matched norms.[9] Patients often sleep during hemodialysis. Mean daytime melatonin levels are increased for patients with CRF (whether on conservative therapy, HD, PD, or post-transplant) versus healthy controls,[92] and the normal nocturnal rise in melatonin concentration seen in healthy controls was reportedly absent in all HD patients and 80% of post-transplant patients.[92] Deficiency in nocturnal pineal synthetic enzyme activity and diminished renal clearance or degradation of melatonin are described as potential etiologies for the lack of nocturnal surge and elevated daytime levels of melatonin, respectively, in patients with renal disease.[92] Vaziri and colleagues[93] demonstrated an attenuation of the normal decline in serum melatonin and little change in its principle metabolite, 6-sulfatoxymelatonin in the morning hours in patients with ESRD, with no significant clearance of either compound with HD. In animal models of CRF using 5/6 nephrectomy, Vaziri and colleagues[94] demonstrated an attenuated nocturnal surge in serum melatonin that was partially restored by the administration of erythropoietin to correct anemia. However, in patients with ESRD, insomnia, delayed sleep onset, and night-time arousals are not directly linked to serum melatonin concentrations, possibly due to the supraphysiologic range that often exists in this population.[95] While altered melatonin physiology may be one contributor to the high prevalence of insomnia in patients with ESRD, multiple other factors are likely to exist, including side effects of various medications, reduced nocturnal sleep drive secondary to daytime naps (i.e., during HD sessions), restless legs symptoms, and prolonged sleep latency from sleep-onset respiratory instability.

MANAGEMENT ISSUES AND CHALLENGES FOR THE FUTURE

Screening for Sleep Disorders

Despite a surprisingly high prevalence, our ability to identify those at highest risk for sleep disorders among patients with ESRD remains limited. Of ESRD patients with "excessively loud snoring," 88% have ODI greater than 15, but so do 38% without, and more than half of ESRD patients with an ODI greater than 15 deny excessively loud snoring by questionnaire.[53] Thus, snoring is not a particularly useful screening tool. Parker and colleagues[9,96] confirmed work done by others to demonstrate that the Epworth Sleepiness Scale (ESS), an often used questionnaire-based method for assessing sleepiness, correlates poorly with the MSLT score (an objective measure of sleepiness used in the laboratory). Patients with ESRD have significantly higher levels of sleepiness by validated questionnaires (Epworth Sleepiness Scale and Visual Analog Scale), but these scores do not correlate with ODI.[53] Questionnaire screening for restless legs syndrome in patients on chronic dialysis is also problematic, with both low sensitivity and specificity.[97] Others have demonstrated that questionnaire-based screening of patients with ESRD for symptoms of sleep apnea is equally inaccurate.[9] One possible practical approach is to assume that all patients have abnormal sleep until proven otherwise and to use screening tools to stratify disease severity. The latter could include limited polysomnography, including nasal pressure-based airflow detection and oximetry (unfortunately not covered by Medicare in the United States, but this limitation does not exist elsewhere), and a restless legs severity questionnaire.

Management Challenges and Sleep Disordered Breathing

Management of sleep and SDB in ESRD poses unique challenges. It seems that everything that could go wrong with the

Table 13–1 Medications for Restless Legs Syndrome and Periodic Limb Movements of Sleep

Agent/Class	Usual Dose (mg)	Dose Adjustment in Renal Failure	Notes/Precautions	Common Side Effects
Dopamine Agonists				
Bromocriptine	1.25 –15 mg qhs	Unknown–liver metabolism predominates	Rarely used for this indication. Rare reports of seizures, serositis/fibrosis, and cardiac arrhythmias	Same as for pergolide
Cabergoline	0.25–2 mg qhs	Unknown	Same as for pergolide	Same as for pergolide
Carbidopa/ levodopa	25/100 mg qhs– 100/400 mg tid	Unknown–no major dose adjustment needed	Higher chance of augmentation phenomena (see text) than other dopamine agonists. Absorption reduced if ingested with iron salts, increased clearance if taken with pyridoxine (B_6)	Dyskinesia, nausea, orthostatic hypotension, hallucination, insomnia
Pergolide	0.05 mg qhs–1 tid	Unknown	Rare reports of serositis/ fibrosis. Rare cardiac arrhythmias	Same as for levodopa, plus somnolence, peripheral edema, nasal congestion
Pramipexole	0.125 mg qhs– 1.5 tid	Renal clearance– very long $t_{1/2}$ in ESRD, start at half tablet of 0.125 mg qhs, increase slowly to minimum necessary dose	Same as for pergolide. Daytime somnolence, "sleep attacks"	Same as for pergolide
Ropinirole	0.25 mg qhs–1 tid	Unknown–liver metabolism predominates	Same as for pergolide	Same as for pergolide
Sedative/Hypnotics				
Clonazepam	0.25–4 mg qhs	Not needed–liver metabolism predominates	Probably best avoided—there are superior medications available	Confusion, somnolence, tolerance
Oxazepam	10–40 mg qhs	Unknown–may need longer time to reach steady state levels in ESRD		Same as for clonazepam
Temazepam	7.5–30 mg qhs	Unknown but has 80%–90% renal clearance		Same as for clonazepam
Triazolam	0.125–0.5 mg qhs	Not needed	Duration of action too short	Same as for clonazepam
Zaleplon	5–20 mg qhs	Unknown–liver metabolism predominates		Same as for clonazepam
Zolpidem	5–20 mg qhs	No dosage adjustment necessary Additional dosing not necessary after HD		Same as for clonazepam

Continued

Table 13–1 Medications for Restless Legs Syndrome and Periodic Limb Movements of Sleep—Cont'd

Agent/Class	Usual Dose (mg)	Dose Adjustment in Renal Failure	Notes/Precautions	Common Side Effects
Opiates				
Codeine	30–180 mg qhs	Decrease dose by 50% for ESRD		Sedation, pruritis, confusion, constipation, nausea
Hydrocodone	5–30 mg qhs	Unknown–6%–20% excreted unchanged in urine		Same as for codeine
Methadone	2.5–30 mg qhs	Recommend low doses due to likely prolonged $t_{1/2}$		Same as for codeine
Morphine	5–30 mg qhs IR, 30 mg qhs–30 mg tid CR	Decrease dose by 50% for ESRD	Controlled–release forms provide longer duration of action	Same as for codeine
Oxycodone	5–10 mg IR, 10 mg qhs–20 mg bid CR	Suggest decreasing dose by 50% in ESRD	Controlled–release forms provide longer duration of action	Same as for codeine
Propoxyphene	150–250 mg qhs	See note to right	AVOID use in patients with renal insufficiency–active metabolite, norpropoxyphene accumulates	Same as for codeine
Tramadol	50–100 mg qhs	Renal excretion occurs, so recommend lowest possible doses. Only 7% removed by HD, so additional dosing not necessary	Potential for augmentation phenomenon	Same as for codeine
Other				
Clonidine	0.1–1 mg qhs	None		Dry mouth, dizziness, constipation, sedation
Ferrous sulfate	325 mg qd–324 mg tid	None	Indicated for patients with serum ferritin levels < 50 mcg/L Consider IV iron if refractory	Constipation, dark stools, nausea
Gabapentin	300–900 mg tid	Renal clearance, dialyzable. 100 qhs –300 tid, with additional 100–200 dose post-HD		Sedation, fatigue, dizziness, somnolence, ataxia

Adapted from Earley CJ: Restless legs syndrome. NEJM 2003; 348:2103-2109. Dosing guidelines should not substitute for clinical judgment. In all cases, lowest initial dose with very gradual titration is recommended because of increased risk for adverse effects from accumulation of active compounds.

sleep system does so in these patients. The effects of weight change and body fluid distribution in the interdialytic interval are not known, but some change in positive airway pressure requirements may occur. Auto-adjusting PAP machines would, in theory, be optimal, but currently available machines do poorly in patients with mixed obstructive and central disease and thus would not be appropriate for many patients with CRF. Bilevel PAP can both stabilize and destabilize breathing in such patients, but some will clearly benefit. Stabilization of respiratory control may be required as an adjunct to support the upper airway; options include additional oxygen (even in the absence of severe desaturations) and cautious use of benzodiazepine hypnotics. Carbon dioxide is a strong stabilizer of periodic breathing, but use of a dead-space mask (with or without PAP) and addition of CO_2 into the PAP circuit remain investigational. Fragmented sleep-wake cycles, an inevitable consequence of napping and excessive time in bed, result in more time spent at the sleep-wake interface, where sleep and breathing are often unstable. This can make falling asleep with PAP quite difficult, and a tight and consistent sleep schedule is critical. Those with predominantly periodic breathing and mild obstruction may gain clinical benefit by sleeping with supplemental nasal oxygen. Nocturnal hemodialysis may improve some of the respiratory abnormality, perhaps by correcting hypocapnia and the resultant periodic breathing and respiratory instability. However, in the reports of patients using this dialysis regimen, sleep quality (arousal index) remained elevated, and the measure of respiration was not nasal pressure, which might have exaggerated the apparent benefit.[66] Nocturnal HD only marginally improves excessive daytime sleepiness.[98] The reality is that the only real option for significant SDB in this population is PAP.

Management Challenges: General

Table 13–2 outlines some of the major challenges faced in the treatment of sleep disorders in patients with renal disease. Periodic limb movements are so common in CRF patients that if persistent even after treating bothersome restless legs, the focus should be on first optimizing SDB management rather than trying to treat "PLM disorder." Iron deficiency and anemia should be managed appropriately. One study of recombinant human erythropoietin therapy in 10 CRF patients to correct anemia found reductions in PLMS, arousals from sleep, and sleep fragmentation, while allowing for more subjectively restorative sleep and improved daytime alertness.[78] A cautious trial of dopaminergics or low-dose opiates may be considered, at the risk of adding to the complexity of the medical management with questionable benefit. Daytime sleepiness/fatigue has numerous causes in ESRD, and after optimizing sleep and dialysis, a cautious trial of a stimulant such as methylphenidate or the wake-promoting drug modafinil could improve quality of life. The latter is now FDA approved as an adjunct to treat persisting daytime symptoms after best current PAP therapy, and most CRF patients with SDB may well qualify. There is, however, no data on efficacy or safety in this population. Napping is common during dialysis and in renal failure patients in general. Excessive napping is disruptive to nocturnal sleep, but a consistently timed mid-afternoon nap of 20 to 40 minutes could allow improved alertness in the late afternoon and evening. Nontraditional methods such as accupoints massage should be rigorously evaluated before acceptance in this population.[99] The implications of high melatonin levels, if any, are unknown.[93, 95]

Management Challenges: The Future

There are numerous unanswered questions in the management of SDB and sleep in CRF. Can more intensive dialysis normalize sleep? From the experience with congestive heart failure, optimizing therapy can improve but does not eliminate the problem. Can appropriate SDB management improve the high mortality in dialysis patients, or can glucose tolerance and blood pressure control be improved? There are little data, and more studies are forthcoming. Does the nocturnal hemodynamic stress inevitably associated with SDB contribute to early renal injury and the development of microalbuminuria? SDB is common and probably pathogenic in preeclampsia (increased risk during pregnancy in those with renal failure), contributing to nocturnal hypertension—could early treatment of disordered breathing reduce this risk or its fetal consequences? The management of SDB in CHF is gaining popularity at least in concept, but the reality is far away outside the research setting. As more patients are referred to sleep centers by cardiologists, we may be able to draw on such experiences for the management of SDB in patients with ESRD. Given the large number of patients and high prevalence of sleep disorders within both of these groups, target-population specific clinics managed by nurse practitioners or clinical nurses and supervised by sleep-medicine trained physicians may be necessary to significantly impact the CRF or CHF populations. Such clinics could be within a heart failure or dialysis program. Laboratory support will also be critical and may require administrative and technical creativity beyond what exists today. Could dialysis centers double as sleep laboratories (at least for diagnostic testing) at night?

There have been a multitude of publications,[100,101] at times redundant, describing the problems of sleep, sleep-disordered breathing, and sleepiness in the end-stage renal failure population. Enough said. Management and outcome trials are long overdue.

Table 13–2 Sleep Medicine: Clinical Challenges in the End-Stage Renal Disease Patient

Insomnia	Always multifactoria—a comprehensive treatment approach is required. Use of sedative-hypnotics without workup is inappropriate.
Excessive daytime sleepiness	Fatigue is so common in patients with ESRD that clinical sleepiness/fatigue scales may have less clinical predictive value. Short of some type of objective sleep-breathing assessment, the contribution of disordered breathing during sleep cannot be estimated.
Restless legs	High probability of abnormal iron status and likely contribution from "uremic toxins." Medications may need adjustment in relation to dialysis. Many antidepressants, especially the serotonin re-uptake inhibitors, may induce or worsen RLS.
Sleep-wake cycle fragmentation	Napping during dialysis will contribute to fragmented nocturnal sleep.
Sleep-disordered breathing	High probability of complexity—obstructive disease and periodic breathing. SDB may contribute to depressed mood. Positive airway pressure may only partially control the disease. Fluctuating weight associated with intermittent dialysis could result in varying positive pressure requirements. Automatic pressure adjusting devices do not work well if there is coexisting periodic breathing.

References

1. Holley JL, Nespor S, Rault R: A comparison of reported sleep disorders in patients on chronic hemodialysis and continuous peritoneal dialysis. Am J Kidney Dis 1992; 19(2):156-161.
2. Parker KP, Bliwise DL, Rye DB, De A: Intradialytic subjective sleepiness and oral body temperature. SLEEP 2000; 23(7): 887-891.
3. Yoshioka M, Ishii T, Fukunishi I: Sleep disturbance of end-stage renal disease. Jpn J Psychiatry Neurol 1993; 47(4):847-851.
4. Veiga J, Goncalves N, Gomes F, et al: Sleep disturbances in end-stage renal disease patients on hemodialysis. Dial Transplant 1997; 26(6):380-384.
5. Mitchell TH, Nolan B, Henry M, et al: Microalbuminuria in patients with non-insulin-dependent diabetes mellitus relates to nocturnal systolic blood pressure. Am J Med 1997; 102:531-535.
6. Walker S, Fine A, Kryger MH: Sleep complaints are common in a dialysis unit. Am J Kidney Dis 1995; 26(5):751-756.
7. Rousseau Y, Haeffner-Cavaillon N, Poignet JL, et al: In vivo intra-cellular cytokine production by leukocytes during haemodialysis. Cytokine 2000; 12:506-517.
8. Hanly P: Sleep apnea and daytime sleepiness in end-stage renal disease. Semin Dial 2004; 17(2):109-114.
9. Kuhlmann U, Becker HF, Birkhahn M, et al: Sleep-apnea in patients with end-stage renal disease and objective results. Clin Nephrol 2000; 53(6):460-466.
10. Parker KP, Bliwise DL, Bailey JL, Rye DB: Daytime sleepiness in stable hemodialysis patients. Am J Kidney Dis 2003; 41(2): 394-402.
11. Bliwise DL, Kutner NG, Zhang R, Parker KP: Survival by time of day of hemodialysis in an elderly cohort. JAMA 2001; 286(21):2690-2694.
12. Benz RL, Pressman MR, Hovick ET, Peterson DD: Potential novel predictors of mortality in end-stage renal disease patients with sleep disorders. Am J Kidney Dis 2000; 35(6):1052-1060.
13. Winkelman JW, Chertow GM, Lazarus JM: Restless legs syndrome in end-stage renal disease. Am J Kidney Dis 1996; 28(3): 372-378.
14. Shepard JW Jr: Hypertension, cardiac arrhythmias, myocardial infarction and stroke in relation to obstructive sleep apnea. Clin Chest Med 1992; 3:437-458.
15. Zoccali C, Mallamaci F, Tripepi G: Traditional and emerging cardiovascular risk factors in end-stage renal disease. Kidney Int 2003; 85:S105-S110.
16. Nieto FJ, Young TB, Lind BK, et al: Association of sleep-disordered breathing, sleep apnea, and hypertension in a large community-based study. Sleep Heart Health study. JAMA 2000; 283:1829-1836.
17. Silverberg DS, Oksenberg A, Iaina A: Sleep related breathing disorders are common contributing factors to the production of essential hypertension but are neglected, underdiagnosed and undertreated. Am J Hypertens 1997; 10:1319-1325.
18. Rosansky SJ, Johnson KL, Hutchinson C, Erdel S: Blood pressure changes during sleep and comparison of daytime and nighttime sleep-related blood pressure changes in patients with chronic renal failure. J Am Soc Nephrol 1993; 4(5):1172-1177.
19. Covic A, Goldsmith DJ: Ambulatory blood pressure monitoring in nephrology: Focus on BP variability. J Nephrol 1999; 12(4): 220-229.
20. Farmer CKT, Goldsmith DJA, Cox J, et al: An investigation of the effect of advancing uraemia, renal replacement therapy and renal transplantation on blood pressure diurnal variability. Nephrol Dial Transplant 1997; 12:2301-2307.
21. Devereux RB, Pickering TG: Relationship between the level, pattern and variability of ambulatory blood pressure and target organ damage in hypertension. J Hypertens 1991; 9(S8): S34-S38.
22. Portaluppi F, Provini F, Cortelli P, et al: Undiagnosed sleep-disordered breathing among male non-dippers with essential hypertension. J Hypertens 1997; 15:1227-1233.
23. Fletcher EC, Bao G, Li R: Renin activity and blood pressure in response to chronic episodic hypoxia. Hypertension 1999; 34(2):309-314.
24. Covic A, Goldsmith DJ, Covic M: Reduced blood pressure variability as a risk factor for progressive left ventricular dilation in hemodialysis patients. Am J Kidney Dis 2000; 35(4):617-623.
25. Zoccali C, Benedetto FA, Tripepi G, et al: Nocturnal hypoxemia, night-day arterial pressure changes and left ventricular geometry in dialysis patients. Kidney Int 1998; 53:1078-1084.
26. Zoccali C, Mallamaci F, Tripepi G: Nocturnal hypoxemia predicts incident cardiovascular complications in dialysis patients. J Am Soc Nephrol 2002; 13:729-733.
27. Timio M, Venanzi S, Lolli S, et al: "Non-dipper" hypertensive patients and progressive renal insufficiency: A three-year longitudinal study. Clin Nephrol 1995; 43:382-387.
28. Poulsen PL, Ebbehoj E, Hansen KW, Mogensen CE: 24–h blood pressure and autonomic function is related to albumin excretion within the normoalbuminuric range in IDDM patients. Diabetologia 1997; 40:718-725.
29. Dinneen SF, Gerstein HC: The association of microalbuminuria and mortality in non-insulin-dependent diabetes mellitus—a systemic overview of the literature. Arch Intern Med 1997; 157:1413-1418.
30. Hogan D, Lurbe E, Salabat MR, et al: Circadian changes in blood pressure and their relationships to the development of microalbuminuria in type 1 diabetic patients. Curr Diab Rep 2002; 2:539-544.
31. Iliescu EA, Lam M, Pater J, Munt PW: Do patients with obstructive sleep apnea have clinically significant proteinuria? Clin Nephrol 2001; 55(3):196-204.
32. Chaudhary BA, Sklar AH, Chaudhary TK, et al: Sleep apnea, proteinuria, and nephrotic syndrome. SLEEP 1988; 11(1):69-74.
33. Sklar AH, Chaudhary BA: Reversible proteinuria in obstructive sleep apnea syndrome. Arch Int Med 1988; 148:87-89.
34. Kinebuchi SI, Kazama JJ, Satoh M, et al: The short-term use of continuous positive airway pressure ameliorates glomerular hyperventilation in patients with obstructive sleep apnea syndrome. Clin Sci 2004 (e-pub).
35. Casserly LF, Chow N, Ali S, et al: Proteinuria in obstructive sleep apnea. Kidney Int 2001; 60(4):1484-1489.
36. Ehlenz K, Firle K, Schneider H, et al: Reduction of nocturnal diuresis and natriuresis during treatment of obstructive sleep apnea (OSA) with nasal continuous positive air pressure (nCPAP) correlates to cGMP excretion. Med Klin 1991; 86(6): 294-296, 332.
37. Kimmel PL, Gavin C, Miller G, et al: Disordered sleep and non-compliance in a patient with end-stage renal disease. Adv Ren Replace Ther 1997; 4(1)55-67.
38. Stepanski E, Faber M, Zorick F, et al: Sleep disorders in patients on continuous ambulatory peritoneal dialysis. J Am Soc Nephrol 1995; 6(2):192-197.
39. Langevin B, Fouque D, Leger P, Robert D: Sleep apnea syndrome and end-stage renal disease. Cure after renal transplantation. CHEST 1993; 103(5):1330-1335.
40. Everson CA, Toth LA: Systemic bacterial invasion induced by sleep deprivation. Am J Physiol Regul Integr Comp Physiol 2000; 278(4):R905-R916.
41. Meier-Ewert HK, Ridker PM, Rifai N, et al: Effect of sleep loss on C-reactive protein, an inflammatory marker of cardiovascular risk. J Am Coll Cardiol 2004; 43(4):678-683.
42. Yokoe T, Minoguchi K, Matsuo H, et al: Elevated levels of C-reactive protein and interleukin-6 in patients with obstructive sleep apnea syndrome are decreased by nasal continuous positive airway pressure. Am J Respir Crit Care Med 2004; 169(2):156-162.

43. Polotsky VY, Li J, Punjabi NM, et al: Intermittent hypoxia increases insulin resistance in genetically obese mice. J Physiol 2003; 552(1):253-264.
44. Tassone F, Lanfranco F, Gianotti L, et al: Obstructive sleep apnoea syndrome impairs insulin sensitivity independently of anthropometric variables. Clin Endocrinol (Oxf) 2003; 59(3): 374-379.
45. Harsch IA, Schahin SP, Radespiel-Troger M, et al: CPAP treatment rapidly improves insulin sensitivity in patients with OSAS. Am J Respir Crit Care Med 2004; 169(2):156-162.
46. Lavie L, Vishnevsky A, Lavie P: Evidence for lipid peroxidation in obstructive sleep apnea. SLEEP 2004; 27(1):123-128.
47. Alberti A, Sarchielli P, Gallinella E, et al: Plasma cytokine levels in patients with obstructive sleep apnea syndrome: A preliminary study. J Sleep Res 2003; 12(4):305-311.
48. Vgontzas AN, Chrousos GP: Sleep, the hypothalamic-pituitary-adrenal axis, and cytokines: Multiple interactions and disturbances in sleep disorders. Endocrinol Metab Clin North Am 2002; 31(1):15-36.
49. Ip MS, Tse HF, Lam B, et al: Endothelial function in obstructive sleep apnea and response to treatment. Am J Respir Crit Care Med 2004; 169(3):348-353.
50. Sklar AH, Riesenberg LA, Silber AK, et al: Postdialysis fatigue. Am J Kidney Dis 1996; 28(5):732-736.
51. Williams SW, Tell GS, Zheng B, et al: Correlates of sleep behavior among hemodialysis patients. The kidney outcomes prediction and evaluation (KOPE) study. Am J Nephrol 2002; 22(1): 18-28.
52. Parker KP, Kutner NG, Bliwise DL, et al: Nocturnal sleep, daytime sleepiness, and quality of life in stable patients on hemodialysis. Health and Quality of Life Outcomes 2003; 1(68): 1-18.
53. Pfister M, Jakob SM, Marti HP, et al: Ambulatory nocturnal oximetry and sleep questionnaire-based findings in 38 patients with end-stage renal disease. Nephrol Dial Transplant 1999; 14(6):1496-1502.
54. Kraus MA, Hamburger RJ: Sleep apnea in renal failure. Adv Perit Dial 1997; 13:88-92.
55. Young T, Palta M, Demsey J, et al: The occurrence of sleep disordered breathing among middle-aged adults. N Engl J Med 1993; 328:1230-1235.
56. Young T, Zaccarro D, Leder R, et al: Prevalence and correlates of sleep disordered breathing in the Wisconsin Sleep Cohort Study. Am Rev Respir Dis 1991; 143:A380.
57. Wadhwa NK, Mendelson WB: A comparison of sleep-disordered respiration in ESRD patients receiving hemodialysis and peritoneal dialysis. Adv Perit Dial 1992; 8:195-198.
58. Kimmel PL, Miller G, Mendelson WB: Sleep apnea syndrome in chronic renal disease. Am J Med 1989; 86(3):308-314.
59. Pressman MR, Benz RL, Schleifer CR, Peterson DD: Sleep disordered breathing in ESRD: Acute beneficial effects of treatment with nasal continuous positive airway pressure. Kidney Int 1993; 43:1134-1139.
60. Zoccali C, Mallamaci F, Tripepi G: Sleep apnea in renal patients. J Am Soc Nephrol 2001; 12:2854-2859.
61. Fletcher EC: Obstructive sleep apnea and the kidney (Editorial). J Am Soc Nephrol 1993; 4(5):1111-1121.
62. Millman RP, Kimmel PL, Shore ET, Wasserstein AG: Sleep apnea in hemodialysis patients: The lack of testosterone effect on its pathogenesis. Nephron 1985; 40:407-410.
63. Fein AM, Niederman MS, Imbriano L, Rosen H: Reversal of sleep apnea in uremia by dialysis. Arch Intern Med 1987; 147: 1355-1356.
64. Hallett M, Burden S, Stewart D, et al: Sleep apnea in end-stage renal disease patients on hemodialysis and continuous ambulatory peritoneal dialysis. ASAIO J 1995; 41(3): M435-M441.
65. Mendelson WB, Wadhwa NK, Greenberg HE, et al: Effects of hemodialysis on sleep apnea syndrome in end-stage renal disease. Clin Nephrol 1990; 33(5):247-251.
66. Hanly PJ, Pierratos A: Improvement of sleep apnea in patients with chronic renal failure who undergo nocturnal hemodialysis. N Engl J Med 2001; 344(2):102-107.
67. Jean G, Piperno D, Francois B, Charra B: Sleep apnea incidence in maintenance hemodialysis patients: Influence of dialysate buffer. Nephron 1995; 71:138-142.
68. Wadhwa NK, Seliger M, Greenberg HE, et al: Sleep related respiratory disorders in end-stage renal disease patients on peritoneal dialysis. Perit Dial Int 1992; 12(1):51-56.
69. Auckley DH, Schmidt-Nowara W, Brown LK: Reversal of sleep apnea hypopnea syndrome in end-stage renal disease after kidney transplantation. Am J Kidney Dis 1999; 34(4):739-744.
70. Soreide E, Skeie B, Kirvela O, et al: Branched-chain amino acid in chronic renal failure patients: Respiratory and sleep effects. Kidney Int 1991; 40(3):539-543.
71. Patel S: Restless legs syndrome and periodic limb movements of sleep: Fact, fad, and fiction. Curr Opin Pulm Med 2002; 8(6): 498-501.
72. Wetter TC, Stiasny K, Kohen R, et al: Polysomnographic sleep measures in patients with uremia and idiopathic restless legs syndrome. Mov Disord 1998; 13(5):820-824.
73. Earley CJ: Restless Legs Syndrome. N Engl J Med 2003; 348: 2103-2109.
74. Aksu M, Bara-Jimenez W: State dependent excitability changes of spinal flexor reflex in patients with restless legs syndrome secondary to chronic renal failure. Sleep Med 2002; 3:427-430.
75. Roger SD, Harris DCH, Stewart JH: Possible relation between restless legs and anemia in renal dialysis patients. Lancet 1991; 1:1551.
76. Yasuda T, Nishimura A, Katsuki Y, Tsuji Y: Restless legs syndrome treated successfully by kidney transplantation: A case report. Clin Transpl 1986:138.
77. Winkelmann J, Stautner A, Samtleben W, Trenkwalder C: Long-term course of restless legs symptoms in dialysis patients after kidney transplantation. Mov Disord 2002; 17(5):1072-1076.
78. Benz RL, Pressman MR, Hovick ET, Peterson DD: A preliminary study of the effects of correction of anemia with recombinant human erythropoietin therapy on sleep, sleep disorders, and daytime sleepiness in hemodialysis patients (SLEEPO study). Am J Kidney Dis 1999; 34:1089-1095.
79. Janzen L, Rich JA, Vericaigne LM: An overview of levodopa in the management of restless legs syndrome in a dialysis population: Pharmacokinetics, clinical trials, and complications of therapy. Ann Pharmacother 1999; 33(1):86-92.
80. Walker SL, Fine A, Kryger MH: L-dopa/carbidopa for nocturnal movement disorders in uremia. Sleep 1996; 19(3):214-218.
81. Trenkwalder C, Stiasny K, Pollmacher T, et al: L-dopa therapy of uremic and idiopathic restless legs syndrome: A double-blind, crossover trial. Sleep 1995; 18(8):681-688.
82. Pieta J, Millar T, Zacharias J, et al: Effect of pergolide on restless legs and leg movements in sleep in uremic patients. Sleep 1998; 21(6):617-622.
83. Tagaya H, Wetter TC, Winkelmann J, et al: Pergolide restores sleep maintenance but impairs sleep EEG synchronization in patient with restless legs syndrome. Sleep Med 2000; 3(1):49-54.
84. Miranda M, Kagi M, Fabres L, et al: Pramipexole for the treatment of uremic restless legs in patients undergoing hemodialysis. Neurology 2004; 62:831-932.
85. Wetter TC: Restless legs syndrome: A review for the renal care professionals. EDTNA ERCA J 2001; 27(1):42-46.
86. Janzen L, Rich JA, Vercaigne LM: An overview of levodopa in the management of restless legs syndrome in a dialysis population: Pharmacokinetics, clinical trials, and complications of therapy. Ann Pharmacother 1999; 33(1):86-92.

87. Read DJ, Feest TG, Nassim MA: Clonazepam: Effective treatment for restless legs syndrome in uremia. Br Med J (Clin Res Ed) 1981; 283(6296):885-886.
88. Braude W, Barnes T: Clonazepam: Effective treatment for restless legs syndrome in uraemia. Br Med J (Clin Res Ed) 1982; 284(6314):510.
89. Wetter TC, Winkelmann J, Eisensehr I: Current treatment options for restless legs syndrome. Expert Opin Pharmacother 2003; 4(10):1727-1738.
90. Thorp ML, Morris CD, Bagby SP: A crossover study of gabapentin in the treatment of restless legs syndrome among hemodialysis patients. Am J Kidney Dis 2001; 38(1):104-108.
91. Sabbatini M, Minale B, Crispo A, et al: Insomnia in maintenance haemodialysis patients. Nephrol Dial Transplant 2002; 17(5):852-856.
92. Viljoen M, Steyn ME, van Rensburg BWJ, Reinach SG: Melatonin in chronic renal failure. Nephron 1992; 60:138-143.
93. Vaziri ND, Oveisi F, Wierszbiezki M, et al: Serum melatonin and 6-sulfatoxymelatonin in end-stage renal disease: Effect of hemodialysis. Artif Organs 1993; 17(9):764-769.
94. Vaziri ND, Oveisi F, Reyes GA, Zhou XJ: Dysregulation of melatonin metabolism in chronic renal insufficiency: Role of erythropoietin-deficiency anemia. Kidney Int 1996; 50: 653-656.
95. Ludemann P, Zwernemann S, Lerchl A: Clearance of melatonin and 6-sulfatoxymelatonin by hemodialysis in patients with end-stage renal disease. J Pineal Res 2001; 31:222-227.
96. Unruh ML, Hartunin MG, Chapman MM, Jaber BL: Sleep quality and clinical correlates in patients on maintenance dialysis. Clin Nephrol 2003; 59(4):280-288.
97. Cirignotta F, Mondini S, Santoro A, et al: Reliability of questionnaire screening restless legs syndrome in patients on chronic dialysis. Am J Kidney Dis 2002; 40(2):302-306.
98. Hanly PJ, Gabor JY, Chan C, Pierratos A: Daytime sleepiness in patients with CRF: Impact of nocturnal hemodialysis. Am J Kidney Dis 2003; 41:403-410.
99. Tsay SL, Rong JR, Lin PF: Acupoints massage in improving the quality of sleep and quality of life in patients with end-stage renal disease. J Adv Nurs 2003; 42:134-142.
100. Wadhwa NK, Akhtar S: Sleep disorders in dialysis patients. Semin Dial 1998; 11:287-297.
101. Parker KP: Sleep disturbances in dialysis patients. Sleep Med Rev 2003; 7(2):131-143.

Chapter 14

The Pediatric Patient with Chronic Kidney Disease

Bradley A. Warady, M.D. • Vimal Chadha, M.D.

Although uncommon in children, chronic kidney disease (CKD) can be a devastating disorder with the potential for serious long-term ramifications (Table 14–1). Reference to CKD includes the spectrum of disease ranging from mild kidney damage with normal solute clearance to end-stage renal disease (ESRD). Despite some basic similarities with the abnormalities seen in adults, CKD in childhood is, in fact, characterized by many unique features not experienced by the adult population. For instance, growth and cognitive development are two of the major characteristics of childhood. Unlike adults who have completed their physiological and intellectual maturation, infants and young children are in the formative phase of their neurodevelopment and physical growth, both of which may be adversely affected by CKD during this particularly vulnerable period. This is especially pertinent because a substantial percentage of the pediatric CKD population develop renal insufficiency very early in life as a result of congenital or inherited disorders (*vide infra*). Additional CKD related clinical manifestations, such as renal osteodystrophy, poor nutrition, anemia, and cardiovascular disease, are also characterized by features unique to the pediatric population. Most significant is that suboptimal management of these and other related issues may be associated with an increased risk for subsequent morbidity and possibly even mortality. This chapter is, in turn, designed to highlight issues associated with the provision of optimal clinical care to children with advanced CKD (or chronic renal insufficiency [CRI]), as defined by a creatinine clearance less than 75 mL/min/1.73m^2), irrespective of the primary renal disorder. It is equally important to mention that this chapter will, on the other hand, not address disease-specific (e.g., renal tubular disease, renal stone disease, nephrotic syndrome) treatment related issues.

DIAGNOSIS AND EVALUATION OF CHRONIC KIDNEY DISEASE

To improve the detection and management of CKD, guidelines have recently been developed by the National Kidney Foundation's Kidney Disease Outcomes Quality Initiative (K/DOQI).[1] The diagnosis of CKD is established based on the presence of kidney damage and level of kidney function (glomerular filtration rate [GFR]), irrespective of the specific type of the underlying kidney disease (diagnosis) (Table 14–2). Kidney damage is defined as structural or functional abnormalities of the kidney, initially without a decreased GFR, which may lead to a decreased GFR over time. Among patients with CKD, the stage of the disease is defined by the level of the GFR, with higher stages (e.g., Stage 5) representing lower levels of GFR (Table 14–3). In the pediatric literature and as noted previously, CRI is defined by a creatinine clearance less than 75 mL/min/1.73m^2, a value that falls within Stage 2 CKD. The rationale for including individuals with a normal GFR within the CKD population is that substantial kidney damage often occurs before the GFR declines and these individuals are at increased risk for adverse outcomes associated with CKD. As the frequency of complications of CKD begin to increase when the GFR falls below 60 mL/min/1.73m^2, individuals with a GFR below this level are characterized as having CKD, even without any other evidence of kidney damage.

Although the level of GFR has been recommended as the primary criterion for defining and staging CKD, an important caveat should be recognized when using these definitions in young children. In children, the normal level of GFR varies according to age, gender, and body size. Whereas the normal GFR in young adults is approximately 120 to 130 mL/min/1.73m^2, the normal value is much lower than this in early infancy, even when corrected for body surface area. It subsequently increases along with the increase in body size for up to 2 years.[2] Hence, the GFR ranges that are used to define the five CKD stages by K/DOQI in Table 14–3 apply only to children 2 years of age and older. The normal range of GFRs at different ages is given in Table 14–4.[2–4]

As per the K/DOQI guidelines, estimates of GFR are the best means of assessing the level of kidney function in children and adolescents in the clinical setting, and the GFR should be estimated from prediction equations that take into account the serum creatinine concentration, the patient's height, and the patient's gender. The Schwartz formulas are, in turn, widely used in pediatric practice.[5–7] The GFR is calculated as follows:

$$C_{Cr}\ (\text{mL/min/1.73m}^2) = 0.55 \times \text{Height (cm)}/S_{Cr}\ (\text{mg/dL})$$

(The constant is 0.45 for infants <1 year of age and 0.7 for adolescent boys)

The validity of these formulas as a means of estimating GFR is compromised in the child with markedly diminished renal function because of the inherent increase in creatinine secretion that occurs in this situation. Alternative methods of assessment, such as the cimetidine clearance[8] or the clearance of cystatin C,[9] may provide the most accurate means of estimating renal function in this select population.

DEMOGRAPHICS

Whereas the exact incidence of CKD in children is not known, the North American Pediatric Renal Transplant Cooperative Study (NAPRTCS) has recently characterized this

Table 14–1 Potential Clinical Consequences of Chronic Kidney Disease in Children

Malnutrition
Growth failure
Anemia
Acidosis
Dyslipidemia
Renal osteodystrophy
Hypertension
Cardiovascular disease

Table 14–2 Definition of Chronic Kidney Disease

1. Kidney damage for ≥ 3 months, as defined by structural or functional abnormalities of the kidney, with or without decreased GFR, manifest by either:
   - Abnormalities in the composition of blood or urine
   - Abnormalities in imaging studies
   - Abnormalities on kidney biopsy
2. GFR < 60 mL/min/1.73m^2 for ≥ 3 months, with or without kidney damage

Table 14–3 K/DOQI Stages of Chronic Kidney Disease

Stage	Description	GFR (mL/min/1.73m^2)
1	Kidney damage with normal or increased GFR	>90
2	Kidney damage with mild decrease in GFR	60–89
3	Moderate decrease in GFR	30–59
4	Severe decrease in GFR	15–29
5	Kidney failure	<15 or dialysis

Table 14–4 Normal GFR in Children and Adolescents

Age (Sex)	Mean GFR ± SD (mL/min/1.73m^2)
1 wk (males and females)	41 ± 15
2–8 wk (males and females)	66 ± 25
>8 wk (males and females)	96 ± 22
2–12 yr (males and females)	133 ± 27
13–21 yr (males)	140 ± 30
13–21 yr (females)	126 ± 22

population.[10] The 2003 annual report has information on 5384 patients with CRI, defined and as mentioned previously as a calculated creatinine clearance of 75 mL/min/1.73m^2 or lower. Sixty-five percent of patients in the CRI registry are males, 62% are white, and 19% are African-Americans. Twenty percent of the CRI patients are less than 24 months of age and 17% are toddlers (2–5 years). Almost one half of the cases are accounted for by patients with the diagnoses of obstructive uropathy (23%), aplasia/hypoplasia/dysplasia (18%), and reflux nephropathy (8%). Apart from focal segmental glomerulosclerosis (FSGS) that accounts for 8% of cases, none of the other primary diseases account for more than 5% of the total population. The prevalence of FSGS among blacks is twice that of the other races combined (16% vs. 6%). Likewise, the registry of the United States Renal Data System (USRDS) has recently revealed that the rate of glomerulonephritis as a primary cause of pediatric renal insufficiency in blacks and other non-white patients has more than doubled over the past 20 years, as have the rates of cystic, hereditary, and congenital diseases.[11]

GROWTH FAILURE

Growth failure is one of the most onerous and visible clinical manifestations of CKD in children, and patients often fail to achieve a final adult height consistent with either population norms or their own genetic potential. According to the NAPRTCS registry, more than one-third of children with CKD are less than the 3rd percentile (standard deviation score [SDS] of −1.88) for height upon entrance to the registry.[10] Overall, patients with CKD are nearly 1.5 SDS below age and sex specific norms for height, while the youngest patients (0–1 year) are the most severely growth retarded portion of the population, with a mean height SDS of −2.35 at baseline.[10] Likewise, the European Study for Nutritional Treatment of Chronic Renal Failure in Childhood found that one third of the height deficit experienced by children at 3 years of age in association with early onset CKD occurs during fetal life and an additional one third during the first postnatal months.[12] This is an important issue since one third of postnatal statural growth overall is attained during the first 2 years of life, and any insult to growth that occurs during this time may have a profound impact on final adult height. The height deficit may be alleviated to a small extent by "catch up growth" in those patients who entered the NAPRTCS registry at 0–1 year of age and who at 2-year follow-up had a mean delta height SDS of 0.67.[10] Pubertal growth is also often adversely affected in the setting of CKD. The onset of puberty is delayed by an average of 2.5 years, the duration of the pubertal growth spurt is 1.6 years shorter in duration than normal, and the pubertal growth spurt is approximately only 50% of that experienced by normal children.[13]

In addition to its negative influence on the achievement of a normal final adult height and the potential association between poor growth and social issues, such as job availability and the ability to find a spouse, poor incremental growth in association with CKD has been associated with an increased risk of morbidity and mortality in children.[14] Furth and associates,[15] utilizing data from the NAPRTCS, demonstrated that children with significant growth failure, as reflected by a height SDS more negative than −2.5 at the time of dialysis initiation (and thus reflective of care provided during the period of CKD), had a significantly increased risk of hospitalization and twofold higher risk of death compared to patients with normal growth (height SDS > −2.5). In a similar manner, analysis of data from the U.S. Renal Data System (USRDS) on 1112 subjects less than 17 years of age revealed that growth failure is associated with a more complicated clinical course and an increased risk of death for children on dialysis.[16]

The more severely growth retarded patients also had more hospital days per month of dialysis and were less likely to attend school full-time.[16] Although these studies do not suggest that poor growth is the immediate cause of poor patient outcomes, growth retardation may possibly serve as a surrogate for suboptimal clinical care in children with CKD. Therefore, delineation of the optimal management of growth retardation in children with CKD may be crucial to the establishment of clinical treatment standards, which may, in turn, reduce the burden of hospitalization and mortality in these patients.

Although multiple factors such as protein energy malnutrition, acidosis, extensive salt and water losses, and secondary hyperparathyroidism may contribute to growth failure, perturbations of the growth hormone/insulin-like growth factor (GH/IGF) axis is the predominant factor contributing to the impaired growth associated with CKD, particularly in those patients outside the period of infancy.[17–22] Normally, growth hormone (GH) release from the pituitary gland is stimulated by growth hormone releasing hormone (GHRH) from the hypothalamus. The GH is bound by GH receptors within the liver with the subsequent production of IGF-1. The majority of IGF-1 is bound to acid labile subunit and insulin growth factor binding protein 3 (IGFBP–3) in a ternary complex, and a portion of the remaining free (bioactive) IGF-1 stimulates cartilogenous growth in bone.[23] In patients with CKD, there is an increased pulsatile release of GH from the pituitary gland due to a less active negative feedback loop to the hypothalamus. In addition, the metabolic clearance rate of GH is reduced, resulting in a rise in the circulating GH concentration.[24,25] However, despite the presence of the elevated GH concentration, GH receptor downregulation within the liver and defects in postreceptor signal transduction result in decreased IGF-1 synthesis by the liver.[26–28] Furthermore, the bioavailability of IGF-1 is reduced as a result of elevated IGF binding proteins (IGFBP). Increased circulating levels of IGFBP-1 and IGFBP-2 are inversely correlated with residual GFR and height[29] and probably contribute directly to the resistance to the anabolic and growth promoting effects of GH and IGF-1.[30] Thus, renal failure is not a state of GH or IGF-1 deficiency but instead a state in which the regulation and bioavailability of components of the GH/IGF/IGFBP system are altered.

Recognition that recombinant human GH (rhGH) treatment improves the height velocity of children with CKD has dramatically changed the therapeutic approach available to correct and/or prevent the growth retardation associated with renal insufficiency.[13,22,31–33] Recombinant GH is approved for the treatment of growth failure in children with CKD at a daily dosage of 0.05 mg/kg given by subcutaneous injection. Children who are Tanner stage I, II, or III and with a height SDS of −1.88 or worse and/or a height velocity SDS more negative than −2.0 are candidates for rhGH treatment.[33] A simple approach to the use of rhGH is provided in Figure 14–1.[34] Preparation is no longer produced. Proper management of malnutrition, correction of acidosis, and control of renal osteodystrophy is essential to maximize growth potential and should always precede treatment with rhGH. It is noteworthy that treatment with rhGH is most effective when prescribed to those with CKD, prior to the need for dialysis,[35] and the treatment response is positively correlated with the initial degree of growth retardation.[13] Whether individualization of the dose can best be guided by IGF-1 levels will soon be studied.

Historically, there has been a concern that the acceleration of growth that results from rhGH treatment during the prepubertal years might be offset by an earlier onset and/or shorter duration of pubertal growth.[36] However, long-term follow-up results of the German Study Group for Growth Hormone Treatment in Chronic Renal Failure has revealed that the onset of the pubertal growth spurt was actually delayed in boys treated with rhGH (although not in girls), and the duration of the growth spurt was no different from controls.[13] Although the prepubertal bone maturation was slightly accelerated in children treated with rhGH, the rhGH induced prepubertal growth stimulation was sufficient to override this effect.[13] Most significant was the finding that those patients who received rhGH grew significantly better than those patients who did not receive rhGH, and only the former group of patients had a normal mean final adult height. Remarkably, despite these results, less than 30% of prepubertal children with CRI in the NAPRTCS registry, who also have a height SDS more negative than −1.88, have received rhGH, a finding that suggests the need for additional education of patients and health care providers.

As mentioned earlier, prior to initiating rhGH therapy, patients should be evaluated for preexisting or worsening osteodystrophy radiographically, along with an assessment of an intact PTH level. Additionally, baseline hip X-rays should be obtained due to the theoretic, increased risk of slipped capital femoral epiphysis and avascular necrosis of the femoral head associated with rhGH therapy. Any limp and/or hip or knee pain should be carefully evaluated. An ophthalmologic evaluation should also take place because of the reported but rare treatment related complication of pseudotumor cerebri. Recent database evaluations have revealed rhGH usage to be safe, as reflected by an adverse event profile no different than that noted in a population of children with CKD and no history of rhGH usage.[37] Finally, the height velocity of patients receiving rhGH should be closely monitored, with the weight related dose modified every 3 to 4 months to maintain the standard dosing regimen. Typically, rhGH is discontinued when the child has closed epiphysis, has achieved a target height percentile, or when adverse events such as severe hyperparathyroidism, pseudotumor cerebri, active neoplasia, or slipped capital femoral epiphysis occurs. If discontinued for reasons other than closed epiphysis, reinstitution of rhGH should be considered, if the height velocity significantly decreases and the reason for discontinuing the drug has resolved.

NEUROLOGIC AND EDUCATIONAL DEVELOPMENT

The majority of brain growth occurs during the first 2 years of life. A seminal report on the developmental outcome of children with CKD during infancy demonstrated a high prevalence of mental dysfunction, microcephaly, and seizures.[38] Thankfully, this has been supplanted by more favorable outcomes resulting from the aggressive treatment of malnutrition, often with the use of supplemental tube feeding, and the avoidance of aluminum-containing compounds.[39,40] Nonetheless, there continues to be evidence that neurologic functioning and development are adversely affected by the uremic state. In some studies, verbal performance and memory skills

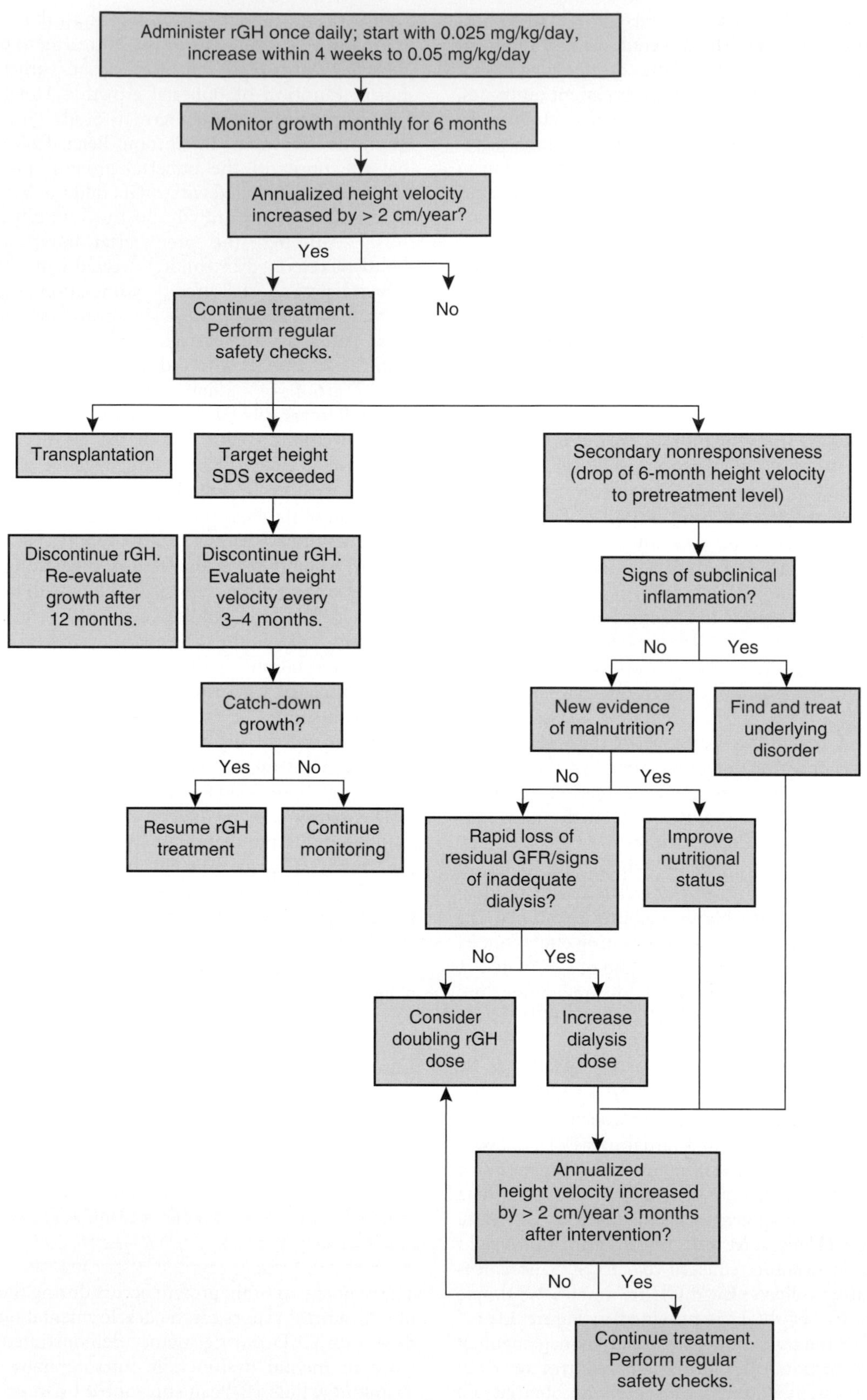

Figure 14–1 Management of rGH therapy.

have been shown to be significantly affected, leading to substantial impairment of school functioning. The duration of renal insufficiency appears to be a factor in neurologic dysfunction, with the worst performance occurring in those with the longest duration of uremia. Nevertheless, the prevalence of neurocognitive impairment, its magnitude, and the specific risk factors that contribute to its development (including metabolic factors) remain largely unknown. To that end, a multicenter, comprehensive prospective study designed to assess the neurocognitive status of children with CKD and risk factors associated with a poor neurocognitive outcome has recently been funded by the National Institutes of Health (NIH) in the United States. This study will include extensive neuropsychological, behavioral, and neuroimaging testing on 600 children over a 5-year period of time. Until this study is completed and we have a better understanding of this complex issue, it is prudent to effectively manage the metabolic derangements and malnutrition associated with CKD aggressively and to enroll active participation of experts in behavioral and developmental pediatrics and neurology for appropriate evaluation and early intervention when deemed necessary.

NUTRITIONAL ISSUES

Protein energy malnutrition is a common problem in patients with CKD and is one of the major contributors to the poor growth seen in these patients, especially during the first few years of life. Since energy intake is the principle determinate of growth during infancy, malnutrition has the most marked negative effect on growth in children with congenital disorders leading to CKD.[41,42] In fact, only in infants has maximizing caloric intake been noted to be an effective means of improving height velocity in association with CKD.[43] As mentioned previously, suboptimal nutrition is also likely to contribute to an impaired neurocognitive outcome in the youngest patients.[44–46] The provision of inadequate nutrition during the period of CKD has resulted in a low body mass index (BMI) in a substantial percentage of children at dialysis initiation, primarily those less than 9 years of age.[11] A low BMI during dialysis has previously been associated with an increased risk for mortality in pediatric patients. Similarly, in a cohort of 1700 children initiating dialysis from 1995 through 1998, the risks of hospitalization and death were two times higher in patients with hypoalbuminemia as compared to those initiating dialysis with a normal serum albumin.[47] Finally, the 2003 annual report of the USRDS has revealed that 49% of pediatric patients start dialysis with a serum albumin level below the test's lower limit; the number drops to 44% for whites but reaches 59% for blacks and 79% for blacks with secondary glomerulonephritis.[48] Thus, the provision of adequate nutrition and the prevention of protein energy malnutrition are necessary to promote optimal growth and development in children with CKD, while hopefully minimizing the physiological and biochemical consequences of uremia.

The assessment of the nutritional status of children with CKD requires the evaluation of multiple indices, as there is no single available measure that alone can assess a patient's nutritional status accurately (Table 14–5).[49] A variety of physical

Table 14–5 Indices Used for Nutritional Assessment

- Nutrient intake estimation
  - dietary recall
  - dietary diary
- Physical measurements
  - weight
  - length/height
  - head circumference
  - skinfold thickness
  - body mass index (BMI)
  - mid-arm circumference (MAC)
  - mid-arm muscle circumference (MAMC)
  - mid-arm muscle area (MAMA)
- Biochemical determinations
  - serum albumin
  - serum prealbumin
  - serum retinol binding protein
  - serum transferrin
  - serum complement fractions
  - serum insulin-like growth factor–1 (IGF–1)
- Special studies
  - protein equivalent of total nitrogen appearance (PNA)
  - Bioelectrical Impedance Analysis (BIA)
  - Dual Energy X-ray Absorptiometry (DEXA)
  - Subjective Global Assessment (SGA)

measurements, anthropometric assessments, and serum studies are routinely performed; special studies such as bioelectrical impedance and DEXA are more often deemed to be research tools in nature. The formula for calculating the normalized protein equivalent of total nitrogen appearance (nPNA) in children, which is reflective of the dietary protein intake, is different from the calculation in adults, as it takes into account the child's anabolic state and the higher nonurea-N excretion.[50] The calculation is as follows:

$$\text{Protein intake (g/kg/day)} = [\text{urea-N excretion (g/kg/day)} \times 15.39] - 0.8$$

The origin of malnutrition in children with CKD is multifactorial (Table 14–6); however, an inadequate voluntary dietary intake is considered a major contributing factor, especially in infants.[51] Nausea and vomiting are common in infants and children with CKD, with delayed gastric emptying and gastroesophageal reflux being detected in as many as 70% of patients with these problems.[52] Medical management with antiemetic medications (metoclopramide, domperidone) and antacids (H-2 blockers, proton-pump inhibitors) or surgical intervention (Nissen fundoplication) is frequently required. Additionally, whey predominant formulas can be used in these patients with resultant benefit because they have been shown to stimulate gastric emptying.[53,54]

Adolescents are the other patient group who appear to be particularly vulnerable to malnutrition due to their poor eating habits. They skip meals, favor fast foods, and in the presence of imposed dietary restrictions, find it difficult to meet the nutritional requirements of normal pubertal growth and development. They may benefit from individualized counseling and from having a special rapport with the renal dietitian.

Table 14–6 Causes of Protein-Energy Malnutrition (PEM) in Children with Chronic Kidney Disease

- Inadequate food intake secondary to
  - anorexia
  - altered taste sensation
  - nausea/vomiting
  - emotional distress
  - intercurrent illness
  - unpalatable prescribed diets
  - impaired ability to procure food because of socioeconomic situation
- Chronic inflammatory state
- Catabolic response to superimposed illnesses
- Possible accumulation of endogenously formed uremic toxins and/or the ingestion of exogenous toxins
- Removal of nutrients during dialysis procedure
- Endocrine causes such as
  - resistance to the actions of insulin and IGF-1
  - hyperglucagonemia
  - hyperparathyroidism

Energy

A number of studies have shown that the majority of pediatric patients with CKD exhibit an inadequate energy intake,[55–59] and the intake progressively decreases with worsening renal failure.[59] In a large, prospective study of growth failure in 120 children between the ages of 18 months and 10 years with CKD, the spontaneous energy intake was less than 80% of the recommended dietary allowance (RDA) for age in greater than 50% of the more than 400 food records obtained, with the poorest results reported in the oldest patients.[60] Whether the energy intake should more appropriately be referenced to height remains unanswered. Nevertheless, since maximizing caloric intake has been noted to be particularly effective in improving height velocity in infants with CKD, with only a rare report of a similar experience in older childen,[17,42,43] the provision of adequate energy intake early in life is clearly most crucial.[61] Infants with CKD requiring fluid restriction, or those who have a poor oral intake, may require a greater caloric density of their milk formula than the standard 20 kcal/oz. Aggressive enteral feeding should be considered if the nutritional intake by the oral route remains suboptimal, despite all attempts at oral supplementation. The use of enteral support has repeatedly resulted in the maintenance or improvement of SD scores for weight and/or height in infants and young children with CKD.[51,62] Nasogastric (NG) tubes, gastrostomy catheters, gastrostomy buttons, and gastrojejunostomy tubes have all been used, with encouraging results, to provide supplemental enteral feeding to children with renal disease. The feeding can be given as an intermittent bolus or, more commonly, by continuous infusion during the night (Figure 14–2).[34]

Current experience suggests that the energy intake of children with CKD should be at least equal to the RDA for normal children of the same chronologic age (Table 14–7).[33,63] Dietary therapy should provide 50% of total calories from primary complex carbohydrates, and the remainder of the non-protein calories should be from fat, with a polyunsaturated/saturated ratio of 2:1. Energy supplementation in excess of the RDA is not recommended in the absence of malnutrition (Figure 14–3).[34]

Protein

Low-protein diets reduce the generation of nitrogenous wastes and inorganic ions that might be responsible for many of the clinical and metabolic disturbances characteristic of uremia. Moreover, low-protein diets decrease the development of hyperphosphatemia, metabolic acidosis, hyperkalemia, and other electrolyte disorders. A large number of clinical trials and experimental studies have examined the impact of dietary protein restriction on the rate of progression to ESRD in adults,[64–70] and indeed, such a diet can retard the progression of renal failure or delay the onset of maintenance dialysis therapy.[71–75] Accordingly, it is recommended that a low-protein diet (0.6 g/kg/day) be considered in adults with significant CKD who are not yet undergoing dialysis.

Pediatricians, on the other hand, are rightly concerned about the potential for harmful effects of severe dietary protein restriction, particularly as it pertains to the growth of infants and young children with CKD. Experimental studies in young animals have, in fact, shown that a decrease in dietary protein intake during the normally rapid period of growth that is sufficient to slow the deterioration of renal function, does adversely affect growth.[65,76] As a result, very few studies of dietary protein restriction have been conducted in children with CKD.[77–80] In one such study, Uauy and associates[79] reported a negative impact of a modest protein restriction on the growth of infants with CKD during the feasibility phase of a multicenter trial. In a seminal 1997 investigation of more than 100 children with CKD, the European Study Group for Nutritional Treatment of Chronic Renal Failure in Childhood found that a reduction in dietary protein intake to a "safe amount" (0.8 to 1.1 g/kg ideal body weight/day) in pediatric patients (2–18 years of age) for 3 years did not interfere with the children's growth, but it also did not influence the progression of renal insufficiency.[80] In conclusion, current data suggest that moderate dietary protein restriction has no beneficial effect in terms of preventing the progression of renal insufficiency, but, on the contrary, such interventions may be associated with a loss of growth velocity, particularly in infants. Thus, current recommendations are to provide 100% of the RDA for healthy children of the same gender and chronologic age (Table 14–7).[33,81] It is advised that at least 50% of the total protein intake come from proteins of high biologic value such as those from milk, eggs, meat, fish, and poultry.

Lipids

Hyperlipidemia is a frequently recognized complication of CKD in children.[82] Uremia is associated with an increase of triglyceride-rich lipoproteins that are atherogenic and likely to increase the risk of cardiovascular disease among children with CKD.[83–85] There is also some evidence that an abnormal lipid status may hasten the progression of renal disease itself.[86] It is important to note that even with a near normal total cholesterol concentration, individual lipoprotein species often

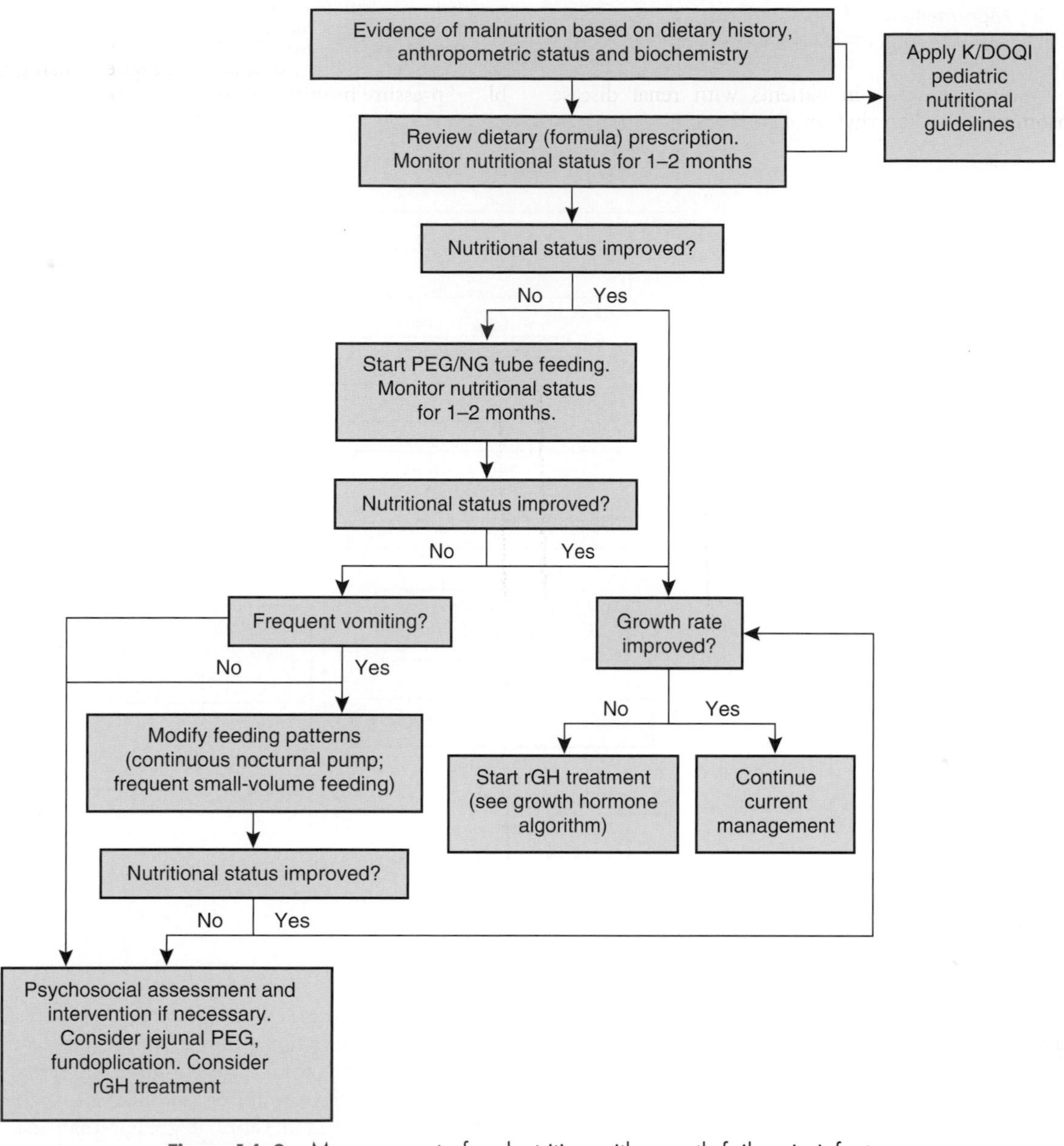

Figure 14–2 Management of malnutrition with growth failure in infants.

Table 14–7 Estimated Energy Allowances and Recommended Dietary Protein (g/kg/day) for Infants and Children with Chronic Kidney Disease[33,81]

	Age (Years)	Energy (kcal/kg/day)	Protein (g/kg/day)
Infants	0.0–0.5	108	2.2
	0.5–1.0	98	1.6
Children	1–3	102	1.2
	4–6	90	1.2
	7–10	70	1.0
Males	11–14	55	1.0
	15–18	45	0.9
	18–21	40*	0.8
Females	11–14	47	1.0
	15–18	40	0.8
	18–21	38*	0.8

*Based on RDA and increased physical activity.

reveal an abnormal pattern, being characterized by a low HDL-cholesterol and high VLDL, IDL, and variable LDL-cholesterol.[87,88] The extent of the abnormality in these values typically parallels the degree of renal impairment. The Friedewald formula, which is commonly used by laboratories to approximate LDL-cholesterol levels as part of a lipid profile, tends to underestimate the true LDL concentration in uremic individuals.[89,90] Plasma ultracentrifugation, available through many commercial laboratories, remains the "gold-standard" technique to measure the various density classes of lipoproteins, while routine, low resolution screening tests in this population may fail to detect dyslipidemia.[86]

The metabolic abnormalities that accompany the dyslipidemia of uremia are complex. Insulin resistance uniformly occurs and is independently associated with disturbances of lipid metabolism.[91] Unlike what occurs in children with nephrotic syndrome, lipoprotein synthesis in patients with

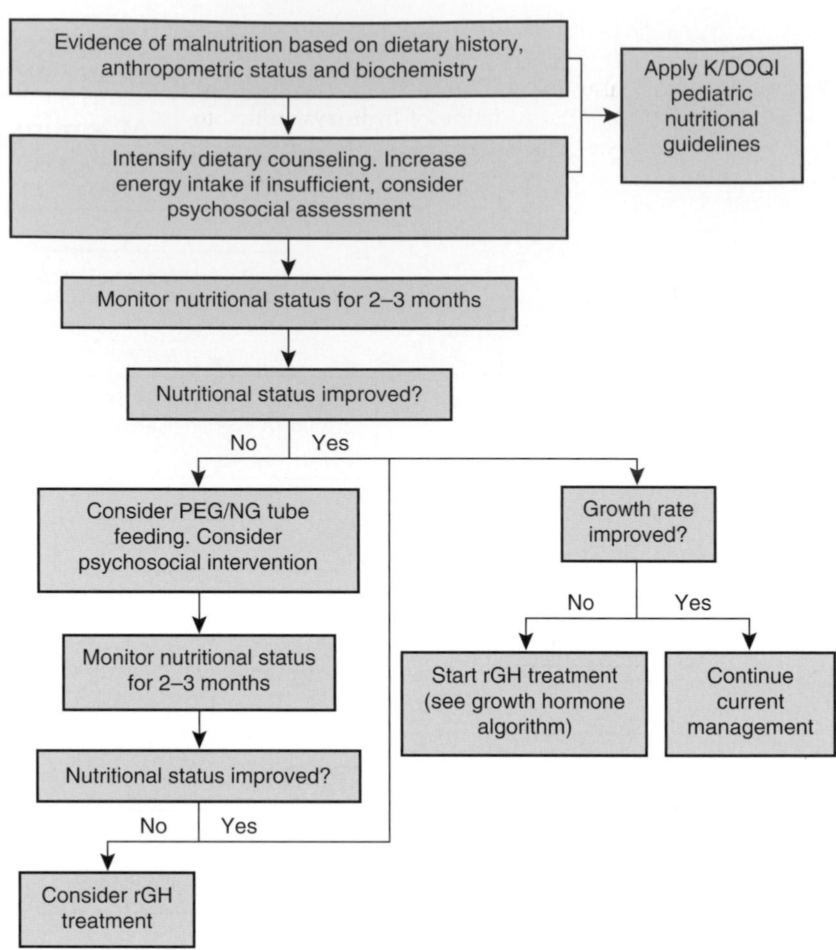

Figure 14–3 Management of malnutrition with growth failure in school children and adolescents.

CKD does not appear to be significantly exaggerated; however, studies consistently demonstrate impaired catabolism of triglyceride-rich lipoproteins.[92] The amount and activity of hepatic triglyceride lipase (HTGL) is decreased in uremic individuals,[93] while decreases in lipoprotein lipase (LPL) function are less consistently noted, despite a clear increase in the concentration of apoC-III, an inhibitor of LPL.[94,95]

The optimal management of dyslipidemia in children with CKD is not clearly defined. Of interest, only 44% of children with ESRD even underwent evaluation of their lipid status in 2001.[48] Treatment of malnutrition related to renal insufficiency is essential and should supersede any potential rise in lipid levels that might result from it. Correction of metabolic acidosis, vitamin D therapy, and correction of anemia with erythropoietin each seem to have some normalizing effect on dyslipidemia in children with renal failure.[96–98] Fish oil has been shown to reduce hypertriglyceridemia in a small group of children with ESRD,[99] and there are reports of statin usage in children with nephrotic syndrome.[100–102] Nevertheless, there is currently not enough data to support the regular long-term usage of the standard lipid lowering therapies such as statins and fibrates in children of all ages, despite their frequent usage in adults. In the absence of substantial safety and efficacy data related to statin therapy in children, the recommended therapeutic approach for children with Stages 2 to 4 CKD generally consists of dietary and lifestyle modifications. In patients with markedly elevated serum triglyceride levels, the dietary carbohydrate intake should be decreased from 50% to 35% of the total caloric intake. The remainder of the nonprotein calories should be supplied as fat with a polyunsaturated to saturated ratio of greater than 2:1. The child should be encouraged to ingest complex carbohydrates in lieu of simple sugars and concentrated sweets and to use unsaturated fats such as oils and margarines from corn, safflower, and soy. Plant stanol esters in the form of dietary supplements reduce intestinal cholesterol absorption and may provide a safe and effective means of reducing serum cholesterol.[103] Lipid-lowering drugs may be used judiciously in selected patients, such as in adolescents with Stage 5 CKD and either an LDL greater than or equal to 130 mg/dL or a combination of a fasting triglyceride level greater than or equal to 200 mg/dL and a non-HDL cholesterol of greater than or equal to 160 mg/dL.[104,105]

Acid-Base and Electrolytes

Infants and children normally have a relatively larger endogenous hydrogen ion load (2–3 mEq/kg) than do adults (1 mEq/kg), and metabolic acidosis is a common manifestation of CKD in children and an important negative influence on growth. Studies performed in adults and children have shown that chronic acidosis is associated with increased oxidation of branched-chain amino acids,[106] increased protein degradation,[107] and decreased albumin synthesis.[108,109] Persistent acidosis also has detrimental effects on bone because it alters the normal accretion of hydroxyapatite into bone matrix and causes bone demineralization as the bone buffers are increasingly used for neutralizing the excess acid load. Thus, it is recommended that the serum bicarbonate level should be maintained at or above 22 mEq/L by supplementing with oral bicarbonate.[33]

Whereas in healthy people the body's sodium balance is maintained by alterations in urinary sodium excretion, sodium requirements in children with CKD are dependent on the underlying kidney disease and the degree of renal insufficiency. Children who have CKD as a result of obstructive uropathy or renal dysplasia are most often polyuric and may experience substantial urinary sodium losses despite advanced degrees of CKD. Signs of sodium depletion are subtle and may include listlessness and hypercalcemia. The growth of these children may also be hampered if ongoing sodium and water losses are not corrected. Fine and associates[110] demonstrated poor weight gain in animals deprived of salt with a resultant decreased extracellular volume, bone mass, and fat mass. In turn, the beneficial effect of sodium and water supplementation on the linear growth of 24 young children with CKD has been reported.[19] In contrast, children with CKD resulting from primary glomerular disease, or those who are oliguric or anuric, typically require sodium and fluid restriction to minimize fluid gain, edema formation, and hypertension. The fluid intake is usually a fraction of the calculated maintenance volume adjusted for the degree of oliguria. A reasonable sodium intake is 3 to 4 g/day, initially. These patients should be advised to avoid processed foods and snacks from fast-food restaurants. The sodium content of other food items should be checked carefully on food labels, and the sodium content of medications may need to be monitored.

Potassium homeostasis in children with CKD is usually unaffected until the glomerular filtration rate falls to less than 10% of normal. However, children with renal dysplasia, post-obstructive renal damage, severe reflux nephropathy, and renal insufficiency secondary to interstitial nephritis, often demonstrate renal tubular resistance to aldosterone action and may manifest hyperkalemia, even when their creatinine clearance is relatively well preserved.[111] The hyperkalemia experienced by these children is exacerbated by volume contraction (and can be particularly common in salt losers), and the majority of the patients respond to salt and water repletion. In patients who are persistently hyperkalemic, dietary potassium intake should be limited. As potassium is infrequently listed on food labels and cannot be tasted, a list of foods rich in potassium such as chocolates, french fries, potato chips, bananas, green leafy vegetables, dried fruits, and orange juice should be provided to patients and their families. Altering the methods of food preparation, such as soaking vegetables before cooking, helps decrease potassium content. In the case of infants and young children being fed milk formula, the potassium content of the formula can be reduced by incorporating the potassium exchange resin sodium polystyrene sulfonate (Kayexalate).[112] Attention should also be paid to medications such as potassium sparing diuretics, cyclosporin, and angiotensin converting enzyme inhibitors, because they may cause or exacerbate hyperkalemia. If constipated, the patient should be treated aggressively as significant quantities of potassium are eliminated through the gastrointestinal route in patients with CKD.

Vitamins and Micronutrients

Vitamins and minerals are essential for normal growth and development, and either a deficiency or an excess amount can prove harmful. Unfortunately, the vitamin and mineral needs of pediatric patients with CKD are not clearly defined and the limited data that are available are derived from patients undergoing maintenance dialysis. Children with CKD are prone to develop vitamin deficiencies because of anorexia and dietary restrictions, while they are also at risk to develop toxic levels of vitamins when the renal clearance is significantly impaired.

The provision of adequate quantities of vitamin B_{12} and folic acid is imperative for effective erythropoiesis. More recently, raised doses of supplemental folic acid (2.5 mg/day) have been suggested by some for children with CKD because folic acid has been shown to decrease the elevated homocysteine level that is commonly seen in patients with renal failure, and this is a potential risk factor for cardiovascular morbidity and mortality.[113,114] Further study of this issue in children is clearly warranted.

Vitamin C is necessary for the formation of collagen. However, an excessive intake of vitamin C in the dialysis population may result in elevated oxalate levels as an end product of vitamin C metabolism and lead to the development of significant vascular complications.[115] Vitamin A levels are reported to be elevated in patients undergoing PD despite the lack of vitamin A supplementation. The elevated levels are a result of the loss of the kidneys' normal ability to excrete vitamin A metabolites.[116] Since elevated levels of vitamin A can be associated with the development of hypercalcemia and complications related to a high calcium-phosphorus product, it is important to avoid the use of vitamin supplements that include vitamin A in patients with Stage 5 CKD. The status of vitamins C and A in children with early stages of CKD has not been well studied.

Since most infant milk formulas, including Similac PM 60/40 are fortified with both water-soluble and fat-soluble vitamins, the majority of infants with CKD receive the dietary reference intakes (DRI) for all vitamins (including vitamin A) by dietary intake alone and do not require vitamin supplementation. The current K/DOQI guidelines recommend an intake of 100% of the DRI for water-soluble vitamins as a reasonable starting point for children undergoing maintenance dialysis therapy. Supplementation should be considered if the dietary intake alone does not meet or exceed the DRI, if measured blood vitamin levels are below normal values, or if clinical evidence of deficiency is present.[33] There are no specific recommendations for children with CKD.

Aluminum, copper, chromium, lead, strontium, tin, and silicon levels have all been noted to be elevated in patients with CKD, reflecting the fact that their clearance is dependent on an adequate glomerular filtration rate.[117,118] Aluminum salts were commonly used in the 1970s and early 1980s as a phosphate binder and were found to cause severe toxicity manifested by encephalopathy with seizures, osteomalacia, and microcytic anemia, even in children with mild renal insufficiency.[119,120] Subsequently, the use of aluminum containing phosphate binders was discontinued. The Growth Failure in

Renal Disease Study[121] showed that serum aluminum levels were elevated only in children taking antacids containing aluminum, which provides 1000 times more aluminum than environmental exposure, which is approximately 3 to 5 mg/day. Aluminum absorption is enhanced by citrate, an important issue for those children with CKD receiving alkali therapy as treatment for metabolic acidosis. Other trace elements have not been as well studied in children; however, zinc levels have been shown to be low in malnourished children and should be monitored and supplemented as necessary.[117] Copper deficiency, although rare, has been associated with ineffective erythropoiesis.

Carnitine

Carnitine is an essential compound in the oxidative process of fatty acids,[122] and the kidney is the major site for its synthesis in humans.[123] Although patients undergoing prolonged dialysis are at risk for carnitine deficiency because carnitine is removed both by hemodialysis and peritoneal dialysis,[124,125] there is little information on the carnitine status of children with CKD. Carnitine has been proposed as a treatment for a variety of metabolic abnormalities in pediatric patients with ESRD, including dyslipidemia and anemia, as well as for treatment of intradialytic hypotension in patients receiving hemodialysis. However, there is currently insufficient evidence to support the routine use of carnitine in either the pediatric CKD or dialysis patient population. Of interest, recent data from the USRDS has revealed that fewer than 2% of pediatric dialysis patients were evaluated for the presence of carnitine deficiency in 2000 to 2001, and only 4% of pediatric patients received supplemental carnitine.[48]

ANEMIA

Anemia is a frequent complication of CKD in children and adults.[126–130] Studies in the adult population have provided substantial evidence that anemia is an important predictor of patient morbidity and mortality. Anemia is strongly associated with cardiovascular disease and is present early in the course of CKD, long before the need for renal replacement therapy arises.[131] The anemia of CKD is associated with a number of physiological abnormalities, including decreased tissue oxygen delivery,[132–134] increased cardiac output, cardiac enlargement, ventricular hypertrophy, congestive heart failure,[135–138] decreased cognition and mental acuity,[139] and impaired immune responsiveness.[140,141] In addition, anemia may play a role in growth retardation and decreased intellectual performance in pediatric patients.[142,143] These poor outcomes stress the importance of anemia management in children with CKD.

Unfortunately, anemia management in children with CKD has received remarkably little study. Data from the 2003 report of the USRDS has revealed that the mean hemoglobin at dialysis initiation in 2001 was only 9.1 g/dL for all pediatric patients (9.3 for whites and 8.9 for blacks), reflective of suboptimal anemia management during the period of CKD.[48] Although the mean hemoglobin varied from state to state, it did not exceed 9.8 g/dL in any of the 50 states.[11] The presence of anemia was most striking in the 0- to 4-year age group and in those who subsequently received chronic hemodialysis.[11] Similarly, the NAPRTCS has revealed that the mean hematocrit (Hct) of children with CRI at entry into the registry is only 33.5%, despite the fact that a hematocrit of 33% to 36% is recommended by K/DOQI. In addition, less than 20% of all children with CRI and followed by NAPRTCS had received recombinant human erythropoietin (rHuEPO) 48 months after the baseline evaluation.[10] A hematocrit less than 33% has also been found to be associated with an accelerated rate of progression towards ESRD in the NAPRTCS registry.[10,144,145] Finally, in a more recent NAPRTCS study, Warady and Ho[146] determined that a hematocrit less than 33% at dialysis initiation was associated with a greater mean number of hospitalization days during the initial year of dialysis as well as with a significantly greater probability for a hospitalization of 30 days or more during that year when compared to patients with an Hct greater than 33%. Most important was the finding that the presence of anemia at dialysis initiation was associated with an estimated 52% greater risk of death.

The anemia present in association with CKD is primarily caused by a decrease in the renal production of erythropoietin.[147] Additional factors that may cause or contribute to anemia include iron deficiency,[148] hyperparathyroidism,[149] acute and chronic inflammatory conditions,[150] aluminum toxicity,[151] folate and vitamin B_{12} deficiency,[152] hypothyroidism,[153] and hemoglobinopathies such as α-thalassemia.[153] In turn, the standard workup of anemia should be initiated when Hgb is less than 11 g/dL (Hct <33%) and initial blood work should include red blood cell indices, reticulocyte count, and iron parameters such as serum iron, total iron binding capacity (TIBC), and serum ferritin. The percent transferrin saturation (TSAT) is calculated as the serum iron × 100 divided by the TIBC. The value and validity of additional diagnostic tests to address the iron status, such as the reticulocyte hemoglobin content and the percent hypochromic red blood cells, awaits further study in pediatrics. When deemed appropriate, testing to evaluate for the possible contribution of the etiologic disorders noted previously should be performed.

Finally, recombinant human erythropoietin (rHuEPO) has been used for the treatment of CKD related anemia since 1986.[154,155] Despite compelling evidence regarding the benefits of rHuEPO, its use in the pediatric CKD population continues to be low, particularly in the context of the severe degree of anemia noted in patients younger than 5 years of age at dialysis initiation.[11] The USRDS has revealed that only 37% of all pediatric patients have received rHuEPO before starting dialysis, and black children were less likely than whites to receive pre-ESRD rHuEPO therapy.[48] The target range for Hgb (Hct) for rHuEPO therapy is 11 to 12 g/dL and 33% to 36%, respectively.[156] Supplemental iron should be administered to maintain a TSAT of greater than or equal to 20% and a serum ferritin level of greater than or equal to 100 ng/mL.[156] While iron is typically provided by the oral route, intravenous iron supplementation can be an efficient means by which iron stores can be enhanced in children with CKD. Levels of TSAT greater than or equal to 50% or serum ferritin greater than or equal to 800 ng/mL are not associated with any further benefit and may require modification of iron therapy. The average dosage of rHuEPO is 150 units/kg/wk given by the subcutaneous route; younger patients (<5 years) frequently require higher doses of up to 300 units/kg/wk given in two to three doses. There are limited data regarding the use of longer acting erythropoietin in children.[157] The response to rHuEPO is monitored by measuring Hgb/Hct every 1 to 2 weeks following the initiation of treatment or following a dose increase or decrease, until a stable target Hgb/Hct and rHuEPO dose have been achieved; monitoring is then recommended to occur every 2 to 4 weeks.

RENAL OSTEODYSTROPHY

Bone disease is a universal complication of CKD, and it encompasses a spectrum of skeletal disorders ranging from the high-turnover lesions of secondary hyperparathyroidism to the low-turnover adynamic bone disease.[158] Although similar factors are involved in the pathogenesis of renal osteodystrophy in adult and pediatric patients with CKD, growth retardation and the development of bone deformities are complications that occur only in children. A number of factors such as disturbances in calcium and phosphorus homeostasis, reduced synthesis of the active form of vitamin D (1,25-dihydroxycholecalciferol), altered metabolism of parathyroid hormone (PTH), and impaired renal clearance of PTH fragments play critical roles in the pathogenesis of renal osteodystrophy.

Over the past decade, the availability of first generation immunometric PTH assays have allowed characterization of the spectrum of renal osteodystrophy in adult and pediatric patients receiving maintenance dialysis therapy.[159–161] Historically, it remained largely unexplained why the concentrations of intact PTH had to remain well above the normal range for healthy individuals (10–65 pg/mL) to maintain normal bone turnover and to prevent the development of adynamic bone disease in adult and pediatric patients treated with dialysis. However, a recent series of studies by D'Amour and associates demonstrated that the first PTH-IMAs detected not only the intact hormone, but also PTH fragments truncated at the amino-terminus, for instance, PTH (7–84).[162–165] The more recently developed second generation immunometric PTH assay (second PTH-IMA) uses a detection antibody raised against the first four amino-terminal amino acids and recognizes only PTH (1–84) and possibly PTH fragments that are truncated at the carboxyl–terminus, but not the PTH (7–84).[166–168] First generation PTH-IMAs thus overestimate the true concentration of PTH (1–84) in serum or plasma, both in patients with ESRD and those with normal renal function, by including PTH (7–84).[164,167,169,170] In patients undergoing dialysis therapy, the PTH concentrations measured with the 1st PTH-IMA are on average 40% to 50% higher than those measured with second PTH-IMA.[166,168–171] Recent data do indicate that one or more PTH (1–84) fragments, such as PTH (7–84), actually antagonize the calcemic actions of PTH (1–84) and may modulate bone metabolism through a receptor distinct from the type I PTH/PTHrP receptor.[168–170,171] Nevertheless, a high degree of correlation ($r = 0.977$) has been observed between the PTH results determined by the first and second PTH-IMAs in patients with ESRD.[167,169,173]

The levels of PTH that are associated with normal rates of bone formation in pediatric patients with different degrees of renal insufficiency before dialysis therapy are not clearly defined. Although additional data on this subject are clearly needed, recent guidelines from K/DOQI have recommended intact PTH values of 30 to 70 pg/mL and 70 to 110 pg/mL in adult patients with CKD Stages 3 and 4, respectively. It is likely that the pediatric work group will soon make similar recommendations.[174]

Although it is well recognized that phosphorus retention in patients with advanced CKD plays a central role in the development and maintenance of secondary hyperparathyroidism (HPT) by causing hypocalcemia and reducing the rate of conversion of 25-hydroxyvitamin D3 to 1,25-dihydroxyvitamin D3,[175] a deficit of calcitriol synthesis has also been shown to be a major factor in the development of HPT.[176,177] In fact, a study involving a large number of adult patients with CKD revealed that HPT developed at a time when the serum calcium and phosphorus were still normal.[178] Thus, the current belief is that calcium, phosphorus, and calcitriol play an integrated role and all are important in the pathogenesis of HPT.

Along the same lines, although dietary phosphorus restriction is the usual first line approach to the management of HPT, phosphorus restriction alone may not be very effective in suppressing PTH, if the calcium intake is inadequate.[178] Apart from having an independent effect on parathyroid gland activity,[178] dietary calcium may also be a signal to upregulate the vitamin D receptor density in the parathyroid glands.[179,180] Thus, the appropriate dietary intakes of calcium, phosphorus, and vitamin D are crucial for the management of HPT in patients with CKD.

Adequate dietary calcium intake during childhood is necessary for the development of optimal peak bone mass.[181] The current recommendation is that patients with CKD should achieve a calcium intake of 100% of the DRI[182] (Table 14–8). Infants and young children usually meet the DRI for calcium with the consumption of adequate volumes of breast milk/formula. Unfortunately, the largest source of dietary calcium for most persons are dairy products which are also rich in phosphorus; in turn, phosphorus restriction universally leads to a decreased calcium intake. In these situations, calcium supplementation may be required as low phosphorus, high calcium foods such as collards, dandelion greens, kale, rhubarb, and spinach usually do not make up a substantial part of a child's diet. Several products fortified with calcium such as fruit juices and breakfast foods are commercially

Table 14–8 Recommended Calcium Intake for Children with Chronic Kidney Disease

Age (Years)	DRI (mg/day)	Recommended Maximum Intake (mg/day)
0.0–0.5	210	420
0.5–1.0	270	520
1–3	500	1000
4–8	800	1600
9–18	1300	2500*

DRI, dietary reference intake.
Recommended maximum intake: preliminary recommendation by a pediatric workgroup developing guidelines for the management of dietary calcium intake in children with CKD.
(From Baker SS, Cochran WJ, Flores CA, et al: Committee on Nutrition, American Academy of Pediatrics, Policy Statement: Calcium requirements of infants, children and adolescents [RE 9904]. Pediatrics 1999; 104: 1152–1157.)

available, and limited studies have suggested that the bioavailability of calcium from these products is at least comparable to that of milk.[183] Calcium can also be supplemented in medicinal forms such as carbonate, acetate, and gluconate salts of calcium that are commonly used as phosphate binders. When used for calcium supplementation alone, ingesting these products between meals maximizes calcium absorption.[184] Chloride and citrate salts of calcium should be avoided as the former may lead to acidosis in patients with CKD, and the latter may enhance aluminum absorption.

On the other hand, excessive calcium intake in conjunction with activated vitamin D analogues can lead to (1) hypercalcemia, (2) adynamic bone disease, and (3) systemic calcification. In the adult K/DOQI guidelines, it is recommended that the elemental calcium intake from phosphate binders should not exceed 1500 mg/day and that the total elemental calcium intake should not exceed 2000 mg/day in an attempt to maintain a normal serum calcium and a calcium × phosphorus product less than 55 mg^2/dL^2.[174] In the absence of definitive pediatric studies, the K/DOQI pediatric work group is likely to recommend a maximal calcium intake of two times the DRI for age, except for ages 9 to 18 years (both genders), where two times the DRI (2600 mg) exceeds the Tolerable Upper Intake Level (UL) of 2500 mg.[182] The serum calcium phosphorus product should probably be kept below 60 mg^2/dL^2 in all but possibly the youngest (<3 years) children who naturally have a "high" serum phosphorus level.

The dietary phosphorus intake in children with CKD should be restricted to less than 800 mg/day if a normal phosphorus level is to be achieved, with recognition that dairy products and high-protein foods are the main sources of dietary phosphorus.[185] However, strict dietary phosphorus restriction is often impractical and ill advised because it may lead to an inadvertent poor protein intake. In addition, extremely low phosphorus diets are typically unpalatable. Although young infants may be effectively managed by a low-phosphorus containing milk formula such as Similac PM 60/40 (Ross Laboratories, OH) and Good Start (Nestlé Company, Switzerland), most other patients require oral intestinal phosphate binders to control hyperphosphatemia. Phosphorus control is particularly difficult in vegetarians because for the same total quantity of dietary protein delivered, the phosphorus content is greater in protein derived from vegetable sources versus animal protein. Whereas food labels rarely state the phosphorus content, chocolates, nuts, dried beans, and cola soft drinks are rich in phosphorus and should be avoided; nondairy creamers and certain frozen nondairy desserts may be used in place of milk and ice cream.

Aluminum hydroxide and carbonate were widely used as phosphate binders in the past, but their use was abandoned once they were found to be associated with severe toxicity in adults and children with renal insufficiency.[119,120] Currently, calcium-containing salts (Table 14–9) such as calcium carbonate and calcium acetate are commonly used as phosphate binders, with the latter often reported to be a more effective binder than the former.[186] To be maximally effective, their intake should coincide with that of meals or snacks. The optimal timing for the administration of binders with tube feedings has not been clearly defined. As noted above, calcium containing phosphate binders also serve as an important source of supplemental calcium. More recently, excessive calcium intake in the form of phosphate binders has been implicated as one of the factors responsible for the development of coronary-artery calcification in young adults who started dialysis as young children.[187–189] These findings have focused attention on calcium and aluminum free phosphate binders such as Sevelamer hydrochloride (RenaGel),[190–192] although no calcium-free phosphate binder is currently approved by the FDA for use in children. On rare occasions and for very restricted periods of time, a closely monitored low-dose (<30 mg/kg/day) of aluminum containing phosphate binders may be tried as a last resort for those patients in whom hyperphosphatemia remains uncontrolled, despite the previously recommended medical/dietary management. Finally, in contrast to the successful pretreatment of milk with ion-exchange resins to decrease potassium content, studies on the pretreatment of milk with calcium acetate to reduce the phosphate content found the procedure ineffective.[193]

In the absence of 1∝-hydroxylation of vitamin D, synthetic 1,25 dihydroxyvitamin D (the active metabolite) or dihydrotachysterol (requires only hepatic hydroxylation for activation) is used in pediatric patients with CKD. These

Table 14–9 Calcium Content of Common Calcium-Based Binders[174]

Compound	Brand Name	Compound Content (mg)	% Calcium	Elemental Calcium (mg)
Calcium acetate	Phoslo	667	25	167
Calcium carbonate	Chooz (Gum)	500	40	200
	TUMS EX	750	40	300
	TUMS Ultra	1000	40	400
	LiquiCal	1200	40	480
	CalciChew	1250	40	500
	CalciMix			
	Oscal 500			
	TUMS 500			
	Caltrate 600	1500	40	600
	NephroCalci			
Calcium citrate	CitraCal		Not recommended	
Calcium acetate/ magnesium carbonate	MagneBind 200	450/200		113
	MagneBind	300/300		76

preparations are often started early in the course of CKD on the basis of an elevation of the intact serum PTH and serum alkaline phosphatase levels. As suggested previously, one of the serious complications associated with the use of these activated vitamin D metabolites is the development of hypercalcemia. Several newer noncalcemic vitamin D analogues, such as paricalcitol (19-nor-1, 25-dihydroxyvitamin D_2)[194] and doxercalciferol (1∝-hydroxyvitamin D_2),[195] selectively depress the parathyroid gland with a lower incidence of hypercalcemia when compared to current agents. Pediatric studies with these medications are currently underway.

CARDIOVASCULAR DISEASE

Systemic atherosclerosis and cardiovascular disease (CVD) are usually viewed as unique problems of adulthood, and adult patients with CKD suffer significantly increased rates of morbidity and mortality secondary to CVD, compared to the general population.[196] Nonetheless, the systemic process of atherogenesis begins during childhood, and many pediatric patients with CKD presumably undergo years of accelerated atherosclerosis as they mature toward later life.[197] To be sure, children with renal insufficiency have a high prevalence of traditional risk factors for CVD. As noted in the NAPRTCS registry, 38% to 78% of these children are hypertensive, and as many as 60% to 90% develop hyperlipidemia.[82] In addition to these traditional risk factors, children with CKD may amplify their cardiovascular risk due to a number of uremia-related factors, including anemia, hyperhomocysteinemia, malnutrition, chronic inflammation, and hyperparathyroidism.[114,198,199] Thus, the combination of traditional and uremia-related risk factors may initiate and accelerate CVD in the pediatric population with CKD. In fact, CVD is now recognized as the second most common cause of death in children with ESRD,[48,85,200,201] and the cardiovascular mortality rate reported in children and young adults on chronic dialysis is almost 1000 times higher than in comparably aged individuals without renal disease.[85]

As mentioned previously, hypertension is a common consequence of CKD and may be a presenting sign in children and adolescents. A significant association between hypertension and progression of CKD in adults has been shown in a recently conducted review of 26 studies by K/DOQI.[202] Similarly, a retrospective analysis of pediatric patients with CRI from the NAPRTCS database demonstrated a high prevalence (48%) of hypertension and a close correlation between hypertension and the progression of renal failure.[203] In the latter study, hypertension predicted the progression of CRI independently of other known risk factors such as baseline kidney function, age, race, and primary kidney disease. The study also revealed that systolic, but not diastolic blood pressure, remained an independent predictor for the progression of renal failure. An earlier study by Wingen and associates[80] has also shown that systolic BP and moderate proteinuria were significant risk factors for the progression of renal failure in children.

The question of whether hypertension is the cause or merely a marker of the progression of renal disease was addressed even before ACE inhibitors became available. Several clinical studies in adults with diabetic nephropathy have demonstrated that lowering BP to the upper normal range[204] or lower[205] results in a slowing of the loss of renal function as well as a simultaneous decrease in proteinuria. A beneficial effect of lowering BP has also been demonstrated in adults with nondiabetic renal diseases.[206] The ACE inhibitors seem to offer better preservation of renal function than other antihypertensive agents,[207] especially in patients with proteinuria.[208] This evidence of renoprotection by ACE inhibitors, as well as their antihypertensive efficacy with few side effects has, in turn, led to the widespread use of these agents in pediatric renal patients despite few published pediatric data. The impact of BP management on the progression of renal failure is, however, currently being examined in a European pediatric multicenter study. In this 3-year trial, children with CRI treated with an ACE inhibitor (ramipril) are randomized to a target BP below the 50th percentile or between the 50th and 95th percentile on the basis of 24-hour ambulatory BP monitoring standards. The results of this trial should become available later this year. Twenty-four–hour ambulatory blood pressure monitoring (ABMP) is being used in the trial because this technique has been found to be superior to clinic BP measurements in predicting end organ damage.[209,210] It is also useful for the detection of abnormal nocturnal BP changes, which are predictive of cardiovascular mortality in patients with CKD.[211] Although limited ABPM data exist presently in pediatrics, its use is likely to become more widespread following the availability of normalized reference values in children[212] and its application in the European study and the U.S. multicenter CKD study.

The number of reviews of cardiac function and structure in children with CKD are limited, but the few that do exist provide in vivo evidence of cardiac morbidity in this population. However, the exact timing of the onset of the cardiovascular abnormalities during the course of CKD in children is not known. It is likely that the pathophysiological processes probably start early, as echocardiographic studies of children have revealed an increased left ventricular mass (LVM) in 22% of children with renal insufficiency, 30% of those treated with dialysis, and 63% of those who have received a kidney transplant.[213] In a cohort of 140 young adult patients from the Netherlands with ESRD onset at age less than 14 years, evidence of increased LVM was found in 47% of males and 39% of females, diastolic dysfunction in 13% and aortic valve calcification in 19% of all patients.[214] An important correlation has also been observed between LVM and decreasing renal function in children with CKD, suggesting that uremia itself may lead to a progressive increase in LVM.[215] It is important as well to note that there is a significant correlation between anemia and CVD because the LVM is reduced in children after correction of anemia with erythropoietin.[216] Another echocardiographic study of children initiating maintenance dialysis (26 HD, 38 PD) showed left ventricular hypertrophy (LVH) in 75% of the children, and the severity of LVH correlated with the duration of renal insufficiency prior to the institution of dialysis.[217] In adults, long-standing cardiac hypertrophy ultimately leads to maladaptive LVH, diastolic and systolic dysfunction, and may eventually lead to cardiac failure and death. Therefore, the LVH that begins during childhood CKD may be a key risk factor for future cardiac disease in young adults with ESRD.

A small autopsy series of children with ESRD or status-post kidney transplantation has also provided evidence of pathologic changes in the intima of the coronary arteries,[218] and the recent cross-sectional studies that detected coronary artery calcification by electron-beam computed tomography in young adults lend support to the possible presence of accelerated coronary artery disease in pediatric/young adult patients with CKD.[187, 188] Despite this growing evidence, congestive heart failure still appears to be much more common in children than atherosclerotic heart disease.[11]

In summary, early evaluation and an aggressive management approach to include effective blood pressure control, anemia management with erythropoietin, control of dyslipidemia, prudent use of calcium salts as phosphorus binding agents, and 1,25 dihydroxyvitamin D3 for secondary hyperparathyroidism are essential to decrease CVD morbidity and mortality. The role of folic acid and anti-inflammatory therapy to treat elevated homocysteine levels and markers of inflammation in children awaits further study.

PREVENTION OF PROGRESSION OF CHRONIC KIDNEY DISEASE

The major health consequences of CKD include not only the progression to kidney failure, but also all of the associated manifestations noted earlier. Recent evidence indicates that these outcomes can be improved by early treatment.[219] Therefore, there is a need to understand the mechanisms involved in the progression of CKD and to determine reliable and early biomarkers that correlate with disease progression. The latter are necessary to follow the early success or failure of applied interventions to preserve renal function and to slow the progression of renal insufficiency.

There is experimental as well as clinical evidence that the response to a loss of renal mass and the subsequent progression to CRI in children is different from that seen in adults. In young animals in whom maturational growth is occurring, injury after renal ablation is often more severe than that seen in adult animals.[220] A reduction in renal mass has been associated with the development of proteinuria and hypertension, both of which are established risk factors for renal disease progression in humans. The presence of glomerular hypertrophy and subsequent glomerulosclerosis is substantial, especially in the deep nephrons of the young rat. This increased sclerosis is postulated to be related to factors unique to the young growing kidney, which is characterized by centripetal growth and differentiation. In humans, a similar response to injury is observed in the juvenile kidney. For example, as many as 33% of children develop microalbuminuria after undergoing unilateral nephrectomy for Wilms' tumor.[221]

As protein leaks through the diseased glomeruli, it injures the tubular cells and thereby causes interstitial inflammation and subsequent fibrosis.[222] Albumin has autocrine and paracrine effects on tubular cells in culture media.[223] The presence of microalbuminuria in adult diabetic patients is associated with a 10-fold higher risk of progression to overt nephropathy.[224] Severe proteinuria is also associated with a faster progression of renal deterioration in adult patients with glomerular diseases,[206] and results from the Modification of Diet in Renal Disease (MDRD) study supports the concept that proteinuria is an independent risk factor for progression of CRI in adults.[225] At the same time, reduction of proteinuria, independent of blood pressure, is associated with a subsequent beneficial effect on progression of CKD in adults.

Although proteinuria is an established biomarker of CKD progression, diseases involving a high filtered load of albumin such as minimal change nephrotic syndrome are not typically associated with the presence of renal insufficiency, suggesting that the assessment of glomerular proteinuria with only albumin may not be optimal. On the other hand, the urinary excretion of IgG and β1-microglobulin predicts the clinical course better than the extent of proteinuria in membranous nephropathy.[225] Evidence of tubular injury and dysfunction, manifested by abnormal amounts of small urinary tubular proteins, may also be useful biomarkers of progression of renal disease. Retinol binding protein (RBP) and *N*-acetylglucosaminidase (NAG) have been shown to be markers of proximal tubular damage and dysfunction. RBP is much more sensitive than NAG for the early detection of tubular impairment.[226] In children with vesicoureteral reflux, evidence of tubular dysfunction as measured by urinary RBP and NAG is frequently noted in patients who have renal scarring, evidence of damage that usually precedes the development of albuminuria. Proteomics and the new methodologies of protein profiling are recent and exciting scientific developments to study urinary proteins and have the potential for identifying clinically useful biomarkers that predict the progression of renal disease.[227] These investigative techniques will be an important component of the multicenter pediatric CKD study.

CONCLUSIONS

In conclusion, the development of CKD during childhood frequently results in a variety of clinical manifestations that can have a lifelong impact on the pediatric patient. To optimize therapy at present, an aggressive diagnostic and management approach designed by a multidisciplinary team is absolutely essential. Future investigative efforts will likely make possible additional therapeutic options to delay or even to prevent the progression of CKD, clearly the desired outcome for children and adults alike.

References

1. Clinical practice guidelines for chronic kidney disease: Evaluation, classification and stratification. National Kidney Foundation. K/DOQI clinical practice guidelines. Am J Kidney Dis 2002; 39:S1–S266.
2. Atiyeh BA, Dabbagh SS, Gruskin AB: Evaluation of renal function during childhood. Pediatr Rev 2001; 17:175–179.
3. Heilbron DC, Holliday MA, Al-Dahwi A, Kogan BA: Expressing glomerular filtration rate in children. Pediatr Nephrol 1991; 5:5–11.
4. Hogg RJ, Furth S, Lemley KV, et al: National Kidney Foundation's Kidney Disease Outcomes Quality Initiative Clinical Practice Guidelines for Chronic Kidney Disease in Children and Adolescents: Evaluation, classification, and stratification. Pediatrics 2003; 111:1416–1421.
5. Schwartz GJ, Haycock GB, Edelmann CM Jr, Spitzer A: A simple estimate of glomerular filtration rate in children derived from body length and plasma creatinine. Pediatrics 1976; 58:259-263.
6. Schwartz GJ, Feld LG, Langford DJ: A simple estimate of glomerular filtration rate in full-term infants during the first year of life. J Pediatr 1984; 104:849–854.
7. Schwartz GJ, Gauthier B: A simple estimate of glomerular filtration rate in adolescent boys. J Pediatr 1985; 106:522–526.

8. Hellerstein S, Berenbom M, Alon US, Warady BA: Creatinine clearance following cimetidine for estimation of glomerular filtration rate. Pediatr Nephrol 1998; 12:49–54.
9. Ylinen EA, Ala-Houhala M, Harmoinen AP, Knip M: Cystatin C as a marker for glomerular filtration rate in pediatric patients. Pediatr Nephrol 1999; 13:506–509.
10. North American Pediatric Renal Transplant Cooperative Study (NAPRTCS) 2003 Annual Report. Rockville, MD, The EMMES Corporation, 2003.
11. United States Renal Data System: 2002 annual data report. Pediatric ESRD. Am J Kidney Dis 2003; 41:S121–S134.
12. Karlberg J, Schaefer F, Hennicke M, et al: Early age-dependent growth impairment in chronic renal failure: European Study Group for Nutritional Treatment of Chronic Renal Failure in Childhood. Pediatr Nephrol 1996; 10:283–287.
13. Haffner D, Schaefer F, Nissel R, et al: Effect of growth hormone treatment on the adult height of children with chronic renal failure. German Study Group for Growth Hormone Treatment in Chronic Renal Failure. N Engl J Med 2000; 343:923–930.
14. Wong CS, Gipson DS, Gillen DL, et al: Anthropometric measures and risk of death in children with end-stage renal disease. Am J Kidney Dis 2000; 36:811-819.
15. Furth SL, Stablein D, Fine RN, et al: Adverse clinical outcomes associated with short stature at dialysis initiation: A report of the North American Pediatric Renal Transplant Cooperative Study. Pediatrics 2002; 109:909–913.
16. Furth SL, Hwang W, Yang C, et al: Growth failure, risk of hospitalization and death for children with end-stage renal disease. Pediatr Nephrol 2002; 17:450–455.
17. Arnold WC, Danford D, Holliday MA: Effects of calorie supplementation on growth in uremia. Kidney Int 1983; 24:205–209.
18. Kuemmerle N, Krieg RJ, Latta K, et al: Growth hormone and insulin-like growth factor in non-uremic acidosis and uremic acidosis. Kidney Int 1997; 58:S102–S105.
19. Parekh RS, Flynn JT, Smoyer WE, et al: Improved growth in young children with severe chronic renal insufficiency who use specified nutritional therapy. J Am Soc Nephrol 2001; 12:2418–2426.
20. Schaefer F, Mehls O: Endocrine and growth disturbances. *In* Barret TM, Avner ED, Harmon WE (eds): Pediatric Nephrology, 4th ed. Baltimore, Lippincott Williams & Wilkins, 1999, pp 1197–1230.
21. Salusky IB, Kuizon BG, Juppner H: Special aspects of renal osteodystrophy in children. Semin Nephrol 2004; 24:69–77.
22. Tonshoff B, Schaefer F, Mehls O: Disturbance of growth hormone-insulin-like growth factor axis in uremia. Pediatr Nephrol 1990; 4:654-662.
23. Roelfsema V, Clark RG: The growth hormone and insulin-like growth factor axis: Its manipulation for the benefit of growth disorders in renal failure. J Am Soc Nephrol 2001; 12:1297-1306.
24. Haffner D, Schaefer F, Girard J, et al: Metabolic clearance of recombinant growth hormone in health and chronic renal failure. J Clin Invest 1994; 93:1163-1171.
25. Tonshoff B, Veldhuis JD, Heinrich U, Mehls O: Deconvolution analysis of spontaneous nocturnal growth hormone secretion in prepubertal children with preterminal chronic renal failure and with end-stage renal disease. Pediatr Res 1995; 37:86–93.
26. Moore LC, Kaskel FJ: Decreased hepatic insulin-like growth factor (IGF)-I and increased IGF binding protein-1 and -2 gene expression in experimental uremia. Endocrinology 1997; 138:938-946.
27. Tonshoff B, Powell DR, Zhao D, et al: Decreased hepatic insulin-like growth factor (IGF-1) and increased IGF binding protein-1 and –2 gene expression in experimental uremia. Endocrinology 1997; 138:938–946.
28. Schaefer F, Chen Y, Tsao T, et al: Impaired JAK-STAT signal transduction contributes to growth hormone resistance in chronic uremia. J Clin Invest 2001; 108:467-475.
29. Tonshoff B, Blum WF, Wingen AM, et al: Serum insulin-like growth factors (IGFs) and IGF binding protein 1, 2 and 3 in children with chronic renal failure: Relationship to height and glomerular filtration rate. J Clin Endocrinol Metab 1995; 80: 2684-2691.
30. Kiepe D, Ulinski T, Powell DR, et al: Differential effects of insulin-like growth factor binding proteins-1, -2, -3 and -6 on cultured growth plate chondrocytes. Kidney Int 2002; 62:1591-1600.
31. Hokken-Koelega AC, Stijnen T, de Muinck K, et al: Placebo-controlled, double-blind, cross-over trial of growth hormone treatment in prepubertal children with chronic renal failure. Lancet 1991; 338:585-590.
32. Fine RN, Kohaut EC, Brown D, Perlman AJ: Growth after recombinant human growth hormone treatment in children with chronic renal failure: Report of a multicenter randomized double-blind placebo-controlled study. Genentech Cooperative Study Group. J Pediatr 1994; 124:374–382.
33. Clinical practice guidelines for nutrition in chronic renal failure. K/DOQI National Kidney Foundation. Am J Kidney Dis 2000; 35:S1–S140.
34. Warady BA, Schaefer F, Alexander SR, et al: Care of the pediatric patient on peritoneal dialysis: Clinical process for optimal outcomes. Baxter Healthcare Corporation, 2004.
35. Wuhl E, Haffner D, Nissel R, et al: Short dialyzed children respond less to growth hormone than patients prior to dialysis. German Study Group for Growth Hormone Treatment in Chronic Renal failure. Pediatr Nephrol 1996; 10:294–298.
36. Kawai M, Momoi T, Yorifuji T, et al: Unfavorable effects of growth hormone therapy on the final height of boys with short stature not caused by growth hormone deficiency. J Pediatr 1997; 130:205–209.
37. Fine RN, Ho M, Tejani A, Blethen S: Adverse events with rhGH treatment of patients with chronic renal insufficiency and end-stage renal disease. J Pediatr 2003; 142:539–545.
38. Rotundo A, Nevins TE, Lipton JM, et al: Progressive encephalopathy in children with chronic renal insufficiency in infancy. Kidney Int 1982; 21:486-491.
39. Warady BA, Belden B, Kohaut E: Neurodevelopmental outcome of children initiating peritoneal dialysis in early infancy. Pediatr Nephrol 1999; 13:759-765.
40. Warady BA: Neurodevelopment of infants with end-stage renal disease: Is it improving? Pediatr Transplant 2002; 6:5-7.
41. Betts PR, Magrath G, White RH: Role of dietary energy supplementation in growth of children with chronic renal insufficiency. Br Med J 1977; 1:416–418.
42. Mehls O, Blum WF, Schaefer F, et al: Growth failure in renal disease. Baillieres Clin Endocrinol Metab 1992; 6:665–685.
43. Sedman A, Friedman A, Boineau F, et al: Nutritional management of the child with mild to moderate chronic renal failure. J Pediatr 1996; 129:S13-S18.
44. Warady BA, Kriley M, Lovell H, et al: Growth and development of infants with end-stage renal disease receiving long-term peritoneal dialysis. J Pediatr 1988; 112:714-719.
45. Geary DF, Haka Iksa K: Neurodevelopmental progress of young children with chronic renal disease. J Pediatr 1989; 84:68-72.
46. Geary DF, Haka Iksa K, Coulter P, et al: The role of nutrition in neurology health and development of infants with chronic renal failure. Adv Perit Dial 1990; 6:252-254.
47. Wong CS, Hingorani S, Gillen DL, et al: Hypoalbuminemia and risk of death in pediatric patients with end-stage renal disease. Kidney Int 2002; 61:630-637.
48. United States Renal Data System: 2003 annual data report. Pediatric ESRD. Am J Kidney Dis 2003; 42:S129–S140.
49. Chadha V, Warady BA: Nutritional management of the child with kidney disease. *In* Kopple JD, Massry SG (eds): Kopple and Massry's Nutritional Management of Renal Disease, 2nd ed. Philadelphia, Lippincott Williams & Wilkins, pp 527–547.

50. Wingen AM, Fabian-Bach C, Mehls O: European Study Group for Nutritional Treatment of Chronic Renal Failure in Childhood. Evaluation of protein intake by dietary diaries and urea-N excretion in children with chronic renal failure. Clin Nephrol 1993; 40:208–215.
51. Rizzoni G, Basso T, Setari M: Growth in children with chronic renal failure on conservative treatment. Kidney Int 1984; 26:52-58.
52. Ravelli AM, Ledermann SE, Bisset WM, et al: Foregut motor function in chronic renal failure. Arch Dis Child 1992; 67: 1343-1347.
53. Fried MD, Khoshoo V, Secker DJ, et al: Decrease in gastric emptying time and episodes of regurgitation in children with spastic quadriplegia fed a whey-based formula. J Pediatr 1992; 120:569-572.
54. Tolia V, Lin CH, Kuhns LP: Gastric emptying using three different formulas in infants with gastroesophageal reflux. J Pediatr Gastroenterol Nutr 1992; 15:297-301.
55. Salusky IB, Fine RN, Nelson P, et al: Nutritional status of children undergoing continuous ambulatory peritoneal dialysis. Am J Clin Nutr 1983; 38:599-611.
56. Holliday MA: Calorie deficiency in children with uremia: Effect upon growth. Pediatrics 1972; 50:590-597.
57. Ratsch IM, Catassi C, Verrina E, et al: Energy and nutrient intake of patients with mild to moderate chronic renal failure compared with healthy children: An Italian multicenter study. Eur J Pediatr 1992; 151:701-705.
58. Kuizon BD, Salusky IB: Growth retardation in children with chronic renal failure. J Bone Miner Res 1999; 14: 1680-1690.
59. Norman LJ, Coleman JE, Macdonald IA, et al: Nutrition and growth in relation to severity of renal disease in children. Pediatr Nephrol 2000; 15:259–265.
60. Foreman JW, Abitol CL, Trachtman H, et al: Nutritional intake in children with renal insufficiency: A report of the Growth Failure in Children with Renal Diseases Study. J Am Coll Nutr 1996; 15:579-585.
61. Foreman JW, Chan JCM: Chronic renal failure in infants and children. J Pediatr 1988; 113:793-800.
62. Claris-Appiani A, Arissino GL, Dacco V, et al: Catch-up growth in children with chronic renal failure treated with long-term enteral nutrition. JPEN 1995; 19:175–178.
63. Kurtin PS, Shapiro AC: Effect of defined caloric supplementation on growth of children with renal disease. J Renal Nutr 1992; 2:13.
64. Kleinknecht C, Salusky IB, Broyer M, et al: Effect of various protein diets on growth, renal function, and survival of uremic rats. Kidney Int 1979; 15:534–542.
65. Salusky IB, Kleinknecht C, Broyer M, et al: Prolonged renal survival and stunting, with protein-deficient diets in experimental uremia. J Lab Clin Med 1981; 21–30.
66. Brenner BM, Meyer TW, Hostetter TH: Dietary protein intake and the progressive nature of kidney disease: The role of hemodynamically mediated glomerular injury in the pathogenesis of progressive glomerular sclerosis in aging, renal ablation and intrinsic renal disease. N Engl J Med 1982:652–659.
67. Klahr S, Levey AS, Beck GJ, et al: The effects of dietary protein restriction and blood-pressure control on the progression of chronic renal disease. Modification of Diet in Renal Disease Study Group. N Engl J Med 1994; 330:877-884.
68. Walser M, Hill S: Can renal replacement be deferred by a supplemented very low protein diet? J Am Soc Nephrol 1999; 10:110–116.
69. Aparicio M, Chauveau P, Precigout VD, et al: Nutrition and outcome on renal replacement therapy of patients with chronic renal failure treated by a supplemented very low protein diet. J Am Soc Nephrol 2000; 11:708–716.
70. Bernhard J, Beaufrere B, Laville M, et al: Adaptive response to a low-protein diet in predialysis chronic renal failure patients. J Am Soc Nephrol 2001; 12:1249–1254.
71. Fouque D, Laville M, Boissel JP, et al: Controlled low protein diets in chronic renal insufficiency: Meta-analysis. BMJ 1992; 304:216–220.
72. Levey AS, Adler S, Caggiula AW, et al: Effects of dietary protein restriction on the progression of advanced renal disease in the Modification of Diet in Renal Disease Study. Am J Kidney Dis 1996; 27:652–663.
73. Pedrini MT, Levey AS, Lau J, et al: The effect of dietary protein restriction on the progression of diabetic and non-diabetic renal diseases: A meta-analysis. Ann Intern Med 1996; 124:627–632.
74. Kasiske BL, Lakatua JD, Ma JZ, et al: A meta-analysis of the effects of dietary protein restriction on the rate of decline in renal function. Am J Kidney Dis 1998; 31:954–961.
75. Levey AS, Greene T, Beck GJ, et al: MDRD Study Group. Dietary protein restriction and the progression of chronic renal disease: What have all the results of the MDRD study shown? J Am Soc Nephrol 1999; 10: 2426–2439.
76. Friedman AL, Pityer R: Benefit of moderate dietary protein restriction on growth in the young animal with experimental chronic renal insufficiency: Importance of early growth. Pediatr Res 1989; 25:509–513.
77. Wingen AM, Fabian-Bach C, Mehls O: European Study Group for Nutritional Treatment of Chronic Renal Failure in Childhood. Multicenter randomized study on the effect of a low-protein diet on the progression of renal failure in childhood: One-year results. Miner Electrolyte Metab 1992; 18: 303-308.
78. Kist-van Holthe tot Echten JE, Nauta J, Hop WC, et al: Protein restriction in chronic renal failure. Archives Dis Child 1993; 68:371–375.
79. Uauy RD, Hogg RJ, Brewer ED, et al: Dietary protein and growth in infants with chronic renal insufficiency: A report from the Southwest Pediatric Nephrology Study Group and the University of California, San Franciso. Pediatr Nephrol 1994; 8:45-50.
80. Wingen AM, Fabian-Bach C, Schaefer F, et al: European Study Group for Nutritional Treatment of Chronic Renal Failure in Childhood. Randomized multicenter study of a low-protein diet on the progression of chronic renal failure in children. Lancet 1997; 349:1117–1123.
81. Food and Nutrition Board, Commission on Life Sciences, National Research Council: Recommended Dietary Allowances, 10th ed. Washington DC, National Academies Press, 1989.
82. Querfeld U: Disturbances of lipid metabolism in children with chronic renal failure. Pediatr Nephrol 1993; 7:749-757.
83. Querfeld U: Under treatment of cardiac risk factors in adolescents with renal failure. Perit Dial Int 2001; 21:S285–S289.
84. Chavers BM, Li S, Collins AJ, et al: Cardiovascular disease in pediatric chronic dialysis patients. Kidney Int 2002; 62:648–653.
85. Parekh RS, Carroll CE, Wolfe RA, Port FK: Cardiovascular mortality in children and young adults with end-stage kidney disease. J Pediatr 2002; 141:162–164.
86. Saland JM, Ginsberg H, Fisher EA: Dyslipidemia in pediatric renal disease: Epidemiology, pathophysiology, and management. Curr Opin Pediatr 2002; 14:197–204.
87. Papadopoulou ZL, Sandler P, Tina LU, et al: Hyperlipidemia in children with chronic renal insufficiency. Pediatr Res 1981; 15:887–891.
88. Zacchello G, Pagnan A, Sidran MP, et al: Further definition of lipid-lipoprotein abnormalities in children with various degrees of chronic renal insufficiency. Pediatr Res 1987; 21:462–465.
89. Friedewald WT, Levy RI, Fredrickson DS: Estimation of the concentration of low-density lipoprotein cholesterol in plasma, without use of the preparative ultracentrifuge. Clin Chem 1972; 18:499–502.
90. Senti M, Pedro-Botet J, Nogues X, et al: Influence of intermediate-density lipoproteins on the accuracy of the Friedewald formula. Clin Chem 1991; 37:1394–1397.

91. Howard BV: Insulin resistance and lipid metabolism. Am J Cardiol 1999; 84:28J–32J.
92. Horkko S, Huttunen K, Kesaniemi YA: Decreased clearance of low-density lipoprotein in uremic patients under dialysis treatment. Kidney Int 1995; 47:1732–1740.
93. Mordasini R, Frey F, Flury W, et al: Selective deficiency of hepatic triglyceride lipase in uremic patients. N Engl J Med 1977; 297:1362–1366.
94. Grtuzmacher P, Marz W, Peschke B, et al: Lipoproteins and apolipoproteins during the progression of chronic renal disease. Nephron 1988; 50:103–111.
95. Moberly JB, Attman PO, Samuelsson O, et al: Apolipoprotein C-III, hypertriglyceridemia and triglyceride-rich lipoproteins in uremia. Miner Electrolyte Metab 1999; 25:258–262.
96. Mak RH: Metabolic effects of erythropoietin in patients on peritoneal dialysis. Pediatr Nephrol 1998; 12:660–665.
97. Mak RH: 1,25-Dihydroxyvitamin D3 corrects insulin and lipid abnormalities in uremia. Kidney Int 1998; 53:1353–1357.
98. Mak RH: Effect of metabolic acidosis on hyperlipidemia in uremia. Pediatr Nephrol 1999; 13:891–893.
99. Goren A, Stankiewicz H, Goldstein R, et al: Fish oil treatment of hyperlipidemia in children and adolescents receiving renal replacement therapy. Pediatrics 1991; 88:265–268.
100. Sanjad SA, al-Abbad A, al-Shorafa S: Management of hyperlipidemia in children with refractory nephrotic syndrome: The effect of statin therapy. J Pediatr 1997; 130:470–474.
101. Matzkies FK, Bahner U, Teschner M, et al: Efficiency of 1-year treatment with fluvastatin in hyperlipidemic patients with nephrotic syndrome. Am J Nephrol 1999; 19:492–494.
102. Wheeler DC: Lipid abnormalities in the nephrotic syndrome: The therapeutic role of statins. J Nephrol 2001; 14:S70–S75.
103. Williams CL, Bollella MC, Strobino BA, et al: Plant stanol ester and bran fiber in childhood: Effects on lipids, stool weight and stool frequency in preschool children. J Am Coll Nutr 1999; 18:572–581.
104. Lambert M, Lupien PJ, Gagne C, et al: Treatment of familial hypercholesterolemia in children and adolescents: Effect of lovastatin. Canadian Lovastatin in Children Study Group. Pediatrics 1996; 97:619–628.
105. Clinical practice guidelines for managing dyslipidemias in chronic kidney disease. K/DOQI National Kidney Foundation. Am J Kidney Dis 2003; 41:S1–S91.
106. Mitch WE, Clark AS: Specificity of the effects of leucine and its metabolites on protein degradation in skeletal muscle. Biochem J 1984; 222:579–586.
107. Movilli E, Bossini N, Viola BF, et al: Evidence for an independent role of metabolic acidosis on nutritional status in hemodialysis patients. Nephrol Dial Transplant 1998; 13:674–678.
108. Uribarri J: Moderate metabolic acidosis and its effects on nutritional parameters in hemodialysis pateints. Clin Nephrol 1997; 48:238–240.
109. Boirie Y, Broyer M, Gagnadoux MF, et al: Alterations of protein metabolism by metabolic acidosis in children with chronic renal failure. Kidney Int 2000; 58:236–241.
110. Fine BP, Antonia TY, Lestrange N, Levine R: Sodium deprivation growth failure in the rat: Alterations in tissue composition and fluid spaces. J Nutr 1987; 117:1623–1628.
111. Schrier RN, Regal EM: Influence of aldosterone on sodium, water, and potassium metabolism in chronic renal disease. Kidney Int 1972; 1:156–168.
112. Bunchman TE, Wood EG, Schenck MH, et al: Pretreatment of formula with sodium polystyrene sulfonate to reduce dietary potassium intake. Pediatr Nephrol 1991; 5:29–32.
113. Schroder CH, de Boer AW, Giesen AM, et al: Treatment of hyperhomocysteinemia in children on dialysis by folic acid. Pediatr Nephrol 1999; 13:583–585.
114. Merouani A, Lambert M, Delvin EE, et al: Plasma homocysteine concentration in children with chronic renal failure. Pediatr Nephrol 2001; 16:805–811.
115. Shah GM, Ross EA, Sabo A, et al: Effects of ascorbic acid and pyridoxine supplementation on oxalate metabolism in peritoneal dialysis patients. Am J Kidney Dis 1992; 20:42–49.
116. Werb R, Clark WF, Lindsay RM, et al: Serum vitamin A levels and associated abnormalities in patients on regular dialysis treatment. Clin Nephrol 1979; 12:63–68.
117. Smythe WR, Alfrey AC, Craswell PW, et al: Trace element abnormalities in chronic uremia. Ann Intern Med 1982; 96: 302–310.
118. Thomson NM, Stevens BJ, Humphrey TJ, et al: Comparison of trace elements in peritoneal dialysis, hemodialysis, and uremia. Kidney Int 1983; 23:9–14.
119. Andreoli SP, Bergstein JF, Sherrard DJ, et al: Aluminum-containing phosphate binders in children with azotemia not undergoing dialysis. N Engl J Med 1984; 310: 1079–1084.
120. Sedman A: Aluminum toxicity in childhood. Pediatr Nephrol 1992; 6:383–393.
121. Chan JCM, McEnery PT, Chinchilli VM, et al: A prospective, double-blind study of growth failure in children with chronic renal insufficiency and the effectiveness of treatment with calcitriol vs dihydrotachysterol. J Pediatr 1994; 124:520–528.
122. Fritz IB: Action of carnitine on long-chain fatty acid oxidation by liver. Am J Physiol 1959; 197:297–304.
123. Englard S, Carnicero HH: gamma-Butyrobetaine hydroxylation to carnitine in mammalian kidney. Arch Biochem Biophys 1978; 190: 361–364.
124. Bartel LL, Hussey JL, Shrago E: Perturbation of serum carnitine levels in human adults by chronic renal disease and dialysis therapy. Am J Clin Nutr 1981; 34:1314–1320.
125. Moorthy A, Rosenblum M, Rajaram R, et al: A comparison of plasma and muscle carnitine levels in patients on peritoneal or hemodialysis for chronic renal failure. Am J Nephrol 1983; 3:205–208.
126. Obrador GT, Ruthazer R, Arora P, et al: Prevalence of and factors associated with suboptimal care before initiation of dialysis in the United Staes. J Am Soc Nephrol 1999; 10:1793-1800.
127. Obrador GT, Roberts T, St Peter WL, et al: Trends in anemia at initiation of dialysis in the United States. Kidney Int 2001; 60:1875-1884.
128. Obrador GT, Arora P, Kausz AT, Pereira BJ: Pre-end-stage renal disease care in the United States: A state of disrepair. J Am Soc Nephrol 1998; 9:S44-S54.
129. United Resource Networks. The anemia of chronic renal insufficiency (CRI). Minneapolis, MN, United Resource Networks, 2002.
130. Kazmi WH, Kausz AT, Kahn S, et al: Anemia: An early complication of chronic renal insufficiency. Am J Kidney Dis 2001; 38:803-812.
131. Collins AJ, Ma JZ, Ebben J: Impact of hematocrit on morbidity and mortality. Semin Dial 2000; 20:345-349.
132. Braumann KM, Nonnast-Daniel B, Boning D, et al: Improved physical performance after treatment of renal anemia with recombinant human erythropoietin. Nephron 1991; 58:129-134.
133. Teehan B, Sigler MH, Brown JM, et al: Hematologic and physiologic studies during correction of anemia with recombinant human erythropoietin in predialysis patients. Pretransplant Proc 1989; 212:63-66.
134. Mayer G, Thum J, Cada EM, et al: Working capacity is increased following recombinant human erythropoietin treatment. Kidney Int 1988; 34:525-528.
135. Harnett JD, Foley RN, Kent GM, et al: Congestive heart failure in dialysis patients: Prevalence, incidence, prognosis and risk factors. Kidney Int 1995; 47:884-890.

136. Cannella G, La Canna G, Sandrini M, et al: Renormalization of high cardiac output and of left ventricular size following long-term recombinant human erythropoietin treatment of anemic dialyzed uremic patients. Clin Nephrol 1990; 34:272-278.
137. Macdougall IC, Lewis NP, Saunders MJ, et al: Long-term cardiorespiratory effects of amelioration of renal anaemia by erythropoietin. Lancet 1990; 335:489-493.
138. Pascual J, Teruel JL, Moya JL, et al: Regression of left ventricular hypertrophy after partial correction of anemia with erythropoietin in patients on hemodialysis: A prospective study. Clin Nephrol 1991; 35:280-287.
139. Stivelman JC: Benefits of anemia treatment on cognitive function. Nephrol Dial Transplant 2000; 15:29-35.
140. Gafter U, Kalechman Y, Ortin JB, et al: Anemia of uremia is associated with reduced in vitro cytokine secretion: Immunopotentiating activity of red blood cells. Kidney Int 1994; 45:224-231.
141. Vanholder R, Van Biesen W, Ringoir S: Contributing factors to the inhibition of phagocytosis in hemodialyzed patients. Kidney Int 1993; 44:208-214.
142. Scigalla P, Bonzel KE, Bulla M, et al: Therapy of renal anemia with recombinant human erythropoietin in children with end-stage renal disease. Contrib Nephrol 1989; 76:227-241.
143. Burke JR: Low-dose subcutaneous recombinant erythropoietin in children with chronic renal failure. Pediatr Nephrol 1995; 9(5):558-561.
144. Neu AM, Ho PL, McDonald RA, Warady BA: Chronic dialysis in children and adolescents. The 2001 NAPRTCS annual report. Pediatr Nephrol 2002; 17:656-663.
145. Lerner GR, Warady BA, Sullivan EK, Alexander SR: Chronic dialysis in children and adolescents. The 1996 annual report of the North American pediatric renal transplant cooperative study. Pediatr Nephrol 1999; 13:404-417.
146. Warady BA, Ho M: Anemia and patient mortality in children on dialysis. Perit Dial Int 2002; 22:S75.
147. Eschbach JW: The anemia of chronic renal failure: Pathophysiology and the effects of recombinant erythropoietin. Kidney Int 1989; 35:134-148.
148. Parker PA, Izard MW, Maher JF: Therapy of iron deficiency anemia in patients on maintenance dialysis. Nephron 1979; 23:181-186.
149. Potasman I, Better OS: The role of secondary hyperparathyroidism in the anemia of chronic renal failure. Nephron 1983; 33:229-231.
150. Adamson JW, Eschbach JW: Management of the anaemia of chronic renal failure with recombinant erythropoietin. Q J Med New Series 1989; 73:1093-1101.
151. Kaiser L, Schwartz KA: Aluminum-induced anemia. Am J Kidney Dis 1985; 6:348-352.
152. Hampers CL, Streiff R, Nathan DG, et al: Megaloblastic hematopoiesis in uremia and in patients on long-term hemodialysis. N Engl J Med 1967; 276:551-554.
153. Eschbach JW: The future of r-HuEPO. Nephrol Dial Transplant 1995; 10(suppl 2):96-109.
154. Winearls CG, Oliver DA, Pippard MJ, et al: Effect of human erythropoietin derived from recombinant DNA on the anaemia of patients maintained by chronic haemodialysis. Lancet 1986; 2:1175-1178.
155. Eschbach JW, Egrie JC, Downing MR, et al: Correction of the anemia of end-stage renal disease with recombinant human erythropoietin: Results of a combined phase I and II clinical trial. N Engl J Med 1987; 316:73-78.
156. Clinical practice guidelines for anemia of chronic kidney disease. K/DOQI National Kidney Foundation. Am J Kidney Dis 2001; 37:S183–S238.
157. De Palo T, Giordano M, Palumbo F, et al: Clinical experience with darbepoietin alfa (NESP) in children undergoing hemodialysis. Pediatr Nephrol 2004; 19:337–340.
158. Goodman WG, Coburn JW, Slatopolsky E, Salusky IB: Renal osteodystrophy in adults and children. *In* Favus MJ (ed): Primer on the Metabolic Bone Diseases and Disorders of Mineral Metabolism, 4th ed. Philadelphia, Lippincott Williams & Wilkins, 1999, pp 347-363.
159. Sherrard DJ, Hercz G, Pei Y, et al: The spectrum of bone disease in end-stage renal failure: An evolving disorder. Kidney Int 1993; 43:436-442.
160. Salusky IB, Ramirez JA, Oppenheim WL, et al: Biochemical markers of renal osteodystrophy in pediatric patients undergoing CAPD/CCPD. Kidney Int 1994; 45:253-258.
161. Mathias RS, Salusky IB, Harmon WH, et al: Renal bone disease in pediatric patients and young adults treated by hemodialysis in a children's hospital. J Am Soc Nephrol 1993; 12:1938-1946.
162. Brossard JH, Cloutier M, Roy L, et al: Accumulation of a non-(1-84) molecular form of parathyroid hormone (PTH) detected by intact PTH assay in renal failure: Importance in the interpretation of PTH values. J Clin Endocrinol Metab 1996; 81:3923-3929.
163. Lepage R, Roy L, Brossard JH, et al: A non-(1-84) circulating parathyroid hormone (PTH) fragment interferes significantly with intact PTH commercial assay measurements in uremic samples. Clin Chem 1998; 44:805-809.
164. Brossard JH, Lepage R, Cardinal H, et al: Influence of glomerular filtration rate on non(1-84) -parathyroid hormone (PTH) detected by intact PTH assays. Clin Chem 2000; 46:697-703.
165. Brossard JH, Yamamoto LN, D'Amour P: Parathyroid hormone metabolites in renal failure: Bioactivity and clinical implications. Semin Dial 2002; 15:196-201.
166. John MR, Goodman WG, Gao P, et al: A novel immunoradiometric assay detects full-length human PTH but not amino-terminally truncated fragments: Implications for PTH measurements in renal failure. J Clin Endocrinol Metab 1999; 84:4287-4290.
167. Gao P, Scheibel S, D'Amour P, et al: Development of a novel immunoradiometric assay exclusively for biologically active whole parathyroid hormone 1-84: Implications for improvement of accurate assessment of parathyroid function. J Bone Miner Res 2001; 16:605-614.
168. Slatopolsky E, Finch J, Clay P, et al: A novel mechanism for skeletal resistance in uremia. Kidney Int 2000; 58: 753-761.
169. Monier-Faugere MC, Geng Z, Mawad H, et al: Improved assessment of bone turnover by the PTH(1-84)/large C-PTH fragments ratio in ESRD patients. Kidney Int 2001; 60:1460-1468.
170. Salomon R, Charbit M, Gagnadoux MF, et al: High serum levels of a non-(1-84) parathyroid hormone (PTH) fragment in pediatric haemodialysis patients. Pediatr Nephrol 2001; 16:1011-1014.
171. Salusky IB, Goodman WG, Kuizon BD, et al: Similar predictive value of bone turnover using first and second generation immunometric PTH assays in pediatric patients treated with peritoneal dialysis. Kidney Int 2003; 63(5):1801–1808.
172. Nguyen-Yamamoto L, Rousseau L, Brossard JH, et al: Synthetic carboxyl-terminal fragments of parathyroid hormone (PTH) decrease ionized calcium concentration in rats by acting on a receptor different from the PTH/PTH-related peptide receptor. Endocrinology 2001; 142:1386-1392.
173. Goodman WG, Juppner H, Salusky IB, Sherrard J: Parathyroid hormone (PTH), PTH-derived peptides, and new PTH assays in renal osteodystrophy. Kidney Int 2003; 63:1–11.
174. Clinical practice guidelines for bone metabolism and disease in chronic kidney disease. National Kidney Foundation–K/DOQI. Am J Kidney Dis 2003; 42:S1–S201.
175. Slatopolsky E, Caglar S, Gradowska L, et al: On the prevention of secondary hyperparathyroidism in experimental chronic renal disease using "proportional reduction" of dietary phosphorus intake. Kidney Int 1972; 2:147.
176. Portale AA, Booth BE, Tsai HC, et al: Reduced plasma concentration of 1,25 dihydroxyvitamin D in children with moderate renal insufficiency. Kidney Int 1982; 21:627– 632.

177. Wilson I, Felsenfeld A, Drezner MK, et al: Altered divalent ion metabolism in early renal failure: Role of 1,25$(OH)_2D_3$. Kidney Int 1985; 7:565–573.
178. Martinez I, Saracho R, Montenegro J, et al: The importance of dietary calcium and phosphorus in the secondary hyperparathyroidism of patients with early renal failure. Am J Kidney Dis 1997; 29:496–502.
179. Russel J, Bar A, Sherwood LM, et al: Interaction between calcium and 1,25-dihydroxyvitamin D3 in the regulation of preproparathyroid hormone and vitamin D receptor messenger ribonucleic acid in avian parathyroids. Endocrinology 1993; 132:2639–2644.
180. Denda M, Finch J, Brown Alex J, et al: 1,25-Dihydroxyvitamin D3 and 22-oxacalcitriol prevent the decrease in vitamin D receptor content in the parathyroid glands of uremic rats. Kidney Int 1996; 50:344–349.
181. Baker SS, Cochran WJ, Flores CA, et al: Committee on Nutrition; American Academy of Pediatrics, Policy Statement: Calcium requirements of infants, children and adolescents (RE 9904). Pediatrics 1999; 104:1152–1157.
182. Food and Nutrition Board, Institute of Medicine: Dietary Reference Intakes for Calcium, Phosphorus, Magnesium, Vitamin D, and Fluoride. Washington DC, National Academies Press, 1997.
183. Andon MB, Peacock M, Kanerva RL, et al: Calcium absorption from apple and orange juice fortified with calcium citrate malate (CCM). J Am Coll Nutr 1996; 15:313–316.
184. Coburn W, Kopple MH, Brickman AS, et al: Study of intestinal absorption of calcium in patients with renal failure. Kidney Int 1973; 3:264–272.
185. Nelson P, Stover J: Nutrition recommendations for infants, children, and adolescents with end-stage renal disease. *In* Gillit D, Stover J (eds): A Clinical Guide to Nutrition Care in End-Stage Renal Disease. Chicago, American Dietetic Association, 1994, pp 79-97.
186. Mai ML, Emmett M, Sheikh MS, et al: Calcium acetate, an effective phosphorus binder in patients with renal failure. Kidney Int 1989; 36:690–695.
187. Goodman WG, Goldin J, Kuizon BD, et al: Coronary-artery calcification in young adults with end-stage renal disease who are undergoing dialysis. N Engl J Med 2000; 342:1478–1483.
188. Oh J, Wunsch R, Turzer M, et al: Advanced coronary and carotid arteriopathy in young adults with childhood-onset chronic renal failure. Circulation 2002; 106:100–105.
189. Salusky IB, Goodman WG: Cardiovascular calcification in end-stage renal disease. Nephrol Dial Transplant 2002; 17:336–339.
190. Bleyer AJ, Burke SK, Dillon M, et al: A comparison of the calcium-free phosphate binder sevelamer hydrochloride with calcium acetate in the treatment of hyperphosphatemia in hemodialysis patients. Am J Kidney Dis 1999; 33:694–701.
191. Goldberg DI, Dillon MA, Slatopolsky EA, et al: Effect of RenaGel, a non-absorbed, calcium- and aluminum-free phosphate binder, on serum phosphorus, calcium, and intact parathyroid hormone in end-stage renal disease patients. Nephrol Dial Transplant 1998; 13: 2303–2310.
192. Mahdavi H, Kuizon BD, Gales B, et al: Sevelamer hydrochloride: An effective phosphate binder in dialyzed children. Pediatr Nephrol 2003; 18:1260–1264.
193. Schroder CH, Swinkels DW, Verschuur R, et al: Studies with pre-treatment of milk with calcium acetate to reduce the phosphate content. Eur J Pediatr 1995; 154:689.
194. Slatopolsky E, Finch J, Ritter C, et al: A new analog of calcitriol, 19-nor-1,25$(OH)_2D_2$ suppresses parathyroid hormone secretion in uremic rats in the absence of hypercalcemia. Am J Kidney Dis 1995; 25:852–860.
195. Tan AU Jr, Levine BS, Mazess RB, et al: Effective suppression of parathyroid hormone by 1 (-hydroxyvitamin D_2 in hemodialysis pateints with moderate to severe secondary hyperparathyroidism. Kidney Int 1997; 51:317–323.
196. Foley RN, Parfrey PS, Sarnak MJ: Clinical epidemiology of cardiovascular disease in chronic renal disease. Am J Kidney Dis 1998; 32:S112–S119.
197. Strong JP, Malcom GT, McMahan CA, et al: Prevalence and extent of atherosclerosis in adolescents and young adults: Implications for prevention from the Pathobiological Determinants of Atherosclerosis in Youth Study. JAMA 1999; 281:727–735.
198. Lilien M, Duran M, Van Hoeck KJ, et al: Hyperhomocyst(e)inaemia in children with chronic renal failure. Nephrol Dial Transplant 1999; 14:366-368.
199. Kang HG, Lee BS, Hahn H, et al: Reduction of plasma homocysteine by folic acid in children with chronic renal failure. Pediatr Nephrol 2002; 17:511-514.
200. Task Force on Cardiovascular Disease. Special report from the National Kidney Foundation. Am J Kidney Dis 1998; 32:1-121.
201. USRDS 1998 Annual Report. Causes of death. Am J Kidney Dis 1998; 32:81-88.
202. Clinical practice for chronic kidney disease: Evaluation, classification, and stratification?Stratification of risk for progression of kidney disease and development of cardiovascular disease. National Kidney Foundation K/DOQI. Am J Kidney Dis 2002; 39:S170–S179.
203. Mitsnefes M, Ho PL, Mcenery PT: Hypertension and progression of chronic renal insufficiency in children: A report of the North American Pediatric Renal Transplant Cooperative Study (NAPRTCS). J Am Soc Nephrol 2003; 14:2618–2622.
204. Mogensen CE: Long-term antihypertensive treatment inhibiting progression of diabetic nephropathy. Br Med J 1982; 285:685–688.
205. Parving H-H, Andersen AR, Smidt UM, Svendsen PAA: Early aggressive antihypertensive treatment reduces the rate of decline in kidney function in diabetic nephropathy. Lancet 1983; 1:1175–1179.
206. Peterson JC, Adler S, Burkart JM, et al: Blood pressure control, proteinuria, and the progression of renal disease. The Modification of Diet in Renal Disease Study. Ann Intern Med 1995; 123:754–762.
207. Kshirsagar AV, Joy MS, Hogan SL, et al: Effect of ACE inhibitors in diabetic and nondiabetic chronic renal disease: A systematic overview of randomized placebo-controlled trials. Am J Kidney Dis 2000; 35:695–707.
208. The GISEN Group (Gruppo Italiano di Studi Epidemiologici in Nefrologia): Randomized placebo-controlled trial of effect of ramipril on decline in glomerular filtration rate and risk of terminal renal failure in proteinuric, non-diabetic nephropathy. Lancet 1997; 349:1857–1863.
209. Mancia G, Parati G: Ambulatory blood pressure monitoring and organ damage. Hypertension 2000; 36:894–900.
210. Sorof JM, Portman RJ: Ambulatory blood pressure measurements. Curr Opin Pediatr 2001; 13:133–137.
211. Liu M, Takahashi H, Morita Y, et al: Non-dipping is a potent predictor of cardiovascular mortality and is associated with autonomic dysfunction in hemodialysis patients. Nephrol Dial Transplant 2003; 18:563–569.
212. Wuhl E, Witte K, Soergel M, et al: German Working Group on Pediatric Hypertension. Distribution of 24-h ambulatory blood pressure in children: Normalized reference values and role of body dimensions. J Hypertens 2002; 20:1995–2007.
213. Johnstone LM, Jones CL, Grigg LE, et al: Left ventricular abnormalities in children, adolescents and young adults with renal disease. Kidney Int 1996; 50:998-1006.
214. Gruppen MP, Groothoff JW, Prins M, et al: Cardiac disease in young adult patients with end-stage renal disease since childhhod: A Dutch cohort study. Kidney Int 2003; 63:1058–1065.
215. Mitsnefes MM, Kimball TR, Witt SA, et al: Left ventricular mass and systolic performance in pediatric patients with chronic renal failure. Circulation 2003; 107:864–868.

216. Morris KP, Skinner JR, Hunter S, Coulthard MG: Cardiovascular abnormalities in end stage renal failure: The effect of anemia or uremia? Arch Dis Child 2000; 71:119-122.
217. Mitsnefes MM, Daniels SR, Schwartz SA, et al: Severe left ventricular hypertrophy in pediatric dialysis: Prevalence and predictors. Pediatr Nephrol 2000; 14:898-902.
218. Pennisi AJ, Heuser ET, Mickey MR, et al: Hyperlipidemia in pediatric hemodialysis and renal transplant patients. Associated with coronary artery disease. Am J Dis Child 1976; 130:957–961.
219. Remuzzi G, Ruggenenti P, Perico N: Chronic renal disease: Renoprotective benefits of renin-angiotensin system inhibition. Ann Intern Med 2002; 136:604-615.
220. Ikoma M, Yoshioka T, Ichikawa I, Fogo A: Mechanism of the unique susceptibility of deep cortical glomeruli of maturing kidneys to serve focal glomerular sclerosis. Pediatr Res 1990; 28:270-276.
221. Di Tullio MT, Casale F, Indolfi P, et al: Compensatory hypertrophy and progressive renal damage in children nephrectomized for Wilm's tumor. Med Pediatr Oncol 1996; 26:325-328.
222. Burton CJ, Walls J: Interstitial inflammation and scarring: Messages from the proximal tubular cells. Nephrol Dial Transplant 1996; 11:1505-1523.
223. Zola C, Benigni A, Remuzzi G: Protein overload activates proximal tubular cells to release vasoactive and inflammatory mediators. Exp Nephrol 1999; 7:420-428.
224. Nelson RG, Knowler WC, Pettitt DJ, et al: Assessment of risk of overt nephropathy in diabetic patients from albumin excretion in untimed urine specimens. Arch Intern Med 1991; 51:1761-1765.
225. Remuzzi G, Ruggenti P, Benigni A: Understanding the nature of renal disease progression. Kidney Int 1997; 51: 2-15.
226. Bernard AM, Vyskocll AA, Mahleu P, Lauwerys RR: Assessment of urinary retinol-binding protein as an index of protein tubular injury. Clin Chem 1987; 33:775-779.
227. Mak RH, Little B, Skoog S, et al: Identification of specific biomarkers in children with primary vesico-ureteric reflux by a proteomics approach. J Am Soc Nephrol 2000; 11:A1983.

Chapter 15

Modality Options for End-Stage Renal Disease Care

Gihad E. Nesrallah, M.D., F.R.C.P.C., F.A.C.P. • Peter G. Blake, M.B., F.R.C.P.C., F.R.C.P.I. • David C. Mendelssohn, M.D., F.R.C.P.C.

Over the last decade, the end-stage renal disease (ESRD) population in the United States and Canada has doubled in size and continues to grow at an alarming rate.[1,2] The exponential rate of growth in the ESRD population has been slowed to some extent by advances in pre-ESRD care, but this should hardly be viewed as reassuring. Projections from the United States Renal Data System (USRDS) database estimate that the ESRD population will exceed 2.2 million by the year 2030 in the United States alone. In 2001, caring for patients with ESRD cost $15.4 billion in U.S. funds, consuming 6.4% of the total Medicare budget.[1] The need for dialysis systems that maximize patient outcomes while controlling cost has never been more apparent.

Transplantation has established itself as the superior mode of renal replacement therapy (RRT), both with respect to outcomes and cost-effectiveness.[3,4] The ESRD population, however, continues to grow out of proportion to the supply of donor organs, thus limiting ESRD management mainly to the realm of the various dialytic therapies. In-center hemodialysis (HD) is the most prevalent and generally the most costly form of RRT in use, consuming the majority of the ESRD budget in most developed countries. Home hemodialysis, though associated with a greater up-front cost, is cost-effective in the long-term when compared to in-center HD.[5] Self-care and home hemodialysis have been estimated to cost 58% as much as in-center HD, and peritoneal dialysis (PD) remains highly cost-effective, costing as little as 53% as much as in-center HD in the United States.[6] In particular, the recent relative decline in utilization of PD in the United States and in Canada remains difficult to understand on the basis of outcomes and cost analysis.[7]

It is reasonable to conclude that the ESRD modality distribution in a given country will have profound and fundamental consequences for patients, stakeholders, and funding bodies. Thus, modality options must be viewed in parallel, on both a systems level and on an individual patient level. It has never been more incumbent upon the nephrology community to devise modality selection and distribution strategies that take into account patient preference, cost, and effectiveness, while keeping pace with current trends in ESRD management. The purpose of this chapter is to outline the relative merits and limitations of the various RRT options from both a patient and system perspectives, to describe the various factors that influence modality selection, and to propose a strategy for delivering cost-effective care to the ESRD population in the years to come.

OPTIONS FOR RENAL REPLACEMENT THERAPY

It is the bias of the authors that there are no perfect ESRD therapies. There has been an unfortunate tendency in the past to cast dialysis therapies in a competitive light. The tragic truth is that all dialysis therapies are burdensome and imperfect, and all these therapies must be improved. Dialysis therapies should be considered as complementary, and suitable patients without contraindications to any form of dialysis therapy should be presented with a menu of choices. Ideally, these informed patients should be encouraged to select the method that suits their personal situation in the least burdensome way.

This section is intended to provide a general overview of the relative merits and shortcomings of the existing ESRD treatment options.

Peritoneal Dialysis

Peritoneal dialysis involves the transport of solutes and water across the peritoneal capillaries and membrane into a dialysate, which has been infused into the peritoneal cavity. Solutes, including uremic wastes, potassium, and acids, diffuse along their concentration gradients into this fluid, and water follows the osmotic gradient created by hypertonic solute, usually glucose, in the dialysate. Solutes are carried along with ultrafiltered water in a process known as *solvent drag*. The net result is translocation of solute and fluid from blood into the dialysate, though transport of both water and solute may occur in the reverse direction, depending on membrane characteristics and dwell time. The dialysate is changed at regular intervals so that these solutes are removed and the concentration and osmotic gradients may be restored.

The two principal techniques are continuous ambulatory peritoneal dialysis (CAPD) and automated peritoneal dialysis (APD). The former involves manual exchanges typically performed every 6 hours, thus four times daily. In CAPD, fluid is always present in the abdominal cavity. APD is usually performed primarily overnight during sleep and requires a cycler machine to automate the fluid exchanges. APD can be further subdivided into continuous cycler peritoneal dialysis (CCPD), which involves the use of daytime dwells and nocturnal intermittent peritoneal dialysis (NIPD) in which exchanges are only performed overnight and the patient is "day-dry." Daytime exchanges and dwells occurring at various intervals, and lasting for various lengths of time, are becoming increasingly common, while NIPD is in decline.

The peritoneal dialysis procedure requires a functioning peritoneal dialysis catheter, of which there are various types. These may either be inserted percutaneously or surgically, and may be placed well in advance and buried in the abdominal wall until they are needed.

PD is usually a chronic, home-based dialysis therapy. Use of PD for acute dialysis in hospital is now rare,[8,9] and hospital-based chronic PD therapy like IPD (intermittent PD) is no longer commonly employed because of high cost, low clearance of uremic toxins, and poor patient outcomes. For purposes of the discussions in this chapter, PD is used to mean chronic, home-based therapy.

Advantages of Home Peritoneal Dialysis

The peritoneal dialysis procedure is fairly simple as compared with hemodialysis and does not require the same level of technical expertise. The equipment is simple and portable, thus making it practical both in the acute and chronic settings. It may be administered around the clock, and reasonable clearances may be obtained, albeit not as efficiently as with hemodialysis. It avoids the use of vascular access catheters, and thus avoids complications such as bleeding (associated with anticoagulation), air embolism, thrombosis, and bacteremia. Because ultrafiltration occurs slowly, there is a lower risk of hypotension, especially in patients with severe heart failure who might not tolerate HD.[10] Thus, PD may also be of potential value to the hemodynamically unstable patient and may also theoretically limit ischemic injury to already failing kidneys in the setting of acute renal failure.

Slow solute and water clearance limit the use of peritoneal dialysis in acute situations such as drug intoxications, life threatening hyperkalemia, and severe pulmonary edema. The insertion of a peritoneal dialysis catheter requires an appropriate peritoneal cavity and abdominal wall, free of malignancy, infection, and adhesions. This is not always feasible in the acute situation, though it is not uncommonly done in the pediatric patient population.[11]

As a home-based therapy, PD is taught to patients and possibly other loved ones or caregivers over a 1- to 2-week training period. For the independent patients, this encourages responsibility for their own care. It offers a more liberal diet than HD and is more flexible in scheduling, which confers advantages to many patients who want to stay employed while on dialysis.

For diabetic patients, PD delays the use of suboptimal vessels for hemodialysis access and provides an intraperitoneal route for insulin administration, which often avoids the need for injections.

Complications and Limitations of Peritoneal Dialysis

In the United States, the hospitalization rate for PD patients is similar to that of HD patients, though their total days in the hospital are greater.[1] Peritoneal dialysis-related complications range from metabolic abnormalities to technical and infectious complications.

The most common symptom noted by patients undergoing peritoneal dialysis is abdominal distension. This is a function of the patient's size and the dwell volume as well as, to some extent, the degree to which the patient has acclimatized to their volume of intra-abdominal fluid. Excessive distension may occur if drainage is inadequate as fluid accumulates in the abdominal cavity. Various abdominal wall hernias are associated with PD, especially with increasing age and body mass index.[12] These may necessitate a technique change (to APD or HD) or occasionally, surgical intervention.

Catheter-related complications include pericatheter leaks, obstruction (inflow or outflow failure), kinking, and pain associated with fluid drainage. Infection of the exit site, tunnel, or peritoneal cavity may occur, and may occasionally require catheter removal or change.[13] While hospitalizations due to hemodialysis-related vascular access-associated infections continue to rise, the reverse has been seen with respect to PD-catheter–associated infections.[1] Metabolic complications of PD include hypernatremia (which may result from frequent exchanges where free-water is lost in excess of sodium, or excessive sodium sieving occurs)[14] and hyperglycemia, due to absorption of dextrose most commonly occurring in diabetic patients.[15]

Finally, protein losses through the peritoneum can be substantial and may preclude the use of peritoneal dialysis in extremely sick and catabolic patients.[16]

PD is a less durable therapy than HD. There are many reasons why a PD patient will eventually transfer to HD, including infection, inadequate dialysis (especially as residual renal function is lost), and failure to thrive.

Hemodialysis

Hemodialysis is the most widely used dialysis modality worldwide. The basic dialysis procedure involves the removal of excess water and solutes from blood passed along a semipermeable membrane within a dialysis filter, as blood is passed through an extracorporeal circuit. Diffusive loss of solute is promoted by the countercurrent passage of a dialysis solution of appropriate electrolyte composition along the opposite side of the semipermeable membrane. Convection, or ultrafiltration, is a process by which water and small solutes dissolved in it are drawn across the membrane by the application of hydrostatic forces.

In its most common form, hemodialysis is a treatment center-based therapy administered three times weekly for periods ranging from 2.5 to 5 hours. Most commonly, it is performed in full-care facilities, including hospitals and freestanding dialysis centers but can also take place in an assisted-care, self-care, or home-based setting, where supervised patients provide varying amounts of their own treatment.

Advantages of Hemodialysis

Hemodialysis is capable of achieving greater small solute clearance and water removal in a shorter period of time than peritoneal dialysis, thus it is more efficient. Rapid clearance is desirable in acute renal failure with its various metabolic derangements, because it is in the setting of intoxication with dialyzable substances and in life-threatening hyperkalemia and pulmonary edema.

Especially for dependent patients, center-based HD allows the responsibility of care to fall on the provider team instead of on the patient and family. The ease of insertion of temporary and semipermanent dialysis catheters makes this an easy option for acute renal failure or for initiation of an unprepared new patient with ESRD.

Complications and Limitations of Hemodialysis

Because HD is an intermittent therapy usually delivered three times per week, many dietary restrictions are necessary. Transportation of patients from where they live to the dialysis facility can be an important challenge.

Setting up and running a hemodialysis unit requires specially trained nurses and technicians and can only be done in specialized centers. It also requires an appropriate water supply, though portable water treatment systems are now widely available. It also usually requires a large capital investment and space for patient treatment and support areas.

Hemodialysis carries with it all the complications of vascular access, including the line insertion and/or surgical procedures and systemic anticoagulation. The high blood flow rates used in a typical hemodialysis procedure require the presence of an adequate cardiac output, occasionally limiting the use of hemodialysis to relatively hemodynamically stable patients and those with reasonable cardiac function.

The hemodialysis procedure is generally well tolerated. Certain conditions may, however, predispose patients to various complications. Patients who begin dialysis with very high blood concentrations of urea and other solutes may experience symptoms related to a rapid drop in serum osmolarity, which can cause cerebral edema. Symptoms can include headache, nausea, vomiting, and in severe cases, seizures, obtundation, and coma. Hypotension is another common hemodialysis complication that results from a rate of intravascular volume removal that exceeds the rate of plasma refilling from the interstitium. This most commonly affects patients with large interdialytic weight gains or impaired cardiac function, as well as those on antihypertensives to control high blood pressure between dialysis treatments. Restless legs, nausea, vomiting, and headache are not uncommon symptoms on dialysis even in the absence of disequilibrium. Leg cramps are quite common, especially when excessive fluid is removed. Less common acute complications include dialyzer reactions, arrhythmias, seizures, hemolysis, and cardiac tamponade.

Home-Based Hemodialysis

In the early days of dialysis in the 1960s and 1970s, home-based hemodialysis was a significant modality. Utilization has dramatically declined to a current rate of only 1% to 2% in the United States and in Canada. This decline was mainly due to technical complexity and caregiver burnout.

However, there is a recent surge in interest in home hemodialysis.[17,18] New patient-friendly machines are being developed by the dialysis industry; these may allow more patients to qualify for and to select home hemodialysis. Home helpers (caregivers) are no longer a requirement.

Conventional home HD utilizes a thrice weekly schedule that mimics intermittent, center-based HD. Recently, the menu of choices has expanded, such that daily (or 5–6 days per week) home HD is attracting increasing attention and excitement.

Home HD shares many advantages of home PD, with flexible diet and scheduling. It is, however, considerably more technically complex. Training requires 4 to 8 weeks, and the complexity precludes its use in many patients. From a health care system perspective, an important advantage is that fewer dialysis nurses and technicians are required to sustain patients on home hemodialysis than on center-based HD, and the capital cost and space requirements are much less. Nephrologists are enthusiastic about an increased role for home HD in the future.[19–21] Delays in approval of adequate public funding of daily home HD in the United States and in Canada are currently limiting the potential growth of these new modalities.

Frequent Hemodialysis Regimens

Frequent HD regimes are ideally suited to the home environment. Daily HD, however, has been successfully applied to an older and sickly center-based population with excellent results.[22] The potential negative financial consequences of this full care, center-based approach are very substantial. The direct cost of daily dialysis is much greater than the cost of thrice weekly, and the incremental requirements for skilled personnel and space are high. At the time of writing, there are no funded programs outside of research settings of which we are aware. Nonetheless, from a theoretic point of view, the comments below apply to both home-based and in-center daily HD.

In 1978, Kjellstrand and associates[23] acknowledged the "unphysiology" of dialysis as a major limitation of the conventional thrice-weekly intermittent hemodialysis regimen. The intermittency of the conventional hemodialysis regimen is associated with large osmotic and fluid shifts, which are insults that are associated with unpleasant symptoms and adverse outcomes, such as left-ventricular hypertrophy. Given that normal kidneys perform so many physiologic functions, and that they do so on a continual basis, it can be understood why the term "renal-replacement therapy" could be viewed by some as an overstatement when applied to conventional, intermittent thrice-weekly hemodialysis.

Frequent dialysis has evolved from the belief that more dialysis treatments per week result in smaller osmotic, electrolyte, and fluid shifts per treatment, while delivering overall more efficient solute clearance. Because of the large volume of distribution of many solutes, they are often cleared from the blood within the first hour of dialysis, with diminishing returns towards the end of a 3- or 4-hour dialysis treatment. This is followed by a rebound phenomenon, where solutes such as urea, for example, redistribute themselves as they shift from the intracellular space to the vascular compartment. Shorter, more frequent dialysis capitalizes on the high rate of solute clearance that is achieved in the first hours of a dialysis and does so twice as frequently as conventional dialysis, removing more uremic waste per unit time and causing less fluctuation in serum levels of various electrolytes and other solutes.

Various terms have been applied to describe frequent dialysis regimens, including "quotidian-" and "hemeral-" dialysis. Frequent dialysis can be delivered in various forms, the most common of which are high-efficiency (hemeral) short-hours daily dialysis and long-hours, slow nocturnal dialysis. Typically these regimens are administered between 5 and 7 days a week. Short-hours daily dialysis typically consists of 1.5- to 2.5-hour runs with blood and dialysate flow rates similar to those used in intermittent HD. Slow nocturnal dialysis is usually given over a 6- to 8-hour period, with slower blood and dialysate flow rates, while the patient sleeps.

The benefits of the various quotidian dialysis regimens are protean and can only be described briefly here. From the patient's perspective, improved quality of life and an improved overall sense of well-being have been universally observed in studies of quotidian dialysis. Rather than spending the better part of each post-dialysis day recovering from their last treatment, quotidian dialysis patients reported no longer feeling "washed-out" after their treatment. On the contrary, many are able to disconnect from their dialysis circuits and immediately go about their regular days' activities.[24] Since these are largely home-based therapies, patients enjoy greater independence and flexibility and are often able to return to work. Because of improved volume control, blood pressure is well-controlled with little or no medication.[25–27] This has been shown to promote regression of left-ventricular hypertrophy, an independent predictor of mortality. Calcium and phosphate balance are more easily regulated, and patients, particularly on long nocturnal dialysis, may actually require phosphate supplementation to maintain a neutral phosphorus balance.[28,29] Patients typically have lower calcium-phosphate products, with less need for calcium-based phosphate binders. Small solute clearance is markedly improved, with less post-dialysis rebound in urea and electrolyte concentrations.[30]

The major limitation to the use of these modalities, at least in the home setting, is that the patient must be able to learn and perform the dialysis procedure either independently or with assistance, thus limiting quotidian dialysis to a smaller subset of the ESRD population. One theoretic disadvantage is direct cost, given that the dialysis materials used must double, and that each dialysis machine is used to treat one patient only instead of the many patients who might be treated with it in a dialysis unit. There is, however, increasing evidence that, in addition to improving all of the previously mentioned biochemical and physiological parameters and quality-of-life, quotidian home dialysis actually results in a net cost savings, even when the large up-front cost of the dialysis machine and its installation are accounted for.[31–33] This is largely attributable to the reduction in nursing costs, drug costs, and fewer hospitalizations.

As growing evidence accumulates, quotidian dialysis therapies may emerge as the treatment of choice for suitable ESRD patients for whom renal transplantation is not immediately available. Also, frequent in-center therapies await further evaluation with respect to efficacy and cost-effectiveness. A recent report shows that patients with high comorbidity have improved outcomes with daily in-center HD compared to conventional HD.[22]

Finally, since most quotidian dialysis studies to date have been small, they have not been adequately powered to assess survival. Theoretically, a treatment that promotes regression of LVH and improves blood pressure, anemia, nutritional status, and the calcium phosphorus product should confer some survival advantage over conventional thrice-weekly dialysis, but larger-scale prospective randomized trials will be needed to confirm this. At the time of this writing, such studies are planned and their findings are eagerly awaited.

Preemptive Renal Transplantation

It is with virtual unanimity that renal transplantation is accepted as the treatment of choice for end-stage renal disease. As compared with dialysis, transplantation has been shown to improve quality of life, reduce mortality, and to reduce the cost of caring for patients with ESRD.[34] With the ever-growing size of the CKD population, there has been an increasing relative shortage of donor organs. This has underlined the need to continue to develop strategies that will improve long-term graft and patient survival, and to do this in a cost-effective manner. Preemptive transplantation offers the potential to improve these important outcomes while containing costs. This section will review evidence for transplantation as a dominant strategy in ESRD care and will present a rationale for vigorously promoting preemptive transplantation where possible.

Survival

Transplantation has long been thought to improve survival in patients with ESRD. Factors that have been shown to impact on long-term patient survival include, but are not limited to, the source of the allograft, patient age, comorbid conditions, gender, race, and degree of immunosuppression. Patients with hypertension, diabetes, advanced age, and those who smoked or received kidneys from cadaveric donors have less favorable outcomes than patients without these factors.[35]

Earlier trials showing improved survival with transplantation were limited by selection bias, since they compared transplant patients with patients still on dialysis, who were presumably older and carried a greater burden of comorbid illness.[35–37] A more recent study attempted to overcome this problem by comparing patients who underwent transplantation with patients awaiting transplantation, groups that are more similar with respect to baseline demographics and comorbidity.[38] This longitudinal survival study, which included over 200,000 patients on dialysis (of whom 23,275 were transplanted), showed that despite a transient increase in early mortality post-transplantation, there was a 42% to 82% reduction in long-term mortality among cadaveric renal transplant recipients as compared with their waiting-list counterparts (Figure 15–1). The survival benefit was greatest in younger patients, Caucasians, and younger patients with diabetes, though elderly patients had improved outcomes with transplantation as well. Comparisons between peritoneal dialysis and hemodialysis transplant recipients have not demonstrated any significant differences.[39]

Quality of Life

Although there are no prospective randomized controlled trials to address the issue of quality of life (QOL) in transplantation, it is generally agreed upon that transplantation offers the best possible QOL of any form or renal-replacement therapy. In one study in which an SF-36 questionnaire was completed by renal transplant recipients, patients on peritoneal dialysis or hemodialysis, and healthy control subjects, transplant patients rated their perception of health higher than either dialysis patient group in six out of eight scales. Transplant patients scored lower on only two and higher on one out of eight scales as compared with healthy subjects.[40] These findings were corroborated in a similar study that also used covariate analysis to control for case-mix.[41] A large meta-analysis that included 218 smaller studies and 14,750 patients found statistically significant pre- to post-transplant improvements in

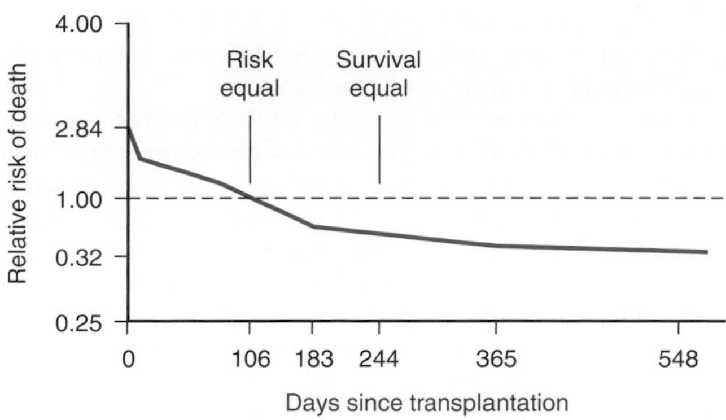

Figure 15–1 Adjusted relative risk of death among 23,275 recipients of a first cadaveric transplant. The reference group was the 46,164 patients on dialysis who were on the waiting list (relative risk, 1.0). Patients in both groups had equal lengths of follow-up since placement on the waiting list. Values were adjusted for age, sex, race, cause of end-stage renal disease, year of placement on the waiting list, geographic region, and time from first treatment for end-stage renal disease to placement on the waiting list.

physical functional QOL, mental health/cognitive status, social functioning, and overall QOL perceptions.[42]

Cost-Effectiveness

USRDS financial data from 2001 (Figure 15–2) depict the relative per-patient per-month costs of incident transplant events, functioning graft care, and dialysis.[1] Despite the increased up-front cost of transplantation, the overall financial benefits are substantial, with graft maintenance costs around one-quarter to one-fifth less than dialysis costs. Given that transplantation provides both improved quality of life and better survival than any other form or renal replacement strategy, and given its lower overall cost, transplantation must be viewed as a dominant strategy. The cost-effectiveness of transplantation is limited only by the donor organ supply.

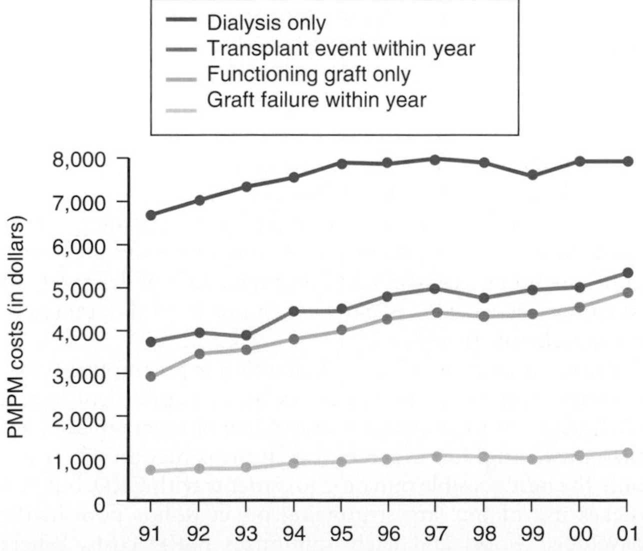

Figure 15–2 PMPM expenditures, by modality: Prevalent patients. (From USRDS Annual Report, 2002.)

Preemptive Transplantation

In the traditional approach to ESRD care, patients with progressive chronic kidney disease would eventually begin some form of dialysis and, if appropriate, would subsequently be evaluated and listed for transplantation. If a patient were fortunate enough to have a suitable and willing living donor, the option of transplantation prior to the initiation of dialysis, that is, preemptive transplantation, exists. In some countries, this concept has been broadened to include the use of cadaveric-donor kidneys. These two strategies differ with respect to their financial and ethical implications, as will be discussed below. Preemptive transplantation rates vary internationally. In Austria, Germany, and Ireland, preemptive transplantation is hardly practiced at all.[43] In the United States, approximately 25% of all live donor transplants are performed prior to initiation of dialysis.[44,45] In Sweden, on the other hand, preemptive transplantation is the standard of care for children and makes up about 70% of all transplants in the pediatric population.

Proposed Benefits and Limitations of Preemptive Transplantation

Preemptive transplantation offers many theoretic advantages. The first and most obvious of these, from the patient perspective, is the potential to avoid dialysis and its associated morbidity and inconvenience. In addition, the patient can avoid vascular access surgery. From a financial perspective, avoiding dialysis spares both the cost of vascular access surgery and the cost of dialysis itself. Preemptive transplantation may also limit the amount of time away from employment, as compared with dialysis, thus conferring an economic advantage to both the patient and to society. One case-control study from the United States compared matched patients who were on dialysis for a minimum of 6 months prior to transplantation, with patients transplanted preemptively. Patients in the preemptive transplant group were more likely to be employed 6 months post-transplant.[46]

Many clinical benefits to preemptive transplantation have been proposed. The most important of these are improved graft and patient survival, which are discussed in more detail in the following section. The potential for improved cardiovascular health (discussed below) and the avoidance of blood transfusion (particularly in hemodialysis) also make preemptive transplantation attractive.

The most frequently cited potential disadvantage to preemptive transplantation is that of noncompliance with immunosuppressive therapy. It has been argued that having never had to suffer the inconvenience and morbidity associated with dialysis, or the unpleasant symptoms associated with advanced chronic kidney disease, such patients might be less inclined to endure the burden of a rigorous drug regimen and its associated side effects. One small study that failed to show any benefit to preemptive transplantation attributed this failure to noncompliance in the preemptive transplant group.[46] Most studies, however, have failed to demonstrate any significant differences in compliance between preemptive and nonpreemptive transplant recipients.[47,48]

Biochemical and Immunologic Factors in Preemptive Transplantation

There are many theoretic reasons why preemptive transplantation may confer both improved patient and graft survival. Patients transplanted before the initiation of dialysis are less likely to have ESRD-related complications, including cardiovascular disease, malnutrition, and chronic inflammation. The associations between these various factors are numerous and complex.

Many biochemical indices have been correlated with adverse outcomes in patients with ESRD. High levels of C-reactive protein, abnormal lipoprotein profiles, and low serum albumin, for example, have all been associated with an increased risk of death in patients on dialysis.[49] Additionally, atherogenic endothelium-related molecules, such as tissue plasminogen activator, von Willebrand factor, endothelin, and homocysteine, for example, are present in higher levels in patients on maintenance hemodialysis than in healthy subjects.[50–53] Because many of these factors increase with time on dialysis, patients who undergo transplantation prior to the initiation of dialysis may theoretically have a lower risk of cardiovascular and renal allograft vascular injury.

Preemptive transplantation has been associated with a lower incidence of acute rejection. A large retrospective cohort study using USRDS data found a 52% reduction in the rate of allograft failure in the first post-transplant year, and further reductions in subsequent years in patients who received preemptive transplantation from a living donor, as compared with matched cohorts who received living donor transplants after the initiation of dialysis. This was partially attributable to reductions in acute rejection episodes and points to the known immunologic differences between dialyzed patients and CKD patients not yet on dialysis.[54] Hemodialysis has, for example, been associated with improvements in T-cell proliferation,[55] as well as changes in cytokine expression, which may thus result in increased rejection rates.[56]

Another fundamental difference between patients who are dialyzed and those who are not is the level of residual renal function (RRF). The idea that RRF may protect the graft from hyperfiltration injury (and vice versa) has been proposed.[57]

Waiting Time on Dialysis: A Strong Predictor of Transplant Outcomes

Although early studies showed favorable outcomes for patients undergoing preemptive transplantation, it was not initially clear whether or not time on dialysis itself independently predicted the poorer outcomes observed in patients transplanted after the initiation of dialysis.[47,58] This was largely because of the inability to exclude selection bias and the possibility that healthier patients had been chosen for preemptive transplantation in earlier studies. In a study by Cosio and associates[59] time on dialysis was found to correlate inversely with patient survival but occurred independently of confounders, such as patient age and comorbid factors. This study, however, also showed that patients who had been on dialysis for longer periods of time had a greater prevalence of left-ventricular hypertrophy (LVH), suggesting that the deleterious effect of a longer time on dialysis was at least, in part, due to the development of LVH, a known independent risk factor for cardiovascular death. In this study, death-censored graft survival was not significantly different between the preemptive and nonpreemptive groups.

A later analysis of data from the USRDS showed not only that time on dialysis was associated with reduced graft and patient survival, but also that death-censored graft survival was worse with increasing time on dialysis.[60] This further strengthened the hypothesis that time on dialysis was an independent predictor of graft loss. This was true for both cadaveric and living donor transplants. This study also showed that the magnitude of the effect of time on dialysis was the same across all major comorbid disease groups, arguing against the view that cumulative disease burden (such as cardiovascular disease) was the main cause of poorer graft survival in patients with longer wait times.

Finally, in an attempt to quantify the impact of time of dialysis on graft and patient survival, Meier-Kriesche and associates[61] analyzed data from 2405 kidney pairs harvested from the same donor and transplanted into one patient with a short waiting time and another with a long waiting time. This controlled for unknown base-line donor characteristics. Using a Cox proportional hazards model, they quantified the risk of time on dialysis on graft function and found overall adjusted 10-year living donor graft survival to be significantly different at 75% and 49% for patients transplanted before 6 months and after 24 months of dialysis, respectively (Figure 15–3). A similar trend was observed for cadaveric transplants (Figure 15–4). Preemptive cadaveric transplantation offered the same graft survival as a living donor transplant done after 24 months of dialysis.

Preemptive Transplantation with a Living Donor

Despite efforts to increase the availability of donor organs worldwide, the supply of cadaveric kidneys has failed to meet the demands of the growing ESRD population. The living donor pool was once restricted to closely-related family members who were more likely to share HLA antigens, thus lowering the risk of rejection. With modern advances in immunosuppressive therapy, HLA compatibility has become less of a limiting factor in long-term graft survival. The living donor pool has been broadened to include not only extended relatives, but also unrelated donors, with long-term outcomes comparable to those seen in living related donor transplants, and superior to cadaveric donor transplants.[62] The living donor pool is, in fact, the most rapidly growing source for renal allografts in the United States.[1]

Kidneys from living donors offer many advantages over grafts from cadaveric donors, including improved long-term graft function and a markedly lower incidence of delayed graft function (DGF). This is partly attributable to differences in warm ischemic time.

Based on current evidence, living donor preemptive transplantation offers outcomes that are at least equivalent to and likely superior to any other known form of renal replacement therapy. Living donor preemptive transplantation offers not only the best possible outcome to patients with CKD, but also makes use of the largest growing organ donor pool in the developed world and likely minimizes ESRD costs. Where possible, it should thus be promoted as the treatment of choice for patients with ESRD.

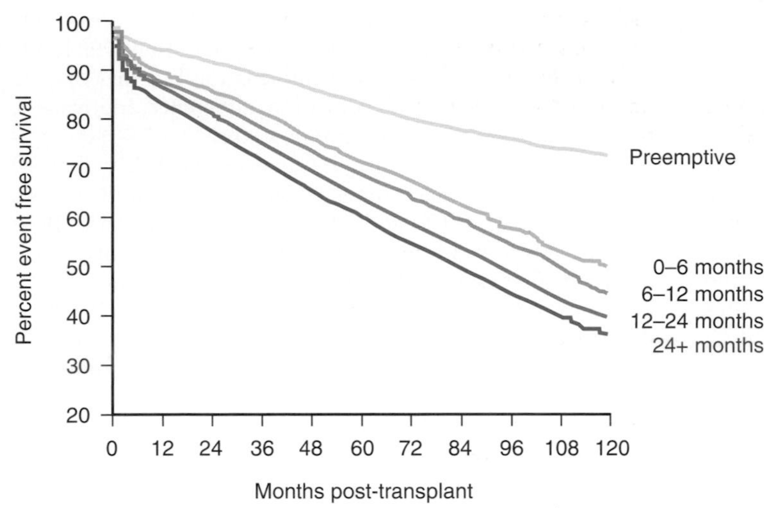

Figure 15-3 Unadjusted graft survival in 21,836 recipients of living transplants by length of dialysis treatment before transplant.

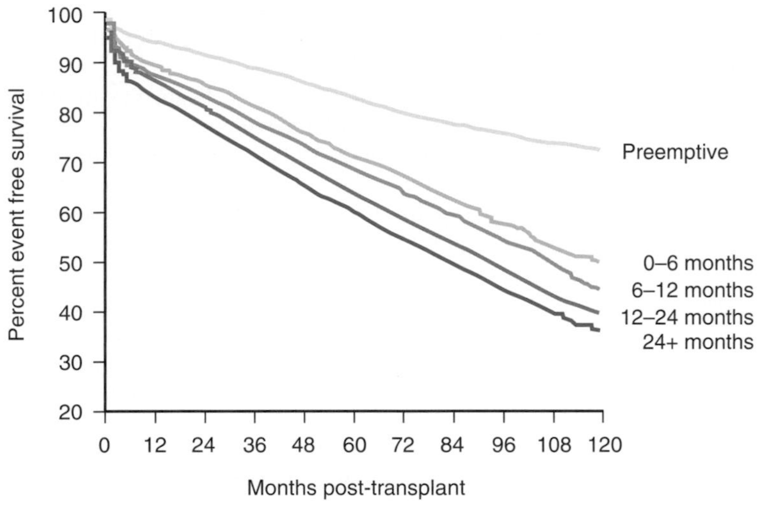

Figure 15-4 Unadjusted graft survival in 56,587 recipients of cadaveric transplants by length of dialysis treatment before transplant.

Preemptive Cadaveric Renal Transplantation

In the case of preemptive cadaveric renal transplantation (PCRT), there are certain logistic concerns that cannot be ignored. The most important of these is that it is often difficult to accurately predict when renal replacement therapy will be required. Owing to the unpredictability of organ availability, it can often be very difficult to time transplant surgery optimally. If the patient is listed for transplantation early, and a cadaveric organ becomes available, then they will have lost many months of native organ function. This also translates to more months of dialysis therapy for a patient already on dialysis who might have otherwise received that organ. From an ethical perspective, this may seem unfair because the patient already on dialysis may be seen as being more "entitled" to receive that same donor kidney. Conversely, one must be prepared to deal with long waiting times, and dialysis may ultimately need to be started before an organ becomes available. This makes it difficult to appropriately time vascular access surgery, or else results in the use of temporary catheters. This, however, may not be much of a problem in countries where the cadaveric donor pool is well matched to the size of the transplantable population. In most developed countries, however, cadaveric kidneys are in short supply, making PCRT not only unethical, but also impractical.

Circumstances have been described in which PCRT may be justifiable. It has, for example, been suggested that growth is better preserved in children who are transplanted early as compared with those treated with chronic dialysis.[63] Some have argued that a patient with dependent family members such as young children should be offered every opportunity to remain employed, and that avoiding dialysis in such a patient justifies PCRT.[43] Others have argued that optimization of HLA matching may be an indication for early listing on the cadaveric donor list. This would allow for highly selective donor matching and would be justified on the basis of improved long-term graft survival.[47]

In countries where the organ supply is more easily met and wait times are estimated to be less than 1 year, PCRT may be a feasible option. Belgium and Austria, for example, have annual cadaveric kidney donor rates equal to the yearly demand. Under these circumstances, it is recommended that patients be listed when the GFR is less than 15 mL/min.[43]

Preemptive Transplantation in Developing Countries

In addition to improved graft and patient survival, preemptive transplantation may offer advantages specific to the developing world.[64] The transmission of infectious diseases is of particular interest. In countries where the incidence of hepatitis B and C is high, a strategy that minimizes blood transfusion is desirable, because liver disease with hepatitis B-antigen positivity, for example, is associated with increased morbidity and mortality in renal transplant patients.[65,66] Other infectious diseases, such as tuberculosis, are more prevalent in dialysis patients as well[67] and are of even greater importance in the developing world. Such infections can complicate, if not preclude, transplantation. Finally, cost is often the greatest barrier to receiving renal replacement therapy in developing countries, and many countries have no publicly funded dialysis system.[68] The cost-effectiveness of preemptive transplantation might make it available to a proportion of the CKD population in countries where financial resources are scarce.

OUTCOMES WITH HEMODIALYSIS AND PERITONEAL DIALYSIS

Modality Comparisons

Any evaluation of the relative merits of HD and PD must, of course, take into account outcome data. Although some comparative studies have addressed hospitalization rates and measures of quality of life, the most frequent and objective end point is patient survival.[69,70]

Methodologic Issues

The complexities of comparative modality studies cannot be well understood without first taking into account methodologic issues. The results are hugely influenced by the type of analysis that is done.

The first and most important point to make is that all existing comparative studies are observational, and most are based on retrospective analyses of large national registry databases. There are no successfully completed randomized controlled trials comparing HD and PD, and none is ever likely to be done, given the stark differences between the two modalities and the consequent unwillingness of most patients to be randomized to one or another. This point was highlighted by the recent thwarted attempt of investigators in the Netherlands to perform a randomized trial.[71] All the evidence that we have is therefore based on suboptimal experimental design with major potential for confounding and bias.

The first methodologic challenge that comparative studies face is the need to correct for the biases in modality selection that occur at the initiation of dialysis. In some countries, such as Italy and Spain, data suggest that PD patients tend to be older with more comorbidity.[72] However, detailed data from the United States and Canada suggest the opposite to be the case in those countries.[73,74] U.S. patients starting PD tend to be younger and to have less comorbidity than their HD counterparts. They are, however, more likely to be Caucasian rather than black, and to be diabetic, both adverse prognostic factors. Other baseline characteristics that are sometimes adjusted for include residual renal function, nutritional measures, body size, and serum albumin. Additional ones that are rarely adjusted for because of lack of information but that may be important include level of education, adherence, motivation, social supports, and socioeconomic status.

With regard to the mortality analysis itself, a variety of other issues arise. Some comparative studies are "intent–to–treat" (ITT) and others are "as treated" (AT). Both approaches are valid and answer related, but distinct, questions. The first asks whether initial modality allocation effects ultimate outcome and so is important to the clinician advising the patient on initial modality selection. The AT analysis is an attempt to answer the fundamental question as to which modality is inherently superior. It is now customary to do both ITT and AT analyses in comparative studies in order to maximize the overall robustness of the analysis, as well as to answer the two distinct questions.[73] Some studies use hybrids of the two methodologies by censoring the ITT analysis at the time of a modality switch.[75] A related but somewhat distinct issue is whether the analysis looks at incident or prevalent dialysis patients. An incident analysis is always preferred.[76] Patterns of early dropout may lead to biases in purely prevalent analyses.

Another important point is when to begin the modality comparison. The first day of dialysis might seem appropriate, but early mortality on dialysis is likely more related to preexisting comorbidity than to the modality chosen. Also, acutely ill patients and urgent starts more often initiate with HD rather than with PD. Accordingly, it is customary to start the comparison 60 or 90 days post-initiation. Waiting longer until 4 or 6 months post-initiation may introduce a bias against PD for reasons that will shortly be discussed. Work by Foley[77] and other authors[74] suggest that this issue has a marked influence on comparative mortality analyses. Again, a good compromise is to perform the analyses at a variety of start points, that is, 0, 60, 90, 120 days, and so forth.[76] Unfortunately, registries such as the USRDS do not have data prior to 90 days post-initiation.

A number of observers have noted that the relative hazards of mortality between HD and PD are not consistent with time. It is therefore misleading to use the Cox proportional hazards model in a comparative analysis, precisely because mortality rates are not "proportional." Foley[77] has argued that the best technique to get around this is to use repeated Cox analyses starting, for example, at 0, 12, 18 months, and so forth. The reasons for this disproportionality are controversial. One is the already mentioned tendency in many centers for urgent, sicker, more acute starts to use HD as initial therapy. This may explain the higher mortality seen with HD early on. Even among more elective starts, there is a clear trend in North America for PD patients to be younger, and to have less comorbid conditions and adjustments for these characteristics may be incomplete.[73] An additional explanation, however, is that superior preservation of residual renal function in PD patients may be playing a role in the first 1 to 3 years on that modality. This is difficult to prove, but the survival advantages of residual function are well recognized and the observation is plausible. Conversely, in later years of PD, more patients are anuric and at greater risk of volume overload, hypertension, and low clearance. In some cases, gradual membrane deterioration occurring with time on PD may also predispose to fluid overload. Another explanation for the trend for long-term HD patients to do relatively better than those on long-term PD, is the possible cumulative atherogenic effect of the peritoneal dialysate glucose.[78]

One more feature of comparative mortality studies that needs to be taken into account is that the results are often outdated by the time they are published. Both HD and PD are constantly changing. Recent changes in HD include more widespread use of high flux membranes, a tendency to deliver higher clearances, the greater use of central catheters as long-term access, and some fall off in the practice of membrane reuse. In PD, recent changes include much greater use of automated cyclers, widespread use of polyglucose solutions, and higher delivered clearances.[79–81] Comparative analyses, based in registry data, are frequently 4 to 8 years out of date by the time they are published.[73,82,83] In the context of changing practices and of apparently declining mortality rates, this places a question on the relevance of the results to contemporary practice.

Results of Comparative Studies

The majority of published data comparing PD and HD mortality has come from the United States and Canada, although there has been some contributions from Europe.[84–86]

A landmark, but flawed study, by Bloembergen and associates[82] from the USRDS, published in 1995, set off the present controversy in this area. This analysis covered a 3-year period in the late 1980s and assigned patients each year to the modality they were using on January 1. On average, this methodology leads to the omission of the first 9 months of time on dialysis, the period when PD does best in comparative studies. Not surprisingly, therefore, the results showed superior survival on HD (Relative Risk [RR] 1.17), particularly in older patients, in females, and in diabetics. A similar analysis covering the early 1990s omitting less of the early time on dialysis, was carried out by Vonesh and associates.[87] This showed that the advantage for HD was of borderline significance, was getting less with time, and was again concentrated in older female diabetics.

Collins and associates[75] used more contemporary data from the mid-1990s to address this issue. A more appropriate ITT analysis of incident dialysis patients was used with censoring occurring after transplantation or modality switch. This study looked at patients beginning 90 days post-initiation of dialysis and covered the 2 subsequent years. This is the period where PD tends to do best and the results showed a substantial advantage for PD in nondiabetics of all ages and also in younger diabetics (Figure 15–5). Only in older female diabetics did HD have the advantage. The contrasting results of the Bloembergen and Collins studies may partly be explained by a change in relative mortality rates between the two modalities over a 10-year period, but it largely reflects the huge influence of the time period after initiation of dialysis that has been covered by the study. Analyses dominated by incident patients always show PD as looking better than those dominated by prevalent or longer-term patients.

In Canada, analyses by Fenton and associates[74,88] from the Canadian Organ Replacement Register (CORR) performed in the early and mid-1990s showed a consistent advantage for PD in all groups except older diabetics. This was the case with both ITT and AT methodologies (Table 15–1). The mortality advantage for PD again tended to lessen with time and by 3 years post-initiation there was no difference. Correction for comorbidity was incomplete in all these United States and Canadian registry-based studies. The Fenton data for Canada had more adjustment for comorbid conditions than did the Collins or Bloembergen studies, but all were limited.

Murphy and associates[76] from Canada used a prospective cohort of almost 1000 patients with detailed comorbidity data to get around this issue. They found that much of the apparent PD survival advantage was removed once more complete adjustment was done, taking into account degree or severity of comorbidity as well as numbers of comorbid conditions.

Comparative mortality data from Denmark and Italy have shown similar patterns of an early advantage for PD followed by a later tendency for HD to do better.[84] New data from the Netherlands showed no difference in survival between PD and HD during the first year but then saw a tendency for HD patients to do better than PD patients, especially those over the age of 60.[86]

By the beginning of the 1st decade of this century, it appeared that some consensus had thus been reached on

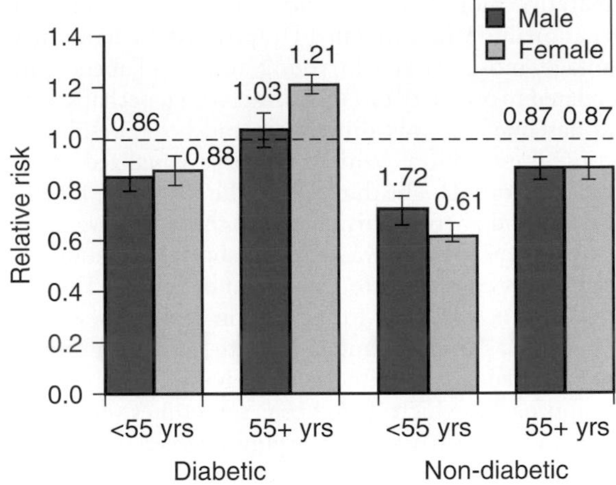

Figure 15–5 Cox regression: Relative risk of CAPD/CCPD versus hemodialysis, all patients (by age, sex, and diabetic status; reference: hemodialysis patients). (From AJ Collins et al: Mortality risks of peritoneal dialysis and hemodialysis. Am J Kidney Dis 1999; 34[6]:1065-1074.)

Table 15–1 Relative Risk of Death with CAPD/CCPD vs. HD in an Analysis of Data from the Canadian Organ Replacement Register

	AT	ITT
All	0.73*	0.93*
Non DM < 65	0.53*	0.84
DM > 65	0.75*	0.95
Non DM 65+	0.76*	0.90
DM 65+	0.88	1.04

* 95% CI < 1.0.

(Adapted from Schaubel et al: Comparing mortality rates on CAPD/CCPD and hemodialysis. The Canadian experience: Fact or fiction? Perit Dial Int 1998; 18[5]:478-484.)

comparative mortality data with a convergence of findings internationally.[89] In general, PD appeared to have an early advantage, most marked in young and nondiabetic patients and related to a variety of factors, including, perhaps, unmeasured baseline case mix differences and better residual renal function preservation. With time, risks equalized and then started to favor HD. The duration of the advantage for PD was least in older diabetics, particularly in those who were female. The advantage for PD was also of shorter duration in the United States compared to Canada and Europe. These findings gave some credence to the notion that PD was particularly suitable as an initial modality with patients subsequently being switched to HD, either electively or as problems arise. This approach, which has been sometimes described as "PD first" has been used to varying degrees in a variety of countries.[90–92]

Recent Analyses

In 2003, however, new analyses based on USRDS data reopened the modality controversy.[73,83] Two papers from the same group looked at over 100,000 incident dialysis patients from the mid-1990s and examined the effect on comparative mortality of the presence or absence of coronary heart disease (CHD) and congestive heart failure (CHF). The analysis was more sophisticated than that of previous USRDS studies in that it used both ITT and AT methodologies. More importantly, it redid the analysis at 6-month intervals to deal with the issue of nonproportional hazards. Of 108,000 patients studied, 87% were on HD and 13% were on PD. At baseline, 26% had overt CHD, 74% did not. Over 2 years, the mortality rate for those with CHD was 34% on HD and 36% on PD, whereas for the larger group without CHD, it was 23% on HD and 18% on PD.[73] However, after adjustment for a variety of baseline demographic, comorbid, and laboratory test characteristics, diabetic patients with CHD had a 23% higher mortality risk than those on PD, whereas those without CHD had a 17% higher risk (Figure 15–6).[73] Among nondiabetics, those with CHD had a 20% higher mortality risk, whereas those without CHD had a 1% lower risk on PD.[73] Results for those with and without CHF were generally similar.[83]

These studies have raised the concern that PD might be problematic in the 25% to 35% of ESRD patients who have clinically overt cardiac disease at initiation, and indeed in diabetic patients in general, also. The notion of PD as a more atherogenic therapy has thus gained some credence.[78] However, the weakness of this type of analysis must be remembered. The completeness of the adjustments for potential confounding factors is always in doubt. Baseline data come from "Medical Evidence Forms" filled in at initiation of dialysis, and the reliability of these has been questioned.[93] No information on the severity, as distinct from the presence and absence, of comorbidity is provided. Furthermore, the data from these studies are already 5 to 7 years old and come from a period when use of antiatherogenic lipid lowering therapy was less common in ESRD patients and when there was less emphasis on glucose sparing strategies in PD in these studies.[73,83] The majority of patients without overt cardiac disease did well on PD.

Recent evidence suggests that PD mortality and technique failure rates in North America continue to fall impressively.[81,94,95] Furthermore, it is uncertain how much these data

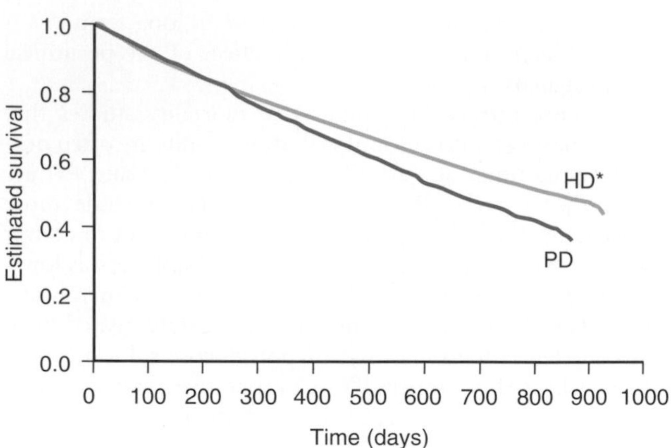

Figure 15–6 Adjusted Cox survival curves for new ESRD patients with coronary artery disease treated with peritoneal dialysis (PD) versus hemodialysis (HD). Adjusted for age at study start, sex, race, cause of ESRD, hypertension, congestive heart failure, peripheral vascular and cerebrovascular disease, tobacco use, chronic lung disease, AIDS, neoplasm, serum albumin, body mass index, hematocrit, estimated GFR, and pre-ESRD erythropoietin use. *P = .0001. (From Ganesh et al: Mortality differences by dialysis modality among incident ESRD patients with and without coronary artery disease. J Am Soc Nephrol 2003; 14[2]:415-424.)

can be extrapolated to ESRD populations outside the United States. Nevertheless, the data do merit attention and should be a "call to arms" to PD practitioners to focus particularly on management of cardiac risk factors and disease in the PD population. Greater use of cardioprotective and lipid lowering medications and more attention to volume status are required. A focus on reducing exposure to the potentially harmful effects of hypertonic glucose by using alternative solutions, especially in patients who are diabetic, obese, or who have overt cardiac disease, would seem desirable.[78]

Conclusion

How do all these data help the clinician when approaching modality selection in the individual patient? All this published evidence is observational, predominantly retrospective, and registry-based and so is prone to confounding. In general, the apparent benefits for one modality over the other in these studies are modest compared to the influence of other larger factors such as age, diabetes, and heart disease. Modality decisions should therefore be based primarily on the personal preferences and social circumstances of the patient concerned. These are of greater relevance to the individual patient. PD may have particular advantages in younger and in nondiabetic patients, but this does not mean all such patients should be directed to PD. Similarly, HD may have apparent advantages in older diabetic patients and in those with overt cardiac disease, but this does not mean that all such patients should be placed on HD. The apparent advantages for one or other modality in these patient subgroups are too modest, are based on evidence that is too unreliable and are too dated to justify such an approach. Rather, the patient should be exposed to information about each modality, and, as far as possible, an informed choice should be made. Regardless of the chosen modality, greater attention should be focused on reducing cardiovascular risks with appropriate medications, lifestyle adjustments, and modifications in the dialysis prescription.

Modality selection in many settings is, of course, complicated by resource issues.[96] In many jurisdictions, the rising cost of ESRD care in general and the lower general cost of PD compared to HD adds an additional complexity to the modality selection process.[91,92] The notion of PD as a preferable initial therapy for many patients with a subsequent elective switch to HD, if problems arise, is an attractive and potentially cost-effective strategy that takes economic data as well as patient outcomes into account and tries to give the patient the best of both modalities.[90] The advent of new home HD modalities also provide opportunities for an integrated home-based approach, using both PD and home HD for provision of renal replacement therapy.[97]

PATIENT ISSUES IN MODALITY SELECTION

Given that (1) all dialysis modalities are imperfect, (2) outcomes are similar with the two dominant forms of treatment (center-based HD and home PD), and (3) costs are lower with home-based dialysis, then it seems reasonable to promote a dialysis modality distribution that reflects these factors. In theory, this would lead to a greater proportion of patients using home dialysis therapies (PD and HD). There are, however, a myriad of factors that interact to cause marked deviations from what one might consider to be an ideal distribution of dialysis modalities.

For the sake of this discussion, we will divide these factors into patient-related factors and system-related factors. In fact, there is often considerable overlap, and in a given patient and/or health care system, many factors may be operating simultaneously.

It is generally agreed that the majority of patients could do either home PD or center-based HD. However, in a minority of patients, there are strong medical or social issues that might cause the provider to recommend, or even insist upon, one form of treatment and not another.

Patient Preference

There is also a general agreement that if a patient has no strong indication for or against a certain form of therapy, that patient preference should be the prime determinant of modality selection. Indeed, recent surveys of nephrologists in Canada, in the United States, and in Europe all show this strong opinion.[19–21, 98]

Allowing patient choice to drive modality selection raises some interesting ethical issues. Utilitarian considerations could be used to justify mandating a less costly form of dialysis for suitable patients. In this way, scarce resources could be used to treat more patients and/or to deliver more expensive and presumably higher quality of care.

On the other hand, the prime imperative in the minds of nephrologists seems to be autonomy in that competent and informed patients should make up their own mind about competing treatment methods, especially when outcomes are not proven to be different. This position is likely strengthened by the realization that forcing patients to take responsibility for a technical, home-based therapy when they do not want to could lead to complications and undermine the likelihood of a successful outcome.

Indeed, there is evidence that empowering patient choice would not lead to an imbalance of modality distribution in favor of more expensive therapies. It has been shown in several studies in Canada, in the United States, and in Europe that patients given appropriate education will choose a method of home dialysis about 50% of the time.[99–102] This has important implications for global costs of dialysis and for modality distribution in most jurisdictions in the Western world.

In practice, the ideal of empowerment of patient choice may not always be a reality. Consider the example of the United States, where more than 90% of its prevalent dialysis patients are on HD and only 8% on PD. Although American nephrologists say that patient preference is the most important determinant of modality decisions,[21,98] recent USRDS Wave II data suggest that only 25% of the selected HD patients recall ever having PD discussed as a modality option.[103] One can speculate that this heavy reliance on HD may be excessive in some regions, limiting patient choice and constraining some patients to treatment regimes that might limit their independence and compromise their lifestyle. Furthermore, this apparent lack of empowerment of patient choice is contrary to ethical principles valued by nephrologists and serves to drive up the overall cost of ESRD care.

The Canadian Society of Nephrology takes on the issue of whether providers should be educating patients in a completely unbiased way and allowing free choice of modality, or whether providers are allowed to promote home dialysis first. The Canadian Society of Nephrology (CSN) policy articulated in a document called "Principles of ESRD Care"[104] states that providers should be encouraging patients to choose less expensive home-based therapies, although they must not be made mandatory.

Medical Factors Affecting Initial Choice of Modality: Indications and Contraindications

Although the list of medical and social contraindications to one form of dialysis is long, in practice most patients will not have an absolute indication or contraindication. It is of interest to note that there are few contraindications to center-based HD, more to home PD (medical and social), and most to home HD (especially social). Indeed, the aging of the dialysis population is a well described phenomenon. Although age per se is not felt to be a contraindication for home dialysis therapies,[19–21] age is associated with many medical and social comorbidities that make home dialysis difficult or impossible. This is one reason why home dialysis has been in decline.

In a prospective cohort study of incident HD and PD patients, the Choices for Healthy Outcomes in Caring for End-Stage Renal Disease (CHOICE) Study Investigators observed significant differences between these groups with respect to comorbidity burden.[105] Using the Index of Coexistent Diseases (ICED) to measure comorbidity across 19 medical conditions, they found that overall, PD patients had fewer and less severe comorbid illnesses at the initiation of dialysis. The incidence and severity of heart failure, arrhythmia, other heart conditions, gastrointestinal disease, respiratory conditions, and physical impairment were substantially lower in PD patients, even after adjusting for other factors affecting modality selection. This finding is corroborated by at least one other recent study.[106] The authors concluded that patients with a heavier burden of illness were less likely to choose (or be chosen for) PD, instead assuming a more dependent role with center-based HD.

To date, no reasonable evidence exists to favor one modality over another on the basis of gender or race. CAPD is generally preferred over hemodialysis in the pediatric patient population for various reasons, including improved nutritional status, higher hematocrit, lower transfusion requirements, better blood pressure control, and avoidance of vascular access, which can be difficult to secure in small children.[107] Peritoneal dialysis has also been associated with better growth indices in infants and young children.[108,109] Children on PD are almost twice as likely to be enrolled in school than their hemodialysis counterparts.[110]

The major medical issues that must be considered by the treatment team are self-explanatory and will not be described in detail. For PD, major medical contraindications include inflammatory bowel disease, ischemic bowel disease, acute diverticulitis, intra-abdominal abcess, colostomy, ileostomy, pregnancy, malnutrition, multiple abdominal adhesions, high grade proteinuria, severe diabetic gastroparesis, severe hypertriglyceridemia, advanced COPD, Le Veen shunt, ascites, ventriculo-peritoneal shunt, and recent renal allograft. Less certain but important considerations include obesity, history of diverticulitis, severe low back pain, hernias, multiple abdominal surgeries, blindness, and hiatus hernia with reflux esophagitis.[111]

For center-based, intermittent HD, the major medical contraindications include inability to secure vascular access, refractory heart failure, prosthetic valve disease, and problems on HD. Other considerations include infectious disease (HIV, hepatitis B or C), and contraindications to heparin use.

Technique Failure and Modality Change

While peritoneal and hemodialysis are not vastly different with respect to long-term patient survival rates, they differ greatly with respect to technique survival. Hemodialysis is a relatively robust therapy. However, technique failure in peritoneal dialysis is a significant issue and has been defined as any situation requiring a switch to hemodialysis for greater than 3 months.[89] This definition excludes patients who have required a short time off PD for peritonitis or a catheter change.

Technique survival in CAPD has improved over the last decade. A Canadian study documented a 20% reduction in technique failure from the 1980s to the 1990s, accounted for largely by lower peritonitis rates.[94] Improvements in sterile technique, including the introduction of Y-transfer sets as well as better patient education are likely major contributors here. Indications for switching from peritoneal dialysis to hemodialysis, as outlined in the NKF-DOQI guidelines, are summarized in Table 15–2.

SYSTEM ISSUES IN MODALITY DISTRIBUTION

There is an astonishing international variation in modality distribution.[1] Countries like Japan utilize peritoneal dialysis (PD) in only 3.9% of dialysis patients, whereas in other countries (Mexico, Hong Kong, New Zealand) it is the dominant modality.

Similarly, dialysis modality distribution is markedly different in Canada and in the United States. Canada is a relatively high user of PD by international standards and had 22.3% of its prevalent patients on this therapy in the year 2000.[2] However, the percent utilization of PD has been falling steadily the past 8 years from a peak of 37.5% in 1992. PD utilization in Canada also varies markedly by province with the highest penetration in New Brunswick at 40.5% and the lowest in Alberta at 17.3% (preliminary 2000 data).

The situation in the United States is such that PD utilization is only 8.4% in 2001 and has fallen each year from a peak of 14.7% in 1993.[1] There is also significant geographic variation, such that network 16 (AK, ID, MT OR, WA) has 12.4% PD utilization, whereas network 2 (NY) has only 6.5%.

There is similar international variation in the use of home hemodialysis. Australia and New Zealand do quite well in this regard with more than 10% of prevalent patients, but most of the rest of the world struggles at around 1% to 2% utilization of home hemodialysis (HD).

Nonmedical Factors and Modality Options

Given that outcomes on hemodialysis and peritoneal dialysis are similar, and that the medical factors described above apply to only a minority of patients, then there must be other important factors that impact on modality decisions for individual patients and, hence, lead to the wide variations in modality utilization described previously. The relative degree

Table 15–2 NKF/DOQI Guidelines: Indications for Switching from Peritoneal Dialysis to Hemodialysis

Consistent failure to achieve a target Kt/V_{Urea} and C_{Cr} when there are no medical, technical, or psychosocial contraindications to HD.
Inadequate solute transport or fluid removal. High transporters may have poor ultrafiltration and/or excessive protein losses (relative contraindication, obviously discovered after initiation and the first PET).
• Unmanageably severe hypertriglyceridemia.
• Unacceptably frequent peritonitis or other PD-related complications.
• Development of technical/mechanical problems.
• Severe malnutrition resistant to aggressive management (relative).

(From United States Renal Data System. The USRDS Morbidity and Mortality Study: Wave 2. Am J Kidney Dis 1998; 32:S67-S85. Copyright 1998, with permission from the National Kidney Foundation.)

to which these nonmedical factors impact upon modality decisions and modality distribution varies from country to country. This section discusses the most important of these factors.

Financial/Reimbursement

In a classic article on nonmedical factors that impact on ESRD modality decisions, Nissenson and associates[112,113] conclude that financial and reimbursement factors stood out as the most important one in nearly every country or region studied. However, it is a complex issue, because physicians and facilities may have different financial interests. Furthermore, there is confusion in discussions about dialysis economics because it is necessary to distinguish the effect of cost from the effect of funding. In the end, it is funding that will impact more on modality decisions.

PD is less costly than center HD in North America and in Europe.[6,114–116] Intermittent home HD is similarly much less costly than center HD, and data suggest that slow nocturnal dialysis is also less costly than center HD.[32]

In some developing countries the least expensive dialysis modality is used predominantly.[117] Often this is PD if the solutions are manufactured locally. Mexico is a good example, with greater than 90% PD utilization. However, some countries like India impose import duties on PD fluid produced elsewhere. This artificially inflates the cost of PD to a level higher than HD, effectively denying a useful therapy to its citizens.

Most Western European nations predominately utilize HD, especially if there is a private or mixed public and private dialysis system.[112,113,118] Publicly funded ESRD delivery systems tend to devote less money to ESRD programs and have higher PD utilization rates but lower ESRD incidence rates. Nations with private funding tend to use HD in more than 90% of cases, possibly because the investment in private ownership of HD facilities produces incentives to keep them full. An additional factor is physician reimbursement systems, which often pay nephrologists more generously for center-based HD. Indeed, in some countries, home-based therapies have no physician fee at all.

In Canada's case, public funding of dialysis services and prohibition of private ownership of facilities has led to relatively high rates of PD utilization. As for the United States, with its high utilization of PD, reimbursement rates for facilities and physicians do not favor either modality. It is therefore not immediately clear why this modality distribution exists. The lack of an existing local PD infrastructure, the less expensive marginal costs of adding an additional patient to a preexisting HD program, and the incentive to keep HD units operating at full capacity are economic explanations that have been advanced.[28] Finally, recent USRDS Wave II data suggest that only 25% of the selected HD patients recall having PD discussed as a modality option, while conversely 68% of PD patients remember discussions regarding HD as an option.[103] One can speculate that the extreme American reliance on HD may be unjustified and contrary to patient preferences.

Resource Availability

Resource limitations can be both capital and human. Lack of capital in underdeveloped countries leads to no public funding of dialysis and very low treatment rates. Similarly, lack of HD facilities or machines can lead to pressures that increase PD utilization. High PD utilization in Canada in the early 1990s was felt to result from centralization of dialysis treatment centers in university centers and excessively tight government control of capital funding of HD expansion.[112] As HD demand exceeded supply in provinces like Ontario, PD utilization rose to levels that were felt by the providers to be beyond reason.[119,120] Lack of trained personnel (physicians, nurses, technologists) can all impact upon available choice of modality.

Social Issues

Many social problems can limit the availability of patients to manage a home dialysis method. Severe poverty and poor hygienic conditions preclude home dialysis therapy. In marginal situations, especially in the elderly who are frail or have many comorbid conditions, support is essential. If support from family members or other loved ones, or from home care nursing, is not available, then home dialysis is not an option. Unsuitable housing and water supply may also contraindicate home dialysis. Drug abuse and/or noncompliance may interfere with the ability of patients to prosper on home dialysis.

On the other hand, living long distances from HD centers can make center HD impossible, and a home dialysis option may be the only viable strategy.

Cultural Habits

It is described that certain ethnic groups share internal values and perceptions that impact on acceptability of a dialysis therapy choice.[112,113] Chinese patients may be more averse to needle puncture and may place more emphasis on the duty and honor of caring for elderly parents. Both factors tend to encourage home PD. Japanese culture seems to prefer receiving care at clinics and hospitals, rather than at home.

Late Referral and Suboptimal Predialysis Care

There seems to be little doubt that late referral to a nephrologist has numerous negative consequences. This topic has been the subject of several recent reviews.[121–126]

The potential benefits of earlier referral include (1) discovery and treatment of reversible causes of renal failure, (2) slowing the rate of decline of progressive renal insufficiency, (3) managing the multiple comorbid conditions and cardiovascular risk factors associated with chronic renal failure, and (4) facilitating efficient entry into ESRD programs of all patients who might benefit.[127,128] Of special significance to policy makers and funders are the observations that it may be possible to increase patient survival,[129–136] increase the use of native AV fistulas,[137–140] achieve better vocational outcomes,[141] increase utilization of more cost-effective home and community-based dialysis modalities,[102,106,142–145] improve quality of life,[146,147] decrease hospital utilization,[130,136,137,139,148] and reduce health care costs.[142,149] Physicians interested in home dialysis should note that patients referred early and adequately educated about dialysis modalities seem more likely to choose home HD or PD.[100–102,112,145,150]

Nephrologists' Attitudes, Opinions, Educational Deficits, and Biases

It is stated that a lack of training and experience of nephrologists and nurses and physician bias impacts upon modality selection.[112] In an attempt to examine nephrologists' opinions and biases, we have done a series of studies in Canada, in the United States, and in the United Kingdom.[19–21] These are published separately, but for the purposes of this chapter, the study data is lumped together in order to highlight the remarkable degree of similarity between them.

We used a very simple survey methodology. We sent a mailed questionnaire to the Canadian Society of Nephrology membership and achieved a 66% response rate. Similarly, we surveyed a random sample of the National Kidney Foundation Council on Dialysis and reported a 47% response rate, and a sampling of the Renal Association of Great Britain and Ireland with a response rate of 63%.

In one set of questions, we asked the physician respondents: What are the most important factors controlling or affecting modality decisions? The single most important factor in all three countries is patient preference. Outcome data is ranked second, costs to the patient and health care system is reported to be a neutral factor, and reimbursement both to facilities and physicians is reported to be not important. This is a survey methodology so there may be limitations in terms of respondents wanting to report socially desirable answers rather than reporting truthfully. Nonetheless, the answers are remarkably similar across three different countries with different modality distributions.

Another question asked of the nephrologist: Suppose you are consulted by a state or province with 10 million people, and you are to give advice to government about planning dialysis systems in the future. No rationing is to occur. Given these seven dialysis modalities, what percent would you assign to each one in an ideal system? Figure 15–7 shows that if the prime criteria was to maximize survival, wellness, and quality of life, a form of HD was recommended for 63%, 67%, and 62% of patients in Canada, in the United States, and in Europe, respectively. Home HD was recommended for 9%, 12%, and 11%, whereas PD was recommended for 37%, 33%, and 38% in the three countries, respectively.

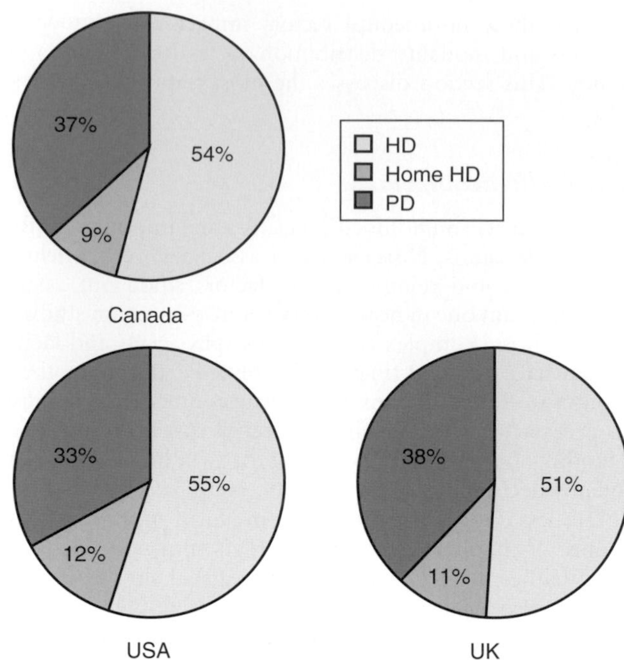

Figure 15–7 Optimal modality distribution recommended by Canadian, American, and European nephrologists based on maximization of survival, wellness, and quality of life.

Figure 15–8 shows results from a similar question, but this time the respondents were asked to maximize outcomes based on the prime criteria of cost-effectiveness. The results changed only slightly. In Canada the HD:PD ratio recommended is now 57:43, in America it is a 60:40 split, and in Europe it is 56:44. Home hemodialysis is now recommended for 12%, 16%, and 10%, respectively. The results are surprisingly similar between these three physician groups who practice in three different countries, with three different health care systems and with three different current PD utilization rates.

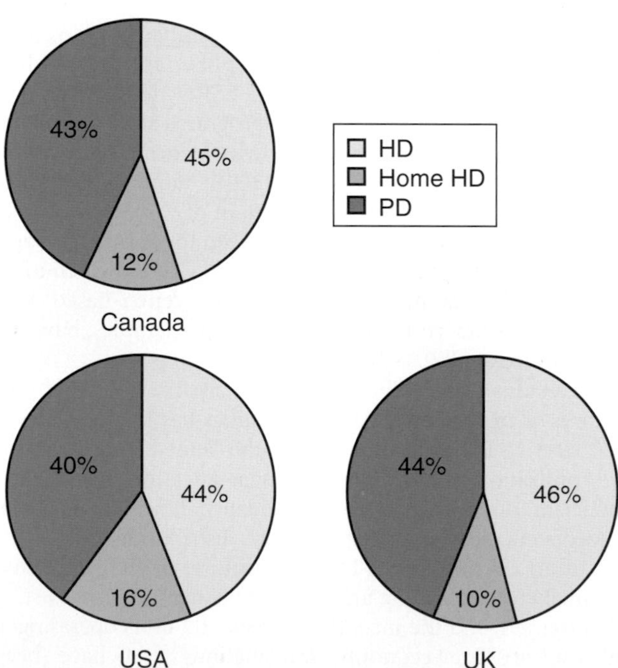

Figure 15–8 Optimal modality distribution recommended by Canadian, American, and European nephrologists based on maximization of cost-effectiveness.

In a subsequent study, we looked specifically at the issue of physician bias.[151] Nephrologists unfamiliar with PD are thought to have a negative attitude toward PD, which is transmitted to patients and impacts on choice. We performed a secondary analysis on our survey database to compare physicians who practice only or mainly hemodialysis, to the physicians who practice only or mainly PD. The hypothesis being tested was that the doctors who practice mainly or only hemodialysis will show marked preferences for HD in their answers, compared to the doctors who practice only or mainly PD. Of the 50 or 60 questions in this survey, Table 15–3 shows only the answers that are statistically significantly different. In other words, most answers are not statistically significantly different. In fact, even in the ones that are statistically different, they are not very different in terms of the number ranking.

Table 15–3 Differences Between Nephrologists Based on Dialysis Practice

	Factor	All or Mainly HD	Both HD and PD (mixed)	All or Mainly PD	P
	No. of respondents	117	232	16	
General factors	Cost to health care system	2.42 ± 0.11	2.78 ±0.07	2.94 ± 0.22	.001*
Patient-Related factors	Cognitive impairment	1.55 ± 0.06	1.84 ± 0.05	2.29 ± 0.18	.0001*
Influencing choice of HD or PD	Poor coordination	1.84 ± 0.06	2.00 ± 0.05	2.47 ± 0.21	.007
	Insufficient IQ	1.91 ± 0.06	2.08 ± 0.05	2.29 ± 0.21	.008
	Poor motor strength	2.09 ± 0.06	2.27 ± 0.05	2.71 ± 0.17	.003
	Age >70	2.67 ± 0.07	2.93 ± 0.05	2.88 ± 0.27	.0001†
	Local availability	2.85 ± 0.10	3.00 ± 0.07	3.59 ± 0.23	.0001*
	Maximum weight	97.8 ± 1.7	101.4 ± 1.1	108.5 ± 3.9	.02*

*Statistical difference between all or mainly HD and all or mainly PD in post hoc analysis.
†Statistical difference between all or mainly HD and mixed type of practice in post hoc analysis.
HD, hemodialysis; *PD,* peritoneal dialysis. (Adapted from Charest AF, Mendelssohn DC: Are North American nephrologists biased against peritoneal dialysis? Perit Dial Int 2001; 21[4]:335-337.)

Age is an example of a difference where hemodialysis doctors feel that greater than 70 years is more of a factor against PD than the PD doctors, but the difference is not large. The biggest difference is related to a weight contraindication to PD. Doctors who do mainly hemodialysis believe that the upper limit for PD should be 98 kg, whereas doctors who do mainly PD say 108 kg.

We then looked again at the optimal system design question. Surprisingly, the hemodialysis doctors and the PD doctors answered these questions very similarly. Concerning the percent PD in the optimal distribution with maximization of survival, wellness and quality of life, 32% was recommended by the HD doctors, whereas 45% was recommended by the PD doctors. Similarly, when framing the question around cost-effectiveness, the recommendations become even more similar with PD utilization suggested at 41% by the HD doctors and at 40% by the PD doctors. Although there is a difference in opinion about optimal modality distribution between nephrologists who do mainly HD compared to those who do mainly PD, the 32% to 45% PD recommendation is 3.5 to 5 times higher than current rates of PD utilization in the United States. An independent published survey of American nephrologists shows very similar results, including emphasis on patient preference in modality decision making, relative underutilization of PD, and no difference between nephrologists who do all HD compared to those familiar with PD.[98]

From the primary and secondary analysis of our surveys, we conclude that nephrologists' attitudes toward PD and home HD are in fact quite positive, and that there is no evidence of significant widespread bias against PD. We acknowledge certain limitations within this survey methodology, but to try to establish the optimal dialysis modality distribution is a very hard question to probe with more rigorous research designs. For example, there will never be a randomized controlled trial of PD versus HD.

A useful guide to medical and nonmedical factors that influence modality selection is shown in Table 15–4. Originally drafted by Hamburger and associates,[152] it has recently been updated and expanded by Shetty and Oreopoulos[111] and presents indications and contraindications to hemodialysis and peritoneal dialysis from the home peritoneal dialysis-perspective.

TIMING THE INITIATION OF DIALYTIC THERAPY IN PATIENTS WITH CHRONIC KIDNEY DISEASE

In everyday clinical practice, nephrologists and their patients are commonly faced with the decision about when to initiate dialysis. On occasion, the decision is straightforward, as in the setting of acute renal failure with acute metabolic or volume-related complications. In the setting of slowly progressive chronic kidney disease, however, the decision-making process is more complex and requires the consideration of several clinical, biochemical, and psychosocial factors.

Absolute Indications for Initiation of Dialysis

The absolute indications for initiation of dialysis are more typically observed in the setting of acute renal failure, and include:

1. Neurologic complications, such as encephalopathy, sensory neuropathy, and motor neuropathy
2. Uremic serositis, including pericarditis and pleuritis
3. Metabolic abnormalities refractory to medical management, including hyperkalemia and metabolic acidosis
4. Volume overload refractory to medical management

When present in the setting of CKD, these complications reflect either an acute or chronic exacerbation in renal function but may also result from failure to recognize pending complications before they occur.

Relative indications for dialysis may be present late in the course of CKD but may also complicate acute renal failure and include symptoms, such as fatigue, weakness, insomnia, anorexia, nausea, vomiting, itching, and weight loss.

To date, no large prospective randomized trials have identified an ideal renal functional threshold at which to initiate renal replacement therapy in patients without uremic symptoms. The many small observational and often retrospective studies that have addressed this question have generated numerous opinions, each focusing on different measures of nutritional status, residual renal function, or clinical parameters. Unfortunately, many of the studies addressing this issue

Table 15–4 Dialysis Modality Selection Guide

Medical Considerations	Demographic Considerations	Psychosocial Considerations
PD Strongly Indicated		
Vascular access difficult to establish	Age 0–5 years	Long way from center
Refractory chronic heart failure		Strong patient preference
Prosthetic valvular disease		Strong need for autonomy, independence, or control
Problems on HD (e.g., severe headache or asthenia post-HD)		
PD Preferred		
Cardiovascular diseases/HTN	Age 6–16 years	Active lifestyle
Chronic disease:		Variable schedule
Known bleeding disorder		Travel
Multiple myeloma		Needle anxiety
Labile diabetes		Demand for flexible diet
HIV positive		
Hepatitis B or C positive		
Transplant candidates		
Transfusion problem (X-match or Jehovah's Witness)		
PD or HD Equally Preferred		
Diabetes mellitus	Both sexes	
Chronic, stable angina	All races	
Peripheral vascular disease	Nursing home residents	
Polycystic kidney disease		
Scleroderma		
PD Not Preferred but Possible with Added Considerations		
Large size (obesity)	Severe depression	
History of diverticulitis	Drug abuse	
Severe low-back pain	Social support needed	
Hernias	Poor compliance	
Multiple abdominal surgeries		
Impaired manual dexterity		
Blindness		
Hiatus hernia with reflux esophagitis		
Questionably Indicated for PD (Relative Contraindications)		
Malnutrition	Chronic poor hygiene	
Multiple abdominal adhesions	Dementia	
Ostomies	Dementia	
Proteinuria >10 g/day	Concern about body image	
Severe diabetic gastroparesis	Homeless	
Severe hypertriglyceridemia	Small home without place to store the supplies	
Advanced COPD		
Ascites		
Patient with patent LeVeen shunt		
Patient with ventriculoperitoneal shunt		
Transplant within 1 month		
Upper limb amputation		
Contraindicated for CAPD		
Severe inflammatory bowel disease	Severe active psychotic disorder or manic-depressive	
Acute active diverticulitis		
Active ischemic bowel disease		
Abdominal abscess	Marked intellectual disability with no helper	
Starting dialysis in the 3rd trimester of pregnancy		

(Modified from Hamburger R et al: A dialysis modality decision guide based on the experience of six dialysis centers. Dial Transplant 1990; 19:66-69.)

have been limited by variations in patient compliance, comorbidity burden, referral-time bias, and starting-time bias.[153]

There has recently been attention focused on an earlier, timely, or healthy start to dialysis.[124,154,155] The argument in favor of an early start begins with the recognition that morbidity and mortality on dialysis is too high and has not been dramatically altered by interventions directed at improving dialysis care. One factor that might contribute to this is that patients become ill while waiting to start dialysis, and that dialysis then becomes a salvage-from-illness type of therapy that does not work very well. Earlier starts might protect against the spontaneous reduction of dietary protein intake associated with late stage progressive CKD, and possible malnutrition (clinical or subclinical) at onset of ESRD, which is known to be an adverse prognosticator. Furthermore, it is noted that many patients start dialysis at a level of residual renal function that corresponds to less clearance of uremic toxins than would be delivered by an adequate dose of dialysis.

Early retrospective work by Bonomini and associates[156,157] recognized significant differences among patients with varying levels of GFR at the initiation of dialysis, showing that an earlier start was associated with improved survival, increased employment, and reduced hospitalization. Nonetheless, proponents of this early start proposition acknowledge the lack of prospective data to validate the hypothesis, but argue forcefully that "although critics of these recommendations may perceive them to be needlessly aggressive, the high morbidity, mortality and costs associated with ESRD call for urgent and bold measures to improve the quality and quantity of life in these patients."[124] To an extent, these arguments influenced some recent North American guidelines about initiation of dialysis.[158,159]

The other side of the dialysis initiation coin is that early dialysis may be more costly and exposes patients to more dialysis-related complications and limitations in lifestyle. Indeed, one study shows only a modest benefit to an early start,[160] four studies have shown no benefit,[131,161–163] and three show worse outcomes.[164–166] Given that it would take a rather large trial to prove any benefit to an early start, the incremental benefit is likely small and would be unlikely to justify the increased cost and inconvenience of an early start approach.

In the absence of any absolute indications, the decision to start dialysis is a dynamic process that largely consists of serial clinical assessments and laboratory investigations. Although it is generally agreed upon that dialysis should be started when significant uremic symptoms develop, there is significant variability in the levels of renal function at which patients will report such symptoms.[162] This observation may partially account for the fact that up to 23% of patients started on dialysis in the United States between 1995 and 1997 began with a GFR of less than 5 mL/min, a level well below any recommended targets.[167] The impact that this may have on outcomes is debatable but serves to illustrate that there may be some value in serially calculating residual renal function through CrCL or GFR formulas in the pre-ESRD setting.

The Importance of Nutritional Status in Patients Starting Dialysis

The relationship between nutritional status at the initiation of dialysis and survival is well established.[168] Progressive chronic renal failure is associated with spontaneously reduced protein intake and a deterioration in nutritional status. This is further exacerbated in patients with protein-losing nephropathies. Low levels of biochemical markers, such as albumin, prealbumin, and creatinine have been associated with adverse outcomes in ESRD patients.[169,170] Fleischmann and associates[171] compared 1346 hemodialysis patients of various levels of body mass index (BMI) and found an inverse relationship between BMI and 1-year survival. Patients with the lowest BMIs also had a greater frequency of hospitalization and lower levels of biochemical markers such as albumin. It has thus been argued that dialysis should be initiated before lean body mass is lost.

When to Initiate Dialysis: Current Guidelines

Many professional organizations have offered guidelines for the initiation of dialysis in asymptomatic patients. Although the various recommendations vary with respect to GFR or nPNA thresholds, there is a general consensus that the focus should be on the overall clinical impression and not on these objective measures. The presence of uremic symptoms should take precedence over any laboratory parameters.

The Canadian Society of Nephrology (Table 15–5) recommends following the glomerular filtration rate (GFR) calculated as the mean of the urea and creatinine clearances determined by 24-hour urine collection.[159] At low levels of GFR, this has been shown to correlate well with inulin clearance, a gold standard for GFR quantification.[172] The CSN argues that the concept of using Kt/V as an estimate of residual renal function is foreign to most nephrologists.[159]

The NKF/DOQI's most current recommendations are largely derived from the peritoneal dialysis literature and were last updated in the year 2000. Applying these recommendations requires a calculation of the residual weekly urea clearance as expressed as renal Kt/V_{urea} , as well as the nPNA, using

Table 15–5 Canadian Society of Nephrology Clinical Practice Guidelines: Initiation of Dialysis

1. When the GFR is less than 120 L/wk per 1.73 m^2 (0.2 mL/s or 12 mL/min), look for symptoms or signs of uremia or evidence of malnutrition. If there is evidence of uremia or if the PNA is 0.8 g/kg per day, or if there is clinical malnutrition (SGA), recommend dialysis. The GFR value of 120 L/wk corresponds to a CCr of approximately 0.3 mL/s or 18 mL/min and a weekly Kt/V of 2.0 (evidence: level IV – case-series with historical controls).
2. If there is no evidence of uremia or malnutrition, increase the frequency of observation to monthly and recommend dialysis when indicated (uremia or malnutrition) (opinion).
3. When the GFR is less than 60 L/wk per 1.73 m^2 (0.1 mL/s or 6 mL/min), recommend initiation of dialysis (opinion).

(Adapted from Churchill DN, et al. The Canadian Society of Nephrology Practice Guidelines, 10 (Suppl 3):S289-S297, 1999.)

methods that have been described extensively.[158] A summary of their recommendations is provided in Table 15–6. A proposed algorithm is presented in Figure 15–9.

The methods proposed by both CSN and NKF/DOQI are not used in routine clinical practice, and the guidelines also show approximate conversions to more widely available markers of renal function like calculated CrCl (Cockcroft Gault formula) or calculated GFR (MDRD formula).

The CSN and NKF/DOQI guidelines recommended thresholds for initiating dialysis are based on very low-level evidence and largely reflect opinion. The more recent Renal Physicians Association (RPA) guidelines reflect that there is insufficient evidence to recommend initiating renal replacement therapy based solely on the specific level of GFR.[173] Instead, the RPA guidelines emphasize the importance of early referral to a CKD program, early counseling about modality options, early referral for transplant assessment, and timely referral for vascular access placement.

INTEGRATED CARE

The epidemic growth rate of ESRD and its attendant enormous costs threaten to outstrip society's ability to pay for it. Modality distribution is an important modifier of dialysis costs. Nephrologists cannot solve the dialysis dilemma of growth and high cost, but they do have an obligation to treat the most patients in the best way possible, for the lowest societal expenditure. In theory, it is possible that there is an optimal dialysis modality distribution, which allows for the treatment of the maximum number of patients, with the highest quality of care and the best possible outcomes, at the lowest cost. Nephrologists must seek to define and promote such an optimal modality distribution.[117,174] In this way, they are credible as advisors to health care policy and funding bodies. Advocating unlimited growth of a dialysis system that is not the most cost-effective will only lead to an inability to influence health care policy decision makers.

Hemodialysis and peritoneal dialysis have traditionally been viewed as competing modalities. Proponents of an integrated care approach to ESRD management, however, maintain that these modalities should rather be viewed as complementary, and that each has its appropriate place in the management of ESRD. This strategy provides each patient with the form of renal replacement therapy that yields the maximum benefit at each stage of their disease.

The Traditional Integrated Care Approach: A Rationale

Arguments in favor of the integrated care approach rest on the following premises[175]:

- Given the freedom to choose, many patients will select a given treatment modality on the basis of lifestyle.
- PD and HD differ in technical and medical terms such that valid arguments exist for using them in a PD first sequence in suitable patients.
- Evidence suggests that patients who have experienced more than one dialytic modality have a survival advantage with a PD first strategy.
- PD is more cost-effective than in-center HD

Traditionally, proponents of the integrated care concept have suggested that hemodialysis and peritoneal dialysis should be presented to patients in an unbiased way so that patient preference would dictate modality selection. Patient education obviously lies central to the self-decision process. One study showed that when provided with adequate information about

Table 15–6 NKF/DOQI Guidelines for Initiation of Dialysis

Guideline 1

When to Initiate Dialysis–Kt/V_{urea} Criterion

Unless certain conditions are met, patients should be advised to initiate some form of dialysis when the weekly renal Kt/V_{urea} (K_rt/V_{urea}) falls below 2.0. The conditions that may indicate dialysis is not yet necessary even though the weekly K_rt/V_{urea} is less than 2.0 are:

1. Stable or increased edema-free body weight. Supportive objective parameters for adequate nutrition include a lean body mass >63%, subjective global assessment score indicative of adequate nutrition and a serum albumin concentration in excess of the lower limit for the lab, and stable or rising.
2. Nutritional indications (see Guideline 2).
3. Complete absence of clinical signs or symptoms attributable to uremia.

A weekly K_rt/V_{urea} of 2.0 approximates a renal urea clearance of 7 mL/min and a renal creatinine clearance that varies between 9 to 14 mL/min/1.73 m^2. Urea clearance should be normalized to total body water (V), and creatinine clearance should be expressed per 1.73 m^2 of body surface area. The GFR, which is estimated by the arithmetic mean of the urea and creatinine clearances, will be approximately 10.5 mL/min/1.73 m^2 when the K_rt/V_{urea} is about 2.0.

Guideline 2

In patients with chronic kidney failure (e.g., GFR <15 to 20 mL/min) who are not undergoing maintenance dialysis, if protein-energy malnutrition (PEM) develops or persists despite vigorous attempts to optimize protein and energy intake, and there is no apparent cause for malnutrition other than low nutrient intake, initiation of maintenance dialysis or a renal transplant is recommended.

(Adapted from National Kidney Foundation, K/DOQI Clinical Practice Guidelines for Peritoneal Dialysis Adequacy, 2000. Am J Kidney Dis 2001; 37[Suppl 1]:S65-S136.)

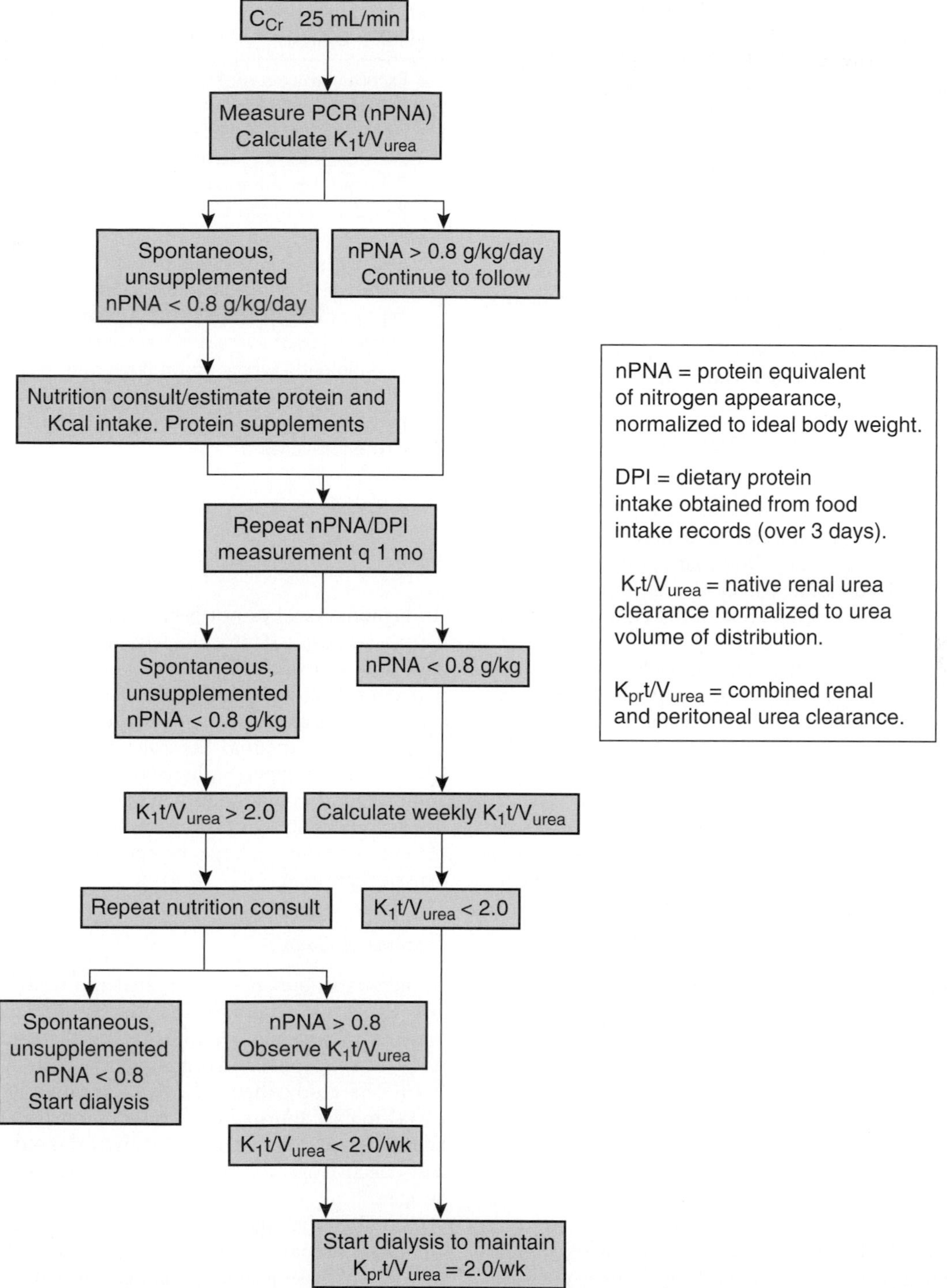

Figure 15–9 An algorithm for initiating dialysis in patients with chronic renal failure. (Adapted from K/DOQI Guidelines 2000: Guidelines for peritoneal dialysis adequacy.)

treatment options, patients were more likely to select CAPD over hemodialysis and were typically satisfied with that decision.[176] Younger patients, especially those who are employed, opt for home-based therapies in favor of in-center HD.[177,178] Home therapies may be preferred over in-center dialysis by the geriatric patient population as well, particularly when adequate education is provided.[179]

With appropriate unbiased predialysis counseling, a greater proportion of patients would thus select PD as the initial modality, thus reaping the proposed benefits of the PD-first approach. The potential benefits of PD over HD are largely confined to the first 2 years on dialysis, and following this period, or following technique failure, patients could switch to HD.[92] This has obvious economic benefits, as well as numerous clinical benefits and implications for quality of life.

Van Biesen and associates[90] published the first-ever large series evaluating the effectiveness of an integrated care approach. In this study, the charts of 223 HD and 194 PD patients were reviewed and assessed for survival in an intention to treat analysis. Patients initially treated with PD, who subsequently switched to HD, had improved survival as compared with those who started with and remained on HD. Of the patients who remained on their initial modality for more than 48 months, PD patients had reduced survival as compared with their matched HD counterparts. Although this study was retrospective, it was concluded that patients who start with PD and switch to HD in a timely fashion, do at least as well as patients initially treated with HD.

Table 15–7 Important Shared Advantages of PD and Home Quotidian Dialysis

- Excellent volume and blood pressure control.
- Patient independence and employment.
- Liberalization of dietary intake.
- Allowance for an incremental dialysis start strategy.
- Reduced risk of hepatitis and other parenteral exposures.
- Reduced erythropoietin requirements.
- Possible reduction in the risk of long-term complications of dialysis, such as amyloidosis.
- Preservation of residual renal function.
- Improved transplant-related outcomes.
- Preservation of vascular access sites (PD only).
- Possible early survival advantage over intermittent HD (PD). Survival advantage with quotidian dialysis seems plausible, but awaits confirmation.
- Cost-effectiveness.

Reformulating the Integrated Care Concept

As we move forward into the new millennium, it is imperative that ESRD management strategies keep pace with evolving technical innovations. The "PD-first" integrated care approach as described earlier, has in several important ways failed to achieve this. A reformulation of this concept has been recently proposed.[97]

First, it is well established that renal transplantation, particularly preemptive transplantation, offers patients the best possible outcomes with respect to survival and quality of life. Unquestionably, transplantation should be promoted as the first-line treatment for ESRD, and any integrated care algorithm should reflect this.

Second, although dialysis-related technologies have advanced over the last decade, technique-changes in PD and conventional thrice-weekly HD have not significantly improved any patient-related outcomes. Emerging home-based hemodialysis therapies such as short daily, and slow nocturnal (collectively known as "quotidian" dialysis therapies) have gained increasing acceptance[17,18] and appear to offer superior intermediate outcomes over conventional in-center thrice-weekly hemodialysis.[17,26,180] Evidence that these therapies are cost-effective has begun to emerge,[31–33] and it is likely that they will soon be accepted as a significant component of dialysis treatment strategies. Indeed, nephrologists believe that home hemodialysis should compromise more than 10% of an optimal modality mix.[19–21] This figure represents much higher utilization than what currently exists in most jurisdictions.

Finally, many of the proposed benefits of a PD first-strategy, however, may apply to quotidian or three times weekly home hemodialysis regimens as well, and both share many potential benefits over in-center HD. These are summarized in Table 15–7 and discussed in detail later. On this basis, it is proposed that all home-based therapies (PD and HD) should be regarded as equivalent, and that these should all be promoted as second-line therapies after preemptive transplantation.

Proposed Benefits of Home-Based Therapies

Survival

A general discussion of survival outcomes comparing PD and HD has been presented earlier in this chapter. To date quotidian hemodialysis has not been studied with respect to mortality advantages. Unfortunately, quotidian dialysis studies have been too small to address this issue. What is known is that quotidian dialysis improves several intermediate outcomes that are associated with an increase in the risk of death. These include anemia, the calcium-phosphorous product, left-ventricular hypertrophy, and nutritional status. It is the authors' opinion that quotidian dialysis will prove to be effective in conferring a survival advantage, but this awaits confirmation in either a large prospective trial or a quotidian dialysis registry.

Treatment Costs

Numerous studies have compared the relative costs of HD and PD.[6,114,115] Although dialysis delivery costs are easily underestimated due to various intangible costs and difficult-to-quantify hospital and organizational costs, it is certain that PD is less costly than HD.[181] A Canadian study estimated CAPD to cost approximately 60% as much as hospital-based hemodialysis.[114] A cost-utility analysis showed PD to be more cost-effective over a 5-year period and across all age groups in Sweden.[96]

Quotidian dialysis has also proven to be cost-effective.[32,33] One cost-comparison study found that despite the up-front cost of purchasing and installing one dialysis machine per patient, and despite a doubling in the cost of disposable materials, short-hours daily and long-hours nocturnal home hemodialysis cost less than conventional in-center dialysis and actually resulted in an increase in quality-adjusted life years.[33] Even if direct costs of daily home hemodialysis are similar to the costs of center-based HD, there are important secondary gains that make them crucial. These include that they do not require new "bricks and mortar" and minimize the capital and operating costs of expanding infrastructure in health care facilities or other locations. Perhaps more important is that they do not rely as much on highly trained dialysis nurses and technicians, who are in short supply in many parts of the world.

Improved Employability

Julius and associates[177] examined a nondiabetic cohort of patients receiving various dialysis modalities. Using logistic regression analysis and controlling for baseline demographic variables, it was found that on CAPD patients were more likely to be employed than their HD counterparts. It should not be inferred that treatment with PD increases employability, but rather that it is possible that patients who are able to perform their own dialysis procedure are more likely to be able to work as well. A study by Garcia-Maldonado[182] evaluated cognitive function using the standardized written test and found that PD patients have better cognitive function than their HD counterparts. PD patients in this study, however, had higher hematocrit levels, which likely accounted for some of the difference.

The freedom and flexibility in treatment schedule offered by home dialysis therapies has also permitted many patients to return to work. In the London Daily/Nocturnal Hemodialysis study, 40% of unemployed patients who switched from conventional in-center dialysis to quotidian dialysis were able to resume full-time employment.[24]

Quality of Life

Patients receiving home-based therapies generally enjoy a higher quality of life (QOL) and greater autonomy than their in-center counterparts. It is intuitively obvious that autonomy impacts on quality of life, but it is not possible to design a prospective study to evaluate this in patients requiring RRT. Autonomy is also important with respect to modality selection. A retrospective series showed that when a program was forced to offer only CAPD (because it could no longer accommodate more hemodialysis patients), quality of life scores were reduced as compared with patients who could choose between HD and CAPD.[183]

It is difficult to assess whether patients prefer PD over HD. One study by De Vecchi and associates[184] attempted this by administering a questionnaire to patients who had experienced both HD and PD for 6 months. Patients were initially allowed to freely choose between PD and HD. A greater proportion of patients had selected CAPD over HD as their initial modality (76% vs. 24%). The reasons for choice of CAPD were: more free time (21%), more freedom (67%), better well-being (44%), less worry (5%); for HD they were: more free time (53%), better well-being (39%), less worry (13%), no need for a peritoneal catheter, and fewer clinical complications (19%). Most patients who had experienced both HD and PD had often switched from one to the other because of technique failure or other complications. Under such circumstances, it is not surprising that patients preferred their current modality.

A discussion on quality of life cannot be complete without addressing the impact of RRT on caregivers. Patients receiving home-based therapies may have varying degrees of dependency on their caregivers, occasionally requiring assistance with all aspects of dialysis delivery, though most quotidian home dialysis patients are independent or minimally assisted. Caregiver burnout is not unheard of and may occasionally necessitate a switch to in-center therapy.

Patients who switch from conventional hemodialysis to quotidian dialysis universally prefer the latter, reporting improved well-being, reduced treatment-associated anxiety, less treatment associated symptoms, such as dizziness and dyspnea. Quotidian dialysis patients may also enjoy an unrestricted diet, which impacts heavily on overall quality of life.[185]

Renal Transplantation

Although long-term graft survival is similar in patients initially treated with PD and HD,[186] PD-treated patients may enjoy certain benefits in the post-transplant period. Delayed graft function (DGF), defined as renal dysfunction requiring renal replacement therapy in the first post-transplant week, is a strong negative predictor of long-term graft function.[187,188] The odds of DGF are lower in patients receiving PD, as is the incidence of oliguria.[189] It has been hypothesized that this could be due to greater hydration in PD patients.[190] The effects of quotidian dialysis on graft function have not yet been explored.

A greater incidence of inadvertent blood loss among HD patients has been associated with greater blood transfusion and erythropoietin requirements when compared with PD.[191] This same study showed a corresponding increase in panel reactive antibodies and increased transplant wait times. Lower blood transfusion rates have also been associated with a lower incidence of hepatitis C among PD patients.[192]

Some have suggested that peritoneal dialysis may indirectly confer some mechanical advantages during ureterovesical anastomosis. Since patients with increased residual renal function are less likely to have atrophic bladders, their anastomoses are theoretically less likely to leak.[193] This, however, has not been evaluated in any scientific way. The potential impact of quotidian dialysis on transplant-related outcomes has not yet been reported.

Preservation of Residual Renal Function

In the early 1990s, Faller and Lameire[194] demonstrated that the loss in total Kt/V in CAPD patients over time was due to a loss of residual renal function (RRF) and not attributable to changes in peritoneal membrane transport characteristics. In this study, the contribution of RRF to the total clearance fell from a predialysis level of 21.6% to less than 3% over a period of 7 years. Subsequent studies have corroborated this finding.[195]

Preserving RRF may be advantageous in many ways. Of greatest significance is the positive impact on survival. The CANUSA study not only demonstrated that the progressive loss in clearance over time was due to the loss of RRF, but that it was specifically the decline in RRF that was associated with decreased patient survival and not the a decline in peritoneal clearance.[196] The ADEMEX and NECOSAD-2 studies reinforced this point, demonstrating that total small solute clearance alone did not predict survival, but that RRF did.[197,198]

The explanation for this finding is not straightforward, as residual renal function may confer numerous metabolic advantages over and above small solute clearance, and hemodynamic factors are likely to be present as well. Extracellular fluid volume (ECFV) control is likely an additional factor. It is well established that cardiovascular mortality is increased in dialysis patients, and that LVH is a major independent predictor of cardiovascular death.[199,200] Residual renal function has recently been associated inversely with the development of

LVH.[201] Higher levels of RRF have also been associated with lesser degrees of ECFV-expansion.[202] The volume-expanded state in patients with low RRF is thus associated with LVH and cardiovascular death. These observations at least partly explain the reduced mortality observed among PD patients as compared with HD patients in the first 2 years on dialysis, when RRF is at its highest.

Improved volume regulation has the added benefit that patients may liberalize their fluid and dietary intake. Indeed, nutritional status tends to be better in patients with preserved RRF. Micronutrient and total caloric intake, for example, is greater in patients with higher levels of renal urea clearance.[203] This has been shown to be associated with improved survival.[204] RRF has also been associated with positive nitrogen balance, reflecting higher dietary protein intake.[205] Other important metabolic effects of RRF include increased middle- and large-molecular weight solute clearance and improved renal endocrine function.[206,207]

Cardiovascular Disease

Cardiovascular disease is the leading cause of mortality among ESRD patients, thus it is imperative that any strategy designed to improve outcomes in this patient population must take cardiovascular risk management into account. In addition to traditional cardiovascular risk factors, one must consider the factors related to kidney failure itself and dialysis. These include hyperhomocysteinemia, anemia, malnutrition, lipoprotein (a), inflammation, and an elevated calcium-phosphorous product.

The relative merits of the various dialytic modalities with respect to cardiovascular disease remains somewhat controversial, and discussions in this area are complex. There are cardiovascular concerns that may relate to PD therapy. The atherogenicity of glucose-based dialysate has been implicated, particularly with respect to its effect on lipid profiles, the production of advanced glycosylation end products, and oxidative stress. Lipoprotein (a), which is also associated with CAD, is markedly elevated in CAPD patients.[208] A recent series documented markedly greater levels of total cholesterol, triglycerides, and lipoprotein (a) and lower HDL levels in PD patients as compared with their HD counterparts.[209] Not surprisingly, both HD and PD patients have elevated LDL levels. Although lipid lowering drugs have proven effective in reducing LDL levels in CAPD patients, no prospective studies to date have conclusively shown any mortality benefits to their use in dialysis populations.

Blood pressure control varies from one dialytic modality to another. One study by Saldanha and associates[210] demonstrated a 7.8% decrease in blood pressure 6 months after switching from HD to PD. This was associated with a drop in ideal body weight, suggesting that improved volume status was a contributing factor. A Japanese survey found systolic blood pressure to be 8 mmHg lower on average in patients on PD versus HD.[211] These findings, however, have not been entirely consistent throughout the literature.[212] Such studies are likely confounded by numerous factors, including aggressiveness with antihypertensive therapy and volume control, as well as the level of residual renal function, though Saldanha's study also documented a reduction in antihypertensive medication in subjects that switched to PD.

Homocysteine levels tend to be high in dialysis patients. A study by Moustapha and associates[213] documented an almost twofold higher level in HD patients versus PD patients. Plasma folate levels were also found to be lower in HD patients, suggesting that folate is removed to a greater degree by HD than by PD. Homocysteine is markedly improved by treatment with both short-daily and long-nocturnal dialysis.[25]

Quotidian dialysis offers a unique approach to cardiovascular risk factor management. Hypertension is unquestionably better controlled with quotidian dialysis than with conventional HD or PD. Quotidian dialysis patients require less antihypertensive medication, and over time even experience regression of left-ventricular hypertrophy.[214,215] Over time, this may translate into an increased survival advantage. Reductions in the calcium-phosphorous product that have been observed in quotidian dialysis have yet to be shown to translate into mortality reduction. Such is also the case with improvements in homocysteine and lipid profiles.

Some have suggested that arrhythmias are more common in conventional HD than in PD. Canziani and associates[216] documented a marked increase in the incidence of severe cardiac arrhythmias in patients treated with PD relative to their HD counterparts. Not surprisingly, these patients also had a greater degree of LVH, a known precipitant of ventricular arrhythmias. Data from the USRDS database have shown that thrice-weekly hemodialysis is associated with greater incidence of sudden cardiac death on Mondays and Tuesdays than on any other days of the week.[217] The supposition here is that following a 72-hour interval between dialysis treatments, electrolyte abnormalities such as hyperkalemia and volume overload are likely to occur. By virtue of its continuous nature, peritoneal dialysis is less likely to expose patients to these insults and is thus not associated with an increase in sudden cardiac death.

Despite these numerous intermodality differences, some clear conclusions can be drawn: (1) quotidian dialysis offers what appears to be the best potential cardiac protection via reductions in LVH, calcium-phosphate product, and blood pressure; and (2) volume control is likely a key factor in preventing LVH and can be achieved to some extent using any modality provided that vigilance is applied.

Anemia Management

It is fairly well-established that treatment of anemia in ESRD improves quality of life, increases exercise capacity, improves sleep disturbances, prevents LVH, and has been associated with improved cognitive function.[218,219] More importantly, hemoglobin levels in excess of current DOQI targets (>12 g/dL) have recently been associated with reduced hospitalization rates, with no increased risk of death, as had previously been thought to be the case.[219]

Hemodialysis patients are constantly faced with modality-associated blood loss; thus, it is not surprising that on average, PD patients achieve their hemoglobin targets more easily than do HD patients. This difference may also be partially accounted for by greater residual renal function, though no study to date has confirmed this. Ultimately, PD patients tend to have higher hemoglobin levels, with reduced erythropoietin requirements resulting in lower anemia management costs. Canadian data from 1998, when most erythropoietin was

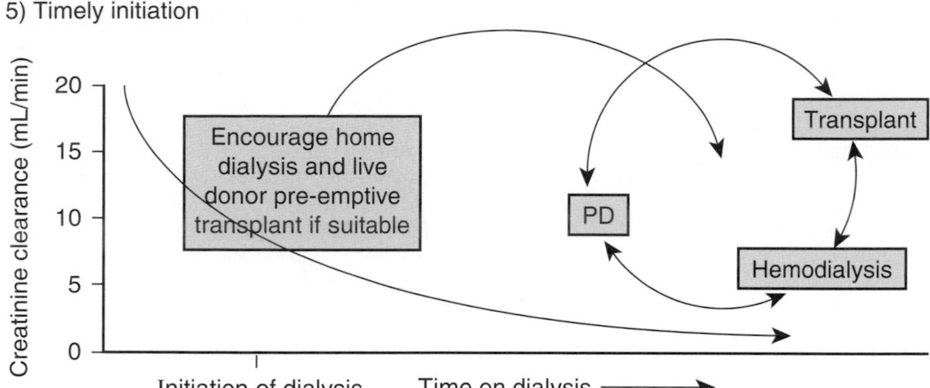

Figure 15–10 A reformulated version of integrated care. (From Mendelssohn DC, Pierratos A: Reformulating the integrated care concept for the new millennium. Perit Dial Int 2002; 22[1]:5-8.)

administered subcutaneously, showed that PD patients received on average 6000 units per week as compared with the 8000 units per week received by their HD counterparts.[220] Additionally, and not surprisingly, the prevalence of intravenous iron preparation usage has been up to nine times greater in HD patients.[220] Quotidian dialysis has also been associated with reduced erythropoietin requirements, and thus substantial cost savings.[27]

THE INTEGRATED CARE CONCEPT REVISITED

In view of the previous discussion, it is apparent that many reasonable arguments favor the use of home peritoneal and home-based quotidian hemodialysis as first-line dialysis therapies for patients who cannot be preemptively transplanted. The approach that is proposed takes into account patient autonomy, important clinical outcomes, including survival and cardiovascular disease, new technologies, and advocates maximizing the use of cost-effective therapies. A proposed algorithm is depicted in Figure 15–10. In summary, a modern integrated care approach should comprise the following principles:

1. Early referral to CKD programs should be promoted, because it is associated with improved outcomes and preservation of renal function.
2. CKD care should include aggressive medical management to delay the progression of chronic renal failure, reduce cardiovascular disease burden, and control the complications of chronic renal failure.
3. Preemptive living donor transplantation should be promoted as the first-line treatment for ESRD.
4. Patients who are not eligible for preemptive transplantation should receive timely, adequate, and unbiased education regarding the complete array of renal replacement therapy options available, including home based hemodialysis and home peritoneal dialysis.
5. Suitable patients should be actively encouraged to select a home-based dialysis modality as their initial therapy.
6. Patients initially treated with home dialysis might be switched to another modality, when and if required.

Based on these concepts, we believe that home hemodialysis is an important option that must be included in public discussions about the optimal dialysis modality distribution at the system level. At the patient level, when it is available, it must be promoted as an excellent initial dialysis choice. Unfortunately, home HD may not be available in many jurisdictions. Perhaps this is why home HD is not always included in discussions about integrated care. Indeed, some recent detailed publications do not even mention home HD.[90,175,193] However, nephrologists believe that home HD is currently underutilized and that it should be a significant part of an optimal modality mix. Where it is not available, nephrologists should advocate locally for adequate funding mechanisms, infrastructure, and other system enhancements in order to increase its availability.

In conclusion, end-stage renal failure modality treatment issues are complex, but fundamental, and affect both costs and outcomes. This chapter has tried to set out the issues in a way that highlights the controversies, that promotes a sound rationale for current clinical decision making, and that sets the stage for future well designed studies.

References

1. United States Renal Data System: USRDS 2003 annual data report: Atlas of end-stage renal disease in the United States. Bethesda, MD, National Institutes of Health, National Institute of Diabetes and Digestive and Kidney Diseases, 2003.
2. Canadian Organ Replacement Registry (CORR): 2001 annual report. Don Mills, Ontario, Canadian Institute for Health Information, 2001.
3. Kalo Z, Jaray J, Nagy J: Economic evaluation of kidney transplantation versus hemodialysis in patients with end-stage renal disease in Hungary. Prog Transplant 2001; 11(3):188-193.
4. Winkelmayer WC, Weinstein MC, Mittleman MA, et al: Health economic evaluations: The special case of end-stage renal disease treatment. Med Decis Making 2002; 22(5): 417-430.

5. Mowatt G, Vale L, Perez J, et al: Systematic review of the effectiveness and cost-effectiveness, and economic evaluation, of home versus hospital or satellite unit haemodialysis for people with end-stage renal failure. Health Technol Assess 2003; 7(2): 1-174.
6. Lee H, Manns B, Taub K, et al: Cost analysis of ongoing care of patients with end-stage renal disease: The impact of dialysis modality and dialysis access. Am J Kidney Dis 2002; 40(3): 611-622.
7. Blake PG, Finkelstein FO: Why is the proportion of patients doing peritoneal dialysis declining in North America? Perit Dial Int 2001; 21(2):107-114.
8. Mehta RL, Letteri JM: Current status of renal replacement therapy for acute renal failure. A survey of U.S. nephrologists. The National Kidney Foundation Council on Dialysis. Am J Nephrol 1999; 19(3):377-382.
9. Hyman A, Mendelssohn DC: Current Canadian approaches to dialysis for acute renal failure in the ICU. Am J Nephrol 2002; 22(1):29-34.
10. Merino JL, Rivera M, Teruel JL, et al: CAPD as treatment of chronic debilitating hemodialysis hypotension. Perit Dial Int 2002; 22(3):429.
11. Vande WJ, Raes A, Castillo D, et al: New perspectives for PD in acute renal failure related to new catheter techniques and introduction of APD. Adv Perit Dial 1997; 13:190-194.
12. Del Peso G, Bajo MA, Costero O, et al: Risk factors for abdominal wall complications in peritoneal dialysis patients. Perit Dial Int 2003; 23(3):249-254.
13. Piraino B: Infectious complications of peritoneal dialysis. Perit Dial Int 1997; 17(suppl 3):S15-S18.
14. Graff J, Fugleberg S, Brahm J, Fogh-Andersen N: Transperitoneal transport of sodium during hypertonic peritoneal dialysis. Clin Physiol 1996; 16(1):31-39.
15. Delarue J, Maingourd C: Acute metabolic effects of dialysis fluids during CAPD. Am J Kidney Dis 2001; 37(1 suppl 2):S103-S107.
16. Burkart JM: Effect of peritoneal dialysis prescription and peritoneal membrane transport characteristics on nutritional status. Perit Dial Int 1995; 15(5 suppl):S20-S35.
17. Pierratos A: Daily hemodialysis: Why the renewed interest? Am J Kidney Dis 1998; 32(6 suppl 4):S76-S82.
18. Kjellstrand C, Ting G: Daily hemodialysis: Dialysis for the next century. Adv Ren Replace Ther 1998; 5(4):267-274.
19. Jassal SV, Krishna G, Mallick NP, Mendelssohn DC: Attitudes of British Isles' nephrologists towards dialysis modality selection: A questionnaire study. Nephrol Dial Transplant 2002; 17(3): 474-477.
20. Jung B, Blake PG, Mehta RL, Mendelssohn DC: Attitudes of Canadian nephrologists toward dialysis modality selection. Perit Dial Int 1999; 19(3):263-268.
21. Mendelssohn DC, Mullaney SR, Jung B, et al: What do American nephologists think about dialysis modality selection? Am J Kidney Dis 2001; 37(1):22-29.
22. Ting GO, Kjellstrand C, Freitas T, et al: Long-term study of high-comorbidity ESRD patients converted from conventional to short daily hemodialysis. Am J Kidney Dis 2003; 42(5): 1020-1035.
23. Kjellstrand CM, Rosa AA, Shideman JR, et al: Optimal dialysis frequency and duration: The "unphysiology hypothesis." Kidney Int Suppl 1978; 8:S120-S124.
24. Heidenheim AP, Muirhead N, Moist L, Lindsay RM: Patient quality of life on quotidian hemodialysis. Am J Kidney Dis 2003; 42(1 suppl):36-41.
25. Nesrallah G, Suri R, Moist L, et al: Volume control and blood pressure management in patients undergoing quotidian hemodialysis. Am J Kidney Dis 2003; 42(1 suppl):13-17.
26. Pierratos A, Ouwendyk M, Francoeur R, et al: Nocturnal hemodialysis: Three-year experience. J Am Soc Nephrol 1998; 9(5):859-868.
27. Woods JD, Port FK, Orzol S, et al: Clinical and biochemical correlates of starting "daily" hemodialysis. Kidney Int 1999; 55(6): 2467-2476.
28. Al Hejaili F, Kortas C, Leitch R, et al: Nocturnal but not short hours quotidian hemodialysis requires an elevated dialysate calcium concentration. J Am Soc Nephrol 2003; 14(9):2322-2328.
29. Lindsay RM, Alhejaili F, Nesrallah G, et al: Calcium and phosphate balance with quotidian hemodialysis. Am J Kidney Dis 2003; 42(1 suppl):24-29.
30. Suri R, Depner TA, Blake PG, et al: Adequacy of quotidian hemodialysis. Am J Kidney Dis 2003; 42(1 suppl):42-48.
31. McFarlane PA, Bayoumi AM, Pierratos A, Redelmeier DA: The quality of life and cost utility of home nocturnal and conventional in-center hemodialysis. Kidney Int 2003; 64(3):1004-1011.
32. McFarlane PA, Pierratos A, Redelmeier DA: Cost savings of home nocturnal versus conventional in-center hemodialysis. Kidney Int 2002; 62(6):2216-2222.
33. Kroeker A, Clark WF, Heidenheim AP, et al: An operating cost comparison between conventional and home quotidian hemodialysis. Am J Kidney Dis 2003; 42(1 suppl):49-55.
34. Kiberd BA: Equitable allocation versus best outcome: Competing economic and ethical strategies in renal transplantation. Ann R Coll Physicians Surg Can 1992; 25(7):446-448.
35. Arend SM, Mallat MJ, Westendorp RJ, et al: Patient survival after renal transplantation: More than 25 years follow-up. Nephrol Dial Transplant 1997; 12(8):1672-1679.
36. Taube DH, Winder EA, Ogg CS, et al: Successful treatment of middle aged and elderly patients with end stage renal disease. Br Med J (Clin Res Ed) 1983; 286(6383):2018-2020.
37. Fauchald P, Albrechtsen D, Leivestad T, et al: Renal replacement therapy in elderly patients. Transpl Int 1988; 1(3):131-134.
38. Wolfe RA, Ashby VB, Milford EL, et al: Comparison of mortality in all patients on dialysis, patients on dialysis awaiting transplantation, and recipients of a first cadaveric transplant. N Engl J Med 1999; 341(23):1725-1730.
39. Snyder JJ, Kasiske BL, Gilbertson DT, Collins AJ: A comparison of transplant outcomes in peritoneal and hemodialysis patients. Kidney Int 2002; 62(4):1423-1430.
40. Khan IH, Garratt AM, Kumar A, et al: Patients' perception of health on renal replacement therapy: Evaluation using a new instrument. Nephrol Dial Transplant 1995; 10(5):684-689.
41. Simmons RG, Abress L: Quality-of-life issues for end-stage renal disease patients. Am J Kidney Dis 1990; 15(3):201-208.
42. Dew MA, Switzer GE, Goycoolea JM, et al: Does transplantation produce quality of life benefits? A quantitative analysis of the literature. Transplantation 1997; 64(9):1261-1273.
43. Vanrenterghem Y, Verberckmoes R: Pre-emptive kidney transplantation. Nephrol Dial Transplant 1998; 13(10):2466-2468.
44. Mange KC, Joffe MM, Feldman HI: Preemptive living donor kidney transplantation in the United States. J Am Soc Nephrol 1998; 9:686A.
45. Mange KC, Weir MR: Preemptive renal transplantation: Why not? Am J Transplant 2003; 3:1336-1340.
46. Katz SM, Kerman RH, Golden D, et al: Preemptive transplantation: An analysis of benefits and hazards in 85 cases. Transplantation 1991; 51(2):351-355.
47. Roake JA, Cahill AP, Gray CM, Gray DW, Morris PJ. Preemptive cadaveric renal transplantation—clinical outcome. Transplantation 1996; 62(10):1411-1416.
48. Papalois VE, Moss A, Gillingham KJ, et al: Pre-emptive transplants for patients with renal failure: An argument against waiting until dialysis. Transplantation 2000; 70(4):625-631.
49. Wanner C, Zimmermann J, Quaschning T, Galle J: Inflammation, dyslipidemia and vascular risk factors in hemodialysis patients. Kidney Int Suppl 1997; 62:S53-S55.
50. Gris JC, Branger B, Vecina F, et al: Increased cardiovascular risk factors and features of endothelial activation and dysfunction in dialyzed uremic patients. Kidney Int 1994; 46(3):807-813.

51. Lariviere R, Lebel M: Endothelin-1 in chronic renal failure and hypertension. Can J Physiol Pharmacol 2003; 81(6):607-621.
52. Ohkuma T, Minagawa T, Takada N, et al: C-reactive protein, lipoprotein(a), homocysteine, and male sex contribute to carotid atherosclerosis in peritoneal dialysis patients. Am J Kidney Dis 2003; 42(2):355-361.
53. Chiarello PG, Vannucchi MT, Vannucchi H: Hyperhomocysteinemia and oxidative stress during dialysis treatment. Ren Fail 2003; 25(2):203-213.
54. Mange KC, Joffe MM, Feldman HI: Effect of the use or nonuse of long-term dialysis on the subsequent survival of renal transplants from living donors. N Engl J Med 2001; 344(10):726-731.
55. Kaul H, Girndt M, Sester U, et al: Initiation of hemodialysis treatment leads to improvement of T-cell activation in patients with end-stage renal disease. Am J Kidney Dis 2000; 35(4): 611-616.
56. Descamps-Latscha B, Herbelin A, Nguyen AT, et al: Balance between IL-1 beta, TNF-alpha, and their specific inhibitors in chronic renal failure and maintenance dialysis. Relationships with activation markers of T cells, B cells, and monocytes. J Immunol 1995; 154(2):882-892.
57. Brenner BM, Milford EL: Nephron underdosing: A programmed cause of chronic renal allograft failure. Am J Kidney Dis 1993; 21(5 suppl 2):66-72.
58. Asderakis A, Augustine T, Dyer P, et al: Pre-emptive kidney transplantation: The attractive alternative. Nephrol Dial Transplant 1998; 13(7):1799-1803.
59. Cosio FG, Alamir A, Yim S, et al: Patient survival after renal transplantation. I. The impact of dialysis pre-transplant. Kidney Int 1998; 53(3):767-772.
60. Meier-Kriesche HU, Port FK, Ojo AO, et al: Effect of waiting time on renal transplant outcome. Kidney Int 2000; 58(3): 1311-1317.
61. Meier-Kriesche HU, Kaplan B: Waiting time on dialysis as the strongest modifiable risk factor for renal transplant outcomes: A paired donor kidney analysis. Transplantation 2002; 74(10): 1377-1381.
62. Alfani D, Pretagostini R, Bruzzone P, et al: Kidney transplantation from living unrelated donors. Clin Transpl 1998:205-212.
63. Turenne MN, Port FK, Strawderman RL, et al: Growth rates in pediatric dialysis patients and renal transplant recipients. Am J Kidney Dis 1997; 30(2):193-203.
64. John AG, Rao M, Jacob CK: Preemptive live-related renal transplantation. Transplantation 1998; 66(2):204-209.
65. Parfrey PS, Forbes RD, Hutchinson TA, et al: The clinical and pathological course of hepatitis B liver disease in renal transplant recipients. Transplantation 1984; 37(5):461-466.
66. Rao KV, Kasiske BL, Anderson WR: Variability in the morphological spectrum and clinical outcome of chronic liver disease in hepatitis B-positive and B-negative renal transplant recipients. Transplantation 1991; 51(2):391-396.
67. Murthy BV, Pereira BJ: A 1990s perspective of hepatitis C, human immunodeficiency virus, and tuberculosis infections in dialysis patients. Semin Nephrol 1997; 17(4):346-363.
68. Correa-Rotter R: The cost barrier to renal replacement therapy and peritoneal dialysis in the developing world. Perit Dial Int 2001; 21(suppl 3):S314-S317.
69. Murphy SW, Foley RN, Barrett BJ, et al: Comparative hospitalization of hemodialysis and peritoneal dialysis patients in Canada. Kidney Int 2000; 57(6):2557-2563.
70. Harris SA, Lamping DL, Brown EA, Constantinovici N: Clinical outcomes and quality of life in elderly patients on peritoneal dialysis versus hemodialysis. Perit Dial Int 2002; 22(4):463-470.
71. Korevaar JC, Feith GW, Dekker FW, et al: Effect of starting with hemodialysis compared with peritoneal dialysis in patients new on dialysis treatment: A randomized controlled trial. Kidney Int 2003; 64(6):2222-2228.
72. Maiorca R, Vonesh EF, Cavalli P, et al: A multicenter, selection-adjusted comparison of patient and technique survivals on CAPD and hemodialysis. Perit Dial Int 1991; 11(2):118-127.
73. Ganesh SK, Hulbert-Shearon T, Port FK, et al: Mortality differences by dialysis modality among incident ESRD patients with and without coronary artery disease. J Am Soc Nephrol 2003; 14(2):415-424.
74. Fenton SS, Schaubel DE, Desmeules M, et al: Hemodialysis versus peritoneal dialysis: A comparison of adjusted mortality rates. Am J Kidney Dis 1997; 30(3):334-342.
75. Collins AJ, Hao W, Xia H, et al: Mortality risks of peritoneal dialysis and hemodialysis. Am J Kidney Dis 1999; 34(6): 1065-1074.
76. Murphy SW, Foley RN, Barrett BJ, et al: Comparative mortality of hemodialysis and peritoneal dialysis in Canada. Kidney Int 2000; 57(4):1720-1726.
77. Foley RN: Comparing the incomparable. *In* Hemodialysis vs. Peritoneal Dialysis in Observational Studies. Peritoneal Dialysis International, 2004 (in press).
78. Davies SJ: Peritoneal dialysis solutions. *In* Pereira BJG, Sayegh M, Blake PG (eds): Chronic Kidney Disease, Dialysis and Transplantation. Burlington, MA, Elsevier, 2004.
79. Perez RA, Blake PG, Jindal KA, et al: Changes in peritoneal dialysis practices in Canada 1996-1999. Perit Dial Int 2003; 23(1): 53-57.
80. Gokal R: Newer peritoneal dialysis solutions. Adv Ren Replace Ther 2000; 7(4):302-309.
81. Guo A, Mujais S: Patient and technique survival in peritoneal dialysis in the United States: Evaluation in large incident cohorts. Kidney Int 2003; 88:S3-S12.
82. Bloembergen WE, Port FK, Mauger EA, Wolfe RA: A comparison of mortality between patients treated with hemodialysis and peritoneal dialysis. J Am Soc Nephrol 1995; 6(2):177-183.
83. Stack AG, Molony DA, Rahman NS, et al: Impact of dialysis modality on survival of new ESRD patients with congestive heart failure in the United States. Kidney Int 2003; 64(3): 1071-1079.
84. Heaf JG, Lokkegaard H, Madsen M: Initial survival advantage of peritoneal dialysis relative to haemodialysis. Nephrol Dial Transplant 2002; 17(1):112-117.
85. Locatelli F, Marcelli D, Conte F, et al: Survival and development of cardiovascular disease by modality of treatment in patients with end-stage renal disease. J Am Soc Nephrol 2001; 12(11): 2411-2417.
86. Termorshuizen F, Korevaar JC, Dekker FW, et al: Hemodialysis and peritoneal dialysis: Comparison of adjusted mortality rates according to the duration of dialysis: Analysis of The Netherlands Cooperative Study on the Adequacy of Dialysis 2. J Am Soc Nephrol 2003; 14(11):2851-2860.
87. Vonesh EF, Moran J: Mortality in end-stage renal disease: A reassessment of differences between patients treated with hemodialysis and peritoneal dialysis. J Am Soc Nephrol 1999; 10(2):354-365.
88. Schaubel DE, Morrison HI, Fenton SS: Comparing mortality rates on CAPD/CCPD and hemodialysis. The Canadian experience: Fact or fiction? Perit Dial Int 1998; 18(5):478-484.
89. Blake PG: Trends in patient and technique survival in peritoneal dialysis and strategies: How are we doing and how can we do better? Adv Ren Replace Ther 2000; 7(4):324-337.
90. Van Biesen W, Vanholder RC, Veys N, et al: An evaluation of an integrative care approach for end-stage renal disease patients. J Am Soc Nephrol 2000; 11(1):116-125.
91. Lai KN, Lo WK: Optimal peritoneal dialysis for patients from Hong Kong. Perit Dial Int 1999; 19(suppl 3):S26-S31.
92. Blake PG: Integrated end-stage renal disease care: The role of peritoneal dialysis. Nephrol Dial Transplant 2001; 16(suppl 5):61-66.
93. Longenecker JC, Coresh J, Klag MJ, et al: Validation of comorbid conditions on the end-stage renal disease medical evidence

report: The CHOICE study. Choices for Healthy Outcomes in Caring for ESRD. J Am Soc Nephrol 2000; 11(3):520-529.
94. Schaubel DE, Blake PG, Fenton SS: Trends in CAPD technique failure: Canada, 1981-1997. Perit Dial Int 2001; 21(4):365-371.
95. Schaubel DE, Fenton SS: Trends in mortality on peritoneal dialysis: Canada, 1981-1997. J Am Soc Nephrol 2000; 11(1):126-133.
96. Sennfalt K, Magnusson M, Carlsson P: Comparison of hemodialysis and peritoneal dialysis: A cost-utility analysis. Perit Dial Int 2002; 22(1):39-47.
97. Mendelssohn DC, Pierratos A: Reformulating the integrated care concept for the new millennium. Perit Dial Int 2002; 22(1):5-8.
98. Thamer M, Hwang W, Fink NE, et al: U.S. nephrologists' recommendation of dialysis modality: Results of a national survey. Am J Kidney Dis 2000; 36(6):1155-1165.
99. Little J, Irwin A, Marshall T, et al: Predicting a patient's choice of dialysis modality: Experience in a United Kingdom renal department. Am J Kidney Dis 2001; 37(5):981-986.
100. Prichard SS: Treatment modality selection in 150 consecutive patients starting ESRD therapy. Perit Dial Int 1996; 16:69-72.
101. Golper TA, Vonesh EF, Wolfson M, et al: The impact of pre-ESRD education on dialysis modality selection. J Am Soc Nephrol 2000; 11:231A.
102. Lameire N, Van Biesen W, Dombros N, et al: The referral pattern of patients with ESRD is a determinant in the choice of dialysis modality. Perit Dial Int 1997; 17(suppl 2):S161-S166.
103. United States Renal Data System: The USRDS Morbidity and Mortality Study: Wave 2. Am J Kidney Dis 1998; 32:S67-S85.
104. Mendelssohn DC: CSN Professional and Public Policy Committee. Principles of end stage renal disease care. Annals RCPSC 1997; 30:271-273.
105. Miskulin DC, Meyer KB, Athienites NV, et al: Comorbidity and other factors associated with modality selection in incident dialysis patients: The CHOICE study. Choices for healthy outcomes in caring for end-stage renal disease. Am J Kidney Dis 2002; 39(2):324-336.
106. Stack AG: Determinants of modality selection among incident U.S. dialysis patients: Results from a national study. J Am Soc Nephrol 2002; 13(5):1279-1287.
107. Baum M, Powell D, Calvin S, et al: Continuous ambulatory peritoneal dialysis in children: Comparison with hemodialysis. N Engl J Med 1982; 307(25):1537-1542.
108. Stefanidis CJ, Hewitt IK, Balfe JW: Growth in children receiving continuous ambulatory peritoneal dialysis. J Pediatr 1983; 102(5):681-685.
109. Ledermann SE, Scanes ME, Fernando ON, et al: Long-term outcome of peritoneal dialysis in infants. J Pediatr 2000; 136(1):24-29.
110. Lerner GR, Warady BA, Sullivan EK, Alexander SR: Chronic dialysis in children and adolescents. The 1996 annual report of the North American Pediatric Renal Transplant Cooperative Study. Pediatr Nephrol 1999; 13(5):404-417.
111. Shetty A, Oreopoulous DG: Peritoneal dialysis: Its indications and contraindications. Dial Transplant 2000; 29:71-77.
112. Nissenson AR, Prichard SS, Cheng IKP: Non-medical factors that impact on ESRD modality selection. Kidney Int 1993; 43(S40):S120-S127.
113. Nissenson AR, Prichard SS, Cheng IKP, et al: ESRD modality selection into the 21st century: The importance of non medical factors. ASAIO J 1997:143-150.
114. Goeree R, Manalich J, Grootendorst P, et al: Cost analysis of dialysis treatments for end-stage renal disease (ESRD). Clin Invest Med 1995; 18(6):455-464.
115. Bruns FJ, Seddon P, Saul M, Zeidel ML: The cost of caring for end-stage kidney disease patients: An analysis based on hospital financial transaction records. J Am Soc Nephrol 1998; 9(5): 884-890.
116. Garella S: The costs of dialysis in the USA. Nephrol Dial Transplant 1997; 12(suppl 1):10-21.
117. McFarlane PA, Mendelssohn DC: A call to arms: Economic barriers to optimal dialysis care. Perit Dial Int 2000; 20(1):7-12.
118. Van Biesen W, Wiedemann M, Lameire N: End-stage renal disease treatment: A European perspective. J Am Soc Nephrol 1998; 9(12 suppl):S55-S62.
119. Blake PG, Mendelssohn DC, Toffelmire EB: New developments in hemodialysis delivery in Ontario, 1995-2000. Nephrol News Issues 2000; 14(11):72-80.
120. Mendelssohn D: Instability in Canadian Medicare: The case of dialysis delivery. Nephrol News Issues 1996; 10(11):37-41.
121. Levin A: Consequences of late referral on patient outcomes. Nephrol Dial Transplant 2000; 15(suppl 3):8-13.
122. Eadington DW: Delayed referral for dialysis: Higher morbidity and higher costs. Semin Dial 1995; 8:258-260.
123. Hood SA, Sondheimer JH: Impact of pre-ESRD management on dialysis outcomes: A review. Semin Dial 1998; 11(3):175-180.
124. Obrador GT, Pereira BJ: Early referral to the nephrologist and timely initiation of renal replacement therapy: A paradigm shift in the management of patients with chronic renal failure. Am J Kidney Dis 1998; 31(3):398-417.
125. Obrador GT, Arora P, Kausz AT, Pereira BJ: Pre-end stage renal disease care in the United States: A state of disrepair. J Am Soc Nephrol 1998; 12:S44-S54.
126. Ismail N, Neyra R, Hakim R: The medical and economical advantages of early referral of chronic renal failure patients to renal specialists. Nephrol Dial Transplant 1998; 13(2):246-250.
127. Mendelssohn DC, Barrett BJ, Brownscombe LM, et al: Elevated levels of serum creatinine: Recommendations for management and referral. CMAJ 1999; 161(4):413-417.
128. Pereira BJ, Burkart JM, Parker TF III: Strategies for influencing outcomes in pre-ESRD and ESRD patients. Am J Kidney Dis 1998; 32(6 suppl 4):S2-S4.
129. Innes A, Rowe PA, Burden RP, Morgan AG: Early deaths on renal replacement therapy: The need for early nephrological referral. Nephrol Dial Transplant 1992; 7:467-471.
130. Ratcliffe PJ, Phillips RE, Oliver DO: Late referral for maintenance dialysis. Br Med J 1984:288.
131. Sesso R, Belasco AG: Late diagnosis of chronic renal failure and mortality on maintenance dialysis. Nephrol Dial Transplant 1996; 11(12):2417-2420.
132. Stack AG: Impact of timing of nephrology referral and pre-ESRD care on mortality risk among new ESRD patients in the United States. Am J Kidney Dis 2003; 41(2):310-318.
133. Kinchen KS, Sadler J, Fink N, et al: The timing of specialist evaluation in chronic kidney disease and mortality. Ann Intern Med 2002; 137(6):479-486.
134. Avorn J, Bohn RL, Levy E, et al: Nephrologist care and mortality in patients with chronic renal insufficiency. Arch Intern Med 2002; 162(17):2002-2006.
135. Jungers P, Massy ZA, Nguyen-Khoa T, et al: Longer duration of predialysis nephrological care is associated with improved long-term survival of dialysis patients. Nephrol Dial Transplant 2001; 16(12):2357-2364.
136. Campbell JD, Ewigman B, Hosokawa M, Van Stone JC: The timing of referral of patients with end stage renal disease. Dial Transplant 1989; 18:660-668.
137. Levin A, Lewis M, Mortiboy P, et al: Multidisciplinary predialysis programs: Quantification and limitations of their impact on patient outcomes in two Canadian settings. Am J Kidney Dis 1997; 29(4):533-540.
138. Arora P, Obrador GT, Ruthazer R, et al: Prevalence, predictors, and consequences of late nephrology referral at a tertiary care center. J Am Soc Nephrol 1999; 10(6):1281-1286.
139. Jungers P, Zingraff J, Page B, et al: Late referral to maintenance dialysis: Detrimental consequences. Nephrol Dial Transplant 1993; 8:1089-1093.
140. Avorn J, Winkelmayer WC, Bohn RL, et al: Delayed nephrologist referral and inadequate vascular access in patients with

advanced chronic kidney failure. J Clin Epidemiol 2002; 55(7): 711-716.
141. Rasgon S, Schwankovsky L, James-Rogers A, et al: An intervention for employment maintenance among blue-collar workers with end-stage renal disease. Am J Kidney Dis 1993; 22:403-412.
142. Schmidt RJ, Domico JR, Sorkin MI, Hobbs G: Early referral and its impact on emergent first dialyses, health care costs, and outcome. Am J Kidney Dis 1998; 32(2):278-283.
143. Diaz-Buxo JA: The importance of pre-ESRD education and early nephrological care in peritoneal dialysis selection and outcome. Perit Dial Int 1998; 18(4):363-365.
144. Wuerth DB, Finkelstein SH, Schwetz O, et al: Patients' descriptions of specific factors leading to modality selection of chronic peritoneal dialysis or hemodialysis. Perit Dial Int 2002; 22(2): 184-190.
145. Gomez CG, Valido P, Celadilla O, et al: Validity of a standard information protocol provided to end-stage renal disease patients and its effect on treatment selection. Perit Dial Int 1999; 19(5):471-477.
146. Sesso R, Yoshihiro MM: Time of diagnosis of chronic renal failure and assessment of quality of life in haemodialysis patients. Nephrol Dial Transplant 1997; 12(10):2111-2116.
147. Caskey FJ, Wordsworth S, Ben T, et al: Early referral and planned initiation of dialysis: What impact on quality of life? Nephrol Dial Transplant 2003; 18(7):1330-1338.
148. Arora P, Kausz AT, Obrador GT, et al: Hospital utilization among chronic dialysis patients. J Am Soc Nephrol 2000; 11(4):740-746.
149. McLaughlin K, Manns B, Culleton B, et al: An economic evaluation of early versus late referral of patients with progressive renal insufficiency. Am J Kidney Dis 2001; 38(5):1122-1128.
150. Golper T: Patient education: Can it maximize the success of therapy? Nephrol Dial Transplant 2001; 16(suppl 7):20-24.
151. Charest AF, Mendelssohn DC: Are North American nephrologists biased against peritoneal dialysis? Perit Dial Int 2001; 21(4):335-337.
152. Hamburger R, Mattern W, Schreiber M, et al: A dialysis modality decision guide based on the experience of six dialysis centers. Dial Transplant 1990; 19:66-69.
153. Churchill DN: An evidence-based approach to earlier initiation of dialysis. Am J Kidney Dis 1997; 30(6):899-906.
154. Nolph KD: Rationale for early incremental dialysis with continuous ambulatory peritoneal dialysis. Nephrol Dial Transplant 1998; 13(suppl 6):117-119.
155. Mehrotra R, Nolph KD: Argument for timely initiation of dialysis. J Am Soc Nephrol 1998; 9(12 suppl):S96-S99.
156. Bonomini V, Albertazzi A, Vangelista A, et al: Residual renal function and effective rehabilitation in chronic dialysis. Nephron 1976; 16(2):89-102.
157. Bonomini V, Feletti C, Scolari MP, Stefoni S: Benefits of early initiation of dialysis. Kidney Int Suppl 1985; 17:S57-S59.
158. II. NKF-K/DOQI Clinical Practice Guidelines for Peritoneal Dialysis Adequacy: Update 2000. Am J Kidney Dis 2001; 37(1 suppl 1):S65-S136.
159. Churchill DN, Blake PG, Jindal KK, et al: Clinical practice guidelines for initiation of dialysis. Canadian Society of Nephrology. J Am Soc Nephrol 1999; 10(suppl 13):S289-S291.
160. Korevaar JC, Jansen MA, Dekker FW, et al: When to initiate dialysis: Effect of proposed U.S. guidelines on survival. Lancet 2001; 358(9287):1046-1050.
161. Roubicek C, Brunet P, Huiart L, et al: Timing of nephrology referral: Influence on mortality and morbidity. Am J Kidney Dis 2000; 36(1):35-41.
162. Ifudu O, Dawood M, Homel P, Friedman EA: Timing of initiation of uremia therapy and survival in patients with progressive renal disease. Am J Nephrol 1998; 18(3):193-198.
163. Ellis PA, Reddy V, Bari N, Cairns HS: Late referral of end-stage renal failure. QJM 1998; 91(11):727-732.
164. Fink JC, Burdick RA, Kurth SJ, et al: Significance of serum creatinine values in new end-stage renal disease patients. Am J Kidney Dis 1999; 34(4):694-701.
165. Beddhu S, Samore MH, Roberts MS, et al: Impact of timing of initiation of dialysis on mortality. J Am Soc Nephrol 2003; 14(9):2305-2312.
166. Traynor JP, Simpson K, Geddes CC, et al: Early initiation of dialysis fails to prolong survival in patients with end-stage renal failure. J Am Soc Nephrol 2002; 13(8):2125-2132.
167. Obrador GT, Arora P, Kausz AT, et al: Level of renal function at the initiation of dialysis in the U.S. end-stage renal disease population. Kidney Int 1999; 56(6):2227-2235.
168. Pifer TB, McCullough KP, Port FK, et al: Mortality risk in hemodialysis patients and changes in nutritional indicators: DOPPS. Kidney Int 2002; 62(6):2238-2245.
169. Lowrie EG, Lew NL: Commonly measured laboratory variables in hemodialysis patients: Relationships among them and to death risk. Semin Nephrol 1992; 12(3):276-283.
170. Avram MM, Mittman N, Bonomini L, et al: Markers for survival in dialysis: A seven-year prospective study. Am J Kidney Dis 1995; 26(1):209-219.
171. Fleischmann E, Teal N, Dudley J, et al: Influence of excess weight on mortality and hospital stay in 1346 hemodialysis patients. Kidney Int 1999; 55(4):1560-1567.
172. van Olden RW, Krediet RT, Struijk DG, Arisz L: Measurement of residual renal function in patients treated with continuous ambulatory peritoneal dialysis. J Am Soc Nephrol 1996; 7(5): 745-750.
173. Bolton WK: Renal physicians association clinical practice guideline: Appropriate patient preparation for renal replacement therapy: Guideline number 3. J Am Soc Nephrol 2003; 14(5):1406-1410.
174. Mendelssohn DC: Reflections on the optimal dialysis modality distribution: A North American perspective. Nephrol News Issues 2002; 16(4):26-30.
175. Davies SJ, Van Biesen W, Nicholas J, Lameire N: Integrated care. Perit Dial Int 2001; 21(suppl 3):S269-S274.
176. Ahlmen J, Carlsson L, Schonborg C: Well-informed patients with end-stage renal disease prefer peritoneal dialysis to hemodialysis. Perit Dial Int 1993; 13(suppl 2):S196-S198.
177. Julius M, Kneisley JD, Carpentier-Alting P, et al: A comparison of employment rates of patients treated with continuous ambulatory peritoneal dialysis vs in-center hemodialysis (Michigan End-Stage Renal Disease Study). Arch Intern Med 1989; 149(4): 839-842.
178. Merkus MP, Jager KJ, Dekker FW, et al: Quality of life in patients on chronic dialysis: Self-assessment 3 months after the start of treatment. The Necosad Study Group. Am J Kidney Dis 1997; 29(4):584-592.
179. Ahmed S, Addicott C, Qureshi M, et al: Opinions of elderly people on treatment for end-stage renal disease. Gerontology 1999; 45(3):156-159.
180. Lindsay RM, Leitch R, Heidenheim AP, Kortas C: The London daily/nocturnal hemodialysis study-study design, morbidity, and mortality results. Am J Kidney Dis 2003; 42(1 suppl): 5-12.
181. Peeters P, Rublee D, Just PM, Joseph A: Analysis and interpretation of cost data in dialysis: Review of Western European literature. Health Policy 2000; 54(3):209-227.
182. Garcia-Maldonado M, Williams C, Smith ZM: Mental performance in CAPD. Adv Perit Dial 1991; 7:105-107.
183. Szabo E, Moody H, Hamilton T, et al: Choice of treatment improves quality of life. A study on patients undergoing dialysis. Arch Intern Med 1997; 157(12):1352-1356.
184. De Vecchi AF, Scalamogna A, Colombini M, et al: Well being in patients on CAPD and hemodialysis. Int J Artif Organs 1994; 17(9):473-477.

185. Spanner E, Suri R, Heidenheim AP, Lindsay RM: The impact of quotidian hemodialysis on nutrition. Am J Kidney Dis 2003; 42(1 suppl):30-35.
186. Maiorca R, Sandrini S, Cancarini GC, et al: Integration of peritoneal dialysis and transplantation programs. Perit Dial Int 1997; 17(suppl 2):S170-S174.
187. Geddes CC, Woo YM, Jardine AG: The impact of delayed graft function on the long-term outcome of renal transplantation. J Nephrol 2002; 15(1):17-21.
188. Cecka JM: The UNOS Scientific Renal Transplant Registry. Clin Transpl 1999:1-21.
189. Bleyer AJ, Burkart JM, Russell GB, Adams PL: Dialysis modality and delayed graft function after cadaveric renal transplantation. J Am Soc Nephrol 1999; 10(1):154-159.
190. Rottembourg J: Residual renal function and recovery of renal function in patients treated by CAPD. Kidney Int Suppl 1993; 40:S106-S110.
191. Page DE, House A: Important cost differences of blood transfusions and erythropoietin between hemodialysis and peritoneal dialysis patients. Adv Perit Dial 1998; 14:87-89.
192. Pereira BJ, Levey AS: Hepatitis C virus infection in dialysis and renal transplantation. Kidney Int 1997; 51(4):981-999.
193. Coles GA, Williams JD: What is the place of peritoneal dialysis in the integrated treatment of renal failure? Kidney Int 1998; 54(6):2234-2240.
194. Faller B, Lameire N: Evolution of clinical parameters and peritoneal function in a cohort of CAPD patients followed over 7 years. Nephrol Dial Transplant 1994; 9(3):280-286.
195. Lysaght MJ, Vonesh EF, Gotch F, et al: The influence of dialysis treatment modality on the decline of remaining renal function. ASAIO Trans 1991; 37(4):598-604.
196. Adequacy of dialysis and nutrition in continuous peritoneal dialysis: Association with clinical outcomes. Canada-USA (CANUSA) Peritoneal Dialysis Study Group. J Am Soc Nephrol 1996; 7(2):198-207.
197. Termorshuizen F, Korevaar JC, Dekker FW, et al: The relative importance of residual renal function compared with peritoneal clearance for patient survival and quality of life: An analysis of the Netherlands cooperative study on the adequacy of dialysis (NECOSAD)-2. Am J Kidney Dis 2003; 41(6): 1293-1302.
198. Paniagua R, Amato D, Vonesh E, et al: Effects of increased peritoneal clearances on mortality rates in peritoneal dialysis: ADEMEX, a prospective, randomized, controlled trial. J Am Soc Nephrol 2002; 13(5):1307-1320.
199. Lameire N, Vanholder RC, Van Loo A, et al: Cardiovascular diseases in peritoneal dialysis patients: The size of the problem. Kidney Int Suppl 1996; 56:S28-S36.
200. Stack AG, Saran R: Clinical correlates and mortality impact of left ventricular hypertrophy among new ESRD patients in the United States. Am J Kidney Dis 2002; 40(6):1202-1210.
201. Wang AY, Wang M, Woo J, et al: A novel association between residual renal function and left ventricular hypertrophy in peritoneal dialysis patients. Kidney Int 2002; 62(2):639-647.
202. Konings CJ, Kooman JP, Schonck M, et al: Fluid status in CAPD patients is related to peritoneal transport and residual renal function: Evidence from a longitudinal study. Nephrol Dial Transplant 2003; 18(4):797-803.
203. Wang AY, Sea MM, Ip R, et al: Independent effects of residual renal function and dialysis adequacy on dietary micronutrient intakes in patients receiving continuous ambulatory peritoneal dialysis. Am J Clin Nutr 2002; 76(3):569-576.
204. Randerson DH, Chapman GV, Farrell PC: Amino acid and dietary status in CAPD patients. *In* Atkins RC, Farrell PC, Thompson N (eds): Peritoneal Dialysis. Edinborough, Churchill Livingstone, 1981, pp 171-191.
205. Bergstrom J, Furst P, Alvestrand A, Lindholm B: Protein and energy intake, nitrogen balance and nitrogen losses in patients treated with continuous ambulatory peritoneal dialysis. Kidney Int 1993; 44(5):1048-1057.
206. Montini G, Amici G, Milan S, et al: Middle molecule and small protein removal in children on peritoneal dialysis. Kidney Int 2002; 61(3):1153-1159.
207. Blake PG: A critique of the Canada/USA (CANUSA) Peritoneal Dialysis Study. Perit Dial Int 1996; 16(3):243-245.
208. Anwar N, Bhatnagar D, Short CD, et al: Serum lipoprotein (a) concentrations in patients undergoing continuous ambulatory peritoneal dialysis. Nephrol Dial Transplant 1993; 8(1):71-74.
209. Kronenberg F, Lingenhel A, Neyer U, et al: Prevalence of dyslipidemic risk factors in hemodialysis and CAPD patients. Kidney Int Suppl 2003; 84:S113-S116.
210. Saldanha LF, Weiler EW, Gonick HC: Effect of continuous ambulatory peritoneal dialysis on blood pressure control. Am J Kidney Dis 1993; 21(2):184-188.
211. Shinzato T, Nakai S, Akiba T, et al: Report of the annual statistical survey of the Japanese Society for Dialysis Therapy in 1996. Kidney Int 1999; 55(2):700-712.
212. Amann K, Mandelbaum A, Schwarz U, Ritz E: Hypertension and left ventricular hypertrophy in the CAPD patient. Kidney Int Suppl 1996; 56:S37-S40.
213. Moustapha A, Gupta A, Robinson K, et al: Prevalence and determinants of hyperhomocysteinemia in hemodialysis and peritoneal dialysis. Kidney Int 1999; 55(4):1470-1475.
214. Chan CT, Floras JS, Miller JA, et al: Regression of left ventricular hypertrophy after conversion to nocturnal hemodialysis. Kidney Int 2002; 61(6):2235-2239.
215. Fagugli RM, Reboldi G, Quintaliani G, et al: Short daily hemodialysis: Blood pressure control and left ventricular mass reduction in hypertensive hemodialysis patients. Am J Kidney Dis 2001; 38(2):371-376.
216. Canziani ME, Cendoroglo NM, Saragoca MA, et al: Hemodialysis versus continuous ambulatory peritoneal dialysis: Effects on the heart. Artif Organs 1995; 19(3):241-244.
217. Bleyer AJ, Russell GB, Satko SG: Sudden and cardiac death rates in hemodialysis patients. Kidney Int 1999; 55(4):1553-1559.
218. Ofsthun N, Labrecque J, Lacson E, et al: The effects of higher hemoglobin levels on mortality and hospitalization in hemodialysis patients. Kidney Int 2003; 63(5):1908-1914.
219. Marsh JT, Brown WS, Wolcott D, et al: RHuEPO treatment improves brain and cognitive function of anemic dialysis patients. Kidney Int 1991; 39(1):155-163.
220. Canadian Organ Replacement Registry. CORR EPREX Study 1998 Report. Toronto, Canadian Institute for Health Information, 1999; 220.

SECTION C

Hemodialysis

Chapter 16

Principles of Hemodialysis

Jane Y. Yeun, M.D. • Thomas A. Depner, M.D.

Hemodialysis is a life-sustaining treatment without which more than a million patients throughout the world would die within a few weeks.[1] This dependence on an extracorporeal blood device is both the fulfillment of hopes by some and the dashing of dreams by others and highlights the need for an in-depth understanding of all aspects of hemodialysis, including the human reactions to it. Before one can configure hemodialysis optimally, one must understand its target, the uremic syndrome. This chapter reviews the physical, chemical, and clinical principles of hemodialysis as they relate to the treatment of uremia, starting with historical milestones and ending with projections for the future. The discussions include brief notes of comparison to other modalities, such as peritoneal dialysis and hemofiltration; these and other topics are abbreviated in this chapter as they are reviewed more extensively in other chapters.

FUNDAMENTAL CONCEPTS

Historical Development

Hemodialysis was originally termed *extracorporeal dialysis* because it was performed outside of the body. Several early pioneers laid the foundation for therapeutic dialysis. Graham[2] (1805–1869), a professor of chemistry in Scotland, invented the fundamental process of separating solutes using semipermeable membranes *in vitro* and coined the word "dialysis." In 1916, Abel[3] in the United States dialyzed rabbits and dogs with a "vividiffusion" device using celloidin membranes and a leech extract called hirudin as an anticoagulant. Abel was the first to apply dialysis to a living organism and to use the term "artificial kidney." In Germany, Georg Haas[4] first used the artificial kidney to dialyze a human in 1924. His attempts were only marginally successful because toxicity from his crude anticoagulant limited his ability to prolong flow in the extracorporeal circuit.

In view of these previous failures, it was not at all certain in 1944 that Willem Kolff's use of extracorporeal dialysis as a human life-saving treatment for patients with renal failure would be successful. Three major advances aided his efforts in the nearly 20 years since Hass's work: the invention of cellophane, the discovery of antibiotics, and the availability of heparin as an anticoagulant. Through his keen interest in kidney failure and his aptitude for mechanics, Kolff[5] and his patients ultimately met with success. Kolff[6–8] is often called the "father of hemodialysis" because his method became accepted as the standard for temporary replacement of kidney function in patients with short-duration acute renal failure.

Attempts to apply hemodialysis to patients who had more prolonged or permanent loss of kidney function were limited because the artery and vein used for blood access had to be tied off after each treatment. In 1960, Belding Scribner,[9] working with Quinton and Dillard at the University of Washington in Seattle, developed a blood access device for repeated dialysis using plastic tubes inserted into the artery and vein. This device, known as the Scribner shunt, and the more permanent arteriovenous (AV) fistulas later introduced by Brescia and Cimino[10] in Italy allowed hemodialysis to be repeated for many years as a life sustaining treatment. For their pioneering work in the field of artificial organs, Kolff and Scribner[11] were granted the prestigious Lasker Clinical Medical Research Award in 2002.

Renal Replacement Therapy

Available Modalities

After the success of hemodialysis, other forms of extracorporeal renal replacement therapy were attempted, including *hemofiltration* and *hemodiafiltration.* These methods rely primarily on convective filtration of the blood instead of diffusion. Several forms of *intracorporeal* dialysis were attempted, including dialysis of the pleura and pericardium, diarrheal therapy, and dialysis of loops of bowel, but the most successful intracorporeal modality has been *peritoneal dialysis.* The most promising renal replacement therapy is *renal transplantation* because it can restore normal or near-normal renal function, including potential functions not yet discovered, with the least inconvenience to the patient.

Hormone Replacement

Modern studies of kidney physiology show that the kidney, like other body organs, has an endocrine function, that is, it produces hormones that act on distant organs.[12] Currently recognized nephrogenic hormones include erythropoietin, thrombopoietin, calcitriol, prostaglandins, and renin. This improved understanding of renal endocrinology led dialysis providers to launch a massive effort to replace erythropoietin and calcitriol, both deficient in patients with kidney failure. The past few years have seen additional advances in endocrine replacement for ESRD patients: (1) the development of darbepoietin, a derivative of erythropoietin with added glycoproteins that reduce the frequency of administration, (2) the development of calcitriol analogues with comparable suppressive effects on the parathyroid gland but lesser effects on gastrointestinal absorption of calcium. See Chapters 14 and 15 for further discussion of hormone replacement.

Psychologic Support

Providers of dialysis have been slow to focus attention on the patient's reaction to kidney loss and dialysis and to develop a better understanding of kidney failure from the patient's perspective. The patient's initial depression on learning about failure of the kidneys, the subsequent denial, often followed by anger and rejection of medical and surgical treatments, and the negative attitude toward renal replacement therapy are now recognized as expected responses that are more intense in younger patients. A common source of frustration for otherwise well-intentioned caregivers, these psychologic reactions to kidney failure and dialysis are undergoing active investigation using quality of life measures developed specifically for dialysis patients. Poor quality of life is associated with higher levels of comorbidity, including malnutrition, anemia, poor quality of sleep, delayed initiation of dialysis, and low level of physical function[13-18] that can adversely impact mortality.[19-21] Because formal psychiatric counseling is considered too expensive for public funding in some countries, it is important for all caregivers to be aware of these stresses and to receive guidance in dealing with them.

Prevention and Management of Medical Complications

Successful management of hemodialysis-dependent patients requires anticipation and prevention of problems rather than simply reacting to crises. Current approaches include attempts to reverse the psychologic effects of kidney loss as discussed previously, preventing anemia and bone disease, monitoring the patient for signs of malnutrition, measuring blood flow in peripheral AV access devices, expecting hypotension during dialysis in patients with concentric ventricular hypertrophy, adjusting medication doses appropriately, and monitoring the quality of dialysate water. Water quality is especially important because the patient is exposed to large volumes that may contain toxic substances, such as aluminum or bacterial endotoxin (see Chapter 5). Several recent publications documenting higher hospitalization rates,[22] morbidity,[23,24] and mortality[25] in patients with chronic kidney failure referred late to nephrologists have highlighted the importance of preemptive care in patients with end-stage renal disease (ESRD). In the United States, the National Kidney Foundation (NKF) has published a series of clinical practice guidelines and practical recommendations, with the ultimate goal of improving the quality of life for dialysis patients.[26-29]

Definitions

Dialysis is the passage of molecules in solution by *diffusion* across a *semipermeable membrane*. Essential elements of this process are a *solvent* containing dissolved *solutes* and the membrane that contains *pores* through which some or all of the solutes move by diffusion (Figure 16–1*A*). The molecular kinetics of diffusion are both solute and membrane specific. Solute characteristics that affect movement across a particular membrane include concentration, molecular weight, shape, charge, and lipid solubility. Membrane characteristics that determine permeability to a particular solute include the average effective pore size; the number, geometry, and distribution of pores within the membrane; membrane surface area and thickness; and surface characteristics, such as charge and hydrophilicity. The solvent itself may also move by diffusion if its chemical activity is not balanced across the membrane. Although solutes may move in both directions across the membrane, it is customary to refer to the compartment containing more vital substances that one wishes to preserve as the *dialyzed compartment* and to the solution in the other, usually larger, compartment as the *dialysate*.

The concept of molecular diffusion is critically important to the definition of dialysis. Solutes pass through the membrane down an *electrochemical gradient* caused primarily by a difference in concentration across the membrane (Figure 16–1*A*). This concentration gradient, which is the driving force for diffusion, may also be dissipated by the dialysis (i.e., the molecular concentration gradient tends to fall with dialysis).

In the absence of an electrochemical gradient, solutes may also pass through pores in the membrane by *filtration*, a process of *convection*. The driving force for filtration is *pressure*, either *hydraulic* or *osmotic*, that is unbalanced across the membrane (Figure 16–1*B*) and independent of dialysis. During filtration, solute passively accompanies the solvent from one compartment to the other, causing no change in solute concentration. Convective movement may occur in the opposite direction to diffusive movement and, even in the same direction, convective movement may interfere with dialysis (i.e., the two fluxes may not be additive when they occur simultaneously).

Hemodialysis means literally "dialysis of the blood." This form of dialysis is distinguished by its location outside the body and by the continuous flow of blood across the dialyzer membrane. Therapeutic hemodialysis is most often used to treat kidney failure by equilibrating the blood against an iso-osmotic dialysate. Vital solutes are added to the dialysate at concentrations designed to mimic those normally maintained by the native kidney (Figure 16–1*A* and Table 16–1). The resulting dialysate is essentially a physiologic salt solution that, in addition to creating a gradient for removal of unwanted solutes, reproduces another vital function of normal kidneys, that of maintaining a constant physiologic concentration of extracellular electrolytes.

Demographics

According to the Centers for Medicare and Medicaid Services, at the end of 2001, there were 406,081 patients in the United States with ESRD.[30] Of these ESRD patients, 28% had func-

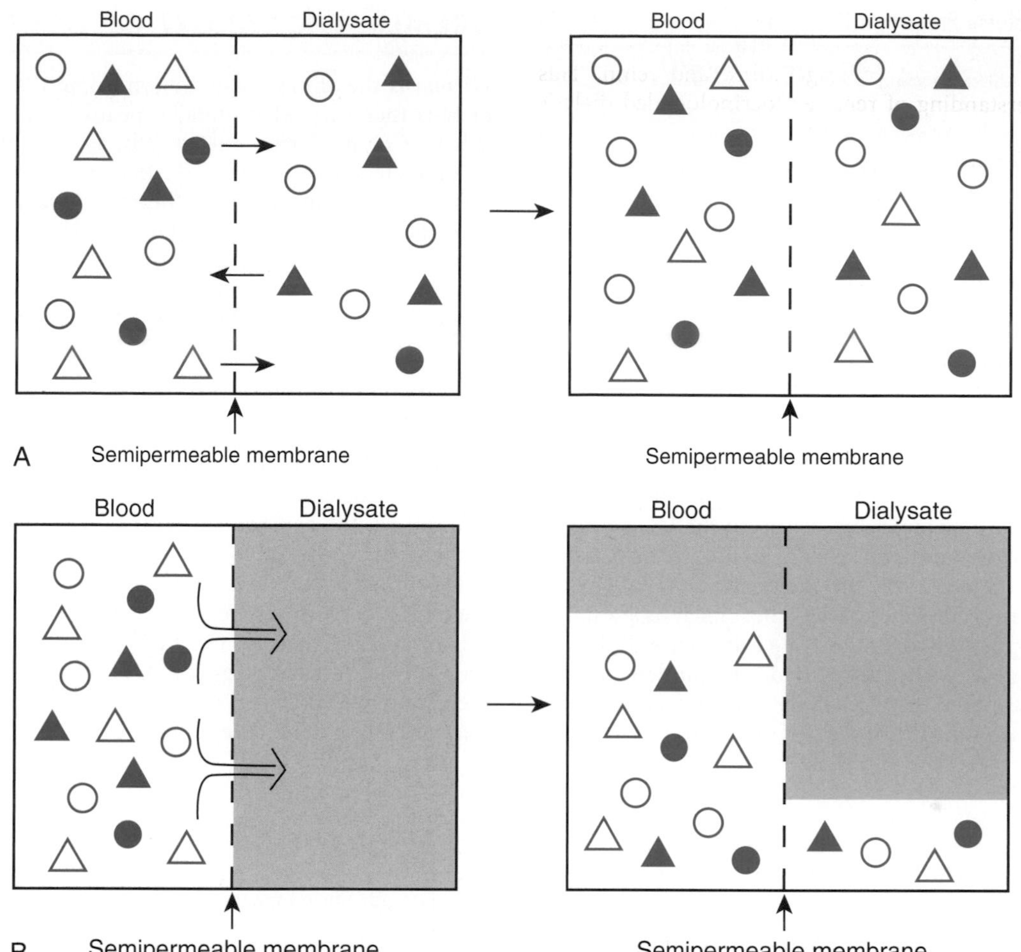

Figure 16–1 ***A,*** Diffusion across a semipermeable membrane. Solutes with higher concentrations in the blood compartment, such as potassium (*solid circles*) and uremic toxins (*open triangles*), diffuse through the membrane into the dialysate compartment. Conversely, solutes with higher concentration in the dialysate, such as bicarbonate (*closed triangles*), diffuse into the blood compartment. Solutes, such as sodium and chloride (*open circles*), with concentrations nearly equivalent in the two compartments, move little across the membrane. ***B,*** Convection across a semipermeable membrane. Hydrostatic pressure applied to the blood compartment causes the solvent to flow across the membrane into the dialysate compartment, bringing along solutes. As a result, for solutes with a sieving coefficient close to 1, there is no change in concentrations in the blood compartment with time.

tioning kidney transplants, whereas the remainder was maintained on dialysis. Both the prevalence and the incidence of ESRD vary greatly with age (Figure 16–2). The high incidence-to-prevalence ratio reflects a high mortality rate, especially in older age groups. The incidence is higher for men (404/million) than for women (280/million) (Figure 16–3), and the disease shows an ethnic predilection for African-Americans and Native Americans (Figure 16–4). The causes of ESRD are listed in Table 16–2. Since 1980, the percentage of patients with diabetic kidney disease has increased from near 0% to 45% of patients initiating dialysis in 2001, primarily because of increased acceptance of diabetic patients into dialysis programs. Before 1980, the reported outcome of diabetic patients receiving long-term hemodialysis was so poor that maintenance hemodialysis was not recommended.[31] Today the mortality rate remains higher than the average, but diabetes mellitus has become the most common cause of ESRD.[30] Mortality rates for patients with diabetic kidney disease also rise with age, but a higher mortality rate is apparent in younger type I diabetic patients, as shown in Figure 16–5.

The cause of the high ESRD mortality documented in the United States, compared with other countries, is controversial.[32] Speculation ranges from delivery of relatively inadequate dialysis or more liberal acceptance of patients in the United States to inadequate records of mortality kept in other countries. Although the survival of dialysis patients has slowly improved in the last 10 years, it remains greater than 20% per year in the United States. Statistics from the United States Renal Data System (USRDS) show a 79% 1-year survival, 65% 2-year survival, and 38% 5-year survival.[30] Causes of death[30] are listed in Table 16–3. Greater than 50% are due to cardiovascular disease, but it is unclear whether the uremic milieu, coexisting medical illnesses, or dialysis itself accounts for the high mortality (see Chapter 12). Seventeen percent of deaths in the United States occurred after voluntary withdrawal of dialysis, presumably because the patient's quality of life was

Table 16–1 Solutes Present in Dialysate

Component	Concentration (mEq/L)
Sodium	135–145
Potassium	0–4.0
Chloride	102–106
Bicarbonate	30–39
Acetate	2–4
Calcium	0–3.5
Magnesium	0.5–1.0
Dextrose	11
pH	7.1–7.3

not sufficient to justify its continuation. This relatively high withdrawal rate probably reflects the ready availability and aggressive approach to initiating dialysis in the United States by all parties involved in that decision, including the patient.

As shown in Figure 16–6, the incidence of ESRD in the United States has steadily increased,[30] most likely as a result of aging of the population and increasing acceptance of dialysis for older patients as part of their Medicare entitlement. The most recent analyses of the USRDS data suggest a leveling off in the rate of rise in the incidence (Figure 16–6).

UREMIA: THE TARGET OF HEMODIALYSIS

Uremia is the clinical state or syndrome that is reversed by dialysis therapy, and it literally means "urine in the blood." Whether or not urine output falls, all patients with uremia accumulate solutes, collectively known as *uremic toxins.* It is this accumulation of solute, the most abundant of which is *urea*, that justified the application of dialysis as a treatment for uremia.[4] From another perspective, the concept of uremia as a state of intoxication by substances normally eliminated by the kidney is supported by the success of therapeutic dialysis.

Clinical Syndrome

Although not all patients exhibit all of the symptoms and signs of uremia, the monotony of the clinical syndrome in patients with widely divergent causes of kidney failure indicates that the syndrome is the consequence of the kidney failure per se, not the underlying disease. Nearly every organ system is involved, but the most highly targeted are the gastrointestinal tract and the central nervous system. Early symptoms include dysgeusia, loss of appetite, nausea, weight loss, inability to concentrate on a mental task, lethargy, daytime sleepiness, pruritus, and menstrual irregularity in women. Unfortunately, these symptoms are not specific. They appear in most patients only at an

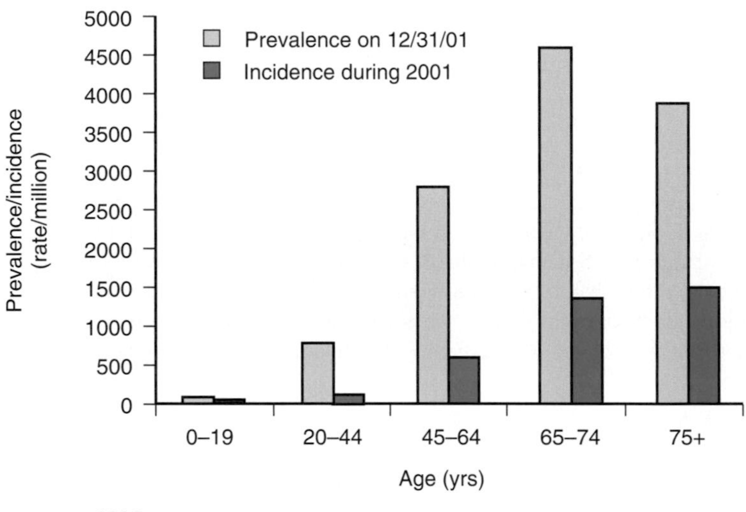

Figure 16–2 Prevalence and incidence of ESRD with age. (Adapted from USRDS: Excerpts from the United States Renal Data System 2003 annual data report. Am J Kidney Dis 2003; 42:S37-S181.)

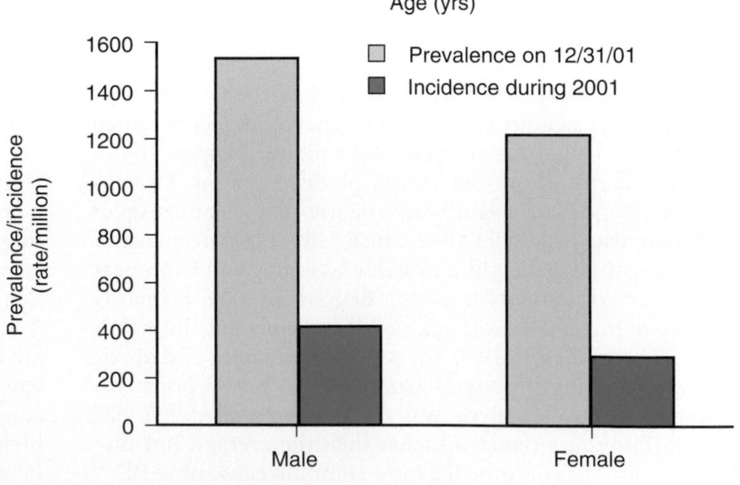

Figure 16–3 Prevalence and incidence of ESRD with sex. (Adapted from USRDS: Excerpts from the United States Renal Data System 2003 annual data report. Am J Kidney Dis 2003; 42:S37-S181.)

Table 16–2 Causes of End-Stage Renal Disease in the United States from 1997 to 2001

Primary Renal Disease	N	% Total
Diabetes mellitus	198,397	43.9
Hypertension	118,463	26.2
Glomerulonephritis	41,218	9.1
Interstitial nephritis/pyelonephritis	16,968	3.8
Cystic/hereditary/congenital diseases	14,509	3.2
Secondary glomerulonephritis/ vasculitis	10,183	2.2
Neoplasms/tumors	8769	1.9
Miscellaneous	18,096	4.1
Unknown	17,862	4.0
Missing data	7561	1.7
All ESRD	452,026	100

Data from USRDS: Excerpts from the United States Renal Data System 2003 annual data report. Am J Kidney Dis 2003; 42:S37-S181.

advanced stage of kidney damage (80% to 90% loss of nephrons). Far advanced symptoms and signs include uremic serositis with pericarditis, once the harbinger of death due to uremia; central nervous system suppression leading to uremic coma; overt peripheral neuropathy; and uremic fetor due to volatile amines emitted in the breath.

Fluid accumulation, which is subtle in most patients, contributes to hypertension that eventually leads to cardiac hypertrophy and diastolic dysfunction. The latter may precipitate congestive heart failure. Because cardiovascular disease is the most common cause of death in hemodialyzed patients, increasing attention has been focused on this aspect of the uremic syndrome and on blood pressure and other risk factors for cardiovascular complications, especially in the early phases of kidney failure (see Chapter 12).

Uremic Toxins

Most of the solutes known to accumulate in uremia (Table 16–4) are low in molecular weight and consequently are dialyzable.

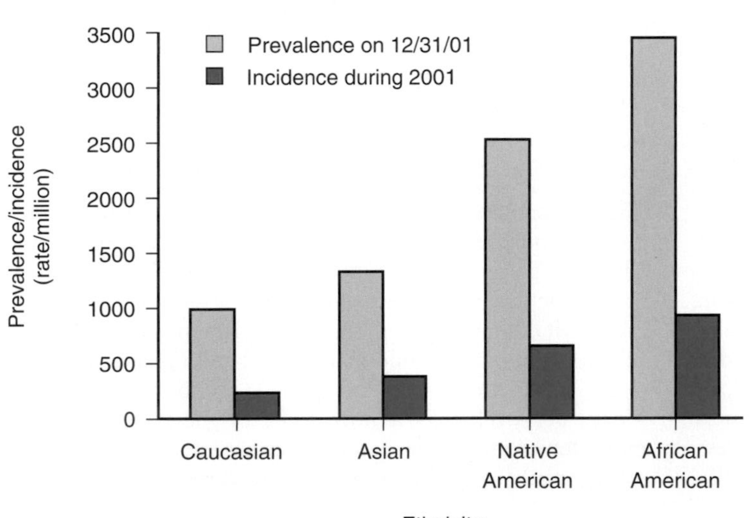

Figure 16–4 Prevalence and incidence of ESRD with ethnicity. (Adapted from USRDS: Excerpts from the United States Renal Data System 2003 annual data report. Am J Kidney Dis 2003; 42:S37-S181.)

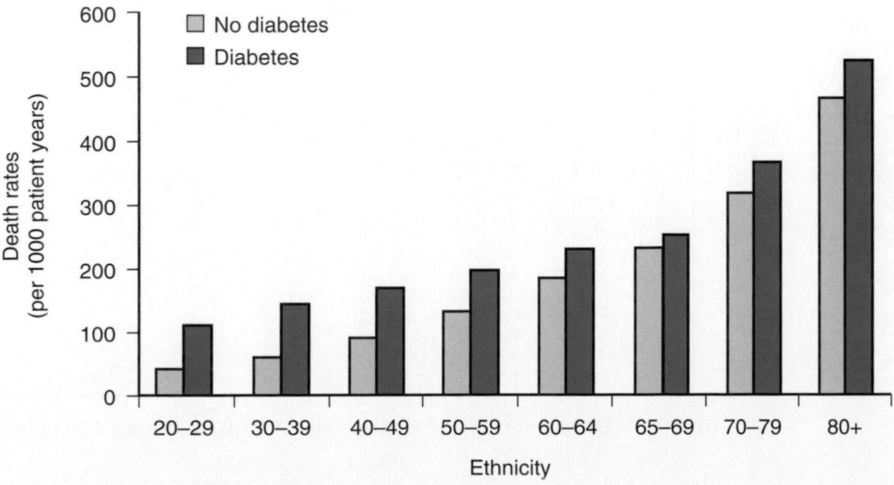

Figure 16–5 Mortality rates for diabetic and nondiabetic patients vary with age. (Adapted from USRDS: Excerpts from the United States Renal Data System 2003 annual data report. Am J Kidney Dis 2003; 42:S37-S181.)

Table 16–3 Causes of Death for Dialysis Patients Aged 45 to 64 by Sex (1999–2001)

	% of Deaths	
Cause of Death	**Male**	**Female**
Cardiovascular disease	50	46
Cardiac arrest	23	22
Acute myocardial infarction	10	8
Cerebrovascular	5	6
Other cardiac	12	10
Infection	15	17
Malignancy	4	3
Other known causes	24	25
Unknown	8	8

Data from USRDS: Excerpts from the United States Renal Data System 2003 annual data report. Am J Kidney Dis 2003; 42:S37-S181.

Some originate from food (e.g., sodium and phosphorus), whereas others are products of metabolism (e.g., urea, uric acid, and hydrogen ion). Routine clinical measurements include serum levels of the electrolytes sodium, potassium, bicarbonate, and chloride; the nitrogenous substances urea, creatinine, and uric acid; and other substances, such as magnesium, calcium, phosphate, and intact parathyroid hormone. Serum pH is not usually measured, but the serum bicarbonate concentration inversely reflects acid accumulation in the patient. Serum aluminum and β_2-microglobulin levels are useful in some patients. Outside of these readily available solute levels, serum levels of the other solutes in Table 16–4 are not clinically useful.

Although urea is a poor marker of native kidney function, it has special significance in ESRD patients because it is the most abundant solute to accumulate and because its accumulation results from both generation (from protein catabolism) and failure of renal excretion. Because urea generation is an index of protein nutrition, monitoring urea levels is potentially doubly important. However, this dual origin of urea complicates interpretation of any measured level, rendering it nearly useless unless additional measurements are taken to identify the relative contributions. Mathematical models of urea kinetics applied to serum urea concentrations measured before and after dialysis treatments allow separation of protein catabolism from the contributions of dialyzer and native kidney function. As discussed in more detail subsequently, this modeling process currently forms the basis for quantifying and prescribing hemodialysis (see Quantifying Hemodialysis).

Other substances proposed as uremic toxins include carbamylated proteins from posttranslational modification by high concentrations of urea and cyanate,[33,34] advanced glycation end products from the Maillard reaction between 3-deoxyglucosone and the terminal NH_2 groups of proteins,[35-37] β_2-microglobulin,[38] uric acid,[39] *p*-cresol,[39,40] parathyroid hormone,[41,42] granulocyte inhibiting proteins,[40] hydrogen ion and metabolic acidosis,[43] homocysteine,[44-46] other organic and phenolic acids,[47] advanced lipoxidation end products,[48,49] and advanced oxidation protein products.[48,49] Some of these substances have been linked with specific diseases:

- β_2-microglobulin and advanced glycation end products with amyloidosis[35,38,50,51]
- Advanced glycation end products and parathyroid hormone with heart disease[36,37,41,42]
- Uric acid, *p*-cresol, and granulocyte inhibiting protein with immune dysfunction[39,40,52]
- Phenolic acids, dicarboxylic acids and guanidines variably with inhibition of erythropoiesis, shortened red blood cell life span, and neurologic symptoms in animals[47,53]
- Both phenolic acids and dicarboxylic acids with impaired protein binding of drugs[47]
- Advanced lipoxidation end products, advanced oxidation protein products, and homocysteine with atherosclerosis[46,48,54]

These substances are thought to evoke their toxicity by (1) progressive bulk accumulation (e.g., β_2-microglobulin and advanced glycation end products), (2) upsetting the oxidation-reduction balance (e.g., uric acid and *p*-cresol), (3) binding to vital signaling and transport proteins (e.g., phenolic acids), (4) altering second messengers, and (5) altering nitric oxide production.[49,55,56] Traditional hemodialysis applied 3 days per week may remove some of these uremic toxins more slowly or not at all because they are larger in size, are not readily available to the dialyzer (sequestered in remote com-

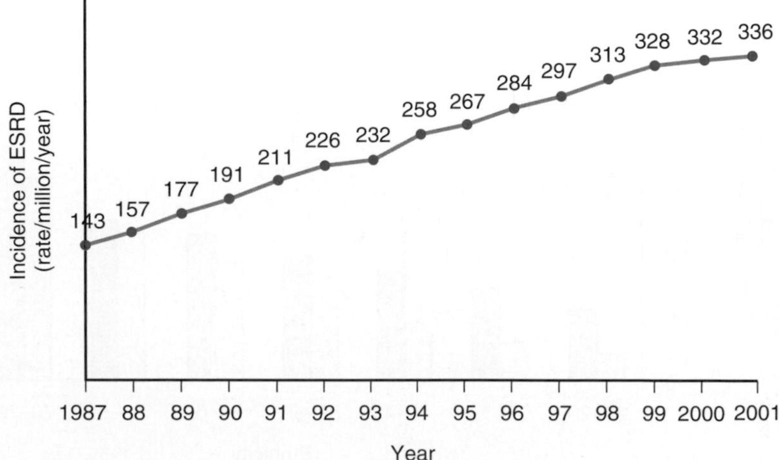

Figure 16–6 Incidence of ESRD in the United States with time. (Adapted from USRDS: Excerpts from the United States Renal Data System 2003 annual data report. Am J Kidney Dis 2003; 42:S37-S181.)

Table 16–4 Solutes That Accumulate in Uremia and Their Proposed Toxicity (If Known)

Solute	Proposed Toxicity
Low molecular weight (<500 daltons)	
Sodium	Volume overload
Potassium	Arrhythmia, muscle weakness
Hydrogen ion (metabolic acidosis)[43]	Degrades protein (activates ubiquitin proteasome); alters vitamin D and parathyroid hormone levels
Urea[65,66]	None
Creatinine	None
Phosphate	Osteodystrophy
Magnesium	Muscle weakness
Uric acid[39]	Disturbs calcitriol production and metabolism; ? immune dysfunction
Guanidines[47]	Immune dysfunction
Hippuric acid[47]	Muscle weakness; neurologic symptoms; decreases drug binding to albumin
Indoxyl sulfate[47]	Displaces drugs bound to albumin; glomerulosclerosis
p-cresol[39]	Immune dysfunction
Oxalic acid[47]	Tissue deposits; inhibits endothelial cell replication and migration
3-carboxyl-4-methyl-5-propyl-2-furanproprionic acid[47]	Displaces drugs bound to albumin; inhibits erythropoiesis; inhibits mitochondrial oxidation
4-hydroxybenzoic acid (phenolic acid)[47]	Platelet dysfunction; shortened red cell survival; neurologic symptoms
Quinolinic acid[47]	Inhibits erythropoiesis; seizures in mice
Homocysteine[44]	Accelerated atherosclerosis
Middle (500–5000 daltons) and high (5000–50,000 daltons) molecular weight	
Parathyroid hormone[41,42]	Inhibits mitochondrial oxidation; hypertrophic cardiomyopathy; cardiac fibrosis; immune dysfunction
β_2-microglobulin[35,38,50,51]	Dialysis amyloidosis
Carbamylated proteins[33,34]	? Accelerated atherosclerosis
Advanced glycation end products[35-37]	Dialysis amyloidosis; accelerated atherosclerosis
Granulocyte inhibitory proteins[40]	Immune dysfunction

Some of the low-molecular-weight solutes behave similarly to middle-molecular-weight solutes because of significant protein binding.

partments),[57] or are protein bound.[58,59] However, if the total duration of hemodialysis or hemodiafiltration is increased and administered over 6 days per week, removal of larger or sequestered molecules and even some protein-bound substances improves significantly.[60-62]

Despite its importance as a measure of dialysis adequacy, urea itself has demonstrated little toxicity in experiments where urea was added to the dialysate to prevent its removal.[63,64] Similarly, although all other solutes mentioned accumulate in kidney failure, their levels are well below that necessary to evoke toxic responses in animals and in humans, even when measured in patients with overt signs of uremia, such as pericarditis or uremic coma.[65,66] Even after decades of research, investigators are unable to identify a single toxin or a group of toxins responsible for the immediate life-threatening uremic syndrome that is quickly reversed by dialysis.[47, 63, 65-69] Because dialysis does little more than remove fluid and dialyzable solutes, the uremic syndrome must result from a rapid accumulation of known and unknown toxins in aggregate, perhaps each at subtoxic levels.

Residual Syndrome

It is now clear that the amount of dialysis necessary to sustain life is not enough to maintain a high quality of life. A challenge to current investigators is the development of techniques for analyzing and treating this "residual syndrome," which affects some patients more than others but reduces the quality of life despite apparently adequate dialysis. At present, several components of the syndrome can be identified, such as anemia, osteodystrophy, dialysis amyloidosis, and accelerated atherosclerosis, some of which are treatable (see Chapters 12 to 15). The proposed uremic toxins discussed previously may account, in part, for the residual syndrome, but, almost certainly, other components remain to be defined.[49,56,58,69] These components include: (1) the cause of inflammation in dialysis patients,[70-73] (2) the cause of malnutrition and accelerated atherosclerosis,[74-78] (3) the role of hyperhomocysteinemia in accelerated atherosclerosis[44,45] and graft thrombosis,[46,79] (4) the role of hyperphosphatemia in cardiovascular disease,[80-82] and (5) the interaction between malnutrition, inflammation, and atherosclerosis.[76-78] The effectiveness of increasing the frequency of dialysis to eliminate the residual syndrome remains to be proven. It is equally possible that the syndrome results from toxins that are poorly dialyzable because of protein binding in the blood or tissues or sequestration of toxins in compartments other than the blood.

Goals of Hemodialysis

The primary goal of hemodialysis is the replacement of renal excretory function. There is no doubt that hemodialysis can sustain life in patients who have no kidney function. Survival for as long as 30 years has been documented for hemodialysis alone, a treatment that does nothing more for the patient than remove solute.[83] Moreover, the molecular weight range of effectively removed solutes was relatively low until recent years when *high-flux* dialysis membranes were introduced.[84] The earlier experience indicates that the most life-threatening toxins are easily dialyzable. Precise goals and standards of dialysis adequacy have been defined, based on outcome studies in large populations, in terms of the clearance of small-molecular-weight, easily dialyzed solutes, the marker for which is urea.[28,85,86]

A prospective interventional study of dialysis adequacy in the late 1970s, the U.S. National Cooperative Dialysis Study (NCDS), provided clear-cut evidence for a level of urea clearance that was inadequate.[87] More recent uncontrolled experience suggests that more dialysis is better for the patient[88-94] (see Chapter 3). Analysis of solute kinetics, however, suggests that the benefit of more dialysis is logarithmically related to the amount of dialysis and that a point may be reached beyond which more dialysis does nothing more than inconvenience the patient, potentially worsening the quality of life.

This theoretical construct was confirmed recently by the National Institutes of Health (NIH)–sponsored Hemodialysis (HEMO) Study, a multicenter prospective clinical trial that randomized 1846 patients to receive hemodialysis with a target equilibrated Kt/V of 1.05 (equivalent to single pool Kt/V of 1.25, the generally accepted minimal standard at the time of the study) versus 1.45 (equivalent to single pool 1.65).[95] The subjects were further randomized to receive dialysis using a high-flux membrane (β_2-microglobulin clearance >20 mL/min) versus a low-flux membrane (clearance <10 mL/min). More dialysis or the use of a high-flux membrane did not reduce mortality, reduce hospitalization rates for infection or cardiovascular disease, or maintain serum albumin levels. Although subgroup analysis showed slightly less first cardiovascular hospitalizations for patients treated with high-flux membranes[95] and slightly lower mortality for women treated with a higher urea clearance,[96] these findings were of borderline significance and must be confirmed by other studies before they can be applied clinically. As with any randomized study, the power of the study diminishes and the probability of error increases exponentially when subgroups are analyzed. For now, hemodialysis patients should receive a urea clearance (Kt/V) of at least 1.2. Whether more frequent dialysis in the form of daily short-duration hemodialysis or daily nocturnal hemodialysis will reduce further mortality or morbidity remains to be determined.

A secondary goal of hemodialysis treatment is the replacement of hormones normally produced by the kidney. Even before dialysis therapy was available, the devastating effects of vitamin D "resistance" were evident, and much was written about renal rickets in children and osteomalacia in adults, even before 1900.[97] When 1,25-dihydroxyvitamin D (calcitriol), an activated form of vitamin D, was isolated in 1969 from renal proximal tubular cells, where it is formed from the precursor 25-hydroxyvitamin D, the puzzle was solved.[98,99] The subsequent synthesis of calcitriol allowed clinical nephrologists to replace this vital hormone[100] and prevent renal osteodystrophy, one of the most devastating long-term complications of renal failure[101] (see Chapter 14). In contrast to bone disease, there was less mystery about the anemia of kidney failure, which was a recognized effect of deficient erythropoietin, a hormone uniquely synthesized by the kidney and responsible for activation of bone marrow erythroid precursors.[102-104] Even before dialysis is necessary, hemoglobin levels begin to decline, causing a syndrome of anemia that has subtle adverse effects on multiple organ systems.[105-107] The synthesis and widespread availability of erythropoietin in the late 1980s and early 1990s removed the transfusion dependency for nearly all patients and improved the quality of life for most patients by raising the average blood hemoglobin concentration[105-107] (Chapter 15). Recent advances in the field of hormone replacement include the availability of (1) calcitriol analogues (e.g., paricalcitol and doxecalciferol that also suppress parathyroid hormone but cause less hypercalcemia) and (2) darbepoietin-α, an erythropoietin derivative with additional glycoproteins attached, conferring a longer half-life (see Chapters 14 and 15).

In addition to the need for dialysis, patients require extensive psychologic and social services support to cope with their own emotional reactions to loss of a vital organ. Nutritional counseling is also important, primarily to limit fluid gains between dialyses, to control hyperphosphatemia (phosphate is removed poorly by standard hemodialysis), to reduce the life-threatening risk of hyperkalemia, and to prevent malnutrition (a major yet potentially reversible risk for morbidity and mortality). Successful treatment and rehabilitation of the whole patient requires intensive initial emotional support and prolonged surveillance of the patient's nutrition.

DIALYSIS

As defined previously, dialysis is a process of diffusion of molecules in solution across a semipermeable membrane. Forces that govern the pattern and rate of diffusion have been defined in precise mathematical terms that include properties of the molecule, the solvent, and the membrane. The salient points of the physics of dialysis are discussed here because a detailed analysis is beyond the scope of this chapter. For detailed analysis of the physical laws that govern dialysis, the reader is referred to formal texts on kinetic modeling.[108-110]

Laws of Diffusion

Diffusion is a consequence of random molecular movements (*molecular kinetics*) that follow the laws of probability and are driven by temperature, pressure, and concentration. Since temperature and pressure are relatively constant during therapeutic dialysis and among dialysis centers (see later), the major clinical variable that affects diffusion is the solute concentration. Fick's law of diffusion, derived from mathematical laws of statistical probability, shows that the rate of diffusion is linearly dependent on the *concentration gradient* (i.e., the driving force for diffusion):

$$J = -(DA/X)\Delta C \qquad (1)$$

J is *solute flux* (mg/min), which, when applied to a membrane, can be viewed as the unidirectional rate of movement of a solute across the membrane (Figure 16–1*A*). ΔC is the concentration gradient across the membrane (mg/mL), A is the membrane area (cm^2), X is the membrane thickness (cm), and D is a constant, called the *coefficient of diffusion* or diffusivity (cm^2/min). The last-mentioned is a measure of the permeability of the membrane material to the measured solute, independent of solute concentration, area, and thickness. Conventionally, a minus sign is placed on the right side of

Equation 1 to indicate that solute moves away from the dialyzed compartment. Equation 1 reflects the intuitive concept that diffusion across a membrane varies directly with the membrane area and solute concentration gradient and inversely with the membrane thickness.

Dividing both sides of Equation 1 by ΔC results in an expression for *solute dialysance*:

$$J/\Delta C = -\text{ dialysance} = -\ DA/X \quad (2)$$

Equation 2 shows that dialysance is always independent of concentration and is constant throughout a static dialysis despite changes in concentration on either side of the membrane. Clinicians rarely use the concept of dialysance, opting instead to describe dialysis in terms of *clearance*. This is reasonable because clearance is derived from measurements only on the blood side of the membrane, where clinical analytic techniques are readily available. The only difference between dialysance and clearance is the substitution of blood side C for ΔC in Equation 2:

$$J/C = -\text{ clearance} = -\ K \quad (3)$$

When the concentration of solute on the dialysate side is 0, $\Delta C = C$, and clearance is equal to dialysance. This condition exists at the start of a dialysis procedure and during all single-pass dialysis (see Hemodialysis). For all other conditions, ΔC is less than C, so clearance is lower than dialysance. Dialysance may also be considered the *unidirectional flux* of solute across the membrane from the blood to the dialysate compartment.

If the *volume of the dialyzed compartment* (*V*) is constant, dividing both sides of Equation 3 by V shows that the fractional rate of change in concentration is constant:

$$(J/V)/C = -\ K/V = -\ k \quad (4)$$

The symbol *k* is called the *rate constant*. The constantly changing term *J/V*, when expressed at any given instant, is dC/dt and therefore (J/V)/C is (dC/C)/dt. The latter can be viewed as the fractional change in concentration over an initial short period of time (*dt*):

$$(dC/C)/dt = -\ K/V = -\ k \quad (5)$$

Equation 5 demonstrates that concentration-dependent diffusion is a *first order process*; that is, despite the minute-to-minute changes in concentration within the dialyzed compartment, the fractional rate of change is constant when the dialysate concentration remains zero. Flux of solute across the membrane, which is the goal of dialysis, is both driven by the concentration and expressed as a change in concentration. When the rate of change is factored by the driving force [(dC/dt)/C)], the resulting fractional rate of change is constant.

The rate constant (k) has units of time^{-1} or a fraction per unit of time and is a function of both the molecular properties of size, shape, charge, and interaction with the membrane, and of the membrane itself, including its surface area, porosity, and thickness. Large molecules, those with complex shapes, and those with an electric charge diffuse less readily across the membrane. Membranes that are more porous, have larger surface, and are thinner favor passage of solutes by diffusion. Although the rate constant is useful to demonstrate the first order concept, it is of less practical value than the expression for clearance depicted in Equation 3.

The difference between the rate constant (k) in Equation 4 and the clearance (K) shown in Equation 3 is *V*, the volume of solute distribution. Equation 3 has the advantage of expressing the dialysis effect as a volume equivalent of solute diffusing across the membrane per unit of time. The volume transferred per unit of time is constant; that is, a milliliter equivalent of solute is transferred per unit of time regardless of how much solute is contained in that milliliter. The rate of diffusion is directly proportional to the membrane surface area, which is constant for any given model of dialyzer.

Effects of Temperature, Pressure, and Molecular Weight

Diffusion is a consequence of molecular motion, which is affected by pressure and heat energy and by molecular mass. The rate of diffusion is proportional to the absolute temperature, which is approximately 273°K at room temperature. Within the range of temperatures experienced in the dialysis center, the proportionate change in absolute temperature (260°K to 280°K) is so small that its influence on diffusion across the dialysis membrane is negligible. More important are the physiologic effects of temperature on blood flow and body water compartmentalization, which have significant effects on solute kinetics within the patient (see Quantifying Hemodialysis). Similarly, pressure effects have little influence on diffusion, within the range of pressures recorded in modern dialyzers.

Molecular mass plays a more significant role in determining the rate of diffusion because at a given temperature and pressure, the heavier molecules move more slowly and collide with the semipermeable membrane less frequently. Small-molecular-weight substances, such as urea and creatinine, diffuse readily across a semipermeable membrane, whereas larger substances, such as β_2-microglobulin or albumin, diffuse slowly or not at all. The larger size of the heavier molecules further impedes diffusion through small pores.

Dialysate

Preparation of the dialysate and its composition are critical to the success of dialysis. For hemodialysis, the solution must be prepared from properly treated water (see Chapter 5) and contain the solutes listed in Table 16–1 in concentrations comparable to those of plasma. Dialysate must have a low concentration of endotoxin to prevent pyrogen reactions in the patient, but, in contrast to peritoneal dialysate (see Chapter 10), sterility is not a requirement because the semipermeable membrane excludes large particles, such as bacteria and viruses. Vital electrolytes and glucose are added to the dialysate to reduce or abolish their concentration gradients, whereas bicarbonate or a bicarbonate precursor is added in higher concentrations to promote accumulation in the patient. Dialysate glucose concentrations are near those of plasma; thus, in contrast to peritoneal dialysis, osmotic forces do not play an important role in removing fluid.

In practice, solute concentrations in the dialysate are fairly standard. The most common concentrations that may be individualized are those for potassium, calcium, and bicarbonate (Table 16–1). In many dialysis centers, the bicarbonate concentration is fixed at 35 or 39 mEq/L. Potassium ranges from 0 to 4 mEq/L, depending on the patient's serum concentration before dialysis. A compelling reason must exist, however, to use dialysate potassium concentrations of 0 or 1 mEq/L because of the dangers associated with a precipitous drop in the serum concentration. In particular, patients on digoxin must be dialyzed against at least 2 mEq/L of potassium. Calcium concentrations vary from 1 to 3.5 mEq/L. At the lower concentration, calcium is removed from the patient, whereas at the higher concentration, calcium diffuses into the patient during dialysis. The concentration of sodium is usually fixed at 140 mEq/L, which is the middle of the normal range in whole plasma. Although the concentration in plasma water is closer to 150 mEq/L, the Gibbs-Donnan effect of negatively charged plasma proteins reduces the sodium concentration in completely equilibrated dialysate closer to 140 mEq/L.[111,112]

HEMODIALYZERS

A *hemodialyzer*, synonymous with *dialyzer*, is often called an "artificial kidney." It is configured to allow blood and dialysate to flow, preferably in opposite directions, through individual compartments, separated by a semipermeable membrane. By convention, blood entering the hemodialyzer is designated *arterial*, whereas blood leaving the hemodialyzer is *venous*. The principal differences among the many available hemodialyzers are the membrane composition, membrane configuration, and membrane surface area. Hemodialyzers affect the efficiency and the quality of dialysis by virtue of their membranes, which determine their K_OA value, and by the rates of blood and dialysate flow, which determine their clearance values (see later discussion of K_OA) (Table 16–5).

Membrane Composition, Configuration, and Surface Area

Composition of the Membrane

Two major classes of membrane material are available commercially: (1) cotton fiber, or *cellulose-based membranes*, and (2) *synthetic membranes*. Cellulose-based membranes range from unmodified cellulose to substituted cellulose membranes. Unmodified cellulose membranes have many free hydroxyl groups, which are thought to be responsible for their bioincompatibility and propensity to activate white blood cells, platelets, and serum complement. In an effort to improve membrane biocompatibility while keeping costs down, the cellulose polymer is treated with acetate and tertiary amino compounds to form a covalent bond with the hydroxyl groups (e.g., cellulose acetate and aminated cellulose—Cellosyn or Hemophan). Further issues of biocompatibility are covered in detail in Chapter 2.

The major polymers in commercial synthetic membranes are polyacrylonitrile, polysulfone, polycarbonate, polyamide, and polymethylmethacrylate. Despite their increased thickness, these membranes can be rendered more permeable than the cellulose membranes, allowing for greater fluid and solute removal. They are also more biocompatible. Because the pore sizes in the synthetic membranes can be made wider, larger-molecular-weight substances, such as β_2-microglobulin, can be removed more efficiently.[113,114] High flux synthetic membranes also clear phosphate more efficiently, although the effect on serum phosphate levels is minimal. Despite their increased cost, synthetic hemodialyzers are increasingly preferred: 50% to 86% of new patients in 1996[115] compared with 36% in 1993 and 15% in 1990.[116]

Table 16–5 Key Factors That Affect the Solute Clearance of a Hemodialyzer

Properties of the Membrane
↑ Membrane porosity
↓ Membrane thickness
↑ Membrane surface area
Properties of the Solute
↓ Molecular weight and size
Shape
↓ Charge
Blood Side
↓ Unstirred blood layer
↑ Blood flow
Dialysate Side
↓ Dialysate channeling and unstirred layer
↑ Dialysate flow
↑ Countercurrent direction of flow

↑, Increases clearance; ↓, decreases clearance.

Plate Versus Hollow Fiber Dialyzers

All current hemodialyzers are constructed with a plastic casing, usually polycarbonate. The *plate dialyzer* is made with flat membrane sheets stacked on top of each other and anchored at the two ends of the casing. Blood and dialysate flow through alternating layers of the membrane in opposite directions. The plate design has been less thrombogenic, requiring less heparin, but the tendency to thrombosis is reduced in more recent models of both plate and hollow-fiber design.[117] The main disadvantages of the plate design are the slightly higher priming volume required to fill the blood compartment (100 to 120 mL) and the expansion of the blood compartment that occurs when transmembrane pressure (TMP) increases during dialysis.

The blood compartment of the *hollow fiber dialyzer* is 60 to 120 mL and does not increase during dialysis. Several thousand of the membrane fibers, each approximately 200 μm in inside diameter, are imbedded in a *potting material*, usually polyurethane, at each end of the casing. The casing closely surrounds the fiber bundle, forcing dialysate to flow between and around each fiber in the direction usually opposite to blood flow. Blood flows to or from the open end of each fiber through a removable *header* attached to the blood tubing. In addition to a lower blood priming volume, the hollow-fiber design increases the area of contact between blood and dialysate, allowing for the most efficient exchange of solutes. Major disadvantages of the hollow-fiber design are thrombosis, and the requirement for a potting compound, which absorbs chemicals used to disinfect newly manufactured dialyzers (ethylene oxide) or reused dialyzers (formaldehyde, peracetic acid, or glutaraldehyde). These chemicals then leach slowly from the material and potentially enter the patient's blood during dialysis (see Chapter 2).

Surface Area Considerations

Most hemodialyzers have a membrane surface area of 0.8 to 2.1 m². As the area increases, the efficiency of the dialyzer increases. To maximize membrane surface area, one can increase the length of the hollow fiber, increase the number of hollow fibers, or decrease the diameter of the hollow fiber while holding other parameters constant.[118] Each of these maneuvers, however, has undesirable effects when carried too far. Increasing the fiber length increases shear rate and magnifies the pressure drop between blood entering and exiting the dialyzer. Increased shear rate increases ultrafiltration, whereas the pressure drop decreases ultrafiltration because the TMP gradient dissipates at the venous end of the dialyzer. Any decrease in ultrafiltration decreases its contribution to solute clearance and offsets the potential advantage of the increased surface area. Increasing the number of hollow fibers increases the volume of extracorporeal blood and may eventually compromise hemodynamic stability. Finally, as the diameter of the hollow fiber decreases, the resistance to blood flow increases and clotting is enhanced. As fibers thrombose, effective surface area for diffusion decreases and solute clearances fall. Because of these adverse consequences, the minimal acceptable internal fiber diameter is 180 μm.[118] The design and geometry of the hollow-fiber dialyzer represent a delicate balance among these factors.

The composition and the thickness of the membrane are usually more important than the surface area in determining dialyzer efficiency. In general, the thinner the membrane, the more efficient the transport of solutes and fluid across the membrane. Because of the high tensile strength of cellulose fibers, cellulose membranes are thinner than synthetic membranes, partially offsetting their inherent low flux.

Effects of Flow on Clearance

Blood Flow

Dialyzer blood flow (Q_b) is driven by a roller pump and generally ranges from 200 to 500 mL/min, depending on the type of vascular access. Blood flow influences the efficiency of solute removal (see Table 16–5).

As Q_b increases, more solute is presented per unit of time to the membrane, and solute removal increases. Urea removal rises steeply as Q_b increases to 300 mL/min, and although urea removal continues to rise as Q_b approaches 400 to 500 mL/min, the slope is less steep. For larger molecular weight substances, removal is slower and more time-dependent rather than flow-dependent because diffusion across the membrane is limited as discussed previously.

Dialysate Flow

Most dialysis centers use a *single pass* of dialysate; that is, the dialysate is discarded after one passage through the dialyzer. For sorbent dialysis, however, only about 5 L of water are used and dialysate is constantly regenerated by cycling through a cartridge system to remove the undesirable solutes (e.g., urea, creatinine, and potassium). Sorbent dialysis is rare because manufacture of the Redy dialysate delivery system stopped in the mid-1990s.

Countercurrent flow maximizes the concentration gradient between blood and dialysate throughout the length of the dialyzer (see Table 16–5). When blood flow and dialysate flow are in the same direction (*co-current*), solute removal decreases by about 10%.

In addition to decreasing boundary layers and streaming effects (see later discussion), increasing Q_d minimizes the accumulation of waste products in dialysate and provides a higher solute gradient between blood and dialysate for optimal diffusion. However, even for highly diffusible solutes, the benefits progressively diminish as the dialysate flow rate is increased above the blood flow rate.

K_OA: Mass Transfer Area Coefficient

K_OA is the product of the *mass transfer coefficient*, K_O, which has units of cm/min, and the membrane area, *A*. K_O is specific for a particular molecule and membrane type, including the membrane's pore size and thickness, but is independent of solute concentration and membrane surface area. It can be considered the solute flux per unit of area per unit of concentration gradient and is equivalent to D/X in Equation 6. Because solute flux per unit of concentration gradient is defined as dialysance, K_O may also be expressed as the dialysance per unit of membrane area. K_OA, which is the *mass transfer area coefficient*, therefore has units of mL/min and is equivalent to the dialysance of a membrane with a fixed area during static dialysis (no flow). In addition to being independent of solute concentration, K_OA is also independent of blood and dialysate flow within certain limits (see later text). Therefore, K_OA is the most specific constant that describes the efficiency of a dialyzer for removal of a particular solute and is the best parameter for comparing dialyzers. Higher values indicate more efficient solute removal.

K_OA has the same units of measurement as clearance and, in practical terms, can be considered the maximum clearance achievable for a particular dialyzer and solute. Maximum clearance is achieved at the beginning of dialysis when blood solute concentrations along the length of the dialyzer are equal (no flow) and dialysate concentration is 0 or, at the opposite extreme, when blood and dialysate flow rates are infinite. Under these two conditions, the only factor governing a solute's clearance is the dialysis membrane.

Conversely, when Q_b and Q_d are finite, the clearance is lower than K_OA because both flow rates govern diffusion, as discussed previously and because of the way clearance is expressed, as the solute removal rate divided by the *inflow concentration*. The net driving force for removal is the *mean concentration gradient* across the membrane, which is a complex function of Q_b and Q_d (see next section). The increase in clearance caused by an increase in Q_b is the result of a flow-dependent increase in the mean concentration gradient across the membrane, driving more solute into the dialysate. Because the inflow concentration does not change with increased Q_b, the conventional measure of clearance as defined previously increases with increasing Q_b.

Relationships Between Flow, K_OA, and Solute Clearance

Because concentrations change logarithmically along the dialyzer membrane, the true mean concentration on either side of the membrane is actually the log mean concentration expressed:

$$\text{log mean } C = (C_{in} - C_{out}) / \ln(C_{in}/C_{out}) \quad (7)$$

where C_{in} and C_{out} represent inflow and outflow solute concentrations. Similarly, the mean gradient or concentration difference across the membrane, which is the driving force for diffusion, is actually the log mean concentration gradient. When flow is countercurrent, the log mean gradient is:

$$[(Cb_{in} - Cd_{out}) - (Cb_{out} - Cd_{in})/ \ln[(Cb_{in} - Cd_{out}) / (Cb_{out}/Cb_{in})] \quad (8)$$

where *Cb* depicts the blood concentration and *Cd* the dialysate concentration, and the subscripts *in* and *out* represent the dialyzer inflow and outflow. A rearrangement of Equation 2 shows that J, the solute flux (removal rate, e.g., in mg/min), can be expressed as the product of K_OA and the concentration gradient:

$$J = \text{Flux} = K_O A(\text{log mean gradient}) \quad (9)$$

Clearance (K_d), as defined for a device with flow, is the flux measured either on the blood side $[Q_b(Cb_{in} - Cb_{out})]$ or on the dialysate side $[Q_d(Cd_{in} - Cd_{out})]$ of the membrane divided by the inflow concentration:

$$K_d = Q_b(Cb_{in} - Cb_{out})/(Cb_{in}) = -Q_d(Cd_{in} - Cd_{out})/(Cb_{in}) \quad (10)$$

Combining Equations 3, 8, 9, and 10 yields a practical equation for calculating K_OA from an instantaneous measurement of solute clearance and both Q_b and Q_d when flow is countercurrent:

$$K_O A = \frac{Q_b \cdot Q_d}{Q_b - Q_d} \ln\left(\frac{Q_d(Q_b - K_d)}{(Q_b(Q_d - K_d)}\right) \quad (11)$$

A rearrangement of Equation 11 gives another practical equation for calculating expected clearance from Q_b, Q_d, and K_OA. This equation eliminates the need to measure blood concentrations to predict the effect of changes in flow on clearance:

$$K_d = Q_b\left[\frac{e^{K_O A \frac{Q_d - Q_b}{Q_d Q_b}} - 1}{e^{K_O A \frac{Q_d - Q_b}{Q_d Q_b}} - \frac{Q_b}{Q_d}}\right] \quad (12)$$

Boundary Layers and Streaming Effects

Despite a rapid flow along the membrane, the solvent tends to adhere to the membrane creating a *boundary layer*, or unstirred layer, that adds to the diffusive pathway on both sides of the membrane.[109] This layer of solvent adjacent to the membrane tends to thin out as flow is increased or as turbulence is produced at the membrane surface. In addition to forming boundary layers, dialysate tends to move along the path of least resistance or channel, leading to nonuniform flow and bypassing some of the membrane area. This *streaming effect* is more pronounced at lower dialysate flow rates, especially in large dialyzers. Both boundary layer and streaming effects cause K_OA (the resistance to solute diffusion across the membrane) to increase as dialysate flow increases,[119] although the effect is less *in vivo* than *in vitro*.[120,121] Recent changes in the shape of hollow fibers and the insertion of inert spacer yarns have improved dialyzer performance further through reducing the effects of channeling and unstirred layers.[122,123] Both effects are less prominent on the blood side of hollow fibers because of the geometric advantages of flow within hollow fibers, the scrubbing effects of red blood cells, and less variance in Q_b.

HEMODIALYSIS

Using dialysis as a form of therapy for the patient vastly complicates this otherwise simple procedure. Factors that complicate the delivery of dialysis include the access device, the patient's compliance with the dialysis prescription and diet, and solute disequilibrium. Developing standards of adequacy requires detailed studies of large populations, with careful attention to the multiple variables that influence outcome, in addition to the dialysis itself. Achieving target solute concentrations in the patient during and between treatments requires complex mathematical models with multiple variables to account for differences among patients, including differences in size and solute generation rate. These factors add considerable complexity to the relatively simple laws of diffusion and flow discussed earlier, so that the solutions to patient problems are often approximations at best.

Types of Clearance

As noted in the discussion of dialysis and depicted in Equation 2, dialyzer clearance is the solute removal rate (flux) factored by the blood inflow concentration. During single-pass dialysis, the flux of urea is directly proportional to the inflow concentration, so that urea clearance tends to be constant despite the fall in blood concentration with time. The simplest type of clearance is the *instantaneous dialyzer clearance*, which can be measured by sampling blood on both sides of the dialyzer while recording Q_b at any instant in time. Although the dialyzer urea clearance tends to remain constant, it may fall during treatment because of loss of surface area from clotting or because of changes in Q_b or Q_d. The *effective clearance*, or *integrated dialyzer clearance*, accounts for these changes by linking the measurement of clearance to the pre-dialysis and post-dialysis blood urea nitrogen (BUN). This clearance is essentially the answer to this question: What average urea clearance would be required to drive the BUN down to the measured post-dialysis value from the measured pre-dialysis value?

The mathematical solution requires a process known as *urea modeling* (see later Quantifying Dialysis). It can be calculated using either a single-compartment or a two-compartment urea kinetic model, entering a pre-dialysis and immediate post-dialysis BUN in the former case and multiple intra-dialysis and post-dialysis BUN in the latter case. In either case, the result is a *dialyzer urea clearance* that is not affected by urea disequilibrium. The integrated dialyzer clearance is often called the *delivered clearance* to distinguish it from the *prescribed clearance*. The latter is simply the expected clearance derived from the dialyzer K_OA and flow rates (see Equation 11).

During dialysis, solutes must diffuse from within the red blood cells and tissues into the blood to reach the dialyzer. Such compartmentalization of body fluids adds complexity to the concept of clearance because different values may be chosen for the denominator of Equation 3. Even for urea, which diffuses easily across cell membranes from tissue to blood, some disequilibrium still develops among the various body compartments during dialysis. As a result, the patient's clearance, or *whole body clearance*, is always less than the dialyzer clearance. Whole body clearance is a virtual clearance (not instantaneously measurable) derived from the pre-dialysis and *equilibrated* post-dialysis BUN. Like dialyzer clearance, it is also a mean clearance integrated over time on dialysis, but it accounts for the presence of solute disequilibrium.

Adding further complexity to the concept of clearance are the frequency and duration of dialysis. Because *residual native kidney clearance* (K_r) exerts most of its effect between dialyses when dialyzer clearance is zero, it cannot be directly added to dialyzer clearance (see Quantifying Hemodialysis). *Intermittent clearance*, as obtained with hemodialysis, is inherently less efficient than the *continuous clearance* of native kidneys or continuous peritoneal dialysis. There are two explanations for this reduced efficiency.

First, although dialyzer clearance is not compromised by an intermittent schedule, total solute removal tends to be reduced because blood solute concentration declines logarithmically and not linearly during dialysis (Figure 16–7).[110, 124, 125] Because solute levels do not change during continuous dialysis, this effect is absent, and solute removal is maximal at all times. Therefore, to reduce solute levels to a similar value, intermittent dialysis must be more intense when averaged over a week of treatment, as shown by the uppermost line in Figure 16–8. This explanation applies even in the absence of solute disequilibrium.

The second explanation applies to the more realistic situation in which solute concentration in the blood compartment is below that in other compartments as solute disequilibrium develops during dialysis. Here again, dialyzer clearance is unaffected, but solute access to the dialyzer is limited (see later further discussion of Solute Disequilibrium). For continuous replacement modalities and native kidney function, the blood solute concentration is stable, and the effect of solute disequilibrium is minimal, so clearances are easy to calculate:

$$\text{Native kidney urea clearance} = K_r = (U_{urea} \times V)/(P_{urea} \times t) \quad (13)$$

$$\text{Peritoneal urea clearance} = (D_{urea} \times V)/(P_{urea} \times t) \quad (14)$$

where U_{urea} is urinary urea concentration, P_{urea} is blood urea concentration, D_{urea} is peritoneal dialysate urea concentration, *t* is time, and *V* is 24-hour urinary volume for Equation 13 and 24-hour dialysate volume for Equation 14. Continuous clearances are easier to calculate but more difficult to measure than intermittent clearances. For hemodialysis, the clinician can take advantage of the dialysis-induced perturbations in urea concentrations to measure clearance and other patient variables that are not readily measurable by other means.

It is apparent from the previous discussion that the clearances measured during intermittent forms of dialysis are not directly comparable to native kidney clearance or clearances measured in patients undergoing continuous dialysis. These observations also help to explain the significant difference between the minimum recommended weekly dose of dialysis (Kt/V) for hemodialysis (1.2 per dialysis × 3 dialyses per week = 3.6/wk) and for peritoneal dialysis (2.0–2.2/wk). To allow a direct comparison, the following formulas adjust for intermittence by calculating the continuous equivalent of intermittent clearance (*equivalent Kt/V or EKR*). For intermittent therapy during a steady state of urea nitrogen balance[126]:

$$EKR_{mean} = \frac{\text{removal rate}}{\text{mean concentration}} = \frac{\text{generation rate}}{\text{mean concentration}} = \frac{G}{TAC} \quad (15)$$

$$EKR_{peak} = \frac{\text{generation rate}}{\text{peak concentration}} = \frac{G}{\text{Av Peak BUN}} \quad (16)$$

G and *TAC* are derived from formal urea modeling. Using Equation 15 and adjusting for time and patient volume, the quantity of hemodialysis necessary to keep a patient's time-averaged BUN constant falls from a weekly Kt/V of 3.6 for thrice-weekly treatments to an EKR of 2.8 for continuous treatment.[127] If mean peak urea is substituted for TAC in Equation 16, the EKR falls to approximately 2.0, consistent with the current clinically accepted minimum adequacy for

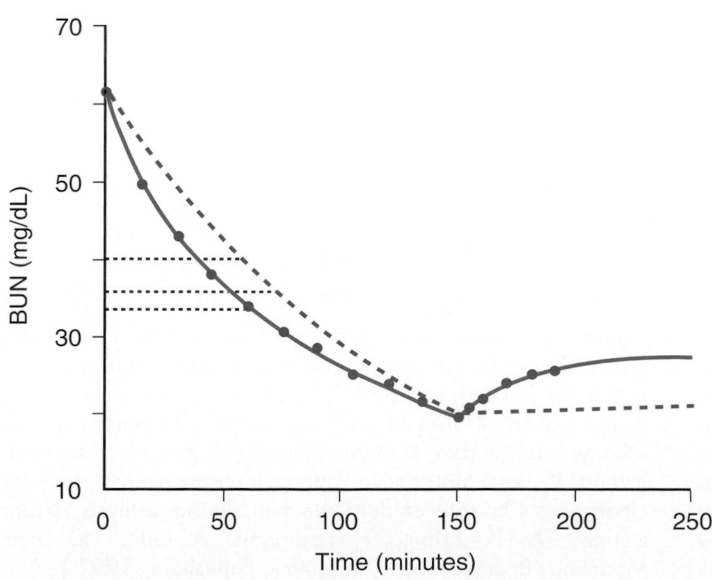

Figure 16–7 Changes in blood urea nitrogen (BUN) concentrations during and after dialysis. Measured BUN levels during and immediately after dialysis fit best into a two-compartment variable-volume mathematical model (*solid line*). The single-compartment variable-volume model (*dashed line*) overestimates BUN levels during the dialysis and fails to predict the rebound. The upper dotted horizontal line at 40 mg/dL is the simple arithmetic mean of the pre-dialysis and the post-dialysis BUN. The middle dotted horizontal line at 36 mg/dL represents the log mean BUN during the treatment, as predicted by the single-compartment model. The lower dotted horizontal line at 34 mg/dL is the true mean BUN, obtained from actual measurements throughout dialysis.

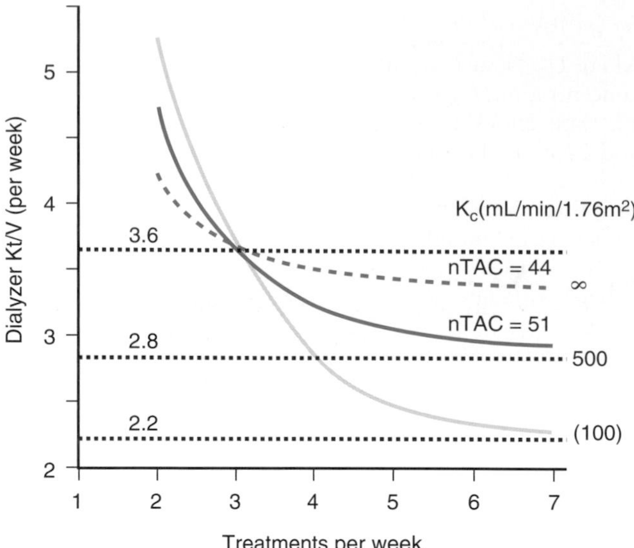

Figure 16–8 Urea kinetics value (Kt/V) required to maintain the same timed average urea concentration (TAC) of urea. To achieve the same mean blood urea nitrogen concentration, the dose of dialysis provided per week may be reduced as the frequency of dialysis increases. The upper solid line shows the required weekly Kt/V for urea based on an intercompartment mass transfer coefficient (K_C) of 500 mL/min. Even a simple single-compartment model with no resistance to diffusion in the patient (*dashed line* = infinite K_C) shows a dependence of weekly Kt/V on dialysis frequency. The discrepancy in weekly Kt/V between intermittent and continuous dialysis is even greater for a theoretic substance that dialyzes as well as urea but exhibits greater disequilibrium within the patient (*dotted line* = K_C of 100 mL/min). (Adapted from Depner TA: Quantifying hemodialysis and peritoneal dialysis: Examination of the peak concentration hypothesis. Semin Dial 1994; 7:315-317. Reprinted with permission of Blackwell Science, Inc.)

peritoneal dialysis[128] (see Chapter 8). Although the EKR_{peak} values calculated using the peak urea concentration (see Equation 16) better matches clinical experience, the argument that peak urea levels mediate uremic toxicity does not naturally follow since urea is relatively nontoxic.[125] Instead the relationship likely reflects a fortuitous difference between the diffusibility of urea and the true uremic toxins. One of the advantages of EKR is allowance of simple arithmetic addition of residual native kidney clearance to dialyzer clearance (see later text).

Quantifying Hemodialysis

Dialysis is a treatment born out of empiricism. Solute mass transport during dialysis was described in precise mathematical terms but only after dialysis was established as a life-sustaining treatment for patients with advanced renal failure. Much of the effort to describe the kinetics of transport has been devoted to determining how to best quantify the amount of dialysis prescribed and delivered. Because it is easy to measure and because the exact uremic toxin(s) are not known, mathematical models of urea kinetics have been used to quantify dialysis.

Mathematical Models of Urea Kinetics

Since urea is a small, highly soluble, yet uncharged molecule with little binding to proteins, it distributes only in aqueous environments and diffuses rapidly among the various body water compartments. The rate of diffusion is so rapid that a single space of distribution (total body water) can be assumed for most approximations. Between dialyses, when urea accumulates at a slow, constant rate and there is ample time for distribution among the compartments, this assumption is reasonable, and the single-pool, or *single-compartment kinetic model*, is appropriate. During dialysis, however, when blood concentrations change rapidly, urea gradients appear. Serum concentrations fall lower than predicted by the single-compartment model during dialysis and rebound after dialysis, as shown in Figure 16–7. Because of this disequilibrium, more complicated mathematical models were developed to better explain the behavior of urea during dialysis.

The *two-compartment model* (Figure 16–9) assumes that the body is divided into two pools of water, with a finite resistance to diffusion between them. The resistance is expressed inversely as the intercompartment mass transfer coefficient (K_C), which is a measure of the average solute conductivity among compartments for the particular solute. K_C is analogous to K_OA, is solute specific, and has units of measurement that are similar to K_OA (mL/min). The mathematical solution

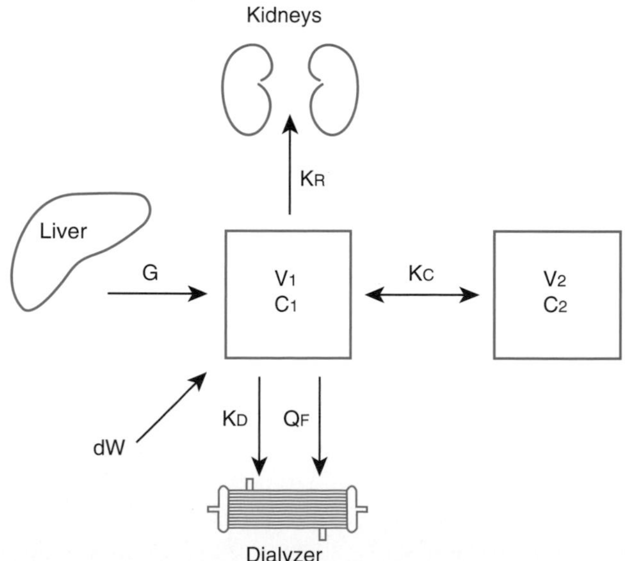

Figure 16–9 Two-compartment, variable-volume urea kinetic model. This model assumes that urea is distributed in two compartments (subscripts 1 and 2). V and C are the volume and concentration of urea in each of the two compartments. *G*, urea generation rate; K_C, intercompartment mass transfer coefficient; K_R, residual native kidney clearance; K_D, dialyzer clearance; Q_F, rate of fluid removal during dialysis. (From Depner TA: Prescribing Hemodialysis: A Guide to Urea Modeling. Boston, Kluwer Academic Publishers, 1991.)

in most cases suggests that the two compartments are the intracellular and extracellular pools separated by cell membranes, but the model does not require this assumption.

For solutes of larger molecular weight, varying charge, and bulkier configuration than urea, disequilibrium among the various compartments is even more pronounced, K_C is lower, and the solute gradients are even larger. Urea is unique in its ability to diffuse across cell membranes, especially the red blood cell membrane, where urea transporters have been found.[129,130] Most other solutes, even in the same range of molecular weight as urea, probably require a more complex kinetic model.

Kt/V$_{urea}$

The greatest lesson learned from the NCDS was that patient outcome correlates best with dialyzer urea clearance (K_d). When the level of any known solute is compared to urea clearance, the latter is better able to predict morbidity and mortality in dialysis populations.[131] To allow comparisons among patients and patient populations, a standard expression of clearance must be used, normalizing variables such as the frequency and duration of dialysis and patient size. Adjustment for size is most conveniently done using the patient's volume of urea distribution (*V*) as the denominator instead of the patient's surface area, commonly used for native kidney clearance. Standards for adequacy are currently available for hemodialysis delivered three times weekly. If K_d/V is multiplied by the duration of each dialysis (*t*), the result ($K_d \times t/V$) is a normalized or fractional clearance expressed per dialysis instead of per unit of time. During dialysis, total clearance is the sum of native kidney clearance and dialyzer clearance ($K_r + K_d = K$), so the fractional clearance per dialysis is more often expressed as *Kt/V*.

Equation 5 shows that simple first-order diffusion across a dialyzer membrane can be expressed as a constant fractional removal rate, if the dialysate concentration remains zero. For hemodialysis with a constant blood flow and a constant single-pass flow of dialysate, fractional solute removal (dC/C) is also constant. Integration and log transformation of Equation 5 gives a powerful expression for the normalized clearance:

$$Kt/V = \ln(C_0/C) \qquad (17)$$

Equation 17 shows that the normalized clearance (Kt/V) can be determined simply by measuring a pre-dialysis BUN (C_0) and a post-dialysis BUN (*C*). This eliminates the need to measure or estimate the dialyzer clearance, the native kidney clearance, the patient's urea volume, or even the duration of each dialysis to obtain this most powerful correlate to patient survival. It also provides an effective *delivered* clearance, because it is derived from measurements of the resulting change in BUN within the patient.

Equation 17 ignores urea generation during hemodialysis (*G*) and the change in volume that invariably occurs due to ultrafiltration (*dV*). These variables have significant effects on Kt/V (changing its value by up to 30%) that can be included in the expression if formal modeling is used to calculate Kt/V:

$$d(CV)/dt = G - (K/V)C \qquad (18)$$

Equation 18 is the mathematical expression of the single pool urea kinetics described earlier. Not only does its solution for the *intra-dialysis* interval give a more accurate measure of Kt/V, but also its *inter-dialysis* solution provides a method for calculating G and V and for expressing urea concentrations (C) at any specific time during the week:

$$C = C_0\left[\frac{V - Bxt}{V}\right]^{\left(\frac{Kr + Kd + B}{B}\right)} + \frac{G}{Kr + Kd + B}\left[1 - \left[\frac{V - Bxt}{V}\right]^{\left(\frac{Kr + Kd + B}{B}\right)}\right] \qquad (19)$$

where *V* is the solute distribution volume after dialysis (mL), and *B* is the rate of change in *V* (mL/min), which is usually negative during dialysis and positive between dialyses.

Residual Clearance

Because native kidney function is continuous and occurs between as well as during dialysis treatments, K_r cannot be simply added to K_d. To do so would grossly underestimate the contribution of K_r to overall excretory function. Two methods have been proposed to combine the two clearances to represent overall excretory function as a single clearance. The first converts the continuous native kidney component to the equivalent of an intermittent clearance, in the form of Kt/V, before addition[108]:

$$Kt/V' = Kt/V + K_r \times 4500/V \qquad (20)$$

Kt/V′ is a new value for Kt/V and approximates the dialyzer clearance required to maintain the same solute levels and therefore the same risk to the patient. The second method is less widely used but is more exact. It essentially converts the intermittent component to an equivalent continuous clearance[126]:

$$EKR = G/TAC \qquad (21)$$

EKR is a combined clearance in mL/min that includes both the dialyzer and the residual clearance components expressed as a continuous clearance. It is calculated from the urea generation rate (*G*) and the mean BUN (*TAC*) obtained from formal urea kinetic modeling. Mathematical subtraction separates the two:

$$EKR_d = EKR - K_r \qquad (22)$$

where EKR_d is the dialyzer component.

Dialysate Methods

The single-pool kinetic model discussed earlier estimates mass balance of urea across the dialyzer from changes in *blood* concentration. It makes several incorrect assumptions that cause the errors shown in Figure 16–7, but the two largest errors are in opposite directions and tend to offset each other.[110] This fortuitous balancing of errors has justified continued use of the single-compartment model to monitor dialysis adequacy. The indirect measurement of urea removal on the blood side, however, has been criticized by some who favor more direct measurements on the *dialysate* side to avoid these errors. However, use of instruments that measure dialysate urea concentrations either continuously (e.g., by urea electrode) or at multiple times intermittently[132-134] is important to ensure the accuracy of the dialysate method.[135] With these instruments, the dialysate curve-fitting method can be used, which is more accurate than the dialysate/volume method.[135] Dialysate monitoring offers additional advantages, including elimination of blood removal from the patient and avoidance of exposure to the patient's blood, eliminating this potential risk to the patients and staff.

Dialysate collection allows a more direct calculation of V from the amount of urea removed during dialysis divided by the change in concentration. Additional adjustments for ultrafiltration and urea generation yield:

$$V = \frac{Q_d C_d t_d - C_0 \Delta V - t_d(G - K_r C_{av})}{C_0 - C_e} \quad (23)$$

where t_d is the duration of dialysis, G is the urea generation rate, ΔV is the change in volume, K_r is the residual urea clearance, C_d is the average dialysate urea concentration, C_{av} is the average serum urea concentration, C_0 is the pre-dialysis BUN, and C_e is the equilibrated post-dialysis BUN. Rearrangement of Equation 23 provides a method that avoids the delay required to measure directly the equilibrated post-dialysis urea concentration:

$$C_e = \frac{C_0 V - Q_d C_d t_d + C_0 \Delta V + t_d(G - K_r C_{av})}{V} \quad (24)$$

eKt/V

C_e obtained from Equation 24 can be used in place of the post-dialysis urea concentration for calculating Kt/V using the single compartment model (spKt/V). This *equilibrated* value for Kt/V, or eKt/V, is always lower than spKt/V but is more realistic because it avoids the rebound error that inflates the single pool value. eKt/V has been called the patient Kt/V because it reflects the actual change in BUN and removal of urea from the patient. A recent large population study showed that eKt/V can be predicted from spKt/V as a function of time on dialysis[136]:

$$\begin{aligned} eKt/V &= spKt/V - 0.6K/V + 0.03 \\ &= spKt/V\,(1 - 0.6/t) + 0.03 \end{aligned} \quad (25)$$

where K/V is spKt/V divided by t in hours. This estimate of eKt/V, when repeated in the same patient, had a lower variance than eKt/V measured using the dialysate method.[136,137] Although eKt/V is a more accurate measure of the dose actually received by the patient and was the target of the HEMO Study, it is not currently used as a yardstick of dialysis because there are no established standards with which to compare measured values.

Volume of Urea Distribution

The total body water volume is equal to the volume of urea distribution (V) and can be calculated using various methods, including indicator dilution,[110] bioimpedance,[138] or averaged V determined from prior kinetic modeling.[110] V is most easily estimated, however, from anthropometric formulas that use the patient's height (cm), weight (kg), sex, and age (years).[139-141] The most commonly used is the Watson formula[139]:

$$\text{Males: } V\,(\text{liters}) = 2.447 - 0.09516 \times \text{age} + 0.1074 \times \text{height} + 0.3362 \times \text{weight} \quad (26)$$

$$\text{Females: } V\,(\text{liters}) = -2.097 + 0.1069 \times \text{height} + 0.2466 \times \text{weight} \quad (27)$$

Equations 26 and 27 were designed to apply to all people with widely differing anatomy, but because V can vary independently of height and weight,[141] the anthropometric estimates of V have a large coefficient of variation.[139] V can be measured more precisely by modeling urea kinetics because the model makes none of the assumptions found in the anthropometric formulas and because repeated modeling further reduces the variance. The resulting modeled V is analogous to V measured by indicator dilution methods, using urea as the indicator. The HEMO Study Group found that kinetically modeled V was consistently 13% to 19% lower than that derived from the Watson equation.[142] It is unclear whether this difference indicates a reduction in total body water or a difference in the volume of water compared to the volume of urea distribution in patients with ESRD.

Urea Generation and Protein Catabolism

In anuric patients, serum urea concentrations reflect urea generation from net protein catabolism and removal of urea by dialysis. Virtually all urea derives from breakdown of amino acids, and, conversely, protein nitrogen is catabolized mostly to urea. Under steady-state conditions, only 10% of amino acid nitrogen is converted to nonurea nitrogenous wastes.[143,144] Furthermore, the net *protein catabolic rate* (PCR) approximates protein intake during a steady state of nitrogen balance. Therefore, the measurement of the *urea generation rate* (G), provided by formal urea modeling, allows an easy estimate of PCR and protein intake. In practice, PCR is usually normalized (divided) by V (PCRn) to allow comparison among patients of different size.

Based on independent detailed studies of two separate groups of patients, one group receiving dialysis[143] and the other with chronic kidney failure not receiving dialysis,[144] the relationship between PCR (g/day) and G (mg/min) can be described with the following equation:

$$PCR = 9.35 \times G + 11 \quad (28)$$

Equation 27 shows that the majority of nitrogen released from excess catabolism of dietary and endogenous protein is converted to urea; only 11 g of protein per day are converted to nonurea nitrogenous compounds, such as creatinine, uric acid, hippurate, and amino acids. The generation of nonurea nitrogenous compounds varies with patient size but not with daily protein intake, whereas the generation of urea depends upon protein intake. Adjusting the production of nonurea nitrogenous compounds for the average body size in these studies, using urea volume, and normalizing the entire expression to V,

$$PCRn = 5420\,(G/V) + 0.17 \quad (29)$$

where PCRn is normalized PCR in g/kg/day and V is the patient's urea volume (total body water) in liters.

The importance of PCR, PCRn, and G cannot be overemphasized. The NCDS showed that a consistently high BUN strongly predicted a poor outcome, but low BUN levels resulting from low urea generation rates (low PCRn) were associated with even higher morbidity and mortality.[145] A subsequent large population study[146] confirmed that patients with low PCRn, and therefore low G, had high morbidity and mortality rates, possibly as a result of severe malnutrition, although other disease states may have suppressed the patients' appetites. These studies illustrate that it is not enough to know the BUN level; one must know how it got there. A low BUN from malnutrition is bad, but a low BUN from vigorous dialysis is good. Urea kinetic modeling allows the clinician to separate nutritional influences from the dialysis effect using urea concentrations sampled immediately before and after dialysis.

Solute Disequilibrium

Solute disequilibrium is defined as a concentration difference or gradient for dissolved solutes among body compartments. This problem develops during dialysis and slowly dissipates over several minutes to hours after the end of dialysis (Figures 16–7 and 16–10). Solute disequilibrium caused by resistance to diffusion across cell membranes is called *diffusion-dependent disequilibrium.* When disequilibrium is caused by differences in blood flow among various vascular beds, it is termed *flow-dependent disequilibrium.*

In the past, diffusion-dependent disequilibrium was thought to be more important. Mathematical models predicted that solute concentration differed among the various compartments but was uniform throughout the blood pool. More recent data suggest that the contribution of diffusion-dependent mechanisms to solute disequilibrium may be less than previously thought.[147-153] Mathematical models have been developed that fully describe urea disequilibrium using purely flow-dependent disequilibrium.[150] These models assume that solutes diffuse instantly between compartments, so the observed gradients are attributed to differences in relative blood flow/volume served by the vascular bed. The relative importance of these two types of disequilibrium remains to be determined. Both predict lower solute concentrations during dialysis than the single-pool model, thus reducing the efficiency of hemodialysis.

Vascular access recirculation may cause a decrease in effective solute clearance[147,154-156] and is a special case of flow-dependent disequilibrium. Access recirculation occurs when blood that has just been dialyzed returns immediately to the dialyzer in the reverse direction through the access device. Multiple causes have been identified, including venous outflow stenosis, central venous stenosis, close proximity of the dialysis needles, and accidental reversal of the arterial and venous needles. Although dialyzer clearance is preserved, total solute removal decreases because the recirculated venous blood dilutes the solute concentration of the incoming arterial blood, thus lowering the solute concentration gradient across the dialyzer membrane. When 100% recirculation exists, all of the dialyzed blood returns to the dialyzer, and the patient derives no benefit from dialysis. Although access recirculation is found in less than 5% of hemodialyses, when it exists, the timing of blood sampling at the end of dialysis is critical to avoid errors in measuring the delivered dialysis dose (Figure 16–10). If blood is sampled immediately at the end of dialysis (Point *A* in Figure 16–10) without slowing the blood pump, the measured urea concentration is significantly lower than the actual arterial concentration. This error leads to a falsely high Kt/V. Sampling the arterial (inflow) blood 10 to 20 seconds after slowing the blood pump at the end of dialysis eliminates dilution from access recirculation (Point *B* in Figure 16–10). Vascular access-related issues are addressed further in Chapter 4.

With a model of *multiple parallel circuits,*[152] differences in blood flowing to various parts of the body have been invoked to explain the differences in solute concentration among these vascular beds during dialysis (Figure 16–11). Blood from the rapidly flowing circuits is exposed to the dialyzer more frequently and dilutes the solute concentration of blood flowing to the dialyzer. This essentially limits the access to the dialyzer of slower-flowing circuits that have higher solute concentrations. Thus, differences in blood flow within the blood pool reduce the solute concentration entering the dialyzer and the average concentration in the patient. This reduces the efficiency of dialysis, decreases solute removal, and invalidates the use of solute concentration in peripheral venous blood for calculating vascular access recirculation.[148,149,153]

Cardiopulmonary recirculation (CPR), present in dialysis patients with AV shunts[151] (see Figure 16–11), is a specific example of one of these multiple parallel circuits. Because the vascular shunt has low resistance and routes blood directly from the arterial to the venous circulation, blood flowing through this circuit returns to the heart at a faster rate. Although the dialyzer clearance is unaffected, the concentration gradient across the dialyzer membrane is reduced by

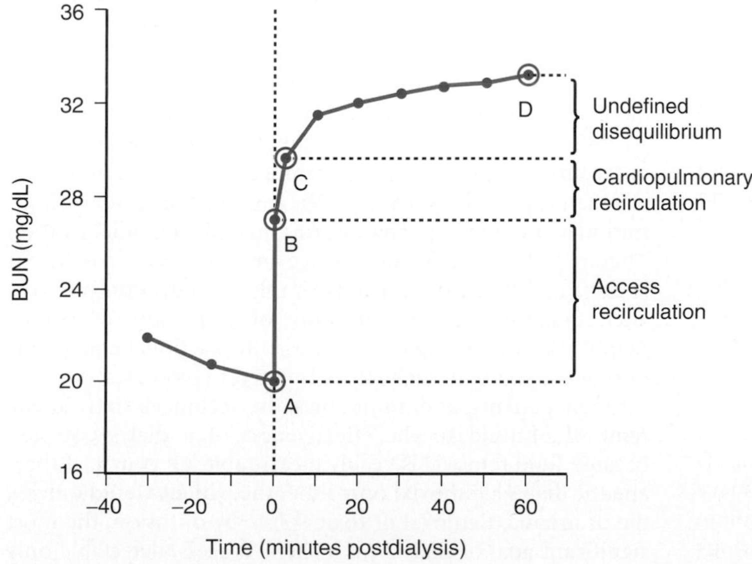

Figure 16–10 Post-dialysis blood urea levels. The post-dialysis blood urea nitrogen (BUN) level is a moving target, so attention to sampling time is needed for consistency and accuracy when measuring both the urea kinetics value and normalized protein catabolic rate. Point A is the immediate post-dialysis sample obtained without taking precaution to prevent the dilution artifact from access recirculation. The sample at point B eliminates this artifact because it is taken from the arterial (inflow) port 10 to 20 seconds after slowing the blood pump at the end of dialysis. Sampling at point C, 2 minutes post-dialysis, eliminates the effects of cardiopulmonary recirculation. At point D, 1 hour post-dialysis, urea equilibration throughout the body is essentially complete. (From Depner TA: Assessing adequacy of hemodialysis: Urea modeling. Kidney Int 1994; 45:1522-1535. Used with permission of Kidney International.)

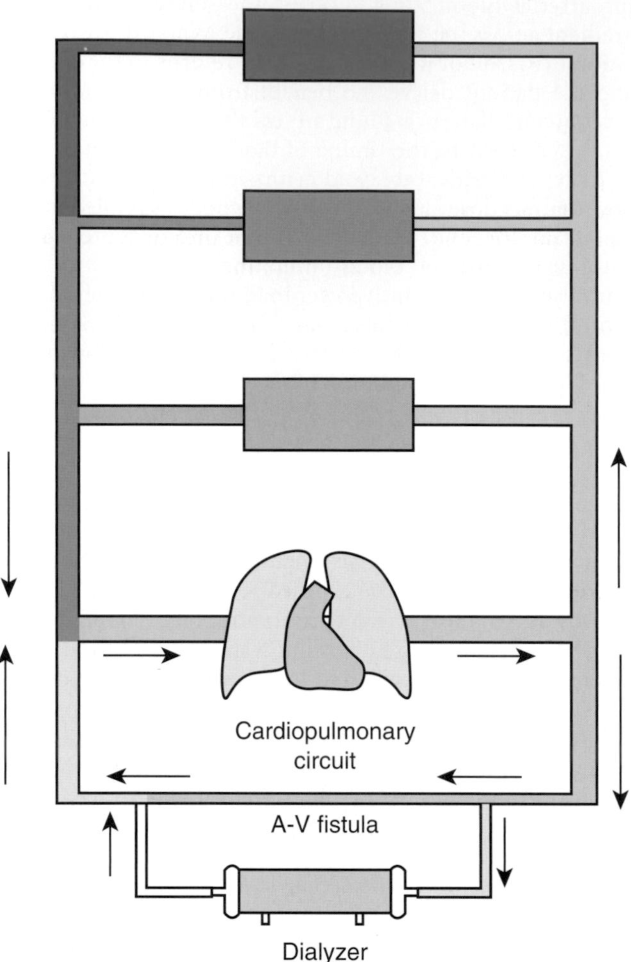

Figure 16–11 Urea disequilibrium as a consequence of differences in regional blood perfusion. Differing simultaneous concentrations of urea throughout the body can develop solely as a consequence of differences in regional blood perfusion, shown here as a parallel arrangement of tissue compartments. Although the consequences are similar to urea disequilibrium resulting from membrane-limited diffusion, the mechanism is entirely different because this model assumes an absence of diffusion barriers. Instead, the rapid changes in blood urea levels at the beginning and end of treatment are caused by the differing blood perfusion rates. Blood in the more rapidly flowing circuits comes into contact with the dialyzer more frequently, so it has a lower urea and solute concentration and essentially dilutes the solute concentration from slower-flowing blood pools. The proximal and most rapidly flowing blood pathway is the cardiopulmonary circuit through the peripheral arteriovenous (AV) access device. (From Depner TA: Approach to hemodialysis kinetic modeling. *In* Henrich WL [ed]: Principles and Practice of Dialysis, 2nd ed. Baltimore, Williams & Wilkins, 1999.)

cardiopulmonary recirculation so that solute removal is impaired. As is evident from Figure 16–10, cardiopulmonary recirculation contributes to the rebound in blood solute (urea) concentration after dialysis is completed, as the various blood compartments equilibrate. Cardiopulmonary recirculation is not present in patients with central venous catheters for vascular access because blood drawn from the central vein is returned to the same vein, and the shunt circuit is absent.

Adequacy of Hemodialysis: Current Recommendations

Before the NCDS, absolute blood urea concentrations were used to monitor the efficacy of dialysis and to determine the frequency of dialysis. Kinetic modeling gained popularity and increasing acceptance after the NCDS reported that both high and low blood urea concentrations were associated with increased mortality,[131,145] highlighting the fact that the absolute blood urea concentration is a poor marker of uremia and dialysis dose. Using absolute blood urea levels risks setting in motion the vicious cycle of providing less dialysis to patients who are malnourished, causing a further reduction in BUN. Assessing dialysis adequacy with kinetic modeling avoids this vicious cycle because kinetic modeling determines the clearance of urea, based on the *change* in urea concentration.

The NCDS data showed that maximal benefit from dialysis was obtained above a Kt/V_{urea} of 1.0 per dialysis administered three times a week.[145] Subsequent data from uncontrolled studies suggested that further benefit may be derived from increasing Kt/V_{urea} to 1.2 or greater[88-94] (see Chapter 3). Based on the available data, the NIH, the Renal Physicians Association, and the NKF established the minimum Kt/V_{urea} at 1.2 per dialysis administered three times a week in their respective consensus conferences.[28,85,86] The HEMO Study results support this minimum Kt/V_{urea} since increasing single pool Kt/V_{urea} from an average of 1.3 to 1.7 did not reduce mortality or morbidity further.[95] The NKF additionally recommended the application of formal urea kinetic modeling (see Quantifying Hemodialysis) for routine quantification of hemodialysis.[28] If formal modeling is not available, simplified formulas should be used.

Filtration and Dialysis

Because fluid nearly always accumulates in patients between therapeutic hemodialyses, net ultrafiltration must be a part of each treatment to maintain fluid balance. In a sense, water is also a toxin that accumulates and must be removed on a regular basis. The mechanism of water removal during hemodialysis is not diffusion but pressure filtration of the blood as it passes through the dialyzer. Although filtration also removes solute, and solute removal by filtration is also a first-order process, the additional clearance from filtration is often less than expected. Conversely, one can remove solute with filtration alone (see later Hemofiltration and Hemodiafiltration Therapy). If no dialysis takes place and the sieving coefficient is close to 1.0, the clearance is simply the filtration rate (see later Quantitative Contribution of Filtration to Solute Removal). The sieving coefficient is the fractional concentration of the solute in dialysate compared to blood water.

Often patients and sometimes the technical staff equate removal of fluid to the effectiveness of a dialysis session because fluid removal is visibly measurable. Of course, if therapeutic dialysis removed only fluid, the patient would quickly die of uremia. Removal of toxic solute by diffusion, the most significant goal of dialysis, is a silent process, detectable only by measuring solute levels in blood or dialysate samples; removal of fluid is easily displayed by modern volume-controlled dialysate delivery systems and is evident from the change in patient weight.

Dialyzer Ultrafiltration Coefficient

The same membrane properties (i.e., thinner, more porous membranes with a large surface area) that improve solute clearance also improve hydraulic fluid removal. In addition, membrane tensile strength plays a role in determining the maximum pressure that can be applied. Dialyzers are rated by their *ultrafiltration coefficient* (K_{Uf}), with units of mL/hr/mmHg. Typical K_{Uf} values for standard and high flux dialyzers are listed in Table 16–6.

Quantitative Contribution of Filtration to Solute Removal

As plasma water moves from the blood compartment to the dialysate, solutes dissolved in plasma follow passively. Convective clearance thus augments diffusive transport, and the contribution can be quantified mathematically. When ultrafiltration is present during dialysis, blood flow into the dialyzer (Q_{bi}) can be expressed as the sum of blood flow out of the dialyzer (Q_{bo}) and the ultrafiltration rate (Q_f):

$$Q_{bi} = Q_{bo} + Q_f \qquad (30)$$

From the previously described definition of dialyzer clearance and considering mass balance, dialyzer clearance (K_d) can be expressed as a function of solute concentrations and blood flow rates through the dialyzer:

$$K_d = J/C_{in} = [(C_{in} \times Q_{bi}) - (C_o \times Q_{bo})]/C_{in} \qquad (31)$$

where J is the solute flux, C_{in} the inlet (arterial) solute concentration, and C_o the outlet (venous) solute concentration. Combining and rearranging Equations 30 and 31 yields the following,

$$K_d = Q_{bi}(C_{in} - C_o)/C_{in} + Q_f(C_o/C_{in}) \qquad (32)$$

Equation 32 shows that dialyzer clearance of a particular solute is the sum of solute clearance in the absence of ultrafiltration ($Q_{bi} = Q_{bo}$) and a fraction of the ultrafiltration rate. At one extreme, when all the solute is removed by diffusion ($C_o = 0$), there is no contribution from ultrafiltration. At the other extreme, when no diffusion is present ($C_{in} = C_o$), the dialyzer clearance is the ultrafiltration rate. This latter case occurs in the setting of hemofiltration (to be discussed further), where all solute clearance results from filtration. During the usual hemodialysis treatment, the contribution of convective clearance to the total dialyzer clearance is small. Even at high rates of ultrafiltration (2 L/hr or 33 mL/min), the relative contribution of ultrafiltration to total urea clearance is only about 10 mL/min or 5%, assuming C_o/C_{in} for urea of 0.3 to 0.4 and dialyzer urea clearance of 200 mL/min.

In clinical practice, outlet solute concentration is rarely measured, limiting the usefulness of Equation 32. With further mathematical manipulation,[110] C_o can be eliminated, yielding:

$$K_d = K_{d0} + Q_f(1 - K_{d0}/Q_{bi}) \qquad (33)$$

where K_{d0} is the dialyzer clearance without ultrafiltration and can be calculated from Q_{bi} and the dialyzer K_OA. Q_f is readily calculated from the weight loss during dialysis divided by the duration of dialysis or directly measured by volume-controlled dialysis machines.

Hemofiltration and Hemodiafiltration Therapy

Up to now, we have discussed the principles of filtration in the context of hemodialysis, using filtration mainly for removing excess fluid, while relying on diffusion for solute removal. Filtration alone can also be used to remove both solute and solvent, so-called *hemofiltration.*[157, 158] As discussed earlier and as evident from Equation 33, in the absence of diffusion, dialyzer clearance is the ultrafiltration rate. Therefore, to achieve solute clearance comparable to that of hemodialysis, large amounts of fluid must be removed, on the order of 30 to 40 L during each treatment, with simultaneous replenishment using a pyrogen-free physiologic salt solution.

The benefits of hemofiltration are improved hemodynamic stability[159,160] and improved removal of larger solutes.[158,161] Larger-molecular substances are removed more effectively by hemofiltration because convection has a greater effect of enhancing the relatively slow diffusive movement of larger molecules compared to small molecules (see earlier discussion

Table 16–6 Characteristic Values for Standard, High-Efficiency, and High-Flux Dialyzers and Hemodialysis

	Standard	High Efficiency	High Flux
Blood flow rate (mL/min)	250	≥350	≥350
Dialysate flow rate (mL/min)	500	≥700	≥700
K_oA urea	300–500	600–1000	Variable
Urea clearance (mL/min)	<200	250–400	Variable
Urea clearance/body weight (mL/min/kg)	<3	>3	Variable
Vitamin B_{12} clearance (mL/min)	30–60	Variable	>100
Ultrafiltration coefficient (mL/hr/mmHg)	3.5–5.0	<15	>15
Membrane	Cellulose	Variable	Variable

of convection and diffusion). In addition, filtration requires a highly permeable (high flux) membrane to achieve the high filtration rates (30 to 40 L per dialysis).[158,161] During filtration, peripheral vascular resistance has been observed to increase, whereas it remains unchanged or decreases during hemodialysis against a bicarbonate-containing or acetate-containing dialysate.[160,162] The reason for the increase is not entirely clear but recent studies have suggested a temperature effect.[163] The increased vascular resistance helps to support the blood pressure during hemofiltration. The primary disadvantage of hemofiltration is the large amount of sterile replacement fluid required, but equipment designed to simplify hemofiltration and produce sterile replacement fluid on-line is under development.[164]

Hemodiafiltration is the combination of hemodialysis and hemofiltration (i.e., addition of dialysate flow to the hemofiltration circuit). Solute removal is accomplished by diffusion and by filtration, but, in contrast to traditional hemodialysis, the filtration component contributes much more because of the higher magnitude of filtration relative to dialysis. Although intermittent hemofiltration and hemodiafiltration are not widely used in the United States for treating ESRD, these two modalities have been adapted for wide use in intensive care units to treat patients with acute renal failure.

Filtration Effects on Blood Pressure, Regional Blood Flow, and Solute Removal

Blood pressure falls as fluid is removed (see Chapter 11), in part, because the normal response of vasoconstriction to fluid removal is impaired in dialysis patients. The use of bioincompatible membranes and acetate as a source of bicarbonate may predispose the patient to vasodilation. To aggravate the situation further, solute removal decreases blood osmolarity, causing slight fluid shifts from the intravascular compartment into the intracellular compartment. In patients at high risk of hypotension during dialysis, separating filtration (*isolated ultrafiltration*) from dialysis may improve their hemodynamic stability.[159,160]

Although theoretically filtration may account for a significant fraction of solute removal during dialysis, in practice it can also interfere with solute removal. The development of intravascular volume depletion during dialysis causes vasoconstriction in the skin and skeletal muscle and shunts blood through other vascular circuits (such as the AV shunt), enhancing flow-related solute disequilibrium.

High-Efficiency, High-Flux Hemodialysis

Initial hemodialyses were limited by low dialyzer membrane permeability, requiring more than 6 hours for each treatment. Although treatment times were shortened to 4 hours or less three times a week as dialyzer design improved, the time spent attached to the dialysis machine was still unacceptable to many patients. The next major advancement came in the late 1980s, when the technical problems with bacteriologic contamination of bicarbonate dialysate, inadequate blood flow, imprecise ultrafiltration control, and continued low dialyzer solute clearance were solved.

The distinction between *high-efficiency* and *high-flux* dialysis is not always made clear, and sometimes these terms are used interchangeably. In essence, both terms address improved solute and fluid clearance compared with standard hemodialysis, taking advantage of higher blood and dialysate flow rates to decrease dialysis time while maintaining an adequate dose. These two therapies are not mutually exclusive and, in fact, frequently overlap (see Table 16–6). The high-efficiency dialyzer contains either a synthetic or a modified cellulose membrane and has a higher clearance of small molecules, such as urea (Table 16–6), compared with a standard dialyzer. The high-flux dialyzer always has a highly permeable synthetic or modified cellulose membrane that removes larger molecules. By their nature, high-flux dialyzers have a higher K_{Uf} compared to high-efficiency dialyzers but not necessarily high urea clearances (see Table 16–6). Conversely, high urea clearance defines high-efficiency dialysis, but the clearance of larger molecules is variable (see Table 16–6).

The advent of substituted cellulose and synthetic membranes improved dialyzer permeability because substituted cellulose membranes can be made thinner to increase porosity and surface area, whereas synthetic membranes can be manufactured with more and larger pores. Both high-efficiency and high-flux dialysis require the use of bicarbonate dialysate and volume-controlled filtration. Standard hemodialysis uses acetate, which the liver and skeletal muscle metabolize to bicarbonate.[165] During high-efficiency and high-flux hemodialysis with acetate, the rate of acetate acquisition exceeded the metabolic ability of the liver and muscle cells, resulting in varying degrees of acidosis[165,166] and leading to peripheral vasodilation and hypotension, which prohibited continuation of the treatment. Substituting bicarbonate for acetate in the dialysate maintains hemodynamic stability, decreases nausea and vomiting, and allows dialysis to proceed. Because the high-efficiency and high-flux dialyzers have a higher K_{Uf}, precise control of ultrafiltration is also mandatory to prevent massive volume depletion (see later Mechanics of Hemodialysis).

The most significant difference is the capability of high-flux dialyzers to remove larger molecules[113,114] because of their greater porosity. Increased β_2-microglobulin removal has reduced the risk of carpal tunnel syndrome in long-term patients treated with high-flux dialysis[38,113,167-169] (see Chapters 13 and 14). Other benefits that derive possibly from removal of large molecules are an improved lipid profile,[167,170-172] a greater response to erythropoietin,[173] a higher leptin removal (leptin is thought to suppress appetite),[174] and perhaps lower mortality and hospitalization rates.[167,168,175] Potential adverse consequences from increased removal of larger molecules, however, include greater removal of drugs, such as vancomycin[176] (see Chapter 19), amino acids,[177] and albumin,[178] although the last-mentioned is disputed.[113] The presence of *back-filtration* during high-flux dialysis has been postulated to increase the risk of exposing patients to endotoxin from the dialysate, although this potential problem has not been clearly demonstrated in clinical studies.[179,180]

Despite the widespread use of these modalities since the 1980s, few comparative data are available. Most of the literature is descriptive[181]; only a few studies have evaluated its efficacy. Despite the shorter duration of dialysis, the urea clearance per dialysis is comparable to that of standard hemodialysis, although the two-compartment model best explains solute removal during treatment with these modalities.[110,182,183] Randomized control or cross-over trials using bicarbonate dialysate found no difference in the incidence of hypotension and intra-dialytic symptoms[113,184,185] or in the control of blood pressure[186] among the three modalities. In studies of a small number of patients treated with high efficiency dialysis, neuropsychological function,[187] mortality, and morbidity[188] are comparable to those for patients treated with standard hemodialysis. The best data available come from the HEMO Study, which detected no difference in mortality or morbidity between patients treated with high-efficiency versus high-flux dialysis.[95]

Limitations to the Delivery of Hemodialysis

High-efficiency dialysis increases solute clearance, but the shorter duration of dialysis decreases efficiency because it accentuates the effects of intermittence and exacerbates solute disequilibrium (see Solute Disequilibrium and Figure 16–7). In addition, as discussed earlier, the shorter duration of high-efficiency hemodialysis may not allow sufficient time to remove larger molecules, such as β_2-microglobulin, for which removal is more time dependent.[113,114] Another potential problem with shortening time is the required increase in the filtration rate.[113,185,189] Most patients can tolerate up to 0.35 mL/min/kg of filtration (1.5 L/hr in a 70-kg person) without developing nausea, cramping, or hypotension.[189] Therefore, an average-sized patient whose weight gain exceeds 4 to 5 kg is a poor candidate for short-duration dialysis and will experience a progressive rise in end-dialysis weight, eventually leading to pulmonary edema. Finally, once patients are accustomed to the shorter time, they are devastated psychologically when their medical condition, such as large fluid gains, inadequate clearance of larger molecules, poorly functioning access, or loss of residual renal function, requires prolonging dialysis time.

Ensuring the adequacy of high-efficiency dialysis is more difficult than for standard dialysis because the myriad of confounding factors already discussed are magnified, including access recirculation, access blood flow, needle positioning, needle size, actual duration of dialysis, compromised dialyzer clearance, and errors in the assumptions made for urea diffusion. Time lost during a high-efficiency dialysis is a larger fraction of the total dialysis time. Factors that decrease actual dialysis time include failure to account for machine downtime caused by alarms, delayed achievement of target Q_b, clotting in the dialyzer requiring a second setup, patient tardiness, and patient noncompliance. Because high-flux and high-efficiency dialyzers are reused, thrombosed hollow fibers that do not reopen during reprocessing may reduce the fiber bundle volume and the surface area for diffusion critically (see Chapter 5). The higher solute removal rate of high-efficiency dialysis further magnifies the differences between the one-compartment and the two-compartment models (see Figure 16–7) by exaggerating the logarithmic decline in urea removal during dialysis and the urea rebound after dialysis.[110,183,190,191] The timing of blood sampling for the post-dialysis BUN becomes even more important (see Figure 16–10), as demonstrated by the average 20% decrease in calculated Kt/V_{urea} if BUN is drawn at 30 minutes instead of immediately after dialysis.[190]

Achieving the desired Q_b is crucial to the success of high-efficiency dialysis. Longer needles and needles with a smaller diameter impede blood flow because resistance is directly proportional to length and inversely related to the fourth power of the needle's inside diameter. An excessively pliable tubing pump segment or low pre-pump pressure invalidates flows reported by the blood pump's RPM meter, as illustrated in Figure 16–12. Not only is the desired Q_b not achieved in this case; health care personnel are also unaware of this problem until urea kinetic study results return. Even if the desired Q_b is achieved, access recirculation is more likely to appear at the higher Q_b used for high-efficiency and high-flux hemodialysis. However, in recent years, the flow variance seems to have diminished due to manufacturing modifications to the tubing pump segment.

Improper needle position with the venous needle abutting the wall causes turbulence and retards the egress of blood

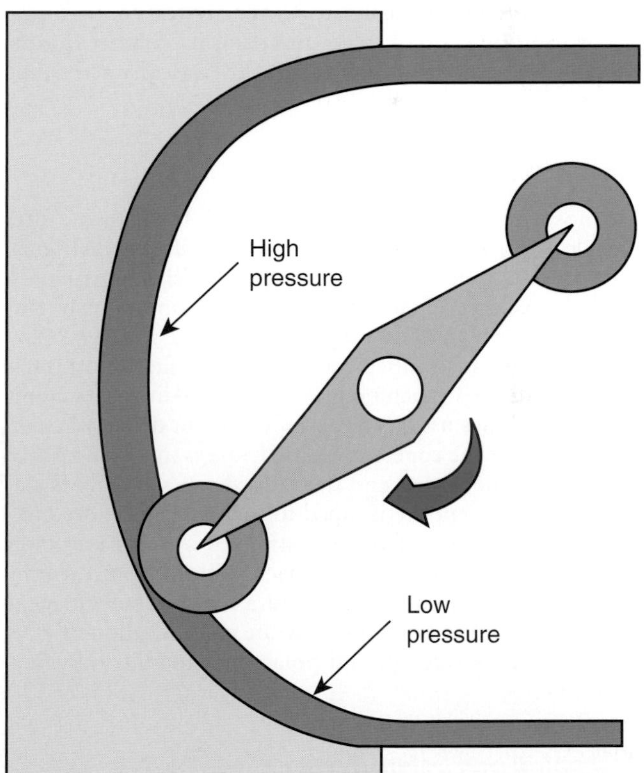

Figure 16–12 Blood flow variance from variable roller pump function. As the roller pump passes along the curved trace and compresses the tubing pump segment, elastic recoil in the tubing behind the roller creates a negative pressure, which refills the tubing with blood. If the pre-pump pressure is too low, the pump segment will not re-expand completely. This incomplete expansion reduces the flow despite no change in the pump speed. (From Depner TA, Rizwan S, Stasi TA: Pressure effects on roller pump blood flow during hemodialysis. ASAIO Trans 1990; 36:M456-M459.)

from the access, promoting recirculation. Placing the arterial and venous needles too closely together at a higher Q_b also creates recirculation. Other important contributors to access recirculation are venous outflow stenosis, arterial insufficiency from atherosclerotic disease in the afferent artery, or stenosis at the inflow anastomosis.

Microbiologic contamination is a risk associated with the use of bicarbonate concentrate because of its potential to support bacterial growth. Recognition of this risk and the subsequent steps taken to prevent contamination have greatly reduced the incidence of pyrogen reactions reported during the early application of high-flux dialysis. Although the risk is theoretically increased by back filtration during high-flux dialysis, few reports of this complication have appeared[179] (see later Dialysate Delivery Systems).

MECHANICS OF HEMODIALYSIS

Twenty to 30 years ago, hemodialysis equipment for a single patient occupied the greater part of an entire room. Now, hemodialysis machines are about the size of a three- to four-drawer filing cabinet and can be transported easily by one person. In addition to the reduction in size, advances have included more reliable dialysate delivery systems, monitoring devices, and automated safety mechanisms. Several on-line devices allow dynamic monitoring of the vascular access, the hematocrit, and the adequacy of the treatment.

Dialysate Delivery Systems

The most commonly used system discards the dialysate after a single passage through the dialyzer (*single-pass* delivery). Most dialysis clinics also use *single-patient delivery* systems in which a machine at each patient station continuously prepares dialysate by mixing a liquid concentrate with a proportionate volume of purified water. To dilute the concentrates safely, the dialysis machine has many built-in safety monitors. Some clinics use a central multi-patient delivery system in which either the concentrated dialysate is mixed in an area away from patient care and then piped to each dialysis station, or the concentrate is piped to each station before mixing. The advantages of these centralized systems are lower patient care costs and less staff back injuries from carrying the individual concentrate jugs, but a major disadvantage is inflexibility in modifying the dialysate concentration of electrolytes, such as calcium and potassium, to suit individual patient needs.

Mechanical and Safety Monitors

The dialysis machine draws up and warms purified water to physiologic temperatures. The heated water then undergoes *deaeration* under vacuum to prevent dissolved air from coming out of solution as negative pressure is applied during dialysis. Air bubbles in the dialysate cause the blood leak detector and the conductivity detector to malfunction. They also "lock" part of the dialysate pathway, increasing channeling and masking parts of the membrane surface area.

The heated and deaerated product water is then mixed with the concentrate to produce dialysate. To ensure proper proportioning, the *conductivity monitor* downstream from the proportioning pump continuously measures the electrical conductivity of the product solution. Because mal-proportioned dialysate may cause severe electrolyte disturbances in the patient, leading to death, the conductivity monitor has a narrow range of tolerance and is usually redundant. Dialysate conductivity may be altered by temperature, the presence of air bubbles, or malfunction of the sensor, usually an electrode. Periodically, the conductivity monitor must be calibrated using standardized solutions or by laboratory measurements of electrolytes in the dialysate.

Since the patient is exposed to 100 to 200 L of dialysate during each treatment, the dialysate must be heated to near body temperature to avoid hypothermia. If the dialysate is too hot, however, protein denaturation (>42°C) and hemolysis (>45°C) occur. In practice, the dialysate temperature is maintained at 36°C to 37°C and falls slightly in transit from the proportioning device to the patient. The *temperature monitor* within the dialysate circuit sets off an alarm if the dialysate temperature is outside of the limits of 36°C to 42°C, and dialysate is pumped directly to the drain, automatically bypassing the dialyzer.

Located after the dialyzer, the *dialysate pump* controls dialysate flow and generates negative dialysate pressure. The dialysate circuit must be able to generate both negative and positive dialysate pressures within the dialyzer because, although many dialyzers require a negative dialysate pressure for filtration, dialyzers with high K_{Uf} or conditions that increase pressure in the blood compartment require a positive dialysate pressure to limit filtration. The dialysate circuitry controls the pressure by variably constricting the dialysate outflow tubing while maintaining a constant flow rate. The dialysate delivery system also monitors the filtration rate, either indirectly by controlling the TMP (*pressure-controlled* ultrafiltration) or directly by controlling the actual filtration (*volume-controlled* ultrafiltration). Earlier dialysate delivery systems used pressure-controlled filtration, requiring dialysis personnel to calculate the TMP, enter the TMP into the machine, closely monitor the filtration rate, and recalculate and adjust the TMP as needed. To prevent excessive fluid removal when using dialyzers with K_{Uf} greater than 6 mL/hr/mmHg, dialysate delivery systems capable of performing volume-controlled filtration are mandatory. Such systems have built-in balance chambers and servomechanisms that accurately control the volume of fluid removed during dialysis once the desired goal is set.[192]

The *blood leak monitor* is situated in the dialysate outflow tubing and is designed to alarm and shut off the blood pump when blood is detected. The presence of blood in the dialysate usually indicates membrane rupture and may be caused by a TMP exceeding 500 mmHg. Although a rare complication, membrane rupture can be potentially life threatening because it allows nonsterile dialysate to come into contact with blood. In this era of dialyzer reuse, the potential for membrane rupture is increased because both bleach and heat disinfection can damage the dialyzer membrane (see Chapter 5). Intravascular hemolysis with hemoglobin in the dialysate may also trigger the blood leak alarm.

Bicarbonate Delivery

Previously, dialysate contained acetate as a source of bicarbonate. The advantages of acetate are the low incidence of bacterial contamination and its ease of storage. Acetate is a hemodynamic stressor, however, during high-efficiency and high-flux dialysis[193-195] (see Chapter 11) because the rate of acetate diffusion into blood often exceeded the metabolic capacity of the liver and skeletal muscle. Acetate accumulation leads to acidosis, vasodilation, and hypotension. The majority of dialysis clinics now use bicarbonate-based dialysate to prevent these complications.

The major complications of bicarbonate dialysate are bacterial contamination and precipitation of calcium and magnesium salts. Gram-negative halophilic rods require sodium chloride or sodium bicarbonate to grow and thus thrive in bicarbonate dialysate.[196,197] When bicarbonate containers are disinfected, these bacteria have a latency period of 3 to 5 days, have an exponential growth phase at 5 to 8 days, and achieve maximum growth at 10 days,[196] compared with a latency of 1 day, exponential growth phase at 2 to 3 days, and maximum growth by 4 days in a contaminated container. Mixing bicarbonate and disinfecting the containers daily help prevent bacterial contamination. Alternatively, commercially available dry powder cartridges can circumvent this problem.

To prevent formation of insoluble calcium and magnesium salts with bicarbonate, the final dialysate is mixed from two separate components: the bicarbonate concentrate and the acid concentrate. The acid concentrate contains all solutes other than bicarbonate and derives its name from the inclusion of a small amount of acetic acid (4 mEq/L in the final dilution). The dialysate delivery system draws up the two components separately and mixes them proportionately with purified water to form the final dialysate. This process minimizes but does not eliminate the precipitation of calcium and magnesium salts, so the dialysate delivery system must be rinsed periodically with an acid solution to eliminate any buildup.

Water Quality

Treatment of the water used to generate dialysate is essential to avoid exposure during dialysis to harmful substances, such as aluminum, chloramine-T, endotoxin, and bacteria. Accumulation of aluminum in the body may cause dialysis dementia, microcytic anemia, and osteomalacia. Chloramine-T, a product of chlorine and organic material, causes acute hemolysis during dialysis. Endotoxin and bacteria cause febrile reactions and hypotension. Good water quality is even more imperative when dialyzers are reused because the blood compartment is exposed to unsterile water and any accompanying bacteria or endotoxin. To avoid these complications, tap water is first softened, then exposed to charcoal to remove contaminants such as chloramine, then filtered to remove particulate matter, and then filtered under high pressure (reverse osmosis) to remove other dissolved contaminants (see Chapter 5).

Blood Circuit Components

The steady flow of blood required for dialysis may be drawn from a central vein, from the ports along the sides of a double-lumen catheter (arterial lumen), and returned through the port at the distal tip (venous lumen). Alternatively, the blood may be drawn from an AV fistula or graft. The blood pump is usually a peristaltic roller pump, which sequentially compresses the pump segment of the blood tubing against a curved rigid track (see Figure 16–12), forcing blood from the tubing. After the roller has passed, the elastic tubing recoils and refills with blood, ready for the next roller. As a result, blood flow through the dialyzer is pulsatile. Most pumps have two or three rollers. The greater the number of rollers, the less pulsatile the flow, but the higher the risk of hemolysis and damage to the pump segment.

The blood pump flowmeter displays flow calculated solely from its speed of rotation (RPM), whereas the actual Q_b is the product of the RPM and the volume of blood forced from the tubing with each revolution. Therefore, the displayed Q_b may be higher than the actual Q_b. As illustrated in Figure 16–12, if the pre-pump pressure is too low, the pump segment will not re-expand completely, leading to a lower blood flow despite no change in the pump speed. This inaccuracy is magnified at higher Q_b if the vascular access is unable to support the desired blood flow.[198] However, because of changes in the manufacturing of blood tubing, the blood pump flowmeter readings may be more accurate.

When the upper or lower limits are exceeded, *pressure monitors* sound an alarm and turn off the blood pump. An arterial pressure monitor should be located proximal to the blood pump and a venous monitor located distal to the dialyzer. Accepted ranges for arterial inflow pressures are −20 to −80 mmHg, but may be as low as −200 mmHg when Q_b is high. Accepted ranges for venous pressures are +50 to +200 mmHg. Kinks in the tubing, improper arterial needle position, hypotension, or arterial inflow stenosis can cause excessively low arterial pressures. High venous pressures should prompt an investigation for blood clotting in the dialyzer, kinking, or clotting in the venous bloodlines, improperly positioned venous needles, infiltration of a venous needle, or venous outflow stenosis. Accurate measurements of both the arterial and venous pressures are essential to determining the TMP. Excessive positive pressures anywhere in the blood compartment may rupture the dialyzer membrane or cause the blood circuit to disconnect. An abrupt fall in pressure anywhere in the blood circuit may signal an accidental disconnection of the blood circuit, which can result in exsanguination if not corrected promptly.

Two other important safety devices, located in the bloodline distal to the dialyzer, are (1) the *venous air trap* and (2) the *air detector*. The venous air trap prevents any air that may have entered the blood circuit through loose connections, improper arterial needle position, or the saline infusion line from returning to the patient. If air is still detected in the venous line after the venous air trap, the machine alarms and turns off the blood pump. Excessive foaming of blood will also trigger the air detector. These safety features prevent air embolism, which carries a high mortality rate, especially when the problem is not immediately recognized.[199]

Computer Controls

As discussed earlier, solute removal during hemodialysis decreases plasma osmolarity, favors fluid shift into the cells, and makes fluid removal more difficult. Increasing the dialysate sodium concentration helps to preserve plasma osmolarity and allows continued fluid removal[200, 201] but may lead to increased thirst, excessive weight gain, and hypertension[200,202] (see Chapter 11). Computer-controlled *sodium modeling* allows the dialysate sodium concentration to change automatically during dialysis according to a preselected profile, usually 150 to 160 mEq/L at the beginning of dialysis to 135 to 140 mEq/L near or at the end of dialysis. Theoretically, this sodium modeling offers the benefit of greater hemodynamic stability while minimizing thirst and inter-dialytic hypertension. To date, a few small studies support this theory,[202-206] but the results are not conclusive.[207,208]

Ultrafiltration modeling, like sodium modeling, provides a variable rate of fluid removal during dialysis, according to a preprogrammed profile (linear decline, stepwise changes, or exponential decline of filtration rate with time). Altering the filtration rate during dialysis theoretically allows time for the blood compartment to refill from the interstitial compartment, leading to improved hemodynamic stability and less cramping. As with sodium modeling, ultrafiltration modeling must be individualized. In fact, the effects of the two are difficult to distinguish because they are often used together.[203,206,207,209]

Anticoagulation

Blood clotting during dialysis is a source of patient blood loss and interferes with solute clearance by decreasing the dialyzer surface area.[210] To prevent clotting, a dose of heparin, the most commonly used anticoagulant in dialysis, is usually given at the start of dialysis (2000–5000 units or 50 units/kg), then continuously infused (1000–1500 units/hr) into the blood circuit before the dialyzer, until 15 to 60 minutes before the end of dialysis.[211] Alternatively, heparin boluses may be given intermittently during dialysis as needed. The bolus method increases nursing time and results in episodes of over-anticoagulation and under-anticoagulation. If the patient is at risk of bleeding, low-dose heparin (bolus of 500 to 1000 units followed by 500 to 750 units/hr)[212,213] or no heparin may be appropriate.[214-218] For heparin-free dialysis, prerinsing the blood circuit with heparinized saline and flushing the dialyzer with 100 mL of 0.9% sodium chloride every 15 to 30 minutes helps prevent clotting. Avoiding blood or platelet transfusions through the circuit is also required to minimize clotting.

Alternatives to heparin anticoagulation include regional citrate anticoagulation,[219-222] low-molecular-weight heparin,[223-230] hirudin,[231-233] prostacyclin,[234-236] dermatan sulfate,[237,238] and serine protease inhibitors.[239, 240] None is in wide use, however, because of complexity, expense, lack of sufficient clinical experience, or equivalency to heparin. Citrate anticoagulation, in particular, may cause hypocalcemia and death if calcium replacement is inadequate[241] and significant metabolic alkalosis if the dialysate bicarbonate concentration is not decreased.[242, 243] In the rare case of confirmed heparin induced thrombocytopenia, low-molecular-weight heparin, hirudin, and citrate anticoagulation have been used with varying success.[244, 245]

On-Line Monitoring of Clearance, Hematocrit, and Access Flow

Urea concentration, hematocrit, and access blood flow may be measured on-line, that is, during the dialysis. Although the equipment and effort are expensive at present, they may prove cost-effective in the long run by improving patient care. Monitoring can minimize the amount of blood drawn and allow more sensitive and frequent assessment of adequacy, control of ultrafiltration, and detection of vascular access stenosis.

Monitoring Clearance

On-line monitoring of urea kinetics may provide the best assessment of urea removal and dialysis adequacy.[246-250] Available monitors include those that sample dialysate continuously or periodically to measure urea concentration[132-134, 251, 252] and those that monitor dialyzer sodium clearance by pulsing the dialysate sodium concentration and measuring conductivity.[253] The on-line methods for monitoring urea kinetics provide Kt/V_{urea} based on whole-body urea clearance, not just dialyzer clearance.

Monitoring Hematocrit

The hematocrit can be measured during dialysis, using either a conductivity method[254] or an optical technique.[255-257] These methods may benefit dialysis patients prone to hypotension and cramping because these symptoms are usually caused by intravascular volume depletion, which is reflected by the degree of hemoconcentration.[256] By monitoring the hematocrit on-line, the filtration rate can be varied during dialysis to minimize the magnitude of hemoconcentration and the occurrence of symptoms during dialysis.[255, 257]

Monitoring Access Flow

Vascular access failure is a major problem, costing mil-lions of health care dollars each year and diminishing the patient's quality of life,[258,259] prompting the National Kidney Foundation to issue management guidelines.[27] If impending access thrombosis can be predicted, the opportunity to intervene with angioplasty or surgery is available to prevent thrombosis and to extend access function. Many techniques have been described, including measuring venous pressures and determining access recirculation. Unfortunately, these techniques have not prevented access thrombosis[258-260] because the venous pressure technique is unable to detect inflow and midgraft stenosis[261] and because access recirculation calculated using peripheral venous blood is actually an artifact of solute disequilibrium.[148,149,152,153,262] The indicator dilution techniques for measuring access blood flow noninvasively during hemodialysis have strong predictive power and may allow timely intervention.[263-268] Observational studies[261,269-273] suggest that an absolute vascular access blood flow of less than 600 mL/min and a 25% decrease in access flow strongly predict vascular access failure within 3 to 12 months. Angioplasty prompted by a decrease in access flow is effective in prolonging fistula survival and preventing thrombosis, but prospective studies of surveillance and angioplasty in arteriovenous grafts have shown mixed results[267, 268, 274-277] (for more details, see Chapter 4). However, because preemptive correction of a stenosis before the access clots is shorter, less expensive, and decreases the risk for a missed dialysis treatment or a temporary dialysis catheter, access surveillance and intervention is still preferred in the absence of conclusive evidence for improved graft survival.[27, 278, 279]

MANAGEMENT OF THE HEMODIALYSIS PATIENT

The general principles of managing the hemodialysis patient are highlighted briefly here because the following chapters provide greater detail on many of these important topics. A typical *hemodialysis prescription* brings together all of the principles discussed so far and includes:

- Duration and frequency of dialysis
- Type of dialyzer
- Blood flow rate
- Dialysate flow rate
- Heparin load and infusion rate
- Amount of fluid to be removed
- Location and type of vascular access
- Dialysate sodium, potassium, calcium, and bicarbonate concentrations

Medication and Diet

Once a patient begins dialysis, the *medications* should be reviewed and adjusted. In particular, the patient should receive vitamin B complex, vitamin C, folic acid supplements, and trace minerals because dialysis removes water-soluble vitamins and trace elements. The major goals are to simplify and to optimize the medication regimen to improve compliance and outcome. Therefore, patients with little urine output should discontinue diuretics, and patients who may benefit from an angiotensin converting enzyme inhibitor should start this medication once dialysis starts. Any medications that may be removed by dialysis or that accumulate in dialysis patients must be adjusted appropriately (see Chapter 19).

The dietitian should meet with the patient on a regular basis to provide feedback and teaching on the *dietary prescription*. Fluid, potassium, and phosphate restrictions are vital to the success of dialysis, given the problems with intra-dialytic hypotension and inefficient removal of phosphate, as discussed earlier. Additionally, adequate protein and calorie intake must be stressed in light of the high morbidity and mortality associated with hypoalbuminemia.[280,281]

Hormonal and Metabolic Disturbances

As management has improved and patients live longer on dialysis, the spectrum of the various *renal osteodystrophies* is changing. The incidence and severity of hyperparathyroid bone disease have decreased as the use of phosphate binders and calcitriol has become routine. Aluminum bone toxicity was an important cause of bone pain and pathologic fractures until the use of aluminum-based phosphate binders declined and water treatment improved. With the advent of high-flux dialyzers, amyloid bone disease is declining. Instead, adynamic bone disease from excessive suppression of parathyroid hormone has emerged, although its clinical significance is still debated[282,283] (see Chapters 13 and 14).

Although replacing erythropoietin in ESRD patients has corrected much of the observed *anemia*, there are still some issues to be resolved (see Chapter 15). The NKF guidelines for treating anemia in patients with ESRD[26] favor administering erythropoietin subcutaneously because of its increased efficacy, supported by the findings of a Veterans Affairs Cooperative Study.[284] The guidelines also suggest using maintenance doses of intravenous iron dextran 50 to 100 mg weekly or every other week to prevent relative iron deficiency. In patients who are anemic despite greater than 150 units/kg/dialysis of erythropoietin and intravenous maintenance iron, evidence for aluminum toxicity, hyperparathyroid bone disease, vitamin deficiency, and inflammation (activation of the acute-phase response) should be sought.[73]

As discussed earlier, *metabolic acidosis* may increase protein and muscle catabolism and is a potential cause of morbidity, but the impact in dialysis patients is debated.[43,285,286] Dialysis does not always correct acidosis completely because the effect of the dialysate on acid/base balance in the patient is complex, the net result of acetate and bicarbonate flux in opposite directions and removal of organic anions.[287] If acidosis is corrected by raising the dialysate bicarbonate concentration, anthropometric parameters improve in both hemodialysis and peritoneal dialysis patients,[288] although the effect on serum albumin is variable.[289] If acidosis cannot be corrected by increasing dialysate bicarbonate, then oral supplementation with bicarbonate should be considered.

Blood Pressure

Both *hypertension* and *hypotension* occur in dialysis patients and pose significant management problems. Blood pressures measured immediately before and during dialysis may not reflect the average pressure between dialyses. Epidemiologic data suggest that blood pressure correlates poorly with mortality in dialysis patients probably because of the confounding effects of severe malnutrition and myocardial failure, which reduce blood pressure and increase mortality risk.[290,291] This association, however, should not engender complacency about blood pressure control in light of the high cardiovascular mortality and widely prevalent left-ventricular hypertrophy in dialysis patients (see Chapter 12).

Intra-dialytic hypotension is associated with significant acute morbidity, including sudden death, and may be a cause of chronic morbidity and mortality when it is recurrent.[292] Hypotension is the result of rapid fluid removal from the blood compartment at a rate faster than refilling from the other fluid compartments, compounded by either a reduced myocardial contractile reserve or inadequate arterial vasoconstriction in response to the blood volume contraction.[293,294] Using a higher dialysate sodium concentration, dialysate sodium modeling, and ultrafiltration modeling during dialysis (see earlier Mechanics of Hemodialysis) may ameliorate the hypotension. However, these maneuvers usually result in increased thirst and greater interdialytic weight gains, thus promulgating the vicious cycle.[295] Additional maneuvers to maintain hemodynamic stability during dialysis include: (1) pharmacologic agents such as midodrine,[296-299] (2) cooling the patient,[296,298] (3) isothermic dialysis using the Fresenius Blood Temperature Monitor,[300] (4) biofeedback devices that prevent excessive blood volume contraction (not yet available in the United States),[301,302] and (5) increasing dialysis frequency, especially nocturnal hemodialysis.[303-306]

Dialysis-Related Complications

Given the excellent predictive value of low blood flows in fistulas and grafts as a signal for impending occlusion and the availability of surveillance techniques, each dialysis clinic should have a vascular access surveillance program in place to decrease the morbidity associated with graft thrombosis[27,307] (see earlier discussion). Ensuring a properly functioning AV graft or fistula minimizes the need for inserting a temporary or permanent dialysis catheter and therefore the risk of catheter-related sepsis. Should a catheter be required, a cuffed and tunneled catheter or a subcutaneous catheter[308-310] is preferable because it lasts longer and has a lower risk of infection compared with a temporary, noncuffed catheter.

Vaccinations against hepatitis B as well as the influenza virus and pneumococcus are important for health care maintenance in dialysis patients because of the increased risk of exposure to hepatitis B and the patients' compromised immune status. Because dialysis patients carrying hepatitis B have a high incidence of hepatitis B e antigenemia,[311] making the disease more contagious, all hepatitis B-naive patients initiating dialysis should receive recombinant hepatitis vaccine. Only 60% to 70% of patients, however, seroconvert on completing the series.[312] Strategies for revaccination, increasing the dose of the vaccine, or changing to the intradermal route of administration may enhance seroconversion[313,314] (see Chapter 18).

Although hemodialysis is much safer now than Kolff's[5] first hemodialysis attempts, the many technical advances have not completely eliminated complications resulting from the dialysis procedure itself (see Chapter 11). Some patients experience anaphylactoid and allergic reactions during the first few minutes of hemodialysis from exposure to the sterilant ethylene oxide, the plasticizers present in the dialyzers, or the less biocompatible dialyzers (see Chapters 2 and 5). Bioincompatible dialyzers activate complement, leukocytes, and platelets and cause chest pain, shortness of breath, and sludging of leukocytes and platelets in the pulmonary vasculature.

Fever during dialysis may be caused by bacterial contamination or endotoxin in the source water or dialysate and by access infection. Rapid removal of solutes may cause symptoms of disequilibrium, including fatigue, light-headedness, and decreased ability to concentrate when mild; and altered mental status, seizures, and death when severe (see Chapter 11). Although many advances have been made during the past three decades of life support with hemodialysis, much remains to be done to improve patients' quality of life.

FUTURE CONSIDERATIONS

More than 30 years of experience have demonstrated that thrice-weekly hemodialysis is not completely successful in reversing the syndrome of uremia. Reasons for this are not entirely clear, but they almost certainly include the residual syndrome (see earlier discussion). Failure to eliminate the residual syndrome may be related to inadequate dialysis, failure of dialysis to reproduce one or more functions of the native kidney, or complications derived from the dialysis treatment itself.

The discovery of dialysis-related amyloidosis and the subsequent identification of β_2-microglobulin as the amyloid precursor represent a major advance in the battle to sustain and maintain a reasonable quality of life over an extended number of years on hemodialysis.[38] Because β_2-microglobulin is a relatively large molecule that is not removed by cellulose membranes, its discovery prompted an investigation into the more permeable high-flux dialysis membranes. Accumulated evidence shows increasingly strong support for the use of synthetic high-flux membranes to prevent clinical progression of dialysis-related amyloidosis.[38]

The ever-changing landscape of the residual syndrome now encompasses adynamic bone disease, uncovered during efforts to improve the understanding and treatment of hyperparathyroid bone disease. Other battle fronts in the effort to improve the quality of life include studies of nutrition; the cause of the acute-phase response in dialysis patients; the complex interaction between the acute-phase response, nutrition, and atherosclerosis[77,78]; and methods to prevent both protein and calorie malnutrition.[75,280] Understanding the mechanisms responsible for accelerated atherosclerosis in dialysis patients may be a key to improving the high mortality from cardiovascular disease.

The HEMO Study suggests that increasing the urea clearance (Kt/V) above 1.3 during three times a week dialysis and enhancing clearance of larger molecular molecules do not correct further the residual syndrome.[95] Instead, preliminary data from daily home hemodialysis show promise in normalizing blood pressure and further correcting the residual syndrome.[304,305] Because goals for future deployment of hemodialysis include reducing the need for travel to and from the dialysis center and shortening the time required for preparation and administration of hemodialysis, home hemodialysis, especially at night or during sleep, has obvious advantages in this regard. Maintaining or improving work conditions for staff managing hemodialysis patients is justifiable in itself but is especially important in dialysis centers where a positive attitude in the staff promotes better tolerance of dialysis by the patient.

References

1. Lysaght MJ: Maintenance dialysis population dynamics: Current trends and long-term implications. J Am Soc Nephrol 2002; 13(suppl 1):S37-S40.
2. Graham T: Osmotic force. Philo Trans R Soc Lond 1854; 144: 177-228.
3. Abel J, Rowntree L, Turner B: On the removal of diffusible substances from the circulating blood of living animals by dialysis. J Pharmacol Exp Ther 1914; 5:275-316.
4. Haas G: Dialysis of the flowing blood in the patient. Klin Wochenschr 1923; 70:1888.
5. Kolff WJ, Berk HT, ter Welle M, et al: The artificial kidney: A dialyser with a great area. 1944 (Classical article). J Am Soc Nephrol 1997; 8(12):1959-1965.
6. Kolff W: First clinical experience with the artificial kidney. Ann Intern Med 1965; 62:608-609.
7. Fishman A, Kroop I, Leiter H, et al: Experiences with the Kolff artificial kidney. Am J Med 1949; 7:15-34.
8. Merrill J, Thorne G, Walter C, et al: The use of the artificial kidney. J Clin Invest 1950; 29:412-424.
9. Quinton W, Dillard D, Scribner BH: Cannulation of blood vessels for prolonged hemodialysis. ASAIO Trans 1960; 6: 104-113.
10. Brescia MJ, Cimino JE, Appel K, et al: Chronic hemodialysis using venipuncture and a surgically created arteriovenous fistula. N Engl J Med 1966; 275:1089-1092.

11. K/DOQI clinical practice guidelines for chronic kidney disease: Evaluation, classification, and stratification. Am J Kidney Dis 2002; 39(2 suppl 1):S1-S266.
12. Lakkis FG, Nassar GM, Badr KF: Hormones and the kidney. *In* Schrier R, Gottschalk C (eds): Diseases of the Kidney. Boston, Little, Brown and Company, 1997, pp 251-292.
13. Walters BA, Hays RD, Spritzer KL, et al: Health-related quality of life, depressive symptoms, anemia, and malnutrition at hemo-dialysis initiation. Am J Kidney Dis 2002; 40(6): 1185-1194.
14. Allen KL, Miskulin D, Yan G, et al: Association of nutritional markers with physical and mental health status in prevalent hemodialysis patients from the HEMO study. J Ren Nutr 2002; 12(3):160-169.
15. Sanner BM, Tepel M, Esser M, et al: Sleep-related breathing disorders impair quality of life in haemodialysis recipients. Nephrol Dial Transplant 2002; 17(7):1260-1265.
16. Fukuhara S, Lopes AA, Bragg-Gresham JL, et al: Health-related quality of life among dialysis patients on three continents: The Dialysis Outcomes and Practice Patterns Study. Kidney Int 2003; 64(5):1903-1910.
17. Caskey FJ, Wordsworth S, Ben T, et al: Early referral and planned initiation of dialysis: What impact on quality of life? Nephrol Dial Transplant 2003; 18(7):1330-1338.
18. Iliescu EA, Coo H, McMurray MH, et al: Quality of sleep and health-related quality of life in haemodialysis patients. Nephrol Dial Transplant 2003; 18(1):126-132.
19. Valderrabano F, Jofre R, Lopez-Gomez JM: Quality of life in end-stage renal disease patients. Am J Kidney Dis 2001; 38(3): 443-464.
20. Knight EL, Ofsthun N, Teng M, et al: The association between mental health, physical function, and hemodialysis mortality. Kidney Int 2003; 63(5):1843-1851.
21. Lowrie EG, Curtin RB, LePain N, et al: Medical outcomes study short form-36: A consistent and powerful predictor of morbidity and mortality in dialysis patients. Am J Kidney Dis 2003; 41(6):1286-1292.
22. Arora P, Kausz AT, Obrador GT, et al: Hospital utilization among chronic dialysis patients. J Am Soc Nephrol 2000; 11(4): 740-746.
23. Winkelmayer WC, Glynn RJ, Levin R, et al: Determinants of delayed nephrologist referral in patients with chronic kidney disease. Am J Kidney Dis 2001; 38(6):1178-1184.
24. Obrador GT, Roberts T, St Peter WL, et al: Trends in anemia at initiation of dialysis in the United States. Kidney Int 2001; 60(5):1875-1884.
25. Metcalfe W, Khan IH, Prescott GJ, et al: Can we improve early mortality in patients receiving renal replacement therapy? Kidney Int 2000; 57(6):2539-2545.
26. NKF-K/DOQI Clinical Practice Guidelines for Anemia of Chronic Kidney Disease: Update 2000. Am J Kidney Dis 2001; 37(1 suppl 1):S182-S238.
27. NKF-K/DOQI Clinical Practice Guidelines for Vascular Access: Update 2000. Am J Kidney Dis 2001; 37(1 suppl 1): S137-S181.
28. NKF-K/DOQI Clinical Practice Guidelines for Hemodialysis Adequacy: Update 2000. Am J Kidney Dis 2001; 37(1 suppl 1): S7-S64.
29. K/DOQI Clinical Practice Guidelines for Chronic Kidney Disease: Evaluation, classification, and stratification. Am J Kidney Dis 2002; 39(2 suppl 1):S1-S266.
30. USRDS: United States Renal Data System. Am J Kidney Dis 2003; 42(6 Pt 6):1-230.
31. Ghavamian M, Gutch CF, Kopp KF, et al: The sad truth about hemodialysis in diabetic nephropathy. JAMA 1972; 222(11): 1386-1389.
32. Hull A, Parker T: Proceedings from the Morbidity, Mortality and Prescription of Dialysis Symposium: Dallas, TX, September 15-17, 1989. Am J Kidney Dis 1990; 15:375-383.
33. Kwan JT, Carr EC, Neal AD, et al: Carbamylated haemoglobin, urea kinetic modelling and adequacy of dialysis in haemodialysis patients. Nephrol Dial Transplant 1991; 6(1):38-43.
34. Davenport A, Jones S, Goel S, et al: Carbamylated hemoglobin: A potential marker for the adequacy of hemodialysis therapy in end-stage renal failure. Kidney Int 1996; 50(4): 1344-1351.
35. Hou FF, Chertow GM, Kay J, et al: Interaction between beta 2 microglobulin and advanced glycation end products in the development of dialysis related-amyloidosis. Kidney Int 1997; 51(5):1514-1519.
36. Odetti P, Cosso L, Pronzato MA, et al: Plasma advanced glycosylation end-products in maintenance haemodialysis patients. Nephrol Dial Transplant 1995; 10(11):2110-2113.
37. Papanastasiou P, Grass L, Rodela H, et al: Immunological quantification of advanced glycosylation end-products in the serum of patients on hemodialysis or CAPD. Kidney Int 1994; 46(1): 216-222.
38. Drueke TB: Dialysis-related amyloidosis. Nephrol Dial Transplant 1998; 13(suppl 1):58-64.
39. De Smet R, Glorieux G, Hsu C, et al: P-cresol and uric acid: Two old uremic toxins revisited. Kidney Int 1997; 62:S8-S11.
40. Cohen G, Haag-Weber M, Horl WH: Immune dysfunction in uremia. Kidney Int 1997; 62:S79-S82.
41. Smogorzewski M, Massry SG: Uremic cardiomyopathy: Role of parathyroid hormone. Kidney Int 1997; 62:S12-S14.
42. Massry SG, Smogorzewski M: Parathyroid hormone, chronic renal failure and the liver. Kidney Int 1997; 62:S5-S7.
43. Bailey JL, Mitch WE: Metabolic acidosis as a uremic toxin. Semin Nephrol 1996; 16(3):160-166.
44. Yeun JY: The role of homocysteine in end-stage renal disease. Semin Dialysis 1998; 11(2):95-101.
45. Bostom AG, Lathrop L: Hyperhomocysteinemia in end-stage renal disease: Prevalence, etiology, and potential relationship to arteriosclerotic outcomes. Kidney Int 1997; 52(1):10-20.
46. Perna AF, Castaldo P, Ingrosso D, et al: Homocysteine, a new cardiovascular risk factor, is also a powerful uremic toxin. J Nephrol 1999; 12(4):230-240.
47. Niwa T: Organic acids and the uremic syndrome: Protein metabolite hypothesis in the progression of chronic renal failure. Semin Nephrol 1996; 16(3):167-182.
48. Horl WH: Hemodialysis membranes: Interleukins, biocompatibility, and middle molecules. J Am Soc Nephrol 2002; 13(suppl 1):S62-S71.
49. Vanholder R, Argiles A, Baurmeister U, et al: Uremic toxicity: Present state of the art. Int J Artif Organs 2001; 24(10):695-725.
50. Miyata T, Oda O, Inagi R, et al: Beta 2-Microglobulin modified with advanced glycation end products is a major component of hemodialysis-associated amyloidosis. J Clin Invest 1993; 92(3): 1243-1252.
51. Niwa T, Katsuzaki T, Momoi T, et al: Modification of beta 2m with advanced glycation end products as observed in dialysis-related amyloidosis by 3-DG accumulating in uremic serum. Kidney Int 1996; 49(3):861-867.
52. Dou L, Cerini C, Brunet P, et al: P-cresol, a uremic toxin, decreases endothelial cell response to inflammatory cytokines. Kidney Int 2002; 62(6):1999-2009.
53. Pawlak D, Koda M, Pawlak S, et al: Contribution of quinolinic acid in the development of anemia in renal insufficiency. Am J Physiol Renal Physiol 2003; 284(4):F693-F700.
54. Vanholder R, Glorieux G, Lameire N: Uraemic toxins and cardiovascular disease. Nephrol Dial Transplant 2003; 18(3): 463-466.
55. Blantz RC, Lortie M, Vallon V, et al: Activities of nitric oxide in normal physiology and uremia. Semin Nephrol 1996; 16(3): 144-150.
56. Vanholder R, De Smet R: Pathophysiologic effects of uremic retention solutes. J Am Soc Nephrol 1999; 10(8):1815-1823.

57. Spalding EM, Chamney PW, Farrington K: Phosphate kinetics during hemodialysis: Evidence for biphasic regulation. Kidney Int 2002; 61(2):655-667.
58. Vanholder R, Smet RD, Glorieux G, et al: Survival of hemodialysis patients and uremic toxin removal. Artif Organs 2003; 27(3):218-223.
59. Dhondt A, Vanholder R, Van Biesen W, et al: The removal of uremic toxins. Kidney Int Suppl 2000; 76:S47-S59.
60. Fagugli RM, De Smet R, Buoncristiani U, et al: Behavior of non-protein-bound and protein-bound uremic solutes during daily hemodialysis. Am J Kidney Dis 2002; 40(2):339-347.
61. Maduell F, Navarro V, Torregrosa E, et al: Change from three times a week on-line hemodiafiltration to short daily on-line hemodiafiltration. Kidney Int 2003; 64(1):305-313.
62. Clark WR, Henderson LW: Renal versus continuous versus intermittent therapies for removal of uremic toxins. Kidney Int Suppl 2001; 78:S298-S303.
63. Merrill J, Legrain M, Hoigne R: Observations on the role of urea in uremia. Am J Med 1953; 14:519-520.
64. Johnson WJ, Hagge WW, Wagoner RD, et al: Effects of urea loading in patients with far-advanced renal failure. Mayo Clin Proc 1972; 47(1):21-29.
65. Bergstrom J, Furst P: Uraemic toxins. *In* Drukker W, Parsons FM, Maher JF (eds): Replacement of Renal Function by Dialysis. Boston, Martinus Nijhoff, 1983, pp 354-390.
66. Mason M, Resnik H, Mino A, et al: Mechanism of experimental uremia. Arch Int Med 1993; 60:312.
67. Vanholder R, Schoots A, Ringoir S: Uremic toxicity. *In* Maher J (ed): Replacement of Renal Function by Dialysis. Dordrecht, Kluwer Academic Publishers, 1989, pp 4-19.
68. Depner TA: The uremic syndrome. *In* Greenberg A (ed): NKF Primer on Kidney Diseases. San Diego, Academic Press, 1994, pp 253-258.
69. Depner TA: Uremic toxicity: Urea and beyond. Semin Dial 2001; 14(4):246-251.
70. Kaysen GA, Stevenson FT, Depner TA: Determinants of albumin concentration in hemodialysis patients. Am J Kidney Dis 1997; 29(5):658-668.
71. Bologa RM, Levine DM, Parker TS, et al: Interleukin-6 predicts hypoalbuminemia, hypocholesterolemia, and mortality in hemodialysis patients. Am J Kidney Dis 1998; 32(1):107-114.
72. Qureshi AR, Alvestrand A, Danielsson A, et al: Factors predicting malnutrition in hemodialysis patients: A cross-sectional study. Kidney Int 1998; 53(3):773-782.
73. Gunnell J, Yeun JY, Depner TA, et al: Acute-phase response predicts erythropoietin resistance in hemodialysis and peritoneal dialysis patients. 1999; 33:63-72.
74. Bergstrom J, Heimburger O, Lindholm B, et al: Elevated serum CRP is a strong predictor of increased mortality and low serum albumin in hemodialysis (HD) patients. J Am Soc Nephrol 1995; 6:573.
75. Yeun JY, Kaysen GA: Factors influencing serum albumin in dialysis patients. Am J Kidney Dis 1998; 32:S118-S125.
76. Kaysen GA, Eiserich JP: Characteristics and effects of inflammation in end-stage renal disease. Semin Dial 2003; 16(6): 438-446.
77. Stenvinkel P, Heimburger O, Paultre F, et al: Strong association between malnutrition, inflammation, and atherosclerosis in chronic renal failure. Kidney Int 1999; 55(5):1899-1911.
78. Pecoits-Filho R, Lindholm B, Stenvinkel P: The malnutrition, inflammation, and atherosclerosis (MIA) syndrome: The heart of the matter. Nephrol Dial Transplant 2002; 17(suppl 11): 28-31.
79. Ducloux D, Pascal B, Jamali M, et al: Is hyperhomocysteinaemia a risk factor for recurrent vascular access thrombosis in haemodialysis patients? (Letter). Nephrol Dial Transplant 1997; 12(9): 2037-2038.
80. Block GA, Hulbert-Shearon TE, Levin NW, et al: Association of serum phosphorus and calcium X phosphate product with mortality risk in chronic hemodialysis patients: A national study. Am J Kidney Dis 1998; 31(4):607-617.
81. Goodman WG, Goldin J, Kuizon BD, et al: Coronary-artery calcification in young adults with end-stage renal disease who are undergoing dialysis. N Engl J Med 2000; 342(20):1478-1483.
82. Block G, Port FK: Calcium phosphate metabolism and cardiovascular disease in patients with chronic kidney disease. Semin Dial 2003; 16(2):140-147.
83. Lundin PA: Prolonged survival on hemodialysis. *In* Maher JF (ed): Replacement of Renal Function by Dialysis. Dordrecht, Kluwer Academic Publishers, 1989, pp 1133-1140.
84. Rockel A, Abdelhamid S, Fliegel P, et al: Elimination of low molecular weight proteins with high flux membranes. Contrib Nephrol 1985; 46:69-74.
85. Consensus Development Conference Panel: Morbidity and mortality of renal dialysis: An NIH consensus conference statement. Ann Intern Med 1994; 121(1):62-70.
86. Renal Physicians Association: Clinical Practice Guideline on Adequacy of Hemodialysis. Washington, DC, Renal Physicians Association, 1993.
87. Lowrie EG, Laird NM, Parker TF, et al: Effect of the hemodialysis prescription of patient morbidity: Report from the National Cooperative Dialysis Study. N Engl J Med 1981; 305: 1176-1181.
88. Charra B, Calemard E, Ruffet M, et al: Survival as an index of adequacy of dialysis. Kidney Int 1992; 41:1286-1291.
89. Owen WFJ, Lew NL, Liu Y, et al: The urea reduction ratio and serum albumin concentration as predictors of mortality in patients undergoing hemodialysis. N Engl J Med 1993; 329: 1001-1006.
90. Collins AJ, Ma JZ, Umen A, et al: Urea index and other predictors of hemodialysis patient survival. Am J Kidney Dis 1994; 23: 272-282.
91. Held PJ, Port FK, Wolfe RA, et al: The dose of hemodialysis and patient mortality. Kidney Int 1996; 50:550-556.
92. Hakim RM, Breyer J, Ismail N, et al: Effects of dose of dialysis on morbidity and mortality. Am J Kidney Dis 1994; 23: 661–669.
93. Parker TF, Husni L, Huang W, et al: Survival of hemodialysis patients in the United States is improved with a greater quantity of dialysis. Am J Kidney Dis 1994; 23:670-680.
94. Yang CS, Chen SW, Chiang CH, et al: Effects of increasing dialysis dose on serum albumin and mortality in hemodialysis patients. Am J Kidney Dis 1996; 27:380-386.
95. Eknoyan G, Beck GJ, Cheung AK, et al: Effect of dialysis dose and membrane flux in maintenance hemodialysis. N Engl J Med 2002; 347(25):2010-2019.
96. Depner TA, Daugirdas JT, Greene T, et al: Dialysis dose and the effect of gender and body size on outcome in the HEMO study. Kidney Int 2004; 65:1386-1394.
97. Lucas RC: On a form of late rickets associated with albuminuria, rickets of adolescents. Lancet 1883; 1:993.
98. Fraser DR, Kodicek E: Unique biosynthesis by kidney of a biological active vitamin D metabolite. Nature 1970; 228(273): 764-766.
99. Lawson DE, Fraser DR, Kodicek E, et al: Identification of 1,25-dihydroxycholecalciferol, a new kidney hormone controlling calcium metabolism. Nature 1971; 230(5291):228-230.
100. Slatopolsky E, Weerts C, Thielan J, et al: Marked suppression of secondary hyperparathyroidism by intravenous administration of 1,25-dihydroxy-cholecalciferol in uremic patients. J Clin Invest 1984; 74(6):2136-2143.
101. Hruska KA, Teitelbaum SL: Renal osteodystrophy. N Engl J Med 1995; 333:166-174.
102. Hurtado A, Merino C, Delgado E: Influence of anoxemia on the hematopoietic activity. Arch Intern Med 1945; 75:284-323.

103. Jacobson LO, Goldwasser E, Gried W, et al: Role of the kidney in erythropoiesis. Nature 1957; 179:633-634.
104. Miyake T, Kung CK, Goldwasser E: Purification of human erythropoietin. J Biol Chem 1977; 252(15):5558-5564.
105. Eschbach JW, Abdulhadi MH, Browne JK, et al: Recombinant human erythropoietin in anemic patients with end-stage renal disease. Results of a phase III multicenter clinical trial. Ann Intern Med 1989; 111(12):992-1000.
106. Evans RW: Recombinant human erythropoietin and the quality of life of end-stage renal disease patients: A comparative analysis. Am J Kidney Dis 1991; 18(4 suppl 1):62-70.
107. Nissenson AR: Epoetin and cognitive function. Am J Kidney Dis 1992; 20(1 suppl 1):21-24.
108. Gotch FA: Kinetic modeling in hemodialysis. *In* Nissenson AR, Fine RN, Gentile DE (eds): Clinical Dialysis, ed 3. Norwalk, CT, Appleton & Lange, 1995, pp 156-188.
109. Colton CK, Lowrie EG: Hemodialysis: Physical principles and technical considerations. *In* Brenner BM, Rector FC Jr (eds): The Kidney. Philadelphia, WB Saunders, 1981, pp 2425-2489.
110. Depner TA: Prescribing Hemodialysis: A Guide to Urea Modeling. Boston, Kluwer Academic Publishers, 1991.
111. Donnan FG: The theory of membrane equilibria. Chem Review 1924; 1:73.
112. Nolph KD, Stoltz ML, Carter CB, et al: Factors affecting the composition of ultrafiltrate from hemodialysis coils. Trans Am Soc Artif Intern Organs 1970; 16:495-501.
113. Locatelli F, Mastrangelo F, Redaelli B, et al: Effects of different membranes and dialysis technologies on patient treatment tolerance and nutritional parameters. The Italian Cooperative Dialysis Study Group. Kidney Int 1996; 50(4): 1293-1302.
114. Leypoldt JK, Cheung AK: Removal of high-molecular-weight solutes during high-efficiency and high-flux haemodialysis. Nephrol Dial Transplant 1996; 11(2):329-335.
115. USRDS: Excerpts from the United States Renal Data System 1998: Annual data report. Am J Kidney Dis 1998; 32(2 suppl 1): S1-S162.
116. USRDS: The USRDS Dialysis Morbidity and Mortality Study (Wave 1). Am J Kidney Dis 1996; 28(3 suppl 2):S58-S78.
117. Taylor JE, Mclaren M, Mactier RA, et al: Effect of dialyzer geometry during hemodialysis with cuprophane membranes. Kidney Int 1992; 42(2):442-447.
118. Mujais SK, Schmidt B: Operating characteristics of hollow fiber dialyzers. *In* Nissenson AR, Fine RN, Gentile DE (eds): Clinical Dialysis. Norwalk, CT, Appleton & Lange, 1995, pp 77-92.
119. Leypoldt JK, Cheung AK, Agodoa LY, et al: Hemodialyzer mass transfer-area coefficients for urea increase at high dialysate flow rates. The Hemodialysis (HEMO) Study. Kidney Int 1997; 51(6):2013-2017.
120. Ouseph R, Ward RA: Increasing dialysate flow rate increases dialyzer urea mass transfer-area coefficients during clinical use. Am J Kidney Dis 2001; 37(2):316-320.
121. Depner TA, Greene T, Daugirdas JT, et al: Dialyzer performance in the HEMO Study: In vivo K_0A and true blood flow determined from a model of cross-dialyzer urea extraction. Kidney Int 2003; submitted.
122. Poh CK, Hardy PA, Liao Z, et al: Effect of spacer yarns on the dialysate flow distribution of hemodialyzers: A magnetic resonance imaging study. ASAIO J 2003; 49(4):440-448.
123. Leypoldt JK, Cheung AK, Chirananthavat T, et al: Hollow fiber shape alters solute clearances in high flux hemodialyzers. ASAIO J 2003; 49(1):81-87.
124. Yeun JY, Depner TA: Complications related to inadequate delivered dose. *In* Mehta R, Lamiere N (eds): Complications of Dialysis—Recognition and Management. New York, Marcel Dekker, 1999.
125. Depner TA: Quantifying hemodialysis and peritoneal dialysis: Examination of the peak concentration hypothesis. Semin Dialysis 1994; 7:315-317.
126. Casino FG, Lopez T: The equivalent renal urea clearance: A new parameter to assess dialysis dose. Nephrol Dial Transplant 1996; 11(8):1574-1581.
127. Depner TA: Benefits of more frequent dialysis: Lower TAC at the same Kt/V. Nephrol Dial Transplant 1998; 13(suppl 6): 20-24.
128. Gotch FA: The current place of urea kinetic modelling with respect to different dialysis modalities. Nephrol Dial Transplant 1998; 13(suppl 6):10-14.
129. Kaplan MA, Hays L, Hays RM: Evolution of a facilitated diffusion pathway for amides in the erythrocyte. Am J Physiol 1974; 226(6):1327-1332.
130. Macey RI, Yousef LW: Osmotic stability of red cells in renal circulation requires rapid urea transport. Am J Physiol 1988; 254(5 Pt 1):C669-C674.
131. Gotch FA, Sargent JA: A mechanistic analysis of the National Cooperative Dialysis Study (NCDS). Kidney Int 1985; 28(3): 526-534.
132. Keshaviah PR, Ebben JP, Emerson PF: On-line monitoring of the delivery of the hemodialysis prescription. Pediatr Nephrol 1995; 9(suppl):S2-S8.
133. Garred LJ: Dialysate-based kinetic modeling. Adv Ren Replace Ther 1995; 2:305-318.
134. Alloatti S, Molino A, Manes M, et al: On-line dialysate urea monitor: Comparison with urea kinetics. Int J Artif Organs 1995; 18:548-552.
135. Depner TA, Greene T, Gotch FA, et al: Imprecision of the hemodialysis dose when measured directly from urea removal. Hemodialysis Study Group. Kidney Int 1999; 55(2): 635-647.
136. Daugirdas JT: Simplified equations for monitoring Kt/V, PCRn, eKt/V, and ePCRn. Adv Ren Replace Ther 1995; 2: 295-304.
137. Daugirdas JT, Depner TA, Gotch FA, et al: Comparison of methods to predict equilibrated Kt/V in the HEMO Pilot Study. Kidney Int 1997; 52(5):1395-1405.
138. Presta E, Segal KR, Gutin B, et al: Comparison in man of total body electrical conductivity and lean body mass derived from body density: Validation of a new body composition method. Metabolism 1983; 32(5):524-527.
139. Watson PE, Watson ID, Batt RD: Total body water volumes for adult males and females estimated from simple anthropometric measurements. Am J Clin Nutr 1980; 33(1):27-39.
140. Hume R, Weyers E: Relationship between total body water and surface area in normal and obese subjects. J Clin Pathol 1971; 24(3):234-238.
141. Chertow GM, Lazarus JM, Lew NL, et al: Development of a population-specific regression equation to estimate total body water in hemodialysis patients. Kidney Int 1997; 51(5):1578-1582.
142. Daugirdas JT, Greene T, Depner TA, et al: Anthropometrically estimated total body water volumes are larger than modeled urea volume in chronic hemodialysis patients: Effects of age, race, and gender. Kidney Int 2003; 64(3):1108-1119.
143. Borah MF, Schoenfeld PY, Gotch FA, et al: Nitrogen balance during intermittent dialysis therapy of uremia. Kidney Int 1978; 14(5):491-500.
144. Cottini EP, Gallina DL, Dominguez JM: Urea excretion in adult humans with varying degrees of kidney malfunction fed milk, egg or an amino acid mixture: Assessment of nitrogen balance. J Nutr 1973; 103(1):11-19.
145. Laird NM, Berkey CS, Lowrie EG: Modeling success or failure of dialysis therapy: The National Cooperative Dialysis Study. Kidney Int 1983; 13:S101-S106.

146. Lowrie EG, Lew NL: Death risk in hemodialysis patients: The predictive value of commonly measured variables and an evaluation of death rate differences between facilities. Am J Kidney Dis 1990; 15:458-482.
147. Depner TA: Assessing adequacy of hemodialysis: Urea modeling. Kidney Int 1994; 45:1522-1535.
148. Depner TA, Rizwan S, Cheer AY, et al: High venous urea concentrations in the opposite arm. A consequence of hemodialysis-induced compartment disequilibrium. ASAIO Trans 1991; 37(3):M141-M143.
149. Tattersall JE, Farrington K, Raniga PD, et al: Haemodialysis recirculation detected by the three-sample method is an artifact. Nephrol Dial Transplant 1993; 8(1):60-63.
150. Schneditz D, Van Stone JC, Daugirdas JT: A regional blood circulation alternative to in-series two compartment urea kinetic modeling. ASAIO J 1993; 39(3):M573-M577.
151. Schneditz D, Kaufman AM, Polaschegg HD, et al: Cardio pulmonary recirculation during hemodialysis. Kidney Int 1992; 42(6):1450-1456.
152. Depner T, Rizwan S, Cheer A, et al: Peripheral urea disequilibrium during hemodialysis is temperature-dependent. J Am Soc Nephrol 1991; 2:321.
153. Van Stone J, Jones M: Peripheral venous blood is not the appropriate specimen to determine recirculation rate. J Am Soc Nephrol 1991; 2:354.
154. Collins DM, Lambert MB, Middleton JP, et al: Fistula dysfunction: Effect on rapid hemodialysis. Kidney Int 1992; 41(5): 1292-1296.
155. Levy SS, Sherman RA, Nosher JL: Value of clinical screening for detection of asymptomatic hemodialysis vascular access stenoses. Angiology 1992; 43(5):421-424.
156. Windus DW, Audrain J, Vanderson R, et al: Optimization of high-efficiency hemodialysis by detection and correction of fistula dysfunction. Kidney Int 1990; 38(2):337-341.
157. Schaefer K, von Herrath D, Pauls A, et al: New insight into hemofiltration. Semin Nephrol 1986; 6(2):161-167.
158. Schaefer K, von Herrath D: Chronic intermittent hemofiltration?the treatment of future? Semin Dialysis 1993; 6:286-287.
159. Fox SD, Henderson LW: Cardiovascular response during hemodialysis and hemofiltration: Thermal, membrane, and catecholamine influences. Blood Purif 1993; 11(4): 224-236.
160. Baldamus CA, Ernst W, Fassbinder W, et al: Differing haemodynamic stability due to differing sympathetic response: Comparison of ultrafiltration, haemodialysis and haemofiltration. Proc Eur Dial Transplant Assoc 1980; 17: 205-212.
161. Kaiser JP, Hagemann J, von Herrath D, et al: Different handling of beta 2-microglobulin during hemodialysis and hemofiltration. Nephron 1988; 48(2):132-135.
162. Donauer J, Bohler J: Rationale for the use of blood volume and temperature control devices during hemodialysis. Kidney Blood Press Res 2003; 26(2):82-89.
163. Donauer J, Schweiger C, Rumberger B, et al: Reduction of hypotensive side effects during online-haemodiafiltration and low temperature haemodialysis. Nephrol Dial Transplant 2003; 18(8):1616-1622.
164. McCarthy JT, Moran J, Posen G, et al: A time for rediscovery: Chronic hemofiltration for end-stage renal disease. Semin Dial 2003; 16(3):199-207.
165. Vinay P, Cardoso M, Tejedor A, et al: Acetate metabolism during hemodialysis: Metabolic considerations. Am J Nephrol 1987; 7(5):337-354.
166. Kaiser BA, Potter DE, Bryant RE, et al: Acid-base changes and acetate metabolism during routine and high-efficiency hemodialysis in children. Kidney Int 1981; 19(1):70-79.
167. Hakim RM: Influence of high-flux biocompatible membrane on carpal tunnel syndrome and mortality. Am J Kidney Dis 1998; 32(2):338-340.
168. Koda Y, Nishi S, Miyazaki S, et al: Switch from conventional to high-flux membrane reduces the risk of carpal tunnel syndrome and mortality of hemodialysis patients. Kidney Int 1997; 52(4):1096-1101.
169. Kuchle C, Fricke H, Held E, et al: High-flux hemodialysis postpones clinical manifestation of dialysis-related amyloidosis. Am J Nephrol 1996; 16(6):484-488.
170. Blankestijn PJ, Vos PF, Rabelink TJ, et al: High-flux dialysis membranes improve lipid profile in chronic hemodialysis patients. J Am Soc Nephrol 1995; 5(9):1703-1708.
171. Goldberg IJ, Kaufman AM, Lavarias VA, et al: High flux dialysis membranes improve plasma lipoprotein profiles in patients with end-stage renal disease. Nephrol Dial Transplant 1996; 11(suppl 2):104-107.
172. Seres DS, Strain GW, Hashim SA, et al: Improvement of plasma lipoprotein profiles during high-flux dialysis. J Am Soc Nephrol 1993; 3(7):1409-1415.
173. Depner TA, Rizwan S, James LA: Effectiveness of low dose erythropoietin: A possible advantage of high flux hemodialysis. ASAIO Trans 1990; 36(3):M223-M225.
174. Coyne DW, Dagogo-Jack S, Klein S, et al: High-flux dialysis lowers plasma leptin concentration in chronic dialysis patients. Am J Kidney Dis 1998; 32(6):1031-1035.
175. Hornberger JC, Chernew M, Petersen J, et al: A multivariate analysis of mortality and hospital admissions with high-flux dialysis. J Am Soc Nephrol 1992; 3(6):1227-1237.
176. Barth RH, DeVincenzo N: Use of vancomycin in high-flux hemodialysis: Experience with 130 courses of therapy. Kidney Int 1996; 50(3):929-936.
177. Ikizler TA, Flakoll PJ, Parker RA, et al: Amino acid and albumin losses during hemodialysis. Kidney Int 1994; 46(3):830-837.
178. Kirschbaum B: The decline in serum albumin after conversion to high flux, high efficiency dialysis. Artif Organs 1994; 18(10): 729-735.
179. Bommer J, Becker KP, Urbaschek R: Potential transfer of endotoxin across high-flux polysulfone membranes. J Am Soc Nephrol 1996; 7(6):883-888.
180. Pereira BJG, Snodgrass BR, Hogan PJ, et al: Diffusive and convective transfer of cytokine-inducing bacterial products across hemodialysis membranes. Kidney Int 1995; 47(2): 603-610.
181. Keshaviah P, Collins A: High efficiency hemodialysis. Contrib Nephrol 1989; 69:109-119.
182. Mactier RA, Madi AM, Allam BF: Comparison of high-efficiency and standard haemodialysis providing equal urea clearances by partial and total dialysate quantification. Nephrol Dial Transplant 1997; 12(6):1182-1186.
183. Smye SW, Dunderdale E, Brownridge G, et al: Estimation of treatment dose in high-efficiency haemodialysis. Nephron 1994; 67(1):24-29.
184. Bergamo Collaborative Dialysis Study Group: Acute intradialytic well-being: Results of a clinical trial comparing polysulfone with cuprophan. Kidney Int 1991; 40(4):714-719.
185. Collins DM, Lambert MB, Tannenbaum JS, et al: Tolerance of hemodialysis: A randomized prospective trial of high-flux versus conventional high-efficiency hemodialysis. J Am Soc Nephrol 1993; 4(2):148-154.
186. Velasquez MT, von Albertini B, Lew SQ, et al: Equal levels of blood pressure control in ESRD patients receiving high-efficiency hemodialysis and conventional hemodialysis. Am J Kidney Dis 1998; 31(4):618-623.
187. Churchill DN, Bird DR, Taylor DW, et al: Effect of high-flux hemodialysis on quality of life and neuropsychological function in chronic hemodialysis patients. Am J Nephrol 1992; 12(6): 412-418.
188. Wauters JP, Bercini-Pansiot S, Gilliard N, et al: Short hemodialysis: Long-term mortality and morbidity. Artif Organs 1986; 10(3):182-184.

189. Ronco C, Brendolan A, Bragantini L, et al: Technical and clinical evaluation of different short, highly efficient dialysis techniques. Contrib Nephrol 1988; 61:46-68.
190. Spiegel DM, Baker PL, Babcock S, et al: Hemodialysis urea rebound: The effect of increasing dialysis efficiency. Am J Kidney Dis 1995; 25(1):26-29.
191. Abramson F, Gibson S, Barlee V, et al: Urea kinetic modeling at high urea clearances: Implications for clinical practice. Adv Ren Replace Ther 1994; 1(1):5-14.
192. Buffaloe GW: Ultrafiltration control. *In* Bosch JP, Stein JH (eds): Contemporary Issues in Nephrology. Hemodialysis: High-Efficiency Treatments. New York, Churchill Livingstone, 1993, pp 79-90.
193. Keshaviah P, Luehmann D, Ilstrup K, et al: Technical requirements for rapid high-efficiency therapies. Artif Organs 1986; 10(3):189-194.
194. Diamond SM, Henrich WL: Acetate dialysate versus bicarbonate dialysate: A continuing controversy. Am J Kidney Dis 1987; 9(1):3-11.
195. Hakim RM, Pontzer MA, Tilton D, et al: Effects of acetate and bicarbonate dialysate in stable chronic dialysis patients. Kidney Int 1985; 28(3):535-540.
196. Ebben JP, Hirsch DN, Luehmann DA, et al: Microbiologic contamination of liquid bicarbonate concentrate for hemodialysis. ASAIO Trans 1987; 33(3):269-273.
197. Bland LA, Ridgeway MR, Aguero SM, et al: Potential bacteriologic and endotoxin hazards associated with liquid bicarbonate concentrate. ASAIO Trans 1987; 33(3):542-545.
198. Depner TA, Rizwan S, Stasi TA: Pressure effects on roller pump blood flow during hemodialysis. ASAIO Trans 1990; 36(3): M456-M459.
199. Manuel MA, Stewart WK, Tulley FM, et al: Air embolism during haemodialysis. Lancet 1972; 1(7749):538.
200. Cybulsky AV, Matni A, Hollomby DJ: Effects of high sodium dialysate during maintenance hemodialysis. Nephron 1985; 41(1):57-61.
201. Swartz RD, Somermeyer MG, Hsu CH: Preservation of plasma volume during hemodialysis depends on dialysate osmolality. Am J Nephrol 1982; 2(4):189-194.
202. Flanigan MJ, Khairullah QT, Lim VS: Dialysate sodium delivery can alter chronic blood pressure management. Am J Kidney Dis 1997; 29(3):383-391.
203. Raja RM, Po CL: Plasma refilling during hemodialysis with decreasing ultrafiltration. Influence of dialysate sodium. ASAIO J 1994; 40(3):M423-M425.
204. Sadowski RH, Allred EN, Jabs K: Sodium modeling ameliorates intradialytic and interdialytic symptoms in young hemodialysis patients. J Am Soc Nephrol 1993; 4(5):1192-1198.
205. Dheenan S, Henrich WL: Preventing dialysis hypotension: A comparison of usual protective maneuvers. Kidney Int 2001; 59(3):1175-1181.
206. Oliver MJ, Edwards LJ, Churchill DN: Impact of sodium and ultrafiltration profiling on hemodialysis-related symptoms. J Am Soc Nephrol 2001; 12(1):151-156.
207. Churchill DN: Sodium and water profiling in chronic uraemia. Nephrol Dial Transplant 1996; 11(suppl 8):38-41.
208. Mann H, Stiller S: Sodium modeling. Kidney Int Suppl 2000; 76:S79-S88.
209. de Vries PM, Olthof CG, Solf A, et al: Fluid balance during haemodialysis and haemofiltration: The effect of dialysate sodium and a variable ultrafiltration rate. Nephrol Dial Transplant 1991; 6(4):257-263.
210. Wei SS, Ellis PW, Magnusson MO, et al: Effect of heparin modeling on delivered hemodialysis therapy. Am J Kidney Dis 1994; 23(3):389-393.
211. Ward RA: Heparinization for routine hemodialysis. Adv Ren Replace Ther 1995; 2(4):362-370.
212. Swartz RD: Hemorrhage during high-risk hemodialysis using controlled heparinization. Nephron 1981; 28(2):65-69.
213. Swartz RD, Port FK: Preventing hemorrhage in high-risk hemodialysis: Regional versus low-dose heparin. Kidney Int 1979; 16(4):513-518.
214. Caruana RJ, Raja RM, Bush JV, et al: Heparin free dialysis: Comparative data and results in high risk patients. Kidney Int 1987; 31:1351-1355.
215. Casati S, Moia M, Graziani G, et al: Hemodialysis without anticoagulants: Efficiency and hemostatic aspects. 1984; 21:102-105.
216. Sanders PW, Taylor H, Curtis JJ: Hemodialysis without anticoagulation. Am J Kidney Dis 1985; 5(1):32-35.
217. Schwab SJ, Onorato JJ, Sharar LR, et al: Hemodialysis without anticoagulation. One-year prospective trial in hospitalized patients at risk for bleeding. Am J Med 1987; 83(3): 405-410.
218. Liboro R, Schwartz AB, Conroy J, et al: Heparin free hemodialysis does not cause fibrin consumptive coagulopathy and maintains alternate pathway complement activation. ASAIO Trans 1990; 36:86-89.
219. Janssen MJ, Huijgens PC, Bouman AA, et al: Citrate versus heparin anticoagulation in chronic haemodialysis patients. Nephrol Dial Transplant 1993; 8(11):1228-1233.
220. Wiegmann TB, MacDougall ML, Diederich DA: Long-term comparisons of citrate and heparin as anticoagulants for hemodialysis. Am J Kidney Dis 1987; 9(5):430-435.
221. Evenepoel P, Maes B, Vanwalleghem J, et al: Regional citrate anticoagulation for hemodialysis using a conventional calcium-containing dialysate. Am J Kidney Dis 2002; 39(2): 315-323.
222. Apsner R, Buchmayer H, Lang T, et al: Simplified citrate anticoagulation for high-flux hemodialysis. Am J Kidney Dis 2001; 38(5):979-987.
223. Schrader J, Stibbe W, Kandt M, et al: Low molecular weight heparin versus standard heparin. A long-term study in hemodialysis and hemofiltration patients. ASAIO Trans 1990; 36(1):28-32.
224. Nurmohamed MT, ten Cate J, Stevens P, et al: Long-term efficacy and safety of a low molecular weight heparin in chronic hemodialysis patients. A comparison with standard heparin. ASAIO Trans 1991; 37:M459-M461.
225. Guillet B, Simon N, Sampol JJ, et al: Pharmacokinetics of the low molecular weight heparin enoxaparin during 48 h after bolus administration as an anticoagulant in haemodialysis. Nephrol Dial Transplant 2003; 18(11):2348-2353.
226. Naumnik B, Borawski J, Mysliwiec M: Different effects of enoxaparin and unfractionated heparin on extrinsic blood coagulation during haemodialysis: A prospective study. Nephrol Dial Transplant 2003; 18(7):1376-1382.
227. Polkinghorne KR, McMahon LP, Becker GJ: Pharmacokinetic studies of dalteparin (Fragmin), enoxaparin (Clexane), and danaparoid sodium (Orgaran) in stable chronic hemodialysis patients. Am J Kidney Dis 2002; 40(5):990-995.
228. Stefoni S, Cianciolo G, Donati G, et al: Standard heparin versus low-molecular-weight heparin. A medium-term comparison in hemodialysis. Nephron 2002; 92(3):589-600.
229. Hainer JW, Sherrard DJ, Swan SK, et al: Intravenous and subcutaneous weight-based dosing of the low molecular weight heparin tinzaparin (Innohep) in end-stage renal disease patients undergoing chronic hemodialysis. Am J Kidney Dis 2002; 40(3):531-538.
230. Lord H, Jean N, Dumont M, et al: Comparison between tinzaparin and standard heparin for chronic hemodialysis in a Canadian center. Am J Nephrol 2002; 22(1):58-66.
231. Fareed J, Callas D, Hoppensteadt DA, et al: Antithrombin agents as anticoagulants and antithrombotics. Implications in drug development. Med Clin North Am 1998; 82(3):569-586.

232. Nowak G, Bucha E, Brauns I, et al: Anticoagulation with r-hirudin in regular haemodialysis with heparin-induced thrombocytopenia (HIT II). The first long-term application of r-hirudin in a haemodialysis patient. Wien Klin Wochenschr 1997; 109(10):354-358.
233. van Wyk V, Badenhorst PN, Kotze HF: The effect of r-hirudin vs. heparin on blood-membrane interactions during hemodialysis. Clin Nephrol 1997; 48(6):381-387.
234. Caruana RJ, Smith MC, Clyne D, et al: Controlled study of heparin versus epoprostenol sodium (prostacyclin) as the sole anticoagulant for chronic hemodialysis. Blood Purif 1991; 9(5-6): 296-304.
235. Maurin N: Antithrombotic management with a stable prostacyclin analogue during extracorporeal circulation. Contrib Nephrol 1991; 93:205-209.
236. Kuzniewski M, Sulowicz W, Hanicki Z, et al: Effect of heparin and prostacyclin/heparin infusion on platelet aggregation in hemodialyzed patients. Nephron 1990; 56(2):174-178.
237. Boccardo P, Melacini D, Rota S, et al: Individualized anticoagulation with dermatan sulphate for haemodialysis in chronic renal failure. Nephrol Dial Transplant 1997; 12(11): 2349-2354.
238. Nurmohamed MT, Knipscheer HC, Stevens P, et al: Clinical experience with a new antithrombotic (dermatan sulfate) in chronic hemodialysis patients. Clin Nephrol 1993; 39(3): 166-171.
239. Akizawa T, Koshikawa S, Ota K, et al: Nafamostat mesilate: A regional anticoagulant for hemodialysis in patients at high risk for bleeding. Nephron 1993; 64(3):376-381.
240. Matsuo T, Kario K, Nakao K, et al: Anticoagulation with nafamostat mesilate, a synthetic protease inhibitor, in hemodialysis patients with a bleeding risk. Haemostasis 1993; 23(3): 135-141.
241. Charney DI, Salmond R: Cardiac arrest after hypertonic citrate anticoagulation for chronic hemodialysis. ASAIO Trans 1990; 36:M217-M219.
242. Kelleher SP, Schulman G: Severe metabolic alkalosis complicating regional citrate hemodialysis. Am J Kidney Dis 1987; 9: 235-236.
243. van der Meulen J, Janssen MJ, Langendijk PN, et al: Citrate anticoagulation and dialysate with reduced buffer content in chronic hemodialysis. Clin Nephrol 1992; 37(1):36-41.
244. O'Shea SI, Ortel TL, Kovalik EC: Alternative methods of anticoagulation for dialysis-dependent patients with heparin-induced thrombocytopenia. Semin Dial 2003; 16(1):61-67.
245. Ouseph R, Ward RA: Anticoagulation for intermittent hemodialysis. Semin Dial 2000; 13(3):181-187.
246. Depner TA, Keshaviah PR, Ebben JP, et al: Multicenter clinical validation of an on-line monitor of dialysis adequacy. J Am Soc Nephrol 1996; 7(3):464-471.
247. Chauveau P, Naret C, Puget J, et al: Adequacy of haemodialysis and nutrition in maintenance haemodialysis patients: Clinical evaluation of a new on-line urea monitor. Nephrol Dial Transplant 1996; 11(8):1568-1573.
248. Rahmati MA, Rahmati S, Hoenich N, et al: On-line clearance: A useful tool for monitoring the effectiveness of the reuse procedure. ASAIO J 2003; 49(5):543-546.
249. Lindsay RM, Sternby J: Future directions in dialysis quantification. Semin Dial 2001; 14(4):300-307.
250. Gotch FA: On-line clearance: Advanced methodology to monitor adequacy of dialysis at no cost. Contrib Nephrol 2002; 137:268-271.
251. Calzavara P, Calconi G, Da Rin G, et al: A new biosensor for continuous monitoring of the spent dialysate urea level in standard hemodialysis. Int J Artif Organs 1998; 21(3):147-150.
252. Argiles A, Ficheux A, Thomas M, et al: Precise quantification of dialysis using continuous sampling of spent dialysate and total dialysate volume measurement. Kidney Int 1997; 52(2): 530-537.
253. Del Vecchio L, Di Filippo S, Andrulli S, et al: Conductivity: On-line monitoring of dialysis adequacy. Int J Artif Organs 1998; 21(9):521-525.
254. Ishihara T, Igarashi I, Kitano T, et al: Continuous hematocrit monitoring method in an extracorporeal circulation system and its application for automatic control of blood volume during artificial kidney treatment. Artif Organs 1993; 17(8): 708-716.
255. Steuer RR, Leypoldt JK, Cheung AK, et al: Reducing symptoms during hemodialysis by continuously monitoring the hematocrit. Am J Kidney Dis 1996; 27(4):525-532.
256. Steuer RR, Leypoldt JK, Cheung AK, et al: Hematocrit as an indicator of blood volume and a predictor of intradialytic morbid events. ASAIO J 1994; 40(3):M691-M696.
257. de Vries JP, Olthof CG, Visser V, et al: Continuous measurement of blood volume during hemodialysis by an optical method. ASAIO J 1992; 38(3):M181-M185.
258. Depner TA: Techniques for prospective detection of venous stenosis. Adv Ren Replace Ther 1994; 1:119-130.
259. Hakim R, Himmelfarb J: Hemodialysis access failure: A call to action. Kidney Int 1998; 54(4):1029-1040.
260. Dember LM, Holmberg EF, Kaufman JS: Value of static venous pressure for predicting arteriovenous graft thrombosis. Kidney Int 2002; 61(5):1899-1904.
261. Bosman PJ, Boereboom FT, Eikelboom BC, et al: Graft flow as a predictor of thrombosis in hemodialysis grafts. Kidney Int 1998; 54(5):1726-1730.
262. Schneditz D, Polaschegg HD, Levin NW, et al: Cardiopulmonary recirculation in dialysis. An underrecognized phenomenon. ASAIO J 1992; 38(3):M194-M196.
263. Depner TA, Krivitski NM: Clinical measurement of blood flow in hemodialysis access fistulae and grafts by ultrasound dilution. ASAIO J 1995; 41(3):M745-M749.
264. Krivitski NM: Theory and validation of access flow measurement by dilution technique during hemodialysis. Kidney Int 1995; 48(1):244-250.
265. Krivitski NM, MacGibbon D, Gleed RD, et al: Accuracy of dilution techniques for access flow measurement during hemodialysis. Am J Kidney Dis 1998; 31(3):502-508.
266. Krivitski NM: Access flow measurement during surveillance and percutaneous transluminal angioplasty intervention. Semin Dial 2003; 16(4):304-308.
267. Tessitore N, Bedogna V, Gammaro L, et al: Diagnostic accuracy of ultrasound dilution access blood flow measurement in detecting stenosis and predicting thrombosis in native forearm arteriovenous fistulae for hemodialysis. Am J Kidney Dis 2003; 42(2):331-341.
268. Schwarz C, Mitterbauer C, Boczula M, et al: Flow monitoring: Performance characteristics of ultrasound dilution versus color Doppler ultrasound compared with fistulography. Am J Kidney Dis 2003; 42(3):539-545.
269. Depner TA, Reasons AM: Longevity of peripheral A-V grafts and fistulas for hemodialysis is related to access blood flow. J Am Soc Nephrol 1996; 7(9):1405.
270. Neyra NR, Ikizler TA, May RE, et al: Change in access blood flow over time predicts vascular access thrombosis. Kidney Int 1998; 54(5):1714-1719.
271. May RE, Himmelfarb J, Yenicesu M, et al: Predictive measures of vascular access thrombosis: A prospective study. Kidney Int 1997; 52:1656-1662.
272. Wang E, Schneditz D, Nepomuceno C, et al: Predictive value of access blood flow in detecting access thrombosis. ASAIO J 1998; 44(5):M555-M558.
273. Paulson WD, Ram SJ, Faiyaz R, et al: Association between blood pressure, ultrafiltration, and hemodialysis graft thrombosis:

A multivariable logistic regression analysis. Am J Kidney Dis 2002; 40(4):769-776.
274. Tordoir JH, Rooyens P, Dammers R, et al: Prospective evaluation of failure modes in autogenous radiocephalic wrist access for haemodialysis. Nephrol Dial Transplant 2003; 18(2): 378-383.
275. Begin V, Ethier J, Dumont M, et al: Prospective evaluation of the intra-access flow of recently created native arteriovenous fistulae. Am J Kidney Dis 2002; 40(6):1277-1282.
276. Ram SJ, Work J, Caldito GC, et al: A randomized controlled trial of blood flow and stenosis surveillance of hemodialysis grafts. Kidney Int 2003; 64(1):272-280.
277. Moist LM, Churchill DN, House AA, et al: Regular monitoring of access flow compared with monitoring of venous pressure fails to improve graft survival. J Am Soc Nephrol 2003; 14(10): 2645-2653.
278. McCarley P, Wingard RL, Shyr Y, et al: Vascular access blood flow monitoring reduces access morbidity and costs. Kidney Int 2001; 60(3):1164-1172.
279. Garland JS, Moist LM, Lindsay RM: Are hemodialysis access flow measurements by ultrasound dilution the standard of care for access surveillance? Adv Ren Replace Ther 2002; 9(2): 91-98.
280. Kopple JD: Effect of nutrition on morbidity and mortality in maintenance dialysis patients. Am J Kidney Dis 1994; 24: 1002-1009.
281. Bergstrom J: Anorexia in dialysis patients. Semin Nephrol 1996; 16(3):222-229.
282. Slatopolsky E, Gonzalez E, Martin K: Pathogenesis and treatment of renal osteodystrophy. Blood Purif 2003; 21(4-5): 318-326.
283. Martin KJ, Gonzalez EA: Strategies to minimize bone disease in renal failure. Am J Kidney Dis 2001; 38(6):1430-1436.
284. Kaufman JS, Reda DJ, Fye CL, et al: Subcutaneous compared with intravenous epoetin in patients receiving hemodialysis. Department of Veterans Affairs Cooperative Study Group on Erythropoietin in Hemodialysis Patients. N Engl J Med 1998; 339(9):578-583.
285. Uribarri J, Levin N, Delmez J, et al: Association of acidosis and nutritional parameters in hemodialysis patients (Abstract). J Am Soc Nephrol 1997; 8:108A.
286. Bergstrom J, Wang T, Lindholm B: Factors contributing to catabolism in end-stage renal disease patients. Miner Electrolyte Metab 1998; 24(1):92-101.
287. Uribarri J, Zia M, Mahmood J, et al: Acid production in chronic hemodialysis patients. J Am Soc Nephrol 1998; 9(1): 114-120.
288. Walls J: Effect of correction of acidosis on nutritional status in dialysis patients. Miner Electrolyte Metab 1997; 23(3-6): 234-236.
289. Brady JP, Hasbargen JA: Correction of metabolic acidosis and its effect on albumin in chronic hemodialysis patients. Am J Kidney Dis 1998; 31(1):35-40.
290. Zager PG, Nikolic J, Brown RH, et al: "U" curve association of blood pressure and mortality in hemodialysis patients. Medical Directors of Dialysis Clinic, Inc. Kidney Int 1998; 54(2):561-569.
291. Port FK, Hulbert-Shearon TE, Wolfe RA, et al: Predialysis blood pressure and mortality risk in a national sample of maintenance hemodialysis patients. Am J Kidney Dis 1999; 33(3):507-517.
292. Schreiber MJ Jr: Clinical case-based approach to understanding intradialytic hypotension. Am J Kidney Dis 2001; 38(4 suppl 4): S37-S47.
293. Nette RW, Krepel HP, van den Dorpel MA, et al: Hemodynamic response to lower body negative pressure in hemodialysis patients. Am J Kidney Dis 2003; 41(4):807-813.
294. Lee PT, Fang HC, Chen CL, et al: High vibration perception threshold and autonomic dysfunction in hemodialysis patients with intradialysis hypotension. Kidney Int 2003; 64(3):1089-1094.
295. Akcahuseyin E, Nette RW, Vincent HH, et al: Simulation study of the intercompartmental fluid shifts during hemodialysis. ASAIO J 2000; 46(1):81-94.
296. Sherman RA: Intradialytic hypotension: An overview of recent, unresolved and overlooked issues. Semin Dial 2002; 15(3): 141-143.
297. Perazella MA: Pharmacologic options available to treat symptomatic intradialytic hypotension. Am J Kidney Dis 2001; 38(4 suppl 4):S26-S36.
298. Hoeben H, Abu-Alfa AK, Mahnensmith R, et al: Hemodynamics in patients with intradialytic hypotension treated with cool dialysate or midodrine. Am J Kidney Dis 2002; 39(1):102-107.
299. Lin YF, Wang JY, Denq JC, et al: Midodrine improves chronic hypotension in hemodialysis patients. Am J Med Sci 2003; 325(5):256-261.
300. Maggiore Q, Pizzarelli F, Santoro A, et al: The effects of control of thermal balance on vascular stability in hemodialysis patients: Results of the European randomized clinical trial. Am J Kidney Dis 2002; 40(2):280-290.
301. Santoro A, Mancini E, Basile C, et al: Blood volume controlled hemodialysis in hypotension-prone patients: Randomized, multicenter controlled trial. Kidney Int 2002; 62(3): 1034-1045.
302. McIntyre CW, Lambie SH, Fluck RJ: Biofeedback controlled hemodialysis (BF-HD) reduces symptoms and increases both hemodynamic tolerability and dialysis adequacy in non-hypotension prone stable patients. Clin Nephrol 2003; 60(2):105-112.
303. Buoncristiani U, Fagugli RM, Pinciaroli MR, et al: Reversal of left-ventricular hypertrophy in uremic patients by treatment with daily hemodialysis (DHD). Contrib Nephrol 1996; 119: 152-156.
304. Pierratos A: Nocturnal home haemodialysis: An update on a 5-year experience. Nephrol Dial Transplant 1999; 14(12): 2835-2840.
305. Pierratos A: Daily hemodialysis: An update. Curr Opin Nephrol Hypertens 2002; 11(2):165-171.
306. Kumar VA, Craig M, Depner TA, et al: Extended daily dialysis: A new approach to renal replacement for acute renal failure in the intensive care unit. Am J Kidney Dis 2000; 36(2):294-300.
307. Depner TA: Hemodialysis access: The role of monitoring. In-line methods. ASAIO J 1998; 44(1):38-39.
308. Schwab SJ, Weiss MA, Rushton F, et al: Multicenter clinical trial results with the LifeSite hemodialysis access system. Kidney Int 2002; 62(3):1026-1033.
309. Levin NW, Yang PM, Hatch DA, et al: Initial results of a new access device for hemodialysis technical note. Kidney Int 1998; 54(5):1739-1745.
310. Moran JE: Subcutaneous vascular access devices. Semin Dial 2001; 14(6):452-457.
311. Kohler H, Arnold W, Renschin G, et al: Active hepatitis B vaccination of dialysis patients and medical staff. Kidney Int 1994; 25:124-128.
312. Peces R, de la Torre M, Alcazar R, et al: Prospective analysis of the factors influencing the antibody response to hepatitis B vaccine in hemodialysis patients. Am J Kidney Dis 1997; 29(2): 239-245.
313. Fabrizi F, Andrulli S, Bacchini G, et al: Intradermal versus intramuscular hepatitis B re-vaccination in non-responsive chronic dialysis patients: A prospective randomized study with cost-effectiveness evaluation. Nephrol Dial Transplant 1997; 12(6): 1204-1211.

314. Vlassopoulos D, Arvanitis D, Lilis D, et al: Complete success of intradermal vaccination against hepatitis B in advanced chronic renal failure and hemodialysis patients. Ren Fail 1997; 19(3): 455-460.

315. Depner TA: Approach to hemodialysis kinetic modeling. *In* Henrich WL (ed): Principles and Practice of Dialysis. Baltimore, Williams & Wilkins, 1999, pp 79-98.

Chapter 17

Vascular Access

Jonathan Himmelfarb, M.D. • Laura M. Dember, M.D. • Bradley S. Dixon, M.D.

HISTORY

The inception of hemodialysis for the treatment of patients with acute renal failure occurred with temporary access to the circulation in 1943.[1] However, the development of hemodialysis therapy for the maintenance treatment of end-stage renal disease (ESRD) required repeated access to the circulation. This became feasible with the introduction of the external arteriovenous Quinton-Scribner shunt in 1960.[2] The pioneering accomplishments of Willem Kolff and Belding Scribner in the development of dialysis were recognized with the Lasker Award for General Medical Research in 2002. The Quinton-Scribner cannula, made of silastic tubing connected to a Teflon cannula, shunt developed frequent problems with thrombosis and infection and typically functioned for a period of months. In 1966, Brescia and colleagues[3] developed the endogenous arteriovenous fistula, which remains the hemodialysis access of choice today. Interpositional bridge grafts were developed in the late 1960s and 70s. Initial grafts consisted of autogenous saphenous veins, bovine carotid arteries, and human umbilical veins. In the late 1970s, synthetic bridge grafts made of expanded polytetrafluoroethylene (ePTFE) were introduced.[4,5] Expanded PTFE can be placed in the majority of patients, are usable within weeks of surgical placement, and are relatively easy to cannulate. Expanded PTFE grafts remain the most frequently utilized graft biomaterial today and continue to be a highly prevalent permanent dialysis access in the United States.

Although the advantages and disadvantages of each type of dialysis access will be discussed later, it is clear that autogenous vein arteriovenous fistulas are preferable to all other currently available vascular access options. Current clinical practice guidelines recommend that patients with chronic kidney disease should be referred to create a primary arteriovenous fistula when the creatinine clearance falls below 25 mL/min, when the serum creatinine level is greater than or equal to 4 mg/dL, or within 1 year of the anticipated need for dialysis therapy.[6]

The use of catheters for hemodialysis access also parallels the history of dialysis. In 1961, Shaldon and colleagues[7] first described femoral artery catheterization for hemodialysis access. Uldall and colleagues[8] first reported the use of guidewire exchange techniques and subclavian vein puncture for placement of temporary dialysis catheters in 1979. In the late 1980s the use of surgically implanted tunneled, cuffed, double-lumen catheters was introduced.[9] Recently, subcutaneous placed vascular ports have been introduced as an alternative to the cuffed tunneled catheter.[10] While the major use of catheters for hemodialysis access is as a bridging device to allow time for maturation of a more permanent access, or for patients who need only temporary vascular access, catheter use as a permanent vascular access in patients for whom all other options have been exhausted is increasing in frequency.[11]

EPIDEMIOLOGY

The rapid growth of end-stage renal failure programs in the United States and worldwide has been accompanied by a tremendous increase in dialysis vascular access-associated morbidity and cost. Indeed, vascular access continues to be referred to as the "Achilles Heel" of the hemodialysis procedure.[12] The creation, maintenance, and replacement of vascular access in hemodialysis patients is recognized as a major source of morbidity and cost within the United States End-Stage Renal Disease Program, with recent estimates that annual costs likely exceed $1 billion within the Medicare program.

There is now compelling evidence that there are large differences in patterns of vascular access usage between Europe and the United States. The Dialysis Outcomes and Practice Patterns Study (DOPPS) compared vascular access use and survival in Europe and the United States.[13] Autogenous arteriovenous fistulas were used by 80% of European patients compared to 24% of prevalent dialysis patients in the United States. Arteriovenous fistula use was significantly associated with male sex, younger age, lower body mass index, absence of diabetes mellitus, and a lack of peripheral vascular disease. However, even after adjustment for these risk factors, there is a 21-fold increased likelihood of arteriovenous fistula use in Europe versus in the United States. A follow-up study from DOPPS suggests that pre-dialysis care by a nephrologist does not account for the substantial variations in the proportion of patients commencing dialysis with an arteriovenous fistula, and the time to fistula cannulation after creation also varies greatly between countries.[14] Enormous facility variation has also been noted within the United States, with the prevalence of arteriovenous fistulas ranging from 0% to 87%.[12] There is also large variation in access type by geographic region, sex, and race within the United States.[15] Thus, practice pattern variations in vascular access are determined by local preference, in addition to patient-related factors.

The importance of vascular access care has been emphasized by data from the United States Renal Data System (USRDS) demonstrating that adjusted relative mortality risk is substantially higher for patients with a central venous catheter compared to an arteriovenous fistula in both diabetic and nondiabetic patient populations (Figure 17–1).[16]

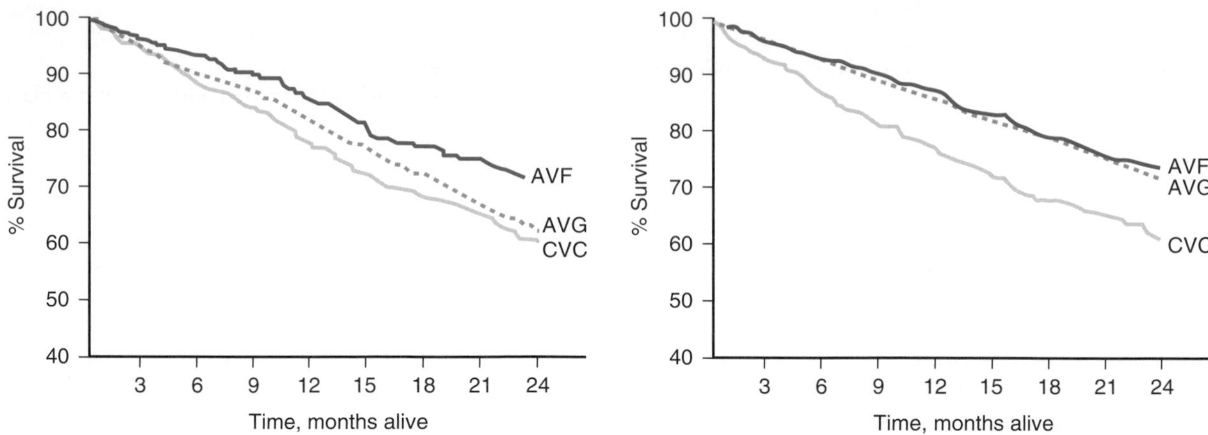

Figure 17–1 Adjusted patient survival based on dialysis access type. *AVF,* arteriovenous fistula; *AVG,* arteriovenous graft; *CVC,* cuffed venous catheter. (Reproduced with permission from Dhingra RK, Young EW, Hulbert-Shearon TE, et al: Type of vascular access and mortality in U.S. hemodialysis patients. Kidney Int 2002; 60:1443-1451.)

For diabetic patients, the use of arteriovenous grafts is also associated with significantly higher mortality risk compared to arteriovenous fistulas. Mortality due to both infectious and cardiovascular causes is implicated.

Data from Medicare and the USRDS indicate that the prevalence of arteriovenous fistula use is increasing in the United States. The increase in fistula placement coincides with the publication of Dialysis Outcome Quality Initiative (DOQI) Guidelines in 1997.[6] However, the K/DOQI clinical practice guidelines recommending that an autologous fistula be placed in 40% of prevalent hemodialysis patients is currently not being met. Furthermore, the use of tunneled catheters as the primary means of hemodialysis access appears to be rising. Thus, considerable challenges remain in attempting to optimize vascular access practice patterns in the future.

CATHETERS

Temporary Dialysis Catheters

Acute hemodialysis refers to the provision of hemodialysis for patients with acute renal failure, for the removal of ingested toxins, and for patients with chronic renal failure who require dialysis but do not have a functioning permanent vascular access. Vascular access requirements for acute hemodialysis are best served by the use of dual-lumen noncuffed temporary catheters. These catheters are made of a variety of materials, including polyurethane, polyethylene, and polytetrafluoroethylene (PTFE). Although temporary dialysis catheters may be placed in a number of anatomic locations, they are most commonly placed in the femoral vein, subclavian vein, or jugular vein. Each of these sites has advantages and disadvantages, depending on the specific clinical circumstances.

In most patients, the femoral vein is the easiest site of catheter insertion and is also associated with a lower risk of life-threatening complications. The major disadvantages are that patients must remain recumbent while the catheter is in place and there is a higher rate of infection. A femoral vein catheter is particularly practical in acute renal failure or after acute intoxications, in which it is anticipated that only one or two dialysis treatments will be necessary. Femoral catheters 24 cm in length are preferable to 15-cm catheters to reduce recirculation.[17] In a patient who is receiving acute hemodialysis because of nonfunction of a renal transplant, the femoral vein site contralateral to the allograft should be cannulated to avoid potential injury to the renal transplant or its vasculature.

For patients who require longer periods of renal replacement (>72 hours but <3 weeks), a noncuffed dialysis catheter placed in the internal jugular vein is preferable. The acute complications associated with both jugular and subclavian line insertions are similar. However, subclavian line insertions are associated with the longer-term complication of subclavian venous stenosis,[18] thereby compromising the potential for permanent vascular access. Catheters inserted under aseptic conditions in either the jugular or subclavian vein may be left in place for up to 3 weeks.

The complication rate associated with either subclavian or jugular catheter insertion is considerably higher than that for femoral line insertion. Complications associated with subclavian or jugular catheter insertion include pneumothorax, arterial puncture, venous puncture, and air embolism. A chest radiograph must be obtained after insertion of either jugular or subclavian lines and before initiation of hemodialysis to exclude the development of a pneumothorax or hemothorax and to confirm that the catheter's position is appropriate. Catheters should be inserted immediately prior to use, and real-time ultrasound-guided venous puncture is recommended for catheter insertion. Infection is the most common complication of dialysis catheters. Careful attention to aseptic technique, including the use of full-body sterile drape can decrease the risk.[19]

Cuffed Venous Catheters

Cuffed tunneled dialysis catheters have the advantage of relatively easy placement and immediate usability. Additionally, cuffed tunneled catheters can be used as a permanent vascular access for those patients who have exhausted all options for placement of an arteriovenous fistula or graft.[11] However, the high rate of infections and thrombotic complications associated with catheter use and the epidemiologic data suggesting higher mortality in patients using catheters make the current trend towards increased prevalence of catheter use in the U.S. dialysis population a disconcerting one. It has been suggested that the use of cuffed venous catheters is "a conundrum" and that we "hate living with them, but can't live without them."[20]

Infections are the most frequent serious complication of cuffed venous catheter use. The importance of sepsis as a cause of mortality in patients with end-stage renal disease has been emphasized because mortality secondary to sepsis is approximately 100- to 300-fold higher in all dialysis patients compared with the general population.[21]

Prospective studies demonstrate that the use of cuffed venous catheters is associated with a high rate of bloodstream infections in hemodialysis patients.[22,23] In most studies, the frequency of catheter-associated bacteremia is approximately 2 to 4 episodes per 1000 patient days, equivalent to 0.7 to 1.5 bacteremias per catheter year. In contrast, the frequency of infections or bacteremias associated with the use of arteriovenous fistulas is approximately 0.05 per patient year.

Catheter-related bacteremia in hemodialysis patients causes serious morbidity and mortality. An important study reported on the poor outcome of attempted catheter salvage (i.e., antibiotic therapy without catheter removal or exchange) in hemodialysis patients.[21] Only 32% of catheters were successfully salvaged, and of the 41 patients with bacteremia (inclusive of those in whom catheters were exchanged and salvage was attempted), 6 patients developed osteomyelitis, 1 patient developed septic arthritis, 4 patients developed infective endocarditis, and 2 patients died. These results underscore the seriousness of catheter-related bacteremia in hemodialysis patients.[24]

There have been reports of successful strategies for dealing with catheter-related bacteremia in hemodialysis patients. In one approach, patients with catheter-related bacteremia were stratified into three groups based on clinical presentation[25]:

1. Patients with minimal septic symptoms and a normal-appearing tunnel and exit site
2. Patients with minimal septic symptoms but with exit site or tunnel infection
3. Patients with severe septic symptoms

Each group received a 3-week course of appropriate antibiotic therapy based on organism identification and antibiotic sensitivity determination. Group 1 underwent catheter exchange over a guide wire, while Group 2 underwent catheter exchange over a guide wire with a creation of a new tunnel. In Group 3, catheters were removed with delayed replacement until defervescence. Utilizing this strategy, reported cure rates were 88%, 75%, and 87%, respectively. Another study compared the results of catheter exchange over a guide wire with catheter removal followed by delayed catheter replacement.[26] Each patient group received 3 weeks of appropriate systemic antibiotic therapy. Infection-free catheter survival time was similar in both groups. In a recent study, these investigators reported on a strategy of attempted catheter salvage by installation of an antibiotic lock solution into the catheter lumen (to eradicate luminal biofilms) in addition to a 3-week course of antibiotics.[27] This protocol was successful in 51% of cases, and overall catheter survival with this strategy was similar to that observed among patients managed with catheter replacement. Several studies have also suggested that the prophylactic application of topical mupirocin or bacitracin to catheter exit sites can markedly reduce catheter-related bacteria, sepsis and can prolong catheter survival.[28–30]

Venous catheters are also subject to frequent episodes of thrombosis requiring either thrombolytic therapy or replacement of the catheter. A prospective randomized, placebo-controlled trial of "mini-dose" warfarin for the prevention of dialysis catheter malfunction, did not demonstrate a significant effect on thrombosis-free catheter survival.[31] The long-term use of cuffed venous catheters may also lead to the development of right atrial thrombi. In a concerning report, intravascular ultrasound prospectively identified the presence of right atrial thrombi in 22% of hemodialysis patients with indwelling venous catheters.[32] In a recent report, large atrial thrombi were associated with a 68% chance of concurrent infection and an overall mortality of 27%.[33] Further research will be required to identify to what extent this poses a risk for hemodialysis patients. The use of cuffed venous catheters also predisposes patients to the development of central venous stenosis. Because subclavian vein stenosis may preclude the subsequent successful placement of ipsilateral arteriovenous fistulas or grafts, the use of subclavian venous catheters is generally contraindicated in dialysis patients unless utilized as a last resort.[18,34–38]

SUBCUTANEOUS PORTS

Vascular access ports are access devices that are entirely implanted into subcutaneous tissue and therefore have no external components. For hemodialysis access, a vascular catheter is inserted into a central vein and then subcutaneously tunneled to connect with the port device. Access to the port is then obtained by the use of specialized needles. Vascular access ports have commonly been adapted for use in oncology and are generally reported to have lower infection and thrombosis rates than traditional cuffed tunneled catheters.

Two hemodialysis port systems have recently been developed and are now in clinical use.[39] The LifeSite hemodialysis access system consists of two separate ports and catheters, one each for aspirating and returning blood during hemodialysis. The catheters are separately tunneled and a 14-gauge needle is inserted into the valve entry site to gain access to the LifeSite port. The LifeSite port is also designed to allow irrigation of the valve with an antimicrobial solution. In initial clinical trials, the LifeSite port has achieved excellent blood flows with a lower catheter-related bacteremia rate than traditional cuffed tunneled catheters.[10]

The Dialock hemodialysis access system also consists of an implantable subcutaneous port, in this case with two separate passages connected to a single lumen vascular catheter. Insertion of a 15-gauge needle opens a septum valve mechanism and provides access to the connecting vascular catheter. Studies using the Dialock access port suggest that excellent blood flows can be achieved with a low catheter-related bacteremia rate.[40]

AUTOGENOUS FISTULAS

Construction

The autogenous arteriovenous fistula is constructed by a surgical anastomosis between an artery and a vein. The exposure of the vein to the arterial blood flow results in dilatation and thickening of the vein wall, a process referred to as maturation. Maturation must be adequate to allow frequent needle cannulation and to support the blood flow of the dialysis circuit. Fistula maturation usually takes 8 to 16 weeks.

Upper extremity fistulas can be created in the forearm or in the upper arm (Figure 17–2). The Brescia-Cimino fistula, created via an anastomosis of the radial artery and cephalic vein at the wrist, was the first type of autogenous fistula described and is the fistula that should be considered initially in a patient who has not had a previous forearm arteriovenous access.[41] Ulnar artery-basilic vein and radial artery-basilic vein anastomoses are additional approaches for creation of a forearm fistula that are used relatively infrequently. In the upper arm, construction of the brachial artery-cephalic vein fistula is the most straightforward from a surgical standpoint. However, because many patients have had multiple prior cannulations of the cephalic vein in the antecubital space, stenoses are often present that preclude use of the vein for an upper arm fistula. An alternative is the brachial artery-basilic vein fistula. Construction of the brachiobasilic fistula requires dissection and subcutaneous tunneling of the basilic vein to reposition it superficially and laterally and thereby enable needle cannulation. Thus, the creation of a brachiobasilic fistula (often referred to as the basilic vein transposition fistula) is relatively laborious, but its use is becoming more widespread due to its favorable short-term and long-term outcomes.[42,43] At most centers, the creation of the anastomosis and the transposition of the vein are performed during a single surgical procedure. Arguments have been made for a two-step procedure in which the vein repositioning is performed several weeks after the anastomosis creation.[44] The potential advantage of the two-step approach is that damage to the vein wall during dissection and tunneling is reduced because of the remodeling that has occurred during the preceding weeks.

Fistulas can be constructed with an end-to-side or a side-to-side vein-artery anastomosis. Advantages of the end-to-side anastomosis include the ability to create a 90-degree rather than an acute-angle anastomosis, reduced likelihood of venous hypertension in the distal extremity, and the ability to bring together vessels that are far apart. Side-to-side anastomoses are technically easier to create and distension of distal veins can be prevented by ligating the vein distal to the anastomosis. However, the acute angle between the vessels that results from a side-to-side anastomosis is associated with increased turbulence that may contribute to stenosis development.[45] End-to-end anastomoses are usually avoided because of the risk of distal extremity ischemia with ligation of the artery.

Advantages of the Autogenous Fistula

Multiple studies indicate that rates of thrombosis and need for salvage procedures are substantially lower for autogenous fistulas than for synthetic grafts.[46–49] Cumulative survival, meaning survival until access abandonment, has also been shown in several analyses to be better for fistulas than grafts, despite aggressive and often successful efforts to restore patency of thrombosed grafts.[47] It should be recognized that many of the studies comparing outcomes of grafts and fistulas did not include primary failures, that is, accesses that fail before ever being used for dialysis. It has been suggested that if primary failures are included in such analyses, the cumulative survival of fistulas and grafts are similar.[42] Nonetheless, there is general

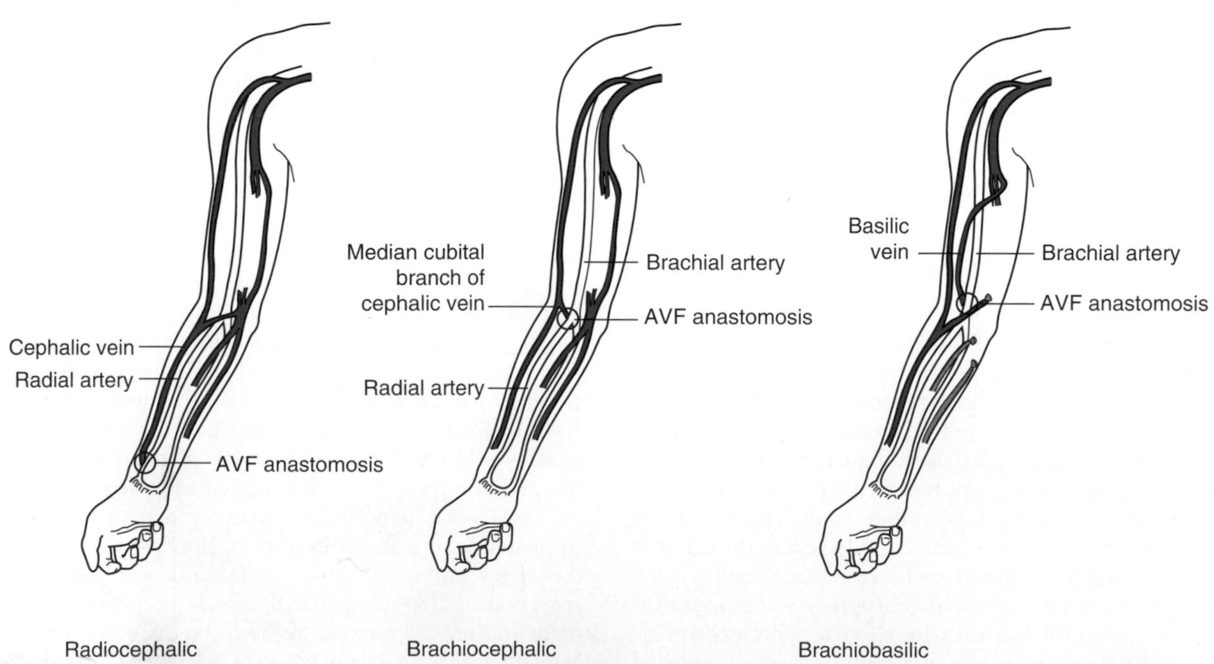

Figure 17–2 Types of autogenous fistulas. (Adapted with permission from Allon M, Robbin ML: Increasing arteriovenous fistulas in hemodialysis patients: Problems and solutions. Kidney Int 2002; 62:1109-1124.)

agreement that once mature, a fistula is much less likely than a graft to require intervention. In addition, infections occur much less frequently in fistulas than in grafts. For these reasons, a concerted effort to increase the prevalence of autogenous fistulas is one of the major recommendations of the National Kidney Foundation K/DOQI Clinical Practice Guidelines.[6]

An additional potential but unproved advantage of the autogenous fistula is that it does not contribute to the chronic inflammatory state evident in a large proportion of patients on maintenance dialysis. With accumulating evidence implicating chronic or recurrent inflammation in the cardiovascular disease of ESRD, it is reasonable to infer that reducing exposure to inflammatory stimuli by using autogenous vessels rather than synthetic material for vascular access may provide benefits that extend beyond access-related events.

Why the Low Prevalence of Autogenous Fistulas?

Despite the recognition of the advantages of the autogenous fistula, only approximately 25% of patients in the United States receive hemodialysis via an autogenous fistula, and nearly 50% are dialyzed with a synthetic graft.[13,46] Two interrelated factors that contribute to the low prevalence of autogenous fistulas are (1) their high rate of early failure and (2) the widespread practice of initially placing a graft rather than attempting construction of an autogenous fistula.

Primary failure of autogenous fistulas occurs as a result of either thrombosis within the first several weeks following surgical creation (early thrombosis) or inadequate maturation of the vein. Series published during the past 10 years report autogenous fistula primary failure rates of 20% to 50%.[50] The wide range of failure rates in these reports likely reflects differences in characteristics of the patients in whom fistula creation was attempted and possibly variation in presurgical evaluation and surgical approaches. Factors found by various investigators to be associated with primary failure include older age, female sex, obesity, diabetes mellitus, black race, and low blood pressure.[51–55] Attempts to identify serologic or other biochemical predictors of fistula failure have not been revealing.

The tendency to place synthetic grafts before attempting autogenous fistula construction has evolved because of the ability to use grafts soon after surgery, the good short-term outcomes in patients with vessels that appear unsuitable for fistula construction, referral of patients to nephrologists when dialysis initiation is imminent rather than earlier in the course of the renal disease, and the technical ease of graft placement relative to fistula creation, particularly when vein transposition is needed.[6,12,50] Although some of these factors are not readily modifiable, marked geographic variations in fistula prevalence that persist after adjustment for demographic characteristics or comorbid conditions suggest that clinical practice patterns are important contributors to the types of accesses created.[56,57] Reports from centers that have implemented multidisciplinary access programs involving nephrologists, vascular surgeons, and dialysis staff suggest that substantial increases in fistula creation attempts can be achieved, and that the higher attempt rates are accompanied by increases in the prevalence of functioning fistulas (Table 17–1).[58,59]

Table 17–1 Components of a Multidisciplinary Autogenous Fistula Program

Team Members
Nephrologists
Dialysis nurses and patient care technicians
Vascular surgeons
Interventional radiologists
Vascular ultrasonographers
Vascular access coordinator
Goals
Early placement of vascular access
Creation of upper arm and transposition fistulas, if radiocephalic fistula not possible
Vascular mapping for identification of suitable vessels
Replacement of failed synthetic grafts with autogenous fistulas
Salvage interventions for fistula maturation failures
Reduction in duration of central venous catheter use
Approaches
Develop consensus regarding goals of program
Prospective tracking of vascular access types and outcomes
Active monitoring of fistula maturation after anastomosis creation
Ongoing education of patients and dialysis facility staff
Ongoing dialogue among team members to modify approaches

Assessment of Vessel Quality

There are several approaches to evaluating vessels preoperatively to identify those that are suitable for fistula creation. The simplest method is physical examination of the veins prior to and after placement of a tourniquet proximally. Although this allows assessment of the diameter of superficial veins, it does not identify proximal stenosis or thrombosis that could interfere with fistula maturation. In addition, physical examination may fail to identify deeper veins that would be suitable if transposed and, thus, could lead to an inappropriate decision to place a graft rather than attempt fistula creation. More information about the vasculature can be obtained with either ultrasonography or venography (i.e., vascular mapping). Ultrasound evaluation of the extremity provides information about vein diameter and the presence of stenosis, thrombosis, and sclerosis. In addition, arterial characteristics can be assessed (e.g., diameter and flow). Vascular mapping with ultrasonography is time-consuming and operator-dependent and is most successful when a specific protocol is followed to ensure uniform measurements and reporting by multiple operators (Table 17–2). Venography also provides information about vessel size and patency and is probably better for identification of stenoses and assessment of central vessel patency than is ultrasound. However, venography does not enable evaluation of arteries, it exposes patients to contrast, and it carries the risk of vein damage from cannulation or phlebitis that could render the vein unsuitable for fistula construction.

Several recent studies have demonstrated increases in rates of attempted fistula creation after implementation of

Table 17–2 Protocol for Vascular Mapping Using Ultrasonography

1. Examine **radial artery** at wrist for flow, peak systolic velocity, quantitative blood flow (should be ≥10 mL/min) and diameter (should be ≥2.0 mm).
2. Examine **ulnar artery** at wrist for flow, peak systolic velocity, quantitative blood flow, and diameter (should be ≥2.0 mm).
3. Examine **brachial artery** just above antecubital fossa for peak systolic velocity, quantitative blood flow, and diameter (should be ≥2.0 mm).
4. Place tourniquet at upper forearm. Examine **cephalic vein** at wrist:
   - Measure diameter at wrist (should be ≥2.5 mm).
   - Follow to elbow, examine for stenoses or occluded segments. Measure diameter at mid and upper forearm.
5. Place tourniquet at upper arm. Examine cephalic vein above elbow:
   - Measure diameter of vein above elbow at low, mid, and upper arm (should be ≥2.5 mm).
   - Follow to shoulder, examine for segmental stenoses or occluded segments.
   - Determine whether vein is superficial for most of its course (within 1 cm of skin).
6. Examine **basilic vein** in upper arm:
   - Measure diameter of vein above elbow at low, mid, and upper arm (should be ≥2.5 mm).
   - Follow to axilla, examine for segmental stenoses or occluded segments.
7. Remove tourniquet. Examine subclavian and internal jugular veins for stenoses or occlusions.

preoperative vascular mapping protocols.[60–63] In most of these studies, the increased rates of fistula creation attempts were accompanied by a reduction in the primary failure rates and, among those studies that reported it, an increase in the fistula prevalence at the center. None of these studies was a randomized, controlled trial, and it is possible that the improvements seen were due to factors other than vascular mapping, such as changes in surgical approaches, better preoperative protection of vessels, or earlier referral for access creation. Thus, although preoperative vascular mapping provides a substantial amount of information about vessel quality, its ultimate impact on fistula outcomes is not yet clear.

Selection of the Location for Autogenous Fistula Creation

In general, it is preferable to use the distal extremity for initial arteriovenous access placement and move to more proximal sites, if necessary, because of access failure. It is also usually preferable to use the nondominant arm to limit the functional disability that might occur with perioperative complications, such as vascular steal syndrome or peripheral neuropathy. Thus, if the forearm vessels appear suitable, a radio-cephalic fistula in the non-dominant arm should be created as the initial access.

Decisions about access type and location are less straightforward, if the forearm vessels do not appear suitable for an autogenous fistula or if a forearm autogenous fistula is created initially but fails. Until recently, the approach in many centers would have been to place a forearm arteriovenous graft. However, with the recognition of the long-term benefits of autogenous fistulas and recent studies suggesting a lower primary failure rate for upper arm than forearm fistulas, some centers will create an upper arm autogenous fistula as an initial access in individuals who do not have suitable forearm vessels.[49] Whether such an approach is preferable to that of initially placing a forearm synthetic graft and subsequently creating an autogenous fistula in the upper arm if the graft fails, is not known. A potential advantage of the latter approach is that alterations in upper arm veins that occur as a result of increased flow via the forearm graft could ultimately enhance the suitability of the upper arm veins for autogenous fistula creation.

Preoperative Preparation for Autogenous Fistula Creation

Because the quality of the vein is so critical to successful autogenous fistula creation, every effort should be made to protect the veins in the extremity that will be used for access creation. Venipuncture for obtaining blood specimens and intravenous catheter placement should be avoided at sites proximal to the planned arteriovenous anastomosis. Fistula creation should be performed many months before vascular access use is required to prevent the need for central venous catheter placement and the associated risk of central vein stenosis. These measures for preserving quality are more feasible for patients undergoing initial access placement than for those who have already had multiple failed accesses.

Pharmacologic Approaches to Improving Autogenous Fistula Outcomes

Several studies have evaluated the efficacy of antiplatelet agents for preventing early thrombosis of autogenous fistulas.[64] Ticlopidine, microencapsulated aspirin, and sulfinpyrazone all appeared effective in small studies. In the largest of these trials, 260 patients were randomized to ticlopidine or placebo starting 3 to 7 days before fistula creation and continued for 28 days after surgery. The rates of fistula thrombosis in the placebo and ticlopidine groups were 19% and 12%, respectively, but this difference was not significant, possibly because of insufficient sample size. A pooled analysis of all placebo-controlled studies of ticlopidine showed a 25% thrombosis rate in the placebo group compared to a 12% thrombosis rate in the ticlopidine group, indicating a statistically significant benefit of ticlopidine. None of the studies of antiplatelet agents reported the proportions of fistulas able to be used for dialysis. Based upon the results of these multiple small studies, a large, multicenter, randomized, placebo-controlled trial is underway to evaluate the effect of clopidogrel on patency and maturation of newly constructed autogenous fistulas.

At present, the understanding of the physiology of vein maturation is limited. Studies in animal models suggest roles for nitric oxide and prostacyclin, but details about the relevant signaling pathways and regulatory influences are scant.[45] Additional investigation of the systemic and local factors involved in vein dilatation and remodeling could lead to the identification of pharmacologic targets for enhancing fistula maturation.

Initial Cannulation of New Fistulas

Premature cannulation of autogenous fistulas predisposes to infiltration and compression of the vein from extravasated blood that can result in fistula thrombosis. Thus, careful examination of the fistula by experienced team members should be performed prior to initial use, and additional time for maturation should be employed, if the fistula appears unsuitable or if initial attempts at use are unsuccessful. Specific recommendations about when to initiate cannulation vary. The K/DOQI guideline is to allow the fistula to mature for 3 to 4 months before initial use.[6] Data from the DOPPS suggest that in some countries, fistula cannulation within 4 to 6 weeks after creation is common and is not associated with reduced fistula survival.[14] Given the substantial long-term benefits of a functioning fistula, it is advisable to exercise caution with regard to early use of new fistulas. However, the risks associated with the extended use of central venous catheters that can accompany cannulation delays should not be discounted.

Salvage of Failing Fistulas

Regular examination of new fistulas should begin early after anastomosis creation to evaluate the maturation process. Two potentially modifiable causes of maturation failure are stenosis of the draining vein and the presence of vein branches that decrease the blood flow through the draining vein. Balloon angioplasty of identified stenoses can enhance maturation as can surgical ligation of vein tributaries.[65,66] Because the use of radiographic contrast may hasten the need for initiation of dialysis, ultrasonography may be preferable to angiography as the diagnostic study for patients who have not yet started dialysis. Surgical superficialization can convert a deep fistula that has matured adequately but is unsuitable for use because of cannulation difficulty, to an effective vascular access.

In many centers, surgical or radiologic thrombectomy of a thrombosed fistula is not attempted because of the technical difficulties and poor outcomes. However, recent reports suggest that with innovative approaches, percutaneous declotting of mature autogenous fistulas can be performed with reasonable success rates.[67–69] Salvage is rarely applied to fistulas that thrombose within the first few weeks after creation; such fistulas are usually abandoned.

Monitoring Mature Fistulas for Stenoses

Stenosis development is less frequent in autogenous fistulas than in synthetic grafts, and the utility of routine monitoring for fistula stenosis has not been established. The methods for monitoring arteriovenous accesses for stenosis are described in the graft section of this chapter. Venous pressure measurement is not as sensitive for fistula stenosis as it is for graft stenosis, in part, because monitoring venous pressure will identify only those stenoses that are downstream of the venous needle. In contrast to grafts, in which the majority of stenoses occur at or near the venous anastomosis, stenoses in fistulas occur anywhere along the length of the draining vein and thus might be upstream of the venous needle. Even if the stenosis is downstream of the venous needle, the development of collateral veins often prevents the venous pressure from increasing substantially. Thus, for monitoring fistulas, a more direct determination of access blood flow (e.g., ultrasound dilution or Doppler ultrasound) is more appropriate than is venous pressure measurement. However, optimal blood flow criteria for confirmatory angiography are still being defined.[70]

Complications of the Autogenous Fistula

Vascular steal syndrome is a potentially devastating complication that can occur with either placement of a synthetic graft or creation of an autogenous fistula. The reduction in perfusion to the distal extremity that results from shunting of blood through the arteriovenous access can produce mild symptoms or irreversible ischemic injury. Steal syndrome occurs predominantly in individuals with underlying vascular disease, and its incidence may be increasing with the growing proportion of elderly and diabetic patients comprising the ESRD population. With a fistula, steal syndrome usually develops gradually over several weeks after creation of the surgical anastomosis as the fistula blood flow increases with progressive vein maturation. In contrast, severe arterial compromise can occur immediately after graft placement. Access ligation is often necessary in severe cases, although banding procedures to reduce, but not eliminate access blood flow, can also be attempted. Banding procedures may result in access thrombosis or fistula maturation failure.

Congestive heart failure is a relatively rare complication resulting from the shunting of blood from the arterial to the venous circulation through either an autogenous fistula or a synthetic graft. It occurs more often with upper arm than forearm accesses because of the greater blood flow in the former. Accurately attributing cardiac failure to access-related high output states can be difficult. If the diagnosis is questionable, demonstration of functional changes, such as decreased heart rate or cardiac output, during manual compression of the access, can be attempted before treating with access banding or ligation.

Aneurysm formation occurs in autogenous fistulas when the vein wall becomes damaged and replaced with tissue that provides less resistance than the contiguous vessel wall. Repetitive cannulation in the same regions of the access and proximal stenosis both predispose to aneurysm formation. Buttonhole cannulation of the exact same two access sites has been suggested to reduce aneurysm formation but may be difficult in practice to achieve. Pseudoaneurysms are usually caused by extravasation of blood after needle removal. Both true aneurysms and pseudoaneurysms can limit sites for needle placement and can rupture if the overlying skin is compromised.

In contrast to synthetic grafts, autogenous fistulas rarely become infected. Antibiotic therapy alone is often sufficient for eradication of fistula infections, although aneurysmal infections may require surgical resection because of intra-aneurysmal stasis or thrombus.

ARTERIOVENOUS GRAFTS

Terminology

In patients for whom an autogenous arteriovenous fistula cannot be constructed by direct anastomosis of adjoining vessels, one option is to interpose a graft that serves as a conduit between the artery and vein. This type of hemodialysis access is referred to as a *non-autogenous access* or an *arteriovenous graft* (AVG).[71] The graft allows for selection of the optimal arterial and venous sites for surgical anastomosis and provides an easy target for cannulation. The graft can be composed of either synthetic material, such as ePTFE, or a biologic material. The latter is referred to as a biograft. The biograft may be an autograft (i.e., from a different site in the same individual, such as the saphenous vein), an allograft (i.e., from a genetically different individual of the same species), or a xenograft (i.e., from a different species, such as a bovine vessel). Allografts are also referred to as homografts, and xenografts are also called heterografts.

Graft Location and Configuration

Depending on the target vessels that are available, there are a number of anatomic variations of arteriovenous graft that can be created. The forearm straight graft typically originates from the radial artery in the forearm and terminates in the cephalic vein at the level of the antecubital fossa. The forearm loop graft typically originates from the brachial artery and terminates in either the cephalic or basilic vein at the level of the antecubital fossa. Most commonly, blood flows through the forearm loop graft from medial (arterial side) to lateral (venous side) in the direction indicated by the extended thumb (Figure 17–3). However, the direction of flow may be reversed in some forearm loop grafts, and the surgeon needs to record this information in the patient's chart at the time of access placement. Arteriovenous grafts placed in the upper arm typically originate from the brachial artery at the antecubital fossa and terminate in the cephalic vein in the upper forearm. If access sites have been exhausted in the arms, then a femoral loop graft may be placed in the leg between the femoral artery and vein. In exceptional circumstances in which other options have been exhausted, heroic types of accesses have been constructed. These include the necklace graft that connects the axillary or subclavian artery to the contralateral jugular or subclavian vein and the arterial interposition graft in which the artery (e.g., subclavian, femoral, or brachial artery) is transected and a loop of graft material is inserted connecting the proximal and distal ends of the transected artery.

Graft Materials

The history leading to the development of modern vascular grafts has been reviewed.[72] The ideal graft material would be biocompatible, nonthrombogenic, easy to cannulate, easy to surgically manipulate, low cost, resistant to infection, and able to withstand multiple cannulations without degeneration or pseudoaneurysm formation.[73] As listed in Table 17–3, many types of materials have been tried, but to date the perfect graft material and design have not been found. Currently, the preferred graft material is expanded polytetrafluoroethylene.

In 1969 Gore discovered that polytetrafluoroethylene (PTFE), the polymer in Teflon invented by DuPont, could be rapidly stretched to create a strong microporous plastic with useful properties. This was called expanded PTFE (ePTFE). Early studies demonstrated that expanded PTFE worked better than woven PTFE for small vessel prosthesis.[74] In 1976, Baker and colleagues[4] reported on the first clinical experience using ePTFE as an arteriovenous graft for hemodialysis patients. Subsequent studies in the late 1970s suggested that

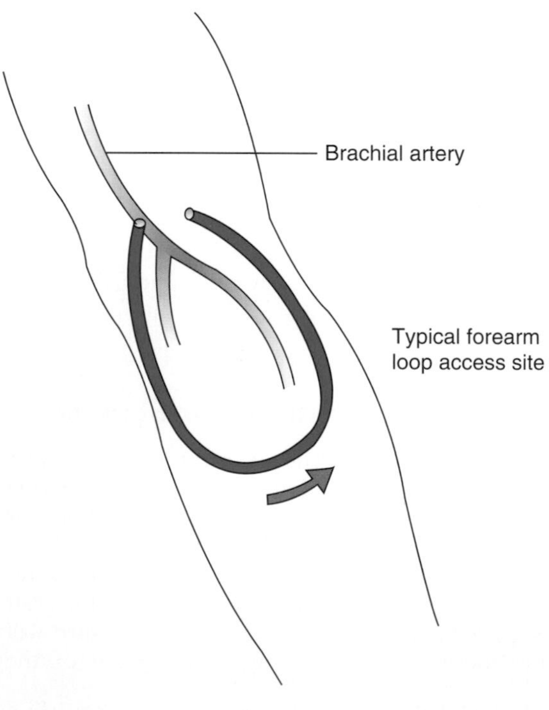

Figure 17–3 Configuration for typical forearm loop graft. (Modified from Kapoian T, Kaufman JL, Nosher J, Sherman RA: Dialysis access and recirculation. *In* Henrich WL [ed]: Dialysis as Treatment of End-Stage Renal Disease, on-line ed, vol. 5. Philadelphia, Current Medicine & Blackwell Science, 1999.)

Table 17–3 Graft Materials

Synthetic Grafts
Dacron velour
Sparks-Mandril graft
Polyurethane (Vectra)
Expanded polytetrafluoroethylene (e.g., Gore-Tex, Impra)
Biografts
Autograft
Saphenous vein
Allograft (cryopreserved or denatured)
Saphenous vein
Femoral vein (CryoVein)
Umbilical vein (Dacron covered)
Xenograft (denatured)
Bovine carotid artery heterograft (e.g., Artegraft)
Bovine mesenteric vein (Procol)

ePTFE was equal to or better than other available synthetic grafts or biografts in terms of long-term patency and had an acceptable complication rate; hence ePTFE rapidly became the preferred choice of many surgeons as graft material for secondary arteriovenous access in hemodialysis patients.[73,75–80] There are several commercial types of ePTFE grafts but the two best known are Gore-Tex and Impra. Both types of ePTFE graft have similar pore size but the Gore-Tex brand is thicker and is reinforced by an external circumferential layer of PTFE not used in Impra grafts. Several randomized controlled trials directly comparing Gore-Tex and Impra hemodialysis grafts have been performed, and there was no significant difference in terms of long-term patency or the rate of complications.[81,82] Some recent experimental studies have suggested that larger pore ePTFE grafts (e.g., 60–90 μm) may have better rates of angiogenesis and graft surface endothelialization.[83,84] However, the available evidence suggests that there is no clinical advantage in terms of long-term patency of such grafts for hemodialysis access.[85]

Polyurethane has also been studied as a vascular access graft.[86–90] Although problems have been reported with some of the polyurethane graft designs,[87,89,90] recent studies have suggested that the polyurethane Vectra graft (Thoratec Lab Corp, CA) is comparable to ePFTE in terms of patency and complications.[86,88] The Vectra graft has an inner and outer porous layer that allows tissue ingrowth and a central core made of Thoralon, which is a self-sealing polyurethane material.[86] The central self-sealing core reportedly allows for earlier graft cannulation after surgery without the problems of bleeding, seroma formation, and thrombosis seen with early cannulation of ePTFE grafts.[86] More information will be needed on this graft. One concern that has been raised is that the Vectra graft is difficult to image by Doppler ultrasound, thus making it difficult to use this technique to look for access stenosis.[91]

Graft Patency

There is a wide variation in the reported long-term patency of ePTFE vascular access grafts. Recent studies demonstrate that primary failure in the United States occurs in half of all new ePTFE grafts within 6 months or less of placement, which is the same as for autogenous fistulas placed in the forearm.[92–95] Synthetic grafts can often be salvaged leading to improved secondary patency rates. The better salvage rate for failed arteriovenous grafts compared to autogenous fistulas leads to nearly equivalent 1- and 2-year rates of secondary patency.[92,94,96–100] This is achieved, however, at the expense of significantly more graft revisions and complications.[92,94,96,99–102] With extended follow-up beyond 2 years most studies demonstrate that autogenous fistulas maintain functional patency longer and with fewer complications than grafts.[13,92,94,97–99,102]

GRAFT COMPLICATIONS

Thrombosis

Thrombosis is the most common graft complication and the most common cause of access failure. Thrombosis has been reported as the cause of 70% to 95% of all graft failures.[47,94,103–107] The rate of graft thrombosis in the literature ranges from about 0.25 to 1.4 thrombotic episodes per patient-year.* The large variation undoubtedly reflects case mix, intensity of access surveillance, and local access management practices. Most recent studies report graft thrombosis rates exceeding 0.5 episodes per patient-year.† As pointed out by Virchow over 150 years ago, the predisposition to thrombosis is dependent on abnormalities in blood flow, blood constituents, and the vessel wall. As applied to the problem of vascular access thrombosis (Table 17–4), abnormalities that predispose to graft thrombosis include: (1) impaired blood flow resulting from vascular stenosis and hematorheological alterations at the graft-vessel anastomosis; (2) vessel wall abnormalities, including the thrombogenic graft-blood interface and endothelial damage or dysfunction; and (3) abnormalities in blood constituents, including acquired or inherited abnormalities in platelet, coagulation, or fibrinolytic pathways. Although most studies have focused on the role of vascular stenosis in graft thrombosis, each of these factors is interrelated, and more than one factor ultimately determines whether thrombosis occurs in a given individual.

Vascular stenosis due to neointimal hyperplasia is the most common underlying cause of access thrombosis. Early surgical studies reported access stenosis in 34% to 63% of

Table 17–4 Predisposing Factors to Graft Thrombosis

Abnormal Blood Flow
Vascular stenosis
Rheologic abnormalities
Abnormal Vessel Wall
Blood-graft interface
Endothelial damage or dysfunction
Abnormal Blood Constituents
Platelets
Coagulation pathway
Fibrinolytic pathway

*References 52,93,94,100-103,105,108-112.

†References 2,93,94,103,105,108,109,111,113,114.

thrombosed grafts.[115] However, more recent angiographic studies find that vascular stenosis exists in over 85% of thrombosed or failing grafts.[47,95,111,116–121] The most common site of stenosis is at the vein-graft anastomosis (Figure 17–4).* Most of the remaining stenoses are found either in the downstream vein or within the body of the graft. Central venous stenosis is seen in at least 3% to 6% of patients in most studies† but may be as frequent as 40% in patients who have had a prior subclavian central catheter for dialysis.[115,126,127] Stenosis also occurs at the artery to graft anastomosis but less frequently than seen in autogenous fistulas. The importance of access stenosis in the pathophysiology of access thrombosis is underscored by the observation that prospective access monitoring to detect and prophylactically treat stenosis decreases the frequency of thrombosis.‡ There are at least two mechanisms whereby stenosis can lead to thrombosis. First, a hemodynamically significant venous stenosis produces a decrease in access flow rate and an increase in intra-access pressure.[128,135–137] The consequence of this is a decrease in the shear rate and altered surface tension at the blood-graft interface leading to an increased interaction of platelets and clotting factors with the surface of the graft.[138] Second, the stenosis itself creates an increase in blood velocity and wall shear stress at the level of the stenosis that can activate platelets and promote platelet adhesion and aggregation.[139,140] Hence, access stenosis with its attendant alterations in blood rheology, platelet activation, and endothelial dysfunction predisposes to thrombosis and is the major underlying cause of access failure.

However, access stenosis is not the sole cause of thrombosis. Access thrombosis has been reported to occur without radiologic evidence of a significant stenosis in up to 15% of grafts.[141] While imaging studies can miss hemodynamically significant stenosis, studies using prospective flow monitoring have also shown that access thrombosis occurs despite having a high access flow rate (over 1000 mL/min) and without a significant change in access flow rate in the preceding months.[125,133,136,142–144] Clinical observation also suggests that many episodes of thrombosis occur in the night often after a preceding dialysis session. This suggests that volume depletion post-dialysis with the resulting hemoconcentration and low cardiac output may predispose to access thrombosis. Thus, other factors likely contribute to the high rate of thrombosis in grafts.[145]

*References 47,95,111,116-120,122.
†References 95,111,116,119,122–125.
‡References 20,95,111,122,128–134.

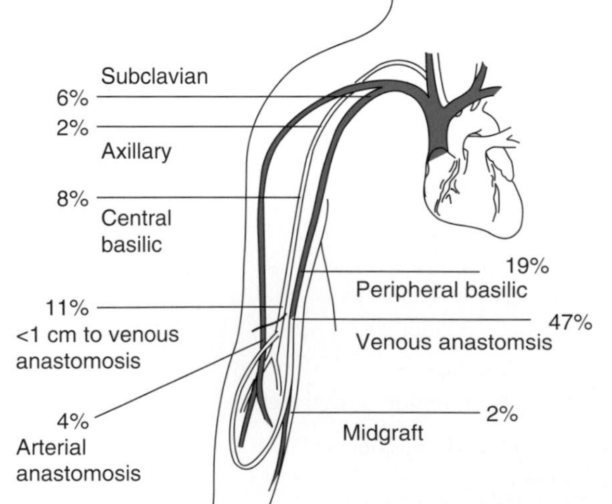

Figure 17–4 Location of stenosis by angiography in failing grafts. (From Kanterman RY, Vesely TM, Pilgram TK, et al: Dialysis access grafts: Anatomic location of venous stenosis and results of angioplasty. Radiology 1995; 195:135-139.)

Acquired or inherited abnormalities in blood constituents, including platelets or components of the coagulation or fibrinolytic pathways, have also been examined as a possible cause of access thrombosis.[145,146] Overall, platelet function has been shown to be impaired and contribute to the hemostatic defect seen in people with ESRD.[146] However, platelet activation by the high shear stress and abnormal luminal surface posed by the arteriovenous graft likely contributes to graft thrombosis. In addition, hemodialysis has been shown to activate platelets and thus could contribute to graft thrombosis.[146,147] Patients with ESRD have evidence for an acquired hypercoagulable state that may underlie the increased risk for atherothrombotic events.[145,146] The prevalence of antiphospholipid antibodies, including anticardiolipin antibodies and to a lesser extent the lupus anticoagulant, is increased in people on hemodialysis.[148,149] Of the antiphospholipid antibodies, the lupus anticoagulant appears to be associated with a higher risk for thrombosis than anticardiolipin antibodies.[150] Several studies have reported an association between the presence of antiphospholipid antibodies and hemodialysis access thrombosis.[151–154] However, this association has not been confirmed in all studies.[149,155,156] Homocysteine is a risk factor for venous and arterial thrombosis.[157,158] Plasma homocysteine levels are elevated in people with end-stage kidney disease, and two studies have reported an association between plasma homocysteine levels and vascular access thrombosis.[159,160] On the other hand, several studies have failed to find an association between plasma homocysteine and access thrombosis.[133,136,161–164] Evidence for the hypercoagulable state includes an activated tissue factor pathway documented by increased circulating tissue factor and factor VII activity as well as evidence for thrombin activation, including increased circulating prothrombin activation fragments (F1+2) and thrombin-antithrombin complexes (TAT).[165–175] Elevated D-dimer levels are also found suggesting increased activation of both the thrombotic as well as the fibrinolytic pathways.[166,172,174–176] Coagulation pathways are also activated by inflammatory stimuli[169,177] that fluctuate with time in people with renal failure.[178,179] Hence, the risk for thrombosis likely will vary depending on inflammatory insults to the patient.[180] Insertion of a vascular access graft itself induces an inflammatory stimulus[179] that may contribute to the enhanced risk of thrombosis compared to an autogenous fistula.

Infection

Infections and their complications account for about 14% of the annual mortality in ESRD patients.[181] Infection of the vascular access graft is a particularly serious complication that can be difficult to manage and has been increasing as a cause of admission for hemodialysis patients.[181] In case series, the percentage of grafts that become infected has been reported to range between 2% and 35%, with most studies reporting rates between 5% and 15% over the duration of the observation.* One report found that the infection rate was

*References 82,93,94,98,99,101,102,107,182–184.

higher in the first year after access placement compared to the second year.[93] The majority of infections are due to *Staphylococcus aureus*.[182,185] Less commonly encountered organisms include *Staphylococcus epidermidis*, Streptococcal species, gram-negative bacteria, and occasionally, candida or other fungal species.[185] Infection or abscess around the graft may present with localized erythema and tenderness over the graft site, but graft infection can also present with fever and systemic symptoms without localized evidence of infection.[186–188] An indium-tagged WBC scan has been used to detect occult graft infections.[186,187,189,190] Serious complications of graft infection include: graft thrombosis, metastatic seeding leading to endocarditis, osteomyelitis, or murantic abcess as well as sepsis and death.[191] Nasal carriage of *S. aureus* has been reported as a risk factor for access infection.[192] Other factors that predispose to graft infection include frequent access surgeries and procedures, poor personal hygiene, intravenous drug abuse, and skin rash or infection.[182] Attention to bactericidal cleansing of the skin and infection control practices at the time of needle insertion in the dialysis unit is an important quality control measure. The use of preoperative vancomycin prior to access surgery has been recommended to decrease the frequency of subsequent post-operative graft infections.[193]

Management of graft infection usually requires excision of the infected graft material and treatment with antibiotics.[182,185,186] Vancomycin with addition of gram-negative coverage, if the patient is septic, is appropriate.[182, 186] However, indiscriminant use of vancomycin has led to an emerging epidemic of vancomycin-resistant organisms. Hence, long-term use of vancomycin should be avoided and alternate antibiotics chosen as soon as the results of antibiotic sensitivity testing are known. A strategy to limit vancomycin use consists of initiating therapy with a first generation cephalosporine and an aminoglycoside until culture and sensitivity results are known and then adjusting the antibiotic regimen accordingly.[186] If alternate access sites are limited and the infection is localized outside the graft, local incision and drainage of the access site without removing the graft can be attempted.[182,188,194] Skin grafting may be required to close the wound over the graft after the infection has resolved. An alternate approach studied recently is to replace the infected prosthetic graft with a biograft that is more resistant to infection.[195–197] If an endovascular source of infection is present, it should be treated for 6 weeks with appropriate intravenous antibiotics to reduce the risk for late sequelas from metastatic seeding.

Arteriovenous Steal

Impaired perfusion of the extremities below the level of the vascular access is a serious and debilitating complication that can occur after placement of either an arteriovenous fistula or graft.[107,198–202] Distal ischemia occurs when the relatively low resistance shunt accommodates more flow than can be delivered by antegrade flow through the inflow artery feeding the fistula.[202] In this case, the fistula also "steals" blood from the artery below the fistula (Figure 17–5). This retrograde flow lowers the perfusion pressure in the distal extremity, and if this falls below a critical level, it will lead to tissue ischemia.

Ischemic monomelic neuropathy, a syndrome characterized by acute pain, weakness, and paralysis of the extremity often in association with sensory loss is a rare complication occurring in patients who get an upper arm access involving the brachial artery.[200,203] It is due to impaired blood supply to nerves in the forearm leading to axonal degeneration without

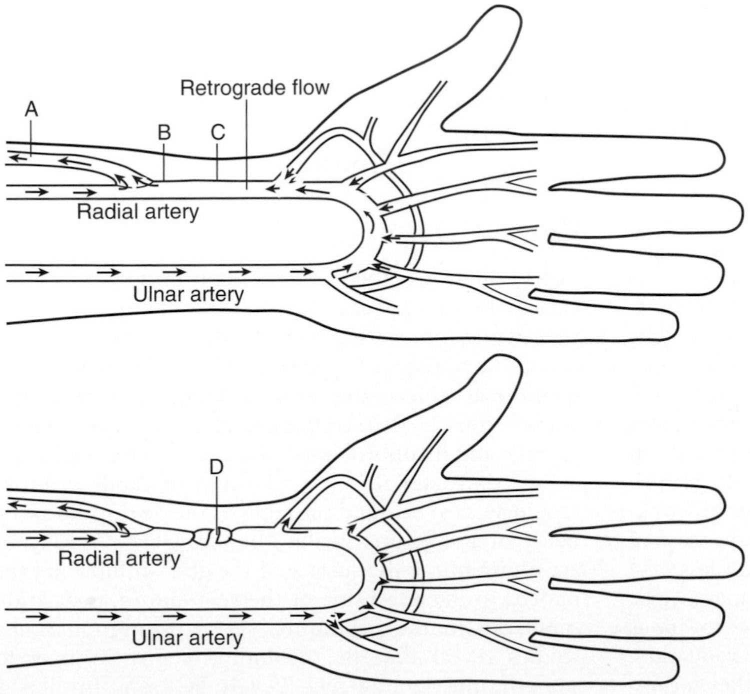

Figure 17–5 Pathogenesis of arteriovenous steal. Steal occurs when the arteriovenous fistula *(A)* receives both antegrade and retrograde *(C)* flow from the radial artery. (*B* is the arteriovenous anastomosis). Steal can be corrected by ligation of the radial artery below the fistula *(D)*. (From Miles AM: Vascular steal syndrome and ischaemic monomelic neuropathy: Two variants of upper limb ischaemia after haemodialysis vascular access surgery. Nephrol Dial Transplant 1999; 14:297-300. By permission of Oxford University Press.)

evidence of ischemic damage to muscle or other tissues in the forearm. In contrast to the classic steal syndrome the radial pulse is usually palpable, and digital pressure is usually greater than 50 mmHg. The patients are typically diabetic, older, and with preexisting neuropathy or vascular disease. Symptoms occur immediately or within hours after access placement in the upper arm and are very difficult to reverse unless the problem is recognized and treated immediately. It is important to recognize the signs and symptoms rapidly at the time of access placement so the access can be ligated before further irreversible damage occurs.[200,203]

Mild symptoms of steal occurring shortly after access placement can be treated symptomatically and observed. In more severe cases, ligation of the access will cure the problem but leaves the patient without an arteriovenous access for dialysis. A number of surgical approaches have been suggested to deal with this problem while leaving the access intact for dialysis.[204] One approach is to decrease flow through the fistula by banding or plicating the fistula until pressure in the hand is measured to be above 50 mmHg.[205,206] This can relieve the symptoms of ischemia, however, most accesses fail shortly after banding due to thrombosis.[198,201,205] An alternate procedure was described by Schanzer and colleagues[207,208] in 1988, in which the artery distal to the fistula is tied off to prevent retrograde flow from stealing blood from the periphery, and then a vein graft is used to place an arterial bypass from the inflow artery above the fistula to a site on the artery just below the ligation. The arterial bypass maintains arterial pressure in the ligated distal artery, thus preventing steal and allowing perfusion of tissue below the fistula. This surgery was later christened the distal revascularization-interval ligation (DRIL) procedure and appears to be quite effective at eliminating steal symptoms while maintaining a functional hemodialysis access.[209,210]

Heart Failure

High output cardiac failure that resolves with closure of the arteriovenous shunt is a well documented but uncommon complication of arteriovenous grafts and autogenous fistulas.[211–214] The greatest risk appears to be in people with an autogenous fistula placed in the upper arm (e.g., brachiocephalic fistula).[211–214] However, high output failure has been reported with ePTFE grafts.[183]

Blood flow in a functional hemodialysis access generally runs between 0.75 to 2.5 liters per minute with occasional patients having blood flows up to 4 or more liters per minute.[92,133,212,214–217] Most patients can maintain this access blood flow over many years without developing clinical evidence of heart failure.[92,218,219] However, this high access flow may contribute to the development of LVH in some patients.[220] Measurement of access blood flow by itself does not identify those with existing or impending high output failure.[212] A drop in heart rate of 7 bpm or more after shunt closure is one sign used to detect a hemodynamically significant shunt (Nicoladoni-Branham's sign) but may be absent in dialysis patients with high output failure.[212,214] A decrease in cardiac output with shunt closure that is significantly less than the measured shunt flow in the unclamped fistula may also be an indication of high output failure due to an arteriovenous shunt.[212] However, this observation needs further validation. If myocardial function cannot be improved by other means, then the arteriovenous shunt may need to be ligated to resolve the high output failure. Banding of the access in an attempt to decrease access flow has been tried but is usually met with limited success either due to inadequate reduction in flow on one hand or access thrombosis on the other.

Aneurysm/Pseudoaneurysm

True aneurysms occur when the vessel wall becomes weak and dilates. Pseudoaneurysms occur due to vessel trauma most commonly at needle puncture sites leading to a localized extravasation of fluid in which the wall is composed of perivascular adventia, fibrous tissue, and hematoma. Most commonly the etiology for these aneurysms is "one site-itis" in which there are frequent repetitive needle sticks into one or two regions of the access. However, infection may also be a cause of aneurysm formation, particularly in biografts. Aneurysms and pseudoaneurysms occur more commonly in biografts than in the currently used reinforced synthetic grafts. Aneurysms and pseudoaneurysms that occur in grafts can be surgically resected and replaced with a new section of graft that preserves the access site for future use.

Venous Hypertension

An increase in venous pressure is a physiologic consequence of all arteriovenous shunts. If the venous valves are incompetent, then retrograde flow may result. In most cases the symptoms are mild and resolve with time. The presence of significant venous hypertension results in dilated veins, swelling of the distal extremity, and bluish discoloration of the skin. Over time, severe and persistent venous hypertension can lead to chronic venostasis changes, such as thickening and discoloration of the skin as well as skin ulceration and pain.[221] A central venous stenosis is the most common etiology for severe venous hypertension occurring after placement of a hemodialysis graft. Angiography of the proximal venous outflow tract and central veins is indicated. If a stenosis is located it can be treated with angioplasty and stenting in an attempt to decrease symptoms and preserve access function.[222–225] In severe cases, the access may need to be ligated to preserve the extremity.

ACCESS STENOSIS

Pathophysiology

Access stenosis is the most common underlying etiology for access thrombosis and failure. The stenotic lesion at the venous anastomosis has been characterized pathologically as a dense neointimal hyperplasia.[226–231] Histochemically, the neointimal thickening consists predominantly of alpha smooth muscle actin containing cells (vascular smooth muscle cells and myofibroblasts) along with associated extracellular matrix material.[226–229,231] Prominent capillary infiltration (angiogenesis) is found throughout the neointima and particularly at the intima-media boundary.[228,229,231] Macrophages are found lining the surface of the graft, infiltrating the graft matrix, in the adventitia of the vein and in association with capillaries in the neointima.[227,229,231] Immunohistochemical studies reveal that the neointima stains strongly for the smooth muscle mitogens PDGF, FGF, insulin-like growth factor and endothelin, the matrix stimulating cytokine TGFβ, and the endothelial mitogens VEGF and FGF.[230,232,233] Indices of increased oxidative stress have been reported within the neointima.[230,233] Increased cellular proliferation is present throughout the lesion in the neointima, media, and adventia.[227,229,231] Proliferation of smooth muscle cells is frequently associated with proliferation of nearby endothelial cells.[227,229,231] In contrast to advanced atherosclerotic lesions, a lipid core and fibrous cap are not seen.[227,229,231] These findings document that vascular access stenosis is a dense lesion characterized by a high rate of proliferation of both vascular smooth muscle and endothelial cells along with abundant extracellular matrix material.

The exact pathophysiology leading to the venous neointimal hyperplasia in arteriovenous grafts is not known but is assumed to involve some of the same processes leading to neointimal hyperplasia seen after arterial injury.[234–236] The predominant localization of stenosis at the graft-vein anastomosis and in the immediate downstream vein suggests that mechanical injury at the time of surgery, the inflammatory reaction to the graft material, venous hypertension, increased turbulence, and altered wall shear stress may all be factors that contribute to neointimal hyperplasia.

MONITORING TO DETECT GRAFT STENOSIS

Longitudinal observational studies have shown that an active access surveillance program can decrease the rate of graft thrombosis and may increase overall access survival.[111,114,128,237] Based on these studies, the guidelines from the National Kidney Foundation/Dialysis Outcomes Quality Initiative (K/DOQI) recommended an organized approach to access surveillance with regular assessment and tracking of access function to detect and treat access stenosis.[114] Several approaches are used for access surveillance (Table 17–5).[114,238] The optimal approach would have a high sensitivity and specificity for the detection of access stenosis, be easy to perform at each dialysis session, and inexpensive. Currently, no surveillance technique has been shown to meet all of these criteria.

Clinical examination of the graft and downstream vein by an experienced observer can detect hemodynamically significant access stenosis, particularly when it occurs at the venous anastomosis or immediate downstream vein.[239] The examination should focus on noting the presence and location of any palpable thrills, the character of the pulse, and the nature of the audible bruit (Table 17–6). Development of significant swelling in the access arm suggests the presence of a central vein stenosis most likely from a prior central catheter or cardiac pacemaker. In the hands of an experienced examiner a careful clinical exam reportedly has a positive predictive value of 92% to detect a hemodynamically significant stenosis.[95,239]

From basic fluid mechanics, access flow rate (Qa) is determined from the pressure drop across the access ($\Delta P = MAP - CVP$) divided by the access resistance (R).

$$Qa = \Delta P \div R = (MAP - CVP) \div R \quad (1)$$

where MAP is the mean arterial pressure and CVP is the central venous pressure. Access stenosis in the range of 50% to 60% leads to an increase in resistance that can be detected by a measurable decrease in access flow rate.[240] Most of the resistance in an arteriovenous access occurs on the arterial side of the access.[215,241,242] In a well functioning graft, resistance on the arterial side of the graft is two to three times that on the venous side of the graft.[215,241,242] Development of a stenosis at the venous anastomosis leads to an increase in the venous resistance such that the venous resistance becomes equal to or greater than the arterial resistance. This leads to an increase in the intra-access venous pressure (P_{IA}) upstream of the stenosis and a decrease in access flow rate. Assuming MAP and cardiac output are constant and there is no change in peripheral shunting through other vascular beds, a decrease in access flow rate or an increase in P_{IA} can be used to detect venous access stenosis.[215,242] When access flow rate significantly falls below the speed of the dialysis blood pump, then recirculation develops and blood from the venous return needle is drawn into the arterial needle (recirculated). Adequate solute clearance during dialysis is then limited by the access flow rate. Hence, measurement of access recirculation, intra-access pressure, and flow rate are all techniques that have been used to detect access stenosis. However, access recirculation only detects critical access stenosis that produces an access flow rate less than the dialyzer blood pump speed, and this may be too late to intervene and prevent access stenosis from leading to thrombosis.[136,243] In addition, measurement of recirculation will miss a critical stenosis that occurs within the body of the graft between the arterial and venous needles.

Table 17–5 Techniques for Access Surveillance to Detect Stenosis

- Clinical exam
- Access recirculation
- Venous pressure
  - Dynamic pressure
  - Static pressure
- Access flow rate
- Direct visualization
  - Doppler ultrasound
  - Angiogram
  - Magnetic resonance angiography

Table 17–6 Clinical Examination to Detect Access Stenosis

Parameter	Normal	Stenosis*
Thrill	Only at arterial anastomosis	At site of stenotic lesion
Pulse	Soft, easily compressible	Water-hammer
Bruit	Low-pitched	High-pitched
	Continuous	Discontinuous
	Diastolic and systolic	Systolic only

*Abnormalities listed are for the two extremes: completely normal and severe stenosis. With lesser degrees of stenosis the findings will be between these two extremes. (From Beathard GA: Physical examination of the dialysis vascular access. Semin Dial 1998; 11:231-236.)

Venous pressure within the access has been used to detect the presence of access stenosis.[238] The simplest technique is to use the venous pressure measured in the post-dialyzer venous drip chamber during dialysis as an index of intra-access pressure. A dynamic venous drip chamber pressure (P_{DC}) greater than 150 mmHg measured 30 minutes into dialysis at a dialyzer pump speed of 200 mL/min is predictive of access stenosis.[111] While monitoring P_{DC} has been shown to detect venous stenosis in grafts and decrease access thrombosis[111,124,242]; its accuracy to detect stenosis and prevent thrombosis is reduced compared to other measures, including intra-access pressure at zero flow or access flow rate.[48,142,242,244,245]

Intra-access venous pressure P_{IA} can be measured directly from a needle inserted into the access.[132,316,325] When normalized for blood pressure (e.g., P_{IA}/MAP, the venous access pressure ratio, VAPR), a VAPR above 0.5 has been shown to have a relatively high sensitivity (81%) and low false-positive rate (20%) for the detection of a 50% diameter stenosis.[242,246] Routine use of intra-access pressure monitoring has been shown to decrease the rate of access thrombosis and prolong access survival compared to historical controls.[128,245] However, two more recent studies have concluded that the VAPR lacked the necessary sensitivity and specificity needed to accurately predict access thrombosis.[247,248] Further study will be needed to sort out the reasons for these discrepancies. In addition, direct measurement of intra-access pressure requires special equipment and is not practical for routine screening.

Using access flow monitoring an access flow of less than 600 mL/min or a 20% decrement in flow that falls below 1000 mL/min has been reported to predict the presence of a greater than 50% stenosis or an increased risk of thrombosis in a graft.[114,135,136,142–144] Several studies have also reported that routine monitoring of access flow rate can decrease the frequency of access thrombosis and overall cost of access management.[129,131,237,245] However, several recent studies that examined the receiver operating characteristic (ROC) curves have questioned whether measurement of access flow rate has the necessary performance characteristics (e.g., sensitivity and specificity greater than 80%) to be a good screening tool to prevent access thrombosis.[247,249,250] Moreover, two recent prospective randomized studies in subjects with established grafts found that routine monthly monitoring of access flow rate led to an increased rate of angioplasty but failed to decrease access thrombosis or prolong graft survival, compared to a control group that received usual graft monitoring.[133,251] In one study, the angioplasty rate in the control group (0.61 per patient year) was already comparatively high, and the baseline thrombosis rate (0.41 per patient year) as well as the overall graft survival rate were much better than generally reported in the United States. This suggests that there may be a threshold rate of angioplasty and that addition of access flow monitoring and additional angioplasty onto an aggressive and successful access monitoring program may not be beneficial.[251]

An alternative to hemodynamic measurements is direct visualization of the access by Duplex ultrasound, angiography, or magnetic resonance angiography (MRA).[238,252–257] An additional advantage of Duplex ultrasound and MRA is that they can provide information on access flow rate.[253,255,256] Several studies have documented the ability of routine Duplex ultrasound monitoring to detect access stenosis and decrease the rate of access thrombosis.[131,133,258] As discussed above, a recent randomized prospective trial also reported that quarterly Duplex ultrasound studies were better than monthly access flow monitoring in detecting access stenosis and preventing access thrombosis. However, overall access survival was not prolonged.[133] Moreover, Duplex ultrasound requires specialized equipment and training and may not be practical for routine monitoring in most dialysis units. Similarly, the use of MRA or angiography are not practical or cost-effective to use for routine access screening but are useful to confirm the suspected stenosis and to plan the appropriate therapeutic intervention.

In summary, careful monitoring of grafts to detect and treat stenosis has been shown to decrease the thrombosis rate at the expense of an increase in the angioplasty rate. Despite this trade-off, a routine monitoring program has been reported to decrease overall access costs and certainly converts the "crisis" of unexpected access thrombosis into a more manageable program of scheduled intervention and treatment. Based on these observations, K/DOQI guidelines recommend an organized approach to access surveillance with regular assessment and tracking of access function to detect and treat access stenosis. At this time, there is no single preferred technique that is low cost and easily performed at each dialysis session and also has the high sensitivity and specificity desired of a screening test. Each hemodialysis unit will need to decide on an approach that works best to fit their needs. Further research and technologic advances are needed in this area. Moreover, despite careful monitoring, access thrombosis and failure will continue to be a problem, and better treatments to prevent and treat graft stenosis and thrombosis are needed.

TREATMENT AND PREVENTION OF GRAFT FAILURE

Graft stenosis detected on routine screening can be treated by either surgical resection or percutaneous transluminal angioplasty. Depending on the site of the stenosis, surgical treatment may consist of an outflow patch graft to widen the venous anastomosis, resection of a stenotic segment, or bypass of the stenosis often requiring anastomosis to a new segment of artery or vein. Angioplasty has become the preferred method in most centers for the initial treatment of access stenosis because it can be done at the time of confirmatory angiography, and it preserves vessels for future surgery.[259,260] The stenotic lesions are denser than typical atherosclerotic lesions and require a higher balloon pressure (up to 20 atm for at least 1–2 minutes) to achieve a satisfactory result (typically defined as <30% stenosis after angioplasty).[259,261] Restenosis occurs rapidly after angioplasty with a median patency of about 6 months.[95,116,122,260] Use of endovascular stents has not been shown to prolong the primary patency after angioplasty of graft stenosis.[262–264] However, stents may be useful in selected situations, such as rapid recurrent re-stenosis, significant elastic recoil after angioplasty or where alterautogenous surgical options are limited.[265] Endovascular stents are also frequently employed to treat central venous stenosis where surgical options are limited.[222–225,266] However, multiple reintervention is often necessary to maintain patency of the central veins. Endovascular stents have been used to treat access complications, such as venous rupture after balloon angioplasty or pseudoaneurysms.[267,268]

If access thrombosis has occurred, percutaneous thrombolysis or surgical thrombectomy is required to restore patency and should be followed by angiography or other imaging technique to detect and treat any underlying stenosis. A crossed-catheter pharmaco-mechanical approach using a thrombolytic agent is most frequently used for percutaneous thrombolysis, but mechanical thrombolysis using saline has also been shown to be effective.[117,119,261,269–272] Percutaneous thrombolysis and surgical thrombectomy have been reported to be similarly effective at restoring short-term patency as long as stenotic regions are identified and treated.[123,273–276] Advantages and disadvantages of both approaches have been debated.[118,277] For both approaches, re-stenosis after thrombosis occurs more rapidly (median patency about 90 days) than after angioplasty for stenosis without thrombosis.[112,118–120,365] Although repeated angioplasty can preserve access function temporarily, access patency tends to decline with each angioplasty.[3] Ultimately, surgical revision or placement of a new access is required in most people who suffer recurrent bouts of graft stenosis and thrombosis.

Given the high costs and patient morbidity associated with treating graft stenosis and thrombosis, increasing attention has been directed to the primary prevention of these complications. Since thrombosis is the ultimate cause of access failure, treatment with anticoagulants and antiplatelet agents have been tried.[150] In uncontrolled trials, anticoagulation with warfarin or heparin has been reported to prolong access survival in people who have had frequent access thrombosis often in association with antiphospholipid antibodies.[151,152] In a small study of 16 people with anticardiolipin antibodies and recurrent thrombosis, the use of warfarin (target INR of 2–3) also produced a small but statistically significant increase in graft survival.[278] However, a recent randomized controlled trial of low dose warfarin, targeting an INR of 1.4 to 1.9, found no benefit (and possible harm) of warfarin over placebo in preventing access thrombosis in subjects who received a new hemodialysis graft.[279] Use of anticoagulants should not be used as a general strategy to prevent graft thrombosis, however, in selected patients with frequent graft thrombosis and known prothrombotic conditions these agents can be considered if the benefit appears to outweigh the risk.

Antiplatelet agents have been examined in randomized controlled trials to prevent graft occlusion.[280,281] In one study, 84 people who received a new graft were randomized to treatment with either aspirin, dipyridamole, aspirin plus dipyridamole, or placebo and found that aspirin alone did not prevent and, in fact, tended to increase the risk of graft thrombosis.[282] Surprisingly, dipyridamole alone or in combination with aspirin was found to decrease the risk of graft thrombosis.[282] Since dipyridamole alone is a weak antiplatelet agent, this suggested that the effect of dipyridamole to inhibit graft thrombosis might be mediated by another mechanism. This concept is currently being tested in a large randomized clinical trial. More recently, the results of the randomized controlled VA Cooperative trial have been reported looking at the effect of the combination of aspirin (325 mg/day) plus clopidogrel (75 mg/day) compared to placebo on graft thrombosis in 200 subjects with prevalent grafts.[283] The study was terminated early due to a twofold increased risk of bleeding in the treatment group without observing any overall benefit of the therapy to reduce graft thrombosis. However, the study did note a trend towards improved graft survival using aspirin plus clopidogrel in the subgroup of subjects who had never suffered an episode of graft thrombosis.[283] Aspirin has also been noted to be associated with a decreased risk of graft thrombosis in two recent prospective observational studies.[251,284] Taken together, the results from randomized controlled trials do not currently support the use of antiplatelet agents to prevent graft thrombosis. However, given the positive results from the observational studies and the benefit of these agents in other arterial vascular diseases, the question of whether an antiplatelet agent can reduce graft thrombosis and prolong graft survival remains unresolved. The question may well be whether the benefit to prevent graft thrombosis will outweigh the increased risk of bleeding.

Fish oil capsules containing omega-3 polyunsaturated fatty acids have been shown in several randomized controlled trials to reduce the risk of atherothrombotic events (i.e., recurrent myocardial infarction and death) in people who have known coronary artery disease.[285,286] In 1990, a small pilot study of fish oil was done in seven hemodialysis patients who had frequent recurrent graft thrombosis and found no effect on graft thrombosis at 6 months, but the study was underpowered.[287,288] Recently, a randomized, double-blind trial of fish oil capsules (4 g/day) compared with a corn oil control was performed in 24 subjects (12 in each group) who received a new ePTFE graft.[289] The study medication was started within 2 weeks after access surgery and follow-up was for 1 year or until access thrombosis developed. A dramatic reduction in the incidence of graft thrombosis was seen in the subjects treated with fish oil (primary patency at 1 year was 14.9% in the control and 75.6% in the fish oil-treated groups).[289] A larger randomized trial of fish oil is needed for confirmation of this effect.

At this time, there is no proven therapy that can delay or prevent graft failure. Many new therapies are on the horizon that offer promise to prevent neointimal hyperplasia and prolong graft survival.[290] Local therapy applied at the vein-graft anastomosis at the time of graft surgery is a new approach that can limit systemic drug toxicity and allow a therapeutic agent to be focused at the major site of neointimal hyperplasia. An example of this therapy is the recent successful trial of an oligonucleotide decoy to the E2F transcription factor applied to vein grafts at the time of coronary artery bypass surgery.[291] A trial of this therapy for dialysis grafts (PREVENT V) is currently underway. Other local therapies applied either to the luminal or advential side of the vein-graft anastomosis are being considered, but concerns regarding impaired healing and aneurysm formation leading to vein rupture will need to be monitored.

Finally, in addition to graft design and pharmacologic therapy, attention to details in surgical placement, graft cannulation, and infection control practices, as well as maintenance of facility access databases to monitor outcomes, are all aspects of routine care that are difficult to quantitate but are likely to contribute to prolonging access survival.

References

1. Kolff WJ, Berk HT: The artificial kidney: A dialyzer with a great area. Acta Med Scand 1944; 117:121.
2. Quinton W, Dillard D, Scribner BH: Cannulation of blood vessels for prolonged hemodialysis. Trans ASAIO 1960; 6:104.
3. Brescia MJ, Cimino JE, Appel K, Hurwich BJ: Chronic hemodialysis using venipuncture and a surgically recreated arteriovenous fistula. N Engl J Med 1966; 275:1089-1092.
4. Baker LD Jr, Johnson JM, Goldfarb D: Expanded polytetrafluoroethylene (PTFE) subcutaneous arteriovenous conduit: An improved vascular access for chronic hemodialysis. ASAIO Trans 1976; 22:382-387.
5. Kaplan MS, Mirahmadi KS, Winer RL, et al: Comparison of "PTFE" and bovine grafts for blood access in hemodialysis patients. ASAIO Trans 1976; 22:388-392.
6. NKF-K/DOQI Clinical Practice Guidelines for Vascular Access 2000 Update. New York, National Kidney Foundation, 2001.
7. Shaldon S, Chianussi L, Higgs B: Hemodialyis by percutaneous catheterization of the femoral artery and vein with regional heparinization. Lancet 1961; 2:75-81.
8. Uldall R, Dyke R, Woods F: A subclavian cannula for temporary vascular access for hemodialyis or plasmapheresis. Dial Transplant 1979; 8:963-968.
9. Schwab SJ, Buller GL, McCann RL, et al: Prospective evaluation of a dacron cuffed hemodialysis catheter for prolonged use. Am J Kidney Dis 1988; 11:166-169.
10. Schwab SJ, Weiss MA, Rushton F, et al: Multicenter clinical trial results with the LifeSite(r) hemodialysis access system. Kidney Int 2002; 62:1026-1033.
11. Blake PG, Huraib S, Wu G, Uldall R: The use of dual-lumen jugular venous catheters as definitive long-term access for hemodialysis. Int J Artif Organs 1990; 13:26-31.
12. Hakim RM, Himmelfarb J: Hemodialysis access failure: A call to action. Kidney Int 1998; 54:1029-1040.
13. Pisoni RL, Young EW, Dykstra DM, et al: Vascular access use in Europe and the United States: Results from DOPPS. Kidney Int 2002; 61:305-316.
14. Rayner HC, Pisoni RL, Gillespie BW, et al: Creation, cannulation, and survival of arteriovenous fistulae: Data from the Dialysis Outcomes and Practice Study. Kidney Int 2003; 63: 323-330.
15. Reddan D, Klassen P, Frankenfield DL, et al: National profile of practice patterns for hemodialysis vascular access in the United States. J Am Soc Nephrol 2002; 13:2117-2124.
16. Dhingra RK, Young EW, Hulbert-Shearon TE, et al: Type of vascular access and mortality in U.S. hemodialysis patients. Kidney Int 2002; 60:1443-1451.
17. LeBlanc M, Fedak S, Morris G, Paganini EP: Blood recirculation in temporary central catheters for acute hemodialysis. Clin Nephrol 1996; 45:315-319.
18. Schwab SJ, Quarles D, Middleton JP, et al: Hemodialysis-associated subclavian vein stenosis. Kidney Int 1988; 33: 1156-1159.
19. Sherertz RJ, Ely EW, Westbrook DM, et al: Education of physicians-in-training can decrease the risk for vascular catheter infection. Ann Intern Med 2000; 132:641-648.
20. Schwab SJ, Beathard GA: The hemodialysis catheter conundrum: Hate living with them, but can't live without them. Kidney Int 1999; 56:1-17.
21. Sarnak MJ, Jaber BL: Mortality caused by sepsis in patients with end-stage renal disease compared with the general population. Kidney Int 2000; 58:1758-1764.
22. Stevenson KB, Hannah EL, Lowder CA, et al: Epidemiology of hemodialysis vascular access infections from longitudinal infection surveillance data: Predicting the impact of NKF-DOQI Clinical Practice Guidelines for Vascular Access. Am J Kidney Dis 2002; 39:549-555.
23. Tokars JI, Light P, Anderson J, et al: A prospective study of vascular access infections at seven outpatient hemodialysis centers. Am J Kidney Dis 2001; 37:1232-1240.
24. Marr KA, Sexton DJ, Conlon PJ, et al: Catheter-related bacteremia and outcome of attempted catheter salvage in patients undergoing hemodialysis. Ann Intern Med 1997; 127:275-280.
25. Beathard GA: Management of bacteremia associated with tunneled-cuffed hemodialysis catheters. J Am Soc Nephrol 1999; 10:1045-1049.
26. Tanriover B, Carlton D, Saddekni S, et al: Bacteremia associated with tunneled dialysis catheters: Comparison of two treatment strategies. Kidney Int 2000; 57:2151-2155.
27. Krishnasami Z, Carlton D, Bimbo L, et al: Management of hemodialyis catheter-related bacteremia with an adjunctive antibiotic lock solution. Kidney Int 2002; 61:1136-1142.
28. Sesso R, Barbosa D, Leme IL, et al: Staphylococcus aureus prophylaxis in hemodialysis patients using central venous catheter: Effect of mupirocin ointment. J Am Soc Nephrol 1998; 9:1085-1092.
29. Johnson DW, MacGinley R, Kay TD, et al: A randomized controlled trial of topical exit site mupirocin application in patients with tunnelled, cuffed haemodialysis catheters. Nephrol Dial Transplant 2002; 17:1802-1807.
30. Lok CE, Stanley KE, Hux JE, et al: Hemodialysis infection prevention with polysporin ointment. J Am Soc Nephrol 2003; 14:169-179.
31. Mokrzycki MH, Jeane-Jerome K, Rush H, et al: A randomized trial of minidose warfarin for the prevention of late malfunction in tunneled, cuffed hemodialysis catheters. Kidney Int 2001; 59:1935-1942.
32. Bolz KD, Fjermeros G, Wideroe TE, Hatlinghus S: Catheter malfunction and thrombus formation on double-lumen hemodialysis catheters: An intravascular ultrasonographic study. Am J Kidney Dis 1995; 25:597-602.
33. Negulescu O, Coco M, Croll J, Mokrzycki MH: Large atrial thrombus formation associated with tunneled cuffed hemodialysis catheters. Clin Nephrol 2003; 59:40-46.
34. Barrett N, Spenser S, McIvor J, Brown EA: Subclavian stenosis: A major complication of subclavian dialysis catheters. Nephrol Dial Transplant 1988; 3:423-425.
35. Cheung AK, Gregory MC: Subclavian vein thrombosis in hemodialysis patients. Trans ASAIO 1985; 31:131.
36. Fant GF, Dennis VW, Quarles D: Late vascular complications of the subclavian dialysis catheter. Am J Kidney Dis 1986; 7:225.
37. Hernandez D, Diaz F, Rufino M, et al: Subclavian vascular access stenosis in dialysis patients: Natural history and risk factors. J Am Soc Nephrol 1998; 9:1507-1510.
38. Khanna S, Sniderman K, Simons M, et al: Superior vena cava stenosis associated with hemodialysis catheters. Am J Kidney Dis 1993; 21:278-281.
39. Moran JE: Subcutaneous vascular access devices. Semin Dial 2001; 14:452-457.
40. Canaud B, Morena M, Leray-Moragues H: Dialock: Results of a French multicenter study. Nephrologie 2001; 22:391-397.
41. Brescia MJ, Cimino JE, Appel K, Hurwich BJ: Chronic hemodialysis using venipuncture and a surgically created arteriovenous fistula. N Engl J Med 1966; 275:1089-1092.
42. Oliver MJ, McCann RL, Indridason OS, et al: Comparison of transposed brachiobasilic fistulas to upper arm grafts and brachiocephalic fistulas. Kidney Int 2001; 60:1532-1539.
43. Coburn MC, Carney WI Jr: Comparison of basilic vein and polytetrafluoroethylene for brachial arteriovenous fistula. J Vasc Surg 1994; 20:896-902.
44. Zielinski CM, Mittal SK, Anderson P, et al: Delayed superficialization of brachiobasilic fistula: Technique and initial experience. Arch Surg 2001; 136:929-932.
45. Konner K, Nonnast-Daniel B, Ritz E: The arteriovenous fistula. J Am Soc Nephrol 2003; 14:1669-1680.

46. System USRD: 1997 annual data report. Bethesda, MD, National Institutes of Health, National Institute of Diabetes and Digestive and Kidney Disease, 1997.
47. Schwab SJ, Harrington JT, Singh A, et al: Vascular access for hemodialysis. Kidney Int 1999; 55:2078-2090.
48. McCarley P, Wingard RL, Shyr Y, et al: Vascular access blood flow monitoring reduces access morbidity and costs. Kidney Int 2001; 60:1164-1172.
49. Dixon BS, Novak L, Fangman J: Hemodialysis vascular access survival: Upper-arm native arteriovenous fistula. Am J Kidney Dis 2002; 39:92-101.
50. Allon M, Robbin ML: Increasing arteriovenous fistulas in hemodialysis patients: Problems and solutions. Kidney Int 2002; 62:1109-1124.
51. Prischl FC, Kirchgatterer A, Brandstatter E, et al: Parameters of prognostic relevance to the patency of vascular access in hemodialysis patients. J Am Soc Nephrol 1995; 6:1613-1618.
52. Culp K, Flanigan M, Taylor L, Rothstein M: Vascular access thrombosis in new hemodialysis patients. Am J Kidney Dis 1995; 26:341-346.
53. Feldman HI, Held PJ, Hutchinson JT, et al: Hemodialysis vascular access morbidity in the United States. Kidney Int 1993; 43:1091-1096.
54. Miller PE, Tolwani A, Luscy CP, et al: Predictors of adequacy of arteriovenous fistulas in hemodialysis patients. Kidney Int 1999; 56:275-280.
55. Feldman HI, Joffe M, Rosas SE, et al: Predictors of successful arteriovenous fistula maturation. Am J Kidney Dis 2003; 42:1000-1012.
56. Hirth RA, Turenne MN, Woods JD, et al: Predictors of type of vascular access in hemodialysis patients. JAMA 1996; 276:1303-1308.
57. Administration, HCFA Health Care Financing. 2000 Annual Report, End Stage Renal Disease Clinical Performances Measures Project. Baltimore, Department of Health and Human Services, Health Care Financing Administration, Office of Clinical Standards and Quality, 2000.
58. Allon M, Bailey R, Ballard R, et al: A multidisciplinary approach to hemodialysis access: Prospective evaluation. Kidney Int 1998; 53:473-479.
59. Lok CE, Oliver MJ: Overcoming barriers to arteriovenous fistula creation and use. Semin Dial 2003; 16:189-196.
60. Silva MB, Hobson RW, Pappas PJ, et al: A strategy for increasing use of autogenous hemodialysis access procedures: Impact of preoperative noninvasive evaluation. J Vasc Surg 1998; 27: 302-308.
61. Allon M, Lockhart ME, Lilly RZ, et al: Effect of preoperative sonographic mapping on vascular access outcomes in hemodialysis patients. Kidney Int 2001; 60:2013-2020.
62. Gibson KD, Caps MT, Kohler TR, et al: Assessment of a policy to reduce placement of prosthetic hemodialysis access. Kidney Int 2002; 59:2335-2345.
63. Patel ST, Hughes J, Mills JL Sr: Failure of arteriovenous fistula maturation: An unintended consequence of exceeding dialysis outcome quality initiative guidelines for hemodialysis access. J Vasc Surg 2003; 38:439-445.
64. Kaufman JS: Antithrombotic agents and the prevention of access thrombosis. Semin Dial 2000; 13:40-46.
65. Turmel-Rodrigues L, Mouton A, Birmele B, et al: Salvage of immature forearm fistulas for haemodialysis by interventional radiology. Nephrol Dial Transplant 2001; 16:2365-2371.
66. Beathard GA, Settle SM, Shields MW: Salvage of the nonfunctioning arteriovenous fistula. Am J Kidney Dis 1999; 33:910-916.
67. Schon D, Mishler R: Salvage of occluded autologous arteriovenous fistulae. Am J Kidney Dis 2000; 36:804-810.
68. Turmel-Rodrigues L, Pengloan J, Rodrigue H, et al: Treatment of failed native arteriovenous fistulae for hemodialysis by interventional radiology. Kidney Int 2000; 57:1124-1140.
69. Haage P, Vorwerk D, Wildberger JE, et al: Percutaneous treatment of thrombosed primary arteriovenous hemodialysis access fistulae. Kidney Int 2000; 57:1169-1175.
70. Tonelli M, Jhangri GS, Hirsch DJ, et al: Best threshold for diagnosis of stenosis or thrombosis within six months of access flow measurement in arteriovenous fistulae. J Am Soc Nephrol 2003; 14:3264-3269.
71. Sidawy AN, Gray R, Besarab A, et al: Recommended standards for reports dealing with arteriovenous hemodialysis accesses. J Vasc Surg 2002; 35:603-610.
72. Wesolowski SA: Foundations of modern vascular grafts. *In* Kaplitt MJ (ed): Vascular Grafts. New York, Appleton-Century-Crofts, 1976, pp 27-49.
73. Johansen K, Lyman D, Sauvage L: Biomaterials for hemodialysis access. Blood Purif 1994; 12:73-77.
74. Matsumoto H, Hasegawa T, Fuse K, et al: A new vascular prosthesis for a small caliber artery. Surgery 1973; 74:519-523.
75. Guillou PJ, Leveson SH, Kester RC: The complications of arteriovenous grafts for vascular access. Br J Surg 1980; 67: 517-521.
76. Kapoian T, Sherman RA: A brief history of vascular access for emodialysis: An unfinished story. Semin Nephrol 1997; 17: 239-245.
77. Veith FJ, Wilson SE, Hobson RW, et al: Vascular access complications and new methods. Trans Am Soc Artif Intern Organs 1982; 28:647-651.
78. Haimov M, Burrows L, Schanzer H, et al: Experience with arterial substitutes in the construction of vascular access for hemodialysis. J Cardiovasc Surg 1980; 21:149-154.
79. Santoro TD, Cambria RA: PTFE shunts for hemodialysis access: Progressive choice of configuration. Semin Vasc Surg 1997; 10:166-174.
80. Tellis VA, Kohlberg WI, Bhat DJ, et al: Expanded polytetrafluoroethylene graft fistula for chronic hemodialysis. Ann Surg 1979; 189:101-105.
81. Hurlbert SN, Mattos MA, Henretta JP, et al: Long-term patency rates, complications and cost-effectiveness of polytetrafluoroethylene (PTFE) grafts for hemodialysis access: A prospective study that compares Impra versus Gore-tex grafts. Cardiovasc Surg 1998; 6:652-656.
82. Kaufman JL, Garb JL, Berman JA, et al: A prospective comparison of two expanded polytetrafluoroethylene grafts for linear forearm hemodialysis access: Does the manufacturer matter? J Am Coll Surg 1997; 185:74-79.
83. Cameron BL, Tsuchida H, Connall TP, et al: High porosity PTFE improves endothelialization of arterial grafts without increasing early thrombogenicity. J Cardiovasc Surg 1993; 34:281-285.
84. Akers DL, Du YH, Kempczinski RF: The effect of carbon coating and porosity on early patency of expanded polytetrafluoroethylene grafts: An experimental study. J Vasc Surg 1993; 18:10-15.
85. Katzman HE: A review of prospective trials to evaluate angioaccess graft materials. *In* Henry ML (ed): Vascular Access for Hemodialysis, vol. 6. Chicago, W. L. Gore & Associates and Precept Press, 1999, pp 263-273.
86. Glickman MH, Stokes GK, Ross JR, et al: Multicenter evaluation of a polytetrafluoroethylene vascular access graft as compared with the expanded polytetrafluoroethylene vascular access graft in hemodialysis applications. J Vasc Surg 2001; 34:465-472.
87. Nakao A, Miyazaki M, Oka Y, et al: Creation and use of a composite polyurethane-expanded polytetrafluoroethylene graft for hemodialysis access. Acta Medica Okayama 2000; 54:91-94.
88. Allen RD, Yuill E, Nankivell BJ, Francis DM: Australian multicentre evaluation of a new polyurethane vascular access graft. Aust N Z J Surg 1996; 66:738-742.
89. Ota K, Nakagawa Y, Kitano Y, et al: Clinical application of modified polyurethane graft to blood access. Artif Organs 1991; 15:449-453.

90. Nakagawa Y, Ota K, Teraoka S, Agishi T: Experimental studies on improved polyester-polyurethane vascular grafts for hemodialysis. ASAIO Trans 1991; 37:M273-M274.
91. Vermeij CG, Smit FW, Elsman BH: Inability to monitor polyurethane haemodialysis vascular access graft by Doppler ultrasound. Nephrol Dial Transplant 2001; 16:1089-1090.
92. Dixon BS, Novak L, Fangman J: Hemodialysis vascular access survival: Upper-arm native arteriovenous fistula. Am J Kidney Dis 2002; 39:92-101.
93. Miller PE, Carlton D, Deierhoi MH, et al: Natural history of arteriovenous grafts in hemodialysis patients. Am J Kidney Dis 2000; 36:68-74.
94. Hodges TC, Fillinger MF, Zwolak RM, et al: Longitudinal comparison of dialysis access methods: Risk factors for failure. J Vasc Surg 1997; 26:1009-1019.
95. Safa AA, Valji K, Roberts AC, et al: Detection and treatment of dysfunctional hemodialysis access grafts: Effect of a surveillance program on graft patency and the incidence of thrombosis. Radiology 1996; 199:653-657.
96. Gibson KD, Gillen DL, Caps MT, et al: Vascular access survival and incidence of revisions: A comparison of prosthetic grafts, simple autogenous fistulas, and venous transposition fistulas from the United States Renal Data System Dialysis Morbidity and Mortality Study (Comment). J Vasc Surg 2001; 34:694-700.
97. Burger H, Kluchert BA, Kootstra G, et al: Survival of arteriovenous fistulas and shunts for hemodialysis. Eur J Surg 1995; 161:327-334.
98. Kalman PG, Pope M, Bhola C, et al: A practical approach to vascular access for hemodialysis and predictors of success. J Vasc Surg 1999; 30:727-733.
99. Kherlakian GM, Roedersheimer LR, Arbaugh JJ, et al: Comparison of autogenous fistula versus expanded polytetrafluoroethylene graft fistula for angioaccess in hemodialysis. Am J Surg 1986; 152:238-243.
100. Palder SB, Kirkman RL, Whittemore AD, et al: Vascular access for hemodialysis: Patency rates and results of revision. Ann Surg 1985; 202:235-239.
101. Churchill DN, Taylor DW, Cook RJ, et al: Canadian hemodialysis morbidity study. Am J Kidney Dis 1992; 19:214-234.
102. Winsett OE, Wolma FJ: Complications of vascular access for hemodialysis. South Med J 1985; 78:513-517.
103. Cinat ME, Hopkins J, Wilson SE: A prospective evaluation of PTFE graft patency and surveillance techniques in hemodialysis access. Ann Vasc Surg 1999; 13:191-198.
104. Palder SB, Kirkman RL, Whittemore AD, et al: Vascular access from hemodialysis: Patency rates and results of revision. Ann Surg 1985; 202:235-239.
105. Rocco MV, Bleyer AJ, Burkart JM: Utilization of inpatient and outpatient resources for the management of hemodialysis access complications. Am J Kidney Dis 1996; 28:250-256.
106. Etheredge EE, Haid SD, Maeser MN, et al: Salvage operations for malfunctioning polytetrafluoroethylene hemodialysis access grafts. Surgery 1983; 94:464-470.
107. Zibari GB, Rohr MS, Landreneau MD, et al: Complications from permanent hemodialysis vascular access. Surgery 1988; 104:681-686.
108. Bosman PJ, Blankestijn PJ, van der Graaf Y, et al: A comparison between PTFE and denatured homologous vein grafts for haemodialysis access: A prospective randomised multicentre trial. The SMASH Study Group. Study of Graft Materials in Access for Haemodialysis. Eur J Vasc Endovasc Surg 1998; 16:126-132.
109. Beathard GA: Thrombolysis versus surgery for the treatment of thrombosed dialysis access grafts. J Am Soc Nephrol 1995; 6:1619-1624.
110. Schuman ES, Gross GF, Hayes JF, Standage BA: Long-term patency of polytetrafluoroethylene graft fistulas. Am J Surg 1988; 155:644-646.
111. Schwab SJ, Raymond JR, Saeed M, et al: Prevention of hemodialysis fistula thrombosis. Early detection of various stenoses. Kidney Int 1989; 36:707-711.
112. Windus DW, Jendrisak MD, Delmez JA: Prosthetic fistula survival and complications in hemodialysis patients: Effects of diabetes and age. Am J Kidney Dis 1992; 19:448-452.
113. Fan PY, Schwab SJ: Vascular access: Concepts for the 1990s. J Am Soc Nephrol 1992; 3:1-11.
114. Initiative: NKF: NKF-DOQI clinical practice guidelines for vascular access. Am J Kidney Dis 1997; 30:S150-S191.
115. Windus DW: Permanent vascular access: A nephrologist's view. Am J Kidney Dis 1993; 21:457-471.
116. Kanterman RY, Vesely TM, Pilgram TK, et al: Dialysis access grafts: Anatomic location of venous stenosis and results of angioplasty. Radiology 1995; 195:135-139.
117. Valji K, Bookstein JJ, Roberts AC, Davis GB: Pharmacomechanical thrombolysis and angioplasty in the management of clotted hemodialysis grafts: Early and late clinical trials. Radiology 1991; 178:243-247.
118. Marston WA, Beathard GA: Surgical management of thrombosed dialysis access grafts. Am J Kidney Dis 1998; 32:168-171.
119. Beathard GA: Mechanical versus pharmacomechanical thrombolysis for the treatment of thrombosed dialysis access grafts. Kidney Int 1994; 45:1401-1406.
120. Glanz S, Bashist B, Gordon DH, et al: Angiography of upper extremity access fistulas for dialysis. Radiology 1982; 143: 45-52.
121. Mennes PA, Gilula LA, Anderson CB, et al: Complications associated with arteriovenous fistulas in patients undergoing chronic hemodialysis. Arch Intern Med 1978; 138: 1117-1121.
122. Turmel-Rodrigues L, Pengloan J, Blanchier D, et al: Insufficient dialysis shunts: Improved long-term patency rates with close hemodynamic monitoring, repeated percutaneous balloon angioplasty, and stent placement. Radiology 1993; 187:273-278.
123. Marston WA, Criado E, Jaques PF, et al: Prospective randomized comparison of surgical versus endovascular management of thrombosed dialysis access grafts (see comments). J Vasc Surg 1997; 26:373-380.
124. Choudhury D, Lee J, Elivera HS, et al: Correlation of venography, venous pressure, and hemoaccess function. Am J Kidney Dis 1995; 25:269-275.
125. Wang E, Schneditz D, Nepomuceno C, et al: Predictive value of access blood flow in detecting access thrombosis. ASAIO J 1998; 44:M555-M558.
126. Schillinger F, Schillinger D, Montagnac R, Milcent T: Post catheterisation vein stenosis in haemodialysis: Comparative angiographic study of 50 subclavian and 50 internal jugular accesses. Nephrol Dial Transplant 1991; 6:722-724.
127. Surratt RS, Picus D, Hicks ME, et al: The importance of preoperative evaluation of the subclavian vein in dialysis access planning (Comment). Am J Roentgenol 1991; 156:623-625.
128. Besarab A, Sullivan KL, Ross RP, Moritz MJ: Utility of intra-access pressure monitoring in detecting and correcting venous outlet stenoses prior to thrombosis. Kidney Int 1995; 47: 1364-1373.
129. McCarley P, Wingard RL, Shyr R, et al: Vascular access blood flow monitoring reduces access morbidity and costs. Kidney Int 2001; 60:1167-1172.
130. Roberts AB, Kahn MB, Bradford S, et al: Graft surveillance and angioplasty prolongs dialysis graft patency. J Am Coll Surg 1996; 183:486-492.
131. Sands JJ, Jabyak PA, et al: Intervention based on monthly monitoring decreases hemodialysis access thrombosis. ASAIO J 1999; 45:147-150.
132. Allon M, Bailey R, Ballard R, et al: A multidisciplinary approach to hemodialysis access: Prospective evaluation. Kidney Int 1998; 53:473-479.

133. Ram SJ, Work J, Caldito GC, et al: A randomized controlled trial of blood flow and stenosis surveillance of hemodialysis grafts. Kidney Int 2003; 64:272-280.
134. Sands JJ, Miranda CL: Prolongation of hemodialysis access survival with elective revision. Clin Nephrol 1995; 44:329-333.
135. Besarab A, Lubkowski T, Frinak S, et al: Detection of access strictures and outlet stenoses in vascular accesses. Which test is best? ASAIO J 1997; 43:M543-M547.
136. Besarab A, Lubkowski T, Frinak S, et al: Detecting vascular access dysfunction. ASAIO J 1997; 43:M539-M543.
137. Tonelli M, Hirsch D, Clark TW, et al: Access flow monitoring of patients with native vessel arteriovenous fistulae and previous angioplasty. J Am Soc Nephrol 2002; 13:2969-2973.
138. Back MR, White RA: Biologic response to prosthetic dialysis grafts. *In* Wilson SE (ed): Vascular Access: Principles and Practice, 4th ed. St. Louis, MO, Mosby, 2002, pp 61-73.
139. Kroll MH, Hellums JD, McIntire LV, et al: Platelets and shear stress (Comment). Blood 1996; 88:1525-1541.
140. Ruggeri ZM: Platelets in atherothrombosis. Nat Med 2002; 8:1227-1234.
141. Schwab SJ: Reducing the risk of hemodialysis access (Comment). Am J Kidney Dis 1999; 34:362-363.
142. Bosman PJ, Boereboom FT, Eikelboom BC, et al: Graft flow as a predictor of thrombosis in hemodialysis grafts. Kidney Int 1998; 54:1726-1730.
143. May RE, Himmelfarb J, Yenicesu M, et al: Predictive measures of vascular access thrombosis: A prospective study. Kidney Int 1997; 52:1656-1662.
144. Neyra NR, Ikizler TA, May RE, et al: Change in access blood flow over time predicts vascular access thrombosis. Kidney Int 1998; 54:1714-1719.
145. Smits JH, van der Linden J, Blankestijn PJ, Rabelink TJ: Coagulation and haemodialysis access thrombosis. Nephrol Dial Transplant 2000; 15:1755-1760.
146. Casserly LF, Dember LM: Thrombosis in end-stage renal disease. Semin Dial 2003; 16:245-256.
147. Windus DW, Santoro S, Royal HD: The effects of hemodialysis on platelet deposition in prosthetic graft fistulas. Am J Kidney Dis 1995; 26:614-621.
148. Garcia-Martin F, De Arriba G, Carrascosa T, et al: Anticardiolipin antibodies and lupus anticoagulant in end-stage renal disease. Nephrol Dial Transplant 1991; 6:543-547.
149. Fabrizi F, Sangiorgio R, Pontoriero G, et al: Antiphospholipid (aPL) antibodies in end-stage renal disease. J Nephrol 1999; 12:89-94.
150. Galli M, Luciani D, Bertolini G, Barbui T: Lupus anticoagulants are stronger risk factors for thrombosis than anticardiolipin antibodies in the antiphospholipid syndrome: A systematic review of the literature. Blood 2003; 101:1827-1832.
151. O'Shea S, Lawson JH, Reddan D, et al: Hypercoagulable states and antithrombotic strategies in recurrent vascular access site thrombosis. J Vasc Surg 2003; 38:541-548.
152. LeSar CJ, Merrick HW, et al: Thrombotic complications resulting from hypercoagulable states in chronic hemodialysis vascular access. J Am Coll Surg 1999; 189:73-81.
153. Brunet P, Aillaud MF, et al: Antiphospholipids in hemodialysis patients: Relationship between lupus anticoagulant and thrombosis. Kidney Int 1995; 48:794-800.
154. Prieto LN, Suki WN: Frequent hemodialysis graft thrombosis: Association with antiphospholipid antibodies. Am J Kidney Dis 1994; 23:587-590.
155. Palomo I, Pereira J, Alarcon M, et al: Vascular access thrombosis is not related to presence of antiphospholipid antibodies in patients on chronic hemodialysis. Nephron 2002; 92:957-958.
156. Chew SL, Lins RL, Daelemans R, et al: Are antiphospholipid antibodies clinically relevant in dialysis patients? Nephrol Dial Transplant 1992; 7:1194-1198.
157. Cattaneo M: Hyperhomocysteinemia, atherosclerosis and thrombosis. Thromb Haemost 1999; 81:165-176.
158. Dennis VW, Robinson K: Homocysteinemia and vascular disease in end-stage renal disease. Kidney Int Suppl 1996; 57:S11-S17.
159. Shemin D, Lapane KL, Bausserman L, et al: Plasma total homocysteine and hemodialysis access thrombosis: A prospective study. J Am Soc Nephrol 1999; 10:1095-1099.
160. Ducloux D, Pascal B, Jamali M, et al: Is hyperhomocysteinaemia a risk factor for recurrent vascular access thrombosis in haemodialysis patients? Nephrol Dial Transplant 1997; 12: 2037-2038.
161. Manns BJ, Burgess ED, et al: Hyperhomocysteinemia, anticardiolipin antibody status, and risk for vascular access thrombosis in hemodialysis patients. Kidney Int 1999; 55:315-320.
162. Bowden RG, Wyatt FB, Wilson R: Homocysteine and vascular access thrombosis in end-stage renal disease patients: A retrospective study. J Nephrol 2002; 15:666-670.
163. Hojs R, Gorenjak M, Ekart R, et al: Homocysteine and vascular access thrombosis in hemodialysis patients. Ren Fail 2002; 24:215-222.
164. Tamura T, Bergman SM, Morgan SL: Homocysteine, B vitamins, and vascular-access thrombosis in patients treated with hemodialysis. Am J Kidney Dis 1998; 32:475-481.
165. Al Saady NM, Leatham EW, Gupta S, et al: Monocyte expression of tissue factor and adhesion molecules: The link with accelerated coronary artery disease in patients with chronic renal failure. Heart 1999; 81:134-140.
166. Ambuhl PM, Wuthrich RP, Korte W, et al: Plasma hypercoagulability in haemodialysis patients: Impact of dialysis and anticoagulation. Nephrol Dial Transplant 1997; 12:2355-2364.
167. Baskin E, Duman O, Besbas N, Ozen S: Hypercoagulopathy in a hemodialysis patient: Are elevations in factors VII and VIII effective? Nephron 1999; 83:180.
168. Gris JC, Branger B, Vecina F, et al: Increased cardiovascular risk factors and features of endothelial activation and dysfunction in dialyzed uremic patients. Kidney Int 1994; 46:807-813.
169. Irish AB, Green FR: Factor VII coagulant activity (VIIc) and hypercoagulability in chronic renal disease and dialysis: Relationship with dyslipidaemia, inflammation, and factor VII genotype. Nephrol Dial Transplant 1998; 13:679-684.
170. Kario K, Matsuo T, Yamada T, et al: Factor VII hyperactivity in chronic dialysis patients. Thromb Res 1992; 67:105-113.
171. Kario K, Matsuo T, Matsuo M, et al: Marked increase of activated factor VII in uremic patients. Thromb Haemost 1995; 73:763-767.
172. Malyszko J, Malyszko JS, Pawlak D, et al: Hemostasis, platelet function and serotonin in acute and chronic renal failure. Thromb Res 1996; 83:351-361.
173. Mercier E, Branger B, Vecina F, et al: Tissue factor coagulation pathway and blood cells activation state in renal insufficiency. Hematol J 2001; 2:18-25.
174. Sagripanti A, Cupisti A, Baicchi U, et al: Plasma parameters of the prothrombotic state in chronic uremia. Nephron 1993; 63:273-278.
175. Tomura S, Nakamura Y, Deguchi F, et al: Coagulation and fibrinolysis in patients with chronic renal failure undergoing conservative treatment. Thromb Res 64:81-90.
176. Vaziri ND, Gonzales EC, Wang J, Said S: Blood coagulation, fibrinolytic, and inhibitory proteins in end-stage renal disease: Effect of hemodialysis. Am J Kidney Dis 1994; 23:828-835.
177. Esmon CT, Taylor FB Jr, Snow TR: Inflammation and coagulation: Linked processes potentially regulated through a common pathway mediated by protein C. Thromb Haemost 1991; 66:160-165.
178. van Tellingen A, Grooteman MP, Schoorl M, et al: Intercurrent clinical events are predictive of plasma C-reactive protein levels in hemodialysis patients. Kidney Int 2002; 62:632-638.

179. Kaysen GA, Dubin JA, Muller HG, et al: The acute-phase response varies with time and predicts serum albumin levels in hemodialysis patients. Kidney Int 2000; 58:346-352.
180. Jurado R, Ribeiro M: Possible role of systemic inflammatory reaction in vascular access thrombosis. South Med J 1999; 92:877-881.
181. United States Renal Data System (USRDS) Annual Data Report: Atlas of end-stage renal disease in the United States. Bethesda, MD, Tertiary USRDS Annual Data Report: Atlas of end-stage renal disease in the United States, 2003.
182. Anderson JE, Chang AS, Anstadt MP: Polytetrafluoroethylene hemoaccess site infections. ASAIO J 2000; 46:S18-S21.
183. Rizzuti RP, Hale JC, Burkart TE: Extended patency of expanded polytetrafluoroethylene grafts for vascular access using optimal configuration and revisions. Surg Gynecol Obstet 1988; 166: 23-27.
184. Tordoir JH, Hofstra L, Leunissen KM, Kitslaar PJ: Early experience with stretch polytetrafluoroethylene grafts for haemodialysis access surgery: Results of a prospective randomised study. Eur J Vasc Endovasc Surg 1995; 9:305-309.
185. Tabbara MR, O'Hara PJ, Hertzer NR, et al: Surgical management of infected PTFE hemodialysis grafts: Analysis of a 15-year experience. Ann Vasc Surg 1995; 9:378-384.
186. Lew SQ, Kaveh K: Dialysis access related infections. ASAIO J 2000; 46:S6-S12.
187. Ayus JC, Sheikh-Hamad D: Silent infection in clotted hemodialyis access grafts. J Am Soc Nephrol 1998; 9:1314-1317.
188. Taylor B, Sigley RD, May KJ: Fate of infected and eroded hemodialysis grafts and autogenous fistulas. Am J Surg 1993; 165:632-636.
189. Palestro CJ, Vega A, Kim CK, et al: Indium-111-labeled leukocyte scintigraphy in hemodialysis access-site infection. J Nucl Med 1990; 31:319-324.
190. Lawrence PF, Dries DJ, Alazraki N, Albo D Jr: Indium 111-labeled leukocyte scanning for detection of prosthetic vascular graft infection. J Vasc Surg 1985; 2:165-173.
191. Butterly DW, Schwab SJ: Dialysis access infections. Curr Opin Nephrol Hypertens 2000; 9:631-635.
192. Yu VL, Goetz A, Wagener M, et al: Staphylococcus aureus nasal carriage and infection in patients on hemodialysis. Efficacy of antibiotic prophylaxis. N Engl J Med 1986; 315:91-96.
193. Zibari GB, Gadallah MF, Landreneau M, et al: Preoperative vancomycin prophylaxis decreases incidence of postoperative hemodialysis vascular access infections (Comment). Am J Kidney Dis 1997; 30:343-348.
194. Bhat DJ, Tellis VA, Kohlberg WI, et al: Management of sepsis involving expanded polytetrafluoroethylene grafts for hemodialysis access. Surgery 1980; 87:445-450.
195. Matsuura JH, Johansen KH, Rosenthal D, et al: Cryopreserved femoral vein grafts for difficult hemodialysis access. Ann Vasc Surg 2000; 14:50-55.
196. Matsuura JH, Rosenthal D, Wellons ED, et al: Hemodialysis graft infections treated with cryopreserved femoral vein. Cardiovasc Surg 2002; 10:561-565.
197. Lin PH, Brinkman WT, Terramani TT, Lumsden AB: Management of infected hemodialysis access grafts using cryopreserved human vein allografts. Am J Surg 2002; 184:31-36.
198. DeCaprio JD, Valentine RJ, Kakish HB, et al: Steal syndrome complicating hemodialysis access (see comments). Cardiovasc Surg 1997; 5:648-653.
199. Haimov M, Baez A, Neff M, Slifkin R: Complications of arteriovenous fistulas for hemodialysis. Arch Surg 1975; 110:708-712.
200. Miles AM: Vascular steal syndrome and ischaemic monomelic neuropathy: Two variants of upper limb ischaemia after haemodialysis vascular access surgery (Editorial) (see comments). Nephrol Dial Transplant 1999; 14:297-300.
201. Morsy AH, Kulbaski M, Chen C, et al: Incidence and characteristics of patients with hand ischemia after a hemodialysis access procedure. J Surg Res 1998; 74:8-10.
202. Wixon CL, Hughes JD, Mills JL: Understanding strategies for the treatment of ischemic steal syndrome after hemodialysis access. J Am Coll Surg 2000; 191:301-310.
203. Wilbourn AJ, Furlan AJ, Hulley W, Ruschhaupt W: Ischemic monomelic neuropathy. Neurology 1983; 33:447-451.
204. Corry RJ, Patel NP, West JC: Surgical management of complications of vascular access for hemodialysis. Surg Gynecol Obstet 1980; 151:49-54.
205. Odland MD, Kelly PH, Ney AL, et al: Management of dialysis-associated steal syndrome complicating upper extremity arteriovenous fistulas: Use of intraoperative digital photoplethysmography. Surgery 1991; 110:664-669.
206. West JC, Bertsch DJ, Peterson SL, et al: Arterial insufficiency in hemodialysis access procedures: Correction by "banding" technique. Transplant Proc 1991; 23:1838-1840.
207. Schanzer H, Schwartz M, Harrington E, Haimov M: Treatment of ischemia due to "steal" by arteriovenous fistula with distal artery ligation and revascularization. J Vasc Surg 1988; 7: 770-773.
208. Schanzer H, Skladany M, Haimov M: Treatment of angioaccess-induced ischemia by revascularization. J Vasc Surg 1992; 16:861-864.
209. Berman SS, Gentile AT, Glickman MH, et al: Distal revascularization-interval ligation for limb salvage and maintenance of dialysis access in ischemic steal syndrome. J Vasc Surg 1997; 26:393-402.
210. Knox RC, Berman SS, Hughes JD, et al: Distal revascularization-interval ligation: A durable and effective treatment for ischemic steal syndrome after hemodialysis access. J Vasc Surg 2002; 36:250-255.
211. Anderson CB, Codd JR, Graff RA, et al: Cardiac failure and upper extremity arteriovenous dialysis fistulas. Case reports and a review of the literature. Arch Intern Med 1976; 136: 292-297.
212. Engelberts I, Tordoir JH, Boon ES, Schreij G: High-output cardiac failure due to excessive shunting in a hemodialysis access fistula: An easily overlooked diagnosis. Am J Nephrol 1995; 15:323-326.
213. Lurie JD, Sox HC: Clinical problem-solving. High on the differential (Comment). N Engl J Med 1997; 337:1377-1381.
214. Young PR Jr, Rohr MS, Marterre WF Jr: High-output cardiac failure secondary to a brachiocephalic arteriovenous hemodialysis fistula: Two cases. Am Surg 1998; 64:239-241.
215. Besarab A, Lubkowski T, Vu A, et al: Effects of systemic hemodynamics on flow within vascular accesses used for hemodialysis. ASAIO J 2001; 47:501-506.
216. O'Regan S, Lemaitre P, Kaye M: Hemodynamic studies in patients with expanded polytetrafluoroethylene (PTFE) forearm grafts. Clin Nephrol 1978; 10:96-100.
217. Polkinghorne KR, Atkins RC, Kerr PG: Native arteriovenous fistula blood flow and resistance during hemodialysis. Am J Kidney Dis 2003; 41:132-139.
218. Kaye M, Baird C, McCloskey B, et al: Two year sequential haemodynamic data on polytetrafluoroethylene (PTFE) grafts used for haemodialysis. Proc Eur Dial Transplant Assoc 1979; 16:266-271.
219. Johnson G Jr, Blythe WB: Hemodynamic effects of arteriovenous shunts used for hemodialysis. Ann Surg 1970; 171: 715-723.
220. Ori Y, Korzets A, Katz M, et al: The contribution of an arteriovenous access for hemodialysis to left ventricular hypertrophy. Am J Kidney Dis 2002; 40:745-752.
221. Wilson SE: Thrombosis, venous hypertension, arterial steal, and neuropathy. *In* Wilson SE (ed): Vascular Access: Principles and Practice, 4th ed. St. Louis, MO, Mosby, 2002, pp 175-188.
222. Haage P, Vorwerk D, Piroth W, et al: Treatment of hemodialysis-related central venous stenosis or occlusion: Results of primary Wallstent placement and follow-up in 50 patients (Comment). Radiology 1999; 212:175-180.

223. Kovalik EC, Newman GE, Suhocki P, et al: Correction of central venous stenoses: Use of angioplasty and vascular Wallstents. Kidney Int 1994; 45:1177-1181.
224. Shoenfeld R, Hermans H, Novick A, et al: Stenting of proximal venous obstructions to maintain hemodialysis access. J Vasc Surg 1994; 19:532-538.
225. Vesely TM, Hovsepian DM, Pilgram TK, et al: Upper extremity central venous obstruction in hemodialysis patients: Treatment with Wallstents. Radiology 1997; 204:343-348.
226. Swedberg SH, Brown BG, Sigley R, et al: Intimal fibromuscular hyperplasia at the venous anastomosis of PTFE grafts in hemodialysis patients. Circulation 1989; 80:1726-1736.
227. Hofstra L, Tordoir JH, Kitslaar PJ, et al: Enhanced cellular proliferation in intact stenotic lesions derived from human arteriovenous fistulas and peripheral bypass grafts. Does it correlate with flow parameters? Circulation 1996; 94:1283-1290.
228. Kelly BS, Heffelfinger SC, Whiting JF, et al: Aggressive venous neointimal hyperplasia in a pig model of arteriovenous graft stenosis. Kidney Int 2002; 62:2272-2280.
229. Rekhter M, Nicholls S, Ferguson M, Gordon D: Cell proliferation in human arteriovenous fistulas used for hemodialysis. Arterioscler Thromb 1993; 13:609-617.
230. Roy-Chaudhury P, Whiting JF, Miller MA, et al: Neointimal hyperplasia and hemodialysis access dysfunction: A pathogenetic role for cytokines, matrix proteins, and specific cell types. *In* Henry ML (ed): Vascular Access for Hemodialysis, 6th ed. Chicago, WL Gore & Associates and Precept Press, 1999, pp 45-53.
231. Roy-Chaudhury P, Kelly BS, Miller MA, et al: Venous neointimal hyperplasia in polytetrafluoroethylene dialysis grafts. Kidney Int 2001; 59:2325-2334.
232. Weiss MF, Scivitarro V, Anderson JM: Oxidative stress and increased expression of growth factors in lesions of failed hemodialysis access. Am J Kidney Dis 2001; 37:970-980.
233. Stracke S, Konner K, Kostlin I, et al: Increased expression of TGF-beta1 and IGF-I in inflammatory stenotic lesions of hemodialysis fistulas. Kidney Int 2002; 61:1011-1019.
234. Sukhatme V: Vascular access stenosis: Prospects for prevention and therapy. Kidney Int 1996; 49:1161-1174.
235. Ross R: Atherosclerosis? an inflammatory disease (see comments). N Engl J Med 1999; 340:115-126.
236. Schwartz SM, deBlois D, O'Brien ER: The intima. Soil for atherosclerosis and restenosis. Circ Res 1995; 77:445-465.
237. Schwab SJ, Oliver MJ, Suhocki P, McCann R: Hemodialysis arteriovenous access: Detection of stenosis and response to treatment by vascular access blood flow. Kidney Int 2001; 59:358-362.
238. Besarab A, Samarapungavan D: Measuring the adequacy of hemodialysis access. Curr Opin Nephrol Hypertens 1996; 5:527-531.
239. Beathard GA: Physical examination of the dialysis vascular access. Semin Dial 1998; 11:231-236.
240. Krivitski NM: Access flow measurement during surveillance and percutaneous transluminal angioplasty intervention. Semin Dial 2003; 16:304-308.
241. Van Stone JC, Jones M, Van Stone J: Detection of hemodialysis access outlet stenosis by measuring outlet resistance. Am J Kidney Dis 1994; 23:562-568.
242. Bosman PJ, Boereboom FT, Smits HF, et al: Pressure or flow recordings for the surveillance of hemodialysis grafts. Kidney Int 1997; 52:1084-1088.
243. Besarab A, Sherman R: The relationship of recirculation to access blood flow. Am J Kidney Dis 1997; 29:223-229.
244. Dinwiddie LC, Frauman AC, Jaques PF, et al: Comparison of measures for prospective identification of venous stenoses. Ann J 1996; 23:593-600.
245. Smits JH, van der Linden J, Hagen EC, et al: Graft surveillance: Venous pressure, access flow, or the combination? Kidney Int 2001; 59:1551-1558.
246. Besarab A, Al-Saghir F, Alnabhan N, et al: Simplified measurement of intra-access pressure. ASAIO J 1996; 42:M682-M687.
247. McDougal G, Agarwal R: Clinical performance characteristics of hemodialysis graft monitoring. Kidney Int 2001; 60:762-766.
248. Dember LM, Holmberg EF, Kaufman JS: Value of static venous pressure for predicting arteriovenous graft thrombosis. Kidney Int 2002; 61:1899-1904.
249. Paulson WD: Blood flow surveillance of hemodialysis grafts and the dysfunction hypothesis (Comment). Semin Dial 2001; 14:175-180.
250. Paulson WD, Ram SJ, et al: Accuracy of decrease in blood flow predicting hemodialysis graft thrombosis. Am J Kidney Dis 2000; 35:1089-1095.
251. Moist LM, Churchill DN, House AA, et al: Regular monitoring of access flow compared with monitoring of venous pressure fails to improve graft survival. J Am Soc Nephrol 2003; 14: 2645-2653.
252. Gadallah MF, Paulson WD, Vickers B, Work J: Accuracy of Doppler ultrasound in diagnosing anatomic stenosis of hemodialysis arteriovenous access as compared with fistulography. Am J Kidney Dis 1998; 32:273-277.
253. Oudenhoven LF, Pattynama PM, de Roos A, et al: Magnetic resonance, a new method for measuring blood flow in hemodialysis fistulae. Kidney Int 1994; 45:884-889.
254. Robbin ML, Oser RF, Allon M, et al: Hemodialysis access graft stenosis: U.S. detection. Radiology 1998; 208:655-661.
255. Sands J, Young S, Miranda C: The effect of Doppler flow screening studies and elective revisions on dialysis access failure. ASAIO J 1992; 38:M524-M527.
256. Sands J, Glidden D, Miranda C: Hemodialysis access flow measurement. Comparison of ultrasound dilution and duplex ultrasonography. ASAIO J 1996; 42:M899-M901.
257. Strauch BS, O'Connell RS, Geoly KL, et al: Forecasting thrombosis of vascular access with Doppler color flow imaging. Am J Kidney Dis 1992; 19:554-557.
258. Martin LG, MacDonald MJ, et al: Prophylactic angioplasty reduces thrombosis in virgin ePTFE arteriovenous dialysis grafts with greater than 50% stenosis: Subset analysis of a prospective randomized study. JVIR 1999; 4:389-397.
259. Schwab SJ, Saeed M, Sussman SK, et al: Transluminal angioplasty of venous stenoses in polytetrafluoroethylene vascular access grafts. Kidney Int 1987; 32:395-398.
260. Beathard GA: The treatment of vascular access graft dysfunction: A nephrologist's view and experience. Adv Ren Replace Ther 1994; 1:131-147.
261. Kidney DD: Radiologic intervention and instrumentation for salvage of hemodialysis access grafts. *In* Wilson SE (ed): Vascular Access: Principles and Practice, 4th ed. St. Louis, MO, Mosby, 2002, pp 155-167.
262. Beathard GA: Gianturco self-expanding stent in the treatment of stenosis in dialysis access grafts. Kidney International. 43:872-877, 1993
263. Hoffer EK, Sultan S, Herskowitz MM, et al: Prospective randomized trial of a metallic intravascular stent in hemodialysis graft maintenance. J Vasc Intervent Radiol 1997; 8:965-973.
264. Quinn SF, Schuman ES, Demlow TA, et al: Percutaneous transluminal angioplasty versus endovascular stent placement in the treatment of venous stenoses in patients undergoing hemodialysis: Intermediate results. J Vasc Intervent Radiol 1995; 6: 851-855.
265. Turmel-Rodrigues LA, Blanchard D, Pengloan J, et al: Wallstents and Craggstents in hemodialysis grafts and fistulas: Results for selective indications. J Vasc Intervent Radiol 1997; 8:975-982.
266. Gray RJ, Horton KM, Dolmatch BL, et al: Use of Wallstents for hemodialysis access-related venous stenoses and occlusions untreatable with balloon angioplasty. Radiology 1995; 195: 479-484.
267. Rundback JH, Leonardo RF, Poplausky MR, Rozenblit G: Venous rupture complicating hemodialysis access angioplasty:

Percutaneous treatment and outcomes in seven patients. Am J Roentgenol 1998; 171:1081-1084.

268. Sapoval MR, Turmel-Rodrigues LA, Raynaud AC, et al: Cragg covered stents in hemodialysis access: Initial and midterm results. J Vasc Intervent Radiol 1996; 7:335-342.
269. Beathard GA, Welch BR, Maidment HJ: Mechanical thrombolysis for the treatment of thrombosed hemodialysis access grafts. Radiology 1996; 200:711-716.
270. Cohen MA, Kumpe DA, Durham JD, Zwerdlinger SC: Improved treatment of thrombosed hemodialysis access sites with thrombolysis and angioplasty. Kidney Int 1994; 46:1375-1380.
271. Cynamon J, Pierpont CE: Thrombolysis for the treatment of thrombosed hemodialysis access grafts. Rev Cardiovasc Med 2002; 3:S84-S91.
272. Valji K, Bookstein JJ, Roberts AC, et al: Pulse-spray pharmacomechanical thrombolysis of thrombosed hemodialysis access grafts: Long-term experience and comparison of original and current techniques. Am J Roentgenol 1995; 164:1495-1500.
273. Beathard GA: Thrombolysis versus surgery for the treatment of thrombosed dialysis access grafts. J Am Soc Nephrol 1995; 6:1619-1624.
274. Polak JF, Berger MF, Pagan-Marin H, et al: Comparative efficacy of pulse-spray thrombolysis and angioplasty versus surgical salvage procedures for treatment of recurrent occlusion of PTFE dialysis access grafts. Cardiovasc Intervent Radiol 1998; 21: 314-318.
275. Sands JJ, Patel S, Plaviak DJ, Miranda CL: Pharmacomechanical thrombolysis with urokinase for treatment of thrombosed hemodialysis access grafts. A comparison with surgical thrombectomy. ASAIO J 1994; 40:M886-M888.
276. Schuman E, Quinn S, Standage B, Gross G: Thrombolysis versus thrombectomy for occluded hemodialysis grafts. Am J Surg 1994; 167:473-476.
277. Beathard GA, Marston WA: Endovascular management of thrombosed dialysis grafts. Am J Kidney Dis 1998; 32:172-175.
278. Valeri A, Joseph R, Radhakrishnan J: A large prospective survey of anti-cardiolipin antibodies in chronic hemodialysis patients. Clin Nephrol 1999; 51:116-121.
279. Crowther MA, Clase CM, Margetts PJ, et al: Low-intensity warfarin is ineffective for the prevention of PTFE graft failure in patients on hemodialysis: A randomized controlled trial. J Am Soc Nephrol 2002; 13:2331-2337.
280. Collaborative overview of randomised trials of antiplatelet therapy. I. Prevention of death, myocardial infarction, and stroke by prolonged antiplatelet therapy in various categories of patients. Antiplatelet Trialists' Collaboration (see comments) [published erratum appears in Br Med J 1994; 308(6943):1540]. Br Med J 1994; 308:81-106.
281. Collaborative overview of randomised trials of antiplatelet therapy. II. Maintenance of vascular graft or arterial patency by antiplatelet therapy. Antiplatelet Trialists' Collaboration (Comment). Br Med J 1994; 308:159-168.
282. Sreedhara R, Himmelfarb J, Lazarus JM, Hakim RM: Antiplatelet therapy in graft thrombosis: Results of a prospective, randomized double-blind study. Kidney Int 1994; 45: 1477-1483.
283. Kaufman JS, O'Connor TZ, Zhang JH, et al: Randomized controlled trial of clopidogrel plus aspirin to prevent hemodialysis access graft thrombosis. J Am Soc Nephrol 2003; 14:2313-2321.
284. Saran R, Dykstra DM, Wolfe RA, et al: Association between vascular access failure and the use of specific drugs: The Dialysis Outcomes and Practice Patterns Study (DOPPS). Am J Kidney Dis 2002; 40:1255-1263.
285. Kris-Etherton PM, Harris WS, Appel LJ, Nutrition C: Fish consumption, fish oil, omega-3 fatty acids, and cardiovascular disease (Comment). [erratum appears in Arterioscler Thromb Vasc Biol 2003; 23(2):e31]. Arterioscler Thromb Vasc Biol 2003; 23:e20-e30, 2003
286. Dietary supplementation with N-3 polyunsaturated fatty acids and vitamin E after myocardial infarction: Results of the GISSI-Prevenzione trial. Gruppo Italiano per lo Studio della Sopravvivenza nell'Infarto miocardico (Comment). [erratum appears in Lancet 2001; 357(9256):642]. Lancet 1999; 354:447-455.
287. Diskin CJ, Stokes TJ, Pennell AT: Pharmacologic intervention to prevent hemodialysis access thrombosis. Nephron 1993; 64:1-26.
288. Diskin CJ, Thomas CE, Zellner CP, et al: Fish oil to prevent intimal hyperplasia and access thrombosis. Nephron 1990; 55: 445-447.
289. Schmitz PG, McCloud LK, Reikes ST, et al: Prophylaxis of hemodialysis graft thrombosis with fish oil: A double-blind, randomized, prospective trial. J Am Soc Nephrol 2001; 13: 184-190.
290. Dzau VJ, Braun-Dullaeus RC, Sedding DG: Vascular proliferation and atherosclerosis: New perspectives and therapeutic strategies. Nat Med 2002; 8:1249-1256.
291. Mann MJ, Whittemore AD, Donaldson MC, et al: Ex-vivo gene therapy of human vascular bypass grafts with E2F decoy: The PREVENT single-centre, randomised, controlled trial. Lancet 1999; 354:1493-1498.
292. Miles AM: Vascular steal syndrome and ischaemic monomelic neuropathy: Two variants of upper limb ischaemia after haemodialysis vascular access surgery. Nephrol Dial Transplant 1999; 14:297-300.

Chapter 18

Biocompatibility of Hemodialysis Membranes

Bertrand L. Jaber, M.D. • Brian J.G. Pereira, M.D., M.B.A.

During hemodialysis (HD), blood comes into contact with several components of the extracorporeal circuit. These include: (1) the dialyzer itself (dialysis membrane, sterilants used during the manufacturing process, and substances that leach from the dialyzer), (2) extracorporeal circuit (temporary vascular access, bloodlines, and cannulas), (3) chemicals used for reprocessing (germicides and cleansing agents), and (4) contaminants in the dialysate. Exposure to each of the above components can result in perturbations of cellular or plasma components of blood. This chapter will restrict its focus on the dialyzer membrane. To date, there is no precise definition of "biocompatibility," which is uniformly agreed upon by nephrologists and bioengineers. In general, a biocompatible dialysis membrane refers to one that elicits little or no reaction from the patient as the result of blood contact with the biomaterials. Reactions resulting from ultrafiltration of fluid or exchanges of electrolytes through the semipermeable membrane are usually excluded from these discussions. This chapter will focus on the alterations in cellular and noncellular elements induced by the blood-membrane interactions during hemodialysis.

BIOMATERIALS USED FOR ARTIFICIAL KIDNEY MEMBRANES

Biomaterials for hemodialysis membranes are broadly classified into unsubstituted cellulose, substituted (modified) cellulose, and synthetic[1] (Table 18–1).

Unsubstituted Cellulose

Cellulose membranes are composed of regenerated cellulose in which the basic structure is a linear chain of glucosan rings with free surface hydroxyl groups. The first hemodialysis membranes that were used clinically in the 1940s were tubes of cellophane, regenerated from cellulose and originally manufactured for sausage casings. Unfortunately, these cellophane tubings were not very stable and leaked frequently, necessitating immediate repair *in situ*. Virtually all hemodialysis membranes used until the late 1960s were made from cellophane or similar materials.

During the 1960s, cuprophan (CU) membranes were developed by regeneration of cellulose using the cuprammonium process (a modification of the process for preparing cellophane). These cuprammonium membranes have been used extensively for hemodialysis since they can be made thin, are mechanically strong, and provide good diffusive transport properties for small solutes. The cuprophan trademarked name has become so popular that the generic terms "cuprophan" and "cuprophane" are frequently used to describe all cuprammonium membranes, even though cuprammonium membranes are manufactured by several other companies and are not all identical.

Regenerated cellulose, predominantly as cuprammonium membranes, continues to be used in more than 50% of all dialyzers throughout the world due to their low cost.[2] In the United States, however, there has been a persistent decline in the use of these membranes, at the expense of an increase in the use of substituted cellulose and synthetic membranes (Figure 18–1).[3] All regenerated cellulose membranes are highly hydrophilic because of the large number of free hydroxyl groups on the cellulose monomer, and they are homogeneous in structure; their porosity is similar throughout the entire membrane thickness. Although the original membranes made, using the cuprammonium process, had low permeability to solutes larger than urea, cuprammonium membranes with high permeability to larger solutes are currently available.

Substituted (Modified) Cellulose

The substitution of the free surface hydroxyl groups on cellulose membranes results in substituted or modified cellulose membranes. Accordingly, substitution of an increasing fraction of the surface free hydroxyl groups with acetyl residues leads to cellulose acetate (CA) or diacetate (80% substitution), and cellulose triacetate (CTA) (100% substitution) membranes, respectively. Cellulose acetate and cellulose triacetate membranes are more hydrophobic than regenerated cellulose membranes because of acetylation of the hydroxyl moieties on the cellulose monomer. Substitution of 1% of the hydroxyl radicals on cellulose with the tertiary amino residue, diethylaminoethyl (DEAE) is the principle behind the manufacture of hemophan membranes.[4–6] All of the above modified cellulose membranes are morphologically homogeneous under scanning electron microscopy. In general, substituted/modified cellulose membranes have substantially less complement activating potential than unsubstituted cellulose membranes. However, to what extent the number of free hydroxyl groups determines the degree of complement activation by cellulose membranes remains controversial and will be discussed subsequently.

A new generation cellulose membrane, excebrane, has recently been developed by covalent binding of synthetic block polymers to the hydroxyl groups on cellulose. In addition to the reduced complement-activating potential, the oleyl alcohol and vitamin E that are incorporated into the synthetic

Table 18–1 Classification of hemodialysis membranes

Biomaterial	Chemical structure	Common name
Cellulose	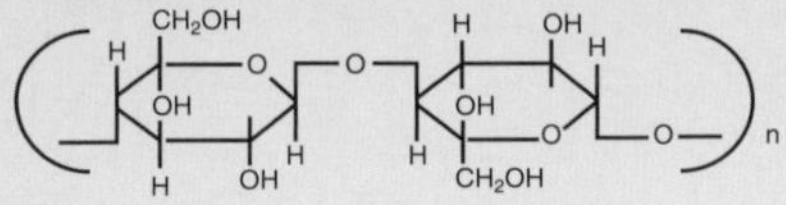 (C_6 glucose rings with CH_2OH, H, OH substituents, linked by –O–)$_n$	Cuprophan
DEAE-substitued cellulose	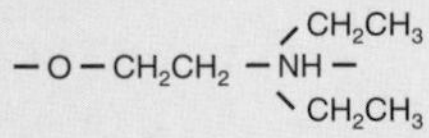 $-O-CH_2CH_2-NH-(CH_2CH_3)(CH_2CH_3)$	Hemophan
Cellulose diacetate and triacetate	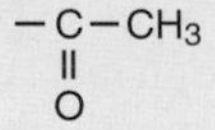 $-C(=O)-CH_3$	CA, CTA
Multi-layer vitamin E–coated cellulose	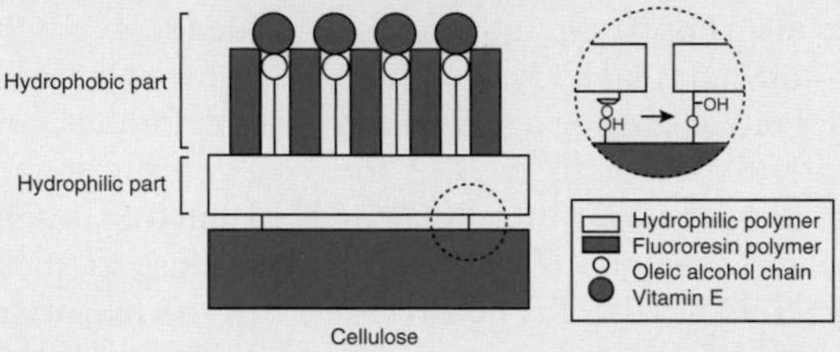 Hydrophobic part; Hydrophilic part; Cellulose; OH → OH; Hydrophilic polymer; Fluororesin polymer; Oleic alcohol chain; Vitamin E	Excebrane
Polysulfone	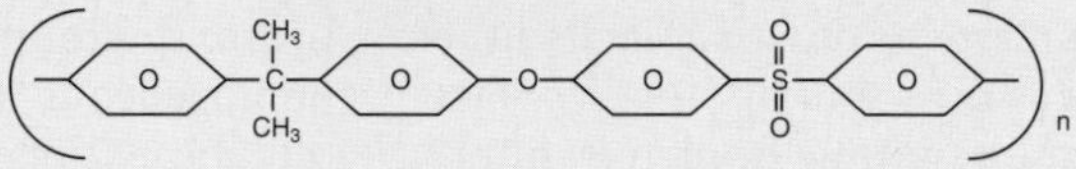 $(-C_6H_4-C(CH_3)_2-C_6H_4-O-C_6H_4-SO_2-C_6H_4-)_n$	F-series Optiflux-series
Polyamide	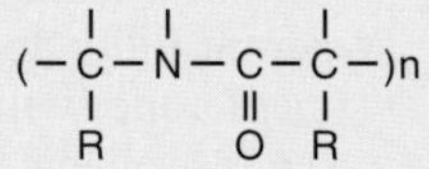 $(-C(R)-N-C(=O)-C(R)-)_n$	Polyflux-series
Polyacrylonitrile and methallyl sulfonate	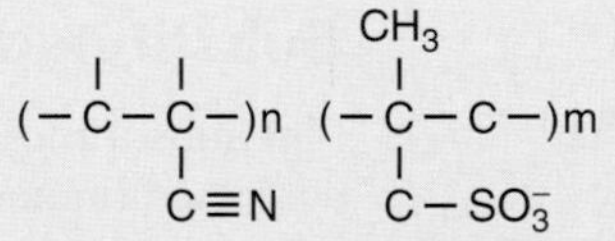 $(-C-C(C{\equiv}N)-)_n\ (-C(CH_3)-C(C-SO_3^-)-)_m$	AN-69
Polyacrylonitrile and methacrylate	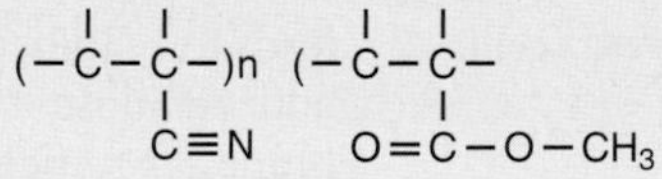 $(-C-C(C{\equiv}N)-)_n\ (-C-C(O{=}C-O-CH_3)-$	PAN
Polymethylmethacrylate	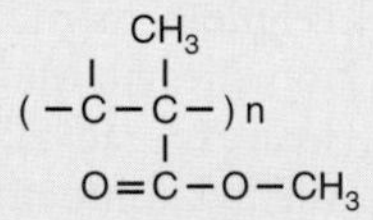 $(-C-C(CH_3)(O{=}C-O-CH_3)-)_n$	PMMA

surface reduce thrombosis and provide antioxidant reserves, respectively.[7,8] Compared with CA and polyamide (PA) membranes, excebrane membranes have been associated with better immune function parameters, as measured by lower IL-6 production levels and less activation of mononuclear cell-Jun N-terminal kinase.[9,10] Although surface modification of CU dialyzers with vitamin E may enhance biocompatibility and improve cytokine levels as well as immune function, the clinical significance of these findings in terms of outcomes is unclear.

Synthetic (Noncellulose) Polymers

Various synthetic membranes were developed during the 1970s primarily for use as hemofilters, although some of them were also used as hemodialysis membranes. AN69 was originally prepared from a copolymer of acrylonitrile and methallyl sulfonate. The latter polymer contains negatively charged ionizable groups. This property was originally deemed desirable for a dialysis membrane because a negatively charged membrane might mimic the glomerular basement

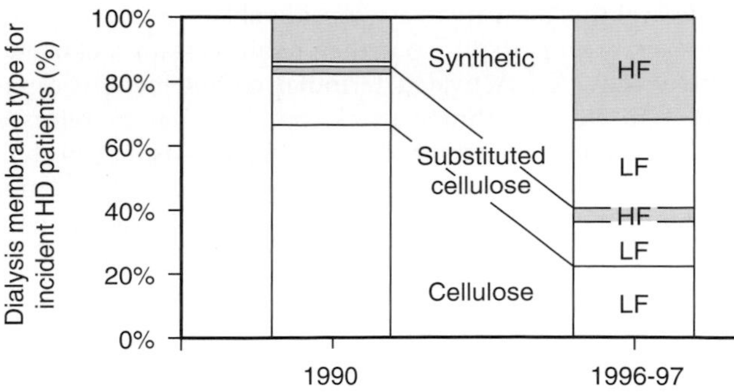

Figure 18–1 Dialysis membrane type used for incident hemodialysis (HD) patients in the United States from year 1990 to 1997. *LF,* low-flux; *HF,* high-flux. (Reprinted with permission from United States Renal Data System. USRDS 1999 annual data report. Bethesda, MD, National Institutes of Health, Diabetes and Digestive and Kidney Diseases, 1999.)

membrane.[11] However, recent studies demonstrate that such negative charges may impart a specific bioincompatible characteristic. The AN69 membrane is also morphologically homogeneous.[12] Polysulfone and polyamide membranes, too, were originally developed for use as hemofilters and were highly asymmetric and hydrophobic. Such membranes required a thick supporting layer to provide mechanical strength to the thin and highly porous inner skin of the hollow fiber. Diffusion rates for small solutes across these membranes were therefore low. Addition of polyvinylpyrrolidone into the manufacturing process[13,14] led to membranes that exhibited high diffusive as well as high convective permeability properties. Such membranes are asymmetric[12,15] but exhibit a sponge- or foam-like structure not the large finger-like pores of the original membranes. Polysulfone membranes with various porosities are now commercially available. Other synthetic membranes in clinical use include polyacrylonitrile (PAN), polymethyl methacrylate (PMMA), polyethersulfone (PES), and polycarbonate.[16] With the exception of polycarbonate, all these synthetic membranes are hydrophobic and tend to adsorb cells and plasma proteins. In contrast, hydrophilic membranes, such as polycarbonate, do not adsorb cells or proteins but activate cells and proteins. However, the manufacturing methods for a given biomaterial can vary between manufacturers and, consequently, the biocompatibility of a given membrane too. Biologic responses elicited by blood-hemodialysis membrane interactions are summarized in Table 18–2.[17]

High flux refers to membranes with larger pore size, which possess high ultrafiltration coefficients (K_{UF}>14 mL/hr/mmHg), and permit clearances of middle molecules (β_2 microglobulin clearance >20 mL/min). Although high-flux dialyzers were originally manufactured with synthetic membranes, cellulose membranes can also be configured to have larger pore sizes, by altering the manufacturing process. Conversely, synthetic membranes can be manufactured as low-flux dialyzers. Dialyzers with cellulose membranes are often termed "conventional" dialyzers because of the modest urea clearances and relatively small pores. However, the urea clearance can be significantly enhanced by larger surface area, and these dialyzers are termed "high efficiency" dialyzers. Given the differences in clearances, flux and biocompatibility characteristics among the many different types of dialyzers, a detailed knowledge of membrane properties is necessary to ensure appropriate dialyzer prescription.

Table 18–2 Biologic Responses Elicited by Blood-Hemodialysis Membrane Interactions

Blood Components	Biologic Responses
Humoral Components	
Complement system	Alternate pathway activation
	Anaphylatoxin (C3a, C5a) production
Coagulation system	Factor XII activation
	Intrinsic pathway activation
	Increased tissue plasminogen activator
Cytokines	Equivocal increased circulating levels
Cellular Components	
Platelets	Platelet activation
	Increased platelet adhesion
	Thrombocytopenia
	Thromboxane A2, adenosine diphosphate (ADP) and platelet factor 4 release
Erythrocytes	Hemolysis (rare)
Neutrophils	Leukopenia
	Increased expression of adhesion molecules
	Degranulation and release of proteolytic enzymes
	Release of reactive oxygen species
	"Exhaustion" and decreased responsiveness to subsequent stimuli
Lymphocytes	T-lymphocyte activation
	Impaired T-lymphocyte proliferative responses
	B-lymphocyte activation
Monocytes	Increased intracellular interleukin-1 mRNA and protein expression
	"Exhaustion" and decreased responsiveness to subsequent stimuli

(Reprinted with permission from Modi GK, Pereira BJG, Jaber BLJ: Hemodialysis in acute renal failure: Does the membrane matter? Semin Dial 2001; 14.)

COMPLEMENT ACTIVATION

Activation of the Complement System by Dialysis Membranes

Since the early 1980s, complement activation has been the standard for assessment of dialysis membrane biocompatibility. Consequently, membranes are often classified as biocompatible or bioincompatible, based on their ability to activate complement. The complement system is comprised of two cascades of plasma proteins that can be sequentially activated by proteolytic enzymes.[18] Activation of either the classic pathway or alternative pathway leads to activation of C_3 and, under conducive conditions, activation of the terminal components (C_5, C_6, C_7, C_8, C_9). Complement activation on cuprophan and cellulose acetate membranes occurs primarily via the alternative pathway (Figure 18–2),[19–22] although the classic pathway may also contribute. The mechanism by which complement activation occurs on other membranes is less certain.

Biologic Activity of Complement Activation Products

Activation of C_3 results in the generation of anaphylatoxin C_{3a} (M_r ~9 kDa),[18] which is usually released into the serum. Larger fragments such as C_{3b} (M_r ~186 kDa) and its degradation product $_iC_{3b}$ are also produced. These larger fragments may also be important because they can modulate cellular functions by interacting with specific cytoplasmic membrane receptors.[23] For example, $_iC_{3b}$ mediates cell adherence[24] and induces the release of intragranular proteolytic enzymes[25] by interacting with complement receptor type 3 (CR_3, Mac_{-1}, or CD_{11b}/CD_{18}) on neutrophil surface. It is important to recognize that assessment of complement activation during hemodialysis, using plasma C_{3a} and C_{5a} as markers, may not adequately reflect its effect, because the larger $_iC_{3b}$ fragment may remain in the plasma and exert its biologic effects, whereas the smaller markers (C_{3a} and C_{5a}) may be lost from the plasma into the dialysate or by adsorption onto the dialysis membrane surface.

Anaphylatoxins C_{3a} and C_{5a} are spasmogenic, increase vascular permeability,[26] release histamine from mast cells,[27] stimulate contraction of smooth muscles,[28] induce degranulation from neutrophils,[29] and promote the transcription and/or release of cytokines from monocytes. Intracoronary bolus infusion of human C_{3a} produces tachycardia, atrioventricular conduction defect, left ventricular failure, and coronary vasoconstriction in animals.[30] Complement C_{5a} induces neutrophil chemotaxis, aggregation,[31–33] attachment to pulmonary endothelial cells, release of leukotriene B_4,[34] oxygen radicals,[35] and intragranular enzymes,[33,36,37] as well as altered expression of cell surface receptors.[38] C_{5a} has also been shown to release β_2-microglobulin from peripheral blood mononuclear cells[39] and stimulate the release of leukotrienes from guinea pig lung strips.[40]

Anaphylatoxins C_{3a} and C_{5a} are degraded by carboxypeptidase N in the serum[41] into $C_{3a\ desArg}$ and $C_{5a\ desArg}$, respectively.

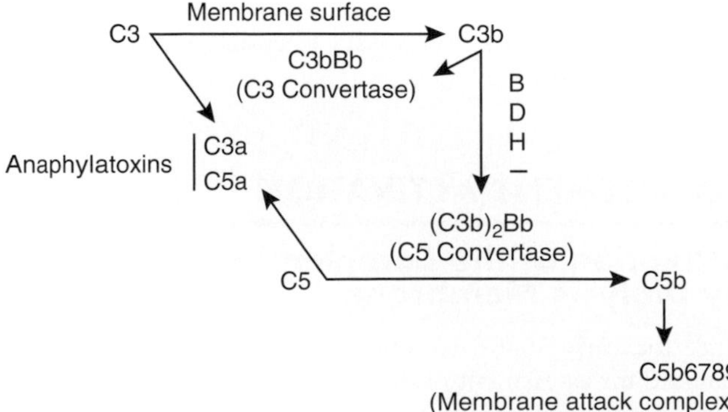

Figure 18–2 Schematic diagram of complement activation via the alternative pathway on the membrane surface. Underlined text inhibits reaction.

The desarginine derivatives are considerably less spasmogenic than their precursors,[41–43] but they retain certain leukocyte-directed activities. Activated terminal complement components (C5b-9 or membrane attack complex) that are released into the plasma are inactivated by binding to plasma S protein to form the SC5b-9 complex. Limited data suggest that terminal complement components activated in association with hemodialysis membranes have biologic activities *in vitro*.[44]

Assays for Complement Activation

Because C3 activation does not necessarily lead to activation of the terminal components and each activated complement product (e.g., C3a, C5a, and C5b-9) has its own biologic activities, ideally, each level of the activation pathway should be assessed.[45] The radioimmunoassays (RIA) for human C3a that are commonly used detect both the anaphylatoxin C3a and $C3a_{desArg}$. Practically all the C3a in clinical plasma samples are in the form of $C3a_{desArg}$. Immunoassays for iC3b are also commercially available. The RIA for C5a also detects both C5a and $C5a_{desArg}$. The membrane attack complex (SC5b-9) can also be quantitated using immunoassays. C3a and C5a can also be assessed by commercially available enzyme-linked immunosorbent assays.[46]

Complement Activation Associated with Different Hemodialysis Membranes

Based on plasma $C3a_{desArg}$ concentrations, cuprophan and unsubstituted cellulose membranes are the most potent complement activators among dialysis membranes (Figure 18–3).[19,47,48] Plasma $C3a_{desArg}$ concentrations usually peak between 10 and 20 minutes after starting dialysis and decline to almost baseline values by the end of the treatment. On a molar basis, plasma $C5a_{desArg}$ and SC5b-9 levels are usually lower than those of $C3a_{desArg}$[19,44,48] because activation of the late components of complement is usually less efficient than that of C3.[49] Binding of C5a to its receptor on neutrophil surfaces may also lower its plasma levels to a modest extent.[25]

Substituted cellulose membranes such as cellulose acetate and hemophan are associated with lower C3a levels than cuprophan.[50] Cellulose triacetate membranes and the synthetic polymer membranes are associated with lower plasma C3a levels than cuprophan or cellulose acetate.[19,44,51,52] Nonetheless, all dialysis membranes in clinical use, without exception, are associated with complement activation, albeit to differing degrees.

Complement activation by cuprophan membrane can be attenuated by either cooling the extracorporeal blood,[53] chelating Mg^{++} in the plasma during citrate hemodialysis,[54] or increasing the amount of heparin in the circuit.[55] Cuprophan membranes reprocessed with formaldehyde or peracetic acid are also associated with less complement activation and leukopenia than new dialyzers.[48,51,56] This reduction is presumably because of the presence of inactive C3 fragments[21] or other proteins on the used membrane surface, which inhibit amplification of the alternative pathway. Cleansing of reprocessed cuprophan membranes with sodium hypochlorite restores complement activation and leukopenia to levels similar to those with new dialyzers.[56] This is presumably because sodium hypochlorite effectively removes the proteins on the membrane surfaces.[21]

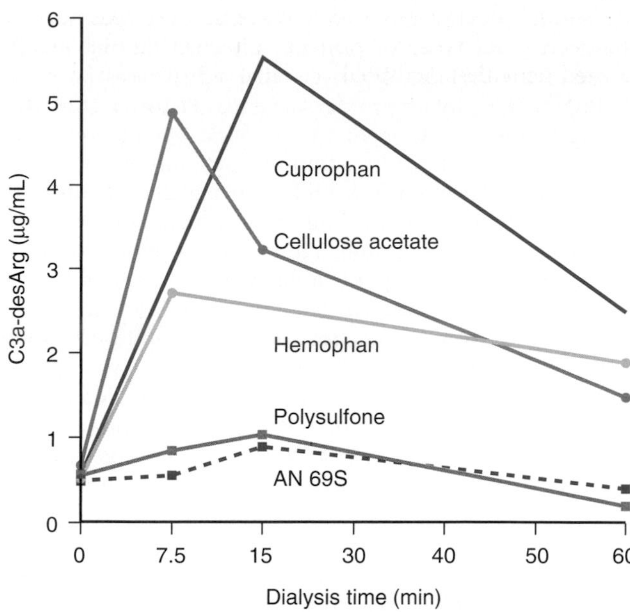

Figure 18–3 C3a generation using different dialysis membranes. Cuprophan: GFS Gambro 12H (1.3 m^2); cellulose acetate: CD4000. CD-Medical (1.4 m^2): Hemophan: GFS Gambro 120 Plus (1.3 m^2); Polysulfone: Fresenius F 60 (1.25 m^2); AN 69S: Filtral 12 (1.3 m^2), Hospal. (Reprinted with permission from Falkenhagen D, Mitzner S, Stange J, Klinkmann H: Biocompatibility: Methodology and evaluation. Contrib Nephrol 1993; 103:34-54.)

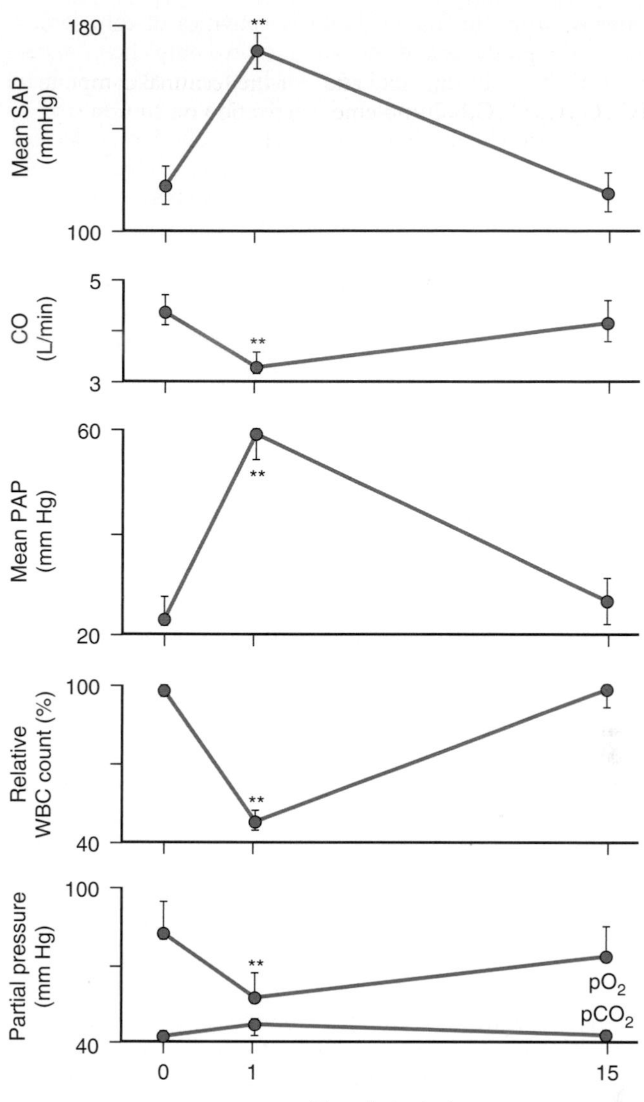

Figure 18–4 Hemodynamic responses to intravenous bolus of 0.7 mL/kg body weight of cuprophan-activated plasma in the swine. *SAP,* systemic arterial pressure; *CO,* cardiac output; *PAP,* pulmonary arterial pressure; **, $p < .01$. (Reprinted with permission from Cheung A, LeWinter M, Chenoweth D: Cardiopulmonary effects of cuprophan-activated plasma in the swine: Role of complement activation products. Kidney Int 1986; 29:799-806.)

In Vivo Consequences of Complement Activation

Animal Models

The acute effects of complement activation or exposure of blood to hemodialysis membranes have been examined in rabbit,[57] sheep,[58–60] and swine[61–63] models. Injection of plasma exposed to cuprophan membranes into animals has variably produced acute peripheral leukopenia, systemic arterial hypoxemia, pulmonary hypertension, increase in mediastinal lymphatic drainage (presumably reflecting an increase in pulmonary interstitial fluid), cardiac arrhythmias, decrease in cardiac output, and fluctuation in systemic arterial pressure.[57,59,61] These changes are apparently initiated by the exposure of blood to cuprophan membranes, which results in complement activation and the formation of anaphylatoxins C3a and C5a. C5a and $C5a_{desArg}$ bind to the neutrophil surface, which along with other activation events (such as alteration in number and configuration of cell surface adhesion molecules and cytoskeleton) induce neutrophil aggregation and attachment to pulmonary endothelial cells, resulting in peripheral leukopenia. Both C3a and C5a constrict the pulmonary blood vessels and cause pulmonary hypertension (Figure 18–4), probably through the release of thromboxanes and/or leukotrienes. These hemodynamic changes occur independently of the accompanying leukoagglutination. Indeed, the hypoxemia is probably caused by airway constriction induced by anaphylatoxins and arachidonic acid metabolites, pulmonary interstitial edema induced by anaphylatoxins, and/or transient lung injury produced by oxygen radicals released from activated neutrophils. Pulmonary leukosequestration or pulmonary hypertension per se does not lead to systemic hypoxemia. It should be emphasized that not all the effects of exposure to dialysis membranes are necessarily due to complement activation, since other blood components, such as the contact proteins, are also altered as a result of membrane exposure.[58,64,65]

Clinical Dialysis

The acute effects of intradialytic complement activation on patients are more controversial. These effects are primarily inferred from the known biologic activities of complement activation products and the fact that the complement system is activated during dialysis. Dialysis-induced peripheral leukopenia has traditionally been attributed to C5a and its ability to modulate neutrophil surface adhesion molecules, although there is evidence that noncomplement factors, such as platelet-activating factors, are also involved. Anaphylatoxins may also cause acute pulmonary hypertension (which has been demonstrated during sham hemodialysis in uremic patients using cuprophan membrane[66]) and contribute to the development of hypoxemia. Because of their ability to release histamine from mast cells, anaphylatoxins may be responsible for some of the allergy-like symptoms on dialysis. Since the spasmogenic properties of anaphylatoxins are markedly diminished when they are degraded to their desarginine derivatives by serum carboxypeptidase, the ability of these peptides to induce acute intradialytic symptoms would not be as great as their plasma levels (as determined by immunoassays) may indicate. However, during hemodialysis, carboxypeptidase activity can decrease.[67] Depending on the magnitude of generation, the rate at which they are inactivated and catabolized, as well as the sensitivity of the end organs, anaphylatoxins may rarely cause anaphylactoid reactions in susceptible individuals. However, some investigators dispute this association.

More recent investigations have concentrated on the potential subacute and chronic effects of complement activation during hemodialysis. Both C5a and iC3b are well known to have neutrophil modulating properties. Stimulation of neutrophils by these complement proteins promotes the release of oxygen radicals[35] and intragranular proteases[25,36,37] from the cells, which may result in catabolism of plasma proteins and injury of other tissues, such as the kidneys. C5a has also been shown to promote the production of cytokines from monocytes[68] and the release of β_2-microglobulin from peripheral blood monocytes,[39] which may contribute to the development of amyloidosis. Definitive demonstration of the roles of complement in clinical problems associated with hemodialysis may require the ability to inhibit its activation. Inhibition of complement activation during hemodialysis using specific inhibitors, such as soluble complement receptor type I (sCR1) has been studied in vitro only.[69] Chelation of divalent cations and the administration of protease inhibitors can also inhibit complement activation, but their effects are relatively nonspecific.

BLEEDING AND CLOTTING ABNORMALITIES

Clotting of blood inside the dialyzer is a problem that has plagued dialysis since the early days of artificial kidney treatment. Although it is very seldom life threatening, it contributes to anemia, reduces the effective surface area of the dialysis membrane for solute transport, and reduces the reuse potential of the dialyzer. Clotting in dialysis circuits is the result of complex protein and cellular interactions, of which we have only a rudimentary understanding.

Activation of Coagulation Proteins

Plasma proteins are adsorbed onto foreign surfaces immediately upon contact with blood, followed by the adhesion of platelets, leukocytes, and, to a lesser extent, erythrocytes.[70,71] The degree and types of proteins adsorbed depend on the nature of the surface. Negatively charged surfaces favor the binding of the contact protein Hageman factor (factor XII), leading to the activation of the intrinsic coagulation pathway[72,73] (Figure 18–5). In addition, high molecular weight kininogen is converted into kinins during the activation of contact proteins.[74] Bradykinin is a potent peptide that increases vascular permeability, diminishes arterial resistance, and mediates a variety of inflammatory responses. The anionic sulfonate domains of the AN69 membrane favors the binding and activation of factor XII, which lead to the subsequent conversion of high molecular weight kininogen to kinins.[72–75] Besides catalyzing the formation of angiotensin II, angiotensin converting enzyme (ACE) also functions as a kininase, which inactivates bradykinin. The use of an ACE inhibitor, therefore, allows the accumulation of bradykinin that is generated as a result of blood contact with the AN69 membrane. Conversion of kininogen to bradykinin by AN69 membrane has been demonstrated in vitro.[65] Intradialytic anaphylactoid reactions have been associated with the use of AN69 membrane and the generation of kinins, especially among those using ACE inhibitors.[75,76]

Activation of either the intrinsic or extrinsic pathway also leads to the conversion of prothrombin to thrombin. Thrombin, in turn, activates platelets.[77] Clinical studies have failed to clearly demonstrate the activation of factor XII during hemodialysis.[78] However, in vitro studies have shown that different dialysis membranes activate Hageman factor to various degrees.[64]

Significant activation of the coagulation cascade leads to overt thrombosis in the extracorporeal circuit. More subtle activation can be detected by a decrease in the half-life of fibrinogen or by an increase in plasma fibrinopeptides.[55,79–81] Fibrinopeptide A (FPA) and fibrinopeptide B (FPB) are fragments cleaved from fibrinogen by thrombin during its activation. Adequate heparinization prevents the cleavage of fibrinogen and, therefore, prevents an increase in plasma FPA

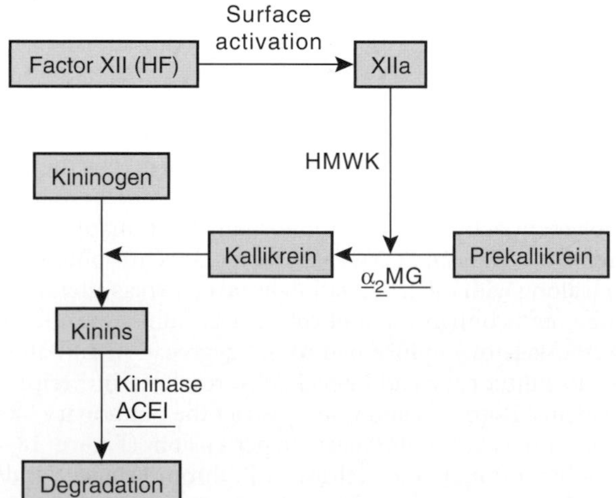

Figure 18–5 Schematic diagram of kinin generation on a negatively charged membrane surface. HF, Hageman factor; *HMWK*, high molecular weight kininogen; *α_2MG*, alpha 2 macroglobulin; *ACEI*, angiotensin converting enzyme inhibitor. Underlined text inhibits reaction.

level.[55,80,81] FPA is usually eliminated by the kidneys and is retained in renal failure.[82] Thus, baseline plasma levels in dialysis patients are usually above normal. Plasma FPA levels have been used as markers of intradialytic clotting. However, the relatively low molecular weight of this peptide (~1.5 kDa) makes it readily removable by most dialysis membranes.[55] This should be taken into consideration when interpreting levels of FPA in the hemodialysis setting.

Under physiologic conditions, activation of the coagulation cascade is counteracted by the simultaneous activation of the fibrinolytic system.[75,83] Plasmin is a major plasma fibrinolytic protein, and its precursor, plasminogen, can be activated by tissue plasminogen activator. Increased plasma concentration of tissue plasminogen activator antigen has been demonstrated during the first hour of hemodialysis with cellulose membranes.[84] This is accompanied by a decrease in the plasma concentration of tissue plasminogen activator inhibitor. The stimuli for the release of the plasminogen activator in this setting are unknown. However, a potential source is the pulmonary vascular bed in response to injury by activated complement and granulocyte proteases. Theoretically, activation of the fibrinolytic system during hemodialysis with cellulose dialyzers could help prevent intradialysis thrombosis.

Adhesion and Activation of Platelets

As in the physiologic clotting process, platelets probably play an integral role in thrombosis of dialyzers. The tendency of platelets to adhere to artificial surfaces depends on the nature of the proteins adsorbed.[70] For example, albumin-coated surfaces are relatively resistant to platelet adhesion. In contrast, surfaces coated with glycoproteins that contain oligosaccharide chains, such as fibrinogen and γ-globulins, promote platelet adhesion. The adhered platelets undergo morphologic changes characterized by pseudopod formation and spreading of the cytoplasm over the foreign surface.[71,85] In response to stimulation by thrombin, mechanical trauma, and other humoral factors, platelets also undergo release reactions.[73,75] A variety of cellular products are thereby released into the circulation, including thromboxane A_2 (TXA_2) and adenosine diphosphate (ADP). These substances promote coagulation by further inducing aggregation and release reactions by platelets. The importance of platelets in thrombosis of dialyzers can be underscored by the effectiveness of antiplatelet agents, such as aspirin and dipyridamole in preventing these events.[86,87] Aspirin is a well-known inhibitor of the cyclooxygenase pathway of arachidonic acid metabolism and the production of TXA_2. Dipyridamole is a cAMP phosphodiesterase inhibitor and increases the level of cAMP, which, in turn, inhibits platelet aggregation induced by ADP. In addition, prostacyclin (PGI_2), a potent stimulator of adenyl cyclase and inhibitor of platelet aggregation, has been successfully used as the sole anticoagulant during hemodialysis.[88–90]

Other intracellular substances released by the activated platelets include platelet factor 4 (PF4) and β-thromboglobulin (β–TG).[91–93] Plasma levels of these substances have been used as specific markers for platelet activation. PF4 is of particular interest because it binds to and neutralizes heparin. Differences in PF4 release may partially account for the differences in heparin requirements during hemodialysis among individual patients. Special caution needs to be exercised to correctly interpret data using these markers. PF4 is normally cleared through binding to the endothelium. Administration of heparin during hemodialysis can increase the plasma concentration of this protein by releasing it from the endothelial cells in the absence of platelet activation.[91] β–TG is normally eliminated by the kidney. Therefore, circulating levels in dialysis patients are often above normal.[92] Nonetheless, an acute increase in plasma β–TG levels above the elevated baseline levels probably reflects platelet activation. When thrombosis is effectively prevented with the use of adequate anticoagulants, such an increase does not occur.[94]

Plasma coagulation proteins, such as thrombin, are known activators of platelets. In addition, platelets can be activated by mechanical disruption during hemodialysis,[95] an event that is probably dependent on the nature of the dialyzer membrane surface and the shear in the blood path. Platelet activating factor released from neutrophils[34,96] and TXA_2 released (from lungs and other tissues) by activated complement[62] can also activate platelets.

Dialyzers appear to differ from each other in their abilities to activate platelets. Hemodialysis with cuprophan dialyzers has been associated with greater thrombocytopenia compared to with PMMA dialyzers.[97] Plasma β–TG levels increase during dialysis with cuprophan but not with polyacrylonitrile.[85,98] Adhesion and morphologic changes of platelets were more profound with cuprophan compared to polycarbonate.[85] It should be noted that several of these clinical studies were not conducted under strict control of experimental conditions, such as heparin dosage and geometry and surface area of the dialyzers. In a well-controlled study in which blood was pumped from the human body through the dialyzers without heparin in a single-pass fashion, hemophan was found to be associated with a lower increase in plasma PF4 than cuprophan.[5] A recent study demonstrated that platelet-activating factor (PAF) is produced during HD with CU and AN69 membrane and may contribute to dialysis-related leukopenia and thrombocytopenia.[99,100]

A recent study comparing the effects of CTA and PS membrane on GPIIb/IIIa (the receptor for fibrinogen that mediates platelet aggregation and adhesion) and platelet activation demonstrated a significant increase in the level of platelet-bound GPIIb/IIIa with PS and not CTA membrane.[101]

Leukocyte-Platelet Aggregation during Hemodialysis

Recent studies have also demonstrated the formation of platelet-leukocyte aggregates during hemodialysis using cuprophan and synthetic membranes.[86,102] Binding between these two cell types is mediated by various adhesion molecules, including GMP140 on platelets and CD15s on leukocytes (Figure 18–6).[103] Presumably, platelet-leukocyte binding facilitates communications and cross-signaling between the two cells, resulting in an enhancement in inflammatory response. More recently, increased platelet-monocyte aggregates with reduced leukocyte P-selectin glycoprotein ligand-1 (PSGL-1) expression in patients with ESRD, irrespective of dialysis modality, was associated with an increased risk of cardiovascular disease, suggesting a novel mechanism by which accelerated atherosclerosis may occur in uremic patients.[104]

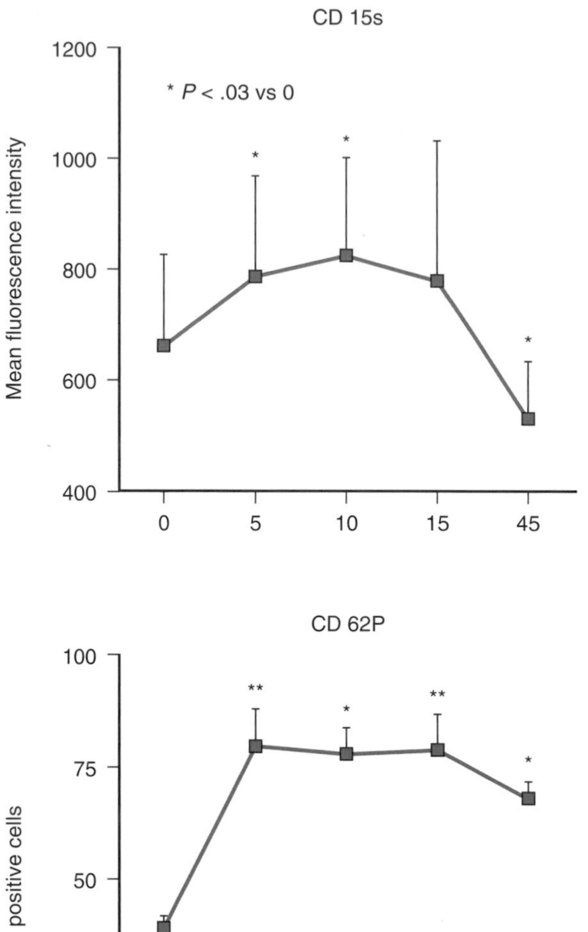

Figure 18–6 Stimulation of whole blood from healthy individuals with autologous normal human serum activated with Sephadex. Expression of CD15s antigen on neutrophils, obtained from four healthy individuals, at different time points of incubation (*upper panel*) and evaluation of platelet-neutrophil aggregates as assessed by CD62P expression on the neutrophils (*lower panel*). (Reprinted with permission from Stuard S, Carreno M-P, Poignet J-L, et al: A major role for CD62P/CD15s interaction in leukocyte margination during hemodialysis. Kidney Int 1995; 48:93-102.)

Assessment of Platelet Activation during Hemodialysis

Several methods have been employed, including:

1. Degree of acute thrombocytopenia, because adhesion of activated platelets on the dialyzer membrane surface, aggregation in the blood, or formation of mural thrombi may result in peripheral thrombocytopenia.[85,97,105]
2. Changes in the morphology of platelets on the dialyzer membrane as examined by electron microscopy.[85]
3. Acute increases in plasma β–TG and PF4 concentrations[5,98] with the caveats noted earlier.
4. Acute increases in plasma TXA_2 concentration.[97] However, it should be noted that platelets are not the only source of TXA_2. The lungs may produce significant amounts of TXA_2 in response to stimulation by the complement anaphylatoxins generated during hemodialysis using cuprophan membrane.[62]

Clinical Consequences of Platelet Activation by Dialysis Membranes

The independent effect of dialysis membranes on clinically significant bleeding abnormalities is incompletely defined. However, although extremely rare, significant thrombocytopenia leading to hemorrhage has been reported following hemodialysis.[106] Further, dialysis with cuprophan membrane is associated with acute dysfunction of platelets, such that the cells become relatively resistant to collagen-induced aggregation and prolonged bleeding time.[85,107] Dialysis with other membranes does not appear to cause such abnormalities. Further, defective platelet adhesiveness and prolonged bleeding time in patients dialyzed with cuprophan has been shown to improve following transfer to polyacrylonitrile membranes.[108] Interestingly, in a retrospective analysis, patients chronically dialyzed with polyacrylonitrile membranes had fewer episodes of arteriovenous fistula thrombosis, leg thrombosis, and fatal pulmonary embolism than those dialyzed with cuprophan membrane.[109] Although definitive conclusions cannot be drawn from these data, they suggest that dialyzers differ from each other in their effects on platelets. However, existing data do not permit the classification of dialysis membrane materials according to their thrombogenic potentials.

The considerations notwithstanding, it should be emphasized that several factors other than the dialysis membranes can affect clotting in the dialyzer circuit. These include dialysis-related factors, such as the type and amount of anticoagulant employed, blood flow rate, geometry of the blood path (including stenosis in the inflow and outflow tracts of the fistula, cannulas, tubing and blood chamber, and blood compartment of the dialyzer), and ultrafiltration rate. In addition, a variety of patient factors, such as hematocrit, number and functional state of the platelets, coagulation proteins, fibrinolytic proteins, and other elements in the blood and endothelium, can also affect clotting in the dialysis circuit.

ERYTHROCYTE ABNORMALITIES

Significant hemolysis during hemodialysis is rare. Several causes of hemolysis associated with the dialysate have been identified, including contamination of the dialysate with chloramine, overheating of dialysate, and dialysate hypotonicity from improper proportioning of the concentrate.[110] Mechanical trauma of blood as it passes through the blood pump is another cause.[111] The dialyzer itself rarely causes hemolysis directly. Theoretically, shearing of erythrocytes at the dialyzer membrane surface or defective dialysis tubing[112,113] produces trauma to the cell. Formaldehyde employed for reuse processing has been incriminated in the development of antibodies directed against the N antigen of erythrocytes.[114–116] These anti-N antibodies are cold agglutinins that can cause hemolysis at low temperatures. Thorough rinsing of the dialyzers to eliminate the formaldehyde prior to reuse or discontinue the use of formaldehyde has markedly diminished the prevalence of anti-N antibodies in the dialysis population.[116] Activation of the terminal components of the complement system leads to the formation of the membrane attack complex. These complexes have been detected on erythrocyte fragments in patients undergoing cardiopulmonary bypass[117] and on neutrophil surfaces in patients undergoing hemodialysis.[44] It is not known whether these complexes increase the fragility of erythrocytes or whether they induce hemolysis during or after hemodialysis. Other causes of hemolysis that may develop during dialysis are reviewed in depth in Chapter 22.

NEUTROPHILS ABNORMALITIES

Hemodialysis-Induced Leukopenia

Leukopenia during hemodialysis has been one of the earliest indices of membrane bioincompatibility. The onset is usually rapid, occurring within the first 2 to 3 minutes and maximum of 10 to 15 minutes.[19,118] Leukocyte counts usually return to normal by the end of dialysis and sometimes exceed the predialysis values. The rebound leukocytosis has been ascribed, in part, to an increase in circulating levels of granulocyte colony-stimulating factor (G-CSF).[119] Neutrophils and other granulocytes are primarily affected. Although granulocytes are readily seen on the dialyzer membrane surface under microscopy,[24, 120] the disappearance of these cells from the circulation is primarily due to sequestration in the pulmonary vasculature. Pulmonary leukosequestration has been demonstrated using radiolabeled cells in clinical studies.[121] Binding of C5a and $C5a_{desArg}$ to their specific receptors has been considered to be the primary mechanism behind dialysis-induced neutropenia. In general, the degree of complement activation correlates closely with the degree of leukopenia.[5,6,48,50,51,53,54,97] Alterations in several other neutrophil surface receptors (such as Mac-1 or CR3, LAM-1, CD15) have also been incriminated in the development and resolution of dialysis-induced leukopenia. Platelet-activating factor and leukotriene B_4 released from the activated neutrophils can further promote cell aggregation.

Transient neutropenia during hemodialysis by itself may be of less significance than the accompanying events, such as the release of reactive oxygen species from stimulated neutrophils and dysfunction of circulating neutrophils. However, the degree of neutropenia may, under some but not all circumstances, serve as a marker of these other events.

Degranulation

Several proteins that are stored in the azurophil and specific granules of neutrophils possess proteolytic, antimicrobial, and/or cell modulating properties. Release of these intracellular constituents (degranulation) in response to specific inflammatory stimuli is essential for host defense.[102] Although neutrophil degranulation during hemodialysis has been well documented,[122–124] the mechanisms that mediate this process have not been elucidated. Based on in vitro degranulating activities of C3a and C5a,[29,36,37] these anaphylatoxins have been postulated to participate in dialysis-induced neutrophil degranulation. However, plasma concentrations of the granular proteins during clinical dialysis do not correlate closely with plasma C3a levels. For example, dialysis with PMMA membranes is associated with lower plasma C3a levels but higher plasma elastase levels than with cuprophan.[122–124] Additional evidence suggests that noncomplement plasma factors also contribute to neutrophil degranulation induced by cuprophan membranes[25] and perhaps other membranes as well (Figure 18–7).[125] Mechanical shearing of the cells possibly plays a role in this phenomenon. In support of this hypothesis, is the observation that clinical dialysis using cuprophan plate dialyzers induced higher plasma levels of elastase and lactoferrin than with hollow fiber dialyzers.[126] Proteolytic enzymes that are released into plasma as a result of neutrophil degranulation may contribute to the protein catabolic state that is observed during clinical dialysis.[127,128]

Release of Reactive Oxygen Species

The release of reactive oxygen species (ROS) is an important mechanism by which neutrophils injure foreign tissues. Clinical studies have shown that cuprophan membranes induced substantially greater ROS production than PMMA membranes (Figure 18–8).[129] One of the mediators in this process is likely to be C5a. The release of ROS by activated neutrophils during dialysis may alter surrounding tissues, such as plasma proteins and lipids.[130] Endothelium that is exposed to activated neutrophils sequestered in the lungs[131] and in the kidneys[132] may potentially be affected as well.

Dysfunction

When neutrophils are activated by hemodialysis membrane, they temporarily lose their ability to respond to subsequent

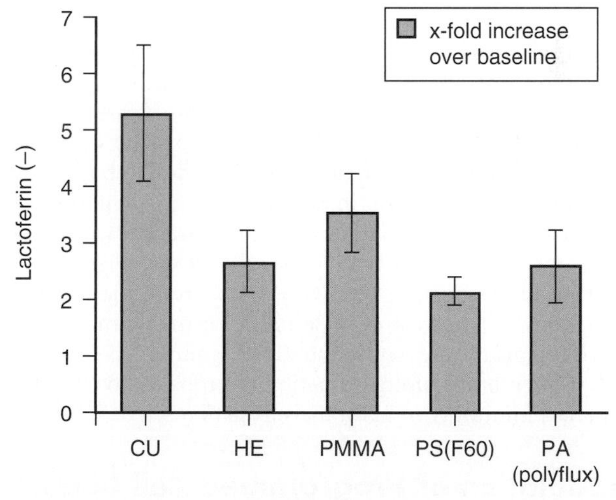

Figure 18–7 Release of lactoferrin from polymorphonuclear cells in the course of dialysis. Data represent the X-fold increase over baseline values in eight patients treated with cuprophan *(CU)*, hemophan *(HE)*, polymethylmethacrylate *(PMMA)*, polysulfone *(PS)*, and polyamide *(PA)*. (Reprinted with permission from Deppisch R, Betz M, Hansch G, et al: Biocompatibility of the polyamide membranes. Contrib Nephrol 1992; 96:26-46.)

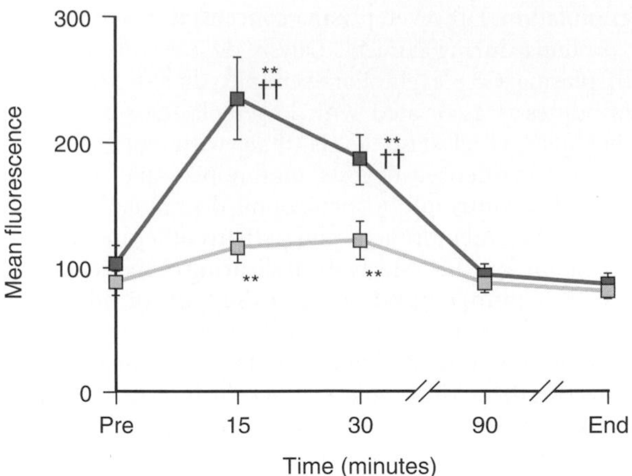

Figure 18–8 Production of whole blood reactive oxygen species from efferent bloodlines during hemodialysis. Whole blood obtained at specified times with either first-use cuprophan (*closed squares*) or first-use PMMA (*open squares*) dialysis membranes. Results are expressed as the log mean fluorescence of dichlorofluorescin diacetate-loaded granulocytes ± standard deviation in 10 patients). °*P* <.05 compared with pre-dialysis; °°*P* <.01 compared with pre-dialysis; ++ *P* <.002, cuprophan versus PMMA at the same time. (Reprinted with permission from Himmelfarb J, Ault K, Holbrook D: Intradialytic granulocyte reactive oxygen species production: A prospective, crossover trial. J Am Soc Nephrol 1993; 4:178-186.)

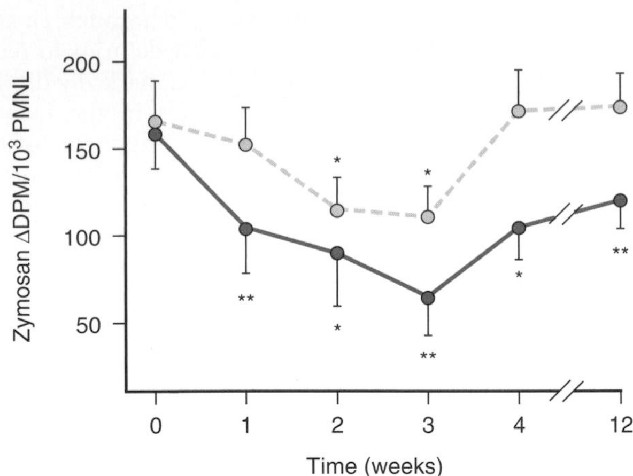

Figure 18–9 Utilization of glucose-1-C^{14} by polymorphonuclear leukocytes (PMNLs) expressed as Δ disintegration per minute (DPM) per 10^3 PMNLs in response to zymosan for patients maintained on hemodialysis with cuprophan (*solid line*) and polysulfone (*dotted line*) dialyzers for 12 weeks after initiation of hemodialysis. **P* <.05. ***P* <.01 from initiation of dialysis. The difference between both groups was statistically significant at all time points (except 2nd week). (Reprinted with permission from Vanholder R, Ringoir S, Dhondt A, Hakim R: Phagocytosis in uremic and hemodialysis patients: A prospective and cross sectional study. Kidney Int 1991; 39:320-327.)

stimuli. The resultant abnormalities include alterations in cell surface receptors, decrease in aggregation and adherence,[133, 134] and defective oxidative metabolism and chemiluminescence.[135, 136] These abnormalities are often above and beyond those observed with uremia per se. An early study showed that although cellulose acetate membranes adversely affected phagocytosis and random motility of neutrophils in vitro, polysulfone membranes did not.[137] In a subsequent study, fifteen incident patients with end-stage renal disease were randomly assigned to initiate dialysis with a low-flux cuprophan or low-flux polysulfone membrane.[138] Although both groups experienced deterioration in neutrophil function upon initiation of chronic hemodialysis, the deterioration with cuprophan was greater than that with polysulfone (Figure 18–9). Neutrophil dysfunction following exposure to dialysis membrane may impair host defense mechanisms when infectious microorganisms are subsequently encountered. Therefore, dialysis membrane bioincompatibility probably contributes to impaired immunity in hemodialysis patients.

Modulation of Programmed Cell Death

Apoptosis, or programmed cell death, is an active form of cell death that is initiated by a number of stimuli and is intricately regulated. Apoptosis in both excessive and reduced amounts has pathologic implications. Evidence suggests that apoptosis may play a role in the pathophysiology of immune dysfunction in uremia.[139] The lifespan and functional activity of neutrophils can be extended in vitro by incubation with pro-inflammatory mediators, such as C5a, IL-1β, and TNF-α[140–143] The generation of these mediators varies between different dialyzer membranes, which results in a differential impact on the fate of circulating neutrophils. During dialysis, the apoptosis-inducing activity of uremic plasma is modulated by the use of dialyzers with different degrees of biocompatibility.[144] Indeed, compared with neutrophils harvested from healthy volunteers and exposed to pre-dialysis uremic plasma samples, a significantly lower proportion of apoptosis was observed in neutrophils exposed to 15-minute plasma samples obtained from patients dialyzed with CU but not with CTA or PS dialyzers (Figure 18–10). By contrast, cells incubated directly with CU membranes undergo accelerated apoptosis.[145] It remains to be determined whether *in vivo*, direct contact with the dialysis membrane is a stronger determinant of the fate of neutrophils than the generation of pro-inflammatory mediators, which may modulate survival pathways.

LYMPHOCYTES AND NATURAL KILLER CELLS

Limited data are available on the effects of dialysis membranes on lymphocytes, probably because significant intradialytic lymphopenia is not a common event, the effects of complement on lymphocytes are less prominent,[146, 147] and the methods of studying lymphocytes are often more complicated. Activation of T lymphocytes during hemodialysis has been detected by changes in cell surface markers, such as interleukin-2 receptor (IL-2R). In the presence of interleukin-1 (IL-1), stimulation of T-lymphocytes by antigens leads to the release of interleukin-2 (IL-2) and the expression of its receptor (IL-2R) on the cell surface. Binding of IL-2 to IL-2R is important in T-cell proliferation and the development of

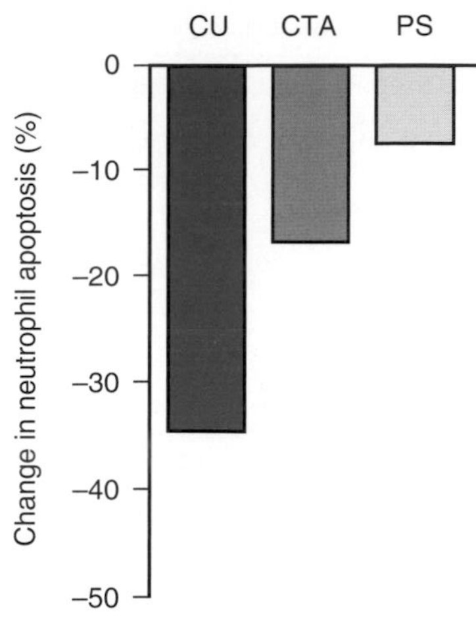

Figure 18–10 Percentage change in neutrophil apoptosis after 24-hour incubation with uremic plasma collected at 15 minutes of dialysis with different dialyzer membranes. Compared with pre-dialysis plasma, in the presence of plasma collected at 15 minutes of dialysis, apoptosis of neutrophils collected from healthy subjects decreased by 35% ($P < .001$), 17% ($P = .11$) and 7% ($P = .80$) in the cuprophan (CU), cellulose triacetate (CTA), and polysulfone (PS) membrane groups, respectively. (Reprinted with permission from Jaber BL, Balakrishnan VS, Cendoroglo M, et al: Apoptosis-inducing activity of uremic plasma during hemodialysis. Blood Purif 1999; 16:325-335.)

functionally active effector T cells.[148] Expression of IL-2R is increased when T-lymphocytes are activated. The high affinity IL-2R receptor is comprised of an α and a β chain. Under certain conditions, the α chain (Tac or p55) is released into the plasma and is known as soluble IL-2R. Plasma soluble IL-2R retains the ability to bind IL-2, thereby reducing the availability of the cytokine to interact with cell surface IL-2R. Elevated plasma level of soluble IL-2R therefore reflects both a state of T-lymphocyte activation and a downregulation of IL-2 effects.

Different dialysis membranes affect T cells differently. Zaoui and colleagues[149] observed that dialysis with cuprophan membranes was associated with greater expression of IL-2R on T-lymphocytes compared to with PMMA membrane. When the cells were stimulated in vitro using phytohemagglutinin, those that had been exposed to cuprophan responded poorly. Others have shown that in vitro proliferation of T-lymphocytes obtained from patients on chronic dialysis with polysulfone membrane was normal but impaired among patients on cuprophan membranes. These data suggest that T-lymphocytes are activated during hemodialysis with cuprophan membranes and, subsequently, become dysfunctional. The mechanism(s) by which T cells are activated by cuprophan membranes is unclear, but it may be related to its ability to activate complement[149] and monocytes.[150] Abnormal T-cell function may predispose dialysis patients to various infections.

Natural killer (NK) cells are normal peripheral leukocytes with cytotoxic activity against tumor cells, microorganism, infected cells, and transplanted tissues. NK cell counts have been shown to increase during chronic clinical dialysis using cuprophan membranes, but their *in vitro* cytotoxic function (against K562 cells) was impaired.[151] *In vitro* studies suggest that different types of dialysis membranes have different effects on NK cell function, with cuprophan faring worse than cellulose acetate or polycarbonate membranes.[152,153] Whether the higher incidence of malignancy among ESRD patients[154, 155] is related to NK cells dysfunction has not been determined.

B-lymphocytes can be activated during dialysis using cuprophan, cellulose acetate, or polysulfone membranes, but not with AN69.[156] The mechanisms behind intradialytic B-cell activation are unknown.

MONOCYTE ACTIVATION

Cytokines are polypeptides with molecular weights of 10 to 45 kDa. These are highly potent molecules, active at picomolar and femtomolar concentrations, and are synthesized by cells in response to infection, inflammation, or trauma.[157–159] There are currently more than a dozen cytokines that have been designated as interleukins.[160] In addition, cytokines, such as tumor necrosis factor, interferon, transforming growth factor, and colony stimulating factors, continue to be known by their original names.[160] In 1983, the Interleukin Hypothesis was proposed, incriminating IL-1 produced during dialysis as the cause of hypotension, fever, and other acute phase responses observed in patients receiving hemodialysis[161] (Table 18–3). Indeed, both studies using *in vitro* models of hemodialysis as well as clinical studies in patients on hemodialysis have demonstrated increased production of a variety of pro-inflammatory cytokines, such as interleukin-1 (IL-1) and tumor necrosis factor (TNF) during hemodialysis.[158,159,162] Over the decade since this hypothesis, a better understanding of the biologic effects of pro-inflammatory cytokines and the close similarities between dialysis-related morbidity and the biologic effects of these cytokines have further strengthened the possibility that cytokines could be involved in dialysis-related symptoms.[158,159,162]

Plasma Cytokine Levels

Pre-dialysis plasma levels of IL-1 and TNF have been shown to be elevated in patients on chronic hemodialysis using cellulose membranes.[163–168] Interestingly, undialyzed patients with ESRD did not show evidence of elevated IL-1 levels,[167] leading to the conclusion that the hemodialysis procedure itself, rather than renal failure, leads to increased IL-1 production. This hypothesis was further strengthened by the observation that hemodialysis with these "bioincompatible" cellulose membranes leads to a further rise in plasma levels of TNF-α[167,169,170] In contrast, dialysis with "biocompatible" membranes, such as PAN, was not associated with a further rise in plasma levels of TNF-α[169,170] In fact, in some studies, plasma levels of TNF-α declined during dialysis with PAN membranes.[170] However, others have failed to show elevated plasma levels of IL-1β or TNF-α before, during, or after a hemodialysis treatment.[171–173]

Pre-dialysis plasma levels of IL-1β and TNF-α in hemodialysis patients have been shown to be higher than those in healthy subjects.[174] However, plasma levels of IL-1β and TNF-α were also elevated in undialyzed patients with chronic kidney disease (CKD) and patients on continuous ambulatory peritoneal dialysis (CAPD), and there were no significant

Table 18–3 Potential Relationship Between the Biologic Effects of Interleukin-1 and Dialysis-Related Morbidity

Biologic Effects of Interleukin-1	Proposed Consequences in Hemodialysis Patients
Fever, sleepiness, anorexia, myalgia, arthralgia, headache, gastrointestinal disturbances, and hypotension	Fever, sleepiness, anorexia, myalgia, arthralgia, headache, gastrointestinal disturbances, and hypotension
Proliferation of vascular smooth muscle cells	Accelerated atherosclerosis
Stimulation of platelet derived growth factor	
Up-regulation of adhesion molecules	
Atherosclerotic plaques	
Synthesis of collagenases	Bone and joint disease
Osteoblast activation	
Suppression of albumin gene expression	Hypoalbuminemia
Increased expression of positive acute phase reactants	Elevated circulating interleukin-6, C-reactive protein and ferritin level
Inhibition of erythropoiesis	Anemia
Suppression of erythrocyte maturation	RHuEPO hyporesponsiveness
Muscle proteolysis	Muscle wasting
	Negative nitrogen balance
Glomerular mesangial cell activation	Loss of residual renal function
Activation of phospholipase A_2 and cyclooxygenase	Delayed recovery from acute renal failure

(Reprinted with permission from Pereira BJ: Balance between pro-inflammatory cytokines and their specific inhibitors in patients on dialysis. Nephrol Dial Transplant 1995; 10:27-32.)

differences in the plasma levels of these cytokines between these patient groups (Fig. 18–11). Similar studies have found elevated plasma levels of TNF-α and IL-6 in both undialyzed patients with Stage 5 CKD as well as those on HD.[167,175] Elevated plasma cytokine levels in patients with CKD could be due to increased production and/or decreased clearance. Indeed, several studies have demonstrated a strong linear correlation between plasma cytokine levels and serum creatinine levels.[174,176] This correlation suggests that the kidney has an important role in the metabolism and/or clearance of these molecules. Further, the fact that the plasma levels of IL-1β and TNF-α were not significantly different between patients with CKD and those receiving CAPD or HD suggests that these dialysis modalities may not significantly affect the clearance of these proteins. Interestingly, studies in septic patients on continuous arteriovenous hemofiltration with PAN membranes have shown that TNF-α is removed from the circulation by adsorption to the membrane and to a lesser extent by ultrafiltration.[177] This suggests that although these proteins may, to some extent, be cleared by dialysis, the clearance may not match the natural excretion by the kidney.

Cytokine Production by Peripheral Blood Mononuclear Cells (PBMC)

PBMC from patients on chronic hemodialysis show signs of mononuclear cell activation. Interleukin-1β is present in the mononuclear cells of patients on dialysis.[164,178–180] In contrast, mononuclear cells isolated from healthy subjects do not contain IL-1β protein or mRNA for IL-1β using northern hybridization or polymerase chain reaction. Even after 24 hours of incubation, there is no evidence of IL-1β synthesis in the mononuclear cells of healthy donors.[181,182] However, incubation of mononuclear cells from patients undergoing chronic HD in the absence of exogenous stimuli results in spontaneous IL-1β production.[178,180] When stimulated with LPS, PBMC produce as much as fivefold more IL-1β compared to mononuclear cells from normal subjects.[164,178–180] Similar results have been reported for the production of TNF-α and IL-6.[183–185]

In vitro studies have shown that when human blood is circulated through a hollow fiber cuprophan membrane, transcription of mRNA for IL-1β is apparent within 2 hours. However, in the absence of endotoxin in the dialysate, there is no translation into IL-1β protein.[186] Similarly, mononuclear cells drawn from the arterial limb of the dialysis circuit in patients on chronic HD contain a small but significant amount of IL-1β and TNF-α.[187,188] However, within 5 minutes of dialysis with a new cuprophan membrane, the mononuclear cells in the blood from the venous limb demonstrate abundant messenger RNA for IL-1β and TNF-α. Interestingly, the mononuclear cells returning to the dialyzer from the arterial side do not show evidence of IL-1β gene expression.[188] A single pass through a cuprophan membrane is apparently sufficient to trigger transcription, and, once activated, the mononuclear cells do not return into the circulation during the course of the dialysis session. In contrast to cuprophan membranes, cytokine genes are not activated by membranes that are weak complement activators, during either in vitro or in vivo dialysis.[186,188]

Thus, in patients on hemodialysis with cellulose membranes, cytokine gene expression takes place in the absence of contaminated dialysate. These cells can either degrade their mRNA without translation into cytokine protein or receive a second signal from ongoing infection or illness, leading to rapid and efficient translation into cytokine protein. However, the most likely source of a second signal is the dialysate (Figure 18–12).[189] In the absence of a second stimulus, it is unclear where the mRNA-primed mononuclear cells exit the circulation during the 5 hours of HD. Certainly, a large pool of cells could be adhering to endothelium, particularly in the lung. Further, receptors on monocytes and adhesion molecules on endothelial cells may attract activated monocytes to the synovium or into other tissues.

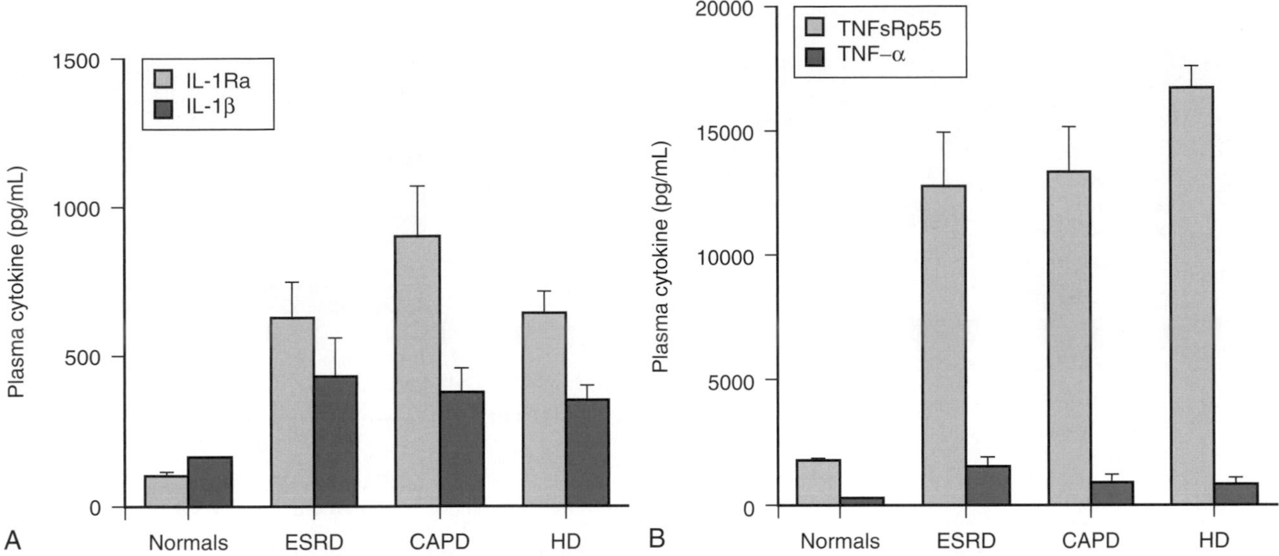

Figure 18–11 ***A,*** Plasma levels of interleukin-1β *(IL-1β)* and interleukin-1 receptor antagonist *(1L-1Ra)* in normals, undialyzed end-stage renal disease *(ESRD)*, continuous ambulatory peritoneal dialysis *(CAPD)*, and hemodialysis *(HD)* patients. Plasma levels of 1L-1β were not significantly different between patient groups and normals. Plasma levels of 1L-1Ra in ESRD (*P* =.03), CAPD (*P* <.001) and HD (*P* =.0004) were significantly higher than those in normals. However, the differences between ESRD, CAPD, and HD were not significant. ***B,*** Plasma levels of tumor necrosis factor α *(TNFα)* and soluble TNF receptor *(TNFsRp55)* in normals, undialyzed end-stage renal disease *(ESRD)* continuous ambulatory peritoneal dialysis *(CAPD)* and hemodialysis *(HD)* patients. Plasma levels of TNF-α were not significantly different between patient groups and normals. Plasma levels of TNFsRp55 in ESRD (*P* <.001), CAPD (*P* <.001), and HD (*P* <.001) were significantly higher than those in normals. However, the differences between ESRD, CAPD, and HD were not significant. (Reprinted with permission from Pereira BJ, Shapiro L, King AJ, et al: Plasma levels of IL-1 beta, TNF alpha and their specific inhibitors in undialyzed chronic renal failure, CAPD and hemodialysis patients. Kidney Int 1994; 45:890-896.)

Cytokine Production as an Index of Transmembrane Passage of Bacterial Products from the Dialysate

The increasing popularity of high-flux as well as high efficiency membranes and the associated risk for backfiltration[190] have raised concerns that patients dialyzed with these membranes may be at a high risk of being exposed to bacterial contaminants in the dialysate.[191] Further, the risk of passage of bacterial products from the dialysate to the blood compartment could potentially be exacerbated by reprocessing of high-flux dialyzers, which has been shown to increase the permeability of the membranes.[192,193] Indeed, the Centers for Disease Control and Prevention (USA) has reported a significant correlation between pyrogen reactions during dialysis and the use of high-flux as well as reprocessed dialyzers.[194] In contrast, others have not found an increased incidence of pyrogen reactions among patients dialyzed with high-flux dialyzers compared to conventional or high-efficiency dialyzers.[195]

The molecular weight of endotoxins is estimated to be approximately 10^6 Da. On the basis of their sizes, endotoxins are not expected to traverse intact dialysis membranes, including high-flux membranes. However, cytokine-inducing products derived from bacteria are not limited to the whole endotoxin particles. The lipid-A portion of endotoxins and other fragments of bacteria, such as muramyl peptides, also possess monocyte-stimulating activities. Indeed, cytokine production by PBMC is a sensitive indicator of the presence of endotoxin.[157] Consequently, several authors have designed in vitro models of HD in which the reverse transfer of cytokine-inducing substances from intentionally contaminated dialysate was used to assess the permeability of different HD membranes to bacterial products (Figure 18–13).[196–200] Using cytokine production as an index of the reverse transfer of bacterial products from the dialysate to blood compartment, several studies have demonstrated that high-flux synthetic membranes, such as polyamide or polysulfone, are less likely to permit the transfer of bacterial products from the dialysate than low-flux cellulose membrane, such as cuprophan or hemophan.[196,199] Further, transmembrane passage of bacterial products has been shown to occur in the absence of backfiltration, suggesting an important role for diffusive transfer of these toxins across dialysis membranes.[196] Synthetic membranes, such as PS and PAN, bind significantly higher amounts of I^{125}-labeled LPS than CU membranes.[201] Hence, it is postulated that the interaction between hydrophobic domains on the synthetic membranes and hydrophobic domains on the bacterial toxins lead to avid adsorption of these toxins on the dialysate side of the membrane and prevent the transfer into the blood compartment.[202] This characteristic could be considered to be another index of biocompatibility.

Clinical Effects of Dialysis-Induced Monocyte Activation

The hypothesis that cytokine production is a contributing cause of several of the acute and chronic metabolic and

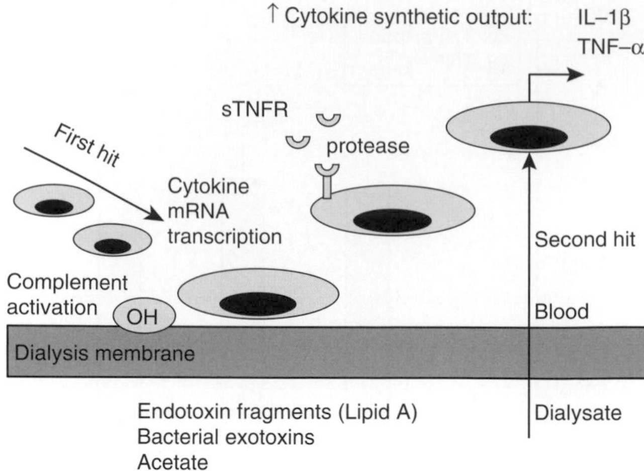

Figure 18–12 Potential mechanisms for cytokine production during dialysis: The double hit hypothesis. Complement activation by dialysis membranes leads to transcription of mRNA for interleukin-1 *(IL-1)* and tumor necrosis factor *(TNF)* in monocytes. In the absence of a "second signal," the mRNA for those cytokines is not translated into protein. The second signal could potentially come from the dialysate, leading to synthesis of IL-1β and TNF-α. Concurrently, proteases cleave the extracellular fragment of the TNF receptors resulting in soluble TNF receptors *(sTNFR)*. Thus, the hemodialysis procedure serves as a stimulus for cytokines such as IL-1β and TNF-α, as well as their specific antagonists. (Reprinted with permission from Pereira BJ, Dinarello CA: Role of cytokines in patients on dialysis. Int J Artif Organs 1995; 18:293-304.)

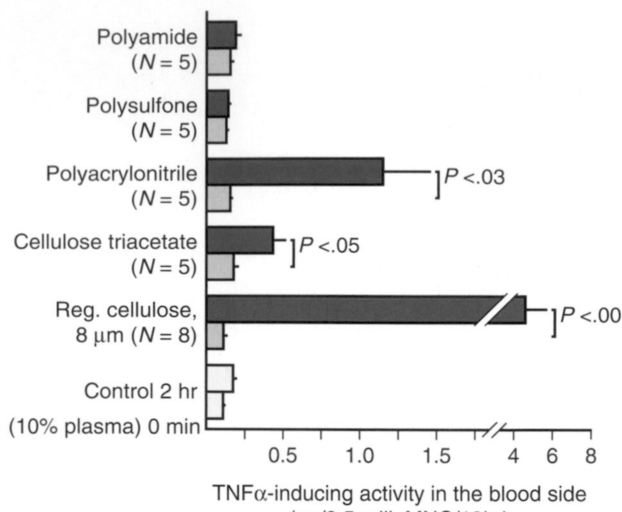

Figure 18–13 Production of TNF-α by human mononuclear cells (MNC) incubated with samples from the blood compartments of the *in vitro* circuits containing 10% plasma in culture medium (MEM), before and after challenge of the dialysate with *P. maltophilia* filtrate (0.2 μg/mL LAL active material. "Control" represents 10% plasma in MEM without contact to the circuit, not preincubated (0′) or preincubated at 37°C for 2 hours. Hatched bars represent the averaged TNF-α–inducing activities of samples drawn at 30 and 60 minutes from the blood side during dialysis sterile tissue culture medium as dialysate. Closed bars depict averaged activities of samples drawn at 90 and 120 minutes from blood side following challenge of the dialysate side with *P. maltophilia* filtrate. Results are expressed as the mean ± SEM of TNF-α–inducing activity (ng/2.5 × 10⁶ MNC/18 hr). (Reprinted with permission from Lonnemann G, Behme TC, Lenzner B, et al: Permeability of dialyzer membranes to TNF alpha-inducing substances derived from water bacteria. Kidney Int 1992; 42:61-68.)

inflammatory changes associated with hemodialysis is based on similar signs and symptoms also observed in (1) healthy volunteers or experimental animals administered cytokines and in (2) diseases, such as rheumatoid arthritis, inflammatory bowel disease, some chronic infections and cancers, and various collagen vascular diseases, where the pathophysiology is largely attributed to enhanced cytokine production.[157–159] Healthy human volunteers administered IL-1β in doses of 10 to 100 ng/kg develop fever, sleepiness, anorexia, myalgia, arthralgia, headache, and gastrointestinal disturbances, and in larger doses (>300 ng/kg), hypotension.[157–159] Likewise, when injected into humans at low concentrations (less than 1μg/kg), TNF-α produces hypotension and leukopenia as well as several metabolic dysfunctions. Indeed, IL-1β and TNF-α are highly synergistic in both animal and in *in vitro* studies and act synergistically in the production of hemodynamic shock.[203] IL-1β and TNF-α also induce a rapid increase in slow wave sleep.[157–159] The similarity between these signs and symptoms observed during experimental administration of pro-inflammatory cytokines and the fever, hypotension, fatigue, somnolence, and other acute phase responses observed during HD, was the basis of the Interleukin Hypothesis.[161] However, the further understanding of the biologic actions of these cytokines has expanded the scope of the role of cytokines in dialysis-related morbidity. In experimental models, cytokines lead to proliferation of vascular smooth muscle cells and stimulation of platelet derived growth factor and atherosclerotic plaques.[157–159] Consequently, cytokines may have a role in the accelerated atherosclerosis and cardiovascular morbidity observed in hemodialysis patients. Further, IL-1β and TNF-α induce osteoblast activation and increase gene expression for phospholipase A_2 and cyclooxygenase.[204] In isolated tissues perfused with IL-1β, prostaglandin E_2 increases rapidly in the perfusate.[205,206] Consequently, cytokines may contribute to various bone, articular, and periarticular diseases. In addition, IL-1β increases the hepatic production of amyloid A (AA), which may contribute to the development of AA amyloidosis. Although amyloid deposits in hemodialysis patients are often composed of $β_2$-microglobulin, AA amyloid is also seen. The presence of macrophages stained positive for IL-1β and TNF-α in chronic renal failure patients' bones that are afflicted with severe $β_2$-microglobulin amyloidosis[207] suggests the possibility that these cytokines also participate in the pathogenesis of this disease as well. IL-1β and TNF-α are also appetite suppressants, but their mechanism of action as anorectic agents is thought to be due to peripheral effects on hepatic metabolism rather than in the central nervous system. Further, IL-1β, TNF-α and IL-6 stimulate hepatic acute phase proteins, such as C-reactive protein, and suppress albumin synthesis, induce muscle proteolysis and a negative nitrogen balance. Taken together, these actions could contribute to the malnutrition observed in dialysis patients. However, to date, a definitive link between dialysis-induced cytokine production and clinical symptoms, signs, or outcomes has not been demonstrated.

As in the case of neutrophils and T-lymphocytes, chronic low-grade activation of monocytes induced by hemodialysis leads to dysfunction of these cells. Monocytes obtained from patients dialyzed with cuprophan membranes for 2 weeks released less IL-1β and TNF-α when stimulated by phytohemagglutinin *in vitro* than cells from patients who were dialyzed using low-flux PMMA membranes.[208] Presumably, this subnormal response would represent a diminished ability of the host to respond appropriately to foreign materials, such as infectious microorganisms.

CLINICAL IMPLICATIONS OF DIALYSIS MEMBRANE BIOCOMPATIBILITY

Hemodialysis-Induced Hypoxemia and Pulmonary Hypertension

A decrease of 10 to 15 mmHg in systemic arterial partial oxygen tension (pO_2) commonly occurs during hemodialysis using cuprophan membrane and acetate dialysate.[57,209,210] This hypoxemia is obviously undesirable for patients with underlying cardiopulmonary diseases. There is little question that acetate dialysate is the major contributor to dialysis-induced hypoxemia, presumably because of the loss of carbon dioxide from blood into dialysate[211] and the metabolism of acetate by the body.[212] Both mechanisms lead to hypoventilation and a decrease in the respiratory quotient. However, there is substantial evidence to support the contribution of membrane bioincompatibility:

1. Patients on mechanical ventilators with constant minute volume and constant inspired oxygen concentration can still develop hypoxemia during hemodialysis.[213]
2. Decrease in pulmonary diffusion capacity (DLCO)[57,214–216] and transthoracic impedance,[215] widening of alveolar-arterial oxygen tension gradient,[209,216] as well as increase in closing volume[57] and dead space to tidal volume ratio,[211] have all been demonstrated during hemodialysis. These aberrations are suggestive of impairment in intrapulmonary gas exchange and cannot be explained by hypoventilation alone.
3. The degree of peripheral leukopenia has been correlated with the degree of hypoxemia.[217]
4. Dialysis using cuprophan membranes has been associated with a larger decrease in diffusion capacity compared to PAN membranes.[218]
5. Replacement of unsubstituted cellulose membranes with PMMA[210] or PAN[209,219] membranes can ameliorate the hypoxemia.
6. During dialysis with cuprophan membranes, replacement of acetate with bicarbonate dialysate does not necessarily abolish the hypoxemia,[217,218] but dialysis using the combination of reused cuprophan membrane and bicarbonate dialysate does.[220]
7. Infusion of cuprophan-activated plasma into humans[215] or experimental animals[61,215] causes hypoxemia.
8. Sham hemodialysis without dialysate in normal human volunteers produces hypoxemia.[221] Therefore, it appears that membrane bioincompatibility does play a role in the development of dialysis-induced hypoxemia. This effect is probably more prominent during the early phase of the treatment, when complement activation and leaching of noxious substances is most intense.

Invasive monitoring of pulmonary arterial pressure has documented the development of pulmonary hypertension during dialysis with cuprophan membranes but not with polycarbonate membranes.[66] In some instances, this hemodynamic derangement can lead to clinical symptoms.[222] In vitro and animal studies described earlier suggest that the mechanisms by which dialysis membrane bioincompatibility causes pulmonary hypertension and hypoxemia involve the activation of complement and other humoral factors. Anaphylatoxins cause smooth muscle contraction[28] and in vivo activation of C3 and/or C5 results in pulmonary hypertension in animals.[63] Anaphylatoxins stimulate the production of thromboxane and leukotrienes, which are potent airway constrictors.[223] In addition, anaphylatoxins increase vascular permeability[26] and may thus cause transient pulmonary interstitial edema. Pulmonary leukosequestration (leukocyte thromboemboli) is likely to be a result of intradialytic complement activation but is unlikely to be the cause of pulmonary hypertension or hypoxemia.

Dialyzer Reactions

Occasionally, severe reactions during hemodialysis can be life threatening. These reactions, by definition, cannot be attributed to the acute loss of fluid, changes in electrolytes, improper composition of dialysate, and malfunctioning of the dialysis machine. The severity and time of onset are variable. The manifestations include various combinations of hypertension or hypotension, dyspnea, coughing, sneezing, wheezing, choking, rhinorrhea, conjunctival injection, headache, muscle cramps, back pain, abdominal pain, chest pain, nausea, vomiting, fever, chills, flushing, urticaria, and pruritus. Death occasionally occurs.[224–236] The term *hypersensitivity reaction* has been used to describe these signs and symptoms. Whether some of these patients are indeed hypersensitive to the offending agents are unclear since the nature and amount of the agents are frequently unknown. Consequently, a more appropriate term is *dialyzer reaction.* Causes of dialyzer reactions are diverse and have been reviewed in detail in Chapter 22.

β_2-Microglobulin (β_2MG) and Amyloidosis

Amyloid deposit containing β_2MG is well recognized as a complication of long erm dialysis.[237,238] The pathogenesis of this disease is unclear, although recent data suggest that some alterations of the β_2MG peptide (e.g., by glycosylation[239] or proteolytic cleavage[240,241]) favor its deposition into tissues. Plasma β_2MG levels in ESRD patients are, in general, markedly elevated to 30 to 60 μg/mL[242–247] compared to those in normal subjects of approximately 1 μg/mL. It is likely that the high plasma concentrations in these patients also promote its deposition. To this end, efforts have been directed to decreasing the plasma β_2MG levels in ESRD patients.

In vitro incubation of PBMC with various types of dialysis membranes in the presence of plasma showed that cuprophan membrane induced the release of more β_2MG than did PMMA or AN69 membrane. Stimulation of mononuclear cells with C5a or IL-1β also enhanced β_2MG release,[39] suggesting that the effect of cuprophan on β_2MG release is mediated both by its ability to activate complement and indirectly by inducing cytokine generation. In contrast, incubation studies performed in the absence of plasma showed that β_2MG release was inhibited to a greater extent by cuprophan (rather than enhanced) compared to hemophan or PAN membranes.[248] β_2MG is also a constituent of neutrophil granules.[249] Theoretically, dialysis membrane induced neutrophil degranulation may also increase plasma β_2MG levels. However, the intragranular content of β_2MG is small, and therefore the contribution of this mechanism to plasma β_2MG increase during dialysis is modest at most. Nonetheless, these experiments indicate that there is a cellular basis for dialysis-induced release of β_2MG. The presence of macrophages in bone tissues afflicted by β_2MG deposits also suggests the possibility that dialysis membrane-induced activated monocytes contribute to the local inflammatory or destructive process.[207]

Whether there is a real increase in total extracellular β_2MG during dialysis using cuprophan membrane has been debated. Some investigators have argued that the apparent increase in plasma β_2MG concentration is due to a hemoconcentration effect as a result of ultrafiltration,[250,251] whereas others have reported a 3% to 15% increase in plasma β_2MG levels despite correction for hemoconcentration.[242,243] Some investigators have failed to demonstrate an increase in plasma β_2MG levels during sham hemodialysis with CU membranes.[251] In contrast, when whole blood was circulated through CU hemofilters in vitro, a 70% increase in plasma β_2MG levels was seen in 15 minutes.[252] Abolishment of the increment by leukocyte depletion in this study further suggested that these cells were the source of the additional β_2MG. The plasma appearance rate of β_2MG has been estimated using radiolabeled β_2MG turnover techniques. A higher plasma appearance rate in the patient would suggest that the enhanced release of this protein by activated leukocytes. Clinical data on this issue have been inconclusive. β_2MG appearance rates in patients dialyzed with cuprophan membrane were 30% to 50% higher than those in normal subjects, but the differences did not reach statistical significance.[244,245] The β_2MG appearance rates in patients dialyzed with AN69 membranes were normal, and were lower than the values for patients dialyzed with CU membranes. However, the differences between AN69 and CU were not statistically significant.[245]

Clinical dialysis with high-flux synthetic membranes decreases plasma β_2MG levels, probably by both membrane adsorption and transfer to the dialysate.[247] Cuprophan membrane induces an increase, whereas high-flux synthetic membranes induce a decrease in plasma β_2MG levels. Hence, one may postulate that patients dialyzed with the latter would suffer from less β_2MG-related amyloidosis. Studies have shown that patients dialyzed with AN69 membrane had less bone cysts and required less decompression surgery for carpal tunnel syndrome than those dialyzed with CU membrane (Figure 18–14).[253–255] These data are suggestive, but not definitive; since they are retrospective, there was overlap between the study groups, and histologic confirmation for β_2MG was not uniformly obtained.

If β_2MG-related amyloidosis in the ESRD patients results only from high plasma β_2MG levels as a result of kidney failure,

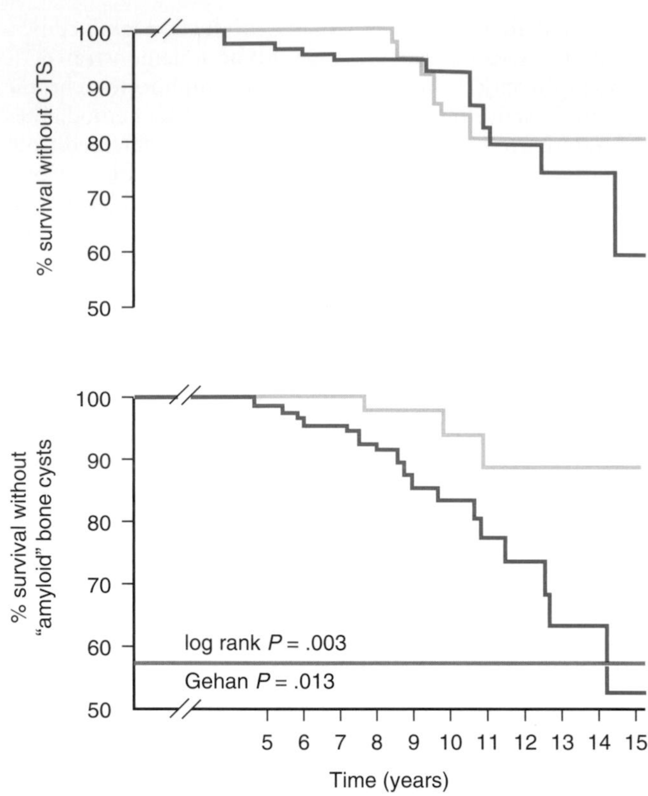

Figure 18–14 Kaplan-Meier survival curves without carpal tunnel syndrome *(CTS)* (upper panel) or without amyloid bone cysts (lower panel) in patients treated exclusively with either AN69 (*thin line*) or cellulose membranes (*thick line*). Survival without amyloid bone cysts is significantly different for the two groups. (Reprinted with permission from van Ypersele de Strihou C, Jadoul M, Malghem J, et al: Effect of dialysis membrane and patient's age on signs of dialysis-related amyloidosis. The Working Party on Dialysis Amyloidosis. Kidney Int 1991; 39:1012-1019.)

it should not be considered as a biocompatibility issue. Decreasing the plasma levels by using high-flux membranes, if it partially prevents β_2MG-related amyloidosis, is an issue of dialysis efficiency and not biocompatibility. However, to the extent that dialysis membrane may increase the release of the peptide from circulating leukocytes[39] and may activate leukocytes such that they promote β_2MG deposition by altering its structural properties[240,241] or potentiate the local inflammatory process in the tissues,[207] β_2MG is a biocompatibility issue. To what extent bioincompatibility contributes to clinical β_2MG amyloid disease is difficult to determine.

Susceptibility to Infection

Deactivation of neutrophils, T lymphocytes, monocytes, and natural killer cells after exposure to the dialysis membrane has been discussed earlier. Hypothetically, this would impair the ability of the leukocytes to subsequently combat infections and malignant cells. Indeed, chronic hemodialysis patients are prone to infections and have a higher incidence of malignancy than the general population.[154,155] Bacterial infections are common, but many of them are at least partially related to anatomic abnormalities, such as vascular access. Nonetheless, dialysis-related immunodeficiency exaggerates the problem. Chronic hemodialysis patients have frequent viral infections, abnormal antibody response to vaccines and hepatitis B viral infection, cutaneous anergy, prolonged graft survival, and altered response to and, perhaps, increased incidence of tuberculosis. These are disorders that are probably due to T-cell dysfunction. Whether this propensity to infections and perhaps malignancy is related to dialysis membrane bioincompatibility is, however, unclear. In a prospective study in which new ESRD patients were started on chronic HD using either CU or PS membrane, the cuprophan group had more significant deterioration of their neutrophil metabolism in response to phagocytic stimuli.[138] In addition, three out of the eight patients in the cuprophan group, and none of the seven patients in the polysulfone group, developed an episode of sepsis during a follow-up period of 20 weeks. However, the sample size in this study was small, precluding definitive conclusions.

Protein Catabolism

Membrane bioincompatibility has been incriminated as a cause of protein catabolism in dialysis patients. There are two potential cellular mechanisms by which this may occur: neutrophil degranulation and release of cytokines from monocytes. Intragranular proteins, such as elastase, are known to be proteolytic enzymes.[102] Elastase released into plasma is usually complexed to plasma α_1-proteinase inhibitor, which limits its functional activity. However, it has been shown that ROS potentiate the effect of elastase on protein degradation, even in the presence of the plasma inhibitor.[256] The simultaneous release of ROS[129] and proteases[122–124] from neutrophils during hemodialysis could therefore damage plasma proteins.[127,128] Another candidate is IL-1β, which is known to induce protein breakdown by releasing prostaglandin E_2.[257]

Using plasma free amino acids as an indicator of protein catabolism, sham HD without dialysate using cuprophan membranes in normal human has been shown to induce more protein catabolism than sham dialysis using AN69 membranes.[258] The enhanced release occurred almost 3 hours after the completion of the dialysis treatments and could be partially inhibited by a cyclooxygenase inhibitor. Based on this latter observation, it would be reasonable to postulate that AN69 membrane induces less monocyte activation and, therefore, it causes less protein catabolism. *In vitro*[259] and clinical[180] data on monokine release by AN69 membrane, however, do not support this hypothesis. A more recent clinical study using a radiolabeled amino acid turnover technique did not suggest an increase in protein catabolism associated with cuprophan membranes.[260] The issue of protein catabolism induced by membrane bioincompatibility is unsettled at present.

Outcomes Among Patients with Acute Renal Failure (ARF)

Activated neutrophils release oxygen radicals and proteolytic enzymes that can injure surrounding cells. Indeed, neutrophils stimulated by C5a, release oxygen radicals, which damage endothelial cells.[35,131] Since neutrophils are activated to release oxygen radicals[129] and proteolytic enzymes[122–124] during hemodialysis, it is possible that they could cause injury to various organs, including the kidneys. In support of this hypothesis is that rats with ischemic ARF and exposed to cuprophan-activated plasma recover renal function at a slower rate compared to those exposed to PAN membrane-treated plasma.[132] Infiltration of the glomeruli by neutrophils could be further demonstrated in the cuprophan group. Zymosan-activated plasma produced similar results as cuprophan-activated plasma. These data suggest that complement fragments mediate the effect of the cuprophan membrane.

In the past decade, several prospective studies have compared the effects of cellulose-derived or synthetic dialyzer membranes on clinical outcomes of patients with ARF. Table 18–4 summarizes the essential attributes of these reports.[17] There are several general limitations inherent to all the studies, as well as individual study limitations that are worthy of mention.

Overall, there were differences in the quality of the studies, the inconsistent randomization process, the absence of a

Table 18–4 Summary of Chronologic Trials Assessing the Impact of Hemodialysis Membranes on Clinical Outcomes in Acute Renal Failure

Authors (Reference)	Year	Trial Type	Dialysis Membrane BCM	Dialysis Membrane BICM	Patients (n) BCM	Patients (n) BICM	APACHE II Score BCM	APACHE II Score BICM	Survival (%) BCM	Survival (%) BICM
Schiffl *et al*[263]	1994	RCT	AN69	CU	26	26	24	24	62	35†
Hakim *et al*[265]	1994	CT	PMMA	CU	37	35	29	29	57	37
Schiffl *et al*[264]	1995	RCT	AN69, PAN	CU	38	38	23	24	63	34†
Kurtal *et al*[266]	1995	CT	PA	CU	25	32	21	23	64	72
Assouad *et al*[267]	1996	RCT	PMMA	CA	26	25	NR	NR	58	64
Himmelfarb *et al*[268]	1998	CT	PMMA, PS	CU, HF	72	81	28	26	57	46†
Jörres *et al*[269]	1999	RCT	PMMA	CU	84	76	24	23	60	58
Gastaldello *et al*[270]	2000	RCT	PS	CA	89*	45	24	23‡	40	51
Albright *et al*[271]	2000	CT	PS	CA	33	33	NR	NR	73	76

RCT, randomized controlled trial; *CT,* controlled trial; *NR,* not reported; *CU,* cuprophan; *HF,* hemophan; *CA,* cellulose acetate; *PS,* polysulfone; *PMMA,* polymethylmethacrylate; *PA,* polyamide; *AN69,* acrylonitrile 69; *PAN,* polyacrylonitrile.
* Patients were randomized to either a low-(n = 41) or high-flux (n = 48) PS dialyzer.
† $P \leq .05$.
‡ Survival was 37% and 42% in the low- and high-flux PS dialyzer group, respectively.
(Reprinted with permission from Modi GK, Pereira BJG, Jaber BLJ: Hemodialysis in acute renal failure: Does the membrane matter? Semin Dial 2001; 14.)

dialyzer blinding process, and the incomplete documentation of statistical procedures, mainly power analyses. In some studies, the comparison of synthetic to substituted rather than unsubstituted cellulose membranes may have confounded the results because these dialyzers are not as bioincompatible. Further, the expected mortality range among those with ARF is very wide, rendering comparison between studies even more difficult. Most studies used the Acute Physiological and Chronic Health Evaluation (APACHE) II scores to define the severity of illness. Although there have been reports of its successful use as a predicative instrument in ARF prognosis,[261] this score is not fully validated to ensure inclusion of all the baseline comorbid conditions.[262] None of the statistical analyses adjusted for the dialysis dose or the center effect. In fact, the dialysis prescription may be an important determinant of outcome, although targets for adequate dialysis in ARF have not yet been established.

In terms of individual study limitations, Schiffl and colleagues[263] originally examined patients with postoperative ARF. This study was criticized on many counts, including the use of dialyzers with different flux characteristics, the subsequent publication of a report inclusive of the authors' original findings[264] and possible imbalance between study groups. In the study by Hakim and colleagues[265] almost 30% of subjects in the synthetic dialyzer group recovered renal function after a single dialysis session, raising once more, the possibility of imbalance between the groups. The study by Kurtal and colleagues[266] was criticized for an imbalance in the etiologies of ARF, which may have confounded the results. Assouad and colleagues[267] reported on their findings in an abstract that did not undergo peer review. Finally, in the original report by Himmelfarb and colleagues[268] dialyzer assignment was made in alternating order, and dialyzer selection as well as treatment practices varied among participating centers.

Three additional trials were published on this issue. Jörres and colleagues[269] reported on a randomized controlled trial (RCT) comparing low-flux CU to PMMA dialyzers and used a pre-defined sample size determination for adequate statistical power. Fourteen-day adjusted survival rates were not different between the two groups. In subgroup analyses, outcomes were not different for oliguric and nonoliguric patients in contrast to other studies, where the benefit of synthetic membranes was more evident in nonoliguric subjects. The study limitations include the exclusion of almost 10% of patients from the original intention-to-treat analysis, outcome assessment at 2 weeks, which may not have been adequate to assess clinical outcomes reliably, and most importantly, the author's handling of dialysis modality switches. Indeed, a significant number of patients who were converted to continuous renal replacement therapy (CRRT) were included in the analysis and counted as alive at 14 days. Nevertheless, the lack of a definite dialyzer benefit in this large randomized study cannot be disregarded. Similarly, Gastaldello and colleagues[270] performed an RCT where patients with ARF were allocated to a low-flux CA, low-flux PS, or high-flux PS dialyzer. This well-conducted study did not detect any effect of membrane type or flux property on mortality or recovery of renal function. Once again, differences in membrane biocompatibility were subtle because no unsubstituted cellulose was used. Finally, Albright and colleagues[271] compared low-flux CA to high-flux PS dialyzers in a relatively small number of patients with ARF. Thirty-day survival was not different between the two groups. In a subgroup analysis of patients confined to the intensive care unit, there was a small benefit in renal recovery in the CA dialyzer group. Unfortunately, as acknowledged by the authors, although the study was originally randomized during the course of patient enrollment, dialyzer assignment was switched over to an alternating order, which might have significantly biased the results.

All the previously mentioned study limitations have precluded a clear answer to the role of membrane biocompatibility in the setting of ARF. The heterogeneity of individual studies reduced the strength of the conclusion. More importantly, the definition of bioincompatible and biocompatible membranes adopted in this analysis assumed that all cellulose-derived and synthetic membranes behaved similarly. Two meta-analyses summarizing all trials published to date, comparing the impact of dialysis membranes on clinical outcomes of patients with ARF receiving HD[272,273] yielded conflicting results. This may be so because these studies were rarely randomized, employed different study designs, collected different data, may have failed to adjust for severity of illness, and may have assessed different end points.[274] Second, because so few of these dialysis membrane trials were randomized, these meta-analyses included nonrandomized controlled trials and observational studies to accrue a larger sample size, and, therefore, to have enough power, to find a clinically and statistically significant difference between two therapies, if one truly exists. In summary, because mortality associated with dialysis-requiring ARF has remained so high, studies comparing dialysis membranes need to be better focused and appropriately powered to answer these questions.

Outcomes Among Patients with Chronic Kidney Failure

Several retrospective studies have examined the association between dialyzer type and clinical outcomes among patients on chronic dialysis. In one such study, patients receiving dialysis with PS dialyzers had an 80% to 90% lower relative risk (RR) of death from all-cause, cardiovascular disease and infection.[275] Although these risks were adjusted for age, gender, race and cause of ESRD, dose of dialysis and flux may have confounded the analysis. Likewise, in a comparison of noncontemporaneous cohorts, other studies have observed a 76% lower RR of death among patients on high-flux PS dialyzers compared with those on cellulose dialyzers.[276] However, differences in the dose of dialysis, flux, and albumin levels in the polysulfone group may have also influenced these results. In a historic prospective cohort study, 2400 prevalent patients on chronic dialysis were followed in the early 1990s until death, transplantation, transfer to peritoneal dialysis, or end of study observation (median duration of 1.4 years).[277] Dialyzers were classified as unsubstituted cellulose, modified cellulose and synthetic, and were used by 66%, 16%, and 18% of patients, respectively. Compared with patients on unsubstituted cellulose dialyzers, patients on modified cellulose and synthetic dialyzers had a 28% lower relative risk of death.[277] The analysis remained robust after adjustment for the dialysis dose.[277] In another study examining the relationship of dialysis membrane and cause-specific mortality, compared with patients dialyzed with unmodified cellulose membranes, the adjusted relative mortality risk from infection was 31% lower and from coronary artery disease was 26% lower for patients dialyzed with modified cellulose and synthetic membranes.[278]

The results of these studies offer support to reported experimental and observational clinical studies that have found that unmodified cellulose membranes may increase the risk for both infection and atherogenesis. However, for several reasons, these conclusions need to be viewed with caution. The fact that the majority of biocompatible dialyzers were also high-flux dialyzers raises the possibility that flux rather than biocompatibility may be the factor that resulted in better outcomes. Also, the possibility that the use of biocompatible dialyzers (which are more expensive) may reflect greater attention to improvements in dialysis technology and commitment of greater resources to patient care, which, in turn, leads to better outcomes, needs to be considered. Whereas further studies are necessary to evaluate the possibility of confounding factors, such as flux properties of membranes, to compare more specific membrane types, and to determine the pathophysiology linking membrane type to cause-specific mortality, the results of a recent multicenter study examining the impact of dialysis dose and use of high-flux dialyzers on clinical outcomes failed to demonstrate a survival advantage to the use of high-flux dialyzers,[279] raising more questions on this controversial issue.

Outcomes in Renal Transplant Recipients

There are few clinical reports that have addressed the impact of biocompatibility of dialyzer membranes on rate of recovery of renal function in the setting of delayed graft function immediately following transplantation. The rationale for these studies was the concern that recovery from delayed graft function, primarily due to ischemic reperfusion injury could be prolonged by the use of unsubstituted cellulose membranes. Valeri[280] first reported on the results of an RCT of 30 patients with delayed graft function following cadaveric renal transplantation who were maintained on HD with either a CU or PMMA dialyzer. Baseline demographic characteristics, including age, gender, and immunosuppresive therapy, were similar between the two groups. The mean number of dialysis sessions and duration of dialysis (in days) were comparable, and no survival outcome was measured. The authors concluded that the dialyzer type had no significant impact on the course of recovery from delayed graft function following cadaveric renal transplant. Romao and colleagues[281] subsequently reported on the results of an RCT involving 53 patients with delayed graft function following cadaveric renal transplantation who were dialyzed with either a CU or PS dialyzer. The performance characteristics of the membranes were not stated. The number of dialysis sessions, oliguric days, and hospital days did not differ between the two groups. The authors framed similar conclusions to the previous study. Woo and colleagues[282] also reported on 42 patients with delayed graft function who were randomly assigned to dialysis with either a CU or PS dialyzer and observed longer duration of ARF in the PS compared to the CU group. The author speculated that PS membranes may in fact delay recovery of renal function in this setting.

It is difficult to draw any definite conclusions from these preliminary studies due to small sample size, overall limited information, and the fact that most of these studies were published in abstract format. In addition, most of these authors assumed that delayed graft function was due to ischemic ATN, although other possibilities, such as acute rejection or drug toxicity, were not appropriately ruled out. This may have confounded the measured outcomes.

References

1. Lyman D: Replacement of renal function by dialysis. *In* Drukker W, Parsons F, Maher J (eds): Membranes. Karger, Basel, 1983, pp 97-105.
2. Lysaght M: Evolution of hemodialysis membranes. Contrib Nephrol 1995; 113:1-10.
3. United States Renal Data System: USRDS 1999 annual data report. Bethesda, MD, National Institutes of Health, Diabetes and Digestive and Kidney Diseases, 1999.
4. Henne W, Duenweg G, Bandel W: A new cellulose membrane generation for hemodialysis and hemofiltration. Artif Organs 1979; 3:466-469.
5. Spencer P, Schmidt B, Samtleben W: Ex vivo model of hemodialysis membrane biocompatibility. Trans Am Soc Artif Intern Organs 1985; 31:495-498.
6. Falkenhagen D, Bosch T, Brown GS, et al: A clinical study on different cellulosic dialysis membranes. Nephrol Dial Transplant 1987; 2:537-545.
7. Galli F, Rovidati S, Chiarantini L, et al: Bioreactivity and biocompatibility of a vitamin E-modified multi-layer hemodialysis filter. Kidney Int 1998; 54:580-589.
8. Galli F, Canestrari F, Buoncristiani U: Biological effects of oxidant stress in haemodialysis: The possible roles of vitamin E. Blood Purif 1999; 17:79-94.
9. Pertosa G, Grandaliano G, Soccio M, et al: Vitamin E-modified filters modulate Jun N-terminal kinase activation in peripheral blood mononuclear cells. Kidney Int 2002; 62:602-610.
10. Girndt M, Lengler S, Kaul H, et al: Prospective crossover trial of the influence of vitamin E-coated dialyzer membranes on T-cell activation and cytokine induction. Am J Kidney Dis 2000; 35:95-104.
11. Anderson S, Garcia D, Brenner B: Renal and systemic mainfestations of glomerular disease. *In* Brenner B, Rector JF (eds): The Kidney, 4th ed. Philadelphia, WB Saunders, 1991, pp 1831-1870.
12. Konstantin P: Newer membranes: Cuprophane versus polysulfone versus polyacrylonitrile. *In* Bosch J, Stein J (eds): Hemodialysis: High Efficiency Treatments. New York, Churchill Livingstone, 1993, pp 63-77.
13. Streicher E, Schneider H: The development of a polysulfone membrane. Contrib Nephrol 1985; 46:1-13.
14. Göhl H, Buck R, Strathmann H: Basic features of the polyamide membranes. Contrib Nephrol 1992; 96:1-25.
15. Radovich J: Composition of polymer membranes for therapies of end-stage renal disease. Contrib Nephrol 1995; 113:11-24.
16. Bonomini V, Berland Y: Dialysis membranes: Structure and predictions. Contrib Nephrol 1995; 113:1-135.
17. Modi GK, Pereira BJG, Jaber BLJ: Hemodialysis in acute renal failure: Does the membrane matter? Semin Dial 2001; 14(5):318-321.
18. Muller-Eberhard H: Complement: Chemistry and pathways. *In* Gallin J, Goldstein I, Snyderman R (eds): Inflammation. New York, Raven Press, 1988, pp 21-54.
19. Chenoweth DE, Cheung AK, Henderson LW: Anaphylatoxin formation during hemodialysis: Effects of different dialyzer membranes. Kidney Int 1983; 24:764-769.
20. Craddock P, Fehr J, Dalmasso A: Hemodialysis leukopenia: Pulmonary vascular leukostasis resulting from complement activation by dialyzer cellophane membranes. J Clin Invest 1977; 59:879-888.
21. Cheung A, Parker C, Janatova J: Analysis of the complement C3 fragments associated with hemodialysis membranes. Kidney Int 1989; 35:576-588.

22. Cheung A, Parker C, Wilcox L: Activation of the alternative pathway of complement by hemodialysis membranes. Kidney Int 1989; 36:257-265.
23. Fearon D, Wong W: Complement ligand-receptor interactons that mediate biological responses. Ann Rev Immunol 1983; 1:243-271.
24. Cheung AK, Hohnholt M, Gilson J: Adherence of neutrophils to hemodialysis membranes: Role of complement receptors. Kidney Int 1991; 40:1123-1133.
25. Cheung A, Paker C, Hohnholt M: B_2 integrins are required for neutrophil degranulation induced by hemodialysis membranes. Kidney Int 1993; 43:649-660.
26. Lepow I, Willms-Kretschmer K, Patrick R: Gross and ultrastructural observations on lesions produced by intradermal injection of human C3a in man. Am J Pathol 1970; 61:13-24.
27. Johnson A, Hugli T, Mulloer-Eberhard H: Release of histamine from mast cells by the complement peptides C3a and C5a. Immunology 1975; 28:1067-1080.
28. Cochrane C, Muller-Eberhard H: The derivation of two distinct anaphylatoxin activities from the third and fifth components of human complement. J Exp Med 1968; 127:371-386.
29. Showell H, Glovsky M, Ward P: Morphological changes in human polymorphonuclear leukocytes induced by Ca3 in the presence and absence of cytochalasin. Int Arch Allergy Appl Immunol 1982; 69:62-67.
30. del Balzo U, Levi R, Polley M: Cardiac dysfunction caused by purified human C3a anaphylatoxin. Proc Natl Acad Sci 1985; 82:886-890.
31. Craddock P, Hammerschmidt D, White J: Complement (C5a)-induced granulocyte aggregation in vitro. J Clin Invest 1977; 60:260-264.
32. Hammerschmidt D, Harris P, Wayland J: Complement-induced granulocyte aggregation in vivo. Am J Pathol 1981; 102:146-150.
33. Yancey K, Hammer C, Harvath L: Studies of human C5a as a mediator of inflammation in normal human skin. J Clin Invest 1985; 75:486-495.
34. Camussi G, Pacitti A, Tetta C: Mechanisms of neutropenia in hemodialysis. Trans Am Soc Artif Intern Organs 1984; 30:364-368.
35. Sacks T, Moldow C, Craddock P: Oxygen radicals mediate endothelial cell damage by complement-stimulated granulocytes. J Clin Invest 1978; 61:1161-1167.
36. Goldstein I, Brai M, Osler A: Lysosomal enzyme release from human leukocytes: Mediation by the alternative pathway of complement activation. J Immunol 1973; 111:33-37.
37. Wright D, Gallin J: Secretory responses of human neutrophils: Exocytosis of specific (secondary) granules by human neutrophils during adherence in vitro and during exudation in vivo. J Immunol 1979; 123:285-294.
38. Arnaout M, Hakim RM, Todd RF, et al: Increased expression of an adhesion-promoting surface glycoprotein in the granulocytopenia of hemodialysis. N Engl J Med 1985; 312:457-462.
39. Zaoui P, Stone W, Hakim R: Effects of dialysis membranes on beta 2-microglobulin production and cellular expression. Kidney Int 1990; 38:962-968.
40. Stimler N, Bach M, Bloor C: Release of leukotrienes from guinea pig lung stimulated by C5ades Arg anaphylatoxin. J Immunol 1982; 128:2247-2252.
41. Bokisch V, Muller-Eberhard H: Anaphylatoxin inactivator of human plasma: Its isolation and characterization as a carboxypeptidase. J Clin Invest 1970; 49:2427-2436.
42. Gerard C, Hugli T: Identification of classical anaphylatoxin as the des-Arg form of the C5a molecule: Evidence of a modulator role for the oligosaccharide unit in human des-Arg C5a. Proc Natl Acad Sci 1981; 78:1833-1837.
43. Hugli T: The structural basis for anaphylatoxin and chemotactic functions of C3a, C4a, and C5a. Crit Rev Immunol 1981; 2:321-366.
44. Deppisch R, Schmitt V, Bommer J, et al: Fluid phase generation of terminal complement complex as a novel index of bioincompatibility. Kidney Int 1990; 37:696-706.
45. Cheung A, Lemke H: Criteria and standardization for biocompatibility. Nephrol Dial Transplant 1994; 9(suppl 2):72-76.
46. Varela M, Kimmel P, Phillips T, et al: Biocompatibility of hemodialysis membranes: Interrelations between plasma complement and cytokine levels. Blood Purif 2001; 19:370-379.
47. Falkenhagen D, Mitzner S, Stange J, Klinkmann H: Biocompatibility: Methodology and evaluation. Contrib Nephrol 1993; 103:34-54.
48. Chenoweth DE, Cheung AK, Ward DM, Henderson LW: Anaphylatoxin formation during hemodialysis: A comparison of new and re-used dialyzers. Kidney Int 1983; 24:770-774.
49. Bhakdi S, Fassbender W, Hugo F: Relative efficiency of terminal complement activation. J Immunol 1988; 141:3117-3122.
50. Ivanovich P, Chenoweth D, Schmidt Rea: Symptoms and activation of granulocytes and complement with two dialysis membranes. Kidney Int 1983; 24:758-763.
51. Hakim R, Fearon D, Lazarus J: Biocompatibility of dialysis membranes: Effects of chronic complement activation. Kidney Int 1984; 26:194-200.
52. Smeby L, Wideroe T, Balstad T, Jorstad S: Biocompatibility aspects of cellophane, cellulose acetate, polyacrylonitrile, polysulfone and polycarbonate hemodialyzers. Blood Purif 1986; 4:93-101.
53. Maggiore Q, Enia G, Catalano C: Effect of blood cooling on cuprophan-induced anaphylatoxin generation. Kidney Int 1987; 32:908-911.
54. MacDougall M, Diedrich D, Wiegmann T: Dissociation of hemodialysis leukopenia and hypoxemia from complement changes during citrate anticoagulation. Kidney Int 1985; 27:166(A).
55. Cheung A, Faezi-Jenkin B, Leypoldt J: Effect of thrombosis on complement activation and neutrophil degranulation during in vitro hemodialysis. J Am Soc Nephrol 1994; 5:110-115.
56. Dumler F, Zasuwa G, Levin N: Effect of dialyzer reprocessing methods on complement activation and hemodialyzer-related symptoms. Artif Organs 1987; 11:128-131.
57. Craddock P, Fehr J, Brigham K: Complement and leukocyte-mediated pulmonary dysfunction in hemodialysis. N Engl J Med 1977; 296:769-774.
58. Lemke H, Eisenhauer T, Krieter D: Generation of bradykinin, hypotension and anaphylactoid shock during hemodialysis. J Am Soc Nephrol 1993; 4:362(A).
59. Walker J, Lindsay R, Peters S: A sheep model to examine the cardiopulmonary manifestations of blood-dialyzer interactions. Am Soc Artif Intern Organs 1983; 6:123-130.
60. Walker J, Lindsay R, Sibbald W: Acute pulmonary hypertension, leukopenia and hypoxia in early hemodialysis. Proc Eur Dial Transplant Assoc 1984; 21:135-142.
61. Cheung A, LeWinter M, Chenoweth D: Cardiopulmonary effects of cuprophan-activated plasma in the swine: Role of complement activation products. Kidney Int 1986; 29:799-806.
62. Cheung A, Baranowski R, Wayman A: The role of thromboxane in cuprophan-induced pulmonary hypertension. Kidney Int 1987; 31:1072-1079.
63. Cheung A, Parker C, Wilcox L: Effects of two types of cobra venom factor on porcine complement activation and pulmonary artery pressure. 1989; 78:299-306.
64. Schulman G, Hakim R, Arias R, et al: Bradykinin generation by dialysis membranes: Possible role in anaphylactic reaction. J Am Soc Nephrol 1993; 3:1563-1569.
65. Lemke H, Fink E: Accumulation of bradykinin generation formed by the AN69- or PAN 17DX-membrane is due to the presence of an ACE-inhibitor in vitro. J Am Soc Nephrol 1992; 3:376(A).

66. Schohn D, Jahn H, Eber M: Biocompatibility and hemodynamic studies during polycarbonate versus cuprophan membrane dialysis. Blood Purif 1986; 4:102-111.
67. McCormick J, Kreutzer D, Keating H: Alterations in activities of anaphylatoxin inactivator and chemotactic factor inactivator during hemodialysis. Am J Pathol 1982; 109:282-287.
68. Schindler R, Gelfand J, Dinarello C: Recombitant C5a stimulates transcription rather than translation of IL-1 and TNF: Priming of mononuclear cells with recombinant C5a enhances cytokine synthesis induced by LPS, IL-1 or PMA. Blood 1990; 76:1631-1635.
69. Cheung A, Parker C, Hohnholt M: Inhibition of complement activation on hemodialysis (HD) membranes by soluble complement receptor type I (sCR1). J Am Soc Nephrol 1993; 3:340(A).
70. Kim S: Platelet adhesion and prevention at blood-polymer interface. Artif Organs 1987; 11:228-236.
71. Marshall J, Ahearn D, Nothum R: Adherence of blood components to dialyzer membranes: Morphological studies. Nephron 1974; 12:157-170.
72. Vroman L, Adams A, Klings M: Interactions among human blood proteins at interfaces. Fed Proc 1971; 30:1494-1502.
73. Salzman E: Role of platelets in blood-surface interactions. Fed Proc 1971; 30:1503-1508.
74. Kozin F, Cochrane C: The contact activation system of plasma: Biochemistry and pathophysiology. *In* Gallin J, Goldstein I, Snyderman R (eds): Inflammation: Basic Principles and Clinical Correlates. New York, Raven Press, 1988, pp 101-120.
75. Colman R, Hirsh J, Marder V, Salzman E (eds): Hemostasis and Thrombosis: Basic Principles and Clinical Practice. Philadelphia, JB Lippincott, 1987.
76. Tielemans C, Goldman M, Vanherweghem J: Immediate hypersensitivity reactions and hemodialysis. Adv Nephrol 1993; 22:401-416.
77. Mohammed S, Whitworth C, Chuang H: Multiple active forms of thrombin: Binding to platelets and effects on platelet function. Proc Natl Acad Sci U S A 1976; 73:1660-1663.
78. Vaziri N, Toohey J, Paule P: Effect of hemodialysis on contact group of coagulation factors, platelets, and leukocytes. Am J Med 1984; 77:437-441.
79. Gasparotto M, Bertoli M, Vertolli U: Biocompatibility of various dialysis membranes as assessed by coagulation assay. Contrib Nephrol 1984; 37:96-100.
80. Wilhelmson S, Asaba H, Gunnarsson B: Measurement of fibrinopeptide A in the evaluation of heparin activity and fibrin formation during hemodialysis. Clin Nephrol 1981; 15:252-258.
81. Wilhelmson S, Ivemark C, Kudryk B: Thrombin activity during hemodialysis: Evaluated by the fibrinopeptide A assay: A comparison between a high and a low heparin dose regimen. Thromb Res 1983; 31:685-693.
82. Lane D, Ireland H, Knight I: The significance of fibrinogen derivatives in plasma in human renal failure. Br J Haematol 1984; 56:251-260.
83. Lindsay R: Practical use of anticoagulant. *In* Drukker W, Parsons F, Maher J (eds): Replacement of Renal Function by Dialysis. Boston, Martinus Nijhoff, 1983, pp 201-222.
84. Speiser W, Wojta J, Korninger C: Enhanced fibrinolysis caused by tissue plasminogen activator release in hemodialysis. Kidney Int 1987; 32:280-283.
85. Sreeharan N, Crow M, Salter M: Membrane effect on platelet function during hemodialysis: A comparison of cuprophan and polycarbonate. Artif Organs 1982; 6:324-327.
86. Lindsay R, Prentice C, Ferguson D: Reduction of thrombus formation on dialyzer membranes by aspirin and RA 233. Lancet 1972; 2(7790):1287-1290.
87. Salter M, Crow M, Donaldson D: Prevention of platelet deposition and thrombus formation on hemodialysis membranes: A double-blind randomized trial of aspirin and dipyridamole. Artif Organs 1984; 8:57-61.
88. Zusman R, Rubin R, Cato A: Hemodialysis using prostacyclin instead of heparin as the sole antithrombotic agent. N Engl J Med 1981; 304:934-939.
89. Smith M, Danviriyasup K, Crow J: Prostacyclin substitution for heparin in long-term hemodialysis. Am J Med 1982; 73:669-678.
90. Caruana R, Smith M, Clyne D: A controlled study of heparin versus epoprostenol sodium (prostacyclin) as the sole anticoagulant for chronic hemodialysis. Blood Purif 1991; 9:296-304.
91. Kaplan K, Owen J: Plasma levels of B-thromboglobulin and platelet factor 4 as indices of platelet activation in vivo. Blood 1981; 57:199-202.
92. Dawes J, Smith R, Pepper D: The release, distributions, and clearance of human B-thromboglobulin and platelet factor 4. Thromb Res 1978; 12:851-861.
93. Nath N, Niewiarowski S, Joist J: Platelet factor 4: Antiheparin protein releasable from platelets: Purification and properties. J Lab Clin Med 1973; 82:754-768.
94. Ireland H, Lane D, Curtis J: Objective assessment of heparin requirements for hemodialysis in human. J Lab Clin Med 1984; 103:643-652.
95. Green D, Santhanam S, Krumlovsky F: Elevated B-thromboglobulin in patients with chronic renal failure. J Lab Clin Med 1980; 95:679-685.
96. Camussi G, Segoloni G, Rotunno M: Mechanisms involved in acute granulocytopenia in hemodialysis: Cell-membrane direct interactions. Int J Artif Organs 1978; 3:123-127.
97. Hakim R, Schafer A: Hemodialysis-associated platelet activation and thrombocytopenia. Am J Med 1985; 78:575-580.
98. Adler A, Berlyne G: B-thromboglobulin and platelet factor-4 levels during hemodialysis with polyacrylonitrile. Am Soc Artif Intern Organs 1981; 4:100-102.
99. Iatrou C, Afentakis N, Antonopoulou S, et al: The production of platelet-activating factor (PAF) during hemodialysis with cuprophane membrane. Does the calcium concentration in the dialysate play any role on it? Int J Artif Organs 1995; 18:355-361.
100. Iatrou C, Afentakis N, Nomikos T, et al: Is platelet-activating factor produced during hemodialysis with AN-69 polyacrylonitrile membrane? Nephron 2002; 91:86-93.
101. Kuragano T, Kuno T, Takahashi Y, et al: Comparison of the effects of cellulose triacetate and polysulfone membrane on GPIIb/IIIa and platelet activation. Blood Purif 2003; 21:176-182.
102. Silber R, Moldow CF: Biochemistry and function of neutrophils, composition of neutrophils. *In* Williams W, Brutler E, Erslev A, Lichtman F (eds): Hematology. New York, McGraw-Hill, 1983, pp 726-734.
103. Stuard S, Carreno M-P, Poignet J-L, et al: A major role for CD62P/CD15s interaction in leukocyte margination during hemodialysis. Kidney Int 1995; 48:93-102.
104. Ashman N, Macey M, Fan S, et al: Increased platelet-monocyte aggregates and cardiovascular disease in end-stage renal failure patients. Nephrol Dial Transplant 2003; 18:2088-2096.
105. Docci D, Turci F, Delvecchio C: Hemodialysis-associated platelet loss: Study of the relative contribution of dialyzer membrane composition and geometry. Int J Artif Organs 1984; 7:337-340.
106. Vicks S, Gross M, Schmitt G: Massive hemorrhage due to hemodialysis-associated thrombocytopenia. Am J Nephrol 1983; 3:30-33.
107. Pavlopoulou G, Perzanowski C, Hakim R: Platelet aggregation studies during dialysis. Kidney Int 1986; 29:221(A).

108. Mingardi G, Vigano G, Massazza M: Polyacrylonitrile membranes for hemodialysis: Long-term effect on primary hemostatis. *In* Smeby L, Jorstad S, Wideroe T (eds): Immune and Metabolic Aspects of Therapeutic Blood Purification Systems., Karger, Basel, 1985.
109. Simon P, Ang K, Cam G: Enhanced platelet aggregation and membrane biocompatibility: Possible influence on thrombosis and embolism in hemodialysis patients. Nephron 1987; 45:172-173.
110. Eschbach J: Hematologic problems of dialysis patients. *In* Drukker W, Parsons F, Maher J (eds): Replacement of Renal Function by Dialysis. Boston, Martinus Nijhoff, 1983, pp 630-645.
111. Blackshear P, Droman F, Steinbach J: Some mechanical effects that influence hemodialysis. Trans Am Soc Artif Intern Organs 1965; 11:112-117.
112. Gault M, Duffett S, Purchase L, Murphy J: Hemodialysis intravascular hemolysis and kinked blood lines. Nephron 1992; 62:267-271.
113. Sweet S, McCarthy S, Steingart R, Callahan T: Hemolytic reactions mechanically induced by kinked hemodialysis lines. Am J Kidney Dis 1996; 27:262-266.
114. Fassbinder W, Pilar J, Scheuermann E: Formaldehyde and the occurrence of anti-N-like cold agglutinins in RDT patients. Proc Eur Dial Transplant Assoc 1976; 13:333-338.
115. Harrison P, Jansson K, Kronenberg H: Cold agglutinin formation in patients undergoing hemodialysis: A possible relationship to dialyzer reuse. Aust N Z J Med 1975; 5:195-197.
116. Lewis K, Dewar P, Ward M: Formation of anti-N-like antibodies in dialysis patients: Effect of different methods of dialyzer rinsing remove formaldehyde. Clin Nephrol 1981; 15:39-43.
117. Salama A, Hugo F, Heinrick D: Deposition of terminal C5b-9 complement complexes on erythrocytes and leukocytes during cardiopulmonary bypass. N Engl J Med 1988; 318:408-414.
118. Kaplow L, Goffinet J: Profound neutropenia during the early phase of hemodialysis. JAMA 1968; 203:1135-1137.
119. Sato H, Ohkubo M, Nagaoka T: Levels of serum colony-stimulating factors (CSFs) in patients on long-term haemodialysis. Cytokine 1994; 6:187-194.
120. Mason R, Zucker W, Bilinsky R: Blood components deposited on used and reused dialysis membranes. Biomater Med Devices Artif Organs 1976; 4:333-358.
121. Dodd N, Gordge M, Tarrant J: A demonstration of neutrophil accumulation in the pulmonary vasculature during hemodialysis. Proc Eur Transplant Assoc 1983; 20:186-189.
122. Horl W, Riegel W, Schollmeyer P: Different complement and granulocyte activation in patients dialyzed with PMMA dialyzers. Clin Nephrol 1986; 25:304-307.
123. Horl W, Schaefer R, Heidland A: Effect of different dialyzers on proteinases and proteinase inhibitors during hemodialysis. Am J Nephrol 1985; 5:320-326.
124. Horl W, Steinhauer H, Riegel W: Effect of different dialyzer membranes on plasma levels of granulocyte elastase. Kidney Int 1988; 33(suppl):S90-S91.
125. Deppisch R, Betz M, Hansch G, et al: Biocompatibility of the polyamide membranes. Contrib Nephrol 1992; 96:26-46.
126. Schaefer R, Heidland A, Horl W: Effect of dialyzer geometry on granulocyte and complement activation. Am J Nephrol 1987; 7:121-126.
127. Heidland A, Horl W, Heller N: Proteolytic enzymes and catabolism: Enhanced release of granulocyte proteinase in uremic intoxication and during hemodialysis. Kidney Int 1983; 24(suppl):S27-S36.
128. Horl W, Heidland A: Evidence for the participation of granulocyte proteinases on intradialytic catabolism. Clin Nephrol 1984; 21:314-322.
129. Himmelfarb J, Ault K, Holbrook D: Intradialytic granulocyte reactive oxygen species production: A prospective, crossover trial. J Am Soc Nephrol 1993; 4:178-186.
130. Maher E, Wickens D, Griffin J: Increased free-radical activity during hemodialysis. Nephrol Dial Transplant 1987; 2:169-171.
131. Till G, Johnson K, Kunke R: Intravascular activation of complement and acute lung injury. J Clin Invest 1982; 69:1126-1135.
132. Schulman G, Fogo A, Gung A, et al: Complement activation retards resolution of acute ischemic renal failure in the rat. Kidney Int 1991; 40:1069-1074.
133. Klempner M, Gallin J, Balow J: The effect of hemodialysis and C5a des arg on neutrophil subpopulations. Blood 1980; 55:777-783.
134. Spagnuolo P, Bass J, Smith M: Neutrophil adhesiveness during prostacyclin and heparin hemodialysis. Blood 1982; 60:924-929.
135. Cohen MS, Elliott DM, Chaplinski T, et al: A defect in the oxidative metabolism of human polymorphonuclear leukocytes that remain in circulation early in hemodialysis. Blood 1982; 60:1283.
136. Wissow L, Covenberg R, Burns R: Altered leukocyte chemiluminescence during dialysis. J Clin Immunol 1981; 1:262-265.
137. Henderson LW, Miller ME, Hamilton RW, Norman ME: Hemodialysis leukopenia and polymorph random mobility?a possible correlation. J Lab Clin Med 1975; 85:191-197 .
138. Vanholder R, Ringoir S, Dhondt A, Hakim R: Phagocytosis in uremic and hemodialysis patients: A prospective and cross sectional study. Kidney Int 1991; 39:320-327.
139. Jaber BL, Cendoroglo M, Balakrishnan VS, et al: Apoptosis of leukocytes: Basic concepts and implications in uremia. Kidney Int 2001; 59(suppl 78):S197-S205.
140. Colotta F, Re F, Polentarutti N, et al: Modulation of granulocyte survival and programmed cell death by cytokines and bacterial products. Blood 1992; 80:2012-2020.
141. Lee A, Whyte MKB, Haslett C: Inhibition of apoptosis and prolongation of neutrophil functional longevity by inflammatory mediators. J Leukoc Biol 1993; 54:283-288.
142. Liles WC, Klebanoff SJ: Regulation of apoptosis in neutrophils: Fast track to death? J Immunol 1995; 155:3289-3291.
143. Perianayagam MC, Balakrishnan VS, King AJ, et al: C5a delays apoptosis of human neutrophils by a phosphatidyl inositol 3-kinase-signaling pathway. Kidney Int 2002; 61:456-463.
144. Jaber BL, Balakrishnan VS, Cendoroglo M, et al: Apoptosis-inducing activity of uremic plasma during hemodialysis. Blood Purif 1999; 16:325-335.
145. Carracedo J, Ramirez R, Martin-Malo A, et al: Nonbiocompatible hemodialysis membranes induce apoptosis in mononuclear cells: The role of G-proteins. J Am Soc Nephrol 1998; 9:46-53.
146. Needleman B, Weiler J, Feldbush T: The third component of complement inhibits human lymphocyte blastogenesis. J Immunol 1981; 126:1586-1591.
147. Hobbs M, Feldbush T, Needleman B: Inhibition of secondary in vitro antibody responses by the third component of complement. J Immunol 1981; 128:1470-1475.
148. Greene W, Bohaleim E, Siekavitz M: Structure and regulation of the human IL-2 receptor. Adv Exp Med Biol 1989; 254:55-60.
149. Zaoui P, Green W, Hakim R: Hemodialysis with cuprophane membrane modulates interleukin-2 receptor expression. Kidney Int 1991; 39:1020-1026.
150. Meuer SC, Hauer M, Kurz P, et al: Selective blockade of the antigen-receptor-mediated pathway of T cell activation in patients with impaired primary immune responses. J Clin Invest 1987; 80:743-749.
151. Zaoui P, Hakim R: Natural killer-cell function in hemodialysis patients. Kidney Int 1993; 43:1298-1305.
152. Kay N, Raij L: Differential effect of hemodialysis membranes on human lymphocyte natural killer function. Artif Organs 1987; 11:165-167.
153. Kay N, Raij L: Immune abnormalities in renal failure in hemodialysis. Blood Purif 1986; 4:120-129.
154. Port F, Ragheb N, Schwartz A: Neoplasms in dialysis patients: A population-based study. Am J Kidney Dis 1989; 14:119-123.

155. Lindner A, Farewell B, Sherrard D: High incidence of neoplasia in uremic patients receiving long term dialysis. Nephron 1981; 27:292-296.
156. Descamps-Latscha B, Herbelin A, Nguyen AT, et al: Soluble CD23 as an effector of immune dysregulation in chronic uremia and dialysis. Kidney Int 1993; 43:878-884.
157. Dinarello CA: Interleukin-1 and interleukin-1 antagonism. Blood 1991; 77:1627-1652.
158. Dinarello C: Cytokines: Agents provocateurs in hemodialysis? Kidney Int 1992; 41:683-694.
159. Dinarello C: Interleukin-1 and tumor necrosis factor and their naturally occurring antagonists during hemodialysis. Kidney Int 1992; 42(suppl 38):S68-S77 .
160. Vilcek J, Le J: Immunology of cytokines: An introduction. *In* Thomson A (ed): The Cytokine Handbook. San Diego, Academic Press, 1991, pp 1-17.
161. Henderson LW, Koch KM, Dinarello CA, Shaldon S: Hemodialysis hypotension: The interleukin-1 hypothesis. Blood Purif 1983; 1:3-8.
162. Pereira BJ, Dinarello CA: Production of cytokines and cytokine inhibitory proteins in patients on dialysis. Nephrol Dial Transplant 1994; 9:60-71.
163. Lonnemann G, Bingel M, Koch KM, et al: Plasma interleukin-1 activity in humans undergoing hemodialysis with regenerated cellulosic membranes. Lymphokine Res 1987; 6:63-70.
164. Luger A, Kovarik J, Stummvoll HK, et al: Blood-membrane interaction in hemodialysis leads to increased cytokine production. Kidney Int 1987; 32:84-88.
165. Bingel M, Lonnemann G, Koch KM, et al: Plasma interleukin-1 activity during hemodialysis: The influence of dialysis membranes. Nephron 1988; 50:273-276.
166. Descamps-Latscha B, Herbelin A, Nguyen AT, et al: Haemodialysis-membrane-induced phagocyte oxidative metabolism activation and interleukin-1 production. Life Supp Sys 1986; 4:349-353.
167. Herbelin A, Nguyen AT, Zingraff J, et al: Influence of uremia and hemodialysis on circulating interleukin-1 and tumor necrosis factor alpha. Kidney Int 1990; 37:116-125.
168. Pereira BJG, King AJ, Falagas ME, et al: Plasma levels of IL-1 , TNFα and their specific inhibitors in undialyzed chronic renal failure. Kidney Int 1994; 45:890-896.
169. Ghysen J, De Plaen JF, van Ypersele de Strihou C: The effect of membrane characteristics on tumour necrosis factor kinetics during haemodialysis. Nephrol Dial Transplant 1990; 5:270-274.
170. Canivet E, Lavaud S, Wong T, et al: Cuprophane but not synthetic membrane induces increases in serum tumor necrosis factor-alpha. Am J Kidney Dis 1994; 23:41-46.
171. Holmes C, Evans R, Ross D, Frankamp P: Plasma IL-1 and TNF levels during high-flux hemodialysis with cellulose triacetate membranes. Kidney Int 1990; 37:301.
172. Powell A, Bland L, Oettinger C, et al: Lack of plasma interleukin-1 beta or tumor necrosis factor-alpha elevation during unfavorable hemodialysis conditions. J Am Soc Nephrol 1991; 2:1007-1013.
173. Davenport A, Crabtree J, Androjna C, et al: Tumour necrosis factor does not increase during routine cuprophane haemodialysis in healthy. Nephrol Dial Transplant 1991; 6:435-439.
174. Pereira BJ, Shapiro L, King AJ, et al: Plasma levels of IL-1 beta, TNF alpha and their specific inhibitors in undialyzed chronic renal failure, CAPD and hemodialysis patients. Kidney Int 1994; 45:890-896.
175. Herbelin A, Urena P, Nguyen A, et al: Elevated circulating levels of interleukin-6 in patients with chronic renal failure. Kidney Int 1991; 39:954-960.
176. Descamps-Latscha B, Herbelin A, Nguyen AT, et al: Imbalance between pro-inflammatory cytokines and their specific inhibitors in chronic renal. J Am Soc Nephrol 1993; 4:343.
177. Cottrell AC, Mehta RL: Cytokine kinetics in septic ARF patients on continuous veno-veno hemodialysis (CVVHD). J Am Soc Nephrol 1992; 3:361.
178. Lonnemann G, Haubitz M, Schindler R: Hemodialysis-associated induction of cytokines. Blood Purif 1990; 8:214-222.
179. Blumenstein M, Schmidt B, Ward RA: Altered interleukin-1 production in patients undergoing hemodialysis. Nephron 1988; 50:277-281.
180. Haeffner-Cavaillon N, Cavaillon JM, Ciancioni C: In vivo induction of interleukin-1 during hemodialysis. Kidney Int 1989; 35:1212-1218.
181. Endres S, Ghorbani R, Lonnemann G, et al: Measurement of immunoreactive interleukin-1 beta from human mononuclear cells: Optimization of recovery, intrasubject consistency and comparison with interleukin-1 alpha and tumor necrosis factor. Clin Immunol Immunopathol 1988; 49:424-438.
182. Endres S, Cannon JG, Ghorbani R, et al: In vitro production of IL-1beta, Il-1alpha, TNF, and IL-2 in healthy subjects: Distribution, effect of cyclooxygenase inhibition and evidence of independent gene regulation. Eur J Immunol 1989; 19:2327-2333.
183. Memoli B, Rampino T, Libetta C, et al: Peripheral blood leukocytes interleukin-6 production in uremic hemodialyzed patients (Abstract). J Am Soc Nephrol 1990; 1:369.
184. Ryan J, Beynon H, Rees AJ, Cassidy MJ: Evaluation of the in vitro production of tumour necrosis factor by monocytes in dialysis patients. Blood Purif 1991; 9:142-147.
185. Oettinger CW, Powell AC, Bland LA, et al: Enhanced release of tumor necrosis factor alpha but not interleukin-1 beta by uremic blood stimulated with endotoxin (Abstract). J Am Soc Nephrol 1990; 1:370.
186. Schindler R, Lonnemann G, Shaldon S, et al: Transcription, not synthesis, of interleukin-1 and tumor necrosis factor by complement. Kidney Int 1990; 37:85-93.
187. Urena P, Gogusev J, Valdovinos R, et al: Transcriptional induction of TNF-alpha in uremic patients undergoing hemodialysis (Abstract). J Am Soc Nephrol 1990; 1:380.
188. Schindler R, Linnenweber S, Shulze M, et al: Gene expression of interleukin-1b during hemodialysis. Kidney Int 1993; 43:712-721.
189. Pereira BJ, Dinarello CA: Role of cytokines in patients on dialysis. Int J Artif Organs 1995; 18:293-304.
190. Peterson J, Hyver S, Cajias J: Backfiltration during dialysis. Semin Dial 1992; 5:13-16.
191. Baurmeister U, Vienken J, Daum V: High-flux dialysis membranes: Endotoxin transfer by backfiltration can be a problem. Nephrol Dial Transplant 1989; 4(suppl 3):89-93.
192. Donahue PR: Dialyzer permeability alteration by reuse. J Am Soc Nephrol 1992; 3:363.
193. Graeber CW, Halley SE, Lapkin RA, et al: Protein losses with reused dialyzers. J Am Soc Nephrol 1993; 4:349.
194. Tokars JI, Alter MJ, Favero MS, et al: National surveillance of hemodialysis associated diseases in the United States. ASAIO J 1990; 39:71-80.
195. Pegues D, Oettinger C, Bland L, et al: A prospective study of pyrogenic reactions in hemodialysis patients using bicarbonate dialysis fluids filtered to remove bacteria and endotoxin. J Am Soc Nephrol 1992; 3:1002-1007.
196. Pereira BJG, Snodgrass BR, Hogan PJ, King AJ: Diffusive and convective transfer of cytokine-inducing bacterial products across hemodialysis membranes. Kidney Int 1995; 47:603-610.
197. Bingel M, Lonnemann G, Shaldon S, et al: Human interleukin-1 production during hemodialysis. Nephron 1986; 43:161-163.
198. Lonnemann G, Binge M, Floege J, et al: Detection of endotoxin-like interleukin-1-inducing activity during in vitro dialysis. Kidney Int 1988; 33:29-35.
199. Lonnemann G, Behme TC, Lenzner B, et al: Permeability of dialyzer membranes to TNF alpha-inducing substances derived from water bacteria. Kidney Int 1992; 42:61-68.

200. Evans RC, Holmes CJ: In vitro study of the transfer of cytokine-inducing substances across selected high-flux hemodialysis. Blood Purif 1991; 9:92-101.
201. Urena P, Herbelin A, Zingraff J, et al: Permeability of cellulosic and non-cellulosic membranes to endotoxins and cytokine production. Nephrol Dial Transplant 1992; 7:16-28.
202. Lonnemann G, Mahiout A, Schindler R, Colton CK: Pyrogen retention by the polyamide membranes. *In* Shaldon S, Koch KM (eds): The Polyamide Membrane. Contrib Nephrol Karger, Basel, 1992; 96:47-63.
203. Okusawa S, Gelfand JA, Ikejima T, et al: Interleukin 1 induces a shock-like state in rabbits: Synergism with tumor necrosis factor and the effect of cyclooxygenase inhibition. J Clin Invest 1988; 81:1162-1172.
204. Raz A, Wyche A, Siegel N, Needleman P: Regulation of fibroblast cyclooxygenase synthesis by interleukin-1. J Biol Chem 1988; 263:3022-3028.
205. Cominelli F, Nast CC, Dinarello CA, et al: Regulation of eicosanoid production in rabbit colon by interleukin-1. Gastroenterology 1989; 97:1400-1405.
206. Schweizer A, Feige U, Fontana A, et al: Interleukin-1 enhances pain reflexes. Mediation through increased prostaglandin E2 levels. Agents Actions 1988; 25:246-251.
207. Ohashi K, Hara M, Kawai R, et al: Cervical discs are most susceptible to beta 2-microglobulin amyloid deposition in the vertebral column. Kidney Int 1992; 41:1646-1652.
208. Zaoui P, Hakim R: The effects of dialysis membrane on cytokine release. J Am Soc Nephrol 1994; 4:1711-1718.
209. DeBacker W, Verpooten G, Borgonjon D: Hypoxemia during hemodialysis: Effects of different membranes and dialysate compositions. Kidney Int 1983; 23:738-743.
210. Hakim R, Lowrie E: Hemodialysis-associated neutropenia and hypoxemia: The effect of dialyzer membrane materials. Nephron 1982; 32:32-39.
211. Dolan M, Whipp B, Davidson W: Hypopnea associated with acetate hemodialysis: Carbon-dioxide-flow dependent ventilation. N Engl J Med 1981; 305:72-75.
212. Oh M, Uribarri J, Del Monte ML, et al: A mechanism of hypoxemia during hemodialysis. Am J Nephrol 1985; 5:366-371.
213. Jones R, Broadfield J, Parsons V: Arterial hypoxemia during hemodialysis for acute renal failure in mechanically ventilated patients: Observations and mechanisms. Clin Nephrol 1980; 14:18-22.
214. Mahajan S, Gardiner H, DeTar B, et al: Relationship between pulmonary functions and hemodialysis induced leukopenia. Trans Am Soc Artif Intern Organs 1977; 23:411-415.
215. Graf H, Stummvoll H, Haber P: Pathophysiology of dialysis related hypoxaemia. Proc Eur Dial Transplant Assoc 1980; 17:155-161.
216. Morrison J, Wilson A, Vaziri N: Determination of pulmonary tissue volume, pulmonary capillary blood flow and diffusing capacity lung before and after hemodialysis. Int J Artif Organs 1980; 3:259-262.
217. Abu-Hamdan D, Desai S, Mahajan S: Hypoxemia during hemodialysis using acetate versus bicarbonate dialysate. 1984; 4:248-253.
218. Fawcett S, Hoenich N, Laker M: Hemodialysis-induced respiratory changes. Nephrol Dial Transplant 1987; 2:161-168.
219. Vaziri N, Barton C, Warner A: Comparision of four dialyzer-dialysate combinations: Effects on blood gases, cell counts, complement contact factors and fibrinolytic system. Contrib Nephrol 1984; 37:111-119.
220. Vanholder R, Pauwels R, Vandenbogaerde JF, et al: Cuprophan reuse and intradialytic changes of lung diffusion capacity and blood gases. Kidney Int 1987; 32:117-122.
221. Bergstrom J, Danielsson S, Freychuss U: Dialysis, ultrafiltration and shamdialysis in normal subjects. Kidney Int 1984; 27:157(A).
222. Agar J, Hull J, Kaplan M: Acute cardiopulmonary decompensation and complement activation during hemodialysis. Ann Intern Med 1979; 90:792-793.
223. Stimler-Gerard N: Immunopharmacology of anaphylatoxin-induced bronchoconstrictor responses. Complement 1986; 3:137-151.
224. Henderson L, Cheung A, Chenoweth D: Choosing a membrane. Am J Kidney Dis 1983; 3:5-20.
225. Foley R, Reeves W: Acute anaphylactoid reactions in hemodialysis. Am J Kidney Dis 1985; 5:132-135.
226. Ogden D: New-dialyzer syndrome. N Engl J Med 1980; 302:1262-1263.
227. Rault R, Silver M: Severe reactions during hemodialysis. Am J Kidney Dis 1985; 5:128-131.
228. Caruana R, Hamilton R, Pearson F: Dialyzer hypersensitivity syndrome: Possible role of allergy to ethylene oxide. Am J Nephrol 1985; 5:271-274.
229. Key J, Nahmias M, Acchiardo S: Hypersensitivity reactions on first-time exposure to cuprophan hollow fiber dialyzer. Am J Kidney Dis 1983; 2:664-666.
230. Popli S, Ing T, Daugirdas J: Severe reactions to cuprophan capillary dialyzers. Artif Organs 1982; 6:312-315.
231. Hakim R, Breilatt J, Lazarus J: Complement activation and hypersensitivity reactions to dialysis membranes. N Engl J Med 1984; 311:878-882.
232. Gutch C, Eskelson C, Ziegler E: 2-Chloroethanol as a toxic residue in dialysis supplies sterlized with ethylene oxide. Dial Transplant 1976; 5:21-25.
233. Villarroel F, Ciarkowski A: A survey on hypersensitivity reactions in hemodialysis. Artif Organs 1985; 9:231-238.
234. Ing T, Daugirdas J, Popli S: First-use syndrome with cuprammonium cellulose dialyzers. Int J Artif Organs 1983; 6:235-239.
235. Nicholls A, Platts M: Anaphylactoid reactions during hemodialysis are due to ethylene oxide hypersensitivity. Proc Eur Dial Transplant 1984; 121:173-177.
236. Poothullil J, Shimizu A, Day R: Anaphylaxis from the product(s) of ethylene oxide gas. Ann Intern Med 1975; 82:58-60.
237. Gorevic P, Casey T, Stone W: Beta-2 microglobulin is an amyloidogenic protein in man. J Clin Invest 1985; 76:2425-2429.
238. Gejyo F, Yamada T, Odani S, et al: A new form of amyloid protein associated with hemodialysis was identified as β2-microglobulin. Biochem Biophys Res Comm 1985; 129:701-806.
239. Miyaya T, Oda O, Inagi R: B2-microglobulin modified with advanced glycation end products is a major component of hemodialysis-associated amyloidosis. J Clin Invest 1993; 92:1243-1252.
240. Ogawa H, Saito A, Ono M: Novel B2-microglobulin and its amyloidogenic predisposition in patients on hemodialysis. Nephrol Dial Transplant 1989; 4(suppl):14-18.
241. Linke R, Hampl H, Lobeck H: Lysine-specific cleavage of B2-microglobulin in amyloid deposits associated with hemodialysis. Kidney Int 1989; 36:675-681.
242. Floege J, Granolleras C, Koch K: Which membrane? Should beta-2 microglobulin decide on the choice of today's hemodialysis membrane? Nephron 1988; 50:177-181.
243. Ritz E, Bommer J: Beta-2-microglobulin-dervied amyloid-problems and perspectives. Blood Purif 1988; 6:61-68.
244. Floege J, Bartsch A, Schulze M: Clearance and synthesis rates of B2-microglobulin in patients undergoing hemodialysis in normal subjects. J Lab Clin Med 1991; 118:153-165.
245. Vincent C, Chanard J, Caudwell V, et al: Kinetics of 125I-beta 2-microglobulin turnover in dialyzed patients. Kidney Int 1992; 42:1434-1443.
246. Floege J, Granolleras C, Bingel M, et al: B2-microglobulin kinetics during hemodialysis and hemofiltration. Nephrol Dial Transplant 1987; 1:223-228.

247. Jorstad S, Smeby L, Balstad T: Removal, generation and adsorption of beta-2-microglobulin during hemofiltration with five different membranes. Blood Purif 1988; 6:96-105.
248. Paczek L, Schaefer R, Heidland A: Dialysis membranes inhibit in vitro release of beta-2-microglobulin from human lymphocytes. Nephron 1990; 56:267-270.
249. Bjerrum O, Bjerrum O, Borregaard N: B2-microglobulin in neutrophils: An intragranular protein. J Immunol 1987; 138:3913-3917.
250. Bergstrom J, Wehle B: No change in corrected B2-microglobulin concentration after cuprophan hemodialysis. Lancet 1987; 1:629.
251. Floege J, Granolleras C, Merscher S: Is the rise in plasma beta-2-microglobulin seen during hemodialysis meaningful? Nephron 1989; 51:6-12.
252. Klinke B, Rockel A, Perschel W: Beta-2-microglobulin adsorption and release in-vitro: Influence of membrane material, osmolality and heparin. Int J Artif Organs 1988; 11:355-360.
253. Chanard J, Bindi P, Lavaud S: Carpal tunnel syndrome and type of dialysis membrane. Br Med 1989; 298(6677):867-868.
254. van Ypersele de Strihou C, Jadoul M, Malghem J, et al: Effect of dialysis membrane and patient's age on signs of dialysis-related amyloidosis. The Working Party on Dialysis Amyloidosis. Kidney Int 1991; 39:1012-1019.
255. Miura Y, Ishiyama T, Inomata A, et al: Radiolucent bone cysts and the type of dialysis membrane used in patients undergoing long-term hemodialysis. Nephron 1992; 60:268-273.
256. Weiss S, Regiani S: Neutrophils degrade subendothelial matrices in the present of alpha-1-proteinase inhibitor: Cooperative use of lysosomal proteinases and oxygen metabolites. Clin Invest 1984; 73:1297-1303.
257. Baracos V, Rodemann HP, Dinarello CA, Goldberg AL: Stimulation of muscle protein degradation by leukocyte pyrogen (interleukin-1). N Engl J Med 1983; 308:553-558.
258. Gutierrez A, Alvestrand A, Wahren J, Bergstrom J: Effect of in vivo contact between blood and dialysis membranes on protein catabolism in humans. Kidney Int 1990; 38:487-494.
259. Lonnemann G, Koch KM, Shaldon S, Dinarello CA: Studies on the ability of hemodialysis membranes to induce, bind, and clear human interleukin-1. J Lab Clin Med 1988; 112:76-86.
260. Lim V, Bier D, Flanigan M: The effect of hemodialysis on protein metabolism: A leucine kinetic study. J Clin Invest 1993; 91:2419-2436.
261. Parker RA, Himmelfarb J, Tolkoff-Rubin N, et al: Prognosis of patients with acute renal failure requiring dialysis: Results of a multicenter study. Am J Kidney Dis 1998; 32:423-443.
262. Fiaccadori E, Maggiore U, Lombardi M, et al: Predicting patient outcome from acute renal failure comparing three general severity of illness scoring systems. Kidney Int 2000; 58:283-292.
263. Schiffl H, Lang SM, Konig A, et al: Biocompatible membranes in acute renal failure: Prospective case-controlled study. Lancet 1994; 344:570-572.
264. Schiffl H, Sitter T, Lang S, et al: Bioincompatible membranes place patients with acute renal failure at increased risk of infection. ASAIO J 1995; 41:M709-M712.
265. Hakim RM, Wingard RL, Parker RA: Effect of the dialysis membrane in the treatment of patients with acute renal failure. N Engl J Med 1994; 331:1338-1342.
266. Kurtal H, von Herrath D, Schaefer K: Is the choice of membrane important for patients with acute renal failure requiring hemodialysis? Artif Organs 1995; 19:391-394.
267. Assouad M, Tseng S, Dunn K, et al: Biocompatibility of dialyzer membranes is important in the outcome of acute renal failure (Abstract). J Am Soc Nephrol 1996; 7:1437.
268. Himmelfarb J, Tolkoff Rubin N, Chandran P, et al: A multicenter comparison of dialysis membranes in the treatment of acute renal failure requiring dialysis. J Am Soc Nephrol 1998; 9:257-266.
269. Jörres J, Gahl GM, Dobis C, et al: Haemodialysis-membrane biocompatibility and mortality of patients with dialysis-dependent acute renal failure: A prospective randomised multicenter trial. Lancet 1999; 354:1337-1341.
270. Gastaldello K, Melot C, Kahn R-J, et al: Comparison of cellulose diacetate and polysulfone membranes in the outcome of acute renal failure: A prospective randomized study. Nephrol Dial Transplant 2000; 15:224-230.
271. Albright RC, Smelser JM, McCarthy JT, et al: Patient survival and renal recovery in acute renal failure: Randomized comparison of cellulose acetate and polysulfone membrane dialyzers. Mayo Clin Proc 2000; 75:1141-1147.
272. Jaber B, Lau J, Schmid CH, et al: Effect of biocompatibility of hemodialysis membranes on mortality in acute renal failure: A meta-analysis. Clin Nephrol 2002; 57:274-282.
273. Subramanian S, Venkataraman R, Kellum JA: Influence of dialysis membranes on outcomes in acute renal failure: A meta-analysis. Kidney Int 2002; 62:1819-1823.
274. Teehan G, Liangos O, Lau J, et al: Dialysis membrane and modality in acute renal failure: Understanding discordant meta-analyses. Semin Dial 2003; 16:356-360.
275. Levin NW, Zasuwa G, Dumler F: Effect of membrane type on causes of death in hemodialysis patients. J Am Soc Nephrol 1991; 2:335.
276. Hornberger J, Chernew M, Petersen J, Garber A: A multivariate analysis of mortality and hospital admissions with high-flux dialysis. J Am Soc Nephrol 1992; 3:1227-1237.
277. Hakim RM, Held PJ, Stannard DC, et al: Effect of the dialysis membrane on mortality of chronic hemodialysis patients. Kidney Int 1996; 50:566-570.
278. Bloembergen WE, Hakim RM, Stannard DC, et al: Relationship of dialysis membrane and cause-specific mortality. Am J Kidney Dis 1999; 33:1-10.
279. Eknoyan G, Beck GJ, Cheung AK, et al: Effect of dialysis dose and membrane flux in maintenance hemodialysis. N Engl J Med 2002; 347:2010-2019.
280. Valeri A: Biocompatible membranes in acute renal failure: A study in post-cadaveric renal transplant acute tubular necrosis. J Am Soc Nephrol 1994; 3:481.
281. Romao JEJ, Abensur H, Castro MCM, et al: Effect of biocompatibility on recovery from acute renal failure after cadaveric renal transplantation (Abstract). J Am Soc Nephrol 1998; 9:181A.
282. Woo Y, King B, Junor B, et al: Dialysis with biocompatible membranes may delay recovery of graft function following renal transplantation. J Am Soc Nephrol 1998; 9:719A.
283. Pereira BJ: Balance between pro-inflammatory cytokines and their specific inhibitors in patients on dialysis. Nephrol Dial Transplant 1995; 10:27-32.

Reprocessing of Hemodialyzers

Bhamidipati V.R. Murthy, M.D., D.M. • Donald A. Molony, M.D.

Reprocessing of hemodialyzers was originally introduced in the 1960s to reduce the expense of coil and Kiil dialyzers.[1, 2] Although the cost of dialyzers decreased with the advent of hollow-fiber dialyzers, a few dialysis centers in the United States continued the practice of multiple uses of dialyzers in the 1960s and 1970s to reduce further the cost of dialysis. In the 1970s, some researchers observed increased biocompatibility of the cellulosic membranes following reprocessing and decreased reactions to the dialyzer membrane or sterilant, thus "justifying" medically the practice of reuse.[3-5] Although these cellulosic dialyzers were designed for single use, reuse continued with little regulation. The Association for Advancement of Medical Instrumentation (AAMI) provided standards and guidelines for dialyzer reprocessing.[6] First provided in 1983, these guidelines have been revised multiple times. Currently, it is mandated by law that the manufacturers of dialyzers label the product, whether it is for single use or for reuse.

Dialyzer reuse is less widespread in Europe and in Asia and is prohibited by law in France and in Japan. Dialyzer reuse has been cited as the reason for the observed difference in mortality between Europe and the United States.[7] While controversies regarding the direction and magnitude of any effect of reuse on morbidity and mortality remain, the predominant factor driving the current practice of reuse of dialyzers in the United States is economic. This chapter will outline the growth of dialyzer reuse in the United States, describe the effect of reuse on solute clearances and biocompatibility, describe the adverse effects of exposure to germicides used for reprocessing of dialyzers, and evaluate the strength of the evidence that dialyzer reuse is associated with adverse patient outcomes.

METHODS OF DIALYZER REPROCESSING

Disinfectants for Reuse

Reuse was originally performed with formaldehyde or formalin as the germicide, using manual techniques.[2] Reuse was initially practiced with Kiil dialyzers. When hollow-fiber dialyzers were introduced, these same methods were adapted for their reuse as well. Formaldehyde remained the only disinfectant in use until the early 1980s for lack of a better alternative, despite the concern of toxicities with formaldehyde. When peracetic acid/hydrogen peroxide mixture (marketed as Renalin) was introduced, it gradually gained ground over the next few years, as shown in Figure 19–1, such that by 1992, peracetic acid was more frequently used than formaldehyde.

Glutaraldehyde is another agent that has been used in place of either of these agents, but the toxicity of glutaraldehyde is greater than that of formaldehyde and, therefore, it has not gained wide acceptance. Currently, only 5% of dialysis centers use glutaraldehyde as the disinfecting agent.[8] Over the last decade, heat has been developed as a disinfectant facilitated by the development of membranes and potting compounds that are heat stable. Initially, a temperature of 105°C was used. This temperature has been reduced to 95°C by performing heat sterilization in the presence of 1.5% citric acid, a method that has proven to be safe and effective. Although pyrogen adverse reactions are significantly reduced with this method of reprocessing, this method is limited to dialysis membranes that are heat resistant and, hence, useful for *polysulfone* dialyzers only.[9]

Bleach has been used as a cleansing agent to improve the appearance of the dialyzer, particularly with formaldehyde, and less often with peracetic acid mixture reprocessing. Although bleach does improve the appearance of the dialyzer, over repeated exposures to bleach modifies the structure of the membrane such that diffusion properties of the dialyzer are altered. These are described in more detail in the section on clearance of solutes with reuse.

Manual Versus Automated Reuse

Until the mid 1980s, reprocessing of dialyzers with either formaldehyde or peracetic acid was accomplished by manual methods only. With the availability of automated systems, most dialysis units have adopted this method because it offers several advantages. Automated systems offer safety to the personnel with less contact with toxic chemicals, decrease the risk of human error, and ensure delivery of the exact specified concentration of the sterilant. They also facilitate proper testing for the integrity of the dialyzer. They ensure proper documentation of the disinfection process, store data for subsequent reference and analysis, and generate appropriate labels for identifying the dialyzers with a given patient. They are also time-efficient because four to eight dialyzers can be processed simultaneously depending on the machine used. The process is reliable and reproducible. Automated machines are available for both formaldehyde and peracetic acid methods of disinfection. The automated machines currently in use perform routinely three major tests on each reprocessed dialyzer. They test the coefficient of ultrafiltration (KUF), the total cell volume (TCV) or percent of total dialyzer surface area that is available for diffusion/ultrafiltration, and the membrane integrity or for the absence of leaks. Although ultrafiltration failure and membrane leaks are rare, decrease in TCV and its effect on solute clearances is still a significant concern with reuse. This is discussed in more detail in the section on clearance of solutes with reuse. For more details of the technology of dialyzer reuse and the sterilants, the reader is referred to the publication *AAMI Standards and Recommended Practices for Dialysis*[6] that should be available at every dialysis unit.

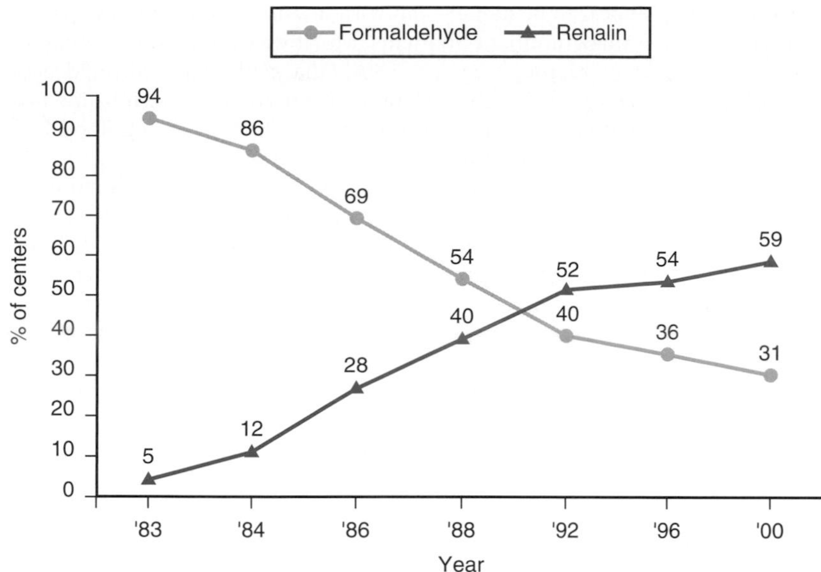

Figure 19–1 Graph showing comparative use of formaldehyde and peracetic acid/hydrogen peroxide mixture (Renalin) for reprocessing of hemodialyzers in the United States. (Modified from Tokars JI, Frank M, Alter MJ, Arduino MJ: National surveillance of dialysis-associated diseases in the United States, 2000. Semin Dial 2002; 15:162–171.)

GROWTH OF DIALYZER REUSE IN THE UNITED STATES

Since its early practice, reuse of dialyzers has had a persistent growth in the United States. In 1976, only 18% of dialysis units reprocessed their dialyzers. A sudden increase in dialyzer reprocessing occurred in the early 1980s with the introduction of composite rate of reimbursement for hemodialysis. With the composite rate remaining constant since its introduction, driven by economics, reuse has grown still further in the United States. In 1982, 43% of dialysis centers reprocessed their dialyzers and, in 1997, 82% of dialysis centers practiced reuse.[8] In recent years, it has stabilized and, in 2000, 80% of centers reprocessed their dialyzers.[8]

Although formaldehyde was the only reprocessing agent available during the 1970s, peracetic acid was introduced as a less toxic alternative in the early 1980s. In 1983, 94% of dialysis centers reprocessed their dialyzers with formaldehyde, 5% with peracetic acid, and less than 1% with glutaraldehyde. Since then, however, use of formaldehyde has steadily and significantly decreased because of the concern of toxicities to patients and personnel. In contrast, use of peracetic acid has consistently increased, replacing formaldehyde in the majority of centers. As shown in Figure 19–1, in the year 2000, only 31% of centers reprocessed their dialyzers with formaldehyde, and 59% of centers reprocessed with peracetic acid.[8] Glutaraldehyde reprocessing had increased to 9% in the early 1990s but subsequently decreased to 5% by 2000.[8] Reprocessing with heated citric acid remains low at 4% in 2000.[8]

Reuse policy is largely dictated by the dialysis unit. However, reuse is medically contraindicated when patients have had a previous reaction to either the germicide or to the cleansing agent. As will be discussed later in the chapter, reuse is not recommended in patients who are carriers of hepatitis B virus because of the risk of transmission to personnel reprocessing the dialyzers. In addition, most units choose to not reuse dialyzers in patients positive for human immunodeficiency virus (HIV) for the same reason. The remaining patients in whom reuse is not medically contraindicated are given a choice whether or not to participate in a reuse program. To understand more fully the differences between patients who choose to participate in reuse and those who do not, an analysis from the Dialysis Mortality and Morbidity Study (DMMS) observed that 8% of patients were not treated with reprocessed dialyzers among 1095 dialysis units that practiced reuse.[10] In 34% of these non-reuse patients, reasons for "no reuse" were not recorded; patient refusal accounted for 26% of patients not on reuse, and hepatitis and other medical conditions accounted for the remaining 40%.[10] Since many of the patients not on reuse in dialysis centers that conducted reuse were excluded from reuse for medical reasons, it would be expected that this subset of patients may represent a sicker subset of patients. Indeed, patients treated with non-reprocessed dialyzers had lower serum albumin levels and received a lesser dose of dialysis.[10] These differences may reflect a sicker population with more severe comorbidities and, hence, one in which it is more difficult to achieve target doses of dialysis, rather than negative effects of treatment with single-use dialyzers.

EFFECT OF DIALYZER REPROCESSING ON SOLUTES CLEARANCE AND PROTEIN LOSSES

Effect of Dialyzer Reuse on Clearance of Uremic Toxins

Guidelines by the Association for Advancement of Medical Instrumentation (AAMI) require that urea clearance of reprocessed dialyzers should be within 10% of the urea clearance by a new dialyzer.[6] However, it is impractical to measure urea clearance before each reuse. Therefore, based on studies by Gotch,[11] showing that a decrease in TCV of reprocessed hollow-fiber dialyzers by 20% decreases the urea clearance by only 10%, the AAMI guidelines recommend that a hollow-fiber dialyzer may be reused until its TCV is 80% or less of the original volume.[6] However, the observations of Gotch[12,13] were based on *in-vitro* studies of "low-flux" dialyzers at low blood flow rates on just a very few of dialyzers and without rigorous statistical analysis. The applicability of these parameters to the dialysis membranes in current practice has not been evaluated and remains unproven.

Clearance of Small Molecular Weight Solutes

Cellulose or substituted cellulose dialyzers

The majority of *in-vitro* and *in-vivo* studies indicate that reprocessing with either formaldehyde (with or without bleach) or peracetic acid does not affect small molecular weight solute (urea or creatinine) clearances of cellulose or substituted cellulose dialyzers. These studies have evaluated the performance of dialyzers by direct measurement of dialyzer clearances after either a small number of reuses (up to 10)[14,15] or large number of reuses (20–30).[16] In one study, the pre-dialysis urea and creatinine concentrations were measured, and no clinically or statistically significant difference between single-use dialyzers and those reprocessed with formaldehyde/bleach up to five times was observed.[17] In a study by Vanholder and colleagues,[18] urea and creatinine clearances and ultrafiltration capacity of cuprophan dialyzers reprocessed with formaldehyde remained unaltered for the small surface area dialyzers (1.0 m^2). However, these investigators observed a small but significant decrease in urea and creatinine clearance for those cuprophan dialyzers tested with the largest surface areas (1.8 m^2). There was a substantial volume loss in these large surface area dialyzers, which may have been the reason for the decrease in dialyzer clearance. In contrast, in a more recent *in-vivo* study of cellulose dialyzers reprocessed with formaldehyde and bleach, Murthy and colleagues[19] observed no such decline in urea or creatinine clearance with reuse.

Reprocessing with peracetic acid does not seem to affect small molecular weight solute clearance of cellulose dialyzers. Vanholder and colleagues[18] observed that reprocessing small or large surface area cuprophan dialyzers with peracetic acid resulted in neither a loss of volume nor a loss of clearance. Likewise, Leypoldt and colleagues[20] observed that the small molecule (urea and phosphate) clearances of low-flux cellulose (TAF175) or substituted cellulose dialyzers (CA210) reprocessed with peracetic acid did not decrease significantly between the 1st and 15th use.

Urea clearances were measured in the HEMO study for several different dialyzer types and for various reprocessing methods on a large number of patients. For low-flux dialyzers (that included cellulose acetate and polysulfone dialyzers), urea clearances decreased by only 1% for every 10 reuses with no significant differences between the various reprocessing methods noted.[21] In the same study, urea clearances of cellulose high-flux dialyzers (CT190G) decreased more with peracetic acid reprocessing than with formaldehyde/bleach reprocessing. However, with either method, the urea clearances of CT190G dialyzers were well above the 90% requirements as estimated from the TCV, for up to 20 reuses.[21]

In summary, neither the small molecule clearances nor the ultrafiltration capacity of cellulose/substituted cellulose dialyzers is affected with reuse, irrespective of the germicide used.

Synthetic dialyzers

With respect to high-flux synthetic dialyzers, the magnitude of the decrease in urea or creatinine clearances with reprocessing appear to be higher than with low-flux cellulose dialyzers. On a small number of patients, Murthy and colleagues[19] observed that reprocessing of F80B dialyzers with formaldehyde decreased the urea clearance from 280 ± 4 mL/min for new dialyzers to 253 ± 7 mL/min after 20 reuses, at a blood flow rate of 400 mL/min. Although the HEMO study observed that the loss of urea clearance of high-flux dialyzers with reuse was much smaller (1.4% decrease for every 10 reuses), this decrease was larger than with substituted cellulose dialyzers for the same reprocessing method.[21] Similarly, peracetic acid reprocessing with or without bleach only modestly affects the urea clearance, as observed in the earlier studies[18,20,22] as well as the more recent HEMO study.[21]

Very limited studies are available on the behavior of other synthetic membranes. Vanholder and colleagues[18] observed that urea clearance of PAN membrane dialyzers reprocessed with formaldehyde decreased from 117 mL/min during the first use to 91 mL/min during the seventh use (22%). Likewise, the ultrafiltration capacity decreased from 1.01 mL/min/mmHg during the first use to 0.41 mL/min/mmHg during the seventh use.[18] Similarly, the same investigators observed that PAN or AN69 dialyzers, reprocessed with peracetic acid, showed a significant decrease of urea and creatinine clearances with reuse, with a concomitant fall of ultrafiltration capacity.[18]

Of all the currently available sterilizing methods used in the reprocessing of dialyzers, heat and citric acid reprocessing has the smallest adverse effect on small molecule clearances. The average decrease in the urea clearance is 1% for every 10 reuses.[21] One of the drawbacks of the physical methods of reprocessing such as heat and citric acid is the limited number of reuses obtainable. Despite improvements in the technique over the years, use of this reprocessing technique is very limited in the United States, where only 4% of centers use this method.[8]

Thus, small molecular weight solute clearances with either cellulose/substituted cellulose or synthetic dialyzers decrease only modestly with reprocessing, with minor differences between different methods. These decreases may be functionally insignificant if a higher dialysis dose is prescribed in units that reprocess dialyzers to account for the temporal decline in clearances with multiple reuses. The clinical implications of changes in clearance of larger molecules will be considered in the next section.

Clearance of Middle Molecular Weight Solutes

β_2 microglobulin (molecular weight 11,800 daltons [Da]) has been used as a convenient marker for assessment of the clearance of solutes in the middle molecular weight range. The HEMO study group has adopted a clearance of β_2 microglobulin of greater than 20 mL/min as a marker of high-flux dialyzers.[21] The β_2 microglobulin clearance of low-flux dialyzers is less than 5 mL/min and remains so with formaldehyde and bleach reprocessing across 20 reuses.[19] In the HEMO study, reprocessing with bleach resulted in a small but statistically significant increase in β_2 microglobulin clearance of these low-flux dialyzers. The increase was more pronounced with non-polysulfone dialyzers (0.52 mL/min per reuse) than with the polysulfone dialyzers (0.25 mL/min per reuse).[21] A similar increase in β_2 microglobulin clearance occurred with peracetic acid and with glutaraldehyde (with bleach) reprocessing, and the rate of increase did not differ significantly from that of formaldehyde.[21]

Several investigators have confirmed the increase in β_2 microglobulin clearance with high-flux polysulfone dialyzers reprocessed with bleach. Kaplan and colleagues[23] observed that during clinical dialysis with polysulfone dialyzers (F80) reprocessed with formaldehyde and bleach, the dialysate β_2 microglobulin concentration increased with increasing number of reuses. The mean dialysate β_2 microglobulin concentration during clinical dialysis with F80 dialyzers reprocessed greater than 10 times (1.54 ± 0.15 mg/L) was significantly higher than that with new F80 dialyzers (1.05 ± 0.13 mg/L) or dialyzers reprocessed greater than 10 times without bleach (0.5 ± 0.15 mg/L).[23] Murthy and colleagues[19] also observed that the plasma β_2 microglobulin clearance of F80B dialyzers reprocessed with formaldehyde and bleach, increased from a mean of 15.8 mL/min for new dialyzers to 35.8 mL/min for dialyzers reused up to 20 times. Similarly, data from the HEMO study show that the β_2 microglobulin clearance with polysulfone dialyzers (F80A and F80B) reprocessed with bleach increased with reuse (Figure 19–2) but when bleach is not employed, the clearance decreased with reuse (Figure 19–3). For F80B dialyzers, the β_2 microglobulin clearance increased from 21.3 mL/min at 0 reuse (new dialyzers) to 49.5 mL/min at 20th reuse with formaldehyde/bleach reprocessing and from 21.3 mL/min at 0 reuse to 41.9 mL/min at 20th reuse with peracetic acid and bleach reprocessing.[21] With peracetic acid reprocessing without bleach, the β_2 microglobulin clearance decreased from 41.1 mL/min at 0 reuse to 36.5 mL/min at tenth reuse.[21]

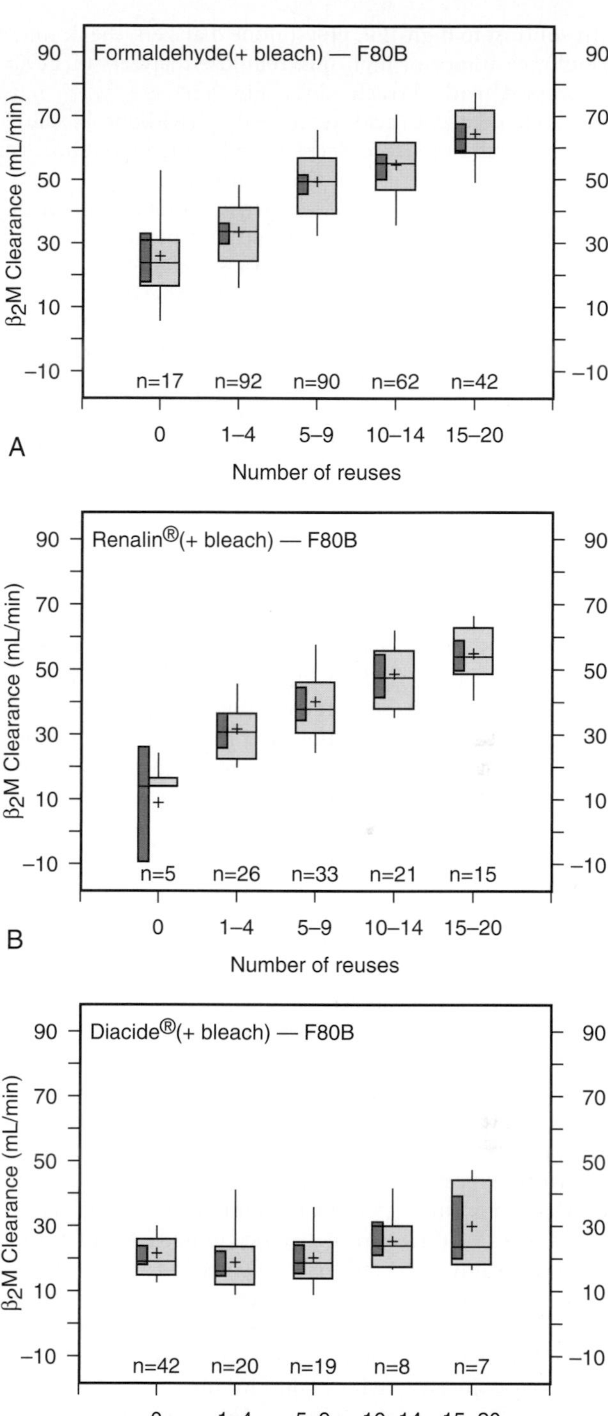

Figure 19–2 Effect of reprocessing using formaldehyde with bleach *(A)*, Renalin with bleach *(B)*, and glutaraldehyde (Diacide) with bleach on β_2M clearance by polysulfone high-flux (F80B) dialyzers. The box and whisker plots show the 10th, 25th, 50th (median), 75th, and 90th percentile values. The plus sign (+) represents the mean and the hatched region represents the 95% confidence interval for the mean. (From Cheung AK, Agodoa LY, Daugirdas JT, et al: Effects of hemodialyzer reuse on clearances of urea and beta-2-microglobulin. The Hemodialysis [HEMO] Study Group. J Am Soc Nephrol 1999; 10:117-127, with permission.)

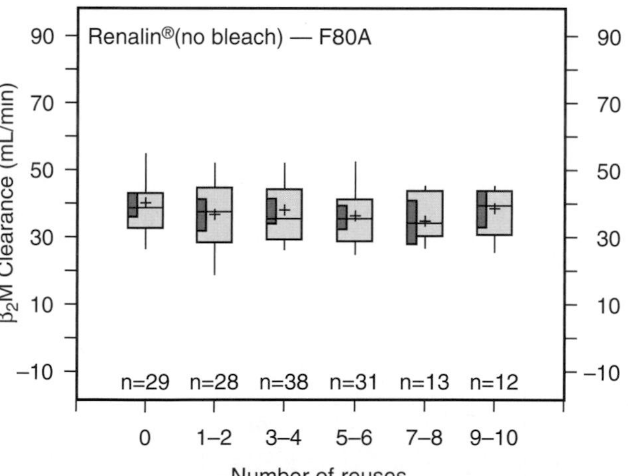

Figure 19–3 Effect of reprocessing using Renalin *without* bleach on β_2M clearance by polysulfone high-flux (F80A) dialyzers. The box and whisker plots show the 10th, 25th, 50th (median), 75th, and 90th percentile values. The plus sign (+) represents the mean and the hatched region represents the 95% confidence interval for the mean. (From Cheung AK, Agodoa LY, Daugirdas JT, et al: Effects of hemodialyzer reuse on clearances of urea and beta-2-microglobulin. The Hemodialysis [HEMO] Study Group. J Am Soc Nephrol 1999; 10:117-127, with permission.)

In contrast to high-flux polysulfone dialyzers, the β_2 microglobulin clearance of high-flux cellulose dialyzers (CT190G) reprocessed with bleach does not increase with reuse. Moreover, peracetic acid reprocessing (without bleach) is associated with a marked decrease in β_2 microglobulin clearance, particularly during the first four reuses.[21]

Studies on the behavior of synthetic membranes other than polysulfone, reprocessed with bleach or peracetic acid, are limited. The principal mechanism of β_2 microglobulin clearance with high-flux polymethyl methacrylate (PMMA) membranes is by adsorption to the dialysis membranes.[24] The efficacy of β_2 microglobulin removal with PMMA is expected to decrease when reprocessed with peracetic acid, because peracetic acid does not strip the membrane of the protein coat formed from an earlier exposure of the membrane to blood. However, during clinical dialysis with PMMA dialyzers, Westhuyzen and colleagues[25] observed that serum β_2 microglobulin concentrations decreased significantly at 15, 60, and 240 minutes into dialysis compared to the pre-dialysis values during the first use, as well as during the second and fourth uses, suggesting an increase in β_2 microglobulin clearance. The dialysate concentrations of β_2 microglobulin increased significantly with reuse from the first to the fourth use. This increased appearance of β_2 microglobulin in the dialysate may have accounted for an increased clearance of β_2 microglobulin during the fourth use of the membrane when compared to its first use. The exact mechanisms underlying this increased clearance into the dialysate are unknown. It is also probable that when reused beyond four times, the β_2 microglobulin removal by these dialyzers may decline. Indeed, Kerr and colleagues[26] observed a decrease in β_2 microglobulin clearance with peracetic acid reprocessed PMMA hemofilters, after the fourth use.

AN69 dialyzers also remove β_2 microglobulin by both adsorption and filtration.[24] *In-vitro* studies observed that reprocessing of these dialyzers with peracetic acid significantly decreased their ability to clear β_2 microglobulin, but bleach reprocessing did not.[24] This observation is consistent with the fact that bleach strips the membrane of the protein coat from a previous exposure to blood, but peracetic acid alone does not. Data on β_2 microglobulin clearance of AN69 dialyzers are limited and are derived from dialyzers reused only a few times. An *in-vivo* study observed that the percent removal of serum β_2 microglobulin by AN69 dialyzers reprocessed with peracetic acid showed no significant decrease up to the fourth use.[25] Whether the removal of serum β_2 microglobulin increases significantly with higher number of reuses of these dialyzers, is a matter of conjecture. In contrast to the PMMA dialyzers, the dialysate concentrations of β_2 microglobulin with AN69 dialyzers did not increase following reprocessing with peracetic acid.[25]

A consistent pattern emerges from the studies discussed above. For polysulfone dialyzers, employing bleach in the reprocessing method with either formaldehyde or peracetic acid as the germicide increases, and reprocessing with peracetic acid alone decreases β_2 microglobulin clearance. A similar but more profound decrease of β_2 microglobulin clearance is observed with high-flux cellulose dialyzers when peracetic acid alone is used but not when bleach is added as a cleansing agent. The mechanism by which bleach increases β_2 microglobulin clearance of polysulfone dialyzers is unclear, but it has been hypothesized that bleach leaches the polyvinyl pyrrolidone (PVP), a copolymer in the membrane, thus increasing the sieving coefficient of the membrane.[27] This has not been proven under actual clinical conditions. The marked decline in β_2 microglobulin clearance of high-flux cellulose dialyzers may be secondary to a protein layer formation that is ineffectively removed by peracetic acid alone.

Protein and/or Albumin Loss

In 1992, with *in-vitro* experiments, Donahue and colleagues[28] showed that the clearance of small (1400 Da) and middle molecular weight (10,000 Da) polymers by polysulfone dialyzers (F60) increased significantly following reprocessing with 1% bleach and formaldehyde, suggesting that reprocessing with bleach alters the membrane permeability of polysulfone dialyzers. Subsequently, Kaplan and colleagues[23] observed that reprocessing of polysulfone dialyzers (F80) with bleach led to a loss of proteins and albumin into the dialysate, and the degree of protein and albumin loss was directly related to the number of times the membrane was reprocessed with bleach (Figure 19–4). The mean dialysate protein concentrations progressively increased from 1.5 mg/dL during the 1st use, to 19.9 mg/dL after 23 to 25 reuses. The mean dialysate protein losses (in the entire spent dialysate) increased progressively from 1.2 g at 1st use to 17.5 g during the 23rd through 25th reuses. In contrast, dialyzers reprocessed without bleach had significantly lower protein losses and did not demonstrate a relationship with reuse. The mean dialysate protein concentrations of the dialyzers with nonbleach reprocessed polysulfone dialyzers after 10 reuses (2.1 mg/dL) were not significantly different from that of the 1st use (dry pack) of the dialyzers (1.5 mg/dL).[23] In addition, Kaplan and

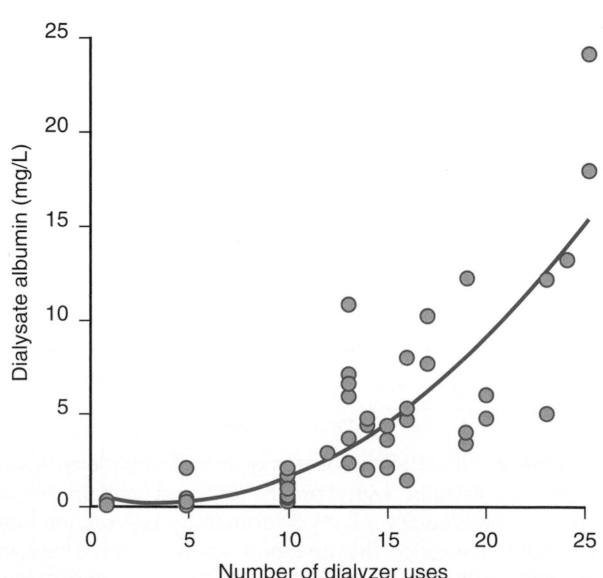

Figure 19–4 Effect of reprocessing of high-flux polysulfone (F80) dialyzers using formaldehyde with bleach on dialysate albumin losses. (From Kaplan AA, Halley SE, Lapkin RA, Graeber CW: Dialysate protein losses with bleach processed polysulfone dialyzers. Kidney Int 1995; 47:573-578. Reprinted with permission.)

colleagues[23] observed that the mean serum albumin levels ranged from 3.5 to 3.6 g/dL during the 6 months prior to discontinuing the bleach from the reprocessing cycle, compared to 3.8 to 3.9 g/dL 3 weeks after discontinuing bleach, in the same patients. These data support the contention that the decrease of serum albumin among these patients may be due to the excessive protein and albumin leak from the dialyzers reprocessed with bleach. Following this study, the manufacturer changed the membrane configuration of F80 dialyzers such that protein leak decreased significantly. Indeed, in a subsequent study, Murthy and colleagues[19] observed that albumin loss from bleach reprocessed F80B dialyzers was negligible for up to 20 reuses. Currently, albumin leak does not seem to be a significant problem anymore with F80B dialyzers reprocessed with bleach.

Protein losses from polysulfone dialyzers (F80) reprocessed with peracetic acid have been shown to be much lower compared to that of dialyzers reprocessed with formaldehyde/bleach. Protein loss after 15 or more uses of polysulfone dialyzers (HF80) reprocessed with peracetic acid was 3.2 ± 1.1 g, a value not significantly different from that with 1st use (dry pack) of the dialyzer.[29]

Reuse and Delivery of Dialysis Prescription

The mortality risk among hemodialysis patients is lower by 7% for each 0.1 increment in delivered Kt/V, and by 11% for each 5% increase in delivered URR.[30] One of the potential reasons for a decreased dialysis adequacy is a decline in dialyzer performance following multiple reuses of dialyzers. In a multicenter study, Sherman and colleagues[12] observed a significantly greater delivered Kt/V (urea) (1.08 vs. 1.02) in centers with low reuse of dialyzers (mean of 4 times) compared to centers with high reuse of dialyzers (mean of 14 times), suggesting a decline in performance of dialyzer with reuse. In 43% of the centers using formaldehyde reprocessing, the difference in Kt/V values between low and high reuses averaged 0.17.[12] However, this study showed a strong center difference, probably related to practices associated with differences in reprocessing techniques. In the context of an increased mortality risk with decreased dose of dialysis, this decline in dialysis dose with reuse was a matter of concern. However, subsequent studies did not confirm this trend. In a prospective study of patients randomized to single use or reuse of cellulose dialyzers with glutaraldehyde and bleach, Pereira and colleagues[31] did not observe a significant difference in URR between groups, over a period of 3 months. In another study using the USRDS data, Agodoa and colleagues[32] observed a higher delivered dose of dialysis as measured by Kt/V (urea) at units that reprocessed dialyzers compared to those that did not (1.22 vs. 1.19). This may be attributable in part to a higher frequency of use of high-flux dialysis among units that reused compared with those that did not (97% vs. 65%), in that study.

Thus, it is encouraging to note that reuse does not, at least, adversely affect the actual delivered dose of dialysis. Although all dialysis units monitor the delivered dialysis dose by measurement of URR or urea kinetic modeling, such measurements are usually performed only on a monthly basis and do not provide timely identification of suboptimal delivered dose from dialysis after many reuses. Dialysis units that practice reuse should be watchful that reuse can adversely affect dialysis adequacy. In such situations, the on-line monitoring systems (blood-side and dialysate-side monitoring of Kt/V) may help assess the efficacy of delivery of dialysis prescription during dialysis with reprocessed dialyzers.

EFFECT OF DIALYZER REPROCESSING ON MEMBRANE BIOCOMPATIBILITY

Complement Activation and Leukopenia

Complement activation and leukopenia during hemodialysis, first described more than 2 decades ago,[33] has now become the benchmark for biocompatibility of dialysis membranes. These changes are observed with cellulose and substituted cellulose dialyzers within the first 30 minutes of dialysis and typically improve to baseline levels prior to the completion of dialysis. These have been shown to be secondary to activation of the complement alternate pathway by these membranes.[4,34] Subsequent investigators have reported an improvement in levels of complement fragments C3a, C3b, and C5a with reprocessed dialyzers compared with first use,[3-5,35] suggesting an improvement of biocompatibility with reprocessing of dialyzers. It has been shown that the reprocessing technique is also important in improving the biocompatibility of the membrane.[3,5,35] Although reprocessing with both formaldehyde and peracetic acid mixture are associated with improvement in complement activation, use of bleach does not provide the same benefit.[15,36] This protective effect is from coating of the membrane surface with the patient's blood proteins after the first use, which is further stabilized with formaldehyde and peracetic acid. Bleach strips the membrane of the protein layer, thus reverting to the original membrane configuration with loss of this acquired "biocompatibility." With the use of more biocompatible membranes such as synthetic polysulfone dialyzers, complement activation and leukopenia during dialysis have decreased significantly even with new dialyzers. Mitigation of complement activation and leukopenia, either with new dialyzers or with reused dialyzers, has not been shown to be associated with improved clinical outcomes.

Anaphylactoid Reactions

First use syndrome

Another advantage of reuse of dialyzers is a decrease in the incidence of "first use syndrome." This first use syndrome was first described in 1978 by Dolovich and colleagues[37] in a hemodialysis patient who was sensitized to ethylene oxide gas that was used for sterilization of blood tubings. These authors investigated whether the acute allergic reactions seen in other patients on hemodialysis might be similarly caused. They reported that in Hamilton, Ontario, 22 of the 27 patients with allergic reactions were positive for ethylene-oxide antibodies.[38] As described since, the syndrome ranges in severity from a mild chest and back pain to hypotension, bronchospasm, and anaphylaxis.[39] A decrease in the incidence of the syndrome with reprocessed dialyzers and preprocessing of dialyzer prior to first use[40] can be explained in part by the reduced content of residual ethylene-oxide in these situations. Interestingly, complement activation is also seen more often with new dialyzers[41] but less often with reprocessed dialyzers.[4]

This led to the confusion in the mid-1980s that the first use syndrome might be due to complement activation. The lack of correlation between the degree of complement activation and the incidence of the syndrome negated this view.[42] It is now believed firmly that first use syndrome is indeed the result of an IgE-mediated reaction to residual ethylene oxide gas. Although ethylene oxide is still used in the dry packs, better manufacturing processes to decrease the content of the gas have decreased significantly the incidence of the syndrome overall.

Reuse Syndromes

Anaphylactoid reactions attributed to reprocessed dialyzers have also been reported. Pegues and colleagues[43] observed 12 episodes of anaphylactoid reactions, all associated with reuse of dialyzers and none with new dialyzers. The sterilant used for reprocessing was peracetic acid with an automated reprocessing system, in this instance. Following termination of reuse, they reported that such episodes ceased to occur. Most of the patients with anaphylactoid reactions were on angiotensin-converting enzyme inhibitors (ACEI). Use of ACEI and AN69 membranes has been implicated in anaphylactoid reactions in dialysis patients.[44-46] These reactions have been attributed to the generation of bradykinin, as these reactions were observed in patients with high plasma bradykinin levels, even in the absence of ACEI but always with use of AN69 membranes.[47] Although not investigated, it is quite possible that anaphylactoid reactions with ACEI and peracetic acid reprocessing may have a similar bradykinin etiology. Interestingly, in an open label study of 406 hemodialysis patients on angiotensin receptor blocker, Losartan, for control of hypertension, Sarache and colleagues[48] observed only two episodes of anaphylactoid reactions over a 6-month period. About a fourth of these patients were dialyzed using AN69 membrane. Furthermore, nine patients who exhibited anaphylactoid reactions with ACEI and AN69 membranes did not have any episodes with Losartan despite continuing to dialyze with the same membrane.[48] These reports lend support to the bradykinin hypothesis because bradykinin levels are significantly less with Losartan compared with ACEI.

Chronic Inflammatory Response

During hemodialysis, blood leukocytes are exposed to the dialyzer membrane and tubing, soluble membrane constituents, complement, and other plasma products activated by the membrane-blood interactions. Leukocytes are also exposed to the bacterial products that diffuse from dialysate to the blood compartment (backfiltration). These interactions stimulate the leukocytes to produce pro-inflammatory cytokines.[49] Several studies in patients on hemodialysis have demonstrated evidence of increased cytokine production by blood leukocytes before and during hemodialysis.[50-52] Henderson and colleagues[49, 53] have hypothesized that hypotension and pyrogen reactions observed in hemodialysis patients and dialysis-related morbidity are secondary to interleukin-1 release by blood-membrane interactions during dialysis. To date, this hypothesis remains unproven, although the symptoms observed with cytokine release are similar to those seen during dialysis reactions.

With respect to reprocessed dialyzers, Lufft and colleagues[54] observed that cytokine-inducing substances, like bacterial products, are retained in the protein layer formed during the first and subsequent uses, despite sterilization of the dialyzer. These products are biologically active in inciting a cytokine release *in vitro*. The bacterial products are likely to gain access to the dialyzer because the water that is used for reprocessing is neither sterile nor pyrogen free. Indeed, pyrogen reactions are more frequently observed among patients treated with reprocessed dialyzers than in patients treated with single use dialyzers.[55] However, these observations are not supported by clinical studies or studies under controlled laboratory conditions. In a single center study, Pereira and colleagues[31] studied plasma cytokine levels in 37 chronic hemodialysis patients randomized to either single use dialyzers or to dialyzers reprocessed with glutaraldehyde and bleach. They observed that levels of plasma IL-1Ra, C3a, lipopolysaccharide binding protein and bactericidal-permeability increasing factor were not significantly different between the two groups at baseline, 15 minutes into dialysis, or at the end of dialysis.[31] Even the endotoxin and IgG stimulated cytokine production by the peripheral blood mononuclear cells (PBMC) were similar in the two groups. In another study, the same investigators performed *in-vitro* dialysis using formaldehyde/bleach or peracetic acid mixture-reprocessed cuprophan dialyzers and compared the cytokine production by unstimulated and endotoxin-stimulated PBMC before and after *in-vitro* dialysis.[56] They observed that after a 3-hour *in-vitro* dialysis, the increase in IL-1α production by unstimulated PBMC was not statistically significant with either new or reprocessed dialyzers. In contrast, a statistically significant increase was observed in IL-1α production by endotoxin-stimulated PBMC with new as well as formaldehyde/bleach reprocessed dialyzers, but the increase with peracetic acid mixture reprocessed dialyzers was not significant. These findings argue against the notion that exposure to reprocessed dialyzers results in enhanced production of pro-inflammatory cytokines. The long-term clinical significance of elevated cytokine levels in dialysis patients is still debated.

Last, chronic kidney disease itself is considered a pro-inflammatory state with higher levels of plasma cytokines and C-Reactive Protein (CRP) levels observed in these patients even before start of dialysis, compared with controls.[50,57,58] Levels are even higher in hemodialysis patients.[57,59-61] While this chronic inflammatory state may be responsible, in part, for the high cardiovascular morbidity and mortality in dialysis patients, no convincing evidence has yet emerged that circulating CRP levels are any higher in patients treated with reprocessed dialyzers or that their cardiovascular morbidity or mortality is higher, compared with patients treated with single use dialyzers.

INFECTIOUS AND CHEMICAL HAZARDS OF DIALYZER REPROCESSING

Introduction

Reprocessing of dialyzers may have some additional direct adverse effects that could result in increases in morbidity, and possibly mortality, for patients on dialysis and adversely affect their quality of life. Some of the major types of adverse effects that have been attributed to reuse include[62]:

- Nosocomial bacterial infections, especially with gram-negative bacteria or non-tuberculous mycobacteria.
- Nosocomial viral infections with hepatitis B, C, and HIV.
- Pyrogenic reactions to preformed bacterial endotoxins.
- Toxic effects from acute exposures to germicides used to reprocess dialyzers.
- Effects after chronic exposures to low levels of germicides.
- Environmental and occupational issues related to reprocessing of dialyzers.

Serious adverse events attributable to reuse are currently identified through voluntary reporting to the Centers for Disease Control (CDC) and through CDC's investigation of adverse event clusters. This method of defining the risks from reprocessing of dialyzers depends on event recognition, proper attribution, and accurate reporting by clinicians. Such methods generally significantly underestimate the full impact of reuse on patient health and quality of life through underestimating the incidence of these adverse events.[63] The true magnitude of the risk and the scope of the adverse effects of dialyzer reuse can be ascertained only by proactively collected data on the entire cohort of dialysis patients.[64] More comprehensive data may be available in the future through a more proactive approach of surveillance as anticipated with the creation of the Dialysis Surveillance Network. The current best evidence available to define the types of potential risks of reuse still relies heavily on the reactive analysis of adverse events.

Current evidence demonstrates that the most common, albeit still remarkably uncommon, adverse events reported in clusters are those related to "nosocomial" infections or to endotoxins elaborated exogenously as a consequence of bacterial contamination.[8,55,65] Accidental exposures to chemical sterilants and/or germicides occur less commonly. Both pyrogenic reactions and first-use-like reactions appear to be related directly to acute exposures to one of the chemicals associated with dialysis, notably the sterilants used in packaging new dialyzers and the germicides that may become adherent to the dialyzer membranes during reprocessing. They are then released during subsequent hemodialysis treatments. Many of the outbreaks of pyrogenic reactions that are subjected to formal root cause investigations are determined to be related to exposure of patients to bacteria or bacterial endotoxins. It is uncertain to what degree pyrogenic reactions related to transient bacteremias are underreported.

Consistent with the rarity of the reported adverse events and with findings that many of these occur because of deviations from the formal AAMI reuse guidelines, the CDC has described reuse of dialyzers as safe if performed with strict adherence to AAMI reuse guidelines.[66,67] Although the current AAMI standards are based on expert opinion and have not been formally validated through rigorous controlled trials, the relative infrequency of both infection related and non-infectious adverse events when these standards are upheld provides relatively strong evidence of their efficacy. It should be emphasized, however, that if protocols based on these standards are breached, then serious nosocomial infections do occur.[65] Furthermore, these AAMI guidelines based on best current opinion and evidence have required modifications in response to the findings from adverse event investigations. Finally, epidemiologic evidence demonstrates that the type of reuse process matters when considering adverse events such as nosocomial transmission of infections, and that automated reprocessing procedures reduce infection transmission and pyrogenic reactions.[68]

A detailed account of the risk of bacterial and viral infections associated with reprocessing of dialyzers is explained in another chapter. This section gives an overview of these risks.

Risks of Infection

Bacterial

Serious bacterial infections remain a major cause for morbidity and mortality in dialysis dependent patients,[65] and this infection rate is influenced by dialyzer reuse. As part of their annual survey of dialysis practices, the CDC have reported from 1986 through 2000 the incidence of pyrogenic reactions associated with dialyzer reprocessing, and a comprehensive analysis of the association of pyrogenic reactions with reuse and the risk factors for this reaction was conducted as part of the 1994 survey.[55] Tokars and colleagues[55] reported in their analysis of the 1994 data that 24% of centers conducting reuse compared to 14% of centers not conducting reuse reported pyrogenic reactions and that 3% of the former and only 1% of the latter reported clusters of these reactions. Both differences were statistically significant. On further analysis of these data, the CDC investigators demonstrated that both reuse and high-flux dialyses were independent predictors of the pyrogenic reactions. The latter is more likely to occur if reprocessing changes membrane characteristics to allow for higher rates of transmembrane flux and, in particular, backflux from the dialysate, of bacteria or endotoxins. The CDC investigators also determined that the increased risk of pyrogenic reactions was associated equally with reprocessing with the germicides formaldehyde or peracetic acid. In the same analysis, the CDC investigators were unable to demonstrate an association between reports of overt sepsis and reuse. For reasons specified above, these analyses are limited by the possibility of ascertainment biases.

An estimate of the risk of sepsis associated with reuse that is less influenced by reporting and ascertainment biases can be obtained from the analysis of the incident dialysis patient cohort assembled for the USRDS case-mix study.[69,70] These investigators conducted a series of analysis of the incidence of sepsis in this representative sample of incident dialysis patients followed prospectively over a 7-year period, where dialysis characteristics such as access type and reuse were determined at baseline. Hospital managed sepsis was defined by ICD-9 codes for a principle admitting diagnosis of sepsis on Medicare claims records submitted upon discharge and, thus, identification of sepsis incidents was not influenced by apriori hypothesis or dependent on voluntary targeted surveillance. Although their conclusions are somewhat limited by the potential impact of misclassification bias and of secular trends in dialysis care during the extended follow-up observation period, these authors provide the first evaluation of the impact of reuse on sepsis risk in a prospectively followed longitudinal cohort. They demonstrated that for the entire cohort of incident hemodialysis patients, assignment to reuse during the baseline period was associated with 28% increase in risk of hospital-managed sepsis.[69] In a separate analysis stratified for the presence or absence of diabetes mellitus, Jaar and colleagues[70] demonstrated that the increased relative risk of sepsis with reuse was largely confined to patients with diabetes. A similar increase risk for non-diabetic patients could not be excluded.

Several hypotheses have been proposed for the possible etiologies of the increased risk of sepsis, bacterial infections without sepsis, and viral infections uniquely attributable to reuse. These include:

- Technical errors, including inadequate sterilization during reprocessing due to either limitations of the effectiveness of germicides at practiced concentrations or inadequate adherence to recommended concentrations.
- Changes in pore size or sieving characteristic of the dialysis membrane that allow for flux of bacteria and virus from the dialysate to the patient's bloodstream.
- Reuse-associated changes in the immune, hematopoietic, or vascular systems or in the nutritional status of patients on dialysis that could otherwise heighten their susceptibility to infection.

Investigations into outbreaks of infections have provided insights into these potential mechanisms. Reports from investigations of clusters of infection episodes have demonstrated clearly that severe sepsis can occur because of human errors with significant adverse effects on patient mortality and morbidity.[65,71-79] A common feature of many of these outbreaks is a "seeding" of the dialysis membranes, o-rings, caps, or other materials with bacteria from contaminated or inadequately purified or sterilized water used in the flushing of and subsequent cleansing of the dialyzers during reprocessing. This problem is then compounded by a failure of the sequential sterilization and storage techniques to ensure adequate sterilization of the dialyzers prior to their next use. Many of the incidents have, as a root cause, a break down in strict adherence to the AAMI reuse guidelines where critical steps in the process of reuse were either violated or by-passed or where concentrations of sterilant known to be inadequate were inadvertently used. A number of the failures in process were, however, defined only after investigations of particular outbreaks of infections revealed inadequacies in the process dictating changes in the AAMI standards. The random rate of occurrence in these incidences and a lack of a defined secular trend in reported outbreaks despite improvements in equipment and techniques support the hypothesis that much of the excess risk of sepsis might be related to human errors, accidents, or some fundamental problem in process yet to be identified.[64]

Two classes of bacteria have been implicated in the majority of dialysis related infectious outbreaks reported to date. Infections with gram-negative bacterial rods, including *Klebsiella* and *Pseudomonas aeruginosa* and *Enterobacter* species have been cultured from water sources and dialysate.[65,80,81] A number of infectious outbreaks traced to nontuberculous mycobacteria have also been identified with associated significant patient morbidity and mortality.[65] Three components are required for these nontuberculous mycobacteria to cause patient morbidity in association with reuse. They have been identified to occur commonly (50% of water samples in 83% of centers in one CDC survey) in the water used for preparation of dialysate and for reprocessing of dialyzers.[82] Patients are exposed to viable organisms either from contamination of the blood side of the dialyzers during reprocessing or across dialysis membranes during dialysis. The former might occur if standard sterilization techniques are inadequate. Evaluation of a number of the early outbreaks in the 1980s revealed that these organisms were relatively resistant to chemical germicides and sufficient concentrations of either formaldehyde or peracetic acid were required to ensure bacterial killing.[82] Patients might be exposed additionally to these organisms if the water quality is substandard *and* if reprocessing of dialyzers alters the exclusion properties of the dialysis membranes sufficiently to allow for flux of viable organisms from dialysate to patient. This problem would be compounded if reprocessed dialyzers exhibit significant dialysate backflux with reuse. Although reprocessing does alter some flux properties of the dialysis membranes, there is no evidence that sterilants currently in use alter membranes sufficiently that in the absence of a frank blood leak, to permit flux of microorganisms from dialyzer to patient occurs.[83,84] Automated reprocessing techniques check for blood leaks and membrane integrity with each reprocessing, thereby ensuring patient safety, if strict adherence to AAMI guidelines is maintained.

Viral Hepatitis and HIV Infections

Through the national dialysis surveillance surveys and other tools, the CDC and others have evaluated the risk of transmission of hepatitis with reuse. The CDC has recommended isolation of hepatitis B patients since the early 1980s for control of the more virulent hepatitis B virus. Isolation procedures were responsible for a substantial reduction in new hepatitis B infections in patients and caregivers even before the introduction of effective hepatitis B vaccines. This risk of new infections has continued to decline despite incomplete vaccination rates.[8] Dialyzers from patients infected with the hepatitis B virus are not reused in the United States. The infectivity of hepatitis C virus and HIV are substantially lower than the infectivity of hepatitis B, and observational studies do not demonstrate an increased risk of new hepatitis C infection in patients on reuse, in the United States.[85] Hence, the CDC does not currently recommend isolation of patients with hepatitis C or HIV when universal precautions are strictly maintained.[86,87] However, in centers in Europe and Asia with high prevalence of hepatitis C infection, higher incidence of hepatitis C infection has been observed.[88] In addition, even a higher transmission rate of hepatitis C infection has been demonstrated in such centers when reuse is practiced. In addition, isolation of hepatitis C positive patients has decreased the incidence of hepatitis C transmission.[88] A prospective study looking at isolation of reprocessing area of dialyzers (to a separate room) in patients positive for hepatitis C infection has resulted in a lower relative risk of transmission of hepatitis C infection.[89] Though not in the United States, the results of these studies suggest that horizontal transmission of hepatitis C infection in dialysis units is a real risk in centers with high prevalence of hepatitis C infection among their patients, and that reuse of dialyzers adds to this risk. In addition, breaks in reuse protocols might put patients at risk and procedures that reduce the opportunity for error improve patient safety. Although hepatitis C transmission in dialysis units in the United States is low, the true incidence in dialysis units can be accurately determined only when active screening on a regular basis in dialysis units is enforced.[85]

Thus, evidence from both observational studies and prospective cohorts reinforces the conclusion that hemodialysis is an intrinsically potentially hazardous therapy and that breakdowns in strict adherence to validated AAMI guidelines leave patients at increased risk of infections with significant morbidities. These same studies demonstrate that when adherence to AAMI guidelines for reprocessing and reuse are ensured, dialysis can be conducted safely. These observational studies, however, do provide for a degree of uncertainty. The true risk of nosocomial infections attributable to reuse can be determined best by automatic and proactive surveillance of all dialysis patients and additional prospective randomized, controlled clinical trials. The potential risks of nontuberculous mycobacterial infections and from hepatitis C warrants continued consideration. Hepatitis C seroconversion rates for incident dialysis patients can be determined only when active screening for hepatitis C is performed.

Toxicity of Long-Term Exposure to Germicides

Germicides used in the reprocessing of dialyzers are toxic products and are, therefore, inherently dangerous. There are four potential consequences of the use of these agents in reprocessing of dialyzers that should be considered when evaluating their toxicity. These are

- Acute accidental exposures of patients to high concentrations of germicides either intravenously from dialyzers or water systems or dermal/inhalation exposures from accidental spills.
- Long-term low dose exposure of patients to germicides from residual concentration of germicides within the dialyzers.
- Acute toxicities of germicides to health care workers.
- Environmental consequence of exposures to germicides.

A number of acute exposures to germicides as noninfectious outbreaks have been reported to the CDC over the last 3 decades. These have involved principally accidents during sterilization of water systems used to prepare and/or deliver dialysate.[90] Formaldehyde was reported to the CDC as the causative agent in an outbreak in 1981.[90] In this case, patients experienced the acute effects of formaldehyde exposure within minutes of initiating dialysis. The acute effects of intravenous formaldehyde include hypotension, cardiovascular collapse, lactic acidosis, respiratory distress, hemolysis, and death.[91] The probable source for the formaldehyde was backflow of water containing formaldehyde from a recycling loop.[90] The frequency of accidental exposures to individual patients from a breakdown in mandated reprocessing procedures and failure to clear germicides from the dialyzers is unknown since recognition of a single major adverse event in a dialysis patient that can be attributed to reuse is difficult. Animal studies and reports from the occupational literature do not examine the effects of intravenous exposure to germicides. Our knowledge about the effect of intravenous exposures comes from the outbreak analyses. Germicides administered intravenously would be expected to result acutely in irritation of the blood vessels from infusion of intermediate amounts of germicides as may occur with incomplete washout after dialyzer reprocessing. Such events have been reported.[90] This is potentially problematic since the usual method to test for residual germicide such as the Schiff test for formaldehyde identifies only concentration greater than 5 ppm and does not protect against release during dialysis of retained reservoirs of germicides.[92]

Another potential acute toxicity to patients on reuse is an increased risk of acute allergic reactions.[90] A higher frequency of acute allergic reactions has also been reported in patients on angiotensin converting enzyme inhibitors and on reuse but is not associated with one particular germicide or another. The increased risk is associated with cleaning of the dialyzers with bleach or hydrogen peroxide during reprocessing, but the exact mechanism of this risk is unknown. This risk is detailed in earlier text.

The long-term consequences of low-dose exposure to germicides (e.g., <5 ppm) is unknown. During the 1970s and 1980s, patients treated with dialyzers reprocessed with formaldehyde were reported to develop cold agglutinins that were thought to increase kidney transplant allograft loss.[93] It was felt that the most likely cause for these cold agglutinins was formation of antibodies to blood group N during reprocessing. Reduction of formaldehyde levels to less than 2 ppm has reduced this problem substantially.[94] However, recent reports suggest that anti-N antibodies and other coombs positive reactions associated with reuse might remain an important toxicity form chronic long-term exposure. Ng and colleagues[95] demonstrated an increased prevalence of anti-N_{form} antibodies and coombs positive reactions in patients on reuse. A chronic low-grade hemolysis due to these antibodies and associated with reuse was assumed to have occurred in any patient whose hematocrit improved when reuse was discontinued.[95]

Health care workers and patients may also be exposed to the toxic effects of germicide concentrations in the ambient air or through dermal contact. Formaldehyde is an OHSA regulated substance. Ventilation of reprocessing area and air quality monitoring for toxic levels are mandated. It is uncertain, however, what constitutes a safe level of a chemical such as formaldehyde. Medical students with normal lung function participating in a gross anatomy laboratory with ventilation up to OHSA standards demonstrated substantial deterioration in pulmonary functions after relatively short periods of exposure. Recovery of their pulmonary functions occurred after exposure was discontinued.[91] Furthermore, formaldehyde has a documented carcinogenic potential that may be important for both health care workers and dialysis patients. In the latter group, an increased risk for carcinogenesis has yet to be demonstrated. This may be due to the relatively long lag time required for development of cancers after toxicant exposure and the relatively shorter life expectancy of current dialysis patients. In the future, as a larger number of these patients are successfully transplanted and treated with long-term immunosuppressant drugs or live longer due to improvements in overall dialysis care, the risk of carcinogenesis might be better defined. The direct toxicities of other germicides to health care workers and patients are less certain and appear to be far less potent.

Thus, in order to achieve adequate killing of bacteria and viruses, germicides for cold sterilization of dialyzers must be inherently toxic substances. The accepted methods of dialyzer reprocessing for reuse are designed to minimize the risks to health care workers and patients by substantially reducing the levels of potential exposures. However, the long-term consequences of low-level exposures remain uncertain. Furthermore, reuse of dialyzers provides opportunities for accidental exposures of patient and/or health care workers to excess quantities of these agents that would not occur in the absence of reuse.

EFFECT ON HOSPITALIZATION AND MORTALITY

Reuse and Hospitalization

Currently, on an average, dialysis patients in the United States experience an inpatient hospital stay of 1.8 days per year.[96] The rate of hospital admissions has decreased by a mere 1% since 1993 for these patients.[97] However, length of hospitalization has decreased by 7% during the same period. Most of the admissions are currently for either cardiovascular or infectious causes, with vascular access related admission having declined by 9% to 14%.[97] Reports on hospitalization rate with the practice of multiple dialyzer use are relatively few. In one of the earliest reports, Kant and colleagues[14] reported no difference in number of hospital days spent per patient when the same patients were transferred from a non-reuse to a reuse dialysis unit. However, this was a single center study with a small study sample and with no ability to either adjust for comorbidities or correct for temporal effects. In another study, the same authors examined the hospitalization rates and length of stay in a larger sample of patients at two centers, Cincinnati, Ohio, and Detroit, Michigan.[98] They observed that either the hospitalization rate (1.63/year and 2.19/year at Cincinnati and Detroit, respectively) or the length of hospitalization stay (14.24 and 22.71 days, respectively) was no different from the contemporary local and national averages.

In a study using Medicare data on over 32,000 prevalent hemodialysis patients in 1989 and 1990 in the United States, Held and colleagues[99] observed that hospital admission rates were significantly higher for patients dialyzed in units that reused dialyzers compared with patients who were dialyzed in units that did not reuse dialyzers. However, this increase in hospitalization rates was observed with either peracetic acid or glutaraldehyde but not formaldehyde reuse (RR 1.11, $p < .01$ for peracetic acid, RR 1.12, $p < .03$ for glutaraldehyde, and RR 1.04, $p = .29$ for formaldehyde).[99] This study had limitations in that it included only *prevalent* patients and that the comorbidity adjustment was limited to a very few covariates. Feldman and colleagues[100] re-analyzed the Medicare data limiting to *incident* patients starting dialysis in 1986 and 1987 in freestanding and hospital-based dialysis units. Their total sample consisted of 27,264 patients. Significant differences were observed between freestanding and hospital-based units. For patients dialyzed in freestanding units that reused dialyzers, there was an 8% increase in hospitalization compared to patients dialyzed in units that did not reuse dialyzers. In addition, an increase in hospitalization was observed with either peracetic acid mixture (11% higher) or formaldehyde (7% higher) but not glutaraldehyde reuse.[100] These differences were not observed among patients dialyzed in hospital-based dialysis units. These findings confirmed those of the earlier study by Held and colleagues[100] referred to earlier. However, the analysis was limited to patients using conventional (low-flux) dialyzers and therefore, not representative of the current practices. In addition, because of limited information in this data set, comorbidity adjustment was limited to age, race, gender, and cause of ESRD.

To overcome the problem of comorbidity adjustment, the same group of investigators used the USRDS case-mix study data where comprehensive information on comorbidity was available at initiation of dialysis. The analysis was restricted to freestanding dialysis units. They observed that among 1491 incident dialysis patients, reuse of dialyzers was associated with a 37% higher hospitalization rate compared with patients treated with single-use dialyzers.[101] Hospitalization rates were 25% higher with formaldehyde reuse and 40% higher with peracetic acid mixture reuse.[101]

Although this data is compelling, a clear cause-and-effect relationship between dialyzer reuse and increased hospitalization cannot be drawn from any of the previously mentioned studies because of inability to control for aspects of care other than reuse, such as adequacy of dialysis, vascular access infections, and so forth. In addition, whether this difference in hospitalization rates with dialyzer reuse and reuse practices persists in the current practice of high-efficiency and high-flux dialyzer use allowing attainment of larger dialysis doses is unclear. Clearly more studies are required in this area to answer definitively these questions.

Reuse and Patient Survival

One of the potential reasons for decreased dialysis adequacy is a decline in dialyzer performance following reprocessing of dialyzers, and any significant decline in dialyzer performance with reuse could result potentially in an increase in overall mortality. In a study using Medicare data for prevalent patients, Held and colleagues[99] observed a 13% increase in mortality among patients treated with dialyzers that were reprocessed with peracetic acid, and a 17% increase in mortality when reprocessed with glutaraldehyde, compared with units that did not practice dialyzer reuse. They observed no significant increase in mortality among patients treated with dialyzers reprocessed with formaldehyde. This was the first study using a national sample that looked at mortality in patients treated with reprocessed dialyzers. The study, however, suffered from certain limitations. The analysis included only dialysis units that predominantly used conventional (low-flux) dialyzers, thus excluding adequate representation of the large number of patients who under current practice use high-flux dialyzers. Hospital-based dialysis units were excluded because of higher comorbidity and a greater variation in case-mix severity among patients treated in these units. Comorbidity adjustment in the statistical analysis was limited and therefore confounding could not be excluded. In addition, the study also suffered from a "survival bias" because only prevalent patients were included.

Feldman and colleagues[102] performed a similar study using Medicare data where they included only *incident* patients who began renal replacement therapy in 1986 and 1987 and followed up until January 31, 1991. They observed that among 27,938 patients, dialysis in freestanding facilities reprocessing dialyzers with peracetic acid mixture was associated with a greater mortality compared with facilities not reprocessing dialyzers (rate ratio 1.10, 95% CI 1.02–1.18).[102] In contrast, survival was not significantly different between facilities reprocessing dialzyers with formaldehyde or glutaraldehyde compared with facilities not reprocessing dialyzers. Among hospital-based facilities, there was no difference in mortality between facilities that reprocessed dialyzers (with any reprocessing method) and those that did not.[102] These findings were similar to those reported by Held and colleagues despite eliminating most of the survival bias. This study also had limitations. First, unit-level data were used, not patient-level data. Second, comorbidity adjustment was limited because of nonavailability of data. Last, certain strong predictors of mortality such as adequacy of dialysis, anemia management and the like were not taken into consideration.

To address the issue of comorbidity adjustment, Feldman and colleagues analyzed patient survival in the USRDS casemix study data set where they analyzed hospitalization rates, as discussed earlier. In this data set, Feldman and colleagues[101] observed that patients treated with reprocessed dialyzers had a 25% higher mortality compared with patients who were not. Comparing the method of reuse, peracetic acid reuse was associated with a 28% increase whereas formaldehyde reuse was associated with a 29% increase in mortality, compared with single-use dialyzers.[101] This study confirms the increase in mortality with reuse in general, and peracetic acid reuse in particular, observed by Held and colleagues. Furthermore, Feldman and colleagues observed an identical increase in mortality with formaldehyde reuse.

Collins and colleagues[103] replicated the earlier study by Held and colleagues with patient-level data, adjusting for comorbidities, and including anemia treatment as well as profit-status of the dialysis units. Again, this analysis was restricted to units using predominantly conventional dialyzers. Seven major comorbidities were included in the analysis. The results showed that when all germicides were combined, significantly lower risks (0.93 CI 0.88–0.98 for each year period) were identified among freestanding units between 1991 and 1993 but not between 1989 and 1990. With profit status as a covariate, there was no significant effect of germicide on mortality in 1989 to 1990 for either type of unit designation (hospital-based or freestanding), but during 1991 to 1993, freestanding units with reuse had a significantly lower associated mortality risk. When hospital-based and freestanding units were combined for analysis, peracetic acid reuse was associated with a 15% higher mortality (RR 1.15, CI 1.01–1.31) compared to non-reuse only in the 1989 to 1990 period. This higher mortality risk was not seen during the 1991 to 1993 period (RR 1.03, CI 0.92–1.15). Formaldehyde and glutaraldehyde did not have any effect on mortality in these studies during either period. The results of this study indicate that the association of reuse practices with mortality vary in different dialysis unit settings. In addition, the mortality risks during the 1991 to 1993 period were significantly lower compared to the earlier period (1989–1990). Multiple explanations can be offered for this observation—a few being an improvement in reuse technique with more reliance on automated method of reuse; use of erythropoietin for anemia treatment on a more regular basis; and, in general, an improved quality of care over the years. Indeed, data from the USRDS suggest that the mean Kt/V has increased from 0.91 in 1986 to 1.37 for prevalent patients in 1996 to 1997, and URR from 63% to 68% during the same period.[104] However, the previous study by Collins and colleagues[105] also suffers from certain limitations. Incident patients were not analyzed separately in this study, and hence, the "survivor advantage" associated with prevalent patients may influence the results. Patient-level and unit-level data were mixed and analyzed using complex statistical analyses. Interpretation of the results of this complex analysis have been questioned. Last, the "center effect" may not be actually due to a difference in reuse technique or germicide used but may depend on other policies of the dialysis units, physician practices, or other unknown confounding variables.

In addition, all of the previous studies collectively have certain limitations. These were restricted to dialysis units using predominantly conventional dialyzers and did not account for differences in dialysis dose. Thus, they exclude a large population of dialysis patients using high-flux dialyzers in whom reuse is almost universal.[8] With more frequent use of high-flux dialyzers in reuse units, a larger dialysis dose could be delivered to patients treated in these units. Indeed, Agodoa and colleagues,[32] using the USRDS data, observed a higher delivered dose of dialysis, as measured by Kt/V urea, at units that reused dialyzers compared to those that did not (Kt/V urea 1.22 vs. 1.19). In addition, the frequency of use of high-flux dialysis was higher among units that reused dialyzers compared with those that did not (97% vs. 65%).[32] Thus, an inability to adjust for flux and dialysis dose seriously limits the applicability of the results of these observational studies to the current dialysis practices. In addition, a lack of random assignment of patients to reuse or non-reuse limits the interpretation with regard to cause-and-effect relationship in these studies. Additionally, data on the Health Care Financing Agency (HCFA) 2728 form are subject to error because of incomplete and inaccurate recording of comorbidities. Indeed, a recent study observed a significant underreporting of comorbidities on the HCFA 2728 Medical Evidence form.[106]

Port and colleagues[107] used DMMS data (waves 1, 3, and 4) collected from dialysis units that were randomly selected and adjusted for demographics, comorbidities, dialysis dose, dialyzer flux, and facility type. They observed that overall, there was no significant difference in the adjusted death rates for patients at facilities that reused dialyzers compared with patients at facilities that did not reuse dialyzers (RR 0.96, 95% CI 0.86–1.08). Among patients who reused dialyzers, there was no significant difference in mortality risk between patients whose dialyzers were reprocessed with peracetic acid (without bleach) and with formaldehyde (with bleach) (RR 1.15 for peracetic acid, 95% CI 0.99–1.30). With regard to the type of membrane, patients treated with reprocessed synthetic membranes and use of bleach had the lowest mortality. When synthetic membranes were separately analyzed, low-flux membranes had a 24% higher relative risk of death compared with high-flux membranes, and no bleach use was associated with a similar 24% higher RR of death ($p = .04$ for both comparisons). Although this study is one of the best that has been conducted so far, it still suffers from limitations such as survival bias. Attribution of patients to dialysis modality (reuse or non-reuse) was done at enrollment into the study, and any subsequent change in modality was not captured.

In a retrospective analysis, Lowrie and colleagues[108] recently analyzed the association of reuse with mortality risk in 71,122 patients treated at dialysis units in the United States, owned by Fresenius Medical Care. Some facilities changed their policy from reuse to single use, and this offered the opportunity to study the effects of reuse and single use in patients treated at these units. In considering cumulative effects of either of the treatment options, a lag analytic strategy was used to model the effects of reuse on mortality, with lag times of 30, 60, 90, and 120 days from the time of switch from reuse to single use. Analyses were adjusted for case-mix and follow-up was 12 months from entry into study. They observed a survival advantage with changing from reuse to single use with benefit improving as the lag time increased (hazard ratio 0.93, $p = .02$ at 6 months, and 0.92, $p = .01$ at 1 year).[108] Again, there are several limitations to this study. Some of these include:

1. Reprocessing method was not taken into consideration.
2. Membrane flux was not modeled.
3. Temporal effects could not be excluded despite the lag time analytic technique.
4. Study was restricted to prevalent patients only.

In addition, the study includes patients treated by a single dialysis provider.

In summary, studies that observed higher patient-mortality rates with reuse had several limitations. In addition, none of these studies have been able to show a direct cause-and-effect relationship between mortality and dialyzer reuse or use of a certain reprocessing technique. Nonetheless, the majority of observational studies are congruent in their findings of effect, indicating a potential for an increased mortality especially when reuse is performed with low flux dialyzers. Some of the more recent studies, however, also observed improved dialysis adequacy in centers that reuse dialyzers.[32] In the setting of falling reimbursement rates for ESRD care in the United States, reuse offers a means to deliver higher quality dialysis with potentially improved outcomes when high-flux dialyzers are used. In this regard, the results of the Hemodialysis Study that observed no additional benefit in survival of hemodialysis patients treated with high-flux dialysis compared with low-flux dialysis are of concern.[109] Experts continue to advocate use of high-flux dialyzers as they offer benefits beyond "flux," such as better biocompatibility, fewer dialysis reactions, and increased clearance of β2-microglobulin, and probably decreased incidence of dialysis-related amyloidosis. It is still unclear whether reuse is associated with a true increase in mortality in hemodialysis patients.

COST-EFFECTIVENESS OF DIALYZER REUSE

Currently, over 350,000 patients are receiving renal replacement therapy for ESRD in the United States.[97] The majority of these patients are supported through the Medicare ESRD Program of the federal government. While ESRD patients accounted for 0.6% of the total Medicare population, treatment cost of ESRD accounted for 6.4% of the total Medicare budget in the year 2001.[97] Thus, ESRD receives a disproportionate funding relative to its prevalence. Moreover, the costs have been rising every year because of increasing incidence of ESRD and longer life expectancy of patients on dialysis and after renal transplantation. For example, in 1991, ESRD expenditure in the United States was $8 billion, with Medicare paying $5.8 billion, the rest coming from non-Medicare sources such as private insurance.[97] By 2001, the costs of the program had risen to $22.8 billion, with Medicare paying $15.4 billion, three times the cost of 1991.[97] During the same period, overall Medicare expenditure increased only two times. To contain the growing costs of the program, the federal government has kept the composite payment rate to dialysis providers constant, thus eroding their returns through inflation. In search of ways of limiting the costs of dialysis, dialysis providers have promoted reuse of dialyzers. Currently 80% of dialysis centers practice reuse.[8] Until recently, a critical cost-effectiveness evaluation of dialyzer reuse has not been undertaken.

In one of the earliest studies done from Canada, a cost-minimization analysis indicated that five uses of a dialyzer might save up to Can$3629 per patient yearly.[110] This would translate into Can$5.8 to $8.9 million annually if all eligible patients in Canada participated in a reuse program.[110] However, this study did not take into account the potential negative health effects of dialyzer reuse. Since this study, the cost of single use dialyzers has significantly decreased, thus narrowing the cost differences between single use and reuse methods. Reuse rates are much lower in Canada at 15%, and even lower in Europe at 10%.[111] In a cost-utility analysis, again from Canada, Manns and colleagues[111] compared single use with multiple uses of high-flux dialyzers. The reuse methods chosen were formaldehyde, and heated citric acid. The cost of formaldehyde reuse was estimated at Can$15.47 per patient per run, and that of heated citric acid was Can$12.66 per patient per run. The measure of effectiveness was quality-adjusted life-years (QALY), obtained from an earlier analysis from Canada.[112] For a dialysis facility with 320 patients, and assuming an average of 13.3 reuses, the 5-year cost of single use dialysis per patient was Can$218,284 and the average number of expected QALYs per patient over a 5-year period was 1.648.[111] For reuse with heated citric acid, per patient, the 5-year cost was estimated at Can$217,073, and the average number of QALYs was 1.644. The incremental cost with single use was Can$299,739 per QALY gained. Given the fact that reuse has not shown to increase mortality, the authors suggested that by switching to reuse, there could be significant cost savings for the payer.[111] In these analyses, formaldehyde method was not cost-effective.

While this is a well-conducted study, extrapolation of this data to the United States is difficult. First, heated citric acid is the least common method of dialyzer reprocessing in the United States; formaldehyde reprocessing is on the decline and peracetic acid is the commonest.[8] An analysis comparing peracetic acid and formaldehyde reuse with single use would be more applicable to the U.S. population. Second, the study assumes no increase in personnel in dialysis units that practice reuse, which is actually not the case in the United States, with centralized reuse being more popular. Last, mortality and hospitalization data were obtained from studies comparing conventional dialyzers. In the United States, conventional dialyzers have largely been replaced with high-flux synthetic dialyzers with over 70% units using exclusively high-flux dialyzers.[8] It is unclear whether the same hospitalization rates would apply to patients dialyzed with reprocessed high-flux dialyzers as well. Nevertheless, this happens to be the best study that is available to date on this subject.

Given the fact that the main benefit of reuse is economic, clearly, a robust cost-effectiveness analysis in the United States is required to answer the question of whether reuse is really worth the cost savings. The federal government continues to benefit indirectly from the ongoing practice of reuse through cost savings experienced by the providers, thus limiting the pressure to raise the composite rate should a cost-effectiveness analysis indicate that single use programs should be implemented universally in the United States.[113] In the absence of data on compromised quality of care when reuse is practiced within accepted guidelines and standards, reuse is likely to continue.

SUMMARY

Reuse of dialyzers has had a persistent growth in the United States since its introduction in the 1960s. Although in 1982, only 43% of dialysis centers reused their dialyzers, currently 80% of the dialysis units practice reuse. Germicides used for disinfecting the reprocessed dialyzers include peracetic acid/hydrogen peroxide mixture, formaldehyde and glutaraldehyde, and, over the last decade, heated citric acid. In addition, bleach is used, predominantly with formaldehyde, to improve the appearance of the dialyzer. Automated machines are more popular than the manual methods of reprocessing of dialyzers. The predominant factor driving the current practice of reuse of dialyzers in the United States is economic. Concern regarding the preservation of integrity of the dialyzer membranes led to several studies on clearance of solutes by reprocessed dialyzers. These reveal that neither the small molecule clearances nor the ultrafiltration capacity of cellulose/substituted cellulose dialyzers are affected with reuse, irrespective of the germicide used. Similarly, small molecule clearances are only modestly affected with reprocessed synthetic dialyzers, and the significance of this decrease is likely clinically insignificant. Middle molecular solute clearances are not significant with low-flux cellulose or synthetic dialyzers and not significantly changed with reprocessing. However, for high-flux polysulfone dialyzers, reprocessing with bleach increases and reprocessing with peracetic acid decreases β_2 microglobulin clearance. Although earlier studies observed heavy protein and albumin losses with high-flux polysulfone dialyzers, a change in the membrane configuration by the manufacturer has essentially taken care of this problem. Despite its effect on clearances, albeit minor, it is encouraging to note that reuse does not adversely affect the delivered dose of dialysis.

Reprocessed dialyzers have been associated with decreased complement activation and leukopenia compared with new dialyzers. However, this mitigation of complement activation and leukopenia has not shown to be associated with improved clinical outcomes. In addition, there is no known evidence that dialysis with reprocessed dialyzers results in enhanced production of pro-inflammatory cytokines or an exaggeration of chronic inflammatory response seen in the uremic environment. Although several episodes of bacterial and viral infections and catastrophic toxicity of chemicals have occurred as a result of reuse, the common feature among most of these episodes is human error leading to a breakdown in strict adherence to the AAMI reuse guidelines.

In large observational studies, hospitalization rates of dialysis patients were 25% higher with formaldehyde reuse and 40% higher with peracetic acid mixture reuse. Because of inability to control for aspects of care other than reuse, a clear cause-and-effect relationship between dialyzer reuse and increased hospitalization cannot be drawn. Some observational studies on large patient populations observed higher patient-mortality rates with reuse, but these studies had several limitations. In addition, none of these studies has been able to show a direct cause-and-effect relationship between mortality and dialyzer reuse or use of a certain reprocessing technique. Some studies also observed improved dialysis adequacy in centers that reuse dialyzers compared with centers that practice single use dialyzers. It is unclear whether reuse is associated with a true increased mortality in hemodialysis patients.

In the setting of falling reimbursement rates for ESRD care in the United States, reuse offers a means to deliver more adequate clearances and potentially thereby improve quality of care with improved outcomes when high-flux dialyzers are used. These dialyzers offer potential benefits beyond "flux" such as better biocompatibility, fewer dialysis reactions, and probably decreased incidence of dialysis-related amyloidosis. Limited cost-effectiveness studies from Canada showed that there could be significant savings per quality-adjusted life year gained by moving from single use to reuse of dialyzers, particularly with heated citric acid reuse. Clearly, a robust cost-effectiveness analysis in the United States is required to answer the question of whether reuse is really worth the cost savings in this society. In the absence of data on compromised quality of care when reuse is practiced within accepted guidelines and standards, reuse is likely to continue.

References

1. Shaldon SH, Silva H, Rosen SM: The technique of refrigerated coil preservation hemodialysis with femoral venous catherization. Br Med J 1964; 2:672–674.
2. Pollard TL, Barnett BMS, Eshbach JW, Scribner BH: A technique for storage and multiple reuse of Kiil dialyzer and blood tubing. ASAIO Trans 1967; 13:24–28.
3. Hakim RM, Lowrie EG: Effect of dialyzer reuse on leukopenia, hypoxemia and total hemolytic complement system. Trans Am Soc Artif Intern Organs 1980; 26:159–164.
4. Chenoweth DE, Cheung AK, Ward DM, Henderson LW: Anaphylatoxin formation during hemodialysis: Comparison of new and re-used dialyzers. Kidney Int 1983; 24:770–774.
5. Stroncek DF, Keshaviah P, Craddock PR, Hammerschmidt DE: Effect of dialyzer reuse on complement activation and neutropenia in hemodialysis. J Lab Clin Med 1984; 104:304–311.
6. AAMI: Reuse of hemodialyzers. AAMI standards and recommended practices, vol. 3. Arlington, VA, Association for the Advancement of Medical Instrumentation, 1995, pp 106–107.
7. Shaldon S: Dialyzer reuse: A practice that should be abandoned. Semin Dial 1993; 6:11–12.
8. Tokars JI, Frank M, Alter MJ, Arduino MJ: National surveillance of dialysis-associated diseases in the United States, 2000. Semin Dial 2002; 15:162–171.
9. Levin NW, Parnell SL, Prince HN, et al: The use of heated citric acid for dialyzer reprocessing. J Am Soc Nephrol 1995; 6:1578–1585.
10. Okechukwu CN, Orzol SM, Held PJ, et al: Characteristics and treatment of patients not reusing dialyzers in reuse units. Am J Kidney Dis 2000; 36:991–999.
11. Gotch FA: Dialyzer transport properties and germicide elution. Proceedings, Seminars on Reuse of Hemodialyzers and Automated and Manual Methods. New York, National Nephrology Foundation, 1984.
12. Sherman RA, Cody RP, Rogers ME, Solanchick JC: The effect of dialyzer reuse on dialysis delivery. Am J Kidney Dis 1994; 24:924–926.

13. Shusterman NH, Feldman HI, Wasserstein A, Strom BL: Reprocessing of hemodialyzers: A critical appraisal (Review). Am J Kidney Dis 1989; 14:81–91.
14. Kant KS, Pollack VE, Cathey M, et al: Multiple use of dialyzers: Safety and efficacy. Kidney Int 1981; 19:728–738.
15. Hoenich NA, Johnston SRD, Buckley P, et al: Hemodialysis reuse: Impact on function and biocompatibility. Int J Artif Organs 1983; 6:261–266.
16. Kaye M, Gagnon R, Mulhearn B, Spergel D: Prolonged dialyzer reuse. Trans Am Soc Artif Intern Organs 1984; 30:491–493.
17. Churchill DN, Taylor DW, Shimizu AG, et al: Dialyzer re-use: A multiple crossover study with random allocation to order of treatment. Nephron 1988; 50:325–331.
18. Vanholder RC, Sys E, DeCubber A, et al: Performance of cuprophane and polyacrylonitrile dialyzers during multiple use. Kidney Int Suppl 1988; 24:S55–S56.
19. Murthy BV, Sundaram S, Jaber BL, et al: Effect of formaldehyde/bleach reprocessing on in vivo performances of high-efficiency cellulose and high-flux polysulfone dialyzers. J Am Soc Nephrol 1998; 9:464–472.
20. Leypoldt JK, Cheung AK, Deeter RB: Effect of hemodialyzer reuse: Dissociation between clearances of small and large solutes. Am J Kidney Dis 1998; 32:295–301.
21. Cheung AK, Agodoa LY, Daugirdas JT, et al: Effects of hemodialyzer reuse on clearances of urea and beta 2-microglobulin. The Hemodialysis (HEMO) Study Group. J Am Soc Nephrol 1999; 10:117–127.
22. Garred LJ, Canaud B, Flavier JL, et al: Effect of reuse on dialyzer efficacy. Artif Organs 1990; 14:80–84.
23. Kaplan AA, Halley SE, Lapkin RA, Graeber CW: Dialysate protein losses with bleach processed polysulfone dialyzers. Kidney Int 1995; 47:573–578.
24. Goldman M, Lagmiche M, Dhaene M, et al: Adsorption of beta 2-microglobulin on dialysis membranes: Comparison of different dialyzers and effects of reuse procedures (Review). Int J Artif Organs 1989; 12:373–378.
25. Westhuyzen J, Foreman K, Battistutta D, et al: Effect of dialyzer reprocessing with Renalin on serum beta-2-microglobulin and complement activation in hemodialysis patients. Am J Nephrol 1992; 12:29–36.
26. Kerr PG, Argiles A, Canaud B, et al: The effects of reprocessing high-flux polysulfone dialyzers with peroxyacetic acid on beta 2-microglobulin removal in hemodiafiltration. Am J Kidney Dis 1992; 19:433–438.
27. Krautzig S, Mahiout A, Koch KM, Lemke HD: Reuse with oxidizing agents leads to a loss of polyvinylpyrrolidone from polysulfone membranes (Abstract). Blood Purif 1994; 12:176.
28. Donahue PR, Ahmad S: Dialyzer permeability alteration by reuse (Abstract). J Am Soc Nephrol 1992; 3:363.
29. Peterson DE, Hyver T, Yeh I, J P: Reprocessing dialyzers with peracetic acid-hydrogen peroxide does not cause substantial protein losses (Abstract). J Am Soc Nephrol 1994; 5:424.
30. Anonymous: NKF-DOQI clinical practice guidelines for hemodialysis adequacy. National Kidney Foundation. Am J Kidney Dis 1997; 30:S15–S66.
31. Pereira BJ, Natov SN, Sundaram S, et al: Impact of single use versus reuse of cellulose dialyzers on clinical parameters and indices of biocompatibility. J Am Soc Nephrol 1996; 7:861–870.
32. Agodoa LY, Wolfe RA, Port FK: Reuse of dialyzers and clinical outcomes: Fact or fiction. Am J Kidney Dis 1998; 32:S88–S92.
33. Kaplow LS, Goffinet JA: Profound neutropenia during the early phase of hemodialysis. JAMA 1968; 203:1135–1137.
34. Cheung AK, Henderson LW: Effects of complement activation by hemodialysis membranes (Review). Am J Nephrol 1986; 6:81–91.
35. Horl WH, Feinstein EI, Wanner C, et al: Plasma levels of main granulocyte components during hemodialysis. Comparison of new and reused dialyzers. Am J Nephrol 1990; 10:53–57.
36. Kuwahara T, Markert M, Wauters JP: Biocompatibility aspects of dialyzer reprocessing: A comparison of 3 re-use methods and 3 membranes. Clin Nephrol 1989; 32:139–143.
37. Dolovich J, Bell B: Allergy to a product(s) of ethylene oxide gas: Demonstration of IgE and IgG antibodies and hapten specificity. J Allerg Clin Immunol 1978; 62:30–32.
38. Dolovich J, Marshall CP, Smith EK, et al: Allergy to ethylene oxide in chronic hemodialysis patients. Artif Organs 1984; 8:334–337.
39. Daugirdas JT, Ing TS: First-use reactions during hemodialysis: A definition of sub-types. Kidney Int Suppl 1988; 24:S37–S43.
40. Charoenpanich R, Pollak VE, Kant KS, et al: Effect of first and subsequent use of hemodialyzers on patient well-being: The rise and fall of a syndrome associated with new dialyzer use. Artif Organs 1987; 11:123–127.
41. Hakim RM, Fearon DT, Lazarus JM: Biocompatibility of dialysis membranes: Effects of chronic complement activation. Kidney Int 1984; 26:194–200.
42. Daugirdas JT, Potempa LD, Dinh N, et al: Plate, coil, and hollow-fiber cuprammonium cellulose dialyzers: Discrepancy between incidence of anaphylactic reactions and degree of complement activation. Artif Organs 1987; 11:140–143.
43. Pegues DA, Beck-Sague CM, Woollen SW, et al: Anaphylactoid reactions associated with reuse of hollow-fiber hemodialyzers and ACE inhibitors. Kidney Int 1992; 42:1232–1237.
44. Tielmans C, Madhoun P, Lenaers M, et al: Anaphylactoid reactions during hemodialysis on AN69 membranes in patients receiving ACE inhibitors. Kidney Int 1990; 38:982–984.
45. Parnes EL, Shapiro WB: Anaphylactoid reactions in hemodialysis patients treated with the AN69 dialyzer. Kidney Int 1991; 40:1148–1152.
46. Brunet P, Jaber K, Berland Y, Baz M: Anaphylactoid reactions during hemodialysis and hemofiltration: Role of associating AN69 membrane and angiotensin I-converting enzyme inhibitors. Am J Kidney Dis 1992; 19:444–447.
47. Veressen L, Fink E, Lemke HD, Vanrenterghem Y: Bradykinin is a mediator of anaphylactoid reactions during hemodialysis with AN69 membranes. Kidney Int 1994; 45:1497–1503.
48. Saracho R, Martin-Malo A, Martinez I, et al: Evaluation of Losartan in Hemodialysis (ELHE) study. Kidney Int Suppl 1998; 68:S125–S129.
49. Pereira BJ, Dinarello CA: Production of pro-inflammatory cytokines and cytokine inhibitory proteins in patients on dialysis. Nephrol Dial Transplant 1994; 9(suppl 2):60–71.
50. Pereira BJ, Poutsiaka DD, King AJ, et al: In vitro production of interleukin-1 receptor antagonist in chronic renal failure, CAPD and HD. Kidney Int 1992; 42:1419–1424.
51. Pereira BJ, King AJ, Falagas ME, Dinarello CA: Interleukin-1 receptor antagonist (IL-1Ra) and index of dialysis-induced interleukin-1 production. Nephron 1994; 67:358–361.
52. Schindler R, Linnenweber S, Schulze M, et al: Gene expression of interleukin-1beta during hemodialysis. Kidney Int 1993; 43:712–721.
53. Henderson LW, Koch KM, Dinarello CA, Shaldon S: Hemodialysis hypotension: The interleukin-1 hypothesis. Blood Purif 1983; 1: 3–8.
54. Lufft V, Mahiout A, Shaldon S, et al: Retention of cytokine-inducing substances inside high-flux dialyzers. Blood Purif 1996; 14:26–34.
55. Tokars JI, Alter MJ, Miller E, et al: National surveillance of dialysis associated diseases in the United States, 1994. ASAIO J 1997; 43:108–119.
56. Pereira BJ, Snodgrass B, Barber G, et al: Cytokine production during *in vitro* hemodialysis with new and formaldehyde or renalin-reprocessed cellulose dialyzers. J Am Soc Nephrol 1995; 6:1304–1308.
57. Haubitz M, Schulze M, Koch KM: Increase of C-reactive protein serum values following hemodialysis. Nephrol Dial Transplant 1990; 5:500–503.

58. Stenvinkel P, Heimburger O, Paultre F, et al: Strong association between malnutrition, inflammation, and atherosclerosis in chronic renal failure. Kidney Int 1999; 55:1899–1911.
59. Docci D, Bilancioni R, Buscaroli A, et al: Elevated serum levels of C-reactive protein in hemodialysis patients. Nephron 1990; 56:364–367.
60. Schindler R, Boenisch O, Fischer C, Frei U: Effect of the hemodialysis membrane on the inflammatory reaction *in-vivo*. Clin Nephrol 2000; 63:452–459.
61. Zimmermann J, Herrlinger S, Pray A, et al: Inflammation enhances cardiovascular risk and mortality in hemodialysis. Kidney Int 1999; 55:648–658.
62. Schoenfeld PY: The technology of dialyzer reuse. Semin Nephrol 1997; 17:321–330.
63. Hudson P: Applying the lessons of high risk industries to health care. Qual Saf Health Care 2003; 12(suppl 1):I7–I12.
64. Ouseph R, Ward RA: Water treatment for hemodialysis: Ensuring patient safety. Semin Dial 2002; 15:50–52.
65. Roth VR, Jarvis WR: Outbreaks of infection and/or pyrogenic reactions in dialysis patients. Semin Dial 2000; 13:92–96.
66. Tokars JI, Arduino MJ, Alter MJ: Infection control in hemodialysis units. Infect Dis Clin North Am 2001; 15:797–812, viii.
67. Favero MS: Requiem for reuse of single-use devices in U.S. hospitals. Infect Control Hosp Epidemiol 2001; 22:539–541.
68. Alter MJ, Favero MS, Miller JK, et al: Reuse of hemodialyzers. Results of nationwide surveillance for adverse effects. JAMA 1988; 260:2073–2076.
69. Powe NR, Jaar B, Furth SL, et al: Septicemia in dialysis patients: Incidence, risk factors, and prognosis. Kidney Int 1999; 55:1081–1090.
70. Jaar BG, Hermann JA, Furth SL, et al: Septicemia in diabetic hemodialysis patients: Comparison of incidence, risk factors, and mortality with nondiabetic hemodialysis patients. Am J Kidney Dis 2000; 35:282–292.
71. Bolan G, Reingold AL, Carson LA, et al: Infections with mycobacterium chelonei in patients receiving dialysis and using processed hemodialyzers. J Infect Dis 1985; 152:1013–1019.
72. Gordon SM, Tipple M, Bland LA, Jarvis WR: Pyrogenic reactions associated with the reuse of disposable hollow-fiber hemodialyzers. JAMA 1988; 260:2077–2081.
73. Lowry PW, Beck-Sague CM, Bland LA, et al: Mycobacterium chelonae infection among patients receiving high-flux dialysis in a hemodialysis clinic in California. J Infect Dis 1990; 161: 85–90.
74. Beck-Sague CM, Jarvis WR, Bland LA, et al: Outbreak of gram-negative bacteremia and pyrogenic reactions in a hemodialysis center. Am J Nephrol 1990; 10:397–403.
75. Vanholder R, Vanhaecke E, Ringoir S: Pseudomonas septicemia due to deficient disinfectant mixing during reuse. Int J Artif Organs 1992; 15:19–24.
76. Flaherty JP, Garcia-Houchins S, Chudy R, Arnow PM: An outbreak of gram-negative bacteremia traced to contaminated O-rings in reprocessed dialyzers. Ann Intern Med 1993; 119: 1072–1078.
77. Jackson BM, Beck-Sague CM, Bland LA, et al: Outbreak of pyrogenic reactions and gram-negative bacteremia in a hemodialysis center. Am J Nephrol 1994; 14:85–89.
78. Rudnick JR, Arduino MJ, Bland LA, et al: An outbreak of pyrogenic reactions in chronic hemodialysis patients associated with hemodialyzer reuse. Artif Organs 1995; 19:289–294.
79. Welbel SF, Schoendorf K, Bland LA, et al: An outbreak of gram-negative bloodstream infections in chronic hemodialysis patients. Am J Nephrol 1995; 15:1–4.
80. Morin P: Identification of the bacteriological contamination of a water treatment line used for haemodialysis and its disinfection. J Hosp Infect 2000; 45:218–224.
81. Arvanitidou M, Vayona A, Spanakis N, Tsakris A: Occurrence and antimicrobial resistance of gram-negative bacteria isolated in haemodialysis water and dialysate of renal units: Results of a Greek multicentre study. J Appl Microbiol 2003; 95:180–185.
82. Carson LA, Bland LA, Cusick LB, et al: Prevalence of nontuberculous mycobacteria in water supplies of hemodialysis centers. Appl Environ Microbiol 1988; 54:3122–3125.
83. Leypoldt JK, Murthy BV, Pereira BJ, et al: Does reuse have clinically important effects on dialyzer function? Semin Dial 2000; 13:281–290.
84. Bland LA, Favero MS, Oxborrow GS, et al: Effect of chemical germicides on the integrity of hemodialyzer membranes. ASAIO Trans 1988; 34:172–175.
85. Murthy BV, Pereira BJ: A 1990s perspective of hepatitis C, human immunodeficiency virus, and tuberculosis infections in dialysis patients. Semin Nephrol 1997; 17:346–363.
86. Jadoul M, Cornu C, van Ypersele de Strihou C: Universal precautions prevent hepatitis C virus transmission: A 54-month follow-up of the Belgian multicenter study. The Universitaires Cliniques St-Luc (UCL) Collaborative Group. Kidney Int 1998; 53:1022–1025.
87. Rao TK: Human immunodeficiency virus infection in end-stage renal disease patients. Semin Dial 2003; 16:233–244.
88. Pereira BJG, Levey AS: Hepatitis C virus infection in dialysis and renal transplantation. Kidney Int 1997; 51:981–999.
89. Pinto dos Santos J, Loureiro A, Cendoroglo M, Pereira BJG: Impact of dialysis room and reuse strategies on the incidence of HCV infection in HD units. Nephrol Dial Transplant 1996; 11:2017–2022.
90. Arduino MJ: CDC investigations of noninfectious outbreaks of adverse events in hemodialysis facilities, 1979–1999. Semin Dial 2000; 13:86–91.
91. Agency for Toxic Substances and Disease Registry: Toxicological effects of formaldehyde: Health effects. Department of Health and Human Services, 2003.
92. Stragier A, Wenderickx D, Jadoul M: Rinsing time and disinfectant release of reused dialyzers: Comparison of formaldehyde, hypochlorite, warexin, and renalin. Am J Kidney Dis 1995; 26:549–553.
93. Kaehny WD, Miller GE, White WL: Relationship between dialyzer reuse and the presence of anti-N-like antibodies in chronic hemodialysis patients. Kidney Int 1977; 12:59–65.
94. Vanholder R, Noens L, De Smet R, Ringoir S: Development of anti-N-like antibodies during formaldehyde reuse in spite of adequate predialysis rinsing. Am J Kidney Dis 1988; 11:477–480.
95. Ng YY, Chow MP, Wu SC, et al: Anti-N-form antibody in hemodialysis patients. Am J Nephrol 1995; 15:374–378.
96. United States Renal Data System: USRDS Annual Data Report, 2002. Bethesda, MD, National Institutes of Health, National Institute of Diabetes and Digestive and Kidney Diseases, 2002.
97. United States Renal Data System: USRDS Annual Data Report, 2003. Bethesda, MD, National Institutes of Health, National Institute of Diabetes and Digestive and Kidney Diseases, 2003.
98. Pollak VE, Kant KS, Parnell SL, Levin NW: Repeated use of dialyzers is safe: Long-term observations on morbidity and mortality in patients with end-stage renal disease. Nephron 1986; 42:217–223.
99. Held PJ, Wolfe RA, Gaylin DS, et al: Analysis of the association of dialyzer reuse practices and patient outcomes. Am J Kidney Dis 1994; 23:692–708.
100. Feldman HI, Bilker WB, Hackett M, et al: Association of dialyzer reuse and hospitalization rates among hemodialysis patients in the U.S. Am J Nephrol 1999; 19:641–648.
101. Feldman HI, Bilker WB, Hackett MH, et al: Association of dialyzer reuse with hospitalization and survival rates among U.S. hemodialysis patients: Do comorbidities matter? J Clin Epidemiol 1999; 52:209–217.
102. Feldman HI, Kinosian M, Bilker WB, et al: Effect of dialyzer reuse on survival of patients treated with hemodialysis. JAMA 1996; 276:620–625.

103. Collins AJ, Ma JZ, Constantini EG, Everson SE: Dialysis unit and patient characteristics associated with reuse practices and mortality: 1989–1993. J Am Soc Nephrol 1998; 9:2108–2117.
104. United States Renal Data System: USRDS Annual Data Report, 1999. Bethesda, MD, National Institutes of Health, National Institute of Diabetes and Digestive and Kidney Diseases, 1999.
105. Kimmel PL, Mishkin GJ: Dialyzer reuse and the treatment of patients with end-stage renal disease by hemodialysis. J Am Soc Nephrol 1998; 9:2153–2156.
106. Longenecker JC, Coresh J, Klag MJ, et al: Validation of comorbid conditions on the end-stage renal disease medical evidence report: The CHOICE study. Choices for Healthy Outcomes in Caring for ESRD. J Am Soc Nephrol 2000; 11:520–529.
107. Port FK, Wolfe RA, Hulbert-Shearon TE, et al: Mortality risk by hemodialyzer reuse practice and dialyzer membrane characteristics: Results from the USRDS dialysis morbidity and mortality study. Am J Kidney Dis 2001; 37:276–286.
108. Lowrie EG, Li Z, Ofsthun N, Lazarus JM: The reuse of dialyzers: Current death risk relationships for patients (Abstract). J Am Soc Nephrol 2003; 14:249A.
109. Eknoyan G, Beck GJ, Cheung AK, et al: Effect of dialysis dose and membrane flux in maintenance hemodialysis. N Engl J Med 2002; 347:2010–2019.
110. Baris E, McGregor M: The reuse of hemodialyzers: An assessment of safety and potential savings. Can Med Assoc J 1993; 148:175–183.
111. Manns BJ, Taub K, Richardson RM, Donaldson C: To reuse or not to reuse? An economic evaluation of hemodialyzer reuse versus conventional single-use hemodialysis for chronic hemodialysis patients. Int J Technol Assess Health Care 2002; 18:81–93.
112. Churchill DN, Torrance GW, Taylor DW, et al: Measurement of quality of life in end-stage renal disease: The time trade-off approach. Clin Invest Med 1987; 10:14–20.
113. Sullivan JD: The economics of dialyzer reuse in ESRD. Nephrol News Issues 2002; 16:32–34, 36, 38.

Chapter 20

Hemodialysis Adequacy

John K. Leypoldt, Ph.D.

THE UREMIC SYNDROME

For approximately 40 years, dialytic therapy has provided successful "long-term" life-sustaining replacement for absent renal function. This is reflected by the fact that many patients have received dialysis over 10 years, and some have survived for more than 25 years.[1,2] In its 2003 annual data report, the United States Renal Data System (USRDS) counted approximately 392,000 Americans with end-stage renal disease (ESRD), of whom 68% (approximately 265,000) were treated by maintenance hemodialysis.[3] Despite this success in treating ESRD, or the "uremic syndrome," with dialysis, our knowledge of what constitutes the uremic toxins is still incomplete and unsatisfactory. Furthermore, the relative amounts of various uremic toxins to remove with dialysis therapy are still unclear.

At its most fundamental level, the *uremic syndrome* is the result of the overall retention of multiple substances that interfere with physiologic and biochemical functions. Retained substances range in size from a molecular weight of less than 300 daltons (e.g., urea) to more than 32,000 daltons (e.g., interleukin-1β). Recent work by the European Uremic Toxin Work Group (EUTox) has classified uremic toxins into three main categories[4]: (1) low molecular weight water-soluble solutes, such as urea and creatinine; (2) molecules defined as middle molecules, that is, those with molecular weights greater than 500 daltons; and (3) low molecular weight solutes that are protein-bound. This categorization of uremic toxins can be helpful in understanding the relationship between the dose of uremic toxin clearance or removal and the adequacy of hemodialysis therapy.

The removal of uremic toxins is one of the major goals of maintenance dialytic therapy; however, one must also remember that the uremic syndrome is defined not only by retention of solutes or toxins, but also by deficiencies of other critical compounds (e.g., bicarbonate, erythropoietin,[5] 1,25-dihydroxycholecalciferol[6]) and certain trace elements (e.g., zinc, carnitine[7,8]). These concerns are also important to consider when defining an adequate hemodialysis therapy prescription.

HEMODIALYSIS ADEQUACY

The most practical, clinically applicable definition of *adequate* dialysis is a treatment regimen that:

- Minimizes short-term and long-term morbidity and mortality
- Is fiscally sound
- Can be routinely delivered
- Provides the patient with an outstanding quality of life (i.e., a balance between the inconvenience of remaining on the dialysis delivery system versus a healthier outcome)

This definition of dialysis adequacy indicates that there are a large number of clinical factors that contribute to an adequate therapy. As noted by others,[9,10] they include blood pressure control, fluid and electrolyte homeostasis, anemia correction, acidosis correction, and adequate toxin removal. A discussion of all of these factors, and their impact on hemodialysis adequacy, is beyond the scope of this review. This chapter will be limited to a discussion of the dose of solute or toxin removal as a measure of adequate dialytic therapy. Which solute to use as a guide continues to be debated; however, it is indisputable that the amount of dialysis matters.[11–19]

The EUTox categorization of uremic toxins, outlined previously, can be used as a guide for understanding the relationship between uremic toxin removal and hemodialysis prescription parameters (Table 20-1). The dose of uremic toxin removal can accordingly be divided into three separate categories: dose of low molecular-weight water-soluble toxins (small molecules), dose of middle molecules, and dose of low molecular-weight protein-bound toxins (protein-bound molecules). It is helpful to identify a marker solute for each category of uremic toxins. The dose of small solute removal or clearance is readily identified with urea and its commonly used dose parameter urea Kt/V (see later). The clearance for such solutes during hemodialysis is relatively high and is limited primarily by the blood flow rate to the dialyzer and the surface area of the hemodialysis membrane. The most common marker solute for middle molecules is β_2-microglobulin, and the dose of middle molecule clearance or removal is proportional to both the surface area and pore size of the hemodialysis membrane. Thus, middle molecules are removed to a significant extent during high flux hemodialysis only. Clearance or removal of protein-bound substances is difficult to quantify, and there is no current marker solute that can generally quantify the removal of such solutes. Marker solutes for protein-bound toxins currently under evaluation include *p*-cresol,[20] indoxyl sulfate, and hippuric acid.[4] It is important to note that the low clearance of such solutes from the body relative to urea is not due to a low permeability or pore size of the hemodialysis membrane but rather to biochemical or physiologic resistances to solute removal.[21]

HISTORICAL BEGINNINGS

Defining an appropriate dose of solute removal during maintenance dialysis therapy has long been a crucial interest, especially as mathematical models or formulations were being

The original chapter from the first edition was written by Titus W. L. Lau, M.D., and William F. Owen, Jr., M.D., and has been revised and updated by John K. Leypoldt, Ph.D.

Table 20–1 Categories of Uremic Toxins, Marker Solutes, Relative Clearances, and Important Hemodialysis (HD) Prescription Parameters

Uremic Toxins	Marker Solute	Relative Clearance	HD Prescription Parameters
Free water soluble	Urea	High	Blood flow rate Dialyzer surface area
Middle molecules	β_2-microglobulin	Low	Dialyzer surface area Membrane pore size
Protein-bound toxins	*p*-cresol	Low	Physiologic resistances (protein-binding & intercompartmental barriers) Treatment frequency

developed to assess the adequacy of hemodialysis. From the observation that uremic neuropathy did not develop in patients receiving peritoneal dialysis, despite higher blood urea nitrogen (BUN) and creatinine concentrations than in patients receiving hemodialysis,[22,23] it was proposed that the peritoneal membrane was able to remove selected uremic toxins of a higher molecular weight than urea with much greater efficiency. This proposal culminated in the *square meter-hour hypothesis*,[24,25] which related the dose of dialysis to the number of hours provided per week and to the surface area of the dialysis membrane. This hypothesis seemed intellectually sound, because the clearance of middle molecules was directly related to membrane surface area. According to this construct, therefore, an adequate dialysis therapy was thought to be related to the dose of middle molecule clearance or removal.

Later, the same investigators devised the *dialysis index*, which is the ratio of the calculated removal of a given molecular species to the minimum clearance of that molecular species necessary to maintain health.[26] In the absence of a pathobiologic and readily measurable molecular species, insufficient dialysis was discerned historically by measuring the motor nerve conduction velocity, electroencephalogram (EEG), and hematocrit, and these laboratory studies were combined with assessments of patient activity, performance level, and dietary intake.

A modest body of evidence suggests that middle molecules may be important in the pathobiology of a number of comorbid conditions observed in patients with ESRD.[27,28] For example, dialysis-associated amyloidosis is characterized by the accumulation of advanced glycation end product-modified β_2-microglobulin, and a small body of evidence suggests that the occurrence of the disease may be attenuated by selected membrane materials, some of which may have higher clearances for β_2-microglobulin (11,800 daltons).[29–31] Further, the characteristic-acquired lipoprotein lipase deficiency of chronic kidney disease[32] may be attenuated by the use of high-flux hemodialysis membranes and, thereby, may decrease the severity of lipid abnormalities.[33]

Despite the enthusiasm for middle molecules, as uremic toxins, to define the adequacy of dialysis, the continued failure to identify such solutes or appropriate marker molecules, which could be used to evaluate their removal, has undermined their clinical utility. Furthermore, outcome studies for ESRD patients treated by dialysis over the past 20 years have primarily used low molecular-weight solutes (e.g., urea) as the surrogate uremic toxin to determine hemodialysis adequacy.[11–19]

The benchmark prospective study of hemodialysis adequacy is the National Cooperative Dialysis Study (NCDS). It was the first randomized trial to examine the effects of dose of small solute removal on patient outcome (morbidity).[11] Note that patient mortality was not a primary outcome parameter in this trial. This interventional trial was designed to evaluate two parameters thought to be critical outcome determinants related to hemodialysis adequacy:

1. Use of the time-averaged concentration (TAC) of BUN as a marker of low molecular-weight solute clearance.
2. Length of each hemodialysis session as a surrogate for the clearance of middle molecules.

The use of dialysis time as a surrogate for middle molecule clearance in this study was an approximation because the removal of large, less readily diffusible solutes is primarily a function of the duration of dialysis, but also depends on hemodialysis membrane surface area. Further, although it is often quoted that dialysis time was used in this study as a surrogate for middle molecule clearance, Wineman[34] has alternatively suggested that dialysis treatment time was selected to assess its importance as a practical hemodialysis prescription parameter.

As for urea or small solute clearance, the time-averaged BUN concentration over a full weekly dialysis cycle (TAC_{urea}) was the measurement selected for quantifying and targeting urea clearance during dialysis, instead of the more conventional and easily measured midweek pre-dialysis BUN. Arguably, the long-term toxicity of ESRD is more likely a function of average "toxin" exposure (TAC_{urea}) than of the peak plasma concentrations (midweek pre-dialysis BUN). This issue is important for the clinician as well, because the midweek pre-dialysis BUN can vary substantially, depending on both the patient's dietary protein intake as well as the amount of hemodialysis.

All patients in the study underwent rigorous and repeated kinetic modeling to achieve the specified TAC_{urea} for their assigned group.[35–37] The final study population consisted of 165 patients, randomized into four different intervention groups (2 × 2 factorial design), and all patient groups received dialysis three times per week. Groups I and III were treated to achieve a TAC_{urea} of 50 mg/dL, whereas groups II and IV were treated to achieve a TAC_{urea} of 100 mg/dL. Groups I and II were assigned the longer duration of hemodialysis, 4.5 to

5.0 hours; groups III and IV had dialysis sessions of 2.5 to 3.5 hours. The designated TAC_{urea} was achieved by variation of the blood and dialysate flow rates and by membrane surface area of the dialyzers. All patients were observed for a minimum of 24 weeks.

The TAC_{urea} proved to be the most important determinant of patient morbidity or withdrawal from the study.[11, 35–39] The proportion of patients not withdrawn for medical reasons or death by 9 months was 89% (group I, long dialysis time) and 94% (group III, short dialysis time) versus 55% and 54%, respectively, for groups II and IV. The duration of dialysis treatment had no effect on patient withdrawal. The TAC_{urea} was also a highly significant determinant of the rate of hospitalization, with fewer hospital admissions occurring in the low TAC_{urea} groups. Also, group I had fewer hospitalizations than group III; similarly, group II had fewer hospitalizations than group IV. However, the effect of the treatment time was statistically significant in the high TAC_{urea} groups (groups II and IV) only.[37,38]

A stepwise, linear logistic regression analysis of the data from the NCDS was performed to determine the effect of multiple treatment variables on the probability of an adverse outcome.[39] Subsequent death, withdrawal from the study, or hospitalization during the first 24 weeks of follow-up was again predicted by the TAC_{urea}.

The second best outcome predictor was the *protein catabolic rate* (PCR),[11,38,39] equivalent to the dietary protein intake for dialysis patients in a steady state.[40] In a subsequent mechanistic analysis of the data from the NCDS, however, it was argued that this statistical association was a consequence of the protocol design (i.e., the PCR was not an independent variable).[41] This lack of independence is most evident when one appreciates that to achieve a predetermined TAC_{urea}, the amount of hemodialysis prescribed must be a function of the PCR. Thus, a higher PCR requires a greater amount of dialysis to achieve the same TAC_{urea}, and vice versa. Hence, any statistical correlation between TAC_{urea} and morbidity will be mirrored similarly by PCR. The design of the NCDS did not set PCR as a study variable. For all study groups, the PCR was permitted to fluctuate between the ranges of 0.8 and 1.4 g/kg/day (an inadequate to an excessive dietary protein intake).

It is apparent from the NCDS results that urea is an appropriate surrogate low molecular-weight solute marker and that the level of its removal predicts patient outcomes. However, several design limitations compromised the study's applicability to the current ESRD patient population and prevalent treatment practices. For example, the NCDS excluded older patients (>60 years of age) and diabetic patients; these patient profiles would exclude the preponderance of current Americans with ESRD.[3,42] Furthermore, participants in the NCDS were treated exclusively with cellulosic hemodialysis membranes that were not reused, so generalization to other increasingly prevalent biocompatible membrane materials[43] may not be appropriate. The follow-up period for the NCDS was 48 weeks or less and therefore did not adequately address more fundamental long-term outcomes, such as mortality. Despite these limitations, the NCDS is the foundation for all subsequent analyses linking hemodialysis adequacy to patient morbidity and mortality and to the use of urea as a surrogate low molecular-weight uremic toxin in the measurement of hemodialysis adequacy.

PRINCIPLES AND METHODS FOR QUANTIFYING THE DOSE OF SMALL SOLUTE REMOVAL DURING HEMODIALYSIS

Many putative uremic toxins are products from protein metabolism.[44] Because it is impossible to measure the large number of water-soluble uremic toxins in routine practice, a derivative of protein catabolism—urea—has emerged as the most popular marker for quantifying the dose of small solute removal. A small and readily dialyzed molecule, urea constitutes 90% of waste nitrogen accumulated in the interdialytic interval.[40] Its measurement is simple, inexpensive, and universally available. Also, the transport properties of urea between body compartments are well studied and thus fairly well understood.[45,46] Most important, its utility as a surrogate for hemodialysis treatment dose and outcomes has been validated, not the least by the NCDS,[11] but also subsequently by other reports.[13–18, 47]

As a result of the mechanistic analysis of the NCDS data, urea Kt/V is the most widely accepted measurement of the dose of small solute removal.[40,41] Indeed, it is often simply called the dose of dialysis, even though it only quantifies the amount of small solute clearance or removal. Although this construct for evaluating the dose of small solute removal enjoys almost universal acceptance, it should be noted that the mechanistic analysis of the NCDS data was an "as treated" analysis not the "intent to treat" analysis that is now universally applied to randomized clinical trials. This expression of the dose of small solute removal can be described as the total cleared volume of urea (Kt) normalized by its distribution volume (V), which is approximately total body water. In turn, K is the dialyzer clearance of urea and is a function of the mass transfer-area coefficient (K_oA) of urea and blood and dialysate flow rates (Q_b and Q_d, respectively). K is reported in L/min, t (hemodialysis treatment time) in minutes, and V in liters. Alternatively, noting that Kt/V is equal to $(Kt \times [urea]_{mean}) / (V \times [urea]_{mean})$, Kt/V approximately expresses the total mass of urea removed during hemodialysis $(Kt \times [urea]_{mean})$ normalized by the mean total amount of urea in the body $(V \times [urea]_{mean})$.

The clinical application of mathematical terms (such as Kt/V), to describe the removal of urea during hemodialysis, is called *urea kinetic modeling*. Nearly all solute kinetic models that apply to hemodialysis are based on the *law of conservation of mass*, which means that the accumulation of any substance in the system is equal to the difference between the input and output. Hence, given adequate knowledge of its rate of accumulation, metabolism, and excretion from the body, virtually any substance can be kinetically modeled. Finally, the accuracy of the model is only as good as the assumptions made to produce the model.

Adapting these principles to urea, we have:

systemic mass accumulation of urea = input/urea mass generated − output/urea mass cleared

expressed in the form of a differential equation:

$$d(V \times C)/dt = G - (K + K_r) \times C \tag{1}$$

where the change in urea mass in the body with time $(d[V \times C] / dt)$ is the result of the difference between net urea generation (G) and total body urea mass cleared by the dialyzer (K) and residual renal function (K_r). Here, C denotes the concentration of urea, and V denotes the volume of distribution of urea.[40]

For most oligoanuric patients with ESRD, the value of such terms changes during and between dialysis treatments. From this simple concept, the single-pool, variable-volume model for urea kinetics has been derived and is the one most often in clinical use. This model assumes that:

1. Urea accumulates in and is removed from a single pool or compartment.
2. This single urea compartment expands in size between hemodialysis treatments (secondary to fluid retention) and diminishes in size with ultrafiltration during hemodialysis.

Formal Urea Kinetic Modeling

Advantages

When rigorously performed, formal urea kinetic modeling is a reproducible, quantitative method for measuring urea removal during hemodialysis. It has several advantages for assessing the adequacy of hemodialysis over alternative methods to measure the delivered dose of hemodialysis. *Assuming a single urea pool of variable-volume, formal urea kinetic modeling is the recommended principle method for measuring hemodialysis dose.* The strengths of formal urea kinetic modeling are that it:

- Can be used to prescribe individual hemodialysis treatment
- Checks for errors in dosage
- Can approximately take into account residual renal function
- Permits calculation of the *normalized protein catabolic rate* (nPCR)

Hemodialysis Prescription

Formal urea kinetic modeling can be utilized as a tool to prescribe individualized hemodialysis treatments to achieve the desired dose of small solute removal during hemodialysis (Kt/V) based on patient-specific parameters, such as (1) body size, (2) residual renal function, and (3) nPCR. To develop a hemodialysis prescription, it is necessary to obtain a dialyzer's urea clearance (K) for a variety of blood and dialysate flows in blood/water. To provide this information, the computational software for urea kinetic modeling uses the manufacturer's K to extrapolate a K_oA value for that dialyzer, which can then be used to calculate urea clearance at different blood and dialysate flow rates.

Ideally, the urea clearance is initially calculated based on the volume from which urea is removed and into which urea is generated as a function nPCR. Further, with computational software, formal urea kinetic modeling calculates the volume of distribution of urea by iteration of two formulas that share common terms. The kinetic determination of V is based on the assumption of a single pool of urea that is coextensive with total body water and that expands during the interdialytic interval from fluid retention and contracts during hemodialysis by ultrafiltration. Assuming a thrice-weekly hemodialysis schedule, the computational software iterates the following two formulas, having shared terms, until unique values are found for Vt and G to satisfy both expressions.

$$Vt = (Qf \times t)/[((C0 - G/(K + Kr - Qf))/(Ct - G/(K + Kr - Qf)))^{Qf/(K+Kr-Qf)} - 1] \quad (2)$$

$$G = [(Kr + \alpha)[C0 - Ct(1 + \alpha\theta/Vt) - (Kr + \alpha)/\alpha)]/[1 - (1 + \alpha\theta/Vt)^{-(Kr + \alpha)/\alpha}] \quad (3)$$

In these equations, Vt is the end dialysis volume; Qf is the rate of volume contraction during dialysis that is calculated from total weight loss during dialysis divided by the length of dialysis, t; G is the interdialytic urea generation rate; K and Kr are the dialyzer and renal urea clearances, respectively; and Ct and C0 are the BUN concentrations at the end and beginning of a dialysis treatment. (Note that C0 in equation 2 is the pre-dialysis BUN concentration from the first hemodialysis session, and C0 in equation 3 is the pre-dialysis BUN concentration from the second hemodialysis session.) Further, α is the rate of interdialytic volume expansion and is calculated by the total interdialytic weight gain divided by the length of the interdialytic interval, θ.[40] With K and V known, the treatment time can be determined easily to achieve the desired Kt/V. Formal urea kinetic modeling supports the derivation of various treatment time and blood flow combinations to achieve a target Kt/V. Thus, the use of formal urea kinetic modeling can guide the hemodialysis care team on which specific parameters of the prescription to modify to achieve the desired hemodialysis dose.

Checking of Dosage Errors

Formal urea kinetic modeling provides a means to check for errors in the delivered dose of hemodialysis, thus offering a necessary quality control mechanism. Formal urea kinetic modeling requires the measurement of pre-dialysis and post-dialysis BUN concentrations, delivered hemodialysis treatment time, and dialyzer clearance of urea (at the blood and dialysate flow rates used). The computer software assumes that all input data are accurate and uses these values to calculate the volume of distribution of urea. In addition, most programs also calculate a volume of distribution based on anthropometric formulas.[48–50] The anthropometric volume of distribution of urea may be calculated by one of several formulas derived from gender-specific estimates of total body water (TBW) in healthy subjects. The most common of these anthropometric formulas, the Watson formula,[49] is shown below:

$$\text{Males: TBW} = 2.447 - (0.09156 \times \text{age}) + (0.1074 \times \text{height}) + (0.3362 \times \text{weight})$$

$$\text{Females: TBW} = -2.097 + (0.1069 \times \text{height}) + 0.2466 \times \text{weight} \quad (4)$$

Because this formula was derived from analyses performed in healthy individuals, their general applicability to patients with ESRD has been questioned. Based on measurements of TBW using single frequency bioelectric impedance (BEI) in ESRD patients, a population-specific equation for calculating total body water was more recently derived by Chertow and associates.[50] Note that the Chertow formula calculates a pre-dialysis, not a post-dialysis value of total body water; thus, it requires a correction before comparison with the other formulas.

All previous anthropometric formulas were based on measurements of TBW using either isotope markers or BEI, and only the Chertow formula was derived in ESRD patients. Recent work by Daugirdas and associates[51] has evaluated the modeled urea distribution volume derived from urea kinetic modeling in a large sample of patients in the HEMO Study. Calculated urea distribution volumes in that study were substantially (15%–20%) lower than the above-referenced anthropometric estimates of TBW. The reasons for these discrepancies are unknown, but these calculated results suggest that the use of anthropometric formulas for predicting TBW may substantially overestimate the urea distribution volume. These authors have also proposed methods to estimate the urea distribution volume from anthropometric formulas for TBW. For example, the modeled urea distribution volume (Vm) can be calculated from the TBW predicted by the Watson formula (Watson V) by the following formula:

$$\text{Vm} = (\text{Watson V}) \times (1.033 \text{ if diabetic}) \times (0.998 \times [\text{age} - 50] \text{ if male}) \times (0.985 \times [\text{age} - 50] \text{ if female}) \times (1.033 \text{ if female}) \times (1.043 \text{ if African American}) \quad (5)$$

Additional equations for predicting the modeled urea distribution volume from the Hume-Weyers and Chertow formulas can also be derived from this recently published work. Although there are no available data to suggest that such modified anthropometric formulas for urea distribution volume are superior to unmodified anthropometric formulas when prescribing hemodialysis, it would seem more valid to use these new modified formulas because they were derived directly from modeled urea distribution volume not from TBW. Only additional studies will permit evaluation of the advantages and disadvantages of these modified formulas.

By comparison of the V derived from formal urea kinetic modeling and that derived from anthropometric data, possible errors related to the hemodialysis procedure may be detected. A discrepancy between these two values should alert the dialysis care team to unappreciated errors in dialysis delivery (Table 20–2). When the kinetically derived V is larger than the anthropometric V, the delivered dose of hemodialysis would be less than the prescribed dose. Alternatively, when the kinetically derived V is less than the expected anthropometric V (used for the initial hemodialysis prescription), the Kt/V may seem inappropriately high. If this erroneous Kt/V is interpreted without consideration of the urea distribution volume, a reduction in the dose of hemodialysis may appear appropriate. However, this reduction in dialysis dose may reduce the delivered hemodialysis dose to an unsafe level and thus compromise the patient's well-being; for example, the hemodialysis dose might be appropriate, but an unappreciated error occurs in the calculation of V.

Because of the enhanced rigor in ascertaining that the delivered dose of hemodialysis is correct and the greater ease with which deficiencies are detected, formal urea kinetic modeling provides the greatest support for continuous quality improvement efforts in the delivery of hemodialysis. Optimal quality improvement efforts require that the processes of care affecting patient outcome be routinely measured, individual deficiencies defined, and corrective steps implemented. Furthermore, formal urea kinetic modeling facilitates the identification of the components in the hemodialysis delivery that were problematic, if the delivered dose has not mirrored the prescribed dose (Table 20–3).

Table 20–2 Reasons for Discrepancies Between the Kinetically Derived and Anthropometric Distribution Volume (V)

Kinetically Derived V Larger Than Anthropometric V
- Low blood flow from the angioaccess
- Inadequate dialyzer performance
- Dialysate flows less than prescribed
- Dialysis machine programmed incorrectly
- Premature completion of treatment
- Pre-dialysis BUN sample drawn after initiation of hemodialysis

Kinetically Derived V Smaller Than Anthropometric V
- Post-dialysis BUN sample drawn from the venous blood line
- Post-dialysis BUN sample drawn in the setting of significant fistula recirculation
- Post-dialysis BUN sample drawn following a very efficient hemodialysis in a patient with a small V (high K/V)
- Post-dialysis BUN sample inadvertently diluted with saline

BUN, blood urea nitrogen.

Residual Renal Function

Formal urea kinetic modeling can account for the contribution of residual renal function to the sum total of the delivered hemodialysis dose. A minority of ESRD patients has significant residual renal function (Kr), but if this remains unaccounted, the actual total urea clearance and the nPCR will be underestimated. Because of the short duration, the effect of residual renal function on total urea clearance during hemodialysis will be small; however, in the relatively long interdialytic period, residual renal function will significantly lower the pre-dialysis BUN concentration.

Graphically, when Kr is zero, the interdialytic rise in BUN concentration is linear. If Kr is greater than 0, the rise in BUN concentration will be more shallow and curvilinear, as a result of continuous renal excretion. Thus, when Kr is greater than 0, less hemodialysis is required to achieve the same pre-dialysis BUN level as when Kr equals 0. The quantitative relationship that relates dialysis dose with and without residual renal function can be defined as:

$$\text{kKr} = \text{Kt} - \text{K}'\text{t} \quad (6)$$

where K and K′ are the dialyzer urea clearances in the absence and presence of residual renal clearance, respectively, and t is the treatment time. Here, k relates Kr to the difference between K and K′ or the decrease in dialysis dose that is possible in the presence of residual renal function to achieve the same predialysis BUN. Therefore, the relationship between the total dialysis dose (KT), the dose provided by the dialyzer (Kt), and the contribution residual renal clearance (kKr), are expressed by:

$$\text{KT/Vt} = \text{Kt/Vt} + \text{kKr/Vt} \quad (7)$$

Since k is a coefficient, not a constant, its value depends on both Kt and Kr; thus, these equations can be solved using only computational software for formal urea kinetic modeling.[40]

Calculation of Normalized Protein Catabolic Rate

Formal urea kinetic modeling permits calculation of PCR and nPCR. The PCR has been shown to be linearly dependent on both the urea generation rate (G) and its distribution volume (Vt):

$$\text{PCR} = 9.35\text{G} + 0.29\text{Vt} \quad (8)$$

Table 20–3 Reasons for Underdelivery of Prescribed Dose of Hemodialysis

Compromised Urea Clearance
- Access recirculation
- Inadequate blood flow from the vascular access
- Inaccurate estimation of dialyzer performance
- Inadequate dialyzer reprocessing
- Dialyzer clotting during dialysis
- Blood pump/dialysate flow calibration errors
- Errors in prescribed blood and dialysate flow rates due to variability in blood pump tubing
- Dialysate flow rate that is inappropriately set too low
- Dialysate flow miscalibration
- Dialyzer leaks

Reductions in Treatment Time
- Inaccurate assessment of effective dialysis time using wristwatches
- Incorrect assumption of continuous treatment time because of failure to account for interruptions
- Premature discontinuation of hemodialysis for staff or unit convenience
- Premature discontinuation of hemodialysis to honor patient request or adherence
- Delay in starting dialysis session due to patient tardiness
- Wrong patient taken off dialysis
- Time on dialysis calculated incorrectly
- Time read incorrectly for initiation or completion of hemodialysis
- Clerical deficiencies

Laboratory or Blood Sampling Errors*
- Dilution of pre-dialysis BUN blood sample with saline
- Pre-dialysis BUN blood sample drawn after the start of dialysis
- Post-dialysis BUN blood sample drawn before the end of dialysis
- Laboratory error due to calibration or equipment problems
- Post-dialysis BUN blood sample drawn more than 5 minutes after dialysis completed

*Apparent underdelivery because of erroneous measurements.

Because urea distribution volumes vary between 30% and 65% of body weight, it is improper to index the PCR simply by dividing PCR by the patient's body weight. Rather, it is necessary to relate PCR to the normalized body weight (nBWT). If we presume that the average volume of urea distribution is 58% of body weight, the patient's weight is converted to an nBWT by the following:

$$nBWt = Vt/0.58 \quad (9)$$

and normalized protein catabolic rate (nPCR) is thus expressed as

$$nPCR = PCR/(Vt/0.58) \quad (10)$$

In patients who are not markedly catabolic or anabolic, the net protein catabolism correlates closely with dietary protein intake.[52–55] Because dietary records and histories are often inaccurate, PCR (calculated as part of formal urea kinetic modeling) provides a more reliable estimate of dietary protein intake. Hence, use of the nPCR enables the dialysis care team to perform longitudinal analysis of the patient's nutritional status and to more soundly guide dietary counseling about protein intake.

Although the NCDS showed that a high nPCR (presumably reflective of a better dietary protein intake) was associated with lower morbidity or lesser likelihood of treatment failure, the design of the study was not ideal to prove conclusively that nPCR was an independent risk factor.[41] However, several subsequent reports have statistically linked laboratory surrogates of nutrition to outcomes in chronic hemodialysis patients.[13,17,47,56,57] For example, a low serum albumin concentration (<3.5 g/dL), a laboratory surrogate of visceral malnutrition, was associated with a relative risk of death of 1.83 and 2.07 for diabetic and nondiabetic ESRD patients, respectively, although this difference was less when adjusted for Kt/V.[58]

In an analysis of 13,473 ESRD patients, the serum albumin concentration was 21 times more powerful a predictor of death than was the dose of hemodialysis. Furthermore, the serum albumin concentration was an independent risk factor, apart from the dose of hemodialysis.[47] This finding is provocative because the serum albumin concentration has been linked to the adequacy of hemodialysis. Although not uniformly observed,[47] a highly significant, positive correlation between the serum albumin concentration and the dose of hemodialysis (Kt/V) has been observed.[56] Certainly, patients who receive inadequate dialysis have a depressed appetite and a diminished protein-caloric intake. Thus, maintaining an adequate dose of hemodialysis may improve nutrition and patient survival.

Disadvantages

The modest disadvantages of formal urea kinetic modeling are logistical. The complexity of the calculations requires the use of computational devices and software. The cost of computer devices and software may not be much, but it remains a consideration for some smaller hemodialysis units. Physical parameters, such as the K and V, are burdensome to measure and monitor, and the actual treatment time can be difficult to determine. In addition, the time required for the dialysis unit staff to accurately collect and process all patient data to support these calculations may be significant in larger hemodialysis centers. Despite these relative limitations, both the Renal Physicians Association (RPA)[54] and the National Kidney Foundation's Dialysis Outcomes Quality Initiative (DOQI)[55] evidence-based clinical practice guidelines agreed that formal urea kinetic modeling is "the most rigorous method for prescribing dialysis treatment and evaluating the consistency with which the prescribed treatment is delivered to the patient."[54]

Alternate Methods of Quantification

Some reports have suggested that only one alternative method of calculating Kt/V (Kt/V *natural logarithm formula*[59]) and one other measurement of the delivered dialysis dose (*urea reduction ratio* [URR][47,60]) should be considered for routine use in clinical dialytic practice.[55]

Kt/V Natural Logarithm Formula

The second-generation logarithm formula,[59] which was proposed based on the variable-volume single-pool urea kinetic model, accounts for urea removed by both diffusive and convective clearance, the latter secondary to ultrafiltration.[55] Urea removal accomplished by convective transport is not associated with a change in the post-dialysis to pre-dialysis BUN ratio. Over a wide range of single-pool, variable volume Kt/V values derived by formal urea kinetic modeling (range 0.7 to 2.1), the second-generation logarithm formula for calculating Kt/V is accurate.[59,61,62] The logarithm formula for calculating Kt/V is:

$$Kt/V = -\ln(R - 0.008 \times t) + (4 - 3.5 \times R) \times UF/W \quad (11)$$

in which ln denotes the natural logarithm, R the post-dialysis to pre-dialysis BUN ratio, t the dialysis session length in hours, UF the ultrafiltration volume in liters, and W the patient's post-dialysis weight in kilograms.

From the aforementioned criteria of accuracy and completeness, the second-generation logarithm formula for calculating Kt/V is the best alternative for dialysis care teams to use, if they cannot perform formal urea kinetic modeling. Although this simplified formula is convenient, its use alone deprives the dialysis care team of the error check function for the delivered hemodialysis dose in contrast to formal urea kinetic modeling. The logarithm calculation of Kt/V does not permit the rigorous, preemptive quantitative analysis of the hemodialysis prescriptions possible with formal urea kinetic modeling. Furthermore, this formula does not allow for calculation of the nPCR. However, an approximation of the nPCR can be derived from a normogram that uses patient-specific parameters and the Kt/V natural logarithm formula.[63]

Urea Reduction Ratio

The URR is calculated simply from the fractional post-dialysis BUN concentration, which equals C_t/C_0, where C_t is the post-dialysis BUN and C_0 the pre-dialysis BUN,[47,60] as

$$URR\,(\%) = 100 \times (1 - C_t/C_0) \quad (12)$$

URR represents the precent of the total urea mass, which is removed from the body during a single hemodialysis treatment, assuming there is no change in urea distribution volume. It can be appreciated that this is a remarkably easy measurement of the dose of hemodialysis. More important, the utility of URR as a measure that correlates with patient mortality has been validated in several clinical studies using different patient databases.[19,47] Therefore, URR is no better or worse than Kt/V in defining mortality risks for hemodialysis patients in epidemiologic studies.

Despite its ease of use, there are limitations to URR as a measure of hemodialysis adequacy. In contrast to formal urea kinetic modeling or the Kt/V natural logarithm formula, URR does not account for the contribution of ultrafiltration to the final delivered dose of hemodialysis.[64,65] As described earlier, although urea is removed with the ultrafiltrate, no change in the plasma concentration occurs. The failure to account for this additional urea removal limits the accuracy of the estimate of dialytic dose, depending on the volume of ultrafiltrate formed.[55] For example, a patient with a large ultrafiltration requirement has a much higher dialytic dose when measured by formal urea kinetic modeling or the natural logarithm formula compared with the same patient with no ultrafiltration requirement. However, the URR will be the same in both these circumstances, if all other parameters for the hemodialysis prescription are equal.

This discrepancy between the dose of small solute removal during hemodialysis delivered in the presence and absence of ultrafiltration and its relationship to URR is illustrated in Figure 20–1. If we assume a 3-hour dialysis session, no residual renal function, and a volume of distribution of urea of 58% body weight, the Kt/V derived using formal urea kinetic modeling is contrasted with the URR.[64] A URR of 65% may correspond to a single-pool Kt/V of as low as 1.1 in the absence of ultrafiltration or can be as high as approximately 1.35 when ultrafiltration of 10% body weight occurs. Furthermore, because the relation between URR and Kt/V is curvilinear, modest decreases in the URR can result in substantial declines in Kt/V, especially in the target range of URR of 65% or higher.

When the URR alone is used, errors in the delivered dose of hemodialysis may be particularly difficult to ascertain. This limitation is a consequence of the inability of URR to support

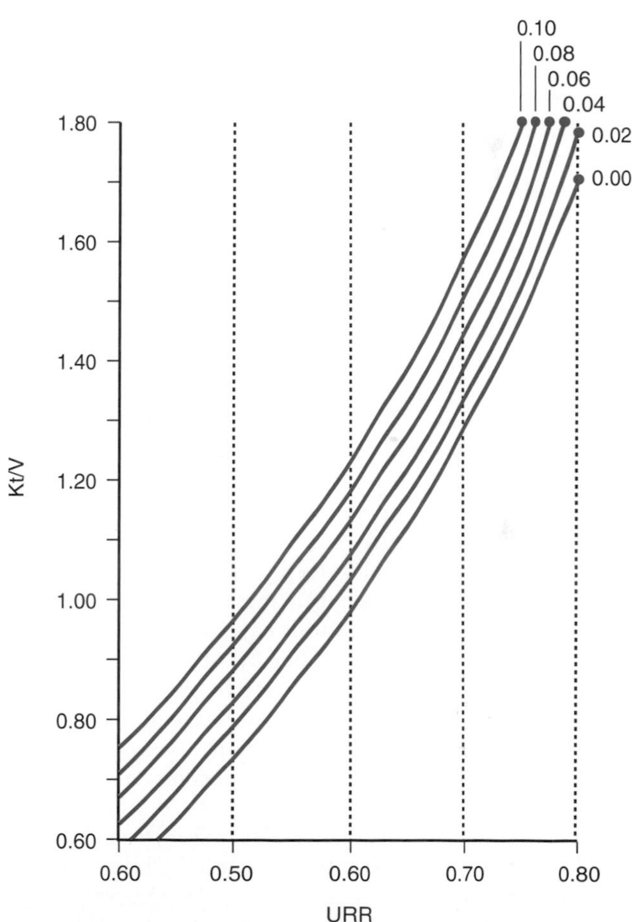

Figure 20–1 Impact of urea clearance secondary to ultrafiltration on Kt/V values. The family of curves is based on the assumption of a 3-hour hemodialysis treatment and the absence of residual renal function. ΔWt is the volume ultrafiltered in liters divided by the patient's estimated dry weight in liters as indicated by the numbers labeling this figure. The greater the ΔWt, the higher the Kt/V for any given urea reduction ratio (URR) value. (From National Kidney Foundation: K/DOQI Clinical Practice Guidelines for Hemodialysis Adequacy, 2000. Am J Kidney Dis 2001; 37[suppl 1]:S7-S64.)

the calculation of V for comparison with anthropometric-derived values. In addition, as noted for the Kt/V calculated by the natural logarithm formula, achieving a target delivered dose of hemodialysis is an empirical exercise involving modification of the various components of the treatment prescription. Similarly, the URR does not support calculations of the nPCR and effectively ignores the contribution of residual renal function to urea clearance. Thus, although the URR is a useful tool to measure the delivered dose of hemodialysis for statistical outcome analyses,[19,47] it lacks sufficient accuracy and detail to routinely provide insight into problems with the dialysis prescription.

Other Methods for Dose Calculation

A variety of alternatives to the Kt/V natural logarithm formula and URR using pre-dialysis and post-dialysis urea concentration has been previously proposed[66–68]; however, there are no demonstrable advantages for using these alternative formulas, and they should be avoided.

The clearance of urea as a surrogate for the clearance of small molecules during hemodialysis can also be quantified by collection of the dialysate.[69] Dialysate-based urea kinetics has been considered by some to be the "gold standard" for dose quantification[69,70]; however, this contention has recently been questioned.[71] The popularity of blood side measurement stems largely from the historical practice of measuring blood levels of different solutes and substances to detect and quantify disease state. Because the current measures of hemodialysis dose are in essence solute removal, quantification of solute removed in the dialysate could potentially provide for a better measure of the effectiveness of treatment. There are several advantages with dialysate side measurements. Direct dialysate quantification bypasses the problem of solute disequilibrium, which occurs at various time points during and after hemodialysis (the double-pool model is discussed later). It also measures patient clearance directly not dialyzer clearance (K). There are several methods by which quantification of solute removed in the dialysate can be made. Either total or fractional dialysate collection techniques[72,73] have previously been proposed, such that the total mass of urea removed can then be calculated. These methods have yet to be used extensively during routine therapy. The advent and application of built-in, online urea sensors in hemodialysis machines permits the automation of dialysate urea quantification and makes this method more feasible than dialysate sampling techniques.[74] Currently available urea sensors are, however, expensive.

Another online measure of clearance utilizes a conductivity probe and does not require a urea sensor. This probe can determine the effective ionic dialysance (D) and permits the calculation of Kt/V at each dialysis session without blood or dialysate sampling at a very low cost.[75–79] Online assessment with this method has been tested against formal urea kinetic, using a 30-minute post-dialysis BUN sample and the *Daugirdas equilibrated Kt/V formula* (see later).[76] In this study, conductivity-derived measurements were found to be accurate and fairly precise, and they compared well with the method of Daugirdas. Hence, with the availability of online assessment that is both clinically useful and affordable, dialysis dose can be measured as often as needed, and immediate remedial steps can be taken to ensure adequate dosing.

Urea Rebound Double-Pool Effects and Recirculation

Physiology of the Double-Pool Model

As described earlier, the simplest model of urea distribution and concentration changes in the anuric hemodialysis patient is the single-pool or "single-compartment" model, which assumes that:

1. Urea is distributed uniformly in a single compartment of volume approximately equal to total body water.
2. The compartment will expand and contract uniformly during and between hemodialysis sessions.

This elementary model yields the single-pool Kt/V, which has proved clinically useful in population studies and has received wide clinical acceptance. However, the actual anatomic distribution of urea consists of plasma, erythrocytes, and interstitial and intracellular water.

Functionally, transfer between these compartments behaves as a diffusive process and can be described by the product of a volumetric mass transfer coefficient and the difference in concentration between the compartments.[40] However, this model omits another physiologic consideration for urea kinetics during and between hemodialysis treatments—the variable distribution of blood flow to various vascular beds and organs. For example, in the anephric patient, approximately 80% of cardiac output is distributed to visceral organs (liver, intestine, heart, and brain), which contain only 30% of TBW. In contrast, only 20% of the cardiac output is distributed to muscle, bone, and skin (primarily muscle), which account for 70% of TBW.[80,81]

During hemodialysis, the clearance of solutes (such as urea) is dependent on dialyzer clearance and the rate at which solutes can be conveyed from all body compartments into the dialyzer. The rapidity with which urea can be transferred from the plasma water compartment into the dialysate can easily exceed its rate of transfer from other compartments into plasma water, thereby giving rise functionally to multiple compartments. This is a fundamental biophysical and practical basis for the double-pool urea kinetic model, which is a more accurate and rigorous description of urea kinetics during hemodialysis.

Specifically, one level of resistance of urea movement is from the intracellular compartment to the extracellular compartment, which is estimated to be approximately 600 to 800 mL/min.[82] This relative resistance to urea movement from the cells across the interstitium and into the blood compartment effectively renders the distribution of urea into at least two pools. This biophysical reality obviously undermines a key assumption made in the formulation of the single-pool model.[83] Perhaps of greater importance is the effect of differential organ perfusion that contributes to this "disequilibrium" of urea removal. Because of the preferential removal of urea from well-perfused, but relatively urea-depleted vascular beds during the course of hemodialysis, no single-pool, variable-volume model for urea kinetics accounts for the different rates of urea transfer between these compartments.

This combination of effects (diffusive resistance and flow-volume disequilibrium) is commonly described by the term *double-pool effects.* As a consequence, after completion of a hemodialysis session, release of the sequestered urea begins and continues for 30 to 60 minutes (post-dialysis urea rebound). The resistance of urea transfer and variable organ perfusion are thought to be the major components of post-dialysis urea rebound.[84–88] The post-dialysis BUN concentrations measured before and after the occurrence of urea rebound vary significantly, such that a lower BUN concentration is observed before rebound than after (Figure 20–2). Thus, the effective delivered dose of dialysis will be overestimated, if this sequestered urea pool is large and not taken into consideration.

Early studies have suggested that the extent of urea rebound varies greatly among patients and is influenced by such variables as the size and the efficiency of the dialyzer. In one study, the mean amount of urea rebound, measured as the percent increase in post-dialysis BUN concentration immediately after dialysis versus 30 minutes post-dialysis, was 170%.[87] In some patients, however, the extent of urea rebound was as great as 45%.[86] The use of dialyzers with high K (efficient, high-flux dialyzers), especially in a patient with a small V, increases the risk of significant double-pool effects.[81,87,89] The extent of post-dialysis urea rebound has been shown by Daugirdas and Schneditz[81] to be primarily a function of K/V. Therefore, the degree of rebound is large in ESRD patients who have a low urea distribution volume, have severely compromised cardiac output, or have suffered intradialytic hypotension.[81,90] On average, the equilibrated Kt/V (the Kt/V calculated using the 30 minutes post-dialysis BUN sample) is approximately 0.2 units less than the single-pool Kt/V.[81,87,91] For most patients, urea rebound is almost complete 15 minutes after discontinuation of hemodialysis; however, for a minority, up to 60 minutes may be required.

Because of the inability to routinely predict which patients will experience significant urea rebound, and in view of the potential deleterious impact of urea rebound on the delivered hemodialysis dose, the double-pool or equilibrated urea kinetic model seems to offer a better estimate of the true dose of hemodialysis. Although the equilibrated model better quantifies intradialytic urea removal, thus resulting in a more precise Kt/V and nPCR,[86,92] the need to obtain a 30- to 60-minute post-dialysis BUN sample makes it impractical in routine clinical practice. To overcome this limitation, several investigators have proposed different formulas to estimate the equilibrated Kt/V (Kt/V_{eq}) from pre-dialysis and immediate (0–20 seconds delayed) post-dialysis blood samples. Formulas have been derived to correct for post-dialysis urea rebound by three independent groups: Smye and associates,[85] Tattersal and associates[93] and Daugirdas and Schneditz.[89] Practical predictions of post-dialysis urea rebound using these formulas are approximately equivalent for thrice-weekly hemodialysis.[94] The Daugirdas-Schneditz rate equation has been verified in small scale studies[70] and in analyses from the pilot phase of the HEMO Study[95]; these are actually two separate formulas, depending on whether the angioaccess is of arterial or venous origin:

$$\text{arterial } Kt/V_{eq} = \text{art } Kt/V_{sp} - (0.6 \times [\text{art } Kt/V_{sp} \div t]) + 0.03 \quad \textbf{(13)}$$

$$\text{venous } Kt/V_{eq} = \text{ven } Kt/V_{sp} - (0.4 \times [\text{ven } Kt/V_{sp} \div t]) + 0.02 \quad \textbf{(14)}$$

where Kt/V_{sp} is the value of calculated Kt/V from single-pool urea kinetic modeling and the units of the $Kt/V_{sp} \div t$ terms are hours^{-1}. These equations are simple to apply during routine hemodialysis because Kt/V_{eq} can be calculated from the previously mentioned equations and single-pool urea kinetic modeling parameters.

The above two formulas are based on the assumption that, if all other variables in the hemodialysis prescription are equal, the urea rebound from a venovenous access is less than with an arteriovenous access.[63,81] These differences are because cardiopulmonary recirculation (see later) is lessened with venovenous sampling, hence, the two formulas for Kt/V_{eq} calculation depend on the blood sampling site.

Recent results from the HEMO Study have verified that the rate of hemodialysis (i.e., $Kt/V_{sp} \div t$) is the single most important predictor of the magnitude of post-dialysis urea

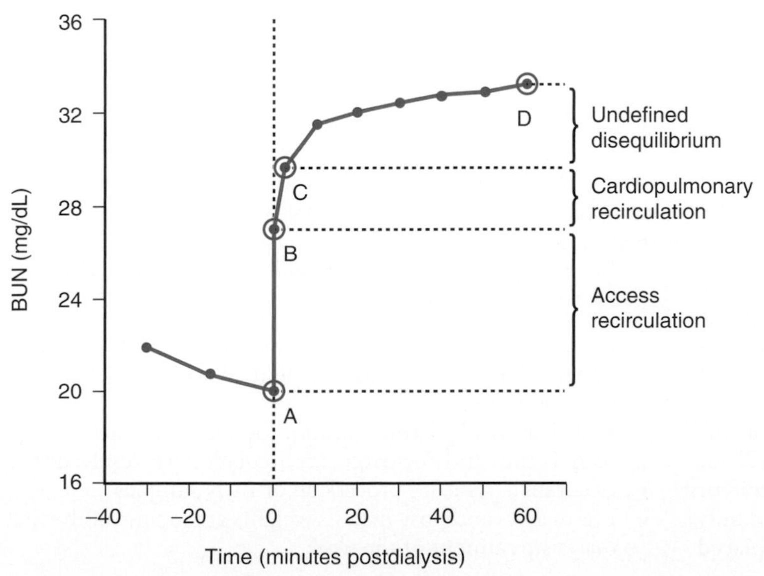

Figure 20–2 Biophysical and kinetic segregation of the components of urea rebound. After the completion of hemodialysis, the blood urea nitrogen (BUN) concentration increases. The increment from point A → B is secondary to access recirculation; from point B → C, secondary to cardiopulmonary recirculation; and point C → D, secondary to flow-volume disequilibrium and/or diffusive impedance of urea (undefined disequilibrium). (From National Kidney Foundation: K/DOQI Clinical Practice Guidelines for Hemodialysis Adequacy, 2000. Am J Kidney Dis 2001; 37[suppl 1]:S7-S64.)

rebound.[96] These results suggest, however, that the coefficients of the Daugirdas-Schneditz rate equation described previously may not always be the most accurate in predicting Kt/V_{eq}. Moreover, this study showed that the optimal coefficients to use in the Daugirdas-Schneditz rate equation depend on when the immediate post-dialysis blood sample is obtained. Based on their studies, these investigators suggested the following equations for general use when the post-dialysis blood sample was obtained 20 seconds after stopping the blood flow rate:

$$\text{arterial } Kt/V_{eq} = \text{art } Kt/V_{sp} - 0.39 \times (\text{art } Kt/V_{sp} \div t) \quad (15)$$

$$\text{venous } Kt/V_{eq} = \text{ven } Kt/V_{sp} - 0.22 \times (\text{ven } Kt/V_{sp} \div t) \quad (16)$$

These equations are potentially important to use in routine clinical practice because they were similar to those used to interpret the outcome results from the HEMO Study (see later).

Although it is increasingly recognized that conversion to an equilibrated model can enhance the accuracy of the measurement of the delivered hemodialysis dose, routine substitution of Kt/V_{eq} for Kt/V_{sp} may be problematic and is not recommended[55] because of the:

1. Impracticality of obtaining a 30- to 60-minute BUN sample after completion of hemodialysis.
2. Uncertainty about the longitudinal validity of the aforementioned formulas for estimation of equilibrated Kt/V for an individual patient.
3. Absence of studies characterizing the dose-response relationship between Kt/V_{eq} and patient outcomes.

Furthermore, it has been proposed that rigorous monitoring of the Kt/V_{sp} and application of the hemodialysis dose recommendations from evidence-based practice guidelines, which are, in turn, derived from appropriate patient outcome studies using single-pool models of urea kinetics,[54,55] ensure patient safety equally as well as the use of double-pool models.[55]

Recirculation

A biophysical variable potentially confounding measurements of the delivered dose of solute removal during hemodialysis is the occurrence of recirculation. During hemodialysis, some of the blood that enters the dialyzer inlet may have flowed from the outlet without first passing through the peripheral capillaries. This flow of previously dialyzed blood from the dialyzer outlet to the inlet is termed "recirculation"[88,97,98]; if it is present, it is a significant contributing factor in urea rebound. It is intellectually useful to consider urea rebound as two temporal phases, an early and a late phase before and after 3 minutes post-dialysis, respectively. In turn, early urea rebound may be segregated into two components, both occurring as a consequence of different types of recirculation. The first component, secondary to blood recirculation within the angioaccess, is termed "access recirculation." The second component of early urea rebound is a consequence of "cardiopulmonary recirculation."[98,99]

Access recirculation occurs when a proportion of the blood returning to the patient through the venous needle or port is immediately drawn back into the arterial needle or port and dialyzed again. Access recirculation commonly occurs when (1) the arterial needle is incorrectly placed downstream of the venous needle, (2) the venous limb of the angioaccess is used for the arterial flow into the dialyzer and vice versa, or (3) the blood pump speed exceeds the flow rate through the fistula (Figure 20–3).[98] The last is usually a result of a critical stenosis in the angioaccess. Without a stenosis, fistula flow rates well exceed 700 mL/min and are unlikely to be superseded by the extracorporeal blood flow rate (Q_b).

Access recirculation begins to resolve immediately upon the completion of hemodialysis, and its effects are completely abolished in a very short time period (10–20 seconds). Therefore, in the presence of access recirculation, a post-dialysis BUN sample obtained either without flushing recirculated blood from the arterial line or within the first 10 to 20 seconds post-hemodialysis, results in an erroneously low BUN concentration, an excessively large Kt/V, URR, and nPCR.

The second component of early urea rebound, *cardiopulmonary recirculation*, is inevitable when an arteriovenous angioaccess is used in hemodialysis.[99] Cardiopulmonary recirculation arises because of the routing of just-dialyzed blood through the veins to the heart and the pulmonary circuit and back to the angioaccess without the passage of this blood through any urea-rich peripheral tissues.[100] Like access recirculation, cardiopulmonary recirculation causes post-dialysis urea rebound that begins approximately 20 seconds after the hemodialysis treatment, and approximately 2 to 3 minutes is required for its dissipation. Similar to access recirculation, improper timing for sampling of the blood for measurement of the post-dialysis BUN concentration causes erroneous results from urea kinetic modeling.[55,101]

Blood Sampling

To calculate Kt/V, using formal urea kinetic modeling requires accurate measures of: pre-dialysis and post-dialysis BUN concentration drawn at the first dialysis treatment of the week, and the pre-dialysis BUN concentration at the following treatment in a thrice-weekly hemodialysis schedule. Urea kinetic modeling, based on two BUN samples obtained on the midweek pre-dialysis and post-dialysis BUN, has been described and validated for accuracy in comparison to classic three-sample urea kinetic modeling.[102]

The accuracy of the calculated Kt/V or URR depends on proper blood sampling techniques for the pre-dialysis and post-dialysis BUN concentrations.[101] These sampling techniques must control for (1) the site of the blood obtained, (2) needle or catheter preparation, (3) blood and dialysate flow rates, (4) ultrafiltration rate, and (5) timing of the blood sampling with respect to the initiation and termination of the hemodialysis treatment.[103]

The ideal and accurate measurement of the Kt/V, URR, and nPCR requires:

- Pre-dialysis BUN concentration be measured before hemodialysis begins and be obtained without dilution of the blood sample[103]
- Post-dialysis BUN concentration be measured after hemodialysis ends and angioaccess recirculation has resolved[104,105]
- Accurate laboratory processing of BUN samples
- Pre-dialysis and post-dialysis weights at the time of the first dialysis treatment of the week

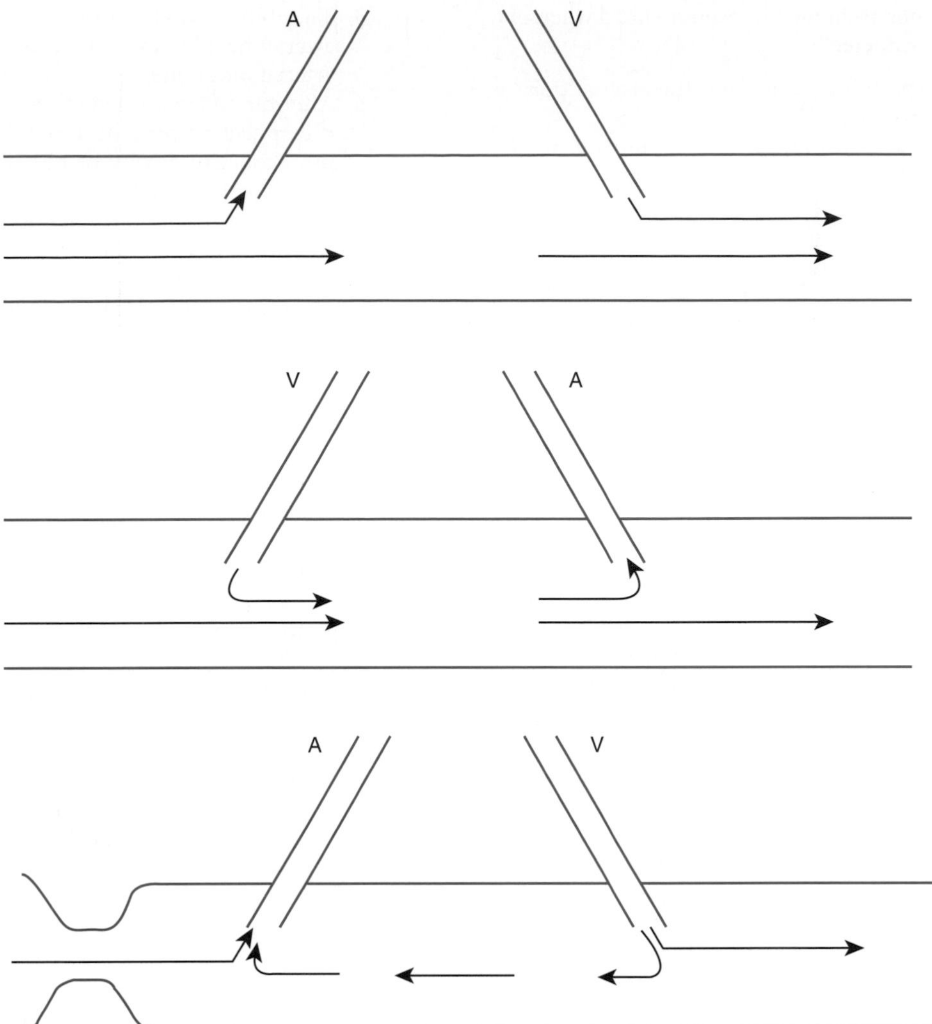

Figure 20–3 Schematic representation of angioaccess recirculation. A and V refer to the arterial and venous paths of blood flow, respectively. *Uppermost panel,* the ideal situation of no access recirculation. *Middle panel,* access recirculation secondary to reversal of the needle placement, so that the blood path is from the venous limb to the arterial limb of the access. *Lower panel,* access recirculation secondary to stenosis of the arterial limb of the access with resultant blood flow that is inadequate to meet the pump speed. (Modified from Tattersall JE, Chamney P, Aldridge C, Greenwood RN: Recirculation and the postdialysis rebound. Nephrol Dial Transplant 1996; 11[suppl 2]:75-80.)

- Actual treatment time (delivered time, not the prescribed time)

The effective clearance of the dialyzer, as calculated from the hemodialysis unit (not the *in vitro* value provided by the manufacturer, which often overestimates the true in vivo value in plasma water).[106]

To calculate the URR requires pre-dialysis and post-dialysis BUN concentrations drawn at the same hemodialysis session. To calculate Kt/V using the simplified Daugirdas formula requires:

- Pre-dialysis and post-dialysis BUN concentration drawn at the same hemodialysis session
- Actual treatment time (delivered time)
- Patient's pre-dialysis and post-dialysis weights

Pre-Dialysis Blood Sampling Procedures

The pre-dialysis BUN must be obtained before dialysis begins to prevent this sample from being affected by the hemodialysis process. Sample dilution by heparin or saline must be avoided, or the pre-dialysis BUN sample will register an artificially low concentration. A recent, evidence-based clinical practice guideline described the best clinical practice for blood sampling. The sampling technique is one utilizing a fistula or graft as follows[55]:

1. Obtain the blood specimen from the arterial needle prior to connecting the arterial blood tubing or flushing the needle. Ensure that no saline or heparin is in the arterial needle.
2. Do not draw sample if the hemodialysis treatment has commenced.

The following sampling technique is recommended when one is utilizing a venous catheter[55]:

1. Withdraw any heparin or saline from the arterial port to prevent dilution of sample.
2. Using sterile technique, withdraw 10 mL of blood from the arterial port of the catheter. Do not discard this specimen, if reinfusion is intended.
3. Connect a new syringe or collection device, and draw the sample for BUN measurement.
4. Optional: Reinfuse the 10 mL of blood withdrawn earlier. Initiate hemodialysis, according to the dialysis unit's protocol.

Post-Dialysis Blood Sampling Procedures

The timing of the acquisition of the post-dialysis sample is especially crucial.[101,103] Immediately upon completion of the hemodialysis treatment, if access recirculation is present, some recirculated blood will be present in the angioaccess. If post-dialysis blood sampling is performed in the presence of recirculated blood, it will dilute the blood sample and give a falsely reduced BUN concentration. This results in an overestimation of the delivered dose of hemodialysis and the nPCR. Subsequently, cardiopulmonary recirculation and the double-pool effects take place to complete the post-dialysis urea rebound.

As described earlier, although the most accurate method to account for these biophysical effects is to wait 30 minutes after completion of dialysis, few patients agree to waiting. An alternative, clinically applicable method that best supports the use of formal urea kinetic modeling is the "slow flow/stop pump sampling technique."[55]

The sampling technique for the post-dialysis BUN concentration is as follows:

I. At the completion of hemodialysis, turn off the dialysate flow (to terminate the hemodialysis process) and decrease the ultrafiltration rate to 50 mL/hr (or to the lowest transmembrane pressure setting).

II. Decrease the blood flow rate to 50 to 100 mL/min for 15 (10–20) seconds. This step is performed to fill the arterial needle and blood tubing with nonrecirculated blood (i.e., to avoid the effect of access recirculation that may be present).

III. Proceed with either of two techniques:

A. *Slow flow technique*

1. Immediately draw the blood sample for measurement of the postdialysis BUN concentration from the arterial needle or port.
2. Stop the blood pump, and complete the patient disconnection procedure according to dialysis unit protocol.

B. *Stop pump technique*

1. After running the blood flow rate at 50 to 100 mL/min for 15 seconds to flush any recirculated blood from the angioaccess, stop the pump immediately.
2. Clamp the arterial line and venous blood lines, and clamp the arterial needle tubing.
3. Take blood sample from the arterial port or the arterial needle tubing after disconnecting from the arterial blood line.
4. After blood is returned to the patient, continue the disconnection procedure according to dialysis unit protocol. Uniformity of blood sampling methods has several advantages:
   a. As technical variability in blood sampling is minimized, the delivered doses of small solute removal during hemodialysis reported are comparable. Alternatively, a similar dose reported by dialysis centers using different blood sampling methods may have varied "actual" dialysis doses and are not comparable.[101]
   b. The single-pool urea kinetic model mandates that the post-dialysis BUN sample be measured without the effects of access recirculation and before significant urea rebound has occurred. The precise timing of the method of blood sampling advocated by the DOQI Hemodialysis Adequacy Work Group meets this requirement.[55]
   c. The recommended formulas for converting the single-pool Kt/V to a double-pool or equilibrated Kt/V value require that the post-dialysis BUN sample be obtained before urea rebound is completed.[95] Therefore, the reproducibility and accuracy of these blood sampling techniques outweigh the potential operational difficulties that may be encountered.

An alternative, widespread method of post-dialysis BUN sampling is the *blood reinfusion technique*,[55] which involves blood sampling after the patient's blood has been completely reinfused. Its relative simplicity has made it a popular technique, with a lower likelihood of operational errors. (The slow flow/stop pump techniques are more demanding technically.)

For blood sampling by the blood reinfusion technique:

1. Using a minimum volume of saline, return the patient's blood until the system is clear. Minimize the amount of saline used so that the post-dialysis BUN concentration is not decreased because of systemic dilution from administered saline. This is a particular concern for patients with a small V. Tapping the dialyzer during blood return, or pinching the lines and releasing to flush the tubing, may permit the use of less saline.
2. Clamp the blood and needle lines. Completely disconnect the patient from the extracorporeal circuit, per the dialysis unit protocol.
3. Using aseptic technique, attach a 10-mL syringe to the arterial needle tubing.
4. Unclamp arterial needle tubing or catheter. Withdraw and reinfuse 5 to 7 mL of blood several times to clear any remaining saline that might dilute the sample.
5. Clamp the arterial needle tubing or catheter after the line is filled with blood.
6. Utilizing a sterile technique, detach the syringe and set it aside.
7. Attach a multiple-sample Luer adapter or a second syringe to the Vacutainer needle holder. Attach whichever of these

devices is used to the end of the arterial fistula needle or catheter. Push the tube onto the holder.

8. Open the clamp on arterial needle tubing or catheter line to collect the post-dialysis BUN sample. Clamp the line when the tube is full. Remove the adapter and needle holder or syringe.
9. Clamp the blood line, and complete the termination procedure per dialysis unit protocol.

It is critical that the dialysis care team appreciate that the doses of hemodialysis measured by this blood sampling method will be systematically lower than those obtained using the slow flow/stop pump sampling techniques, even when the actual delivered dose of hemodialysis is the same.[107] Because variable amounts of urea rebound will have occurred owing to differences in the timing of blood reinfusion and sampling, the measured dialysis dose with the slow flow/stop pump sampling technique will be higher than that with the reinfusion sampling technique. Therefore, continuous quality improvement initiatives, which contrast the delivered dose of hemodialysis and nPCR between patients and facilities as clinical performance measurements, must not trivialize the potential for apparent differences arising from the blood sampling method alone.[101]

Uniformity of Dose Quantification and Blood Sampling

As implied from the earlier discussions, the method of drawing the pre-dialysis and especially post-dialysis BUN samples can affect the results of the Kt/V or URR measurement independent of the hemodialysis dose. A survey of 202 units across North America estimates that 5% of the centers have errors in their pre-dialysis sampling method, and up to 40% of the units surveyed have potential faults in their post-dialysis sampling method.[108] Adoption of the same method of hemodialysis dose quantification (either Kt/V or URR) for all patients in a given facility can enhance consistency and enable meaningful comparison of data for a given patient over time, between different patients in the same center, and among different hemodialysis facilities.[101]

In the absence of such uniformity in measurement, longitudinal comparisons of delivered doses of small solute removal during hemodialysis cannot be made. However, the adoption of one method of hemodialysis dose quantification does not preclude the use of another method as a supplementary measurement for some or all patients. Nevertheless, the dialysis facility must adopt a single, consistent, and comparable measurement of the dose of hemodialysis. For example, if a center uses URR as the principal measurement of the delivered dose of hemodialysis, this can be supplemented episodically by the more precise measure of Kt/V derived from formal urea kinetic modeling. Similarly, a dialysis facility that uses single-pool Kt/V can supplement this with a measurement of the equilibrated Kt/V.

Frequency of Dose Measurement

Numerous outcome studies have correlated the dose of small solute removal with patient morbidity and mortality.[11,14–16,18,19,47] It is clear that the outcome of the ESRD population receiving hemodialysis can be improved with a selected minimum dose of small solute removal during hemodialysis. As such, the dose of small solute removal during hemodialysis must be measured on a regular basis to ensure dialysis adequacy. Clinical signs and symptoms alone are not reliable indicators of hemodialysis adequacy.

The evidence suggests that measurement of hemodialysis dose should be performed monthly. This recommendation is based on the observation that most hemodialysis outcome studies have relied on monthly measurements.[11,14,19,47] Measurements performed less frequently may compromise the timeliness with which deficiencies in the delivered hemodialysis dose are detected and hence may delay implementation of corrective steps. Because most dialysis facilities schedule their patients to undergo monthly blood-based biochemical evaluations with monthly reporting of the institutional results, monthly measurement of the delivered hemodialysis dose is pragmatic.

The frequency of small solute dose measurements should be increased if:

1. Patients are noncompliant (i.e., if they often miss treatment or sign off prematurely).
2. Problems are noted in the delivery of hemodialysis (i.e., poor blood flow, treatment interruptions, clotting of the dialyzer).
3. The delivered dose varies widely in the absence of prescription changes.
4. The hemodialysis prescription has been modified.

When the use of online (real-time) measurement of dialysis dose becomes available extensively, dose of dialysis can be ascertained for every treatment and correction can be made immediately.

DEFINING AND DELIVERING AN ADEQUATE DOSE OF HEMODIALYSIS

Guideline Recommendations

In 1993, the Renal Physicians Association (RPA) released the first evidence-based, clinical practice guidelines on the adequacy of hemodialysis.[54] This document defined adequate hemodialysis as the "recommended quantity of hemodialysis delivered which is required for adequate treatment of ESRD such that patients receive full benefit of hemodialysis therapy." At the time of its release, the only randomized, prospective controlled trial that provided evidence for the required dose of hemodialysis was the NCDS.[11] As detailed earlier, reanalysis of the primary data from this trial showed that single-pool Kt/V values below 0.8 were associated with a relatively high rate of morbidity, whereas Kt/V values between 1.0 and 1.2 were associated with a relatively lower rate of morbidity.[41]

Extrapolating from the NCDS to current dialysis practice is problematic because of major differences in patient mix and dialysis practice since the performance of the trial. Because of the paucity of definitive literature at the time of the RPA's Clinical Guidelines on Adequacy of Hemodialysis, a supplementary clinical decision analysis was performed using available data.[107] The initial analysis used a probabilistic model to assess how variables in the dialysis prescription affect a patient's *quality-adjusted life expectancy* (QALE). In a complementary analysis, lifetime costs and QALE were modeled to determine the "marginal cost-effectiveness of the components of the dialysis prescription."[109]

On the basis of these analyses, the RPA recommended that, "the delivered dose Kt/V should be at least 1.2." In the analysis by Hornberger[107] the QALE continued to increase to a tested Kt/V level of 2.0; at Kt/V values of 1.4 and greater, a rapid increase in cost was noted secondary to the increased costs of the delivery of hemodialysis, which offset the savings achieved by fewer hospitalizations. Thus, the RPA made a final recommendation that balanced the patient's QALE with marginal cost-effectiveness of the dialysis dose.

Since the publication of the RPA's Clinical Practice Guideline, several reports have suggested greater mortality benefit associated with a higher minimum dose of hemodialysis.[15,16,18,19,110] However, most of these reports were observational, retrospective analyses from self-selected dialysis centers. Some of the limitations include the following:

1. Comparison of patient outcomes to uncontrolled historical standards[18,110]
2. Lack of randomization[15,19]
3. Lack of standardization in the blood sampling method[15,19]
4. Use of relatively broad categories of Kt/V or URR for analysis[15,19,47]
5. Major differences in clinical practice and patient behaviors in other countries compared with those in the United States[110]

For example, Hakim and associates[16] performed a prospective study to increase the Kt/V of 130 patients from 0.8 to 1.3 over a 4-year period (1988 to 1991). Concurrent with this increase, they reported a reduction in gross annual mortality from 22.8% in 1988 to 9.1% in 1991. The standardized mortality rate and the hospitalization rate were also reduced. However, this was not a randomized controlled trial, and several factors during the course of the study period varied simultaneously with the dose of hemodialysis. The study did not define dose, because the only comparisons made were between Kt/V of 0.8 (known to be inadequate since the NCDS) and 1.3 (which is above the minimum set by the RPA's Clinical Practice Guidelines). Furthermore, not all study results suggest an improved survival with delivered hemodialysis doses higher than Kt/V of 1.2 or URR of 65%.[19,47] A retrospective analysis of data from the USRDS, which used both single-pool (sp) and double-pool (dp) urea kinetic models, found no improvement in survival for a categoric Kt/V_{sp} of 1.2 to 1.4 or a Kt/V_{dp} of 1.0 to 1.2.[111]

From a literature review in this area of hemodialysis care since the publication of the RPA's Clinical Practice Guidelines, the DOQI Hemodialysis Adequacy Work Group[55] recommended the following:

1. In the absence of definite and consistent evidence, the minimum dose of delivered hemodialysis, as recommended, should remain unchanged.
2. The present literature does not support the definition of an optimal dose of hemodialysis.[55] Specifically, "the dialysis care team should deliver a Kt/V of at least 1.2 (single-pool, variable-volume) for both adult and pediatric hemodialysis patients. For those using the URR, the delivered dose should be equivalent to a Kt/V of 1.2, that is, an average URR of 65%. URR can vary substantially as a function of fluid removal, however."[55]

In determining the minimum dose of hemodialysis, as measured by the URR, we note that the relationship between URR and Kt/V is greatly affected by the extent of the ultrafiltration.[64,65] Thus, the required URR to achieve the minimum adequate Kt/V of 1.2 can vary substantially as a function of fluid removal (see Figure 20–1).

It is clear that many ESRD patients do not receive their prescribed dose of hemodialysis. Some studies have suggested that only 50% of the ESRD patients in the United States actually received their prescribed hemodialysis dose.[14,19,112] As discussed later, URR cannot be prescriptive, but it does offer a valid single point in time analysis of the delivered dose of hemodialysis. A representative national survey of 6000 ESRD patients revealed that in 1995 only 59% of the patients surveyed received a URR of 65% or higher. A variety of factors may compromise the delivery of the prescribed dose.[14,112–115] These factors may be categorized into those that (1) compromise urea clearance, (2) reduce the hemodialysis treatment time, or (3) result in errors in blood sampling. Again, these problems in the delivered dose of hemodialysis result in a discrepancy between the V derived from urea kinetic modeling and the V derived from anthropometric values (see Tables 20–2 and 20–3). A continuous quality improvement initiative that uses formal urea kinetic modeling can readily detect these problems in the delivered hemodialysis dose.

To prevent the delivered dose of hemodialysis from declining to values below the recommended minimum dose, practitioners should prescribe doses of dialysis that are above these minimum values. In the HEMO Study, in which rigorous implementation and measurements of the hemodialysis prescription were executed, the 90% confidence interval for the single-pool Kt/V of 1.3 is 0.1 unit (personal communication, T. Greene, 1995). As such, the DOQI Hemodialysis Adequacy Work Group[55] suggests that *the prescribed minimum Kt/V should be 1.3.* For the URR, the HEMO Study observed a 90% confidence interval of 4% (Greene, 1995). Therefore, *for those using URR, a minimum target URR of 70% should be set.*[55]

To achieve a desired Kt/V, K and V can be derived by various means and the treatment time, t, then determined. As such, Kt/V is prescriptive but URR is not. In contrast to the Kt/V, means to increase the URR are subject to the preferences of the dialysis physician and are executed by trial and error. Specifically, an arbitrary estimate of the blood or dialysate flow rates, or the duration of treatment needed to achieve the target URR, is prescribed and a follow-up URR is obtained. However, when a series of normograms is used, the URR can be correlated to an extrapolated Kt/V, and this value is used to guide modification of the appropriate components of the hemodialysis prescription.[63]

Patients with Diabetes Mellitus

Collins and associates[15] suggested that diabetic patients with ESRD may experience an approximate 40% reduction in their odds of risk of death, if the minimum delivered single-pool Kt/V is increased from 1.0 to 1.2 to 1.4 or greater. However, this finding has not been observed uniformly in other studies of diabetic patients with ESRD.[19,111] Therefore, this discrepancy makes it difficult to routinely recommend a higher minimum dose of hemodialysis for diabetic patients.

Race and Gender

Several observational analyses have reported that although African-Americans with ESRD often receive less than the minimum appropriate dose of hemodialysis (as recommended by the RPA and DOQI),[116,117] they have an improved survival rate compared with whites.[47,117] Despite knowledge of the cause of death, the basis of the improved survival for African-Americans is unclear. Potential explanations include:

1. The selection of healthier African-Americans for maintenance dialysis
2. Misdiagnosis or misclassification of the cause of ESRD among African-Americans
3. Improved nutrition among African-Americans
4. African-Americans have better quality of life on dialysis and thus adopt fewer deleterious health-related behaviors
5. Relatively less susceptibility to the deleterious effects of inadequate hemodialysis[117]

It is important to realize that all previous analyses of the relationship between the dose of hemodialysis and patients' mortality risk were derived by statistically aggregating all patient subgroups (race, gender, diabetes), on the assumption that their sensitivity is equivalent. Using a database of 18,144 representative ESRD patients (from Fresenius Medical Care), the analysis suggests that the previous clinical assumption of no difference in the odds of risk of death among different racial groups and genders by URR is incorrect.[19,47,118] White patients, particularly white females, are much more affected by the mortal risk of lower URR values than African-Americans (Figure 20–4). This differential racial sensitivity to lower hemodialysis doses, as measured by the URR, is not explained by differences in patients' ages. It may not be a case of differential sensitivity to dialysis dose, but, simply, that URR is inadequate as a measure of hemodialysis dose. African-Americans were observed to have greater weight and TBW and higher serum albumin and serum creatinine levels.

The TBW is related to both URR and nutrition because TBW is calculated using patient weight and not directly measured. A change in TBW causes the two predictors (URR and nutrition) to bring about changes in contrasting direction.

The nutrition-derived effect of urea distribution volume may supersede its mortality impact by way of URR. These findings underscore the limitation of URR and Kt/V because measures of the adequacy of hemodialysis suggest that quality assurance efforts in this domain of care must be dynamic and reiterative to reflect the rapidly evolving knowledge base in dialysis care. However, there is no evidence that African-Americans should receive less dialysis than Caucasians.

Twice-Weekly Hemodialysis

Twice-weekly hemodialysis is usually inadequate, unless there is a significant amount of residual renal function, that is, a glomerular filtration rate (GFR) of 5 mL/min or greater. Because residual renal function declines with time, the presence of a significant amount of residual renal function at the initiation of maintenance hemodialysis mandates serial monitoring of renal function, if the patient is undergoing twice-weekly hemodialysis. Such diligence can guide the appropriate addition of a third-weekly hemodialysis treatment, if renal function declines further. Unless the patient's residual renal function can be monitored serially and regularly, patients should start a thrice-weekly hemodialysis schedule from the onset.[55]

Are the Current Measures Appropriate Predictors of Survival?

The clearance of urea normalized to the volume of distribution of urea (Kt/V) and the URR are the current standards upon which clinical guidelines and regulation on hemodialysis adequacy in the United States are based. As stated earlier, any clinically meaningful measure of the dose of dialysis must be relevant to patient outcome. The urea kinetic concepts of Kt/V and URR have been correlated variously to morbidity and mortality outcomes in past years (Table 20–3). It does appear that these mathematical constructs are useful and relevant to patient outcome.*

However, recent reports suggest clinical problems and paradoxes when medical outcome is considered in terms of Kt/V or URR. First, Kopple and associates[121] reported progressive deterioration of survival among patients grouped by weight-for-height percentile. URR decreased progressively with increasing weight-for-height percentile, so that the lightest patients had both the highest URR and death risk. Taken by themselves, one may conclude from these data that higher clearance (as measured by URR) leads to undernutrition and increased risk of death.

A second report by Chertow and associates[122] described increasing mortality risk when URR was above 70%, producing a reverse J curve to the URR death risk profile. He then measured TBW (by bioelectric impedence) and adjusted URR for TBW and showed improved survival across the entire range of TBW adjusted URR.[122] Low TBW (giving rise to a high unadjusted URR) reflected low lean body mass and poor nutritional status, thus contributing to greater risk of death. The reverse J curve profile has also been reported in the past, although no satisfactory answers availed at the time that it was published. Patients with a URR above 70% (urea ratio, 3.4) and Kt/V above 1.25 were associated with higher mortality risk.[119,123]

The mortality risk of low URR appears to affect African-Americans and males less significantly.[118] As is known, African-Americans and males have higher body mass, suggesting that the effect of URR on survival is altered by body mass. Serum concentration of creatinine is favorably associated with survival in dialysis patients, and African-Americans and males tend to have higher levels. Statistical adjustment for differences in serum creatinine concentration negates the survival advantage of African-Americans receiving hemodialysis.

Using data from a USRDS special study (of 8591 patients), Wolfe and associates[124] reported their findings on the relationship between dose of hemodialysis (Kt/V), body size, and mortality. Kt/V and body size measure were both independently and significantly related to mortality after adjustment for patient characteristics and comorbid conditions.[124] It was concluded that Kt/V (as a measure of dialysis dose) and body size (as proxy for nutrition) are clinically important predictors of mortality.

---

*References 11,15,16,18,19,47,118–120.

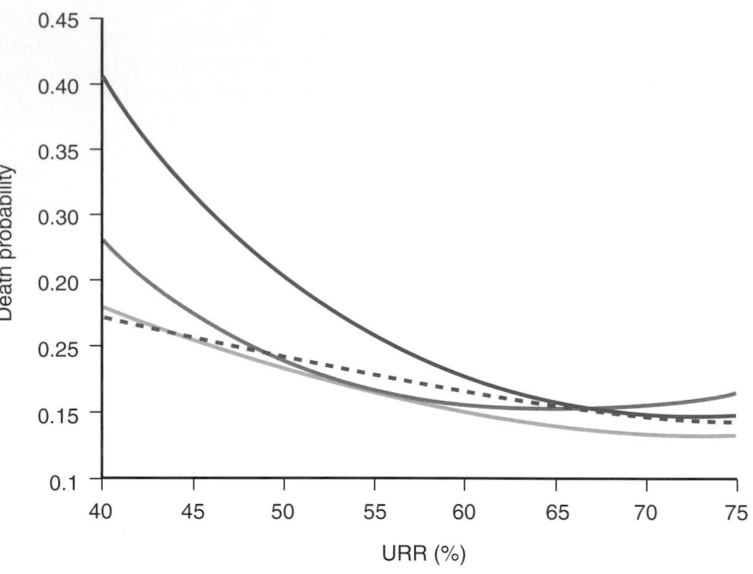

Figure 20–4 Age-adjusted death probability for patients with end-stage renal disease as a function of urea reduction ratio (URR). *Key:* Top curve, white females; second *(solid)* curve, white males; third *(dotted)* curve, black males; bottom curve, black females. The URR is expressed as a second-order variable.[118] Again, white females and males exhibited a greater sensitivity to the mortal effects of URR values less than those recommended by the Renal Physicians Association (RPA) and Dialysis Outcomes Quality Initiative (DOQI) Clinical Practice Guidelines on hemodialysis adequacy.

These observations suggest that the present urea kinetic construct for dialysis dose, Kt/V or URR, whereby one measure (the urea clearance product, K × t) is divided by another (V, a proxy of lean body mass and nutrition) may be flawed. Increasing V diminishes Kt/V, generally associated with higher mortality risk, but a larger V by itself is associated with better nutritional status and, hence, better outcome (lower mortality risk).

Lowrie and associates,[125] analyzing data from more than 17,000 patients using the Fresenius Medical Care database, demonstrated improving death odds with increasing Kt alone (not corrected for V). Similar favorable findings were noted with increasing body size (measured here as BSA, TBW, body weight, and body mass index) whether adjusted or not for Kt. Patients with smaller body size needed higher Kt/V to achieve the same level of risk. Thus, dividing Kt by V failed to "normalize" treatment across all classes of body size as it was intended to; instead, it accentuated the differences. Additional analyses by these same investigators have confirmed and extended these concepts, using an even larger database.[126]

The fundamental premise that V is assumed to be an inert receptacle for urea is not true—the reason why the seemingly contradictory rise in mortality risk as Kt/V or URR is very high. Some patients with small body size have both higher mortality and URR or Kt/V (i.e., lower body mass permits higher URR but contributes to greater mortality). This paradox can be resolved, if we disaggregate Kt/V into two separate measures of outcome: (1) dialysis exposure and (2) body mass. Indexing treatment to body size gives rise to confusing discrepancies of patient outcome. The Lowrie[125] report suggested that Kt may be a better outcome predictor, and the minimum clearance (Kt) threshold is 40 to 45 L per treatment for female patients and 45 to 50 L per treatment for male patients. This was inferred from retrospective data, and the possibility that higher values may yield incremental benefit must be considered. The consideration of Kt as a dose parameter for evaluating dialysis adequacy has both scientific and clinical merit; recent work confirms its comparability to Kt/V in epidemiologic studies.[127]

PRINCIPLES AND METHODS FOR QUANTIFYING THE DOSE OF MIDDLE MOLECULE REMOVAL DURING HEMODIALYSIS

Duration of Treatment

It has been suggested that the duration of the hemodialysis session is an independent measure of hemodialysis adequacy, separate from either Kt/V or URR. The proponents of dialysis duration as a unique measure of hemodialysis adequacy propose that extending the length of hemodialysis disproportionately increases the clearance of uremic toxins for which urea is not a good surrogate (e.g., middle molecules). Because of their size, middle molecules are less dependent on diffusive clearance than urea, if a conventional low-flux dialyzer is used. Acknowledging that urea is only a marker solute for uremic toxins, treatment time becomes a crude surrogate for the clearance of these molecules. Therefore, a longer duration for hemodialysis may enhance patient survival[13,128,129] and, thus, offer an alternative measure not accounted for by urea-based kinetic modeling alone.

A second potential advantage of longer hemodialysis sessions is the greater ease of establishing intravascular euvolemia. If the estimated dry weight is defined as the post-dialysis weight that correlates with intravascular euvolemia, routinely achieving this weight may reduce the risk of cardiovascular complications, especially from hypervolemia and hypertension.[129,130] Both the ultrafiltration volume and the rate of ultrafiltration greatly affect blood pressure,[131,132] such that large ultrafiltration volumes or rapid ultrafiltration can result in hypotension, cramps, or both. These symptoms are a frequent cause of the premature discontinuation of hemodialysis,[112,114,133] which, in turn, may lead patients to finish the treatment without achieving their true estimated dry weight. With a typical interdialytic weight gain, the cycle is repeated at the next dialysis, such that the patient is chronically hypervolemic. This cycle may be further exaggerated by the physiologically incorrect clinical practice of routinely relying on hypotension or cramps to define estimated dry weight.[134–138]

All of these events may be confounded further by the deleterious effect of antihypertensive medications on the patient's intradialytic blood pressure.[139] Because some investigators have reported improved patient survival in the setting of greatly improved blood pressure control associated with increased dialysis treatment times,[129] it has been suggested that this is a causal relationship. Therefore, extending the duration of hemodialysis sessions has been advocated as a means of minimizing intradialytic hypotension and cramps, thus improving the likelihood of achieving the patient's dry weight.[55]

Despite these clinically sound arguments, there are no clinical outcomes data to support a minimum time for hemodialysis treatment. The few studies that have attempted to statistically examine this issue are compromised by reliance on the prescribed instead of the delivered dialysis time.[11,47] Held and associates[19] reported that prescribed treatment time was not statistically significant in explaining mortality when adjusted for dose of dialysis. A similar conclusion was published in an earlier study.[123] When dose of dialysis was maintained, hemodialysis time did not affect survival. Further studies are needed to ascertain whether actual delivered treatment time is a predictor of mortality. As described previously, however, the accuracy of the single-pool, variable-volume model of urea kinetics becomes increasingly compromised with shorter dialysis times, so that the delivered dose of hemodialysis becomes increasingly overestimated.[55] Therefore, some groups have recommended that irrespective of the delivered dose of hemodialysis, the dialysis time should not be shortened to less than 2.5 hours,[15] especially if single-pool urea kinetic modeling is used.

Calculation of Beta-2-Microglobulin Clearances

An alternative method for evaluating middle molecule removal during hemodialysis is by direct evaluation of the clearance of a given marker solute in the middle molecular weight range. The middle molecule that has historically been used as a marker is vitamin B_{12}, and calculated in vitro dialyzer clearances of vitamin B_{12} are an independent predictor survival among chronic hemodialysis patients.[140] Dialyzer clearances for this solute, however, can be accurately evaluated *in vitro* only; thus, determination of vitamin B_{12} clearance as an in vivo marker of middle molecule clearance is problematic because of its extensive binding to plasma proteins. The causative role of β_2-microglobulin in the pathogenesis of dialysis-related amyloidosis[31] and its ready measurement in the plasma of ESRD patients have resulted in the common use of β_2-microglobulin as a marker solute for evaluating the clearance of middle molecules.

Kinetic modeling of β_2-microglobulin during hemodialysis follows the same general principles as those described previously for urea. When modeling β_2-microglobulin, however, different simplifying assumptions are required. Assuming a single compartment model,[141] the following assumptions are reasonable:

1. β_2-microglobulin is uniformly distributed in a single compartment that approximates extracellular fluid volume. This assumption neglects post-dialysis rebound of β_2-microglobulin.
2. Fluid removed during hemodialysis treatment originates entirely from the extracellular fluid space.
3. The amount of β_2-microglobulin generated intradialytically can be neglected.
4. There is no residual renal nor extrarenal clearance of β_2-microglobulin.

Based on these assumptions, equation (1) can be integrated over the intradialytic period. From that solution, the following equation was derived to calculated mean dialyzer clearance of β_2-microglobulin (K_{b2m}) during the hemodialysis session from pre-dialysis and post-dialysis concentrations, C(0) and C(t), respectively:

$$K_{b2m} = Qf\ (1 - \ln\ (C(t)/C(0))/\ln\ [1 + Qf \times t/V\ [t]]) \quad \mathbf{(17)}$$

where Qf is the ultrafiltration rate determined as the difference between the pre-dialysis and post-dialysis body weights divided by t, the treatment time, and V(t) is an estimate of extracellular fluid volume post-dialysis. Equation (17) was used to evaluate dialyzer clearances of β_2-microglobulin to define the flux intervention in the HEMO Study and to examine the effect of reuse on dialyzer clearances of β_2-microglobulin.[142] Although valuable for certain purposes, the estimates of dialyzer clearance provided by equation (17) are likely inaccurate because this model neglects post-dialysis rebound of β_2-microglobulin.[143] Further work is needed to provide practical equations for calculating dialyzer clearances of β_2-microglobulin, which account for post-dialysis rebound.

RESULTS FROM THE HEMO STUDY

The HEMO Study was a prospective, randomized, multicenter clinical trial designed to study the effects of the dose of small solute removal (defined in this trial as "dialysis dose") and membrane flux on hemodialysis patient morbidity and mortality. Patients were randomized using a 2 × 2 factorial design to a target eKt/V of either 1.05 of 1.45 and to the use of either low-flux or high-flux membranes. Entry criteria included a thrice-weekly treatment regimen, age 18 to 80 years, residual renal urea clearance less than 1.5 mL/min/35 L of urea volume, and anticipated ability to achieve a target eKt/V of 1.45 during a 4.5-hour hemodialysis session. Between 1995 and 2001, 1846 patients were randomized in 72 dialysis units affiliated with 15 clinical centers in the United States. More details on the study design and implementation have been reported elsewhere.[144,145] The primary outcome was patient death from any cause. Several secondary outcomes were also evaluated.

Randomized patients were, in general, similar to national data from the United States. There was a slight predominance of women, 63% African-Americans, and 45% of the patients were diabetic. Table 20–4 shows selected treatment characteristics during the follow-up period of study for each intervention group. Duration of treatment, blood flow rate, and all parameters related to urea clearance or removal were greater

Table 20–4 Characteristics of Treatments During HEMO Study Follow-Up (Values are Mean ± SD)

Treatment Variable	Standard Dose Group	High-Dose Group	Low-Flux Group	High-Flux Group
Duration of dialysis (min)	190 ± 23	219 ± 23	206 ± 28	203 ± 27
Blood flow rate (mL/min)	311 ± 51	375 ± 32	344 ± 53	341 ± 54
Urea clearance (mL/min)	218 ± 25	251 ± 18	233 ± 27	236 ± 28
spKt/V	1.32 ± 0.09	1.71 ± 0.11	1.51 ± 0.22	1.52 ± 0.22
eKt/V	1.16 ± 0.08	1.53 ± 0.09	1.34 ± 0.21	1.34 ± 0.21
Urea reduction ratio (%)	66.3 ± 2.5	75.2 ± 2.5	70.6 ± 5.1	70.9 ± 5.1
β_2-microglobulin clearance (mL/min)	18.9 ± 19.0	18.3 ± 16.8	3.4 ± 7.2	33.8 ± 11.4

in the high dose than in the standard dose group. Dialyzer clearance of β_2-microglobulin was higher in the high-flux than in the low-flux group. There were no differences in urea clearance parameters in the flux groups or β_2-microglobulin clearances in the dose groups.

Table 20–5 shows the primary analyses of mortality.[145] Patient mortality was lower for younger patients, females than males, African-Americans than all other races, nondiabetics than diabetics, patients who had been treated for shorter periods before the enrollment into the study, patients with higher serum albumin levels, and patients with lower comorbidity (ICED) scores. These results were similar to those expected from prior studies. In contrast, neither the dose intervention nor the flux intervention had a significant effect on all-cause mortality. Kaplan-Meier survival curves for the dose and flux interventions are shown in Figures 20–5 and 20–6, respectively. The 95% confidence intervals were relatively large, suggesting that either intervention may have had an effect on mortality, but the size of the effect was too small to be detected in a trial of this size. Of interest, however, the effect of the flux intervention on two main secondary outcomes, death due to cardiac causes and first hospitalization or death due to cardiac causes, showed a statistically significant reduction in risk of 20% ($P = .04$) and 13% ($P = .05$), respectively.[145,146]

The results for interactions of the treatment interventions with seven of the prespecified baseline characteristics are shown in Tables 20–6 and 20–7 for the dose and flux interventions on the primary outcome, respectively. The interaction of the dose intervention with gender was significant ($P = .014$), only before considering the Bonferroni correction for multiple comparisons, however. Women randomized to the high dose group had a lower mortality rate than women randomized to the standard dose group (relative risk or RR = 0.81, $P = .02$), whereas men randomized to the high dose group had a nonsignificant trend for a higher mortality rate than men randomized to the standard dose group (RR = 1.16, $P = .16$). Although mean body sizes were different between men than women, the RR of mortality for the high vs. standard dose groups remained lower in women than in men after adjustment for the modeled urea volume or with other size parameters, including body weight and body-mass index. The interaction of the dose intervention with race was of borderline significance ($P = .06$); thus, race will need further consideration in additional analyses. Indeed, it appeared that the effect of gender was predominantly driven by the greater response to the higher dose in non–African-American females than in African-American females. Further details of these analyses have been recently reported.[147] No other interaction within the dose intervention for the primary outcome (all-cause mortality) was significant. It is important to emphasize that there was no interaction of dose with age, diabetes, or comorbidity, as suggested in certain previous studies.[15]

The interaction of the flux intervention and pre-study years on dialysis was statistically significant ($P = .005$), even after considering the Bonferroni correction for multiple comparisons. Thus, patients who had been previously treated for more than 3.7 years and were randomized to the high-flux group had a lower mortality rate than such patients randomized to the low-flux group (RR = 0.68, $P = .001$). In contrast, in patients who had been previously treated for less than 3.7 years and were randomized to high-flux hemodialysis had a nonsignificant trend for a higher mortality rate than those randomized to the low-flux hemodialysis (RR = 1.05, $P = .55$). Further analyses of these data did not find a difference in the effect of high-flux hemodialysis on mortality between patients with less than 0.24 mL/min versus greater than 0.24 mL/min of residual renal clearance. It should be noted, however, that more than half of the patients entering the HEMO Study had no residual renal clearance.[145] Thus, it does not follow that these outcomes can be explained by differences in residual renal clearances. Finally, it should be pointed out that the effect of

Table 20–5 Primary Cox Regression Analysis of All-Cause Mortality in the HEMO Study

Predictor Variable	Relative Risk of Death (95% CI)	P Value
High dose	0.96 (0.84-1.10)	.53
High flux membrane	0.92 (0.81-1.05)	.23
Age (per 10-year increase)	1.41 (1.33-1.50)	<.001
Female gender	0.85 (0.73-0.98)	.02
Black race	0.77 (0.55-0.91)	.002
Diabetes	1.29 (1.11-1.50)	.001
Pre-study years on dialysis (per 1-year increase)	1.04 (1.02-1.06)	<.001
Baseline ICED score (per 1-unit increase)	1.37 (1.25-1.50)	<.001
Baseline serum albumin (per 0.5 g/dL increase)	0.51 (0.43-0.62)	<.001

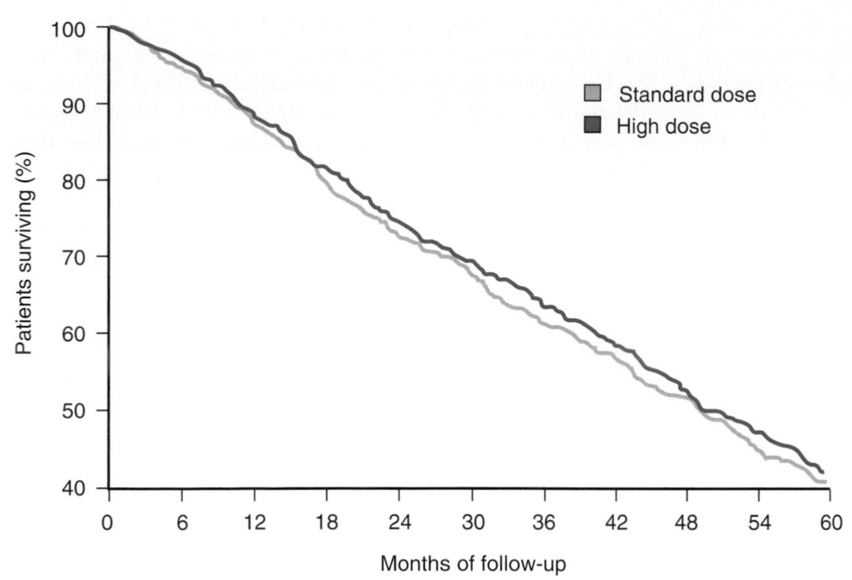

No. at risk										
Standard dose	854	759	630	524	451	382	315	253	197	149
High dose	857	753	637	538	470	399	327	266	219	166

Figure 20–5 Kaplan-Meier survival curves for the dose intervention in the HEMO Study. The curves are adjusted for the prespecified baseline factors. Mortality in the high-dose group was 4% lower (P = .53) than that in the standard dose group.

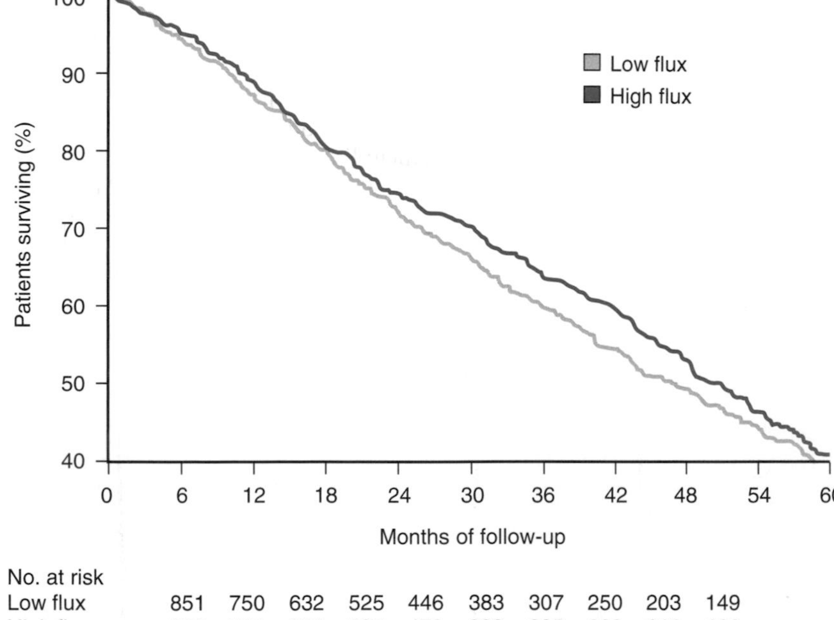

No. at risk										
Low flux	851	750	632	525	446	383	307	250	203	149
High flux	860	761	635	537	473	399	335	269	212	160

Figure 20–6 Kaplan-Meier survival curves for the flux intervention in the HEMO Study. The curves are adjusted for the prespecified baseline factors. Mortality in the high-flux group was 8% lower (P = .23) than that in the low-flux group.

high flux hemodialysis on patient mortality was considerably weakened when the years on dialysis during the follow-up phase were combined with the pre-study years of dialysis in those analyses. Further details of these analyses have been recently reported.[146] No other interaction with the flux intervention in the primary analysis was statistically significant.

FUTURE TRENDS

The findings from the HEMO Study that increasing the dose of small solute removal or the use of high-flux membranes during thrice-weekly hemodialysis therapy is unlikely to produce improved patient outcomes provides numerous challenges to the dialysis community. Two of these major challenges, discussed later, are: (1) the effect of the HEMO Study results on current treatment guidelines and (2) the importance of using and developing new markers for assessing hemodialysis adequacy for treatment schedules other than thrice weekly.

Although it is not the purpose of this review to propose new treatment recommendations, a major challenge to the dialysis community is whether current practice guidelines for hemodialysis should be altered, based on the results from the HEMO Study. One could argue that there is justification for keeping these guidelines unaltered, based on the primary outcome of that study. If, however, one considers the possibility that the study was underpowered to perform analyses on various subgroups of patients, then it may be appropriate to revisit several aspects of the guidelines.

Let us examine a few such considerations. The K/DOQI 2000 Guidelines recommend that spKt/V be used to guide the dose of small solute removal. Because the HEMO Study used eKt/V dosing parameter to guide therapy, however, one could argue that eKt/V should be used to monitor therapy. This is not necessarily the case, as illustrated in Tables 20–8 and 20–9. Table 20–8 compares the relationship between spKt/V and eKt/V for the standard dose group in the HEMO Study, using the new rate equation developed in that study, as described previously.[96] Remember that mean achieved spKt/V and eK/V values in the standard dose group were 1.32 and 1.16, respectively (Table 20–4). If a target value for spKt/V is chosen as 1.32, for example, then only some of the patients would receive an eKt/V of 1.16 or greater, depending on treatment time. On the contrary, if instead a target spKt/V of 1.4 is chosen, then virtually all patients treated for greater than 2.5 hours would achieve an eKt/V of 1.16 or greater. Thus, an alternative strategy for achieving at least an eKt/V of 1.16 is to deliver a spKt/V of 1.4, unless treatment time is less than 2.5 hours. Since 2.5 hours was the minimum allowed during the HEMO Study, this would seem to also be an acceptable approach for achieving a minimum delivered dose of small solute removal. Indeed, this dose target for small solute removal is equivalent to that recommended by the European Best Practice Guidelines for Hemodialysis.[148] Similar considerations suggest that a spKt/V of 1.8 could be used to deliver a dose of small solute removal equivalent to that in the high dose group of the HEMO Study (Table 20–9).

Considering recent evidence discussed earlier regarding the effect of body size, gender, and membrane flux on patient outcome, one can also argue that patients of low body weight (or body mass index) and females should be treated with a dose of small solute removal higher than that delivered to the standard dose group of the HEMO Study. Since the evidence for these effects are only suggestive from a statistical perspective, it can be argued that the data do not support such a recommendation. To err on the conservative side, however, that is, to do no harm to the patient, delivering a higher dose to such

Table 20–6 Effects of Seven Prespecified Baseline Factors on the Response to High Dose (All-Cause Mortality)

Factor	Subgroup	Relative Risk (95% CI)	P Value for Interaction
Age	=58 years	0.95 (0.74-1.12)	.92
	>58 years	0.97 (0.82-1.13)	
Gender	Men	1.16 (0.94-1.43)	.014
	Women	0.81 (0.68-0.97)	
Race	Non-black	1.13 (0.91-1.39)	.06
	Black	0.87 (0.73-1.03)	
Diabetes	Nondiabetic	0.90 (0.74-1.09)	.35
	Diabetic	1.02 (0.85-1.22)	
Pre-study years of dialysis	=3.7 years	1.03 (0.88-1.22)	.12
	>3.7 years	0.83 (0.66-1.04)	
ICED Score	=2	0.92 (0.70-1.22)	.96
	>2	0.93 (0.76-1.15)	
Serum albumin	=3.6 g/dL	0.89 (0.75-1.06)	.16
	>3.6 g/dL	1.08 (0.88-1.32)	

Table 20–7 Effects of Seven Prespecified Baseline Factors on the Response to High Flux (All-Cause Mortality)

Factor	Subgroup	Relative Risk (95% CI)	P Value for Interaction
Age	=58 years	0.98 (0.76-1.26)	.26
	>58 years	0.92 (0.79-1.08)	
Gender	Men	1.03 (0.84-1.26)	.27
	Women	0.88 (0.74-1.06)	
Race	Non-black	1.04 (0.84-1.28)	.24
	Black	0.88 (0.74-1.04)	
Diabetes	Nondiabetic	0.95 (0.78-1.15)	.87
	Diabetic	0.93 (0.77-1.11)	
Pre-study years of dialysis	=3.7 years	1.05 (0.89-1.24)	.005
	>3.7 years	0.68 (0.53-0.86)	
ICED Score	=2	0.95 (0.72-1.24)	.94
	>2	0.93 (0.76-1.09)	
Serum albumin	=3.6 g/dL	0.91 (0.76-1.09)	.65
	>3.6 g/dL	0.97 (0.79-1.19)	

Table 20–8 Effect of Treatment Time on the Relationship Between spKt/V and eKt/V for HEMO Study Standard Dose Group

spKt/V	Treatment Time (Hrs)	eKt/V
1.32	2.0	1.06
1.32	2.5	1.11
1.32	3.0	1.15
1.32	3.5	1.17
1.32	4.0	1.19
1.32	4.5	1.21
1.40	2.0	1.13
1.40	2.5	1.18
1.40	3.0	1.22
1.40	3.5	1.24
1.40	4.0	1.26
1.40	4.5	1.28

Table 20–9 Effect of Treatment Time on the Relationship Between spKt/V and eKt/V for HEMO Study High Dose Group

spKt/V	Treatment Time (Hrs)	eKt/V
1.71	2.0	1.38
1.71	2.5	1.44
1.71	3.0	1.49
1.71	3.5	1.52
1.71	4.0	1.54
1.71	4.5	1.56
1.80	2.0	1.45
1.80	2.5	1.52
1.80	3.0	1.57
1.80	3.5	1.56
1.80	4.0	1.58
1.80	4.5	1.60

patients would appear prudent. Similar reasoning holds when considering whether to employ high-flux hemodialysis. The data in this case are stronger and appear to support the use of high-flux hemodialysis therapy, especially for patients who have been treated for some time on hemodialysis. Others have even suggested that these data support the use of even higher-flux membranes or the use of adsorption devices to remove other middle molecules. These suggestions require further study.

The HEMO Study has expanded the definition of hemodialysis adequacy as described by the K/DOQI Guidelines to include the consideration of the dose of middle molecule removal. As other treatment schedules for hemodialysis, such as short daily and nocturnal, are increasingly being considered, one must question whether treatment adequacy can be defined only by considering the dose of small solute and middle molecule removal. The previous discussion regarding the EUTox categorizations of uremic toxins suggests that consideration of protein-bound uremic toxins may also be necessary in such definitions. Indeed, recent work suggests that clearances of protein-bound solutes are greater during daily hemodialysis than during thrice-weekly hemodialysis.[149] Alternatively, the use of other dose parameters, such as the standard urea Kt/V parameter defined by Gotch[150] and its relationship to protein-bound uremic toxin removal, are of high interest. The definition of treatment adequacy for dialysis patients remains the most significant challenge to the dialysis community, as long as dialysis remains far less efficient than the native kidneys.

References

1. Owen WF, Madore F, Brenner BM: An observational study of cardiovascular characteristics of long-term end-stage renal disease survivors. Am J Kidney Dis 1996; 8:931-936.
2. Scribner BH: Forward to the fourth edition. *In* Jacobs C, Kjellstrand CM, Koch KM (eds): Replacement of Renal Function by Dialysis. Dordrecht, Kluwer Academic, 1996, p v-vi.
3. US Renal Data System: Excerpts from the USRDS 2003 Annual Data Report: Atlas of end-stage renal disease in the United States. Am J Kidney Dis 2003; 42(suppl 5):S1-S230.
4. Vanholder R, De Smet R, Glorieux G, et al: The European Uremic Toxin Work Group (EUTox): Review on uremic toxins: Classification, concentration, and interindividual variability. Kidney Int 2003; 63:1934-1943.
5. Eschbach JW, Adamson JW: Anemia of end-stage renal disease (ESRD). Kidney Int 1985; 28:1-5.
6. Mawer EB, Taylor CM, Backhouse J, et al: Failure of formation of 1,25-dihydroxycholecalciferol in chronic renal insufficiency. Lancet 1973; 1:626-628.
7. Mahajan SK: Zinc metabolism in uremia. Int J Artif Organs 1988; 11:223-228.
8. Golper TA, Ahmad S: L-carnitine administration to hemodialysis patients: Has its time come? Semin Dial 1992; 5:94-98.
9. Hull AR: Predictors of the excessive mortality rates of dialysis patients in the United States. Curr Opin Nephrol Hypertens 1994; 3:286-291.
10. Santoro A: Confounding factors in the assessment of delivered hemodialysis dose. Kidney Int 2000; 58(suppl 76):S19-S27.
11. Lowrie EG, Laird NM, Parker TF, Sargent JA: Effect of the hemodialysis prescription of patient morbidity: Report from the National Cooperative Dialysis Study. N Engl J Med 1981; 305:1176-1181.
12. The National Cooperative Dialysis Study. Kidney Int 1983; 23(suppl 13):S1-S122.
13. Lowrie EG, Lew NL: Death risk in hemodialysis patients: The predictive value of commonly measured variables and an evaluation of death rate differences between facilities. Am J Kidney Dis 1990; 15:458-482.
14. Acchiardo SR, Hatten KW, Ruvinsky MJ, et al: Inadequate dialysis increases gross mortality rate. ASAIO J 1992; 38:M282-M285.
15. Collins AJ, Ma JZ, Umen A, Keshaviah P: Urea index and other predictors of hemodialysis patient survival. Am J Kidney Dis 1994; 23:272-282.
16. Hakim RM, Breyer J, Ismail N, Schulman G: Effects of dose of dialysis on morbidity and mortality. Am J Kidney Dis 1994; 23:661-669.
17. Lowrie EG: Chronic dialysis treatment: Clinical outcome and related processes of care. Am J Kidney Dis 1994; 24:255-266.
18. Parker TF III, Husni L, Huang W, et al: Survival of hemodialysis patients in the United States is improved with a greater quantity of dialysis. Am J Kidney Dis 1994; 23:670-680.
19. Held PJ, Port FK, Wolfe RA, et al: The dose of hemodialysis and patient mortality. Kidney Int 1996; 50:550-556.
20. Vanholder R, De Smet R, Lesaffer G: P-Cresol: A toxin revealing many neglected but relevant aspects of uraemic toxicity. Nephrol Dial Transplant 1999; 19:2813-2815.
21. Lesaffer G, De Smet R, Lamiere N, et al: Intradialytic removal of protein-bound toxins: Role of solute characteristics and of dialyzer membrane. Nephrol Dial Transplant 2000; 15:50-57.
22. Tenkhoff H, Shilipetan G, Boen ST: One year's experience with home peritoneal dialysis. Trans Am Soc Artif Intern Organs 1965; 11:11-14.
23. Tenkhoff H, Curtis FK: Experience with maintenance peritoneal dialysis in the home. Trans Am Soc Artif Intern Organs 1970; 16: 90-99.
24. Scribner BH: Discussion. Trans Am Soc Artif Intern Organs 1965; 11:29.
25. Babb AL, Popovich RP, Christopher TG, Scribner BH: The genesis of the square meter-hour hypothesis. Trans Am Soc Artif Intern Organs 1971; 17:81-91.
26. Babb AL, Strand MJ, Uvelli DA, et al: Quantitative description of dialysis treatment: A dialysis index. Kidney Int Suppl 1975; 2: 23-29.
27. Gotch FA, Sargent JA, Peters JH: Studies on the molecular etiology of uremia. Kidney Int Suppl 1975; 3:276-279.
28. Lowrie EG, Steinberg SM, Galen MA, det al: Factors in the dialysis regimen which contribute to alterations in the abnormalities of uremia. Kidney Int 1976; 10:409-422.
29. van Ypersele de Strihou C, Jadoul M, Malghem J, et al: Effect of dialysis membrane and patient's age on signs of dialysis-related amyloidosis. The Working Party on Dialysis Amyloidosis. Kidney Int 1991; 39:1012-1019.
30. Koch KM: Dialysis-related amyloidosis. Kidney Int 1992; 41: 1416-1429.
31. Floege J, Ketteler M: β_2-microglobulin-derived amyloidosis: An update. Kidney Int 2001; 59(suppl 78):S164-S171.
32. Attman PO, Alaupovic P: Lipid abnormalities in chronic renal insufficiency. Kidney Int Suppl 1991; 31:S16-S23.
33. Seres DS, Strain GW, Hashim SA, et al: Improvement of plasma lipoprotein profiles during high-flux dialysis. J Am Soc Nephrol 1993; 3:1409-1415.
34. Wineman RJ: Rationale of the National Cooperative Dialysis Study. Kidney Int 1983; 23(suppl 13):S8-S10.
35. Lowrie EG, Laird NM, Henry RR: Protocol for the National Cooperative Dialysis Study. Kidney Int Suppl 1983; 13:S11-S18.
36. Sargent JA: Control of dialysis by a single-pool urea model: The National Cooperative Dialysis Study. Kidney Int Suppl 1983; 13: S19-S25.
37. Parker TF, Laird NM, Lowrie EG: Comparison of the study groups in the National Cooperative Dialysis Study and a description of morbidity, mortality, and patient withdrawal. Kidney Int Suppl 1983; 13:S42-S49.

38. Harter HR: Review of significant findings from the National Cooperative Dialysis Study and recommendations. Kidney Int Suppl 1983; 13:S107-S112.
39. Laird NM, Berkey CS, Lowrie EG: Modeling success or failure of dialysis therapy: The National Cooperative Dialysis Study. Kidney Int Suppl 1983; 13:S101-S106.
40. Gotch FA: Kinetic modeling in hemodialysis. *In* Nissenson AR, Fine RN, Gentile DE (eds): Clinical Dialysis. Norwalk, CT, Appleton & Lange, 1995, pp 156-188.
41. Gotch FA, Sargent JA: A mechanistic analysis of the National Cooperative Dialysis Study (NCDS). Kidney Int 1985; 28:526-534.
42. US Renal Data System, USRDS 1998 Annual Data Report. Bethesda, MD, The National Institutes of Health, National Institute of Diabetes and Digestive and Kidney Diseases, 1998.
43. Tokars JI, Frank M, Alter MJ, Arduino MJ: National surveillance of dialysis-associated diseases in the United States, 2000. Semin Dial 2002; 15:162-171.
44. Vanholder R, Van Loo A, Dhondt AM, et al: Second symposium on uraemic toxicity. Summary of a symposium held in Gent, Belgium, 22-24 September 1994. Nephrol Dial Transplant 1995; 10:414-418.
45. Brahm J: Urea permeability of human red cells. J Gen Physiol 1983; 82:1-23.
46. Cheung AK, Alford MF, Wilson MM, et al: Urea movement across erythrocyte membrane during artificial kidney treatment. Kidney Int 1983; 23:866-869.
47. Owen WF Jr, Lew NL, Liu Y, et al: The urea reduction ratio and serum albumin concentration as predictors of mortality in patients undergoing hemodialysis. N Engl J Med 1993; 329:1001-1006.
48. Hume R, Weyers E: Relationship between total body water and surface area in normal and obese subjects. J Clin Pathol 1971; 24: 234-238.
49. Watson PE, Watson ID, Batt RD: Total body water volumes for adult males and females estimated from simple anthropometric measurements. Am J Clin Nutr 1980; 33:27-39.
50. Chertow GM, Lazarus JM, Lew NL, et al: Development of a population-specific regression equation to estimate total body water in hemodialysis patients. Kidney Int 1997; 51:1578-1582.
51. Daugirdas JT, Greene T, Depner TA, et al: The Hemodialysis (HEMO) Study: Anthropometrically estimated total body water volumes are larger than modeled urea volume in chronic hemodialysis patients: Effects of age, race, and gender. Kidney Int 2003; 64:1108-1119.
52. Sargent J, Gotch F, Borah M, et al: Urea kinetics: A guide to nutritional management of renal failure. Am J Clin Nutr 1978; 31: 1696-1702.
53. Sargent JA, Gotch FA: Mathematic modeling of dialysis therapy. Kidney Int Suppl 1980; 10:S2-S10.
54. Renal Physician's Association: Clinical practice guideline working committee. *In* Clinical Practice Guideline on Adequacy of Hemodialysis. Clinical Practice Guideline, No. 1. Dubuque, IA, Kendall/Hunt, 1996.
55. National Kidney Foundation: K/DOQI Clinical Practice Guidelines for Hemodialysis Adequacy, 2000. Am J Kidney Dis 2001; 37(suppl 1):S7-S64.
56. Flanigan MJ, Lim VS, Redlin J: The significance of protein intake and catabolism. Adv Ren Replace Ther 1995; 2:330-340.
57. Owen WF: Nutritional status and survival in end-stage renal disease patients. Miner Electrolyte Metab 1998; 24:72-81.
58. Keane WF, Collins AJ: Influence of co-morbidity on mortality and morbidity in patients treated with hemodialysis. Am J Kidney Dis 1994; 24:1010-1018.
59. Daugirdas JT: Second generation logarithmic estimates of single-pool variable volume Kt/V: An analysis of error. J Am Soc Nephrol 1993; 4:1205-1213.
60. Lowrie EG, Lew NL: The urea reduction ratio (URR): A simple method for evaluating hemodialysis treatment. Contemp Dial Nephrol 1991; 1:11-19.
61. Daugirdas JT: Rapid methods of estimating Kt/V: Three formulas compared. ASAIO Trans 1990; 36:M362-M364.
62. Flanigan MJ, Fangman J, Lim VS: Quantitating hemodialysis: A comparison of three kinetic models. Am J Kidney Dis 1991; 17: 295-302.
63. Daugirdas JT: Simplified equations for monitoring Kt/V, PCRn, eKt/V, and ePCRn. Adv Ren Replace Ther 1995; 2:295-304.
64. Depner TA: Estimation of Kt/V from the urea reduction ratio for varying levels of dialytic weight loss: A bedside graphic aid. Semin Dial 1993; 6:242.
65. Sherman RA, Cody RP, Rogers ME, Solanchick JC: Accuracy of the urea reduction ratio in predicting dialysis delivery. Kidney Int 1995; 47:319-321.
66. Basile C, Casino F, Lopez T: Percent reduction in blood urea concentration during dialysis estimates Kt/V in a simple and accurate way. Am J Kidney Dis 1990; 15:40-45.
67. Jindal KK, Manuel A, Goldstein MB: Percent reduction in blood urea concentration during hemodialysis (PRU). A simple and accurate method to estimate Kt/V urea. ASAIO Trans 1987; 33: 286-288.
68. Daugirdas JT: Linear estimates of variable-volume, single-pool Kt/V: An analysis of error. Am J Kidney Dis 1993; 22:267-270.
69. Garred LJ: Dialysate-based kinetic modeling. Adv Ren Replace Ther 1995; 2:305-318.
70. Bankhead MM, Toto RD, Star RA: Accuracy of urea removal estimated by kinetic models. Kidney Int 1995; 48:785-793.
71. Depner TA, Greene T, Gotch FA, et al: The Hemodialysis Study Group: Imprecision of the hemodialysis dose when measured directly from urea removal. Kidney Int 1999; 55:635-647.
72. Ing TS, Yu AW, Wong FK, et al: Collection of a representative fraction of total spent hemodialysate. Am J Kidney Dis 1995; 25: 810-812.
73. Raj DS, Tobe S, Saiphoo C, Manuel MA: Quantitating dialysis using two dialysate samples: A simple, practical and accurate approach for evaluating urea kinetics. Int J Artif Organs 1997; 20: 422-427.
74. Depner TA, Keshaviah PR, Ebben JP, et al: Multicenter clinical validation of an on-line monitor of dialysis adequacy. J Am Soc Nephrol 1996; 7:464-471.
75. Del Vecchio L, Di Filippo S, Andrulli S, et al: Conductivity: On-line monitoring of dialysis adequacy. Int J Artif Organs 1998; 21: 521-525.
76. Di Filippo S, Andrulli S, Manzoni C, et al: On-line assessment of delivered dialysis dose. Kidney Int 1998; 54:263-267.
77. Di Filippo S, Manzoni C, Andrulli S, et al: How to determine ionic dialysance for the online assessment of delivered dialysis dose. Kidney Int 2001; 59:774-782.
78. Kuhlmann U, Goldau R, Samadi N, et al: Accuracy and safety of online clearance monitoring based on conductivity variation. Nephrol Dial Transplant 2001; 16:1053-1058.
79. McIntyre CW, Lambie SH, Taal MW, Fluck RJ: Assessment of hemodialysis adequacy by ionic dialysance: Intra-patient variability of delivered treatment. Nephrol Dial Transplant 2003; 18: 559-562.
80. Schneditz D, Van Stone JC, Daugirdas JT: A regional blood circulation alternative to in-series two compartment urea kinetic modeling. ASAIO J 1993; 29:M573-M577.
81. Daugirdas JT, Schneditz D: Overestimation of hemodialysis dose depends on dialysis efficiency by regional blood flow but not by conventional two pool urea kinetic analysis. ASAIO J 1995; 41: M719-M724.
82. Heineken FG, Evans MC, Keen ML, Gotch FA: Intercompartmental fluid shifts in hemodialysis patients. Biotechnol Progr 1987; 3:69-73.
83. Cappello A, Grandi F, Lamberti C, Santoro A: Comparative evaluation of different methods to estimate urea distribution volume and generation rate. Int J Artif Organs 1994; 17:322-330.
84. Daugirdas JT: Bedside formulas for Kt/V. A kinder, gentler approach to urea kinetic modeling. ASAIO Trans 1989; 35:336-338.

85. Smye SW, Evans JH, Will E, Brocklebank JT: Paediatric haemodialysis: Estimation of treatment efficiency in the presence of urea rebound. Clin Phys Physiol Meas 1992; 13:51-62.
86. Abramson F, Gibson S, Barlee V, Bosch JP: Urea kinetic modeling at high urea clearances: Implications for clinical practice. Adv Ren Replace Ther 1994; 1:5-14.
87. Leblanc M, Charbonneau R, Lalumiere G, et al: Postdialysis urea rebound: Determinants and influence on dialysis delivery in chronic hemodialysis patients. Am J Kidney Dis 1996; 27:253-261.
88. Kaufman AM, Schneditz D, Smye S, et al: Solute disequilibrium and multicompartment modeling. Adv Ren Replace Ther 1995; 2:319-329.
89. Daugirdas JT: Estimation of equilibrated Kt/V using unequilibrated postdialysis BUN. Semin Dial 1995; 8:283-284.
90. George TO, Priester-Coary A, Dunea G, et al: Cardiac output and urea kinetics in dialysis patients: Evidence supporting the regional blood flow model. Kidney Int 1996; 50:1273-1277.
91. Spiegel DM, Baker PL, Babcock S, et al: Hemodialysis urea rebound: The effect of increasing dialysis efficiency. Am J Kidney Dis 1995; 25:26-29.
92. Stegeman CA, Huisman RM, de Rouw B, et al: Determination of protein catabolic rate in patients on chronic intermittent hemodialysis: Urea output measurements compared with dietary protein intake and with calculation of urea generation rate. Am J Kidney Dis 1995; 25:887-895.
93. Tattersall JE, DeTakats D, Chamney P, et al: The post-hemodialysis rebound: Predicting and quantifying its effect on Kt/V. Kidney Int 1996; 50:2094-2102.
94. Smye SW, Tattersall JE, Will EJ: Modeling the postdialysis rebound: The reconciliation of current formulas. ASAIO J 1999; 45:562-567.
95. Daugirdas JT, Depner TA, Gotch FA, et al: Comparison of methods to predict equilibrated Kt/V in the HEMO Pilot Study. Kidney Int 1997; 52:1395-1405.
96. Daugirdas JT, Greene T, Depner TA, et al: Factors affecting postdialysis rebound in serum urea concentrations, including the rate of dialysis: Results from the HEMO Study. J Am Soc Nephrol 2004; 15:194-203.
97. Sherman RA, Levy SS: Rate-related recirculation: The effect of altering blood flow on dialyzer recirculation. Am J Kidney Dis 1991; 17:170-173.
98. Tattersall JE, Chamney P, Aldridge C, Greenwood RN: Recirculation and the postdialysis rebound. Nephrol Dial Transplant 1996; 11(suppl 2):75-80.
99. Schneditz D, Kaufman AM, Polaschegg HD, et al: Cardiopulmonary recirculation during hemodialysis. Kidney Int 1992; 42:1450-1456.
100. Depner TA, Rizwan S, Cheer AY, et al: High venous urea concentrations in the opposite arm: A consequence of hemodialysis-induced compartment disequilibrium. ASAIO Trans 1991; 37:M141-M143.
101. Owen WF Jr, Meyer KB, Schmidt G, Alfred H: Methodological limitations of the ESRD Core Indicators Project: An ESRD network's experience with implementing an ESRD quality survey. Medical Review Board of the ESRD Network of New England. Am J Kidney Dis 1997; 30:349-355.
102. Depner TA, Cheer A: Modeling urea kinetics with two vs. three BUN measurements. A critical comparison. ASAIO Trans 1989; 35:499-502.
103. Lai YH, Guh JY, Chen HC, Tsai JH: Effects of different sampling methods for measurement of post dialysis blood urea nitrogen on urea kinetic modeling derived parameters in patients undergoing long-term hemodialysis. ASAIO J 1995; 41:211-215.
104. Sherman RA, Matera JJ, Novik L, Cody RP: Recirculation reassessed: The impact of blood flow rate and the low-flow method reevaluated. Am J Kidney Dis 1994; 23:846-848.
105. Daugirdas JT, Burke MS, Balter P, et al: Screening for extreme postdialysis urea rebound using the Smye method: Patients with access recirculation identified when a slow flow method is not used to draw the postdialysis blood. Am J Kidney Dis 1996; 28: 727-731.
106. Saha LK, Van Stone JC: Differences between KT/V measured during dialysis and KT/V predicted from manufacturer clearance data. Int J Artif Organs 1992; 15:465-469.
107. Hornberger JC: The hemodialysis prescription and quality-adjusted life expectancy. Renal Physicians Association Working Committee on Clinical Guidelines. J Am Soc Nephrol 1993; 4: 1004-1020.
108. Beto JA, Bansal VK, Ing TS, Daugirdas JT: Variation in blood sample collection for determination of hemodialysis adequacy. Council on Renal Nutrition National Research Question Collaborative Study Group. Am J Kidney Dis 1998; 31:135-141.
109. Hornberger JC: The hemodialysis prescription and cost effectiveness. Renal Physicians Association Working Committee on Clinical Guidelines. J Am Soc Nephrol 1993; 4:1021-1027.
110. Lindsay RM, Henderson LW: Adequacy of dialysis. Kidney Int Suppl 1988; 24:S92-S99.
111. Gotch FA, Levin NW, Port FK, et al: Clinical outcome relative to the dose of dialysis is not what you think: The fallacy of the mean. Am J Kidney Dis 1997; 30:1-15.
112. Delmez JA, Windus DW: Hemodialysis prescription and delivery in a metropolitan community. The St. Louis Nephrology Study Group. Kidney Int 1992; 41:1023-1028.
113. Sargent JA: Shortfalls in the delivery of dialysis. Am J Kidney Dis 1990; 15:500-510.
114. LeFebvre JM, Spanner E, Heidenheim AP, Lindsay RM: Kt/V: Patients do not get what the physician prescribes. ASAIO Trans 1991; 37:M132-M133.
115. Sehgal AR, Snow RJ, Singer ME, et al: Barriers to adequate delivery of hemodialysis. Am J Kidney Dis 1998; 31:593-601.
116. Sherman RA, Cody RP, Solanchick JC: Racial differences in the delivery of hemodialysis. Am J Kidney Dis 1993; 21:632-634.
117. Price DA, Owen WF Jr: African-Americans on maintenance dialysis: A review of racial differences in incidence, treatment, and survival. Adv Ren Replace Ther 1997; 4:3-12.
118. Owen WF Jr, Chertow GM, Lazarus JM, Lowrie EG: Dose of hemodialysis and survival: Differences by race and sex. JAMA 1998; 280:1764-1768.
119. Goldwasser P, Mittman N, Antignani A, et al: Predictors of mortality in hemodialysis patients. J Am Soc Nephrol 1993; 3:1613-1622.
120. McClellan WM, Soucie JM, Flanders WD: Mortality in end-stage renal disease is associated with facility-to-facility differences in adequacy of hemodialysis. J Am Soc Nephrol 1998; 9: 1940-1947.
121. Kopple JD, Zhu X, Lew NL, Lowrie EG: Body weight-for-height relationships predict mortality in maintenance hemodialysis patients. Kidney Int 1999; 56:1136-1148.
122. Chertow GM, Owen WF, Lazarus JM, et al: Exploring the reverse J-shaped curve between urea reduction ratio and mortality. Kidney Int 1999; 56:1872-1878.
123. Capelli JP, Kushner H, Camiscioli T, et al: Factors affecting survival of hemodialysis patients utilizing urea kinetic modeling. A critical appraisal of shortening dialysis times. Am J Nephrol 1992; 12:212-223.
124. Wolfe RA, Ashby VB, Daugirdas JT, et al: Body size, dose of hemodialysis, and mortality. Am J Kidney Dis 2000; 35:80-88.
125. Lowrie EG, Chertow GM, Lew NL, et al: The urea (clearance × dialysis time) product (Kt) as an outcome-based measure of hemodialysis dose. Kidney Int 1999; 56:729-737.
126. Lowrie EG, Li Z, Ofsthun N, Lazarus JM: Body size, dialysis dose and death risk relationships among hemodialysis patients. Kidney Int 2002; 62:1891-1897.
127. O'Conner AS, Leon JB, Sehgal AR: The relative predictive ability of four different measures of hemodialysis dose. Am J Kidney Dis 2002; 40:1289-1294.

128. Held PJ, Levin NW, Bovbjerg RR, et al: Mortality and duration of hemodialysis treatment. JAMA 1991; 265:871-875.
129. Charra B, Calemard E, Ruffet M, et al: Survival as an index of adequacy of dialysis. Kidney Int 1992; 41:1286-1291.
130. Charra B, Calemard M, Laurent G: Importance of treatment time and blood pressure control in achieving long-term survival on dialysis. Am J Nephrol 1996; 16:35-44.
131. Rozich JD, Smith B, Thomas JD, et al: Dialysis-induced alterations in left ventricular filling: Mechanisms and clinical significance. Am J Kidney Dis 1991; 17:277-285.
132. Skroeder NR, Jacobson SH, Lins LE, Kjellstrand CM: Acute symptoms during and between hemodialysis: The relative role of speed, duration, and biocompatibility of dialysis. Artif Organs 1994; 18:880-887.
133. Rocco MV, Burkart JM: Prevalence of missed treatments and early sign-offs in hemodialysis patients. J Am Soc Nephrol 1993; 4:1178-1183.
134. Kinet JP, Soyeur D, Balland N, et al: Hemodynamic study of hypotension during hemodialysis. Kidney Int 1982; 21:868-876.
135. Jahn H, Schohn D, Schmitt R: Hemodynamic modifications induced by fluid removal and treatment modalities in chronic hemodialysis patients. Blood Purif 1983; 1:80-89.
136. de Vries JP, Kouw PM, van der Meer NJ, et al: Non-invasive monitoring of blood volume during hemodialysis: Its relation with post-dialytic dry weight. Kidney Int 1993; 44:851-854.
137. De Vries JP, Bogaard HJ, Kouw PM, et al: The adjustment of post dialytic dry weight based on non-invasive measurement of extracellular fluid and blood volumes. ASAIO J 1993; 39:M368-M372.
138. Fishbane S, Natke E, Maesaka JK: Role of volume overload in dialysis-refractory hypertension. Am J Kidney Dis 1996; 28: 257-261.
139. Sulkova S, Valek A: Role of antihypertensive drugs in the therapy of patients on regular dialysis treatment. Kidney Int Suppl 1988; 25:S198-S200.
140. Leypoldt JK, Cheung AK, Carroll CE, et al: Effect of dialysis membranes and middle molecule removal on chronic hemodialysis patient survival. Am J Kidney Dis 1999; 33:349-355.
141. Leypoldt JK, Cheung AK, Deeter RB: Single compartment models for evaluating β_2-microglobulin clearance during hemodialysis. ASAIO J 1997; 43:904-909.
142. Cheung AK, Agodoa LY, Daugirdas JT, et al: Effects of hemodialyzer reuse on clearances of urea and β_2-microglobulin. The Hemodialysis (HEMO) Study Group. J Am Soc Nephrol 1999; 10:117-127.
143. Leypoldt JK, Cheung AK, Deeter RB: Rebound kinetics of β_2-microglobulin after hemodialysis. Kidney Int 1999; 56: 1571-1577.
144. Eknoyan G, Levey AS, Beck GJ, et al: The HEMO Study Group: The Hemodialysis (HEMO) Study: Rationale for selection of interventions. Semin Dial 1996; 9:24-33.
145. Eknoyan G, Beck GJ, Cheung AK, et al: The Hemodialysis (HEMO) Study Group: Effect of dialysis dose and membrane flux in maintenance hemodialysis. N Engl J Med 2002; 347:2010-2019.
146. Cheung AK, Levin NW, Greene T, et al: Effects of high-flux hemodialysis on clinical outomes: Results of the HEMO Study. J Am Soc Nephrol 2003; 14:3251-3263.
147. Depner T, Daugirdas J, Greene T, et al: The Hemodialysis (HEMO) Study Group: Effect of gender and body size on outcome in the HEMO Study. 2004 (In review).
148. European Best Practice Guidelines for Haemodialysis (Part 1). Nephrol Dial Transplant 2002; 17(suppl 7):1-109.
149. Fagugli RM, De Smet R, Buoncristiani U, et al: Behavior of non-protein bound and protein-bound uremic solute during daily hemodialysis. Am J Kidney Dis 2002; 40:339-347.
150. Gotch FA: The current place of urea kinetic modelling with respect to different dialysis modalities. Nephrol Dial Transplant 1998; 13(suppl 6):10-14.

Chapter 21

Nosocomial Infections in Hemodialysis Units

Jerome Tokars, M.D., M.P.H. • Miriam J. Alter, Ph.D. • Matthew J. Arduino, M.S., Dr.P.H. • Martin S. Favero, Ph.D.

Of the patients with end-stage renal disease (ESRD) treated by maintenance hemodialysis in the United States, 91% are on hemodialysis.[1] Chronic hemodialysis patients are at high risk for infection because the process of hemodialysis requires vascular access for prolonged periods. In an environment where multiple patients receive dialysis concurrently, repeated opportunities exist for person-to-person transmission of infectious agents, directly or indirectly via contaminated devices, equipment and supplies, environmental surfaces, or hands of personnel. Furthermore, hemodialysis patients are immunosuppressed, which increases their susceptibility to infection, and they require frequent hospitalizations and surgery, which increases their opportunities for exposure to nosocomial infections. This chapter describes (1) the major infectious diseases that can be acquired in the dialysis center setting, (2) the important epidemiologic and environmental microbiologic considerations, and (3) infection control strategies.

CONTAMINANTS IN HEMODIALYSIS SYSTEMS

Gram-negative water bacteria are commonly found in water supplies used for hemodialysis. Under certain circumstances, these microorganisms can persist and multiply in aqueous environments associated with hemodialysis equipment. These bacteria can adhere to surfaces and form biofilms (glycocalyces), which are virtually impossible to eradicate.[2–4] Control strategies are designed to not eradicate bacteria but to reduce their concentration to relatively low levels and to prevent their regrowth.

Although certain genera of gram-negative water bacteria (e.g., *Achromobacter, Acinetobacter, Alcaligenes, Aeromonas, Burkholderia, Flavobacterium, Pseudomonas, Ralstonia, Serratia*, and *Xanthomonas*) are most commonly encountered, virtually any bacterium that can grow in water can be a problem in a hemodialysis unit. Several species of nontuberculous mycobacteria may also contaminate water treatment systems, including *Mycobacterium chelonae, M. abscessus, M. fortuitum, M. gordonae, M. mucogenicum* (formerly *MCLO*), *M. scrofulaceum, M. kansaii, M. avium*, and *M. intracellulare*; these microorganisms do not contain bacterial endotoxin but are comparatively resistant to chemical germicides.[5–7]

Gram-negative water bacteria can multiply even in water containing relatively small amounts of organic matter, such as water treated by distillation, softening, deionization, or reverse osmosis, reaching levels of 10^5 to 10^7 microorganisms/mL[8]; these levels are not associated with visible turbidity. When treated water is mixed with dialysis concentrate, the resulting dialysis fluid is a balanced salt solution and growth medium almost as rich in nutrients as conventional nutrient broth.[8,9] Gram-negative water bacteria growing in dialysis fluids can reach levels of 10^8 to 10^9 microorganisms/mL, which produce visible turbidity.

Bacterial growth in water used for hemodialysis depends on the types of water treatment system used, dialysate distribution systems, dialysis machine type, and method of disinfection[5,6,10] (Table 21–1). Each component is discussed separately.

Water Supply

Municipal water may be derived from either surface or ground waters, both of which may be contaminated with bacteria and endotoxin (Table 21–1). Endotoxin is particularly likely to be present in surface waters, is not substantially removed by conventional municipal water treatment processes, and may cause pyrogenic reactions.[11] Disinfectants such as chlorine and combined chlorine (monochloramine) reduce the numbers of but do not eliminate bacteria in municipal water.

Water Treatment Systems

Water used for the production of dialysis fluid must be treated to remove chemical and microbial contaminants. The Association for the Advancement of Medical Instrumentation (AAMI) has published guidelines for the chemical and bacteriologic quality of water used to prepare dialysis fluid (Table 21–2)[12] Some components of the water treatment system may allow amplification of water bacteria. For example, ion exchangers such as water softeners and deionizers do not remove endotoxins or bacteria and provide sites for significant bacterial multiplication.[13] Granular activated carbon adsorption media (i.e., carbon filters) are used to remove certain organic chemicals and available chlorine from water, but they also significantly increase the level of water bacteria and do not remove bacterial endotoxins.

A variety of filters are marketed to control bacterial contamination in water and dialysis fluids. Most are inadequate, especially if they are not routinely disinfected or changed frequently. Particulate filters, commonly called prefilters, operate by depth filtration and do not remove bacteria or bacterial endotoxins. These filters can become colonized with gram-negative water bacteria, resulting in higher levels of bacteria and endotoxin in the filter effluent. Absolute filters, including the membrane types, temporarily remove bacteria from passing water. However, some of these filters tend to clog, and gram-negative water bacteria can "grow through" the filter

Table 21–1 Factors Influencing Microbial Contamination in Hemodialysis Systems

Factors	Comments
Water supply	
Source of community water	
Groundwater	Contains endotoxin and bacteria
Surface water	Contains high levels of endotoxin and bacteria
Water treatment at dialysis center	
None	Not recommended
Filtration	
Prefilter	Particulate filter to protect equipment; does not remove microorganisms
Absolute filter (depth or membrane)	Removes bacteria but, unless changed frequently or disinfected, bacteria will accumulate and grow through filter; acts as significant reservoir of bacteria and endotoxin
Activated carbon filter	Removes organics and available chlorine or chloramine; significant reservoir of water bacteria and endotoxin
Water treatment devices	
Ion-exchange softener, deionization	Softeners and deionizers are significant reservoirs of bacteria and neither remove endotoxin
Reverse osmosis	Removes bacteria and endotoxin, but must be disinfected; operates at high water pressure
Ultraviolet light	Kills some bacteria, but there is no residual, and ultraviolet-resistant bacteria can develop
Ultrafilter	Removes bacteria and endotoxin; operates on normal line pressure; can be positioned distal to deionizer; must be disinfected
Water and dialysate distribution system	
Distribution pipes	
Size	Oversized diameter and length decrease fluid flow and increase bacteria reservoir for both treated water and centrally prepared dialysate
Construction	Rough joints, dead ends, and unused branches can act as bacterial reservoirs
Elevation	Outlet taps should be located at highest elevation to prevent loss of disinfectant
Storage tanks	Undesirable because they act as reservoir of water bacteria; if present, must be routinely scrubbed and disinfected
Dialysis machines	
Single-pass	Disinfectant should have contact with all parts of machine that are exposed to water or dialysis fluid
Recirculating single-pass, or recirculating (batch)	Recirculating pumps and machine design allow for massive contamination levels if not properly disinfected. Overnight chemical germicide treatment recommended.

Table 21–2 Association for the Advancement of Medical Instrumentation (AAMI) Microbiologic and Endotoxin Standards for Dialysis Fluids

Type of Hemodialysis Fluid	Maximum Contaminant Level Total Heterotrophs (CFU/mL)	Maximum Contaminant Level Endotoxin (EU/mL)
Water used to prepare dialysate, rinse dialyzers, or prepare dialyzer disinfectant	200	2
Conventional dialysate	2000/200*	No standard/2†
Ultrapure dialysate	0.1	0.03
Dialysate for infusion	ND‡	0.03

*2000 is the current standard; 200 is the proposed standard.
†There is no current standard for endotoxin; 2 is the proposed standard.
‡Not detectable by routine methods—limit is 1 CFU/1000 L.

matrix and colonize the downstream surface of the filters within a few days. Further, absolute filters do not reduce levels of endotoxin in the effluent water. These types of filters should be changed regularly in accordance with the manufacturer's directions and disinfected in the same manner and at the same time as the dialysis system.

Ultraviolet irradiation is sometimes used to reduce bacterial contamination in water, but this approach is not recommended.[8] Certain populations of gram-negative water bacteria are far more resistant to and may survive ultraviolet radiation. In recirculating dialysis systems, repeated exposures to ultraviolet radiation are used to ensure adequate disinfection; however, this approach allows progressive removal of sensitive microorganisms and multiplication of ultraviolet-resistant microorganisms. In addition, bacterial endotoxins are not affected.

Reverse osmosis is an effective water treatment modality that is used in 97% of U.S. hemodialysis units.[14] Reverse osmosis possesses the singular advantage of being able to remove both bacterial endotoxins and bacteria from supply water. However, low numbers of gram-negative and nontuberculous mycobacteria water bacteria can either penetrate this barrier or, by other means, colonize the downstream portion of the reverse osmosis unit. Consequently, reverse osmosis systems must be disinfected routinely.

We recommend a water treatment system that produces chemically adequate water while avoiding high levels of microbial contamination. The components in the following sequence are well suited for treatment of hard water[15]: (1) a set of prefilters, (2) a softener, (3) carbon adsorption tanks (at least two in series are recommended), (4) a particulate filter, (5) a reverse osmosis unit, (6) a deionization unit, and (7) an ultrafilter. As the water passes through these components, it becomes progressively more pure chemically, but the level of bacterial contamination increases. Therefore, an ultrafilter is included as the final component to remove bacteria and bacterial endotoxin. The ultrafilter contains membranes similar to those in a reverse osmosis unit but is operated at ordinary waterline pressure. Additional source water treatment devices may be added to this system, depending on the chemical quality of the municipal water. If this system is adequately disinfected, the microbial content of water should be well within the recommended guidelines.

Distribution Systems

Water that has passed through the water treatment system (product water) may be distributed to individual dialysis machines where it is combined with dialysate concentrate. Alternately, it may be combined with concentrate in a central location and the resulting dialysis fluid supplied to individual machines. Plastic pipes (usually polyvinyl chloride) are used to distribute water or dialysis fluid to dialysis machines. The use of pipes with a diameter larger than necessary slows the fluid velocity and increases the wetted surface area available for microbial colonization. Increased surface area also results from using pipes that are longer than needed. Gram-negative bacteria in fluids remaining in pipes overnight can multiply rapidly and colonize the wetted surfaces of the pipes, producing bacterial populations and endotoxin in quantities proportional to the volume and surface area. Such colonization results in the formation of a protective biofilm, which is difficult to remove and protects the bacteria from disinfection.[16]

Routine disinfection of the water or dialysate distribution system should be performed at least weekly.[17] However, the AAMI Standards and recommendations, which are consensus documents, do not specify a schedule for disinfection other than suggest that routine disinfection should be conducted. In many instances, microbiologic monitoring can be used to determine frequency of disinfection of the water distribution system.[18,19]

To prevent disinfectant from draining from pipes by gravity before contact time is adequate, distribution systems should be designed with all outlet taps at equal elevation and at the highest point of the system. Furthermore, the system should be free of rough joints, dead-end pipes, and unused branches and taps. Fluid trapped in such stagnant areas can serve as a reservoir for bacteria that are later inoculated into the distribution system.[20]

Storage tanks greatly increase the volume of fluid and surface area of the distribution system. If used, they should be drained frequently, cleaned (including scrubbing of the sides of the tank to remove bacterial biofilm), and disinfected. Also, an ultrafilter distal to the storage tank is recommended.

Hemodialysis Machines

In the 1970s, most dialysis machines were of the recirculating or recirculating single-pass type; their design contributed to relatively high levels of gram-negative bacterial contamination in dialysis fluid. Currently, virtually all centers in the United States use single-pass hemodialysis machines. Single-pass machines tend to respond to adequate cleaning and disinfection procedures and, in general, have lower levels of bacterial contamination in their dialysis fluid than do recirculating machines. Levels of contamination in single-pass machines depend primarily on the bacteriologic quality of the incoming water and on the method of machine disinfection.[8,21]

A frequent error in disinfecting single-pass systems is introduction of the disinfectant in the same manner and through the same port as the dialysate concentrate. By so doing, the pipes and tubing carrying incoming water or dialysate are not disinfected and may act as a reservoir for bacteria. To ensure adequate disinfection of a single-pass machine, the disinfectant must reach all parts of the system's fluid pathways.

Disinfection of Hemodialysis Systems

Routine disinfection of isolated components of a dialysis system frequently produces inadequate results. Consequently, the total dialysis system (water treatment system, distribution system, and dialysis machine) should be included in the disinfection procedure.

Chlorine-based disinfectants, such as sodium hypochlorite solutions, are convenient and effective in most parts of the dialysis system when used at the manufacturer's recommended concentration. Also, the test for residual available chlorine to confirm adequate rinsing is simple and sensitive. However, because chlorine is corrosive, it is usually rinsed from the system after a short (20–30 min) exposure time. The rinse water invariably contains gram-negative water bacteria that can multiply to significant levels, if the system is permitted to stand overnight. Therefore, chlorine disinfectants are best used just before the start-up of the dialysis system rather than at the end of the day. In centers dialyzing patients in multiple shifts, it may be reasonable to disinfect with sodium hypochlorite between shifts (this may not be necessary with some single-pass machines, if the levels of bacterial contamination are within AAMI limits) and with another disinfectant (formaldehyde, peroxyacetic acid, or glutaraldehyde) at the end of the day.

Aqueous formaldehyde, peroxyacetic acid, or glutaraldehyde solutions produce good disinfection results.[22,23] These products are not as corrosive as hypochlorite solutions and can be allowed to remain in the dialysis system for long periods when the system is not operational, thereby preventing regrowth of bacteria. Formaldehyde has good penetrating characteristics but is considered an environmental hazard and potential carcinogen and has irritating qualities that may be objectionable to staff members.[24] The U.S. Environmental Protection Agency (EPA) has reduced the allowable amount of formaldehyde that can be discharged into the wastewater stream, which has reduced the use of this disinfectant in the dialysis community. Commercial tests (e.g., Formalert, Organon Teknika, Durham, NC) are available and can detect residual formaldehyde in water at concentrations as low as 1 part per million. Peroxyacetic acid and glutaraldehyde are commercially available and are designed for use with dialysis machines; both are good germicides when used according to the manufacturer's recommendations.

Some dialysis systems use hot-water disinfection for the control of microbial contamination. In this type of system, water heated to greater than 80°C (176°F) is passed through all proportioning, distribution, and patient-monitoring devices at the end of the day. These systems are excellent for controlling bacterial contamination.

Monitoring of Water and Dialysis Fluid

Microbiologic and endotoxin standards for water and dialysis fluids (Table 21–2)[3,12,25–27] were originally based on the results of culture assays performed during epidemiologic investigations and should be used as broad guidelines rather than absolute standards. These standards are in the process of being revised based on new data on the effects of the microbial quality of hemodialysis fluids on chronic inflammatory response syndrome and anemia management in dialysis patients.[28–32]

Water samples should be collected from a source as close as possible to where water enters the dialysate concentrate-proportioning unit. Water samples should be collected at least monthly and repeated when bacteriologic counts exceed 200 colony forming units per milliliter (CFU/mL) and/or endotoxin activity exceeds 2 EU/mL (Table 21–2) or when changes have been made in the disinfection procedure, the water treatment system, or the water distribution system. Dialysis fluid samples should be collected during or at the termination of dialysis from a source close to where the dialysis fluid either enters or leaves the dialyzer. Dialysis fluid samples should also be collected at least once monthly and repeated when the recommended levels for microbial or endotoxin contamination are exceeded (Table 21–2), when pyrogenic reactions are suspected, or when changes are made in the water treatment system or disinfection protocol. If centers reprocess dialyzers for reuse on the same patient, water used to rinse dialyzers and prepare dialyzer disinfectants should also be assayed at least monthly.

Specimens should be assayed within 30 minutes or refrigerated at 4°C and assayed within 24 hours of collection. Conventional laboratory procedures such as the pour plate, spread plate, or membrane filter technique can be used. Calibrated loops should not be used because they sample a small volume and are inaccurate. Although standard methods agar, blood agar, and trypticase soy agar were once considered equivalent, it has since been shown that a portion of the gram-negative bacterial flora of bicarbonate dialysis fluid and water have special growth requirements. Microorganisms found in bicarbonate dialysis fluid require a small amount of sodium chloride, and those found in processed water may require a nutrient poor medium. Consequently, to cover both conditions needed, trypticase soy agar is the currently recommended medium; however, one may also use standard plate count, standard methods, or soybean-casein digest agars along with commercially available samplers. Blood agar should not be used for this purpose. The assay should be quantitative, not qualitative, and a standard technique for enumeration should be used. Colonies should be counted with the aide of a magnifying device after 48 hours of incubation at 35° to 37°C.[3,12,25–27,33] Total viable counts (standard plate counts) are the objective of the assays.

In an outbreak investigation, the assay may need to be both qualitative and quantitative; also, detection of nontuberculous mycobacteria in water may be desirable. In such instances, plates should be incubated for 5 to 14 days.

DIALYSIS-ASSOCIATED PYROGENIC REACTIONS

Gram-negative bacterial contamination of dialysis water or components can cause pyrogenic reactions. Pyrogenic reactions are defined as objective chills (visible rigors) or fever (oral temperature 37.8°C [100°F] or higher) or both in a patient who was afebrile (oral temperature up to 37.0°C [98.6°F]) and had no signs or symptoms of infection before the dialysis treatment.[24] Depending on the type of dialysis system and level of contamination, fever and chills may start 1 to 5 hours after dialysis is initiated. Other symptoms may include hypotension, headache, myalgia, nausea, and vomiting. Pyrogenic reactions can occur with or without bacteremia; because presenting signs and symptoms may not be different in these two instances, blood cultures are necessary.

During the 1990s, an annual average of 20% of the hemodialysis centers in the United States reported at least one pyrogenic reaction in the absence of septicemia in patients undergoing dialysis.[14] Pyrogenic reactions without bacteremia can result from either the passage of bacterial endotoxin (lipopolysaccharide) in the dialysis fluid across the dialyzer membrane[34,35] or the transmembrane stimulation of cytokine production in the patient's blood by endotoxins in the dialysis fluid.[36,37] In other instances, endotoxins can enter the bloodstream directly with fluids that are contaminated with gram-negative bacteria.[38,39] The signs and symptoms of pyrogenic reactions without bacteremia generally abate within a few hours after dialysis has been stopped. If gram-negative bacterial sepsis is associated, fever and chills may persist, and hypotension is more refractory to therapy.[11,38]

When a pyrogenic reaction occurs, the following steps are recommended: (1) a careful physical examination to rule out other causes of chills and fever (e.g., pneumonia, vascular access infection, urinary tract infection); (2) blood cultures, other diagnostic tests (e.g., chest radiograph), and cultures as clinically indicated; (3) collection of dialysis fluid from the dialyzer (downstream side) for quantitative and qualitative bacteriologic assays; and (4) recording of the incident in a log or other permanent record. Determining the cause of these episodes is important because they may be the first indication of a remediable problem.

The higher the level of bacteria and endotoxin in dialysis fluid, the higher the probability that they will pass through the dialysis membrane or stimulate cytokine production. In an outbreak of febrile reactions among patients undergoing dialysis, the attack rates were directly proportional to the level of bacterial contamination in the dialysis fluid.[8] Prospective studies also demonstrated a lower pyrogenic reaction rate among patients when they underwent dialysis with dialysis fluid that had been filtered and from which most bacteria had been removed, compared with patients who underwent dialysis with dialysis fluid that was highly contaminated (mean 19,000 CFU/mL).[40–42]

Among seven outbreaks of bacteremia and pyrogenic reactions not related to dialyzer reuse investigated by the Centers of Disease Control (CDC), inadequate disinfection of the water distribution or storage system was implicated in three (Table 21–3). The most recent outbreaks occurred at centers using dialysis machines having a port to dispose of dialyzer priming fluid (waste handling option).[43,44] One-way valves in the waste handling option had not been maintained, checked for competency, or disinfected as recommended, allowing backflow from the drain and contamination of the port.

Hemodialyzer Reuse

Since 1976, the percentage of chronic dialysis centers in the United States that reported reuse of disposable hollow-fiber dialyzers has increased steadily[44]; the largest increase (126%) occurred during 1976 to 1982, from 18% to 43%, and the highest percentage (82%) was reported in 1997. In 2001, reuse of dialyzers was reported by 76% of centers (CDC, unpublished data).

In 1986, the AAMI's guidelines for reusing hemodialyzers[45] were adopted by the U.S. Public Health Service (USPHS) and later became the Centers for Medicare and Medicaid Services (CMS) regulations. In general, dialyzer reuse appears to be safe if performed according to strict and established protocols. Dialyzer reuse has not been associated with transmission of hepatitis B virus (HBV) or hepatitis C virus (HCV) infection but has been associated with pyrogenic reactions[46] (Table 21–3). These adverse events may be the result of the use of incorrect concentrations of chemical germicides or the failure to maintain standards for water quality. Manual reprocessing of dialyzers that does not include a test for membrane integrity, such as the air-pressure leak test, may fail to detect membrane defects and may be a cause of pyrogenic reactions.[46]

Some procedures used to reprocess hemodialyzers generally constitute high-level disinfection rather than sterilization.[3,47] There are several liquid germicides commonly used for high-level disinfection of dialyzers. Formaldehyde is a chemical solution obtained from chemical supply houses and is not formulated specifically for dialyzer disinfection. There are chemical germicides specifically formulated for this purpose (e.g., peracetic acid and glutaraldehyde-based products) that are approved by the U.S. Food and Drug Administration (FDA) as sterilants for reprocessing hemodialyzers. In 2001, a peracetic acid formulation was used by 62% of centers that reused dialyzers, formaldehyde by 29%, and glutaraldehyde by 5%; 4% of centers used a heat process (CDC, unpublished data).

In 1983, most centers in the United States used 2% aqueous formaldehyde with a contact time of approximately 36 hours for high-level disinfection of disposable dialyzers.[48] In 1982, a center using this regimen experienced an outbreak of infections caused by nontuberculous mycobacteria.[5] It subsequently was shown that the 2% formaldehyde regimen was not effective against nontuberculous mycobacteria. Rather, a regimen of 4% formaldehyde with a minimum contact time of 24 hours is required to inactivate high numbers of these microorganisms and is recommended as a minimum solution for disinfection of dialyzers.[3,46,47] A similar outbreak of systemic mycobacterial infections in five dialysis patients, resulting in two deaths, occurred when high-flux dialyzers were contaminated with mycobacteria during manual reprocessing and were then disinfected with a commercial dialyzer disinfectant prepared at a concentration that did not ensure complete inactivation of mycobacteria.[7] These two outbreaks of infection in dialysis patients emphasize the need to use dialyzer disinfectants at concentrations that are effective against the more chemically resistant microorganisms, such as mycobacteria.

Outbreaks of pyrogenic reactions have often resulted from reprocessing dialyzers with water that did not meet AAMI standards (Table 21–3). In most instances, the water used to rinse dialyzers or to prepare dialyzer disinfectants exceeded allowable AAMI microbial or endotoxin standards because the water distribution system was not disinfected frequently, the disinfectant was improperly prepared, or routine microbiologic assays were improperly performed.

High-Flux Dialysis and Bicarbonate Dialysate

High-flux dialysis uses dialyzer membranes with hydraulic permeabilities 5 to 10 times greater than those of conventional dialyzer membranes. There is concern that bacteria or endotoxin in the dialysate may penetrate these highly permeable high-flux dialyzer membranes.

Another concern is that high-flux dialysis requires the use of bicarbonate rather than acetate dialysate. Acetate dialysate is prepared from a single concentrate with a high salt molarity (4.8 M) that cannot support the growth of most bacteria. Bicarbonate dialysate, however, must be prepared from two concentrates, an acid concentrate with a pH of 2.8 that is not conducive to bacterial growth and a bicarbonate concentrate with a relatively neutral pH and a salt molarity of 1.2 M. Because the bicarbonate concentration will support rapid bacterial growth,[49] its use can increase bacterial and endotoxin concentrations in the dialysate and theoretically may contribute to an increase in pyrogenic reactions, especially when it is used during high-flux dialysis.

Some of this concern appeared justified by the results of surveillance data during the 1990s that showed a significant

Table 21–3 Outbreaks of Dialysis-Associated Illnesses Investigated by the Centers for Disease Control and Prevention

Description (Reference)	Cause(s) of Outbreak	Corrective Measure(s) Recommended
Bacteremia, Fungemia, or Pyrogenic Reactions Not Related to Dialyzer Reuse		
Pyrogenic reactions in 49 patients[11]	Untreated city water contained high levels of endotoxin	Install reverse osmosis system
Pyrogenic reactions in 45 patients[20]	Inadequate disinfection of fluid distribution system	Increase disinfection frequency and germicide contact time
Pyrogenic reactions in 14 patients; 2 bacteremias; 1 death[4]	Reverse osmosis water storage tank contaminated with bacteria	Remove or properly disinfect and maintain storage tank
Pyrogenic reactions in 6 patients; 7 bacteremias[149]	Inadequate disinfection of water distribution system and dialysis machines; improper microbial assay procedure	Use correct microbial assay procedure; disinfect water distribution system and dialysis machines according to manufacturer's recommendations
Bacteremia in 35 patients with central vein catheters[150]	Central vein catheters used as primary access; median duration of infected catheters was 311 days; improper aseptic techniques	Use central vein catheters only when necessary; use appropriate aseptic techniques when inserting and performing catheter care
3 pyrogenic reactions and 10 bacteremias in patients treated on machines with a port for disposal of dialyzer priming fluid (waste handling option or WHO)[151]	Incompetent valve allowing backflow from drain to the WHO; bacterial contamination of the WHO	Routine maintenance, disinfection, and check for valve competency of the WHO
Bacteremia in 10 patients treated on machines with a port for disposal of dialyzer prime[152]	Incompetent valve allowing backflow from drain to the WHO; bacterial contamination of the WHO	Routine maintenance, disinfection, and check for valve competency of the WHO
Outbreak of pyrogenic reactions and gram-negative bacteremia in 11 patients (4 with bacteremia)[17]	Water distribution system and machines were not routinely disinfected or according to manufacturer's instructions. Water and dialysate samples were cultured using calibrated loop and blood agar plates—results were always recorded as no growth	Disinfect machines according to manufacturer's instructions; include water distribution system in the weekly disinfection of the RO system.
Phialemonium curvatum access infections in 4 hemodialysis patients; 2 of these patients died of systemic disease. (CDC, unpublished data)	Observations at the facility noted some irregularities in site prep for needle insertion. All affected patients have synthetic grafts. One environmental culture was positive for *P. curvatum* (condensate pan of HVAC serving the dialysis facility)	Review infection control practices; clean and disinfect HVAC system where water accumulates. Perform surveillance on all patients.
Bacteremia/Pyrogenic Reactions Related to Dialyzer Reuse		
Mycobacterial infections in 27 patients[5]	Inadequate concentration of dialyzer disinfectant	Increase formaldehyde dialyzer disinfectant concentration to 4%
Mycobacterial infection in 5 high-flux dialysis patients; 2 deaths[7]	Inadequate concentration of dialyzer disinfectant	Use higher disinfectant concentration and more frequent disinfection of water treatment system
Bacteremia and pyrogenic reactions in 6 patients[153]	Dialyzer disinfectant diluted to improper concentration	Use disinfectant at recommended dilution and verify concentration
Bacteremia in 6 patients (CDC unpublished data)	Inadequate concentration of dialyzer disinfectant; water used for reuse did not meet AAMI standards	Use AAMI quality of water; ensure proper germicide concentration in dialyzer
Bacteremia and pyrogenic reactions in 6 patients[154]	Inadequate mixing of dialyzer disinfectant	Thoroughly mix disinfectant and verify proper concentration
Bacteremia in 33 patients at two dialysis centers[39,155]	Dialyzer disinfectant created holes in dialyzer membrane	Change disinfectant (removed from marketplace by manufacturer)

Description (Reference)	Cause(s) of Outbreak	Corrective Measure(s) Recommended
	Bacteremia/Pyrogenic Reactions Related to Dialyzer Reuse—cont'd	
Bacteremia in 6 patients; all blood isolates had similar plasmid profiles[156]	Dialyzers contaminated during removal and cleaning of headers with gauze; staff not routinely changing gloves; dialyzers not processed for several hours after disassembly and cleaning	Do not use gauze or similar material to remove clots from header; change gloves frequently; process dialyzers immediately after rinsing and cleaning
Pyrogenic reactions in 3 high-flux dialysis patients[157]	Dialyzer reprocessed with two disinfectants; water used for reuse did not meet AAMI standards	Do not disinfect dialyzers with multiple germicides; more frequent disinfection of water system
Pyrogenic reactions in 14 high-flux dialysis patients; 1 death[158]	Dialyzers rinsed with city water; water for reuse did not meet AAMI standards	Do not rinse or clean dialyzers with city water; disinfect water treatment system more frequently
Pyrogenic reactions in 18 patients[51]	Dialyzers rinsed with city water containing high levels of endotoxin; water used for reuse did not meet AAMI standards	Do not rinse or clean dialyzers with city water; disinfect water treatment system more frequently
Pyrogenic reactions in 22 patients[159]	Water for reuse did not meet AAMI standards; improper microbial assay technique	Use correct microbial assay procedure; disinfect water distribution system
	Transmission of Viral Agents	
26 patients seroconverted to HBsAg positive during a 10-month period[160]	Leakage of coil dialyzer membranes and use of recirculating bath dialysis machines	Separation of HBsAg-positive patients and equipment from other patients
19 patients and 1 staff seroconverted to HBsAg positive during a 14-month period[96]	No specific cause determined; false-positive HBsAg results caused some susceptible patients to be dialyzed with infected patients	Laboratory confirmation of HBsAg-positive results; strict adherence to glove use and use of separate equipment
24 patients and 6 staff seroconverted to HBsAg positive during a 10-month period[91]	Staff not wearing gloves; surfaces not properly disinfected; improper handling of needles/sharps resulting in many staff needlesticks	Separation of HBsAg-positive patients and equipment from other patients; proper precautions by staff (e.g., gloves; handling of needles/sharps)
13 patients and 1 staff seroconverted to HBsAg positive during a 1-month period[95]	Extrinsic contamination of intravenous medication being prepared adjacent to area where blood work was handled	Separate medication preparation area and blood processing for diagnostic tests
10 patients seroconverted to HBsAg positive in 1 month[161]	Extrinsic contamination of multidose medication vial shared by HBsAg-positive and HBsAg-susceptible patients	No sharing of supplies, equipment, and medications between patients
8 patients seroconverted to HBsAg positive during a 5-month period (CDC, unpublished data)	Sporadic screening for HBsAg; HBsAg carriers not separated; major bleeding incident with environmental contamination	Monthly screening of patients for HBsAg; separation of positive patients with dedicated equipment and staff; vaccination of all susceptibles
7 patients seroconverted to HBsAg positive during a 3-month period[92]	Same staff caring for HBsAg-positive and HBsAg-negative patients	Separation of HBsAg-positive patients from other patients; same staff should not care for HBsAg-positive and HBsAg-negative patients on same shift
8 patients seroconverted to HBsAg-positive during 1 month[148]	Not consistently using pressure transducer filters; same members staff cared for HBsAg-positive and -negative patients on same shift	Use pressure transducer filters and replace after each use; same staff members should not care for HBsAg-positive and HBsAg-negative patients on same shift

continued

Table 21–3 Outbreaks of Dialysis-Associated Illnesses Investigated by the Centers for Disease Control and Prevention—cont'd

Description (Reference)	Cause(s) of Outbreak	Corrective Measure(s) Recommended
	Transmission of Viral Agents	
14 patients seroconverted to HBsAg positive during a 6-week period[93]	Failure to review results of admission and monthly HBsAg testing; inconsistent handwashing and use of gloves; adjacent clean and contaminated areas; <20% of patients vaccinated	Proper infection control precautions for dialysis units; routine review of serologic testing; hepatitis B vaccination of all patients
7 patients seroconverted to HBsAg positive during a 2-month period[93]	Same staff members cared for HBsAg-positive and HBsAg-negative patients on same shift; common medication and supply carts were moved between stations, and multidose vials were shared. No patients were vaccinated.	Dedicated staff for HBsAg-positive patients; no sharing of medication or supplies between any patients; centralized medication and supply areas; hepatitis B vaccination of all patients
4 patients seroconverted to HbsAg positive during a 3-month period[93]	Transmission appeared to occur during hospitalization at an acute care facility	Hepatitis B vaccination of all patients
11 patients seroconverted to HbsAg positive during a 3-month period[93]	Staff, equipment, and supplies were shared between HBsAg-positive and HBsAg-negative patients. No patients were vaccinated.	Dedicated staff for HbsAg-positive patients; no sharing of medication or supplies between any patients; hepatitis B vaccination of all patients.
2 patients seroconverted to HbsAg positive during a 4-month period[101]	Same staff members cared for HBsAg-positive and HBsAg-negative patients; no patients were vaccinated.	Dedicated staff for HbsAg-positive patients; hepatitis B vaccination of all patients.
36 patients with liver enzyme elevations consistent with non-A, non-B hepatitis[162]	Environmental contamination with blood	Monthly liver enzyme screening; proper precautions (i.e., use of gloves) by staff
35 patients with liver enzyme elevations consistent with non-A, non-B hepatitis during a 22-month period; 82% of probable cases were anti-HCV positive[163]	Inconsistent use of infection control precautions, especially handwashing and glove use	Strict compliance to aseptic technique and dialysis center precautions
HCV infection developed in 7/41 (17.1%) patients; shift specific attack rates of 29%–36%[164]	Multidose vials left on top of machine and used by multiple patients; routine cleaning and disinfection of surfaces and equipment between patients not routinely done; arterial line for draining prime waste draped into bucket that was not routinely cleaned between patients	Strict compliance with infection control precautions recommended for all dialysis patients; routine HCV testing
HCV infection developed in 5/75 (6.6%) patients[165]	Sharing of equipment and supplies between chronically infected and susceptible patients; gloves not routinely used; clean and contaminated areas not separated	Strict compliance with infection control precautions recommended for all dialysis patients
HCV infection developed in 3/23 (13%) patients[166]	Supply carts moved between stations and contained both clean supplies and blood-contaminated items. Medications prepared in same area used for disposal of used injection equipment	Strict compliance with infection control precautions recommended for all dialysis patients

association between use of high-flux dialysis and reporting of pyrogenic reactions among patients during dialysis.[50] However, a prospective study of pyrogenic reactions in patients receiving more than 27,000 conventional, high-efficiency, or high-flux dialysis treatments with a bicarbonate dialysate containing high concentrations of bacteria and endotoxin found no association between pyrogenic reactions and the type of dialysis treatment.[51] Although there seem to be conflicting data on the relationship between high-flux dialysis and pyrogenic reactions, centers providing high-flux dialysis should ensure that dialysate meets AAMI microbial standards (Table 21–2).

OTHER BACTERIAL INFECTIONS

The annual mortality rate among hemodialysis patients is 23%, and infections are the second most common cause, accounting for 14% of deaths.[1] Septicemia (11% of all deaths) is the most common infectious cause of mortality. In studies published during 1997 to 2000 that evaluated rates of bacterial infections in hemodialysis outpatients, bacteremia occurred in 0.6% to 1.7% of patients per month and vascular access infections (with or without bacteremia) in 1.3% to 7.2% of patients per month.[52–60] A review of four studies published during 2002 estimated that 1.8% of hemodialysis patients have vascular access associated bacteremia each month, amounting to 50,000 cases nationally per year.[61]

Because of the importance of bacterial infections in hemodialysis patients, the CDC initiated an ongoing surveillance project in 1999.[62] All U.S. hemodialysis centers treating outpatients are eligible to enroll. Only bacterial infections associated with hospital admission or intravenous antimicrobial receipt are counted; since infections treated with outpatient oral antimicrobials are excluded, this system likely detects only the more severe infections. During 1999 to 2001, 109 centers reported data. Rates of infection per 100 patient months were 3.2 for all vascular access infections (including access infections both with and without bacteremia), 1.8 for vascular-access associated bacteremia, 1.3 for wound infections not related to the vascular access, 0.8 for pneumonias, and 0.3 for urinary tract infections. Among patients with fistulas or grafts, wounds were the most common site of infection. Among patients with hemodialysis catheters, infections of the vascular access site were most common.

In a study of 27 French hemodialysis centers, 28% of 230 infections in hemodialysis patients involved the vascular access, whereas 25% involved the lung, 23% the urinary tract, 9% the skin and soft tissues, and 15% other or unknown sites.[58] Thirty-three percent of infections involved either the vascular access site or were bacteremias of unknown origin, many of which might have been caused by occult access infections. Thus, the vascular access site was the most common site for infection but accounted for only one-third of infections.

Bacterial pathogens causing infection can be either exogenous (i.e., acquired from contaminated dialysis fluids or equipment) or endogenous (i.e., caused by invasion of bacteria present in or on the patient). Exogenous pathogens have caused numerous outbreaks, most of which resulted from inadequate dialyzer reprocessing procedures (e.g., contaminated water or inadequate disinfectant) or inadequate treatment of municipal water for use in dialysis. During 1995 to 1997, four outbreaks were traced to contamination of the waste drain port on one type of dialysis machine.[43] Recommendations to prevent such outbreaks are published elsewhere.[63]

Contaminated medication vials are also a potential source of bacterial infection for patients. In 1999, an outbreak of Serratia liquefaciens bloodstream infections and pyrogenic reactions among hemodialysis patients was traced to contamination of vials of erythropoietin. These vials, which were intended for single use, were contaminated by repeated puncture to obtain additional doses and by pooling of residual medication into a common vial.[64]

Vascular Access Infections

Access site infections are particularly important because they can cause disseminated bacteremia or loss of the vascular access. Local signs of vascular access infection include erythema, warmth, induration, swelling, tenderness, breakdown of skin, loculated fluid, or purulent exudates.[53,56,62,65] In the CDC surveillance project, rates of access-associated bacteremia per 100 patient months were 1.8 overall and varied by access type: 0.25 for fistulas, 0.53 for grafts, 4.8 for permanent (tunneled, cuffed) catheters, and 8.7 for temporary (nontunneled, noncuffed) catheters.[62]

Vascular access infections are caused (in descending order of frequency) by *Staphylococcus aureus* (32%–53% of cases), coagulase-negative staphylococci (CNS; 20%–32%), gram-negative bacilli (10%–18%), nonstaphylococcal gram-positive cocci (including enterococci; 10%–12%), and fungi (< 1%).[62] The proportion of infections caused by *S. aureus* is higher among patients with fistulas or grafts, and the proportion caused by CNS is higher among patients dialyzed through catheters.

The primary risk factor for access infection is access type, with catheters having the highest risk for infection; grafts intermediate; and native arteriovenous (AV) fistulas the lowest.[55,62,66] Other potential risk factors for vascular access infections include: (1) location of the access in the lower extremity; (2) recent access surgery; (3) trauma, hematoma, dermatitis, or scratching over the access site; (4) poor patient hygiene; (5) poor needle insertion technique; (6) older age; (7) diabetes; (8) immunosuppression; and (9) iron overload.[53,56,67–69]

Based on the relative risk of both infectious and noninfectious complications, it is recommended that native arteriovenous fistulas be used more commonly and hemodialysis catheters less commonly; a goal of no more than 10% of patients maintained with permanent catheter-based hemodialysis treatments is recommended.[53,56,67–70] To minimize infectious complications, patients should be referred early for creation of an implanted access, thereby decreasing the time dialyzed through a temporary catheter. Additionally, permanent catheters should be used only in patients for whom implanted access is impossible. During 1995 to 2001, the percentage of patients dialyzed through fistulas increased from 22% to 30%, with most of the increase occurring since 1999.[44] (CDC, unpublished data). During the same period, use of grafts decreased from 65% to 44% of patients, and use of catheters increased from 13% to 25%; however, the rate of increase in catheter use appears to be slowing.

Recommendations for preventing vascular access infections have been developed by the National Kidney Foundation[70] and the CDC[71] and recently summarized.[72] Selected recommendations for preventing hemodialysis-catheter associated infection include: (1) not using antimicrobial prophylaxis before insertion or during the use of the catheter; (2) not routinely replacing the catheter; (3) using sterile technique (cap, mask, sterile gown, large sterile drapes, and gloves) during catheter insertion; (4) limiting use of noncuffed catheters to 3 to 4 weeks; (5) using the catheter solely for hemodialysis unless there is no alternative; (6) restricting catheter manipulation and dressing changes to trained personnel; (7) replacing catheter-site dressing at each dialysis treatment or if damp, loose, or soiled; (8) disinfecting skin before catheter insertion and dressing changes (a 2% chlorhexidine-based preparation is preferred); and (9) ensuring that catheter-site care is compatible with the catheter material.

In hemodialysis patients, the Infectious Diseases Society of America has recommended treatment with nasal mupirocin in documented *S. aureus* carriers who have a catheter-related bloodstream infection with *S. aureus* and continue to need the hemodialysis catheter.[73] Otherwise, the routine use of nasal mupirocin in patients with hemodialysis catheters is not recommended by either CDC or the National Kidney Foundation.[70,71]

Antimicrobial Resistant Bacteria

Hemodialysis patients have been in the forefront of the epidemic of antimicrobial resistance, especially vancomycin resistance. One of the earliest reports of vancomycin-resistant enterococci (VRE) was from a renal unit in London, England, in 1988.[74] The prevalence of VRE stool colonization among dialysis patients has varied from 2.4% at three centers in Indianapolis, IN,[75] to 9.5% at a university hospital in Baltimore, MD.[76] In one center with a prevalence of 9%, three patients developed VRE infections in 1 year.[77] Among enterococci causing bloodstream infections in hemodialysis patients, 0% to 5% have been reported to be resistant to vancomycin.[62,78,79]

Vancomycin resistance in staphylococci has also been reported in dialysis patients. Five of the first six U.S. patients identified with vancomycin intermediate-resistant *S. aureus* infections required dialysis.[80] Additionally, the first patient found to be infected with a fully vancomycin resistant *S. aureus* strain was a chronic hemodialysis patient; vancomycin-resistant *S. aureus* was isolated from a foot wound and temporary catheter exit site.[81]

For certain patients, including those infected or colonized with Methicillin-resistant *Staphylococcus aureus* (MRSA) or VRE, contact precautions are used in the inpatient hospital setting. However, contact precautions are not recommended in hemodialysis units for patients infected or colonized with pathogenic bacteria for several reasons. First, although contact transmission of pathogenic bacteria is well-documented in hospitals, similar transmission has not been well-documented in hemodialysis centers. Transmission might not be apparent in dialysis centers, possibly because it occurs less frequently than in acute-care hospitals or results in undetected colonization rather than overt infection. Also, because dialysis patients are frequently hospitalized, determining whether transmission occurred in the inpatient or outpatient setting is difficult. Second, contamination of the patient's skin, bedclothes, and environmental surfaces with pathogenic bacteria is likely to be more common in hospital settings (where patients spend 24 hours a day) than in outpatient hemodialysis centers (where patients spend approximately 10 hours a week). Third, the routine use of infection control practices recommended for hemodialysis units, which are more stringent than the *standard precautions* routinely used in hospitals, should prevent transmission by the contact route.

HEPATITIS B VIRUS

HBV is the microbe that is most efficiently transmitted in the dialysis setting. Recommendations for the control of hepatitis B in hemodialysis centers were first published in 1977[82] and, by 1980, their widespread implementation was associated with a sharp reduction in incidence of HBV infection among both patients and staff members.[83] In 1982, hepatitis B vaccination was recommended for all susceptible patients and staff members.[84] However, outbreaks of both HBV and HCV infections continue to occur among chronic hemodialysis patients. Hepatitis A and E viruses, which are spread by the fecal-oral route and rarely by blood, have not been associated with hemodialysis.

Epidemiology

During the early 1970s, HBV infection was endemic in dialysis units and outbreaks were common. Subsequently, the incidence and prevalence of HBV infection among chronic hemodialysis patients in the United States have dramatically declined, and, by 2001, was 0.05% and 0.9%, respectively.[85] (CDC, unpublished data, 2001) Only 2.9% of all centers reported patients with newly acquired infections, however, 26.5% of centers provided dialysis to one or more chronically infected patients (CDC, unpublished data, 2001).

The chronically infected person is central to the epidemiology of HBV transmission. HBV is transmitted by percutaneous (i.e., puncture through the skin) or permucosal (i.e., direct contact with mucous membranes) exposure to infectious blood or to body fluids that contain blood. All HBsAg positive persons are infectious, but those who are also positive for hepatitis B e antigen (HBeAg) circulate HBV at high titers in their blood (10^{8-9} virions/mL).[86,87] With virus titers this high in blood, body fluids containing serum or blood can also contain high levels of HBV and are potentially infectious. Furthermore, HBV at titers of 10^{2-3} virions/mL can be present on environmental surfaces in the absence of any visible blood and still cause transmission.[86,88,89]

HBV is relatively stable in the environment and remains viable for at least 7 days on environmental surfaces at room temperature.[86,88,89] HBsAg has been detected in dialysis centers on clamps, scissors, dialysis machine control knobs, and doorknobs.[90] Thus, blood-contaminated surfaces that are not routinely cleaned and disinfected represent a reservoir for HBV transmission. Dialysis staff members can transfer virus to patients from contaminated surfaces by their hands or gloves or through use of contaminated equipment and supplies.

Most HBV infection outbreaks among hemodialysis patients (Table 21–3) were caused by cross-contamination to patients via (1) environmental surfaces, supplies (e.g., hemostats, clamps), or equipment that were not routinely disinfected after each use; (2) multiple dose medication vials and intravenous solutions that were not used exclusively for one patient; (3) medications for injection that were prepared in areas adjacent to areas where blood samples were handled; and (4) staff members who simultaneously cared for both HBV-infected and susceptible patients.[91–96] Once the factors that promote HBV transmission among hemodialysis patients were identified, recommendations for control were published in 1977.[82] These recommendations included: (1) serologic surveillance of patients (and staff members) for HBV infection, including monthly testing of all susceptible patients for HBsAg; (2) isolation of HBsAg-positive patients in a separate room; (3) assignment of staff members to HBsAg-positive patients and not to HBV-susceptible patients during the same shift; (4) assignment of dialysis equipment to HBsAg-positive patients that is not shared by HBV-susceptible patients; (5) assignment of a supply tray to each patient (regardless of serologic status); (6) cleaning and disinfection of nondisposable items (e.g., clamps, scissors) before use on another patient; (7) glove use whenever any patient or hemodialysis equipment is touched and glove changes between each patient (and station); and (8) routine cleaning and disinfection of equipment and environmental surfaces.

The segregation of HBsAg-positive patients and their equipment from HBV-susceptible patients resulted in 70% to 80% reductions in incidence of HBV infection among hemodialysis patients.[97–99] The success of isolation practices in preventing transmission of HBV infection is linked to other infection control practices, including routine serologic surveillance and routine cleaning and disinfection. Frequent serologic testing for HBsAg detects patients recently infected with HBV quickly so isolation procedures can be implemented before cross-contamination can occur. Environmental control by routine cleaning and disinfection procedures reduces the opportunity for cross-contamination, either directly from environmental surfaces or indirectly by hands of personnel.

Despite the current low incidence of HBV infection among hemodialysis patients, outbreaks continue to occur in chronic hemodialysis centers. Investigations of these outbreaks have documented that HBV transmission resulted from failure to use recommended infection control practices, including: (1) failure to routinely screen patients for HBsAg or routinely review results of testing to identify infected patients; (2) assignment of staff members to the simultaneous care of infected and susceptible patients; and (3) sharing of supplies, particularly multiple dose medication vials, among patients.[93] In addition, few patients had received hepatitis B vaccine. National surveillance data have demonstrated that independent risk factors among chronic hemodialysis patients for acquiring HBV infection include the presence of more than one HBV-infected patient in the hemodialysis center who is not isolated, as well as a less than 50% hepatitis B vaccination rate among patients.[100]

HBV infection among chronic hemodialysis patients has also been associated with hemodialysis provided in the acute-care setting.[93,101] Transmission appeared to stem from chronically infected HBV patients who shared staff members, multiple dose medication vials, and other supplies and equipment with susceptible patients. These episodes were recognized when patients returned to their chronic hemodialysis units, and routine HBsAg testing was resumed. Transmission from HBV-infected chronic hemodialysis patients to patients undergoing hemodialysis for acute renal failure has not been documented, possibly because these patients are dialyzed for short durations and have limited exposure. However, such transmission could go unrecognized because acute renal failure patients are unlikely to be tested for HBV infection.

Other risk factors for acquiring HBV infection include injection drug use, sexual and household exposure to an HBV-infected contact, exposure to multiple sexual partners, male homosexual activity, and perinatal exposure. Dialysis patients should be educated about these other risks and, for those patients chronically infected with HBV, informed that their sexual partners and household contacts should be vaccinated against hepatitis B.[102]

Screening and Diagnostic Tests

Several well-defined antigen-antibody systems are associated with HBV infection, including HBsAg and antibody to HBsAg (anti-HBs); hepatitis B core antigen (HBcAg) and antibody to HBcAg (anti-HBc); and HBeAg and antibody to HBeAg (anti-HBe). Serologic assays are commercially available for all of these except HBcAg because no free HBcAg circulates in blood. One or more of these serologic markers are present during different phases of HBV infection (Table 21–4).[103] HBV infection can also be detected, using qualitative or quantitative tests for HBV DNA. These tests are not FDA-approved and are most commonly used for patients being managed with antiviral therapy.[97,98,104,105]

The presence of HBsAg is indicative of ongoing HBV infection and potential infectiousness. In newly infected persons, HBsAg is present in serum 30 to 60 days after exposure to HBV and persists for variable periods. Transient HBsAg positivity (lasting < 18 days) can be detected in some patients during vaccination.[106,107] Anti-HBc develops in all HBV infections, appearing at onset of symptoms or liver test abnormalities in acute HBV infection, rising rapidly to high levels, and persisting for life. Acute or recently acquired infection can be distinguished by presence of the immunoglobulin M (IgM) class of anti-HBc, which persists for approximately 6 months.

In persons who recover from HBV infection, HBsAg is eliminated from the blood, usually in 23 months, and anti-HBs develops during convalescence. The presence of anti-HBs indicates immunity from HBV infection. After recovery from natural infection, most persons will be positive for both anti-HBs and anti-HBc, whereas only anti-HBs develops in persons who are successfully vaccinated against hepatitis B. Persons who do not recover from HBV infection and become chronically infected remain positive for HBsAg (and anti-HBc), although a small proportion (0.3% per year) eventually clear HBsAg and might develop anti-HBs.[108]

In some persons, the only HBV serologic marker detected is anti-HBc (i.e., isolated anti-HBc). Among most asymptomatic persons in the United States tested for HBV infection, an average of 2% (range: < 0.1%–6%) test positive for isolated anti-HBc[109]; among injecting-drug users, however, the rate is 24%.[110] In general, the frequency of isolated anti-HBc is directly related to the frequency of previous HBV infection in the population and can have several explanations. This pattern can occur after HBV infection among persons who have recovered but whose anti-HBs levels have waned or among persons who failed to develop anti-HBs. Persons in the latter category include those who circulate HBsAg at levels not detectable by current commercial assays. However, HBV DNA

Table 21–4 Interpretation of Serologic Test Results for Hepatitis B Virus Infection

Serologic Markers				Interpretation
HBsAg*	**Total Anti-HBc†**	**IgM‡ Anti-HBc**	**Anti-HBs§**	
–	–	–	–	Susceptible, never infected
+	–	–	–	Acute infection, early incubation¶
+	+	+	–	Acute infection
–	+	+	–	Acute resolving infection
–	+	–	+	Past infection, recovered and immune
+	+	–	–	Chronic infection
–	+	–	–	False positive (i.e., susceptible), past infection, or low-level chronic infection
–	–	–	+	Immune if titer is ≥ 10 mIU/mL

*Hepatitis B surface antigen.
†Antibody to hepatitis B core antigen.
‡Immunoglobulin M.
§Antibody to hepatitis B surface antigen.
¶Transient HBsAg positivity (lasting ≤18 days) might be detected in some patients during vaccination.

has been detected in less than 10% of persons with isolated anti-HBc, and these persons are unlikely to be infectious to others except under unusual circumstances involving direct percutaneous exposure to large quantities of blood (e.g., transfusion).[111] In most persons with isolated anti-HBc, the result appears to be a false positive. Data from several studies have demonstrated that a primary anti-HBs response develops in most of these persons after a three-dose series of hepatitis B vaccine.[112,113] No data exist on response to vaccination among hemodialysis patients with this serologic pattern.

A third antigen, HBeAg, can be detected in serum of persons with acute or chronic HBV infection. The presence of HBeAg correlates with viral replication and high levels of virus (i.e., high infectivity). Anti-HBe correlates with the loss of replicating virus and with lower levels of virus. However, all HBsAg-positive persons should be considered potentially infectious, regardless of their HBeAg or anti-HBe status.

HEPATITIS C VIRUS

Epidemiology

Data are limited on current incidence and prevalence of HCV infection among chronic hemodialysis patients. In 2001, 62% of centers reported that they tested patients for antibody to HCV (anti-HCV) (CDC, unpublished data). In the centers that tested, the reported incidence was 0.29% and prevalence was 8.6% (range among ESRD networks, 5.7%–11.9%). Twelve percent of centers reported newly acquired HCV infections among patients. Higher incidence rates have been reported from cohort studies of hemodialysis patients in the United States (less than 1%–3%) and in Europe (3%–10%).[114–120] Higher prevalences (10%–36%) have also been reported from studies of patients in individual facilities.[114,121]

HCV is most efficiently transmitted by direct percutaneous exposure to infectious blood, and like HBV, the chronically infected person is central to the epidemiology of HCV transmission. Risk factors associated with HCV infection among hemodialysis patients include blood transfusions from unscreened donors and years on dialysis.[114,121] The number of years on dialysis is the major risk factor independently associated with higher rates of HCV infection. As the time patients spent on dialysis increased, their prevalence of HCV infection increased from an average of 12% for patients receiving dialysis less than 5 years to an average of 37% for patients receiving dialysis more than 5 years.[114,121–123]

These studies, as well as investigations of dialysis-associated outbreaks of hepatitis C, indicate that HCV transmission occurs most likely because of inadequate infection control practices. During 1999 to 2000, CDC investigated three outbreaks of HCV infection among patients in chronic hemodialysis centers (CDC, unpublished data, 1999 and 2000). In two of the outbreaks, multiple transmissions of HCV occurred during periods of 16 to 24 months (attack rates: 6.6%–17.5%), and seroconversions were associated with receiving dialysis immediately after a chronically infected patient. Multiple opportunities for cross-contamination among patients were observed, including: (1) equipment and supplies that were not disinfected between patient use; (2) use of common medication carts to prepare and distribute medications at patients' stations; (3) sharing of multiple dose medication vials, which were placed at patients' stations on top of hemodialysis machines; (4) contaminated priming buckets that were not routinely changed or cleaned and disinfected between patients; (5) machine surfaces that were not routinely cleaned and disinfected between patients; and (6) blood spills that were not cleaned up promptly. In the third outbreak, multiple new infections clustered at one point in time (attack rate: 27%), suggesting a common exposure event. Multiple opportunities for cross-contamination from chronically infected patients were also observed in this unit. In particular, supply carts were moved from one station to another and contained both clean supplies and blood-contaminated items, including small biohazard containers, sharps disposal boxes, and used vacutainers containing patients' blood.

Other risk factors for acquiring HCV infection include injection drug use, exposure to an HCV-infected sexual partner or household contact, multiple sexual partners, and perinatal exposure.[124,125] The efficiency of transmission in settings involving sexual or household exposure to infected contacts is low, and the magnitude of risk and the circumstances under which these exposures result in transmission are not well defined.

Screening and Diagnostic Tests

FDA-licensed or approved anti-HCV screening test kits being used in the United States comprise three immunoassays: two enzyme immunoassays (EIA) and one enhanced chemiluminescence immunoassay (CIA).[126] FDA-licensed or approved supplemental tests include a serologic anti-HCV assay, the strip immunoblot assay (Chiron RIBA HCV 3.0 SIA, Chiron Corp., Emeryville, CA), and nucleic acid tests (NAT) for HCV RNA (including reverse transcriptase polymerase chain reaction [RT-PCR] amplification and transcription mediated amplification [TMA]).

Anti-HCV testing includes initial screening with an immunoassay. If the screening test is positive, an independent supplemental test with high specificity should be performed to verify the results. Among hemodialysis patients, the proportion of false-positive screening test results averages approximately 15%.[126] For this reason, not relying exclusively on anti-HCV screening-test–positive results to determine whether a person has been infected with HCV is critical. Table 21–5 describes the interpretation of HCV testing results for both screening and diagnosis.

For routine HCV testing of hemodialysis patients, the anti-HCV screening immunoassay is recommended and, if positive, supplemental anti-HCV testing using RIBA. RIBA is recommended rather than a NAT because it is a serologic assay and can be performed on the same serum or plasma sample collected for the screening anti-HCV assay. In addition, certain situations exist in which the HCV RNA result can be negative in persons with active HCV infection. As the titer of anti-HCV increases during acute infection, the titer of HCV RNA declines.[127] Thus, HCV RNA is not detectable in certain persons during the acute phase of their hepatitis C, but this finding can be transient and chronic infection can develop.[128] In addition, intermittent HCV RNA positivity has been observed among persons with chronic HCV infection.[129–131] Therefore, the significance of a single negative HCV RNA result is unknown, and the need for further investigation or follow-up is determined by verifying anti-HCV status. In addition, detection of HCV RNA requires that the serum or plasma sample be collected and handled in a manner suitable for NAT and that testing be performed in a laboratory with facilities established for this purpose (test MMWR). Although in rare instances, detection of HCV RNA might be the only evidence of HCV infection, a recent study conducted among almost 3000 hemodialysis patients in the United States found that only 0.07% were HCV RNA positive but anti-HCV negative (CDC, unpublished data).

Table 21–5 Interpretation of Test Results for Hepatitis C Virus Infection

Anti-HCV-Positive

- An anti-HCV-positive result is defined as anti-HCV screening-test-positive and recombinant immunoblot positive (RIBA) or nucleic acid test (NAT) positive; or anti-HCV screening-test-positive, NAT negative, RIBA positive.
  - An anti-HCV-positive result indicates past or current HCV infection.
  - An HCV RNA-positive result indicates current (active) infection, but the significance of a single HCV RNA negative result is unknown; it does not differentiate intermittent viremia from resolved infection.
  - All anti-HCV positive persons should receive counseling and undergo medical evaluation, including additional testing for the presence of virus and liver disease.
  - Anti-HCV testing generally does not need to be repeated, once a positive anti-HCV result has been confirmed.

Anti-HCV-Negative

- An anti-HCV negative result is defined as anti-HCV screening-test-negative*; or anti-HCV screening-test-positive, RIBA negative; or anti-HCV screening-test-positive, NAT negative, RIBA negative.
  - An anti-HCV negative person is considered uninfected.
  - No further evaluation or follow-up for HCV is required, unless recent infection is suspected or other evidence exists to indicate HCV infection (e.g., abnormal liver enzyme levels in immunocompromised persons or persons with no other etiology for their liver disease).

Anti-HCV-Indeterminate

- An indeterminate anti-HCV result is defined as anti-HCV screening-test-positive, RIBA indeterminate; or anti-HCV screening-test-positive, NAT negative, RIBA indeterminate.
  - An indeterminate anti-HCV result indicates that the HCV antibody status cannot be determined.
  - Can indicate a false positive anti-HCV screening test result, the most likely interpretation in those at low risk for HCV infection; such persons are HCV RNA negative.
  - Can occur as a transient finding in recently infected persons who are in the process of seroconversion; such persons usually are HCV RNA positive.
  - Can be a persistent finding in persons chronically infected with HCV; such persons are usually HCV RNA positive.
  - If NAT is not performed, another sample should be collected for repeat anti-HCV testing (≥1 month later).

Anti-HCV, antibody to hepatitis C virus.
*Interpretation of screening immunoassay test results based on criteria provided by the manufacturer.
(From Centers for Disease Control and Prevention. Guidelines for laboratory testing and result reporting of antibody to hepatitis C virus. MMWR Morb Mortal Wkly Rep 2003; 52[No. RR-3]:1–15.)

HEPATITIS DELTA VIRUS

Delta hepatitis is caused by the hepatitis delta virus (HDV), a defective virus that causes infection only in persons with active HBV infection. The prevalence of HDV infection is low in the United States, with rates of less than 1% among HBsAg-positive persons in the general population and greater than 10% among HBsAg-positive persons with repeated percutaneous exposures (e.g., injecting-drug users, persons with hemophilia).[132] Areas of the world with high endemic rates of HDV infection include southern Italy, parts of Africa, and the Amazon Basin.

Few data exist on the prevalence of HDV infection among chronic hemodialysis patients, and only one transmission of HDV between such patients has been reported in the United States.[133] In this episode, transmission occurred from a patient who was chronically infected with HBV and HDV to an HBsAg-positive patient after a massive bleeding incident; both patients received dialysis at the same station.

HDV infection occurs either as a co-infection with HBV or as a superinfection in a person with chronic HBV infection. Co-infection usually resolves, but superinfection frequently results in chronic HDV infection and severe disease. High mortality rates are associated with both types of infection. A serologic test that measures total antibody to HDV is commercially available.

HUMAN IMMUNODEFICIENCY VIRUS (HIV) INFECTION

During 1985 to 2001, the percentage of U.S. hemodialysis centers that reported providing chronic hemodialysis for patients with HIV infection increased from 11% to 37%, and the proportion of hemodialysis patients with known HIV infection increased from 0.3% to 1.5%[44] (CDC, unpublished data, 2001). HIV is transmitted by blood and other body fluids that contain blood. No patient-to-patient transmission of HIV has been reported in U.S. hemodialysis centers. However, such transmission has been reported in other countries; in one case, HIV transmission was attributed to mixing of reused access needles and inadequate disinfection of equipment.[134] HIV infection is usually diagnosed with assays that measure antibody to HIV, and a repeatedly positive EIA test should be confirmed by Western blot or another confirmatory test.

PREVENTING TRANSMISSION OF INFECTIONS AMONG CHRONIC HEMODIALYSIS PATIENTS

Preventing transmission among chronic hemodialysis patients of blood-borne viruses and pathogenic bacteria from both recognized and unrecognized sources of infection requires implementation of a comprehensive infection control program. The components of such a program include infection control practices specifically designed for the hemodialysis setting, including routine serologic testing and immunization, surveillance, and training and education. CDC has published recommendations describing these components in detail.[135]

The infection control practices recommended for hemodialysis units (Table 21–6) will reduce opportunities for patient-to-patient transmission of infectious agents, directly or indirectly via contaminated devices, equipment and supplies, environmental surfaces, or hands of personnel. These practices should be carried out routinely for all patients in the chronic hemodialysis setting because of the increased potential for blood contamination during hemodialysis and because many patients are colonized or infected with pathogenic bacteria.

Such practices include additional measures to prevent HBV transmission because of the high titer of HBV and its ability to survive on environmental surfaces (Table 21–6). It is the potential for environmentally mediated transmission of HBV, rather than internal contamination of dialysis machines, that is the focus of infection control strategies for preventing HBV transmission in dialysis centers. For patients at increased risk for transmission of pathogenic bacteria, including antimicrobial-resistant strains, additional precautions might also be necessary in some circumstances. Furthermore, surveillance for infections and other adverse events is required to monitor the effectiveness of infection control practices, as well as training and education of both staff members and patients to ensure that appropriate infection control behaviors and techniques are carried out.

In each chronic hemodialysis unit, policies and practices should be reviewed and updated to ensure that infection control practices recommended for hemodialysis units are implemented and rigorously followed. Intensive efforts must be made to educate new staff members and reeducate existing staff members regarding these practices. Readers should consult the CDC recommendations for details on these practices.[135] The following is a summary of selected issues.

Routine Testing

All chronic hemodialysis patients should be routinely tested for HBV and HCV infection and the results promptly reviewed so that potential episodes of transmission can be identified quickly and patients appropriately managed based on their testing results. Test results (positive and negative) must be communicated to other units or hospitals when patients are transferred for care. Routine testing for HDV or HIV infection for purposes of infection control is not recommended.

Before admission to the hemodialysis unit, the HBV serologic status (i.e., HBsAg, total anti-HBc, and anti-HBs) of all patients should be known. For patients transferred from another unit, test results should be obtained before the patients' transfer. If a patient's HBV serologic status is not known at the time of admission, testing should be completed within 7 days. The hemodialysis unit should ensure that the laboratory performing the testing for anti-HBs can define a 10 mIU/mL concentration to determine protective levels of antibody.

Routine HCV testing should include use of both a screening immunoassay to test for anti-HCV and supplemental or confirmatory testing with an additional, more specific assay. Use of NAT for HCV RNA as the primary test for routine screening is not recommended because few HCV infections will be identified in anti-HCV negative patients. However, if alanine aminotransferase (ALT) levels are persistently abnormal

Table 21–6 Recommended Infection Control Practices for Hemodialysis Units

Infection Control Precautions for All Patients

- Wear disposable gloves when caring for the patient or touching the patient's equipment at the dialysis station; remove gloves and wash hands between each patient or station.
- Items taken into dialysis station should either be disposed of, dedicated for use only on a single patient, or cleaned and disinfected before taken to a common clean area or used on another patient.
    - Nondisposable items that cannot be cleaned and disinfected (e.g., adhesive tape, cloth-covered blood pressure cuffs) should be dedicated for use only on a single patient.
    - Unused medications (including multiple dose vials containing diluents) or supplies (syringes, alcohol swabs, etc.) taken to the patient's station should be used only for that patient and should not be returned to a common clean area or used on other patients.
- When multiple dose medication vials are used (including vials containing diluents), prepare individual patient doses in a clean (centralized) area away from dialysis stations and deliver separately to each patient. Do not carry multiple dose medication vials from station to station.
- Do not use common medication carts to deliver medication to patients. Do not carry medication vials, syringes, alcohol swabs, or supplies in pockets. If trays are used to deliver medication to individual patients, they must be cleaned between patients.
- Clean areas should be clearly designated for the preparation handling and storage of medications and unused supplies and equipment. Clean areas should be clearly separated from contaminated areas where used supplies and equipment are handled. Do not handle and store medications or clean supplies in the same or an adjacent area to that where used equipment or blood samples are handled.
- Use external venous and arterial pressure transducer filters/protectors for each patient treatment to prevent blood contamination of the dialysis machines' pressure monitors. Change filters/protectors between each patient treatment, and do not reuse them. Internal transducer filters do not need to be changed routinely between patients.
- Clean and disinfect the dialysis station (chairs, beds, tables, machines, etc.) between patients.
    - Give special attention to cleaning control panels on the dialysis machines and other surfaces that are frequently touched and potentially contaminated with patients' blood.
    - Discard all fluid and clean and disinfect all surfaces and containers associated with the prime waste (including buckets attached to the machines).
- For dialyzers and blood tubing that will be reprocessed, cap dialyzer ports and clamp tubing. Place all used dialyzers and tubing in leak-proof containers for transport from station to reprocessing or disposal area.

Schedule for Routine Testing for Hepatitis B Virus (HBV) and Hepatitis C Virus (HCV) Infections

Patient Status	On Admission*	Monthly	Semi-Annual	Annual
All patients	HBsAg,[†] Anti-HBc (total)[†] Anti-HBs,[†] Anti-HCV, ALT[†]			
HBV susceptible, including nonresponders to vaccine		HBsAg		
Anti-HBs positive (=10 mIU/mL), anti-HBc negative				Anti-HBs
Anti-HBs and anti-HBc positive		No additional HBV testing needed		
Anti-HCV negative		ALT	Anti-HCV	

*Results of HBV testing should be known before the patient begins dialysis.
[†]HBsAg = hepatitis B surface antigen; Anti-HBc = antibody to hepatitis B core antigen; Anti-HBs = antibody to hepatitis B surface antigen; Anti-HCV = antibody to hepatitis C virus; ALT = alanine aminotransferase.

Hepatitis B Vaccination

- Vaccinate all susceptible patients against hepatitis B.
- Test for anti-HBs 1–2 months after last dose
    - If anti-HBs is <10 mIU/mL, consider patient susceptible, revaccinate with an additional three doses, and retest for anti-HBs.
    - If anti-HBs is >10 mIU/mL, consider immune, and retest annually.
        - Give booster dose of vaccine if anti-HBs declines to <10 mIU/mL and continue to retest annually

Management of HBsAg-Positive Patients

- Follow infection control practices for hemodialysis units for all patients.
- Dialyze HBsAg-positive patients in a separate room using separate machines, equipment, instruments, and supplies.
- Staff members caring for HBsAg-positive patients should not care for HBV susceptible patients at the same time (e.g., during the same shift or during patient changeover).

(From Centers for Disease Control and Prevention. Recommendations for preventing transmission of infections among chronic hemodialysis patients. MMWR Morb Mortal Wkly Rep 2001; 50[No.RR-5]:1–43.)

in anti-HCV negative patients in the absence of another etiology, testing for HCV RNA should be considered. Blood samples collected for NAT should not contain heparin, which interferes with the accurate performance of this assay.

Hepatitis B vaccination is an essential component of prevention in the hemodialysis setting. All susceptible patients and staff should receive hepatitis B vaccine. Susceptible patients who have not yet received hepatitis B vaccine, are in the process of being vaccinated, or have not adequately responded to vaccination should continue to be tested regularly for HBsAg. Detailed recommendations for vaccination and follow-up of hemodialysis patients have been published elsewhere.[135]

Management of Infected Patients

HBV

HBsAg-positive patients should undergo dialysis in a separate room designated only for HBsAg-positive patients. They should use separate machines, equipment, and supplies, and, most importantly, staff members should not care for both HBsAg-positive and susceptible patients on the same shift or at the same time. Dialyzers should not be reused on HBsAg-positive patients. Because HBV is efficiently transmitted through occupational exposure to blood, reprocessing dialyzers from HBsAg-positive patients might place HBV-susceptible staff members at increased risk for infection.

HBV chronically infected patients (i.e., those who are HBsAg positive, total anti-HBc positive, and IgM anti-HBc negative) are infectious to others and are at risk for chronic liver disease. They should be counseled regarding preventing transmission to others, their household and sexual partners should receive hepatitis B vaccine, and they should be evaluated (by consultation or referral, if appropriate) for the presence or development of chronic liver disease according to current medical practice guidelines. Persons with chronic liver disease should be vaccinated against hepatitis A, if susceptible.

HBV chronically infected patients do not require any routine follow-up testing for purposes of infection control. However, annual testing for HBsAg is reasonable to detect the small percentage of HBV-infected patients who might lose their HBsAg.

HCV

HCV transmission within the dialysis environment can be prevented by strict adherence to infection control precautions recommended for all hemodialysis patients (Table 21–6). Although isolation of HCV positive patients is not recommended, routine testing for ALT and anti-HCV is important for monitoring the potential for transmission within centers and ensuring that appropriate precautions are being properly and consistently used. Furthermore, HCV-positive patients can participate in dialyzer reuse programs. Unlike HBV, HCV is not transmitted efficiently through occupational exposures. Thus, reprocessing dialyzers from HCV-positive patients should not place staff members at increased risk for infection.

HCV-positive persons should be evaluated (by consultation or referral, if appropriate) for the presence or development of chronic liver disease according to current medical practice guidelines. They should also receive information concerning how they can prevent further harm to their liver and prevent transmitting HCV to others.[136,137] Persons with chronic liver disease should be vaccinated against hepatitis A, if susceptible.

HDV

Because HDV depends on an HBV-infected host for replication, prevention of HBV infection will prevent HDV infection in a person susceptible to HBV. Patients known to be infected with HDV should be isolated from all other dialysis patients, especially those who are HBsAg positive.

HIV

Infection control precautions recommended for all hemodialysis patients are sufficient to prevent HIV transmission between patients. HIV-infected patients do not have to be isolated from other patients or dialyzed separately on dedicated machines. In addition, they can participate in dialyzer reuse programs. Because HIV is not transmitted efficiently through occupational exposures, reprocessing dialyzers from HIV-positive patients should not place staff members at increased risk for infection.

Bacterial

Contact transmission can be prevented by hand hygiene,[138] glove use, and disinfection of environmental surfaces. Infection control precautions recommended for all hemodialysis patients are adequate to prevent transmission for most patients infected or colonized with pathogenic bacteria, including antimicrobial-resistant strains. However, additional precautions should be considered for treatment of patients who might be at increased risk for transmitting pathogenic bacteria. Such patients include those with either an infected skin wound with drainage that is not contained by dressings (the drainage does not have to be culture positive for MRSA or VRE or any specific pathogen) or fecal incontinence or diarrhea uncontrolled with personal hygiene measures. For these patients, consider using the following additional precautions[135]:

1. Staff members treating the patient should wear a separate gown over their usual clothing and remove the gown when finished caring for the patient.
2. Dialyze the patient at a station with as few adjacent stations as possible (e.g., at the end or corner of the unit).

Vancomycin is used commonly in dialysis patients, in part, because vancomycin can be conveniently administered to patients when they come in for hemodialysis treatments. Prudent antimicrobial use is an important component of the CDC recommendations for preventing the spread of vancomycin resistance.[139] This guideline states that vancomycin is *not* indicated for therapy (chosen for dosing convenience) of infections due to β-lactam-sensitive gram-positive microorganisms in patients with renal failure. Depending on the situation, alternative antimicrobials (e.g., cephalosporins) with dosing intervals greater than 48 hours, which would allow post-dialytic dosing, could be used. Recent studies suggest that cefazolin given three times a week in the dialysis unit provides adequate blood levels and could be used to treat many infections in hemodialysis patients.[140,141]

Disinfection, Sterilization, and Environmental Hygiene

Good cleaning, disinfection, and sterilization procedures are important components of infection control in the hemodialysis center. The procedures do not differ from those recommended for other health care settings,[142,143] but the high potential for blood contamination makes the hemodialysis setting unique. Additionally, the need for routine aseptic access of the patient's vascular system makes the hemodialysis unit more akin to a surgical suite than to a standard hospital room. Medical items are categorized as critical (e.g., needles and catheters), which are introduced directly into the bloodstream or normally sterile areas of the body; semicritical (e.g., fiberoptic endoscopes), which come in contact with intact mucous membranes; and noncritical (e.g., blood pressure cuffs), which touch only intact skin.[138,142]

Cleaning and housekeeping in the dialysis center have two goals: to remove soil and waste on a regular basis, thereby preventing the accumulation of potentially infectious material, and to maintain an environment that is conducive to good patient care. Crowding of patients and overtaxing of staff members may increase the likelihood of microbial transmission. Adequate cleaning may be difficult if there are multiple wires, tubes, and hoses in a small area. There should be enough space to move completely around each patient's dialysis station without interfering with the neighboring stations. Where space is limited, elimination of unneeded items; orderly arrangement of required items; and removal of excess lengths of tubes, hoses, and wires from the floor can improve accessibility for cleaning. Because of the special requirements for cleaning in the dialysis center, staff should be specially trained in this task.

After each patient treatment, frequently touched environmental surfaces, including external surfaces of the dialysis machine, should be cleaned (with a good detergent) or disinfected (with a detergent germicide). It is the cleaning step that is important for interrupting the cross-contamination transmission routes. Antiseptics, such as formulations with povidone-iodine, hexachlorophene, or chlorhexidine, should not be used, because these are formulated for use on skin and are not designed for use on hard surfaces.

There is no evidence that medical waste is any more infectious than residential waste or has caused disease in the community.[144] Wastes from a hemodialysis center that are actually or potentially contaminated with blood should be considered infectious and handled accordingly. Eventually, these items of solid waste should be disposed of properly in an incinerator or sanitary landfill, depending on state or local laws.

Standard protocols for sterilization and disinfection are adequate for processing any items or devices contaminated with blood. Historically, there has been a tendency to use "overkill" strategies for instrument sterilization or disinfection and housekeeping protocols. This is not necessary. The floors in a dialysis center are routinely contaminated with blood, but the protocol for floor cleaning is the same as for floors in other health care settings. Usually, this involves the use of a good detergent-germicide; the formulation can contain a low- or intermediate-level disinfectant.

Blood-borne viruses, such as HBV and HIV, are inactivated by any standard sterilization systems such as standard steam autoclave cycles of 121°C (249.8°F) for 15 minutes, ethylene oxide gas,[142] and low-temperature hydrogen peroxide gas plasma.[145] Large blood spills should be cleaned to remove visible material, and then, the area should receive low- to intermediate-level disinfection after the directions of the germicide manufacturer.

Blood and other specimens, such as peritoneal fluid, from all patients should be handled with care. Peritoneal fluid can contain high levels of HBV and should be handled in the same manner as the patient's blood. Consequently, if the center performs peritoneal dialysis, the same criteria for separating HBsAg-positive patients who are undergoing hemodialysis apply to those undergoing peritoneal dialysis.

HBV has not been grown in tissue cultures, and without a viral assay system, studies on the precise resistance of this virus to various chemical germicides and heat have not been performed. However, the resistance of HBV to heat and chemical germicides may approach that of some other viruses and bacteria but certainly not that of the bacterial endospore or the tubercle bacillus. Further, studies have shown that HBV is not resistant to commonly used high-level and intermediate-level disinfectants.[146,147]

Blood contamination of venous pressure monitors has been implicated in HBV transmission.[148] Therefore, venous pressure transducer filters should be used; these filters should not be reused.

In single-pass artificial kidney machines, the internal fluid pathways are not subject to contamination with blood. Although the fluid pathways that exhaust dialysis fluid from the dialyzer may become contaminated with blood in the event of a dialyzer leak, it is unlikely that this blood contamination will reach a subsequent patient. Therefore, disinfection and rinsing procedures should be designed to control contamination with bacterial rather than blood-borne pathogens.

For dialysis machines that use a dialysate recirculating system (such as some ultrafiltration control machines and those that regenerate the dialysate), a blood leak in a dialyzer, especially a massive leak, can result in contamination of a number of surfaces that will contact the dialysis fluid of subsequent patients. However, the procedures that are normally practiced after each use—draining of the dialysis fluid, subsequent rinsing, and disinfection—will reduce the level of contamination to below infectious levels. In addition, an intact dialyzer membrane will not allow passage of bacteria or viruses. Consequently, if a blood leak does occur with either type of dialysis machine, the standard disinfection procedure used for machines in the dialysis center to control bacterial contamination will also prevent transmission of blood-borne pathogens.

References

1. U.S. Renal Data System 2002 Annual Data Report: Atlas of end-stage renal disease in the United States. Bethesda, MD, National Institutes of Health, National Institute of Diabetes and Digestive and Kidney Diseases, 2002, pp 15–564.
2. Favero MS, Carson LA, Bond WW, Petersen NJ: Pseudomonas aeruginosa: Growth in distilled water from hospitals. Science 1971; 173(999):836–838.
3. Favero MS, Bland LA: Microbiologic principles applied to reprocessing hemodialyzers. *In* Deane N, Wineman RJ, Bemis JA (eds): Guide to Reprocessing of Hemodialyzers. Boston, Martinus Nijhoff, 1986, pp 63–73.

4. Favero MS, Petersen NJ, Boyer KM, et al: Microbial contamination of renal dialysis systems and associated health risks. Trans Am Soc Artif Intern Organs 1974; 20A:175–183.
5. Bolan G, Reingold AL, Carson LA, et al: Infections with mycobacterium chelonei in patients receiving dialysis and using processed hemodialyzers. J Infect Dis 1985; 152:1013–1019.
6. Carson LA, Bland LA, Cusick LB, et al: Prevalence of nontuberculous mycobacteria in water supplies of hemodialysis centers. Appl Environ Microbiol 1988; 54:3122–3125.
7. Lowry P, Beck-Sague CM, Bland L, et al: Mycobacterium chelonae infections among patients receiving high-flux dialysis in a hemodialysis clinic, California. J Infect Dis 1990; 161:85–90.
8. Favero MS, Petersen NJ, Carson LA, et al: Gram-negative water bacteria in hemodialysis systems. Health Laboratory Science 1975; 12:321–334.
9. Bland LA, Favero MS: Microbial contamination control strategies for hemodialysis systems. Oakbrook Terrace, IL, Joint Commission on Accreditation of Healthcare Organizations, Plant, Technology, and Safety Management Series 3, 1989, pp 30–36.
10. Carson LA, Bland LA, Cusick LB, et al: Factors affecting endotoxin levels in fluids associated with hemodialysis procedures. *In* Watson SW, Levin J, Novitsky TJ (eds): Detection of Bacterial Endotoxins with the Limulus Amebocyte Lysate Test. New York, Alan R. Liss, 1987, pp 223–234.
11. Hindman SH, Favero MS, Carson LA, et al: Pyrogenic reactions during haemodialysis caused by extramural endotoxin. Lancet 1975; 2:732–734.
12. Association for the Advancement of Medical Instrumentation. American National Standard. Hemodialysis systems. Arlington, VA, AAMI, 1992.
13. Stamm JM, Engelhard WE, Parsons JE: Microbiological study of water-softener resins. Applied Microbiology 1969; 18:376–386.
14. Tokars JI, Miller ER, Alter MJ, Arduino MJ: National surveillance of dialysis-associated diseases in the United States, 1996. Atlanta, GA, Centers for Disease Control and Prevention, 1998, pp 1–59.
15. Favero MS: Microbiological contaminants. Proceedings of the Association for the Advancement of Medical Instrumentation Technology Assessment Conference: Issues in hemodialysis. Arlington, VA, AAMI, 1981, pp 30–33.
16. Anderson RL, Holland BW, Carr JK, et al: Effect of disinfectants on pseudomonads colonized on the interior surface of PVC pipes. Am J Public Health 1990; 80:17–21.
17. Jackson BM, Beck-Sague CM, Bland LA, et al: Outbreak of pyrogenic reactions and gram-negative bacteremia in a hemodialysis center. Am J Nephrol 1994; 14(2):85–89.
18. Arduino MJ: Microbiologic quality of water used for hemodialysis. Contemp Dial Nephrol 1996; 17:17–19.
19. Arduino MJ: What's new in water treatment standards for hemodialysis? Contemp Dial Nephrol 1997; 18:21–24.
20. Petersen NJ, Boyer KM, Carson LA, Favero MS: Pyrogenic reactions from inadequate disinfection of a dialysis fluid distribution system. Dialysis and Transplantation 1978; 7:52, 57–60.
21. Favero MS, Carson LA, Bond WW, Petersen NJ: Factors that influence microbial contamination of fluids associated with hemodialysis machines. Applied Microbiology 1974; 28:822–830.
22. Petersen NJ, Carson LA, Doto IL, et al: Microbiologic evaluation of a new glutaraldehyde-based disinfectant for hemodialysis systems. Trans Am Soc Artif Intern Organs 1982; 28:287–290.
23. Townsend TR, Wee SB, Bartlett J: Disinfection of hemodialysis machines. Dialysis and Transplantation 1985; 14:274–287.
24. Centers for Disease Control and Prevention. Occupational exposures to formaldehyde in dialysis units. Mor Mortal Wkly Rep 1986; 35(24):399–401.
25. Favero MS, Petersen NJ: Microbiologic guidelines for hemodialysis systems. Dialysis and Transplantation 1977; 6:34–36.
26. Bland LA, Favero MS: Microbiologic and endotoxin considerations in hemodialyzer reprocessing. Arlington, VA, AAMI Standards and Recommended Practices 1993; 3(3):293–300.
27. Association for the Advancement of Medical Instrumentation. American National Standard. Water treatment equipment for hemodialysis applications. Arlington, VA, ANSI/AAMI RD62, 2001.
28. Baz M, Durand C, Ragon A, et al: Using Ultrapure water in hemodialysis delays carpal tunnel syndrome. Int J Artif Organs 1991; 14(11):681–685.
29. Lonnemann G: Chronic inflammation in hemodialysis: The role of contaminated dialysate. Blood Purif 2000; 18(3):214–223.
30. Lonnemann G, Koch KM: Efficacy of ultra-pure dialysate in the therapy and prevention of haemodialysis-associated amyloidosis. Nephrol Dial Transplant 2001; 16(suppl 4):17–22.
31. Canaud B, Bosc JY, Leray H, et al: Microbiologic purity of dialysate: Rationale and technical aspects. Blood Purif 2000; 18(3):200–213.
32. Schiffl H, Lang SM, Bergner A: Ultrapure dialysate reduces dose of recombinant human erythropoietin. Nephron 1999; 83(3): 278–279.
33. Arduino MJ, Bland LA, Aguero SM, et al: Comparison of microbiologic assay methods for hemodialysis fluids. J Clin Microbiol 1991; 29:592–594.
34. Gazenfeldt-Gazit E, Eliahou HE: Endotoxin antibodies in patients on maintenance hemodialysis. Israel J Med Sci 1969; 5:1032–1036.
35. Laude-Sharpe M, Caroff M, Simard L, et al: Induction of IL-1 during hemodialysis: Transmembrane passage of intact endotoxins (LPS). Kidney Int 1990; 38:1089–1094.
36. Henderson LW, Koch KM, Dinarello CA, Shaldon S: Hemodialysis hypotension: The interleukin hypothesis. Blood Purif 1983; 1:3–8.
37. Port FK, VanDeKerkhove KM, Kunkel SL, Kluger MJ: The role of dialysate in the stimulation of interleukin-1 production during clinical hemodialysis. Am J Kidney Dis 1987; 10:118–122.
38. Kantor RJ, Carson LA, Graham DR, et al: Outbreak of pyrogenic reactions at a dialysis center: Association with infusion of heparinized saline solution. Am J Med 1983; 74:449–456.
39. Murphy J, Parker T, Carson L, et al: Outbreaks of bacteremia in hemodialysis patients associated with alteration of dialyzer membranes following chemical disinfection (Abstract). ASAIO Journal 1987; 16:51.
40. Gordon SM, Oettinger CW, Bland LA, et al: Pyrogenic reactions in patients receiving conventional, high-efficiency, or high-flux hemodialysis treatments with bicarbonate dialysate containing high concentrations of bacteria and endotoxin. J Am Soc Nephrol 1992; 2:1436–1444.
41. Pegues DA, Oettinger CW, Bland LA, et al: A prospective study of pyrogenic reactions in hemodialysis patients using bicarbonate dialysis fluids filtered to remove bacteria and endotoxin. J Am Soc Nephrol 1992; 3:1002–1007.
42. Oliver JC, Bland LA, Oettinger CW, et al: Bacteria and endotoxin removal from bicarbonate dialysis fluids for use in conventional, high-efficiency, and high-flux dialysis. Artif Organs 1992; 16:141–145.
43. Centers for Disease Control and Prevention. Outbreaks of gram-negative bacterial bloodstream infections traced to probable contamination of hemodialysis machines: Canada, 1995; United States, 1997; and Israel, 1997. Mor Mortal Wkly Rep 1998; 47:55–59.
44. Tokars JI, Frank M, Alter MJ, Arduino MJ: National surveillance of dialysis-associated diseases in the United States, 2000. Semin Dial 2002; 15(3):162–171.
45. Association for the Advancement of Medical Instrumentation. American National Standard. Reuse of hemodialyzers. Arlington, VA, ANSI/AAMI RD47, 1993.

46. Bland L, Alter M, Favero M, et al: Hemodialyzer reuse: Practices in the United States and implication for infection control. ASAIO Journal 1985; 31:556–559.
47. Favero MS: Distinguishing between high-level disinfection, reprocessing, and sterilization. Association for the Advancement of Medical Instrumentation, Reuse of Disposables: Implications for quality health care and cost containment.Technology assessment report No.6. Arlington, VA, AAMI, 1983, pp 19–23.
48. Alter MJ, Favero MS, Miller JK, et al: National surveillance of dialysis-associated diseases in the United States, 1988. ASAIO Journal 1990; 36:107–118.
49. Bland LA, Ridgeway MR, Aguero SM, et al: Potential bacteriologic and endotoxin hazards associated with liquid bicarbonate concentrate. ASAIO Journal 1987; 33:542–545.
50. Tokars JI, Miller E, Alter MJ, Arduino MJ: National surveillance of dialysis-associated diseases in the United States, 1995. Atlanta, GA, U.S. Department of Health and Human Services, 1998.
51. Gordon S, Tipple M, Bland L, Jarvis W: Pyrogenic reactions associated with the reuse of processed hollow-fiber hemodialyzers. JAMA 1988; 260:2077–2081.
52. Bloembergen WE, Port FK: Epidemiological perspective on infections in chronic dialysis patients. Adv Ren Replace Ther 1996; 3(3):201–207.
53. Bonomo RA, Rice D, Whalen C, et al: Risk factors associated with permanent access-site infections in chronic hemodialysis patients. Infect Control Hosp Epidemiol 1997; 18(11):757–761.
54. Dobkin JF, Miller MH, Steigbigel NH: Septicemia in patients on chronic hemodialysis. Ann Intern Med 1978; 88(1):28–33.
55. Hoen B, Paul-Dauphin A, Hestin D, Kessler M: EPIBACDIAL: A multicenter prospective study of risk factors for bacteremia in chronic hemodialysis patients. J Am Soc Nephrol 1998; 9(5): 869–876.
56. Kaplowitz LG, Comstock JA, Landwehr DM, et al: A prospective study of infections in hemodialysis patients: Patient hygiene and other risk factors for infection. Infect Control Hosp Epidemiol 1988; 9(12):534–541.
57. Keane WF, Shapiro FL, Raij L: Incidence and type of infections occurring in 445 chronic hemodialysis patients. Trans Am Soc Artif Intern Organs 1977; 23:41–47.
58. Kessler M, Hoen B, Mayeux D, et al: Bacteremia in patients on chronic hemodialysis: A multicenter prospective survey. Nephron 1993; 64(1):95–100.
59. Stevenson KB, Adcox MJ, Mallea MC, et al: Standardized surveillance of hemodialysis vascular access infections: 18-month experience at an outpatient, multifacility hemodialysis center. Infect Control Hosp Epidemiol 2000; 21(3):200–203.
60. Tokars JI, Light P, Armistead N, et al: Vascular access infections among hemodialysis outpatients. Am J Kidney Dis 2001; 37:1232–1240.
61. Tokars JI: Bloodstream infections in hemodialysis patients: Getting some deserved attention. Infect Control Hosp Epidemiol 2002; 23(12):713–715.
62. Tokars JI, Miller ER, Stein G: New national surveillance system for hemodialysis-associated infections: Initial results. Am J Infect Control 2002; 30(5):288–295.
63. Tokars JI, Alter MJ, Arduino MJ: Nosocomial infections in hemodialysis units: Strategies for control. *In* Jacobsen H, Striker G, Klahr S (eds): The Principles and Practice of Nephrology. St. Louis, Mosby, 1995, pp 337–357.
64. Grohskopf LA, Roth VR, Feikin DR, et al: Serratia liquefaciens bloodstream infections from contamination of epoetin alfa at a hemodialysis center. N Engl J Med 2001; 344(20):1491–1497.
65. Padberg FT Jr, Lee BC, Curl GR: Hemoaccess site infection. Surgery, Gynecology, and Obstetrics 1992; 174:103–108.
66. Stevenson KB, Hannah EL, Lowder CA, et al: Epidemiology of hemodialysis vascular access infections from longitudinal infection surveillance data: Predicting the impact of NKF-DOQI clinical practice guidelines for vascular access. Am J Kidney Dis 2002; 39(3):549–555.
67. Besarab A, Bolton WK, Browne JK, et al: The effects of normal as compared with low hematocrit values in patients with cardiac disease who are receiving hemodialysis and epoetin. N Engl J Med 1998; 339(9):584–590.
68. Fan PY, Schwab SJ: Vascular access: Concepts for the 1990s. J Am Soc Nephrol 1992; 3(1):1–11.
69. Powe NR, Jaar B, Furth SL, et al: Septicemia in dialysis patients: Incidence, risk factors, and prognosis. Kidney Int 1999; 55(3):1081–1090.
70. National Kidney Foundation. K/DOQI clinical practice guidelines for vascular access, 2000. Am J Kidney Dis 2001; 37(suppl 1):S137–S181.
71. Centers for Disease Control and Prevention. Guidelines for the prevention of intravascular catheter-related infections. MMWR Morb Mortal Wkly Rep 2002; 51(No.RR-10):1–29.
72. Berns JS, Tokars JI: Preventing bacterial infections and antimicrobial resistance in dialysis patients. Am J Kidney Dis 2002; 40(5):886–898.
73. Mermel LA, Farr BM, Sherertz RJ, et al: Guidelines for the management of intravascular catheter-related infections. Clin Infect Dis 2001; 32(9):1249–1272.
74. Uttley AH, George RC, Naidoo J, et al: High-level vancomycin-resistant enterococci causing hospital infections. Epidemiol Infect 1989; 103(1):173–181.
75. Brady JP, Snyder JW, Hasbargen JA: Vancomycin-resistant enterococcus in end-stage renal disease. Am J Kidney Dis 1998; 32(3):415–418.
76. Roghmann MC, Fink JC, Polish L, et al: Colonization with vancomycin-resistant enterococci in chronic hemodialysis patients. Am J Kidney Dis 1998; 32(2):254–257.
77. Fishbane S, Cunha BA, Mittal SK, et al: Vancomycin-resistant enterococci in hemodialysis patients is related to intravenous vancomycin use. Infect Control Hosp Epidemiol 1999; 20(7):461–462.
78. Dopirak M, Hill C, Oleksiw M, et al: Surveillance of hemodialysis-associated primary bloodstream infections: The experience of ten hospital-based centers. Infect Control Hosp Epidemiol 2002; 23(12):721–724.
79. Taylor G, Gravel D, Johnston L, et al: Prospective surveillance for primary bloodstream infections occurring in Canadian hemodialysis units. Infect Control Hosp Epidemiol 2002; 23(12):716–720.
80. Fridkin SK: Vancomycin-intermediate and -resistant Staphylococcus aureus: What the infectious disease specialist needs to know. Clin Infect Dis 2001; 32(1):108–115.
81. Chang S, Sievert DM, Hageman JC, et al: Infection with vancomycin-resistant Staphylococcus aureus containing the vanA resistance gene. N Engl J Med 2003; 348(14): 1342–1347.
82. Centers for Disease Control and Prevention. Hepatitis: Control measures for hepatitis B in dialysis centers. HEW Publication No.[CDC] 78-8358 (Viral Hepatitis Investigations and Control Series). Atlanta, GA, Centers for Disease Control and Prevention, 1977.
83. Alter MJ, Favero MS, Petersen NJ, et al: National surveillance of dialysis-associated hepatitis and other diseases, 1976 and 1980. Dialysis and Transplantation 1983; 12:860–865.
84. Centers for Disease Control. Recommendations of the Immunization Practices Advisory Committee(ACIP): Inactivated hepatitis B virus vaccine. MMWR Morb Mortal Wkly Rep 1982; 31:317–322, 327–328.
85. Tokars JI, Miller ER, Alter MJ, Arduino MJ: National surveillance of dialysis-associated diseases in the United States, 1997. Semin Dial 2000; 13(2):75–85.

86. Alter HJ, Seeff LB, Kaplan PM, et al: Type B hepatitis: The infectivity of blood positive for e antigen and DNA polymerase after accidental needlestick exposure. N Engl J Med 1976; 295(17): 909–913.
87. Shikata T, Karasawa T, Abe K, et al: Hepatitis B e antigen and infectivity of hepatitis B virus. J Infect Dis 1977; 136:571–576.
88. Bond WW, Favero MS, Petersen NJ, et al: Survival of hepatitis B virus after drying and storage for one week. Lancet 1981; 1:550–551.
89. Favero MS, Bond WW, Petersen NJ, et al: Detection methods for study of the stability of hepatitis B antigen on surfaces. J Infect Dis 1974; 129(2):210–212.
90. Favero MS, Maynard JE, Petersen NJ, et al: Hepatitis-B antigen on environmental surfaces (Letter). Lancet 1973; 2:1455.
91. Snydman DR, Bryan JA, Macon EJ, Gregg MB: Hemodialysis-associated hepatitis: Report of an epidemic with further evidence on mechanisms of transmission. Am J Epidemiol 1976; 104:563–570.
92. Niu MT, Penberthy LT, Alter MJ, et al: Hemodialysis-associated hepatitis B: Report of an outbreak. Dialysis and Transplantation 1989; 18:542–555.
93. Centers for Disease Control and Prevention. Outbreaks of hepatitis B virus infection among hemodialyis patients—California, Nebraska, and Texas, 1994. MMWR Morb Mortal Wkly Rep 1996; 45:285–289.
94. Alter MJ, Ahtone J, Maynard JE: Hepatitis B virus transmission associated with a multiple-dose vial in a hemodialysis unit. Ann Intern Med 1983; 99:330–333.
95. Carl M, Francis DP, Maynard JE: A common-source outbreak of hepatitis B in a hemodialysis unit. Dialysis and Transplantation 1983; 12:222–229.
96. Kantor RJ, Hadler SC, Schreeder MT, et al: Outbreak of hepatitis B in a dialysis unit, complicated by false positive HBsAg test results. Dialysis and Transplantation 1979; 8:232–235.
97. Anonymous. Decrease in the incidence of hepatitis in dialysis units associated with prevention programme: Public health laboratory survey. BMJ 1974; 4:751–754.
98. Najem GR, Louria DB, Thind IS, Lavenhar MA, Gocke DJ, Baskin SE et al. Control of hepatitis B infection. The role of surveillance and an isolation hemodialysis center. JAMA 1981; 245:153-157.
99. Alter MJ, Favero MS, Maynard JE: Impact of infection control strategies on the incidence of dialysis-associated hepatitis in the United States. J Infect Dis 1986; 153:1149–1151.
100. Tokars JI, Alter MJ, Miller E, et al: National surveillance of dialysis associated diseases in the United States, 1994. ASAIO Journal 1997; 43:108–119.
101. Hutin YJ, Goldstein ST, Varma JK, et al: An outbreak of hospital-acquired hepatitis B virus infection among patients receiving chronic hemodialysis. Infect Control Hosp Epidemiol 1999; 20(11):731–735.
102. Centers for Disease Control and Prevention. Hepatitis B virus: A comprehensive strategy for eliminating transmission in the United States through universal childhood vaccination. Recommendations of the Immunization Practices Advisory Committee (ACIP). MMWR Morb Mortal Wkly Rep 1991; 40(No. RR-13):1–25.
103. Hoofnagle JH, Di Bisceglie AM: Serologic diagnosis of acute and chronic viral hepatitis. Semin Liver Dis 1991; 11(2):73–83.
104. Dienstag JL, Schiff ER, Wright TL, et al: Lamivudine as initial treatment for chronic hepatitis B in the United States. N Engl J Med 1999; 341(17):1256–1263.
105. Lai C-L, Chien R-N, Leung NWY, et al: Asia Hepatitis Lamivudine Study Group. A one-year trial of lamivudine for chronic hepatitis B. N Engl J Med 1998; 339:61–68.
106. Kloster B, Kramer R, Eastlund T, et al: Hepatitis B surface antigenemia in blood donors following vaccination. Transfusion 1995; 35(6):475–477.
107. Lunn ER, Hoggarth BJ, Cook WJ: Prolonged hepatitis B surface antigenemia after vaccination. Pediatrics 2000; 105(6):E81.
108. McMahon BJ, Alberts SR, Wainwright RB, et al: Hepatitis B-related sequelae. Prospective study in 1400 hepatitis B surface antigen-positive Alaska native carriers. Arch Intern Med 1990; 150(5):1051–1054.
109. Hadler SC, Murphy BL, Schable CA, et al: Epidemiological analysis of the significance of low-positive test results for antibody to hepatitis B surface and core antigens. J Clin Microbiol 1984; 19(4):521–525.
110. Levine OS, Vlahov D, Koehler J, et al: Seroepidemiology of hepatitis B virus in a population of injecting drug users. Association with drug injection patterns. Am J Epidemiol 1995; 142(3): 331–341.
111. Silva AE, McMahon BJ, Parkinson AJ, et al: Hepatitis B virus DNA in persons with isolated antibody to hepatitis B core antigen who subsequently received hepatitis B vaccine. Clin Infect Dis 1998; 26(4):895–897.
112. McMahon BJ, Parkinson AJ, Helminiak C, et al: Response to hepatitis B vaccine of persons positive for antibody to hepatitis B core antigen. Gastroenterology 1992; 103(2):590–594.
113. Lai C-L, Lau JY, Yeoh E-K, et al: Significance of isolated anti-HBc seropositivity by ELISA: Implications and the role of radioimmunoassay. J Med Virol 1992; 36:180–183.
114. Niu MT, Coleman PJ, Alter MJ: Multicenter study of hepatitis C virus infection in chronic hemodialysis patients and hemodialysis center staff members. Am J Kidney Dis 1993; 22(4): 568–573.
115. Fabrizi F, Lunghi G, Guarnori I, et al: Incidence of seroconversion for hepatitis C virus in chronic haemodialysis patients: A prospective study. Nephrol Dial Transplant 1994; 9(11):1611–1615.
116. Fabrizi F, Martin P, Dixit V, et al: Acquisition of hepatitis C virus in hemodialysis patients: A prospective study by branched DNA signal amplification assay. Am J Kidney Dis 1998; 31(4):647–654.
117. Pinto dos Santos J, Loureiro A, Cendoroglo N, Pereira BJG: Impact of dialysis room and reuse strategies on the incidence of hepatitis C virus infection in haemodialysis units. Nephrol Dial Transplant 1996; 11:2017–2022.
118. Forns X, Fernandez-Llama P, Pons M, et al: Incidence and risk factors of hepatitis C virus infection in a haemodialysis unit. Nephrol Dial Transplant 1997; 12(4):736–740.
119. McLaughlin KJ, Cameron SO, Good T, et al: Nosocomial transmission of hepatitis C virus within a British dialysis centre. Nephrol Dial Transplant 1997; 12(2):304–309.
120. Petrosilla N, Gilli P, Serraino D, et al: Prevalence of infected patients and understaffing have a role in hepatitis C virus transmission in dialysis. Am J Kidney Dis 2001; 35(5):1004–1010.
121. Sivapalasingam S, Malak SF, Sullivan JF, et al: High prevalence of hepatitis C infection among patients receiving hemodialysis at an urban dialysis center. Infect Control Hosp Epidemiol 2002; 23(6):319–324.
122. Hardy NM, Sandroni S, Danielson S, Wilson WJ: Antibody to hepatitis C virus increases with time on hemodialysis. Clin Nephrol 1992; 38(1):44–48.
123. Selgas R, Martinez-Zapico R, Bajo MA, et al: Prevalence of hepatitis C antibodies (HCV) in a dialysis population at one center. Perit Dial Int 1992; 12:28–30.
124. Alter MJ: The epidemiology of acute and chronic hepatitis C. Clinics in Liver Disease 1997; 1:559–568.
125. Alter MJ: Prevention of spread of hepatitis C. Hepatology 2002; 36(5 suppl 1):S93–S98.
126. Centers for Disease Control and Prevention. Guidelines for laboratory testing and result reporting of antibody to hepatitis C virus. MMWR Morb Mortal Wkly Rep 2003; 52(No. RR-3):1–15.
127. Busch MP, Kleinman SH, Jackson B, et al: Committee report. Nucleic acid amplification testing of blood donors for transfusion-transmitted infectious diseases: Report of the

Interorganizational Task Force on nucleic acid amplification testing of blood donors. Transfusion 2000; 40(2):143–159.

128. Williams IT, Gretch D, Fleenor M, et al: Hepatitis C virus RNA concentration and chronic hepatitis in a cohort of patients followed after developing acute hepatitis C. *In* Margolis HS, Alter MJ, Liang TJ, Dienstag JL (eds): Viral Hepatitis and Liver Disease. Atlanta, GA, International Medical Press, 2002, pp 341–344.
129. Alter MJ, Margolis HS, Krawczynski K, et al: The natural history of community-acquired hepatitis C in the United States. N Engl J Med 1992; 327:1899–1905.
130. Thomas DL, Astemborski J, Rai RM, et al: The natural history of hepatitis C virus infection: Host, viral, and environmental factors. JAMA 2000; 284(4):450–456.
131. Larghi A, Zuin M, Crosignani A, et al: Outcome of an outbreak of acute hepatitis C among healthy volunteers participating in pharmacokinetics studies. Hepatology 2002; 36(4 pt 1): 993–1000.
132. Hadler SC, Fields HA: Hepatitis delta virus. *In* Belshe RB (ed): Textbook of Human Virology. St. Louis, MO, Mosby, 1991, pp 749–765.
133. Lettau LA, Alfred HJ, Glew RH, et al: Nosocomial transmission of delta hepatitis. Ann Intern Med 1986; 104(5):631–635.
134. Velandia M, Fridkin SK, Cardenas V, et al: Transmission of HIV in dialysis centre. Lancet 1995; 345(8962):1417–1422.
135. Centers for Disease Control and Prevention. Recommendations for preventing transmission of infections among chronic hemodialysis patients. MMWR Morb Mortal Wkly Rep 2001; 50(No.RR-5):1–43.
136. Centers for Disease Control and Prevention. Recommendations for prevention and control of hepatitis C virus (HCV) infection and HCV-related chronic disease. MMWR Recommendations and Reports 1998; 47(RR-19):1–39.
137. National Institutes of Health. Chronic hepatitis C: Current disease management. Bethesda, MD, National Institute of Diabetes and Digestive and Kidney Diseases, 2000, pp 1–21.
138. Boyce JM, Pittet D: Guideline for hand hygiene in health-care settings. Recommendations of the Healthcare Infection Control Practices Advisory Committee and the HICPAC/SHEA/APIC/IDSA Hand Hygiene Task Force. Am J Infect Control 2002; 30(8):S1–S46.
139. Centers for Disease Control and Prevention. Recommendations for preventing the spread of vancomycin resistance. MMWR Morb Mortal Wkly Rep 1995; 44(No. RR-12):1–13.
140. Fogel MA, Nussbaum PB, Feintzeig ID, et al: Use of cefazolin in chronic hemodialysis patients: A safe and effective alternative to vancomycin. Am J Kidney Dis 1998; 32(3):401–409.
141. Marx MA, Frye RF, Matzke GR, Golper TA: Cefazolin as empiric therapy in hemodialysis-related infections: Efficacy and blood concentrations. Am J Kidney Dis 1998; 32(3):410–414.
142. Favero MS, Bond WW: Chemical disinfection of medical and surgical materials. *In* Block SS (ed): Disinfection, Sterilization and Preservation, 4th ed. Philadelphia, Lea & Febiger, 1991, pp 617–641.
143. Favero MS, Bolyard EA: Microbiologic considerations. Disinfection and sterilization strategies and the potential for airborne transmission of bloodborne pathogens. Surg Clin North Am 1995; 75(6):1071–1089.
144. Centers for Disease Control and Prevention. Recommendations for prevention of HIV transmission in health-care settings. MMWR Morb Mortal Wkly Rep 1987; 36:1S–18S.
145. Roberts C, Antonoplos P: Inactivation of human immunodeficiency virus type 1 (HIV-1), hepatitis A virus (HAV), respiratory syncytial virus (RSV), vaccinia virus, herpes simplex virus type 1 (HSV-1), and poliovirus type 2 by hydrogen peroxide gas sterilization. Am J Infect Control 1998; 26: 94–101.
146. Bond WW, Favero MS, Petersen NJ, Ebert JW: Inactivation of hepatitis B virus by intermediate- to high-level disinfectant chemicals. J Clin Microbiol 1983; 18:535–538.
147. Sattar SA, Tetro J, Springthorpe VS, Giulivi A: Preventing the spread of hepatitis B and C viruses: Where are germicides relevant? Am J Infect Control 2001; 29(3):187–197.
148. Centers for Disease Control and Prevention. Outbreak of hepatitis B in a dialysis center. Epidemic Investigation Report EPI 91-17. Atlanta, GA, Centers for Disease Control and Prevention, 1993.
149. Centers for Disease Control and Prevention. Pyrogenic reactions and gram-negative bacteremia in patients in a hemodialysis center. Epidemic Investigation Report EPI 91-37. Atlanta, GA, Centers for Disease Control and Prevention, 1991.
150. Centers for Disease Control and Prevention. Bacteremia in hemodialysis patients. Epidemic Investigation Report EPI 92-10. Atlanta, GA, Centers for Disease Control and Prevention, 1992.
151. Jochimsen EM, Frenette C, Delorme M, et al: A cluster of bloodstream infections and pyrogenic reactions among hemodialysis patients traced to dialysis machine waste-handling option units. Am J Nephrol 1998; 18(6):485–489.
152. Wang S, Levine RB, Carson LA, et al: An outbreak of gram-negative bacteremia in hemodialysis patients traced to hemodialysis machine waste drain ports. Infect Control Hospital Epidemiol 1999; 20:746–751.
153. Centers for Disease Control and Prevention. Clusters of bacteremia and pyrogenic reactions in hemodialysis patients—Georgia. Epidemic Investigation Report EPI 86-65. Atlanta, GA, Centers for Disease Control and Prevention, 1987.
154. Beck-Sague CM, Jarvis WR, Bland LA, et al: Outbreak of gram-negative bacteremia and pyrogenic reactions in a hemodialysis center. Am J Nephrol 1990; 10:397–403.
155. Centers for Disease Control. Bacteremia associated with reuse of disposable hollow-fiber hemodialyzers. MMWR Morb Mortal Wkly Rep 1986; 35:417–418.
156. Welbel SF, Schoendorf K, Bland LA, et al: An outbreak of gram-negative bloodstream infections in chronic hemodialysis patients. Am J Nephrol 1995; 15:1–4.
157. Centers for Disease Control and Prevention. Pyrogenic reactions in patients undergoing high-flux hemodialysis—California. Epidemic Investigation Report EPI 86-80. Atlanta, GA, Centers for Disease Control and Prevention, 1987.
158. Centers for Disease Control and Prevention. Pyrogenic reactions in hemodialysis patients on high-flux hemodialysis—California. Epidemic Investigation Report EPI 87-12. Atlanta, GA, Centers for Disease Control and Prevention, 1987.
159. Rudnick JR, Arduino MJ, Bland LA, et al: An outbreak of pyrogenic reactions in chronic hemodialysis patients associated with hemodialyzer reuse. Artif Organs 1995; 19:289–294.
160. Snydman DR, Bryan JA, London WT, et al: Transmission of hepatitis B associated with hemodialysis: Role of malfunction (blood leaks) in dialysis machines. J Infect Dis 1976; 134(6):562–570.
161. Alter MJ, Ahtone J, Maynard JE: Hepatitis B virus transmission associated with a multiple-dose vial in a hemodialysis unit. Ann Intern Med 1983; 99:330–333.
162. Centers for Disease Control and Prevention. Non-A, non-B hepatitis in a dialysis center, Nashville, Tennessee. Epidemic Investigation Report EPI 78-96. Phoenix, AZ, Centers for Disease Control and Prevention, 1979.
163. Niu MT, Alter MJ, Kristensen C, Margolis HS: Outbreak of hemodialysis-associated non-A, non-B hepatitis and correlation with antibody to hepatitis C virus. Am J Kidney Dis 1992; 19:345–352.
164. Centers for Disease Control and Prevention. Possible ongoing transmission of hepatitis C virus in a hemodialysis unit.

Epidemic Investigation Report EPI 99-38. Atlanta, GA, Centers for Disease Control and Prevention, 1999.

165. Centers for Disease Control and Prevention. Transmission of hepatitis C virus among hemodialysis patients. Epidemic Investigation Report EPI 2000. Atlanta, GA, Centers for Disease Control and Prevention, 2000.

166. Centers for Disease Control and Prevention. Transmission of hepatitis C virus in a hemodialysis unit. Epidemic Investigation Report EPI 2000-64. Atlanta, GA, Centers for Disease Control and Prevention, 2000.

Chapter 22

Acute Complications Associated with Hemodialysis

Orfeas Liangos, M.D. • Brian J.G. Pereira, M.D., M.B.A. • Bertrand L. Jaber, M.D.

Since first successfully performed in 1945,[1] hemodialysis (HD) has become a routine procedure. However, despite significant improvements in HD equipment and improvement in patient monitoring, acute complications can still occur during the therapy. This chapter will review acute complications that are encountered during or are directly related to HD. The chronic complications of dialysis have been extensively reviewed elsewhere.[2,3]

DIALYSIS REACTIONS

Adverse reactions occurring during HD may be caused by the exposure of patient blood to surface components of the extracorporeal circuit including the dialyzer, tubing, as well as other compounds used in the manufacturing and sterilization processes. This interaction between the patient's blood and the extracorporeal system can lead to various adverse reactions that can range in severity from mild to life-threatening anaphylactic/anaphylactoid reactions (Table 22–1).[4]

LIFE-THREATENING ANAPHYLACTIC/ ANAPHYLACTOID REACTIONS

Anaphylaxis is the result of an immunoglobulin E (IgE)-mediated acute allergic reaction in a sensitized patient, whereas anaphylactoid reactions result from the direct release of mediators by host cells. Symptoms typically develop within the first 5 minutes of dialysis initiation, although they may be delayed by up to 20 minutes. The severity can range from mild to life threatening and can encompass a burning or heat sensation throughout the body or at the access site, dyspnea, chest pressure or tightness, angioedema/laryngeal edema, acral or oral paresthesias, rhinorrhea, lacrimation, sneezing or coughing, flushing, pruritus, nausea/vomiting, abdominal cramps, and diarrhea. A history of atopy, elevated total serum IgE, eosinophilia, and the use of angiotensin converting enzyme (ACE) inhibitors as well as, but less frequently, angiotensin receptor blockers predispose the patient to such reactions.[5,6] The etiology of dialysis reactions (DR) is diverse and requires prompt investigation to help prevent further reactions.

Leachables

Allergy to Ethylene Oxide: "First Use Syndrome"

Ethylene oxide (ETO), the dialyzer manufacturer's gas sterilant, can cause DR by acting as a hapten through binding to albumin. Specific IgE antibodies against ETO conjugated to human serum albumin (HSA) have been detected using a radioallergosorbent test (RAST).[7] However, only two-thirds of patients with such reactions have circulating IgE antibodies against ETO-HSA, whereas one-third do not. Circulating levels of anti-ETO-HSA IgE antibodies can be detected in up to 10% of patients with no prior history of DR.[8] The potting compound used to anchor the hollow fibers in the dialyzer housing acts as a reservoir for ETO and may impede its washout from the dialyzer. ETO may still be detectable after long periods of thorough rinsing of the dialyzer.[9] Furthermore, delayed entry of ETO into the priming fluid has also been observed, and dialyzer reprocessing prior to first use has reduced the incidence of these reactions.[4] Testing for ETO-specific IgE antibodies may be helpful if an ETO allergy is suspected.[10] Once the diagnosis has been confirmed or is highly suspected, ETO-sterilized dialyzers should be replaced with gamma- or steam-sterilized dialyzers. A recent survey suggests that allergic reactions to ETO have become less frequent.[11]

Dialyzer's Reuse Reactions: "Reuse Syndromes"

Most residual ETO is washed out of the dialyzer during "first use" and with subsequent reprocessing. Thus, reuse reactions are more likely to be due to other agents, such as the germicides used for dialyzer reprocessing. Commonly used germicides include formaldehyde, glutaraldehyde, and peracetic acid/hydrogen peroxide. Formaldehyde is a known allergen, and life-threatening reactions have been observed in HD patients in whom the RAST to formaldehyde was positive.[6,12] Exposure may also result from residual formaldehyde after disinfection of the water supply system.[13]

Other Leachables

Isopropyl myristate used in the solution spinning process of hollow fiber fabrication, isocyanates found in the potting compound, and nonendotoxin LAL-reactive material believed to be cellulose in nature and found during rinsing of cellulose hollow-fiber dialyzers have also been suspected to cause DR.[4]

Membrane Bioincompatibility

Evidence to support the hypothesis that life-threatening reactions follow complement activation during dialysis with unsubstituted cellulose membranes has been disputed.[4] Indeed, although complement activation does occur during dialysis, it does not prove causality because severe anaphylaxis results in complement activation.[14] However, it is possible that

Table 22–1 Development, Management, and Prevention of Dialysis Reactions

Dialysis Reaction	Onset During Hemodialysis	Etiology	Course of Action	Prevention
Life-threatening anaphylactic/anaphylactoid	5-20 minutes	Ethylene oxide (first-use dialyzer syndrome) Germicide (reuse dialyzer syndrome) AN69 dialyzer and ACE inhibitor interaction Renalin dialyzer reuse and ACE inhibitor interaction Medications (parenteral iron, heparin)	Stop hemodialysis Do not return blood to patient Epinephrine Corticosteroids Antihistamines	Rinse dialyzer before use Use gamma/steam sterilized dialyzer Discontinue dialyzer reuse Avoid AN69 dialyzer with ACE inhibitor Discontinue reuse with renalin Use test dose for parenteral iron
Non-life threatening	20-40 minutes	Complement activation	Continue hemodialysis	Use noncellulose dialyzer membrane
Pyrogen	Anytime	Endotoxin/bacterial contamination	Stop hemodialysis if hypotension present Blood cultures Antibiotics Antipyretics	Preventive strategies (Table 22–3)

secondary or concomitant release of complement fragments may amplify an IgE-mediated ETO reaction, for instance, by enhancing release of histamine or other mediators.[15]

Bradykinin-Mediated Reactions

Polyacrylonitrile (PAN) is a negatively charged synthetic membrane, which is composed of a copolymer of acrylonitrile and an aryl sulfonate.[16] In the 1990s, severe anaphylactoid reactions were reported in patients dialyzed with PAN membranes who were also taking ACE inhibitors.[17,18] Binding of Hageman factor (Factor XII) to a negatively charged membrane leads to formation of kallikrein from prekallikrein and the subsequent release of kinins (i.e., bradykinin) from kininogen. Although cuprophan and polymethyl methacrylate (PMMA) membranes display an ability to activate factor XII, PAN activates it to a greater extent.[19] Bradykinin, a molecule with a very short half-life, in turn, activates production of prostaglandin and histamine release, with subsequent vasodilatation and increased vascular permeability.[20] ACE inactivates bradykinin and, therefore, ACE inhibitors can prolong the biologic activities of bradykinin, which are highly calcium-dependent.[4]

Several anaphylactoid reactions have also been reported in patients dialyzed with bleach reprocessed polysulfone (PS) membranes and treated with ACE inhibitors.[21] These reactions ceased once the use of bleach was discontinued. Furthermore, a cluster of anaphylactoid reactions was observed in patients dialyzed with different membranes who were also taking ACE inhibitors.[22] Hydrogen peroxide/peracetic acid was the reprocessing agent used, and the reactions abated once reprocessing was discontinued, despite continued use of ACE inhibitors.[23]

Dialysate Factors

The use of acetate dialysate has been implicated in DR, and proposed mechanisms include interleukin 1 (IL-1) production by monocytes and prostaglandin/adenosine-mediated mechanisms.[4] Conversely, bicarbonate dialysate is highly susceptible to bacterial contamination, and bacterial products present in the dialysate can diffuse across both high-flux and low-flux membranes[24,25] (see "Bacterial Contamination"). Further, reprocessing of dialyzers, particularly with bleach, can increase the likelihood of reverse transfer of bacterial products from the dialysate to blood.[24] These bacterial products can induce cytokine release by monocytes and, consequently, pyrogen reactions (PR). Although PR during dialysis are reported with a high frequency in dialysis units that use high-flux or reprocessed dialyzers,[26] some authors suggest that they do not cause life-threatening reactions.[27]

Drug-Induced Reactions

Iron Dextran

Dextran, a mixture of synthetic glucose polymers has been associated with systemic reactions.[28] Anaphylactic reactions to iron dextran are due to this compound and occur in 0.6% to 1% of recipients.[4] The incidence of anaphylactic reactions is expected to rise, in view of the increasing need for parenteral iron therapy in erythropoietin-treated HD patients who suffer from absolute or functional iron deficiency.[29] The precise mechanisms responsible for dextran-induced anaphylactoid reactions are elusive, but there seems to be dose-dependent basophil histamine release that may account for the cardiovascular collapse.[4] Due to this dose-related toxicity, iron dextran should always be initiated as a 0.5- to 1-mg test dose, with staff available to respond to reactions. If the test dose is uneventful, a course of therapy can then be given safely (i.e., 100-200 mg/dialysis session for 10 doses).[30] Intravenous iron gluconate or saccharate are alternatives for patients with severe iron deficiency anemia who are allergic to iron dextran.[31]

Heparin

Patients rarely exhibit hypersensitivity to heparin formulations but usually respond by substituting beef with pork heparin or vice versa.[4] Heparin reduces aldosterone secretion by a direct action on the adrenal gland, leading to hyperkalemia. It is not clear, however, whether this effect is due to heparin or its preservative chlorbutol.[32] The resultant hyperkalemia may be clinically-significant in patients with underlying chronic kidney disease.[33] However, this phenomenon has not been studied in the dialysis population, and heparin-associated complications are mainly related to bleeding (see "Hemorrhage") of thrombocytopenia (see "Hematologic Complications").

Desferrioxamine

Desferrioxamine therapy for aluminum or iron chelation can produce hypotension during dialysis or rare allergic reactions, gastrointestinal disturbances, loss of vision, auditory toxicity, bone pain, or exacerbation of aluminum encephalopathy.[34]

Treatment and Prevention

The treatment of severe anaphylactic and anaphylactoid reaction is similar and requires immediate cessation of HD without returning the extracorporeal blood to the patient's circulation. Antihistamines (H_1- and H_2-antagonists), epinephrine, corticosteroids, and respiratory support should be provided, if needed.[35] Specific preventive measures include rinsing the dialyzer immediately before first use, substituting ETO with gamma- or steam-sterilized dialyzers, and avoiding PAN membranes in patients on ACE inhibitors.

MILD REACTIONS

Mild reactions consisting of chest/back pain often occur 20 to 40 minutes after initiation of HD. They are not characterized by anaphylactic or allergic reactions, and dialysis can usually be continued. Symptoms usually abate after the 1st hour, suggesting a relation to the degree of complement activation.[36] Indeed, these reactions decrease with the use of substituted and reprocessed unsubstituted cellulose membranes, particularly when bleach has been omitted from the reuse procedure.[4] Some studies suggest that the incidence of chest/back pain parallels the degree of complement activation and increases with larger surface-area dialyzers.[4] However, a randomized crossover study comparing two similar size unsubstituted cellulose and PAN dialyzers showed no difference in these reactions between the two membranes, in spite of differences in complement activation.[37] Treatment with oxygen and analgesics is usually sufficient, and preventive measures include automated cleansing of new dialyzers or using non-cellulose membranes.

MICROBIAL CONTAMINATION

Naturally occurring water bacteria commonly found in HD water systems include gram-negative bacteria (GNB) such as *Pseudomonas* species and nontuberculous mycobacteria. GNB release endotoxin or lipopolysaccharide (LPS) and other bacterial products, and nontuberculous mycobacteria are highly resistant to germicides.[4] Several factors that are operative during dialysis place patients at risk for exposure to bacteria and/or bacterial products, including contaminated water or bicarbonate dialysate, improperly sterilized dialyzers, and cannulation of infected grafts or fistulas.

Bicarbonate-containing solutions are highly susceptible to bacterial contamination.[4] If stored for too long, sodium bicarbonate breaks down to sodium carbonate, which, along with glucose contained in the dialysate, constitute a growth medium for bacteria. When GNB reach excessively high concentrations in the dialysate, serious health risks to patients, including PR with or without bacteremia can result.[38] Indeed, outbreaks of clusters of infection in HD patients have been ascribed to bacterial contamination (Table 22–2). The passage of endotoxin from the dialysate into the blood can occur by diffusion or convection. The use of high-flux dialyzers, especially those reprocessed with bleach (which increases the permeability), increases the risk of passage of endotoxin, particularly lipid A (~2000 Da), the active moiety of LPS, from dialysate into blood. LPS interacts with plasma LPS Binding Protein (LBP) and mediates cytokine production by interacting with the monocyte CD14 receptor.[39] The subsequent release of pyrogenic cytokines, such as interleukin-1, and tumor necrosis factor produce a transient febrile reaction.

Reprocessing of dialyzers has become a common practice in the United States because of decreased cost, improved biocompatibility, and fewer patient symptoms.[4] However, despite general safety of the procedure, PR and bacteremia may supervene. Reprocessing involves rinsing, cleaning, testing, and sterilizing hollow-fiber dialyzers. PR due to reprocessing have been attributed to improper disinfection procedures, inadequate potency of the solution used to disinfect the dialyzer, and inadequate measures to disinfect the O-rings of dialyzers with removable headers.[4] In a survey by the Centers for Disease Control (CDC) and Prevention in the United States, the incidence of PR in the absence of septicemia was reported by 19% of U.S. dialysis centers.[26] Furthermore, the use of high-flux dialyzers (especially in conjunction with bicarbonate dialysate) and reprocessed dialyzers was associated with an increased incidence of PR.[26] Finally, intradialytic hypotension can also cause transient mesenteric ischemia that may be sufficient to damage the gastrointestinal mucosa and lead to bacterial and/or LPS translocation.[39]

Pyrogenic reactions should be entertained after septicemia has been ruled out. Careful examination of the dialysis access is warranted and blood cultures should be obtained. Treatment of PR includes antipyretics, empiric broad-spectrum antibiotics, discontinuation of ultrafiltration whenever hypotension is present, and selective hospitalization. An outbreak of

Table 22–2 Reactions/Infections Related to Microbial Contamination of Dialysis Fluids

Causative Agents	Identifiable Sources of Contamination	Manifestations
Bacterial Products		
Lipopolysaccharide	Backfiltration from bicarbonate/glucose dialysate High-flux dialysis Highly reprocessed dialyzers Gut translocation following intradialytic hypotension	PR without bacteremia
Microcystis aeruginosa exotoxin (Microcystin-LR)	Carbon filters contaminated by blue-green algae	Acute hepatic necrosis
Bacteria	O-rings	PR with bacteremia
Klebsiella pneumoniae	Hose connected to water spray device	
Pseudomonas species	Cross-contamination by technician's gloves	
Xanthomonas maltophilia	Cross-contamination of blood tubing by ultrafiltrate waste bag	
Citrobacter freundii	Low levels of disinfectant	
Acinetobacter species	Inadequate mixing of disinfectant with tap water	
Enterobacter species	Inadequate potency of disinfectant despite standard measures	
Bacillus species		
Achromobacter		
Mycobacteria	Inadequate potency of disinfectant despite standard measures	PR with mycobacteremia
Mycobacterium chelonae abscessus		Soft tissue infection Arteriovenous graft infection
Yeast		
Rhodotorula glutinis	Drain of hemodialysis machines	Unknown

PR, pyrogen reaction.

bacteremia among several patients, involving a similar organism should prompt thorough search for bacterial contaminants of the dialysis equipment.

Strategies for the prevention of PR are summarized in Table 22–3 and start with strict adherence to the Association for the Advancement of Medical Instrumentation (AAMI) standards. In an era of high-flux dialysis and reuse, some authors believe that these recommendations are too liberal and that sterile, pyrogen-free dialysis fluids be used.[40] Although this approach may offer clear advantages to patients, skepticism with regards to cost remains an unresolved issue, and data to support its benefit are currently lacking.

BLOODLINE TOXICITY

Particle Spallation

Bloodline components may enter the circulation by spallation, which is the release of silicone (not used in the United States) or polyvinyl chloride (PVC) particles, induced by the roller pump.[41,42] Studies of the bioengineering aspects of spallation indicate that the origin of these particles is from cracks in the pump insert material near the point of flexing caused by the repeated compression/relaxation of the tubing by the rollers.[42] With current high-flux technology demanding high pump speed performances, spallation is more likely to occur. Quantitative studies indicate that the majority of particles released are less than 5μm in diameter and that the greatest release of particles occurs during the 1st hour of pumping.[43] Even though silicone has been largely replaced by PVC, the problem of spallation persists.[43] Loading of animals with PVC or silicone particles induces IL-1 and prostanoid secretion by macrophages,[44,45] and ascribed clinicopathologic effects include hepatomegaly, granulomatous hepatitis and hypersplenism.[42] Silicon-related toxicity with plasma levels greater than 2 mg/L has been described in two dialysis patients.[46] Although it was not thought to be related to dialysis-related contamination, the syndrome was characterized by perforating folliculitis and aberrant hair growth.[46] Future bioengineering advances aimed at improving bloodline biocompatibility are warranted, including newer design of roller and pump segments and internal coating of PVC tubing.

Leachables

The flexibility of PVC is achieved by the addition of a plasticizer, di(2-ethylhexyl) phthalates (DEHP).[47] Phthalates are physically linked but not bound to PVC and hence may leach from the tubing matrix into the circulation. DEHP has been recovered from plasma and erythrocytes that were stored in plastic tubes.[42] Although there is no clear evidence to confirm its toxicity, DEHP can bind to plasma lipids and lipoproteins, and significant tissue levels have been recovered at autopsy.[42] Furthermore, a hepatitis-like syndrome and necrotizing dermatitis have been reported in association with PVC exposure.[42] In the dermatologic literature, contact dermatitis due to DEHP exposure has been described.[48]

Leachability studies of a newer plasticizer, trimellitate from blood tubing demonstrate a lower release when compared to DEHP.[49] Of note, the AAMI standards do not enforce leachability and spallation study requirements from manufacturers of bloodline tubing and dialysis equipment.

Table 22–3 Strategies for Prevention of Bacterial Contamination

Strict adherence to AAMI standards	Type of Fluid	Microbial Count	Endotoxin
	Water products	< 200 CFU/mL	<2 EU
	Dialysate	< 2000 CFU/mL	No standard
	Reprocessed dialyzers	No growth	—
Appropriate germicide	4% Formaldehyde*		
	1% Formaldehyde heated to 40°C*†		
	Glutaraldehyde†		
	Hydrogen peroxide/peracetic acid mixture (Renalin)*†		
	Heat sterilization (105°C for 20 hours) for reprocessing of polysulfone membranes†		
Wash and rinse the vascular access arm with soap and water.			
Prior to cannulation, inspect vascular access for local signs of inflammation.			
Scrub the skin with povidone iodine or chlorhexidine; allow to dry out for 5 minutes prior to cannulation.			
Record temperature prior and at the end of dialysis.			
When central delivery systems are used:			
	Clean and disinfect connecting pipes regularly.		
	Remove residual bacteria or endotoxin by additional filtration.		
When single-patient proportioning dialysis machines are used:			
	Freshly prepare bicarbonate dialysate on a daily basis.		
	Discard unused solutions at the end of each day.		
	Containers should be rinsed and disinfected with fluids that meet AAMI standards, and air-dried prior to dialysate preparation.		

AAMI, Association for the Advancement of Medical Instrumentation; *CFU,* colony forming unit.
*A minimum of 11- or 24-hour exposure to peracetic acid or formaldehyde is required, respectively.
†These germicides are all equivalent or superior to 4% formaldehyde.

CARDIOVASCULAR COMPLICATIONS

Hypotension

Intradialytic hypotension requiring medical intervention occurs in 10% to 30% of treatments.[50] Although it may be frequently asymptomatic, it can also be accompanied by a severe compromise of vital organ perfusion resulting in loss of consciousness, seizures, and even death. Associated vomiting may be complicated by aspiration.

The pathogenesis of intradialytic hypotension is multifactorial. Ultrafiltration rate, total volume of fluid removed, a reduced plasma refilling rate coupled with impaired compensatory physiologic responses to hypovolemia play a major role. An altered nitric oxide versus endothelin balance has recently been implied in the pathogenesis of dialysis induced hypotension.[51] Although an ultrafiltration rate of greater than 0.35 mL/kg/min will produce hypotension in most patients,[52] slower ultrafiltration rates, with up to a 20% decrease in plasma volume are generally well tolerated.[53] Failure of the normal compensatory responses to hypovolemia, which include central redistribution of the blood volume and increase in peripheral vascular resistance, are frequent mechanisms in hypotensive episodes. Patient-related factors include autonomic dysfunction (i.e., baroreflex impairment and alteration of heart rate responses), particularly in elderly and diabetic patients, use of anti-hypertensive medications, structural heart disease, cardiac arrhythmias, bacterial sepsis, hemorrhage, intradialytic venous pooling, increase in core body temperature, ingestion of food during dialysis and anemia. Dialysis associated L-carnitine deficiency may also contribute to intradialytic hypotension.[54] In addition, "sympathetic failure" due to a lack of appropriate rise in plasma norepinephrine levels during HD may be a manifestation of baroreflex dysfunction.[55] The decreased sensitivity of the renin-angiotensin, adrenergic, and arginine vasopressine systems could also contribute to inadequate vasoactive responses to HD-induced hypovolemia.[56]

Immediate management of intradialytic hypotension consists of restoration of vital organ perfusion by placing the patient in a Trendelenburg's position while preventing aspiration and augmentation of the circulating blood volume through infusion of isotonic normal saline, hypertonic agents, and reduction/cessation of ultrafiltration.

Cardiovascular instability and intradialytic hypotension can also be reduced with the use of bicarbonate dialysate, volumetric control of ultrafiltration, increased dialysate sodium concentration, better assessment of patient's "dry weight" using bioelectric impedance or vena caval ultrasound, and the use of cooler temperature dialysis.[57] Sodium modeling also reduces hypotensive episodes.[58] The use of salt-poor albumin offers no advantage to normal saline but costs more. On-line blood volume monitoring techniques have been used to control intradialytic hypotensive episodes, but their effectiveness is controversial.[59,60] Other preventive strategies include (1) correction of anemia and hypoalbuminemia, (2) withdrawal of antihypertensive drugs before dialysis, (3) avoiding food before and during dialysis, (4) counseling patients regarding weight gain, (5) treatment of congestive heart failure and arrhythmias, and (6) search for other causes such as pericardial effusion. Finally, the pre-dialysis use of midodrine, a selective $alpha_1$-adrenergic receptor agonist, is effective and safe in reducing the severity and frequency of hypotensive episodes.[61] Other pharmacologic options include the use of L-carnitine and setraline.[62,63]

Hypertension

Intradialytic and immediate postdialytic hypertension also constitute an important risk factor for cardiovascular mortality, the leading cause of mortality in HD patients. Time-averaged blood pressure measurements correlate better with postdialysis than with predialysis blood pressure, and dialysis patients often fail to show the normal "nocturnal dip" in blood pressure.[64,65] In a recent study, elevated postdialysis pulse pressure was associated with a 12% increase in the hazard for death, whereas postdialysis systolic blood pressure was inversely related to mortality.[66]

Although volume control is still the mainstay of blood pressure management in dialysis patients, blood pressure control is not achieved despite fluid removal in up to 50% of patients.[67] Preexisting hypertension, volume depletion, hypokalemia-induced increased renin-angiotensin secretion,[68] hypercalcemia-induced increased inotropism and vascular tone,[69] and increased sympathetic tone during rapid ultrafiltration, especially among young patients with kidneys *in situ*,[70] have all been associated with volume-independent hypertension in HD.[71] The chronic administration of recombinant human erythropoietin (rHuEPO) has also been associated with hypertension. This effect may be mediated by rheologic mechanisms as well as humoral factors, such as elevation in resting and agonist-stimulated cytoplasmic calcium concentration, increased endothelin production, upregulation of tissue renin and angiotensinogen expression, and a possible change in vascular tissue prostaglandin production.[72]

If signs or symptoms of volume contraction are lacking, it is justified to reduce the dry weight by 0.5 kg, observe the clinical response, and reevaluate periodically. Increases in dialysis or ultrafiltration time and/or frequency may facilitate volume removal. Atrial natriuretic peptide measurements indicate that a substantial fraction of patients with dialysis-refractory hypertension are not at their "true dry weight."[73]

Changing the administration of rHuEPO from the intravenous to the subcutaneous route has been associated with improved blood pressure control in hypertensive dialysis patients.[74]

Cardiac Arrhythmias

Intradialytic atrial and ventricular arrhythmias are common in HD patients, and the etiology is often multifactorial. Frequently encountered underlying conditions include ischemic or hypertensive heart disease, left ventricular hypertrophy and/or dysfunction, uremic pericarditis, silent myocardial ischemia, and conduction system calcification.[75–78] In addition, acute and chronic alterations in fluid, electrolyte, and acid/base homeostasis, may enhance the arrhythmogenic properties of digitalis preparations, antiarrhythmic and other drugs,[76] or simply increase myocardial oxygen delivery or consumption, such as in intradialytic hypotension or volume overload, respectively.

Measures to prevent arrhythmias include the use of bicarbonate dialysate and careful attention to dialysate potassium and calcium levels. Use of zero potassium dialysate should be discouraged due to arrhythmogenic potential, and potassium modeling may be useful.[79] In patients on digitalis, intracellular potassium shifts during dialysis should be minimized. Serum digoxin levels should be regularly monitored and the need for the drug regularly reassessed. Dialysate calcium levels of 3.5 mEq/L have been associated with cardiac ectopy.[80] By contrast, a calcium dialysate of 2.5 mEq/L has been associated with a prolonged QT interval.[81] QT dispersion, a measure of the variation in QT interval length on a standard 12-lead electrocardiogram, appears to reflect on the inhomogeneity in ventricle repolarization and has been used to predict risk of malignant cardiac arrhythmia. In HD patients, QT dispersion correlates with left ventricular hypertrophy, and mass and has been shown to improve following kidney transplantation.[82,83]

Similar to the general population, HD patients who develop atrial fibrillation have an increased risk for thromboembolic complications and may benefit from anticoagulation.[84]

Sudden Death

Based on data from the United States Renal Data System, 42% of dialysis patient deaths were documented as sudden or cardiac in origin, with 22% of deaths related to cardiac arrests and arrhythmia.[85] An excess mortality (approximately 20% of all deaths occurring per week) was found on Mondays for patients dialyzing on Mondays, Wednesdays, and Fridays and similarly on Tuesdays for patients dialyzing on Tuesdays, Thursdays, and Saturdays. No excess mortality on a particular day of the week was found in patients on peritoneal dialysis. These observational studies suggest that the cause of death may be due to the discontinuous nature of HD.[85] Elevations of cardiac troponin T[86] and elevations of serum phosphate and calcium phosphate product[87] have also been associated with an increased risk of death in dialysis patients.

Patients who sustain a cardiac arrest in the dialysis facility tend to be older and are more likely to have diabetes mellitus and a dialysis catheter for vascular access. They also tend to have had a recent hospitalization and often experience a blood pressure drop prior to the cardiac arrest.[88] There has been particular interest in the occurrence of ventricular ectopic activity in HD patients and risk factors such as age, left ventricular hypertrophy or dysfunction, and electrolyte disturbances have been entertained. A clear relationship to cardiovascular outcomes, however, has not been shown to date.

Considering that a variety of psychotropic drugs have been linked to reports of iatrogenic prolongation of the QT interval, cardiac arrhythmia, and sudden death in the general population,[89] a thorough drug history is warranted when investigating sudden cardiac arrest. This is critical because numerous psychotropic drugs that enter the market may not undergo thorough post-marketing pharmacokinetic studies in dialysis patients.

In the acute management of intradialytic cardiac arrest, other catastrophic intradialytic events need to be ruled out. The prompt recognition and treatment of life-threatening hyperkalemia and the identification and correction of technical errors, such as air embolism, unsafe dialysate composition, overheated dialysate, line disconnection, or sterilant in the dialyzer have to be sought and ruled out. Air in the dialysate, grossly hemolyzed blood, and hemorrhage due to line disconnection may be immediately detected. However, if no obvious cause is identifiable, blood should not be returned to the patient, particularly if the arrest occurred immediately upon initiation of dialysis. Complaints of burning at the access site prior to arrest might indicate an exposure to formaldehyde. If the event occurred during dialysis and a problem with dialysate composition is unlikely, blood may be returned to the patient, blood and dialysate samples should be immediately sent for electrolyte analysis, the dialyzer and bloodlines should be saved for later analysis, and the dialysis machine should be replaced until all of its safety features have been thoroughly evaluated for possible malfunction, which will be discussed later. The management of cardiopulmonary arrest during dialysis should follow the guidelines for cardiopulmonary resuscitation.

Dialysis-Associated Steal Syndrome (DASS)

While the construction of an arteriovenous fistula or graft for HD access frequently results in reduction of blood flow to the hand,[90] clinically significant or symptomatic ischemia is much more infrequent. Once it becomes symptomatic, however, it can lead to critical limb ischemia and amputation, particularly in patients with peripheral vascular disease and/or diabetes mellitus.[91–93] Fistulas or grafts are classified as small, if their diameter is less than 75% of the diameter of the feeding artery, and large, if they are greater than 75%. Blood flow in the artery located distal to a small fistula/graft remains orthodirectional, whereas larger fistulas/grafts cause retrograde flow in the distal artery, thus leading to a steal syndrome.[94] DASS has been reported in 1% and 6% of patients with radiocephalic fistulas and grafts, respectively.[95] Symptoms of numbness, pain, and weakness of the hand may appear or worsen during HD, and clinical findings include coolness of the distal arm, diminished pulses, acrocyanosis, and, rarely, gangrene. Symptomatic DASS should be differentiated from other causes of painful limbs, including dialysis-associated muscle cramps, coexistent polyneuropathy, and entrapment mononeuropathies, such as the carpal tunnel syndrome associated with dialysis-related amyloidosis. The syndrome of acute ischemic monomelic mononeuropathy following the creation of an arm access has been described,[92] and rapidly progressing acral gangrene may also be caused by calciphylaxis.[96]

The evaluation of a painful hand includes pulse oximetry,[97] plethysmography,[95] doppler flows, and arteriography.[92] The treatment of DASS depends on its clinical severity and the anatomy of the access. The simplest and most effective treatment is ligation of the venous outflow of the fistula/graft.[98] However, this procedure results in the elimination of a site for vascular access and the immediate need to construct another. Ipsilateral distal revascularization-interval ligation[91] is a surgical treatment that preserves vascular access patency and relieves clinical steal symptoms in about 90% of patients.[99] Narrowing or "banding" of the fistula/graft to reduce flow[100] can also be used. Intraoperative digital plethysmography[95] or duplex sonography[101] may be useful for an early diagnosis or for intraoperative guidance in the correction of DASS. Percutaneous luminal angioplasty or laser recanalization is reserved for patients with inflow or outflow arterial disease.[92,102]

A different DASS that may be of clinical significance was recently reported in dialysis patients with an arteriovenous fistula who received myocardial revascularization with an ipsilateral mammary artery bypass graft. These patients developed a significant reduction in coronary bypass blood flows and myocardial perfusion that was manifest during dialysis.[103]

NEUROLOGIC COMPLICATIONS

Muscle Cramps

Prolonged involuntary muscle contractions or cramps that occur late in HD and typically involve the legs are the most common acute neuromuscular complications observed during dialysis. They occur in 5% to 20% of treatments[104] and frequently lead to premature discontinuation of dialysis. Electromyography performed during HD demonstrates tonic muscle electrical activity, steadily increasing throughout dialysis in those who develop cramps, as opposed to a steady decline in those who do not.[105] Furthermore, a subset of patients have elevated predialysis serum creatine phosphokinase levels during periods of cramping.[106]

The pathogenesis of intradialytic cramps is unknown. Plasma volume contraction and progressive hypoosmolality induced by HD are the two most important predisposing factors.[107] Hypomagnesemia, L-carnitine, and vitamin C and E deficiencies have also been incriminated.

The acute management of cramps is directed at increasing the plasma osmolality. Parenteral infusion of 23.5% hypertonic saline (15–20 mL), 25% mannitol (50–100 mL), or 50% dextrose in water (25–50 mL) has been shown to be equally effective.[108] Dextrose in water is preferred because compared to the other agents, it neither causes flushing during infusion nor leads to increased thirst, interdialytic fluid intake and, therefore, fluid overload, but it may cause transient hyperglycemia. The use of midodrine may reduce cramps in patients with concomitant symptomatic intradialytic hypotension.[109]

Preventive measures include dietary counseling to reduce excessive interdialytic weight gains. In patients without clinical signs of fluid overload, it is reasonable to increase the dry weight by 0.5 kg and observe the clinical response. In those patients who do not respond to the above measures, 5 mg of enalapril twice weekly has been shown to be effective, presumably by inhibiting angiotensin II-mediated thirst.[110] Oral quinine sulfate (325 mg) at the initiation of HD has been shown to significantly reduce the incidence of muscle cramps.[111] However, quinine sulfate is currently not approved as an over-the-counter product for the prevention of cramps and is only available by prescription.[112] The association of quinine with the hemolytic uremic syndrome and the lack of the U.S. Food and Drug Administration's (FDA) approval, however, should discourage its use. The use of sodium gradient HD is effective in minimizing intradialytic hypoosmolality and preventing hypotension. Different sodium modeling strategies, such as starting from a dialysate sodium concentration of 145 to 155 mEq/L and decreasing linearly exponentially or step-wise to 135 to 140 mEq/L,[107,113] have yielded similar clinical results.[114] The use of an intradialytic blood volume ultrafiltration feedback control system has been associated with a lower incidence of cramps.[115] Finally, stretching exercises during dialysis, targeting the affected muscle groups may be beneficial.[113] Both L-carnitine[116] as well as creatine monohydrate[117] are effective pharmacotherapies in decreasing the frequency of muscle cramps.

Headache

Both historic and contemporary data indicate that dialysis-associated headache is common and occurs in about 60% to 70% of patients.[118,119] The symptoms may resemble migraines, tension headaches, or a combination of both.

The etiology of dialysis headache is unknown. It may be a subtle manifestation of the dialysis disequilibrium syndrome (DDS) and, in the past, may have been related to the use of acetate dialysate. The incidence of headaches seems to be lower with reused than with new dialyzers, with longer than with shorter conventional dialysis treatments, with dialysate containing glucose than with a glucose-free dialysate, and in patients undergoing short daily hemodialysis.[120] Furthermore, headaches may be a manifestation of caffeine withdrawal, caused by an acute intradialytic drop in blood caffeine levels in heavy coffee drinkers.[113]

The treatment of dialysis headache consists of oral analgesics (acetaminophen). Preventive measures include a reduction in the blood flow rate during the early part of dialysis. Coffee ingestion during dialysis may also be beneficial.

Restless Legs Syndrome (RLS)

With 20% to 40% prevalence in patients with end-stage renal disease, restless legs syndrome (RLS) is much more common than in the general population (5%).[121] It has been associated with premature discontinuation of dialysis ("sign-offs").[122] RLS is characterized by deep paresthesias, drawing and crawling sensations in the calves and legs, occasionally bordering on pain at the same site, which occur exclusively during rest and inactive seated or recumbent wakefulness.[123] Movement of the legs yields prompt relief of the symptoms, thus RLS may be responsible for premature discontinuation of a dialysis treatment. Insomnia, anxiety, and mild depression are frequent accompanying symptoms, whereas neurologic and electromyographic testing is generally unremarkable. RLS has to be differentiated from peripheral neuropathy in which paresthesias are constant and not relieved by activity. The exact cause of RLS is unknown but uremic toxins have been implied in its etiology. RLS and insomnia are frequently encountered in severely uremic patients and are relieved within a few weeks of initiating dialysis therapy.[123] RLS symptoms also improve after kidney transplantation.[124] Iron deficiency anemia, vascular insufficiency, chronic lung disease, and caffeine abuse have all been implicated in the pathogenesis of this syndrome.[123]

Short acting benzodiazepines, opiates, and carbamazepine have all been reported to be effective therapies but have the potential for tolerance and abuse. A small randomized, controlled trial recently reported on the effectiveness of gabapentin 200 to 300 mg given after dialysis.[125] Levodopa/carbidopa has also been used with some success.[121] A nonpharmacologic approach with transcutaneous electric nerve stimulation is reserved for refractory cases, but experience is limited.[123] In a nondialysis population, pramipexole, a dopamine receptor agonist, has also been associated with good outcomes.[126]

Dialysis Disequilibrium Syndrome (DDS)

DDS still represents a clinical problem in patients with acute renal failure and end-stage renal disease (ESRD) initiating HD, particularly with use of large surface area, high-flux dialyzers and shorter dialysis time. Risk factors include young age, severe azotemia, low dialysate sodium concentration, and preexisting neurologic disorders, such as recent stroke, head trauma, subdural hematoma, or malignant hypertension.[127] Use of dialysis machines with volumetric control, bicarbonate dialysate, sodium modeling, and earlier initiation of renal replacement therapy has reduced the incidence of DDS.

Minor symptoms include restlessness, headache, nausea, vomiting, blurred vision, muscle twitching, disorientation, tremor, and hypertension. But major symptoms including obtundation, seizures, coma, cardiac arrhythmias, or death may occur. DDS usually occurs towards the end of dialysis and may be delayed by up to 24 hours. This syndrome is usually self-limited but full recovery may take several days. DDS is a clinical diagnosis, and electroencephalography (EEG) is usually nonspecific, whereas cerebral edema is a consistent finding on computerized tomographic scanning (CT-scan). The differential diagnosis includes intracranial hemorrhage, ischemic or hemorrhagic stroke, and Wernicke's encephalopathy.[128]

The pathogenesis of DDS, although not fully understood, is largely thought to be due to cerebral edema.[2] The classic hypothesis includes the development of a transient osmotic disequilibrium due to more rapid removal of urea from blood than from cerebrospinal fluid (CSF), leading to an osmotic disequilibrium and subsequent cerebral edema. An alternative hypothesis is the development of paradoxical CSF acidosis during HD, which is aborted by slower dialysis.[127] Other implemented factors include intracerebral accumulation of endogenous osmotic solutes such as inositol, glutamine, and glutamate.[2]

Preventive measures include shorter and more frequent dialysis using small surface area dialyzers, hypernatric dialysate, reduction in blood flow, and individual intradialytic sodium modeling. Continuous mannitol infusions during dialysis or the prophylactic use of anticonvulsants are not recommended.

Seizures

HD-associated seizures are typically generalized and easily controlled. They occur in less than 10% of chronically dialyzed patients and may be more frequent in acutely dialyzed patients.[129] Focal neurologic symptoms indicate a localized neurologic disease such as an intracranial hemorrhage and warrant further evaluation. Other causes for seizures include

DDS, uremic encephalopathy, acute aluminum intoxication, hypertensive encephalopathy, hypoglycemia, alcohol withdrawal, cerebral anoxia due to sustained intradialytic hypotension (i.e., from cardiac arrhythmias, hypersensitivity reaction, sepsis, or hemorrhage), hyperosmolality due to hypernatremia, hypocalcemia, use of epileptogenic drugs (i.e., theophylline, meperidine, β-lactams), and brain retention of contrast. Recombinant Human Erythropoietin (rHuEPO) therapy has also been implicated as a cause for seizures during dialysis, typically in patients with preexisting hypertension.

Treatment of established seizures requires cessation of dialysis, maintenance of airway patency, and investigation for metabolic abnormalities. Intravenous diazepam or clonazepam, and phenytoin may be required. Intravenous administration of 50% dextrose in water should be administered if hypoglycemia is suspected. In children with HD-associated seizures, the prophylactic use of diazepam appears to be more effective than phenobarbital.[130]

Acute Aluminum Neurotoxicity

Acute aluminum neurotoxicity may occur because of aluminum contamination of dialysate following administration of desferrioxamine resulting in higher aluminum levels. It may also follow the concomitant administration of oral aluminum-based phosphate binders and citrate compounds, which enhance aluminum absorption in the small intestine and increase solubility and uptake of aluminum by the central nervous system.[131] The acute onset of this syndrome comprises agitation, confusion, seizures, myoclonic jerks, coma, and death. Plasma aluminum levels are typically greater than 500 μg/L, and highly suggestive EEG findings include multifocal bursts of slow or delta wave activity and frequent spikes. The CT-scan is usually normal. Acute aluminum neurotoxicity of adult patients leads to death in most of the patients despite chelation therapy. The administration of low-dose (5 mg/kg) desferrioxamine 5 hours prior to the start of HD has been shown to be uneventful.[132]

The classical aluminum intoxication syndrome has a more chronic course characterized by "dialysis dementia," osteomalacia, microcytic anemia, and elevated plasma aluminum levels.

HEMATOLOGIC COMPLICATIONS

Leukopenia

Intradialytic leukopenia has been one of the earliest indices of membrane bioincompatibility. The onset is usually rapid and peaks at 10 to 15 minutes.[133,134] Neutrophils and other granulocytes are primarily affected. The leukocyte count usually returns to normal by the end of dialysis and may exceed the predialysis values. This rebound leukocytosis has been ascribed in part to demargination of leukocytes from the vascular wall as well as from a recruitment of neutrophils from the bone marrow following an increase in circulating levels of granulocyte colony-stimulating factor.[135] Although granulocytes are readily seen on the dialyzer membrane surface under microscopy,[136,137] the disappearance of these cells from the circulation is primarily due to sequestration in the pulmonary vasculature. Pulmonary leukosequestration has been demonstrated using radiolabeled cells in clinical studies.[138] Binding of C5a to neutrophil cell-surface specific receptors is the primary underlying mechanism, and the degree of complement activation correlates closely with the degree of leukopenia.[139–141]

Intradialytic Hemolysis

Hemolysis associated with hemodialysis is rare (Table 22–4) and is most often caused by chemical contaminants, hypotonic or overheated dialysate,[142] or kink or manufacturing defects of the bloodline tubing.[142,143] Oxidative stress may also incease the RBC membrane fragility through lipid peroxidation, resulting in hemolysis.[144]

Whereas arterial limb negative pump pressures of less than −350 mmHg can cause mild hemolysis in a clinical setting,[145] in experimental studies, pressures as low as −720 mmHg failed to cause hemolysis.[146] The use of smaller gauge cannulas has been associated with significant hemolysis.[147] Other mechanical factors within the circuitry that may result in hemolysis include the varying geometry of the dialyzer inlet chamber.[148]

The most common chemical contaminants that cause hemolysis are chloramines, monochloramines, dichloramines, and trichloramines, which form when chlorine and ammonium are added to the municipal water supply as disinfectants.[149] These compounds can cause oxidative injury to RBC, resulting in methemoglobinemia and acute hemolysis.[150] Copper contamination leads to similar oxidative stress. Deionization and reverse osmosis do not effectively remove these contaminants. Adsorption through granular activated carbon[151] or neutralization of the dialysis fluid with ascorbic acid, a reducing compound, can prevent complications from chloramine.[150] The AAMI guidelines indicate a maximum chloramine content of 0.1 mg/L in dialysis water, compared with the 4 mg/L maximum concentration allowed in drinking water, according to the Environmental Protection Agency (EPA).[152]

Nitrate and nitrite intoxication can occur in home HD patients who use well water contaminated with urine from domesticated animals, resulting in methemoglobinemia and hemolysis.[153] The AAMI guidelines recommend a maximum nitrate concentration of 2 mg/L for dialysis water, compared with the 10 mg/L maximum concentration allowed in drinking water.[152]

The retention of formaldehyde and hydrogen peroxide during dialyzer reprocessing has been associated with hemolysis.[154,155] Formaldehyde is a potent reducing agent that impairs RBC metabolism by inhibiting glycolysis[154] and may act as a hapten that induces hemolysis by formaldehyde-induced anti-N-like cold agglutinins.[156]

Finally, drug-induced hemolysis, particularly in patients with glucose-6-phosphate dehydrogenase (G6PD) deficiency, microangiopathic hemolytic anemia (e.g., quinine sulfate), hypophosphatemia, hypersplenism, and insufficient dialysis are rare causes that need to be considered.[150]

Patients with methemoglobinemia usually complain of nausea, vomiting, hypotension, and cyanosis, and oxygen therapy does not improve black-colored blood present in the extracorporeal circuit. Copper contamination should be suspected in the presence of skin flushing, abdominal pain, and/or diarrhea.

The diagnosis of acute hemolysis is self-evident when grossly translucent hemolyzed blood is observed in the

Table 22–4 Causes of Intradialytic Hemolysis

Mechanisms of Injury	Etiologies
Traumatic fragmentation	Dialyzer roller pump Excessive suction at arterial access site Single-needle dialysis High blood flow through a small needle Kinked dialysis catheter/tubing Right atrial subclavian catheter
Thermal	Overheated dialysate > 47°C Dialysate <35°C, activation of anti-N cold agglutinin (formaldehyde)
Osmolar	Hypoosmolar dialysate Hyperosmolar dialysate
Oxidative injury	Chloramines Nitrite/nitrate Copper Drugs (quinine sulfate)
Reducing injury	Formaldehyde
Interference with cellular thiols	Copper
Interference with iron uptake	Aluminum
Inhibition of RBC glycolysis	Formaldehyde
G6PD deficiency	Exacerbated by oxidants (quinine sulfate)
2,3-DPG deficiency	Hypophosphatemia
Drug-induced microangiopathy	Quinine sulfate

G6PD, Glucose-6-phosphate dehydrogenase; *2,3-DPG*, 2,3-diphosphoglycerate.

tubing. Evaluation should include reticulocyte count, haptoglobin, lactate dehydrogenase, blood smear for schistocytes or Heinz bodies, Coombs' test, and measurement of methemoglobin. Bone marrow examination may occasionally be indicated. More importantly, analysis of tap water for chloramines and metal contaminants and thorough analysis of the dialysis procedure for clues of increased blood turbulence and mechanical RBC injury are recommended.

Thrombocytopenia

Heparin-induced thrombocytopenia (HIT) has increasingly been recognized as an important clinical problem in dialysis patients. Type-I HIT is characterized by the development of mild thrombocytopenia, where the platelet count rarely drops to less than 100,000/µL. Heparin can be usually continued and the thrombocytopenia resolves spontaneously. By contrast, type-II HIT results in more severe thrombocytopenia, is IgG-antibody mediated,[157] and is characterized by arterial and venous thromboses and dialysis circuit clotting[158] as well as a hemorrhagic propensity. The antibodies are directed against the complex of heparin and platelet factor IV.[159,160] Among chronic dialysis patients the prevalence of HIT is around 4%.[159,161]

The diagnosis of type-II HIT is complex and depends on multiple criteria, including the degree, rapidity and time of onset of thrombocytopenia, the presence of thrombosis, and resolution of the symptoms after cessation of heparin.[159,160] The presence of heparin antibodies only acts as an adjunct to the diagnosis.

The treatment of this syndrome includes complete withdrawal of all heparin products, including flush solutions and catheter locks, the use of heparinoids such as argatroban or danaparoid,[162] or direct thrombin inhibitors such as lepirudin, a biosynthetic hirudin analogue. Low molecular weight heparin is contraindicated. Lepirudin can be used as a 0.1 to 0.2 mg/kg IV bolus administered 5 minutes before starting HD, with an aPTT goal 1-hour into dialysis of 1.5 to 2.0 times normal.[163,164] Among patients with HIT who have indwelling dialysis catheters, at the end of dialysis, the venous and arterial ports of the catheter can be filled with lepirudin (1 mg/mL), according to the volumes indicated on the catheter.[165]

Transient thrombocytopenia may also result from blood-membrane interactions and reaches a nadir 1 hour after starting dialysis, with a platelet count declining to less than $100{,}000/mm^3$.[140] Thrombocytopenia may also be secondary to other drugs used during dialysis such as vancomycin, quinine sulfate, or desferrioxamine.[166,167,168]

Hemorrhage

Bleeding complications are commonly related to anticoagulation. Heparin confounds the uremic bleeding tendency, which is due to platelet dysfunction, abnormal platelet-vessel wall interaction, alteration of blood rheology and platelet adhesion secondary to anemia, and abnormal production of nitric oxide.[169,170] An increased incidence of spontaneous bleeding episodes has been reported in HD patients, particularly bleeding at specific sites such as gastrointestinal arteriovenous malformation, colonic ulcera of the Dieulafoy-type, subdural hematoma, retroperitoneal bleeding, uremic hemopericardium, hemorrhagic pleural effusion, hemoptysis, subcapsular hepatic hematoma, ocular anterior chamber hemorrhage, and skin hemorrhages, including petechiasis, ecchymosis, and subungual splinter hemorrhages.[2,77,171–173] Rupture of native, cystically transformed kidneys with retroperitoneal hematoma formation has also been described.[174]

Despite its limitations, the bleeding time is the best indicator of hemorrhagic tendency in dialysis patients. Local treatment of the hemorrhage and treatment/reversal of uremic platelet dysfunction are both needed. Strategies to achieve improvement in platelet function include an increase in rHuEPO dose or RBC transfusions to achieve a hematocrit greater than 30% in order to improve rheologic platelets-vessel wall interactions, intravenous conjugated estrogens at 0.6 mg/kg/day for 5 consecutive days, intravenous/subcutaneous 1-deamino-8-D-arginine vasopressin (DDAVP) at 0.3 µg/kg over 15 to 30 minutes, and/or intravenous infusion of cryoprecipitate. For patients experiencing severe bleeding, particularly when related to anticoagulation, it is advisable to consider heparin-free dialysis, using normal saline flushes every 15 to 30 minutes with ultrafiltration adjustments,[175] regional heparin or citrate anticoagulation,[176] and heparin modeling or prostacyclin.[177] It is important to note that heparin free dialysis may cause a stimulation of the coagulation system, increased fibrinogen consumption, and accelerated dialyzer hollow-fiber clotting.[178] The use of low-molecular weight heparin in HD has recently been proposed due to its convenient dosage regimen and lower impact on blood lipid levels, although bleeding complications are still possible.[179] Similarly, the use of lepirudin in dialysis patients with type-II HIT has also been associated with bleeding complications.[180]

In patients scheduled to undergo elective surgery or invasive procedures, it is recommended that aspirin be stopped a week earlier, the dose of anticoagulants be reduced to minimum and hematocrit maintained above 30%. In some cases, DDAVP and/or estrogens may also be required.

PULMONARY COMPLICATIONS

Hypoxemia

Transient hypoxemia during HD occurs in up to 90% of patients and is defined by a drop in arterial PaO_2 by 5 to 30 mm Hg, which reaches a nadir between 30 and 60 minutes, and returns to normal within 60 to 120 minutes following discontinuation of dialysis.[181] This mild reduction becomes clinically significant only when significant structural cardiopulmonary disease is present. The use of supplemental oxygen during dialysis improves arterial oxygen tension, but neither carbon dioxide tension nor breathing patterns are altered by this intervention.[182] Transient hypoxia is more common when dialyzers with high complement activating potential (unsubstituted cellulose) and acetate dialysate are used.[183,184] This may be mediated by complement activation following blood exposure to the free hydroxyl groups of cellulose membranes, with subsequent margination of leukocytes in the pulmonary vasculature.[2] Acetate dialysate may lead to loss of carbon dioxide in the dialyzer and, thus, result in hypocapnia and consequent compensatory hypoventilation. Use of bicarbonate dialysate (>35 mEq/L) may lead to hypoventilation and hypoxia by way of metabolic alkalosis.[2]

For diagnosing hypoxia during dialysis, arterial bloodline oxygen tension accurately correlates with systemic arterial blood and can conveniently be used in patients with an arteriovenous fistula or graft.[185]

Substituting acetate with bicarbonate dialysate at a concentration of less than 37 mEq/L, intradialytic oxygen supplementation, particularly in high risk patients, maintaining optimal hematocrit values to maximize blood's oxygen carrying capacity and sequential ultrafiltration followed by HD, particularly in patients with fluid overload can ameliorate dialysis-associated hypoxemia. In addition, the use of dialyzers with lower complement activating potential, such as synthetic, substituted cellulose, or reprocessed unsubstituted cellulose dialyzers could further reduce the likelihood of hypoxemia during HD. Finally, the use of cold dialysate may reduce intradialytic hypoxic episodes.[186]

TECHNICAL MALFUNCTIONS

Air Embolism

The incidence of air embolism, a potentially fatal complication, has decreased significantly due to improvements in dialysis machine safety monitors. The segment of the extracorporeal circuit that is most vulnerable to air entry is the pre-pump tubing segment, where significant subatmospheric pressures of up to 250 mm Hg can occur. Air can also originate from intravenous infusions circuits, especially with glass bottled intravenous solutions, air bubbles from the dialysate, and central venous catheters.[187] Furthermore, the use of high blood flow rates may allow rapid entry of large volumes of air despite small leaks.

Clinical manifestations depend on the volume of air introduced, the site of introduction, the patient's position, and the speed at which air is introduced.[188] The volume of air required to produce clinical manifestations varies due to above factors, and is partly dependent on preexisting cardiovascular or pulmonary disease. Microbubbles of air introduced at a slow rate dissolve in the blood and are better tolerated than macrobubbles. In the sitting position, air entry through a peripheral vein may bypass the heart and cause emboli into the cerebral circulation.[189] The acute onset of seizures and coma in the absence of precedent symptoms, such as chest pain or dyspnea, is highly suggestive of air embolism. If the patient is supine, air introduced through a central venous line will be trapped in the right ventricle where it forms foam, interfering with cardiac output and, if large enough, leads to obstructive shock. Dissemination of microemboli into the pulmonary vasculature occurs. In this event, dyspnea, dry cough, chest tightness, or respiratory arrest can also occur. Further passage of air across the pulmonary capillary bed can lead to embolization to a major cerebral or coronary artery. Foam may be visible in the extracorporeal tubing, and cardiac auscultation reveals a peculiar churning sound. In the Trendelenburg's position, air emboli migrate to the lower extremity venous circulation, resulting in ischemia, due to increased outflow resistance. Clinical manifestations include acrocyanosis, paresthesia and pain, and, unless peripheral vascular disease coexists, the outcome is usually favorable.

Once the diagnosis is suspected, the first step is to clamp the venous bloodline and stop the blood pump. For right heart air emboli, the patient is immediately placed in a recumbent position on the left side with the chest and head tilted downward. Cardiorespiratory support includes the administration of high-flow oxygen and endotracheal intubation and mechanical ventilation as needed. Aspiration of air from the ventricle by a percutaneously inserted needle or right atrial dialysis catheter can be attempted. If available, consideration should be given to hyperbaric oxygenation, where the patient undergoes decompression at a rate that allows the dissolved air to be expired through the lungs without coming out of solution.[190,191]

Preventive measures depend primarily on dialysis machines equipped with venous air bubble traps and foam detectors located just distal to the dialyzer and venous pressure monitor at the venous end. The detector is attached to a relay switch that simultaneously activates an alarm, shuts off the blood pump, and clamps the venous bloodline if air is detected. Therefore, dialysis should never be performed in the presence of an inoperative air detection alarm system. Glass bottles containing intravenous solutions should be avoided since they create vacuum effects that can permit air entry into the extracorporeal system. Further, dialysis catheters should be aspirated for blood return and flushed with saline prior to connection. Dialyzers rinsing with saline should fill up all compartments and remove air bubbles. Finally, in order to remove dissolved air, heating and degassing of dialysis water, particularly in winter months, is accomplished by exposing heated water (34°–39°C) to high negative pressure during the purification process.[192]

Blood Loss

Blood loss during HD can result from malfunction of the dialysis circuitry or internal or external hemorrhage of the patient that is caused or worsened by anticoagulation given during dialysis. The latter has been discussed previously. Technical complications are arterial or venous needle disengagement, bloodline disconnection, femoral or central line dialysis catheter perforation or dislodgment, or rupture of a dialysis membrane with or without malfunction of the blood leak detector. Clinical findings include hypotension, loss of consciousness, and cardiac arrest, sometimes within minutes of starting HD.[193]

Blood loss can also occur following traumatic insertion of a dialysis catheter that results in a rapidly expanding, painful hematoma. Intrapericardial blood loss can lead to chest, shoulder, or neck pain[194]; back, flank, groin, or lower abdominal quadrant pain/distention can result from retroperitoneal bleeding.[195] Management of acute blood loss includes the immediate discontinuation of HD, pressure application for local hemostasis, hemodynamic support, oxygen administration, and blood transfusion may be needed for severe blood loss.

Incorrect Dialysate Composition

Incorrect dialysate composition occurs as a result of technical or human errors. There are two types of dialysate solution delivery systems. With central delivery, the solution used for the whole dialysis unit is produced by one machine by mixing liquid concentrate with purified water and offers the advantage of reduced equipment and labor cost. With the individual system, each dialysis machine proportions its own dialysate liquid concentrate with purified water, permitting the modification of dialysate composition for a given patient. Because the primary solutes constituting the dialysate are electrolytes, the degree of dialysate concentration will be reflected by its electrical conductivity. Therefore, proper proportioning of concentrate-to-water can be achieved by a meter, which continuously measures the conductivity of the dialysate solution as it is being fed to the dialyzer. Life-threatening electrolyte and acid-base abnormalities are avoidable if the conductivity alarm is functioning properly and the alarm limits are set correctly. However, in dialysis machines that are equipped with conductivity-controlled mixing systems, the system automatically changes the mixing ratio of the concentrates until the dialysate solution conductivity falls within the set limits. This may inadvertently lead to dialysate without any bicarbonate, with apparently acceptable conductivity. Therefore, if conductivity-controlled systems are used, it is safer to also check the dialysate pH prior to dialysis. Conductivity monitors can fail or can be improperly adjusted due to human error. However, it is important to add human monitoring of dialysate composition before every treatment, whenever a machine has been sterilized, moved about, and whenever a new concentrate is used. Furthermore, many nonstandardized solutions are available, some of which may be used with an inappropriate proportioning system. Therefore, it is essential that the supplies match the machine proportioning ratio for which they were prepared to obtain the appropriate final dialysate composition.

Dysnatremias

Since disturbances in renal water handling cannot occur in anephric dialysis patients, the etiology and management of dysnatremias is limited to factors related to dialysis and interdialytic fluid and electrolyte intake.

Hypernatremia

Hypernatremia can result from a faulty dialysate concentrate composition or an incorrect concentrate to water ratio, and dysfunction of conductivity monitors or alarms.[52] This results in water shifts from the intracellular to the extracellular fluid compartment and leads to cell shrinking. Symptoms include profound thirst, headache, nausea and vomiting, seizures, coma, and death.[171] Aggressive treatment is mandatory, because mortality from acute severe hypernatremia (Na > 160 mEq/L) is greater than 70%.[196] Management includes cessation of dialysis, hospitalization, and infusion of 5% dextrose in water and HD with a different dialysis machine, particularly if conductivity monitoring malfunction is suspected. The dialysate sodium level should be 2 mEq/L lower than the plasma, and isotonic saline should be concurrently infused. Dialysis against a dialysate sodium level that is 3 to 5 mEq/L lower than plasma may increase the risk of disequilibrium. Ultrafiltration with equal volume replacement with normal saline is another option.

Hyponatremia

Failure to add concentrate, inadequate concentrate/water ratio, and conductivity monitor or alarm malfunction can cause hyponatremia. Hyponatremia can also occur during the course of dialysis with a proportioning system, if the concentrate container runs dry and the conductivity set limits are inappropriate. Acute hypoosmolality causes hemolysis with hyperkalemia and hemodilution of all plasma constituents due to massive transfer of water from dialysate in the blood, leading to water intoxication.[197] Symptoms include restlessness, anxiety, pain in the vein injected with the hypotonic hemolyzed blood, chest pain, headache, nausea, and occasional severe abdominal/lumbar cramps.[171] Pallor, vomiting, and seizures may be observed. Treatment of dialysis-induced hypoosmolality consists of clamping the bloodlines and discarding the hemolyzed blood in the extracorporeal circuit. High-flow oxygen and cardiac monitoring because of hyperkalemia and potential myocardial injury are imperative.[171] Dialysis should be restarted without delay, with a new batch of dialysate, new dialyzer, and low dialysate potassium.[171] Anticonvulsants are indicated for seizures, and blood transfusions may be needed for severe anemia.

The susceptibility of dialysis patients to complications due to rapid correction of hyponatremia by dialysis against a high sodium dialysate is poorly understood. Transient urea disequilibrium has been implied as a protective factor against cerebral water loss during rapid correction of extracellular osmolality during dialysis.[198] Even in the most acute symptomatic hyponatremic patient, a cautious approach is warranted, where a correction of sodium concentration by no more than 1 to 2 mEq/L/hr should be achieved.[199] Continuous renal replacement therapies have been used successfully for such a gradual correction of serum osmolality.[200]

Dyskalemias

Life-threatening hyperkalemia is not a common problem in dialysis patients and, if it occurs, is often caused by inadequate dialysis or dietary indiscretion. In healthy subjects, over 90% of the daily dietary potassium load is usually excreted by the kidneys. Anuric dialysis patients are able to excrete significant amounts of potassium via extrarenal potassium excretion, primarily in the colon. This mode of excretion depends on the stool volume and is minimal if constipation exists.[201] The use of fludrocortisone, a mineralocorticoid, has been proposed for enhancing colonic potassium secretion.[202] Despite a typically low dialysate potassium concentration of 1 to 3 mEq/L, potassium removal is limited due to its large distribution in the intracellular compartment of over 90% of total body potassium. A quantitative study of potassium removal over 4 hours of dialysis with a 1 mEq/L dialysate potassium concentration in hyperkalemic (serum potassium level 5–6 mEq/L) patients resulted in a mean potassium removal of 107 mEq per treatment. However, the serum levels rose back to over 5 mEq/L after reaching a nadir of 3.5 mEq/L.[203] The findings confirm our current understanding of the kinetics of potassium removal by dialysis, which does not follow single pool kinetics due to the delayed release of intracellular potassium. This underscores the relative inefficiency of a high serum to dialysate potassium gradient and illustrates why the use of potassium-free dialysate should be discouraged. The latter may precipitate cardiac arrhythmias, reduce dialysis efficiency through arteriolar vasoconstriction and small solute compartmentalization and limit correction of acidosis, by impairing bicarbonate diffusion into the blood compartment.[204–206] Potassium modeling and longer HD treatments have been suggested to avoid severe rebound.[207] Finally, with regards to the effects of packed RBC (PRBC) transfusion on potassium balance, various studies suggest that the potassium load per unit of PRBC transfused is 5 to 7 mEq for units stored 14 and 21 days, respectively,[208] and therefore, intradialytic PRBC transfusion should not be discouraged.

Severe hypokalemia induced by HD can occur despite the use of dialysate potassium concentration higher than serum.[209] This is due to rapid correction of acidosis that leads to intracellular shift of potassium. Overall, unless significant losses as a result of vomiting, diarrhea, or nasogastric suction are present, hypokalemia is not generally considered to be a problem in HD patients. Patients with marginal total body potassium stores (due to gastrointestinal losses) and metabolic acidosis, however, are prone to life-threatening hypokalemia during HD, where intradialytic potassium losses combined with intracellular shifts due to correction of acidosis may acutely precipitate life-threatening muscle weakness or cardiac arrhythmias, particularly in patients treated with digoxin.

Acid-Base Disturbances

HD patients have an alkali requirement of 240 mEq/treatment, taking into account daily acid generation and intradialytic losses of organic anions, which are bicarbonate precursors.[210] The physiology of acid-base disturbances in anephric patients on dialysis differs from that in subjects with functioning kidneys and is primarily governed by dialysis.

Metabolic Acidosis

A decrease in serum bicarbonate of greater than 4 mEq/L suggests the presence of a new metabolic acidosis.[210] Although acute intradialytic metabolic acidosis can occur due to improper mixing of concentrates or failure of pH monitors,[211] other causes that need to be ruled out include diabetic or alcoholic ketoacidosis, lactic acidosis, toxic ingestions, increased protein catabolism, progressive loss of residual renal function, and dilutional acidosis.[210,212] A transient acidosis during the 1st hour of acetate dialysis because of intradialytic bicarbonate losses that have not yet been compensated for by the metabolism of acetate by muscle mitochondria[213] has been described.

The patients typically present with acute onset of hyperventilation during HD. Severe metabolic acidosis is treated by correcting the underlying cause and administering HD with appropriate dialysate concentrate. Although dialysate bicarbonate levels of 35 to 38 mEq/L are adequate in most circumstances, excessive correction of severe metabolic acidosis (bicarbonate < 10 mEq/L) may lead to paradoxical acidification of the CSF and increased lactic acid formation by tissues.[213]

Metabolic Alkalosis

In anephric patients, elimination of excess base does not occur and the high concentration of bicarbonate in standard dialysate usually maintains the alkalosis. However, with acetate dialysis, net alkali loss will occur when plasma bicarbonate is greater than 26 to 28 mEq/L.[214] The presence of metabolic alkalosis is suggested by a rise in plasma bicarbonate by 4 to 5 mEq/L from its usual value.[214] A blood gas may be warranted to assess the respiratory response. The most common cause of metabolic alkalosis in HD patients is hydrochloric acid loss as a result of vomiting or nasogastric suction and is usually seen in the intensive care unit setting or endogenous and exogenous sources of added alkali. Such alkali or alkali precursors include sodium bicarbonate, calcium carbonate or acetate, citrate (blood products), lemon consumption, alkalinizing agents, lactate (Ringer's solution), acetate (TPN solutions), and connection of the bicarbonate concentrate to the wrong port.[214,215] The combination of sodium polystyrene sulfonate (Kayexalate) and aluminum hydroxide can lead to absorption of alkali that is normally neutralized in the small intestine.[216] Usually, removal of the alkali source is sufficient, and H_2-receptor antagonist or gastric H^+/K^+ ATPase inhibitors may be successful if gastric acid loss is present. If dialytic support is required for the rapid correction of this acid-base disorder, the dialysate composition may be altered by replacing alkali with chloride,[217] substituting bicarbonate with acetate dialysate,[218] using acid dialysate,[219] or using hydrochloric acid infusion during dialysis with citrate buffer.[220] Conventional bicarbonate dialysis or dialysis using lower dialysate bicarbonate levels (25–30 mEq/L) is probably as effective.[221]

Severe metabolic alkalosis due to HD is rare and may be due to error in dialysate concentrates,[222] reversed connection of bicarbonate and acid concentrate containers to the entry ports of the dialysis machine[223] or malfunction of the pH monitor. Furthermore, severe metabolic alkalosis can occur with regional citrate HD[224] and following continuous renal replacement therapies in the setting of acute renal failure.[225,226]

Respiratory Alkalosis

Due to the lack of a renal compensatory response,[214] acute respiratory acid-base disorders are more likely to cause mixed acid-base disorders that may be severe and life threatening.

During HD, despite losses of carbon dioxide into the dialysate, respiratory alkalosis does not occur.[227] However, anxiety, stroke, sepsis, and hepatic failure or pregnancy may be precipitating factors for hyperventilation and result in respiratory alkalosis. A hyperventilation syndrome has been described in a patient on continuous ambulatory peritoneal dialysis (CAPD), which disappeared once the patient was switched over to HD.[228]

Respiratory Acidosis

The concomitance of respiratory acidosis and renal failure is common in the intensive care unit setting. REDY sorbent dialysis is a dialysate regenerating system, requiring only 6 L of dialysate compared to 120 L for a standard 4-hour dialysis treatment.[229] The system contains a sorbent cartridge that has three different layers that participate in the detoxification process. Although it offers some advantages over HD, REDY sorbent dialysis can cause acute hypercapnia.[230] Indeed, during dialysate regeneration, the breakdown of urea by urease that occurs in the second layer generates NH_4^+ and HCO_3^-. The third layer consisting of zirconium phosphate is a cation exchanger that exchanges Na^+ and H^+ for NH_4^+. Hence, carbonic acid is formed when HCO_3^- combines with H^+.

Carbon dioxide is then usually eliminated by the lungs. However, the excess of carbon dioxide may be limited in patients with underlying pulmonary disease, resulting in hypercapnia and a superimposed or worsening respiratory acidosis.[229]

Last, despite the theoretic possibility of a decrease in respiratory drive due to bicarbonate supplementation during dialysis, a study of intubated patients with ARF who were undergoing HD showed that the decrease in respiratory drive correlated with the ultrafiltration volume rather than with the reversal of the metabolic acidosis.[231]

Chemical Contaminants

The "hard water syndrome" used to occur when untreated tap water containing high levels of dissolved minerals was used for dialysate preparation. It manifests an hour after start of dialysis and symptoms include nausea, vomiting, hypertension, extreme weakness and lethargy (due to hypercalcemia), and warm sensation to the skin (due to hypermagnesemia).[232] Acute pancreatitis may be observed.[233] Currently, the water used for dialysate preparation is treated with deionization and reverse osmosis to control levels of divalent cations and remove trace elements that may be present. However, in some rural areas, the mineral content of the water is very high, and the hard water syndrome can occur during home HD despite seemingly adequate pretreatment of the water source.[234] The diagnosis is confirmed by establishing elevated dialysate water calcium and magnesium levels. Treatment is supportive and dialysis should be stopped and restarted with properly treated water.

Metal contaminants that induce acute hemolysis include copper, zinc, and aluminum (see "Intradialytic Hemolysis"). Intoxications with other metals such as lead and nickel may also occur.[171] Fluoride is a trace element that may accumulate in HD patients and deposit in bone.[235,236] Its contribution to renal osteodystrophy, however, is unclear.

When dialysate water purification is based on deionizing (DI) systems utilizing ion exchange resins, fluoride contamination of dialysate can occur once deionizing columns are exhausted. Acute fluoride poisoning may follow, manifesting primarily by gastrointestinal symptoms and life-threatening hyperkalemia due to potassium channel blockade, leading to significant extracellular potassium leakage.[237] A case of acute fluoride poisoning that occurred in a dialysis unit in Illinois in 1993 was reported to the CDC.[13] DI systems were used during unit remodeling when the incident occurred. Periodic testing of dialysis water supply for fluoride content, maintenance of and familiarity of the health care team with deionizing systems are necessary to prevent these events.

Temperature Monitor Malfunction

Heating of the dialysate assists in the degassing and improves the mixing of water with dialysate concentrate. The internal controls of the thermostat are set up by the manufacturer to limit the dialysate temperature to 33° to 39°C. Malfunction of the thermostat in the dialysis machine can result in the production of excessively cool or hot dialysate. Accidental use of cool dialysate is not dangerous and has beneficial hemodynamic effects, although it may cause shivering and/or hypothermia. Overheated dialysate, especially when temperatures above 51°C are reached, can cause immediate hemolysis and life-threatening hyperkalemia.[171] Lower temperatures of 47° to 51°C may cause up to a 48-hour delay in the onset of hemolysis.[238]

If the dialysate temperature rises to 51°C, dialysis must be stopped immediately and the blood in the system discarded. The patient should be monitored and treated for hyperkalemia and transfused as necessary. Dialysis may be resumed to treat hyperkalemia and to cool the patient by using a dialysate temperature of 34°C. To prevent this potentially catastrophic complication, visual and audible alarms are mandatory, as is a dialysate bypass for drainage, required with high-temperature alarms.

Milder thermal imbalances may be caused or worsened by ultrafiltration such that a reduction in blood volume has to be accompanied by relative cooling in order to achieve thermal energy homeostasis and avoid heat accumulation.[239]

MISCELLANEOUS COMPLICATIONS

Post-Dialysis Fatigue Syndrome

Common nonspecific symptoms of fatigue and malaise are observed in about 33% of patients.[193,240] The incidence of this syndrome has decreased since glucose-free acetate-containing solutions were replaced by glucose/bicarbonate dialysate.[241] Reduced cardiac output, peripheral vascular disease, depression, poor conditioning, postdialysis hypokalemia or hypoglycemia, mild uremic encephalopathy, neuropathy, or myopathy and blood membrane interactions may be contributing factors. Randomized, double-blind, controlled studies failed to show improvement by exchange of cuprophane with PS membranes[242,243] but showed that high ultrafiltration rates and low dialysate sodium concentration predispose to postdialysis fatigue.[244] On-line predilution hemofiltration has been shown to be more effective than ultrapure high-flux HD.[245] Malaise has also been ascribed to carnitine deficiency, which is important for muscle metabolism, and L-carnitine supplementation has been shown to improve postdialysis well-being.[116]

Pruritus

Pruritus is a common finding among dialysis patients and often multifactorial and difficult to treat. Xerosis, hypercalcemia, and hyperphosphatemia (resulting in calcium phosphate crystal deposition in the skin), hyperparathyroidism, inadequate dialysis,[246] and female gender[247] are all risk factors for this vexing problem. Some, but not all, studies have observed elevated plasma histamine and serotonin levels and increased mast cell proliferation in the skin.[248] Use of antihistamine agents and 5-HT3 receptor antagonists do not affect these levels.[248] Two clinical trials failed to demonstrate any benefit from the use of ondansetron for pruritus in dialysis patients.[249,250]

In many cases, pruritus is more severe during or after dialysis and may be an allergic manifestation to heparin, ETO, formaldehyde, or acetate.[27] The exchange of formaldehyde as the germicide during reuse and the use of gamma-sterilized dialyzers, and switching over to bicarbonate dialysate has been associated with cessation of itching.[27] Anecdotal reports suggest a likelihood of itching with cuprophan and new dialyzers compared to substituted cellulose and reused dialyzers.[193] Eczematous reactions to antiseptic solutions used to clean the vascular access site, rubber glove components (thiuram), nickel in the puncture needles, epoxy of the glue at the tube-needle joint, or the collophane of glues used to maintain needles should be considered.[251]

Therapeutic strategies include the use of both emollients and antihistamine agents, oral activated charcoal, ultraviolet therapy and sunbathing, ketotifen (a mast cell stabilizer), rHuEPO therapy, topical capsaicin,[252,253] essential fatty acid replacement,[254] and short term use of daily oral naltrexone.[255] Finally, the dialysis prescription and adequacy should always be assessed.

Priapism

Priapism occurs either during or 2 to 7 hours following dialysis in about 0.5% of male patients[256] and is characterized by a painful erection that is unrelated to sexual activity. A causal relationship to an increase in blood viscosity due to heparin,[257,258] high hematocrit, rHuEPO[259] and androgen therapy[260,261] as well as dialysis-induced hypoxemia, hypovolemia due to excessive ultrafiltration, particularly in black males with sickle cell trait,[256] and the use of prazosin[262] have all been implicated in the pathogenesis of this condition. Treatment includes immediate aspiration and irrigation of the corpora cavernosa.[263] Metaraminol has been used for irrigation in one report.[264] A dorsal penile block with 1% xylocaine without epinephrine and intravenous sedation can be given for pain control, but opiates are also effective. Surgical treatment consists of creating a shunt for drainage of the corpora cavernosa.[263] Permanent erectile dysfunction frequently results but can be treated with implantable cavernosal prostheses.[171]

Hearing and Visual Loss

The exact role of HD in hearing disturbances is unclear. Hearing loss in HD patients has been reported.[265,266] One study reported a hearing loss incidence of 41%, 15%, and 53% in the low, middle, and high frequency ranges, respectively.[267] In the same study, the low frequency hearing improved in 38% and worsened in 10% of patients after a single dialysis session.[267] Hearing impairment may improve following transplantation.[268] Advanced age, elevated plasma viscosity, and prior gentamicin administration are confounding factors of high frequency loss.[267] However, more recent investigations showed no acute change in audiometric parameters after HD but demonstrated a higher prevalence of hearing loss in patients with chronic kidney failure.[269,270] Acute hearing loss during HD may be due to bleeding in the inner ear as a consequence of heparinization or hair cell injury of the cochlea from edema (endolymphatic hydrops).[171] Finally, ototoxicity has been reported following desferrioxamine therapy,[271] isoniazid,[272] and amikacin.[273]

Visual loss is rare during HD and may be caused by central retinal vein occlusion,[274] precipitation of acute glaucoma,[275] ischemic optic neuropathy associated with intradialytic hypotension,[276,277] or Purtscher's-like retinopathy due to leukoembolization.[278] Desferrioxamine also causes ocular toxicity, and serial audiovisual monitoring may be required with chronic chelation therapy.[271]

Last, a recent outbreak of sudden onset of visual and hearing impairment 7 to 24 hours after a maintenance hemodialysis treatment in one center was caused by aged cellulose acetate dialyzers with patient exposure to cellulose acetate degradation products.[279]

Digoxin Toxicity

HD patients are particularly prone to complications associated with the use of digoxin (see "Cardiac Arrhythmias"). This compound has a narrow therapeutic window and, despite careful monitoring of drug levels, digoxin-induced arrhythmias can occur especially when coexistent with hypercalcemia, hypokalemia, and hypomagnesemia. A syndrome consisting of recurrent abdominal pain associated with use of digoxin can occur shortly after dialysis, particularly following marked ultrafiltration, and has been ascribed to digoxin-induced transient mesenteric ischemia.[276] Once digoxin intoxication has occurred, hemoperfusion with charcoal and antidigoxin antibodies are necessary for treatment due to inadequate clearance by dialysis. Adequate digoxin clearance of 145 mL/min has been achieved utilizing a commercially available β-2-microglobulin adsorption column (Lixelle, BM-01).[280]

References

1. Kolff WJ: Lasker Clinical Medical Research Award. The artificial kidney and its effect on the development of other artificial organs. Nat Med 2002; 8(10):1063–1065.
2. Lazarus JM, Denker BM, Owen WFJ: Hemodialysis. *In* Brenner BM (ed). The Kidney, 5th ed. Philadelphia, W.B. Saunders Company, 1996, p 2424–2506.
3. Gokal R, Hutchison A: Dialysis therapies for end-stage renal disease. Semin Dial 2002; 15(4):220–226.
4. Jaber BL, Pereira BJG: Dialysis reactions. Semin Dial 1997; 10: 158–165.
5. Saracho R, Martin-Malo A, Martinez I, et al: Evaluation of the Losartan in Hemodialysis (ELHE) Study. Kidney Int Suppl 1998; 68:S125–S129.
6. Bousquet J, Maurice F, Rivory JP, et al: Allergy in long-term hemodialysis. J Allergy Clin Immunol 1988; 81:605–610.
7. Dolovich J, Marshall CP, Smith EKM, et al: Allergy to ethylene oxide in chronic hemodialysis patients. Artif Organs 1984; 8: 334–337.
8. Dolovich J, Marshall CP, Smith EKM, et al: Allergy to ethylene oxide in chronic hemodialysis patients. Artif Organs 1985; 8: 334–337.
9. Ing TS, Daugirdas JT: Extractable ethylene oxide from cuprammonium cellulose plate dialyzers: Importance of potting compound. Trans Am Soc Artif Intern Organs 1986; 32: 108–110.
10. Purello D'Ambrosio F, Savica V, Gangemi S, et al: Ethylene oxide allergy in dialysis patients. Nephrol Dial Transplant 1997; 12(7): 1461–1463.
11. De Filippi C, Piazza V, Efficace E, et al: Dialysis hypersensitivity: A fading problem? Blood Purif 1998; 16(2):66–71.
12. Bousquet J, Michel FB: Allergy to formaldehyde and ethylene oxide. Clin Rev Allergy 1991; 9:357–370.
13. Arduino MJ: CDC investigations of noninfectious outbreaks of adverse events in hemodialysis facilities, 1979–1999. Semin Dial 2000; 13(2):86–91.
14. Van der Linden PW, Hack CE, Kerckhaert JA, et al: Preliminary report: Complement activation in wasp-sting anaphylaxis. Lancet 1990; 336:904–906.
15. Del Balzo U, Polley MJ, Levi R: Cardiac anaphylaxis. Complement activation as an amplification system. Circ Res 1989; 65:847–857.
16. Lysaght MJ: Evolution of hemodialysis membranes. *In* Bonomini V, Berland Y (eds). Contrib Nephrol Basel Karger, 1995, p 1–10.
17. Tielemans C, Madhoun P, Lemars M, et al: Anaphylactoid reactions during hemodialysis on AN69 membranes in patients receiving ACE inhibitors. Kidney Int 1990; 38:982–984.
18. Verresen L, Waer M, Vanrenterghem Y, Michielsen P: Angiotensin converting enzyme inhibitors and anaphylactoid reactions to high flux membrane dialysis. Lancet 1990; 336:1360–1362.
19. Schulman G, Arias R, Diehl S, et al: A comparison of the ability of dialysis membranes to activate Hageman factor (HF) (Abstract). Kidney Int 1986; 29:224.
20. Gavras I: Bradykinin-mediated effects of ACE inhibition. Kidney Int 1992; 42:1020–1029.
21. Schmitter L, Sweet S: Anaphylactic reactions with the addition of hypochlorite to reuse inpatients maintained on reprocessed polysulfone hemodialyzers and ACE inhibitors (Abstract). ASAIO Trans 1993; 39:75.
22. Control USCFD: Update. Acute allergic reactions associated with reprocessed hemodialyzers, Virginia. MMWR Morb Mortal Wkly Rep 1989; 38:873–874.
23. Pegues DA, Beck-Sague CM, Woollen SW, et al: Anaphylactoid reactions associated with reuse of hollow-fiber hemodialyzers and ACE inhibitors. Kidney Int 1992; 42:1232–1237.
24. Sundaram S, Barrett TW, Meyer KB, et al: Transmembrane passage of cytokine-inducing bacterial products across new and reprocessed polysulfone dialyzers. J Am Soc Nephrol 1996; 7: 2183–2191.
25. Urena P, Herbelin A, Zingraff J, et al: Permeability of cellulosic and non-cellulosic membranes to endotoxin subunits and cytokine production during in vitro haemodialysis. Nephrol Dial Transplant 1992; 7:16–28.
26. Tokars JI, Alter MJ, Favero MS, et al: National surveillance of dialysis associated diseases in the United States, 1992. ASAIO 1994; 40:1020–1031.
27. Salem M, Ivanovich PT, Ing TS, Daugirdas JT: Adverse effects of dialyzers manifesting during the dialysis session. Nephrol Dial Transplant 1994; 9(suppl):127–137.
28. Hedin H, Richter W: Pathomechanisms of dextran-induced anaphylactoid/anaphylactic reactions in man. Int Arch Allergy Appl Immunol 1982; 68:122–126.
29. Hörl WH, Cavill I, Macdougall IC, et al: How to diagnose and correct iron deficiency during rHuEPO therapy. Nephrol Dial Transplant 1996; 11:246–250.
30. Van Wyck DB: Iron dextran in chronic renal failure. Semin Dial 1991; 4:112–114.
31. Sunder-Plassmann G, Hörl WH: Safety of intravenous injection of iron saccharate in haemodialysis patients. Nephrol Dial Transplant 1996; 11:1797–1802.
32. Sequeira SJ, McKenna TJ: Chlorbutol, a new inhibitor of aldosterone biosynthesis identified during examination of heparin effect on aldosterone production. J Clin Endocrinol Metab 1986; 63:780–784.
33. Phelps KR, Oh MS, Carroll HJ: Heparin-induced hyperkalemia: Report of a case. Nephron 1980; 25:254–258.
34. Felsenfeld AJ: When and how should desferrioxamine be used in chronic dialysis. Semin Dial 1990; 3:8–20.
35. Bochner BS, Lichtenstein LM: Anaphylaxis. New Engl J Med 1991; 324:1785–1790.
36. Daugirdas JT, Ing TS: First use reactions during hemodialysis: A definition of subtypes. Kidney Int 1988; 24:S37–S43.
37. Collins DM, Lambert MB, Tannenbaum JS, et al: Tolerance of hemodialysis: A randomized prospective trial of high-flux versus conventional high-efficiency hemodialysis. J Am Soc Nephrol 1993; 4:148–154.
38. Bland LA, Favero MS, Arduino MJ: Should hemodialysis fluid be sterile? Semin Dial 1993; 6:34–36.
39. Jaber BL, Pereira BJG: Inflammatory mediators in sepsis: Rationale for extracorporeal therapies. Am J Kidney Dis 1996; 28(suppl 3):S35–S49.
40. Henderson L: Should hemodialysis fluid be sterile? Semin Dial 1993; 6:26–27.
41. Leong A, Sy-Disney ATS, Gove DW: Spallation and migration of silicone from blood pump tubing in patients on hemodialysis. N Engl J Med 1982; 306:135–140.
42. Hoenich NA: Spallation and plasticizer release from hemodialysis blood tubing: A cause of concern? Semin Dial 1991; 4: 227–230.
43. Hoenich NA, Thompson J, Varini E, et al: Particle spallation and plasticizer (DEHP) release from extracorporeal circuit tubing material. Int J Artif Organs 1990; 13:55–62.
44. Bommer J, Gemsa D, Waldherr R, et al: Plastic filing from dialysis tubing induces prostanoid release from macrophages. Kidney Int 1984; 26:331–337.
45. Bommer J, Weinreich J, Lovett PA, et al: Particles from dialysis tubing stimulate interleukin-1 secretion by macrophages. Nephrol Dial Transplant 1990; 5:208–213.
46. Saldanha LF, Gonick HC, Rodriguez HJ, et al: Silicon-related syndrome in dialysis patients. Nephron 1997; 77(1):48–56.
47. Rockel A, Klinke B, Hertel J, et al: Allergy to dialysis materials. Nephrol Dial Transplant 1989; 4:646–652.
48. Sugiura K, Sugiura M, Hayakawa R, et al: A case of contact urticaria syndrome due to di(2-ethylhexyl) phthalate (DOP) in work clothes. Contact Dermatitis 2002; 46(1):13–16.

49. Flaminio LM, De Angelis L, Ferazza M, et al: Leachability of a new plasticizer tri(2-ethyl-hexyl) trimellitate from haemodialysis tubing. Int J Artif Organs 1988; 11:435–441.
50. Levin NW, Kupin WL, Zasuwa G, Venkatt KK: Complications during hemodialysis. *In* Clinical Dialysis, 2nd ed. Norwalk, CT, Appleton & Lange, 1990, p172–201.
51. Raj DS, Vincent B, Simpson K, et al: Hemodynamic changes during hemodialysis: Role of nitric oxide and endothelin. Kidney Int 2002; 61(2):697–704.
52. Ronco C, Brendolan A, Bragantini L, et al: Technical and clinical evaluation of different short, highly efficient dialysis techniques. Contrib Nephrol 1988; 61:46–68.
53. Stiller S, Thommes A, Konigs F, et al: Characteristic profiles of circulating blood volume during dialysis therapy. Trans Am Soc Artif Intern Organs 1989; 35:530–532.
54. Ahmad S, Robertson HT, Golper TA, et al: Multicenter trial of L-carnitine in maintenance hemodialysis patients. II. Clinical and biochemical effects. Kidney Int 1990; 38(5):912–918.
55. Daugirdas JT: Dialysis hypotension: A hemodynamic analysis. Kidney Int 1991; 39:233–246.
56. Heintz B, Reiners K, Gladziwa U, et al: Response of vasoactive substances to reduction of blood volume during hemodialysis in hypotensive patients. Clin Nephrol 1993; 39:198–204.
57. Maggiore Q: Isothermic dialysis for hypotension-prone patients. Semin Dial 2002; 15(3):187–190.
58. Acchiardo DR, Hayden AJ: Is Na^+ modeling necessary in high-flux dialysis? ASAIO Trans 1991; 37:M135–M137.
59. Tonelli M, Astephen P, Andreou P, et al: Blood volume monitoring in intermittent hemodialysis for acute renal failure. Kidney Int 2002; 62(3):1075–1080.
60. Leypoldt JK, Lindsay RM: Hemodynamic monitoring during hemodialysis. Adv Ren Replace Ther 1999; 6(3):233–242.
61. Perazella M: Efficacy and safety of midodrine in the treatment of dialysis–associated hypotension. Expert Opin Drug Saf 2003; 2:37–47.
62. Pezerella M: Pharmacologic options available to treat symptomatic intradialytic hypotension. Am J Kidney Dis 2001; 38 (suppl 4):S26–S36.
63. Eknoyan G, Latos D, Lindberg J: Practice recommendations for the use of L-carnitine in dialysis-related carnitine disorder National Kidney Foundation Carnitine Consensus Conference. Am J Kidney Dis 2003; 41:868–876.
64. Baumgart P, Walger P, Gemen S, et al: Blood pressure elevation during the night in chronic renal failure, hemodialysis and after renal transplantation. Nephron 1991; 57:293–298.
65. Horl M, Horl W: Hemodialysis-associated hypertension: Pathophysiology and therapy. Am J Kidney Dis 2002; 39:227–244.
66. Klassen P, Lowrie E, Reddan D, et al: Association between pulse pressure and mortality in patients undergoing maintenance hemodialysis. JAMA 2002; 287:1548–1555.
67. Cheigh JS, Milite C, Sullivan JF, et al: Hypertension is not adequately controlled in hemodialysis patients. Am J Kidney Dis 1992; 5:453–459.
68. Fellner SK: Intradialytic hypertension II. Semin Dial 1993; 6: 371–373.
69. Sica DA, Harford AM, Zawada ET: Hypercalcemic hypertension in hemodialysis. Clin Nephrol 1984; 22:102–104.
70. Zucchelli P, Santoro A, Zuccala A: Genesis and control of hypertension in hemodialysis patients. Semin Nephrol 1988; 8:163–168.
71. Raine AEG, Roger SD: Effects of erythropoietin on blood pressure. Am J Kidney Dis 1991; 18:S76–S83.
72. Vaziri ND: Cardiovascular effects of erythropoietin and anemia correction. Curr Opin Nephrol Hypertens 2001; 10:633–638.
73. Fishbane S, Natke E, Maesaka JK: Role of volume overload in dialysis-refractory hypertension. Am J Kidney Dis 1996; 28: 257–261.
74. Navarro J, Teruel J, Marcen R, Ortuno J: Improvement of erythropoietin-induced hypertension in hemodialysis patients changing the administration route. Scand J Urol Nephrol 1995; 29:11–14.
75. Bailey RA, Kaplan AA: Intradialytic cardiac arrhythmias: I. Semin Dial 1994; 7:57–58.
76. Kant KS: Intradialytic cardiac arrhythmias: II. Semin Dial 1994; 7:58–60.
77. Rutsky, EA, Rostand SG: Pericarditis in end-stage renal disease: Clinical characteristics and management. Semin Dial 1989; 2: 25–30.
78. Derfler K, Kletter K, Balcke P, et al: Predictive value of thallium-201-dipyridamole myocardial stress scintigraphy in chronic hemodialysis patients and transplant recipients. Clin Nephrol 1991; 36:192–202.
79. Redaelli B, Locatelli F, Limido D, et al: Effect of a new model of hemodialysis potassium removal on the control of ventricular arrhythmias. Kidney Int 1996; 50(2):609–617.
80. Nishimura M, Nakanishi T, Yasui A, et al: Serum calcium increases the incidence of arrhythmias during acetate hemodialysis. Am J Kidney Dis 1992; 19:149–155.
81. Nappi SE, Virtanen VK, Saha HH, et al: QTC dispersion increases during hemodialysis with low-calcium dialysate. Kidney Int 2000; 57(5):2117–2122.
82. Yildiz A, Akkaya V, Tukek T, et al: Increased QT dispersion in hemodialysis patients improve after renal transplantation: A prospective-controlled study. Transplantation 2001; 72(9): 1523–1526.
83. Howse M, Sastry S, Bell G: Changes in the corrected QT interval and corrected QT dispersion during haemodialysis. Postgrad Med J 2002; 78:273–275.
84. Vazquez E, Sanchez-Perales C, Borrego F, et al: Influence of atrial fibrillation on the morbido-mortality of patients on hemodialysis. Am Heart J 2000; 140(6):886–890.
85. Bleyer AJ, Russell GB, Satko SG: Sudden and cardiac death rates in hemodialysis patients. Kidney Int 1999; 55(4):1553–1559.
86. Lowbeer C, Gutierrez A, Gustafsson SA, et al. Elevated cardiac troponin T in peritoneal dialysis patients is associated with CRP and predicts all-cause mortality and cardiac death. Nephrol Dial Transplant 2002; 17(12):2178–2183.
87. Ganesh SK, Stack AG, Levin NW, et al: Association of elevated serum PO(4), Ca x PO(4) product, and parathyroid hormone with cardiac mortality risk in chronic hemodialysis patients. J Am Soc Nephrol 2001; 12(10):2131–2138.
88. Karnik JA, Young BS, Lew NL, et al: Cardiac arrest and sudden death in dialysis units. Kidney Int 2001; 60(1):350–357.
89. Witchel H, Hancox J, Nutt D: Psychotropic drugs, cardiac arrhythmia, and sudden death. J Clin Psychopharmacol 2003; 23:58–77.
90. Kwun KB, Schanzer H, Finkler BA, et al: Hemodynamic evaluation of angioaccess procedures for hemodialysis. Vasc Surg 1979; 13:170–177.
91. Schanzer H, Skladany M, Haimov M: Treatment of angioaccess-induced ischemia by revascularization. J Vasc Surg 1992; 16(6): 861–864; discussion 4–6.
92. Valji K, Hye RJ, Roberts AC, et al: Hand ischemia in patients with hemodialysis access grafts: Angiographic diagnosis and treatment. Radiology 1995; 196(3):697–701.
93. Redfern AB, Zimmerman NB: Neurologic and ischemic complications of upper extremity vascular access for dialysis. J Hand Surg Am 1995; 20(2):199–204.
94. Barnes RW: Hemodynamics for the vascular surgeon. Arch Surg 1980; 115:216–223.
95. Odland MD, Kelly PH, Ney AL, et al: Management of dialysis associated steal syndrome complicating upper extremity arteriovenous fistulas: Use of intraoperative digital photoplethysmography. Surgery 1991; 110(4):664–669; discussion 9–70.
96. Tamura M, Hiroshige K, Osajima A, et al: A dialysis patient with systemic calciphylaxis exhibiting rapidly progressive visceral ischemia and acral gangrene. Intern Med 1995; 34(9):908–912.

97. Halevy A, Halpern Z, Negri M, et al: Pulse oximetry in the evaluation of the painful hand after arteriovenous fistula creation. J Vasc Surg 1991; 14(4):537–539.
98. Corry RJ, Patel NP, Natvarlal P, West JC: Surgical management of complications of vascular access for hemodialysis. Surg Gynecol Obstet 1980; 151:49–54.
99. Knox RC, Berman SS, Hughes JD, et al: Distal revascularization-interval ligation: A durable and effective treatment for ischemic steal syndrome after hemodialysis access. J Vasc Surg 2002; 36(2):250–255; discussion 6.
100. Jain KM, Simoni EJ, Munn JS: A new technique to correct vascular steal secondary to hemodialysis grafts. Surg Gynecol Obstet 1992; 175(2):183–184.
101. Aschwanden M, Hess P, Labs KH, et al: Dialysis access-associated steal syndrome: The intraoperative use of duplex ultrasound scan. J Vasc Surg 2003; 37(1):211–213.
102. Zwaan M, Weiss HD, Gothlin JH, et al: Initial clinical experience with a new pulsed dye laser device in angioplasty of limb ischemia and shunt fistula obstructions. Eur J Radiol 1992; 14(1):72–76.
103. Gaudino M, Serricchio M, Luciani N, et al: Risks of using internal thoracic artery grafts in patients in chronic hemodialysis via upper extremity arteriovenous fistula. Circulation 2003; 107(21):2653–2655.
104. Benna P, Lacquaniti F, Triolo G, et al: Acute neurologic complications of hemodialysis. Ital J Neurol Sci 1981; 2:53–57.
105. Howe RC, Wombolt DG, Michie DD: Analysis of tonic muscle activity and muscle cramps during hemodialysis. J Dial 1978; 2: 85–99.
106. Hernando P, Caramelo C, Lopez Garcia D, Hernando L: Muscle cramps: A cause of elevated creatinine kinase levels in hemodialysis patients. Nephron 1990; 55:231–232.
107. Canzanello VJ, Burkart JM: Hemodialysis-associated muscle cramps. Semin Dial 1992; 5:299–304.
108. Canzanello VJ, Hylander-Rossner B, Sands RE, et al: Comparison of 50% dextrose water, 25% mannitol, and 23.5% saline for the treatment of hemodialysis-associated muscle cramps. ASAIO Trans 1991; 37:649–652.
109. Cruz DN, Mahnensmith RL, Perazella MA: Intradialytic hypotension: Is midodrine beneficial in symptomatic hemodialysis patients? Am J Kidney Dis 1997; 30(6):772–779.
110. Oldenburg B, MacDonald GJ, Shelley S: Controlled trial of enalapril in patients with chronic fluid overload undergoing dialysis. Br Med J 1988; 296:1089–1091.
111. Kaji DM, Ackad A, Nottage WG, Stein RM: Prevention of muscle cramps in haemodialysis patients by quinine sulfate. Lancet 1976; 2:66–67.
112. Register F: Drug products for the treatment and/or prevention of nocturnal leg muscle cramps for over-the-counter human use; final rule: Department of Health and Human Services; 1994. Report No.: 21 CFR part 310.
113. Bregman H, Daugirdas JT, Ing TS: Complications during hemodialysis. *In* Daugirdas JT, Ing TS (eds): Handbook of Dialysis, 2nd ed. Boston, Little, Brown and Company, 1994, p149–168.
114. Sadowski RH, Allred EN, Jabs K: Sodium modeling ameliorates intradialytic and interdialytic symptoms in young hemodialysis patients. J Am Soc Nephrol 1993; 4:1192–1198.
115. Basile C, Giordano R, Vernaglione L, et al: Efficacy and safety of haemodialysis treatment with the Hemocontrol biofeedback system: A prospective medium-term study. Nephrol Dial Transplant 2001; 16(2):328–334.
116. Ahmad S, Robertson HT, Golper TA, et al: Multicenter trial of L-carnitine in maintenance hemodialysis patients. II. Clinical and biochemical effects. Kidney Int 1990; 38:912–918.
117. Chang CT, Wu CH, Yang CW, et al: Creatine monohydrate treatment alleviates muscle cramps associated with haemodialysis. Nephrol Dial Transplant 2002; 17(11):1978–1981.
118. Bana DS, Yap AU, Graham JR: Headache during hemodialysis. Headache 1972; 12:1–14.
119. Antoniazzi AL, Bigal ME, Bordini CA, et al: Headache and hemodialysis: A prospective study. Headache 2003; 43(2):99–102.
120. Andre MB, Rembold SM, Pereira CM, Lugon JR: Prospective evaluation of an in-center daily hemodialysis program: Results of two years of treatment. Am J Nephrol 2002; 22(56): 473–479.
121. Janzen L, Rich JA, Vercaigne LM: An overview of levodopa in the management of restless legs syndrome in a dialysis population: Pharmacokinetics, clinical trials, and complications of therapy. Ann Pharmacother 1999; 33(1):86–92.
122. Winkelman J, Chertow G, Lazarus J: Restless legs syndrome in end stage renal disease. Am J Kidney Dis 1996; 28:372–378.
123. Krueger BR: Restless legs syndrome and periodic movements of sleep. Mayo Clin Proc 1990; 65:999–1006.
124. Winkelmann J, Stautner A, Samtleben W, Trenkwalder C: Long-term course of restless legs syndrome in dialysis patients after kidney transplantation. Mov Disord 2002; 17(5):1072–1076.
125. Thorp ML, Morris CD, Bagby SP: A crossover study of gabapentin in treatment of restless legs syndrome among hemodialysis patients. Am J Kidney Dis 2001; 38(1):104–108.
126. Montplaisir J, Nicolas A, Denesle R, Gomez-Mancilla B: Restless legs syndrome improved by pramipexole: a double-blind randomized trial. Neurology 1999; 23:938–943.
127. Arieff AI: Dialysis disequilibrium syndrome: Current concepts on pathogenesis and prevention. Kidney Int 1994; 45: 629–635.
128. Ihara M, Ito T, Yanagihara C, Nishimura Y: Wernicke's encephalopathy associated with hemodialysis: Report of two cases and review of the literature. Clin Neurol Neurosurg 1999; 101(2):118–121.
129. Swartz RD: Hemodialysis-associated seizure activity. *In* Nissenson AR, Fine RN (eds): Dialysis Therapy, 2nd ed. Philadelphia St. Louis, Hanley & Belfus, Inc. Mosby – Year Book, 1993, p 113–116.
130. Sonmez F, Mir S, Tutuncuoglu S: Potential prophylactic use of benzodiazepines for hemodialysis-associated seizures. Pediatr Nephrol 2000; 14(5):367–369.
131. Alfrey AC: Aluminum neurotoxicity. *In* Nissenson AR, Fine RN (eds): Dialysis Therapy, 2nd ed. Philadelphia, Hanley & Belfus, 1993, p 275–277.
132. Barata JD, D'Haese PC, Pires C, et al: Low-dose (5 mg/kg) desferrioxamine treatment in acutely aluminum-intoxicated haemodialysis patients using two drug administration schedules. Nephrol Dial Transplant 1996; 11(1):125–132.
133. Chenoweth DE, Cheung AK, Henderson LW: Anaphylatoxin formation during hemodialysis: Effects of different dialyzer membranes. Kidney Int 1983; 24:764–769.
134. Kaplow L, Goffinet J: Profound neutropenia during the early phase of hemodialysis. JAMA 1968; 203:1135–1137.
135. Sato H, Ohkubo M, Nagaoka T: Levels of serum colony-stimulating factors (CSFs) in patients on long-term haemodialysis. Cytokine 1994; 6:187–194.
136. Cheung AK, Hohnholt M, Gilson J: Adherence of neutrophils to hemodialysis membranes: Role of complement receptors. Kidney Int 1991; 40:1123–1133.
137. Mason R, Zucker W, Bilinsky R: Blood components deposited on used and reused dialysis membranes. Biomat Med Dev Art Org 1976; 4:333–358.
138. Dodd N, Gordge M, Tarrant J: A demonstration of neutrophil accumulation in the pulmonary vasculature during hemodialysis. Proc Eur Transplant Assoc 1983; 20:186–189.
139. Ivanovich P, Chenoweth D, Schmidt R: Symptoms and activation of granulocytes and complement with two dialysis membranes. Kidney Int 1983; 24:758–763.
140. Hakim RM, Schafer AI: Hemodialysis-associated platelet activation and thrombocytopenia. Am J Med 1985; 78:575–580.

141. Hakim R, Fearon D, Lazarus J: Biocompatibility of dialysis membranes: Effects of chronic complement activation. Kidney Int 1984; 26:194–200.
142. From the Centers for Disease Control and Prevention. Multistate outbreak of hemolysis in hemodialysis patients–Nebraska and Maryland, 1998. JAMA 1998; 280(15):1299–3000.
143. Duffy R, Tomashek K, Spangenberg M, et al: Multistate outbreak of hemolysis in hemodialysis patients traced to faulty blood tubing sets. Kidney Int 2000; 57(4):1668–1674.
144. Weinstein T, Chagnac A, Korzets A, et al: Haemolysis in haemodialysis patients: Evidence for impaired defense mechanisms against oxidative stress. Nephrol Dial Transplant 2000; 15(6):883–887.
145. Twardowski ZJ: Safety of high venous and arterial line pressures during hemodialysis. Semin Dial 2000; 13(5):336–337.
146. Chambers SD, Ceccio SL, Annich GA, Bartlett RH: Extreme negative pressure does not cause erythrocyte damage in flowing blood. ASAIO J 1999; 45(5):431–435.
147. De Wachter DS, Verdonck PR, De Vos JY, Hombrouckx RO: Blood trauma in plastic haemodialysis cannulae. Int J Artif Organs 1997; 20(7):366–370.
148. Yang MC, Lin CC: Influence of design of the hemodialyzer inlet chamber on red blood cell damage during hemodialysis. ASAIO J 2001; 47(1):92–96.
149. Perez-Garcia R, Rodriguez-Benitez P: Chloramine, a sneaky contaminant of dialysate. Nephrol Dial Transplant 1999; 14(11): 2579–2582.
150. Eaton JW, Leida MN: Hemolysis in chronic renal failure. Semin Nephrol 1985; 5:133–139.
151. Ward DM: Chloramine removal from water used in hemodialysis. Adv Ren Replace Ther 1996; 3(4):337–347.
152. Amato L: Clinical Symptoms of Inadequately Treated Water for Hemodialysis. *In* Water Quality for Dialysis, 3rd ed. AAMI Dialysis Monograph Series (3rd ed): 1998.
153. Salvadori M, Martinelli F, Comparini L, et al: Nitrate induced anaemia in home dialysis patients. Proceedings of the European Dialysis & Transplant Association-European Renal Association 1985; 21:321–325.
154. Orringer EP, Mattern WD: Formaldehyde-induced hemolysis during chronic hemodialysis. New Engl J Med 1976; 294:1416–1420.
155. Gordon SM, Bland LA, Alexander SR, et al: Hemolysis associated with hydrogen peroxide at a pediatric dialysis center. Am J Nephrol 1990; 10(2):123–127.
156. Ng YY, Chow MP, Wu SC, et al: Anti-Nform antibody in hemodialysis patients. Am J Nephrol 1995; 15:374–378.
157. Kelton JG, Sheridan D, Santos A, et al: Heparin-induced thrombocytopenia: Laboratory studies. Blood 1988; 72:925–930.
158. Pham PT, Miller JM, Demetrion G, Lew SQ: Clotting by heparin of hemoaccess for hemodialysis in an end-stage renal disease patient. Am J Kidney Dis 1995; 25:642–647.
159. Reilly RF: The pathophysiology of immune-mediated heparin-induced thrombocytopenia. Semin Dial 2003; 16(1):54–60.
160. Finazzi G, Remuzzi G: Heparin-induced thrombocytopenia: Background and implications for haemodialysis. Nephrol Dial Transplant 1996; 11(11):2120–2122.
161. Yamamoto S, Koide M, Matsuo M, et al: Heparin-induced thrombocytopenia in hemodialysis patients. Am J Kidney Dis 1996; 28:82–85.
162. Neuhaus TJ, Goetschel P, Schmugge M, Leumann E: Heparin-induced thrombocytopenia type II on hemodialysis: switch to danaparoid. Pediatr Nephrol 2000; 14(8–9):713–716.
163. Vanholder R, Camez A, Veys N, et al: Pharmacokinetics of recombinant hirudin in hemodialyzed end-stage renal failure patients. Thromb Haemost 1997; 77:650–655.
164. Wittkowsky AK, Kondo LM: Lepirudin dosing in dialysis-dependent renal failure. Pharmacotherapy 2000; 20(9):1123–1128.
165. Patel V, Snyder J, Shopnick R: Successful use of low dose r-hirudin (Refludan) for recurrent dialysis catheter thrombosis in a patient with heparin induced thrombocytopenia. Thromb-Haemost 1999; 82:1205–1206.
166. Walker JA, Sherman RA, Eisinger R: Thrombocytopenia associated with intravenous desferrioxamine. Am J Kidney Dis 1985; 4:254–256.
167. Walker RW, Heaton A: Thrombocytopenia due to vancomycin. Lancet 1985; 1:932.
168. Gottschall JL, Neahring B, McFarland JG, et al: Quinine-induced immune thrombocytopenia with hemolytic uremic syndrome: Clinical and serological findings in nine patients and review of literature. Am J Hematol 1994; 47:283–289.
169. Remuzzi G: Bleeding in renal failure. Lancet 1988; i:1205–1208.
170. Remuzzi G, Rossi EC: Hematologic consequences of renal failure. *In* Brenner BM (ed): The Kidney. Philadelphia, W.B. Saunders Company, 1996, p 2170–2186.
171. Blagg C: Acute complications associated with hemodialysis. *In* Maher J (ed): Replacement of Renal Function by Dialysis: A Textbook of Dialysis, 3rd ed. Dordrecht, Holland, Kluwer Academic, 1989, p 750–771.
172. Yoon W, Kim JK, Kim HK, et al: Acute small bowel hemorrhage in three patients with end-stage renal disease: Diagnosis and management by angiographic intervention. Cardiovasc Intervent Radiol 2002; 25(2):133–136.
173. Nozoe T, Kitamura M, Matsumata T, Sugimachi K: Dieulafoy-like lesions of colon and rectum in patients with chronic renal failure on long-term hemodialysis. Hepatogastroenterology 1999; 46(30):3121–3123.
174. Carlson CC, Holsten SJ, Grandas OH: Bilateral renal rupture in a patient on hemodialysis. Am Surg 2003; 69(6):505–507.
175. Schwab SJ, Onorato JJ, Sharar LR, Dennis PA: Hemodialysis without anticoagulation. One year prospective trial in hospitalized patients at risk for bleeding. Am J Med 1987; 83: 405–410.
176. Lohr JW, Slusher S, Diederich D: Safety of regional citrate hemodialysis in acute renal failure. Am J Kidney Dis 1989; 13: 104–107.
177. Caruana RJ, Smith MC, Clyne D, et al: A controlled study of heparin versus epoprostenol sodium (prostacyclin) as the sole anticoagulant for chronic hemodialysis. Blood Purif 1991; 9: 296–304.
178. Romao JE Jr, Fadil MA, Sabbage E, Marcondes M: Haemodialysis without anticoagulant: Haemostasis parameters, fibrinogen kinetic, and dialysis efficiency. Nephrol Dial Transplant 1997; 12(1):106–110.
179. Gerlach AT, Pickworth KK, Seth SK, et al: Enoxaparin and bleeding complications: A review in patients with and without renal insufficiency. Pharmacotherapy 2000; 20(7): 771– 775.
180. Muller A, Huhle G, Nowack R, et al: Serious bleeding in a haemodialysis patient treated with recombinant hirudin. Nephrol Dial Transplant 1999; 14(10):2482–2483.
181. Patterson RW, Nissenson AR, Miller J, et al: Hypoxemia and pulmonary gas exchange during hemodialysis. J Appl Physiol: Respiratory, Environmental & Exercise Physiology 1981; 50: 259–264.
182. Yap JC, Wang YT, Poh SC: Effect of oxygen on breathing irregularities during haemodialysis in patients with chronic uraemia. Eur Respir J 1998; 12(2):420–425.
183. Cardoso M, Vinay P, Vinet B, et al: Hypoxemia during hemodialysis: A critical review of the facts. Am J Kidney Dis 1988; 11:281–297.
184. Munger MA, Ateshkadi A, Cheung AK, et al: Cardiopulmonary events during hemodialysis: Effects of dialysis membranes and dialysate buffers. Am J Kidney Dis 2000; 36(1):130–139.
185. Nielsen AL, Thunedborg P, Brinkenfeldt H, et al: Assessment of pH and oxygen status during hemodialysis using the arterial blood line in patients with an arteriovenous fistula. Blood Purif 1999; 17(4):206–212.

186. Hegbrant J, Sternby J, Larsson A, et al: Beneficial effect of cold dialysate for the prevention of hemodialysis-induced hypoxia. Blood Purif 1997; 15(1):15–24.
187. Keshaviah PR, Luehmann D, Shapiro FL, Comty CM: Investigation of the Risks and Hazards Associated with Hemodialysis Devices. Technical report: Food and Drug Administration, Department of Health, Education and Welfare, 1980.
188. O'Quin RJ, Lakshminarayan S: Venous air embolism. Arch Intern Med 1982; 142:2173–2176.
189. Yu AS, Levy E: Paradoxical cerebral air embolism from a hemodialysis catheter. Am J Kidney Dis 1997; 29(3):453–455.
190. Baskin SE, Wozniak RF: Hyperbaric oxygenation in the treatment of hemodialysis associated air embolism. N Engl J Med 1975; 293:184–185.
191. Dunbar EM, Fox R, Watson B, Akrill P: Successful late treatment of venous air embolism with hyperbaric oxygen. Postgrad Med J 1990; 66:469–470.
192. Butler BD: Biophysical aspects of gas bubbles and blood. Med Instrum 1985; 19:59–62.
193. Abuelo JG, Shemin D, Chazan JA: Acute symptoms produced by hemodialysis: A review of their causes and associations. Semin Dial 1993; 6:59–69.
194. Barton BR, Hermann G, Weill RI. Cardiothoracic emergencies associated with subclavian hemodialysis catheters. JAMA 1983; 250:2660–2662.
195. Sharp KW, Spees EK, Selby LR, et al: Diagnosis and management of retroperitoneal hematomas after femoral vein cannulation for hemodialysis. Surgery 1984; 95:90–95.
196. Covey CM, Arieff AI: Disorders of sodium and water metabolism and their effects on the central nervous system. *In* Brenner BM, Stein JH (eds): Contemporary Issues in Nephrology. New York, Churchill-Livingstone, 1978, p 212–241.
197. Said R, Quintanilla A, Levin N, Ivanovich P: Acute hemolysis due to profound hypoosmolality. A complication of hemodialysis. J Dial 1977; 1:447–452.
198. Oo TN, Smith CL, Swan SK: Does uremia protect against the demyelination associated with correction of hyponatremia during hemodialysis? A case report and literature review. Semin Dial 2003; 16(1):68–71.
199. Sterns RH, Silver SM: Hemodialysis in hyponatremia: Is there a risk? Semin Dial 1990; 3:3–4.
200. Bender FH: Successful treatment of severe hyponatremia in a patient with renal failure using continuous venovenous hemodialysis. Am J Kidney Dis 1998; 32(5):829–831.
201. Ahmed J, Weisberg LS: Hyperkalemia in dialysis patients. Semin Dial 2001; 14(5):348–356.
202. Imbriano LJ, Durham JH, Maesaka JK: Treating interdialytic hyperkalemia with fludrocortisone. Semin Dial 2003; 16(1): 5–7.
203. Blumberg A, Roser HW, Zehnder C, Muller-Brand J: Plasma potassium in patients with terminal renal failure during and after haemodialysis; relationship with dialytic potassium removal and total body potassium. Nephrol Dial Transplant 1997; 12(8):1629–1634.
204. Redaelli B, Sforzini S, Bonoldi L, et al: Potassium removal as a factor limiting the correction of acidosis during dialysis. Proc EDTA 1983; 19:366–371.
205. Cupisti A, Galetta F, Caprioli R, et al: Potassium removal increases the QTc interval dispersion during hemodialysis. Nephron 1999; 82(2):122–126.
206. Dolson GM, Adrogue HJ: Low dialysate [K+] decreases efficiency of hemodialysis and increases urea rebound. J Am Soc Nephrol 1998; 9(11):2124–2128.
207. Spital A, Sterns RH: Potassium homeostasis in dialysis patients. Semin Dial 1988; 1:14–20.
208. Ketchersid TL, Van Stone JC: Dialysate potassium. Semin Dial 1991; 4:46–51.
209. Wiegand CF, Davin TD, Raij L, Kjellstrand CM: Severe hypokalemia induced by hemodialysis. Arch Intern Med 1981; 141:167–170.
210. Gennari FJ, Rimmer JM. Acid-base disorders in end-stage renal disease: Part I. Semin Dial 1990; 3:81–85.
211. Navarro JF, Mora-Fernandez C, Garcia J: Errors in the selection of dialysate concentrates cause severe metabolic acidosis during bicarbonate hemodialysis. Artif Organs 1997; 21(9):966–968.
212. Mirza BI, Sahani M, Leehey DJ, et al: Saline-induced dilutional acidosis in a maintenance hemodialysis patient. Int J Artif Organs 1999; 22(10):676–678.
213. Ross EA, Nissenson AR: Acid-base and electrolyte disturbances. *In* Daugirdas JT, Ing TS (eds): Handbook of Dialysis, 2nd ed. Boston, Little, Brown & Company, 1994, p 401–415.
214. Gennari HJ, Rimmer JM: Acid-base disorders in end-stage renal disease: Part II. Semin Dial 1990; 3:161–165.
215. de Precigout V, Larroumet N, Combe C, et al: Correction of a metabolic alkalosis induced by lemon consumption by acetate-free biofiltration (Letter). Nephrol Dial Transplant 1993; 8(10): 1184–1185.
216. Madias NE, Levey AS: Metabolic alkalosis due to absorption of "non-absorbable" antacids. Am J Med 1983; 74:155–158.
217. Swartz RD, Jacobs JF: Modified dialysis for metabolic alkalosis. Ann Intern Med 1978; 88:432–433.
218. Asensio Sanchez MJ, del Pozo Hernando LJ, Asensio Sanchez VM, et al: Severe metabolic alkalosis during hemodialysis. Anales de Medicina Interna 1991; 8(4):179–180.
219. Gerhardt RE, Koethe JD, Glickman JD, et al: Acid dialysate correction of metabolic alkalosis in renal failure. Am J Kidney Dis 1995; 25(2):343–345.
220. McDonald BR, Steiner RW: Rapid infusion of HCl during citrate dialysis to counteract alkalosis. Clin Nephrol 1990; 33(5): 255–256.
221. Hsu SC, Wang MC, Liu HL, et al: Extreme metabolic alkalosis treated with normal bicarbonate hemodialysis. Am J Kidney Dis 2001; 37(4):E31.
222. Bouvier P, Hecht M, Sibai R, et al: Severe metabolic alkalosis due to error of dialysis concentration. Nephrologie 1993; 14(3): 155–156.
223. Sethi D, Curtis JR, Topham DL, Gower PE: Acute metabolic alkalosis during haemodialysis. Nephron 1989; 51(1):119–120.
224. Kelleher SP, Schulman G: Severe metabolic alkalosis complicating regional citrate hemodialysis. Am J of Kidney Dis 1987; 9(3):235–236.
225. Davenport A, Worth DP, Will EJ: Hypochloraemic alkalosis after high-flux continuous haemofiltration and continuous arteriovenous haemofiltration with dialysis. Lancet 1988; 1(8586):658.
226. Mehta R MB, Gabbai F, Pahl M, et al: A randomized clinical trial of continuous versus intermittent dialysis for acute renal failure. Kidney Int 2001; 60:1154–1163.
227. Tolchin N, Roberts JL, Hayashi J, Lewis EJ: Metabolic consequences of high mass-transfer hemodialysis. Kidney Int 1977; 11:366–378.
228. Kenamond TG, Graves JW, Lempert KD, Moss AH: Severe recurrent alkalemia in a patient undergoing continuous cyclic peritoneal dialysis. Am J Med 1986; 81:548–550.
229. Shapiro WB: The current status of sorbent hemodialysis. Semin Dial 1990; 3:40–45.
230. Hamm L, Lawrence G, DuBose JT: Sorbent regeneration hemodialysis as a potential cause of acute hypercapnia. Kidney Int 1982; 21:416–418.
231. Huang CC, Tsai YH, Lin MC, et al: Respiratory drive and pulmonary mechanics during haemodialysis with ultrafiltration in ventilated patients. Anaesth Intensive Care 1997; 25(5):464-470.
232. Freeman RM, Lawton RL, Chamberlain MA: Hard-water syndrome. N Engl J Med 1967; 276:1113–1118.
233. Evans DB, Slapak M: Pancreatitis in the hard water syndrome. Br Med J 1975; 3(748).
234. Mulloy AL, Mulloy LL, Weinstein RS: Hypercalcemia due to hard water used for home hemodialysis (see comments). South Med J 1992; 85(11):1131–1133.

235. Erben J, Hajakova B, Pantucek M, Kubes L: Fluoride metabolism and renal osteodystrophy in regular dialysis treatment. Proc Eur Dial Transplant Assoc Eur Renal Assoc 1985; 21:421–425.
236. Bello VA, Gitelman HJ: High fluoride exposure in hemodialysis patients. Am J Kidney Dis 1990; 15:320–324.
237. McIvor M, Baltazar RF, Beltran J, et al: Hyperkalemia and cardiac arrest from fluoride exposure during hemodialysis. Am J Cardiol 1983; 51:901–902.
238. Berkes SL, Kahn SI, Chazan JA, Garella S: Prolonged hemolysis from overheated dialysate. Ann Intern Med 1975; 83:363–364.
239. Schneditz D, Rosales L, Kaufman AM, et al: Heat accumulation with relative blood volume decrease. Am J Kidney Dis 2002; 40(4):777–782.
240. Parfrey PS, Vavasour HM, Henry S, et al: Clinical features and severity of nonspecific symptoms in dialysis patients. Nephron 1988; 50:121–128.
241. Van Stone JC, Cook J: The effect of bicarbonate dialysate in stable chronic hemodialysis patients. Dial Transplant 1979; 8:703–709.
242. Group BCDS: Acute intradialytic well-being: Results of a clinical trial comparing polysulfone with cuprophan. Kidney Int 1991; 40:714–719.
243. Sklar AH, Beezhold DH, Newman N, et al: Postdialysis fatigue: Lack of effect of a biocompatible membrane. Am J Kidney Dis 1998; 31(6):1007–1010.
244. Sklar A, Newman N, Scott R, et al: Identification of factors responsible for postdialysis fatigue. Am J Kidney Dis 1999; 34(3):464–470.
245. Altieri P, Sorba GB, Bolasco PG, et al: On-line predilution hemofiltration versus ultrapure high-flux hemodialysis: A multicenter prospective study in 23 patients. Sardinian Collaborative Study Group of On-Line Hemofiltration. Blood Purif 1997; 15(3):169–181.
246. Osman Y, Poh-Fitzpatrick MB: Dermatologic disorders associated with chronic renal failure. Semin Dial 1988; 1:86–90.
247. Szepietowski JC, Sikora M, Kusztal M, et al: Uremic pruritus: A clinical study of maintenance hemodialysis patients. J Dermatol 2002; 29(10):621–627.
248. Weisshaar E, Dunker N, Domrose U, et al: Plasma serotonin and histamine levels in hemodialysis-related pruritus are not significantly influenced by 5-HT3 receptor blocker and antihistaminic therapy. Clin Nephrol 2003; 59(2):124–129.
249. Murphy M, Reaich D, Pai P, et al: A randomized, placebo-controlled, double-blind trial of ondansetron in renal itch. Br J Dermatol 2003; 148(2):314–317.
250. Ashmore SD, Jones CH, Newstead CG, et al: Ondansetron therapy for uremic pruritus in hemodialysis patients. Am J Kidney Dis 2000; 35(5):827–831.
251. Weber M, Schmutz JL: Hemodialysis and the skin. Contr Nephrol 1988; 62:75–85.
252. Weisshaar E, Dunker N, Gollnick H: Topical capsaicin therapy in humans with hemodialysis related pruritus. Neurosci Lett 2003; 345(3):192–194.
253. Feinstein EI: The skin. *In* Daugirdas JT, Ing TS (eds): Handbook of Dialysis, 2nd ed. Boston, Little, Brown & Company, 1994, p 583–589.
254. Peck LW: Essential fatty acid deficiency in renal failure: Can supplements really help? J Am Diet Assoc 1997; 97(10 suppl 2): S150–S153.
255. Peer G, Kivity S, Agami O, et al: Randomised crossover trial of naltrexone in uraemic pruritus. Lancet 1996; 348(9041):1552–1554.
256. Singhal PC, Lynn RI, Scharschmidt LA: Priapism and dialysis. Am J Nephrol 1986; 6(5):358–361.
257. Duggan ML, Morgan CJ: Heparin: A cause of priapism? S Med J 1970; 63:1131–1134.
258. Port FK, Fiegel P, Hecking E, et al: Priapism during regular haemodialysis. Lancet 1974; 2:1287–1288.
259. Brown JA, Nehra A: Erythropoietin-induced recurrent veno-occlusive priapism associated with end-stage renal disease. Urology 1998; 52(2):328–330.
260. Fassbinger W, Frei U, Issantier R, et al: Factors predisposing to priapism in haemodialysis patients. Proc Euro Dial Transplant 1977; 12:380–386.
261. Sombolos K, Zoumbaridis N, Mavromatidis K, Natse T: Effect of androgen administration or the action of exogenous erythropoietin in hemodialysis patients. Am J Kidney Dis 1992; 19(1):94.
262. Nakamura N, Takaesu N, Arakaki Y: Priapism in haemodialysis patient due to prazosin? Brit J Urol 1991; 68(5):551–552.
263. O'Brien WM, O'Connor KP, Lynch JH: Priapism: Current concepts. Ann Emerg Med 1989; 18:980–983.
264. Branger B, Ramperez P, Oules R, et al: Metaraminol for haemodialysis-associated priapism (Letter). Lancet 1985; 1(8429):641.
265. Rizvi SS, Holmes RA: Hearing loss from haemodialysis. Arch Otolaryngol 1980; 106:751–756.
266. Kligerman AB, Solangi KB, Ventry IM, et al: Hearing impairment associated with chronic renal failure. Laryngoscope 1981; 91:583–592.
267. Gatland D, Tucker B, Chalstrey S, et al: Hearing loss in chronic renal failure-hearing threshold changes following haemodialysis. J Roy Soc Med 1991; 84:587–589.
268. Mitschke H, Schmidt P, Zazgorlik J, et al: Effect of renal transplantation on uraemic deafness: A long-term study. Audiology 1977; 16:530–534.
269. Ozturan O, Lam S: The effect of hemodialysis on hearing using puretone audiometry and distortion-product otoacoustic emissions. ORL J Otorhinolaryngol Relat Spec 1998; 60(6):306–313.
270. Serbetcioglu MB, Erdogan S, Sifil A: Overall no adverse effect of a single session of hemodialysis on hearing abilities. Nephron 2001; 87(3):286.
271. Olivieri NF, Buncic JR, Chew E, et al: Visual and auditory neurotoxicity in patients receiving subcutaneous deferrioxamine infusions. N Engl J Med 1986; 314:869–873.
272. Altiparmak MR, Pamuk ON, Pamuk GE, et al: Is isoniazid ototoxic in patients undergoing hemodialysis? Nephron 2002; 92(2):478–480.
273. Saxena AK, Panhotra BR, Naguib M: Sudden irreversible sensory-neural hearing loss in a patient with diabetes receiving amikacin as an antibiotic-heparin lock. Pharmacotherapy 2002; 22(1):105–108.
274. Barton CH, Vaziri ND: Central retinal vein occlusion associated with hemodialysis. Am J Med Sci 1979; 277:39–47.
275. Jaeger P, Morisod L, Wauters JP, Faggioni R: Prevention of glaucoma during hemodialysis by mannitol and acetazolamide. N Engl J Med 1980; 303:702.
276. Servilla KS, Groggel GC: Anterior ischemic optic neuropathy as a complication of hemodialysis. Am J Kidney Dis 1986; 8:61–63.
277. Sabeel A, Al-Hazzaa SA, Alfurayh O, Mikkonen P: The dialysed patient who turned blind during a haemodialysis session. Nephrol Dial Transplant 1998; 13(11):2957–2958.
278. Arora N, Lambrou FHJ, Stewart MW, et al: Sudden blindness associated with central nervous symptoms in a hemodialysis patient. Nephron 1991; 59:490–492.
279. Hutter JC, Kuehnert MJ, Wallis RR, et al: Acute onset of decreased vision and hearing traced to hemodialysis treatment with aged dialyzers. JAMA 2000; 283(16):2128–2134.
280. Tsuruoka S, Osono E, Nishiki K, et al: Removal of digoxin by column for specific adsorption of beta(2)-microglobulin: A potential use for digoxin intoxication. Clin Pharmacol Ther 2001; 69(6):422–430.

Daily Hemodialysis

Andreas Pierratos, M.D., F.R.C.P.C. • Phil McFarlane, M.D., F.R.C.P.C. • Christopher Chan, M.D., F.R.C.P.C.

The quest for a solution to the problem of poor outcomes and low quality of life for patients with end-stage renal disease (ESRD) has led to an increased interest in daily hemodialysis.[1] Two distinct forms of daily dialysis have emerged (Figure 23–1). The first is characterized by frequent short treatments, with dialysis typically performed for 2 to 4 hours. The second is a nightly form, with treatments lasting 6 to 8 hours and performed while the patient sleeps. In both cases, treatments are performed five to seven times a week. Hybrid forms of varying frequency and length have also been used. In addition, some have chosen daily hemo(dia)filtration with an aim to increase middle molecule clearance.[2,3]

The term *quotidian* hemodialysis has been proposed to categorize any form of dialysis performed on a daily basis. The term *hemeral* has been suggested for the short daily form and *nocturnal* for the long overnight form. Other names in use include *short daily* hemodialysis and *daily (home) nocturnal* hemodialysis. Last, the term *intensive* hemodialysis has been proposed for any method whose length or frequency exceeds that of conventional hemodialysis.[4] Daily dialysis is not new; DePalma[5] first reported the benefits of short daily hemodialysis in 1969. Overnight dialysis at home was pioneered by Shaldon in 1968, with Uldall[6,7] reporting the use of daily home nocturnal hemodialysis in 1994. The number of publications in this area has increased in recent years, reflecting an increasing interest in these intensive dialysis techniques.[8] In the following chapter, we will discuss the available evidence suggesting that quotidian dialysis can improve outcomes in selected patients.

DIALYSIS TECHNIQUE

Although all hemodialysis machines can be used for quotidian hemodialysis, several new machines have been developed specifically for this purpose, and existing machines have been adapted for the specific needs of home hemodialysis.[2,9] Short daily hemodialysis can be done at an in-center facility or at home using high blood and dialysate flow to achieve maximal efficiency. Nocturnal hemodialysis thrice a week or every other night can be performed in-center or at home but quotidian nocturnal hemodialysis is typically not performed in-center.[10] For home treatments, the patient or a family member is trained in the technique. For quotidian nocturnal hemodialysis, blood flow is 200 to 300 mL/min, and dialysate flow is 100 to 300 mL/min. With this modality, a high dialysis dose can be delivered even through single needle systems. No data exist on how dialyzers should be selected for quotidian dialysis, with existing programs using low- and high-flux membranes and some programs using pediatric size dialyzers in adult patients.[10] Dialyzer reprocessing has been used in quotidian programs, with delays in reprocessing of up to 1 week allowed in home programs.[11] The starting dialysate for short daily hemodialysis is similar to that used in conventional hemodialysis. Dialysate composition in quotidian nocturnal hemodialysis must be tailored for each patient, because the effect of intensive hemodialysis on calcium-phosphate balance and acid-base status can vary between individuals. The typical dialysate has a bicarbonate level of 28 to 35 mEq/L, calcium of 3.3 ± 0.2 mEq/L (1.6 ± 0.1 mmol/L), and phosphorus of 1.6±0.9 mg/dL (0.5 ± 0.3 mmol/L). Dialysate calcium, if desired, can be adjusted through the addition of calcium chloride powder in the "acid" concentrate by the patient. Sodium phosphate can be added to either the acid or bicarbonate concentrate for patients requiring supplementation. In the absence of a commercially available preparation, oral Fleet Phospho-Soda or Fleet enema can be used. Heparin dose on both methods is similar to conventional hemodialysis. Water for dialysate is usually purified using reverse osmosis systems and carbon filters. Local water quality can require the use of deionizers, and some programs have chosen to use ultra-pure dialysate for quotidian dialysis.[12,13]

Live Remote Monitoring

Several centers have been remotely monitoring patients "live" while on home nocturnal hemodialysis through a telephone or an Internet connection, usually dependent on whether a call from the patient's home is a local phone call to the monitoring center.[14–16] Current technology allows for the monitoring of machine functions, such as alarms and pump speeds. Biologic monitoring (e.g., heart rate, blood pressure) will require further innovations. While some programs and patients have touted the extra safety associated with remote monitoring, other programs have many patients performing these techniques without remote monitoring systems, without complications to this point.

Dialysis Access

Access for quotidian dialysis has been established through central venous catheters and arteriovenous fistulas or grafts. Single needle systems have been used in some home nocturnal hemodialysis programs, decreasing the number of cannulations and providing improved safety in scenarios where a needle is inadvertently removed during a nocturnal dialysis treatment.[17] Many quotidian dialysis programs access arteriovenous fistulae through the buttonhole technique, where cannulation occurs at the same site each day, allowing for the development of a subcutaneous track that aids the accurate

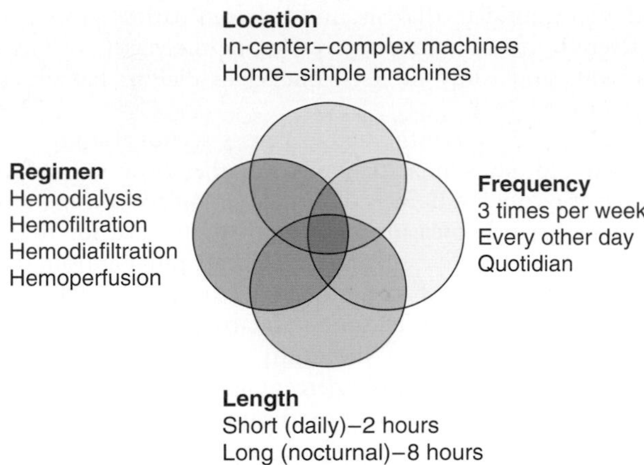

Figure 23–1 Available blood-based dialysis modalities.

placement of needles. Once a track has developed, noncutting needles are used at buttonhole sites, helping preserve the tracks, and improving patient comfort during cannulation.[18] Meticulous attention to hygiene is pivotal when the buttonhole technique is utilized, with aseptic removal of scabs and cleansing of the site required prior to cannulation. Evidence of lower fistula complication rates on daily hemodialysis has been reported by Quintaliani and associates[19] and Woods and associates,[20] but no prospectively collected data has been published. The long-term use of central venous catheters has also been demonstrated but published data are again insufficient. Given our current understanding, an arteriovenous fistula is the preferred access for quotidian dialysis, with grafts or central venous catheters used in patients where a fistula is not feasible.

Safety

Controversy remains about when a partner is required for home hemodialysis modalities, and whether the partner needs to be trained in the technique. Most home programs do not require a partner for hemeral or nocturnal techniques. As patients are expected to be sleeping during nocturnal treatments, extra safety precautions have been developed for this modality. In order to prevent air embolism in the case of accidental central venous catheters disconnection, the InterLink system has been utilized, allowing dialysis to be performed through the pre-slit diaphragm of the catheter cap.[10] A plastic nondisposable clamshell-locking box around the catheter-tubing connection can prevent an accidental separation. Blood or dialysate leaks are sensed by moisture sensors placed strategically on the floor and an "enuresis alarm" is taped on both arterial and venous needles.

Patient Selection/Training

A wide variety of people have been selected for quotidian dialysis. In many cases (especially in home programs), patients have selected themselves, in hope of realizing clinical or lifestyle benefits. In other cases, patients were selected to address problems related to hemodynamic instability, uncontrolled hypertension, congestive heart failure, refractory electrolyte or calcium-phosphate metabolism issues, malnutrition, or poor quality of life.[21] The main selection criteria for home hemodialysis training are the ability and willingness to learn the technique. Patients living in small housing will require extra support from their program, usually through more frequent supply deliveries. Contraindication to heparin precludes the use of nocturnal hemodialysis but not short daily hemodialysis. Serious comorbid conditions and hemodynamic instability such as heart failure, ascites, and symptomatic coronary artery disease have not been contraindications for daily hemodialysis. Indeed, patients with these conditions may be especially well suited for quotidian hemodialysis. Incident ESRD patients are excellent candidates for daily hemodialysis and can be trained for home modalities. It is speculated that about 20% of the current dialysis population could be trained for home hemodialysis using the current dialysis machines. Training for home dialysis lasts an average of 6 weeks for previously untrained patients,[22,23] with shorter periods for patients already trained to perform self-care hemodialysis. Longer training in a self-care environment allows patients with marginal ability to master the technique over a longer period of time. It is hoped that new or modified dialysis machines will be simpler to operate, thereby allowing more patients to be trained.[2,3]

Kinetics/Dialysis Dose: Solute Removal

The similarity of the patient mortality rates between peritoneal dialysis and conventional thrice-weekly hemodialysis, despite the differences in dialysis dose as quantified by urea Kt/V,[25] has led some to conclude that continuous or frequent dialysis offers better clinical outcomes at an equivalent Kt/V.[25] Assuming that outcomes are mainly related to the dialysis dose, several attempts have been made to create a universal renal toxin clearance metric applicable to all dialysis modalities and residual renal function. These include the EKR (equivalent kidney urea clearance) proposed by Casino and Lopez,[26] the normalized Kt/V proposed by Depner,[27] and the standard Kt/V (stdKt/V) proposed by Gotch.[28] The traditional measurement of dialysis dose by calculating Kt/V assumes that uremic toxicity correlates to time-averaged urea concentration. EKR makes similar assumptions. StdKt/V is based on the mid-week pre-dialysis urea levels, whereas the normalized Kt/V is based on the time-averaged concentration of a theoretical molecule with larger molecular weight than urea. The last two measures therefore favor daily hemodialysis, which is characterized by lower pre-dialysis urea levels. The stdKt/V is commonly used to measure urea dialysis dose and has been expanded to measure the clearance of larger molecules.[29] The calculation of these values is complex and cannot be easily done at the bedside, but they can be used to calculate the appropriate single pool Kt/V for the daily dialysis regimens.

The recently published HEMO study did not demonstrate a decrease in mortality when dialysis dose was increased above the level suggested in the Dialysis Outcome Quality Initiative (DOQI) guidelines.[30] The DOQI guidelines suggest a conventional dialysis dose of 1.2 spKt/V per session or 2.0 stdKt/V per week. This is equivalent to a daily session 0.38 equilibrated Kt/V (eKt/V), which can be delivered by shorter total dialysis duration per week than when using conventional hemodialysis. By choosing to maintain the same weekly hemodialysis duration but perform treatments daily, the weekly stdKt/V increases to about 3.[31] Quotidian nocturnal hemodialysis can provide a higher dose of dialysis than any other outpatient dialysis modality (spKt/V about 2.0 per daily session or weekly stdKt/V of more than 5).[10,29,31–33]

The removal of larger molecules is dependent on the permeability of the dialysis membranes, length of dialysis, and last, on the presence of convective transport as part of ultrafiltration or hemofiltration. Increase in the frequency of dialysis plays a significant role in the removal of molecules diffusing slowly across the intercompartmental barriers.[34] Large molecule clearance by short daily hemodialysis is increased only modestly if the calculation is based on the time-averaged concentration[35] but substantially when stdKt/V is used.[29] The clearance of large molecules increases significantly by nocturnal hemodialysis irrespective of the method of calculation, since it combines both long duration and high frequency.[29,35] This is exemplified by the enhanced β_2 microglobulin removal by this method which is fourfold that of conventional hemodialysis, leading to lower serum β_2 microglobulin levels.[36] Large molecule removal by short daily hemo(dia)filtration approaches the levels of daily nocturnal hemodialysis despite the shorter dialysis time.[3,29] Quotidian nocturnal hemofiltration would presumably provide the highest dose of large molecule removal.

Floridi and associates[37] have found that advanced glycated end-product (AGE) levels are significantly lower on short daily hemodialysis compared with conventional HD. Friedman and associates[38] have also found that patients on nocturnal hemodialysis have significantly lower total homocysteine levels compared with those on conventional HD. Lower levels of both parameters may lead to decreased cardiovascular morbidity and mortality on daily hemodialysis. It is unclear whether the decrease in circulating levels of these solutes is related to increased removal, decreased production, or increased extrarenal catabolism.

Finally, it is likely that some of the putative benefits of daily hemodialysis are mediated by improvements in hemodynamic parameters or by decreased fluctuations of other biologic parameters. A measure of such fluctuation is the time average deviation (TAD), which Lopot[39] has proposed as an index of physiologic treatment and reflects the variation of the urea values around its time-averaged concentration. The use of this parameter as a predictor of clinical outcomes has not yet been validated.

QUALITY OF LIFE

ESRD reduces both length and quality of life. The quality of life on conventional hemodialysis is equivalent to that seen in patients with hepatocellular carcinoma, or a second recurrence of breast cancer.[40,41]

A variety of studies have quantified the impact of quotidian dialysis on quality of life, using disease independent instruments, such as the Medical Outcomes Study Short-Form Health Survey-36 (MOS SF-36), the Sickness Impact Profile (SIP), the Nottingham Health Profile, the Beck Depression Index, or instruments specific for renal disease such as the Kidney Disease Quality of Life (KDQOL).[42–44] Techniques used to generate utility scores such as the standard gamble and the time trade-off technique have also been used.[45] Unique measures such as the time to recovery after a dialysis session have also been examined.[46] Comparisons have been made prospectively and retrospectively, within patient groups before and after quotidian dialysis, and between patient groups on different forms of hemodialysis. Despite the variety of measurements and study designs, quotidian dialysis has always been favored.

Quality of life was estimated in a cross-sectional study of 43 demographically similar patients on either conventional in-center or quotidian home nocturnal hemodialysis using utility scores, which measure a patient's preference for health states and are usually expressed on a scale ranging from 0 (a health state equivalent to death) to 1 (equivalent to the best imaginable health).[47] When the standard gamble technique is used to elicit preferences, the utility score can be calculated after determining the highest percentage chance of immediate death that a patient would agree to gamble against for perfect health (SG utility = 1, highest change of immediate death willing to gamble against for perfect health). In this study, utility scores were significantly higher in the intensively dialyzed group (0.77 vs. 0.53). The utility scores for patients on conventional dialysis were similar to those previously published, but the quotidian nocturnal group scores were similar to those seen in kidney transplant recipients, which mirrors anecdotal reports of patients removing themselves from transplant waiting lists in favor of home quotidian hemodialysis.[48] Although utility scores provide a global measure of quality of life through examination of patient preferences for health states, they do not provide insights into why quality of life has changed. For this information we must look at studies that used metrics that quantify quality of life in a variety of different domains.

In a study of 18 patients before and after conversion to quotidian home nocturnal hemodialysis, the mean SIP total score improved significantly from 14 to 10, primarily driven by improvements in Eating and Household Management scores. SF-36 scores also improved, with significant changes in Social Functioning (mean score 54 to 80) and Physical Functioning (mean 61 to 69), and there was a significant reduction in Beck Depression Index scores as well.[42,44] Similarly, in a study of patients switched from conventional to short daily dialysis (at that same weekly urea Kt/V), improvements were seen in SF-36 and Nottingham health index scores, which were primarily driven by improvements in mental health, vitality, and energy.[49] In a study of 11 hemeral, 12 nocturnal, and 22 conventional hemodialysis patients, quotidian dialysis was better tolerated and was associated with preserved quality of life over 18 months of follow-up, while patients on conventional hemodialysis suffered a significant decline in quality of life over the study period.[46] Thus, quotidian hemodialysis is associated with an improved quality of life in selected patients. These results are even more striking when one considers the additional time required for quotidian treatments, the medicalization of the home setting, and additional demands on patients performing home modalities. It appears that global improvements in quality of life reflect a broad impact of quotidian hemodialysis on physical, mental, and social parameters.

CARDIOVASCULAR PARAMETERS

Clinical Improvements

Blood pressure (BP) control is improved with short daily hemodialysis and nocturnal hemodialysis.[10,20,50] Most patients do not require the use of anti-hypertensive medications. Indeed, in a prospective crossover study involving short daily nocturnal home hemodialysis (SDHD),[51] BP control improved, the need for anti-hypertensive medication fell, and left ventricular mass index decreased during the 6 months of SDHD. Although the exact mechanism leading to the fall in BP with SDHD is unknown, a decrease in extracellular fluid (ECF) volume may be an important contributing factor.[51] Similar blood pressure control can be achieved with nocturnal hemodialysis. The Toronto experience has consistently reported the normalization of BP with this modality.[14] Chan and associates[33] reported on the restoration of normal blood pressure in 28 patients on NHD who were followed for 3 years after conversion from CHD to home NHD. Left ventricular mass index also declined significantly from 147 to 122 g/m^2. A control cohort of home conventional hemodialysis patients did not show any change in BP or left ventricular geometry over this time period. Additionally, there was no difference in post dialysis ECF volume, as measured by bioelectrical impedance. We hypothesize that less fluctuation of ECF volume due to the quotidian frequency of dialysis or the lower average ECF volume may be relevant to the enhanced BP control. Most recently, Nesrallah and associates[50] presented evidence that ECF volume control is less important in the BP improvement while on nocturnal hemodialysis as compared to short daily hemodialysis. Removal or decreased production of neurohormonal or humoral parameters is also conceivable and will be addressed later.

The effect of converting ESRD patients with impaired left ventricular systolic function has also been studied. Six patients with depressed left ventricular ejection fraction (< 40%) were converted to NHD and were followed for 3.2 years. Again, this cohort of patients had a significant improvement in BP control with a marked increase in left ventricular ejection fraction from a mean of 28% to 41% without any change in the post dialysis ECF volume.[52]

Mechanistic Analyses

The dramatic influence of intensive hemodialysis on BP control offers an opportunity for more rigorous mechanistic analyses of the hemodynamic changes conferred by daily dialysis.

Our group performed hemodynamic, neurohormonal, and vascular responsiveness testing in 18 ESRD patients before, and at 1 and 2 months after conversion from conventional hemodialysis to nocturnal hemodialysis.[53] In this prospective cohort study, nocturnal hemodialysis resulted in lower BP while maintaining similar stroke volume and cardiac output. Total peripheral resistance (TPR) fell significantly from 1967 to 1499 dyne/sec/cm^{-5} implicating that the hypotensive effect of NHD is mediated through a reduction in an elevated TPR rather than a fall in intravascular volume. Brachial artery responsiveness to reactive hyperemia (endothelial function) and to sublingual nitroglycerine (vascular smooth muscle cell function) was also assessed. Patients demonstrated a significant increase in endothelium dependent vasodilation with an increase in brachial artery response to hyperemia from −3% on CHD to 5% after 1 month of NHD and +8% after 2 months. The endothelium independent response was augmented similarly over the same time period. These observations are the first to suggest a sustained time dependent improvement in vascular responsiveness with nocturnal hemodialysis.

Zilch and associates[54] found decrease in sympathetic activity on short daily hemodialysis. Decrease in Brain Natriuretic Peptide (BNP) on short daily hemodialysis was reported by Odar-Cederlof and associates.[55]

ERYTHROPOIETIN (EPO) DOSE AND ANEMIA CONTROL

Anemia is associated with poor uremia control and is an established cardiovascular risk factor in patients with end-stage renal disease. A decrease in erythropoietin (EPO) dose of about 30% to 40% and an increase in hemoglobin on daily hemodialysis has been reported by most groups,[20,21,56,57] but negative or equivocal results have also been reported.[10,49,58] We conducted a controlled cohort study to test the hypotheses that augmenting the dose and frequency of dialysis by daily nocturnal hemodialysis would improve the hemoglobin (Hb) concentration and decrease EPO requirement. Sixty-three patients on NHD and 32 self-care patients on conventional hemodialysis were studied.[59] There were no differences in baseline iron indices between the two groups. After transfer from CHD to NHD, there were significant improvements in Hb concentration, despite a fall in EPO requirement. In contrast, the CHD cohort had no change in EPO requirement. There was a higher percentage of patients who did not require EPO in the NHD cohort (24% vs. 3%). Enhancing uremia clearance by NHD resulted in an improvement in Hb and a fall in EPO requirement. Anemia is associated with poor uremia control and is an established cardiovascular risk factor in patients with end-stage renal disease. Further prospective studies are required to elucidate the mechanisms and clinical impact of improving anemia management in patients undergoing nocturnal or daily hemodialysis.

CALCIUM, PHOSPHORUS METABOLISM, AND BONE DISEASE

There is a recent interest in phosphate kinetics[60] with accumulating evidence that improving phosphate control prevents increases in vascular calcifications with implications on cardiovascular mortality.[61] Phosphate removal by conventional hemodialysis is inadequate, sustaining hyperphosphatemia and an elevated calcium phosphate product, which have been linked to increased mortality.[62] Phosphate is difficult to remove due to the slow mobilization of phosphate from the deep tissues during dialysis, resulting in an early decline in the serum phosphate levels during hemodialysis treatments and a loss of the serum to dialysate concentration gradient. Serum phosphate levels rebound during the last hour of dialysis and after the end of dialysis.[63] Therefore, the length of dialysis is the major determinant of phosphate removal.

Short Daily Hemodialysis

There has been only minimal effect of short daily hemodialysis on serum phosphate or the dose of the phosphate binders needed.[49] Dialysate phosphate reflecting phosphate removal increases after conversion to short daily hemodialysis, suggesting that increased phosphate intake as a result of improving appetite prevents a substantial decrease in the serum phosphate levels or the dose of phosphate binders.[64,65]

Quotidian Nocturnal Hemodialysis

The weekly phosphate removal by nocturnal hemodialysis is twice as high as by conventional hemodialysis (4.8 ± 1.7 g vs. 2.2 ± 0.6 g).[66] In some reports, all patients discontinue phosphate binders within 1 week of initiating daily nocturnal hemodialysis and are on an unrestricted phosphate diet. More than 50% of patients require the addition of sodium phosphate into the dialysate at average 1.6 ± 0.9 mg/dL (0.5 ± 0.3 mmol/L). This results in serum phosphate levels within normal limits both pre- and post-dialysis. Use of daily nocturnal hemodialysis has led to the dissolution of tumoral extraosseous calcifications in one patient.[67] Oral calcium intake may be insufficient to balance calcium loss in the dialysate, therefore, periodic bone densitometry may be required in patients receiving nocturnal hemodialysis. Average dialysate calcium of 3.3 ± 0.2 mEq/L (1.6 ± 0.1 mmol/L) was used in one center. By increasing dialysate calcium the serum parathyroid hormone (PTH) was significantly suppressed, from 580 ± 590 ng/mL (61 ± 62 pmol/L) to 228 ± 295 ng/mL (24 ± 31 pmol/L)after 6 months. Preliminary results from bone biopsies showed that 9 out of 15 patients on daily nocturnal home hemodialysis had low bone turnover.[68] This may indicate that a lower dialysate calcium (i.e., 2.5 mEq/L) than was used thus far may be preferable. More studies are needed to establish the criteria for the adjustment of the dialysate calcium levels. The role of vitamin D analogues is unclear, as is the target PTH level for patients on daily nocturnal home hemodialysis.

NUTRITION

Several studies on quotidian hemodialysis have reported improvement in nutritional aspects, including improved appetite and weight gain. Galland and associates[69] described an increase in albumin, prealbumin, cholesterol, body weight, and lean body mass upon conversion to short daily hemodialysis, although Kooistra[49] did not find an increase in serum albumin over 6 months. Spanner and associates[70] reported a trend towards higher protein equivalent of total nitrogen appearance (nPNA), on both short and nocturnal hemodialysis arms of their study, but found an increase in serum albumin and arm circumference in the short daily hemodialysis group only. Although amino acid losses in the dialysate are expected to be higher on quotidian and particularly on the nocturnal regimen,[71] total body nitrogen, as measured by *in vivo* neutron activation analysis, remained stable over 2 years of nocturnal hemodialysis.[72] In our center, body weight significantly increased in 48 patients on nocturnal hemodialysis 78 ± 18 to 80 ± 18 kg over an average of 2 years. More data are needed on the effect of daily dialysis on nutritional parameters.

SLEEP

The prevalence of sleep abnormalities is high in ESRD, and they are associated with poor quality of life[73] and higher mortality.[74] Sleep studies were done prior to and after 14 patients were enrolled in the first quotidian nocturnal hemodialysis project in Toronto.[75] In seven patients with sleep apnea, conversion to nocturnal hemodialysis normalized the frequency of apnea/hypopnea episodes from 46 ± 19 to 9 ± 9 per hour, and the lowest oxygen saturation during sleep significantly increased from 89 ± 2% to 94 ± 2%. Nocturnal hemodialysis did not have an effect on daytime sleepiness when measured prior to and after the conversion to daily nocturnal hemodialysis in the first 24 patients enrolled in the same project.[76] The effect of short daily hemodialysis on sleep apnea is unknown.

The mechanistic impact of nocturnal hemodialysis on nocturnal cardiac autonomic outflow has recently been examined. Our group performed heart rate variability analysis in nine ESRD patients while on conventional hemodialysis and 6 to 15 months after conversion to nocturnal hemodialysis during stage II sleep. Nocturnal hemodialysis significantly reduced the duration of nocturnal hypoxemia and restored the normal balance between sympathetic and parasympathetic modulation of heart rate.[77]

SURVIVAL

No hard data have been published on patient survival. Woods and associates[20] reported an 80% survival over 5 years on 70 patients treated with short daily hemodialysis. Nocturnal hemodialysis in the Toronto Program demonstrated, similarly, an 85% survival over 5 years.[78] Hospitalization rates of patients on daily hemodialysis were reported to be lower than conventional hemodialysis in a retrospective study on a limited number of patients[44] as well as in a prospective study comparing two cohorts of patients on conventional and nocturnal hemodialysis.[79] Although survival in these studies is higher than expected, it is not possible to separate the effect of intensive dialysis on survival from case-mix bias.

HEALTH ECONOMICS

Local restraints in finances, staffing, physical facilities, and the availability of home programs usually dictate access to quotidian dialysis. Modality-specific costs of dialysis such as the costs of membranes, dialysate, and tubing increase in proportion to the number of treatments. As staff salary and benefits and overhead expenses account for up to a half of conventional dialysis costs, a quotidian home dialysis program can leverage savings in theses areas to offset increased modality costs. In-center quotidian hemodialysis programs must either rely upon savings in areas such as hospital admissions and medications or accept incremental costs for their additional benefits. Even if quotidian dialysis is more effective, the acceptability of additional dialysis costs is controversial, because the costs of conventional dialysis is already considered to be near the maximum that society is willing to bear.

To date, the best comparative costing data come from studies comparing home quotidian hemodialysis techniques with conventional in-center hemodialysis. Based on modeling of data derived from retrospective costing studies, Mohr and associates[44] calculated savings of US$12,500 (18%) for in-center short daily hemodialysis and US$15,600 (23%) for home hemodialysis. Dialyzer reuse as well as the use of remote monitoring for nocturnal hemodialysis can affect the overall cost.[80] Financial data were also published by Robers.[81]

A prospective descriptive cost analysis by McFarlane and associates[79] showed that home nocturnal hemodialysis was associated with total health care costs that were about CAN$13,000/patient/year, lower than conventional in-center hemodialysis. Nocturnal hemodialysis significantly reduced staffing and overhead costs, which compensated for significantly higher costs for dialysis materials, laboratory tests, and capital items. In a cost-utility study performed on the same population, home nocturnal hemodialysis was the economically "dominant" method, with both lower costs and higher effectiveness as measured by quality of life.[47] In contrast, a study by Kroeker and associates[45] found no significant differences between the costs of conventional in-center and either home quotidian nocturnal or hemeral hemodialysis. However, in a retrospective cost comparison of each study patient from the prior year, total annual costs fell by $7171 per patient in those converted to short daily hemodialysis and by $12,782 per patient in those converted to home nocturnal hemodialysis, compared with a rise by $2247 in those who remained on in-center hemodialysis.[45]

These studies suggest that home quotidian dialysis modalities reduce total health care costs. The impact on costs of in-center quotidian dialysis programs remains to be established. In addition, the reduction of hospitalization costs and medications such as EPO and vitamin D analogues is realized at the societal level but often not at the level of the dialysis program. Indeed, in the United States, some of these cost savings may adversely affect the local budgets of dialysis programs. This disparity highlights the fact that the method of funding dialysis programs may need to be adjusted in order to support quotidian dialysis programs, especially when those programs have been found to be cost-effective at the societal level.

SHORT DAILY HEMODIALYSIS VERSUS NOCTURNAL HEMODIALYSIS

Short daily hemodialysis provides a higher dose of dialysis than conventional hemodialysis, and quotidian nocturnal hemodialysis provides a higher dose still. The advantages of nocturnal methods include increased clearance of small and large molecules, added hemodynamic stability, improvement of sleep apnea, improved phosphate control and secondary hyperparathyroidism, lower burden of dialysis during the day, higher dialysis access fault tolerance, and free diet. The advantages of short daily methods include lower risk of deficiency syndromes, less exposure to the dialysis membrane and possibly poor dialysate quality, lower risk of accidental dialysis needle disconnection, and less sleep disturbance by the dialysis procedure.

The only study comparing the two methods was conducted in London, Ontario, and was recently published.[82] This was a prospective nonrandomized study comparing a group of 11 patients on short daily hemodialysis, 12 patients on nightly hemodialysis, and matched control subjects on conventional hemodialysis. The differences in the dialysis dose and phosphate control among the methods were confirmed as described earlier.[83] Quality of life parameters were better preserved in both daily modalities compared to conventional HD,[46] as was the control of hypertension.[50] The short daily HD group fared better in relationship to some of the nutritional parameters.[70] Furthermore, the overall cost of the treatment was higher in nocturnal compared with short daily HD. When the cost during the year prior to the conversion was taken into account, the savings were higher in the nocturnal HD group.[45] The limitations of the study include the small sample size, the lack of randomization, and higher preexisting comorbidity in the nocturnal HD group. Case-mix differences may also account for the differences in nutritional parameters and cost between the two modalities and point to the need for further studies. At this point, the choice of the daily modality at home depends on patient preference and facility experience.

DAILY HEMOFILTRATION VERSUS DAILY HEMODIALYSIS

The role of hemofiltration as an alternative modality is evolving. The merits of hemofiltration are discussed in a different chapter of this book. Hemofiltration and hemodiafiltration can be performed thrice weekly or daily and can be used for short or long treatments. Based on published reports to this point, the clinical benefits of daily hemofiltration are similar to daily hemodialysis[2,3] and are related to the schedule rather than to the technique. There is laboratory evidence of increased removal of large molecules leading to a decrease in the pre-dialysis levels of β_2 microglobulin.[3] The added effect on middle molecule removal and the relationship to clinical outcomes need further studies.

OBSTACLES/FUTURE

Despite the interest in daily hemodialysis, the penetration of these modalities is low, because few dialysis programs offer them. Many obstacles have restricted availability of these modalities. The infrastructure for home hemodialysis is poor in many areas, and many patients are initially reluctant to undergo hemodialysis at home.[84] Experienced staff will require retraining in order to be prepared for the different clinical issues that arise in intensively dialyzed patients. Even if funding for in-center quotidian dialysis programs is adequate, other restrictions such as the availability of space and staff may limit the ability of a program to offer quotidian dialysis.

To overcome these obstacles, a series of steps will need to be taken. Improvements should be made to home dialysis infrastructure through the education of health professionals, administrators, and payers. Stakeholders such as clinicians and patient organizations should continue to advocate for improved resources for quotidian programs in the home and in-center settings. Larger programs can assist smaller ones to offer quotidian dialysis by providing technical support, staff education, and patient training. The possibility of an increase in home hemodialysis market share may encourage the industry to develop hemodialysis machines that are simpler to operate and quicker to set up.

The need for data collection on dialysis was recognized by the National Institutes of Health.[85,86] Funds for a pilot prospective randomized, controlled study were granted in 2003. The study will allow comparison of conventional hemodialysis to either short daily hemodialysis or daily nocturnal hemodialysis over at least 1 year. The study is expected to be completed by 2008. The results may lead to a larger prospective randomized, controlled study or may provide enough justification for adequate funding of daily hemodialysis. The need for a randomized study has been debated as representing either a necessary step towards proper funding or a cause of an unnecessary delay for the implementation of a method that has been universally supported by all the nonrandomized studies published to date.

In conclusion, daily hemodialysis in the form of short daily or long nocturnal hemodialysis seems to provide significant benefits to selected patients with ESRD, and these modalities should be considered in suitable patients. Through advocacy and education, more dialysis programs should be able to offer quotidian hemodialysis to patients who are expected to benefit from more intensive dialysis techniques.

References

1. Pierratos A: Daily hemodialysis: Why the renewed interest? (See comments). Am J Kidney Dis 1998; 32(6 suppl 4):S76–S82.
2. Zimmerman DL, Swedko PJ, Posen GA, Burns KD: Daily hemofiltration with a simplified method of delivery. ASAIO J 2003; 49(4):426–429.
3. Maduell F, Navarro V, Torregrosa E, et al: Change from three times a week on-line hemodiafiltration to short daily on-line hemodiafiltration. Kidney Int 2003; 64(1):305–313.
4. Chertow GM: "Wishing don't make it so": Why we need a randomized clinical trial of high-intensity hemodialysis. J Am Soc Nephrol 2001; 12(12):2850–2853.
5. DePalma JR, Pecker EA, Maxwell MH: A new automatic coil dialyser system for "daily" dialysis. Proc EDTA 1969; 6:26–34.
6. Shaldon S: Independence in maintenance haemodialysis. Lancet 1968; 1(7541):520.
7. Uldall PR, Francoeur R, Ouwendyk M: Simplified nocturnal home hemodialysis (SNHHD). A new approach to renal replacement therapy. J Am Soc Nephrol 1994; 5:428.
8. Kjellstrand CM, Ing T: Daily hemodialysis: History and revival of a superior dialysis method. ASAIO J 1998; 44(3):117–122.
9. Twardowski ZJ: PHD(R): The technological solution for daily haemodialysis? Nephrol Dial Transplant 2003; 18(1):19–23.
10. Pierratos A, Ouwendyk M, Francoeur R, et al: Nocturnal hemodialysis: Three-year experience (See comments). J Am Soc Nephrol 1998; 9(5):859–868.
11. Pierratos A, Francoeur R, Ouwendyk M: Delayed dialyzer reprocessing for home hemodialysis. Home Hemodial Int 2000; 4:51–54.
12. Francoeur R, Digiambatista A: Technical considerations for short daily home hemodialysis and nocturnal home hemodialysis. Adv Ren Replace Ther 2001; 8(4):268–272.
13. Mehrabian S, Morgan D, Schlaeper C, et al: Equipment and water treatment considerations for the provision of quotidian home hemodialysis. Am J Kidney Dis 2003; 42(suppl 1): 66–70.
14. Pierratos A: Nocturnal home haemodialysis: An update on a 5-year experience. Nephrol Dial Transplant 1999; 14(12): 2835–2840.
15. Hoy CD: Remote monitoring of daily nocturnal hemodialysis. Hemodialysis Int 2001; 4:8–12.
16. Heidenheim AP, Leitch R, Kortas C, Lindsay RM: Patient monitoring in the London Daily/Nocturnal Hemodialysis Study. Am J Kidney Dis 2003; 42(suppl 1):61–65.
17. Pierratos A: Daily hemodialysis: An update. Curr Opin Nephrol Hypertens 2002; 11(2):165–171.
18. Twardowski ZJ, Kubara H: Different sites versus constant sites of needle insertion into arteriovenous fistulas for treatment by repeated dialysis. Dial Transplant 1979; 8:978–980.
19. Quintaliani G, Buoncristiani U, Fagugli R, et al: Survival of vascular access during daily and three times a week hemodialysis. Clin Nephrol 2000; 53(5):372–377.
20. Woods JD, Port FK, Orzol S, et al: Clinical and biochemical correlates of starting "daily" hemodialysis. Kidney Int 1999; 55(6): 2467–2476.
21. Ting GO, Kjellstrand C, Freitas T, et al: Long-term study of high-comorbidity ESRD patients converted from conventional to short daily hemodialysis. Am J Kidney Dis 2003; 42(5): 1020–1035.
22. Ouwendyk M, Leitch R, Freitas T: Daily hemodialysis: A nursing perspective. Adv Ren Replace Ther 2001; 8(4):257–267.
23. Leitch R, Ouwendyk M, Ferguson E, et al: Nursing issues related to patient selection, vascular access, and education in quotidian hemodialysis. Am J Kidney Dis 2003; 42(suppl 1):56–60.
24. Schaubel DE, Fenton SS: Trends in mortality on peritoneal dialysis: Canada, 1981–1997. J Am Soc Nephrol 2000; 11(1): 126–133.
25. Gotch FA: Modeling the dose of home dialysis. Home Hemodial Int 1998; 2:37–40.
26. Casino FG, Lopez T: The equivalent renal urea clearance: A new parameter to assess dialysis dose. Nephrol Dial Transplant 1996; 11(8):1574–1581.
27. Depner TA: Daily hemodialysis efficiency: An analysis of solute kinetics. Adv Ren Replace Ther 2001; 8(4):227–235.
28. Gotch FA: The current place of urea kinetic modelling with respect to different dialysis modalities. Nephrol Dial Transplant 1998; 13(suppl 6):10–14.
29. Leypoldt JK, Jaber BL, Lysaght MJ, et al: Kinetics and dosing predictions for daily haemofiltration. Nephrol Dial Transplant 2003; 18(4):769–776.
30. Eknoyan G, Beck GJ, Cheung AK, et al: Effect of dialysis dose and membrane flux in maintenance hemodialysis. N Engl J Med 2002; 347(25):2010–2019.
31. Suri R, Depner TA, Blake PG, et al: Adequacy of quotidian hemodialysis. Am J Kidney Dis 2003; 42(suppl 1):42–48.
32. Goldfarb-Rumyantzev AS, Cheung AK, Leypoldt JK: Computer simulation of small-solute and middle-molecule removal during short daily and long thrice-weekly hemodialysis. Am J Kidney Dis 2002; 40(6):1211–1218.
33. Chan CT, Floras JS, Miller JA, et al: Regression of left ventricular hypertrophy after conversion to nocturnal hemodialysis. Kidney Int 2002; 61(6):2235–2239.
34. Pierratos A: Effect of therapy time and frequency on effective solute removal. Semin Dial 2001; 14(4):284–288.
35. Clark WR, Leypoldt JK, Henderson LW, et al: Quantifying the effect of changes in the hemodialysis prescription on effective solute removal with a mathematical model. J Am Soc Nephrol 1999; 10(3):601–609.
36. Raj DS, Ouwendyk M, Francoeur R, Pierratos A: Beta(2)-microglobulin kinetics in nocturnal haemodialysis. Nephrol Dial Transplant 2000; 15(1):58–64.
37. Floridi A, Antolini F, Galli F, et al: Daily haemodialysis improves indices of protein glycation. Nephrol Dial Transplant 2002; 17(5):871–878.
38. Friedman AN, Bostom AG, Levey AS, et al: Plasma total homocysteine levels among patients undergoing nocturnal versus standard hemodialysis. J Am Soc Nephrol 2002; 13(1): 265–268.

39. Lopot F, Valek A: Time-averaged concentration? time-averaged deviation: A new concept in mathematical assessment of dialysis adequacy. Nephrol Dial Transplant 1988; 3(6): 846–848.
40. Wong JB, Koff RS, Tine F, Pauker SG: Cost-effectiveness of interferon-alpha 2b treatment for hepatitis B e antigen-positive chronic hepatitis B. Ann Intern Med 1995; 122(9): 664–675.
41. Hillner BE, Smith TJ: Efficacy and cost effectiveness of adjuvant chemotherapy in women with node-negative breast cancer. A decision-analysis model. N Engl J Med 1991; 324(3): 160–168.
42. Brissenden JE, Pierratos A, Ouwendyk M, Roscoe JM: Improvements in quality of life with nocturnal hemodialysis. J Am Soc Nephrol 1998; 9:168A.
43. McPhatter LL, Lockridge RSJ, Albert J, et al: Nightly home hemodialysis: Improvement in nutrition and quality of life. Adv Ren Replace Ther 1999; 6(4):358–365.
44. Mohr PE, Neumann PJ, Franco SJ, et al: The case for daily dialysis: Its impact on costs and quality of life. Am J Kidney Dis 2001; 37(4):777–789.
45. Kroeker A, Clark WF, Heidenheim AP, et al: An operating cost comparison between conventional and home quotidian hemodialysis. Am J Kidney Dis 2003; 42(suppl 1):49–55.
46. Heidenheim AP, Muirhead N, Moist L, Lindsay RM: Patient quality of life on quotidian hemodialysis. Am J Kidney Dis 2003; 42(suppl 1):36–41.
47. McFarlane PA, Bayoumi AM, Pierratos A, Redelmeier DA: The quality of life and cost utility of home nocturnal and conventional in-center hemodialysis. Kidney Int 2003; 64(3): 1004–1011.
48. Laupacis A, Keown P, Pus N, et al: A study of the quality of life and cost-utility of renal transplantation. Kidney Int 1996; 50(1): 235–242.
49. Kooistra MP, Vos J, Koomans HA, Vos PF: Daily home haemodialysis in the Netherlands: Effects on metabolic control, haemodynamics, and quality of life. Nephrol Dial Transplant 1998; 13(11):2853–2860.
50. Nesrallah G, Suri R, Moist L, et al: Volume control and blood pressure management in patients undergoing quotidian hemodialysis. Am J Kidney Dis 2003; 42(suppl 1):13–17.
51. Fagugli RM, Reboldi G, Quintaliani G, et al: Short daily hemodialysis: Blood pressure control and left ventricular mass reduction in hypertensive hemodialysis patients. Am J Kidney Dis 2001; 38(2):371–376.
52. Chan C, Floras JS, Miller JA, Pierratos A: Improvement in ejection fraction by nocturnal haemodialysis in end-stage renal failure patients with coexisting heart failure. Nephrol Dial Transplant 2002; 17(8):1518–1521.
53. Chan C, Harvey PJ, Picton P, et al: Short-term blood pressure, noradrenergic, and vascular effects of nocturnal home hemodialysis. Hypertension 2003; 42(5): 925–931.
54. Zilch O, Vos PF, Oey LP, et al: Daily dialysis reduces peripheral vascular resistance and sympathetic activity. J Am Soc Nephrol 2001; 12:280A.
55. Odar-Cederlof IE, Bjellerup P, Juhlin-Dannfelt A, et al: Brain natriuretic peptide (BNP) in plasma reflects left ventricular (LV) dysfunction in hemodialysis (HD) patients and decreases with daily dialysis. J Am Soc Nephrol 2001; 12:404A.
56. Fagugli RM, Buoncristiani U, Ciao G: Anemia and blood pressure correction obtained by daily hemodialysis induce a reduction of left ventricular hypertrophy in dialysed patients. Int J Artif Organs 1998; 21(7):429–431.
57. Vos PF, Zilch O, Kooistra MP: Clinical outcome of daily dialysis. Am J Kidney Dis 2001; 37(1 suppl 2):S99–S102.
58. Rao M, Muirhead N, Klarenbach S, et al: Management of anemia with quotidian hemodialysis. Am J Kidney Dis 2003; 42(1 Pt 2):18–23.
59. Schwartz D, Pierratos A, Richardson RMA, et al: Impact of nocturnal home hemodialysis on anemia management in patients with end-stage renal disease. J Am Soc Nephrol 2003; 14:498A.
60. Gotch FA, Panlilio F, Sergeyeva O, et al: A kinetic model of inorganic phosphorus mass balance in hemodialysis therapy. Blood Purif 2003; 21(1):51–57.
61. Chertow GM, Burke SK, Raggi P: Sevelamer attenuates the progression of coronary and aortic calcification in hemodialysis patients. Kidney Int 2002; 62(1):245–252.
62. Block GA, Hulbert-Shearon TE, Levin NW, Port FK: Association of serum phosphorus and calcium x phosphate product with mortality risk in chronic hemodialysis patients: A national study. Am J Kidney Dis 1998; 31(4):607–617.
63. DeSoi CA, Umans JG: Phosphate kinetics during high-flux hemodialysis. J Am Soc Nephrol 1993; 4(5):1214–1218.
64. Traeger J, Galland R, Ferrier ML, Delawari E: Optimal control of phosphatemia by short daily hemodialysis. J Am Soc Nephrol 2002; 13:410A–411A.
65. Lugon JR, Andre MB, Duarte ME, et al: Effects of in-center daily hemodialysis upon mineral metabolism and bone disease in end-stage renal disease patients. Sao Paulo Med J 2001; 119(3): 105–109.
66. Mucsi I, Hercz G, Uldall R, et al: Control of serum phosphate without any phosphate binders in patients treated with nocturnal hemodialysis. Kidney Int 1998; 53(5):1399–1404.
67. Kim SJ, Goldstein M, Szabo T, Pierratos A: Resolution of massive uremic tumoral calcinosis with daily nocturnal home hemodialysis. Am J Kidney Dis 2003; 41(3):E12.
68. Pierratos A, Hercz G, Sherrard DJ, et al: Calcium, phosphorus metabolism and bone pathology on long term nocturnal hemodialysis. J Am Soc Nephrol 2001; 12:274A.
69. Galland R, Traeger J, Arkouche W, et al: Short daily hemodialysis rapidly improves nutritional status in hemodialysis patients. Kidney Int 2001; 60(4):1555–1560.
70. Spanner E, Suri R, Heidenheim AP, Lindsay RM: The impact of quotidian hemodialysis on nutrition. Am J Kidney Dis 2003; 42(suppl 1):30–35.
71. Ikizler TA, Flakoll PJ, Parker RA, Hakim RM: Amino acid and albumin losses during hemodialysis. Kidney Int 1994; 46(3): 830–837.
72. Pierratos A, Ouwendyk M, Rassi M: Total body nitrogen increases on nocturnal hemodialysis. J Am Soc Nephrol 1999; 10(9):299A.
73. Sanner BM, Tepel M, Esser M, et al: Sleep-related breathing disorders impair quality of life in haemodialysis recipients. Nephrol Dial Transplant 2002; 17(7):1260–1265.
74. Benz RL, Pressman MR, Hovick ET, Peterson DD: Potential novel predictors of mortality in end-stage renal disease patients with sleep disorders. Am J Kidney Dis 2000; 35(6): 1052–1060.
75. Hanly PJ, Pierratos A: Improvement of sleep apnea in patients with chronic renal failure who undergo nocturnal hemodialysis. N Engl J Med 2001; 344(2):102–107.
76. Hanly PJ, Gabor JY, Chan C, Pierratos A: Daytime sleepiness in patients with CRF: Impact of nocturnal hemodialysis. Am J Kidney Dis 2003; 41(2):403–410.
77. Chan CT, Hanly P, Gabor J, et al: Impact of nocturnal hemodialysis on the variability of heart rate and duration of hypoxemia during sleep. Kidney Int 2004; 65(2):661–665.
78. Pierratos A: Daily nocturnal home hemodialysis. Kidney Int 2004; 65(5):1975–1986.
79. McFarlane PA, Pierratos A, Redelmeier DA: Cost savings of home nocturnal versus conventional in-center hemodialysis. Kidney Int 2002; 62(6):2216–2222.
80. Mohr PE: The economics of daily dialysis. Adv Ren Replace Ther 2001; 8(4):273–279.
81. Robers S: Cost of daily hemodialysis. ASAIO J 2001; 47(5): 459–461.

82. Lindsay RM: Introduction. Am J Kidney Dis 2003; 42(suppl 1): 3–4.
83. Lindsay RM, Henderson LW: Adequacy of dialysis. Kidney Int Suppl 1988; 24:S92–S99.
84. Nissenson AR: Daily hemodialysis: Challenges and opportunities in the delivery and financing of end-stage renal disease patient care. Adv Ren Replace Ther 2001; 8(4):286–292.
85. Briggs JP: Evidence-based medicine in the dialysis unit: A few lessons from the USRDS and from the NCDS and HEMO trials. Semin Dial 2004; 17(2):136–141.
86. NIH: Frequent hemodialysis clinical trials. From *http://grants1.nih.gov/grants/guide/rfa-files/RFA-DK-03-005.html*, 2003.

Chapter 24

Hemofiltration and Hemodiafiltration for End-Stage Renal Disease

Zhongping Huang, Ph.D. • Dayong Gao, Professor • Lee W. Henderson, M.D., F.A.C.P. • William R. Clark, M.D.

Hemodialysis (HD) has been the primary treatment mode in the management of patients with end-stage renal disease (ESRD) for the past 40 years. In this therapy, the countercurrent flow of blood and dialysate creates gradients for diffusive solute removal across a semipermeable membrane. The hollow fiber dialyzer membranes used for HD are manufactured specifically with diffusion-enhancing characteristics, such as a thin wall structure and a narrow inner diameter.[1] The removal of low-molecular weight (MW) nitrogenous waste products during HD is very effective. However, the limitations of diffusion become increasingly evident as uremic toxin MW increases.[2] Although the use of membranes with high water permeability or adsorptivity may be beneficial,[3] the clearance of middle and large MW compounds is limited by the fundamental dominance of diffusion in HD.

Many variables comprise the dialysis prescription, but factors influencing urea clearance represent the most important prescriptive consideration for many clinicians. Indeed, for both HD patients and those treated with peritoneal dialysis (PD), urea Kt/V or a derivative parameter assumes a prominent role in the assessment of both therapy prescription and delivery. Although generally not considered a uremic toxin *per se*, urea is assumed to be representative of the broad class of low MW nitrogenous compounds from a kinetic perspective.[4] Studies from the late 1970s and early 1980s, performed with dialyzers having very limited middle molecule clearance capabilities, suggested patient survival was more dependent on changes in small solute clearance than on middle molecule clearance.[5,6] Consequently, interest in urea-based therapy quantification developed and its use increased, beginning in the late 1980s.[7] Subsequently, several retrospective clinical trials published in the mid-1990s demonstrated a direct relationship between delivered urea-based HD dose and survival.[8–11] Moreover, one prospective trial and several retrospective studies suggested a similar relationship between total (i.e., peritoneal plus renal) clearance and survival for PD-treated patients.[12–14] By the end of the last decade, the notion that survival in dialysis patients was directly tied to the extent of small solute removal had become nearly axiomatic, and specific urea-based dosing guidelines were in place for both HD and PD.[15,16]

However, two prospective, randomized studies published in 2002 challenged this axiom. In the American HEMO Study,[17] outcome-related effects of increasing delivered dose significantly beyond a level considered to be standard of care were assessed in approximately 1800 patients. In addition, the effect of treatment with high-flux dialyzers versus lower permeability high-efficiency dialyzers on patient survival was studied. In the HEMO trial, neither the high-dose nor the high-flux intervention resulted in a significant survival advantage. In PD, the **Ade**quacy of Dialysis in **Mex**ico (ADEMEX) Study[18] also failed to confirm a survival benefit for increasing dose delivery in a clinically relevant dose range for this therapy. These studies call into question the utility of small solute clearance parameters, both for quantifying dialysis dose and predicting survival. Moreover, the results of these two landmark studies provide compelling evidence that the conventional approach of managing chronic dialysis patients with either conventional (thrice-weekly) HD or PD has a limited ability to influence patient outcome favorably. Thus, the evaluation of alternative dialytic approaches is urgently needed for the ESRD population.[19]

Alternative therapies that may improve ESRD patient outcome include continuous-flow PD,[20] daily therapies,[21–23] sorbent-based systems,[24] and convective therapies. The last category, which is comprised of hemofiltration (HF) and hemodiafiltration (HDF), is the focus of this review.

CONVECTIVE SOLUTE REMOVAL

The determinants of convective solute removal differ significantly from those of diffusion. Convective solute removal is determined primarily by the sieving properties of the membrane used and the ultrafiltration rate.[25] The mechanism by which convection occurs is termed *solvent drag*. If the molecular dimensions of a solute are such that transmembrane passage to some extent occurs, the solute is swept ("dragged") across the membrane in association with ultrafiltered plasma water. Thus, the rate of convective solute removal can be modified either by changes in the rate of solvent (plasma water) flow or by changes in the mean effective pore size of the membrane. As discussed later, the blood concentration of a particular solute also influences its convective removal rate.

Both the water and solute permeability of an ultrafiltration membrane are influenced by the phenomena of secondary membrane formation[26] and concentration polarization.[27] The exposure of an artificial surface to plasma results in the nonspecific, instantaneous adsorption of a layer of proteins, the composition of which generally reflects that of the plasma itself. Therefore, plasma proteins such as albumin, fibrinogen, and immunoglobulins form the bulk of this secondary membrane. Moreover, the plasma total protein concentration also influences this phenomenon. This layer of proteins, by serving as an additional resistance to mass transfer, effectively reduces both the water and solute permeability of an extracorporeal membrane. Evidence of this is found in comparisons of solute sieving coefficients determined before and after exposure of a membrane to plasma or other protein-containing solution.[28–31]

Although concentration polarization primarily pertains to plasma proteins, it is distinct from secondary membrane formation. Concentration polarization specifically relates to ultrafiltration-based processes and applies to the kinetic behavior of an individual solute. Accumulation of a solute that is predominantly or completely rejected by a membrane used for ultrafiltration of plasma occurs at the blood compartment membrane surface. This surface accumulation causes the solute concentration just adjacent to the membrane surface (i.e., the submembranous concentration) to be higher than the bulk (plasma) concentration. In this manner, a submembranous (high) to bulk (low) concentration gradient is established, resulting in "backdiffusion" from the membrane surface out into the plasma. At steady state, the rate of convective transport to the membrane surface is equal to the rate of backdiffusion. The polarized layer of solute is the distance defined by the gradient between the submembranous and bulk concentrations. This distance (or thickness) of the polarized layer, which can be estimated by mass balance techniques, reflects the extent of the concentration polarization process.

By definition, concentration polarization is applicable in clinical situations in which relatively high ultrafiltration rates are used. Conditions that promote the process are high ultrafiltration rate (high rate of convective transport), low blood flow rate (low shear rate or membrane "sweeping" effect), and the use of post-dilution (rather than pre-dilution) replacement fluids (increased local solute concentrations).[32]

The extent of the concentration polarization determines its effect on actual solute removal. In general, the degree to which the removal of a rejected solute is influenced is directly related to that solute's extent of rejection by a membrane. In fact, concentration polarization may actually enhance the removal of uremic toxins falling in the low MW protein category that otherwise would have minimal convective removal.[33] This is explained by the fact that the pertinent blood compartment concentration subjected to the ultrafiltrate flux is the high submembranous concentration primarily rather than the much lower bulk concentration.

On the other hand, the use of very high ultrafiltration rates in conjunction with other conditions favorable to solute polarization may significantly impair overall membrane performance. The relationship between ultrafiltration rate and transmembrane pressure (TMP) is linear for relatively low ultrafiltration rates, and the positive slope of this line defines the ultrafiltration coefficient of the membrane. However, as ultrafiltration rate further increases, this curve eventually reaches a plateau.[34] At this point, fouling of the membrane with denatured proteins may occur and an irreversible decline in solute and water permeability of the membrane ensues. Therefore, the ultrafiltration rate (and associated TMP) used for a convective therapy with a specific membrane needs to fall on the initial (linear) portion of the UFR versus TMP relationship with avoidance of the plateau region.

Convective solute removal can be quantified in the following manner[35]:

$$N = (1 - \sigma)J_V\,C_M.$$

In this equation, N is the convective flux (mass removal rate per unit membrane area), J_V is the ultrafiltrate flux (ultrafiltration rate normalized to membrane area), C_M is the mean intramembrane solute concentration, and σ is the reflection coefficient, a measure of solute rejection. As Werynski and Waniewski have explained,[35] the parameter ($1-\sigma$) can be viewed as the membrane resistance to convective solute flow. If σ equals 1, no convective transport occurs while a value of 0 implies no resistance to convective flow. Of note, C_M is the average of the filtrate-side and blood-side solute concentrations, with the latter represented by the submembranous concentration rather than the bulk phase concentration. Therefore, this parameter is significantly influenced by the effect of concentration polarization.

CONVECTIVE RENAL REPLACEMENT THERAPIES

Hemofiltration Versus Ultrafiltration

The convective therapies used in the management of ESRD patients are HF and HDF. Although ultrafiltration is a fundamental aspect of convective therapies, it is useful to differentiate between this process and HF. Ultrafiltration (UF) is the extracorporeal removal of plasma water by application of a transmembrane pressure gradient. Although useful for volume removal in the management of "isolated" fluid overload,[36] UF is not effective as a blood cleansing modality based on the following:

1. The concentrations of small solutes not rejected appreciably by an HF membrane are effectively the same in the ultrafiltrate and the plasma water.
2. Although net mass removal from the body is achieved in the ultrafiltrate, the fraction of the total body solute mass removed is the same as the fractional removal of plasma water.
3. Since fractional mass removal of solute and plasma volume reduction occur proportionately, small solute concentrations in the plasma do not change significantly in isolated UF.

On the other hand, the ultrafiltrate concentrations of larger solutes having restricted transmembrane passage are less than their simultaneous plasma water concentrations due to partial or complete rejection by the membrane. Thus, fractional mass removal in the ultrafiltrate is proportionately less than plasma volume reduction, resulting in a net increase in the blood concentrations of larger sized molecules.

On the other hand, HF involves the simultaneous removal of plasma water by UF and replacement with a buffered electrolyte solution (replacement or substitution fluid).[37] Since the ultrafiltration rate used in HF may be as high as 400 mL/min, one obvious function of the replacement fluid in HF is volume preservation in the patient. The difference between this (absolute) ultrafiltration rate and the replacement fluid rate is the net ultrafiltration (weight loss) rate. However, the use of replacement fluid differentiates HF from isolated UF and accounts for the fact that the former is a blood cleansing modality and the latter is not. In HF, replacement fluid administration results in the dilution of nonfiltered toxins remaining in the bloodstream and an associated reduction in blood concentrations. This dilution phenomenon accounts for HF's effectiveness as a renal replacement therapy.

Post-Dilution HF

The location of replacement fluid delivery in the extracorporeal circuit during HF has a significant impact on solute removal and therapy requirements[32] (Figure 24–1). Replacement fluid can be delivered to the arterial blood line prior to the hemofilter (pre-dilution mode) or to the venous line after the hemofilter (post-dilution mode). In post-dilution HF, the relationship between solute clearance and ultrafiltration rate is relatively straightforward.[38] In this situation, solute clearance is determined primarily by and related directly to the solute's sieving coefficient and the ultrafiltration rate. (Sieving coefficient is defined as the ratio of the solute concentration in the filtrate to the simultaneous plasma concentration.) For a given solute, the extent to which it partitions from the plasma water into the red blood cell mass and the rate at which it is transported across red blood cell membranes also influence clearance. For example, the volume of distribution of both urea and creatinine includes the red blood cell water. However, while urea movement across red blood cell membranes is very fast, the movement of creatinine is significantly less rapid. Furthermore, red blood cell membranes are completely impermeable to many uremic toxins. A prominent example of this is the low MW protein toxin class, for which the volume of distribution is the extracellular fluid. These observations lead to the obvious conclusion that hematocrit also influences solute clearance in HF. Finally, through its effect on secondary membrane formation and concentration polarization (see earlier text), plasma total protein concentration is also a determinant of solute clearance in HF.

For a given volume of replacement fluid over the entire MW spectrum of uremic toxins, post-dilution HF provides higher solute clearance than does pre-dilution HF. As discussed below, the relative inefficiency of the latter mode is related to the dilution-related reduction in solute concentrations, which decreases the driving force for convective mass transfer. Despite its superior efficiency with respect to replacement fluid utilization, post-dilution HF is limited inherently by the attainable blood flow rate. More specifically, the ratio of the ultrafiltration rate to the plasma flow rate delivered to the filter, termed the filtration fraction, is the limiting factor. In general, a maximal filtration fraction of 50% usually guides prescription in post-dilution HF. At filtration fractions beyond this value, concentration polarization and secondary membrane effects become prominent and may impair hemofilter performance.

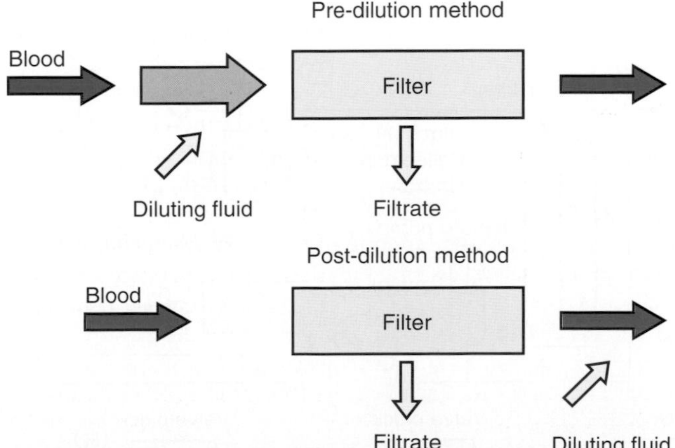

Figure 24–1 Pre-dilution versus post-dilution hemofiltration. (From Henderson LW: Pre vs. post dilution hemofiltration. Clin Nephrol 1979; 11:120–124. Reprinted with permission.)

For a hypothetical patient with a hematocrit of 35% and a vascular access capable of delivering a blood flow rate of 350 mL/min, the above filtration fraction limit implies a maximal ultrafiltration rate of 114 mL/min or a total ultrafiltrate volume of approximately 27 L for a 4-hr treatment. For a given filtration fraction, a higher blood flow rate or a lower hematocrit enables attainment of a higher ultrafiltration rate.

In the early clinical application of HF, because replacement fluid was infused generally as a terminally sterilized solution from bags, volumes rarely surpassed 20 L per treatment.[41–43] (As an exception, see the following description of the pre-dilution system described by Henderson and colleagues in the mid-1970s.) This limitation resulted in post-dilution as the predominant mode when HF was performed prior to the last decade. However, the technology of on-line production by sequential ultrafiltration of dialysate[44–46] has allowed significantly larger volumes of replacement fluid to be used in HF. This ready availability of replacement fluid and the resultant capability to employ ultrafiltration rates as high as 400 mL/min permits attainment of clearances in pre-dilution that far surpass maximal achievable clearances in post-dilution HF.[47] Thus, as discussed below, the predominant mode used in contemporary HF is pre-dilution.

Pre-Dilution HF

From a mass transfer perspective, the use of pre-dilution has several potential advantages over post-dilution. First, in contemporary on-line HF, the blood flow and replacement fluid rates typically are similar.[47] As such, both hematocrit and blood total protein concentration are reduced significantly prior to the entry of blood into the hemofilter. This effective reduction in the red cell and protein content of the blood attenuates the secondary membrane and concentration polarization phenomena described earlier, resulting in improved mass transfer.[48] Pre-dilution also favorably impacts mass transfer due to augmented flow in the blood compartment, with the pre-filter mixing of blood and replacement fluid effectively doubling the blood compartment flow rate. This achieves a relatively high membrane shear rate, which also reduces solute-membrane interactions. Finally, pre-dilution may also enhance mass transfer for some compounds by creating concentration gradients that induce solute movement out of red blood cells.[48] The above mass transfer benefits must be weighed against the predictable dilution-induced reduction in plasma solute concentrations, one of the driving forces for convective solute removal. The extent to which this reduction occurs is determined mainly by the ratio of the replacement fluid rate to the blood flow rate, which may be as high as unity in contemporary on-line HF. However, the ultrafiltration rate afforded by such a high replacement fluid rate allows the dilution-related loss of efficiency to be overcome.

Hemodiafiltration

Although considerable enthusiasm for HF existed in the late 1970s and early 1980s, its popularity waned subsequently for several reasons. As indicated earlier, logistic and cost considerations limited replacement fluid volumes to approximately 20 L or less per treatment. Urea clearances obtained with such volumes were substantially less than those achieved with HD. The increasing focus on urea-based quantification of dialysis therapy in the 1980s only served to accentuate the relatively low urea clearances in HF.[7]

A solution to this problem was actually published by two different groups in 1978. Leber and colleagues[49] described a system employing simultaneous HF and HD with a polyacrylonitrile (RP6) dialyzer. The operating parameters included a blood flow rate of 200 mL/min, dialysate flow rate range of 200 to 900 mL/min, and ultrafiltration rate range of approximately 40 to 60 mL/min. The replacement fluid was lactate-based and administered post-filter from bags while the dialysate was acetate-based. Relative to pure HF at an ultrafiltration rate of 55 to 60 mL/min, diffusive removal provided by a dialysate flow rate of 900 mL/min increased urea and creatinine clearance by approximately threefold. Kunitomo and colleagues[50] also described a similar post-dilution system employing a high-permeability polymethyl methacrylate dialyzer.

As was the case for HF, the introduction of on-line technology broadened significantly the capabilities of HDF. In the initial characterization of on-line HDF by Canaud and colleagues[46] (Figure 24–2), proportioned dialysate was first ultrafiltered to produce ultrapure dialysate. A portion of this stream was diverted and subjected to a second ultrafiltration step to produce replacement fluid, delivered in the post-dilution mode. The ultrafiltration rate was approximately 70 mL/min, resulting in an exchange volume of 16 L per treatment. As HDF therapy has evolved, ultrafiltration rates and exchange volumes have increased and are now approximately 100 mL/min and 20 to 25 L/session, respectively.[52–54] However, the general approach of using ultrafiltration to generate ultrapure dialysate and replacement fluid sequentially, a process termed "cold sterilization," remains intact.

FACTORS INFLUENCING LOW-MOLECULAR WEIGHT PROTEIN REMOVAL IN HEMOFILTRATION AND HEMODIAFILTRATION

The low MW protein (LMWP) class (Table 24–1) is a relatively large MW class of uremic toxins whose clearance is enhanced by the use of convective blood purification therapies.[33] As noted previously, concentration polarization and secondary membrane effects are relatively important considerations for these solutes. Röckel and colleagues[26] investigated the effect of secondary membrane formation on low MW pro-

Table 24–1 Uremic Toxins

Molecule	MW (kDa)	Toxicity
Urea	0.06	Unclear
Adrenomedullin	6	Hypotension
CIP	8.5	Chemotaxis inhibition
C_3a	8.9	AP activation
PTH	9	Osteodystrophy; ? other
AGE-peptides	<10	Various
AGE-proteins	>10	Various
C_5a	11	AP activation
β_2M	11.8	Amyloidosis
Leptin	16	Malnutrition
Myoglobin	17	Tubular damage
Factor D	23	AP activation
GIP I	28	Granulocyte inhibition
Carbamylated proteins	Various	? anemia

Adapted with permission from Clark WR, Gao D: Low-molecular weight proteins in end-stage renal disease: Potential toxicity and dialytic removal mechanisms. J Am Soc Nephrol 2002; 13:S41–S47.

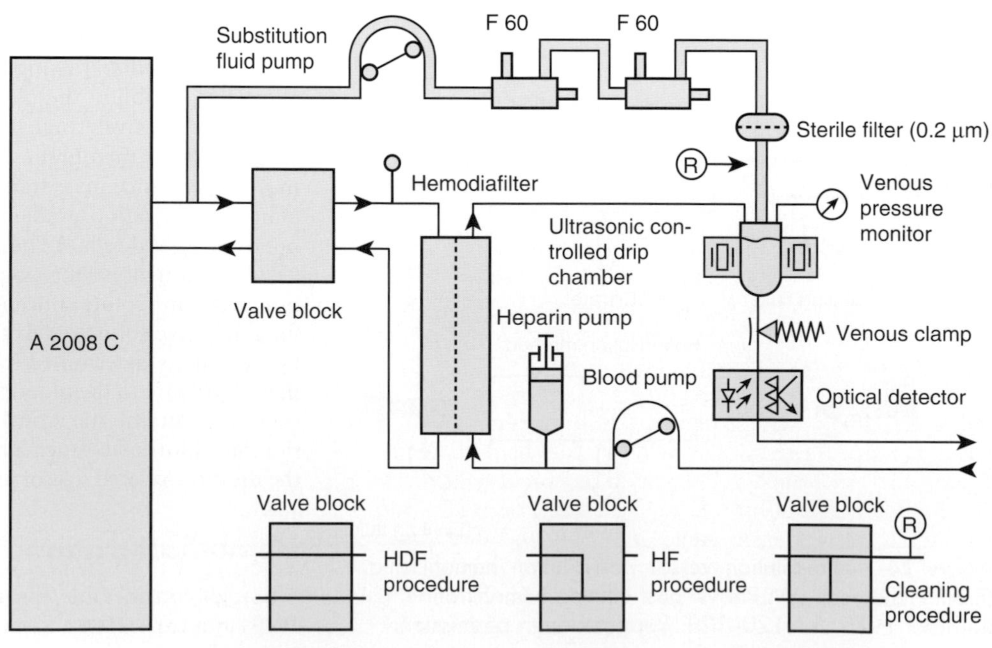

Figure 24–2 System for on-line preparation of ultrapure dialysate and replacement fluid. (From Canaud B, Nguyen QV, Lagrarde C, et al: Clinical evaluation of a multipurpose dialysis system adequate for hemodialysis or for post-dilution hemofiltration/ hemodiafiltration with on-line preparation of substitution fluid from dialysate. Contrib Nephrol 1985; 46:184–186. Reprinted with permission, (C) 1985 S. Karger AG, Basel)

tein sieving coefficient (SC) values during clinical hemofiltration with a high-flux polysulfone hemofilter. These investigators measured *in vivo* sieving coefficients for several solutes in this category, ranging in molecular weight from 12 kDa (β2M) to 55 kDa (prealbumin). Sieving coefficient determinations were made in the first 10 min (peak SC: PSC) and at treatment times of 20 and 180 min. For each protein, a significant decrease was observed between the PSC and the 20-min value. This effect was directly proportional to protein molecular weight such that after 20 min of treatment, no measurable filtration of solutes of MW greater than 30 kDa was evident.

For equivalent ultrafiltration rates up to 110 mL/min (with Q_B = 300 mL/min), several investigators have shown that post-dilution HDF is superior to pre-dilution HDF with respect to removal of LMW proteins in the 12 to 33 kDa range.[27,55,56] As discussed previously, the benefit of the post-dilution mode is explained by the thicker polarized boundary layer (relative to the pre-dilution mode), and the associated high concentration submembranous protein upon which the convective forces act. Because the degree of polarization is directly proportional to the degree of rejection, the relative benefit of the post-dilution mode generally increases as LMWP molecular weight increases. Unfortunately, these same considerations also apply to albumin removal. As such, from the perspective of large solute removal, post-dilution HDF requires a balance to be struck between the optimization of LMWP removal while minimizing albumin losses (see later text).

CLINICAL CHARACTERIZATION OF CONTEMPORARY CONVECTIVE MODALITIES

Hemofiltration

Before addressing more recent applications of HF, the first formal application of HF by Henderson and colleagues is discussed. After laboratory experiments demonstrating proof of concept, these investigators reported their clinical experiences, which were groundbreaking in two respects. First, it was the first clinical description of hemofiltration, which they actually termed "hemodiafiltration."[34] In this landmark original work, the pre-dilution system employing blood flow, ultrafiltration, and replacement fluid rates all of about 200 mL/min was characterized, particularly with respect to middle molecule clearances. In a separate report, Henderson and colleagues[41] also first described in detail the on-line production of sterile, non-pyrogenic replacement fluid by ultrafiltration with an Amicon polysulfone filter. The general approach of cold sterilization used in this latter study was the foundation for subsequently developed on-line fluid generation systems, which continue to be used today for both HF and HDF.

Over the past several years, Altieri and colleagues[57–60] from Italy have clearly defined the clinical capabilities of on-line HF. In a multi-center trial involving 23 patients,[57] these investigators first performed a clinical comparison of high-flux HD and on-line pre-dilution HF. The HD arm consisted of ultrapure dialysate and the same high permeability dialyzer (polyamide membrane) used in the HF arm. The HF treatment parameters included a mean blood flow rate of 372 mL/min and a mean substitution fluid rate of 327 mL/min, resulting in a total substitution fluid volume of 68.5 L per treatment. With respect to intradialytic symptoms, the HF arm was associated with a significantly reduced rate of hypotension, hypertension, arrhythmia, cramps, headache, and nausea, relative to the HD arm. Moreover, the incidence of interdialytic cramps, arthralgia, headache, and fatigue was significantly lower in the HF arm.

A comparison of solute kinetics in the two arms was also performed. Although delivered urea Kt/V was significantly greater in the HD than in the HF arm (mean, 1.4 and 1.1, respectively), no difference in normalized protein catabolic rate (nPCR) was observed. In a subgroup of 18 patients, a regression analysis of nPCR versus Kt/V was performed for both the HD phase and HF arms, the latter occurring after patients had been stabilized on HF for 3 months. The slope of the regression line was significantly higher for the HF arm than the HD arm. Thus, for a given increase in urea Kt/V, the resultant increase in nPCR was greater during the HF phase. One explanation for this finding is the relatively greater removal of middle molecular weight anorectic compounds[61] by HF than HD.

In another Italian study of 24 patients comparing high-flux HD and on-line pre-dilution HF,[60] the same authors used a crossover design (HF-HD-HF) and attempted to achieve equality in the two arms with respect to delivered Kt/V and treatment duration. Similar to the first study, an on-line generation system was used to prepare the ultrapure dialysate for the HD and substitution fluid for HF, and the same highly permeable membrane (polyamide) was used in both phases. However, attainment of an equivalent Kt/V in the two arms required a significantly higher mean blood flow rate of 421 mL/min in HF versus 307 mL/min in HD. Moreover, the surface areas of the dialyzer in the HF and HD arms were 2.0 and 1.4 m^2, respectively.

The primary aim of the study was achieved in that delivered urea Kt/V was the same in all three phases of the study (mean 1.3). In the HF phases, this was associated with a mean substitution fluid rate and volume (317 mL/min and 69.6 L per treatment, respectively), which closely approximated the values from the first study. Significant differences in the occurrence of intradialytic events, including hypotension, cramps, and need for volume repletion, were observed in both HF arms relative to the HD arm. Likewise, in the interdialytic period, the prevalence of hypotension and fatigue was lower in the HF arms.

Hemodiafiltration

Maduell and colleagues[52] reported the clinical effects of transitioning patients from low-substitution volume ("soft") HDF to on-line HDF, which allowed a much higher substitution fluid volume to be used. Both modalities were performed in the post-dilution mode, which has been nearly the exclusive mode for HDF until very recently (see later text). In the low-volume arm, the mean substitution fluid rate was 22 mL/min, resulting in a mean total substitution volume of 4.1 L per treatment. The mean blood and dialysate flow rates were 402 and 654 mL/min, respectively. In the on-line arm, each patient continued to use the same high-flux dialyzer and, on average, the dialysate flow rate was not significantly changed. However, the mean blood flow rate modestly, but significantly, increased to 434 mL/min versus 402 mL/min in the previous phase. As far as prescription parameters, the major difference between the two arms was the significantly higher mean substitution fluid rate of 121 mL/min, corresponding to a mean total substitution volume of 22.5 L per treatment.

Several clinical benefits were observed during the 12-month follow-up after the therapy change. During soft-HDF and after 12 months of on-line HDF, mean single-pool urea Kt/V increased significantly from 1.35 to 1.52. Based on a comparison at the same time points, anemia parameters also improved, with a significant increase in hematocrit (32.2% vs. 34.0%) and a significant decrease in weekly mean erythropoietin requirements (3861 vs. 3232 U) (Figure 24–3). Finally, a sustained decrease in mean pretreatment serum β2-microglobulin from 27.4 mg/L during soft-HDF to 24.2 mg/L after 12 months of on-line HDF was also observed.

The above β2-microglobulin kinetic results reported by Maduell and colleagues have been corroborated recently by Lin and colleagues[62] in Taiwan. These investigators treated 58 patients over a mean period of 7.9 months with on-line post-dilution HDF according to the following prescription parameters: blood flow rate, 300 mL/min; dialysate flow rate, 500 mL/min; 1.8 m^2 polysulfone dialyzer; and total substitution fluid volume per treatment, 20 to 22 L. At baseline prior to HDF therapy, these patients received high-flux HD using similar blood and dialysate flow rates and the same dialyzer. Use of HDF resulted in a significantly higher mean β2-microglobulin reduction rate of 76% compared with 61% during HD. This greater degree of depuration resulted in a significantly lower mean pretreatment serum β2-microglobulin (22.2 mg/L vs. 34.8 mg/L during HD). Moreover, in a subgroup of nine patients receiving at least 12 months of HDF, a significant negative inverse correlation between HDF duration (in months) and pretreatment serum β2-microglobulin concentration was observed.

Although it is tempting to regard the results as seemingly intuitive, it is important to note that the clinical data regarding the effect of on-line HDF on serum pretreatment β2-microglobulin concentration are not entirely consistent. Employing the same high-flux dialyzer, Ward and colleagues[63] compared LMWP clearance and removal during HD and on-line post-dilution HDF (mean 21 L substitution fluid volume per treatment). Although mean dialyzer β2-microglobulin clearance was significantly higher during HDF (61 mL/min vs. 38 mL/min in HD), the effect on pretreatment β2-microglobulin concentration was not significant. Two potential explanations for this somewhat surprising finding were offered by the investigators. First, it is possible that the clearance provided by "internal filtration" (Starling's flow) during high-flux HD is greater than previously considered.[64] Under normal operating conditions of high-flux HD, the large axial pressure drop that occurs in such highly permeable membranes typically results in pressures in a certain portion of the distal (venous) end of the fibers that are less than the corresponding dialysate compartment pressure. This results in the routine occurrence of backfiltration of dialysate during high-flux HD. Although the combination of significant backfiltration and contaminated dialysate may be problematic,[65] this internal filtration circuit is actually beneficial from a large molecule clearance perspective by providing a significant convective component to total clearance. Patient-related mass transfer limitations represent the second potential explanation for this finding. Under standard dialysis conditions, the rate-limiting step for the removal of uremic toxins is not at the level of the dialyzer but rather within the patient's body.[66] Specifically, relatively slow transfer of β2-microglobulin and similar compounds within various compartments in the body, hinders delivery of solute out of the body. With solute delivery to the dialyzer impaired in such a manner, an increase in extracorporeal *clearance* has little effect on extracorporeal *removal*.[67] Despite this failure to find a significant impact on pretreatment β2-microglobulin concentration, Ward and colleagues did observe a significantly greater mean percent reduction in the plasma concentration of a larger middle molecule, complement Factor D (22 kDa), during HDF versus HD (33% vs. –2%, respectively).

Daily Convective Therapies

Due to its greater volume removal capabilities and more favorable solute kinetic profiles relative to thrice-weekly HD, daily HD therapy is considered by many experts to be superior to standard HD. Indeed, multiple small studies demonstrating benefits in such parameters as blood pressure control, anemia

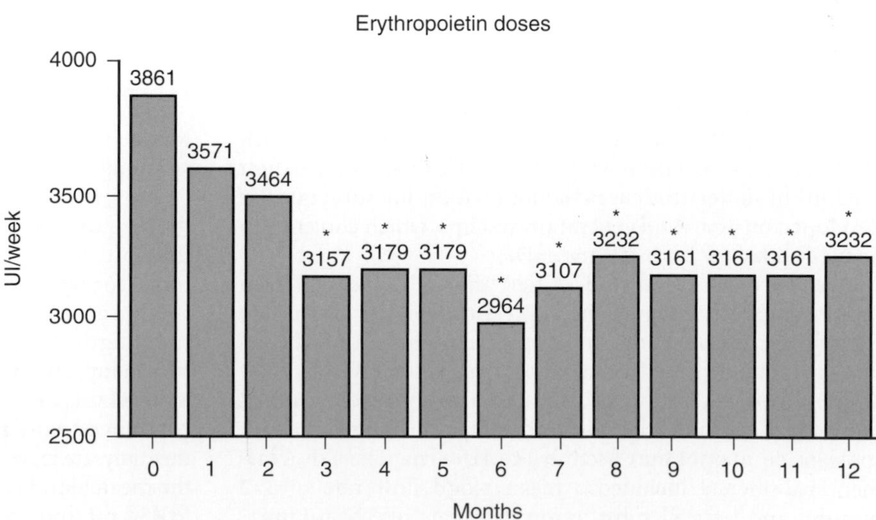

Figure 24–3 Effect of conversion from "soft" hemodiafiltration to on-line hemodiafiltration on erythropoietin requirements. (From Maduell F, del Pozo C, Garcia H, et al: Change from conventional hemodiafiltration to on-line hemodiafiltration. Nephrol Dial Transplant 1999; 14: 1202–1207. Reprinted with permission.)

markers, and nutritional status have appeared in the literature over the past few years.[68–71] Data from these studies have been sufficiently convincing that the National Institutes of Health in the United States is funding a multicenter study to explore further the potential clinical effects of daily HD.

As suggested, significant benefits are derived from performing dialysis therapy on a daily basis. When HD is performed only thrice-weekly, pretreatment solute concentrations increase to relatively high levels due to the long interdialytic intervals. Consequently, diffusive transmembrane concentration gradients are relatively high at the start of therapy. However, efficient depuration results in a relatively rapid dissipation of the concentration gradient, along with the driving force for diffusive removal. Thus, the latter part of a conventional HD treatment is relatively inefficient with respect to solute removal. Therapy delivery on a more frequent basis over shorter duration is advantageous because treatment is truncated before the inefficient phase (i.e., the low solute concentration period) is reached.[72]

A pioneer in the field of on-line convective therapies, Dr. Ledebo,[73] has recently suggested that a daily convection-based therapy approximates native kidney function most closely. However, only a small body of clinical experience with such an approach exists currently. Canaud and colleagues[74] prescribed daily on-line post-dilution HF to a series of ESRD patients more than a decade ago. A mean ultrafiltrate volume of 20.8 L per treatment and blood flow rate of 482 mL/min were prescribed. Despite the brevity of the study (1 week), a significant 35% decrease in the mean pre-treatment β2-microglobulin concentration from 39 to 25 mg/L was observed. More recently, Maduell and colleagues[75] evaluated the clinical effects of transitioning eight ESRD patients from thrice-weekly on-line HDF to a 6-month period of short daily on-line HDF. The ranges for the prescription parameters, which did not differ between the two arms, were: blood flow rate, 350 to 560 mL/min; substitution fluid rate, 80 to 150 mL/min; and dialysate flow rate, 800 mL/min minus the substitution fluid rate. Although mean treatment duration was shorter in the daily arm (133 min vs. 274 min in thrice-weekly arm), total weekly treatment duration was not significantly different (822 vs. 798 min in daily and thrice weekly arms, respectively). Despite this, urea EKR[76] and standard urea Kt/V,[77] two "continuous-equivalent" clearance measurements that allow for comparisons of therapies of differing frequency, both increased significantly by a mean of 26% and 48%, respectively, in the daily HDF phase (Figure 24–4). This finding is consistent with the argument concerning the kinetic benefits of daily therapy.

Maduell and colleagues[75] also quantified the differences in the clearance and removal of larger molecular weight uremic toxins in the two arms. Although the weekly percent solute removal of urea and creatinine increased significantly by 51% and 55%, respectively, this same parameter increased to an even greater extent for the larger molecules evaluated. Indeed, for osteocalcin (MW, 5.8 kDa), β2-microglobulin (11.8 kDa), myoglobin (17.2 kDa), and prolactin (23 kDa), the increase ranged from 67% to 75% (Figure 24–5). Specifically for β2-microglobulin, the mean pretreatment concentration decreased significantly by approximately 15% from a baseline concentration of 29.5 mg/L. Associated with these improvements in solute removal parameters were favorable changes in a number of cardiac parameters defined by echocardiography. After both 3 and 6 months of daily HDF therapy, significant decreases in interventricular septal thickness, left ventricular mass, and left ventricular mass index relative to baseline were observed.

Finally, Zimmerman and colleagues[78] have reported recently their experience with a novel delivery system for daily HF. In 11 patients treated at baseline with thrice-weekly high-flux HD, these investigators assessed the clinical effects of a 4-week treatment period of daily HF. In this approach, substitution fluid was provided as terminally sterilized fluid from bags in volumes generally ranging from 10 to 20 L, depending on the dose requirement and size of an individual patient. The mean treatment duration and substitution volumes were 132

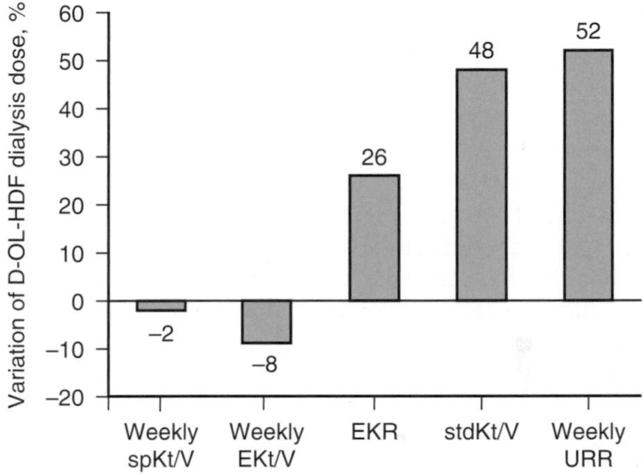

Figure 24–4 Effect of conversion from thrice-weekly on-line hemodiafiltration to daily on-line hemodiafiltration on urea clearance markers. (From Maduell F, Navarro V, Torregrosa E, et al: Change from three times a week on-line hemodiafiltration to short daily on-line hemodiafiltration [D-OL-HDF]. Kidney Int 2003; 64:305–313. Reprinted with permission.)

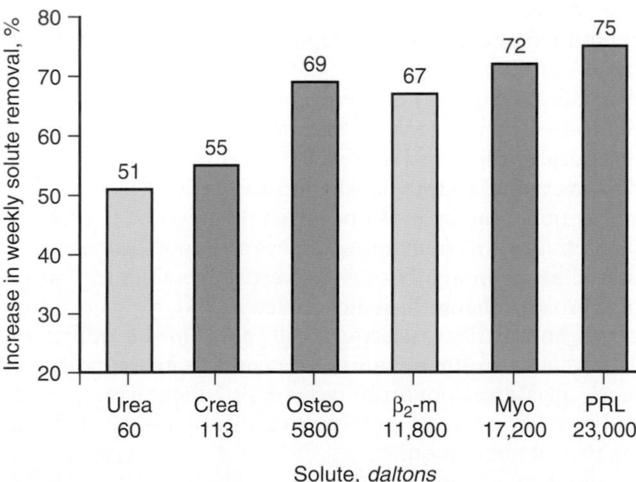

Figure 24–5 Effect of conversion from thrice-weekly on-line hemodiafiltration to daily on-line hemodiafiltration on solute removal parameters. (From Maduell F, Navarro V, Torregrosa E, et al: Change from three times a week on-line hemodiafiltration to short daily on-line hemodiafiltration. Kidney Int 2003; 64:305–313. Reprinted with permission.)

min and 11.6 L, respectively, in the daily HF phase of the study. Despite the relatively short duration of the daily HF phase, blood pressure control improved significantly, with mean arterial pressure decreasing from 96 to 86 mm Hg. In addition, mean pre-treatment β2-microglobulin decreased from 22.9 to 19.2 mg/L.

RECENT DEVELOPMENTS

In the next few years, several areas of interest in the convective therapies are likely to be explored. One of the emerging developments is the use of "mixed" dilution HDF rather than the traditional mode of post-dilution only. One approach to achieve mixed dilution was described originally for hemofiltration by Shaldon and colleagues[79] and later adapted by Collins and colleagues[80] in the form of a customized device. Effectively, the use of combined, simultaneous pre-dilution and post-dilution HDF also achieves the same end.[81,82] As described by Pedrini and colleagues,[82] use of the mixed mode avoids high transmembrane pressures, which are typically associated with high filtration fraction and membrane fouling. In addition, relative to post-dilution alone, mixed mode HDF may also result in less albumin loss, as suggested by a recent comparison of pre-dilution and post-dilution HF.[83] Another recently described approach to disrupt membrane fouling and concentration polarization and, thus, attenuate albumin losses is "push-pull" HDF.[84] In this therapy, repetitive application of positive and negative transmembrane pressure effectively achieves this disruption.

SUMMARY AND CONCLUSIONS

Recently performed outcome studies caution clinicians not to be over reliant on urea-based dosing parameters in the management of ESRD patients on maintenance dialysis. More importantly, these studies suggest that new dialytic approaches are needed to improve survival in ESRD patients. One approach that may influence survival favorably is broader application of convective therapies. The widespread availability of on-line systems for the preparation of ultrapure dialysate and sterile, non-pyrogenic replacement fluid allows the convective therapies to have solute clearance capabilities that surpass those of HD and PD. At present, outcome data demonstrating a clear benefit for convective therapies over conventional therapies do not exist. However, it is expected that results from comparative studies assessing this possibility will be forthcoming. For the convective therapies to flourish on a broad global scale, issues related to cost, regulatory concerns, and patient selection will need to be addressed. Nevertheless, in the opinion of the authors, these modalities represent a great opportunity for ESRD therapy to advance and meet the needs of an increasingly complex and challenging patient population.

References

1. Clark WR, Hamburger RJ, Lysaght MJ: Effect of membrane composition and structure on performance and biocompatibility in hemodialysis. Kidney Int 1999; 56:2005–2015.
2. Henderson LW: The problem of peritoneal membrane area and permeability. Kidney Int 1973; 3:409–410.
3. Clark WR, Macias WL, Molitoris BA, Wang NHL: Plasma protein adsorption to highly permeable hemodialysis membranes. Kidney Int 1995; 48:481–487.
4. Vanholder R, De Smet R, Glorieux G, et al: European Uremic Toxin Work Group (EUTox): Review on uremic toxins: Classification, concentration, and interindividual variability. Kidney Int 2003; 63:1934–1943.
5. Lowrie EG, Steinberg SM, Galen MA, et al: Factors in the dialysis regimen which contribute to alternations in the abnormalities of uremia. Kidney Int 1976; 10:409–422.
6. Lowrie EG, Laird NM, Parker TF, Sargent JA: Effect of the hemodialysis prescription on patient morbidity: Report from the National Cooperative Dialysis Study. N Engl J Med 1981; 305:1176–1181.
7. Gotch FA, Sargent JA: A mechanistic analysis of the National Cooperative Dialysis Study. Kidney Int 1985; 28:526–534.
8. Owen WF, Lew NL, Liu Y, et al: The urea reduction ratio and serum albumin concentration as predictors of mortality in patients undergoing hemodialysis. N Engl J Med 1993; 329:1001–1006.
9. Parker TF, Husni L, Huang W, et al: Survival of hemodialysis patients in the United States is improved with a greater quantity of dialysis. Am J Kidney Dis 1994; 23:67–680.
10. Collins AJ, Ma JZ, Umen A, Keshaviah P: Urea index and other predictors of hemodialysis survival. Am J Kidney Dis 1994; 23:272–282.
11. Hakim RM, Breyer J, Ismail N, Schulman G: Effects of dose of dialysis on morbidity and mortality. Am J Kidney Dis 1994; 23:661–669.
12. CANADA-USA (CANUSA) Peritoneal Dialysis Study Group: Adequacy of dialysis and nutrition in continuous peritoneal dialysis: Association with clinical outcomes. J Am Soc Nephrol 1996; 7:198–207.
13. Teehan B, Schleifer C, Brown J, et al: Urea kinetic analysis and clinical outcomes on CAPD: A five year longitudinal study. Adv Perit Dial 1990; 6:181–185.
14. Genestier S, Hedelin G, Schaffer P, Faller B: Prognostic factors in CAPD patients: A retrospective study of a 10-year period. Nephrol Dial Transplant 1995; 10:1905–1911.
15. NKF-DOQI Clinical Practice Guidelines for Hemodialysis Adequacy: Update 2000. Am J Kidney Dis 2001; 37(suppl 1):S7–S64.
16. NKF-DOQI Clinical Practice Guidelines for Peritoneal Dialysis Adequacy: Update 2000. Am J Kidney Dis 2001; 37(suppl 1):S65–S136.
17. Eknoyan G, Beck GJ, Cheung AK, et al: Effect of dialysis dose and membrane flux in maintenance hemodialysis. N Engl J Med 2002; 347:2010–2019.
18. Paniagua R, Amato D, Vonesh EF, et al: Effects of increased peritoneal clearances on mortality rates in peritoneal dialysis: ADEMEX, a prospective, randomized, controlled trial. J Am Soc Nephrol 2002; 13:1307–1320.
19. Clark WR, Winchester JW: Middle molecules and small molecular weight proteins in ESRD: Properties and strategies for their removal. Adv Renal Replace Ther (in press).
20. Diaz-Buxo J: Continuous flow peritoneal dialysis: Clinical applications. Blood Purif 2002; 20:36–39.
21. Ting G: The strategic role of daily hemodialysis in managed care in the United States. Semin Dial 2000; 13:385–388.
22. Pierratos A: Nocturnal home haemodialysis: An update on a 5-year experience. Nephrol Dial Transplant 1999; 14:2835–2840.
23. Heidenheim AP, Muirhead N, Moist L, Lindsay RM: Patient quality of life on quotidian hemodialysis. Am J Kidney Dis 2003; 42(suppl 1):36–41.
24. Morena MD, Guo D, Balakrishnan VS, et al: Effect of a novel adsorbent on cytokine responsiveness to uremic plasma. Kidney Int 2003; 63:1150–1154.

25. Henderson LW: Biophysics of ultrafiltration and hemofiltration. *In* Jacobs C (ed): Replacement of Renal Function by Dialysis, 4th ed. Dortdrecht, Kluwer Academic Publishers, 1996, pp 114–118.
26. Rockel A, Hertel J, Fiegel P, et al: Permeability and secondary membrane formation of a high flux polysulfone hemofilter. Kidney Int 1986; 30:429–432.
27. Kim S: Characteristics of protein removal in hemodiafiltration. Contrib Nephrol 1994; 108:23–37.
28. Ofsthun NJ, Zydney AL: Importance of convection in artificial kidney treatment. Contrib Nephrol 1994; 108:53–70.
29. Bosch T, Schmidt B, Samtleben W, Gurland H: Effect of protein adsorption on diffusive and convective transport through polysulfone membranes. Contrib Nephrol 1985; 46:14–22.
30. Langsdorf LJ, Zydney AL: Effect of blood contact on the transport properties of hemodialysis membranes: A two-layer model. Blood Purif 1994; 12:292–307.
31. Morti SM, Zydney AL: Protein-membrane interactions during hemodialysis: Effects on solute transport. ASAIO J 1998; 44: 319–326.
32. Henderson LW: Pre vs post dilution hemofiltration. Clin Nephrol 1979; 11:120–124.
33. Clark WR, Gao D: Low-molecular weight proteins in end-stage renal disease: Potential toxicity and dialytic removal mechanisms. J Am Soc Nephrol 2002; 13:S41–S47.
34. Clark WR, Gao D: Properties of membranes used for hemodialysis therapy. Semin Dial 2002; 15:1–5.
35. Werynski A, Waniewski J: Theoretical description of mass transport in medical membrane devices. Artif Organs 1995; 19:420–427.
36. Silverstein ME, Ford CA, Lysaght MJ, Henderson LW: Treatment of severe fluid overload by ultrafiltration. N Engl J Med 1974; 291:747–751.
37. Henderson LW, Colton CK, Ford CA, Lysaght MJ: Kinetics of hemodiafiltration. II. Clinical characterization of a new blood cleansing modality. J Lab Clin Med 1975; 85:372–391.
38. Colton CK, Henderson LW, Ford C, Lysaght MJ: Kinetics of hemodiafiltration. I. In vitro transport characteristics of a hollow-fiber blood ultrafilter. J Lab Clin Med 1975; 85:355–371.
39. Clark WR, Gao D: Determinants of small solute clearance in hemodialysis. Semin Dial (in press).
40. Maack T, Johnson V, Kau ST, et al: Renal filtration, transport, and metabolism of low-molecular weight proteins: A review. Kidney Int 1979; 16:251–270.
41. Quellhorst E: New trends in blood purification. Life Support Syst 1983; 1:207–216.
42. Quellhorst E, Scheunemann B, Hildebrand U: Hemofiltration: An improved method of treatment for chronic renal failure. Contrib Nephrol 1985; 44:194–211.
43. Baldamus CA, Quellhorst E: Outcome of long-term hemofiltration. Kidney Int 1985; 17 (suppl):S41–S46.
44. Henderson LW, Beans E: Successful production of sterile pyrogen-free electrolyte solution by ultrafiltration. Kidney Int 1978; 14:522–525.
45. Shaldon S, Beau MC, Deschodt G, et al: Economic preparation of sterile non-pyrogenic infusate for hemofiltration. Dial Transplant 1983; 12:792–793.
46. Canaud B, Nguyen QV, Lagrarde C, et al: Clinical evaluation of a multipurpose dialysis system adequate for hemodialysis or for post-dilution hemofiltration/hemodiafiltration with on-line preparation of substitution fluid from dialysate. Contrib Nephrol 1985; 46:184–186.
47. Ledebo I: Principles and practice of hemofiltration and hemodiafiltration. Artif Organs 1998; 22:20–25.
48. Ofsthun NJ, Colton CK, Lysaght MJ: Determinants of fluid and solute removal rates during hemofiltration. *In* Henderson LW, Quellhorst EA, Baldamus CA, Lysaght MJ (eds): *Hemofiltration.* Berlin, Springer-Verlag, 1986, pp 18–39.
49. Leber HW, Wizemann V, Goubeaud G, et al: Simultaneous hemofiltration/hemodialysis: An effective alternative to hemofiltration and conventional hemodialysis in the treatment of uremic patients. Clin Nephrol 1978; 9:115–121.
50. Kunitomo T, Kirkwood RG, Kumazawa S, et al: Clinical evaluation of postdilution dialysis with a combined ultrafiltration (UF)?hemodialysis (HD) system. Trans Am Soc Artif Intern Organs 1978; 24:169–177.
51. Ledebo I: On-line hemodiafiltration: Technique and therapy. Adv Renal Replace Ther 1999; 6:195–208.
52. Maduell F, del Pozo C, Garcia H, et al: Change from conventional hemodiafiltration to on-line hemodiafiltration. Nephrol Dial Transplant 1999; 14:1202–1207.
53. Canaud B, Bosc JY, Leray-Moragues H, et al: On-line hemodiafiltration: Safety and efficacy in long-term clinical practice. Nephrol Dial Transplant 2000; 15(suppl 1):60–67.
54. Wizemann V, Lotz C, Techert F, Uthoff S: On-line hemodiafiltration vs. low-flux haemodialysis: A prospective, randomized study. Nephrol Dial Transplant 2000; 15(suppl 1):43–48.
55. Ono M, Taoka M, Takagi T, et al: Comparison of types of on-line hemodiafiltration from the standpoint of low-molecular weight protein removal. Contrib Nephrol 1994; 108:38–45.
56. Ahrenholz P, Winkler RE, Ramlow W, et al: On-line hemodiafiltration with pre- and post-dilution: A comparison of efficacy. Int J Artif Organs 1997; 20:81–90.
57. Altieri P, Sorba GB, Bolasco PG, et al: On-line predilution hemofiltration versus ultrapure high-flux hemodialysis: A multi-center prospective study in 23 patients. Blood Purif 1997; 15:169–181.
58. Altieri P, Sorba G, Bolasco P, et al: Pre-dilution haemofiltration?the Sardinian studies: Present and future. Nephrol Dial Transplant 2000; 15(suppl 2):55–59.
59. Bolasco P, Altieri P, Sorba G, et al: Adequacy in pre-dilution haemofiltration: Kt/V or infusion volume? Nephrol Dial Transplant 2000; 15(suppl 2):60–64.
60. Altieri P, Sorba G, Bolasco P, et al: Predilution haemofiltration? the Second Sardinian Multicentre Study: Comparisons between haemofiltration and haemodialysis during identical Kt/V and session times in a long-term cross-over study. Nephrol Dial Transplant 2001; 16:1207–1213.
61. Anderstam B, Mamoun A, Sodersten P, Bergstrom J: Middle-sized molecule fractions isolated from uremic ultrafiltrate and normal urine inhibit ingestive behavior in the rat. J Am Soc Nephrol 1996; 7:2453–2460.
62. Lin CL, Yang CW, Chiang CC, et al: Long-term on-line hemodiafiltration reduces predialysis beta–2-microglobulin levels in chronic hemodialysis patients. Blood Purif 2001; 19:301–307.
63. Ward RA, Schmidt B, Hullin J, et al: A comparison of on-line hemodiafiltration and high-flux hemodialysis: A prospective clinical study. J Am Soc Nephrol 2000; 11:2344–2350.
64. Ofsthun NJ, Leypoldt JK: Ultrafiltration and backfiltration during hemodialysis. Artif Organs 1995; 19:1143–1161.
65. Lonneman G: Dialysate bacteriological quality and the permeability of dialyzer membranes to pyrogens. Kidney Int 1993; suppl 41:S195–S200.
66. Clark WR, Leypoldt JK, Henderson LW, et al: Quantifying the effect of changes in the hemodialysis prescription on effective solute removal with a mathematical model. J Am Soc Nephrol 1999; 10:601–610.
67. Clark WR, Henderson LW: Renal vs continuous vs intermittent therapies for removal of uremic toxins. Kidney Int 2001; 59(suppl 78):S298–S303.
68. Fagugli RM, Reboldi G, Quintaliani G, et al: Short daily hemodialysis: Blood pressure control and left ventricular mass reduction in hypertensive hemodialysis patients. Am J Kidney Dis 2001; 38:371–376.
69. Galland R, Traeger J, Arkouche W, et al: Short daily hemodialysis and nutritional status. Am J Kidney Dis 2001; 37(1 suppl 2): S95–S98.

70. Pierratos A: Nocturnal home haemodialysis: An update on a 5-year experience. Nephrol Dial Transplant 1999; 14:2835–2840.
71. Raj DS, Charra B, Pierratos A, Work J: In search of ideal hemodialysis: Is prolonged frequent dialysis the answer? Am J Kidney Dis 1999; 34:597–610.
72. Depner TA: Benefits of more frequent dialysis: Lower TAC at the same Kt/V. Nephrol Dial Transplant 1998; 13(suppl 6):20–24.
73. Ledebo I: Does convective therapy applied daily approach renal blood purification? Kidney Int 2001; 59(suppl 78):S286–S291.
74. Canaud B, Assounga A, Kerr P, et al: Failure of a daily haemofiltration programme using a highly permeable membrane to return β2-microglobulin concentrations to normal in haemodialysis patients. Nephrol Dial Transplant 1992; 7:924–939.
75. Maduell F, Navarro V, Torregrosa E, et al: Change from three times a week on-line hemodiafiltration to short daily on-line hemodiafiltration. Kidney Int 2003; 64:305–313.
76. Casino FG, Lopez T: The equivalent renal urea clearance: A new parameter to assess dialysis dose. Nephrol Dial Transplant 1996; 11:1574–1591.
77. Gotch FA: The current place of urea kinetic modeling with respect to different dialysis modalities. Nephrol Dial Transplant 1998; 13(suppl 6):10–14.
78. Zimmerman DL, Swedko PJ, Posen GA, Burns KD: Daily hemofiltration with a simplified method of delivery. ASAIO J 2003; 49:426–429.
79. Shaldon S, Beau MC, Deschodt G, Mion C: Mixed hemofiltration: 18 months experience with ultrashort treatment time. Trans Am Soc Artif Organs 1981; 27:610–612.
80. Krieter DH, Falkenhain S, Chalabi L, et al: Prospective cross-over comparison of mid-dilution HDF: Nephros OLpur™ MD 190 diafilter versus post-dilution HDF (Abstract). J Am Soc Nephrol 2003; 14:501A.
81. Hillion D, Haas T, Pertuiset N, Uzan M: Pre-postdilution hemofiltration. Blood Purif 1995; 13:241–245.
82. Pedrini LA, de Christofaro V, Pagliari B, Sama F: Mixed pre-dilution and post-dilution online hemodiafiltration compared with traditional infusion modes. Kidney Int 2000; 58:2155–2165.
83. Santoro A, Canova C, Mancini E, et al: Protein loss in on-line hemofiltration. Blood Purif (in press).
84. Shinzato T, Miwa M, Nakai S, et al: Alternate repetition of short fore- and backfiltrations reduces convective albumin loss. Kidney Int 1996; 50:432–435.

SECTION D

Peritoneal Dialysis

Chapter 25

Peritoneal Physiology

Olof Heimbürger, M.D., Ph.D.

In patients with chronic renal failure, waste products, which normally are excreted in the urine, accumulate in the blood resulting in uremic intoxication, and the obvious goal of dialysis treatment is to remove "uremic toxins" (including water) from the patient. Peritoneal dialysis (PD) utilizes dialysis fluid infused into the peritoneal cavity and a system of biologic membranes—the peritoneal barrier—for this purpose. Whereas the artificial hemodialysis membrane has well characterized, reproducible, solute and fluid transport characteristics, the peritoneum is not really a membrane but rather a complex structure of living tissues with different transport characteristics, which, furthermore, will differ between patients, a fact that will affect the fluid and solute transport kinetics of PD as well as dialysis efficiency in PD patients. In addition, the transport characteristics of the peritoneal membrane may not be constant in an individual patient but may be altered with time due to effects of the dialysis procedure or the dialysis fluids, in response to various physiologic reactions or due to pharmacologic effects of different drugs.

THE PERITONEAL ANATOMY

The peritoneal cavity is the largest serosal cavity in the body with a surface area of approximately 1 to 2 m^2. Although the peritoneal area is commonly suggested to be similar to the body surface area, recent studies suggest that the anatomic surface area of the peritoneum may be only about 50% of the body surface area in adults.[1–3] Peritoneum etymologically means "wrapped tightly around," which is a good description of the arrangement of this serous membrane that consists of two parts: the parietal peritoneum that covers the abdominal wall and the diaphragm and the visceral peritoneum that covers the intra-abdominal viscera.[4] The parietal peritoneum represents a smaller portion (approximately 10% to 20%) of the total peritoneal surface area[1,2] and receives its blood supply from the vasculature of the abdominal wall. The visceral peritoneum represents the larger part (approximately 80% to 90%) of the total peritoneal surface area[2] and receives its blood supply via the mesenteric vessels. However, it should be pointed out that it is the functional peritoneal surface area that is important not the anatomic surface area.[5] The functional area will be related to the surface area of the capillaries in the peritoneal interstitium, the capillary density, and the spatial arrangement of these capillaries.[3,5] In addition, the peritoneal cavity is only a potential space under normal conditions and the functional contact area between the peritoneum and the dialysis fluid in the peritoneal cavity during PD will be lower than the anatomic area.[6] In particular, functional area of the visceral peritoneum is reduced due to the incomplete contact and poor mixing in small fluid compartments within pockets of the visceral peritoneum. In mice, less than half of the peritoneal surface is in contact with a large volume of solution in the peritoneal cavity, but the contact area could be improved by shaking of the animal, and, particularly, by adding dioctyl sodium sulfosuccinate (a surface-tension lowering agent).[6]

HISTOLOGY

The Mesothelium

The surface of the peritoneal cavity is lined by a single layer of mesothelial cells (fixed to a continuous basement membrane) that under normal physiologic conditions are covered with a thin (5 μm) film of peritoneal fluid that is kept in place by numerous microvilli.[4] The microvilli and the peritoneal fluid have a lubricating function to prevent formation of adhesions and to allow the free movement of the visceral organs during respiration, peristalsis, and body movement.[4] The peritoneal fluid contains protein, electrolytes, cells (mainly macrophages, lymphocytes, and desquamated mesothelial cells), and has a high content of phospholipids that are secreted in from the mesothelium by the formation of lamellar bodies, similar to the production of surfactant from type II pneumocytes.[7]

The mesothelial cells may modulate the peritoneal microcirculation by secretion of vasodilators like PGE_2 and nitric oxide as well as vasoconstrictors, such as endothelin,[8] and, furthermore, the mesothelial cells have an important role in the initiation of the local immune response regulating leukocyte infiltration via the secretion of chemokines and expression of adhesion molecules.[9,10] Mesothelial cells have a capacity to produce tissue plasminogen activator (tPA), and the mesothelium normally expresses high fibrinolytic activity.[8,11] However, the mesothelium also have antifibrinolytic capacity by synthesis of fibrinolytic inhibitors like plasminogen activator inhibitor 1 (PAI-1) and PAI-2, and the balance between the synthesis of fibrinolytic and agents in mesothelial cells will determine their capacity to promote fibrin degradation. Under normal conditions the fibrinolytic activity strongly dominates, but the balance may change completely during inflammation when the antifibrinolytic activity of the mesothelium will dominate, and furthermore, the mesothelium may also exhibit procoagulant activity with expression of tissue factor (which is markedly upregulated in mesothelial cells during inflammation).[8] Thus, the mesothelium plays an important role in regulation of the balance between fibrinolytic and procoagulant activity in the peritoneal cavity.

The underlying basement membrane is a very thin laminar network containing collagen type IV, proteoglycans, and glycoproteins such as laminin, and allows macrophages and lymphocytes to pass through it, whereas fibroblasts cannot pass this basement membrane.[8] The thin mesothelial cell layer and their basement membrane seem to offer very little resistance to the transport of small and large solutes, in vitro or in vivo.[3,12] Thus, the mesothelium does not seem to have any major impact on the transport across the peritoneal barrier.

The Interstitium

Beneath the mesothelium lies the interstitial tissue, comprising of an amorphous ground substance or gel-like extracellular matrix interlaced with collagenous, reticular, and elastic fibers, adipocytes, fibroblasts, and granular material, and containing blood capillaries, nerves, and lymphatic vessels.[13–15] The collagen fibers constitute the largest component of the space between the cells in the peritoneum and form a fibrous skeleton in the interstitium.[15] The collagen fibers bind via β1-integrins to fibroblasts and other cells in the tissue.[16] The interstitial ground substance may be subdivided into a colloid-rich and a water-rich phase, the two phases being in equilibrium with each other.[3,12,14] The colloid-rich phase contains several different glycosaminoglycans (GAG), including hyaluronan (HA, which is the major component). All GAGs except HA are covalently bound to a protein backbone forming proteoglycans (the combination of a GAG and a protein), for example, chondroitin sulphate, dermatan sulphate, keratan sulphate, and heparan sulphate. The GAGs are polyanionic, have low isoelectric points, and, consequently, the interstitial ground substance has a high density of negative colloidal charge at physiologic pH.[14] Water and small solutes can easily enter the colloid-rich phase, whereas macromolecules are excluded from large parts of this phase. In a complex manner, the interstitium may act as a mucopolysaccharide hydrogel, penetrated with more or less continuous channels of free fluid.[3] Whereas small solutes may pass through interstitial matrix hydrogels without much hindrance, the diffusion of macromolecules may be markedly retarded.[5,15] However, it is important to remember that the capillary wall determines the amount of solutes that are transported from blood to interstitium, and both the interstitium and the capillary wall need to be taken into account for the description of the peritoneal transport process.

In general, changes in aggregation and hydration of the ground substance in interstitial tissues affect the physicochemical properties and the functional characteristics of the interstitium,[14] but it is at present not established exactly how peritoneal dialysis may affect the functional characteristics of the peritoneal interstitial tissues.[12]

The Capillary Wall

The microvascular exchange vessels in the peritoneal membrane consist of both true capillaries (diameter 5–6 μm) and postcapillary venules (diameter 7–20 μm),[5] and the capillary wall is considered to be the major transport barrier for transperitoneal exchange of fluid and solutes during peritoneal dialysis. The peritoneal capillaries belong to the continuous type (in which endothelial cells form a continuous layer enwrapped in a negatively charged glycocalix),[5,17,18] which functionally restrict solute exchange to less than 0.1% of the total capillary surface area (= the small pores, see later).[3,19] The peritoneal capillaries behave functionally as having a heteroporous structure, with a small number of large pores (radius 200–400 Å) through which macromolecules are filtered due to convective flow and a large number of "small pores" (radius 40–65 Å), which are impermeable for macromolecules larger than albumin (molecular weight 69,000 Dalton) but do not restrict the passage of small solutes.[17,18,20] In addition, "ultra-small" pores (radius 4–6 Å) were postulated to be involved in the water flow induced by the osmotic effect of low molecular weight osmotic agents, for example, glucose[17,20,21] (Figure 25–1). The anatomic correlate of the water channels was later demonstrated to be aquaporin-1, a protein 28 KDa intramembrane protein shown to be one of the water channels in human proximal tubular cells in the kidney as well as in various nonfenestrated epithelia.[22,23] Aquaporin-1 has been demonstrated in peritoneal endothelial cells, at mRNA protein, and functional levels.[24–26] The anatomic correlates to the small pores are possibly the interendothelial clefts.[5,17,20] The three-dimensional structure of the interendothelial clefts has been described in detail.[27] However, the morphologic counterpart to the large pores is not established, although it most likely corresponds to larger interendothelial gaps.[5,17,20] Though there has been considerable controversy about the mechanism of macromolecular transport through the endothelium and the potential role of vesicular transport (transcytosis), it is now established that the quantitative role of transcytosis is negligible.[28,29]

The three-pore concept of transcapillary exchange[18] has been successfully applied by Rippe and associates[17,30–33] to model the peritoneal transport of small solutes and macromolecules as well as the peritoneal fluid transport, supporting the view that the capillary wall is the main resistance for transperitoneal fluid and solute transport.

PERITONEAL BLOOD FLOW

The mesenteric blood flow is generally supposed to be about 10% of cardiac output.[34] The effective peritoneal blood flow, that is, the blood flow to the capillaries that are directly involved in peritoneal transport, cannot be directly measured.[35] Indirect estimations suggest that the effective peritoneal blood flow may vary from 20 to 40 mL/min (using

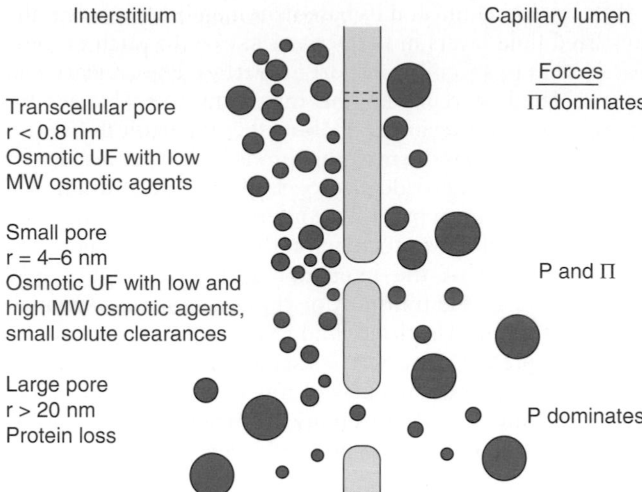

Figure 25–1 The three-pore model of peritoneal capillary permselectivity, including the transcellular pore (aquaporin-1), the small pore (the interendothelial clefts), and the large pores (possibly large interendothelial clefts). Small circles represent small solutes and large circles represent proteins. The forces are: Π, osmotic pressure and P, hydrostatic pressure. Crystalloid osmotic pressure induced by glucose is very efficient through the transcellular pores, and about 50% of the ultrafiltered fluid will pass through the aquaporins when glucose is used as an osmotic agent in PD. (From Flessner MF: Peritoneal transport physiology: Insights from basic research. J Am Soc Nephrol 1991; 2:122-135, with permission.)

estimations of the maximal possible ultrafiltration rate) to more than 100 mL/min (based on the measurements of the clearance of gases).[36,37] The effective peritoneal blood flow is generally not believed to limit the clearance of small solutes during peritoneal dialysis[37,38] because the diffusive mass transport coefficient for urea is approximately 20 mL/min. Also, tracer disappearance from small plastic chambers glued to the serosa was not reduced with a 30% decrease in blood flow and only to a minor degree with no blood flow (in dead rats).[39,40] However, this issue is still controversial, and there are some observations indicating that peritoneal urea clearance may be blood flow limited.[12,35,41] Recently, Rosengren and Rippe[42] reported that a reduction of blood flow by 40% (caused by bleeding of rats) resulted in a decreased transport of glucose and ^{51}Cr-EDTA by 13% and 24%, respectively. They concluded that there is to some extent a blood flow limitation of peritoneal transport, but that the level of blood flow limitation is much smaller than in other organs. Note that the diffusion rate of small solutes theoretically will not be proportional to the blood flow, but to the square root of perfusion rate, which to a large extent may explain the small change in transport with marked alterations in blood flow.[43]

Vasodilators have been shown to increase peritoneal clearances due possibly to increase in the capillary surface area due to vasodilatation and recruitment of capillaries.[35,44] Furthermore, changes in the distribution of the blood flow may possibly also affect the peritoneal transport rate.

PERITONEAL LYMPHATICS

The Anatomy of Peritoneal Lymphatics

About 4% of the mesothelial surface area is reported to be covered by lymphatic vessels,[45] but the major part of the lymphatic drainage is considered to occur via the lymphatic stomata in the diaphragmatic part of the peritoneum.[46,47] The diaphragmatic lymphatic stomata, that were first described by von Recklinghausen[48] in 1862, are small openings (diameter 4–12 μm) that are formed by intercellular junctions between both mesothelial cells and lymphatic endothelial cells, and opens directly into underlying lymphatic lacunae.[45–47] It is through these specific openings that large particles like erythrocytes and bacteria can directly leave the peritoneal cavity. The underlying lymphatic plexuses (which in humans are situated mainly on the muscular portion of the diaphragm) intercommunicate directly with the plexuses on the pleural surface via intercommunicating vessels.[46] After leaving the diaphragm, the lymph is drained via the large collecting ducts associated with the internal thoracic vessels to reach the venous circulation via the right lymphatic duct.[46] The lymphatic drainage of the peritoneal cavity is to a large extent dependent on the periodic compression and release of the lymphatic vessels caused by the movements of the diaphragm during respiration.[46,49]

In addition to the lymphatic vessels the diaphragmatic part of the peritoneum, subserosal lymphatic vessels can also be found in other parts of the peritoneal cavity, including the omentum,[46] and, furthermore, local lymphatic vessels are also present in the tissues surrounding the peritoneal cavity, although their role in peritoneal transport seem to be minor under normal conditions.[46]

The Importance of Lymphatic Flow for Peritoneal Fluid Absorption

The disappearance of a macromolecular marker from the peritoneal cavity has often wrongly been used to estimate lymph flow from the peritoneal cavity during peritoneal dialysis. It is now well established that the peritoneal absorptive flow of fluid and solutes is comprised of two different pathways[12,50,51]: (1) direct lymphatic absorption (mainly via the lymphatic stomata in the diaphragm, and, to a lesser extent, through visceral lymphatic pathways,[51] and (2) fluid absorption into tissues.[17,52] Studies using tracer appearance in plasma have demonstrated that the direct lymphatic flow represents about 20% of the fluid absorptive flow from the peritoneal cavity in clinically stable CAPD patients.[53–55] See "fluid absorption" below for a more detailed discussion.

PERITONEAL LOCAL REACTION TO INFECTION

The peritoneal host defense reaction to infection is a complex network of interactions between mesothelial cells, peritoneal macrophages (PMø), infiltrating neutrophils, monocytes and other inflammatory cells, and orchestrated by the secretion of vasoactive substances, cytokines, chemokines, growth factors as well as components of extracellular matrix.[8,9] The initiation, resolution, and repair process of inflammation in the peritoneal cavity are very complex processes, which presently are under intense study, and the regulation of these processes is starting to be understood.[8–10,56,57]

The initial inflammatory activation by bacteria entering the peritoneal cavity is likely to occur on the mesothelial surface, where mesothelial cells together with PMø have an important role in the initiation of the local immune response.[9] The mesothelial cells are able to contribute to the massive neutrophil influx by generation of chemokines like CXCL8 (previously called interleukin-8), a process that is amplified by the PMø-derived cytokines tumor necrosis factor α (TNFα) and interleukin (IL)-1β[9,58,59]; and the mesothelial cells are also capable of expression of adhesion molecules like ICAM-1, VCAM-1, and PECAM-1 as well as integrins, which may promote leukocyte attachment to the mesothelial cells.[8] The PMø produced TNFα and IL-1a are thought to be key mediators in the activation of mesothelial cells.[9] The mesothelial cells are the principal source of IL-6 in the peritoneal cavity and synthesize large amounts of IL-6 upon inflammatory challenge.[60] However, mesothelial cells do not express the cognate IL-6 receptor and therefore they initially are unresponsive to IL-6. There is a rapid accumulation of neutrophils within the peritoneal cavity during the first 12 to 24 hours, however, after a few days the neutrophils are replaced by a more sustained population of monocytes and lymphocytes.[10] In fact, this temporal switch in the recruitment of leucocytes (which is under a complex regulation) determines whether or not the infection is cleared.[61,62] Liberation of the soluble IL-6 receptor (SIL-6R) from the initial neutrophils allows for the formation of the IL-6 and SIL-6R complex, that allows IL-6 responsiveness in cell types (including mesothelial cells) lacking the cognate IL-6 receptor.[61] The IL-6 and SIL-6R complex will downregulate the expression of CXCL8 and other neutrophil-activating chemokines, and the SIL-6R may also directly promote MCP-1 expression resulting in the more sustained mononuclear leukocyte infiltration.[10] In addition, the release of oncostatin M from the infiltrating neutrophils will have a synergistic effect with the SIL-6R for the temporal switch from neutrophil influx to mononuclear cell recruitment as oncostatin M suppresses IL-1β-mediated expression of CXCL8.[56] Interferon-γ (IFN-γ) also has an important role in this process by control of both the initial neutrophil recruitment independently of IL-6 (through regulation of chemokine expression) as well as the neutrophils clearance phase by regulating local IL-6 levels.[57,63] The neutrophils will, to a large extent, undergo apoptosis and then be phagocytized by mononuclear cells.[63] This transition from the recruitment of neutrophils (typically associated with innate immunity) to the leukocytes typically associated with acquired immunity is considered to facilitate the successful resolution on the inflammatory reaction.[10]

PERITONEAL TRANSPORT PHYSIOLOGY

Barriers to Transperitoneal Exchange

The peritoneum is a complex structure of at least five different resistance barriers coupled in a series: (1) the unstirred fluid layer in the capillaries, (2) the capillary wall (endothelium and basement membrane), (3) the interstitial space, (4) the mesothelium and its basement membrane, and (5) the unstirred fluid layers in the peritoneal cavity.[64] Each of these barriers has its specific transport properties. The capillary wall is considered to represent the major transport barrier for transperitoneal exchange,[17,20] but the interstitium is also important, whereas the mesothelium is highly permeable.[17,20] The mucopolysaccharide hydrogel of the interstitium will exclude solutes from part of the interstitial water volume and force solutes to follow a tortuous path,[12] and, furthermore, the negative charge of the interstitial ground substance may markedly retard the transport of charged molecules through the interstitium.[14] Unstirred fluid layers in the peritoneal cavity may represent transport resistances for the diffusion of small solutes[12,65] but are likely of much less importance than the interstitium as the diffusibility is much less in the interstitium compared to the stagnant fluid layers.[3,66]

Modeling of Peritoneal Transport

To completely model the peritoneal transport process, all transport barriers, and their specific transport characteristics, should be taken into account as well as the distribution of the capillaries within the peritoneal interstitium. This will result in very complex models that are difficult to apply in the clinical situation, and, at present, even complex models fail to predict ultrafiltration with better accuracy than simpler models.

Single-membrane models have been used to estimate transport parameters in clinical peritoneal dialysis.[67–73] In the single-membrane models, the peritoneal barrier is regarded as a single membrane separating the well-mixed blood and dialysate compartments. The single-membrane models will work very well to describe the transport of small solutes (up to the size of small proteins like β2-microglobulin) from plasma to dialysate, but they will not work as well for the description of dialysate to plasma transport, and in particular, they cannot correctly describe the osmotic fluid transport when a high molecular solute (e.g., icodextrin) is used as osmotic agent.[5] The distributed model by Dedrick and Flessner[74–76] takes into account the distribution of capillaries in the interstitium and should be preferred from a theoretical point of view. However, the simpler three-pore model by Rippe and associates,[30–32] which takes into account the three pore systems in the capillary wall (see earlier text), is still as accurate in predicting both fluid and solute transport during clinical peritoneal dialysis, using both small molecular weight as well as macromolecular osmotic agents[30,32,77] (Figure 25–2). Also, a model describing the peritoneum as two heteroporous membranes in series (presumably the capillary wall and the interstitium) has been developed.[78] The detailed description of the different models lies outside the scope of the present chapter.

Fluid Transport

Ultrafiltration

The intraperitoneal dialysate volume over time curves during a peritoneal dialysis exchange are characterized by three phases: (1) initial *net ultrafiltration* (rate and duration is depending on the osmotic pressure of the solution); (2) *dialysate isovolemia* (during which ultrafiltration is counterbalanced by fluid absorption); and (3) *net fluid absorption* (independent on the osmolality of the solution)[79] (Figure 25–3).

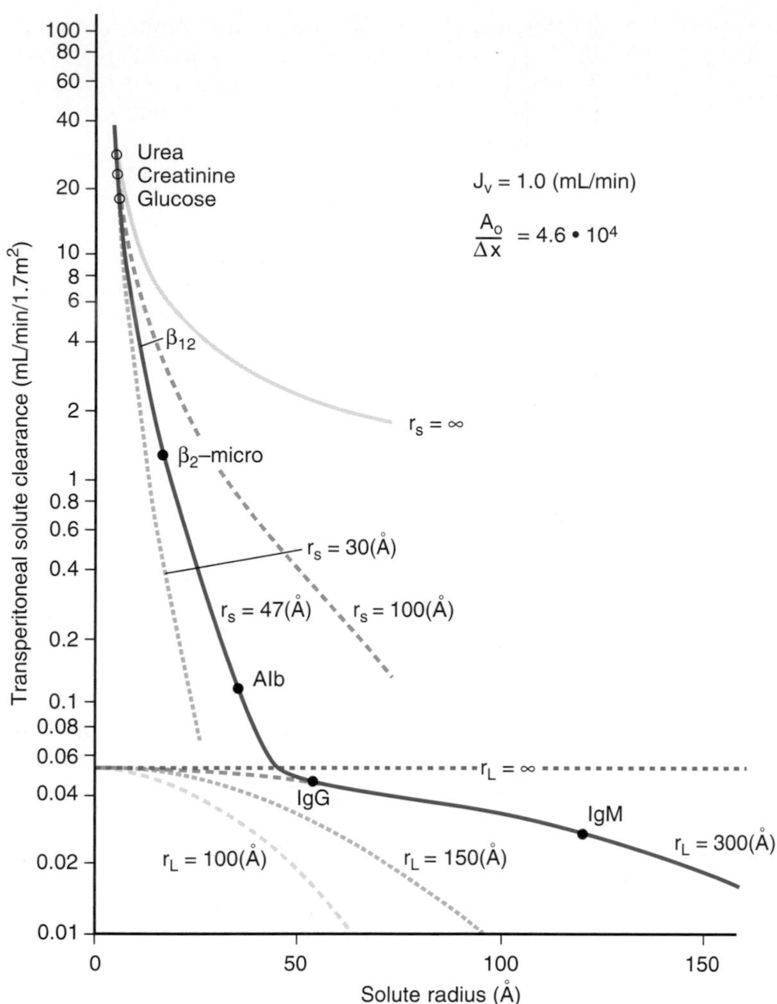

Figure 25–2 Semilogarithmic plot of transperitoneal unidirectional clearances versus molecular radius. The solid line represents the theoretic clearances simulated for a small pore radius of 47 Å, a large pore radius of 300 Å, a pore area over unit diffusion distance ($A_0/\Delta x$) of 45,000, and a total blood to peritoneal cavity filtration rate at 1 mL/min/1.73 m^2 body surface area. (From Rippe B, Krediet RT: Peritoneal physiology-transport of solutes. *In* Gokal R, Nolph KD (eds): The Textbook of Peritoneal Dialysis. Dordrecht, Kluwer Academic Publishers, 1994, pp 69-113, with permission.)

Ultrafiltration in peritoneal dialysis is achieved by the application of a high concentration of an osmotic agent (usually glucose) in the dialysate, resulting in a high osmotic pressure gradient across the peritoneal barrier.[12,13,80] However, the osmotic pressure gradient over the peritoneal barrier decreases rapidly due to the absorption of the osmotic agent, when small solutes like glucose, amino acids, or glycerol, are used as osmotic agents. When a large molecular solute, for example, icodextrin, is used as osmotic agent the absorption of the osmotic agent is much slower, resulting in a much longer lasting osmotic gradient and positive net ultrafiltration.

Applying the thermodynamic theory of volume transport through selective membranes to the peritoneal membrane, the ultrafiltration rate (QU) is directly proportional to the ultrafiltration coefficient (L_pA), which, in turn, represents the product of the hydraulic conductance (L_p) and the effective surface area (A).[13,31,80,81] The ultrafiltration rate is therefore described as:

$$QU = L_pA\left(\Delta P - \sigma_{prot}\Delta\pi_{prot} - \sum_{i=1}^{n}\sigma_i\Delta\pi_i\right) \quad (1)$$

where ΔP is the hydrostatic pressure gradient, σ_{prot} is the reflection coefficient for total protein, $\Delta\pi_{prot}$ is the colloid osmotic pressure difference caused by the plasma proteins, and the third term within the parentheses represents the sum of all effective crystalloid osmotic pressure gradients across the peritoneal barrier.[31,82,83] Note that this equation is a simplification that applies to the capillary wall and, for the full description of the total process, also local effects in peritoneal tissue (e.g., the distribution capillaries in the interstitium, interstitial tissue pressure gradients) will have an impact on the ultrafiltration rate. Thus, the ultrafiltration induced when glucose is used as osmotic agent in PD, is dependent on the osmotic pressure difference for glucose, the hydraulic conductance (L_p), the surface area (A), and the reflection coefficient for glucose (σ_g)[31,82,83] A wide range of values for the ultrafiltration coefficient (L_pA) has been reported in the literature due to that markedly different values of σ_g have been estimated.[13,68,69,84,85] The reason for these discrepancies is that σ_g in several studies have been calculated as $\sigma_g = 1 - S_g$ (where S_g is the "lumped" glucose sieving coefficient for the whole peritoneal membrane), which is true for homogeneous membranes. However, as the peritoneal membrane is a heteroporous membrane, the relationship between σ_g and S_g may vary.[31] In fact, one of the most convincing arguments for the heteroporous character of the peritoneal membrane is that the direct determinations of L_pA for the peritoneal membrane

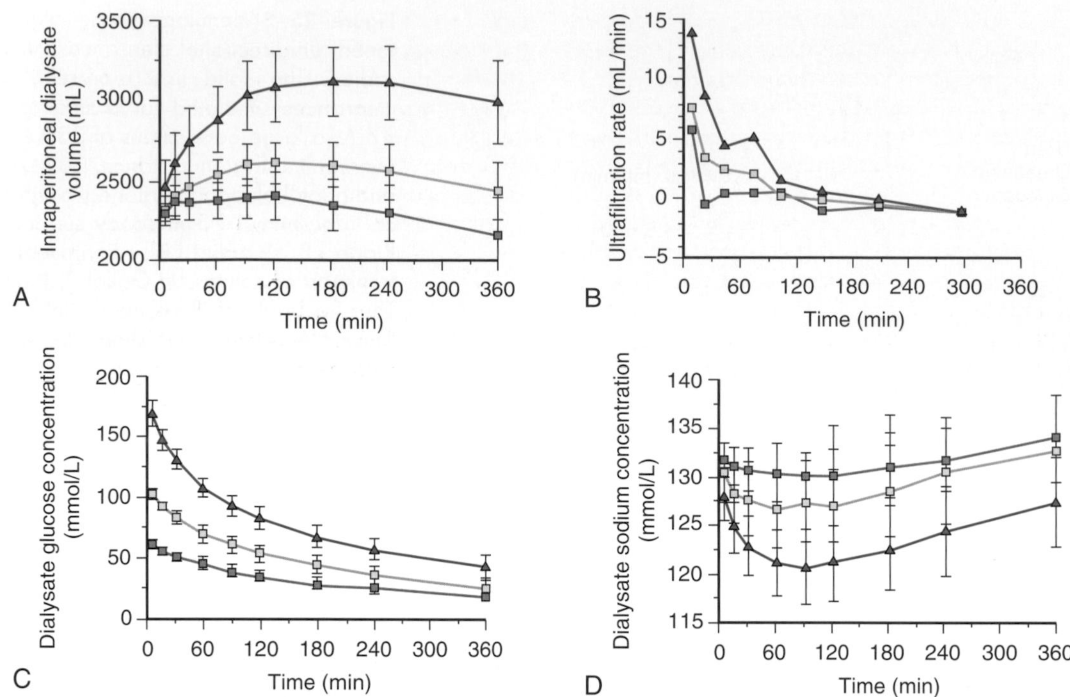

Figure 25–3 Intraperitoneal dialysate volume ***(A)***, net ultrafiltration rate ***(B)***, dialysate glucose concentration ***(C)***, and dialysate sodium concentration ***(D)*** versus time, during a 6-hour dwell study with an exchange of 2 L of 1.36% (■), 2.27% (□), and 3.86% (▲) glucose solution (mean ± SD). The intraperitoneal dialysate volumes were assessed from the dilution of the tracer (radioiodinated human serum albumin) with a correction applied for the elimination of the tracer. Note that when hypertonic 3.86% glucose dialysis solution is used, there is a marked dip in dialysate sodium concentration due to dilution of the dialysate by the ultrafiltrate. The sodium concentration in the ultrafiltrate is much less than the sodium concentration in plasma due to sodium sieving as about half of the ultrafiltered fluid will pass through the aquaporins. (From Heimbürger O, Waniewski J, Werynski A, et al: A quantitative description of solute and fluid transport during peritoneal dialysis. Kidney Int 1992; 41:1320-1332, with permission.)

(assuming $\sigma_{albumin}$ = 0.9) in cats and rats (scaled to humans using the scaling factor $BW^{0.7}$) yielded an L_pA value of approximately 0.1 mL/min.mmHg, which, in turn, yielded a σ_g of approximately 0.02.[82,83] These values are well in agreement with the reported initial ultrafiltration rate of 10 to 20 mL/min with 3.86% glucose solution.[68,69,79,86]

For the peritoneal barrier, the total σ of a solute is equal to the sum of the product of σ and the fractional hydraulic conductivity α for each set of pores. Thus, when applying the three-pore model for the peritoneal membrane the total σ for a solute will be given by the equation:

$$\sigma = \alpha_A \times \sigma_A + \alpha_S \times \sigma_S + \alpha_L \times \sigma_L \quad (2)$$

where subscripts A, S, and L denote aquaporins, small pores, and large pores, respectively. As the aquaporins are impermeable for glucose, σ_A =1 for glucose across the aquaporins, whereas the relative osmotic efficiency of glucose is much less across the small pores (σ_S = 0.03) and negligible across the large pores (σ_L approximately 0).[32] During normal conditions, the aquaporins account only for a small fraction (approximately 2%) of the LpA, and they will play a minor role in fluid transport, whereas the small pores account for about 90% of LpA. However, when applying a high crystalloid osmotic pressure over the membrane by using a small molecular osmotic agent, the importance of the aquaporins for fluid transport markedly increases. As α × σ will be quite similar for the aquaporins (0.02 × 1 = 0.02), and the small pores (0.90 × 0.03 = 0.027) about half of the ultrafiltration will pass through the aquaporins resulting in marked sieving of solutes.[32] (For the large pores α × σ will approximately be zero as σ_L is approximately 0.)

Fluid Absorption

During peritoneal dialysis, ultrafiltration is partly counterbalanced by the peritoneal fluid absorption (Q_A).[31,87–89] Thus, the net change in dialysate volume (V_D) is equal to:

$$\frac{dV_D}{dt} = Q_U - Q_A \quad (3)$$

Because Q_A is considered to be a bulk flow, it can be estimated by the disappearance rate (K_E) of a macromolecular marker applied in the dialysate (see reference 89 for a detailed discussion).

Pathways for Peritoneal Absorptive Flow

The peritoneal absorptive flow consists of two different pathways[12,17,50-52]: (1) direct lymphatic absorption (via lymphatic stomata mainly in the diaphragm, and, to a lesser extent, through visceral lymphatic pathways[51]) and (2) fluid absorption into tissues (where the fluid is absorbed into the capillaries due to the Starling forces, whereas the macromolecules are absorbed slowly via local lymphatics[17,52]). Sieving of macromolecules is assumed to be negligible with the direct lymphatic absorption, and with the second pathway (fluid absorption into tissues), sieving of macromolecules at the site of the mesothelium is considered to be negligible from a practical point of view. Thus, the macromolecular disappearance rate from the peritoneal cavity may be used as an estimate of the peritoneal bulk absorptive flow[89] because it is mainly dependent on the two components of peritoneal absorption, which both are considered to be bulk flows.[52,89] When the fluid, which has entered the peritoneal interstitial tissue compartment, is absorbed across the capillary wall (due to the Starling forces), sieving of macromolecules should occur at the site of the capillary wall. It is generally agreed that almost no protein may enter the plasma compartment directly through the capillary wall (although direct capillary uptake of radioiodinated human serum albumin, RISA, has been demonstrated under certain conditions[18,90]). The macromolecules that have entered the interstitial tissue compartment may thus accumulate in the interstitial tissue compartment before they are slowly absorbed by local lymphatics.[52]

The peritoneal absorptive flow is independent of the intraperitoneal osmotic pressure[91] and thus not influenced by ultrafiltration induced by the osmotic agent in the dialysate (i.e., osmotic pressure-driven convective flow). On the other hand, the peritoneal fluid and protein absorption rate in animal experiments have been shown to be directly proportional to the intraperitoneal hydrostatic pressure.[92] Studies by Flessner and associates[52,93,94] of tissue concentration profiles of RISA and labelled IgG (absorbed from the peritoneal cavity in rats) strongly support the notion that hydrostatic pressure-driven convection is the most likely mechanism driving the fluid and protein transport into adjacent tissues. It may seem puzzling that osmotic pressure-driven convection during dialysis and hydrostatic pressure-driven convection are considered to go simultaneously in different directions through the peritoneal barrier without any major interaction. However, this apparent paradox may be explained by the nonhomogenous nature of the peritoneal barrier, where different parts have different vascularization, hydrostatic pressure gradients, and so forth.[5,50,52] Furthermore, osmotic pressure-driven convection will only take place close to the capillaries, whereas the major part of the peritoneal surface area will allow hydrostatic pressure-driven convection in the opposite direction.[52]

The Relative Importance of Lymphatic Absorption and Absorption into Adjacent Tissues

The relative contribution of the two different components of peritoneal absorptive flow (lymphatic absorption and absorption into tissues) has been controversial.* In fact, the disappearance rate of a macromolecular marker has previously been assumed to provide an estimate of the lymphatic absorption rate in peritoneal dialysis patients.[95] However, several studies have shown that the plasma appearance rate of a macromolecular marker is on average only about 10% to 20% of its disappearance rate from the peritoneal dialysate (in clinically stable CAPD patients[53–55, 96] as well as in animals[94,97,98]). Furthermore, studies in animals have demonstrated that a major part of the lost marker accumulates inside the tissues adjacent to the peritoneal cavity, mainly in the liver, diaphragm, and anterior abdominal wall.[66,93,94,97,99] Thus, the interstitial adjacent tissues may serve as a reservoir for RISA from which it is slowly absorbed into local lymphatic vessels.[12,52,94,99]

Theoretically, it is also possible that RISA transport is delayed in lymph nodes compared to the fluid accompanying RISA in the lymphatic vessels.[47] However, trapping in lymph nodes have not been found to be of major importance,[100] and, furthermore, this would not explain the high tissue concentrations of macromolecular tracers reported by Flessner and associates[93,94] from studies in the rat.

Solute Transport

During peritoneal dialysis solutes are transported bidirectionally through the peritoneal barrier mainly by diffusion (due to the concentration gradient between blood and dialysate) and, to a lesser extent, by convection into the peritoneal cavity (due to hydrostatic pressure differences and the osmotic disequilibrium caused by the osmotic agent).[13,79] Also, the solute transport accompanying the convective fluid absorption from the peritoneal cavity (into the surrounding tissues and to blood via the lymphatics; see earlier mention) needs to be taken into account.[13,54,74,97]

Diffusion Transport

Diffusive transport through a membrane is driven by the concentration gradient over the membrane. If diffusion is unrestricted, the solute transfer rate (J_S) is proportional to the concentration gradient between dialysate and plasma (ΔC), the solute's diffusion constant (D, which is inversely proportional to the solutes radius), the surface area available for diffusion (A), and inversely proportional to the diffusion distance (Δ_x)[3]:

$$J_S = \frac{D}{\Delta_x} A\Delta C \tag{4}$$

The ratio of the solute's diffusion constant to the diffusion distance (D/Δ_x) is called permeability (P) and the product of P and surface area is usually denoted permeability surface area product (PS), which in PD has also been denoted diffusive mass transport coefficient (K_{BD}), mass transfer coefficient (MTC), or mass transfer area coefficient (MTAC). Thus, $PS=K_{BD}=MTC=MTAC$. Inserting PS into equation 4 yields the following description of diffusive solute transfer rate for a solute can across the peritoneal barrier:

$$J_S = PS\Delta C \tag{5}$$

However, as the peritoneal barrier behaves as a porous structure, the diffusion of a solute may be restricted by the pore passage; the solute has to hit the pore entrance area and the solute may also be restricted by interaction due to friction with the pore wall.[3] The diffusion through the peritoneal barrier will therefore be restricted, and a restriction factor (A/A_0) need to be introduced (where A denotes equal to the apparent

*References 12,17,47,50,52,95.

pore surface area and A_0 the total cross-sectional pore surface area), and inserting this into equation 4 yields:

$$J_S = \frac{DA}{\Delta x}\Delta C = \frac{DA_0}{\Delta x}\frac{A}{A_0}\Delta C \quad (6)$$

From this it follows that the diffusion rate over the peritoneal membrane for a solute will be governed by the solute's diffusion constant (D), the restriction factor (A/A_0), the concentration gradient (ΔC), and the term A_0/Δ_x, that represents the unrestricted pore area over unit the diffusion distance.[3] Because A_0 and Δ_x cannot usually be determined, A_0/Δ_x will be central term describing the membranes diffusive properties. Knowing A_0/Δ_x, the PS can be calculated for different solutes using their diffusion constants (based on the solute radius).[3] Also, when PS is known for one solute, A_0/Δ_x can be estimated and used to estimate PS for other solutes.

PS Under Standard Conditions

Several authors have estimated PS for various small solutes and proteins under standard conditions. The PS values for different solutes decrease with increasing molecular weight, and there seems to be a good agreement between the results from different studies, with reported PS for: urea about 18 mL/min, creatinine 10 mL/min, glucose 11 mL/min, inulin 4 mL/min, β_2-microglobulin 1.2 mL/min, albumin 0.12 mL/min, IgG 0.06 mL/min, and $\alpha 2$-macroglobulin 0.02 mL/min.[3,101,102] The variation in PS from different studies seems to be largest for urea, which is not surprising because dialysate urea concentration is close to equilibration with plasma concentration after 4 hours; the estimated value of PS for urea will be highly dependent on the estimation procedure, in particular, the model applied for PS estimation,[70] and whether or not urea concentrations in plasma are corrected for plasma protein content.[103]

Convective Transport

The magnitude of convective transport is determined by the ultrafiltration rate (J_V) through the peritoneal membrane, the average solute concentration within the membrane (CM, which for low flow rates is equal to the average of dialysate and plasma concentration), and the sieving coefficient (S, describing the fraction of the solute, which passes through the membrane with the water flow; $0 \le S \le 1$). The rate of solute flow through the membrane, J_S, due to diffusion and osmotic-pressure induced convection, can be described as:

$$J_S = PS\Delta C + SJ_V C_M \quad (7)$$

Note that solutes are also transported from the peritoneal cavity due to the peritoneal fluid absorption (J_A, vide supra), which is considered to be a bulk flow.[52,89,104] Thus, the intraperitoneal solute mass will decrease with a term proportional to J_A and C_D. The net solute flow to the peritoneal cavity (Q_S) is equal to[105]:

$$Q_S = PS\Delta C + SJ_V C_M - J_A C_D \quad (8)$$

For the peritoneal barrier, the sieving coefficient for small solutes will be dependent of the fraction of ultrafiltration that passes through small and large pores in relation to the total ultrafiltration flow (through aquaporins, small pores and large pores), because no solutes will pass through the aquaporins and the convective passage of small solutes through the other pores will not be subject to any sieving.

Importance of Different Parts of the Peritoneum for Peritoneal Transport

Different parts of the peritoneal barrier may have different transport characteristics. These differences will influence the relative importance of different parts of the peritoneum on the total solute and fluid transport through the peritoneal barrier. In particular, the permeability, distribution, and surface area of the capillaries within different parts of the peritoneal membrane may have an impact on the relative importance of different parts of the peritoneal membrane for the overall fluid and solute transport.[41] Furthermore, the mixing of dialysate may be different in different parts of the peritoneal cavity, with particularly poor mixing in pockets of the visceral peritoneum, which may decrease solute transport in regions of the peritoneal cavity where mixing is poor.[6] This is likely one reason why studies of peritoneal transport after evisceration suggests that the hollow viscera may play only a minor role in the overall peritoneal transport as evisceration was found to reduce absorption of urea, creatinine, glucose, and inulin only by about 10% to 20% despite removal of approximately 60% of the peritoneal surface area during experimental peritoneal dialysis in rats.[106] After evisceration the contact between dialysate and the membrane is likely to be improved in some areas due to redistribution of fluid to areas not accessible to the dialysate prior to evisceration.[41]

The parietal peritoneum seems to have only a minor role in peritoneal solute transport, because shielding of the parietal wall with plastic patches did not affect the overall peritoneal transport of urea, creatinine, glucose, or inulin.[106]

The role of different parts of the peritoneal membrane for lymphatic absorption has been studied by Rippe and associates[107] by measuring the peritoneal to plasma clearance of ^{125}I-RISA in rats after evisceration, or after sealing the diaphragm or the anterior abdominal wall with histoacrylate glue, compared to control rats. They concluded that lymphatic absorption mainly occurs (60%) via diaphragmatic pathways, whereas about 30% occurs via visceral lymphatic pathways and just a small fraction passes through parietal tissue pathways. On the other hand, the total bulk fluid absorption from the peritoneal cavity (as assessed by the disappearance of RISA) decreased markedly after sealing of the anterior abdominal wall, indicating that the anterior abdominal wall plays an important role in peritoneal fluid absorption.[107] This is in agreement with the studies by Flessner and associates[93,94,97] demonstrating that a significant portion (28%) of the tracer leaving the peritoneal cavity is absorbed into the anterior abdominal wall resulting in local tracer accumulation within the tissues of the anterior abdominal wall.

Tests to Assess Peritoneal Transport

There are several tests available for the assessment of peritoneal transport characteristics. There are commercial computer programs available to assess basic peritoneal transport parameters and to predict effects of various treatment schedules on peritoneal small solute clearances and ultrafiltration.[33,108–111] In general, the results will be closely dependent on the quality of data used for calculations or put into the computer. In particular, if only long dwells are used and the solutes are close to equilibration, it will be impossible to calculate transport characteristics (see later text). The lab methods may also be very important for the results, and, in particular, creatinine levels in dialysate measured with the Jaffé method must be corrected for the interference with high concentrations of glucose in dialysate.[112] Sodium levels should preferably be measured with flame photometry because ion-selective electrode measurements may give different results.[113]

Diffusive Mass Transport Coefficients

For small solutes, the diffusive mass transport coefficient PS ($=K_{BD}$=MTC=MTAC, see previous text) can be assessed with high accuracy using equation 8, if the sieving coefficients and the volume flow is known. If there are no large volume changes, PS can easily be determined using the solute concentrations in dialysate at the beginning (C_{D1}) and in the end of a dwell (C_{D2}), the solute concentration in plasma (C_P)[3,114,115]:

$$PS = \frac{\overline{V}}{t_2 - t_1} \ln \frac{C_P - C_{D1}}{C_P - C_{D2}} \qquad (9)$$

Where t_1 and t_2 are start and end of the exchange, respectively, and $\overline{V}$ is the average volume during the exchange. This equation has been widely used for the estimation of PS but should only be used when there is a low ultrafiltration rate. Also, it is important to note that the result is closely dependent on the difference between solute concentration in dialysate and plasma at the end of the dwell. Therefore, when using this method, solute concentration in plasma (C_P) should be preferably recalculated to achieve the concentration in plasma water (C_{PW}) by correcting for plasma protein and lipid content to avoid overestimation of PS.[115] This can be done using the equation[103]:

$$C_{PW} = C_P \frac{1}{1 - V_{Lip} - 0.000718 \cdot C_{Prot}} \qquad (10)$$

where V_{lip} is the fractional volume for lipids (often approximated to 0.016) and C_{prot} is the concentration of total protein (often approximated to 65g/L) in plasma. However, for solutes that are almost equilibrated at the end of an exchange, this method should still not be used, because small random errors in solute concentration will result in large variations in PS. Instead, a shorter dwell time (when the solute concentrations are not equilibrated between dialysate and plasma) should be used for estimation of PS.

There are also much more sophisticated methods to estimate PS for small solutes, but results agree quite well bearing the limitations of different methods in mind. Presently, computer software is available for the calculation of PS.[33,108–111]

The Peritoneal Equilibration Test

The most widely used approach to evaluate peritoneal transport characteristics in individual patients is to measure the dialysate to plasma solute concentration ratio (D/P) for particular solutes during an exchange with conventional peritoneal dialysis fluid (Figure 25–4).[79] This procedure (which was first proposed by Verger[116]) has been standardized in the peritoneal equilibration test (PET) by Twardowski and associates[112] and has won wide acceptance as a routine method to assess clinically important alterations in peritoneal transport characteristics. The PET procedure is standardized as regards sampling procedures, duration of dwell, evaluation of the results, and so forth.[112,117,118] Briefly, the overnight dialysate is drained and 2 L of 2.27% glucose dialysis fluid are infused. The original PET description included several dialysate samples,[112] but usually, the procedure is simplified and dialysate samples are taken after infusion, and then after 2 and 4 hours, at which time the dialysate is drained and the volume recorded. A blood sample is drawn at 2 hours dwell time. Usually, the dialysate drainage volume (used as a measure of ultrafiltration capacity), D/P for creatinine, and D/D_0 (dialysate concentration/initial dialysate concentration) for glucose are compared to standard values. The D/P for creatinine and D/D_0 for glucose from the PET will be closely related to the diffusive mass transport coefficient for these solutes.[119] The patients are usually classified according to D/P creatinine at 4 hours using Twardowski's initial classification into high transporters (above mean + 1 SD), high average transporters (between mean and mean + 1 SD), low average transporters (between mean and mean − 1 SD), and low transporters (below mean −1 SD) (Table 25–1). High and high average transporters have more rapid equilibration of creatinine and poorer net ultrafiltration due to more rapid glucose absorption, whereas low average and low transporters will have lower solute transport, resulting in slow glucose absorption and high net ultrafiltration but low peritoneal clearances for creatinine and larger and larger solutes. Usually, Twardowski's initial limits[112,117] are used to define transport groups, although most studies show an average creatinine D/P equilibration rate that is more rapid than in the study of Twardowski.[120–122]

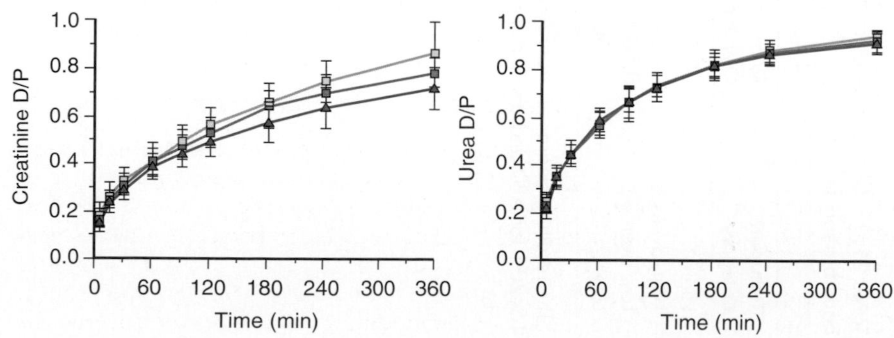

Figure 25–4 Dialysate to plasma equilibration curves (mean ± SD) for creatinine and urea during a 6-hour dwell study with an exchange of 2 liters of 1.36% (■), 2.27% (□), and 3.86% (▲) glucose solution. (From Heimbürger O, Waniewski J, Werynski A, et al: Dialysate to plasma solute concentrations (D/P) versus peritoneal transport parameters in CAPD. Nephrol Dial Transplant 1994; 9:47-59, with permission.)

Table 25–1 Characteristics of the Four Different Peritoneal Solute Transport Groups as Classified by D/P Creatinine After 4 Hours of a Peritoneal Equilibration Test[112]

				Standard CAPD 2 L x 4/24 hr[101, 120]		APD Compared to CAPD[122a]	
Transport Category	**D/P Creatinine[112,117]**	**A_0/Δ_x[108] (cm/1.73 BSA)**	**Ultrafiltration[118,119]**	**Kt/V**	**Creatinine Clearance**	**Kt/V[a]**	**Creatinine Clearance***
High	>0.81	>30,000	↓↓	=	↑↑	↑↑	↑↑
High average	0.65–0.81	23,600–30,000	↓	=	↑	↑↑	↑↑
Low average	0.50–0.65	17,200–23,600	↑	=	↓	↑↑	=–↑
Low	<0.50	<17,200	↑↑	=	↓↓	↑	=–↓

*The resulting clearances from APD will, of course, be strongly dependent on the APD prescription. The table is based on an APD prescription with a total dialysis fluid volume of about 15–20 L for APD and a wet day with an additional daytime exchange.

Recently, it has been suggested to use 3.86% glucose solution instead of 2.27% glucose solution for the PET because it will give a better estimate of ultrafiltration capacity because the ultrafiltration rate is higher and the discrimination between patients better. Thus, the net ultrafiltration will be less dependent on variations in residual volume between the start and end of the dwell, and the use of more hypertonic solution also makes it possible to use decrease in dialysate sodium as an additional parameter to identify patients with poor ultrafiltration.[123-128] When hypertonic 3.86% glucose dialysis solution is used, there is a marked dip in dialysate sodium concentration due to sieving of sodium as about half of the ultrafiltered fluid will pass through the aquaporins (see earlier text) (Figure 25–3). In patients with normal transport characteristics, the decrease in dialysate sodium is marked during the first 60 minutes, then it decreases slightly to reach its lowest value after approximately 90 minutes and thereafter the dialysate sodium concentration increased due to sodium diffusion from plasma.[79]

PET is a simple procedure and easy to perform, the standard values are well established, and it does not require any complicated calculations. On the other hand, the D/P and D/D0 results are rather sensitive to laboratory errors (only three samples are used), and the net ultrafiltration (measured as drained minus infused volume) is sensitive to variation in the intraperitoneal residual dialysate volume (due to incomplete drainage). Furthermore, PET does not provide any details of the peritoneal transport process. However, a commercial computer software program (PD-Adequest™) has been developed using results from the PET and the preceding overnight exchange to allow for calculation of basic transport parameters and to simulate the effects of changes in treatment schedules in individual patients.[33,111] The PET has also been modified by using more frequent sampling and adding a tracer to the dialysate to allow for more detailed analysis of changes in intraperitoneal volume.[129]

The D/P values generated by the PET procedure show an excellent correlation with the diffusive mass transport coefficient PS for small solutes, and PS as well as D/P for creatinine and PS as well as D/D0 for glucose can be used to identify patients with loss of ultrafiltration capacity due to increased diffusive transport.[124] When using 2 L of 4.25%/3.86 % glucose solution for the PET, it was suggested to define *loss of ultrafiltration capacity* as a net ultrafiltration below 400 mL after 4 hours.[125]

Personal Dialysis Capacity Test (PDC)

The personal dialysis capacity test involves urine, blood, and dialysate sampling. The patient collects urine and dialysate during a standardized CAPD-day using a special exchange schedule, with two short (2 to 3 hours) and two medium long exchanges (4 to 6 hours), each with two different glucose solutions, and one long overnight exchange. A sample is taken from each bag and the volume of each bag is measured, to give the variation in net ultrafiltration and solute equilibration with time, with the two glucose-based dialysis fluids.[108,110,130,131] The data are put into a special software program, Personal Dialysis Capacity (PDC™), based on the three-pore model of peritoneal transport and calculates the following transport parameters (in addition to adequacy parameters and residual renal function): (1) area parameter ($Ao/\Delta x$), determining the diffusion capacity of small solutes, and indirectly, the hydraulic conductance of the membrane (LpA); (2) reabsorption rate of fluid from the peritoneal cavity to the blood after peak time, when the glucose gradient has dissipated; and (3) large pore fluid flow, which determines the loss of proteins to the PD-fluid. The $Ao/\Delta x$ is a more general parameter than PS for a specific solute and can be also used to classify the patients into similar transport groups as the PET (Table 25–1). Because the PDC is based on five different determinations of dialysate concentration, it should have better and more reliable classification of individual patient's transport rate, if a correct sampling procedure has been carried out.[110,130,131]

Effluent Soluble Markers of the Peritoneal Membrane

In addition to solutes originating from the circulation, the drained peritoneal dialysate also contains substances that are locally produced or released from the surrounding tissues or from cells released into the dialysate. These substances include lubricants and surface tension-lowering substances, such as phospholipids, various cytokines, growth factors, chemokines, and prostanoids as well as constituents of the extracellular matrix (e.g., glycosaminoglycans and procollagen peptides), and also coagulation, fibrinolytic, and antithrombogenic substances.[132] Some of these substances have been measured in effluent dialysate to better understand to the local intraperitoneal immune system and the local reaction to complications like peritonitis, and the concentrations of some of these substances have also been used as markers of the peritoneal membrane status in apparently stable PD patients. However, it should be noted that the interindividual variation is very large even in clinically stable patients without overt complications, and surprisingly little data are available on the long-term evolution of these markers in patients treated with PD. It should also be stressed that appearance rate (i.e., the amount of solute in the drained bag multiplied with the drained volume and divided by time) should be used when comparing patients, and not the concentration, if there is a marked interpatient variation in drained volume or dwell time. Otherwise, the marker concentration may vary due to differences in dilution due to, for example, differences in infused volume or in net ultrafiltration.

The most widely used marker of membrane status in clinical studies has been the dialysate effluent concentration of cancer antigen 125 (CA125).[133] CA125 is a 220 kD glycoprotein produced by mesothelial cells, and the CA125 level in dialysate increases linearly with dwell time and correlates with the number of mesothelial cells in the effluent. Patients on long-term PD have low levels of dialysate CA125[134] as well as patients with peritoneal sclerosis. Based on these observations, CA125 has been suggested to be a marker of the mesothelial cell mass or turnover in stable CAPD patients.[133] Increased levels of dialysate CA125 have widely been used as a marker of improved biocompatibility of new PD solutions and effluent levels of CA125 consistently increase with the use of more biocompatible dialysis solutions in clinical studies.[135,136] However, the interpatient variation in dialysate CA125 is large, and it is not completely clear exactly what it represents. Therefore, the CA125 levels in dialysate effluent need to be interpreted with some caution.

Another interesting effluent candidate marker of peritoneal membrane health status during long-term PD is hyaluronan (HA), which is an important constituent of the interstitial tissue and is produced by mesothelial cells and fibroblasts. HA is involved in several physiologic processes, such as tissue repair and wound healing. The fraction of HA that is produced by mesothelial cells forms a coat on the mesothelial cells together with other glycosaminoglycans and phospholipids. HA concentration increases with intraperitoneal inflammation and decreases with use of more biocompatible PD solutions.[136,137] The procollagen peptides, procollagen-1-C-terminal peptide and procollagen-3-N-terminal peptide, are produced locally by fibroblasts and mesothelial cells during the synthesis of collage 1 and 3, respectively, and have also been measured in dialysate as potential markers of local collagen synthesis,[135,136] but it is not completely clear what the levels represent.

Other potentially important markers are the central proinflammatory cytokine interleukin-6 (IL-6) and its soluble receptor (sIL-6R) due to their central role in the regulation of intraperitoneal inflammation.[10] Vascular endothelium growth factor (VEGF) is also a potentially interesting marker, because it enhances vascular permeability and angiogenesis, and it is upregulated in peritoneal capillary endothelium in long-term PD patients.[138] Interestingly, both IL-6 and VEGF decrease with the use of more biocompatible solutions.[137]

Factors Affecting Peritoneal Transport

A number of factors have been shown to influence peritoneal transport, possibly by altering the underlying physiologic conditions that govern the exchange rate between blood plasma and dialysate. In particular, vasodilatory factors have been shown to increase peritoneal clearances due possibly to an increase in capillary surface area available for transperitoneal exchange.[139]

Temperature

Klapp[140] reported in the beginning of the last century that heating the anterior abdominal wall resulted in increased fluid absorption from the peritoneal cavity, whereas the opposite effect was noted with cooling of the abdominal wall. The effect of increased temperature was possibly mediated via local vasodilation because local hyperemia could be observed at the serosal as well as parietal peritoneum.[140] An increase in dialysate temperature will also result in an increased solute transport, in addition to the increased fluid absorption.[141]

Intraperitoneal Hydrostatic Pressure

The intraperitoneal hydrostatic pressure is the driving force for convective movement of fluid and solutes into the adjacent tissues.[52] The hydrostatic pressure increases with increasing intraperitoneal dialysate volume[142-144] and varies with body position; the pressure is higher in sitting and standing than in supine position.[142] The intraperitoneal hydrostatic pressure seems to increase in almost linear fashion with increased and infused dialysis volume in PD patients,[142,143] but a study in rats using a larger variation in infused dialysate volume shows that this relationship, in fact, seems to be exponential.[144]

The increased intraperitoneal pressure results in increased fluid absorption,[145] mainly due to increased fluid absorption into adjacent tissues and not to increased lymphatic absorption because the peritoneum to plasma clearance of a radioactive tracer was unchanged when the intraperitoneal pressure was increased in a study in rats.[146] In agreement with these findings, Durand and associates[147,148] reported on a negative correlation between net ultrafiltration and intraperitoneal pressure at the end of a 2-hour dwell in stable CAPD patients.

Dialysate Volume

In a systematic study of infused dialysate volumes between 0.5 and 3 liters in 10 stable PD patients, Keshaviah and associates[149] found that PS for urea, creatinine, and glucose increased in an almost linear fashion between 0.5 and 2 L infused volume, its values almost doubling over this range. Between 2 and 3 L infused dialysate volume there was only a small increase in PS values.[149] However, infused volumes yielding maximum urea PS were found to increase with increasing body surface area.[149] The authors attributed the increase in PS to a more effective contact between dialysate and the peritoneal surface area.[149] Krediet and associates[150] studied the effect of a 3-L exchange compared to a 2-L exchange with 1.36% glucose solution and reported on significantly higher PS for creatinine, kanamycin, and inulin with the larger volume, but no difference in PS for urea, lactate, glucose, β2-microglobulin, albumin, or IgG was found. However, the net ultrafiltration relative to the volume at 5 minutes was lower at almost all occasions due to a markedly increased fluid absorption rate with the 3-L exchange volume, possibly related to an increased intraperitoneal hydrostatic pressure.[150]

The Effect of Body Posture on Peritoneal Transport

The effect of upright body position have been addressed in a few studies showing a slightly slower D/P equilibration as well as a decreased net ultrafiltration rate in sitting or standing compared to recumbent position.[151,152] The slightly slower transport rates are due likely to a decreased contact between dialysate and the peritoneal membrane in sitting position as ultrasound investigation revealed that the bulk of the dialysate was found in the subumbilical region of the peritoneal cavity,[151] and the reduced net ultrafiltration is due to an increased peritoneal fluid absorption due to an increased hydrostatic pressure in upright position compared to supine position.[152] Upright position will also increase the hydrostatic pressure gradient over the anterior abdominal wall, where a large part of the convectively induced peritoneal absorption takes place.[52]

Effect of Dialysate Composition on Peritoneal Transport

Several factors related to the peritoneal dialysis solutions per se may also affect peritoneal transport, for example, hyperosmolality, type and concentration of osmotic agent applied, pH, type of buffer, buffer concentration, glucose degradation products, and other contaminants.

Glucose Concentration and Osmolality

As hyperosmolality is a known vasodilatory factor,[153] it is reasonable to expect that hyperosmolality may induce changes in peritoneal transport rates. The use of a 7% glucose solution for peritoneal dialysis in uremic patients was associated with an increased solute clearance (compared to 1.5% glucose solution), which exceeded the possible contribution of convective transport,[154,155] and similar effects have been found in animal studies. In contrast, the clinical use of the presently available hypertonic 3.86% (anhydrous glucose, corresponding to 4.25% of hydrous glucose) dialysis solutions does not seem to affect the peritoneal diffusive transport characteristics in peritoneal dialysis patients.[79]

In addition, during heat sterilization and storage of glucose containing peritoneal dialysis solutions, several toxic glucose degradation products (GDPs) are formed, for example, formaldehyde, 3-deoxyglucosone, 3,4-Dideoxyglucosone-3-ene, and several other low molecular weight aldehydes.[156-159] Although GDPs do not seem to have any major acute effect on peritoneal transport in the concentration found in currently used peritoneal dialysis solutions, these pollutants are likely involved in the evolution of the changes in peritoneal structure and function observed in the long-term PD patients.[160]

Alternative Osmotic Agents

In general, osmotic agents with a lower molecular weight compared to glucose, for example, amino acids and glycerol, will be absorbed more rapidly than glucose, resulting in a shorter period of positive net ultrafiltration than with glucose solutions of the same osmolality.[161-163] Although the use of the presently available 1.1% amino acids solution does not seem to affect peritoneal transport using the PET,[164] they seem to slightly increase peritoneal solute transport and blood flow in a detailed study,[165] and hypertonic 2.7% amino acid solution has also been reported to be associated with slightly increased peritoneal transport rates.[163,166]

Several large molecular weight osmotic agents, such as starch, glucose polymers, dextran, gelatine, albumin, and polypeptides, have been used in experimental studies.[167] Since the capillary wall is easily permeable to water and small solutes but restricts the passage of large molecular weight solutes, the osmotic effect of colloid during peritoneal dialysis is much more prolonged than the osmotic effect of small solutes. Therefore, even with a relatively low osmolality, the colloid osmotic pressure may ensure the sustained osmotic transport of water.[168] Note that the main osmotic effect of the polymers will occur over the small pores, and sodium sieving will thus not be observed.[77] Thus, the presently used 7.5% icodextrin solution is in fact hypo-osmolar compared to plasma, but will result in a sustained net ultrafiltration for more than 14 hours due to the sustained colloid osmotic gradient.[77] The icodextrin-based solution does not affect peritoneal solute transport characteristics,[169] but the large osmotic fluid flow through the small pores will result in increased clearance of sodium, as well as of low molecular proteins like β2-microglobulin and leptin.[77,169,170]

Effect of pH and Different Buffers on Peritoneal Transport

Conventional glucose-based dialysis solutions were reported to be vasoactive (when applied directly to capillaries) with an initial transient vasoconstriction (for less than 2 minutes) followed by a maximal vasodilatation sustained during the whole study period.[171,172] The high osmolality or high concentration of buffers, acetate, or lactate, were indicated as possible factors.[171,172] The unphysiologically low pH in traditional dialysis fluids is also considered to be vasoactive and may thus theoretically influence the vascular responses in the peritoneum during dialysis. A few studies have been conducted to assess the effect of pH per se on peritoneal transport. However, the low pH in dialysis fluids was not found to induce distinguishable vasoactive responses in the peritoneum[172] or to affect the peritoneal solute transport characteristics in rats[173,174] or humans.[175,176]

Acetate, lactate, and bicarbonate have been used as buffers in peritoneal dialysis solutions. As pH, and other factors, may also differ between solutions with different buffers, it is difficult to assess the possibly independent effects of pH and buffer on peritoneal transport. Furthermore, the long-term effects of the dialysis solution on peritoneal transport seem to differ between similar solutions produced by different manufacturers,[177,178] and it is possible that differences in their production processes may have resulted in differences between the solutions, for example, in different content of GDPs.

Acetate was previously used as a buffer in dialysis fluids. However, although acetate buffered solutions seem to have no effect on peritoneal UFC in short-term studies,[179] long-term use of acetate is associated with high frequency of ultrafiltration capacity failure[177,180,181] and has, furthermore, been suggested to be implicated in the aetiology of encapsulating peritoneal sclerosis.[182]

Because of the side effects of acetate solutions, lactate was for many years the almost exclusively used buffer in commercially available peritoneal dialysis solutions. Recently, bicarbonate solutions have been introduced, and the transport does not seem to differ to a major extent in clinical studies between lactate, bicarbonate/lactate, or pure bicarbonate solutions.[175,183]

Pharmacologic Effects on Peritoneal Transport

Several drugs and hormones have been reported to alter peritoneal transport rates.[35,44,139,184] The results of many of these studies must, however, be interpreted with caution because the experimental conditions are not always standardized, and several other factors may also have been altered by the experimental conditions. Also, accurate determinations of dialysate volume are often lacking.[185]

Vasoactive Drugs

Intravenous administration of norepinephrine significantly decreases peritoneal clearances, whereas dopamine increases the peritoneal solute transport rate, possibly due to vasodilation caused by stimulation of mesenteric dopamine receptors.[184] In general, vasodilatory drugs have been reported to increase peritoneal transport,[35,44,139,186,187] for example, theophylline, furosemide, hydralazine, and sodium nitroprusside (a nitric oxide donor) have all been reported to augment peritoneal clearances—an effect that is possibly related to an increased peritoneal capillary surface area. On the other hand, splanchnic vasoconstrictors, like norepinephrine,[188] generally tend to decrease peritoneal clearances.[139]

Changes in Peritoneal Transport During Peritonitis

Peritonitis is associated with several changes in peritoneal transport. A fall in ultrafiltration capacity (UFC) is often noted during peritonitis,[189–191] but this alteration is transient and UFC usually returns to normal within less than 1 month.[189,192]

The decreased UFC is most commonly associated with increased small solute transport and rapid glucose absorption and, consequently, loss of the osmotic driving force.[189,191] In addition, the peritoneal fluid absorption is markedly increased.[108,193] Detailed studies of peritoneal fluid absorption have not been performed, but it is likely that the increase in fluid absorption is due to both increased lymphatic flow and increased convective fluid transport into adjacent tissues.[101]

The increased small solute transport seems to be related to an increased peritoneal capillary surface area, probably due to inflammatory recruitment of microvessels.[32,108] This effect is likely, to a large extent, mediated nitric oxide (NO) and both endothelial nitric oxide synthase (eNOS) and inducible nitric oxide synthase (iNOS), which have been demonstrated to be markedly upregulated in a rat model of acute peritonitis with poor ultrafiltration and increased small solute transport.[194] Also, the structural changes, the increased solute transport, and the poor ultrafiltration were much less pronounced in eNOS knockout mice.[195]

Furthermore, peritonitis is associated with markedly increased protein losses in dialysate,[108,189–191] indicating an increase in the number or size of the large pores.[108] The intraperitoneal production of prostaglandins (e.g., PGE2 and PGI2) is increased during peritonitis.[190] As the increased peritoneal protein loss during peritonitis correlates with the increased dialysate concentration of prostanoids, and, furthermore, as the increased protein loss partly may be inhibited by indometacin,[190] it may be suggested that the increased peritoneal protein loss during peritonitis is mediated, at least partly, by the vasoactive prostaglandins.[190]

Changes in Water and Solute Transport with Time on PD

Changes in peritoneal solute transport are common after initiation of peritoneal dialysis. Several studies using the PET have reported on a significant increase in 4-hour D/P creatinine from the PET after 6 months of CAPD compared to initial results obtained during the first 2 weeks of CAPD, whereas ultrafiltration was rather stable.[196–199] It has also been reported that in patients with initially high solute transport, transport rate may, in fact, decrease.[199,200]

Changes in Peritoneal Transport with Long-Term Peritoneal Dialysis

In the majority of patients treated with CAPD for up to 3 years, the peritoneal UFC as well as small solute transport characteristics seem to be relatively stable,[199,201,202] although several studies demonstrate a tendency toward increasing diffusive mass transport coefficients for small solutes as well as a tendency toward decreasing net UF.[196,198,199,202-204] However, individual patients may behave markedly different; some patients demonstrate increased diffusive solute transport and decreased ultrafiltration, whereas other patients show opposite patterns.

In patients treated with PD for 4 years or more, the tendency toward decreasing ultrafiltration and increasing small solute transport is evident in almost all prospective studies.[196,205] In contrast, macromolecule transport (as assessed by protein clearances) has been reported to be stable or to decrease with time on CAPD[204,206–208] indicating a stable or decreased peritoneal permeability for macromolecules.

However, the interpretation of most studies (and, in particular, the cross-sectional studies) of peritoneal transport with time may suffer from methodologic fallacy in that patients with "inadequate" peritoneal transport will drop out, so that both high transporters (insufficient fluid removal) and low transporters (insufficient small solute clearances) may drop out, resulting in selection bias.

Loss of Ultrafiltration Capacity (UFC)

With time on PD there is an increasing risk of developing loss of UFC, with a markedly higher incidence among patients treated with acetate-containing dialysis solutions.[180,196,205] Using the standard lactate-based solutions, the risk of developing permanent loss of UFC (using a clinical definition) increases markedly with time on CAPD being 9% after 48 months and 35% after 72 months of PD.[196]

There are several pathophysiologic mechanisms behind ineffective fluid removal due to permanent loss of UFC (Table 25–2). Increased transport of small solutes with rapid glucose absorption is the most common mechanism observed in CAPD patients with impaired UFC.* The rapid glucose absorption results in rapid loss of the osmotic driving force (glucose gradient) and, consequently, a rapid decline in ultrafiltration rate. However, detailed kinetic analyses of patients with UFC due to rapid diffusive transport also show that the remaining osmotic gradient cannot induce water flow as effectively as in patients with normal UFC, indicating a decreased osmotic conductance of the peritoneal membrane.[72,211]

A selective decrease in ultrafiltration in patients with normal diffusive glucose transport has also been reported in some

Table 25–2 Suggested Causes of Ineffective Fluid Removal in CAPD

A) Obstructed outflow and increased residual dialysate volume
B) Loss of residual renal function
C) Subcutaneous leakage
D) Loss of ultrafiltration capacity due to:
1. Increased solute transport (most common mechanism)
2. Reduced efficiency of the osmotic gradient (Impaired transcellular water transport or reduced UF coefficient) (not uncommon)
3. "Hypopermeable peritoneum" with decreased water transport or decreased surface area (rare)
4. Increased peritoneal fluid absorption (probably rare)

*References 126,127,196,207,209,210.

CAPD patients (with loss of UFC), who also had a minor decline of dialysis sodium concentration when using hypertonic glucose solution.[127,128,212] This may imply a decreased hydraulic conductivity of the peritoneal membrane, and it was suggested that these alterations may be due to decreased transcellular water transport (deficient aquaporin-mediated ultrafiltration) and that this may be an additional cause of UFC failure. However, this finding needs to be interpreted with caution because when the ultrafiltration rate is low, a reduction of dialysate sodium due to dilution of dialysate by ultrafiltrate will not occur to the same degree. Sodium sieving will always be markedly reduced when ultrafiltration is poor, even when the aquaporin function is normal.[213] An alternative explanation to the normal glucose transport without decline of dialysate sodium could be a combination of selective changes in the peritoneal ultrafiltration coefficient due to a reduced surface area in combination with increased membrane permeability. This would result in unchanged diffusive solute transport in combination with reduced ultrafiltration coefficient across both transcellular water pores (aquaporins) and small pores.[123]

Loss of peritoneal surface area with slow solute transport due to fibrosis and the formation of adhesions have been reported during the late stage of encapsulating peritoneal sclerosis (EPS, previously called sclerosing encapsulating peritonitis) in a few cases.[209] However, detailed studies in four patients developing EPS, showed increasing PS in three of the patients,[214] suggesting that loss of UFC associated with increased solute transport in these patients was an early sign that preceded the development of more overt signs of EPS. Thus, initially, EPS seems to be associated with increased peritoneal solute transport, which later is followed by formation of adhesions and finally encapsulation of the intestinal loops, resulting in slow peritoneal solute transfer due to loss of the surface area.[209] However, slow solute transport seems to be an extremely rare cause of UFC loss, and only a few cases have been reported.

Increased peritoneal fluid absorption has also been reported as the cause of UFC loss.[127,207] The increase in peritoneal fluid absorption in these patients is not due to increased lymphatic absorption but to increased fluid absorption into the peritoneal interstitial tissue, indicating changes in the interstitial tissue fluid hydraulic conductivity.[55] The mechanisms behind these changes are not clear.

Relation Between Peritoneal Transport Characteristics and Clinical Outcome

Peritoneal transport characteristics have a major impact on the clinical management and outcome in peritoneal dialysis patients. The patients' peritoneal small solute transport characteristics will have a major impact on the optimal dialysis prescription as regards ultrafiltration and small solute clearances. Furthermore, a high peritoneal transport rate has been identified as an important risk factor for both PD technique failure and mortality.[120,215–218]

Although the reasons for this are not established, several different mechanisms may contribute. At first, there is an association between a high peritoneal transport rate and comorbidity, including diabetes, cardiovascular disease, and chronic inflammation (with elevated plasma levels of CRP and IL-6).[215,219-223] Second, high transporters have a more rapid glucose absorption and, thus, an impaired fluid and sodium removal and have a high risk to chronic fluid overload,[218,224-226] which in itself is associated with LVH and LV dysfunction in PD patients[227] and may potentially cause immune activation because of bacterial or endotoxin translocation in patients with severe gut edema as a result of severe volume overload.[228,229] In contrast, although a low fluid removal may result in low urea clearance, peritoneal small solute clearances are usually not lower in high transporters. During standard CAPD, the Kt/V urea is not different between transport groups, and creatinine clearance is usually higher in high transporters.[101,230]

Because there is a close relationship between the peritoneal transport characteristics of solutes of different molecular weight up to the size of albumin[30,101] (Figure 25–2), it is not surprising that high transporters also exhibit increased protein losses and that these patients have more severe hypoalbuminemia than patients with lower D/P ratios.[216,231,232] It is interesting to note that the low serum albumin levels are already present in high transporters before the initiation of PD,[233] indicating that another mechanism, such as inflammation, may also contribute. Furthermore, a large influx of glucose absorbed from the dialysate may suppress appetite,[216,234] although Davies and associates[235] reported that calories derived from the dialysate in CAPD patients did seem to reduce appetite in PD patients. The low albumin levels and increased glucose absorption in high transporters lead to the hypothesis that a high transport state will lead to malnutrition, which, in turn, may affect clinical outcome. However, except from low serum albumin levels, high transporters do not seem to be more malnourished as regards other nutritional parameters.[120,232] Furthermore, there were no signs of change in any nutritional parameter in high transporters in a longitudinal study of nutritional parameters.[236]

It is striking that the relation between peritoneal transport rate and serum albumin[120] and some other nutritional markers was seen already at start of CAPD.[236] Therefore, it is likely that the relation between peritoneal transport and some nutritional parameters seen in some studies, in fact, are due to a relation between peritoneal transport and the malnutrition, inflammation, and atherosclerosis (MIA)-syndrome.[237] High peritoneal transport characteristics may thus be another feature of the MIA syndrome.[237]

Moreover, it is important to note that the etiology and clinical features of high transporters may be different. It has recently been suggested that there may be two distinct types of high transporters.[238,239] The Early *Inherent Type* is found in patients who show signs of high PSTR from the beginning of PD. These patients are typically inflamed (systemically and intraperitoneally) and have a high prevalence of comorbidities, low RRF, and high mortality. The Late *Acquired Type* occurs in patients who develop high transport rate over time on PD, perhaps due mainly to local structural changes in the peritoneal membrane as a consequence of the continuous exposure to bioincompatible PD solutions, resulting in an increased vascular surface.[239] These patients do not necessarily have higher prevalence of inflammation or comorbidities, such as diabetes mellitus and cardiovascular disease. In addition, other patients may perhaps exhibit an increase in transport rate over time on PD because of the development of clinical complications, resulting in increasing inflammation. The relative importance of the two main types of high transporters and their contribution to the poor clinical outcome of high transport patients is not known.

CHANGES IN PERITONEAL MORPHOLOGY WITH TIME ON PD

During the last 15 years, several small studies have demonstrated marked changes in peritoneal morphology in patients treated with PD, including mesothelial denudation, submesothelial thickening and fibrosis, and vascular changes with vascular basement membrane reduplications.[240-243] More recently, vascular changes with subendothelial hyalinization and neoangiogenesis,[244-246] as well as accumulation of advanced glycation end products (AGEs) in the peritoneum[244,247] have been reported, factors which also were related to functional changes with increasing peritoneal solute transport.

Recently, the first results were reported from The Peritoneal Biopsy Registry reporting the analysis of biopsies from the parietal peritoneum in 130 PD patients and compared them to peritoneal biopsies from normal individuals and uremic subjects not treated with PD.[248] The most dramatic changes were the marked increase in the submesothelial compact zone (which approximately equals the interstitium), which was 50 μm in normal subjects, 150 μm in hemodialysis patients, and 270 μm in PD patients. The thickness increased markedly with time on PD from 180 μm in patients treated with PD for less than 2 years to a median value of 700 μm in patients treated for more than 97 months[248] (Figure 25-5). Vascular changes with progressive subendothelial hyalinization and luminal narrowing or obliteration were seen in 56% of the PD patients and increased with time on PD. Patients with membrane failure had higher submesothelial thickness and also a higher density of blood vessels, which correlated with the degree of fibrosis.[248]

In a few patients that had been treated with PD for several years, progressive peritoneal fibrosis with development of encapsulating peritoneal sclerosis (previously called sclerosing encapsulating peritonitis) have also been reported. This is a frightening complication with fibrotic thickening of the peritoneal membrane, formation of adhesions, and in the last phase encapsulation of the intestinal loops and formation of an intestinal cocoon.[182]

Pathophysiologic Considerations

Potentially Causative Factors

The pathogenetic mechanisms behind the structural and functional alterations in the peritoneal membrane are not clear, but both bioincompatibility of the peritoneal dialysis solutions and the effect of peritonitis have been discussed. Davies and associates[198] reported that recurrences or clusters of peritonitis as well as the cumulative dialysate leukocyte count were related to increased D/P creatinine and reduced UFC, whereas D/P creatinine and UFC were stable in patients with no or single isolated peritonitis episodes. Furthermore, the relationship between peritonitis and high solute peritoneal transport rate is not evident in studies of patients with loss of UFC, where most studies have failed to demonstrate any relation between the number of peritonitis episodes and loss of UFC.[207,210] Although numerous studies have demonstrated the bioincompatibility of the presently used peritoneal dialysis solutions in vitro, and bioincompatibility has been extensively discussed as a cause of changes in peritoneal solute transport,[160,249] there are little clinical data demonstrating such a relationship, except from the relation between loss of UFC and the use of acetate as buffer. However, it should be noted that until recently, almost all standard peritoneal dialysis solutions have had similar composition and biocompatibility. Recently, much attention has focused on the relatively high content of reactive carbonyls in the conventional PD solutions.[159,160,250] These reactive carbonyls are particularly of interest because they are more potent promoters of formation of advanced glycation end products (AGEs)

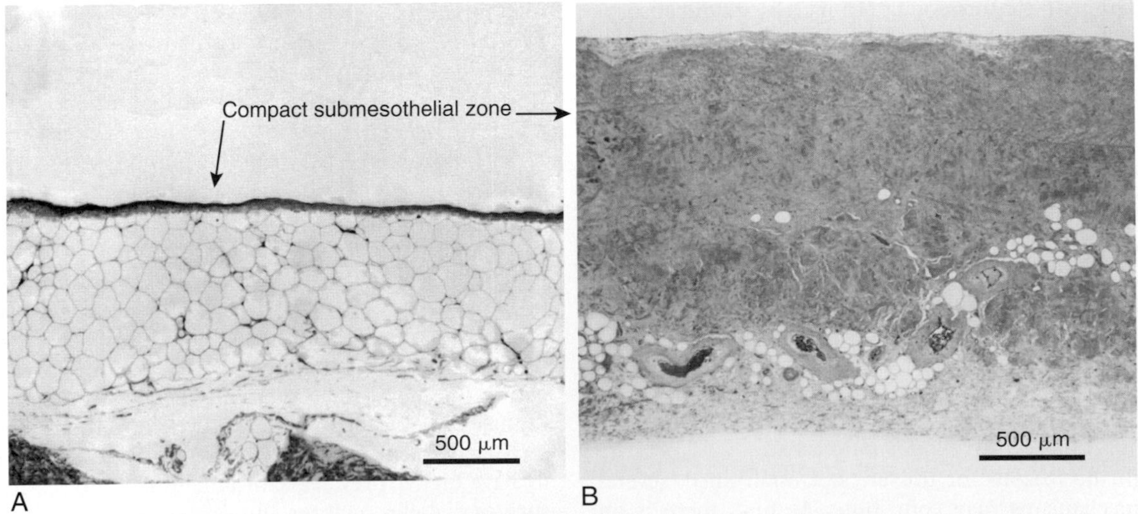

Figure 25–5 Parital peritoneal biopsies from a normal individual ***(A)*** and from a patient who had been treated with PD for 9 years ***(B)***. Note the marked expansion of the submesothelial compact zone in *B*. (From Williams JD, Craig KD, Topley N, et al: Morphological changes in the peritoneal membrane of patients with renal disease. J Am Soc Nephrol 2002; 13:470-479.)

than glucose itself.[250] The potential pathogenetic role of carbonyls and AGEs in the changes of peritoneal function are supported by the facts that increased AGE content has been found in the peritoneum of long-term PD patients and was furthermore associated with increased peritoneal small solute transport.[244,247] Furthermore, it was recently reported that patients with increasing small solute transport (as assessed from the PET) with time on PD, had a higher glucose exposure compared to patients with stable peritoneal membrane transport.[251]

Physiologic Mechanisms

The mechanism(s) by which small solute transport increases in patients with poor ultrafiltration and increased small solute transport is not yet understood. It has been suggested that the cause of the increased small solute transport rate is an increase in peritoneal vascular surface area due to neoangiogenesis, which has been demonstrated in the peritoneal membrane.[138,244–246,248] However, if this was the only explanation, the protein losses should also be increased among these patients due to the larger vascular surface area. However, it is possible that the markedly expanded interstitium (submesothelial compact zone) retard macromolecular transport more than small solute transport, resulting in an increased small solute transport and normal macromolecular transport (M. Flessner, personal message).

In reduced osmotic conductance (reduced osmotic efficiency of glucose) observed in many patients, it has been suggested that this is due to decreased transcellular water transport (deficient aquaporin-mediated ultrafiltration).[127,128,212] However, this is still not established, and the aquaporin expression was, in fact, reported to be normal in a long-term PD patients with poor ultrafiltration attributed to impaired transcellular water transport.[252] Furthermore, computer simulations have demonstrated that sodium sieving will always be markedly reduced when ultrafiltration is poor, even when the aquaporin function is normal.[213] Therefore, further research is needed to establish the pathophysiologic mechanisms behind the reduced osmotic conductance in many PD patients with poor ultrafiltration.

Devuyst[253] has suggested a model where the increased reactive carbonyls (due to uremia and the carbonyls in the PD fluid) will amplify the AGE formation in the peritoneal membrane. The carbonyls and AGEs will have several effects, including stimulation of peritoneal cells to produce vascular endothelial growth factor (VEGF), which will stimulate neoangiogenesis and interact with endothelial cells to produce endothelial nitric oxide synthase (eNOS), which is markedly increased in long-term PD patients[138] and will cause vasodilation as well as further stimulate neoangiogenesis. Nitric oxide (NO) is a crucial regulator of vascular tone and permeability, and the finding that eNOS knockout mice, to a large extent, were protected against the structural and functional changes induced by acute peritonitis[195] underscores the importance of NO in the pathophysiology of peritoneal membrane dysfunction. The correlation seen between submesothelial fibrosis and neoangiogenesis suggests that these two processes are related.[245,248] It is in this context of interest that uremia per se and the binding of VEGF to the extracellular matrix will induce the release of basic fibroblast growth factor (bFGF), which has fibrotic as well as angiogenetic effects.[253] Furthermore, inflammatory cytokines like IL-6 may also stimulate neoangiogenesis and fibrosis.

However, even if much progress has been made during the last few years, very little is still known about which factors will be most important in causing the long-term changes in the peritoneal membrane structure and function, or which basic mechanisms are involved in the evolution of these alterations. Much further research is clearly needed in this area.

References

1. Esperanca MJ, Collins DL: Peritoneal dialysis efficiency in relation to body weight. J Pediatr Surg 1966; 1:162-169.
2. Rubin J, Clawson M, Planch A, et al: Measurements of peritoneal surface area in man and rat. Am J Med Sci 1988; 295: 453-458.
3. Rippe B, Krediet RT: Peritoneal physiology-transport of solutes. *In* Gokal R, Nolph KD (eds): The Textbook of Peritoneal Dialysis. Dordrecht, Kluwer Academic Publishers, 1994, pp 69-113.
4. Bouchet Y, Voilin C, Yver R: The peritoneum and its anatomy. *In* Bengmark S (ed): The Peritoneum and Peritoneal Access. London, Wright, 1989, pp 1-13.
5. Rippe B, Rosengren BI, Venturoli D: The peritoneal microcirculation in peritoneal dialysis. Microcirculation 2001; 8: 303-320.
6. Flessner MF, Lofthouse J, Zakaria ER: Improving contact area between the peritoneum and intraperitoneal therapeutic solutions. J Am Soc Nephrol 2001; 12:807-813.
7. Dobbie JW, Lloyd JK: Mesothelium secretes lamellar bodies in a similar manner to type II pneumocyte secretion of surfactant. Perit Dial Int 1989; 9:215-219.
8. Nagy JA: Peritoneal membrane morphology and function. Kidney Int 1996; 50(suppl 56):S2-S11.
9. Topley N, Davenport A, Li F-K, et al: Activation of inflammation and leukocyte recruitment into the peritoneal cavity. Kidney Int 1996; 50:S17-S21.
10. Hurst SM, Wilkinson TS, McLoughlin RM, et al: IL-6 and its soluble receptor orchestrate a temporal switch in the pattern of leukocyte recruitment seen during acute inflammation. Immunity 2001; 14:705-714.
11. Whitaker D, Papadimitriou JM, Walters MNI: The mesothelium: Its fibrinolytic properties. J Pathol 1982; 136:291-299.
12. Flessner MF: Peritoneal transport physiology: Insights from basic research. J Am Soc Nephrol 1991; 2:122-135.
13. Lysaght MJ, Farrell PC: Membrane phenomena and mass transfer kinetics in peritoneal dialysis. J Membrane Sci 1989; 44:5-33.
14. Haljamäe H: Anatomy of the interstitial tissue. Lymphology 1978; 11:128-132.
15. Flessner MF: The role of extracellular matrix in transperitoneal transport of water and solutes. Perit Dial Int 2001; 21(suppl 3):S24-S29.
16. Rubin K, Gullberg D, Tomasini-Johansson B: Molecular recognition of the extracellular matrix by cell surface receptors. *In* Comper WD (ed): Extracellular Matrix. The Netherlands, Harwood Academic Publishers, 1996, pp 262-309.
17. Rippe B, Zakaria ER: Lymphatic versus non-lymphatic fluid absorption from the peritoneal cavity as related to the peritoneal ultrafiltration capacity and sieving properties. Blood Purif 1992; 10:189-202.
18. Rippe B, Haraldsson B: Transport of macromolecules across microvascular walls: The two-pore theory. Physiol Rev 1994; 74:163-219.
19. Pappenheimer JR, Renkin EM, Borrer LM: Filtration, diffusion and molecular sieving through peripheral capillary membranes.

A contribution to pore theory of capillary permeability. Am J Physiol 1951; 167:13-46.
20. Rippe B, Stelin G: How does peritoneal dialysis remove small and large molecular weight solutes? Transport pathways: Fact and myth. *In* Khanna R, Nolph KD, Prowant BF, et al (eds): Advances in Peritoneal Dialysis (vol 6). Toronto, Peritoneal Dialysis Bulletin, 1990, pp 13-18.
21. Rippe B, Carlsson O: Role of transcellular water channels in peritoneal dialysis. Perit Dial Int 1999; 19(suppl 2):S95-S101.
22. Preston GM, Carroll TP, Guggino WB, et al: Appearance of water channels in Xenopus oocytes expressing red cell CHIP 28 protein. Science 1992; 256:385-387.
23. Agre P, Preston GM, Smith BL, et al: Aquaporin CHIP: The archetypal molecular water channel. Am J Physiol 1993; 265: F463-F476.
24. Carlsson O, Nielsen S, Zakaria ER, et al: In vivo inhibition of transcellular water channels (aquaporin-1) during acute peritoneal dialysis in rats. Am J Physiol 1996; 271:H2254-H2262.
25. Pannekeet MM, Mulder JB, Weening JJ, et al: Demonstration of aquaporin-CHIP in peritoneal tissue of uremic and CAPD patients. Perit Dial Int 1996; 16(suppl 1):S54-S57.
26. Devuyst O, Nielsen S, Cosyns JP, et al: Aquaporin-1 and endothelial nitric oxide synthase expression in capillary endothelia of human peritoneum. Am J Physiol 1998; 275: H234-H242.
27. Bundgaard M: The three-dimensional organization of tight junctions in a capillary endothelium revealed by serial-section electron microscopy. J Ultrastruct Res 1984; 88:1-17.
28. Rosengren BI, Carlsson O, Rippe B: Transendothelial transport of low-density lipoprotein and albumin across the rat peritoneum in vivo. Effects of transcytosis inhibitors NEM and filipin. J Vasc Res 2002; 39:230-237.
29. Rippe B, Rosengren BI, Carlsson O, et al: Transendothelial transport: The vesicle controversy. J Vasc Res 2002; 39:375-390.
30. Rippe B, Stelin G: Simulations of peritoneal solute transport during CAPD. Applications of two-pore formalism. Kidney Int 1989; 35:1234-1244.
31. Stelin G, Rippe B: A phenomenological interpretation of the variation in dialysate volume with dwell time in CAPD. Kidney Int 1990; 38:465-472.
32. Rippe B, Stelin G, Haraldsson B: Computer simulations of peritoneal fluid transport in CAPD. Kidney Int 1991; 40:315-325.
33. Vonesh EF, Rippe B: Net fluid absorption under membrane transport models of peritoneal dialysis. Blood Purif 1992; 10: 209-226.
34. Lanciault G, Jacobson ED: The gastrointestinal circulation. Gastroenterology 1976; 71:851-873.
35. Korthuis RJ, Granger DN: Role of the peritoneal microcirculation in peritoneal dialysis. *In* Nolph KD (ed): Peritoneal Dialysis. Dordrecht, Kluwer Academic Publishers, 1989, pp 28-47.
36. Grzegorzewska AE, Antoniewitz K: An indirect estimation of effective peritoneal capillary blood flow in peritoneally dialyzed uremic patients. Perit Dial Int 1993; 13(suppl 2):S39-S40.
37. Grzegorzewska AE, Antoniewitz K: Effective peritoneal capillary blood flow and peritoneal transfer parameters. *In* Khanna R, Nolph KD, Prowant BF, et al (eds): Advances in Peritoneal Dialysis (vol 9). Toronto, Peritoneal Publications, 1993, pp 8-11.
38. Aune S: Transperitoneal exchange: II. Peritoneal blood flow estimation by hydrogen gas clearance. Scand J Gastroenterol 1970; 5:99-104.
39. Kim M, Lofthouse J, Flessner MF: Blood flow limitations of solute transport across the visceral peritoneum. J Am Soc Nephrol 1997; 8:1946-1950.
40. Kim M, Lofthouse J, Flessner MF: A method to test blood flow limitation of peritoneal-blood solute transport. J Am Soc Nephrol 1997; 8:471-474.
41. Flessner MF, Dedrick RL: Role of the liver in small-solute transport during peritoneal dialysis. J Am Soc Nephrol 1994; 5:116-120.
42. Rosengren BI, Rippe B: Blood flow limitations in vivo of small solute transfer during peritoneal dialysis in rats. J Am Soc Nephrol 2003; 14:1599-1604.
43. Waniewski J, Werynski A, Lindholm B: Effect of blood perfusion on diffusive transport in peritoneal dialysis. Kidney Int 1999; 56:707-713.
44. Felt J, Richard C, McCaffrey C, et al: Peritoneal clearances of creatinine and inulin during dialysis in dogs: Effects of splanchnic vasodilators. Kidney Int 1979; 16:459-469.
45. Verger C: Peritoneal ultrastructure (with special reference to chronic renal failure alterations). *In* Bengmark S (ed): The Peritoneum and Peritoneal Access. London, Wright, 1989, pp 14-23.
46. Barrowman JA, Granger DN: Lymphatic drainage of the peritoneal cavity. *In* Bengmark S (ed): The Peritoneum and Peritoneal Access. London, Wright, 1989, pp 85-93.
47. Khanna R, Mactier RA: Role of lymphatics in peritoneal dialysis. Blood Purif 1992; 10:163-172.
48. von Recklinghausen F: Zur Fettresorption. Arch Pathol Anat Physiol Klini Med 1863; 26:172.
49. French JE, Florey HW, Morris B: The absorption of particles by the lymphatic of the diaphragm. Q J Exp Physiol 1960; 45:88.
50. Shockley TR, Ofsthun NJ: Pathways for fluid loss from the peritoneal cavity. Blood Purif 1992; 10:115-121.
51. Zakaria ER, Simonsen O, Rippe A, Rippe B: Transport of tracer albumin from peritoneum to plasma: role of diaphragmatic, visceral, and parietal lymphatics. Am J Physiol 1996; 270: H1549-H1556.
52. Flessner MF: Net ultrafiltration in peritoneal dialysis: Role of direct fluid absorption into tissue. Blood Purif 1992; 10: 136-147.
53. Daugirdas JT, Ing TS, Gandhi VC, et al: Kinetics of peritoneal fluid absorption in patients with chronic renal failure. J Lab Clin Med 1980; 95:351-361.
54. Rippe B, Stelin G, Ahlmén J: Lymph flow from the peritoneal cavity in CAPD patients. *In* Maher JF, Winchester JF (eds): Frontiers in Peritoneal Dialysis. New York, Field, Rich and Associates, 1986, pp 24-30.
55. Heimbürger O, Waniewski J, Werynski A, et al: Lymphatic absorption in CAPD patients with loss of ultrafiltration capacity. Blood Purif 1995; 13:327-339.
56. Hurst SM, McLoughlin RM, Monslow J, et al: Secretion of oncostatin M by infiltrating neutrophils: Regulation of IL-6 and chemokine expression in human mesothelial cells. J Immunol 2002; 169:5244-5251.
57. Robson RL, McLoughlin RM, Witowski J, et al: Different regulation of chemokine production in human peritoneal mesothelial cells: IFN-γ controls neutrophil migration across the mesothelium in vitro and in vivo. J Immunol 2001; 167:1028-1038.
58. Zemel D, Krediet RT, Koomen GCM, et al: Interleukin 8 during peritonitis in patients treated with CAPD: An in vivo model of acute inflammation. Nephrol Dial Transplant 1994; 9:169-174.
59. Zemel D, Imholz ALT, de Waart DR, et al: The appearance of tumor necrosis factor-α and soluble TNF-receptors I and II in peritoneal effluent during stable and infectious CAPD. Kidney Int 1994; 46:1422-1430.
60. Witowski J, Jörres A, Williams JD, et al: Superinduction of IL-6 synthesis in human peritoneal mesothelial cells is related to the induction and stabilization of IL-6 mRNA. Kidney Int 1996; 50:1212-1223.
61. Jones SA, Horiuchi S, Topley N, et al: The soluble interleukin-6 receptor: Mechanisms of production and implications in disease. FASEB J 2001; 15:43-58.
62. Bellingan GJ, Caldwell H, Howie SEM, et al: In vivo fate of the inflammatory macrophage during the resolution of inflammation. J Immunol 1996; 157:2577-2585.
63. McLoughlin RM, Witowski J, Robson RL, et al: Interplay between IFN-γ and IL-6 signalling governs neutrophil trafficking and

apoptosis during acute inflammation. J Clin Invest 2003; 112: 598-607.
64. Nolph KD: Peritoneal anatomy and transport physiology. *In* Maher JF (ed): Replacement of Renal Function by Dialysis, 3rd ed. Dordrecht, Kluwer Academic Publishers, 1989.
65. Leypoldt JK: Interpreting peritoneal membrane osmotic reflection coefficients using a distributed model of peritoneal transport. *In* Khanna R, Nolph KD, Prowant BF, et al (eds): Advances in Peritoneal Dialysis (vol 9). Toronto, Peritoneal Publications, 1993, pp 3-7.
66. Flessner MF, Dedrick RL, Schultz JS: A distributed model of peritoneal-plasma transport: Analysis of experimental data in the rat. Am J Physiol 1985; 248:F413-F424.
67. Randerson DH, Farrell PC: Mass transfer properties of the human peritoneum. ASAIO J 1980; 3:140-146.
68. Pyle WK, Moncrief JW, Popowich RP: Peritoneal transport evaluation in CAPD. *In* Moncrief JW, Popowich RP (eds): CAPD Update. New York, Masson Publishing, 1981, pp 35-53.
69. Pyle WK: Mass Transfer in Peritoneal Dialysis. PhD thesis, University of Texas at Austin, University Microfilms International, Ann Arbor, MI, 1982.
70. Waniewski J, Werynski A, Heimbürger O, et al: A comparative analysis of mass transfer models in peritoneal dialysis. ASAIO Trans 1991; 37:65-75.
71. Waniewski J, Werynski A, Heimbürger O, et al: Simple membrane models for peritoneal dialysis. Evaluation of diffusive and convective solute transport. ASAIO J 1992; 38:788-796.
72. Waniewski J, Heimbürger O, Werynski A, et al: Osmotic conductance of the peritoneum in CAPD patients with permanent loss of ultrafiltration capacity. Perit Dial Int 1996; 16:488-496.
73. Waniewski J, Heimbürger O, Werynski A, et al: Simple models for fluid transport in peritoneal dialysis. Int J Artif Organs 1996; 19:455-466.
74. Flessner MF, Dedrick RL, Schultz JS: A distributed model of peritoneal-plasma transport: Theoretical considerations. Am J Physiol 1984; 246:R597-R607.
75. Dedrick RL, Flessner MF, Collins JM, et al: Is the peritoneum a membrane? ASAIO J 1982; 5:1-8.
76. Dedrick RL, Flessner MF, Collins JM, et al: A distributed model of peritoneal transport. *In* Maher JF, Winchester JF (eds): Frontiers in Peritoneal Dialysis. New York, Field, Rich and Associates, 1986, pp 31-36.
77. Rippe B, Levin L: Computer simulations of ultrafiltration profiles for an icodextrin-based peritoneal fluid in CAPD. Kidney Int 2000; 57:2546-2556.
78. Venturoli D, Rippe B: Transport asymmetry in peritoneal dialysis: Application of a serial heteroporous peritoneal membrane model. Am J Physiol 2001; 280:F599-F606.
79. Heimbürger O, Waniewski J, Werynski A, et al: A quantitative description of solute and fluid transport during peritoneal dialysis. Kidney Int 1992; 41:1320-1332.
80. Henderson LW, Leypoldt JK: Ultrafiltration with peritoneal dialysis. *In* Nolph KD (ed): Peritoneal Dialysis, Dordrecht, Kluwer Academic Publishers, 1989, pp 117-132.
81. Smeby LC, Widerøe TE, Jörstad S: Individual differences in water transport during continuous peritoneal dialysis. ASAIO J 1981; 4:17-27.
82. Zakaria ER, Rippe B: Osmotic barrier properties of the rat peritoneal membrane. Acta Physiol Scand 1993; 149:355-364.
83. Rippe B, Perry MA, Granger DN: Permselectivity of the peritoneal membrane. Microvasc Res 1985; 29:89-102.
84. Ronco C, Feriani M, Chiaramonte S, et al: Pathophysiology of ultrafiltration in peritoneal dialysis. Perit Dial Int 1990; 10: 119-126.
85. Morgenstern BZ: Equilibration testing: Close, but not quite right. Pediatr Nephrol 1993; 7:290-291.
86. Lindholm B, Heimbürger O, Waniewski J, et al: Peritoneal ultrafiltration and fluid reabsorption during peritoneal dialysis. Nephrol Dial Transplant 1989; 4:805-813.
87. Mactier RA, Khanna R, Twardowski Z, et al: Role of peritoneal cavity lymphatic absorption in peritoneal dialysis. Kidney Int 1987; 32:165-172.
88. Mactier RA, Khanna R, Twardowski Z, et al: Contribution of lymphatic absorption to loss of ultrafiltration and solute clearances in continuous ambulatory peritoneal dialysis. J Clin Invest 1987; 80:1311-1316.
89. Waniewski J, Heimbürger O, Park MS, et al: Methods for estimation of peritoneal dialysate volume and reabsorption rate using macromolecular markers. Perit Dial Int 1994; 14:8-16.
90. Haraldsson B: Diffusional transport of albumin from the interstitium to blood across small pores in the capillary walls of rat skeletal muscle. Acta Physiol Scand 1988; 133:63-71.
91. Nolph KD, Mactier R, Khanna R, et al: The kinetics of ultrafiltration during peritoneal dialysis: The role of lymphatics. Kidney Int 1987; 32:219-226.
92. Zink J, Greenway CV: Control of ascites absorption in anesthetized cats: Effects of intraperitoneal pressure, protein, and furosemide diuresis. Gastroenterology 1977; 73:1119-1124.
93. Flessner MF, Fenstermacher JD, Blasberg RG, et al: Peritoneal absorption of macromolecules studied by quantitative autoradiography. Am J Physiol 1985; 248:H26-H32.
94. Flessner MF, Dedrick RL, Reynolds JC: Bidirectional peritoneal transport of immunoglobulin in rats: Tissue concentration profiles. Am J Physiol 1992; 263:F275-287.
95. Mactier RA, Khanna R: Peritoneal lymphatics. *In* Gokal R, Khanna R, Krediet RT, et al (eds): Textbook of Peritoneal Dialysis. Dordrecht, Kluwer Academic Publishers, 2000, pp 173-192.
96. Spencer PC, Farrell PC: Solute and water transfer kinetics in CAPD. *In* Gokal R (ed): Continuous Ambulatory Peritoneal Dialysis. Edinburgh, Churchill Livingstone, 1986, pp 38-55.
97. Flessner MF, Parker RJ, Sieber SM: Peritoneal lymphatic uptake of fibrinogen and erythrocytes in the rat. Am J Physiol 1983; 244:H89-H96.
98. Tran L, Rodela H, Hay JB, et al: Quantification of lymphatic drainage of the peritoneal cavity in sheep: Comparison of direct cannulation techniques with indirect methods to estimate lymph flow. Perit Dial Int 1993; 13:270-279.
99. Flessner MF, Dedrick RL, Reynolds JC: Bidirectional peritoneal transport of immunoglobulin in rats: Compartmental kinetics. Am J Physiol 1992; 262:F275-287.
100. Adair TH: Studies of lymph modification by lymph nodes. Microcirc Endothelium Lymph 1985; 2:257-269.
101. Heimbürger O: Peritoneal transport in patients treated with continuous peritoneal dialysis. PhD thesis, Department of Renal Medicine. Stockholm, Karolinska Institutet, 1994.
102. Krediet RT, Koomen GCM, Koopman MG, et al: The peritoneal transport of serum proteins and neutral dextrane in CAPD patients. Kidney Int 1989; 35:1064-1072.
103. Waniewski J, Heimbürger O, Werynski A, et al: Aqueous solute concentrations and evaluation of mass transport coefficients in peritoneal dialysis. Nephrol Dial Transplant 1992; 7:50-56.
104. Krediet RT, Struijk DG, Koomen GCM, et al: The disappearance of macromolecules from the peritoneal cavity during continuous ambulatory peritoneal dialysis (CAPD) is not dependent on molecular size. Perit Dial Int 1990; 10:147-152.
105. Waniewski J, Heimbürger O, Park MS, et al: Bidirectional solute transport in peritoneal dialysis. Perit Dial Int 1994; 14: 327-337.
106. Rubin J, Jones Q, Planch A, et al: The minimal importance of the hollow viscera to peritoneal transport during peritoneal dialysis in the rat. ASAIO Trans 1988; 34:912-915.
107. Zakaria ER, Simonsen O, Rippe A, et al: Transport of tracer albumin from peritoneum to plasma: Role of diaphragmatic, visceral and parietal lymphatics. Am J Physiol 1996; 270:H1549-H1556.
108. Haraldsson B: Assessing the peritoneal dialysis capacities of individual patients. Kidney Int 1995; 47:1187-1198.

109. Flessner MF: Computerized kinetic modeling: A new tool in the quest for adequacy in peritoneal dialysis. Perit Dial Int 1997; 17:581-585.
110. Rippe B: Personal dialysis capacity. Perit Dial Int 1997; 17(suppl 2): S131-S134.
111. Vonesh EP, Lysaght MJ, Moran J, et al: Kinetic modeling as a prescription aid in peritoneal dialysis. Blood Purif 1991; 9: 246-270.
112. Twardowski ZJ, Nolph KD, Khanna R, et al: Peritoneal equilibration test. Perit Dial Bull 1987; 7:138-147.
113. La Milia V, Di Filippo S, Crepaldi M, et al: Spurious estimations of sodium removal during CAPD when [Na]+ is measured by Na electrode methodology. Kidney Int 2000; 58:2194-2199.
114. Garred LJ, Canaud B, Farrell PC: A simple model for assessing peritoneal mass transfer in chronic ambulatory peritoneal dialysis. ASAIO J 1983; 6:131-137.
115. Waniewski J, Werynski A, Heimbürger O, et al: Simple models for description of small-solute transport in peritoneal dialysis. Blood Purif 1991; 9:129-141.
116. Verger C, Brunschvicg O, Le Charpentier Y, et al: Peritoneal structure alterations on CAPD. *In* Gahl GM, Kessel M, Nolph KD (eds): Advances in Peritoneal Dialysis. Amsterdam, Excerpta Medica, 1981, pp 10-15.
117. Twardowski ZJ: Clinical value of standardized equilibration tests in CAPD patients. Blood Purif 1989; 7:95-108.
118. Twardowski Z: Peritoneal equilibration test: Meaning and relevance. *In* La Greca G, Ronco C, Feriani M, et al (eds): Peritoneal Dialysis. Milano, Wichtig Editore, 1991, pp 101-107.
119. Heimbürger O, Waniewski J, Werynski A, et al: Dialysate to plasma solute concentrations (D/P) versus peritoneal transport parameters in CAPD. Nephrol Dial Transplant 1994; 9:47-59.
120. Churchill DN, Thorpe KE, Nolph KD, et al: Increased peritoneal membrane transport is associated with decreased patient and technique survival for continuous peritoneal dialysis patients. J Am Soc Nephrol 1998; 9:1285-1292.
121. Harty JC, Goldsmith DJA, Boulton H, et al: Limitations of the peritoneal equilibration test in prescribing and monitoring dialysis therapy. Nephrol Dial Transplant 1995; 10:252-257.
122. Blake P, Burkart JM, Churchill DN, et al: Recommended clinical practices for maximizing peritoneal dialysis clearances. Perit Dial Int 1996; 16:448-456.
122a. Durand PY, Freida P, Issad B, Chanlian J: How to reach optional creatinine clearance in automated peritoneal dialysis. Perit Dial Int 1996; 16(suppl 1): S167-S170.
123. Rippe B: How to measure ultrafiltration failure: 2.27% or 3.86% glucose? Perit Dial Int 1997; 17:125-128.
124. Heimbürger O, Tranæus A, Park MS, et al: Relationships between peritoneal equilibration test (PET) and 24 h clearances in CAPD (Abstract). Perit Dial Int 1992; 12(suppl 2):S12.
125. Mujais S, Nolph KD, Gokal R, et al: Evaluation and management of ultrafiltration problems in peritoneal dialysis. Perit Dial Int 2000; 20(suppl 4):S5-S21.
126. Krediet RT, Lindholm B, Rippe B: Pathophysiology of peritoneal membrane failure. Perit Dial Int 2000; 20(suppl 4):S22-S42.
127. Ho-dac-Pannekeet MM, Atasever B, Struijk DG, et al: Analysis of ultrafiltration failure in peritoneal dialysis patients by means of standard peritoneal permeability analysis. Perit Dial Int 1997; 17:144-150.
128. Smit W, Langedijk MJ, Schouten N, et al: A comparison between 1.36% and 3.86% glucose solution for the assessment of peritoneal membrane failure. Perit Dial Int 2000; 20:734-741.
129. Pannekeet MM, Imholz ALT, Struijk DG, et al: The standard peritoneal permeability analysis: A tool for the assessment of peritoneal permeability characteristics in CAPD patients. Kidney Int 1995; 48:866-875.
130. Haraldsson B: Optimization of peritoneal dialysis prescription using computer models of peritoneal transport. Perit Dial Int 2001; 21(suppl 3):S148-S151.
131. Johnsson E, Johansson AC, Andréasson BI, et al: Unrestricted pore area is a better indicator of peritoneal function than PET. Kidney Int 2000; 58:1773-1779.
132. Krediet RT: Biologic markers in peritoneal effluent: Are they useful? *In* Ronco C, Dell'Aquila R, Rodighiero MP (eds): Peritoneal Dialysis Today. Basel, Karger, 2003, pp 30-37.
133. Krediet RT: Dialysate cancer antigen125 concentration as marker of peritoneal membrane status in patients treated with chronic peritoneal dialysis. Perit Dial Int 2001; 21:560-567.
134. Ho-dac-Pannekeet MM, Hiralall JK, Struijk DG, et al: Longitudinal follow-up of CA125 in peritoneal effluent. Kidney Int 1997; 51:888-893.
135. Jones S, Holmes CJ, Krediet RT, et al: Bicarbonate/lactate-based peritoneal dialysis solution increases cancer antigen 125 and decreases hyaluronic acid levels. Kidney Int 2001; 59:1529-1538.
136. Rippe B, Simonsen O, Heimbürger O, et al: Long-term clinical effects of a peritoneal dialysis fluid with less glucose degradation products. Kidney Int 2001; 59:348-357.
137. Cooker LA, Luneburg P, Holmes CJ, et al: Interleukin-6 levels decrease in effluent from patients dialyzed with bicarbonate/lactate-based peritoneal dialysis solutions. Perit Dial Int 2001; 21(suppl 3):S102-S107.
138. Combet S, Miyata T, Moulin P, et al: Vascular proliferation and enhanced expression of endothelial nitric oxide synthase in human peritoneum exposed to long-term peritoneal dialysis. J Am Soc Nephrol 2000; 11:717-728.
139. Korthuis RJ, Granger DN: Peritoneal dialysis: An analysis of factors which influence peritoneal mass transport. *In* Bengmark S (ed): The Peritoneum and Peritoneal Access. London, Wright, 1989, pp 24-41.
140. Klapp R: Über Bauchfellresorption. Mitt Grenzgeb Med Chir 1902; 10:254-282.
141. Gross M, McDonald HPJ: Effect of dialysate temperature and flow rate on peritoneal clearance. JAMA 1967; 202:215-217.
142. Twardowski ZJ, Prowant BF, Nolph KD, et al: High volume, low frequency continuous ambulatory peritoneal dialysis. Kidney Int 1983; 23:64-70.
143. Gotloib L, Mines M, Garmizo L, et al: Hemodynamic effects of increasing intraabdominal pressure in peritoneal dialysis. Perit Dial Bull 1981; 1:41-43.
144. Park MS, Heimbürger O, Bergström J, et al: Evaluation of an experimental rat model for peritoneal dialysis: Fluid and solute transport characteristics. Nephrol Dial Transplant 1994; 9: 404-412.
145. Imholz ALT, Koomen GCM, Struijk DG, et al: Effect of an increased intraperitoneal pressure on fluid and solute transport during CAPD. Kidney Int 1993; 44:1078-1085.
146. Zakaria ER, Rippe B: Peritoneal fluid and tracer albumin kinetics in the rat. Effects of increases in intraperitoneal hydrostatic pressure. Perit Dial Int 1995; 15:118-128.
147. Durand PY, Chanliau J, Gamberoni J, et al: Intraperitoneal pressure, peritoneal permeability and volume of ultrafiltration in CAPD. *In* Khanna R, Nolph KD, Prowant BF, et al (eds): Advances in Peritoneal Dialysis, vol 8. Toronto, Peritoneal Dialysis Bulletin, 1992, pp 22-25.
148. Durand PY, Chanliau J, Gambéroni J, et al: Intraperitoneal hydrostatic pressure and ultrafiltration volume in CAPD. *In* Khanna R, Nolph KD, Prowant BF, et al (eds): Advances in Peritoneal Dialysis vol 9. Toronto, Peritoneal Dialysis Bulletin, 1993, pp 46-48.
149. Keshaviah P, Emerson PF, Vonesh EF, et al: Relationship between body size, fill volume, and mass transfer area coefficient in peritoneal dialysis. J Am Soc Nephrol 1994; 4:1820-1826.
150. Krediet RT, Boeschoten EW, Struijk DG, et al: Differences in the peritoneal transport of water, solutes and proteins between dialysis with two- and with three-litre exchanges. Nephrol Dial Transplant 1988; 3:198-204.
151. Curatola G, Zoccali C, Crucitti S, et al: Effect of posture on peritoneal clearance in CAPD patients. Perit Dial Int 1988; 8:58-59.

152. Imholz ALT, Koomen GCM, Voorn WJ, et al: Day-to-day variability of fluid and solute transport in upright and recumbent position during CAPD. Nephrol Dial Transplant 1998; 13: 146-153.
153. Folkow B, Neil E: Circulation. New York, Oxford University Press, 1971, pp 399-416.
154. Henderson LW: Peritoneal ultrafiltration dialysis: Enhanced urea transfer using hypertonic peritoneal dialysis fluid. J Clin Invest 1966; 45:950-955.
155. Henderson LW, Nolph KD: Altered permeability of the peritoneal membrane using hypertonic peritoneal dialysis fluid. J Clin Invest 1969; 48:992-1001.
156. Henderson IS, Couper IA, Lumsden A: Potentially irritant glucose metabolites in unused CAPD fluid. *In* Maher JF, Winchester JF (eds): Frontiers in Peritoneal Dialysis. New York, Field, Rich and Associates, 1986, pp 261-264.
157. Nilsson-Thorell CB, Muscalu N, Andrén AHG, et al: Heat sterilization of fluids for peritoneal dialysis gives rise to aldehydes. Perit Dial Int 1993; 13:208-213.
158. Wieslander AP, Andrén A, Martinson E, et al: Toxicity of effluent peritoneal dialysis fluid. *In* Khanna R, Nolph KD, Prowant BF, et al (eds): Advances in Peritoneal Dialysis (vol 9). Toronto, Peritoneal Publications, 1993, pp 31-35.
159. Lindén T, Forsbäck G, Deppisch R, et al: 3,4-dideoxyglucosone-3-ene (3,4-DGE), a cytotoxic glucose degradation product in fluids for peritoneal dialysis. Kidney Int 2002; 62:697-703.
160. Musi, B: Biocompatibility of peritoneal dialysis fluids: Impact of glucose degradation products, pH and buffer choice on peritoneal transport and morphology in the rat. PhD thesis, Dept of Nephrology. Lund, Lund University, 2003.
161. Lindholm B, Werynski A, Bergström J: Kinetics of peritoneal dialysis with glycerol and glucose as osmotic agents. ASAIO Trans 1987; 33:19-27.
162. Lindholm B, Werynski A, Bergström J: Peritoneal dialysis with amino acid solutions: Fluid and solute transport kinetics. Artif Organs 1988; 12:2-10.
163. Park MS, Heimbürger O, Bergström J, et al: Peritoneal transport during dialysis with amino acid-based solution. Perit Dial Int 1993; 13:280-288.
164. Jones M, Hagen T, Boyle CA, et al: Treatment of malnutrition with 1.1% amino-acid peritoneal dialysis solution: Results of a multicenter outpatient study. Am J Kidney Dis 1998; 32:761-769.
165. Douma CE, de Waart DR, Struijk DG, et al: Effect of amino acid based dialysate on peritoneal blood flow and permeability in stable CAPD patients: A potential role for nitric oxide? Clin Nephrol 1996; 45:295-302.
166. Waniewski J, Werynski A, Heimbürger O, et al: Effect of alternative osmotic agents on peritoneal transport. Blood Purif 1993; 11:248-264.
167. Heimbürger O, Lindholm B: New solutions for peritoneal dialysis. *In* Falkenhagen D, Klinkman H, Piskin E, et al (eds): Blood–Material Interaction. Glaskow, International Faculty for Artificial Organs, 1998, pp 129-136.
168. Mistry C, Mallick NP, Gokal R: Ultrafiltration with an isosmotic solution during long peritoneal dialysis exchanges. Lancet 1987; 2:178-182.
169. Ho-dac-Pannekeet MM, Schouten N, Langendijk MJ, et al: Peritoneal transport characteristics with glucose polymer based dialysate. Kidney Int 1996; 50:979-986.
170. Pecoits-Filho R, Mujais S, Lindholm B: Future of icodextrin as an osmotic agent in peritoneal dialysis. Kidney Int 2002; 62(suppl 81):S80-S87.
171. Miller FN, Nolph KD, Joshua IG, et al: Hyperosmolality, acetate, and lactate: Dilatory factors during peritoneal dialysis. Kidney Int 1981; 20:397-402.
172. Miller FN, Nolph KD, Patrick DH, et al: Microvascular and clinical effects of altered peritoneal dialysis solutions. Kidney Int 1979; 15:630-639.
173. Grzegorzewska AE, Moore HL, Chen TC, et al: Peritoneal transfer during maximal hyperosmotic ultrafiltration in the rat. ASAIO J 1993; 39:66-70.
174. Musi B, Carlsson O, Rippe A, et al: Effects of acidity, glucose degradation products, and dialysis fluid buffer choice on peritoneal solute and fluid transport in rats. Perit Dial Int 1998; 18:303-310.
175. Heimbürger O, Waniewski J, Wang T, et al: Peritoneal transport with lactate 40 mmol/l (L) vs. bicarbonate/lactate (BL) dialysis fluid (Abstract). J Am Soc Nephrol 1998; 9:192A.
176. Nolph KD, Rubin J, Wiegman DL, et al: Peritoneal clearances with three types of commercially available peritoneal dialysis solutions. Nephron 1979; 24:35-40.
177. International Cooperative Study (second report): A survey of ultrafiltration in continuous ambulatory peritoneal dialysis. Perit Dial Bull 1984; 4:137-142.
178. International Cooperative Study (third report): A survey of ultrafiltration in continuous ambulatory peritoneal dialysis. *In* Khanna R, Nolph KD, Prowant B, et al (eds): Advances in Peritoneal Dialysis (vol 1). Toronto, Toronto University Press, 1985, pp 79-86.
179. Katirtzoglou A, Digenis GE, Kontesis P, et al: Is peritoneal ultrafiltration influenced by acetate or lactate buffers? *In* Maher JF, Winchester JF (eds): Frontiers in Peritoneal Dialysis. New York, Field, Rich and Associates, 1986, pp 270-273.
180. Slingeneyer A, Canaud B, Mion C: Permanent loss of ultrafiltration capacity of the peritoneum in long-term peritoneal dialysis: An epidemiological study. Nephron 1983; 33:133-138.
181. Faller B, Marichal JF: Evolution of ultrafiltration in CAPD according to the dialysis fluid buffer. *In* Maher JF, Winchester JF (eds): Frontiers in Peritoneal Dialysis. New York, Field, Rich and Associates, 1986, pp 274-278.
182. Kawaguchi Y, Kawanishi H, Mujais S, et al: Encapsulating peritoneal sclerosis: Definition, etiology, diagnosis and treatment. Perit Dial Int 2000; 20(suppl 4):S43-S55.
183. Feriani M, Dissegna D, La Greca G, et al: Short-term clinical study with bicarbonate-containing peritoneal dialysis solution. Perit Dial Int 1993; 13:296-301.
184. Hirszel P, Maher JF: Pharmacological alteration of peritoneal transport rates. *In* Nolph KD (ed): Peritoneal Dialysis. Dordrecht, Kluwer Academic Publishers, 1989, pp 184-198.
185. Maher JF, Hirszel P, Larich M: An experimental model for study of pharmacological and hormonal influences on peritoneal dialysis. Contrib Nephrol 1979; 17:131-138.
186. Steinhauer HB: Pharmacological manipulation of peritoneal transport in CAPD. Clin Nephrol 1988; 30(suppl 1):S29-S33.
187. Nolph KD, Ghods AJ, Brown PA, et al: Effects of intraperitoneal nitroprusside on peritoneal clearances in man with variations of dose, frequency of administration and dwell times. Nephron 1979; 24:114-120.
188. Hirszel P, Lasrich M, Maher JF: Augmentation of peritoneal mass transport by dopamine: Comparison with norepinephrine and evaluation of pharmacologic mechanisms. J Lab Clin Med 1979; 94:747-754.
189. Krediet RT, Zuyderhoudt MJ, Boeschoten EW, et al: Alterations in the peritoneal transport of water and solutes during peritonitis in continuous ambulatory peritoneal dialysis patients. Eur J Clin Invest 1987; 17:43-52.
190. Steinhauer HB, Schollmeyer P: Prostaglandin-mediated loss of proteins during peritonitis in continuous ambulatory peritoneal dialysis. Kidney Int 1986; 29:584-590.
191. Verger C, Luger A, Moore HL, et al: Acute changes in peritoneal transport properties with infectious peritonitis and mechanical injury. Kidney Int 1983; 23:823-831.
192. Widerøe TE, Smeby LC, Mjåland S, et al: Long-term changes in transperitoneal water transport during continuous ambulatory peritoneal dialysis. Nephron 1984; 38:238-247.
193. Krediet RT, Arisz L: Fluid and solute transport across the peritoneum during continuous ambulatory peritoneal dialysis. Perit Dial Int 1989; 9:15-25.

194. Combet S, van Landschoot M, Moulin P, et al: Regulation of aquaporin-1 and nitric oxide synthase isoforms in rat model of acute peritonitis. J Am Soc Nephrol 1999; 10:2185-2196.
195. Ni J, Moulin P, Gianello P, et al: Mice that lack endothelial nitric oxide synthase are protected against functional and structural modifications induced by acute peritonitis. J Am Soc Nephrol 2003; 14:3205-3216.
196. Heimbürger O, Wang T, Lindholm B: Alterations in water and solute transport with time on peritoneal dialysis. Perit Dial Int 1999; 19(suppl 2):S83-S90.
197. Rocco MV, Jordan JR, Burkart JM: Changes in peritoneal transport during the first month of peritoneal dialysis. Perit Dial Int 1995; 15:12-17.
198. Davies SJ, Bryan J, Phillips L, et al: Longitudinal changes in peritoneal kinetics: The effects of peritoneal dialysis and peritonitis. Nephrol Dial Transplant 1996; 11:498-506.
199. Blake PG, Abraham G, Sombolos K, et al: Changes in peritoneal membrane transport rates in patients on long term CAPD. *In* Khanna R, Nolph KD, Prowant BF, et al (eds): Advances in Peritoneal Dialysis (vol 5). Toronto, University of Toronto Press, 1989, pp 3-7.
200. Lo W-K, Bredolan A, Prowant BF, et al: Changes in the peritoneal equilibration test in selected chronic peritoneal dialysis patients. J Am Soc Nephrol 1994; 4:1466-1474.
201. Randerson DH, Farrell PC: Long-term peritoneal clearance in CAPD. *In* Atkins RC, Thomson NM, Farrell PC (eds): Peritoneal Dialysis. Edinburgh, Churchill Livingstone, 1981, pp 23-29.
202. Selgas R, Fernandez-Reyes MJ, Bosque E, et al: Functional longevity of the human peritoneum: How long is continuous peritoneal dialysis possible? Results of a prospective medium long-term study. Am J Kidney Dis 1994; 23:64-73.
203. Struijk DG, Krediet RT, Koomen GCM, et al: A prospective study of peritoneal transport in CAPD patients. Kidney Int 1994; 45:1739-1744.
204. Kush RD, Hallett MD, Ota K, et al: Long-term continuous ambulatory peritoneal dialysis. Mass transfer and nutritional and metabolic stability. Blood Purif 1990; 8:1-13.
205. Davies SJ, Phillips L, Griffiths AM, et al: What really happens to patients on long-term peritoneal dialysis? Kidney Int 1998; 54:2207-2217.
206. Pollock CA, Ibels LS, Caterson RJ, et al: Continuous ambulatory peritoneal dialysis, eight years of experience at a single center. Medicine 1989; 68:293-308.
207. Heimbürger O, Waniewski J, Werynski A, et al: Peritoneal transport in CAPD patients with permanent loss of ultrafiltration capacity. Kidney Int 1990; 38:495-506.
208. Krediet RT, Boeschoten EW, Zuyderhoudt FMJ, et al: Peritoneal transport characteristics of water, low-molecular weight solutes and proteins during long-term continuous ambulatory peritoneal dialysis. Perit Dial Bull 1986; 6:61-65.
209. Verger C, Larpent L, Celicout B: Clinical significance of ultrafiltration failure in CAPD. *In* La Greca G, Chiarmonte S, Fabris A, et al (eds): Peritoneal Dialysis. Milan, Wichtig Editore, 1985, pp 91-94.
210. Pollock CA, Ibels LS, Hallett MD, et al: Loss of ultrafiltration in continuous ambulatory peritoneal dialysis (CAPD). Perit Dial Int 1989; 9:107-110.
211. Smit W, van den Berg N, Schouten N, et al: Free water transport in fast transport status: A comparison between CAPD peritonitis and long-term PD. Kidney Int 2004; 65:298-303.
212. Monquil MCJ, Imholz ALT, Struijk DG, et al: Does transcellular water transport contribute to net ultrafiltration failure during CAPD? Perit Dial Int 1995: 42-48.
213. Rippe B, de Arteaga J, Venturoli D: Aquaporins are unlikely to be affected in marked ultrafiltration failure: Results from a computer simulation. Perit Dial Int 2001; 21(suppl 3):S30-S34.
214. Krediet RT, Struijk DG, Boeschoten EW, et al: The time course of peritoneal transport kinetics in continuous ambulatory peritoneal dialysis patients who develop sclerosing peritonitis. Am J Kidney Dis 1989; 13:299-307.
215. Chung SH, Chu WS, Lee HA, et al: Peritoneal transport characteristics, comorbid diseases and survival in CAPD patients. Perit Dial Int 2000; 20:541-547.
216. Heaf J: CAPD adequacy and dialysis morbidity: Detrimental effect of a high equilibration rate. Ren Fail 1995; 17:575-587.
217. Davies SJ, Phillips L, Russell GI: Peritoneal solute transport predicts survival on CAPD independently of residual renal function. Nephrol Dial Transplant 1998; 13:962-968.
218. Wang T, Heimbürger O, Waniewski J, et al: Increased peritoneal permeability is associated with decreased fluid and small solute removal and higher mortality in CAPD patients. Nephrol Dial Transplant 1998; 13:1242-1249.
219. Pecoits-Filho R, Araujo MR, Lindholm B, et al: Plasma and dialysate IL-6 and VEGF concentrations are associated with high peritoneal solute transport rate. Nephrol Dial Transplant 2002; 17:1480-1486.
220. Davies SJ, Phillips L, Naish PF, et al: Quantifying comorbidity in peritoneal dialysis patients and its relationship to other predictors of survival. Nephrol Dial Transplant 2002; 17: 1085-1092.
221. Chung SH, Heimbürger O, Stenvinkel P, et al: Association between inflammation and changes in residual renal function and peritoneal transport rate during the first year of dialysis. Nephrol Dial Transplant 2001; 16:2240-2245.
222. Heimbürger O, Wang T, Chung SH, et al: Increased peritoneal transport rate from an early peritoneal equilibration test (PET) is related to inflammation, cardiovascular disease and mortality (Abstract). J Am Soc Nephrol 1999; 10:315A.
223. Cueto-Manzano AM, Correa-Rotter R: Is high peritoneal transport rate an independent risk factor for CAPD mortality? Kidney Int 2000; 57:314-320.
224. Wang T, Waniewski J, Heimbürger O, et al: A quantitative analysis of sodium transport and removal during peritoneal dialysis. Kidney Int 1997; 52:1609-1616.
225. Konings CJAM, Kooman JP, Schonck M, et al: Fluid status, blood pressure, and cardiovascular abnormalities in patients on peritoneal dialysis. Perit Dial Int 2002; 22:477-487.
226. Konings CJAM, Kooman JP, Schonck M, et al: Fluid status in CAPD patients is related to peritoneal transport and residual renal function: Evidence from a longitudinal study. Nephrol Dial Transplant 2003; 18:797-803.
227. Koc M, Toprak A, Tezcan H, et al: Uncontrolled hypertension due to volume overload contributes to higher left ventricular mass index in CAPD patients. Nephrol Dial Transplant 2002; 17:1661-1666.
228. Niebauer J, Volk H-D, Kemp M, et al: Endotoxin and immune activation in chronic heart failure: A prospective cohort study. Lancet 1999; 353:1838-1842.
229. Anker SD, Coats AJ: Cardiac cachexia: A syndrome with impaired survival and immune and neuroendocrine activation. Chest 1999; 115:836-847.
230. Tzamaloukas AH, Murata GH, Piraino B, et al: Peritoneal urea and creatinine clearances in continuous ambulatory peritoneal dialysis patients with different types of peritoneal solute transport. Kidney Int 1998; 53:1405-1411.
231. Blake PG, Flowerdew G, Blake RM, et al: Serum albumin in patients on continuous ambulatory peritoneal dialysis: Predictors and correlations with outcomes. J Am Soc Nephrol 1993; 3:1501-1507.
232. Harty JC, Boulton H, Venning MC, et al: Is peritoneal permeability an adverse risk factor for malnutrition in CAPD patients? Miner Electrolyte Metab 1996; 22:97-101.
233. Margetts PJ, McMullin JP, Rabbat CG, et al: Peritoneal membrane transport and hypoalbuminemia: Cause or effect? Perit Dial Int 2000; 20:14-18.

234. Nolph KD, Moore HL, Prowant B, et al: Continuous ambulatory peritoneal dialysis with a high flux membrane. ASAIO J 1993; 39:904-909.
235. Davies SJ, Russel L, Bryan J, et al: Impact of peritoneal absorption of glucose on appetite, protein catabolism and survival in CAPD patients. Clin Nephrol 1996; 45:194-198.
236. Szeto CC, Law MC, Wong TYH, et al: Peritoneal transport status correlates with morbidity but not longitudinal change of nutritional status of continuous ambulatory peritoneal dialysis patients: A 2-year prospective study. Am J Kidney Dis 2001; 37:329-336.
237. Stenvinkel P, Chung SH, Heimbürger O, et al: Malnutrition, inflammation and atherosclerosis in peritoneal dialysis patients. Perit Dial Int 2001; 21(suppl 3): S157-S162.
238. Chung SH, Heimburger O, Stenvinkel P, et al: Association between residual renal function, inflammation and patient survival in new peritoneal dialysis patients. Nephrol Dial Transplant 2003; 18:590-597.
239. Pecoits-Filho R, Stenvinkel P, Wang AYM, et al: Chronic inflammation in peritoneal dialysis: The search for the Holy Grail? Perit Dial Int 2004; 24:327-339.
240. Honda K, Nitta K, Horita S, et al: Morphological changes in the peritoneal vasculature of patients on CAPD with ultrafiltration failure. Nephron 1996; 72:171-176.
241. Dobbie JW: Morphology of the peritoneum in CAPD. Blood Purif 1989; 7:74-85.
242. Pollock CA, Ibels LS, Caterson RJ, et al: Peritoneal morphology on maintenance dialysis. Am J Nephrol 1989; 9:198-204.
243. Di Paolo N, Sacchi G, De Mia M, et al: Morphology of the peritoneal membrane during continuous ambulatory peritoneal dialysis. Nephron 1986; 44:204-211.
244. Honda K, Nitta K, Horita S, et al: Accumulation of advanced glycation end products in the peritoneal vasculature of continuous ambulatory peritoneal dialysis patients with low ultrafiltration. Nephrol Dial Transplant 1999; 14:1541-1549.
245. Mateijsen MA, van der Wal AC, Hendriks PM, et al: Vascular and interstitial changes in the peritoneum of CAPD patients with peritoneal sclerosis. Perit Dial Int 1999; 19:517-525.
246. Numata M, Nakayama M, Nimura S, et al: Association between an increased surface area of peritoneal microvessels and a high peritoneal transport rate. Perit Dial Int 2003; 23:116-122.
247. Nakayama M, Kawaguchi Y, Yamada K, et al: Immunohistochemical detection of advanced glycosylation end products in the peritoneum and its possible pathophysiological role in CAPD. Kidney Int 1997; 51:182-186.
248. Williams JD, Craig KD, Topley N, et al: Morphological changes in the peritoneal membrane of patients with renal disease. J Am Soc Nephrol 2002; 13:470-479.
249. Jörres A, Williams JD, Topley N: Peritoneal dialysis solution biocompatibility: Inhibitory mechanisms and recent studies with bicarbonate-buffered solutions. Perit Dial Int 1997; 17(suppl 2):S42-S46.
250. Wieslander A, Lindén T, Musi B, et al: Exogenous uptake of carbonyl stress compounds promoting AGE formation from peritoneal dialysis fluids. *In* D'Angelo A, Favaro S (eds): Advanced Glycation End Products in Nephrology. Basel, Karger, 2001, pp 82-89.
251. Davies SJ, Phillips L, Naish PF, et al: Peritoneal glucose exposure and changes in membrane solute transport with time on peritoneal dialysis. J Am Soc Nephrol 2001; 12:52-58.
252. Goffin E, Combet S, Jamar F, et al: Expression of aquaporin-1 (AQP1) in long-term peritoneal dialysis patients with impaired transcellular water transport. Am J Kidney Dis 1999; 33:383-388.
253. Devuyst O: New insight in the molecular mechanisms regulating peritoneal permeability. Nephrol Dial Transplant 2002; 17:548-551.

Peritoneal Dialysis Access

Elias D. Thodis, M.D. • Vassilis Vargemezis, M.D. • Dimitrios G. Oreopoulos, M.D., Ph.D., F.R.C.P.C., F.A.C.P.

PERITONEAL DIALYSIS ACCESS

After peritoneal dialysis (PD) was recognized as an effective renal replacement, we have had great increases in our knowledge of the clinical and basic science of continuous peritoneal dialysis therapies. However, peritoneal access is still a challenge in our day-to-day practice. The provision of safe and reliable access to the peritoneal cavity is vital to the CAPD patient. The catheter is the patient's lifeline to the peritoneal dialysis membrane.[1]

A good peritoneal catheter should provide adequate rates of solution inflow and outflow, and its design should minimize infection at the skin exit site and should allow successful resolution of peritonitis if it occurs. Finally, it should be safely implantable without major surgery.

Most centers have reduced technique failure, mainly through improved connection technology and cumulative experience acquired by the involved team. The literature does not provide a definite answer concerning the most preferable access, method of implantation, and exit-site care protocol. The individual center's performance effect will always be a confounding variable. On the other hand, the search for evidence-based recommendations faces a major difficulty, namely the small number of randomized, controlled studies and the lack of statistical power of small population studies. However promising, advances in PD technology deserve the close attention of all nephrologists.[2]

This chapter describes the catheters and implantation techniques, which have been used for chronic peritoneal dialysis (CPD) and some of the complications that have arisen from them. Also, it discusses the complication related to the catheters and the implantation and certain difficulties that may arise during their treatment.

Anatomy of the Abdominal Wall and Peritoneum

A working knowledge of the anatomy of the anterior abdominal wall and peritoneal cavity is necessary for an understanding of the various techniques of catheter placement and is vital for those undertaking this procedure.[3,4]

The skin of the anterior abdominal wall is of moderate thickness and is relatively mobile on the underlying fascia and muscle. Most incisions for catheter insertion are relatively short and exposure is equally good whichever their direction.

The skin, fascia, muscles, and parietal peritoneum of the anterior abdominal wall are innervated segmentally largely from the anterior primary rami of spinal nerves T6 to L1. A well-infiltrated field block around the terminal branches of these nerves as they pass medially towards the incision will provide good local anesthesia down to the peritoneum, which in the thin patient is an obvious layer, but in the obese is lost in a thick, fatty panniculus.

The main muscles of the anterior abdominal wall are four. Three of them: the external oblique, the internal oblique, and the transversus abdominis, pass from their various origins as separate, fleshy muscle bellies in a predominantly medial direction. The major vessels and nerves pass downward and medially in the neurovascular plane, between the transversus abdominus and the internal oblique muscles.

The rectus sheath appears as an elliptical tube with a strong anterior wall. The weaker posterior wall only extends to just below the level of the umbilicus. Supplying the rectus muscle and firmly adherent to its posterior surface are the epigastric vessels. These are easily damaged, particularly during a lateral approach for catheter insertion.

In obese patients there may be a variable amount of preperitoneal fat. The peritoneum is usually a bluish, almost avascular membrane, underneath which bowel or omentum can be seen to move with respiration. In a patient who has had previous peritoneal dialysis or who has had previous surgery, the peritoneum may be thicker and sometimes slightly vascular. Adhesions between the intra-abdominal contents and the parietal peritoneum may be encountered when operating through the scar tissue of previous incisions.[5]

The peritoneal cavity is a large potential space. Conventionally, it is divided into the greater and lesser sacs with the root of the transverse mesocolon dividing the greater sac into the supracolic and infracolic compartments. The intraperitoneal portion of the dialysis catheter should lie wholly in this lower compartment, potentially in contact with the small bowel, greater omentum, transverse and sigmoid colon, and the reproductive organs in the female. If the peritoneal cavity is filled with fluid, the omentum tends to float because of its fat content, as do those parts of the bowel that have a mesenteric attachment. Theoretically, if the tip of a dialysis catheter is well positioned in the most dependent part of the pelvis and the peritoneal cavity is full of fluid, it should be relatively unobstructed by these other intraperitoneal structures.

The peritoneum itself is a single layer of mesothelial cells supported by a basement membrane, which rests upon a bed of connective tissue varying in thickness according to the site. The peritoneum is divided into the visceral layer that covers those parts of the bowel and parenchymal organs that hang by a mesentery within the peritoneal cavity and the parietal layer that covers the walls of the cavity itself.[3,6,7]

Development of Peritoneal Catheters

The ideal catheter should be simple, safe and long-lasting, with a minimal rate of access-related complications and rapid dialysate flows.

Ganter[8] and Putnam[9] made the first attempts to gain access to the peritoneal cavity for dialysis. Although it was recognized that potentially the peritoneum was an effective dialyzing membrane, attempts to use it for this purpose were frustrated by the lack of a useful access device.

Palmer and Quinton[10] were the first to use silicone rubber catheters to provide prolonged access to the peritoneal cavity. Palmer's catheter used a long subcutaneous tunnel, which diminished the risk of sepsis. Several patients dialyzed successfully for long intervals between infections.

In 1964 Gutch[11] made a major step forward in creating a permanent peritoneal access when he noted less irritation of the peritoneum and lower protein losses with silicon rubber catheters, compared to those made with polyvinyl.

In 1968 Tenckhoff and Schechter[12] published the results of their studies on a new catheter, which was an improved version of the Palmer catheter. The intra-abdominal flange was replaced by a Dacron cuff, the subcutaneous tunnel was shortened, and it had a second, external cuff to decrease the length of the catheter sinus tract. The intraperitoneal segment was kept open-ended and the size of the side holes was 0.5 mm to prevent tissue suction. To avoid excessive bleeding and to assist easy penetration, the catheter was inserted through the midline.

The Tenckhoff catheter became the gold standard of peritoneal access. Few complications were reported in patients treated by periodic peritoneal dialysis. Even today, more than 30 years later, the Tenckhoff catheter in its original form is the most widely used catheter type. Some of the original recommendations for catheter insertion, such as an arcuate subcutaneous tunnel with downward directions of both intraperitoneal and external exits, are still considered to be important elements of catheter implantation.[13-15]

A number of subcutaneous and intraperitoneal variations have been proposed as better devices. The catheter may be single- or double-cuffed with a straight or curled intraperitoneal portion and will be described later on in this chapter.

Catheter Design and Insertion: General Principles

Before describing individual catheters, it is worth reviewing some of the general principles of catheter design and use. The catheter can be considered in three parts, each with a separate function. These are the extra-abdominal, subcutaneous, and intraperitoneal sections. It is in the last section that catheters vary so widely (Figure 26–1).

The extra-abdominal section, which protrudes from the skin exit site, needs to be at least 10 cm long for easy handling and have enough length in reserve to permit trimming if a split occurs at the connector site. The subcutaneous section permits a degree of freedom in the siting of the catheter exit at a convenient place on the anterior abdominal wall. In catheters with a single preperitoneal cuff, the subcutaneous tunnel varies in length and is open at the exit site. In two-cuff catheters, this open part of the tunnel is relatively short between the exit site and the subcutaneous cuff. The deep part of the tunnel is then blind at both ends between the subcutaneous and preperitoneal cuffs. In the absence of sepsis the subcutaneous tunnel becomes lined by a downgrowth of epidermal cells. Ideally, the subcutaneous part of the catheter should be designed and implanted in such a way as to avoid skin exit-site infections, superficial cuff erosion, and tunnel infections.[1,13,14]

The short transmural section of catheter that passes through the abdominal wall muscles or the linea alba, and which then perforates the peritoneum, has three functions: to provide a mechanical anchorage, a water-tight peritoneal seal, and a further antibacterial seal. All three can be served by a single cuff just superficial to the peritoneum and deep to the overlying structures. The fibrous tissue ingrowth bonds the catheter to muscle and fascia strongly enough to prevent its displacement by traction. When the cuff is routed obliquely through the tissues, this bond will stabilize the intraperitoneal section of the catheter in a direction pointing towards the pelvis. At this level, the cuff also produces fibrosis immediately adjacent to the peritoneum, forming an effective fluid seal. The transmural section should be implanted to prevent catheter extrusion, early and late dialysate leaks and incisional hernias.

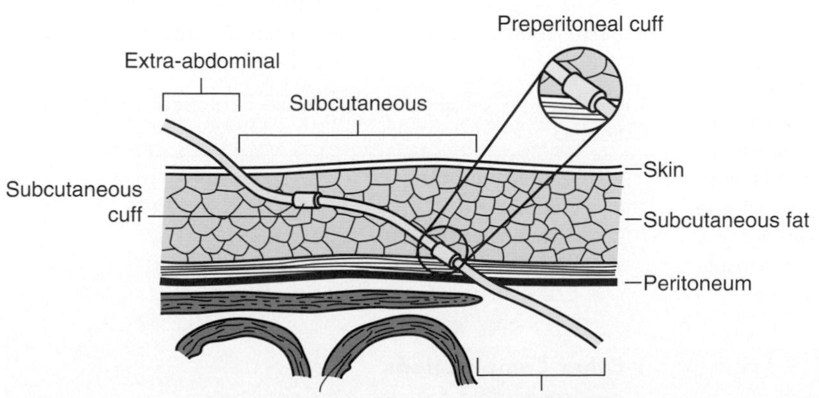

Figure 26–1 Functional parts of a peritoneal catheter and the abdominal wall with adjacent tissues.

Types of Catheters

Peritoneal Catheters Categorized as Acute or Chronic

Acute catheters

The catheter design for acute PD and chronic PD differs significantly. Acute PD catheters are straight and relatively rigid with a conduit about 3 mm in diameter and 25 to 30 mm in length without any protective Dacron cuff. It can be placed at the bedside under local anesthesia with a tiny skin incision with the tip of the scalpel. It is used immediately after implantation. It is not recommended to be left in situ for longer than 3 days. With prolonged use, it is associated with significant risk of peritonitis, malfunction, and bowel perforation. Acute PD is still used in the management of acute and chronic renal failure in many developing countries.[12,13]

All acute catheters have the same basic design: a straight or slightly curved, relatively rigid tubing with numerous side holes at the distal end. A metal stylet or flexible wire over which the catheter slides is used to guide insertion.

Acute peritoneal dialysis can also be carried out through a semi-rigid catheter implanted at bedside using a Tenckhoff trocar Seldinger technique or by laparoscopic insertion. The incidence of complications related to peritoneal access (such as hemorrhage, bowel injury) vary from center to center.[16-19]

Because acute catheters do not have cuffs to protect against bacterial migration, the incidence of peritonitis increases prohibitively beyond 3 days of use. Also, the risk of bowel perforation increases with duration of use. If extended dialysis is necessary, the acute catheter must be removed periodically and replaced by a new catheter in a different location.

Implantation of Acute Peritoneal Dialysis Catheters

Planning the access implantation, which is part of an integrated approach to renal replacement therapy and pre-dialysis care, begins with careful patient preimplantation evaluation. Such evaluation includes search for any herniation, or weakness of the abdominal wall, which can be corrected before or preferably at the time of the implantation, determination of the exit site by an experienced member of the PD team, bladder emptying, and the administration of prophylactic antibiotics just as in any abdominal surgery.

The acute peritoneal catheter is placed blindly into an abdomen that has been pre-filled with fluid. Insertion is guided by a sharpened stylet or by flexible guidewire. Examples of acute catheters with stylets are the Stylocath (Abbott Laboratories North Chicago, ID) and the Trocath (Baxter Healthcare, Deerfield, IL). An acute catheter designed to be inserted over a flexible guidewire is available from Cook Co. (Bloomington, IN).[17,19]

The incidence of complications is increased in patients with ileus or adhesions from previous abdominal surgery. Placement is also difficult in comatose or uncooperative patients who cannot tense their abdominal wall during insertion of the catheter or the prefilling needle. Surgical or peritoneoscopic placement of a chronic peritoneal catheter should be considered for such patients.

Procedure

Either a midline or a lateral abdominal entry site can be chosen. The midline site is about 3 cm below the umbilicus. The lateral site is just lateral to the border of the rectus muscle, on a line between the umbilicus and the anterior superior iliac spine. On the right, the lateral site is approximately at McBurney's point. The left lateral site is considered preferable because it avoids the cecum. When choosing an insertion site, avoid areas of previous catheter insertion or scars by at least 2 to 3 cm. The bladder must be empty, because a full bladder can be penetrated inadvertently by the stylet during insertion. The abdomen should be carefully examined to exclude the presence of massive enlargement of the liver, spleen, bladder, or other organs and *to* exclude other remarkable pathology (e.g., abdominal carcinomatosis).[3,18]

Complications of Acute Catheter Insertion (Table 26–1)

Pain

An experienced and skilled operator, either a physician or a surgeon, in a dedicated room, under sterile conditions, must implant the catheter. Pain which is due mainly to dialysis-related complications, is seen in 56% to 75% of patients with the first use of a catheter.[12-14] It occurs because of low dialysis pH, overdistension, low and high temperature of dialysate, free abdominal air, and peritonitis. Pain may occur during flow, dwelling, and outflow of dialysis solution. Outflow pain is caused by the entrapment of omentum in the catheter during the siphoning action of fluid drainage. Constant pain indicates pressure effects on intra-abdominal organs and often produces continuous rectal or low back pain. This may need adjustment in catheter position. In a small percentage of patients, catheter tip irritation of abdominal viscera causes pain. It is relieved with plain water enema. Pain during catheter insertion can be alleviated by adequate local anesthesia and sedation.[16]

Bleeding

After catheter insertion, bloody outflow appears in 30% of cases.[20,21] The reasons for bleeding after rigid catheter insertion are (1) pre-peritoneal placement of the catheter; (2) injury to minor capillaries in parietal peritoneum, subcutaneous space, or mesentery; and (3) puncture of major intra-abdominal vessels.

The treatments usually required for minor bleeding are (1) pressure application over catheter entry side, (2) suitable pursestring suture, (3) rapid exchange of dialysate without dwell to clear the effluent and prevents catheter block, (4) heparin 1000 IU/L of dialysate that minimizes the risk of

Table 26–1 Complications of Acute Peritoneal Dialysis (PD) Catheters

- Abdominal pain
- Bleeding
- Pericatheter dialysis solution leak
- Viscus perforation
- Catheter malfunction/poor drainage
- Infections/Peritonitis

Other Complications

- Loss of rigid catheter in the peritoneum
- Extraperitoneal space penetration

catheter block (intraperitoneal heparin is not absorbed in sufficient amount to influence systemic coagulation), (5) the use of room temperature dialysate that may slow or stop capillary bleeding, and (6) fresh blood transfusion; removal of rigid catheter may be required in some patients. Persistent significant bleeding (hemoglobin in effluent >5 g/dL) not only causes blood loss, but it also causes blockage of catheter due to blood clot and is a source of infection.[22]

Pericatheter Dialysis Solution Leak

Pericatheter leak occurs in 14% to 36% of patients after acute PD catheter insertion.[13,20,21] The predisposing factors are (1) frequent manipulation of catheter to improve drainage, (2) catheter not properly secured to skin, and (3) presence of high intra-abdominal pressure due to ascites or polycystic kidney disease. Rarely, fluid may leak into the pleural cavity through a congenital or traumatic defect in the diaphragm. The management of early leak includes temporary discontinuation of PD and supine low volume PD. Catheter replacement may be required if it persists.[23]

Viscus Perforation

Bowel injury

Bowel injury occurs in 0.1% to 1.3% of all procedures.[24,25] It is a rare but serious complication. The predisposing factors are: previous abdominal surgery with peritoneal adhesions, distention of bowel with gas, and paralytic ileus. Minor injury is harmless, but significant injury can cause turbid outflow because of fecal contamination of the peritoneum. The injury also results in poor outflow and can cause watery diarrhea. Filling the peritoneal cavity adequately with dialysis fluid and withdrawing the stylet as soon as the peritoneum is punctured prevents any injury to bowel.

Broad-spectrum antibiotics with anaerobic cover should be started empirically and later modified according to culture and sensitivity. Laparotomy may be required for the repair of gut injury along with removal of the catheter.

Bladder injury

Bladder injury occurs when the bladder is full during catheter insertion and if the stylet is not withdrawn after piercing the peritoneum and the bladder comes beneath the stylet. This complication manifests as suprapublic swelling, and the patient may pass hemorrhagic PD fluid per urethra. The outflow by PD catheter may be poor and hemorrhagic.[24]

Catheter Malfunction/Poor Drainage

Catheter malfunction usually results in poor dialysate inflow and outflow. The reasons for poor dialysate flow are kinked catheter, fibrin or blood clot, omental wrapping, catheter tip migration, loculation of fluid in the peritoneal cavity because of previous peritoneal adhesion, and neurogenic distended urinary bladder. The incidence of acute peritoneal catheter malfunction has been reported to be 12% to 28% in various studies.[26]

Infections/Peritonitis

Exit-site infection is a rare complication of acute peritoneal dialysis. The incidence of peritonitis is about 2.5% of all dialyses when stylet catheter is used. The incidence is almost doubled when the duration of dialysis is longer than 60 hours. The incidence of positive culture in the absence of clinical infection is as high as 10% to 30%.[22,27]

Other Complications

Loss of a part or all of the rigid catheter has been reported following its manipulation with the trocar in place.[3,28,29] Its distal end may be amputated after intra-abdominal kinking of the catheter, followed by manipulation. However, the presence of broken catheters within the abdominal cavity does not cause symptoms or ill-effects. During laparoscopy, broken catheters have been found lying freely in the peritoneal cavity without causing a peritoneal reaction, or have been found walled off by mesentery without an inflammatory reaction. On routine postmortem examination, Stein[30] discovered such a catheter in a patient who had had previous peritoneal dialysis. Exploration to retrieve the catheter is unnecessary because laparotomy is more hazardous than leaving the catheter in a severely ill patient. The incidence of catheter loss into the peritoneal cavity has been greatly reduced since the introduction of a design that incorporates a metal disc with a central hole; this not only allows the catheter to pass through the wall but also holds the catheter snugly to the skin of the abdominal wall.[26] The incidence of the accidental penetration of the extraperitoneal space is low varying between 0.5% and 1.3%. In this situation the fluid may become trapped, resulting in poor dialysate drainage.[32,33]

Chronic Peritoneal Dialysis Catheters: General Principles

Chronic peritoneal catheters are constructed from silicone rubber or polyurethane and have one or two Dacron cuffs. Like acute catheters, most chronic catheters have numerous side holes at the distal end of the intraperitoneal part. The silicone rubber or polyurethane surface promotes development of squamous epithelium in the subcutaneous "tunnel" next to the catheter, at the exit site, and within the abdominal wall. The presence of this epithelium increases resistance to bacterial penetration of the tissue near the skin exit and peritoneal entry sites. The Dacron cuffs provoke a local inflammatory response that progresses to form fibrous and granulation tissue within one month. This fibrous tissue serves to fix the catheter cuff in position and to prevent bacterial migration from the skin surface or from the peritoneal cavity (in cases of peritonitis) past the cuff into the subcutaneous tunnel (Table 26–2).

The intraperitoneal segment has multiple 0.5 mm perforations in the 3 to 9 cm terminal part. The variety of catheter lengths permits one to choose an appropriate catheter for every patient size.[1,17,19]

Several modifications have been made to the intraperitoneal sections of various catheters with the aim of obtaining an unrestricted flow of dialysate to and from the peritoneal cavity. This flow is most efficient if the catheter tip lies deep within the pelvis. When the peritoneal cavity is full of dialysate, the mobile parts of the bowel and omentum, although restrained to some extent by their mesenteric attachments, tend to float upon a fluid sump. During run-out, this sump drains under the influence of a positive intra-

Table 26–2 Specifications, Materials, Design of Catheter Types

Catheter	Material	No. of Cuffs	Segment between Cuffs	Intra-Abdominal Segment	Features
Standard Tenckhoff	Silicone	1–2	Usually straight	Straight-coiled	?
Swan-neck arcuate	Silicone	1–2	Arcuate	Straight-coiled	Beads on sites of deep cuff
Missouri	Silicone	1–2	Arcuate 150°–170°	Straight-coiled	Intraperitoneal flange
Toronto-Western	Silicone	2	Straight	Straight	Bead-flange intraperitoneal disc
Moncrief-Popovich	Silicone	2	Arcuate	Straight-coiled	Extra-large external cuff
Ash Advantage	Silicone	2	Straight	T-shaped made of long grooves or	?
Cruz	Polyurethane	2	"Pail handle"	Two 90° angles on different planes	?

abdominal pressure coupled with a syphon effect produced by the difference in height between the catheter tip and the empty dialysis bag. Typically, an outflow rate will begin at 100 to 150 mL/min and then decrease gradually towards the end of the run-out period as the catheter side-holes are occluded by the intra-abdominal contents. A small residual volume is always left behind. The outflow may become obstructed at any time if bowel or omentum surrounds the catheter before drainage is complete. This is more likely if the catheter tip becomes displaced from the pelvis into the upper abdomen. Several modifications have been made to the end of the Tenckhoff catheter, all with the object of stabilizing the tip in the lower quadrant. Thus, catheter design and insertion of the intraperitoneal section is aimed at the prevention of one- or two-way obstruction, dislodgement from the pelvis and wrapping by omentum.

Catheters are soft, flexible, and atraumatic to bowel. Catheters are available with barium impregnated either throughout or as a radiopaque stripe to assist in the radiologic localization of the intra-abdominal section.

In order to eliminate the "shape memory" that tends to extrude the external cuff if a straight catheter is forced in an arcuate tunnel, the "swan-neck catheter" was introduced.[34] This catheter has a permanent bend between the cuffs and is placed with both the internal and external part directed downwards. The intra-abdominal part may be straight or curled. Curled or coil catheters reduce discomfort by minimizing the "jet effect" caused by the high flow of dialysate, and potentially are less prone to migration.[35] Several other catheters, designed to prevent obstruction and migration, for example, the Column disk catheter and the Ash catheter[36] are not in use anymore. The Cruz catheter has a larger inner diameter allowing high flow rates and faster bag exchanges.[37] This catheter, in contrast to most others, is made of polyurethane, a material with greater strength, allowing thinner walls. Unlike silicone, polyurethane is degraded by alcohol and iodine. Repeated exposure of the catheter to these agents may result in crack development.[28,38] The Gore-tex catheter, developed to prevent exit-site infection, did not fulfill this expectation.[39] Likewise, the results of silver-impregnated catheters have been disappointing.[40,41]

Chronic peritoneal catheters and fixed in position, are not restricted to a 3-day period of use as are the uncuffed acute catheters. Usually peritonitis can be treated successfully without catheter removal.[19]

There are no long-term controlled studies that suggest the superiority of any one catheter over all the others. Any new catheter must compete with the long-term experience of the Tenckhoff catheter.

Whatever type of catheter is chosen, at best one can expect a 3-year catheter survival rate of 80%. The minimum acceptable catheter survival rate is regarded as 50% at 12 months.[38] A good survival rate seems to depend more on a good insertion technique and meticulous care than on the catheter device chosen. The implantation should be performed by a competent experienced operator under strict sterile conditions. Exit-site care and attention to detail is of paramount importance.

Usually a chronic catheter is implanted by surgical dissection in the operating room. Effective and safe techniques exist for bedside placement, using guidewire and dilators or peritoneoscopy. When it is anticipated that the patients will need peritoneal dialysis for longer than a few days, a chronic catheter should be placed initially, avoiding the necessity for periodic replacement of acute catheters.

Chronic Peritoneal Dialysis Catheter Types (Figure 26–2)

Straight and Coiled Tenckhoff Catheter

The Tenckhoff catheter was the first catheter to enter widespread clinical use, and it is available from several manufacturers in a range of lengths and cuff positions. It remains the most commonly used and has become a standard for comparison with other catheters. The "chronic catheter" consists of a silicone rubber tube of 2.6 mm internal diameter and 5 mm external diameter bonded to two 1 cm cuffs. The intraperitoneal portion varies in length from 6.5 to 19.5 cm, with numerous 0.5 mm perforations in the terminal 2.5 to 9.5 cm. This wide range of lengths permits one to select an appropriate catheter for patients of every stature. The standard length distal to the superficial cuff is 20 cm, which leaves an external segment of approximately 10 cm; an acute catheter, available with a single cuff in a range of lengths, has now been adopted widely for chronic use and is considered by some clinicians to reduce the incidence of exit-site infections.[42,43]

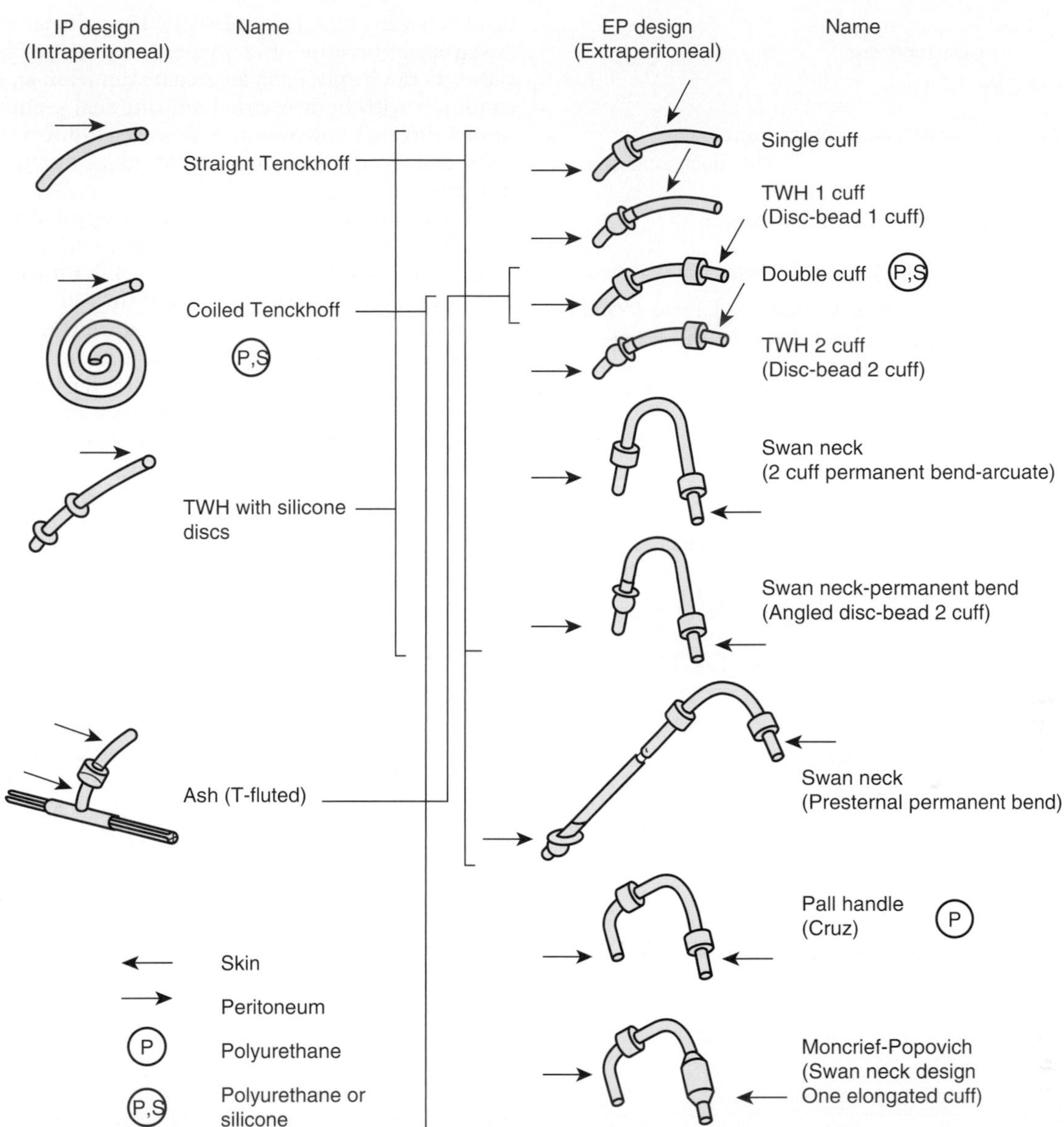

Figure 26–2 Currently available chronic peritoneal catheters showing combinations of intraperitoneal and extraperitoneal designs. Intraperitoneal *(IP)* designs appear on the left, and extraperitoneal *(EP)* designs appear on the right. The letters in circles indicate material of construction: *P* = polyurethane; *P, S* = polyurethane or silicone. (From Gokal R, Khanna R, Krediet R, Nolph K: Textbook of Peritoneal Dialysis, 2nd ed. , Kluwer, 2000.)

The coiled Tenckhoff catheter differs from the straight in having a coiled, 18.5 cm long perforated distal end. As mentioned earlier, the coiled catheter reduces inflow infusion "jet effect" and pressure discomfort. All Tenckhoff catheters have a barium-impregnated radiopaque strip to assist in its radiologic visualization.

The standard Tenckhoff catheter almost always allows easy inflow of fluid. However, effective drainage of the abdomen may be variable and difficult. To minimize outflow obstruction, a number of alternative catheters have been devised (Figures 26–2, 26–3, and 26–4). The curled Tenckhoff catheter provides an increased bulk of tubing to separate the parietal and visceral layers of the peritoneum. Flow into and out of the catheter tip is more protected, and there are more side holes for outflow.[44]

Toronto Western Hospital (TWH) or Oreopoulos-Zellerman Catheter

In an attempt to stabilize the Tenckhoff catheter in the pelvis and to prevent viscera from interfering with fluid drainage, Oreopoulos and colleagues[45] attached two flat silicone rubber discs to the catheter tip. Further developments of this design have become known as the Oreopoulos-Zellerman or Toronto Western Hospital (TWH) catheters. These are available in two forms, TWH1 and TWH2 (Figures 26–2 and 26–3). The former has the dimensions of an adult Tenckhoff catheter with two thin flat Silastic discs 5 cm apart attached to the end of the intra-abdominal section. The latter has an additional modification consisting of a Dacron disc plus a silicone rubber bead

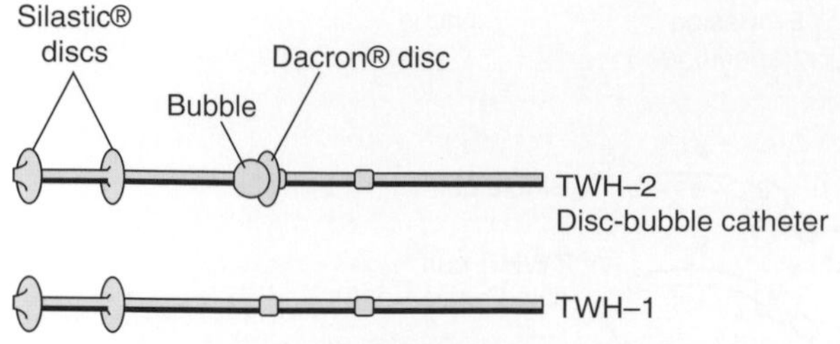

Figure 26–3 The Oreopoulos-Zellerman or Toronto Western Hospital catheter showing the silastic discs. (With kind permission of Kluwer Academic Publishers.)

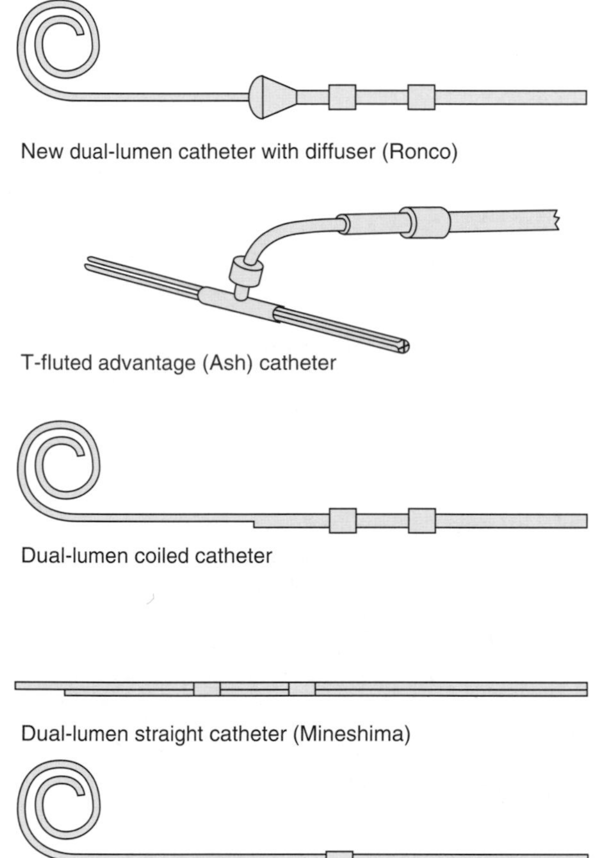

Figure 26–4 Different catheter designs for CFPD.

in series with the preperitoneal cuff. The incorporation of a disc just superficial to the peritoneal closure is an attempt to prevent late dialysate leaks by producing a greater area of peritoneal sealing. The bead adjacent to the disc provides a groove to assist in a tight peritoneal closure. This method of fixing the deep cuff is different from that of the Tenckhoff catheters, in which the deep cuff rests entirely in the rectus muscle.

Swan-Neck Catheters

The swan-neck catheter is now the second most frequently used catheter. Swan-neck catheters feature a permanent bend between cuffs (Figure 26–2)[46] The catheter was dubbed "swan-neck" because of its shape. As a result of this design, catheters can be placed in an arcuate tunnel in an unstressed condition with both external and internal segments of the tunnel directed downward. A downward-directed exit, two cuffs, and an optimal sinus length reduce exit/tunnel infection rates.

A major improvement was in the intercuff shape; the distance between cuffs was shortened from 8.5 cm to 5 cm in swan-neck 2 and to 3 cm in swan-neck 3 catheters, and the bend was increased from 80° to 170° to 180° arc angle. The catheters are supplied with short or long intraperitoneal segments, selected according to patient size and insertion site, to secure the catheter-tip position in the true pelvis.[46,47] Because in several patients infusion pain occurred due to a "jet effect" and/or tip pressure on the peritoneum, the intraperitoneal segment of the catheters, was modified replacing a straight segment with a coiled one (swan-neck coiled). These catheters were introduced in January 1990 and within a month swan-neck straight catheters were phased out.[48]

Swan-Neck Missouri Straight

The swan-neck Missouri catheter has a flange and bead circumferentially surrounding the catheter just below the internal cuff; the flange and bead are slanted approximately 45° relative to the axis of the catheter. The catheters for left and right tunnels are mirror-images of each other. A swan-neck Missouri 2 catheter with a 5 cm intercuff distance is used in average to obese people. The intraperitoneal segment is 21.5 cm long in the swan-neck Missouri 2 long catheters. A swan-neck Missouri 3 catheter with a 3 cm intercuff distance is used in lean to average persons[46,48] (Figure 26–2).

Swan-Neck Missouri Coiled

The intraperitoneal segment in all swan-neck coiled catheters is 34 cm from the bead to the tip of the coil. Swan-neck Missouri 2 coiled catheters with the 5 cm intercuff distance are used in average to obese people. Swan-neck Missouri 3 coiled catheters with 3 cm intercuff distance are used in lean to average persons. The catheters for left and right tunnels are mirror-images of each other.[46] The overall survival times for straight and coiled swan-neck Missouri catheters are not significantly different, but none of the patients experienced infusion or pressure pain with coiled catheters, whereas this complication was seen in several patients, who had catheters with straight intraperitoneal segments.[48] Swan-neck catheters are also available in smaller sizes for children and infants.[49]

Pail-Handle (Cruz) Catheter

This catheter has two right-angle bends: one to direct the IP portion parallel to the parietal peritoneum and one to direct the subcutaneous portion downward toward the skin exit site. It is available only in polyurethane. Its clinical benefits have not been well defined. Its larger internal diameter and position of the coil near the parietal peritoneum allows more rapid outflow than standard silicone catheters, and its shape facilitates placement in obese patients (see Figure 26–2).

Presternal Swan-Neck Peritoneal Catheter

The presternal peritoneal dialysis catheter is composed of two flexible (silicon rubber) tubes, which are connected end-to-end at the time of implantation. The implanted abdominal tube constitutes the intraperitoneal catheter segment and a part of the intramural segment (Figure 26–2). The distal end of the abdominal tube located in the peritoneal cavity is coiled and the central bore with multiple small side perforations that provides for fluid delivery into and drainage from the peritoneal cavity. The proximal end of the abdominal tube carries a polyester cuff to be located in the rectus muscle also the tubing is provided with a flange circumferentially surrounding the tubing just below the cuff and a bead adjacent to the flange. As in the swan-neck Missouri catheter, the flange and bead are slanted at an angle of about 45°. During implantation, the proximal part of the abdominal tube is trimmed to the desired length. After implantation, the proximal end of the abdominal tube extends a few centimeters from the cuff and is provided with a connector made of titanium. The connector is coupled to the distal part of the thoracic tube at the time of implantation. The thoracic tube constitutes the remaining part of the intramural segment and the external catheter segment. The distal-end bore of the thoracic tube communicates with the proximal-end bore of the abdominal tube through the titanium connector. The tube carries two porous cuffs: a superficial cuff and a middle or central cuff. The tube between the cuffs has a permanently bent section (swan-neck feature) defining an arc angle of 180°. Both tubes have a radiopaque barium stripe that helps achieve proper alignment of the tubes during implantation. The stripe is also useful during insertion and postimplantation care, facilitating recognition of catheter twisting. The distal part of the thoracic tube is trimmed to the desired length during implantation.[50,51]

The swan-neck presternal catheter is available for children and infants. Tubing diameter is smaller for pediatric patients.[52]

Moncrief-Popovich Catheter and Implantation Technique

Moncrief and Popovich designed their new catheter, made of silicone rubber, with several important structural changes that differ from Tenckhoff catheter.[50] The changes and the reasons for the changes are as follows: (1) a coiled internal segment, (2) an arcuate bend in the subcutaneous segment similar to the swan-neck Missouri catheter designed by Twardowski and colleagues,[45] and (3) two Dacron cuffs. The external Dacron cuff, however, is elongated to 2.5 cm, and the ends of the cuff are tapered longer than the internal one.

This catheter is similar to the standard swan-neck Tenckhoff, except that the external cuff is much longer. When the catheter is first implanted with 1.000 Units of heparin instilled, the external segment is buried subcutaneously (Initially there is no exit site) for a period of 4 to 8 weeks or longer to allow tissue ingrowth into the external cuff in a sterile environment. Subsequently, a small incision is made in the skin through which the external segment of the catheter is brought out.[52]

Ash (Advantage) Catheter

The Advantage catheter contains a straight portion that is held adjacent to the parietal peritoneum assuring a stable position, without extrusion of the deep cuff or exit site erosion.[53] The intraperitoneal portion contains a short, perpendicular cylinder connected to two limbs with external grooves (flutes) to carry fluid into the catheter from the upper and lower abdomen. The catheter may be placed by a dissective or a peritoneoscopic technique. Due to the apposition of the grooved portion of this catheter against the parietal peritoneum and the T-shape of the catheter, the deep cuff of this catheter is "fixed" in position, and outward migration of the catheter is impossible. Following placement of this catheter in 18 patients, with up to 4 years of follow-up, no catheter developed exit site erosion, exit infection pericatheter hernia, or pericatheter leaks[54] (Figures 26–2 and 26–4).

Catheters Designed for Continuous Flow Peritoneal Dialysis (CFPD)

In 1965 James Shinaberger[55] reported a series of patients treated with CFPD. He used two peritoneal catheters inserted acutely at opposite ends of the peritoneal cavity, 3 L of sterile intraperitoneal dialysate regenerated by an external twin-coil dialyzer in 100 L of dialysate. Dialysate flow rates ranged from 120 to 300 mL/min. Clearances of urea varied from 46 to as high as 125 mL/min! Over the next 2 decades, other groups attempted to reproduce this technique and met with mixed success.[56-62] Ash[63] has designed a catheter with a T-shape configuration in order to maximally separate the tips of the two lumens.[64] This catheter offers promise in CFPD but has not yet been tested clinically (Figure 26–4).[65]

Ronco and colleagues[66] designed a novel catheter for CFPD equipped with a thin-walled silicone diffuser used to gently infuse the inflow dialysate into the peritoneum (Figure 26–4). The holes on the round-tapered diffuser are positioned to allow dialysate to perpendicularly exit 360° from the diffuser, thereby reducing trauma to the peritoneal walls and allowing the dialysate to mix into the peritoneum. The fluid is then drained through the second lumen, whose tip is positioned in the lower pelvis.

CRITICAL COMPARISON OF CATHETER DESIGN

Facing so many different options, which catheter should one choose? Early studies favored the double-cuff over the single-cuff Tenckhoff catheters, because they gave better catheter survival, longer time to the first peritonitis episode, and fewer exit-site infections. Previous ISPD consensus opinion also supported the choice of double-cuffed Tenckhoff catheters. Searching for evidence-based, level A studies, Lewis and colleagues[67] carried out a prospective controlled, randomized study that confirmed such benefits. However, Eklund and colleagues[68] found no difference in the number of peritonitis episodes, exit-site infections, or in catheter survival between single- and double-cuff Tenckhoff catheters[67-72, 96-100] (Table 26–3).

A controversy over coiled or straight catheters also justified some controlled, randomized studies. Theoretically, the coiled catheter would offer less infusion/pressure pain, better flow, less catheter migration, and omental wrapping. A pair of studies gave no conclusive answers, with inconsistent results.[69,70]

Other variations of the intraperitoneal portion of the catheter, such as silicone discs perpendicular to the catheter

Table 26–3 Randomized, Controlled Studies on Catheter Type and Implantation Methodology

Catheter Type	Group (first author)	Patients (n)	Outcome
Double vs. single-cuff	Lewis, 1997[67]	40 (pediatric)	More peritonitis-related catheter loss in single-cuff catheters
	Eklund, 1997[68]	60	Similar peritonitis/exit-site rate and survival
Coil vs. straight	Nielsen, 1995[69]	72	Better survival and fewer mechanical complications
	Akyol, 1990[70]	39	Similar outcomes
Swan-neck vs. Tenckhoff	Lye, 1996[71]	40	Fewer exit-site infections, less catheter-tip migration; similar survival
	Eklund, 1995[72]	40	Similar outcomes
Surgical vs. peritoneoscopic implantation	Cadallah, 1999[96]	148	Less peritonitis, less leakage, better survival
	Tsimoyiannis, 2000[97]	50	No leak or tip migration with peritoneoscopy
	Wright, 1999[98]	50	Similar outcomes
Moncrief technique vs. conventional	Park, 1998[99]	60	Less catheter-related peritonitis, similar survival
	Dasgupta, 1998[100]	39	Fewer exit-site infections, better catheter survival

(Toronto-Western-Hospital catheter) designed to avoid catheter-tip migration, and T-fluted catheters that promised better flow and also less migration, have not shown any consistent advantage over the standard Tenckhoff. Concerning the subcutaneous pathway, some have reported fewer exit-site/tunnel infections with the permanently bent catheters such as the swan-neck and presternal swan-neck catheter. Although this benefit seems promising, several studies[71,72] found no difference in catheter survival between the swan-neck and the straight Tenckhoff catheters. Therefore, the choice of catheter should be based on the experience of the centers.

Catheters with deep cuffs or larger IP portions, such as the Toronto Western and Missouri models, require surgical dissection for placement, whereas standard Tenckhoff-type catheters and the T-fluted catheter can be placed blindly or peritoneoscopically. The Toronto Western catheter, by design, has increased attachment to the abdominal wall, and thus is more difficult to remove. Preliminary data on the new Moncrief-Popovich catheter and technique suggest a reduced incidence of peritonitis but no decrease in exit-site infection.

It was hoped that polyurethane, because it is a stronger and smoother material than silicone, would reduce the formation of biofilm. However, it has not been shown that polyurethane catheters have a lower incidence of recurrent peritonitis, outflow obstruction, or mechanical failure; indeed, they may be more susceptible to damage by chemicals, such as alcohol and polyethylene glycol, and to disruption of the bond between the catheter and its cuffs.

Catheter selection is difficult for patients in high risk for early catheter failure, including those who are known to have intra-abdominal adhesions, who may have had previous difficulties with catheters, or who may be obese with a lax abdominal musculature.

CHRONIC CATHETER-PLACEMENT PROCEDURES

The few absolute surgical contraindications to CAPD, particularly when considering the anatomy of the abdominal wall or previous abdominal procedures within it, are listed in Table 26–4. Relative contraindications include previous extensive pelvic or low abdominal surgery, where it is anticipated that much of the infracolic compartment will be involved by adhesions. In such patients, who are otherwise good candidates for treatment by CAPD, it may be advantageous to perform a small laparotomy to assess the peritoneal cavity or to undertake peritoneoscopy, which is also useful in assessing complications during CAPD.[73] Wu and colleagues[74] suggested that extensive colonic diverticulosis may be a relative contraindication because, in the elderly, it is related to a high mortality from diverticular perforations.

Patient Assessment

Complications may arise from the presence of a hernia that should be identified at the initial patient assessment. This may be repaired in one procedure with catheter insertion. Where hernia defects are large, any use of the catheter should be delayed until a sound surgical repair has been carried out.

Table 26–4 Surgical Contraindications to CAPD

Absolute Contraindications

1. Absence of anterior abdominal wall? prune belly syndrome
2. Severe peritoneal adhesions
3. Sclerosing peritonitis
4. Inflammatory bowel disease
5. Sepsis of anterior abdominal wall
6. Large unrepairable herniae of abdominal wall

Relative Contraindications to CAPD

Pleuroperitoneal leak	Blindness
Low-back problems	Crippling arthritis
Polycystic kidneys	Amputations
Ileostomy	Poor motivation
Colostomy	Overt psychosis
Nephrostomy	Severe pulmonary impairment
Obesity	Hyperlipidemia

Elderly patients have an increased incidence of cholelithiasis and diverticulosis of the colon; The latter is more common in patents with polycystic disease.[75] While both of these conditions may remain asymptomatic during CAPD, an episode of acute cholecystitis or diverticulitis may well mimic an episode of primary peritonitis. When considering the differential diagnosis of peritonitis, one should assess patients over the age of 60 years for these conditions. This can be performed conveniently by ultrasound and flexible sigmoidoscopy. In patients with proven diverticular disease, constipation should be prevented by the adoption of a high residue diet.

Polycystic kidneys may appear to occupy considerable space in the peritoneal cavity, however, in practice this usually does not limit the volume of fluid exchanges. Brown and colleagues[76] and Khanna and colleagues[77] have drawn attention to the symptomatic exacerbation of peripheral vascular disease in patients starting CAPD. Thus, one should consider doing corrective vascular surgery or angioplasty on patients with symptoms of arterial disease before starting CAPD.

Preparation for Catheter Insertion

Before proceeding with catheter insertion, one should demonstrate the technique to the patient, who should be familiar with the catheter as well as with the various connections and lines that will be used. It is important to determine with the patient's own preference concerning the catheter exit site, which should be above or below the belt line, easily accessible and in a direct line of sight. Obviously, skin creases should be avoided, and it is wise to mark the preferred site for easy reference in the operating theater. Thin individuals may wish to avoid a midline insertion, where the cuff can cause discomfort, particularly during sexual activity.[78]

The abdominal wall hair should be clipped from the xiphisternum to the symphysis pubis. The bowel should be empty before catheter insertion and this may be assisted by the administration of an enema. Also, the patient should be asked to empty the bladder as completely as possible. The choice of anesthesia may be dictated by the patient's age, medical condition, or the likely extent of the surgical dissection. In adults who have not had previous abdominal surgery, either local or general anesthesia is acceptable and the patient's preference can be noted. Some discomfort is inevitable during insertion under local anesthesia, but this can be minimized by the administration of a hypnotic or analgesic agent before operation. However, the patient must be informed of what to expect, particularly as one needs some co-operation during certain parts of the procedure. An open insertion is the procedure of choice in patients who previously have undergone a low abdominal procedure.[1,18,19]

Catheters should be inserted by trained personnel-using a strict aseptic technique. Although closed medical insertion can be accomplished at the bedside, access and lighting are often less than ideal. It is strongly recommended that all catheters are inserted under operating theater conditions, where diathermy, suction, and good lighting are available.

Chronic Catheters-Placement Procedures

There are four options for placement or chronic peritoneal catheters: (1) surgical placement by dissection, (2) blind placement using the Tenckhoff trocar, (3) blind placement using a guidewire, and (4) minitrocar placement using peritoneoscopy. The larger catheters, such as the Toronto Western and Missouri models, must be placed surgically. Straight and curled Tenckhoff catheters, with or without a swan-neck section, may be placed by any technique.[17]

Immediately before implantation, the catheter is removed from the sterile peel pack and immersed in sterile saline. Dacron cuffs and the Dacron[79] flange are gently squeezed to remove air.[46] Thoroughly wetted cuffs provide markedly better tissue ingrowth compared to unwetted, air-containing cuffs.[31,80]

Surgical Implantation

This, the most popular method for placement of chronic peritoneal catheters, begins with either extensive local anesthesia or light general anesthesia. There are two general approaches: the lateral and the paramedian. Either can be used with any of the catheters, although usually Toronto Western and Missouri catheters are placed using the paramedian technique.

General anesthesia is avoided, if possible, because it predisposes patients to vomiting and constipation and requires voluntary coughing during the postoperative period as a part of pulmonary atelectasis prevention; coughing, vomiting, and straining markedly increase infra-abdominal pressures and predispose patients to abdominal leaks.[81]

A 3- to 4-cm transverse incision is made through the skin and the subcutaneous tissue. The peritoneum is identified, lifted, and opened using a 1- to 2-cm incision. The space between the anterior abdominal wall and the mass of bowel and omentum is identified.

The catheter is threaded on a long, blunt stiffening stylet. About 1 cm of catheter is left beyond the tip of the stylet to protect the bowel. The edges of the opening are lifted. The catheter is inserted through the opening and introduced into the opposite deep pelvis if there is no resistance. The patient may feel some pressure on the bladder or rectum. When the catheter with stylet is about half to three-quarters inserted, the stylet is removed and the catheter continues to be pushed into the pelvis.[31]

After proper positioning of the catheter tip, the peritoneum is closed tightly around the catheter below the level of the deep cuff using a running lock stitch. The incidence of subsequent leakage will depend largely on the care and skill used to fashion this suture line.

The skin exit site must be selected. The location can be estimated by laying the outer part of the catheter over the skin, accommodating for a V bend to direct the exit toward the patient's feet.

The skin exit site should be exactly 2 cm from the superficial cuff to allow proper epithelialization of the tract down toward this cuff.

A tunneling tool is then passed subcutaneously from below the primary incision to the skin exit site. The skin is nicked over the tool to create the exit site, and the catheter is pulled through the tunnel by attachment to the tunneling tool.

Seldinger (Guidewire) and Peel-Away Sheath

This technique may be used to insert a straight and coiled Tenckhoff catheters as well as a swan-neck Tenckhoff straight and coiled catheters. The pre-insertion patient preparation is similar to that described for rigid catheter insertion. The procedure may be done with[82] or without[83-86] prefilling the abdomen with dialysis solution. Prefilling of the abdomen is accomplished through a temporary peritoneal catheter.[31]

In the "dry" method a 2-cm incision is made and the "dry" abdomen is entered with an l8-gauge needle, for example, the Verres needle as used for laparoscopy. A guidewire is passed through the needle and the needle is withdrawn. The introducer (dilator) with sheath is passed over the guidewire. The Tenckhoff or swan-neck Tenckhoff catheter, stiffened by a partially inserted blunt stiffening stylet, is then directed down into the sheath.[85,86] As the cuff advances, the sheath is split by pulling tabs on its opposing sides. By further splitting and retraction, the sheath is removed from its position around the catheter. The subcutaneous tunnel is then created as in surgical placement. With this technique, the incidence of early leaks is very low. However, it has the risk of viscus perforation and improper placement of catheter.

Peritoneoscopic Technique

Ash[53,87] developed the use of peritoneoscopy for peritoneal catheter placement. Tenckhoff and Swan-neck Tenckhoff (straight and coiled) catheters may be implanted with this technique. Like blind insertion, it is performed through a single abdominal puncture. No fluid is instilled before insertion of the cannula and the trocar into the abdomen through the medial or lateral border of the rectus. The trocar is removed, and the scope is inserted through the cannula. After assuring the intraperitoneal location by observing motion of glistening surfaces, the scope is removed and 600 cm^3 of air placed in the peritoneal cavity with the patient in the Trendelenburg position. The scope is reinserted, and, during continuous observation, scope, quill, and cannula are advanced into the clearest space and most open direction between the parietal and visceral peritoneum. Following this, the scope and cannula are removed and the Quill catheter guide is left in place. The next step involves the dilation of the Quill and musculature to approximately 0.5 cm. The catheter follows the path previously viewed by the peritoneoscope as directed by the Quill guide. As long as the Quill guide stays in position, the catheter will advance into the desired place. The catheter is advanced on a stylet and is "dilating" its way until the cuff arrives and stops at the muscular layer. Placing the cuff in the musculature can be accomplished using a pair of hemostats advancing the cuff within the Quill guide. Thereafter, the Quill guide is removed, hydraulic function of the catheter checked, the tunnel made subcutaneously using a trocar, and the catheter brought out through the exit site, similar to the surgical insertion technique.[35,88,89]

Its originator reported excellent results with this technique. More recently Copley and colleagues[90] reported 1183 patient-months experience with 135 double-cuff, swan-neck, coiled catheters inserted peritoneoscopically over a 40-month period. Actuarial life-table analysis showed that, at the end of the 40-month follow-up, 62% of the catheters were expected to survive. Twenty-eight patients (20.6%) experienced catheter-related infections and there were five leaks (3.7%). Mechanical complications were recorded in 10 patients (7.4%) due to catheter migration (9 patients) and to preperitoneal placement (1 patient).

Blind Placement Using the Tenckhoff Trocar (Figure 26–5)

This method is still used to place straight and curved Tenckhoff catheters, although less frequently, than are other methods.[19]

- A 2- to 3-cm skin incision is made and blunt dissection carried out down to the fascia. A plastic tube or needle is inserted in the peritoneal cavity, which is then filled with dialysis solution as for acute catheter placement. The plastic tube is removed.
- The patient is asked to tense the abdomen, and the abdominal wall is penetrated in a perpendicular direction using the Tenckhoff trocar. This 6-mm–diameter trocar is surrounded by two half-cylinders which, in turn, are surrounded by an

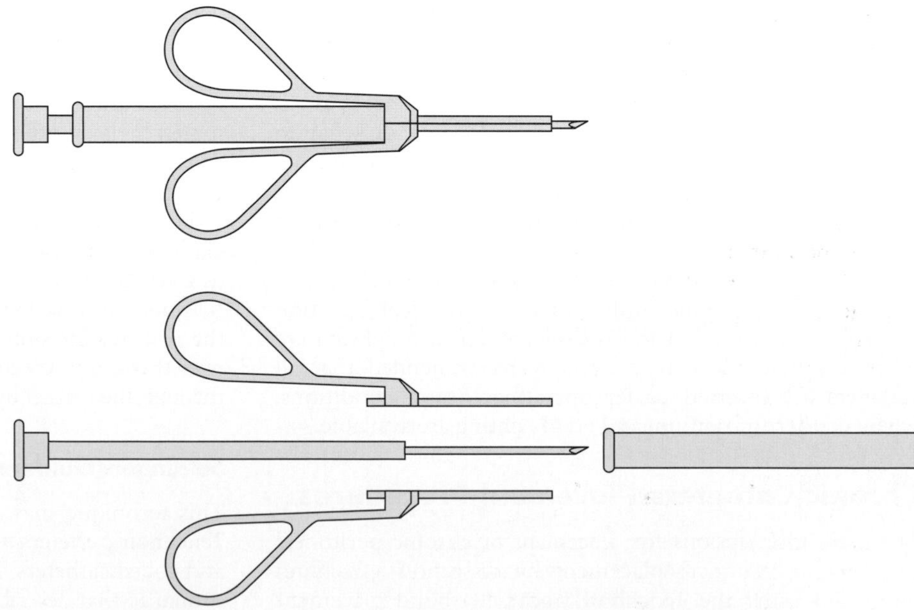

Figure 26–5 The Tenckhoff catheter introducer, fully assembled *(above)* and with parts separated *(below)*. (From Khanna R, Nolph K, Oreopoulos DG (eds): Essentials of Peritoneal Dialysis, Dordrecht, the Netherlands, Kluwer, 1993, p 57.)

external housing. After insertion of the entire device, the trocar is removed, leaving the half-cylinders in place within the housing. Peritoneal fluid should now well up into the housing.

- An obturator is inserted into the cuffed peritoneal catheter to reinforce it, stopping 2 to 3 cm short of the tip, leaving the catheter with a soft, pliable, leading end. The housing is aimed caudad at the left lower quadrant, and the stiffened catheter is inserted through the housing into the abdomen until the cuff comes to rest against the narrowed "shoulder" of the half-cylinders. The cuff is now near the outer surface of the abdominal wall.
- The housing and half-cylinders are removed carefully from around the cuff and catheter, leaving the cuff next to the abdominal wall on the outer rectus sheath.
- Creation of the subcutaneous tunnel and exit site then proceeds as for surgical implantation.[17,31]

Procedure for Placement of the T-Fluted Catheter

The initial placement steps are the same as for Tenckhoff catheters, up to the step where the dilators are removed and the dilated plastic catheter guide is left in place. Then the T-fluted catheter, with the two limbs folded forward, is inserted into a special spiral-shaped guide that also incorporates a steel tube with wings to aid in cuff implantation.

This catheter may be placed surgically, laparoscopically, or peritoneoscopically. Both limbs fold forward to fit the catheter within a large Quill guide, which can then be advanced through a smaller Quill guide placed peritoneoscopically or by blind puncture.[3,17]

External Cuff Extrusion

The main cause of cuff extrusion is placement of the external segment of the catheter in any shape other than its natural design with the subcutaneous cuff too close to the exit. If the cuff is not infected it should be left alone; however, the cuff usually becomes infected during extrusion and requires systemic antibiotics or even surgical intervention. If there is no peritonitis or deep cuff infection, the catheter may be saved, at least for some time, by shaving off the infected cuff.[91] Ultrasound examination of the tunnel is valuable in detecting collections around the catheter in the tunnel. Cuff infection responds to therapy slowly, if at all, and a complete cure is unlikely. Local care has to be aggressive. Deroofing the sinus tract and cuff shaving have been practiced with some success.[92] Others find these measures ineffective.[93] Catheter replacement and removal can be done in one step if there is no active peritonitis.

Comparison of Various Implantation Techniques

Although each catheter and placement technique has had its advocates, comparative clinical trials have been few and limited in scope and seldom have employed randomized controls (Table 26–3).

Maher and colleagues[94] compared, retrospectively, two types of Tenckhoff catheter insertion, the guidewire method and the surgical method. Poor drainage requiring catheter removal was more common with catheters inserted by the guidewire (6/23 vs. 1/32). Dialysate leakage requiring temporary cessation of dialysis was seen less often with catheters inserted with the guidewire (7/21 vs. 16/32) surgical method. Dialysate leakage in the guidewire group was usually subcutaneous into the scrotum or abdominal wall (5/7 patients), while leakage was through the incision in the group. No episodes of catheter-related infection were seen in either group.

Ash[53] did a literature review of the frequency of complications according to the technique of catheter placement. Catheters placed peritoneoscopically had the lowest incidence of all complications—6%, 2%, and 1%—for infection, outflow obstruction, and leak, respectively. Blind placement of double-cuff Tenckhoff catheters resulted in a higher average complication rate—16%, 22%, and 10%—as did surgical placement, 25%, 17% and 13%, although some studies of both of these techniques reported much better success.[95] For the curled, double-cuff Tenckhoff catheter, peritoneoscopic placement again seemed to have a lower complication rate than blind or surgical placement. However, only about 10% of all centers placed catheters peritoneoscopically, and those centers had extensive experience.

Cuffs

In a retrospective analysis, Twardowski and colleagues[34] observed that the rates of exit-site infection were similar for single- and double-cuff catheters (55% vs. 46%, respectively), but that the infections with single-cuff catheters were more resistant to treatment as estimated by the duration of treatment for each cuff type (5.7% vs. 1.6%).

Smith[101] compared the incidence of peritonitis, exit-site infection, and catheter tunnel infection in relation to the number of PD catheter cuffs. Tunnel infections were considerably less frequent with double-cuff catheters than with single-cuff catheters (one episode per 60.45 vs. 24.2 patient-months). Peritonitis and exit-site infections were similar for the two types of catheters.

The U.S. National CAPD Registry[102] reported a significant difference in length of catheter survival with respect to cuff types, for example, catheters using a single cuff located in the deep fascia had a shorter survival than double-cuff catheters where the cuff is located in the subcutaneous tissue (relative risk = 1.4). They found no difference with respect to survival between catheters with a double cuff versus those with a subcutaneously placed single cuff. Exit-site infections were more frequent in patients using a single, subcutaneously placed cuff (13%) than in patients using a double cuff (7%).

In a prospective study, Piraino and colleagues[103] investigated the location of the exit site in relationship to the belt line as a risk factor for catheter function and loss. The percentage of catheters that became infected and required removal was the same for catheters exiting above, below, or on the belt line, suggesting that exit-site location is not an important determinant of infection rate or catheter outcome.

Postoperative Use of Peritoneal Dialysis Catheters

The aim of the postoperative dialysis regimen should be to minimize the risk of fluid leak. However, patients may come to catheter insertion in a variety of clinical states, some having an urgent need for dialysis. In some, the procedure may be wholly elective, when it is performed well before dialysis is necessary and when there is no immediate reason to use the catheter. Then sufficient time can be taken for adequate wound healing and cuff fibrosis before the institution of peritoneal dialysis. These patients rarely have trouble with immediate catheter use.

Conversely, a number of patients will present in acute or chronic renal failure, who are strong candidates for peritoneal dialysis but who need dialysis immediately after catheter insertion. Several groups[104,105] have considered the use of 2 L fluid cycles immediately after operation in these patients that is associated with an unacceptable incidence of postoperative fluid leakage, particularly in elderly patients who have poor tissues. Also, it occurs more frequently after open insertion. All patients require some form of break in regimen, and opinion varies widely as to how this is best achieved. Most units have developed their own particular schedules.

Afterward the insertion on the patient is attached to a cycler to perform additional exchanges. Each liter of dialysis solution contains 1000 units of heparin. One-half or 1 L volumes of dialysis solutions are used for the first supine peritoneal dialysis. Usual cycler settings are: 10 min fill time, 0 min dwell, and 12 min outflow. In spite of clear dialysate in the first post-implantation washout, the dialysate usually is blood-tinged during the first cycler exchange. No-dwell exchanges are continued until the dialysate is clear. If immediate peritoneal dialysis is needed, the patient continues on a cycler in the strict supine position with dwell time prolonged to 30 to 40 min. **Instead of using the cycler, exchanges can be done manually if trained nurses are available.** In addition, the patient may be maintained on hemodialysis using the temporary access before peritoneal dialysis training can be started, or may require hemodialysis because of catheter malfunction.

Prophylactic Antimicrobial Drugs

It has been recorded that early colonization at the exit-site has a detrimental effect on the quality of healing and catheter-related infections complications.[106,107]

The use of prophylactic antibiotics at the time of PD-catheter insertion is controversial. The recent 1998 ISPD guidelines state that it is prudent to use antibiotics and suggest the use of antistaphylococcal antibiotics.[108] Epidemiologic data show that gram positive bacilli and especially *Staphylococcus aureus* is the most common cause of exit-site infection, difficult to treat, and if results in peritonitis is likely to lead to significant morbidity and catheter loss. Regarding antibiotic prophylaxis after PD catheter placement, there have been three randomized, prospective trials. Two showed a benefit using cefuroxime (1.5 gr IV, 250 mg IP) or gentamycin (1.5 mg/Kgr/IV).[109,110]

In both cases the incidence of peritonitis was lower ($p < .001$) in the 1st month after insertion. In contrast, Lye and colleagues[100] found no benefit using gentamicin (80 mg IV) and cephazolin (500 mf IP). Although staphylococcal infections predominate in those untreated, gram-negative infections have also been reported.[109-112] Thus, although the ISPD recommendation is for an antistaphylococcal antibiotic, it seems more prudent to use an antibiotic that also has gram-negative coverage (e.g., cephazolin). During the last 10 years there have been several studies on the use of local antibiotics mupirocin applied to the exit-site to prevent *Staph. aureus* infections. Bernardini and colleagues[112] (1995), Thodis and colleagues[113] (1998), Casey and colleagues[114] (2000), Utley and colleagues[115] (2001), and Boer and colleagues[116] (2002) found that applying mupirocin at the exit-site as local care, recorded a significant decrease in *Staph. aureus* catheter-related infections (exit-site, tunnel infections, and peritonitis).

Catheter Break-In and Catheter Care

The break-in period for a peritoneal catheter is the time between catheter insertion and routine catheter use. During this period, every effort is made to avoid leakage of fluid around the new catheter.[1,3,117]

Because of the risks of leakage, wound dehiscence, and hernia formation, a break-in period of at least 2 weeks is recommended after catheter insertion. In practice, the time allocated for break-in varies because the urgency for peritoneal dialysis differs from patient to patient. Short break-in periods are associated with increased risks of leakage. Straining during defecation or coughing should be minimized if possible, because both increase intra-abdominal pressure and therefore the chance of herniation and leakage. If one encounters difficulty with inflow, first try simple interventions, including bowel stimulation, clot dislodgement, and brisk ambulation. Often catheter obstruction soon after implantation is due to a clot or fibrin plugs and may respond to flushing. If unsuccessful, heparin or a thrombolytic agent (tissue plasminogen activator or streptokinase) can be used. In countries where Urokinase is not available (United States), the imminent availability of recombinant urokinase is anticipated.

Acute Catheters

In situations requiring acute dialysis, often the patient already is confined to bed and dialysis can begin immediately. Initially, exchange volumes of 500 mL, with 1- to 2-hr dwells, should be used, increasing to exchanges to 1000 mL after the first four exchanges. Unless leakage or discomfort occurs, the volume may be further increased after day 1 or 2. Patients may experience restriction of diaphragmatic excursions and respiratory distress if the volume of exchanges is increased too rapidly, and therefore respiratory function should be assessed periodically, especially in the intensive-care setting.[17,18]

Chronic Catheters

For patients requiring chronic dialysis, the planning can be done over a period of a few weeks. If necessary, intermittent peritoneal dialysis may be started after the initial few days with low volumes (500 to 1000 mL). Exchange volumes may be increased in two to three dialysis sessions to 2000 mL. The patient should remain supine for most of the dialysis period, and activity during dialysis must be restricted. In practice on intermittent peritoneal dialysis schedule of 20 h per session, two or three times a week, during a 2-week period, is sufficient to allow wound healing. Alternatively, symptoms can be managed with regular hemodialysis. In the ideal situation, the catheter should be inserted 4 to 6 weeks before use. Flushes with 1000 mL of 1.5% dextrose solution and 250 units of heparin should be done at time of insertion, then on return to the nursing unit, and again at 24 hours. **Flushing should be**

continued at weekly intervals to maintain catheter patency until dialysis is commenced. Data from the Moncrief-Popovich technique, in which the catheter remains buried without flushing for some weeks, suggest that flushing at weekly intervals may not always be necessary, but to date no trials have been done to answer this question.[31,44]

COMPLICATIONS OF CATHETER INSERTION

Hemorrhage

Intraperitoneal hemorrhage may arise from trauma to omental or mesenteric vessels while manipulating the catheter tip into the pelvis. During a closed insertion, this is usually recognized as heavy bloodstaining of the draining fluid. If a significant hemorrhage is obvious, it is safer to create adequate access to obtain hemostasis and to ensure bowel viability. This situation is easier to deal with during an open insertion, when the patient may already be under general anesthesia or at least it is available. Usually the site of trauma is known and bleeding can be controlled once with a small extension to the wound with adequate retraction. Once the peritoneal cavity is cleared of clot by lavage and suction, catheter insertion can continue. Occasionally intraperitoneal bleeding may occur from a vessel severed during the division of adhesions or omentectomy.

A significant extraperitoneal bleed may occur from the inferior epigastric vessels. If it is difficult to control the bleeding, these vessels should be underrun with a ligature above and below the site of trauma.[3,31,118]

Hemorrhage may occur or be recognized only postoperatively after catheter insertion. If the bleeding is intraperitoneal, it will arise from one of the sources earlier mentioned and present with bloodstaining of the dialysate effluent. If it is slight and the patient can be supported with a zero or minimal blood transfusion, conservative management is indicated. This policy should not be pursued in the presence of heavy bloodstaining clots or a significant transfusion requirement, in which case the patient should be returned to operating theater.

Extraperitoneal bleeding may be obvious with a leak of blood from the wound edge or an enlarging hematoma there. A skin edge bleed can be controlled with additional sutures under local anesthesia. A large wound hematoma should be explored and the source of bleeding arrested. The hematoma needs to be evacuated to prevent postoperative discomfort plus the risk of wound sepsis.

Perforated Viscus

Intra-abdominal perforation is a well recognized hazard of the closed insertion of intermittent PD catheters.[119] A similar incidence (1% or 2%) might be expected using the closed insertion technique for Tenckhoff catheters. The most common injuries appear to be bowel perforation[120] and bladder laceration/perforation,[121] the latter a particular risk in the presence of chronic urinary outflow obstruction. If in doubt about the bladder, it is wise to insert a catheter before the insertion. Perforation of viscera by erosion of the peritoneal catheter is well recognized but rare.[122] This complication is facilitated by peritonitis, an empty peritoneal cavity, the use of steroids, or the presence of vasculitis.[123]

Urine in the peritoneal cavity, because it is irritating, may give rise to the signs of peritonitis. A small laceration will close spontaneously if the bladder is drained with a urethral catheter. A large laceration should be repaired formally and the bladder drained. If this complication is recognized during the insertion procedure, it is probably best to delay peritoneal catheter insertion because of the risk of contamination of the catheter by organisms from the bladder.

The risk of bowel perforation is higher in patients with intra-abdominal adhesions from previous surgery or peritonitis. The most common mechanism of injury is advancement of the catheter against resistance into a bowel loop that has been fixed in the peritoneal cavity by adhesions. However, damage may occur at any of several stages during catheter insertion, and it may be recognized during or after the procedure.[119,122]

It is also possible to pass the peritoneal catheter into or through the lumen of the bowel. This may be recognized after insertion when dilute bowel content is returned with the dialysis run-out. After catheter insertion, perforation can present in a variety of ways. The patient, without developing abdominal signs, may pass large volumes of dialysate per rectum. Alternatively, the run-out may be cloudy and contain mixed bacterial organisms with the signs of a mixed-organism peritonitis. Several courses of action are possible. In the absence of clinical signs and in the hope of avoiding a laparotomy, the catheter may be left on free drainage for 7 to 10 days to allow an intraperitoneal track to form. Then it may be withdrawn and the peritoneum allowed to settle for a further 3 weeks before attempting reinsertion of the catheter. In established peritonitis, laparotomy should be done immediately to remove the catheter and repair the bowel. This course of action may also become necessary if conservative management fails. As a general guide, conservative management is more likely to succeed if the laceration is small or if the small bowel is involved rather than the large bowel. Clinical assessment is the most useful guide to the management of bowel perforation.

Catheter-Related Complications

Fluid Leak

Pericatheter leakage, which is most frequent immediately after insertion, is seen in 7% to 24% of patients.[122] Most postoperative catheter leakage can be prevented by observing a break-in period of about 2 weeks, during which the wound can heal and ingrowth of fibrous tissue can anchor the Dacron cuffs. When peritoneal dialysis is started without a break-in period, we recommend a reduction of the dialysate volume (500–1000 mL in adults) for the initial period. Usually leakage can be managed by cessation of peritoneal dialysis for about 2 weeks.[1,26,124,125]

Early fluid leak is defined as the appearance of dialysate through the catheter insertion wound or from the catheter exit site after insertion during the break-in period. In contrast, later leaks present after a period of successful CAPD. In addition to the signs described, they may present as an edematous swelling of the lower abdominal wall without fluid appearing at the skin surface. In both cases the leak arises from the peritoneal closure around the catheter.[3,19]

Some series have divided leaks into early and late. Ponce and colleagues[126] reported an overall incidence of 27% with 9 out of 10 being early leaks, and Francis and colleagues[127] reported an overall incidence of 25% with 14 out of 31 being early leaks.

The type of catheter and mode of insertion appear to have a profound influence on the incidence of this complication. Other factors that may be important (Table 26–5) include the strength of tissues around the closure site and the speed with which healing progresses. Olcott and colleagues[128] reported that 75% of their patients who developed a dialysate leak were taking steroids. Ponce and colleagues[126] suggested that this complication was more common among patients older than 60 years of age, females, and in second or subsequent catheter insertions. The type of break-in regimen also helps determine the early leak rate. Khanna and colleagues[104] suggested that, to avoid early leaks, one should delay the commencement of CAPD for 2 weeks after catheter insertion. No early leaks were reported in this large series, although 7% of patients developed late leaks.

The risk of early fluid leak can be minimized by careful suture technique and avoidance of PD for 7 days, except for an initial 24-hour period of low volume short-dwell cycles. If patients do develop an early leak, PD should be stopped and the peritoneum left empty for 1 to 2 weeks before restarting dialysis. In an established leak unresponsive to conservative management, the catheter should be removed, the wound closed, and a new catheter inserted through an alternative site. Usually late leaks require catheter replacement, although a few may respond to conservative manoeuvres, such as temporary discontinuation of CAPD or conversion to CCPD.

Catheter Obstruction

Obstruction is one of the most common hazards with peritoneal catheters. Usually it occurs early after insertion and presents as a one-way obstruction (outflow obstruction) or occasionally as a two-way obstruction (inflow/outflow obstruction). The overall incidence of both hazards varies widely depending on the type of catheter and the insertion technique used.

One-way obstruction

One-way obstruction presents when PD fluid runs into the peritoneal cavity but only drains slowly or does not drain at all. The defect may occur suddenly in a catheter that has been working normally, or the obstruction may be gradual and thus may be mistaken for the loss of ultrafiltration.

The most common cause of obstruction is catheter migration from the pelvis into the upper quadrants (Table 26–6). Here the catheter tip and side perforations are surrounded by the viscera and omentum and cannot drain the fluid, which accumulates within the lower abdomen. Interestingly, not all catheters that migrate suffer from outflow disturbances. In a small series of Tenckhoff catheters, Oreopoulos and colleagues[45] determined radiologically that tip migration had occurred in 15% of catheters 1 month after implantation. Rottembourg and colleagues[129] performed routine radiology every 3 months on 48 straight Tenckhoff catheters implanted with a closed technique. Catheter displacement occurred in 7, 5, and 2 catheters at 0 to 3, 3 to 6, and 6 to 12 months, respectively.

Table 26–5 Patients at Risk from Early Leak

- Age over 60 years
- Poor abdominal musculature
- Previous treatment with steroids
- Extended incision
- Other recent abdominal incisions
- Previous early leak
- Second or subsequent catheter insertion through the same incision

Table 26–6 Causes and Management of "One-Way" Obstruction Cause

Cause	Action
Constipation	Relief of constipation
Fibrin	1 Flushing with syringe "Milking" transfer set Manual pressure to dialysis bag 2 1000–2000 UI heparin to PD fluid 3 Streptokinase
Displaced catheter tip	Reposition tip by Fogarty catheter Sterile trocar Peritoneoscopy Catheter replacement

Usually one-way obstruction due to malposition is an early complication that occurs in 1% to 28% of CAPD patients.[122]

The management of one-way obstruction depends upon the cause. A plain abdominal film will show the position of the catheter tip. Cannulography may be of value when one requires information about the potential space around the catheter. If simple measures fail and if the catheter tip lies in the pelvis, it may be useful to instill heparin or streptokinase (5000 U in 2–4 mL into PD catheter with clamping) to clear catheters blocked by fibrin.[104,130]

Among the procedures that have been used to reposition displaced catheters, a Fogarty catheter can be passed intraluminally to move the tip of a Tenckhoff catheter,[131] or a sterile bent trocar is used to manipulate the catheter.[132] However, this was successful only when initial function had been good for over 3 weeks. Jaques and colleagues[133] achieved a higher success rate with this procedure under radiologic control. Peritoneoscopy has also been used in a limited number of patients[134] to relocate malfunctioning catheters without surgical intervention. Unfortunately, the application of these techniques in any center is limited by local expertise. Also, the manipulation of catheters using intraluminal instruments risks visceral damage as well as bacterial contamination of the peritoneal cavity.[135]

Usually, catheter obstruction can be relieved with patience, observation, mobilization of the patient and the administration of enemas to stimulate peristaltic forces. In a few cases, persisting obstruction of outflow was relieved by manipulation of the catheter with a semiflexible probe under fluoroscopic guidance.[108,122]

Total obstruction

Total catheter obstruction occurs when fibrin or blood clots fill the lumen. The cause of the obstruction may be determined by cannulography[69,122] with or without air contrast. Most patients with two-way obstruction require operative management. When the catheter has become incarcerated in adhesions, one should attempt to estimate the volume of the peritoneal cavity that remains. Occasionally, this revealed only by sharp dissection and digital palpation. Rarely, one may find that the whole of the peritoneal cavity is occluded and that CAPD must be discontinued.

Forcing 20 to 50 mL of dialysate into the catheter lumen with a syringe may relieve the obstruction. Sometimes intraluminal heparin is useful, and finally, fibrinolytic agents such as urokinase may dissolve the clot.[122]

Catheter Migration

The reasons for catheter migration are complex. Colombi and Giancela[132] suggest that the curve imparted to the catheter in the subcutaneous tunnel places the silicone rubber under strain. This produces pressure and damage to surrounding tissue while the catheter attempts to achieve a position of less strain, ultimately leading to a lateral deviation of the intraperitoneal section. Other causes of catheter displacement are an unduly long intraperitoneal catheter section or omental wrapping of the catheter. Occlusion of the catheter perforations by a full rectum or bladder, and a "ball-valve" obstruction of the lumen by fibrin and clot can also reduce the outflow.

Other Complications of Peritoneal Catheters

Genital Oedema

Edema of the labia majora or scrotum and penis is a distressing complication of PD.[136] Early reports suggested that up to 10% of CAPD patients would experience genital edema,[137–139] although more recently authors have reported a lower incidence of this complication.[140,141] It appears that women have a much lower incidence of genital edema than men. This disparity may be due to the fact that more often the processus vaginalis is patent in males; alternatively, labial swelling may not be as noticeable as swelling over the penis and scrotum. On the other hand, rarely dialysate may dissect through the pouch of Douglas, the vaginal vault, or even travel through the fallopian tubes and present as leakage through the vagina.[142–144]

The passage of dialysate through an open processus vaginalis produces a hydrocele, and, if the peritoneal lining of the processus is breached by fluid, this may lead to massive scrotal and penile edema. In the female, labial edema may develop through a similar mechanism.

King[145] was the first to describe intermittent scrotal swelling in an elderly man who developed 1 month after the initiation of CAPD. Eventually, he had surgical correction of a bilateral hydrocele, which increased and decreased in size with dialysate flow. Alexander and Tank[146] drew attention to the importance of identifying a patent processus during catheter insertion in children using peritoneography. These patients may need ligation of the processus at the time of catheter insertion.

On clinical examination the patient should stand. Asymmetry of the abdomen may indicate dialysis leak into the abdominal wall. Moreover, when the dialysate has dissected superficially, the abdominal wall may look pale and boggy.

Treatment of genital oedema

The risk of any of the above complications in a CAPD patient relates to the incidence of a patent processus vaginalis at the time of commencement of CAPD or the ease with which a closed processus recanalises during treatment. In adults the risk of this complication is low and requires no particular measures, apart from a careful search for overt or incipient inguinal hernia before catheter insertion. Once the complication has occurred, conservative measures are unlikely to be successful.

Treatment of actual genital edema includes bed rest, scrotal elevation if symptomatic, and the use of frequent low-volume exchanges by cycler, if possible.[137] In the case of abdominal wall leaks, cessation of PD for 1 or 2 weeks or conversion of nocturnal PD (with dry days) for 2 weeks may permit the leak to close.[130] Many or most patients can resume CAPD.[138]

Some workers have infiltrated the catheter cuff *in situ* with fibrin glue to stop pericatheter leakage.[96]

Peritoneo-Vaginal Leak

In certain circumstances the fallopian tubes can act as conduits for the antegrade passage of dialysate or the retrograde passage of uterine contents. Khanna and colleagues[104] described three woman who had a bloody PD effluent in association with menstrual bleeding and one woman who had a leakage of dialysate per vagina and went on to develop *Candida peritonitis*. In this latter case the leak was stopped by bilateral tubal ligation during an operation for catheter replacement. Occasionally, retrograde bleeding can also give rise to eosinophilic peritonitis.[148] Repetitive episodes of peritonitis have been reported in association with menstruation, which culminated in an episode of Candida peritonitis. Diaz-Buxo and colleagues[149] reported a rare instance of vaginal leakage of dialysate caused by the late erosion of a Tenckhoff catheter leading to a persistent peritoneo-vaginal fistula.

In instances of fungal peritonitis in women, one should consider the possibility of a vaginal leak. In an established leak, if one were to pursue CAPD safely, a surgical correction by tubal ligation would be required. However, if subsequent transplantation is likely, a women may elect conversion to hemodialysis in the hope of a later pregnancy.

References

1. Gokal A, Ash SR, Helfrich GB, et al: Peritoneal catheters and exit-site practices: Toward optimum peritoneal access. Perit Dial Int 1993; 13:29–39.
2. Official Report from the International Society for Peritoneal Dialysis: Peritoneal catheters and exit-site practices toward optimum peritoneal access: 1998 update. Perit Dial Int 1998; 18:11–33.
3. Veitch P: Surgical aspects of CAPD. *In* Gokal R (ed): Continuous Ambulatory Peritoneal Dialysis. Churchill Livingstone, 1986, pp 110–144.
4. Dobbie JW: Pathology of the peritoneum. *In* Bengmark S (ed): The Peritoneum and Peritoneal Access. Wright, 1989, pp 42–52.
5. Francis DMA, Donnelly PK, Veitch PS, et al: 1984 Surgical aspects of continuous ambulatory peritoneal dialysis? 3 years experience. Br J Surg 71:225–229.
6. Putnam TJ: The living peritoneum as a dialysing membrane. Am J Physiol 1923; 63:548–565.
7. Gutch CF: Peritoneal dialysis. Trans Am Soc Artif Intern Organs 1964; 10:406–407.

8. Ganter E: Uber die besietigung giftiger staffe aus dem blute durch dialyse. Munch Med Weschr 1923; 70:1478–1480.
9. Putnam TJ: The living peritoneum as a dialysing membrane. Am J Physiol 1923; 63:548–565.
10. Palmer RH, Quinton WE: Prolonged peritoneal dialysis for chronic renal failure. Lancet 1964; 1:700–702.
11. Gutch CF: Peritoneal dialysis. Trans Am Soc Artif Intern Organs 1964; 10:406–407.
12. Tenckhoff J, Schechter HA: Bacteriologically safe peritoneal access device. Trans Am Soc Artif Intern Organs 1968; 14:181–187.
13. Ash SR: Peritoneal access devices and placement techniques. *In* Nisenson AR, Fine RN (eds): Dialysis Therapy, 2nd ed. St. Louis, Mosby, 1993.
14. Ash SR: Chronic peritoneal dialysis catheters: Overview of design, placement, and removal procedures. Semin Dial 2003; 16(4):323.
15. Vaamonde CA, Michael UF, Melzger RA, et al: Complications in acute peritoneal dialysis. J Chronic Dis 1975; 28:637–659.
16. Bargman JM: Noninfectious complications of peritoneal dialysis. *In* Gokal R, Nolph KD (eds): The Textbook of Peritoneal Dialysis. Dordrecht, Kluwer Academic, 1994.
17. Popovich RP, Moncrief JW, Decherd JE, et al: The definition of a novel portable wearable equilibrium peritoneal technique (Abstract). ASAIO J 1976; 5:64.
18. American College of Physicians: Clinical competence in acute peritoneal dialysis. Health and Public Policy Committee. Ann Intern Med 1988; 108:763–765.
19. Ash SR, Daugirdas JT: Peritoneal access devices. *In* Daugirdas JT, Blake PG, Ing TS (eds): Handbook of Dialysis. Dordrecht, Kluwer Academic, 2001, pp 309–343.
20. Valk TW, Swartz RD, Hsu CH: Peritoneal dialysis in acute renal failure: Analysis of outcome and complications. Dial Transplant 1980; 9:48–54.
21. Maher JF, Schreiner GE: Hazards and complications of dialysis. N Eng J Med 1965; 273:370–377.
22. Agarwal S: Acute peritoneal dialysis: Practical aspects. Ind J Nephrol 2000; 10:27–28.
23. Song JH, Kim GA, Lee SW, Kim M: Clinical outcomes of immediate full volume exchange one year after peritoneal catheter implantation for CARD. Perit Dial Int 2000; 20:194–199.
24. Simkin EP, Wright FK: Perforating injuries of the bowel complicating peritoneal catheter insertion. Lancet 1968; 1:64–66.
25. Mathew M, Padma G, Suresh S, et al: Pericatheter leak in chronic peritoneal dialysis. Ind J Perit Dial 2001; 4:32–385.
26. Padma G, Edwin B, Suresh S, et al: Permanent peritoneal dialysis catheter malfunction: Our experience. Ind J Perit Dial 2000; 3:22–24.
27. Prasad N, Gupta A, Mathew M, Abraham G: Access-related complications in peritoneal dialysis in developing countries. Adv Ren Rep Ther 2002; 9(2):144–148.
28. Yata N, Ishikura K, Hataya H, et al: Peritoneal dialysis catheter-related complications. Nippon Jinzo Gakkai Shi 2003; 45(4):378–380.
29. Henderson LW: Peritoneal dialysis. *In* Massry SG, Sellers AL (eds): Clinical Aspects of Uremia and Dialysis. Springfield, IL, Charles C. Thomas, 1976, p 574.
30. Stein MF Jr: Intraperitoneal loss of dialysis catheter. Ann Intern Med 1969; 71:869–870.
31. Twardowski ZJ, Nichols WK: Peritoneal dialysis access and exit-site including surgical aspects. *In* Gokal R, Khanna R, Krediet R, Nolph K (eds): Textbook of Peritoneal Dialysis, 2nd ed. Dordrecht, Kluwer Academic, 2000, pp 307–361.
32. Maher JF, Schreiner GE: Hazards and complications of dialysis. N Engl J Med 1965; 273:370–377.
33. Vargemezis V, Passadakis P, Thodis E, et al: Late perforation of bladder as a complication of an unused straight Tenckhoff catheter. Perit Dial Int 1988; 8:55.
34. Twardowski ZJ, Nolph KD, Khanna R, et al: The need for "swan-neck" permanently bent arcuate peritoneal catheter. Peril Dial Bull 1985; 5:219–223.
35. Swartz R, Messana J, Rocher L, et al: The curled catheter: Dependable device for percutaneous peritoneal access. Perit Dial Int 1990; 10:231–235.
36. Ash SR, Daugirdas JT: Peritoneal access devices. *In* Daugirdas JT, Ing TS (eds): Handbook of Dialysis. Boston, Little Brown, 1994, pp 275–300.
37. Cruz C: Cruz catheter implantation technique and clinical results. Perit Dial Int 1994; 14:S59–S63.
38. Gokal A, Ash SR, Helfrich GB, et al: Peritoneal catheters and exit-site practices: Toward optimum peritoneal access. Peril Dial Int 1993; 13:29–39.
39. Ogden DA, Bernavente G, Wheeler D, et al: Experience with the right angle GORE-TEX: Peritoneal dialysis catheter. *In* Khanna R, Nolph KD, Prowant B, et al (eds): Advances in Continuous Ambulatory Peritoneal Dialysis. Toronto, Peritoneal Dialysis Bulletin Inc, 1986, pp 155–159.
40. Pommer W, Brauner M, Westphale HJ, et al: The effect of a silver device in preventing catheter-related infections in peritoneal dialysis patients: Silver Ring Prophylaxis at the Catheter Exit Study. Am J Kidney Dis 1998; 32:752–760.
41. Boeschoten EW: Continuous ambulatory peritoneal dialysis. *In* Gokal R, Khamma R, Krediet R, Nolph K (eds): Textbook of Peritoneal Dialysis, 2nd ed. Dordrecht, Kluwer Academic, 2000, pp 387–418.
42. Tenckhoff J, Schechter H: A bacteriologically safe peritoneal access device. Trans Am Soc Artif Intern Organs 1968; 14:181–187.
43. Diaz-Buxo JA, Geissinger WT: Single versus double Tenckhoff catheters: Perit Dial Bull 1984; 4:100.
44. Ash SR, Nichols WK: Placement, repair and removal of chronic peritoneal catheters. *In* Gokal R, Nolph KD (eds): Textbook of Peritoneal Dialysis. Boston, Kluwer Academic, 1994.
45. Oreopoulos DG, Izatt S, Zellerman G, et al: A prospective study of the effectiveness of three permanent peritoneal catheters. Proc Clin Dial Transplant Forum 1976; 6:96– 100.
46. Twardowski ZJ, Nichols WK, Khanna R, Nolph KD: Swan-neck Missouri peritoneal dialysis catheters: Design, insertion, and break-in (Video). Columbia, MO, University of Missouri, Academic Support Center, 1993.
47. Twardowski ZJ, Prowant BF, Khanna R, et al: Long-term experience with swan neck Missouri catheters. ASAIO Trans 1990; 36:M491–M494.
48. Twardowski ZJ, Prowant BF, Nichols WK, et al: Six year experience with swan neck catheter. Peril Dial Int 1992; 12:384–389.
49. Sieniawska M, Blaim M, Warchol S: Swan-neck presternal catheter (SNPC) for CAPD in children. Perit Dial Int 1993; 13(suppl l):S22.
50. Twardowski ZJ, Nichols WK, Nolph KD, Khanna R: Swan neck presternal peritoneal dialysis catheter. Proceedings of the ISPD Meeting, Thessaloniki, Greece, October 1-4, 1992. Perit Dial Int 1993; 13(suppl 2):S130–S132.
51. Twardowski ZJ, Nichols WK, Khanna R, Nolph KD: Swan neck presternal peritoneal dialysis catheter: Design, insertion, and break-in (Video). Columbia, MO, University of Missouri, Academic Support Center, 1993.
52. Twardowski ZJ, Prowant BF, Pickett B, et al: Four-year experience with swan neck presternal peritoneal dialysis catheter. Am J Kidney Dis 1996; 27:99–105.
53. Ash SR: Chronic peritoneal dialysis catheter: Effect of catheter design, materials and location. Semin Dial 1990; 3:39–46.
54. Ash SR: Experience with a new catheter design. Twenty-first Conference on Dialysis proceedings. New Orleans, LA, February 19-21, 2001, pp 303–305.
55. Shinaberger JH, Shear L, Barry KG: Peritoneal-extracorporeal recirculation dialysis: A technique for improving efficiency of peritoneal dialysis. Investig Urol 1965; 2:555–565.

56. Lange K, Treser G, Mangalat J: Automatic continuous high flow rate peritoneal dialysis. Arch Klin Med 1968; 214:201– 206.
57. Stephen RL, Atkin-Thor E, Kolff WJ: Recirculating peritoneal dialysis with subcutaneous catheter. Trans Am Soc Artif Intern Organs 1976; 22:575–585.
58. Raja RM, Kramer MS, Rosenbaum JL: Recirculation peritoneal dialysis with sorbent Redy cartridge. Nephron 1976; 16:134–142.
59. Gordon A, Lewin AJ, Maxwell MH, Morales ND: Augmentation of efficiency by continuous flow sorbent regeneration peritoneal dialysis. Trans Am Soc Artif Intern Organs 1976; 22:599–604.
60. Warden GD, Maxwell G, Stephen RL: The use of reciprocation peritoneal dialysis with a subcutaneous peritoneal catheter in end-stage renal failure in diabetes mellitus. J Surg Res 1978; 24:495–500.
61. Kabtitz C, Stephen RL, Jacobsen SC, et al: Reciprocating peritoneal dialysis. Dial Transplant 1978; 7:211– 214.
62. Kraus MA, Shasha SM, Nemas M, et al: Ultrafiltration peritoneal dialysis and recirculating peritoneal dialysis with a portable kidney. Dial Transplant 1983; 12:385–388.
63. Ash SR, Janle EM: Continuous flow-through peritoneal dialysis: Comparison of efficiency to IPD, TPD and CAPD in an animal model. Perit Dial Int 1997; 17:365–372.
64. Ronco C, Gloukhoff A, Dell'Aquila R, Levin NW: Catheter design for continuous flow peritoneal dialysis. Blood Purif 2002; 20:40–44.
65. Amerling R, Glezerman I, Savransky E, et al: Continuous flow peritoneal dialysis: Principles and applications. Semin Dial 2003; 16(4):335–340.
66. Ronco C, Levin NW, Dell'Aquila R, Sergeyeva O: New dual-lumen catheter with diffuser for continuous flow peritoneal dialysis. J Am Soc Nephrol 2002; 13:1A.
67. Lewis MA, Smith T, Postlewaite RJ, et al: A comparison of double-cuffed with single-cuffed Tenckhoff catheters in the prevention of infection in pediatric patients. Adv Perit Dial 1997; 13:274–276.
68. Eklund B, Honkanen E, Kyllonen L, et al: Peritoneal dialysis access: Prospective randomised comparison of single-cuff and double-cuff straight Tenckhoff catheters. Nephrol Dial Transplant 1997; 12:2664–2666.
69. Nielsen PK, Hemmingsen C, Friss SU, et al: Comparison of straight and curled Tenckhoff peritoneal dialysis catheters implanted by percutaneous technique: A prospective randomised study. Perit Dial Int 1995; 15:18–21.
70. Akyol AM, Porteous C, Brown MW: A comparison of two types of catheters for continuous peritoneal dialysis. Perit Dial Int 1990; 10:63–66.
71. Lye WC, Kour NW, van der Straaten JC, et al: A prospective randomised comparison of swan neck, coiled and straight Tenckhoff catheters in patients on CAPD. Perit Dial Int 1996; 16(suppl 1):333–335.
72. Eklund BH, Honkanen EO, Kard AR, et al: Peritoneal dialysis access: Prospective randomised comparison of swan neck and Tenckhoff catheters. Peril Dial Int 1995; 15:353– 356.
73. Cunningham JT, Tucker CT: Peritoneoscopy in chronic peritoneal dialysis: Use in evaluation and management of complications. Gastrointest Endosc 1983; 29:47–50.
74. Wu G, Khanna R, Vas S, Oreopoulos DG: Is extensive diverticulosis of the colon a contraindication to CAPD? Perit Dial Bull 1983; 3:180-183.
75. Scheff RT, Zucherman G, Harter H, et al: Diverticular disease in patients with chronic renal failure due to polycystic kidney disease. Ann Intern Med 1980; 92:202–204.
76. Brown PM, Johnston KW, Fenton SSA, Cattran DC: Symptomatic exacerbation of peripheral vascular disease with chronic ambulatory peritoneal dialysis. Clin Nephrol 1981; 16:258–261.
77. Khanna R, Oreopoulos DG, Dombros N, et al: Continuous ambulatory peritoneal dialysis after 3 years: Still a promising treatment. Perit Dial Bull 1981; 1:24–34.
78. Dequidt C, Vijt D, Veys N, Van Biesen W: Bed-side blind insertion of peritoneal dialysis catheters. EDTNA ERCA J 2003; 29(3):137–139.
79. U.S. Renal Data System: USRDS 1992 Annual Data Report, VI. Catheter-related factors and peritonitis risk in CAPD patients. Am J Kidney Dis 1992; 5(suppl 2):48–54.
80. Poirier VL, Daly BDT, Dasse KA, et al: Elimination of tunnel infection. *In* Maher JF, Winchester JF (eds): Frontiers in Peritoneal Dialysis. Proceedings of the III International Symposium on Peritoneal Dialysis, New York, Washington, DC, 1984. New York, Field, Rich and Assoc, 1986, pp 210–217.
81. Twardowski ZJ, Khanna R, Nolph KD, et al: Intraabdominal pressure during natural activities in patients treated with continuous ambulatory peritoneal dialysis. Nephron 1986; 44:129–135.
82. Gonzales AR, Goltz GM, Eaton CL, et al: The peel away method for insertion of Tenckhoff catheter (Abstract). Am Soc Nephrol 1983; 16:119A.
83. Updike S, O'Brien M, Peterson W, Zimmerman S: Placement of catheter using pacemaker-like introducer with peel-away sleeve (Abstract). Am Soc Nephrol 1984; 17:87A.
84. Updike S, Zimmerman S, O'Brien M, Peterson W: Peel-Away sheath technique for placing peritoneal dialysis catheters (Video). School of Nursing, University of Wisconsin, Madison, WI, Television Studio, 1984.
85. Zappacosta AR, Perras ST, Closkey GM: Seldinger technique for Tenckhoff catheter placement. ASAIO Trans 1991; 37:13–15.
86. Zappacosta AR: Seldinger technique for placement of the Tenckhoff catheter (Video). Bryn Mawr Hospital, 1984.
87. Ash SR, Nichols WK: Placement, repair, and removal of chronic peritoneal catheters. *In* Gokal R, Nolph KD (eds): Textbook of Peritoneal Dialysis. Dordrecht, Kluwer Academic, 1994, pp 315–333.
88. Yun EJ, Meng MV, Brennan TV, et al: Novel microlaparoscopic technique for peritoneal dialysis catheter placement. Urology 2003; 61(5): 1026–1028.
89. Tarcoveanu E, Bradea C, Florea L, et al: Laparoscopic management of peritoneal dialysis catheters. Chirurgia (Bucur) 2002; 97(3):293–296.
90. Copley JB, Lindberg JS, Back SN, Tapia NP: Peritoneoscopic placement of swan neck peritoneal dialysis catheters. Perit Dial Int 1996; suppl 1:S330–S332.
91. Nichols WK, Nolph KD: A technique for managing exit site and cuff infection in Tenckhoff catheters. Perit Dial Bull l983; 3(suppl 4):S4–S5.
92. Gadallah MF, Pervez A, el-Shahawy MA, et al: Peritoneoscopic versus surgical placement of peritoneal dialysis catheters: A prospective randomised study on outcome. Am J Kidney Dis 1999; 33:118–122.
93. Scalamogna A, Castelnovo C, Dc Vecchi A, Ponticelli C: Exit-site and tunnel infections in continuous ambulatory peritoneal dialysis. Am J Kidney Dis 1991; 28:674–677.
94. Piraino B, Bernardini J, Peitzman A, Sorkin M: Failure of peritoneal catheter cuff shaving to eradicate infection. Perit Dial Bull 1987; 7:179–182.
95. Maher ER, Stevens J, Murphy C, Brown EA: Comparison of two methods of Tenckhoff catheter insertion. Nephron 1988; 48:87–88.
96. Liberek T, Chmielewski M, Lichodziejewska–Niemierko M, et al: Survival and function of Tenckhoff peritoneal dialysis catheter after surgical or percutaneous placement: One centre experience. Int J Artif Organs 2003; 26(2):174–175.
97. Gadallah MF, Pervez A, el-Shahawy MA, et al: Peritoneoscopic versus surgical placement of peritoneal dialysis catheters: A prospective randomised study of outcome. Am J Kidney Dis 1999; 33:118–122.

98. Tsimoyiannis EC, Siakas P, Glantzounis G, et al: Laparoscopic placement of the Tenckhoff catheters for peritoneal dialysis. Surg Laparosc Endosc Percutan Tech 2000; 10:218–221.
99. Wright MJ, Beleed K, Johnson BF, et al: Randomised prospective comparison of laparoscopic and operative peritoneal dialysis catheter insertion. Perit Dial Int 1999; 19:372–375.
100. Park MS, Yim AS, Chung SH, et al: Effect of prolonged subcutaneous implantation of peritoneal catheter on peritonitis rate during (APD): A prospective randomised study. Blood Purif 1998; 16:171–178.
101. Dasgupta MK, Fox S, Card J, et al: Catheter survival is improved by the use of Moncrief-Popovich catheters. J Am Soc Nephrol 1998; 9:190A.
102. Smith C: CAPD: One cuff vs. two cuff catheters in reference to incidence of infection. *In* Maher JF, Winchester JF (eds): Frontiers in Peritoneal Dialysis. New York, Field, Rich and Assoc, 1986, pp 181–182.
103. Lindblad AS, Novak JW, Nolph KD: Continuous ambulatory peritoneal dialysis in the USA. Section 7. Special reports, 1987. E. Complications of peritoneal catheters. Dordrecht, Kluwer Academic, 1989, pp 157–166.
104. Piraino B, Bernardini J, Johnston JR, Sorkin ML: Exit-site location does not influence peritoneal catheter infection rate. Perit Dial Int 1989; 9:127–129.
105. Khanna R, Oreopoulos DG, Dombros N, et al: Continuous ambulatory peritoneal dialysis after 3 years: Still a promising treatment. Perit Dial Bull 1981; 1:24–34.
106. Mallonga ET, Van Coevorden F, Boeschoten E W, et al: Surgical problems in continuous ambulatory peritoneal dialysis (CAPD). Neth J Surg 1982; 34(3):117–122.
107. Twardowski ZJ, Prowant BF: Exit-site healing post catheter implantation. Perit Dial Int 1996; 16(suppl 3):51–70.
108. Vychytil A, Lorenz M, Schneider B, et al: New strategies to prevent S. aureus infections in peritoneal dialysis patients. J Am Soc Nephrol 1998; 9:669–676.
109. Gokal R, Alexander S, Ash S, et al: Peritoneal catheters and exit-site practices toward optimum peritoneal access: 1998 update. Perit Dial Int 1998; 18:11–33.
110. Wikdahl AM, Engman U, Stemayr BG, Sorensen JG: One dose cefuroxime IV and IP reduces microbial growth in PD patients after catheter insertion. Nephrol Dial Transplant 1997; 12: 157– 160.
111. Bennett-Jones DN, Martin J, Barratt AJ, et al: Prophylactic gentamicin in the prevention of early exit-site infections and peritonitis in CAPD. Adv Perit Dial 1988; 4:147– 150.
112. Lye WC, Lee EJC, Tan CC: Prophylactic antibiotics in the insertion of Tenckhoff catheters. Scand J Urol Nephrol 1992; 26:177–180.
113. Bernardini J, Lutes R, Johnston JR, et al: Randomized trial of rifampin versus mupirocin to prevent S. aureus infections in PD patients (Abstract). Perit Dial Int 1995; 15(1):517.
114. Thodis E, Bhaskaran S, Passadakis P, et al: Decline in S. aureus exit site infection and peritonitis in CAPD patients by local application of mupirocin ointment at the catheter exit site. Peril Dial Int 1998; 18:261–270.
115. Casey M, Taylor J, Clinard P, et al: Application of mupirocin cream at the exit-site reduces exit-infections and peritonitis in peritoneal dialysis patients. Perit Dial Int 2000; 20(5):566–574.
116. Uttley L, Smart B, Hutchinson A, Gokal R: Decrease in infections with the introduction of mupirocin cream at the catheter exit-site (Abstract). Perit Dial Int 2001; 21(suppl 2):86.
117. Boer WH: Daily nasal and exit-site mupirocin application greatly reduces the S. aureus peritonitis rates without causing mupirocin resistance (Abstract). Perit Dial Int 2001; 21(suppl 2):122.
118. Khanna R: Is a break-in period necessary following peritoneal catheter insertion(A break-in period is recommended. Semin Dial 1992; 5:197.
119. Clark KR, Forsythe JLR, Rigg KM, et al: Surgical aspects of chronic peritoneal dialysis in the neonate and infant under 1 year of age. J Pediatr Surg 1992; 27:780.
120. Simkin EP, Wright FK: Perforating injuries of the bowel complicating peritoneal catheter insertion. Lancet 1968; 1:64–66.
121. Devine H, Oreopoulos DG, Izatt S, et al: The permanent Tenckhoff catheter for CAPD. Can Med Assoc J 1975; 113:219–221.
122. Francis DMA, Schofield I, Veitch PS: Abdominal hernias in patients treated with continuous ambulatory peritoneal dialysis. Brit J Surg 1982; 69:409.
123. Diaz-Buxo JA: Mechanical complications of chronic peritoneal dialysis catheters. Semin Dial 1991; 4:106–111.
124. Bustos E, Rotellar C, Mazzoni J, et al: Clinical aspects of bowel perforation in patients undergoing continuous ambulatory peritoneal dialysis. Semin Dial 1994; 7:355.
125. Hirsch DJ, Jindal KK: Late leaks in peritoneal dialysis patients. Nephrol Dial Transplant 1990; 6:670.
126. Joffe P: Peritoneal dialysis catheter leakage treated with fibrin glue. Nephrol Dial Transplant 1993; 8:474.
127. Ponce SP, Pierratos A, Izatt S, et al: Comparison of the survival and complications of three permanent peritoneal dialysis catheters. Perit Dial Bull 1982; 2:82–86.
128. Francis DMA, Donnelly PK, Veitch PS, et al: Surgical aspects of continuous ambulatory peritoneal dialysis: 3 years experience. Brit J Surg 1984; 71:225–229.
129. Olcott C, Feldman CA, Coplon NS, et al: Continuous ambulatory peritoneal dialysis: Technique of catheter insertion and management of associated surgical complications. Am J Surg 1983; 146:98–102.
130. Rottembourg J, Jacq D, Vonlamhen M, et al: Straight or curled Tenckhoff peritoneal catheter for continuous ambulatory peritoneal dialysis (CAPD). Perit Dial Bull 1981; 1:123–124.
131. Palacios M, Schley W, Dougherty JS: Use of streptokinase to clear peritoneal catheters. Dial Transplant 1982; 1:172–174.
132. Grefberg N, Danielson BG, Nilsson P, Wahlberg J: Comparison of two catheters for peritoneal access in patients undergoing continuous ambulatory peritoneal dialysis (CAPD). Scand J Urol Nephrol 1983; 17(3):343–346.
133. Colombi A, Gianella C: Straight implantation of the Tenckhoff catheter for continuous ambulatory peritoneal dialysis. *In* Legrain M (ed): Continuous Ambulatory Peritoneal Dialysis. Amsterdam, Excerpta Medica, 1980, p 69–75.
134. Jaques P, Richey W, Maudel S: Tenckhoff peritoneal dialysis catheter: Cannulography and manipulation. Am J Roentgenology 1980; 135:83–86.
135. Korten G, Arendt R, Brugmann E, Klein B: Relocation of a peritoneal catheter without surgical intervention. Perit Dial Bull 1983; 3:46.
136. Ogunc G: Malfunctioning peritoneal dialysis catheter and accompanying surgical pathology repaired by laparoscopic surgery. Perit Dial Int 2002; 22(4):454–462.
137. Bargman JM: Non-infectious complications of peritoneal dialysis. *In* Gokal R, Khanna R, Krediet R, Nolph K (eds): Textbook of Peritoneal Dialysis, 2nd ed. Great Britain, Kluwer Academic, 2000, p 609–646.
138. Kopecky R, Funk M, Kreitzer P: Localized genital edema in patients undergoing continuous ambulatory peritoneal dialysis. J Urol 1985; 134:880–884.
139. Beaman M, Fechally J, Smith B, Walls J: Anterior abdominal wall leakage in CAPD patients: Management by intermittent peritoneal dialysis (Letter). Perit Dial Bull 1985; 5:81–82.
140. Cooper JC, Nicholls AJ, Simms JM, et al: Genital oedema in patients treated by continuous ambulatory peritoneal dialysis: An unusual presentation of inguinal hernia. Br Med J 1983; 286:1923–1924.
141. Abraham G, Blake PG, Mathews RE, et al: Genital swelling as a surgical complication of continuous ambulatory peritoneal dialysis. Surg Gynecol Obstet 1990; 170:306–308.

142. Tzamaloukas AH, Gibel LJ, Eisenberg B, et al: Scrotal edema in patients on CAPD: Causes, differential diagnosis and management. Dial Transplant 1992; 21:581–590.
143. Caporale N, Perez D, Alegre S: Vaginal leak of peritoneal dialysate liquid. Perit Dial Int 1991; 11:284–285.
144. Whiting M, Smith N, Agar J: Vaginal peritoneal dialysate leakage per fallopian tubes (Letter). Perit Dial Int 1995; 15:85.
145. Bradley A, Mamtora H, Pritchard N: Transvaginal leak of peritoneal dialysate demonstrated by CT peritoneography. Br J Radiol 1997; 70:652–653.
146. King C: Hydrocele: A complication of CAPD. Nephrology Nurse 1981; 3:37–39.
147. Alexander SR, Tank ES: Surgical aspects of continuous ambulatory peritoneal dialysis in infants, children and adolescents. J Urol 1982; 127:501–504.
148. Litnerland J, Gibson M, Sambrook P, et al: Investigation and treatment of poor drains of dialysate fluid associated with anterior abdominal wall leaks in patients on chronic ambulatory peritoneal dialysis. Nephrol Dial Transplant 1992; 7:1030–1034.
149. Gokal R, Ramos JM, Ward MK, Kerr DNS: Eosinophilic peritonitis in CAPD. Clin Nephrol 1981; 15:328–330.
150. Diaz-Buxo JA, Burgess P, Walker PJ: Peritoneovaginal fistula: Unusual complication of peritoneal dialysis. Perit Dial Bull 1983; 3:142–143.

Peritoneal Dialysis Solutions

Simon J. Davies, M.D., F.R.C.P.

The last 15 years have seen an encouraging trend in the development of peritoneal dialysis (PD) solutions. As our understanding of how the peritoneal membrane works and how this changes with time on therapy is combined with a clearer view of the issues that face patients requiring renal replacement therapy, new solutions have been devised to address these problems. This, in turn, has both driven and been driven by competition within industry with the result that an increasing number of randomized trials are now performed (Figure 27–1), which, in addition to testing product benefit, they teach us clinicians much about how this therapy works and how to improve it. Hopefully, this is just the beginning.

What are the characteristics of the ideal peritoneal dialysis solution? At the very least, it must do the job of dialysis treatment. This includes the removal of water-soluble toxins, maintenance of electrolyte and acid base status, and the removal of salt and water. This in itself might not be so simple. For example, the physiology of the peritoneal membrane turns out to be more complex than originally thought, with different pathways and mechanisms for solute and water removal, respectively. As a result, the ability to create both osmotic gradients with small osmolytes and oncotic gradients with larger, potentially charged molecules is desirable. Given the chance, however, the clinician would like to do more. Solution development opens up the opportunity for therapy, for example, not just maintenance of electrolyte balance but its very manipulation such that, especially in combination with other drug treatments, specific problems associated with renal failure might be treated. Indeed, the peritoneal cavity offers an alternative method of drug delivery that is already being exploited in nonrenal failure patients.[1–3]

It is also important that solutions used in peritoneal dialysis do no harm to the patient. The literature now indicates that this has not been the case to date, with evidence of both local (e.g., membrane damage) and systemic problems (e.g., obesity) that can be attributed to PD solutions. This issue, termed *biocompatibility*—although "bio*in*compatibility" is perhaps more accurate—has assumed increasing importance in the last few years. The difficulty facing development of solutions in this area is that it may take many years for problems of biocompatibility to develop and, by the same token, studies of many years' duration to demonstrate the benefits of new fluids. This is a problem in a therapy that is used by only 130,000 patients worldwide, which, for many, is relatively short-term.

This chapter will discuss PD solutions under a number of headings, ranging from electrolyte and acid-base homeostasis, through alternative osmotic agents to newer biocompatible fluids. In each case the clinical need for the solution type will be discussed, followed by description and rationale of their formulation, evidence of clinical benefit, and, finally, a discussion of any problems and limitations associated with their use. The chapter will conclude with a discussion of potential future developments, some of which are undergoing clinical trials, others under investigation in animal models.

SOLUTIONS FOR CALCIUM AND MAGNESIUM HOMEOSTASIS

Clinical Need

Patients treated with peritoneal dialysis can be in negative, positive, or equal calcium balance. This has led to the development of PD solutions with a variety of calcium concentrations (Table 27–1), which enable the clinician to control the excretion of these ions, so that, in turn, it is possible to utilize additional therapeutic measures (e.g., phosphate binders and vitamin D analogues), to maintain Ca^{++} and Mg^{++} homeostasis.[4] In general, patients with hypocalcemia in whom hyperphosphatemia is well controlled a dialysate fluid containing a relatively high concentration of calcium will be required. Low calcium dialysate will be needed for the patient in whom there is a need to use larger oral doses of calcium containing phosphate binder, and these were originally designed to enable clinicians to use this as opposed to the more efficient but toxic aluminum containing binders. However, growing concerns over vascular calcification in the dialysis population and its association with increased mortality[5–8] have led to greater concern and, thus, emphasis in controlling the plasma calcium phosphate product and the avoidance of episodes of hypercalcemia. With the development of newer alternative phosphate binders, for example, resins, such as sevelamer (Renagel), hypercalcemia can be minimized further.[9] The impact of calcimimetics in this field is not yet known, although it seems likely that this development will only increase the need for flexibility in controlling calcium losses. The purpose of using a lower magnesium concentration is in the prevention of hypermagnesemia,[4,10] which may itself worsen metabolic bone disease. Reducing magnesium levels, at least in principle, also enable the clinician to prescribe magnesium containing phosphate binders.

Solution Description

It can be seen from Table 27–1 that solutions can be divided broadly into high (above normal ionized calcium concentration, typically greater than 1.5 mmol/L and low calcium concentration, ranging from 1.0 mmol/L down to zero. Usually the difference in the cation concentration is compensated for by a change in the chloride content, although some solutions have also been designed to reduce magnesium content as patients with renal failure can develop hypermagnesemia.

High calcium solutions are designed to keep the patient close to equal balance for calcium by minimizing dialysate losses. By setting the concentration above the normal ionized Ca^{++} concentration in the blood (e.g., dialysate: 1.75 mmol/L vs. plasma: 1.2 mmol/L), this is achieved, although the loss of calcium in the dialysate due to convection will modify this. Typically, when using 1.36% exchanges calcium balance will be achieved at a calcium concentration of 1.38 mmol/L, whereas at 2.27% and 3.86% glucose exchanges this will be at 1.7 and 2.2 mmol/L Ca^{++}, respectively.[11]

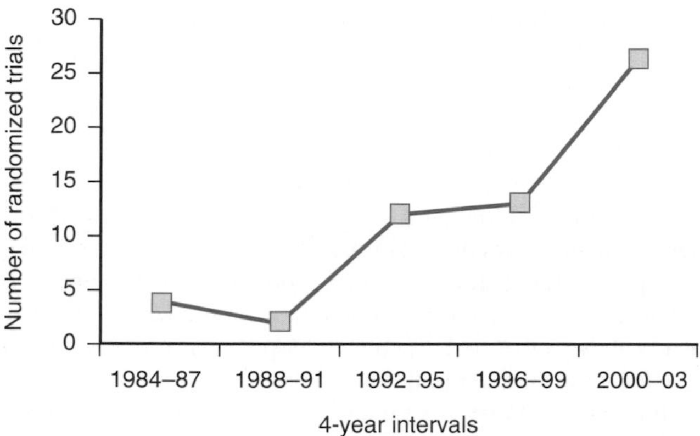

Figure 27–1 Increase in the number of randomized clinical trials involving peritoneal dialysis solutions over the last 20 years.

Evidence of Clinical Benefit

Patients commencing dialysis treatment are often in negative calcium balance due to accrued metabolic bone disease and poor nutritional status, and the ability of the clinician to prescribe a dialysis regime that prevents further calcium loss is important. Testimony to the efficacy of this approach is the relatively high proportion of patients who, when treated with calcium 1.75 mmol solution in combination with calcium containing phosphate binders, develop hypercalcemia.[12,13] The concentration of Mg^{++} in these solutions is set at the lower end of the normal range for plasma. This is because there is a tendency for this ion to accumulate in dialysis patients. There is evidence that patients using these solutions can develop mild hypermagnesemia, which appears to be of no apparent clinical significance.[10] Magnesium intoxication has not been reported.

The ability of low calcium solutions to achieve negative calcium balance has also been confirmed by cross-sectional studies,[4,14–16] and their clinical efficacy in reducing the incidence of hypercalcemia in patients using calcium containing phosphate binders only is well established in longitudinal studies.[4,12,13,17–21] With the increasing evidence of the detrimental effect of vascular calcification on survival in PD patients and the poor outcome of individuals with adynamic bone, itself associated with hypoparathyroidism due, at least in part, to hypercalcemia, it would seem sensible to favor the use of lower rather than higher dialysate calcium concentrations. Dialysate with lower magnesium concentration has been shown in clinical studies to resolve hypermagnesemia[22] and is associated with normal magnesium levels in plasma.[10]

Table 27-1 Summary of the Composition of the Principle Dialysis Solutions Commercially Available

Solution Type	Electrolytes (mmol/L)					Buffer (mmol/L)	
and Name	Sodium	Calcium	Magnesium	Chloride	Lactate	Bicarbonate	pH
Glucose sol'n							
Gemini 10[a]	132	1.75	0.25	96	40	—	5.5
Gambrosol trio[a]	131–133	1.31–1.38	0.24–0.26	95.2–95.4	39–41	—	5.5–6.5
CAPD/DPCA 2-4[b]	134	1.75	0.5	103.5	35	—	5.5
CAPD/DPCA 10-12[b]	134	1.0	0.5	102	35	—	5.5
CAPD/DPCA 17-12[b]	134	1.25	0.5	102.5	35	—	5.5
Balance 1.25 Calcium[b]	134	1.25	0.5	102.5	35		7.0
Balance 1.75 Calcium[b]	134	1.75	0.5	101.5	35	—	7.0
Dianeal PD1[c]	132	1.75	0.75	102	35	—	5.5
Dianeal PD2[c]	132	1.75	0.25	96	40	—	5.5
Dianeal PD4[c]	132	1.25	0.25	95	40	—	5.5
Physioneal 35[c]	132	1.75	0.25	101	10	25	7.4
Physioneal 40[c]	132	1.25	0.25	95	15	25	7.4
Amino acid sol'n							
Nutrineal[c]	132	1.25	0.25	105	40		6.7
Icodextrin sol'n							
Extraneal[c]	133	1.75	0.25	96	40		5.1

Electrolyte, buffer, and pH formulations are shown for the three worldwide manufacturers of PD solutions ([a]Gambro, [b]Fresenius, and [c]Baxter). To convert from mmol to mEq for calcium and magnesium, multiply by 2. Where a range is indicated, this reflects the variability due to different solution combinations derived from a multicompartment bag when reconstituting to obtain varying glucose concentrations.

There are no published clinical trials comparing the efficacy of different dialysate solutions in relation to calcium and magnesium homeostasis in children, although calcium balance studies have been performed.[23] The physiology and clinical problems as outlined above are essentially the same in children as in adults, with the added concern of adequate growth and particular emphasis in avoiding aluminum bone disease.[24] Current guidelines favor the use of low calcium concentration fluids[25] to enable concurrent use of calcium containing phosphate binders. Data from the pediatric national registries would indicate that maintenance of growth on peritoneal dialysis in children is reasonable using this strategy.[26,27]

Problems

As might be anticipated, a small proportion of patients treated with lower calcium concentration solutions will experience a rise in PTH levels,[19,28] and, equally, occasional patients will develop hypomagnesemia when using a lower concentration of this cation.[29] Clinicians need to be aware of this potential but entirely predictable problem, by adjusting the oral dose of calcium containing phosphate, vitamin D analogues, and, in the near future, calcimimetics, in response to their monitoring of parathyroid hormone, calcium phosphate product, and markers of bone turnover. Particular care should be taken in using very low, or even zero, calcium concentration solutions, which should be used as a short-term measure only in the treatment of severe hypercalcemia, for example, preparation for parathyroidectomy, because long-term use runs the risk of developing a significant negative calcium balance. Nevertheless, judicial use of the lower calcium containing fluids should reduce the problems of hypercalcemia thought to be etiologic in vascular calcification.

SOLUTIONS FOR ACID-BASE BALANCE

Clinical Need

In replacing the functions of the kidney, there is a requirement to provide buffering capacity to enable excretion of hydrogen ions, continuously produced as a consequence of human metabolism.[30] Peritoneal dialysis fluid must, therefore, contain a buffer in a greater concentration than it is in plasma to ensure net flow across the peritoneal membrane into the patient. There are essentially two issues related to the choice of PD solution that need to be considered in this regard: first, the concentration of buffer required to maintain optimal acid-base status of the patient, and this will be the principal focus of this section. Second, there are issues of biocompatibility that will be dealt with in more detail under the section on biocompatible fluids. Briefly, the buffers that have been employed in PD solutions have changed and continue to change as the therapy develops. Initially, acetate was employed, but this was abandoned following strong circumstantial evidence that it was an etiologic factor in the development of sclerosing peritonitis. Subsequently, lactate has been widely employed, which once it has entered the patient, is metabolized rapidly to bicarbonate.[31] More recently, primarily for reasons of patient comfort and biocompatibility, pH neutral bicarbonate solutions have been developed (see later text), although there is potential for superior acid-base control using bicarbonate under special conditions, for example, in children or patients with liver disease.

The efficacy of dialysis treatment in controlling acid-base balance and, in particular, preventing the development of metabolic acidosis is usually assessed from measurement of the plasma bicarbonate (or CO_2) concentration.[32] In contrast to hemodialysis patients, who tend to have a fluctuating acid-base status, such that they are frequently relatively acidotic prior to the treatment sessions, patients treated with peritoneal dialysis are usually in a steady state. Typically, 70% of PD patients have a plasma bicarbonate in the normal range, about 12% have low level indicating acidosis, and the remainder have mild degrees of alkalosis. In CAPD patients but not APD patients, there is a modest effect of peritoneal solute transport status on plasma bicarbonate, such that low transport is associated with a tendency for lower levels and vice versa. In both modalities, lower bicarbonate levels appear, at least in part, to be due to inadequate dialysis dose. It should also be remembered that buffering capacity is increased by the oral ingestion of drugs, such as calcium carbonate, also used as a phosphate binder, and sodium bicarbonate. Although the need to achieve adequate buffering capacity is not in doubt, the optimal target for plasma bicarbonate, as will be seen, is not so clear. The need to achieve stable and adequate control of acid-base status in the pediatric population is more important than the adult population.[33] Poorly controlled acidosis is an important reason for poor growth in children with renal failure. The ability of peritoneal dialysis to provide steady state control of acidosis is one reason why this is becoming a preferred treatment modality in pediatric practice.[27,34,35]

Solution Description

The range of buffer types and concentrations that are commercially available are summarized in Table 27–1. Lactate concentrations vary between 35 and 40 mmol/L. Some years ago manufacturers changed from using the racemic mixture, D(−) and L(+) lactate to the L(+) isomer form only. This is of no clinical consequence because the metabolism of both isomers is equally efficient in the human. Bicarbonate containing fluids might be either solely this buffer, at a buffering capacity similar to conventional lactate solutions (buffering capacity is the same mol for mol), or contain a mixture of bicarbonate (e.g., 25 mmol/L) and lactate (e.g., 15 mmol/L). The rationale for this latter choice is that a bicarbonate solution of 40 mmol/L is supraphysiologic and may cause local changes in the microcirculation of the peritoneal membrane. This concern is based from the observation that pure bicarbonate solution is associated with significantly more abdominal pain than the mixture.[36] This argument will be developed further when discussing the relative merits of these solutions and their biocompatibility.

Evidence of Clinical Benefit

The combination of bicarbonate obtained from dialysate lactate and the oral phosphate binder calcium carbonate has been demonstrated to achieve normal, steady state acid-base status in the vast majority of peritoneal dialysis patients.[32] There is good evidence, however, that not only is prevention of acidosis beneficial in peritoneal dialysis patients, but also maintaining higher plasma bicarbonate, albeit within the normal range. In one prospective study of acid-base status, comparison was made between the formulation lactate 35 mmol/L with lactate 40 mmol/L.[37] In this study further attempts were made to make the lactate 35 mmol/L group more acidotic by avoiding calcium carbonate and the lactate 40 mmol/L group more alkalotic by coprescribing sodium bicarbonate. Between-group separation was achieved, such that plasma bicarbonate levels were 23 ± 0.3 and 27.2 ± 0.3 mmol/L at 1 year, that is, both within normal limits. Patients randomized to the high lactate treatment had fewer hospital admissions and gained lean body mass as determined from anthropometrics. In another randomized study, patients who had been acidotic on conventional fluids had better clinical outcomes, if their treatment was supplemented with oral sodium bicarbonate.[38] It seems, therefore, that patients on PD are better maintained with a bicarbonate level in the upper part of the normal range.

In adults, a bicarbonate-only solution, containing 33 mmol/L when compared to lactate 40 mmol/L did not result in adequate buffering capacity.[39] For mixed solutions, there is no clear evidence that substituting bicarbonate for lactate at a high equivalent buffering capacity (40 mmol/L) results in superior acid-base balance in CAPD patients—indeed the mix of bicarbonate to lactate does not seem to matter.[40] However, for solutions with a lower buffering capacity, when patients are switched from an all lactate (35 mmol/L) to a 25 mmol bicarbonate to 10 mmol lactate mix, there is a significant improvement in plasma bicarbonate (24.4 to 26.1 mmol/L), such that a higher proportion of patients had a value within the normal range.[41] Both these solution combinations (bicarbonate 25 mmol/L, lactate 10 or 15 mmol/L) are effective in controlling acid-base in APD patients, although when using the 25:10 combination, there was a significant fall (~1.26 mmol/L) in the plasma bicarbonate after switch from standard lactate (40 mmol/L) solutions. Patients switched from lactate 40 mmol/L to the 25:15 mix were significantly more likely to achieve plasma bicarbonate in the normal range.[42]

A recent study comparing lactate (35 mmol/L, pH 5.5) with a pure bicarbonate-buffered PD solution (34 mmol/L, pH 7.4) in children suggests that this is safe in the short term,[43] and current recommendations are in favor of using bicarbonate solutions in this patient group.[25] The additional benefits of bicarbonate containing solutions, which by definition are also pH neutral, are of reduced infusion pain,[36,42] and potential benefits to membrane function and host defenses will be discussed under the section on biocompatibility.

Potential Problems

There is a tendency for some patients (approximately 17%) to run bicarbonate levels above the normal range, usually when combining high buffering capacity solutions with oral calcium carbonate. Although reported, this has not been demonstrated to result in detriment to the patient with any certainty.[29] This problem is likely to become less of an issue as clinicians move toward using alternative phosphate binders. Failure to achieve adequate control of acidosis will be uncommon with commercially available solutions. By increasing the dialysis dose in anuric patients, using bicarbonate 25/lactate 15 mmol/L mix, particularly if on APD, and the careful use of oral sodium bicarbonate should always be avoidable. Bicarbonate solutions are not associated with any increase in peritonitis and may be associated with a slight improvement in ultrafiltration in the long term.[44,45]

GLUCOSE AND GLUCOSE-POLYMER SOLUTIONS

Clinical Need

Ultrafiltration is an essential component of peritoneal dialysis treatment. Apart from the need to remove water to maintain stable fluid status, it is required for the convective component of solute removal. This is proportionally more important for solutes that have a low concentration gradient between blood and dialysate, such as sodium or calcium,[11,46] and for larger molecules, such as β–2 microglobulin, that diffuse relatively slowly compared to their mass transport by convection.[47]

There is also increasing evidence that the ability to obtain adequate ultrafiltration has relevance to clinical outcomes that is currently more convincing than for the achievable variability in peritoneal solute clearance.[48] At present, this is from observational cohort studies only and, in some aspects, only indirect, although the weight of evidence is impressive. First, a number of observational studies have found that in CAPD patients high solute transport is associated with worse outcomes, in terms of both patient and technique survival.[49–52] One likely explanation of this association is the negative relationship between peritoneal ultrafiltration capacity and increasing solute transport when glucose is used as the osmotic agent, such that in longer exchanges there may even be a net reabsorption of fluid during a dialysis exchange. Other studies have related achieved peritoneal fluid and sodium removal (they are tightly coupled in CAPD patients) to either patient or technique survival.[53,54] More recently, the European Automated Peritoneal Dialysis Outcomes Study has found that inability to achieve more than a predefined 750 mL of daily ultrafiltration in anuric patients was associated with worse survival.[55]

There has also been considerable progress in our understanding of the mechanisms of fluid removal across the peritoneal membrane.[56] There are essentially two pathways of water transport that will work differently with different types of osmotic agent (Figure 27–2). There are water specific pathways, known to correspond to aquaporin channels situated in the endothelium, which are highly efficient but require an osmotic gradient best achieved with small osmolytes, such as glucose.[57,58] There is also a larger set of pores or channels, responsible for allowing the removal of solutes, such as creatinine, that also enable water removal. These are less efficient when using low molecular solutes, such as glucose, than the aquaporins, because they readily permit transport of the osmolyte into the patient, resulting both in a much reduced reflection coefficient but also a drop in the osmotic gradient with time during the dwell. This is why patients with high solute transport have less good ultrafiltration with glucose. When a larger molecule is used, for example albumin or a polyglucose (e.g., icodextrin, Extraneal), a sustained ultrafiltration can be achieved during a long dwell because it will remain in the peritoneal cavity for a much longer period.[59,60] In fact, under these circumstances, the larger the number of these pores potentially the better, because the achieved ultrafiltration will be proportional to their area. Furthermore, it is possible to achieve net ultrafiltration without creating an

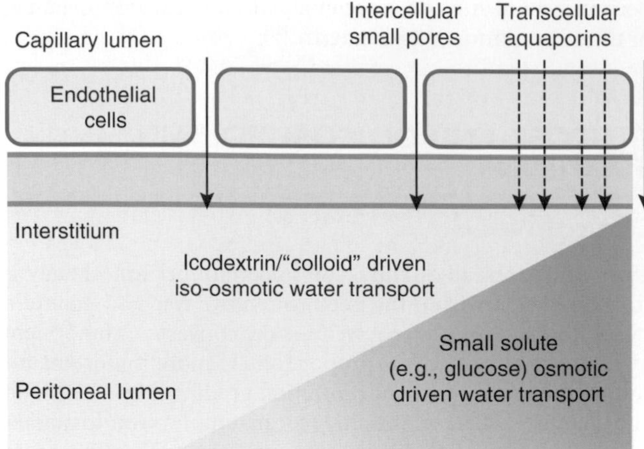

Figure 27–2 There are two pathways for ultrafiltration. First, a water-exclusive, high-efficiency transcellular pathway, due to the presence of aquaporins present in the vascular endothelium, which requires an osmotic gradient. Second, an intercellular pathway that is less efficient but still contributes half of the ultrafiltration because it represents the majority of the total pore area. Small osmolytes, such as glucose, amino acids, and glycerol, act across both pathways but require an osmotic gradient. Large molecules, such as icodextrin, are able to exert a "colloidal" gradient across the intercellular pathway.

osmotic pressure because large molecules, by virtue of their size, have colligative properties that will drive convective flow without the need for an osmotic gradient. In the case of albumin, which also has an electric charge, this is a true *oncotic* pressure, a term that is frequently applied to any large molecule, such as a polyglucose, albeit that this is strictly incorrect.

To summarize, therefore, peritoneal physiology dictates the different types of solution that will be required to achieve the best ultrafiltration. There is a need for *both* small osmotic agents to generate short term, efficient, predominantly aquaporin mediated ultrafiltration and larger molecules that can achieve long dwell fluid removal, with properties more similar to albumin, the naturally occurring oncotic agent.

There is another reason why an alternative to glucose may be required: the avoidance of the metabolic complications of excessive peritoneal absorption of glucose. Obesity is a well-recognized complication of PD, as is associated hyperinsulinemia and lipid abnormalities.[61–63] Longitudinal studies have shown that patients on PD tend to gain fat weight and that this weight gain is associated with a worsening lipid profile.[61,64] With an increasing proportion of dialysis patients being diabetics, who do not always appear to enjoy the same benefit from PD as is seen in nondiabetics,[65] the importance of glycemic control is in need of receiving increased attention.

Solution Description

Glucose

Glucose containing dialysate solutions have been manufactured in three strengths for many years. The concentrations are 1.36%/1.5%, 2.27%/2.5%, and 3.86%/4.25% (the alternative values represent the anhydrous/hydrated form), and these result in fluids with an osmolality of 344–347, 395–398 and 483–486 mOsmol/L, respectively. They enable the clinician and patient to vary the dialysis prescription so as to titrate peritoneal fluid removal and thus maintain the desired dry weight.

Glucose Polymer

Icodextrin is the only polyglucose and thus the only large molecular weight solution commercially available. It is currently formulated to be iso-osmotic with plasma (284 mOsmol/L) at a concentration of 7.5%, with a sodium concentration of 133 mmol/L and a lactate concentration of 40 mmol/L. As its name implies, it consists of several glucose molecules tagged together since they are found in starch, from which it is manufactured (Figure 27–3). Although the prefix to the name ("ico") implies 20 glucose building blocks per molecule, it is, in fact, a poly-dispersed mixture of the glucose polymers (range 2 → 1000 units) found in starch that has been refined to remove the smaller fractions, which would otherwise cross the peritoneal membrane more readily and accumulate or be metabolized by the patient. As it is, a significant proportion of the starches do enter the circulation, where they are metabolized eventually to maltose by circulating amylase.[66,67] In patients using icodextrin for one exchange per day, steady state of these metabolites is reached within 2 weeks. They do, however, contribute to the osmolality of the plasma, resulting in a variable degree of isosmotic hyponatremia, usually about 2 to 5 mmol/L lower than the patient's pretreatment plasma sodium.[68] The maltose cannot be metabolized in the circulation of humans, which lacks maltase, although this enzyme is present in the kidney and intracellularly throughout the body. There is no evidence to date that maltose accumulates within patients treated with icodextrin.

Evidence of Clinical Benefit

Glucose Solutions

Glucose is a highly effective osmotic agent that was well established in the use of intermittent peritoneal dialysis before the inception of CAPD and APD. Its undisputed efficacy

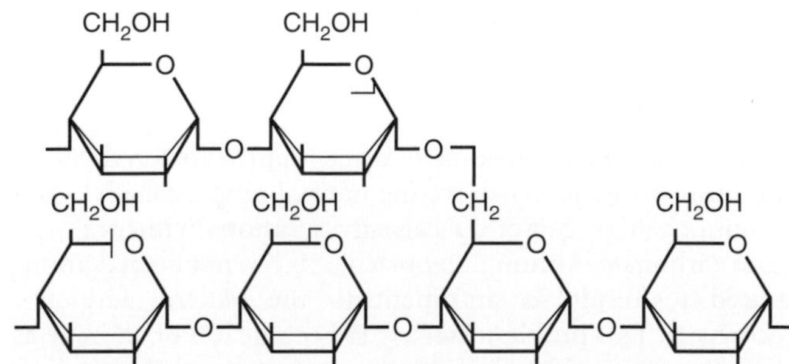

Figure 27–3 Icodextrin has a polyglucose structure found in starch; the number of subunits range from 2 to 1000. Ninety percent of the linkages between subunits are of the a 1-4 type. The majority fraction, accounting for approximately 50%, comprises 30–120 subunits, with a molecular weight range of 5–20,000 Daltons.

combined with its low cost means that it is always likely to have a role in this treatment modality. Carefully conducted single dwell studies have confirmed that the initial ultrafiltration rate across the peritoneum is directly proportional to the initial glucose osmotic gradient.[69] Glucose solutions have also become the standard for assessing peritoneal membrane function. Generally, using a standardized 4-hour dwell period, patients achieving more than 200 mL of ultrafiltration using a glucose 2.27%/2.5% (standard peritoneal equilibration test)[70,71] or more than 400 mL with a glucose 3.86%/4.25% exchange (simplified standardized permeability analysis)[72] will be able to obtain sufficient overall daily ultrafiltration.[73] Values below this indicate relative ultrafiltration failure, although this might not manifest clinically until the residual urine volume of the patient has become critically low.

Glucose dialysate also has the potential of being an important calorie source for patients who are malnourished. Adequate calorie intake appears to be important in maintaining nitrogen balance, especially in long-term PD patients,[74] and it should be remembered that when the dialysis dose is increased, there is inevitably an increase in delivered calories from this route, which may be of help in maintaining nutrition in the malnourished.[75]

Glucose Polymer

There is now considerable clinical experience with icodextrin, a PD solution that has been subjected to more randomized clinical trials than any other (see summary Table 27–2). Used as salvage therapy, in patients with clinically inadequate ultrafiltration, it can extend the life of PD treatment.[76] When used on a daily basis for the long exchange (overnight in CAPD and during the daytime in APD patients), it results in net ultrafiltration that is equivalent to that achieved using 2.27% to 3.86% glucose, depending on length of dwell and peritoneal membrane function.[77] Generally, the longer the dwell the more ultrafiltration will be obtained, although there is rarely any value in extending beyond 14 hours. On average, it is slightly more effective in patients with high solute transport, in keeping with its proposed mechanism of action across the small pores, although there is considerable individual variability. As a rule of thumb, icodextrin will achieve significantly better ultrafiltration than glucose 2.27% in patients with high or high average solute transport characteristics (D/P creatinine ration at 4 hours >0.64),[78] and this is why this has been the main comparator solution used in the randomized studies. As a result of better convection, icodextrin will also remove more sodium when compared to glucose 2.27%.[79] The diffusive removal of sodium, however, is not so well optimized. The length of the dwell ensures that there is time for equilibration, but the sodium gradient is compromised, partly because the concentration of sodium in the dialysate is 133 mmol/L (compared to 132 mmol/L in conventional glucose solutions) but also because patients on icodextrin develop a relative hyponatremia, which influences sodium removal throughout the rest of the day. Nevertheless, provided better ultrafiltration is obtained, icodextrin will achieve better overall sodium losses.

There is now evidence that this improved fluid removal translates into changes in weight, fluid status, and body composition. In a large randomized trial comparing icodextrin with glucose 2.27% over 12 months, a divergence in weight was observed, such that weight gain was prevented in the patients treated with icodextrin.[78] This could have, of course, been due to either fat of fluid gain in the glucose treated patients or the opposite, including loss of lean body mass in the icodextrin treated group. More detailed studies in smaller patient groups, using more sophisticated techniques, such as bioelectric impedance, isotope dilution methods, and DEXA scan, have shown that weight loss in patients randomized to icodextrin lose fluid from the extracellular compartment.[80,81] In one such study, conducted over 6 months, there was also a weight gain in the patients randomized to glucose, supporting the findings of the 12-month study cited earlier. This weight gain was not fully explained by increases in fluid status, implying that there was also an additional increase in body fat.[81]

This latter observation emphasizes the metabolic advantages in utilizing icodextrin when compared to the more hypertonic glucose solutions. In nondiabetic subjects, the hyperinsulinemia associated with the continuous use of glucose containing solutions is significantly improved by the use of icodextrin, and this is associated with an improvement in insulin sensitivity.[82] In diabetic subjects, a recent randomized study has shown that diabetic control is improved in treatment regimes that include icodextrin and amino acids.[83] Gastric emptying, which is delayed in PD patients and may be responsible for lack of appetite, is less marked when using icodextrin than glucose.[84] The effect of icodextrin on lipid profiles has been variable, although there is evidence that they can improve when using icodextrin.[85] The reason for these discrepancies may well reflect the fact that many PD patients are already receiving lipid-lowering treatment when they commence icodextrin.[81] This may also be the explanation for the lack of effect on blood pressure observed in these studies, which might be expected to have fallen following reduction in the extracellular fluid volume. With the exception of one single center, open study,[86] randomized studies have not shown a significant effect on blood pressure.[80,81] Blood pressure control in these studies has been good in both randomized groups, which were designed to give maximum freedom to the clinician in terms of antihypertensive drug prescription.

Apart from extending life of therapy, avoiding some of the detrimental metabolic effects of glucose and improving both achieved ultrafiltration and fluid status, there is evidence that use of icodextrin improves the quality of life of PD patients. In the short term (13 weeks), patients randomized to icodextrin reported better physical and mental health status than those using standard glucose.[87]

Potential Problems

Glucose Solutions

The problems associated with using glucose solutions are threefold. First, there is issue of local tissue damage to the peritoneum, which will be discussed later under bioincompatibility. Second, there are the unwanted systemic metabolic effects, which have largely been dealt with. Third, there is a more general problem associated with the use of any osmotic agent that relies substantially upon its effects across the aquaporins to achieve ultrafiltration. Precisely because this mechanism of ultrafiltration is water exclusive, solutes, such as sodium, that are dependent on convective for their loss may not in fact be removed so efficiently due to their sieving by

Table 27–2 Summary of Randomized Controlled Trials Establishing the Safety and Efficacy of Icodextrin

Author, Year, Reference	n	Length	Comparator fluid (Design)	Comment
Mistry, 1994[77]	I: 106 G: 103	6 months	1.36% or 3.86%	MIDAS study: Ultrafiltration compared to 1.36% was 3.5 times greater for 8-hour and 5.5 times greater for 12-hour dwell length and equivalent to that achieved with 3.86% exchanges.
Gokal, 1995[171]				Using icodextrin for the long dwell in CAPD does not increase the rate of peritonitis or alter the outcome of peritonitis. Peritonitis does not affect uptake of icodextrin from the peritoneum.
Posthuma, 1997[172]	I: 11 G: 12	12 months	2.27%	Icodextrin enhances ultrafiltration during the daytime dwell in CCPD patients, increasing convective clearance of creatinine.
Postuma, 1997 & 1998[68,173]	I: 19 G: 19	12 months	2.27%	Icodextrin preserved the daytime dwell ultrafiltration in CCPD patients during peritonitis. Serum icodextrin metabolites increased during icodextrin use, accounted for the osmolar gap and associated hyponatremia, but remained stable during peritonitis.
Plum, 2002[79]	I: 20 G: 19	12 weeks	2.27%	Icodextrin produced increased, sustained ultrafiltration during the long dwell period, increasing (convective) clearance and sodium removal in APD patients. No effect on residual function.
Wolfson, 2002[78]	I: 90 G:85	4 weeks	2.27%	Efficacy study showing icodextrin increases UF in long dwell preventing fluid reabsorption. Greatest comparative benefit to glucose observed with higher solute transport.
Wolfson, 2002[78]	I: 175 G:112	52 weeks	2.27%	Safety study showing a significant difference in body weight between groups (lower with icodextrin, gain with glucose) when compared to baseline.
Guo, 2002[87]	I: 58 G:35	13 weeks	2.27%	Peritoneal dialysis patients treated with icodextrin experienced substantial quality of life improvement at 13 weeks after the start of treatment, in particular, improvement of patients' mental health, general health, and symptoms, such as muscle spasms or twitching, cramps during an exchange or treatment, cramps after an exchange or treatment, itchy skin, and faintness or dizziness.
Konings, 2003[80]	I: 22 G:18	4 months	1.36%) (Open-label RCT)	Patients randomized to icodextrin experienced a large increase in UF, reduction in extracellular fluid volume, left ventricular mass and weight, and a small but significant reduction in urine volume. No changes in glucose group. No changes in BP or CRP.
Davies, 2003[81]	I: 28 G:22	6 months	2.27% (Double-blind RCT)	Icodextrin patients achieved greater ultrafiltration, sodium removal, weight loss, and a reduction in extracellular fluid volume. Weight in glucose patients increased without increase in body water suggesting fat gain. Residual renal function better preserved in the icodextrin group. No change in BP, CRP, or lipid profiles.
Ota, 2003[174]	18	3 months	1.36% (Open, crossover)	Confirms better UF in Japanese PD patients with icodextrin. Peritoneal absorption of fluid ranges between 36% and 42%.

G, glucose; *I*, icodextrin. See Table 27–3 for randomized trials combining icodextrin and amino acids.

these pores. When APD is used with multiple short exchanges using hypertonic glucose, there might be quite efficient ultrafiltration but insufficient time for the diffusive component of sodium loss to occur. This leads to relatively poor sodium losses in APD patients, despite apparently good ultrafiltration, an issue the prescribing clinician should be aware of.[88] There is some evidence to suggest that APD patients have less good blood pressure control, perhaps for this reason,[89] and certainly anuric APD patients with poor ultrafiltration (< 750 mL/day) seem, by whatever mechanism, to have worse clinical outcomes.[55] Optimizing daytime ultrafiltration, for example, with icodextrin, can ameliorate the problem.[88]

Glucose Polymers

As discussed, there is absorption of glucose polymer fractions across the peritoneum, which results in a number of potential problems that the clinician needs to be aware of. First, these polymers and their metabolites reach a steady state in plasma between 1 and 2 weeks of treatment. The slight hyperosmolality that they cause, combined with its associated hyponatremia, do not appear to have any clinical adverse effects. It does result in some reduction in the efficacy of icodextrin as an ultrafiltration agent, however, and patients who initially report very high ultrafiltration volumes may see a modest reduction with time. The presence of icodextrin and its metabolites in plasma can also interfere with some analytical methods. For example, certain blood sugar measuring devices that employ glucose oxidase will overestimate the blood sugar,[90,91] whereas the usual method for determining plasma amylase in the diagnosis of pancreatitis is unreliable due to its underestimation.[92,93]

The other potential problem with the use of icodextrin is the development of allergies and sterile peritonitis. Skin rashes are well described and appear to be due to an allergic reaction to starch.[94] Usually these are mild, localized, and typically occur on the palm of the hand. In most cases they are transient, and the patients can put up with them until they resolve over a few weeks. Occasionally (1%–3% of patients), the patient develops an exfoliating dermatitis that is often generalized and can be quite severe causing erythroderma.[95] In these situations the icodextrin should be withdrawn and not reintroduced since the problem will recur. Sterile peritonitis has also been described in patients using icodextrin, and mini-epidemics of this problem have been described.[96] At least one of these outbreaks was found to be due to contamination of the icodextrin solution by proteoglycans, the product of bacterial cell walls that were contaminating the refining of raw product. Typically, patients with this problem have a sterile peritonitis that does not respond to antibiotics, which on differential white cell count is associated either with raised eosinophils or mononuclear cells but not neutrophils.[97] The patient is not usually unwell and the problem responds very rapidly to withdrawal of the product. Although this problem has been identified and largely put right by tightening the quality controls of fluid production, isolated cases of icodextrin-associated sterile peritonitis are occasionally reported. Importantly, however, none of the controlled trials (summarized in Table 27–2) have reported a higher incidence of peritonitis using icodextrin.

Concern has been expressed that too rapid ultrafiltration induced by icodextrin might precipitate a significant fall in residual renal function. There is certainly increasing evidence that episodes of volume depletion, intentional or otherwise, are associated with a fall in urine volume.[98] The majority of randomized trials using icodextrin have not shown any significant differences in the effect of icodextrin compared to glucose. In the detailed study in which icodextrin was compared to glucose 1.36% solution, a very large increase in average ultrafiltration (from 744 to 1670 mL/day) was associated with a fall in urine volume (1131 to 913 mL/day).[80] In contrast, the change and between-group difference in ultrafiltration, typically 400 mL/day, was more modest in patients selected for greater risk of fluid-related problems (urine volume <750 mL, high or high average solute transport), using glucose 2.27% as the comparator fluid. In this study residual function was better preserved in patients randomized to icodextrin, despite a similar average reduction in extracellular fluid volume.[81] The conclusion that should be drawn is that sudden large increases in ultrafiltration should be avoided in PD patients (by whatever fluid regime), and that provided icodextrin is introduced carefully, it is possible to achieve the desired effect safely.

AMINO-ACID SOLUTIONS

Clinical Need

It is well recognized that many patients on dialysis treatment are, or become, malnourished.[99] It is also known, especially for peritoneal dialysis patients, that malnutrition is an independent predictor of poor survival.[55,100] The causes of malnutrition are, however, complicated. Reduction in renal function is associated with a spontaneous fall in appetite,[101] which does to some extent improve following the commencement of dialysis treatment,[102] although this is certainly reduced once residual renal function is lost.[103] There is also evidence that positive nitrogen balance is better maintained in the short term when protein intake is high, although in longer-term PD patients, it may be that adequate calories derived from carbohydrate are important.[104] It is increasingly clear, however, that protein-calorie malnutrition is also influenced by comorbid disease, in particular, cardiovascular atheromatous disease when associated with an inflammatory state.[105] PD patients with increasing comorbidity, now known to be the dominant determinate of survival on dialysis report reduced dietary protein and calorie intake for a given small solute clearance[106] and generally fail to improve their intake following an increase in delivered dialysis dose.[75] In patients who cannot or will not eat, it is tempting to try an alternative approach to delivering nutrition, hence the development of amino-acid containing solutions.

There is, however, perhaps another equally important clinical need for an amino-acid solution, an alternative low molecular weight osmolyte to glucose, for reasons both discussed previously and in further detail below, when considering biocompatibility.

Solution Description

The only commercially available dialysate fluid containing amino acid is a 1.1% solution (see Table 27–1 for description) that exerts sufficient osmotic force to give an average ultrafiltration equivalent, or a little more, to that achieved with glucose 1.36%. It contains 87 mmol/L of amino acids the majority of which (61%) are essential amino acids.

This is not the only amino acid solution that has been formulated over the last few years and several different formulations have been evaluated. The aims of solution design have been to give the patient sufficient nitrogen in the form of amino acids to at least replace the nitrogen losses associated with both peritoneal amino acid (3–4 g/day) and protein losses (4–15 g/day), and, if possible, to normalize the plasma amino-acid profile that is associated with uremia and acidosis. In the early stages of solution development, a number of different amino acid concentrations were investigated, ranging from 1.0% to 2.7% in concentration, to establish their osmotic effectiveness, effects on membrane function, absorption profiles, and their potential for inducing acidosis.[107–109] Typically 72% to 82% of amino acids are absorbed, with a peak in amino acid concentrations in the plasma occurring by 1 hour. The higher concentration solutions (e.g., 2.7%) resulted in increased estimates of solute mass transfer indicating a vasodilatatory effect on the peritoneal membrane,[110] possibly mediated by locally generated prostanoids or nitric oxide.[111] They also resulted in nonphysiologically high concentrations of amino acids and were thus abandoned. Even the 1.1% solution has a small but detectable effect on peritoneal blood flow resulting in a small but significant increase in small solute transport.[110] Earlier amino-acid formulations resulted in excessive acidosis due to the catabolism of lycine, arginine, and methionine, which when replaced by anionic amino acids was largely prevented.[112]

Evidence of Clinical Benefit

Initial balance studies were able to establish that the nitrogen absorbed in the form of amino acids from a single daily dwell of 1.1% solution is sufficient to counterbalance the losses associated with amino acid and protein in the daily dialysis effluent. The typical amount of amino acids adsorbed per day is 18 g, which, if compared to oral protein, would represent about one quarter, typically 0.3 g/kg, of the daily recommended intake.[107,113] One advantage of this method of delivery is that it avoids the phosphate load associated with the equivalent dietary protein and thus the need for phosphate binders. Furthermore, improvement but not normalization of the plasma amino acid profile has been reported.[114] Thus, the primary aims of solution design are largely successful. However, to provide convincing evidence of clinical benefit, three things are further required. First, demonstration that nitrogen from amino acid absorbed from the peritoneal cavity can be incorporated into somatic protein. Second, that patients with impaired nutrition can show an improvement, and third, if possible, that this translates into improved clinical outcomes (see Table 27–3 for summary of studies).

Detailed studies employing ^{15}N-glycine, $^{2}H_3$ leucine, and ^{13}C leucine have shown that of the total amino acid dose, 55% is absorbed by 1 hour and 80% by 5 hours; about half (48%) is utilized for protein synthesis, whereas a significant proportion (16%) is oxidized as an energy source during the dwell period.[115,116] By giving the patient an oral calorie meal at the same time as the amino acid solution is used, the proteolysis that occurs during this period can be reduced by 25%.[116] Amino acids delivered via the peritoneal cavity can, therefore, be incorporated into protein, and where possible patients should be encouraged to consume a calorie rich meal or snack, typically 600 kcal, during the course of the exchange.

Several randomized controlled trials have been performed to evaluate the safety and efficacy of amino-acid solutions in PD patients with varying degrees of nutritional status. Summarized in Table 27–3, along with open studies describing clinical experience, these have given mixed, although generally encouraging, results. Smaller earlier studies evaluating precursors to the current commercially available solution failed to demonstrate clear benefit and noted variable beneficial or no effects on plasma lipid profiles. A later multicenter study of malnourished patients studied for just 3 months demonstrated an increase in circulating IGF in patients randomized to amino-acid solution, suggesting an increase in protein synthesis.[117] In a subgroup of patients with a plasma albumin below 35 g/L at the start of the study, those randomized to amino acids had increases in the plasma prealbumin and transferrin levels but no increase in mid-arm muscle circumference (MAMC). In contrast, those with albumin levels above 35 g/L at baseline showed fewer changes in plasma proteins (these deteriorated in the glucose group) but did experience an increase in MAMC if using amino acids. The only long-term (3 years) randomized study of amino acid solutions was performed in malnourished Chinese PD patients and did examine clinical outcomes, although was probably not sufficiently powered to detect a difference in patient survival.[118] Of the 60 patients randomized, both groups had similar mortality, hospitalization duration, serial C-reactive protein levels, and drop-out rates during the study. Patients using amino acids had an improvement in triglyceride levels and more stable biochemical markers of nutrition (e.g., albumin, total cholesterol), combined with an increase in the appearance of nitrogen and a reported increase in dietary protein intake. Anthropometrics improved, especially in women in the amino acid treated group, but composite nutritional scores were no different.

In summary, the true benefits of amino-acid solutions used in malnourished patients remain equivocal. Certainly they are absorbed and utilized in healthy PD patients, but it is likely that their relatively disappointing effect in malnourished patients reflects the underlying difficulty of reversing this problem in dialysis patients in whom comorbidity, combined with associated inflammation, is blunting the therapeutic effect. The potential benefit to lipid profiles is also variably reported. It is perhaps more logical to use amino-acid solution as part of a dialysis regime that prevents the use and complications associated with heavy use of glucose solutions, for example, in improving glycemic control in diabetics,[83] improving gastric emptying,[84] preventing fat gain and associated hypertriglyceridemia, and even membrane preservation (see later), with a hope that protein-calorie malnutrition may be prevented to some extent.

Potential Problems

The most common side effect seen in patients using amino-acid solutions is increased nausea and anorexia. The former may be reported in association with the very slight odor that some patients detect or reflect the modest increase on plasma urea levels that might be observed. In these circumstances there may be symptomatic benefit from increasing the dialysis dose. Some patients will develop mild evidence of

Table 27–3 Summary of Clinical Trials Examining Safety and Efficacy of Amino-Acid Solutions

Author, Year, Reference	n	Length	Trial Design	Comments
Bruno, 1989[109]	6	6 months	Open-label, cross-over	1% AA solution. Nitrogen balance became positive and patients gained weight. Lipid profiles improved significantly, and AA profiles became more normal.
Young, 1989[175,176] Dibble, 1990 [177]	8	12 weeks	Open, non-randomized	Malnourished patients (albumin <35 g/L). 1% solution. Lipids improved (LDL cholesterol fell). Modest benefit in nutrition only. No changes were seen in body weight, body fat, arm muscle circumference, fasting plasma glucose, insulin, growth hormone, triglyceride, nonesterified fatty acids, or HDL cholesterol.
Faller, 1995[178]	15	3 months	Open, non-randomized	Evaluation of a 1.1% solution. Albumin and transferring improved significantly. Plasma urea but not bicarbonate increased.
Kopple, 1995[115]	19	20 days	Open, non-randomized	Detailed inpatient nitrogen balance studies in malnourished patients. 1.1% solution made nitrogen balance significantly more positive.
Jones, 1997[112]	12	14 days	Randomized, cross-over	Study to evaluate a modified 1.1% AA formula containing reduced lysine, arginine, and methionine to reduce acidosis. Despite a good total protein/nitrogen intake, bicarbonate was higher with modified solution.
Mirsa, 1997[179]	18	6 months	Randomized, cross-over	The use of 1.1% AA, although clinically safe and without side effects, had no effect on the dyslipidemia in these CAPD patients.
Jones, 1998[113]	20	2–3 days	Open-label, cross-over	Using a 1.1% solution daily loss of AAs and proteins into dialysate more than offset by gains absorbed from one exchange; such net gains exceeded losses in all patients studied.
Jones, 1998[117]	AA:54 G: 51	3 months	Randomized, open-label	1–2 exchanges daily of 1.1% AA solution is safe and provides nutritional benefit for malnourished PD patients (anthropometrics and insulin-like growth factor) while improving plasma phosphate levels.
Grzegorzewska, 1999[119]	8	6 months	Open, non-randomized	Overnight administration of 1.1% solution using concomitant antacids to avoid acidosis. Relatively well-nourished CAPD patients resulted in increased serum concentration of AAs without changes in other nutritional parameters.
Plum, 1999[180]	10	6 hour dwell	Randomized, cross-over	1.0 % bicarbonate buffered solution compared to both bicarbonate and lactate buffered glucose (1.5%). Reduced serum glucose concentrations were found with AA solution, but bicarbonate buffering (34 mmol/L) did not change blood acid-base status combined with either glucose or AAs.
Qamar, 1999[120]	7	3 months	Randomized, cross-over	Only randomized study in children. Caloric intake increased and protein intake improved. Appetite and total body nitrogen increased in at least half the children during AA dialysis. Total plasma protein and albumin concentrations did not change significantly.
Van, 2002[84]	61	Single dwell	Randomized, cross-over	PD patients have impaired gastric emptying even when empty of dialysate fluid. This is worse with glucose instilled than either AA or icodextrin.
Marshall, 2003[83]	8	72 hours	Randomized, cross-over	Glycemic control (both concentration and variability determined from continuous measurements) was improved in insulin-dependent diabetics with a dialysis regime that included AA and icodextrin.
Li, 2003[118]	60	3 years	Randomized, open-label	Long-term administration of amino acid dialysate is well tolerated, tends to improve nutritional status in high-risk patients, especially women, but does not alter patient survival.

AA, amino acid solution.

metabolic acidosis, manifested by a fall in the plasma bicarbonate.[109,115,119,120] This can almost always be corrected by adjusting the dialysate buffer in the remaining exchanges, adding sodium bicarbonate or calcium carbonate to the medications, or again increasing dialysis dose, as a negative relationship between plasma bicarbonate levels and urea clearance has been reported.[32] It is strongly advised that the product be used in combination with expert dietetic support to ensure that the solution supplements rather than replaces adequate total calorie intake.

BIOCOMPATIBLE SOLUTIONS

Clinical Need

The degree of "biocompatibility" of a treatment might be considered as its lack of interference with normal physiologic function, although at the same time achieving the desired therapeutic effect. It has been formally defined as the ability of a material, device, or system to perform without a clinically significant host response in a specific application.[121] As already discussed, the instillation of high glucose concentrations within the peritoneal cavity undoubtedly affects systemic physiology in a fashion that can be considered bio*in*compatible. The purpose of this section, however, is to discuss biocompatibility of PD solutions locally within the peritoneal cavity and specifically their interaction with the peritoneal membrane, specifically its biology and function. The need to develop biocompatible solutions derives from several strands of evidence which, although largely circumstantial, taken together make a very powerful case. These lines of evidence include the intrinsically bioincompatible nature of standard fluids, including their established in vitro and ex vivo toxicity, and the demonstration of both functional and morphologic changes to the peritoneal membrane that culminate in ultrafiltration failure and, in the worst cases, sclerosing encapsulating peritonitis.

Bioincompatibility of Standard Fluids

This can be conveniently divided into short-term toxicity, associated with low pH, high osmolality and the use of lactate as buffer, and long-term toxicity due to the damaging effects of glucose, either because of direct cellular toxicity, the formation of glucose degradation products as a consequence of the sterilization procedure, or the formation of advanced glycosylation end products within the membrane or systemic circulation.

The short-term effects of bioincompatibility result in infusion pain, experienced by many patients but considerably variable in severity, combined with cellular toxicity shown in both in vitro and ex vivo studies.[36] Because of the insistence by regulatory authorities throughout the world to heat sterilize PD solutions, this has to be performed at low pH to prevent gross caramelization of glucose. As a result, for the first 45 minutes or so of a dialysis exchange the intra-abdominal fluid is at an unphysiologically low pH, which causes a fall in the intracellular pH of local cell populations (macrophages, mesothelial cells), that is potentiated in its toxicity by the presence of lactate.[122] This results in repeated damage to the local host-defense mechanism and the mesothelial cell lining of the luminal surface of the membrane that is thought to have a protective and modulatory role in membrane damage and prevention of inflammation.[123,124] This damage is always exacerbated when solutions of higher osmolality are used.

Standard dialysis fluids also contain glucose degradation products (GDPs), which along with glucose are thought to contribute more to the long-term bioincompatibility of these solutions.[125] Generally, these molecules, which are highly reactive and toxic to cells, are formed from the nonenzymic autocatabolism of glucose within the dialysate during sterilization that is accelerated by heat and slowed down at low pH. The exception might be acetaldehyde, which also results from catabolism of lactate. Extended shelf life will also increase their concentration in dialysate, especially if the storage has been at room temperature or even higher. (Anders Wieslander, personal communication, data awaiting publication.) The list of culprits is growing steadily (Table 27–4), and some, in particular, are thought to be especially toxic (e.g., 5-hydroxy-methyl-2-furaldehyde). However, long-term toxicity might also result from glucose exposure by at least two other mechanisms: the intracellular toxicity of high glucose concentrations resulting in hypoxia due to excess metabolism via the sorbitol pathway, and the formation of advanced glycosylation end products (AGEs), resulting in damage to extracellular and intracellular proteins.[126] This latter mechanism is, again, nonenzymic and is thought to occur in situ within the peritoneal membrane where glucose concentration may be very high, simulating an extreme diabetic milieu.

Functional and Morphologic Changes to the Membrane

There is now convincing evidence from longitudinal studies that peritoneal membrane function changes with time on treatment. There is considerable variability between patients, but the overall pattern is one of increasing rates of small solute transport and reductions in the ultrafiltration capacity of the peritoneal membrane.[103,127,128] The latter is mostly explained

Table 27–4 Glucose Degradation Products (GDPs) Found in Commercial Dialysate Fluids and Markers Used to Identify Systemic GDP and Advanced Glycosylation End Products (AGEs)

Glucose Degradation Products
Acetaldehyde[181–185]*
Formaldehyde[142,183]*
Glyoxal[142,153,183,186,187]*
Methylglyoxal[142,153,183,185–187]*
3-Deoxyglucasone[188]
3,4-Dideoxy-glucasone-3-ene[188]
5-Hydroxy-methyl-2-furaldehyde[142,184,189,190]*
2-Furaldehyde[183,190]
Systemic Markers of GDPs and AGE Formation
Plasma fluorescence[185]
Nepsilon-carboxymethyllysine[153]
Imidazolone[191]
Pyrraline[185,192]
Pentosidine[153]

* Significantly reduced in biocompatible dual- or triple-bag systems.

by the increases in solute transport, which accelerates the rate of glucose absorption across the peritoneal membrane, thus causing earlier loss of the osmotic gradient during any dwell. This rise in the solute transport rate is thought to reflect an increase in the effective peritoneal surface area, such as would occur with increasing vascularity of the membrane. There is now, however, increasing evidence that a second process is contributing to loss in ultrafiltration capacity with time on treatment. This process results in a reduction in the osmotic conductance of water convection—literally less ultrafiltration for a given osmotic gradient—that might result either from altered hydraulic conductance of the membrane or impaired aquaporin function, or both.[129,130]

These functional alterations in the membrane are associated with important morphologic changes with time on treatment. Although it is difficult to perform longitudinal studies of membrane morphology, data from the Peritoneal Biopsy Registry have built a convincing picture of what appears to happen.[131–133] The two overwhelming abnormalities observed with increasing severity when associated with time on treatment have been thickening of the submesothelial compact zone and the development of a diabetiform occlusive vasculopathy of the small arterioles and venules (Figure 27–4). There was a modest increase in vessel numbers, although it should be remembered that it is the capillary circulation that is responsible for the bulk of solute diffusion, and further examination of this aspect of morphology is still awaited. Other studies have reported increased capillary vessels, and this has also been reported consistently in animal models of PD solution exposure.[134]

How can these morphologic changes be linked to functional changes of the membrane? There are only two studies, so far, linking morphology and function, but both show that worse membrane damage is associated with worse function, in one case a link between high solute transport and sclerosis,[135] the other with increased area of microvessels.[134] This supports the concept that increasing small solute transport results from a greater vascular surface area. Although intuitively it seems logical to assume that increasing thickness of the submesothelial compact zone might reduce solute transport, it is possible to conceive of a situation in which the interstitium enables faster transport of small solutes, including water, because its structure is disrupted and yet offers resistance to convective movement of water, which is a quite different process at a molecular level.

Solution Description

The ideal biocompatible solution would have a physiologic pH, use bicarbonate as its buffer, contain no GDPs, be isosmotic, and only contain osmotic agents in concentrations that are not toxic to human tissue. No such single solution can

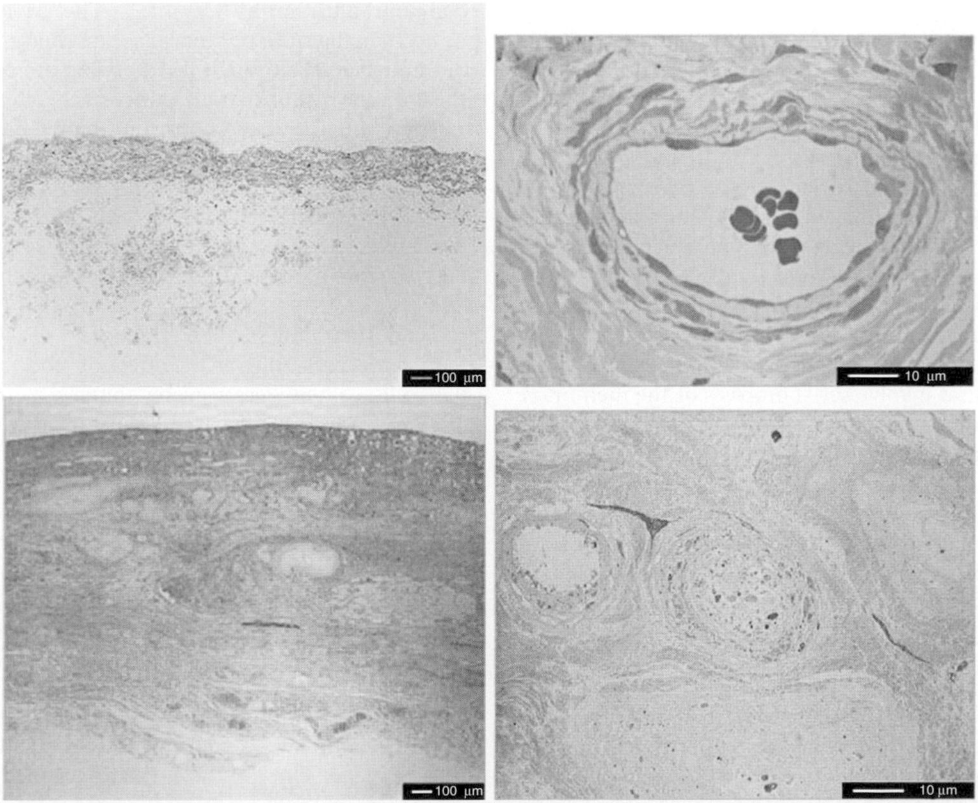

Figure 27–4 Images from the Peritoneal Biopsy Registry showing the two most striking abnormalities found in long-term peritoneal dialysis, thickening of the submesothelial compact zone (left lower panel compared to upper) and an obliterative diabetiform vasculopathy (right lower compared with upper panel). (Photographs shown courtesy of Professor John Williams, Cardiff, UK.)

exist, however, because without the presence of an osmotic gradient, short-term ultrafiltration, which will always be needed, cannot be achieved. Nevertheless, solutions are now available that go some considerable way toward meeting these objectives. As already discussed, glucose can be avoided by using either amino-acid solutions or polyglucose (icodextrin), and the latter is also isosmotic with plasma and contains less GDP than conventional glucose 1.36% solutions.[136]

The development of pH neutral solutions has necessitated a different approach, however, with the use of dual or triple compartment dialysate bag technology. In each case the principle underlying this approach is the same, although different manufacturers have come up with differing designs. By using more than one compartment during the manufacturing process, it is possible to do two things. First, it is possible to confine the glucose to a compartment that has a very low pH (optimally ~3.5), such that during the sterilization process the formation of GDPs is minimized. Second, when the two components of the dialysis fluid are brought together, just prior to instillation by the patient? performed by manually breaking a small septum? the final solution can be made to have a normal pH. This general model can be developed to enable the predominant buffer to be bicarbonate by separating this from magnesium during storage, so as to prevent its precipitation. Alternatively, by utilizing a third compartment, the potential number of recombinations can be increased, enabling all three glucose concentrations to be obtained from the same bag, for example, Gambrosol Trio.

Evidence of Clinical Benefit

A considerable number of studies have demonstrated that normal pH, low GDP solutions result in reduced cellular toxicity in vitro as well as improved function of cell populations derived from dialysate effluent when examined ex vivo.[137–141] Mesothelial cell layers when grown in culture as a monolayer, similar to that seen on the surface of the peritoneal membrane, may be physically damaged by scratching with a needle. Their subsequent ability to regrow to confluence is inhibited by standard high GDP solution but unaffected by low GDP fluids.[142] There is, however, a problem when it comes to demonstrating the benefit of these solutions in the prevention of long-term functional and morphologic changes to the peritoneum. Studies that involve serial biopsies of the membrane are difficult to justify on ethical and practical grounds, and both functional and morphologic changes take many years to develop which, when combined with high drop-out rates, mean that they are not financially viable. Furthermore, the equipoise of many clinicians is such that the justification for the use of biocompatible fluids can be made on *a priori* grounds and if cost implications were not an issue, that it would be unacceptable to randomize patients to bioincompatible solutions.

Nevertheless, this difficulty has led to another approach, namely the use of biomarkers within peritoneal dialysis effluent that act as surrogate measures of peritoneal damage or integrity. The example most studied is the cancer antigen, CA 125, which is a product of mesothelial cells usually used to track the bulk of tumors derived from this cell type. It has been demonstrated that CA 125 is present in dialysate effluent in concentrations that imply its local production, and it is argued that its relative concentration reflects a changes in viability and thus integrity of the mesothelial cell layer.[143] Randomized trials of all the normal pH, lower GDP biocompatible solutions have shown that they are associated with a relative increase in the dialysate concentrations of CA 125, implying their greater biocompatibility in vivo as well as underlining the role GDPs appear to have in adversely affecting mesothelial cell function.[144–146] The benefit appears to be independent of the buffer type used. Other markers that have been investigated include hyaluronan and procollagen peptides, thought to represent interstitial damage or turnover, respectively, the inflammatory cytokines interleukin-6 (IL-6) and tumour necrosis factor (TNFα), and vascular endothelial growth factor (VEGF). In each case the biocompatible solutions have been associated with evidence of better preservation of the interstitium, reduced inflammation (Il-6 but not TNFα), and reduced production of VEGF.[140,145]

Although there is no clear evidence as yet that biocompatible solutions preserve membrane function for longer than conventional fluids, there are apparent clinical benefits. Bicarbonate-lactate neutral pH solution has been demonstrated to reduce infusion pain compared to either lactate or bicarbonate-only solutions.[36,45] Because bicarbonate-only solution was associated with more pain than the mixed buffer solution (although still less than lactate only low pH solutions) is of interest. One possible explanation is that supraphysiologic concentrations, which are required in a bicarbonate only solution, result in hyperemia of the peritoneal vasculature. Bicarbonate-lactate solution in a 12-month randomized study was also associated with a significant increase in the achieved daily ultrafiltration by 150 mL.[147] The explanation for this is not certain, because peritoneal solute transport characteristics did not change, although it is possible there was an improvement on the osmotic conductance of the membrane.

There are also data supporting better biocompatibility of icodextrin and amino-acid solutions when compared to conventional glucose containing fluids. Ex vivo studies of macrophages derived from the effluent following an icodextrin exchange show better phagocytosis compared to those derived from glucose effluent, and mesothelial cells in culture also have better function and viability when exposed to icodextrin rather than glucose,[148–150] although concern has been expressed over the effect of icodextrin on mesothelial cells, albeit less severe than hypertonic glucose.[151] Similarly, amino acid based solutions also show better biocompatibility than glucose solutions, with demonstration in both in vitro and ex vivo studies improved phagocytosis of macrophage and a reduction in the secretion of inflammatory cytokines, presumably due to the lack of glucose or GDP toxicity.[152] Compared to conventional glucose solutions, GDP concentrations in icodextrin and amino acid solutions are significantly reduced, especially in the latter case, such that in both cases single dwell studies show a net loss of AGEs demonstrated by the time-dependent appearance of these compounds into the dialysate effluent, presumably due to their removal from the circulation or peritoneal membrane.[153] One study evaluating a neutral, bicarbonate compared to lactate buffered amino acid solution suggests that this is more biocompatible.[154] Data awaiting publication would suggest that adverse changes in membrane occurring in anuric APD patients are, to some extent, ameliorated by use of icodextrin (Davies, et al. European Automated

Peritoneal Dialysis Outcome Study, American Society of Nephrology, Philadelphia, 2003).

Potential Problems

As would be hoped, there are few, if any, problems associated with the use of more biocompatible solutions (with the exception of specialized solution specific issues discussed previously). Peritonitis rates, if anything, are reported as being lower than with conventional fluids, supporting the in vitro and ex vivo observations of improved cellular function of the innate immune system.[155] Due to their dual or triple compartment bag design, they are perhaps a little more complex for patients to use than conventional fluids, and some patients are said to not be able to manage this. In each case, however, they have been designed with safety in mind so that patients cannot infuse a solution that might be harmful. Their benefit in APD is not fully established, although it would be anticipated that with the short night-time exchanges during which pH does not fully normalize, their advantages would be greater. There is recently published evidence confirming the safety and efficacy of bicarbonate-lactate solution in two short-term prospective open-label studies evaluating 25/10 mmol and 25/15 mmol mixes, respectively. In each case, when compared to the 35 and 40 mmol lactate solution, respectively, patient reported less infusion pain, although no specific data on biocompatibility (e.g., membrane markers) have yet been published.[42]

FUTURE DEVELOPMENTS

It can be seen from the previous that, although significant advances in solution design have been made, there remains room for further improvements. In addition, there is still a lack of evidence that those improvements already made will actually translate into perceived clinical benefit, such as improved technique and patient survival rates or better health status/quality of life. A number of potential areas are considered.

Optimization of Ultrafiltration of Sodium Removal

Although the presence of sodium sieving is a good sign in a PD patient, because it is evidence of efficient ultrafiltration induced by small osmolytes via the aquaporin pathway, it results in a potential deficit between sodium and water removal (see Figure 27–2). As discussed previously, this is maximal when a regime employs short exchanges, such as APD, and may result in worse blood pressure control, poor fluid status, and contribute to the poor survival seen in APD patients achieving low fluid losses.[88,89] Optimizing sodium removal is also an attractive way of improving blood pressure control, especially when residual renal function has dropped off. As discussed previously, sodium removal is dependent mainly on convective losses, although diffusion plays a significant part.[46] There are, therefore, essentially two strategies available for increasing sodium loss: increasing ultrafiltration or enhancing diffusion with the use of low sodium dialysate fluids. Combining these processes by using the long exchange, to allow time for the diffusion to occur, also makes sense. For example, combining a low molecular weight osmolyte (e.g., glucose, glycerol, or amino acid) with icodextrin will increase ultrafiltration that enables sodium to follow due to the long dwell time. This approach has already been shown, by combining icodextrin with glucose, to significantly enhance ultrafiltration.[193] Studies using low sodium dialysates have been performed and have also shown to increase sodium removal, although their beneficial effects have been variable.[156–159] Some have reported improvements in blood pressure and echocardiographic parameters, whereas others have observed worrying side effects. There is clearly room for further research on both safety and efficacy.

Optimizing Biocompatibility

As indicated earlier, the evidence that improved biocompatibility of dialysate solutions results in preservation in either preservation of membrane function or the prevention of membrane morphology is keenly awaited. So far, the main target of improving long-term biocompatibility has been the creation of low GDP solutions. Further understanding of the mechanisms of how they act and which are important can only enhance this approach. However, at least two other mechanisms of glucose toxicity, intracellular hypoxia via the sorbitol pathway and non-GDP dependent AGE formation, and probably more, exist. This invites alternative strategies, and several have been proposed that are either undergoing animal testing or clinical evaluation. These include the use of pyruvate as an alternative buffer,[160,161] glycerol as an alternative low molecular weight osmolyte,[162,163] or different combinations of existing dialysate fluids during the 24-hour period to achieve a period of glucose free treatment, often referred to as *portfolio* approach.[164]

A Drug Delivery System?

The concept that PD solutions may also act as the vehicle for drug delivery is not a new one. As already mentioned, the delivery of cytotoxic therapy directly to the peritoneal cavity is already being evaluated and used clinically.[1–3,165] In dialysis patients both desferrioxamine, used as an aluminum chelating agent,[166] and erythropoietin[167,168] have been administered via the intraperitoneal route. Antibiotics for the treatment of peritonitis and insulin for the treatment of diabetic patients have been standard therapy for many years. However, more potentially exciting possibilities might be considered in an attempt to preserve or enhance peritoneal membrane function. For example, the intraperitoneal injection of hyaluronan, in an attempt to replace the dialysate losses and thus the integrity of the interstitium, has been performed in experimental animals.[169, 170]

References

1. Mohamed F, Marchettini P, Stuart OA, Sugarbaker PH: Pharmacokinetics and tissue distribution of intraperitoneal paclitaxel with different carrier solutions. Cancer Chemother Pharmacol 2003; 23:23.
2. Mohamed F, Marchettini P, Stuart OA, et al: A comparison of hetastarch and peritoneal dialysis solution for intraperitoneal chemotherapy delivery. Eur J Surg Oncol 2003; 29:261-265.
3. Mohamed F, Stuart OA, Sugarbaker PH: Pharmacokinetics and tissue distribution of intraperitoneal docetaxel with different carrier solutions. J Surg Res 2003; 113:114-120.

4. Hutchinson AJ, Were AJ, Boulton HF, et al: Hypercalcaemia, hypermagnesaemia, hyperphosphataemia and hyperaluminaemia in CAPD: Improvement in serum biochemistry by reduction in dialysate calcium and magnesium concentrations. Nephron 1996; 72:52-58.
5. Locatelli F, Bommer J, London GM, et al: Cardiovascular disease determinants in chronic renal failure: Clinical approach and treatment. Nephrol Dial Transplant 2001; 16:459-468.
6. Kronenberg F, Mundle M, Langle M, Neyer U: Prevalence and progression of peripheral arterial calcifications in patients with ESRD. Am J Kidney Dis 2003; 41:140-148.
7. Stompor T, Pasowicz M, Sullowicz W, et al: An association between coronary artery calcification score, lipid profile, and selected markers of chronic inflammation in ESRD patients treated with peritoneal dialysis. Am J Kidney Dis 2003; 41:203-211.
8. Wang AY, Wang M, Woo J, et al: Cardiac valve calcification as an important predictor for all-cause mortality and cardiovascular mortality in long-term peritoneal dialysis patients: A prospective study. J Am Soc Nephrol 2003; 14:159-168.
9. Letizia C, Mazzaferro S, De Ciocchis A, et al: Poly[allylamine hydrochloride] (RenaGel): A noncalcemic phosphate binder for the treatment of hyperphosphatemia in chronic renal failure. Am J Kidney Dis 1997; 29:66-71.
10. Saha HH, Harmoinen AP, Pasternack AI: Measurement of serum ionized magnesium in CAPD patients. Perit Dial Int 1997; 17: 347-352.
11. Simonsen O, Venturoli D, Wieslander A, et al: Mass transfer of calcium across the peritoneum at three different peritoneal dialysis fluid Ca2+ and glucose concentrations. Kidney Int 2003; 64: 208-215.
12. Armstrong A, Beer J, Noonan K, Cunningham J: Reduced calcium dialysate in CAPD patients: Efficacy and limitations. Nephrol Dial Transplant 1997; 12:1223-1228.
13. Johnson DW, Rigby RJ, McIntyre HD, et al: A randomized trial comparing 1.25 mmol/l calcium dialysate to 1.75 mmol/l calcium dialysate in CAPD patients. Nephrol Dial Transplant 1996; 11:88-93.
14. Bender FH, Bernardini J, Piraino B: Calcium mass transfer with dialysate containing 1.25 and 1.75 mmol/L calcium in peritoneal dialysis patients. Am J Kidney Dis 1992; 20:367-371.
15. Montenegro J, Saracho R, Aguirre R, Martinez I: Calcium mass transfer in CAPD: The role of convective transport. Nephrol Dial Transplant 1993; 8:1234-1236.
16. Piraino B, Bernardini J, Holley J, et al: Calcium mass transfer in peritoneal dialysis patients using 2.5 mEq/l calcium dialysate. Clin Nephrol 1992; 37:48-51.
17. Bernardini J, Piraino B: Low calcium dialysate increases the tolerance to vitamin D in peritoneal dialysis. Contrib Nephrol 1991; 89: 190-198.
18. Weinreich T, Passlick Deetjen J, Ritz E: Low dialysate calcium in continuous ambulatory peritoneal dialysis: A randomized controlled multicenter trial. The Peritoneal Dialysis Multicenter Study Group. Am J Kidney Dis 1995; 25:452-460.
19. Duncan R, Cochrane T, Bhalla C, et al: Low calcium dialysate and hyperparathyroidism. Perit Dial Int 1996; 16(suppl 1):S499-S502.
20. Chagnac A, Ori Y, Weinstein T, et al: Hypercalcemia during pulse vitamin D3 therapy in CAPD patients treated with low calcium dialysate: The role of the decreasing serum parathyroid hormone level. J Am Soc Nephrol 1997; 8:1579-1586.
21. Hutchison AJ, Turner K, Gokal R: Effect of long-term therapy with 1.25 mmol/L calcium peritoneal dialysis fluid on the incidence of peritonitis in CAPD. Perit Dial Int 1992; 12:321-323.
22. Hutchison AJ, Merchant M, Boulton HF, et al: Calcium and magnesium mass transfer in peritoneal dialysis patients using 1.25 mmol/L calcium, 0.25 mmol/L magnesium dialysis fluid. Perit Dial Int 1993; 13:219-223.
23. Sieniawska M, Roszkowska Blaim M, Wojciechowska B: The influence of dialysate calcium concentration on the PTH level in children undergoing CAPD. Perit Dial Int 1996; 16(suppl 1): S567-S569.
24. Mathias R, Salusky I, Harman W, et al: Renal bone disease in pediatric and young adult patients on hemodialysis in a children's hospital. J Am Soc Nephrol 1993; 3:1938-1946.
25. Schroder CH: The choice of dialysis solutions in pediatric chronic peritoneal dialysis: Guidelines by an ad hoc European committee. Perit Dial Int 2001; 21:568-574.
26. Alexander SR, Donaldson LA, Sullivan EK: CAPD/CCPD for children in North America: The NAPRTS experience. *In* Fine RN, Alexander SR, Warady BA (eds): CAPD/CCPD in Children. Boston, Kluwer Academic Publishers, 1998.
27. Kaiser BA, Polinsky MS, Stover J, et al: Growth of children following the initiation of dialysis: A comparison of three dialysis modalities. Pediatr Nephrol 1994; 8:733-738.
28. Weinreich T, Ritz E, Passlick Deetjen J: Long-term dialysis with low-calcium solution (1.0 mmol/L) in CAPD: Effects on bone mineral metabolism. Collaborators of the Multicenter Study Group. Perit Dial Int 1996; 16:260-268.
29. Tattersall JE, Dick C, Doyle S, et al: Alkalosis and hypomagnesaemia: Unwanted effects of a low-calcium CAPD solution. Nephrol Dial Transplant 1995; 10:258-262.
30. Mehrotra R, Kopple JD, Wolfson M: Metabolic acidosis in maintenance dialysis patients: Clinical considerations. Kidney Int 2003; Suppl 88:13-25.
31. Heimburger O, Mujais S: Buffer transport in PD. Kidney Int 2003; Suppl 88:37-42.
32. Mujais S: Acid base profile in patients on PD. Kidney Int 2003; Suppl 88:26-36.
33. Brewer ED: Pediatric experience with intradialytic parenteral nutrition and supplemental tube feeding. Am J Kidney Dis 1999; 33:205-207.
34. Honda M, Kamiyama Y, Kawamura K, et al: Growth, development and nutritional status in Japanese children under 2 years on continuous ambulatory peritoneal dialysis. Pediatr Nephrol 1995; 9:543-548.
35. Turenne MN, Port FK, Strawderman RL, et al: Growth rates in pediatric dialysis patients and renal transplant recipients. Am J Kidney Dis 1997; 30:193-203.
36. Mactier RA, Sprosen TS, Gokal R, et al: Bicarbonate and bicarbonate/lactate peritoneal dialysis solutions for the treatment of infusion pain. Kidney Int 1998; 53:1061-1067.
37. Stein A, Moorhouse J, Iles Smith H, et al: Role of an improvement in acid-base status and nutrition in CAPD patients. Kidney Int 1997; 52:1089-1095.
38. Szeto CC, Wong TY, Chow KM, et al: Oral sodium bicarbonate for the treatment of metabolic acidosis in peritoneal dialysis patients: A randomized placebo-control trial. J Am Soc Nephrol 2003; 14:2119-2126.
39. Cancarini GC, Faict D, De Vos C, et al: Clinical evaluation of a peritoneal dialysis solution with 33 mmol/L bicarbonate. Perit Dial Int 1998; 18:576-582.
40. Coles GA, O'Donoghue DJ, Pritchard N, et al: A controlled trial of two bicarbonate-containing dialysis fluids for CAPD? final report. Nephrol Dial Transplant 1998; 13:3165-3171.
41. Otte K, Gonzalez MT, Bajo MA, et al: Clinical experience with a new bicarbonate (25 mmol/L)/lactate (10 mmol/L) peritoneal dialysis solution. Perit Dial Int 2003; 23:138-145.
42. Dratwa M, Wilkie M, Ryckelynck JP, et al: Clinical experience with two physiologic bicarbonate/lactate peritoneal dialysis solutions in automated peritoneal dialysis. Kidney Int Suppl 2003; 88:S105-S113.
43. Schmitt CP, Haraldsson B, Doetschmann R, et al: Effects of pH-neutral, bicarbonate-buffered dialysis fluid on peritoneal transport kinetics in children. Kidney Int 2002; 61:1527-1536.
44. Coles GA, Gokal R, Ogg C, et al: A randomized controlled trial of a bicarbonate- and a bicarbonate/lactate-containing dialysis solution in CAPD (See comments). (Published erratum

appears in Perit Dial Int 1997; 17(3):223). Perit Dial Int 1997; 17:48-51.
45. Tranaeus A: A long-term study of a bicarbonate/lactate-based peritoneal dialysis solution? clinical benefits. The Bicarbonate/ Lactate Study Group. Perit Dial Int 2000; 20:516-523.
46. Wang T, Waniewski J, Heimburger O, et al: A quantitative analysis of sodium transport and removal during peritoneal dialysis. Kidney Int 1997; 52:1609-1616.
47. Waniewski J, Wang T, Heimburger O, et al: Discriminative impact of ultrafiltration on peritoneal protein transport. Perit Dial Int 2000; 20:39-46.
48. Paniagua R, Amato D, Vonesh E, et al: Effects of increased peritoneal clearances on mortality rates in peritoneal dialysis: ADEMEX, a prospective, randomized, controlled trial. J Am Soc Nephrol 2002; 13:1307-1320.
49. Davies SJ, Phillips L, Russell GI: Peritoneal solute transport predicts survival on CAPD independently of residual renal function. Nephrol Dial Transplant 1998; 13:962-968.
50. Churchill DN, Thorpe KE, Nolph KD, et al: Increased peritoneal membrane transport is associated with decreased patient and technique survival for continuous peritoneal dialysis patients. J Am Soc Nephrol 1998; 9:1285-1292.
51. Wang T, Heimbürger O, Waniewski J, et al: Increased peritoneal permeability is associated with decreased fluid and small-solute removal and higher mortality in CAPD patients. Nephrol Dial Transplant 1998; 13:1242-1249.
52. Chung SH, Heimburger O, Stenvinkel P, et al: Influence of peritoneal transport rate, inflammation, and fluid removal on nutritional status and clinical outcome in prevalent peritoneal dialysis patients. Perit Dial Int 2003; 23:174-183.
53. Jager KJ, Merkus MP, Dekker FW, et al: Mortality and technique failure in patients starting chronic peritoneal dialysis: Results of the Netherlands Cooperative Study on the Adequacy of Dialysis. NECOSAD Study Group. Kidney Int 1999; 55: 1476-1485.
54. Ates K, Nergizoglu G, Keven K, et al: Effect of fluid and sodium removal on mortality in peritoneal dialysis patients. Kidney Int 2001; 60:767-776.
55. Brown EA, Davies SJ, Rutherford P, et al: Survival of functionally anuric patients on automated peritoneal dialysis: The European APD Outcome Study. J Am Soc Nephrol 2003; 14:2948-2957.
56. Rippe B: A three-pore model of peritoneal transport. Perit Dial Int 1993; 13(suppl 2):S35-S38.
57. Pannekeet MM, Mulder JB, Weening JJ, et al: Demonstration of aquaporin-CHIP in peritoneal tissue of uremic and CAPD patients. Perit Dial Int 1996; 16(suppl 1):S54-S57.
58. Yang B, Folkesson HG, Yang J, et al: Reduced osmotic water permeability of the peritoneal barrier in aquaporin-1 knockout mice. Am J Physiol 1999; 276:C76-C81.
59. Ho-dac-Pannekeet MM, Schouten N, Langendijk MJ, et al: Peritoneal transport characteristics with glucose polymer based dialysate. Kidney Int 1996; 50:979-986.
60. Rippe B, Levin L: Computer simulations of ultrafiltration profiles for an icodextrin-based peritoneal fluid in CAPD. Kidney Int 2000; 57:2546-2556.
61. Little J, Phillips L, Russell L, et al: Longitudinal lipid profiles on CAPD: Their relationship to weight gain, comorbidity, and dialysis factors. J Am Soc Nephrol 1998; 9:1931-1939.
62. Heimburger O, Stenvinkel P, Berglund L, et al: Increased plasma lipoprotein(a) in continuous ambulatory peritoneal dialysis is related to peritoneal transport of proteins and glucose. Nephron 1996; 72:135-144.
63. Lameire N, Matthys D, Matthys E, Beheydt R: Effects of long-term CAPD on carbohydrate and lipid metabolism. Clin Nephrol 1988; 30(suppl 1):S53-S58.
64. Johansson AC, Samuelsson O, Haraldsson B, et al: Body composition in patients treated with peritoneal dialysis. Nephrol Dial Transplant 1998; 13:1511-1517.
65. Vonesh EF, Moran J: Mortality in end-stage renal disease: A reassessment of differences between patients treated with hemodialysis and peritoneal dialysis. J Am Soc Nephrol 1999; 10:354-365.
66. Burke RA, Moberly JB, Patel H, et al: Maltose and isomaltose in uremic plasma following icodextrin administration. Adv Perit Dial 1998; 14:120-123.
67. Moberly JB, Mujais S, Gehr T, et al: Pharmacokinetics of icodextrin in peritoneal dialysis patients. Kidney Int Suppl 2002; S23-S33.
68. Posthuma N, ter Wee PM, Donker AJ, et al: Serum disaccharides and osmolality in CCPD patients using icodextrin or glucose as daytime dwell. Perit Dial Int 1997; 17:602-607.
69. Krediet RT, Zuyderhoudt FMJ, Boeschoten EW, Arisz L: The relationship between peritoneal glucose absorption and body fluid loss by ultrafiltration during continuous ambulatory peritoneal dialysis. Clin Nephrol 1987; 27:51-55.
70. Twardowski ZJ, Nolph KD, Khanna R, et al: Peritoneal equilibration test. Perit Dial Bull 1987; 7:138-147.
71. Davies SJ, Brown B, Bryan J, Russell GI: Clinical evaluation of the peritoneal equilibration test: A population-based study. Nephrol Dial Transplant 1993; 8:64-70.
72. Ho-dac-Pannekeet MM, Atasever B, Struijk DG, Krediet RT: Analysis of ultrafiltration failure in peritoneal dialysis patients by means of standard peritoneal permeability analysis. Perit Dial Int 1997; 17:144-150.
73. Davies SJ: Montoring of long-term membrane function. Perit Dial Int 2001; 21:225-230.
74. Bergstrom J, Furst P, Alvestrand A, Lindholm B: Protein and energy intake, nitrogen balance and nitrogen losses in patients treated continuous ambulatory peritoneal dialysis. Kidney Int 1993; 44:1048-1057.
75. Davies SJ, Phillips L, Russell L, et al: An analysis of the effects of increasing delivered dialysis treatment to malnourished peritoneal dialysis patients. Kidney Int 2000; 57:1743-1754.
76. Wilkie ME, Plant MJ, Edwards L, Brown CB: Icodextrin 7.5% dialysate solution (glucose polymer) in patients with ultrafiltration failure: Extension of CAPD technique survival. Perit Dial Int 1997; 17:84-87.
77. Mistry CD, Gokal R, Peers E: A randomized multicenter clinical trial comparing isosmolar icodextrin with hyperosmolar glucose solutions in CAPD. MIDAS Study Group. Multicenter investigation of icodextrin in ambulatory peritoneal dialysis. Kidney Int 1994; 46:496-503.
78. Wolfson M, Piraino B, Hamburger RJ, Morton AR: A randomized controlled trial to evaluate the efficacy and safety of icodextrin in peritoneal dialysis. Am J Kidney Dis 2002; 40:1055-1065.
79. Plum J, Gentile S, Verger C, et al: Efficacy and safety of a 7.5% icodextrin peritoneal dialysis solution in patients treated with automated peritoneal dialysis. Am J Kidney Dis 2002; 39:862-871.
80. Konings CJ, Kooman JP, Schonck M, et al: Effect of icodextrin on volume status, blood pressure and echocardiographic parameters: A randomized study. Kidney Int 2003; 63:1556-1563.
81. Davies SJ, Woodrow G, Donovan K, et al: Icodextrin improves the fluid status of peritoneal dialysis patients: Results of a double-blind randomized controlled trial. J Am Soc Nephrol 2003; 14:2338-2344.
82. Amici G, Orrasch M, Da Rin G, Bocci C: Hyperinsulinism reduction associated with icodextrin treatment in continuous ambulatory peritoneal dialysis patients. Adv Perit Dial 2001; 17:80-83.
83. Marshall J, Jennings P, Scott A, et al: Glycemic control in diabetic CAPD patients assessed by continuous glucose monitoring system (CGMS). Kidney Int 2003; 64:1480-1486.
84. Van V, Schoonjans RS, Struijk DG, et al: Influence of dialysate on gastric emptying time in peritoneal dialysis patients. Perit Dial Int 2002; 22:32-38.
85. Bredie SJ, Bosch FH, Demacker PN, et al: Effects of peritoneal dialysis with an overnight icodextrin dwell on parameters of glucose and lipid metabolism. Perit Dial Int 2001; 21:275-281.

86. Woodrow G, Oldroyd B, Stables G, et al: Effects of icodextrin in automated peritoneal dialysis on blood pressure and bioelectrical impedance analysis. Nephrol Dial Transplant 2000; 15: 862-866.
87. Guo A, Wolfson M, Holt R: Early quality of life benefits of icodextrin in peritoneal dialysis. Kidney Int Suppl 2002; S72-S79.
88. Rodriguez-Carmona A, Fontan MP: Sodium removal in patients undergoing CAPD and automated peritoneal dialysis. Perit Dial Int 2002; 22:705-713.
89. Ortega O, Gallar P, Carreno A, et al: Peritoneal sodium mass removal in continuous ambulatory peritoneal dialysis and automated peritoneal dialysis: Influence on blood pressure control. Am J Nephrol 2001; 21:189-193.
90. Wens R, Taminne M, Devriendt J, et al: A previously undescribed side effect of icodextrin: Overestimation of glycemia by glucose analyzer. Perit Dial Int 1998; 18:603-609.
91. Oyibo SO, Pritchard GM, McLay L, et al: Blood glucose overestimation in diabetic patients on continuous ambulatory peritoneal dialysis for end-stage renal disease. Diabet Med 2002; 19:693-696.
92. Anderstam B, Garcia-Lopez E, Heimburger O, Lindholm B: Determination of alpha-amylase activity in serum and dialysate from patients using icodextrin-based peritoneal dialysis fluid. Perit Dial Int 2003; 23:146-150.
93. Wang R, Leesch V, Turner P, et al: Kinetic analysis of icodextrin interference with serum amylase assays. Adv Perit Dial 2002; 18:96-99.
94. Valance A, Lebrun-Vignes B, Descamps V, et al: Icodextrin cutaneous hypersensitivity: Report of 3 psoriasiform cases. Arch Dermatol 2001; 137:309-310.
95. Goldsmith D, Jayawardene S, Sabharwal N, Cooney K: Allergic reactions to the polymeric glucose-based peritoneal dialysis fluid icodextrin in patients with renal failure. Lancet 2000; 355:897.
96. MacGinley R, Cooney K, Alexander G, et al: Relapsing culture-negative peritonitis in peritoneal dialysis patients exposed to icodextrin solution. Am J Kidney Dis 2002; 40:1030-1035.
97. Glorieux G, Lameire N, Van Biesen W, et al: Specific characteristics of peritoneal leucocyte populations during sterile peritonitis associated with icodextrin CAPD fluids. Nephrol Dial Transplant 2003; 18:1648-1653.
98. Gunal AI, Duman S, Ozkahya M, et al: Strict volume control normalizes hypertension in peritoneal dialysis patients. Am J Kidney Dis 2001; 37:588-593.
99. Young GA, Kopple JD, Lindholm B, et al: Nutritional assessment of continuous ambulatory peritoneal dialysis patients: An international study. Am J Kidney Dis 1991; 17:462-471.
100. Churchill DN, Taylor DW, Keshaviah PR: Adequacy of dialysis and nutrition in continuous peritoneal dialysis: Association with clinical outcome. J Am Soc Nephrol 1996; 7:198-207.
101. Kopple JD, Greene T, Chumlea WC, et al: Relationship between nutritional status and the glomerular filtration rate: Results from the MDRD study. Kidney Int 2000; 57:1688-1703.
102. McCusker FX, Teehan BP, Thorpe KE, et al: How much peritoneal dialysis is required for the maintenance of a good nutritional state? Kidney Int 1996; 50(suppl 56):S56-S61.
103. Davies SJ, Phillips L, Griffiths AM, et al: What really happens to people on long-term peritoneal dialysis? Kidney Int 1998; 54:2207-2217.
104. Bergström J, Fürst P, Alvestrand A, Lindholm B: Protein and energy intake, nitrogen balance and nitrogen losses in patients treated with continuous ambulatory peritoneal dialysis. Kidney Int 1993; 44:1048-1057.
105. Stenvinkel P, Heimburger O, Paultre F, et al: Strong association between malnutrition, inflammation, and atherosclerosis in chronic renal failure. Kidney Int 1999; 55:1899-1911.
106. Davies SJ, Russell L, Bryan J, et al: Comorbidity, urea kinetics and appetite in continuous ambulatory peritoneal dialysis: Their interrelationship and prediction of survival. Am J Kidney Dis 1995; 26:353-361.
107. Goodship TH, Lloyd S, McKenzie PW, et al: Short-term studies on the use of amino acids as an osmotic agent in continuous ambulatory peritoneal dialysis. Clin Sci (Lond) 1987; 73:471-478.
108. Jones MR, Martis L, Algrim CE, et al: Amino acid solutions for CAPD: Rationale and clinical experience. Miner Electrolyte Metab 1992; 18:309-315.
109. Bruno M, Bagnis C, Marangella M, et al: CAPD with an amino acid dialysis solution: A long-term, cross-over study. Kidney Int 1989; 35:1189-1194.
110. Park MS, Heimburger O, Bergstrom J, et al: Peritoneal transport during dialysis with amino acid-based solutions. Perit Dial Int 1993; 13:280-288.
111. Steinhauer HB, Lubrich-Birkner I, Kluthe R, et al: Effect of amino acid based dialysis solution on peritoneal permeability and prostanoid generation in patients undergoing continuous ambulatory peritoneal dialysis. Am J Nephrol 1992; 12:61-67.
112. Jones M, Kalil R, Blake P, et al: Modification of an amino acid solution for peritoneal dialysis to reduce risk of acidemia. Perit Dial Int 1997; 17:66-71.
113. Jones MR, Gehr TW, Burkart JM, et al: Replacement of amino acid and protein losses with 1.1% amino acid peritoneal dialysis solution. Perit Dial Int 1998; 18:210-216.
114. Jones CH, Smith M, Henderson MJ, et al: Fasting plasma amino acids are not normalized by 12-month amino acid-based dialysate in CAPD patients. Perit Dial Int 1999; 19:174-177.
115. Kopple JD, Bernard D, Messana J, et al: Treatment of malnourished CAPD patients with an amino acid based dialysate. Kidney Int 1995; 47:1148-1157.
116. Delarue J, Maingourd C, Objois M, et al: Effects of an amino acid dialysate on leucine metabolism in continuous ambulatory peritoneal dialysis patients. Kidney Int 1999; 56:1934-1943.
117. Jones M, Hagen T, Boyle CA, et al: Treatment of malnutrition with 1.1% amino acid peritoneal dialysis solution: Results of a multicenter outpatient study. Am J Kidney Dis 1998; 32:761-769.
118. Li FK, Chan LY, Woo JC, et al: A 3-year, prospective, randomized, controlled study on amino acid dialysate in patients on CAPD. Am J Kidney Dis 2003; 42:173-183.
119. Grzegorzewska AE, Mariak I, Dobrowolska-Zachwieja A, Szajdak L: Effects of amino acid dialysis solution on the nutrition of continuous ambulatory peritoneal dialysis patients. Perit Dial Int 1999; 19:462-470.
120. Qamar IU, Secker D, Levin L, et al: Effects of amino acid dialysis compared to dextrose dialysis in children on continuous cycling peritoneal dialysis. Perit Dial Int 1999; 19:237-247.
121. Holmes C, Faict D: Peritoneal dialysis solution biocompatibility: Definitions and evaluation strategies. Kidney Int Suppl 2003; 88:S92-S98.
122. Liberek T, Topley N, Jorres A, et al: Peritoneal dialysis fluid inhibition of polymorphonuclear leukocyte respiratory burst activation is related to the lowering of intracellular pH. Nephron 1993; 65:260-265.
123. Jörres A, Topley N, Steenweg L, et al: Inhibition of cytokine synthesis by peritoneal dialysate persists throughout the CAPD cycle. Am J Nephrol 1992; 12:80-85.
124. McGregor SJ, Topley N, Jorres A, et al: Longitudinal evaluation of peritoneal macrophage function and activation during CAPD: Maturity, cytokine synthesis and arachidonic acid metabolism. Kidney Int 1996; 49:525-533.
125. Musi B, Carlsson O, Rippe A, et al: Effects of acidity, glucose degradation products, and dialysis fluid buffer choice on peritoneal solute and fluid transport in rats. Perit Dial Int 1998; 18:303-310.
126. Nakayama M, Kawaguchi Y, Yamada K, et al: Immunohistochemical detection of advanced glycosylation end-products in the peritoneum and its possible pathophysiological role in CAPD. Kidney Int 1997; 51:182-186.

127. Davies SJ, Bryan J, Phillips L, Russell GI: Longitudinal changes in peritoneal kinetics: The effects of peritoneal dialysis and peritonitis. Nephrol Dial Transplant 1996; 11:498-506.
128. Struijk DG, Krediet RT, Koomen GCM, et al: A prospective study of peritoneal transport in CAPD patients. Kidney Int 1994; 45:1739-1744.
129. Smit W, Schouten N, van den Berg JW, et al: Analysis of the prevalence and causes of ultrafiltration failure during long-term peritoneal dialysis: A cross-sectional study. Perit Dial Int 2003; 23 (In press).
130. Krediet RT, Van Esch S, Smit W, et al: Peritoneal membrane failure in peritoneal dialysis patients. Blood Purif 2002; 20:489-493.
131. Williams JD, Craig KJ, Topley N, et al: Morphologic changes in the peritoneal membrane of patients with renal disease. J Am Soc Nephrol 2002; 13:470-479.
132. Devuyst O, Topley N, Williams JD: Morphological and functional changes in the dialysed peritoneal cavity: Impact of more biocompatible solutions. Nephrol Dial Transplant 2002; 17:12-15.
133. Williams JD, Craig KJ, Topley N, Williams GT: Peritoneal dialysis: Changes to the structure of the peritoneal membrane and potential for biocompatible solutions. Kidney Int 2003; 63:158-161.
134. Numata M, Nakayama M, Nimura S, et al: Association between an increased surface area of peritoneal microvessels and a high peritoneal solute transport rate. Perit Dial Int 2003; 23:116-122.
135. Honda K, Nitta K, Horita S, et al: Morphological changes in the peritoneal vasculature of patients on CAPD with ultrafiltration failure. Nephron 1996; 72:171-176.
136. Dawnay AB, Millar DJ: Glycation and advanced glycation end-product formation with icodextrin and dextrose. Perit Dial Int 1997; 17:52-58.
137. Topley N, Kaur D, Petersen MM, et al: In vitro effects of bicarbonate and bicarbonate-lactate buffered peritoneal dialysis solutions on mesothelial and neutrophil function. J Am Soc Nephrol 1996; 7:218-224.
138. Topley N, Kaur D, Petersen MM, et al: Biocompatibility of bicarbonate buffered peritoneal dialysis fluids: Influence on mesothelial cell and neutrophil function. Kidney Int 1996; 49: 1447-1456.
139. MacKenzie RK, Holmes CJ, Moseley A, et al: Bicarbonate/lactate- and bicarbonate-buffered peritoneal dialysis fluids improve ex vivo peritoneal macrophage TNF alpha secretion. J Am Soc Nephrol 1998; 9:1499-1506.
140. Cooker LA, Luneburg P, Holmes CJ, et al: Interleukin-6 levels decrease in effluent from patients dialyzed with bicarbonate/lactate-based peritoneal dialysis solutions. Perit Dial Int 2001; 21:S102-S107.
141. Mackenzie RK, Jones S, Moseley A, et al: In vivo exposure to bicarbonate/lactate- and bicarbonate-buffered peritoneal dialysis fluids improves ex vivo peritoneal macrophage function. Am J Kidney Dis 2000; 35:112-121.
142. Morgan LW, Wieslander A, Davies M, et al: Glucose degradation products (GDP) retard remesothelialization independently of d-glucose concentration. Kidney Int 2003; 64:1854-1866.
143. Krediet RT: Evaluation of peritoneal membrane integrity. J Nephrol 1997; 10:238-244.
144. Jones S, Holmes CJ, Krediet RT, et al: Bicarbonate/lactate-based peritoneal dialysis solution increases cancer antigen 125 and decreases hyaluronic acid levels. Kidney Int 2001; 59:1529-1538.
145. Rippe B, Simonsen O, Heimburger O, et al: Long-term clinical effects of a peritoneal dialysis fluid with less glucose degradation products. Kidney Int 2001; 59:348-357.
146. Jones S, Holmes CJ, Mackenzie RK, et al: Continuous dialysis with bicarbonate/lactate-buffered peritoneal dialysis fluids results in a long-term improvement in ex vivo peritoneal macrophage function. J Am Soc Nephrol 2002; 13:S97-S103.
147. Coles GA, Gokal R, Ogg C, et al: A randomized controlled trial of a bicarbonate- and a bicarbonate/lactate-containing dialysis solution in CAPD. Perit Dial Int 1997; 17:48-51.
148. Barre DE, Chen C, Cooker L, Moberly JB: Decreased in vitro formation of AGEs with extraneal solution compared to dextrose-containing peritoneal dialysis solutions. Adv Perit Dial 1999; 15:12-16.
149. Cooker LA, Holmes CJ, Hoff CM: Biocompatibility of icodextrin. Kidney Int Suppl 2002; S34-S45.
150. Posthuma N, ter Wee PM, Donker AJ, et al: Assessment of the effectiveness, safety, and biocompatibility of icodextrin in automated peritoneal dialysis. The Dextrin in APD in Amsterdam (DIANA) Group. Perit Dial Int 2000; 20:S106-S113.
151. Gotloib L, Wajsbrot V, Shostak A: Icodextrin-induced lipid peroxidation disrupts the mesothelial cell cycle engine. Free Radic Biol Med 2003; 34:419-428.
152. Brulez HF, Dekker HA, Oe PL, et al: Biocompatibility of a 1.1% amino acid-containing peritoneal dialysis fluid compared to a 2.27% glucose-based peritoneal dialysis fluid. Nephron 1996; 74:26-32.
153. Ueda Y, Miyata T, Goffin E, et al: Effect of dwell time on carbonyl stress using icodextrin and amino acid peritoneal dialysis fluids. Kidney Int 2000; 58:2518-2524.
154. Jorres A, Gahl GM, Ludat K, et al: In vitro biocompatibility evaluation of a novel bicarbonate-buffered amino-acid solution for peritoneal dialysis. Nephrol Dial Transplant 1997; 12:543-549.
155. Pecoits-Filho R, Tranaeus A, Lindholm B: Clinical trial experiences with physioneal. Kidney Int 2003; Suppl 83:124-132.
156. Vande Walle J, Raes A, Castillo D, et al: Advantages of HCO3 solution with low sodium concentration over standard lactate solutions for acute peritoneal dialysis. Adv Perit Dial 1997; 13:179-182.
157. Nakayama M, Yokoyama K, Kubo H, et al: The effect of ultra-low sodium dialysate in CAPD. A kinetic and clinical analysis. Clin Nephrol 1996; 45:188-193.
158. Amici G, Virga G, Da Rin G, et al: Low sodium concentration solution in normohydrated CAPD patients. Adv Perit Dial 1995; 11:78-82.
159. Freida P, Issad B, Allouache M: Impact of a low sodium dialysate on usual parameters of cardiovascular outcome of anuric patients during APD. Perit Dial Int 1998; 18:124.
160. Brunkhorst R, Mahiout A: Pyruvate neutralizes peritoneal dialysate cytotoxicity: Maintained integrity and proliferation of cultured human mesothelial cells. Kidney Int 1995; 48:177-181.
161. Zhou FQ: Advantages of pyruvate over lactate in peritoneal dialysis solutions. Acta Pharmacol Sin 2001; 22:385-392.
162. de Fijter CW, Verbrugh HA, Oe PL, et al: The effect of glycerol-containing peritoneal dialysis fluid on peritoneal macrophage function in vivo. Adv Perit Dial 1991; 7:154-157.
163. Van Biesen W, Faict D, Boer W, Lameire N: Further animal and human experience with a 0.6% amino acid/1.4% glycerol peritoneal dialysis solution. Perit Dial Int 1997; 17:S56-S62.
164. Vardhan A, Zweers MM, Gokal R, Krediet RT: A solutions portfolio approach in peritoneal dialysis. Kidney Int 2003; Suppl 88:114-123.
165. Young A, Gilbert J, Sherman M, et al: Intraperitoneal chemotherapy: A prolonged infusion of 5-fluorouracil using a novel carrier solution. Br J Nurs 1996; 5:539-543.
166. Mazzaferro S, Pasquali M, Ballanti P, et al: Treatment of aluminum intoxication: A new scheme for desferrioxamine administration. Nephrol Dial Transplant 1994; 9:1431-1434.
167. Schroder CH, Rusthoven E, Monnens LA: Intraperitoneal administration of erythropoietin. Pediatr Nephrol 2000; 14:84-85.
168. Rusthoven E, van de Kar NC, Monnens LA, Schroder CH: Long-term effectiveness of intraperitoneal erythropoietin in children on NIPD by administration in small bags. Perit Dial Int 2001; 21:196-197.
169. Breborowicz A, Polubinska A, Pawlaczyk K, et al: Intraperitoneal hyaluronan administration in conscious rats: Absorption, metabolism, and effects on peritoneal fluid dynamics. Perit Dial Int 2001; 21:130-135.

170. Moberly JB, Sorkin M, Kucharski A, et al: Effects of intraperitoneal hyaluronan on peritoneal fluid and solute transport in peritoneal dialysis patients. Perit Dial Int 2003; 23:63-73.
171. Gokal R, Mistry CD, Peers EM: Peritonitis occurrence in a multicenter study of icodextrin and glucose in CAPD. MIDAS Study Group. Multicenter investigation of icodextrin in ambulatory dialysis. Perit Dial Int 1995; 15:226-230.
172. Posthuma N, ter Wee PM, Verbrugh HA, et al: Icodextrin instead of glucose during the daytime dwell in CCPD increases ultrafiltration and 24-h dialysate creatinine clearance. Nephrol Dial Transplant 1997; 12:550-553.
173. Posthuma N, ter Weel PM, Donker AJ, et al: Icodextrin use in CCPD patients during peritonitis: Ultrafiltration and serum disaccharide concentrations. Nephrol Dial Transplant 1998; 13: 2341-2344.
174. Ota K, Akiba T, Nakao T, et al: Peritoneal ultrafiltration and serum icodextrin concentration during dialysis with 7.5% icodextrin solution in Japanese patients. Perit Dial Int 2003; 23:356-361.
175. Young GA, Dibble JB, Hobson SM, et al: The use of an amino-acid-based CAPD fluid over 12 weeks. Nephrol Dial Transplant 1989; 4:285-292.
176. Young GA, Dibble JB, Taylor AE, et al: A longitudinal study of the effects of amino acid-based CAPD fluid on amino acid retention and protein losses. Nephrol Dial Transplant 1989; 4:900-905.
177. Dibble JB, Young GA, Hobson SM, Brownjohn AM: Amino-acid-based continuous ambulatory peritoneal dialysis (CAPD) fluid over twelve weeks: Effects on carbohydrate and lipid metabolism. Perit Dial Int 1990; 10:71-77.
178. Faller B, Aparicio M, Faict D, et al: Clinical evaluation of an optimized 1.1% amino-acid solution for peritoneal dialysis. Nephrol Dial Transplant 1995; 10:1432-1437.
179. Misra M, Reaveley DA, Ashworth J, et al: Six-month prospective cross-over study to determine the effects of 1.1% amino acid dialysate on lipid metabolism in patients on continuous ambulatory peritoneal dialysis. Perit Dial Int 1997; 17:279-286.
180. Plum J, Erren C, Fieseler C, et al: An amino acid-based peritoneal dialysis fluid buffered with bicarbonate versus glucose/bicarbonate and glucose/lactate solutions: An intraindividual randomized study. Perit Dial Int 1999; 19:418-428.
181. Cooker LA, Luneburg P, Faict D, et al: Reduced glucose degradation products in bicarbonate/lactate-buffered peritoneal dialysis solutions produced in two-chambered bags. Perit Dial Int 1997; 17:373-378.
182. Cooker LA, Choo CG, Luneburg P, et al: Effect of icodextrin peritoneal dialysis solution on cell proliferation in vitro. Adv Perit Dial 1999; 15:17-20.
183. Ishikawa N, Miyata T, Ueda Y, et al: Affinity adsorption of glucose degradation products improves the biocompatibility of conventional peritoneal dialysis fluid. Kidney Int 2003; 63:331-339.
184. Sundaram S, Cendoroglo M, Cooker LA, et al: Effect of two-chambered bicarbonate lactate-buffered peritoneal dialysis fluids on peripheral blood mononuclear cell and polymorphonuclear cell function in vitro. Am J Kidney Dis 1997; 30:680-689.
185. Zeier M, Schwenger V, Deppisch R, et al: Glucose degradation products in PD fluids: Do they disappear from the peritoneal cavity and enter the systemic circulation? Kidney Int 2003; 63:298-305.
186. Schalkwijk CG, Posthuma N, ten Brink HJ, et al: Induction of 1,2-dicarbonyl compounds, intermediates in the formation of advanced glycation end-products, during heat-sterilization of glucose-based peritoneal dialysis fluids (In process citation). Perit Dial Int 1999; 19:325-333.
187. Miyata T, Horie K, Ueda Y, et al: Advanced glycation and lipidoxidation of the peritoneal membrane: Respective roles of serum and peritoneal fluid reactive carbonyl compounds. Kidney Int 2000; 58:425-435.
188. Wieslander AP: Cytotoxicity of peritoneal dialysis fluid: Is it related to glucose breakdown products? Nephrol Dial Transplant 1996; 11:958-959.
189. Usta MF, Tuncer M, Baykal A, et al: Impact of chronic renal failure and peritoneal dialysis fluids on advanced glycation end product and iNOS levels in penile tissue: An experimental study. Urology 2002; 59:953-957.
190. Koksal IT, Usta MF, Akkoyunlu G, et al: The potential role of advanced glycation end product and iNOS in chronic renal failure-related testicular dysfunction: An experimental study. Am J Nephrol 2003; 23:361-368.
191. Nakamura S, Tobita K, Tachikawa T, et al: Immunohistochemical detection of an AGE, a ligand for macrophage receptor, in peritoneum of CAPD patients. Kidney Int 2003; 63:152-157.
192. Mizuiri S, Miyata S, Sakai K, et al: Effect of intraperitoneal administration of heparin on advanced glycation end-products in CAPD (In process citation). Perit Dial Int 1999; 19:361-365.
193. Jenkins SB, Wilkie ME: An exploratory study of a novel peritoneal combination dialysate (1.36+ACU-glucose/7.5+ACU-icodextrin), demonstrating improved ultrafiltration compared to either component studied alone. Perit Dial Int 2003; 23(5): 475-480.

Chapter 28

Peritoneal Dialysis Prescription and Adequacy

Peter G. Blake, M.B., F.R.C.P.C., F.R.C.P.I. • Rita Suri, M.D., F.R.C.P.C.

Since the late 1980s, efforts have been made to apply to peritoneal dialysis (PD) the principles of quantification and prescription of dialytic dose originally established for hemodialysis (HD) by the National Cooperative Dialysis Study and other subsequent publications.[1-3] Over this period, numerous attempts were made to validate this approach by investigating whether measures of small solute clearance are associated with, or are predictive of, patient well-being and survival on PD.[4-6] Initial controversy seemed to have been, at least partly, resolved by large cohort studies from North America and Italy, published in the mid-1990s. These showed a clear association between small solute clearances received and subsequent clinical outcomes, including survival.[7,8] These findings gave rise in a number of countries to influential guidelines proposing relatively high solute clearance targets.[9,10] This, in turn, altered the practice of PD significantly in many jurisdictions.[11,12] However, the recent publication of the results of the first large randomized, controlled trials looking at the effects of raising clearance have brought into question the validity of this approach in PD and have certainly undermined existing guidelines.[13,14] Analogous results in the large randomized, controlled HEMO trial have lead to a similar questioning of the validity of the model in HD as well.[15] The result is that the whole "adequacy of dialysis" field is now in a state of flux.[16]

In this chapter, the standard adequacy indices used in PD will be defined, and the methods by which they are measured will be addressed. The strategies used in clinical practice to raise PD dose will be reviewed. The literature assessing the effectiveness of raising clearance in PD will then be critically evaluated. Special attention will be given to the value of residual renal function (RRF). Evidence-based recommendations will be proposed.

Alternative aspects of PD adequacy will then be reviewed with particular attention to nutritional factors and volume status in PD patients.

PERITONEAL DIALYSIS ADEQUACY INDICES

Small solute clearance in PD is measured using either urea clearance, normalized to total body water (Kt/V), or creatinine clearance, normalized to body surface area (CrCl). In each case, clearance includes a dialytic and a residual renal component. The latter is particularly important in PD because it accounts for a greater proportion of the overall clearance achieved than is typically the case in HD, and because it appears to persist longer in PD patients.[17,18] It should be remembered, however, that generally it is only the dialytic component that can be modified by the prescribing physician.

The dialytic component is calculated by measuring the urea and creatinine content of a 24-hour collection of dialysate effluent. These values are then divided by the serum urea and creatinine levels, respectively, to give the urea and creatinine clearance (Boxes 28–1 and 28–2). Dialysate creatinine levels need to be corrected for the high dialysate glucose content, which interferes with the assay used in many laboratories. The timing of the serum urea and creatinine samples is not important in continuous ambulatory peritoneal dialysis (CAPD) because levels do not vary significantly during the day. In automated peritoneal dialysis (APD), however, there may be a 10% or greater variation in serum urea and creatinine from a trough value after the patient finishes cycling in the morning to a peak value before the patient resumes cycling in the evening. It is thus recommended that serum samples be taken approximately half way through the noncycling period, which, in practice for most patients, means the mid afternoon. The renal component of urea and creatinine clearance is calculated in the same manner with a 24-hour urine collection, except that, in the case of creatinine clearance, an average of residual renal urea and creatinine clearance is typically used. This is because unmodified creatinine clearance substantially overestimates the true glomerular filtration rate.

The dialysate and residual renal component of clearance are added to give a total clearance, which is normalized to body water (V) to give Kt/V, or to 1.73 m^2 body surface area to give CrCl (see Tables 28–1 and 28–2). The value for V is estimated using anthropometric formulas, such as those of Watson or Hume, based on age, sex, height, and weight.[19,20] Estimates of V from the Watson formulas, when compared to a gold standard, such as deuterium oxide dilution, are, on average, slightly low but the discrepancy varies substantially from patient to patient, especially in the obese.[21] Nevertheless, because most of the clinical literature is based on a V calculated from the Watson equations, and because they have the advantage of simplicity, they remain the current method of choice. In children, the Mellits-Cheek formulas are used.[22] The value for body surface area is similarly estimated using the du Bois formulas.[23] In general, the edema free body weight should be used in the formulas to calculate V and body surface area.[9,10] In the case of patients who have lost a substantial amount of body weight due to malnutrition, it is suggested that the desirable rather than the actual body weight be used in these formulas. This desirable or "normal" body weight can be obtained from the National Health and Nutrition Evaluation Survey tables. These tables give the median body weight of North Americans of the same age, sex, height, and frame as the patient and are regularly updated. It can be

Table 28–1 Formulas Required to Calculate Urea Clearance Normalized to Body Water (Kt/V) and Normalized Protein Equivalent of Nitrogen Appearance (nPNA)

Kt/V

Kt/V per week = 7 (daily peritoneal Kt/V plus daily renal Kt/V)

$$\text{Daily Peritoneal Kt} = \frac{\text{24-hr dialysate urea content}}{\text{serum urea}}$$

$$\text{Daily renal Kt} = \frac{\text{24-hr urine urea content}}{\text{serum urea}}$$

According to Watson and colleagues[19]:

V (in males) = 2.447 – 0.09516(A) + 0.1704(H) + 0.3362(W)

V (in females) = –2.097 – 0.1069(H) + 0.02466(W)

where A = age (yr)
H = height (cm)
W = weight (kg)

nPNA

According to Bergstrom and colleagues[95]:

PNA (g/day) = 13 + 7.31 (daily dialysate plus urine urea content*) + daily dialysate plus urine protein content*

or

PNA (g/day) = 19 + 7.62 (daily dialysate plus urine urea content*)

The first formula is preferred because it requires urine and dialysate protein losses to be specifically measured rather than estimated.

$$\text{nPNA} = \frac{\text{PNA}}{\text{standardized or desired body weight (kg)}}$$

*Measured in g/day.
PNA, protein equivalent of nitrogen appearance.

argued, however, that they are applicable only to a North American population. The use of the desirable body weight to normalize clearance values avoids the situation where malnourished emaciated patients have a misleadingly high, normalized clearance value and, conversely, one where obese patients have a misleadingly low value. Both Kt/V and CrCl values are conventionally expressed as weekly, rather than daily, clearances to facilitate comparisons with HD.

It has been observed that there is substantial intraindividual variation when repeated clearance measurements are done in the same patient on the same prescription.[24] The variation is particularly marked for the renal component of clearance. Some of this variation may be accounted for by inevitable inaccuracies in collections of dialysate and urine, but some undoubtedly represent genuine day-to-day variation in urinary volume, peritoneal ultrafiltration, and degree of equilibration, consequent upon alterations in hydration, fluid intake, timing of exchanges, and tonicity of peritoneal fluids used.

Dialysate collections may be cumbersome because of the relatively high volumes involved. In CAPD, it is feasible for the patient to bring the entire effluent collection to the clinic. This volume is then measured either in the clinic or in the laboratory, and a representative aliquot is taken for urea and creatinine measurement after appropriate mixing. In the case of APD, the dialysate volumes involved are typically greater. Many centers train patients to record or measure cycler effluent volumes in the home, using the machine reading, and then to take a representative aliquot of the effluent into the clinic for measurement of urea and creatinine levels.

Typically, the residual renal component of clearance declines gradually toward zero over the first 2 to 3 years on PD, but there is great variation. Total clearance will therefore tend to decrease if the dialysis prescription is not modified (Figure 28–1). This was commonplace until relatively recently but, as a result of influential publications and

Table 28–2 Formulas Required to Calculate Creatinine Clearance Normalized to Body Surface Area (CrCl) and Lean Body Mass

$$\text{CrCl} = \text{creatinine clearance} \times \frac{1.73}{\text{body surface area (m}^2)}$$

Creatinine clearance = 7 (daily peritoneal plus daily renal creatinine clearance)

$$\text{Daily peritoneal creatinine clearance} = \frac{\text{24-hr dialystate creatinine content*}}{\text{serum creatinine}}$$

$$\text{Daily renal creatinine clearance} = \frac{\text{24-hr urine creatinine content}}{\text{serum creatinine} \times 2} + \frac{\text{24-hr urine area content}}{\text{serum urea} \times 2}$$

Body surface area (according to *du Bois and colleagues*[23]):

Log A = 0.415 Log W + 0.725 Log H + 1.8564

where A = body surface area (cm^2)
H = height (cm)
W = weight (kg)

Lean body mass (kg) (according to *Keshaviah and colleagues*[25]) = 7.38 + 0.029 (creatinine production [mg/day])

Creatinine production (mg) = Creatinine excretion + creatinine degradation

Creatinine excretion (mg/day) = 24-hr dialysate creatinine* content (mg) Plus 24-hr urine creatinine content (mg)

Creatinine degradation (mg/day) = 0.38 (serum creatinine [mg/dL]) (body weight [kg])

*Corrected for dialysate glucose content by a formula specific to each laboratory.

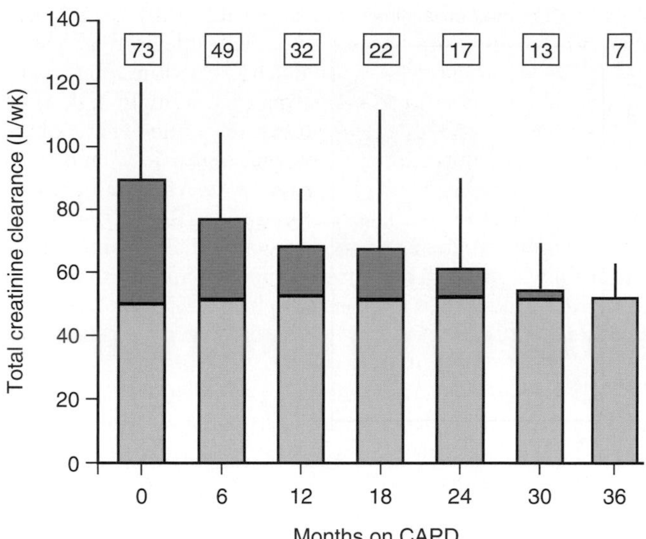

Figure 28–1 Changes in clearance with time in standard CAPD. (Modified from Blake PG, Balaskas EV, Izatt S, Oreopoulos DG: Is total creatinine clearance a good predictor of clinical outcomes in continuous ambulatory dialysis? Perit Dial Int 1992; 12:353-358.)

guideline recommendations, alterations in the dialytic prescription have become common.

Notwithstanding this, total weekly Kt/V values achieved in PD are typically half to two-thirds of those on HD. This might suggest substantial under-dialysis, but it must be remembered that the efficiency, in terms of small solute removal of clearance delivered continuously, is much greater than that of a similar quantity of clearance delivered intermittently.[25,26] Also, continuous modalities avoid the substantial disequilibria of intermittent ones. Furthermore, continuous modalities may be at a relative advantage because peak levels of uremic toxins are theoretically lower for a given clearance than is the case with intermittent modalities. This concept underlies the "Peak Concentration Hypothesis" of Keshaviah and colleagues,[25] which proposes that peak rather than mean levels of small solutes are the determinant of uremic toxicity (Figure 28–2). Recently, driven by the interest in models of daily HD, as well as in PD, a number of investigators have attempted to define indices or methodologies that allow more realistic comparison of intermittently and continuously delivered clearance.[27] None of these has been clearly validated, but there is some evidence that urea clearances, corrected to take into account the frequency of dialytic delivery, are associated with similar patient survival rates. As will be subsequently shown, such indices generally give equal weight to peritoneal and renal clearance, but recent trials suggest that this is not a valid approach.[13,14]

PERITONEAL EQUILIBRATION TEST (PET)

Before discussing peritoneal clearances any further, it is important to have an understanding of the PET and what it measures.[28] The PET is a simple clinical method for assessing the differences in the rapidity with which urea, creatinine, and other solutes diffuse across the peritoneal membrane in different patients. Classically, this involves measurement of dialysate and plasma urea and creatinine levels during a 4-hour duration, 2 L, 2.5% dextrose dwell done under standard conditions. Equilibration curves are constructed based on dialysate to plasma ratios for urea and creatinine, and patients are classified as low, low average, high average, or high transporters with cutoff values being defined by the frequency distribution for the population in the original study by Twardowski[28] (Figure 28–3). Those with values greater than one standard deviation above the mean are classified as high transporters, and those between the mean and one standard deviation above the mean are classified as high average. Those below the mean are classified as low and low average in the same manner. Patients who are high transporters equilibrate quickly and so dialyze well, but they tend to ultrafiltrate poorly because their osmotic gradient for glucose dissipates relatively rapidly. These patients might be expected to do better with short dwell times as in APD. However, any long duration day dwells may be largely resorbed and so, if one is

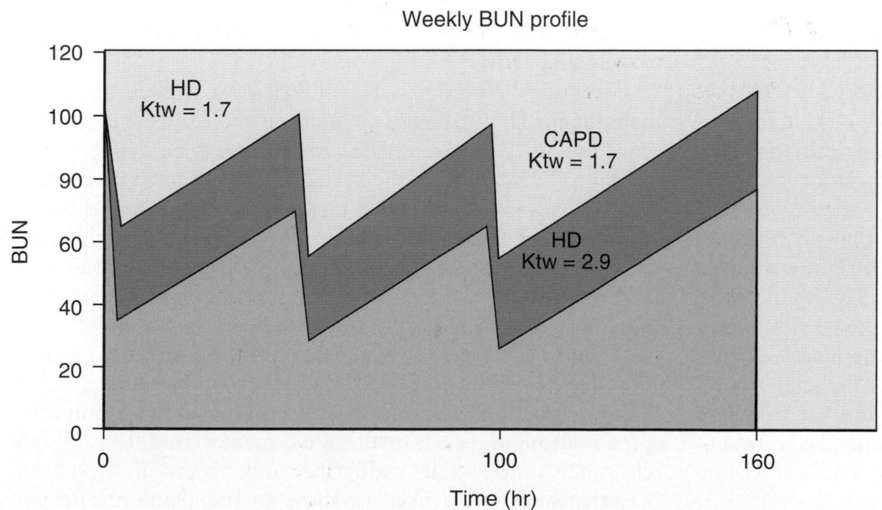

Figure 28–2 Peak concentration hypothesis. (Redrawn from Keshaviah PR, Nolph KD, Van Stone JC: The peak concentration hypothesis: A urea kinetic approach to comparing the adequacy of CAPD and hemodialysis. Perit Dial Int 1989; 9: 257-260.)

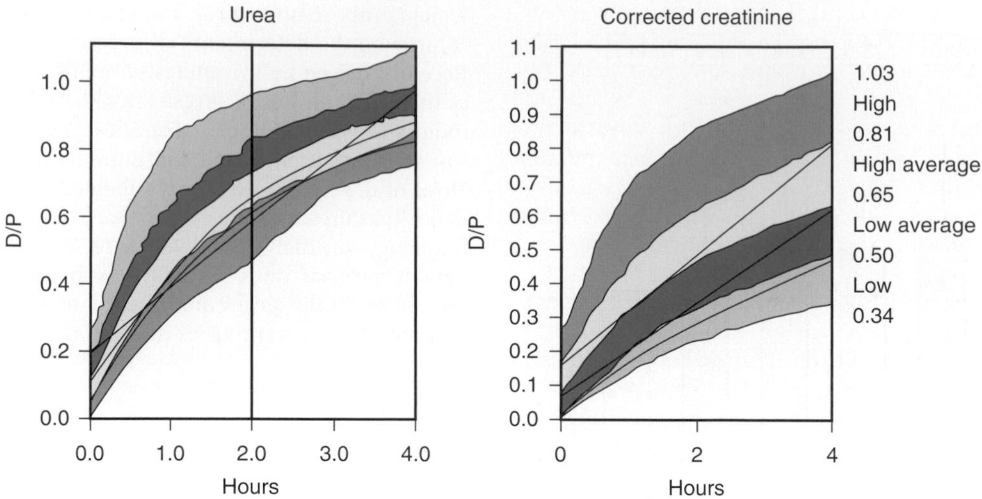

Figure 28–3 Peritoneal equilibration curves. (From Twardowski ZJ, Nolph KD, Khanna R, et al: Peritoneal equilibration test. Perit Dial Bull 1987; 7:138-147.)

required, it should be of short duration or, alternatively, be replaced by the polyglucose solution, icodextrin.[29] In contrast, low transporters ultrafiltrate well but equilibrate slowly and, consequently, large dwell volumes and long dwell times may be more effective. In general, in CAPD patients, urea clearance is much less affected by PET status than is creatinine clearance. This is because a greater than 90% urea equilibration will usually occur, regardless of transport status, with the long dwell times that are typical of CAPD. This is not the case for creatinine equilibration, which may show a twofold to threefold difference between low and high transporters, even after a 4- to 6-hour dwell (see Figure 28–3). In APD, where dwells are typically 1 to 2 hours or less in duration, both urea and creatinine equilibration will vary substantially with PET status and hence, this is a critical determinant of the clearances achieved. As will be seen, this is an important consideration in prescribing APD. Notwithstanding all of this, it should be said that the constraints imposed on achieving clearances in patients with different peritoneal transport characteristics are often not apparent until residual renal function is lost.

CLEARANCES AND OUTCOMES IN PD

Initial studies carried out in the late 1980s and early 1990s to look at the influence of small solute clearance on outcome in PD were small and, in retrospect, methodologically naive.[4,5] Results varied with some showing good correlation between clearance and outcomes and others finding little or no relationship.[4,5,30,31] It soon became apparent in the early studies that, in the context of a relatively uniform CAPD prescription, variations in clearance were due primarily to changes in residual renal function.[4] In subsequent analyses, the need to separate out peritoneal and renal clearance became more evident. In addition, analyses had to take into account the tendency of residual clearance to decline with time, and so frequent remeasurement of clearance indices was required, as were statistical methodologies that attributed outcomes to recent, rather than remote, measurements.

Canada–USA (CANUSA) was a large prospective cohort study of 680 incident CAPD patients done in multiple centers in Canada and in the United States.[7] Follow-up was for 2 years, and the investigators found an impressive association between clearance received and a number of outcomes, including survival. In particular, for every extra 0.1 Kt/V a patient received, the relative risk of dying fell by 6%, and for every extra 5 L a week CrCl, the risk fell by 7%. Maiorca and colleagues[8] found an association between weekly Kt/V values greater than 1.96 and subsequent survival in a cohort of 86 prevalent Italian CAPD patients followed over 3 years. These two studies had a major influence on the U.S. National Kidney Foundation Dialysis Outcomes Quality Initiative (K/DOQI) guidelines published in 1997 and revised in 2000.[9] These K/DOQI guidelines recommended a weekly Kt/V of 2.0 for those on CAPD with modestly higher targets of 2.2 and 2.1 for those on "day dry" APD and on APD with day dwells, respectively. The rationale behind the higher targets for the APD modalities is that they are slightly more intermittent than CAPD and, as already mentioned, intermittency decreases the efficiency of any given amount of delivered clearance.[25,26] The corresponding CrCl targets were 60, 63, and 66 liters a week for CAPD, "day dry" APD and APD with day dwells, respectively.[9]

Criticism of the CANUSA and Maiorca studies and of the consequent DOQI targets focused on the concern that residual function was severely confounding interpretation of the evidence.[32] The bulk of the variation in delivered clearance in CANUSA was due to declining residual function and not to variations in peritoneal clearance, which was left relatively constant. Neither the CANUSA nor the Maiorca studies were able to show any independent effect of peritoneal clearance on outcome.[33] In a sense, all that was shown was that more residual renal function was associated with superior survival, a not unexpected finding given the associated benefits of native kidney function, such as better volume control, superior preservation of nutritional status, greater middle molecule clearance, and renal endocrine and metabolic function. Clearly, there was a need to show an independent effect of peritoneal clearance on outcome, if the expense and inconvenience of increasing dialytic dose was to be justified. The proponents of the new targets would have argued that peritoneal clearance and residual renal clearance are, at least partly, interchangeable and that existing studies, coming from an era of uniform prescription, did not have a sufficient range of peritoneal clearance to detect the supposed beneficial effect on outcomes. Subsequent data from the late 1990s, when there was greater variation in peritoneal prescribing, continued, however, to show no independent effect of peritoneal clearance and outcomes.[12,34] It was clear that randomized, controlled trials were required.

The first two randomized trials addressing this issue appeared in 1997 and 2000 and came from the United Kingdom and Hong Kong, respectively.[35,36] Harty and colleagues[35] used 2:1 randomization of 68 CAPD patients with 42 CAPD patients receiving a 0.5 liter increase in their 1.5% dextrose dwell volumes only. Follow-up was for 1 year, but tolerance of the greater volumes was poor with 12 of the 42 not accepting the increase and only 17 completing the year. No difference in survival was identified but the study was severely underpowered. Mak and colleagues[36] randomized 82 prevalent CAPD patients to 3 × 2 L dwells as compared to 4 × 2 L dwells with 1 year follow-up. Again, there was no difference in survival, but this study was also significantly underpowered.

The ADEMEX study, published in 2002, is the largest randomized trial ever done in PD.[13] Almost 1000 incident and prevalent Mexican PD patients were randomized to receive either the standard 4 × 2 L CAPD prescription or an augmented prescription designed to achieve 60 L per week peritoneal CrCl. This study was well designed and carried out. Baseline characteristics of the two groups were almost identical, both in terms of demographics, comorbidity, baseline peritoneal clearance, and residual function. This study was large enough to have the power to detect a 20% increase in mortality, equivalent to a 4% absolute difference in 1-year survival. As one would expect, not all of the intervention group reached the demanding peritoneal clearance target of 60 L a week, but separation between the two groups was substantial (Table 28–3). Survival was identical between the two groups and, furthermore, there was no difference between subgroups, designated

Table 28–3 Weekly Kt/V and CrCl Values in ADEMEX

	Standard Group	High Clearance Group
Peritoneal Kt/V	1.62	2.13
Total Kt/V	1.80	2.27
Peritoneal CrCl	46 L	57 L
Total CrCl	53 L	63 L

Kt/V, urea clearance, normalized to body water; *CrCl*, creatinine clearance, normalized to body surface area.

by age, sex, diabetes, body size, and presence or absence of residual function (Figure 28–4). This impressively negative study had no major flaws and deals with exactly the range of doses that can be delivered in clinical practice.[11] One objection to the study was the claim that it was carried out in Mexican patients only and might not be applicable to populations elsewhere. In 2003, however, Lo and colleagues[14] reported another large randomized trial comprising 320 incident CAPD patients from six centers in Hong Kong who were randomized to high, normal, and low Kt/V prescriptions of greater than 2.0, 1.7 to 2.0, and 1.5 to 1.7 per week, respectively. In this study, the Kt/V target took into account residual function as well as peritoneal clearance, and so the high target was less demanding. The baseline characteristics of the three groups did, unfortunately, vary somewhat in that, for example, the sex distribution, the age, and the body size differed substantially across these groups. Follow-up was 2 years and, again, there was no survival benefit for the high clearance group, as compared to the other two. The low clearance group did a little worse in terms of erythropoietin requirements and study withdrawals, but the fact that this was an open-label study makes the latter finding hard to interpret.[14] Overall, the Lo study appeared to support the ADEMEX finding that high clearance PD prescriptions do not improve outcomes.

Another criticism of ADEMEX, and implicitly of the Lo study, was that both comprised populations with relatively lower rates of cardiovascular disease as compared to those seen in North America and Western Europe.[37] In the case of

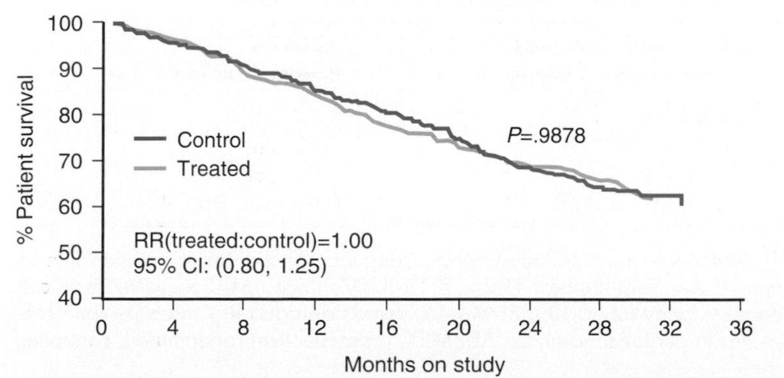

Figure 28–4 Survival in ADEMEX study. (From Paniagua R, Amato D, Vonesh E, et al: Effects of increased peritoneal clearances on mortality rates in peritoneal dialysis: ADEMEX, a prospective, randomized, controlled trial. J Am Soc Nephrol 2002; 13:1307-1320.)

ADEMEX, patients with overt cardiac disease were excluded, and in Hong Kong the prevalence of this complication in PD patients is relatively low to begin with. However, 60% of deaths in the ADEMEX study were cardiovascular in etiology, and this did not differ between the two groups. Another concern relates to the possibility of noncompliance in the intervention groups in these studies. This is always an issue in any study, or real-life situation, that requires the patient to deliver a treatment. Analyses based on blood work from ADEMEX, however, suggest that the extra dialytic dose was generally delivered. An additional issue raised regarding ADEMEX was the finding that, although the absolute number of deaths did not differ across the two groups, those attributed to congestive heart failure and uremia, hyperkalemia, and acidosis were significantly more frequent in the control group. Similarly, there were more dropouts attributed to uremia in the control group. Overinterpretation of these findings should be avoided, however. ADEMEX was, by its nature, an open-label study and there is a strong possibility that physicians classifying the etiology of deaths and withdrawals from the study would be more likely to designate those in the control group as being due to uremia or volume overload.

Residual skepticism about these two large and impressive controlled trials should also be tempered because the findings do not differ from those of the CANUSA[7] and Rocco and colleagues'[12] studies. Each of these studies, a randomized, controlled trial, a prospective cohort study, and a retrospective analysis, respectively, showed a very similar effect of residual renal function on survival, and each showed no effect of peritoneal clearance (Table 28–4). There is a convincing consistency about these findings. Accordingly, apart from some reservations about unreservedly applying the results to patients with overt cardiac disease, it seems unreasonable to not accept the findings of ADEMEX and of Lo and colleagues as valid and highly relevant. There is now a broad consensus that guideline groups need to reconvene and revise existing recommendations.

NEW RECOMMENDATIONS

A reasonable approach might be to use the dialytic dose received by the control group in the ADEMEX study, perhaps with a modest increment for safety, as the new minimum target Kt/V.[13] This would, therefore, be about 1.7 peritoneal per week or 45 to 50 L per week CrCl. There is no longer justification for the old policy of adding peritoneal and residual renal clearance together because the two are clearly not interchangeable in their implications for patient outcomes. Residual clearance should be treated as a precious bonus to be protected but should not be part of a clearance target. A target Kt/V value of 1.7 peritoneal is, with a bit of effort, feasible in almost all patients. In most, it will not require prescriptions that unreasonably disrupt the already impaired quality of life of dialysis patients.

The justification for having both CrCl and Kt/V targets also needs to be questioned. There is no evidence from any of the randomized, controlled trials that one index is any better than the other in predicting outcome. The apparent superiority of CrCl in some previous prospective and retrospective studies is merely a mark of the fact that CrCl gives greater weight to residual renal clearance.[30] A reasonable approach, for simplicity, might be to have a single peritoneal Kt/V target. The evidence for having separate targets for CAPD and APD was never strong and introduces an unnecessary degree of complexity. All of these PD modalities are relatively continuous, compared to three times weekly HD, for example. There is also no convincing need for different targets by transport type either, especially when CrCl is taken out of consideration.

If "incremental" or "early start" PD is practiced with patients being initiated on dialysis while residual function is still substantial, there is justification for a lower peritoneal prescription, such as two to three CAPD exchanges daily or "day dry," low-volume APD.[38] If the residual function exceeds 2 mL/min, a peritoneal Kt/V of 1.2 per week would likely be sufficient in that the total Kt/V in such a case would still easily exceed the old K/DOQI targets.

Trials of higher peritoneal clearances than 1.7 per week might still be indicated if patients have persisting uremic type symptoms, and, particularly, if there is coexisting cardiovascular disease, but expectations for a beneficial effect would have to be guarded and alternative diagnoses and treatments considered.

WHY HIGHER CLEARANCES DO NOT HELP?

Why is high clearance PD not more successful in improving quality and quantity of life? Similar questions are being asked

Table 28–4 Relative Risks for Mortality by Peritoneal and Renal Clearance Indices in Three Major Studies

Type of Study	CANUSA Prospective Cohort	Rocco and Colleagues Retrospective Analysis	ADEMEX Randomized Trial
Peritoneal CrCl	1.04 (ns)	0.90 (ns)	1.03 (ns)
Renal CrCl	0.83 (p = .001)	0.60 (p <0.001)	0.89 (p = .013)
Peritoneal Kt/V	1.00 (ns)	1.00 (ns)	1.00 (ns)
Renal Kt/V	0.68 (p <.001)	0.88 (p = 0.003)	0.94 (p = .005)

ns, not significant. (Adapted from Canada-USA [CANUSA] Peritoneal Dialysis Study Group: Adequacy of dialysis in nutrition in continuous peritoneal dialysis: Association with clinical outcomes. J Am Soc Nephrol 1996; 7:198-207; Rocco M, Souci JM, Pastan S, McClellan WM: Peritoneal dialysis adequacy and risk of death. Kidney Int 2000; 58:446-457; and Paniagua R, Amato D, Vonesh E, et al: Effects of increased peritoneal clearances on mortality rates in peritoneal dialysis: ADEMEX, a prospective, randomized, controlled trial. J Am Soc Nephrol 2002; 13:1307-1320.)

about high clearance HD in the aftermath of the equally negative HEMO study. A number of possible answers need to be considered.[16]

One is that relative to the clearance provided by normal kidneys, the levels being tested in these trials are very low. Comparisons of 4 to 6 mL as compared to 6 to 8 mL a week, as was done in ADEMEX, seem very modest if 100 mL/min or more is considered to be normal. Proponents of this point of view argue that dialysis will significantly improve survival only if substantially greater clearances are delivered, as might be the case with daily or nocturnal HD.[39] An alternative view is that survival in ESRD is primarily determined by associated comorbidity and not by variations in dialytic dose. Once frank uremia is prevented by a baseline amount of dialysis, incremental survival requires not more clearance but rather a more successful strategy for preventing and treating cardiovascular disease and infection, the two great killers of dialysis patients.[16]

Others still argue that the small solute clearance is the wrong "yardstick" and that middle molecule clearance has been neglected or that indices of volume control may be more important. These theories may be correct, but the HEMO study gives little support to the middle molecule hypothesis and no new dogma should be accepted unreservedly without more convincing proof.[15]

Last, the notion that high clearance PD is doing no harm and that patients should therefore be given "the benefit of the doubt" also needs to be addressed. Not only is high-dose PD more costly, but it is also potentially onerous for patients.[40] Larger dwell volumes in the ADEMEX and other studies were associated with mechanical symptoms leading to dropout, hernias, and so forth.[13] More exchanges may increase the risk of peritonitis, and there is evidence that patient noncompliance also results.[41] Cycler prescriptions with 2, 3, or more day dwells may also impair quality of life. Furthermore, increases in dialytic dose generally lead to more peritoneal glucose exposure and absorption, and there is a growing body of evidence that this is deleterious, not only to the peritoneal membrane but also, more critically, to the patient's cardiovascular risk profile.[42,43]

STRATEGIES TO INCREASE PERITONEAL CLEARANCE

Notwithstanding recent skepticism concerning the benefits of augmented PD prescriptions, it will still be necessary to prescribe more than the conventional 4 × 2 L CAPD or 10 L per night APD regimens to bring many patients above the proposed 1.7 peritoneal Kt/V target.[44]

In CAPD, an increase in dwell volume from 2 to 2.5 L is the least disruptive approach, is usually well tolerated, and leads to approximately a 20% increase in peritoneal clearance.[44] The need to use 3-L volumes should be noticeably less with future lower Kt/V targets. The alternative strategy of adding a fifth exchange is less attractive because it is more expensive and disruptive of a lifestyle and because it is associated with increased noncompliance.[40,41] If this strategy is chosen, however, the most effective way to add the extra exchange would be to use a night exchange device to break up the long nocturnal dwell.[45]

APD is increasingly the chosen option for PD patients.[11] The addition of a day dwell is the most effective way to increase clearances with this modality. This is particularly so in the patient who is "day dry," where the resulting increase in clearance is often 30% to 35%.[44] If a day dwell is already being used, the addition of a second one will also have a substantial effect, provided that each is in place for at least 4 hours to allow good solute equilibration. Strategies based on using the cycler as a "docking station" reduce the cost and inconvenience of adding a second day dwell, although they do require the patient to return to the cycler to do the exchange.[46] A manual "double bag" exchange is an alternative for the patient who does not wish to return to the cycler. If there is just 1 long day dwell, fluid resorption may be a problem. In this situation, an early drain after 4 to 8 hours may be an option that increases ultrafiltration, preserves clearance, and even enhances lifestyle in that many patients prefer being "empty" for at least some of the day. An alternative approach to maintaining ultrafiltration is to introduce the polyglucose solution, icodextrin, for the long day dwell.[29] This approach is also useful for the long nocturnal dwell in CAPD.

Alternative methods of raising clearance in APD are to increase the number of cycles per treatment session. Typically, this effect starts to plateau out once the number of cycles exceeds about seven per 9-hour cycling session.[44,47] This number may be a little higher for high transporters, but the cost of more than seven cycles per night is also a factor.[40] Lengthening the cycler time is also somewhat effective in increasing clearance, but, again, there are lifestyle constraints. Larger dwell volumes may also help; that is, 4 × 2.5 L give better clearance than 5 × 2 L. The effect is modest and some argue that the rise in intraperitoneal pressures with higher volumes may impair ultrafiltration.[48]

Measurement of peritoneal clearance should be carried out once the new PD patient stabilizes on the initial prescription. It would seem appropriate to measure clearance every 6 months, as part of a general check on the prescription that the patient is doing.[9,10] Measurement should also be repeated soon after any prescription change and in the event of any unexpected or unexplained change in clinical status. Residual renal and urinary volume should be measured at the same time as peritoneal clearance. However, if the patient is on an "incremental" PD prescription with an initial low peritoneal clearance, residual renal clearance should be measured at 2-month intervals to avoid missing a decline in residual function and consequent "under-dialysis."[38]

MAINTENANCE OF RESIDUAL RENAL FUNCTION

One lesson that PD practitioners have learned in the past decade is the impressive value of preservation of even very modest amounts of residual renal function. Thus, in the CANUSA study, an extra 5 L a week creatinine clearance, which is equivalent to 0.5 mL/min glomerular filtration rate, was associated with a 7% increase in survival.[7] Similarly, a 250-mL increment in urine volume was associated with a 36% decrease in relative risk of death. When both renal clearance and urine volume were added to the same Cox model, the urinary volume appeared to be the stronger predictor of survival.[33] Other studies have shown that RRF is a crucial factor in maintenance of good volume, cardiac status, control of hyperphosphatemia and that it may also decrease the risk of malnutrition.[49-51]

Of course, all of this may not be cause and effect. It is plausible that preserved renal function may be a marker of general well-being, of less systemic inflammation, or just of an earlier stage in the evolution of ESRD.[52] However, the possibility that better preserved function enhances survival through its effects on volume status, middle molecule clearance, metabolism, or nutrition is also quite conceivable.

Regardless, the preservation of residual function would seem to be a priority. A recent randomized, controlled trial showed that angiotensin converting enzyme inhibition and, in particular, ramipril 5 mg daily, was associated with better retention of residual function and lower probability of anuria.[53] This study, based on 60 CAPD patients in Hong Kong, with no other indication to be on an angiotensin converting inhibitor, showed a small but significant effect with a 1 mL/min greater clearance at 12 months and a 42% lower chance of development of anuria.

In another randomized, controlled trial, Medcalf and colleagues[54] randomized 61 incidence PD patients to either furosemide 250 mg/day or no diuretic. Urine volume was better maintained at 1 year in the furosemide group with a difference of just over 350 mL/day. Urine sodium excretion was also enhanced and volume status appeared better in that percentage of body water by bioimpedance rose in the control group but stayed constant in the treatment group.

Both ACE inhibitors and high dose furosemide appear to be safe interventions in PD patients and this evidence that they are reasonably effective in maintaining urinary clearance and volume, respectively, would appear to justify their routine use. Other strategies to consider in preserving residual renal function are to avoid, as much as possible, volume depletion, the use of aminoglycosides, nonsteroidal anti-inflammatories, and radiologic contrast. When the latter has to be used, renoprotection with intravenous saline and administration of acetylcysteine should be considered, if residual renal function is still significant.[55]

NUTRITION

The influence of nutrition on outcomes and survival in dialysis patients has long been appreciated. A variety of nutritional indices predict survival in PD patients. These include serum albumin, subjective global assessment, lean body mass, and other indices of creatinine production, total body nitrogen, a variety of other composite nutritional indices, and, in some studies, protein intake.[7,8,56-58]

The mechanism of this association of nutrition and survival is not clear. A crucial issue is whether it represents cause and effect or just association. In other words, is the poor nutrition the proximate cause of the inferior outcomes, or are they both common consequences of underlying comorbid conditions that are the true cause of the patients' poor survival? Traditionally, nutrition and clearances have been linked together with the theory being that inadequate clearances lead to poor protein intake, which, in turn, leads to malnutrition and premature death.[13] This theory stems from the general observation that degree of uremia and appetite for protein are closely correlated and also from the suggestion in the 1980s that Kt/V and protein intake were closely associated.[54] However, this paradigm has been shown to be an oversimplification. The original observations relating clearance and protein intake were confounded by the phenomenon of "mathematical coupling."[60,61] More significantly, there is now a greater awareness that much of the malnutrition seen in dialysis patients is independent of dialytic dose.[62]

Contributors to impaired nutritional status in PD patients can be divided into those that are found in ESRD in general and those that are specific to PD (Table 28–5). The former include inflammation, metabolic acidosis, impaired protein anabolism, and uremic anorexia. The latter include the obligatory dialysate protein losses and some of the impairment of gastric emptying.

The greatest area of interest, recently, with regard to the etiology of malnutrition in renal failure has been in the notion that persistent inflammation is a critical underlying factor. Inflammation, as indicated by elevated serum C-reactive protein (CRP) and interleukin-6 levels, is present, usually without any clinically obvious cause, in as many as 30% to 60% of dialysis patients.[63-66] Most importantly, it is associated with decreased survival in ESRD patients. It has been associated in some studies with progressive atherosclerosis, giving rise to the concept of the "malnutrition inflammation atherosclerosis," or MIA, syndrome.[63,67] Inflammation has also been shown to account for much of the hypoalbuminemia seen in both PD and HD patients, an effect mediated through decreased hepatic albumin production, consequent on a chronically "turned on" acute phase response.[68]

Table 28–5 Factors Contributing to Malnutrition in PD Patients

General ESRD-Related Causes	PD Specific Causes
Uremic anorexia	Dialysate protein losses
Inadequate dialysis	Impaired gastric emptying (present in ESRD but worse in PD)
Systemic inflammation	Anorexic effect of dialysis glucose absorption
General comorbidity	Peritonitis episodes
Gastrointestinal comorbidity (e.g., gastritis, ulcers, constipation, diabetic gastropathy)	
Metabolic acidosis	
Growth hormone resistance	
IGF-I resistance	
Medication side effects (e.g., oral iron, phosphate binders)	
Socioeconomic deprivation	
Poor dietary habits (e.g., previous low protein diets)	
Decreased activity	
Depression	

Why ESRD patients should have chronically stimulated immune responses is unclear. Initial theories proposed a role for the bioincompatible aspects of dialysis, such as the blood membrane interaction in hemodialysis and the dialysis solution peritoneal membrane interaction in PD.[63-65] However, the finding that inflammation is equally common in patients with advanced renal failure prior to initiation of dialysis argues against this being the major cause.[67] Another possibility is that the inflammation is directly related to renal failure per se and the associated impaired clearance of cytokines.[69] However, there is no clear proportionality between clearances and inflammation, and so this cannot be more than a modest part of the overall explanation. Coexistent comorbid conditions, in particular, cardiovascular disease, may be a critical player in cytokine activation, though which is the cause and which is the consequence are unknown.

Management of the inflammation of ESRD has not been very successful. The cardiology literature varyingly suggests roles for statins, aspirin, and even angiotensin converting enzyme inhibitors in suppressing inflammation, but there is little evidence as to how effective these strategies are in ESRD.[70–74]

Numerous studies in recent years testify to the contributory role of acidosis to the impaired nutritional status of renal failure.[75-77] The mechanism here is increased breakdown of muscle protein due to activation of the ubiquitin-proteasome proteolytic system.[76,77] In PD patients, acidosis tends to be less of an issue because the continuous nature of the dialysis usually ensures good maintenance of serum bicarbonate.[78] Interestingly, two recent randomized trials have shown that supplementation to increase the serum bicarbonate to levels that are in the high normal to alkalotic range improves nutritional parameters modestly in PD patients.[79,80] Oral sodium bicarbonate should therefore be considered in the small minority of PD patients with a serum bicarbonate level less than 25 mmol/L. More aggressive use of bicarbonate is probably not justified by the available data. The introduction of bicarbonate based PD solutions will have only a very mild effect on serum bicarbonate levels.[81]

Another important factor in the malnutrition of ESRD is impaired anabolism. The etiology of this relates to uremia being a state of resistance to a number of hormones involved in nutrition and metabolism, most notably insulin, growth hormone (GH), and insulin-like growth factor one (IGF-I).[82-84] The etiology of this state of resistance is complex and multifactorial. Some theories have implicated high levels of GH and IGF binding proteins or abnormalities of GH and IGF receptors, whereas others focus on post-receptor mechanisms.[82-84] Whatever the etiology, the consequence of this is that nitrogen supplements are frequently not effectively anabolized in renal failure and may just result in increased levels of blood urea. Strategies to deal with this include administration of recombinant GH, recombinant IGF-I, and anabolic steroids.[85-87] All these approaches are, however, constrained by concerns about side effects.

Obligatory protein losses in PD average 8 to 9 g/day, about half of which is accounted for by albumin.[88] This is the primary cause of the hypoalbuminemia seen in PD patients.[56,68,89] Protein losses increase in the presence of peritonitis and generally tend to be greater in those with high transport status.[56,69] Losses are not generally influenced by dialysate flow rates, but they may be less in patients who are left "dry" for part of the day. No convincing method of decreasing dialysate protein losses has been identified.

Suboptimal protein intake is a frequent feature in PD patients.[7,13] The widely quoted protein intake PNA target of 1.2 g/kg body weight/day is based on observations made in younger, healthier patients than those typically seen in contemporary PD programs.[90] Even more modest targets of 0.9 to 1.0 g/kg/day are often not achieved.[91] Some of this reflects the decreased activity, the comorbidity, and the general poor health of many patients. However, an additional factor is the impaired gastric emptying seen in many PD patients.[92,93] This is more marked in diabetics and seems, at least in part, to be related to the dialysate glucose content.[92]

DIAGNOSIS OF MALNUTRITION

High awareness of the frequency and significance of malnutrition is important. Basic history taking and clinical examination with assessment of food intake, appetite, weight, fat stores, and muscle mass should be routine practice in the evaluation of PD patients. Some of this can be formalized in the technique of subjective global assessment.[7] Regular evaluations by a experienced dietitian are also important with particular regard to assessment of nutrient intake. Low serum levels of urea, potassium, and phosphate are all suggestive of poor nutritional intake. Urea kinetics can be used to estimate the normalized protein equivalent of nitrogen appearance (nPNA), a surrogate for protein intake in a stable patient.[94] The rationale here is that urea generation and excretion in the stable patient is proportional, in a predictable manner, to protein intake. A variety of formulas have been used to estimate protein intake from urea and other nitrogen losses. Some are taken from the chronic renal failure or hemodialysis literature, whereas others were derived directly from PD patients (see Table 28–2).[91,95,96] The best validated are those of Bergstrom.[95] Normalization of the calculated protein intake is typically done using desirable rather than actual body weight because the latter can be misleading if there is marked malnutrition or obesity.[9,10,98] Desirable body weight can be taken from standardized tables based on age, sex, height, and body frame. Simple estimates of body composition can be performed using creatinine excretion in dialysate and urine to estimate lean body mass.[99] Formulas for this take into account extrarenal creatinine degradation as well as level of serum creatinine. Estimates based on these measurements have been shown to be predictive of outcomes.[7,57] More sophisticated methods of assessing body composition include bioelectric impedance, DEXA, and total body nitrogen measurements.[58,100–102]

Serum albumin is now recognized to be a poor measure of nutrient intake in the PD patient but a low value, along with a high CRP level, may be a clue to ongoing inflammation.[68] The other major contributor to hypoalbuminemia in this setting is high peritoneal transport status and the associated dialysate protein losses.[56,90]

MANAGEMENT OF MALNUTRITION

Malnutrition is a frustrating complication of ESRD because it is frequently not amenable to correction. A multidisciplinary approach is preferred involving the dietitian, the nurse, and the social worker as well as the physician.[9,10] Attention to social, economic, and educational factors is important. Medications should be reviewed, looking particularly at those, such as oral iron, phosphate binders, and nonsteroidal anti-inflammatories, which may be irritating to the stomach. Comorbidities, such as poor dentition, gastrointestinal disease, and depression should be looked for and addressed. Counseling concerning the importance of protein intake is essential, but frequently patients cannot achieve the recommended targets of 1.0 to 1.2 g/kg/day, and, in these situations, it is important that more modest increments be encouraged.[9,10] Indeed, there is evidence that patients can go into nitrogen balance at lower levels of protein intake.[91]

Identification and correction of under-dialysis is an important aspect of managing malnutrition but, as already mentioned, this is now understood to be a less significant contributor than was thought to be the case in the past. However, peritoneal Kt/V values less than 1.7 in the presence of malnutrition should be considered an indication for increasing clearance. Oral sodium bicarbonate supplements should also be considered if the serum bicarbonate is low.[78,79] If symptoms are suggestive of impaired gastric emptying, a trial of a promotility agent, such as domperidone, should be considered.[93] There may also be a role for empiric use of antacid agents, such as protein pump inhibitors or histamine antagonists. Identification and treatment of *Helicobacter pylori* infection may also help.[103] If elevated serum CRP levels indicate the presence of inflammation, a search for a primary cause may be made, but a specific treatable entity is uncommonly identified and, more often, there is nothing definitive or just generalized comorbidity.[65]

Trials of protein and/or nitrogen supplements are commonly carried out even though there is little evidence that this approach is effective in improving clinical outcomes in ESRD patients. If oral supplements are not of benefit, consideration should be given to using intraperitoneal amino acids. Modest benefits have been demonstrated for these in clinical trials.[104-106] They have been shown to improve nitrogen balance and, in some studies, to induce an anabolic response and to ameliorate hypoalbuminemia. However, substantial improvement to clinical outcomes has not been demonstrated. Care has to be taken to ensure that intraperitoneal amino acids do not induce uremia or acidosis. For this reason, use is limited to one 2- or 2.5-L bag of 1.1% amino acids daily, given at the same time as ingestion of an energy source. Feeding by gastrostomy tube has occasionally been attempted in adults with ESRD but is more frequently done in children. This intervention can be successfully carried out in patients on PD but complications are significant, and, again, there is little evidence of long-term benefit.[107]

Approaches based on improving anabolism have also been studied. One randomized trial done in both HD and PD patients showed benefits for the use of anabolic steroids.[87] This trial was small but still showed important functional improvements in the patients receiving the intervention. The anabolic effects of recombinant GH and of IGF-I have also been demonstrated in a number of studies, but their use is not practical in view of concerns about side effects and high costs.[85,86]

If all these approaches are ineffective and the patient is clinically failing, a trial of HD may be worth considering. Some patients improve after such a switch, but there is often no change.

VOLUME STATUS IN PD

The importance of achieving optimal volume status in both PD and HD patients has been emphasized recently for a number of reasons. First, the failure of an approach based on small solute clearance to reduce ESRD mortality substantially has encouraged investigators to look at other approaches to improving outcomes.[13,14,16] Second, the increasing realization that dialysis, as presently practiced, is not normalizing blood pressure in most patients has caused concern, given that cardiovascular disease is the commonest cause of death in these patients.[108,109] The notion that hypertension usually reflects inadequately managed volume status and may be contributing to adverse cardiovascular outcomes has therefore become popular.[109,110]

In PD patients, there is some evidence that volume status is even less well controlled than in HD patients.[111,112] This is most likely to be the case after residual renal function is lost.[51] As a consequence of all this, an International Society of Peritoneal Dialysis Committee published recommendations on management of volume status in 1999.[113]

Much of the literature on fluid overload in PD deals with the differential diagnosis of problems with the peritoneal membrane for which the term *ultrafiltration failure* (UFF) is commonly used. However, it should be emphasized that UFF is not the only cause of fluid overload in PD patients. Indeed in the early years of PD, UFF is relatively uncommon and other causes should be sought.

Nonmembrane causes of fluid overload are shown in Table 28–6. Excess salt and water intake and declining urine output are often major contributing factors. In some patients, noncompliance with the PD exchanges or inappropriate selection of dialysis solution strengths contributes to the problem. Mechanical complications that impair peritoneal fluid drainage may also be an issue. These lead to greater residual volumes and consequent fluid resorption. Examples include poorly functioning catheters, peritoneal leaks, loculations in the peritoneal cavity, and even hernias. Hyperglycemia may also contribute by decreasing the glucose osmotic gradient driving ultrafiltration.[113]

Careful history taking, physical examination, and inspection of dialysis records should help to identify these nonmembrane causes of UFF. In some situations, direct observation of dialysate drainage, assessment of residual volume and contrast peritoneography may be helpful.[113]

ULTRAFILTRATION FAILURE (UFF)

The term *ultrafiltration failure* (UFF) is best used to refer to cases of clinical fluid overload in which membrane dysfunction is identified as the primary cause of the problem. The classic definition is a net ultrafiltration volume of less than 400 mL at the end of the standard 2-L, 4-hour duration 4.25% dextrose dwell.[114]

The commonest cause of this, known as type I UFF, is where equilibration across the membrane is so rapid that the osmotic gradient for glucose dissipates before adequate ultra-

Table 28-6 Causes of Fluid Overload

Membrane Causes	Nonmembrane Causes
Type I—high effective membrane area	Excess salt and water intake
Type II—inadequate effective membrane area	Marked decline in urine output
Type III—excessive peritoneal fluid absorption	Noncompliance with PD prescriptions
Other types:	Inappropriate choice of solution tonicity
Impaired aquaporin function	Peritoneal leak (abdominal wall, retroperitoneum, perineum)
Impaired hydraulic conductance	Poor catheter function with resulting high residual volume
	Hyperglycemia—inadequate osmotic gradient

filtration has had time to occur. Rapid transport status is present from the initiation of PD in a minority of patients, whereas, in others, it appears with time. Thus, the cumulative incidence of UFF in one study was 2.6% after 1 year on PD, rising to 9.5% after 2 years, and to 30.9% after 6 years. This cumulative rise in incidence is partly related to the tendency for peritoneal transport to increase significantly in many patients. It is, however, frequently made more overt by the simultaneous tendency to lose residual renal function over the same time course.

The causes of the increase in peritoneal transport that tends to occur with time, has been a focus of research interest. Pathologically, there is an association of decreased ultrafiltration with submesothelial fibrosis, vasculopathic changes, and neovascularization.[116] The latter is believed to be the most significant finding in that vascular proliferation increases the effective peritoneal surface area and so results in more rapid transport.

The most popular hypothesis is that exposure to hypertonic glucose is the key factor in this process. Analogous pathologic and functional changes occur in diabetic animal models. There is a plausible pathway by which glucose and glucose degradation production (GDPs) in PD solution induce vascular endothelial growth factor (VEGF), which, in turn, promotes neovascularization through the action of nitric oxide.[117,118] De Vriese and colleagues[119] have, for example, shown that anti-VEGF antibodies can prevent much of the deterioration of ultrafiltration in animal models of PD.

Recently, Davies and colleagues[42] have strengthened this glucose related hypothesis by showing that patients who develop increased transport characteristics tend to have been exposed to more hypertonic glucose exchanges in their early years on PD, as compared to other patients who maintain relatively stable membrane transport. Glucose exposure may not be the only factor, however. The Davies' study also found that patients with stable peritoneal transport were more likely to have maintained their residual renal function for longer.[42] This may be association or it may be cause and effect. It is possible that some factor associated with residual renal function is protective for the peritoneal membrane. Chung and colleagues[120] have speculated that systemic inflammation might be such a factor. As previously discussed, systemic activation of cytokines can be detected in approximately half of all PD patients. Chung and colleagues[120] have shown that these patients are more likely to show increases in peritoneal transport in the first year on PD. The same patients are more likely to show faster declines in residual renal function.[52] The evidence for this hypothesis, is, as yet, not as strong as for the dialysate glucose mechanism.

Other bioincompatible features of PD solutions may contribute to peritoneal membrane damage. The glucose degradation products that arise during glucose sterilization may, in addition to stimulating VEGF production, also give rise to advanced glycosylation end products, which may themselves damage membrane function.[117,118] Other potential PD solution-related factors include low pH and lactate. Evidence for these is less convincing. The contribution of cumulative episodes of peritonitis to membrane function is relatively controversial with different studies yielding contrasting results.[121] The consensus at this stage is that mild peritonitis causes little permanent damage to the membrane, but severe peritonitis may be a contributor.

Type II UFF is much less common. In this condition, peritoneal transport of small solute as well as of water, actually decreases. This reflects a loss of peritoneal surface area. Most often, this is seen in the context of peritoneal adhesions acquired during severe peritonitis or after surgical complications. The available surface area for dialysis is too small and neither solute nor water transport is adequate. Some investigators have proposed that type II UFF may be a harbinger of encapsulating peritoneal sclerosis, but many cases of this condition show high rather than low transport characteristics in the early stages.[122]

Type III UFF is where lymphatic reabsorption of fluid from the peritoneal cavity is large enough to impair ultrafiltration. Peritoneal fluid absorption from the cavity occurs by two routes.[123] One is direct lymphatic absorption, occurring predominantly through diaphragmatic stomata. The other is hydrostatic pressure driven absorption of fluid across the peritoneal membrane into, predominantly, the tissues of the anterior abdominal wall. From here, the fluid is gradually resorbed, either by the lymphatics or directly into the systemic capillaries. The total fluid absorption by the two routes is difficult to measure but is thought to approximate 1 to 2 mL/min or 60 to 120 mL/hr. The main variation is thought to be in the direct lymphatic flow component. If this is significantly above the normal range, it is likely to become a clinical problem, especially if salt and water intake is high or urine volume is minimal. The proportion of cases of UFF due to this cause is unclear, but, in one review, Heimburger and colleagues[121] found that two of nine cases had high fluid resorption as the principal abnormality. In other cases, however, it may be a contributory factor.[114] In general, it is a diagnosis of exclusion because most PD units do not routinely measure peritoneal lymphatic flow or fluid absorption. Recent work by Fussholler and colleagues[124] suggests that peritoneal lymphatic flow does increase somewhat with time on PD.

Less common causes of UFF include aquaporin dysfunction and impaired hydraulic conductance of water by membrane.[123,125] The diagnosis of these is discussed in more detail in the "Physiology of PD" chapter. In practice, these conditions will only be suspected when UFF occurs in the presence of relatively well maintained peritoneal transport and even then, it is not easy to differentiate them from type III UFF. One clue to aquaporin dysfunction is a loss of the normal sodium sieving that occurs when hypertonic PD solutions are used.[114] However, this finding is not truly specific for aquaporin related problems.

Investigation of fluid overload and UFF should follow the broad sequence outlined in the algorithms from the 1999 ISPD recommendations (Figure 28–5).[113] These emphasize history taking, clinical examination, inspection of dialysis records, and observation of catheter drainage. If a diagnosis is not then apparent, a PET using 4.25% dextrose is indicated and will allow a formal diagnosis of UFF to be made. The equilibration characteristics shown in the PET will then allow the UFF to be divided into the three distinct categories. Of course, many cases are multifactorial with, for example, a mixture of a membrane and a mechanical problem or perhaps a combination of excess lymphatic drainage issue and high salt intake.

MANAGEMENT OF FLUID OVERLOAD

Management of fluid overload includes general and specific measures.[113] The general approach applicable to all cases is to review salt and water intake and to ensure the patient is making appropriate choices of dialysate tonicity and is avoiding excessively long duration dwells, such as which may occur with the nocturnal dwell of CAPD or the daytime dwell of APD. An additional aspect of the general approach is to maximize urinary output using loop diuretics and angiotensin converting enzyme inhibitors.[53,54] Recent randomized, controlled trials are helpful in this regard. Medcalf and colleagues[54] have shown in a small placebo-controlled trial that furosemide 250 mg/day is associated with better preservation of urinary volume. Similarly, Szeto and colleagues[53] have shown in a randomized, controlled open-label study that ramipril 5 mg daily is associated with better preservation of renal clearance and with a lower probability of progression to anuria. These medications can easily be prescribed and are generally safe in the PD population, although the risk of volume depletion and disorders of serum potassium must be kept in mind.

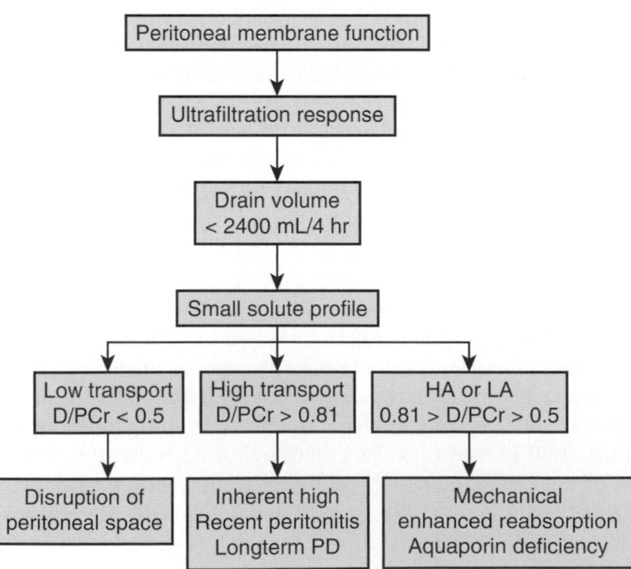

Figure 28–5 Management of fluid overload. (From Mujais S, Nolph K, Gokal R, et al: Evaluation and management of ultrafiltration problems in peritoneal dialysis. International Society for Peritoneal Dialysis Ad Hoc Committee on Ultrafiltration Management in Peritoneal Dialysis. Perit Dial Int 2000; 20[suppl 4]:S43-S55.)

More specific management measures depend on the cause of the fluid overload. Mechanical problems, such as leaks, hernias, and malfunctioning catheters will need surgical interventions. Noncompliance with the prescription, excess salt, and water intake, or inappropriate choice of solution tonicity require educational interventions. Glycemic control may need attention.

In the case of type I UFF, long duration dwells are a particular problem. They can be avoided in CAPD by using a night exchange device to split up the nocturnal dwell or, alternatively, a cycler based APD prescription can be introduced. The long day dwell in APD can be avoided by doing an extra exchange, either manually or from the cycler, midway through the day, or by simply draining the daytime fluid after 3 to 6 hours and leaving the patient "dry" until cycling commences again.[34] The decision as to which of these strategies should be followed will depend on the patient's lifestyle and clearance requirements.

An alternative approach is to continue with the long dwell in CAPD or APD but to instead use the polyglucose solution, icodextrin.[29] Icodextrin does not diffuse across the peritoneal membrane and so remains an effective osmotic agent, inducing ultrafiltration for many hours. Use of icodextrin is limited only by cost and by concerns that more than one dwell per 24-hour period might lead to accumulation of metabolites with unknown consequences. Wilkie and colleagues[126] have shown that icodextrin can prolong technique survival significantly in patients with UFF. Data from this study have been used to show that icodextrin, despite its expense, is a cost-effective intervention.[127]

In type II UFF, general measures may be tried, but PD is rarely viable because clearance and ultrafiltration are both compromised.

General measures are also the focus in management of type III UFF. Specific agents to decrease peritoneal lymphatic flow, such as lecithin, have been proposed but evidence to support their use has not been convincing.[128] Patients with type III UFF can also be maintained on PD because the problem is frequently moderate in severity and not progressive. Simply switching to APD may deal effectively with the fluid retention.

GLUCOSE SPARING STRATEGIES

The concept of glucose sparing strategies has become popular in recent time for two main reasons. First, the evidence that hypertonic glucose exposure is damaging to the peritoneal membrane has become stronger.[42,117,118] Second, and perhaps more significantly, there is a concern that systemic absorption of glucose from the dialysate has an adverse effect on the cardiovascular risk profile in that it may promote hyperglycemia, hyperlipidemia, hyperinsulinemia, and obesity. Glucose sparing strategies include the use of alternative nonglucose solutions, such as icodextrin and amino acids. However, it may also involve consideration of strategies that reduce the need for more hypertonic glucose. These include salt and water restriction and use of loop diuretics and ACE inhibitors to maintain or increase urine output.

Glucose sparing strategies are very attractive, and, although the evidence to justify them is circumstantial rather than conclusive, it seems prudent to follow them as far as is feasible. However, they should not be considered as a justification to leave volume overload and hypertension inadequately treated. The adverse effects of hypertension and fluid overload are likely more immediate than those of excess glucose exposure. However, a general approach of optimizing volume status while avoiding excess glucose exposure would be ideal.

CONCLUSION

An approach to optimizing PD adequacy involves prescribing the modality with attention to clearances, maintenance of good nutrition, and achievement of normal volume status. Such an integrated strategy is more likely to be successful than was the previous paradigm, which was largely limited to small solute clearance. Such an approach may also be helpful in improving the cardiovascular risk profile of these vulnerable patients.

References

1. Teehan BP, Schleifer CR, Sigler MH, Gilgore GS: A quantitative approach to the CAPD prescription. Perit Dial Bull 1985; 5:152-156.
2. Keshaviah PR, Nolph KD, Prowant B, et al: Defining adequacy of CAPD with urea kinetics. Adv Perit Dial 1990; 6:173–177.
3. Lowrie EG, Laird NM, Parker TF, Sargent JA: Effect of the hemodialysis prescription on patient morbidity: Report from the National Cooperative Dialysis Study. N Engl J Med 1981; 305: 1176–1181.
4. Blake PG, Sombolos K, Abraham G, et al: Lack of correlation between urea kinetic indices and clinical outcomes in CAPD patients. Kidney Int 1991; 39:700–706.
5. Teehan BP, Schleifer CR, Brown JM, et al: Urea kinetic analysis and clinical outcome on CAPD. A five-year longitudinal study. Adv Perit Dial 1990; 6:181–185.
6. Lameire NH, Vanholder R, Veyt D, et al: A longitudinal five-year survey of urea kinetic parameters in CAPD patients. Kidney Int 1992; 42:426–432.
7. Canada-USA (CANUSA) Peritoneal Dialysis Study Group: Adequacy of dialysis in nutrition in continuous peritoneal dialysis: Association with clinical outcomes. J Am Soc Nephrol 1996; 7:198–207.
8. Maiorca R, Brunori G, Zubani R, et al: Predictive value of dialysis adequacy and nutritional indices for mortality and morbidity in CAPD and HD patients. A longitudinal study. Nephrol Dial Transplant 1995; 10:2295–2305.
9. National Kidney Foundation. K/DOQI Clinical practice guidelines for peritoneal dialysis adequacy. Am J Kidney Dis 2001; 37(suppl 1):S65–S136.
10. Blake PG, Bargman J, Bick J, et al: Clinical practice guidelines of the Canadian Society of Nephrology for PD Adequacy and Nutrition. J Am Soc Nephrol 1999; 10(suppl 13):S311–S321.
11. Perez RA, Blake PG, Jindal KA, et al: Canadian Organ Replacement Register: EPREX study group changes in peritoneal dialysis practices in Canada 1996-1999. Perit Dial Int 2003; 23:53–57.
12. Rocco M, Souci JM, Pastan S, McClellan WM: Peritoneal dialysis adequacy and risk of death. Kidney Int 2000; 58:446–457.
13. Paniagua R, Amato D, Vonesh E, et al: Effects of increased peritoneal clearances on mortality rates in peritoneal dialysis: ADEMEX, a prospective, randomized, controlled trial. J Am Soc Nephrol 2002; 13:1307–1320.
14. Lo WK, Ho YW, Li CS, et al: Effect of Kt/V on survival and clinical outcome in a randomized prospective study. Kidney Int 2003; 64:649–656.
15. Eknoyan G, Beck GJ, Cheung AK, et al: Hemodialysis (HEMO) Study Group. Effect of dialysis dose and membrane flux in maintenance hemodialysis. N Engl J Med 2002; 19(347):2010–2019.
16. Blake PG: Adequacy of dialysis revisited. Kidney Int 2003; 63: 1587–1599.
17. Rottembourg J: Residual renal function and recovery of renal function in patients treated by CAPD. Kidney Int 1993; 40:S106–S110.
18. Moist LM, Port FK, Orzol SM, et al: Predictors of loss of residual renal function among new dialysis patients. J Am Soc Nephrol 2000; 11:556–564.
19. Watson PE, Watson ID, Batt RD: Total body water volumes for adult males and females estimated from simple anthropometric measurements. Am J Clin Nutr 1980; 33:27–39.
20. Hume R, Weyers E: Relationship between total body water and surface area in normal and obese subjects. J Clin Pathol 1971; 24: 234–238.
21. Wong KC, Xiong XW, Kerr PG, et al: Kt/V in CAPD by different estimations of V. Kidney Int 1995; 48:563–569.
22. Mellits ED, Cheek DB: The assessment of body water and fatness from infancy to adulthood. Monogr Soc Res Child Dev, Serial 140 1970; 35:12–26.
23. du Bois D, du Bois EF: A formula to estimate the approximate surface area if height and weight be known. Arch Intern Med 1916; 17:863–971.
24. Rodby RA, Firanek CA, Cheng YG, Korbet SM: Reproducibility of studies of peritoneal dialysis adequacy. Kidney Int 1996; 50: 267–271.
25. Keshaviah PR, Nolph KD, VanStone JC: The peak concentration hypothesis: A urea kinetic approach to comparing the adequacy of CAPD and hemodialysis. Perit Dial Int 1989; 9:257–260.
26. Depner TA: Quantifying hemodialysis and peritoneal dialysis: Examination of the peak concentration hypothesis. Semin Dial 1994; 7:315–317.
27. Gotch FA: The current place of urea kinetic modelling with respect to different dialysis modalities. Nephrol Dial Transplant 1998; 13(s6):10–14.
28. Twardowski ZJ, Nolph KD, Khanna R, et al: Peritoneal equilibration test. Perit Dial Bull 1987; 7:138–147.
29. Mistry CD, Gokal R, Peers E: A randomized multicenter clinical trial comparing isosmolar icodextrin with hyperosmolar glucose solutions in CAPD. Kidney Int 1994; 46:496–503.
30. Blake PG: Creatinine is the best molecule to target adequacy of peritoneal dialysis. Perit Dial Int 2000; 20(suppl 2):S65–S69.
31. Goodship TH, Pablick-Deetjen J, Ward MK, Wilkinson R: Adequacy of dialysis and nutritional status in CAPD. Nephrol Dial Transplant 1993; 8:1366–1371.
32. Blake PG: A critique of the Canada/USA (CANUSA) Peritoneal Dialysis Study. Perit Dial Int 1996; 16:243–245.
33. Bargman JM, Thorpe KE, Churchill DN, et al: Relative contribution of residual renal function and peritoneal clearance to adequacy of dialysis: A reanalysis of the CANUSA study. J Am Soc Nephrol 2001; 12:2158–2162.
34. Diaz-Buxo JA, Lowrie EG, Lew NL, et al: Associates of mortality among peritoneal dialysis patients with special reference to peritoneal transport states and solute clearance. Am J Kidney Dis 1999; 33:523–534.
35. Harty J, Boulton H, Venning M, Gokal R: Impact of increasing dialysis volume on adequacy targets: A prospective study. J Am Soc Nephrol 1997; 8:1304–1310.
36. Mak SK, Wong PN, Lo KY, et al: Randomized prospective study of the effect of increased dialytic dose on nutritional and clinical

outcome in continuous ambulatory peritoneal dialysis patients. Am J Kidney Dis 2000; 36:105–114.
37. Churchill DN: The ADEMEX Study: Make haste slowly. J Am Soc Nephrol 2002; 13:1415–1418.
38. Tzamaloukas AH: Incremental initiation of PD: Current practice. Adv Perit Dial 1999; 15:175–178.
39. Lindsay RM, Leitch R, Heidenheim AP, et al: The London Daily/Nocturnal Hemodialysis Study? study design, morbidity and mortality results. Am J Kidney Dis 2003; 42(suppl 1):5–12.
40. Blake PG, Floyd J, Spanner E, Peters K: How much extra does "adequate" peritoneal dialysis cost? Perit Dial Int 1996; 16(suppl 1): S171–S175.
41. Blake PG, Korbet SM, Blake RM, et al: A multicenter study of non-compliance with continuous ambulatory peritoneal dialysis in U.S. and Canadian patients. Am J Kidney Dis 2000; 35:506–514.
42. Davies SJ, Philips L, Naish PF, Russell GI: Peritoneal glucose exposure and changes in membrane solute transport with time on peritoneal dialysis. J Am Soc Nephrol 2001; 12:1046–1051.
43. Holmes CJ, Shockley TR: Strategies to reduce glucose exposure in PD patients. Perit Dial Int 2000; 20(suppl 2):S37–S41.
44. Blake P, Burkart JM, Churchill DN, et al: Recommended clinical practices for maximizing peritoneal dialysis clearances. Perit Dial Int 1996; 16:448–456.
45. Page DE: CAPD with a night-exchange device is the only true CAPD. Adv Perit Dial 1998; 14:60–63.
46. Diaz-Buxo JA: Enhancement of peritoneal dialysis: The PD Plus concept. Am J Kidney Dis 1996; 27:92–98.
47. Perez RA, Blake PG, McMurray S, et al: What is the optimal frequency of cycling in automated peritoneal dialysis? Perit Dial Int 2000; 20:548–556.
48. Durand PY, Chanliau J, Kessler M: Intraperitoneal pressure/volume effects on peritoneal transport in automated peritoneal dialysis. Contrib Nephrol 1999; 129:54–61.
49. Jones MR: Etiology of severe malnutrition: Results of an international cross-sectional study in continuous ambulatory peritoneal dialysis patients. Am J Kidney Dis 1994; 23:412–420.
50. Wang AY, Woo J, Sea MM, et al: Hyperphosphatemia in Chinese peritoneal dialysis patients with and without residual renal function: What are the implications? Am J Kidney Dis 2004; 43:712–720.
51. Wang AY, Wang M, Woo J, et al: A novel association between residual renal function and left ventricular hypertrophy in peritoneal dialysis patients. Kidney Int 2002; 62:639–647.
52. Chung SH, Heimburger O, Stenwinkel P, et al: Association between residual renal function, inflammation and patient survival in new peritoneal dialysis patients. Nephrol Dial Transplant 2003; 18:590–597.
53. Li PK, Chow KM, Wong TY, et al: Effects of an angiotensin-converting enzyme inhibitor on residual renal function in patients receiving peritoneal dialysis. Ann Intern Med 2003; 139:105–112.
54. Medcalf JF, Harris KP, Walls J: Role of diuretics in the preservation of residual renal function in patients on CAPD. Kidney Int 2001; 59:1128–1133.
55. Tepel M, van der Giet M, Schwarzfeld C, et al: Prevention of radiographic-contrast-agent-induced reductions in renal function by acetylcysteine. N Engl J Med 2000; 343:180–184.
56. Blake PG, Flowerdew G, Blake RM, Oreopoulos DG: Serum albumin in patients on continuous ambulatory peritoneal dialysis: Predictors and correlations with outcomes. J Am Soc Nephrol 1993; 3:1501–1507.
57. Perez RA, Blake PG, Spanner E, et al: High creatinine excretion predicts a good outcome in peritoneal dialysis patients. Am J Kidney Dis 2000; 36:362–367.
58. Pollock CA, Ibels LS, Allen BJ, et al: Total body nitrogen as a prognostic marker in maintenance dialysis. J Am Soc Nephrol 1995; 6:82–88.
59. Lindsay RM, Spanner E: A hypothesis: The protein catabolic rate is dependent on the type and amount of treatment in dialyzed uremic patients. Am J Kidney Dis 1989; 13:382–389.
60. Harty J, Farragher B, Venning M, Gokal R: Urea kinetic modelling exaggerates the relationship between nutrition and dialysis in CAPD patients (The hazards of cross sectional analysis). Perit Dial Int 1995; 15:105–109.
61. Blake PG: The problem of mathematical coupling: How can statistical artifact and biological causation be separated when relating protein intake to clearance in predialysis and dialysis patients? Perit Dial Int 1997; 17:431–434.
62. Bergstrom J, Lindholm B: Malnutrition, cardiac diseases and mortality: An integrated point of view. Am J Kidney Dis 1998; 32: 834–841.
63. Stenvinkel P, Heimburger O, Wang T, et al: Are there two types of malnutrition in chronic renal failure? Evidence for relationships between malnutrition, inflammation and atherosclerosis (MIA syndrome). Nephrol Dial Transplant 2000; 15:953–960.
64. Noh H, Lee SW, Kang SW, et al: Serum C-reactive protein: A predictor of mortality in CAPD patients. Perit Dial Int 2000; 20:345–348.
65. Herzig KA, Purdie DM, Chang W, et al: Is C-reactive protein a useful predictor of outcome in peritoneal dialysis patients? J Am Soc Nephrol 2001; 12:814–821.
66. Fine A: Relevance of C-reactive protein levels in peritoneal dialysis patients. Kidney Int 2002; 61:615–620.
67. Stenvinkel P, Heimburger O, Paultre F, et al: Strong association between malnutrition, inflammation and atherosclerosis in chronic renal failure. Kidney Int 1999; 55:1899–1911.
68. Yeun JY, Kaysen GA: Acute phase proteins and peritoneal dialysate in albumin loss are the main determinants of serum albumin in peritoneal dialysis patients. Am J Kidney Dis 1997; 30:923–927.
69. Memoli B, Postiglione L, Ciancaruso B, et al: Role of different dialysis membranes in the release of interleukin-6-soluble receptor in uremic patients. Kidney Int 2000; 58:417–424.
70. Ridker PM, Cushman M, Stampfer MJ, et al: Inflammation, aspirin, and the risk of cardiovascular disease in apparently healthy men. N Engl J Med 1997; 336:973–979.
71. Ridker PM, Rifai N, Clearfield M, et al: Measurement of C-reactive protein for the targeting of statin therapy in the primary prevention of acute coronary events. N Engl J Med 2001; 344: 1959–1965.
72. Stenvinkel P, Andersson P, Wang T, et al: Do ACE-inhibitors suppress tumor necrosis factor-alpha production in advanced chronic renal failure? J Intern Med 1999; 246:503–507.
73. Seliger SL, Weiss NS, Gillen DL, et al: HMG-CoA reductase inhibitors are associated with reduced mortality in ESRD patients. Kidney Int 2002; 61:297–304.
74. Chang JW, Yang WS, Min WK, et al: Effects of simvastatin on high-sensitivity C-reactive protein and serum albumin in hemodialysis patients. Am J Kidney Dis 2002; 39:1213–1217.
75. Mitch WE: Malnutrition: A frequent misdiagnosis for dialysis patients. J Clin Invest 2002; 110:437–439.
76. May RC, Bailey JL, Mitch WE, et al: Glucocorticoids and acidosis stimulate protein and amino acid catabolism in vivo. Kidney Int 1996; 49:679–683.
77. Bailey JL, Wang W, England BK, et al: The acidosis of chronic renal failure activates muscle proteolysis in rats by augmenting transcription of genes encoding proteins of the ATP-dependent ubiquitin-proteasome pathway. J Clin Invest 1996; 97:1447–1453.
78. Mujais S: Acid-base profile in patients on PD. Kidney Int 2003; 63:s26–s36.
79. Stein A, Moorhouse J, Iles-Smith H, et al: Role of an improvement in acid-base status in CAPD patients. Kidney Int 1997; 52: 1089–1095.
80. Szeto CC, Wong TY, Chow KM, et al: Oral sodium bicarbonate for the treatment of metabolic acidosis in peritoneal dialysis patients: A randomized placebo-controlled study. J Am Soc Nephrol 2003; 14:2119–2126.
81. Coles GA, O'Donoghue DJ, Pritchard N, et al: A controlled trial of two bicarbonate-containing dialysis fluids for CAPD–final report. Nephrol Dial Transplant 1998; 13:3165–3171.

82. Blake PG: Growth hormone and malnutrition in dialysis patients. Perit Dial Int 1995; 15:210–216.
83. Ding H, Gao XL, Hirschberg R, et al: Impaired actions of insulin-like growth factor 1 on protein synthesis and degradation in skeletal muscle of rats with chronic renal failure. Evidence for a post receptor defect. J Clin Invest 1996; 97:1064–1075.
84. Ding H, Qing DP, Kopple JD: IGF-1 resistance in chronic renal failure: Current evidence and possible mechanisms. Kidney Int 1997; 62:s45–s47.
85. Ikizler TA, Wingard RL, Breyer JA, et al: Short-term effects of recombinant human growth hormone in CAPD patients. Kidney Int 1994; 46:1178–1183.
86. Fouque D, Peng SC, Shamir E, Kopple JD: Recombinant human insulin-like growth factor 1 induces an anabolic response in malnourished CAPD patients. Kidney Int 2000; 57:646–654.
87. Johansen KL, Mulligan K, Schambelan M: Anabolic effects of nandrolone decanoate in patients receiving dialysis: A randomized controlled trial. JAMA 1999; 281:1275–1281.
88. Blumenkrantz MJ, Gahl GM, Kopple JD, et al: Protein losses during peritoneal dialysis. Kidney Int 1981; 19:694–704.
89. Malhotra D, Tzamaloukas AH, Murata GH, et al: Serum albumin in continuous peritoneal dialysis: Its predictors in relationship to urea clearance. Kidney Int 1996; 50:243–249.
90. Blumenkrantz MJ, Kopple JD, Moran JK, et al: Nitrogen and urea metabolism during continuous ambulatory peritoneal dialysis. Kidney Int 1981; 20:78–82.
91. Bergstrom J, Furst P, Alvestrand A, Lindholm B: Protein and energy intake, nitrogen balance and nitrogen losses in patients treated with continuous ambulatory peritoneal dialysis. Kidney Int 1993; 44:1048–1057.
92. Van V, Schoonans RS, Struijk DG, et al: Influence of dialysate on gastric emptying time in peritoneal dialysate patients. Perit Dial Int 2001; 21:275–281.
93. Ross EA, Koo LC: Improved nutrition after the detection and treatment of occult gastroparesis in nondiabetic dialysis patients. Am J Kidney Dis 1998; 31:62–66.
94. Bargman JM: The rationale and ultimate limitations of urea kinetic modeling in the estimation of nutritional status. Perit Dial Int 1996; 16:347–351.
95. Bergstrom J, Heimburger O, Lindholm B: Calculation of the protein equivalent of total nitrogen appearance from urea appearance. Which formulas should be used? Perit Dial Int 1998; 18:467–473.
96. Kopple JD, Gao XL, Qing DP: Dietary protein, urea nitrogen appearance and total nitrogen appearance in chronic renal failure and CAPD patients. Kidney Int 1997; 52:486–494.
97. Mandolfo S, Zucchi A, Cavalieri D'Oro L, et al: Protein nitrogen appearance in CAPD patients: What is the best formula? Nephrol Dial Transplant 1996; 11:1592–1596.
98. Harty JC, Boulton H, Curwell J, et al: The normalized protein catabolic rate is a flawed marker of nutrition in CAPD patients. Kidney Int 1994; 44:103–109.
99. Keshaviah PR, Nolph KD, Moore HL, et al: Lean body mass estimation by creatinine kinetics. J Am Soc Nephrol 1994; 4: 1475–1485.
100. Bhatla B, Moore H, Emerson P, et al: Lean body mass estimation by creatinine kinetics, bioimpedance and dual energy x-ray absorptiometry in patients on continuous ambulatory peritoneal dialysis. ASAIO J 1995; 41:M442–M446.
101. De Fijter WM, de Fijter CW, Oe PL, et al: Assessment of total body water and lean body mass from anthropometry, Watson formula, creatinine kinetics, and body electrical impedance compared with antipyrine kinetics in peritoneal dialysis patients. Nephrol Dial Transplant 1997; 12:151–156.
102. Nielsen PK, Ladefoged J, Olgaard K: Lean body mass by dual energy x-ray absorptiometry (DEXA) and by urine and dialysate creatinine recovery in CAPD and predialysis patients compared to normal subjects. Adv Perit Dial 1994; 10:99–103.
103. Mak SK, Loo CK, Wong AM, et al: Efficacy of a 1-week course of proton-pump inhibitor based triple therapy for eradicating Heliobacter pylori in patients with and without chronic renal failure. Am J Kidney Dis 2002; 40:576–581.
104. Jones M, Hagen T, Boyle CA, et al: Treatment of malnutrition with 1.1% amino acid peritoneal dialysis solution: Result of a multicenter outpatient study. Am J Kidney Dis 1998; 32:761–769.
105. Kopple JD, Bernard D, Messana J, et al: Treatment of malnourished CAPD patients with an amino acid based dialysate. Kidney Int 1995; 47:1148–1157.
106. Li FK, Chan LYY, Woo JCY, et al: A 3-year, prospective randomized controlled study on amino acid dialysate in patients on CAPD. Am J Kidney Dis 2003; 42:173–183.
107. Fein PA, Madane SJ, Jorden A, et al: Outcome of percutaneous endoscopic gastrostomy feeding in patients on peritoneal dialysis. Adv Perit Dial 2001; 17:148–152.
108. Levey A, Beto JA, Coronado BE, et al: Controlling the epidemic of cardiovascular disease in chronic renal disease: What do we know? What do we need to learn? Where do we go from here? National Kidney Foundation Task Force on Cardiovascular Disease. Am J Kidney Dis 1998; 32:853–906.
109. Khandelwal M, Kothari J, Krishnan M, et al: Volume expansion and sodium balance in peritoneal dialysis patients. Part I: Recent concepts in pathogenesis. Adv Perit Dial 2003; 19:36–43.
110. Charra B, Bergstrom J, Scribner BH: Blood pressure control in dialysis patients: Importance of the lag phenomenon. Am J Kidney Dis 1998; 32:720–724.
111. Enia G, Mallamaci F, Benedetto F, et al: Long-term CAPD patients are volume expanded and display more severe left ventricular hypertrophy than haemodialysis patients. Nephrol Dial Transplant 2002; 16:1459–1464.
112. Konings C, Kooman J, Schonck M, et al: Fluid status, blood pressure, and cardiovascular abnormalities in patients on peritoneal dialysis. Perit Dial Int 2002; 22:477–487.
113. Mujais S, Nolph K, Gokal R, et al: Evaluation and management of ultrafiltration problems in peritoneal dialysis. International Society for Peritoneal Dialysis Ad Hoc Committee on Ultrafiltration Management in Peritoneal Dialysis. Perit Dial Int 2000; 20(suppl 4):S43–S55.
114. Ho-dac-Pannekeet MM, Atasever B, Struijk DG, Krediet RT: Analysis of ultrafiltration failure in peritoneal dialysis patients by means of standard peritoneal permeability analysis. Perit Dial Int 1997; 17:144–150.
115. Heimburger O, Waniewski J, Wreynski A, et al: Peritoneal transport in CAPD patients with permanent loss of ultrafiltration capacity. Kidney Int 1990; 38:495–506.
116. Williams JD, Craig KJ, Topley N, et al: Morphologic changes in the peritoneal membrane of patients with renal disease. J Am Soc Nephrol 2002; 13:470–479.
117. De Vriese AS, Mortier S, Lameire NH: What happens to the peritoneal membrane in long term peritoneal dialysis? Perit Dial Int 2001; 21(suppl 3):S9–S18.
118. Devuyst O: New insights in the molecular mechanisms regulating peritoneal permeability. Nephrol Dial Transplant 2002; 17:548–551.
119. De Vriese AS, Tilton RG, Stephan CC, Lameire NH: Vascular endothelial growth factor is essential for hyperglycemia-induced structural and functional alterations of the peritoneal membrane. J Am Soc Nephrol 2001; 12:1734–1741.
120. Chung SH, Heimburger O, Stenvinkel P, et al: Influence of peritoneal transport rate, inflammation, and fluid removal on nutritional status and clinical outcome in prevalent peritoneal dialysis patients. Perit Dial Int 2003; 23:174–183.
121. Heimburger O, Wang T, Lindholm B: Alterations in water and solute transport with time on peritoneal dialysis. Perit Dial Int 1999; 19(suppl 2):S83–S90.
122. Kawaguchi Y, Kawanishi H, Mujais S, et al: Encapsulating peritoneal sclerosis: Definition, etiology, diagnosis and treatment.

International Society for Peritoneal Dialysis Ad Hoc Committee on Ultrafiltration Management in Peritoneal Dialysis. Perit Dial Int 2000; 20(suppl 4):S43–S55.

123. Krediet RT, Lindholm B, Rippe B: Pathophysiology of peritoneal membrane failure. Perit Dial Int 2000; 20(suppl 4):S22–S42.

124. Fussholler A, zur Neiden S, Grabensee B, Plum J: Peritoneal fluid and solute transport: Influence of treatment time, peritoneal dialysis modality and peritonitis incidence. J Am Soc Nephrol 2002; 13:1055–1060.

125. Monquil MC, Imholz AL, Struijk DG, Krediet RT: Does impaired transcellular water transport contribute to net ultrafiltration failure during CAPD? Perit Dial Int 1995; 15:42–48.

126. Wilkie ME, Plant MJ, Edwards L, Brown CB: Icodextrin 7.5% dialysis solution (glucose polymer) in patients with ultrafiltration failure: Extension of CAPD technique survival. Perit Dial Int 1997; 17:84–87.

127. Weijnen TJ, van Hamersvelt HW, Just PM, et al: Economic impact of extended time on peritoneal dialysis as a result of using polyglucose: The application of a Markov chain model to forecast changes in the development of the ESRD programme over time. Nephrol Dial Transplant 2003; 18:390–396.

128. Chan H, Abraham G, Oreopoulos DG: Oral lecithin improves ultrafiltration in patients on peritoneal dialysis. Perit Dial Int 1989; 9:203–205.

129. Blake PG, Balaskas EV, Izatt S, Oreopoulos DG: Is total creatinine clearance a good predictor of clinical outcomes in continuous ambulatory dialysis? Perit Dial Int 1992; 12:353–358.

Chapter 29

Peritoneal Dialysis-Related Infections

Cheuk-Chun Szeto, M.D., M.R.C.P. • Philip Kam-Tao Li, M.D., F.R.C.P., F.A.C.P.

Peritoneal dialysis (PD) related infections are serious complications in PD patients.[1–3] The classification of PD-related infections is summarized in Table 29–1. Complications resulting from peritonitis and catheter infections include catheter loss,[4,5] transfer to hemodialysis, either permanent or temporary, hospitalization, and death.[6–12] Peritonitis is probably the most important cause of technique failure in PD patients.[2,3] In Hong Kong, over 16% of the deaths in patients being treated with PD are secondary to peritonitis.[13] Similarly, 18% of the infection-related mortality in PD patients are results of peritonitis in the United States.[14]

During the early phase of the development of PD, peritonitis was common. For example, Rubin and colleagues[15] reported a rate of 1 episode per 1.9 patient-months at risk. The incidence of peritonitis decreased markedly over the following decade, largely as a result of improvements in connection technology.[16–17] More recently reported peritonitis rates are lower than 1 episode per 20 patient-months at risk.[18–20] However, there has been little reduction in the peritonitis rates over the past 10 years, and PD-related infection remains a major problem in dialysis practice.

PD infections result in technique failure, hospitalization, pain, and inconvenience to the patient. Less often, the consequence is death or peritoneal fibrosis. An understanding of the pathogenesis and management of PD is essential for the health care worker caring for these patients. Prevention of infection is critical to the success of a PD program.

PERITONITIS

Pathogenesis

The common causes of PD-related peritonitis are summarized in Table 29–2. Despite the advances in PD system connectology, contamination at the time of the PD exchange remains a major cause of peritonitis.[4,21] The following exchange practices are associated with peritonitis[22, 23]:

- Touching the connection
- Dropping the tubing on the floor or table
- Not wearing a mask during the exchange
- Performing the exchange in an atmosphere filled with dust or animal hair

Holes in the catheter or tubing and accidental disconnections are obvious but uncommon causes of PD-related peritonitis.[24]

Organisms that are commonly grown from specimens in contamination-related peritonitis are coagulase-negative staphylococci (CNS) and diphtheroids (*Corynebacterium*).[20,23,25] Nasal carriers of *Staphylococcus aureus* often have *S. aureus* on their hands and at the exit sites, which can lead to peritonitis through either touch contamination during connections or catheter-related infection. Careful hand washing with a disinfectant followed by thorough drying of the hands is critical in reducing the risk of infection.[23] In addition, organisms found in the oral cavity, such as streptococci, may cause peritonitis, if a mask is not worn during an exchange or may occur via transient bacteremia (for example, after a dental procedure).

Approximately 15% to 20% of peritonitis episodes are caused by catheter infection,[4,8,12] especially those due to *S. aureus* or *Pseudomonas aeruginosa.* Exit site infections can spread to involve the catheter tunnel and then the peritoneum.[8,26,27] Such infections are often refractory or relapsing.[28] In addition, there is substantial seasonal variation in the incidence of dialysis-related peritonitis, with peak incidence in the months that are hot and humid.[29–31] A warm and humid climate favors the accumulation of sweat and dirties around catheter exit site, and therefore the growth and colonization of bacteria.

Peritonitis, particularly in patients with multiple episodes of infection, is not uncommonly caused by the release of planktonic bacteria from biofilm on the walls of catheters.[32] In fact, bacteria can form biofilm on the walls of catheters within 48 hours of their placement. These bacteria within the slime layer are resistant to both host defenses and many antibiotics[33] and may be the cause of recurrent peritonitis.[34–36] This hypothesis is supported by the observation that catheter exchange, after dialysis effluent clears up, is effective in preventing the relapse of peritonitis.[37,38] However, biofilm is present in most patients undergoing PD after the catheter is in place for a time and, in many cases, do not result in peritonitis.[39] Peritoneal immune defenses are important in preventing peritonitis related to biofilm (see later text).[40]

Gram-negative bacteria that cause PD-related peritonitis, especially in the absence of known contamination or a catheter infection, are generally considered to originate from the bowel.[25] Similar to the spontaneous bacterial peritonitis in patients with liver cirrhosis, most of the cases of gram-negative PD-related peritonitis are due to transmural movement of bacteria rather than to perforation.[41,42] Constipation,[43,44] diarrhea,[45,46] and diverticular disease may predispose to such an event. Gastric acid inhibitors may also predispose to gram-negative peritonitis.[47] Intra-abdominal disease, such as appendicitis, cholecystitis, or ischemic colitis, may also result in enteric peritonitis.[48,49]

Traditionally, polymicrobial peritonitis is believed to be caused by the perforation of internal viscus, and surgical exploration is often recommended.[50,51] The latest guideline for the management of dialysis-related peritonitis by the International Society of Peritoneal Dialysis also recommends

Table 29–1 Classification of Peritoneal Dialysis-Related Infections

Catheter linfections	Peritonitis
• Exit-site infections	• Catheter-related
• Tunnel infections	• Non–catheter-related

Table 29–2 Causes of Peritonitis

Etiology	
• Contamination	
• Catheter-related	
• Enteric	
• Bacteremia	
• Gynecologic	
Common Organisms	
Bacteria	80%–90%
• *S. epidermidis*	30%–45%
• *S. aureus*	10%–20%
• *Streptococcus* species	5%–10%
• *E. coli*	5%–10%
• Other gram-negative species	5%
• *Pseudomonas* species	5%
• Others	<5%
• Mycobacterium	<1%
Fungus	<1%~10%
Culture Negative	5%~20%

early consideration of surgical exploration for polymicrobial peritonitis.[52] However, this recommendation is based on reports early after the invention of peritoneal dialysis.[50,51,53] Recent reports show that most of the patients with dialysis-related polymicrobial peritonitis responded to antibiotic therapy.[54–57] Surgical exploration is only needed in a small selected group of patients.

Peritonitis may follow colonoscopy with polypectomy,[49,58] hysteroscopy,[59] endoscopy with sclerotherapy,[60] and dental procedures.[61] Peritonitis following dental procedures is most likely related to transient bacteremia. Vaginal leak of dialysate,[62,63] the use of intrauterine devices,[64,65] and endometrial biopsy[66] are other recognized causes of peritonitis. Because of the risk of peritonitis related to such procedures, antibiotic prophylaxis administered prior to any such procedure is necessary.

Host Defense Mechanisms of the Peritoneal Cavity

Uremia per se causes a wide spectrum of defects in the immunologic defense against infection, which is beyond the scope of this chapter. Both humoral and cellular factors participate in the local peritoneal defense processes against peritonitis.[67] Theoretically, bacteria entering the peritoneal cavity are digested by peritoneal macrophages and neutrophils. Individual variation in the phagocyte function may partly account for interindividual differences in the incidence of peritonitis.[68] Here, we will discuss only the relationship between abnormalities in peritoneal defense mechanisms and the frequency of peritonitis, as well as the effect of dialysate on peritoneal defense mechanisms.[68–70]

Humoral Immunity

Opsonization of bacteria takes place when immunoglobulin G (IgG) molecules bind to specific epitopes on bacterial surface antigens via the antigen-binding site of the IgG molecule. In addition, microbial cell surface activates the complement system, either directly via interaction with microbial polysaccharides through the alternate pathway or indirectly via interaction with IgG or IgM bound to bacteria through the classic pathway. C3b formed during C3 cleavage by either pathway is deposited on the bacterial surface and augments phagocytosis. Other activated complement compounds contribute to recruitment of neutrophils by chemotaxis. In vivo, both IgG and C3b are important opsonins. Phagocytic cells, either neutrophil or macrophage, have specific surface receptors for the Fc region of the IgG molecule as well as C3b. The opsonized microbe is ingested via receptor-mediated phagocytosis.[70] Phagocytosis is further amplified by fibronectin, which has binding sites for both macrophages and bacteria. For example, there is evidence that fibronectin augments the phagocytosis of *S. aureus.*[70]

The concentrations of IgG, complement, and fibronectin in normal peritoneal fluid are similar to those in the normal serum. In peritoneal dialysis effluent, however, these values are reduced by 100- to 1000-fold,[71,72] even after several hours of dwell time. This dilutional effect severely compromises the humoral immunity within the peritoneal cavity. In comparison, the low levels of IgG and complement in the ascitic fluid of cirrhotic patients are associated with a high incidence of spontaneous bacterial peritonitis.[73] In patients receiving CAPD, an inverse relationship between either peritoneal opsonic activity or IgG concentration and frequency of CAPD peritonitis has been reported.[40] However, this finding is not universally observed,[70] and peritoneal IgG levels failed to prospectively predict the risk for peritonitis.[74] In addition, IgG levels in spent dialysate vary markedly over time in any given patient,[74] and the opsonic activity in a given sample of spent dialysate against different strains of *Staphylococcus epidermidis* is also inconsistent.[75]

The opsonic activity of spent dialysate against gram-negative bacteria is substantially lower than that against gram-positive bacteria.[40] In fact, both IgG and C3b have different affinities for gram-negative and gram-positive organisms. This may account, at least in part, for the greater severity of the gram-negative peritonitis. Fibronectin has opsonic activity against gram-positive organisms,[70] especially *S. aureus,* but apparently not against gram-negative bacteria. Low concentrations of fibronectin in the spent dialysate has been found to be a risk factor of PD-related peritonitis.[71] Fibrinogen polymerizes to fibrin in the spent dialysate during episodes of peritonitis. In addition to the effect on bacterial biofilm, intraperitoneal administration of urokinase enhances opsonic activity of spent dialysate against *S. aureus,*[76] probably due to splitting of the fibrin strands.

Cellular Immunity

The leukocyte count in peritoneal dialysis effluent is 100- to 1000-fold less than in normal peritoneal fluid.[69] The differential leukocyte counts in uninfected spent dialysate vary greatly among patients but remain stable over time in a given individual.[77] In general, macrophages predominate in spent dialysate, lymphocyte percentages may vary between 2% and 84%, and neutrophils are usually 5% to 10%.[77] However, baseline peritoneal leukocyte count is not associated with the risk of CAPD peritonitis.[77]

Resident peritoneal macrophages, believed to originate from blood monocytes, constitute the first line of defense against bacterial invasion of the peritoneal cavity. In the early stages of peritonitis, both polymorphonuclear cells and macrophage migrate intraperitoneally from the systemic circulation as well as the interstitial matrix of the peritoneal membrane. Compared to cells from normal individuals, blood neutrophils from CAPD patients exhibit decreased binding of C5a, decreased chemotaxis, and impaired opsonic activity.[69] The oxidative metabolism of blood polymorphonuclear cells is adversely affected by low serum albumin levels.[78]

In CAPD patients, phagocytic capacity of peritoneal macrophages incubated in culture media (i.e., not dialysis effluent) is normal.[67] Bacterial killing capacity of peritoneal macrophages studied in dialysate-free media has been reported as either normal[67] or slightly decreased.[79] However, the oxidative metabolism of macrophages from noninfected spent dialysate is lower than that of macrophages from normal peritoneal fluid[69] but higher than that of peripheral blood monocytes.[79]

The oxidative metabolism of peritoneal macrophages is impaired in CAPD patients with frequent peritonitis.[72] Moreover, peritoneal macrophages, in comparison to blood monocytes, exhibit increased binding capacity of C5a (a chemotactic factor) and expression of Fc receptors, HLA-DR (Ia) antigens and CD14 antigens (which binds bacterial lipopolysaccharide). Taken together, these findings suggest that peritoneal macrophages are activated in CAPD patients.[80] Long-term CAPD may also have adverse effects on Fc-receptor-mediated phagocytosis and adhesion of polymorphonuclear cells and macrophages to endothelial cells.[81] Similar to peritoneal macrophage, T lymphocytes in peritoneal cavity, both helper and suppressor, appear to be activated in CAPD patients.[72] An increased percentage of blood and peritoneal T-suppressor cells has been associated with frequent peritonitis in isolated case reports.[82]

Mesothelial cells lining the serosal surface of the peritoneal membrane represent another important cell line in the defense against peritonitis and containment of infection within the peritoneal cavity.[83] The vital interaction between mesothelial cells and peritoneal macrophages early in the course of peritonitis occurs via cell–cell interaction, secretion of cytokines (both pro- and anti-inflammatory), prostaglandins, growth factors and fibrinolytic factors, and expression of adhesion proteins affecting leukocyte traffic.[83]

Cytokines

A panel of cytokines are synthesized by mesothelial cells, peritoneal macrophages, and lymphocytes, representing an important component of the immunologic defense against peritonitis. Activated macrophages release tumor necrosis factor alpha (TNF-α) early in the course of peritonitis,[83] whereas other cytokines, including interleukin (IL)-1b, IL-8, and IL-6 are released later.[68] Both IL-8 and IL-6 are synthesized by mesothelial cells and are stimulated by IL-1b and TNF-α. IL-8 plays a role in the recruitment of leukocytes, whereas IL-6 may modulate the inflammatory response by inhibiting the transcription of other cytokines.[83,84]

Lymphocytes activated by IL-1b and TNF-α release IL-2 and interferon-gamma (IFN-γ). The latter enhances macrophage bactericidal activity, whereas IL-1b stimulates prostaglandin E2 (PGE2) release from macrophages and mesothelial cells. PGE2 has a negative feedback effect on IL-1b production. In addition, IL-6, IL-8, and PGE2 modulate the synthesis of IL-1a and IL-1b.

Effects of PD Solutions on Peritoneal Defense

The effects of CAPD solutions on peritoneal defense mechanisms are related to the dilution, high osmolality, low pH, lactate, and heat sterilization of the dialysate. In addition to the dilutional effects on humoral defense mechanisms, decreased density of peritoneal macrophages reduces the phagocyte-bacterium encounter and thus bacterial killing.[69] Both sustained high dialysate osmolality and low dialysate pH suppress peritoneal neutrophil and macrophage functions.[85] Although dialysate pH rises rapidly after intraperitoneal infusion and reaches blood pH by 30 minutes, the dialysate infusion period carries a high risk of bacterial entry at the same time that peritoneal defenses are compromised by low dialysate pH.

Lactate in commercial dialysate preparations appears to have independent adverse effects on peritoneal inflammatory cell function, specifically affecting macrophages, polymorphonuclear cells, mesothelial cells, and fibroblasts.[86] The development of peritoneal dialysis solutions containing non-lactate buffers may augment peritoneal defense mechanisms. The cytotoxicity of bicarbonate-based dialysate appears to be less than that of lactate-based dialysate. However, polymorphonuclear cell function studied in vitro after incubation in bicarbonate-based dialysate remains deficient.[87] Pyruvate-based dialysate has fewer adverse effects on macrophage and polymorphonuclear cell function than does lactate-based dialysate.[88] Finally, heat sterilization of the dialysate causes a decrease in the adhesion of leukocytes to endothelial cells.[89]

Presentation

Patients with peritonitis usually present with cloudy dialysis effluent and abdominal pain.[15,90–92] The severity of illness varies widely, depending on the etiologic microorganism.[12,93] For example, *S. epidermidis* or diphtheroids often cause minimal abdominal pain. On the other hand, virulent organisms, such as *S. aureus, P. aeruginosa,* and fungi, often cause severe abdominal pain and, not uncommonly, diarrhea. In general, fever indicates systemic sepsis. Hypotension indicates severe peritonitis.[93,94]

Diagnosis

Although most practicing nephrologists can diagnose PD-related peritonitis on clinical ground, the diagnosis needs to be confirmed by an effluent white blood cell (WBC) count, which should exceed 100 cells/μL (i.e., 0.1×10^9 cells/L), with more than 50% neutrophil. In the absence of peritonitis, the effluent WBC count is less than 25 cells/μL with primarily mononuclear cells.[95–100] If the patient is already taking antibiotics, a WBC count of 50 cells/μL or greater is suggestive of peritonitis. If the specimen is obtained after a short dwell time or in the absence of a dwell, the percentage of neutrophil (>50%) is a more sensitive marker than total WBC count.[98,99]

Occasionally, patients with peritonitis present with abdominal pain without cloudy effluent.[95,100] Koopmans and colleagues[100] reported that in 6% of peritonitis episodes, the effluent WBC count is initially less than 100 cells/μL. The effluent becomes cloudy in most cases within a few hours. It is possible that patients who present with pain and the absence of cloudy effluent has delayed intraperitoneal cytokine response to the infection, signifying an underlying immunologic abnormality.[100] In the future, the application of diagnostic strip may enhance early diagnosis of peritonitis prior to the onset of cloudy effluent.[101]

The differential diagnosis for infectious peritonitis includes eosinophilic peritonitis, chemical peritonitis, pancreatitis, chylous ascites, intra-abdominal malignancy, and hemoperitoneum. In eosinophilic peritonitis, a large number of eosinophil is present in the effluent. It usually occurs early in the course of PD, resolves spontaneously, and is usually not associated with infection.[102–106] The mechanism is generally believed to be allergic reaction to the plasticizers on the dialysis tubing, and the eosinophilia generally resolves spontaneously within 2 to 6 weeks.

Intraperitoneal administration of generic vancomycin[107,108] and amphotericin[109] can cause chemical peritonitis, which mimics bacterial infection. Recently, cases of sterile chemical peritonitis have been attributed to icodextrin.[110] The episodes are characterized by mild abdominal discomfort, cloudy effluent only with icodextrin dialysates, dialysate leukocytosis with a predominance of macrophages and sterile cultures, and the absence of systemic symptoms.

A patient receiving PD who has pancreatitis may present with abdominal pain and cloudy peritoneal fluid, but cultures of the fluid are sterile and the effluent amylase concentration should be greater than 100 μ/L.[111–114] Chylous ascites is a rare cause of sterile cloudy effluent, and the effluent WBC count is normal.[115,116] Patients with intra-abdominal malignancy may also have cloudy effluent, and the diagnosis can be established by cytologic evaluation.[117,118]

Treatment of Peritonitis

Initial Evaluation

In patient presenting with possible peritonitis, evaluation should include close questioning about a history of possible touch contamination, compliance in sterile dialysis technique, recent procedures that may have led to peritonitis, and change in bowel habits, either diarrhea or constipation. The physician should review any history of peritonitis to assess for the possibility of recurrent peritonitis with the same organism or previous infection with a methicillin-resistant organism. In addition to the usual physical examination, one must carefully assess the exit site and tunnel for edema, erythema, tenderness, and discharge. The effluent should be examined, and specimens should be collected for cell count, differential count, Gram stain, and culture. The Gram stain result, if positive, is helpful in guiding the choice of antibiotic therapy.[119] Rapid institution of treatment once the appropriate assessment is completed is essential.

Despite a careful history, physical examination, and Gram stain of the effluent, frequent empirical treatment of peritonitis has to be initiated in the absence of appropriate diagnostic information. An arbitrary decision regarding antibiotic therapy must be made after considering the likely causative organisms.[52,120,121] As discussed earlier, the application of diagnostic strip may enhance early diagnosis of peritonitis prior to the onset of cloudy effluent.[101]

Evolving Trend of Empirical Therapy

There is a growing consensus for a standardized approach, which combines the continuation of peritoneal dialysis with intraperitoneal administration of antibiotics. Such an approach has been further emphasized in the 2000 update of the Advisory Committee on Peritoneal Dialysis (a subcommittee of the ISPD).[122]

In their 1993 recommendations, the Ad Hoc Committee advocated (1) the use of vancomycin to treat gram-positive infections; (2) the use of ceftazidime or aminoglycoside to cover the gram-negative organisms as first-line agents; and (3) empirical therapy, if an organism has not been identified on Gram stain at presentation.[120] Since the publication of that report, however, increasing numbers of vancomycin-resistant microorganisms have emerged, a trend that has been particularly evident in larger hospitals. Vancomycin resistance has been associated with resistance to other penicillins and aminoglycosides, thus presenting a treatment dilemma. Many of the second-line antimicrobial agents that could be used have not been proven to be effective in therapeutic trials.

With increasing numbers of vancomycin-resistant microorganisms, the use of vancomycin is discouraged for prophylaxis, for routine use, and for use in oral form against *Clostridium difficile* enterocolitis.[123–125] The major concern is that the vancomycin resistance will be transmitted to staphylococcal strains, creating a situation of major epidemiologic importance. In fact, a case of vancomycin-resistant, CNS peritonitis in a patient being treated with CAPD has been reported.[126] This situation has prompted the Ad Hoc Committee to move away from the use of vancomycin as a first-line therapy, and in 1996 the ISPD subcommittee on peritonitis has reverted to recommending use of first-generation cephalosporins in large doses for all cases.[127] Recent study shows that there is no significant difference in clinical response or relapse rate between vancomycin and cefazolin as the initial antibiotic for gram-positive peritonitis.[128] Furthermore, empirical treatment with intraperitoneal cefazolin was as effective as vancomycin for *S. epidermidis* peritonitis, despite a high prevalence of methicillin resistance.[129]

On the other hand, many authorities continue to advocate vancomycin as the first-line therapy in spite of the concern on VRE. For example, Sandoe and colleagues[130] found that at least 50% of cases of peritonitis due to CNS would not be adequately treated with a cephalosporin. The reasons given for continuing to use vancomycin were the low prevalence of VRE and a high prevalence for CNS methicillin resistance. In short, each program should assess the local patterns of sensitivity and methicillin resistance before a decision is made whether to use vancomycin or cephalosporin for initial therapy of peritonitis. If, however, the patient has a history of frequent methicillin-resistant staphylococcal infections or seems seriously ill, vancomycin, along with a second drug for gram-negative coverage, is still a good choice. In addition, for the patient who is allergic to penicillin and cephalosporins, vancomycin remains a good alternative.

In their 1996 recommendations, the Ad Hoc Committee Recommendations involved the use of a combination of a first-generation cephalosporin and an aminoglycoside.[127] However, there is some evidence suggesting a more rapid loss of residual renal function in patients receiving aminoglycosides.[131] Since residual renal function is an independent predictor of patient survival,[132] there has been a growing concern to avoid routine use of aminoglycoside so as to preserve residual renal function. As a result, in their 2000 recommendations, the Ad Hoc Committee recommended ceftazidime, instead of an aminoglycoside, as empirical therapy for coverage of gram-negative organisms in patients with significant residual renal function,[122] which was arbitrarily defined as a daily urine output of 100 mL or more. Although empirical monotherapy of broad-spectrum antibiotic is an attractive alternative, and certain success has been reported from the use of cefepime[133] and imipenem-cilastatin,[134] the evidence is preliminary, and empirical combination antibiotics remain the standard of practice.

Figure 29–1 is an algorithm for the assessment and antibiotic therapy of peritonitis. Table 29–3 lists the agents and dosages. As shown, empirical treatment depends on the patient's residual urine output. This approach prevents unnecessary use of vancomycin and lessens the risk of the development of vancomycin-resistant organisms, and also avoids unnecessary exposure to aminoglycosides, which may adversely affect the residual renal function. The rationale for using the recommended large dose of a first-generation cephalosporin is that the organisms are, in fact, "sensitive" to the drug because of the high local level achieved at the site of the infection (i.e., within the peritoneal cavity).

Table 29–3 Empirical Initial Therapy for Peritoneal Dialysis-Related Peritonitis, Stratified for Residual Urine Volume

	Residual Urine Output	
Antibiotic	<100 mL/day	>100 mL/day
Cefazolin or cephalothin	1 g/bag daily or 15 mg/kg BW/bag daily	20 mg/kg BW/bag daily
Ceftazidime	1 g/bag daily	20 mg/kg BW/bag daily
Gentamicin, tobramycin, netilmicin	0.6 mg/kg BW/bag daily	Not recommended

BW, body weight. (Modified from Keane WF, Bailie GR, Boeschoten E, et al: Adult peritoneal dialysis-related peritonitis treatment recommendations: 2000 update. Perit Dial Int 2000; 20:396-411.)

Once-Daily Antibiotic Therapy

Another major change in the Ad Hoc Committee Recommendations in 2000 is the routine application of once-daily intraperitoneal antibiotics.[52] Once-daily therapy has the advantage of ease of use by patient and staff, both in hospital and at home. More importantly, there are theoretical advantages to administering aminoglycosides as a single dose in a long-dwell exchange.[135] Aminoglycosides given as a single daily dose may result in less ototoxicity and nephrotoxicity[135–139] and improved bacterial killing in association with prolonged post-antibiotic effect. In a pharmacokinetic study by Low and colleagues,[140] intraperitoneal (IP) gentamicin 0.6 mg/kg was given in one exchange with a 6-hour dwell. Intraperitoneal drug levels were high throughout the dwell but negligible thereafter. Serum levels remained low.

Lai and colleagues[135] studied the efficacy of once-daily IP cefazolin and gentamicin for treatment of peritonitis. Of the 14 episodes of gram-negative peritonitis in the series, 6 were due to *Pseudomonas* and required alteration in therapy. In spite of the change in therapy, catheter removal was eventually needed in 3 of the cases. One third of the non–*Pseudomonas* gram-negative infections required alteration of therapy. Bailie

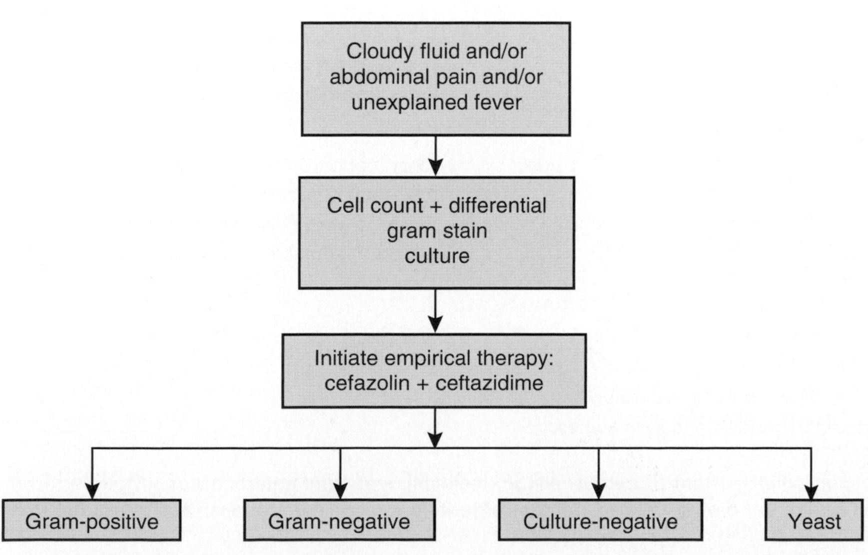

Figure 29–1 Algorithm of the initial assessment and therapy for peritoneal dialysis infections.

and colleagues[141] used once daily gentamicin (in combination with an initial dose of vancomycin) and reported resolution of two-thirds of the non–*Pseudomonas* gram-negative peritonitis episodes in their patients. The "nonresponder" organisms include *Acinetobacter* and *Alcaligenes* species. These results show that gentamicin given in one exchange per day provides adequate coverage for gram-negative organisms for most of the peritonitis episodes.

Although the Ad Hoc Committee recommends the use of once-daily intraperitoneal cefazolin and ceftazidime, there is, at best, incomplete evidence for this practice. In the study of once-daily IP cefazolin and gentamicin by Lai and colleagues,[135] all 19 episodes of gram-positive peritonitis resolved, with only one infection due to *S. aureus* requiring modification of the initial therapy. The organisms in 3 episodes of *S. epidermidis* in this study were shown by sensitivity testing to be resistant to both gentamicin and cefazolin yet responded to therapy with these agents. In another study reported by Goldberg and colleagues[142] once-daily IP cefazolin for the initial treatment of PD-related peritonitis was at least as effective as the historical control of a vancomycin-based regimen. However, it is important to note that episodes of peritonitis with associated catheter infection were excluded from both of the studies, accounting, in part, for the excellent results.

Therapy for Specific Organisms

Gram-positive Microorganisms

The therapy for gram-positive peritonitis is outlined in Table 29–4. Peritonitis episodes due to CNS, *S. aureus*, and *Streptococcus* are distinctly different in presentation, pathogenesis, and outcome. Therapy must therefore be individualized.

Coagulase-Negative Staphylococci For CNS, the first-generation cephalosporins are usually sufficient. If, however, the organism is methicillin-resistant *S. epidermidis* (MRSE), vancomycin or clindamycin should be used. Cefazolin tends to be less effective than vancomycin for the treatment of MRSE peritonitis. In a study by Vas and colleagues[143] there was no difference in cure rates for the two agents in treatment of CNS that were methicillin-sensitive (92% for vancomycin vs. 100% for cefazolin). For MRSE, however, the cure rate was 73% for vancomycin and only 45% for cefazolin.

Inadequate treatment of CNS peritonitis, for example, with once-weekly vancomycin in a patient with residual renal function, is not an infrequent cause of relapsing infection.[144] CNS exit site infection does not usually lead to peritonitis, and exit site infection is rarely a concern in the pathogenesis of CNS peritonitis.[8,28] However, CNS may exist within a biofilm of bacterial exopolysaccharides encasing the intra-abdominal portion of the catheter, frequently in conjunction with a healthy appearing exit site or tunnel.[145]

Recurrent peritonitis must be treated aggressively. To prevent further relapse of peritonitis, the catheter may be replaced as a single procedure after the dialysis effluent clears up with antibiotics.[146–148] Alternatively, the use of fibrinolytic agents, such as urokinase (5000 units in 5 mL normal saline injected into the catheter with the abdomen drained and allowed to dwell for 2 hours), is successful in approximately 50% of the patients with recurrent CNS peritonitis.[149–152] In a randomized study, Williams and colleagues[150] found that catheter replacement was superior to urokinase in preventing further relapse. Thrombolytic therapy should be reserved for infections for which no other cause or complication is evident (e.g., tunnel infection) and probably should be limited to CNS or culture-negative infection.

Staphylococcus aureus *S. aureus* is the major cause of exit site and tunnel infections and is also an important cause of peritonitis.[153] Patients with *S. aureus* peritonitis often have severe abdominal pain, require hospitalization, and may require catheter removal for resolution, especially when a concomitant tunnel infection is present.[28,93] *S. aureus* peritonitis occurs predominantly in patients who have a history of *S. aureus* catheter infections. Patients who have *S. aureus* colonization in the nares,[154–156] on the skin,[157] or at the peritoneal catheter exit site[157–159] are at particular risk of developing *S. aureus*

Table 29–4 Treatment Strategies After Identification of Gram-Positive Organism on Culture

Enterococcus	*Staphylococcus aureus*	Other Gram-Positive Organism (Coagulase-Negative Staphylococcus)
At 24 to 48 Hours		
• Stop cephalosporins • Start ampicillin 125 mg/L/bag • Consider adding aminoglycoside • If ampicillin-resistant, start vancomycin or clindamycin	• Stop ceftazidime or aminoglycoside, continue cefazolin • Add rifampin 600 mg/day, oral • If MRSA, start vancomycin or clindamycin	• Stop ceftazidime or aminoglycoside, continue cefazolin • If MRSE and clinically not responding, start vancomycin or clindamycin
Duration of Therapy		
• 14 days	• 21 days	• 14 days
At 96 Hours		
• If no improvement, reculture and evaluation for exit-site or tunnel infection, catheter colonization, etc. • Choice of final therapy should always be guided by antibiotic sensitivities.		

VRE, vancomycin-resistant enterococcus; *MRSA*, methicillin-resistant *S. aureus; MRSE*, methicillin-resistant enterococcus. (Modified from Keane WF, Bailie GR, Boeschoten E, et al: Adult peritoneal dialysis-related peritonitis treatment recommendations: 2000 update. Perit Dial Int 2000; 20:396-411.)

peritonitis. Even one positive nose culture increases the risk of *S. aureus* peritonitis.[154,160]

After empirical therapy and once the organism is identified as *S. aureus*, its sensitivity to methicillin will dictate further choice of antibiotics. If the organism is sensitive to methicillin, cefazolin should be continued. We prefer adding rifampin (600 mg/day) orally to the IP cephalosporin in all cases of *S. aureus* peritonitis. Vancomycin and cefazolin have similar efficacy in the treatment of methicillin-sensitive *S. aureus* peritonitis. For example, Vas and colleagues[142] reported that 58% of cases of *S. aureus* peritonitis resolved with vancomycin treatment and 67% with cefazolin. The cure rate for *S. aureus* peritonitis is relatively low because concomitant catheter infections are common. As a result, removal of the catheter should be considered early, if a concomitant exit site or tunnel infection is present.

If methicillin-resistant *S. aureus* (MRSA) is isolated from dialysis effluent, rifampin should be added, and the cephalosporins should be replaced by vancomycin. The vancomycin (up to 2 g IP, depending on body weight) may be repeated every 5 to 7 days. To avoid inadequate treatment, therapeutic drug monitoring and more frequent vancomycin dosage may be needed in selected cases with substantial residual renal function. Unfortunately, MRSA peritonitis is always difficult to treat and frequently requires catheter removal.[161,162]

Streptococci A respiratory, cutaneous, digestive, or urinary tract infection precedes Streptococcal peritonitis episode in 25% of patients.[163] It is our experience that most cases of peritonitis caused by *Streptococci* have satisfactory response to 2-week course of IP cefazolin. Alternatively, 90% of cases respond to ampicillin, which appear to be more effective than vancomycin.[163] In some cases, Streptococcal species cause a severe form of peritonitis,[163–167] and shock followed by death may occur within a short time.[165]

Enterococci In contrast to *Streptococcus viridans*, the occurrence of enterococcus peritonitis has not been decreased with the use of disconnect systems, probably because enterococcal infection is related more to a bowel source than to contamination or bacteremia.[163] As a rule, enterococcal infection does not respond to cephalosporins. Peritonitis due to enterococcus is severe and has a slower response to antibiotics,[163] partly as a result of the current Ad Hoc Committee Recommendation of cephalosporins as initial therapy. Although still fairly uncommon in patients undergoing PD, VRE peritonitis has been reported by Troidle and colleagues[168] VRE peritonitis is associated with previous hospitalization and antibiotic use (particularly cephalosporins and vancomycin) and has a high mortality rate even with catheter removal.

Gram-Negative Microorganisms

Peritonitis due to gram-negative organisms is often associated with fever, nausea, vomiting, and abdominal pain. The care of gram-negative peritonitis is summarized in Table 29–5. Good results have been reported with either IP aminoglycoside or ceftazidime.[169] Alternatively, quinolones, which have the advantage of convenient oral administration, can be used with acceptable results.[170]

Pseudomonas and Stenotrophomonas Recent antibiotic therapy is the major risk factor of Pseudomonas peritonitis.[171] Patients with immunosuppression are also at higher risk for Pseudomonas peritonitis.[172,173] If the effluent culture reveals a *Pseudomonas* infection, especially one due to *P. aeruginosa*, the ceftazidime should be continued, and a second antipseudomonal agent should be added to the regimen. In general, IP gentamicin or oral ciprofloxacin are reasonable choices. One needs to look carefully for evidence of catheter infection. Exit site infection and recent antibiotic therapy are associated with poor therapeutic response to antibiotics.[171] When therapeutic response is suboptimal, early catheter removal may help preserve the peritoneum for further peritoneal dialysis. Elective catheter exchange after clear up of PDE may also reduce subsequent relapse.[171]

Stenotrophomonas maltophilia (formerly *Pseudomonas* or *Xanthomonas maltophilia*), a common environmental organism, is the cause of 1.5% of all peritonitis episodes.[174] Recent bacterial peritonitis with broad-spectrum antibiotics therapy was the major risk factor. The outcome was poor with medical treatment alone. Treatment should consist of two antibiotics, such as ceftazidime and cotrimoxazole. However, fungal peritonitis was a common consequence, probably related to the prolonged course of antibiotics.[174] Most, if not

Table 29–5 Treatment Recommendations If a Gram-Negative Organism Is Identified on Culture at 24 to 48 Hours

Single Gram-Negative Organism	*Pseudomonas/Stenotrophomonas*	Multiple Gram-Negative and/or Anderobes
At 24 to 48 Hours		
• Stop cefazolin • Continue ceftazidime or aminoglycoside • Adjust antibiotics according to sensitivity	• Stop cefazolin, continue ceftazidime • If urine <100 mL/day, add aminoglycoside • If urine >100 mL/day, add ciprofloxacin 500 mg p.o. b.i.d. or piperacillin 4 gm IV q12 hours or sulfamethoxazole/trimethoprim 1–2 DS/day or aztreonam load 1 g/L; maintenance dose 250 mg/L IP/bag	• Continue cefazolin and ceftazidime • Add metronidazole 500 mg q8 hours p.o., IV, or rectally • If no change in clinical status, consider surgical intervention
Duration of Therapy		
• 14 days	• 21 days	• 14 days

IV, intravenously; *DS*, double strength; *IP*, intraperitoneally. (Modified from Keane WF, Bailie GR, Boeschoten E, et al: Adult peritoneal dialysis-related peritonitis treatment recommendations: 2000 update. Perit Dial Int 2000; 20:396-411.)

all, patients eventually required removal of catheter, either because the effluent failed to clear up or because of secondary peritonitis.

Acinetobacter *Acinetobacter* is a ubiquitous bacterial species that causes peritonitis when peritoneal host defenses are suppressed from previous peritonitis episodes.[175] As a result, peritonitis due to *Acinetobacter* frequently occurs within a few months of a previous episode of peritonitis due to another organism and is infrequently associated with catheter infection.[175,176] Treatment with ampicillin-sulbactam or imipenem-cilastatin may have a better response rate than the conventional regimen.[175,176] However, relapse peritonitis is common, and change of therapy from PD to hemodialysis is needed in 17% of the cases.[176]

Enteric and Polymicrobial Peritonitis Polymicrobial peritonitis is a serious complication in peritoneal dialysis patients and is present in 6% to 11% of all peritonitis episodes.[54–57] Traditionally, perforation of internal viscus and underlying gastrointestinal pathology are believed to be the cause, but many cases may be due to touch contamination or catheter infection. Response to antibiotics is excellent when only gram-positive organisms are isolated from dialysis fluid, which accounts for approximately one third of the polymicrobial peritonitis episodes.[57] The presence of fungus, anaerobes, and *Pseudomonas* species in dialysis fluid are independent predictors of poor response to antibiotic therapy. Pooled analysis of four case series[54–57] shows that less than 6% of the polymicrobial peritonitis have a surgical cause. Although it is possible that some of the cases with underlying surgical pathology responded to conservative management and were not identified, the finding suggests that surgical pathology that needs aggressive surgical intervention is uncommon. A careful examination of the organisms isolated may help identify patients who need catheter removal or surgical intervention.

Intra-abdominal abscess is an uncommon complication of PD-related peritonitis, occurring in 0.7% of all peritonitis episodes. Abscess is more common following *P. aeruginosa*, *Candida albicans*, and polymicrobial peritonitis.[177,178] Persistent fever, abdominal tenderness, and peripheral leukocytosis despite antibiotic therapy and catheter removal are all consistent with this diagnosis, which can then be confirmed by CT scan or ultrasonography. The abscesses require drainage.

Fungal Organisms

Fungal peritonitis occurs in patients undergoing PD at the rate of 0.01 to 0.19 episodes per dialysis-year, accounting for 3% to 6% of episodes.[7,179–182] Over 70% of the episodes of fungal peritonitis are caused by *Candida* species.[182, 183] Recent antibiotic therapy, frequent episodes of bacterial peritonitis, and immunosuppression are the major risk factors of fungal peritonitis.[180,184] Patients are often severely ill with marked abdominal tenderness.[183,185,186]

The management approach of fungal peritonitis is outlined in Box 29–1. It is imperative to remove the catheter, if there is no improvement after 4 to 5 days of adequate therapy. The outcome is generally poor, with only 37% patients managed to continue PD.[183] Conversion to long-term hemodialysis is needed in 14% of patients, and mortality is 44%. Many clinicians still believe that catheter removal is indicated immediately after identification of a fungal infection by Gram stain or culture.[184,187] In an uncontrolled trial, Goldie and colleagues[180] found that mortality at 1 month was 15% in patients in whom the catheter was removed within a week of diagnosis but 50% in those in whom the catheter was left in place.

Mycobacterium Peritonitis

Tuberculous peritonitis is rarely seen in peritoneal dialysis patients in the Western world, but is more common in Asian countries. Contrary to the common belief, the WBCs in the effluent are predominantly polymorphonuclear cells, and an acid-fast bacilli stain of an effluent specimen is generally negative.[188] Abnormal chest radiograph findings and ascitic fluid lymphocytosis could only identify 33% and 37% of the cases, respectively.[189] Conventional microbiologic diagnostic methods are slow and may not be sensitive enough for establishing a diagnosis in a timely manner. Standard antituberculous chemotherapy is highly effective,[188,189] although ultrafiltration failure may occur, if PD is continued.[190] Advanced age and delayed initiation of therapy are associated with higher mortality rates.[189]

Culture-negative Peritonitis

In approximately 14% to 20% of episodes that meet the criteria for peritonitis on the basis of cell count, culture of the effluent results in no growth of organisms. Most of the culture-negative peritonitis could be explained by recent antibiotic therapy or technical problems during dialysate culture.[191] Placing 5 mL of the effluent into trypticase soy broth-blood culture bottles (aerobic and anaerobic) decreases the rate of negative culture results to 25% compared with a 50-mL centrifugation culture technique, for which the rate is 42%. On the other hand, approximately 75% of patients presenting with peritonitis, when tested for the presence of antibiotics (some taken surreptitiously), have sterile cultures. In cases of no growth, repeated culture of the effluent results in identification of an organism in about one-third of episodes.

The management approach of patients with culture-negative peritonitis is summarized in Table 29–6. Most authorities suggest that if a patient is clinically improving after 4 to 5 days of therapy, and there is no suggestion of gram-negative organisms from Gram stain of the effluent, only cefazolin should be continued. Recent peritonitis and antibiotic therapy are associated

Box 29–1 Treatment Recommendations If Yeast or Other Fungus Is Identified on Gram Stain or Culture

At 24 to 48 Hours
- Flucytosine, loading dose 2 g p.o.; maintenance 1 g p.o.; and
- Fluconazole 200 mg p.o. or intraperitoneally, daily

At 4 to 7 Days
- If clinical improvement, duration of therapy 4 to 6 weeks
- If no clinical improvement, remove catheter and continue therapy for 7 days

(Modified from Keane WF, Bailie GR, Boeschoten E, et al: Adult peritoneal dialysis-related peritonitis treatment recommendations: 2000 update. Perit Dial Int 2000; 20:396-411.)

Table 29-6 Treatment Strategies If Peritoneal Dialysis Fluid Cultures Are Negative at 24 to 48 Hours or Not Performed

If Clinical Improvement	If No Clinical Improvement
• Discontinue ceftazidime or aminoglycoside • Continue cefazolin	• Repeat cell count, Gram stain and culture • If culture positive, adjust therapy accordingly • If culture negative, continue antibiotics, consider infrequent pathogens and/or catheter removal
Duration of Therapy	
• 14 days	• 14 days

(Modified from Keane WF, Bailie GR, Boeschoten E, et al: Adult peritoneal dialysis-related peritonitis treatment recommendations: 2000 update. Perit Dial Int 2000; 20:396-411.)

with poor treatment response.[191] Early catheter removal is recommended in this group of patients.

Reassessment After 48 Hours of Therapy

Most patients with PD-related peritonitis show considerable clinical improvement within 2 days of starting antibiotics. Occasionally, symptoms persist beyond 48 to 96 hours. At 96 hours, if a patient has not shown definitive clinical improvement, a reevaluation is essential. Dialysis effluent cell counts, Gram stain, and cultures should be repeated. Antibiotic removal techniques may be used in an attempt to maximize culture yield. Catheter removal should be considered if the response to antibiotic therapy is poor after 96 hours.

One should be aware of the presence of unusual organisms, such as mycobacteria, fungi, or fastidious organisms, which require specific cultures and the potential of surgical disorders. If *S. aureus* and *P. aeruginosa* peritonitis are related to catheter or tunnel infection, catheter removal should be considered.

Special Considerations

Refractory and Relapsing Peritonitis

Refractory peritonitis is generally defined as episodes in which the effluent remains cloudy after 5 days, despite appropriate antibiotic therapy. Recurrent or *relapsing* peritonitis, defined as a second episode of peritonitis with the same organism within 2 to 4 weeks of the end of antibiotic therapy[21] may also be due to catheter biofilm without clinically obvious involvement of the catheter tunnel. Catheter removal should be considered in most cases of refractory peritonitis. Catheter exchange after dialysis effluent clears up is also effective in preventing the relapse of peritonitis.[37,38]

Peritonitis in Patients Undergoing Automated Peritoneal Dialysis (APD)

As in CAPD peritonitis, the majority of APD peritonitis episodes are caused by gram-positive bacteria. In a randomized study comparing continuous cyclic PD (CCPD) with CAPD using a Y-connector, peritonitis rates were lower with the former (0.51 and 0.94 per dialysis year at risk, respectively).[192] Holley and colleagues,[193] using case controls, also found peritonitis rates to be lower in patients undergoing CCPD than in patients undergoing CAPD using Y-connectors (0.3 vs. 0.5 per dialysis year at risk, respectively). Rates may be lower with CCPD because of longer dwell times, which result in improved peritoneal macrophage functioning and opsonic activity, thereby leading to better host defense.[194] Leaving the peritoneal cavity free of fluid during the day time (dry days), as in nocturnal intermittent PD, offers no further improvement in peritoneal macrophage functioning.[195]

The choice of first-line antibiotics in CAPD also applies to APD. In many centers, during peritonitis, APD patients are changed to a CAPD schedule because it is then easier to evaluate the clinical course using standardized procedures for obtaining dialysate for cell count and culture and sensitivity. Furthermore, the recommendations for antibiotic treatment are based mainly on data obtained using CAPD and limited experience in APD.[196] If patients stay on APD, antibiotics can be given continuously or intermittently. Because the bactericidal action of aminoglycosides is dose-dependent, once-daily administration of aminoglycosides is recommended. Vancomycin can be given intermittently because of its unique pharmacokinetic properties. With all other antibiotics, the dose in APD can only be extrapolated from pharmacokinetic studies in CAPD, because no such studies are available in APD patients.

There is a limited report on the clinical outcome of peritonitis in APD patients.[197] Attention should be given to an adequate dwell time of at least 4 hours to allow absorption of antibiotic agents. An interesting option for treatment of peritonitis in APD patients is oral administration of antibiotics. However, pharmacokinetic studies are lacking and this route of administration can therefore be recommended in uncomplicated episodes only due to coagulase-negative *staphylococci.* As with CAPD, adjustments for APD prescription may be needed in patients who experience altered ultrafiltration during episodes of peritonitis.

Peritoneal Lavage

As discussed previously, fresh dialysis solutions have detrimental effect on the local peritoneal defense mechanisms.[198] Rapid-exchange peritoneal lavage is therefore not advisable in the management of peritoneal infection. After two to three in-and-out exchanges that remove inflammatory products and lessen abdominal pain, CAPD should be resumed with usual long-dwell exchanges. Ejlersen and colleagues[199] reported poor outcome in patients treated with 24 hours of initial lavage. Peritoneal lavage, however, is still indicated prior to surgical exploration in cases of fecal peritonitis.

Nevertheless, ultrafiltration problem is common during acute peritonitis because peritoneal permeability is increased during an episode of peritonitis.[200] The dwell time may therefore have to be shortened or the dialysate dextrose level increased. The use of dialysate containing icodextrin in this situation has been shown to improve ultrafiltration.[201]

Catheter Removal

Infections are the cause of catheter removal in approximately 85% of cases.[4] *S. aureus* and *Pseudomonas* species are the common organisms responsible for the greatest catheter loss.[153,171]

It is usually suggested that after an episode of severe peritonitis that requires catheter removal, peritoneal dialysis can be resumed after a minimum of 3 weeks. In a series of 100 CAPD patients with catheter removed for severe peritonitis, catheter was successfully reinserted, and peritoneal dialysis was resumed in 51 cases, and 45 of them required additional dialysis exchanges or hypertonic dialysate to compensate for the loss of solute clearance or ultrafiltration, although there was no significant change in dialysis adequacy or nutritional status.[202] Eleven patients were changed to long-term hemodialysis within 8 months after their return to CAPD. An early assessment of peritoneal function after catheter reinsertion is therefore advisable.[202]

On the other hand, if a catheter is removed for catheter infection or relapsing or recurrent peritonitis with clear effluent, it can be placed simultaneously.[146–148,203] It is critical that the effluent WBC count be less than 200 cells/L before one can proceed with simultaneous removal and replacement of a catheter.[146,204–206] Data suggest that this is feasible procedure that decreases costs and minimizes the use of temporary hemodialysis. If the peritonitis can be transiently cleared, in a patient with relapsing *Pseudomonas* peritonitis, simultaneous removal and replacement of the catheter may be feasible.[171,205] Simultaneous removal and reinsertion of catheters is also a safe and effective method for the treatment of refractory exit site infection.[207] However, this approach is less successful for fungal, which generally requires some time off PD.

Complications

Peritonitis results in a marked increase in effluent protein losses, which may contribute to the protein malnutrition of PD patients.[208–210] More importantly, ultrafiltration problem is common during acute peritonitis because peritoneal permeability is increased during an episode of peritonitis.[200] The pH of the effluent falls, especially in the presence of gram-negative peritonitis, and results in a further impairment of neutrophil activity.[211] These physiologic changes in the peritoneal membrane are usually transient.[209,212] However, after an episode of severe peritonitis, an increase in solute transport and loss of ultrafiltration may occur, resulting in a hyperpermeable membrane and permanent loss of ultrafiltration capability.[202,213] This process is probably proportional to the extent of inflammation and the number of peritonitis episodes.[214]

The final stage of this process is peritoneal fibrosis, sometimes referred to as sclerosing encapsulating peritonitis (SEP).[213,215] SEP is possibly more common in Japan, and the condition is present in 0.9% of patients undergoing PD.[216] The peritonitis rate among patients who experienced SEP was 3.3 times higher than that among the rest of the patients. Peritoneal fibrosis is a severe complication of PD. In addition to ultrafiltration failure, the patient becomes progressively malnourished because of recurrent partial intestinal obstruction from encasement of the bowel. PD cannot be continued, and this complication is frequently lethal, despite conversion to long-term hemodialysis.

CATHETER INFECTIONS

Colonization of the PD catheter exit site with bacteria may lead to infection of the catheter exit site, which may further spread along the subcutaneous tunnel of the catheter to the inner cuff and, subsequently, to the peritoneum, resulting in tunnel infection and peritonitis, respectively. Catheter infection generally encompasses both exit site and tunnel infections and occurs at an incidence of around 1 episode per 20 patient-months of treatment. However, reported figures vary considerably because definitions have not been standardized in the literature.[14,217] In general, *S. aureus* and *P. aeruginosa* are the most common, and infection with either of these two organisms is difficult to resolve and commonly results in peritonitis and catheter loss.* However, the prevalence of individual organism varies markedly in different centers. Lye and colleagues[219] reported that 77% of all catheter infections is caused by *S. aureus* and 11% caused by *Pseudomonas* species. In our center in Hong Kong, 46% of all catheter infections is caused by staphylococcal species, 28% caused by *Pseudomonas* species, and 13% caused by other gram-negative bacteria (our unpublished data).

Box 29–2 Classification of Exit-Site Appearance in Peritoneal Dialysis

Perfect
Good
Equivocal
Infected
- acute
- chronic

Definitions

An exit site infection is present, if there is purulent discharge at the peritoneal catheter exit site with or without erythema.[220–222] The presence of induration and tenderness indicate poor prognosis.[222] Isolated erythema can represent either skin irritation or an early infection. The classification of catheter exit site appearance is summarized in Box 29–2.[223] The classification of catheter exit site appearance forms the basis of management as presented in a regimen adopted in 1998 by the report of the Committee on Catheter and Exit Site Practices of the International Society of Peritoneal Dialysis (ISPD).[224]

A catheter tunnel infection is defined as the presence of pain, tenderness, erythema, induration, or any combination of these signs and symptoms present over the subcutaneous tunnel of the catheter. Nevertheless, catheter tunnel infections are commonly occult and often only detected by ultrasonography of the subcutaneous catheter tunnel.[26, 227-228] Tunnel infections occasionally occur in the absence of an exit site infection.[26,27,225–227] However, it is present in approximately half of all exit site infections as detected by the use of ultrasonography. The infection can involve the outer-cuff, the inter-cuff, or the inner-cuff of the catheter.[26,27,226–228] As the infection spreads along the tunnel toward the peritoneum, the risk of peritonitis increases.[26,227]

Risk Factors

The major risk factor in *S. aureus* catheter infections is carriage of *S. aureus*.[154,229–231] Approximately 50% of new and prevalent

*References 8,27,28,43,204,218.

PD patients are *S. aureus* carriers.[229,230] In approximately one third of them, repeat cultures revealed carriage of the same phage type; in 16%, either only one culture was positive or subsequent culture was positive but showed a change in phage type with time.[230] Patients who were *S. aureus* carriers had significantly higher incidences of *S. aureus* exit site infections, tunnel infections, and peritonitis than patients who were not carriers.[154,229–231]

Intravenous (IV) antibiotics given at the time of catheter insertion reduce infection risk.[4] Tunnel infections are probably more common in diabetic patients.[232] Immunosuppressed patients are at increased risk for catheter infections.[233] A downward-directed catheter exit site is associated with easier-to-treat infections, with fewer episodes of catheter-related peritonitis.[4]

Treatment

The treatment of exit site infections is summarized in Box 29–3 and in Figure 29–2.[218] Intensified local care with chlorhexidine or diluted hydrogen peroxide is often used together with systemic antibiotic therapy.[71,72] Mupirocin or gentamicin ophthalmic solution is sometimes used without concomitant systemic antibiotics for an exit site with an equivocal appearance or when only erythema is present.[224,234,235]

Box 29–3 Treatment Options for Catheter Exit-Site Infection

- Intensified local care
- Local antibiotics
- Systemic antibiotics
- Tunnel or cuff revision
- Catheter removal

Oral antibiotic therapy for catheter infection should be tailored according to the specific organism identified. *S. aureus* catheter infections are treated with antibiotics, such as penicillinase-resistant penicillin or trimethoprim-sulfamethoxazole.[222,224,236] Exit site care is intensified. Rifampin may have activity within bacterial biofilm and can be used as additional therapy, although it should not be used alone. Oral antibiotics appear to be as efficacious as parenteral agents.[222] In view of the growing concern about vancomycin-resistant enterococci, this agent should not be used to treat exit site or tunnel infections unless the infecting organism is methicillin resistant.[161]

Prolonged antibiotic therapy (over 2 weeks) is often necessary for *S. aureus* catheter infections.[237] Effectiveness of antibiotic therapy for *S. aureus* tunnel infections may be assessed

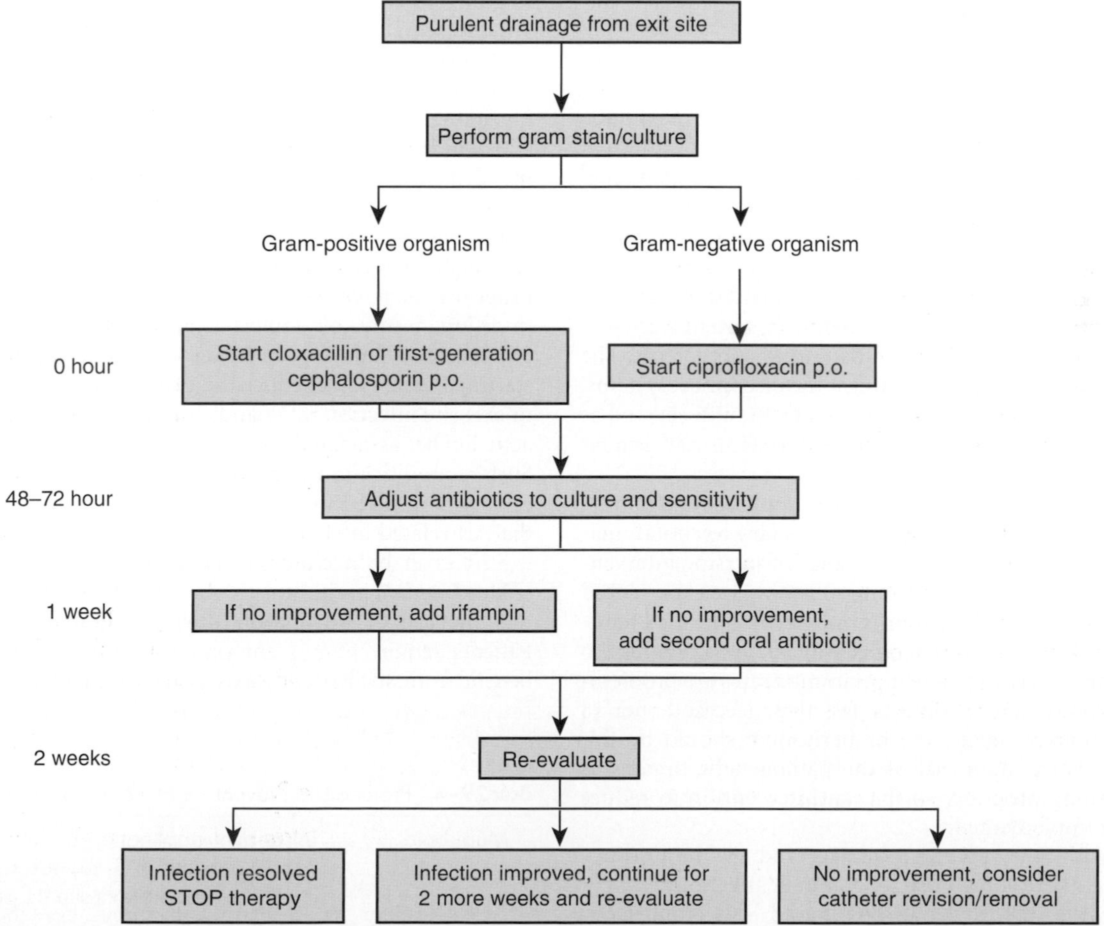

Figure 29–2 Flow chart for diagnosis and management of exit-site infections. (From Keane WF, Bailie GR, Boeschoten E, et al: Adult peritoneal dialysis-related peritonitis treatment recommendations: 2000 update. Perit Dial Int 2000; 20:396-411.)

and further therapeutic decision guided by repetitive ultrasonography of the tunnel.[233] In a study of deep tunnel infection without peritonitis caused by *S. aureus*,[233] sonographic examination of the tunnel was performed every second week. If the hypoechogenic area around the cuff decreases for 30% or more, conservative treatment with antibiotic therapy had an 85% success rate. In cases without sonographic improvement (less than 30% decrease in the pericatheter fluid collection 2 weeks after therapy), the failure rate for antibiotic therapy was high, and catheter removal is recommended.

Antibiotic therapy is generally prescribed for bacterial colonization or collection around the catheter external cuff. Surgical revision of the exit site and tunnel, with removal of the external cuff and exposure of the infectious portion of the catheter tunnel may be considered.[236,238,239] However, the procedure is associated with a risk of immediate peritonitis and should not be attempted without systemic antibiotics coverage. Revision of the tunnel and exit site is contraindicated, if the deep cuff is involved or if simultaneous peritonitis is present. If the inner cuff is involved with the infection, as demonstrated by ultrasonography of the tunnel, the catheter should be removed because peritonitis is likely to develop within weeks in untreated cases.[26] In addition, if the response to antibiotics is inadequate, it is appropriate to replace the catheter in a single procedure.

PREVENTION

There are several approaches to reduce the risk of peritonitis. First, the risk of touch contamination at the time of the exchange has decreased owing to the improvement in connection technology. Peritonitis rate is improved after the introductions of various disconnect systems.[18–20] The fundamental concept of the disconnect system is "flush-before-fill," which carries with it any contaminating bacteria introduced during connection.[240] Results from the Y-set disconnect systems consistently give lower peritonitis rates than standard spike set.[241,242] Previous study found that Y-set disconnect system was cost-effective and had a lower peritonitis rate as compared to the conventional spike system.[18] Amongst the disconnect systems, double-bag had a better peritonitis rate than Y-set and is better accepted by patients.[19,20] The two systems had similar incidences of exit site infection.

Careful selection of patients and an emphasis on training also diminish the rate of peritonitis secondary to contamination. Prowant[243] outlines the importance of nursing intervention in the prevention of peritonitis. Training by experienced nurses is the key to keep peritonitis rates low. Continued monitoring of peritonitis rates is necessary in a dialysis program so that intervention can be made if peritonitis rates are problematic.[244] Peritonitis rates should be less than 1 episode per 18 patient-months; a higher rate of peritonitis should be followed by a critical appraisal of the pathogenetic organisms and the training program, so that an intervention to reduce rates can be implemented.

Patients with *S. aureus* nasal carriage and all immunosuppressed patients are at high risk for *S. aureus* infections.[159,233,245] The rate of such infections may be reduced with prophylactic antibiotics. Antibiotic prophylaxis with mupirocin applied at the exit site[246] or intranasally[247–249] or with oral rifampin[250] reduces the risk of *S. aureus* catheter infection. The protocol to prevent *S. aureus* infection is outlined in Box 29–4. In general, we prefer mupirocin because rifampin prophylaxis is associated with side effects and may result in resistant organisms.[246–250] Repetitive courses are needed if either intranasal mupirocin or rifampin is used, because recolonization is frequent.[159,248–250] Alternatively, a randomized controlled trial found that a regimen of one single-strength tablet of trimethoprim-sulfamethoxazole on alternate days resulted in fewer staphylococcal peritonitis episodes, especially of those due to *S. aureus*, with the most prominent effect during the first 3 months of therapy.[159] Without prophylaxis, the rates of *S. aureus* exit site infection are about 0.3 to 0.4 episodes per year at risk.[251,252] Prophylaxis reduces the rate to less than 50% of this average.[28,246–250] Long-term use of prophylaxis also reduces *S. aureus* peritonitis secondary to catheter infection.[28,156] However, we have to be aware of the potentials for developing resistance with long-term prophylaxis.

Antibiotics given at the time of catheter insertion have been found to decrease catheter-related peritonitis and catheter infections. In general, single-dose cefazolin immediately before catheter insertion is sufficient. However, Gadallah and colleagues[253] found that single-dose vancomycin is superior to single-dose cefazolin in reducing the risk for postoperative peritonitis, and vancomycin should be considered in high-risk cases. Prophylactic antibiotic therapy with adequate coverage of gram-negative organism is recommended prior to colonoscopy or similar interventions because the procedure can lead to gram-negative peritonitis.

The use of povidone-iodine ointment at the exit site prevents exit site infections during the first 20 weeks of PD. Catheter immobilization, proper location of the exit site, sterile wound care immediately after placement of the catheter, and avoidance of trauma are all preventive measures recommended by most authorities.[254] Downward-pointing exit site locations, suggested as a method of reducing exit site infections, decrease the risk of catheter-related peritonitis.[4,255] Although new catheter designs or modifications have been proposed as a means of reducing peritonitis from catheter insertion, results of clinical trial are largely disappointing. Subcutaneous burying of the distal catheter segment prior to starting PD does not reduce the risk of contracting peritonitis or exit-site infection,[256,257] and delayed use of the catheter may actually be associated with a greater risk of infection.[257] Surface modification of catheters with ion beam implantation of silver produced no clinical effect with respect to reducing dialysis-related infections.[258]

Studies in both children and adults have shown that the risk of *Candida* peritonitis can be reduced with prescription of oral nystatin or fluconazole during antibiotic therapy.[259–262] Patients requiring frequent or prolonged antibiotic therapy benefit from such prophylaxis. Since oral nystatin is safe and

Box 29–4 Protocols to Prevent *Staphylococcus aureus* Infection

Mupirocin	Intranasal application bid for 5 days every month in S. aureus carriers; or Daily at the exit-site as part of routine care
Rifampin	300 mg bid for 5 days every 12 weeks

inexpensive, we advocate routine prescription of oral nystatin during empirical antibiotic treatment for PD-related peritonitis.

The success of peritoneal dialysis depends, in part, to the prevention and treatment of peritoneal dialysis associated infections.[263] The need to prevent and treat the infections also requires resources like cost relating to double-bag system, the prophylactic and the therapeutic antibiotics as well as the cost in removing the catheter, the need to switch to hemodialysis, and the need to reinsert another catheter.[264] With good prevention and treatment of peritoneal dialysis infections, we can help in reducing a lot of patient morbidity and even mortality in relation to the problem.

References

1. Piraino B: Peritonitis as a complication of peritoneal dialysis. J Am Soc Nephrol 1998; 9:1956-1964.
2. Oreopoulos DG, Tzamaloukas AH: Peritoneal dialysis in the next millennium. Adv Ren Replace Ther 2000; 7:338-346.
3. Szeto CC, Wong TY, Leung CB, et al: Importance of dialysis adequacy in mortality and morbidity of Chinese CAPD patients. Kidney Int 2000; 58:400-407.
4. Golper TA, Brier ME, Bunke M, et al: Risk factors for peritonitis in long-term peritoneal dialysis: The Network 9 peritonitis and catheter survival studies. Academic Subcommittee of the Steering Committee of the Network 9 Peritonitis and Catheter Survival Studies. Am J Kidney Dis 1996; 28:428-436.
5. Steinberg SM, Cutler SJ, Nolph KD, Novak JW: A comprehensive report on the experience of patients on continuous ambulatory peritoneal dialysis for the treatment of end-stage renal disease. Am J Kidney Dis 1984; 4:233-241.
6. Ataman R, Burton PR, Gokal R, et al: Long-term CAPD? some U.K. experience. Clin Nephrol 1988; 30(suppl 1):S71-S75.
7. Pollock CA, Ibels LS, Caterson RJ, et al: Continuous ambulatory peritoneal dialysis. Eight years of experience at a single center. Medicine (Baltimore) 1989; 68:293-308.
8. Piraino B, Bernardini J, Sorkin M: The influence of peritoneal catheter exit-site infections on peritonitis, tunnel infections, and catheter loss in patients on continuous ambulatory peritoneal dialysis. Am J Kidney Dis 1986; 8:436-440.
9. Woodrow G, Turney JH, Brownjohn AM: Technique failure in peritoneal dialysis and its impact on patient survival. Perit Dial Int 1997; 17:360-364.
10. Piraino B, Bernardini J, Sorkin M: Catheter infections as a factor in the transfer of continuous ambulatory peritoneal dialysis patients to hemodialysis. Am J Kidney Dis 1989; 13:365-369.
11. Nissenson AR, Gentile DE, Soderblom RE, et al: Morbidity and mortality of continuous ambulatory peritoneal dialysis: Regional experience and long-term prospects. Am J Kidney Dis 1986; 7:229-234.
12. Bunke CM, Brier ME, Golper TA: Outcomes of single organism peritonitis in peritoneal dialysis: Gram negatives versus gram positives in the Network 9 Peritonitis Study. Kidney Int 1997; 52:524-529.
13. Szeto CC, Wong TY, Chow KM, et al: Are peritoneal dialysis patients with and without residual renal function equivalent for survival study? Insight from a retrospective review of the cause of death. Nephrol Dial Transplant 2003; 18:977-982.
14. Bloembergen WE, Port FK: Epidemiological perspective on infections in chronic dialysis patients. Adv Ren Replace Ther 1996; 3:201-207.
15. Rubin J, Rogers WA, Taylor HM, et al: Peritonitis during continuous ambulatory peritoneal dialysis. Ann Intern Med 1980; 92:7-13.
16. Levey AS, Harrington JT: Continuous peritoneal dialysis for chronic renal failure. Medicine (Baltimore) 1982; 61:330-339.
17. Rotellar C, Black J, Winchester JF, et al: Ten years' experience with continuous ambulatory peritoneal dialysis. Am J Kidney Dis 1991; 17:158-164.
18. Li PK, Chan TH, So WY, et al: Comparisons of Y-set disconnect system (Ultraset) versus conventional spike system in uremic patients on continuous ambulatory peritoneal dialysis: Outcome and cost analysis. Perit Dial Int 1996; 16(suppl 1): S368-S370.
19. Li PK, Szeto CC, Law MC, et al: Comparison of double-bag and Y-set disconnect systems in continuous ambulatory peritoneal dialysis: A randomised prospective multi-center study. Am J Kidney Dis 1999; 33:535-540.
20. Li PK, Law MC, Chow KM, et al: Comparison of clinical outcome and ease of handling in two double-bag systems in continuous ambulatory peritoneal dialysis: A prospective randomized controlled multi-center study. Am J Kidney Dis 2002; 40:373-380.
21. British Society for Antimicrobial Chemotherapy: Diagnosis and management of peritonitis in continuous ambulatory peritoneal dialysis. Lancet 1987; 1:845-849.
22. Macia M, Vega N, Elcuaz R, et al: Neisseria mucosa peritonitis in CAPD: Another case of the nonpathogenic Neisseriae infection. Perit Dial Int 1993; 13:72-73.
23. Miller TE, Findon G: Touch contamination of connection devices in peritoneal dialysis: A quantitative microbiologic analysis. Perit Dial Int 1997; 17:560-567.
24. Rubin J, McElroy R: Peritonitis secondary to dialysis tubing contamination among patients undergoing continuous ambulatory peritoneal dialysis. Am J Kidney Dis 1989; 14:92-95.
25. Shemin D: Gram negative rod peritonitis in peritoneal dialysis. Semin Dial 1997; 10:38-45.
26. Plum J, Sudkamp S, Grabensee B: Results of ultrasound-assisted diagnosis of tunnel infections in continuous ambulatory peritoneal dialysis. Am J Kidney Dis 1994; 23:99-104.
27. Piraino B, Bernardini J, Sorkin M: A five-year study of the microbiologic results of exit site infections and peritonitis in continuous ambulatory peritoneal dialysis. Am J Kidney Dis 1987; 10:281-286.
28. Gupta B, Bernardini J, Piraino B: Peritonitis associated with exit site and tunnel infections. Am J Kidney Dis 1996; 28:415-419.
29. Correa-Rotter R: The cost barrier to renal replacement therapy and peritoneal dialysis in the developing world. Perit Dial Int 2001; 21(suppl 3):S314-S317.
30. Chan MK, Chan CY, Cheng IK, Ng WS: Climatic factors and peritonitis in CAPD patients. Int J Artif Organs 1989; 12: 366-368.
31. Szeto CC, Chow KM, Wong TY, et al: Climatic influence on the incidence of peritoneal dialysis-related peritonitis. Perit Dial Int (In press).
32. Finkelstein ES, Jekel J, Troidle L, et al: Patterns of infection in patients maintained on long-term peritoneal dialysis therapy with multiple episodes of peritonitis. Am J Kidney Dis 2002; 39: 1278-1286.
33. Gagnon RF, Richards GK, Obst G: The modulation of rifampin action against Staphylococcus epidermidis biofilms by drug additives to peritoneal dialysis solutions. Perit Dial Int 1993; 13(suppl 2):S345-S347.
34. al-Wali W, Baillod R, Brumfitt W, Hamilton-Miller JM: Differing prognostic significance of reinfection and relapse in CAPD peritonitis. Nephrol Dial Transplant 1992; 7:133-136.
35. Beaman M, Solaro L, Adu D, Michael J: Peritonitis caused by slime-producing coagulase negative staphylococci in continuous ambulatory peritoneal dialysis. Lancet 1987; 1:42.
36. Dasgupta MK, Kowalewaska-Grochowska K, Costerton JW: Biofilm and peritonitis in peritoneal dialysis. Perit Dial Int 1993; 13(suppl 2):S322-S325.
37. Schroder CH, Severijnen RS, de Jong MC, Monnens LA: Chronic tunnel infections in children: Removal and replacement

of the continuous ambulatory peritoneal dialysis catheter in a single operation. Perit Dial Int 1993; 13:198-200.
38. Swartz R, Messana J, Reynolds J, Ranjit U: Simultaneous catheter replacement and removal in refractory peritoneal dialysis infections. Kidney Int 1991; 11:213-216.
39. Swartz R, Messana J, Holmes C, Williams J: Biofilm formation on peritoneal catheters does not require the presence of infection. ASAIO Trans 1991; 37:626-634.
40. Keane WF, Comty CM, Verbrugh HA, Peterson PK: Opsonic deficiency of peritoneal dialysis effluent in continuous ambulatory peritoneal dialysis. Kidney Int 1984; 25:539-543.
41. van der Reijden HJ, Struijk DG, van Ketel RJ, et al: Fecal peritonitis in patients on continuous ambulatory peritoneal dialysis: An end-point in CAPD? Adv Perit Dial 1988; 4:198-203.
42. Schweinburg FB, Seligman AM, Fine J: Transmural migration of intestinal bacteria. N Engl J Med 1976; 242:747-751.
43. de Vecchi AF, Maccario M, Braga M, et al: Peritoneal dialysis in nondiabetic patients older than 70 years: Comparison with patients age 40 to 60 years. Am J Kidney Dis 1998; 31:479-490.
44. Singharetnam W, Holley JL: Acute treatment of constipation may lead to transmural migration of bacteria resulting in gram negative, polymicrobial or fungal peritonitis. Perit Dial Int 1996; 16:423-425.
45. Wood CJ, Fleming V, Turnidge J, et al: Campylobacter peritonitis in continuous ambulatory peritoneal dialysis: Report of eight cases and a review of the literature. Am J Kidney Dis 1992; 19:257-263.
46. Orr KE, Wilkinson R, Gould FK: Salmonella enteritis causing CAPD peritonitis. Perit Dial Int 1993; 13:164.
47. Caravaca F, Ruiz-Calero R, Dominguez C: Risk factors for developing peritonitis caused by microorganisms of enteral origin in peritoneal dialysis patients. Perit Dial Int 1998; 18:41-45.
48. Kaplan RA, Alon U, Hellerstein S, et al: Unusual causes of peritonitis in three children receiving peritoneal dialysis. Perit Dial Int 1993; 13:60-63.
49. Harwell CM, Newman LN, Cacho CP, et al: Abdominal catastrophe: Visceral injury as a cause of peritonitis in patients treated by peritoneal dialysis. Perit Dial Int 1997; 17:586-594.
50. Morduchowicz G, van Dyk DJ, Wittenberg C, et al: Bacteremia complicating peritonitis in peritoneal dialysis patients. Am J Nephrol 1993; 13:278-280.
51. Rubin J, Oreopoulos DG, Lio TT, et al: Management of peritonitis and bowel perforation during chronic peritoneal dialysis. Nephron 1976; 16:220-225.
52. Keane WF, Bailie GR, Boeschoten E, et al: Adult peritoneal dialysis-related peritonitis treatment recommendations: 2000 update. Perit Dial Int 2000; 20:396-411.
53. Tzamaloukas AH, Obermiller LE, Gibel LJ: Peritonitis associated with intra-abdominal pathology in continuous ambulatory peritoneal dialysis patients. Perit Dial Int 1992; 13(suppl 2):S335-S337.
54. Holley JL, Bernardini J, Piraino B: Polymicrobial peritonitis in patients on continuous peritoneal dialysis. Am J Kidney Dis 1992; 19:162-166.
55. Kiernan L, Finkelstein FO, Kliger AS, et al: Outcome of polymicrobial peritonitis in continuous ambulatory peritoneal dialysis patients. Am J Kidney Dis 1995; 25:461-464.
56. Kim GC, Korbet SM: Polymicrobial peritonitis in continuous ambulatory peritoneal dialysis patients. Am J Kidney Dis 2000; 36:1000-1008.
57. Szeto CC, Chow KM, Wong TY, et al: Conservative management of polymicrobial peritonitis complicating peritoneal dialysis: A series of 140 consecutive cases. Am J Med 2002; 113:728-733.
58. Ray SM, Piraino B, Holley J: Peritonitis following colonoscopy in a peritoneal dialysis patient. Perit Dial Int 1990; 10:97-98.
59. Li PK, Leung CB, Leung AKL, et al: Post-hysteroscopy fungal peritonitis in a patient on continuous ambulatory peritoneal dialysis. Am J Kidney Dis 1993; 21:446-448.
60. Barnett JL, Elta G: Bacterial peritonitis following endoscopic variceal sclerotherapy. Gastrointest Endosc 1987; 33:316-317.
61. Kiddy K, Brown PP, Michael J, et al: Peritonitis due to Streptococcus viridans in patients receiving continuous ambulatory peritoneal dialysis. Br Med J 1985; 290:969-970.
62. Swartz RD, Campbell DA, Stone D, Dickinson C: Recurrent polymicrobial peritonitis from a gynecologic source as a complication of CAPD. Perit Dial Bull 1983; 3:32-33.
63. Coward RA, Gokal R, Wise M, et al: Peritonitis associated with vaginal leakage of dialysis fluid in continuous ambulatory peritoneal dialysis. Br Med J 1982; 284:1529.
64. Korzets A, Chagnac A, Ori Y, et al: Pneumococcal peritonitis complicating CAPD: Was the indwelling intrauterine device to blame? Clin Nephrol 1991; 35:24-25.
65. Stuck A, Seiler A, Frey FJ: Peritonitis due to an intrauterine device in a patient on CAPD. Perit Dial Bull 1986; 6:158-159.
66. Piraino B, Rasool A, Bernardini J: Iatrogenic peritonitis. Perit Dial Int 1998; 18(suppl 1):S34.
67. Verbrugh HA, Keane WF, Hoidal JR, et al: Peritoneal macrophages and opsonins: Antibacterial defense in patients undergoing chronic peritoneal dialysis. J Infect Dis 1983; 147: 1018-1029.
68. Coles GA, Lewis SL, Williams JD: Host defense and effects of solution on peritoneal cells. *In* Gokal R, Nolph KD (eds): The Textbook of Peritoneal Dialysis. Dordrecht, Kluwer, 1994, pp 503-528.
69. Lewis S, Holmes S: Host defense mechanisms in the peritoneal cavity of continuous ambulatory peritoneal dialysis patients. First of two parts. Perit Dial Int 1991; 11:14-21.
70. Holmes S, Lewis S: Host defense mechanisms in the peritoneal cavity of continuous ambulatory peritoneal dialysis patients II: Humoral defense. Perit Dial Int 1991; 11:112-117.
71. Goldstein CS, Garrick RE, Polin RA, et al: Fibronectin and complement secretion by monocytes and peritoneal macrophages in vitro from patients undergoing continuous ambulatory peritoneal dialysis. J Leukoc Biol 1986; 39:457-464.
72. Davies SJ, Suassuna J, Ogg CS, Cameron JS: Activation of immunocompetent cells in the peritoneum of patients treated with CAPD. Kidney Int 1989; 36:661-668.
73. Runyon BA: Low protein concentration ascitic fluid is predisposed to spontaneous bacterial peritonitis. Gastroenterology 1986; 91:1343-1346.
74. Coles GA, Minors SJ, Horton JK, et al: Can the risk of peritonitis be predicted for new continuous ambulatory peritoneal dialysis (CAPD) patients? Perit Dial Int 1989; 9:69-72.
75. Bennett-Jones DN, Yewdall VM, Gillespie CM, et al: Strain differences in the opsonisation of Staphylococcus epidermidis. Perit Dial Int 1989; 9:333-339.
76. Davies SJ, Yewdall VM, Ogg CS, Cameron JS: Peritoneal defense mechanisms and Staphylococcus aureus in patients treated with continuous ambulatory peritoneal dialysis (CAPD). Perit Dial Int 1990; 10:135-140.
77. Holmes CJ, Lewis SL, Kubey WY, Van Epps DE: Comparison of peritoneal white blood cell parameters from continuous ambulatory peritoneal dialysis patients with a high or low incidence of peritonitis. Am J Kidney Dis 1990; 15:258-264.
78. Nagai T, Kuriyama M, Kawada Y: Oxidative metabolism of polymorphonuclear leukocytes in continuous ambulatory peritoneal dialysis. Perit Dial Int 1997; 17:167-174.
79. Peterson PK, Gaziano E, Suh HJ, et al: Antimicrobial activities of dialysate-elicited and resident human peritoneal macrophages. Infect Immun 1985; 49:212-218.
80. Lewis SL, Norris PJ, Holmes CJ: Phenotypic characterization of monocytes and macrophages from CAPD patients. ASAIO Trans 1990; 36:M575-M577.
81. Carcamo C, Fernandez-Castro M, Selgas R, et al: Long-term continuous ambulatory peritoneal dialysis reduces the expression of CD11b, CD14, CD16, and CD64 on peritoneal macrophages. Perit Dial Int 1996; 16:582-589.

82. Giacchino F, Pozzato M, Formica M, et al: Lymphocyte subsets assayed by numerical tests in CAPD. Int J Artif Organs 1984; 7: 81-84.
83. Topley N, Williams JD: Role of the peritoneal membrane in the control of inflammation in the peritoneal cavity. Kidney Int Suppl 1994; 48:S71-S78.
84. Topley N: The cytokine network controlling peritoneal inflammation. Perit Dial Int 1995; 15(7 suppl):S35-S39.
85. Duwe AK, Vas SI, Weatherhead JW: Effects of the composition of peritoneal dialysis fluid on chemiluminescence, phagocytosis, and bactericidal activity in vitro. Infect Immun 1981; 33: 130-135.
86. Ing TS, Zhou XJ, Yu AW, et al: Lactate-containing peritoneal dialysis solutions. Int J Artif Organs 1993; 16:688-693.
87. Scambye HT, Peterson FG, Wang P: Bicarbonate is not the ultimate answer to the bioincompatibility problems of CAPD solution. Adv Perit Dial 1992; 8:42-46.
88. Mahiout AM, Brunkhorst R: Pyruvate anions neutralize peritoneal dialysate cytotoxicity. Nephrol Dial Transplant 1995; 10: 391-394.
89. Jonasson P, Wieslander A, Braide M: Heat-sterilized PD fluid blocks leucocyte adhesion and increases flow velocity in rat peritoneal vessels. Perit Dial Int 1996; 16(suppl 2):S137-S140.
90. Nolph KD, Sorkin M, Rubin J, et al: Continuous ambulatory peritoneal dialysis: Three-year experience at one center. Ann Intern Med 1980; 92:609-613.
91. Vas SI: Microbiologic aspects of chronic ambulatory peritoneal dialysis. Kidney Int 1983; 23:83-92.
92. Spencer RC: Infections in continuous ambulatory peritoneal dialysis. J Med Microbiol 1988; 27:1-9.
93. Kim D, Tapson J, Wu G, et al: Staph aureus peritonitis in patients on continuous ambulatory peritoneal dialysis. Trans Am Soc Artif Intern Organs 1984; 30:494-497.
94. Tzamaloukas AH, Murata GH, Fox L: Death associated with Pseudomonas peritonitis in malnourished elderly diabetics on CAPD. Perit Dial Int 1993; 13:241-242.
95. Korzets Z, Korzets A, Golan E, et al: CAPD peritonitis: Initial presentation as an acute abdomen with a clear peritoneal effluent. Clin Nephrol 1992; 37:155-157.
96. Gould IM, Casewell MW: The laboratory diagnosis of peritonitis during continuous ambulatory peritoneal dialysis. J Hosp Infect 1986; 7:155-160.
97. Brahm M: A simple diagnostic method of peritonitis in patients on CAPD. J Urol Nephrol 1984; 18:223-225.
98. Flanigan M, Freeman RM, Lim VS: Cellular response to peritonitis among peritoneal dialysis patients. Am J Kidney Dis 1985; 6:420-424.
99. Riera G, Bushinsky D, Emmanouel DS: First exchange neutrophilia: An index of peritonitis during chronic intermittent peritoneal dialysis. Clin Nephrol 1985; 24:5-8.
100. Koopmans JG, Boeschoten EW, Pannekeet MM, et al: Impaired initial cell reaction in CAPD-related peritonitis. Perit Dial Int 1996; 16(suppl 1):S362-S367.
101. Cropper E, Coleclough S, Griffiths S, et al: Rapid diagnosis of peritonitis in peritoneal dialysis patients. J Nephrol 2003; 16:379-383.
102. Chan MK, Chow L, Lam SS, Jones B: Peritoneal eosinophilia in patients on continuous ambulatory peritoneal dialysis: A prospective study. Am J Kidney Dis 1988; 11:180-183.
103. Piraino BM, Silver MR, Dominguez JH, Puschett JB: Peritoneal eosinophils during intermittent peritoneal dialysis. Am J Nephrol 1984; 4:152-157.
104. Humayun HM, Ing TS, Daugirdas JT, et al: Peritoneal fluid eosinophilia in patients undergoing maintenance peritoneal dialysis. Arch Intern Med 1981; 141:1172-1173.
105. Gokal R, Ramos JM, Ward MK, Kerr DN: Eosinophilic peritonitis in continuous ambulatory peritoneal dialysis (CAPD). Clin Nephrol 1981; 15:328-330.
106. Chandran PK, Humayun HM, Daugirdas JT, et al: Blood eosinophilia in patients undergoing maintenance peritoneal dialysis. Arch Intern Med 1985; 145:114-116.
107. Charney DI, Gouge SF: Chemical peritonitis secondary to intraperitoneal vancomycin. Am J Kidney Dis 1991; 17:76-79.
108. Wang AYM, Li PK, Lai KN: Comparison of intraperitoneal administration of two preparations of vancomycin in causing chemical peritonitis. Perit Dial Int 1996; 16:172-174.
109. Benevent D, El Akoum N, Lagarde C, et al: Danger of the intraperitoneal administration of amphotericin B during continuous ambulatory peritoneal dialysis. Presse Med 1984; 13: 1844.
110. Tintillier M, Pchet JM, Christophe JL, et al: Transient sterile chemical peritonitis with icodextrin: Clinical presentation, prevalence, and literature review. Perit Dial Int 2002; 22:534-537.
111. Caruana RJ, Wolfman NT, Karstaedt N, Wilson DJ: Pancreatitis: An important cause of abdominal symptoms in patients on peritoneal dialysis. Am J Kidney Dis 1986; 7:135-140.
112. Gupta A, Yuan ZY, Balaskas EV, et al: CAPD and pancreatitis: No connection. Perit Dial Int 1992; 12:309-316.
113. Pannekeet MM, Krediet RT, Boeschoten EW, Arisz L: Acute pancreatitis during CAPD in The Netherlands. Nephrol Dial Transplant 1993; 8:1376-1381.
114. Burkart J, Haigler S, Caruana R, Hylander B: Usefulness of peritoneal fluid amylase levels in the differential diagnosis of peritonitis in peritoneal dialysis patients. J Am Soc Nephrol 1991; 1:1186-1190.
115. Humayun HM, Daugirdas JT, Ing TS, et al: Chylous ascites in a patient treated with intermittent peritoneal dialysis. Artif Organs 1984; 8:358-360.
116. Porter J, Wang WM, Oliveira DB: Chylous ascites and continuous ambulatory peritoneal dialysis. Nephrol Dial Transplant 1991; 6:659-661.
117. Bargman JM, Zent R, Ellis P, et al: Diagnosis of lymphoma in a continuous ambulatory peritoneal dialysis patient by peritoneal fluid cytology. Am J Kidney Dis 1994; 23:747-750.
118. Bagnis C, Gabella P, Bruno M, et al: Cloudy dialysate due to adenocarcinoma cells in a CAPD patient. Perit Dial Int 1993; 13:322-323.
119. Bezerra DA, Silva MB, Caramori JS, et al: The diagnostic value of Gram stain for initial identification of the etiologic agent of peritonitis in CAPD patients. Perit Dial Int 1997; 17:269-272.
120. Keane WF, Everett ED, Golper TA, et al: Peritoneal dialysis-related peritonitis treatment recommendations. 1993 update. The Ad Hoc Advisory Committee on Peritonitis Management. International Society for Peritoneal Dialysis. Perit Dial Int 1993; 13:14-28.
121. Tranaeus A, Heimburger O, Lindholm B: Peritonitis in continuous ambulatory peritoneal dialysis (CAPD): Diagnostic findings, therapeutic outcome and complications. Perit Dial Int 1989; 9:179-190.
122. Keane WF, Bailie GR, Boeschoten E, et al: Adult peritoneal dialysis-related peritonitis treatment recommendations: 2000 update. Perit Dial Int 2000; 20:396-411.
123. Centers for Disease Control and Prevention. Staphylococcus aureus with reduced susceptibility to vancomycin? United States, 1997. JAMA 1997; 278:891-892.
124. Centers for Disease Control and Prevention. Update: Staphylococcus aureus with reduced susceptibility to vancomycin? United States, 1997. Morb Mortal Wkly Rep 1997; 46:813-815.
125. Tabaqchali S: Vancomycin-resistant Staphylococcus aureus: Apocalypse now? Lancet 1997; 350:1644-1645.
126. Schwalbe RS, Stapleton JT, Gilligan PH: Emergence of vancomycin resistance in coagulase-negative staphylococci. N Engl J Med 1987; 316:927-931.
127. Keane WF, Alexander SR, Bailie GR, et al: Peritoneal dialysis-related peritonitis treatment recommendations: 1996 update. Perit Dial Int 1996; 16:557-573.

128. Khairullah Q, Provenzano R, Tayeb J, et al: Comparison of vancomycin versus cefazolin as initial therapy for peritonitis in peritoneal dialysis patients. Perit Dial Int 2002; 22:339-344.
129. Ariano RE, Franczuk C, Fine A, et al: Challenging the current treatment paradigm for methicillin-resistant Staphylococcus epidermidis peritonitis in peritoneal dialysis patients. Perit Dial Int 2002; 22:335-338.
130. Sandoe JA, Gokal R, Struthers JK: Vancomycin-resistant enterococci and empirical vancomycin for CAPD peritonitis. Perit Dial Int 1997; 17:617-618.
131. Shemin D, Maaz D, St Pierre D, et al: Effect of aminoglycoside use on residual renal function in peritoneal dialysis patients. Am J Kidney Dis 1999; 34:14-20.
132. Szeto CC, Lai KN, Wong TY, et al: Independent effects of residual renal function and dialysis adequacy on nutritional status and patient outcome in continuous ambulatory peritoneal dialysis (CAPD). Am J Kidney Dis 1999; 34:1056-1064.
133. Li PK, Ip M, Law MC, et al: Use of intra-peritoneal (IP) cefepime as monotherapy in the treatment of CAPD peritonitis. Perit Dial Int 2000; 20(2):232-234.
134. Lui SF, Cheng AB, Leung CB, et al: Imipenem/cilastatin sodium in the treatment of continuous ambulatory peritoneal dialysis-associated peritonitis. Am J Nephrol 1994; 14:182-186.
135. Lai MN, Kao MT, Chen CC, et al: Intraperitoneal once-daily dose of cefazolin and gentamicin for treating CAPD peritonitis. Perit Dial Int 1997; 17:87-89.
136. Chong TK, Piraino B, Bernardini U: Vestibular toxicity due to gentamicin in peritoneal dialysis patients. Perit Dial Int 1991; 11:152-155.
137. Vas SI: Single daily dose of aminoglycosides in the treatment of continuous ambulatory peritoneal dialysis peritonitis. Perit Dial Int 1993; 13(suppl 2):S355-S356.
138. Raz R, Adawi M, Romano S: Intravenous administration of gentamicin once daily versus thrice daily in adults. Eur J Clin Microbiol Infect Dis 1995; 14:88-91.
139. Gendeh BS, Said H, Gibb AG, et al: Gentamicin ototoxicity in continuous ambulatory peritoneal dialysis. J Laryngol Otol 1993; 107:681-685.
140. Low CL, Bailie GR, Evans A, et al: Pharmacokinetics of once-daily IP gentamicin in CAPD patients. Perit Dial Int 1996; 16: 379-384.
141. Bailie GR, Haqqie SS, Eisele G, et al: Effectiveness of once-weekly vancomycin and once-daily gentamicin, intraperitoneally, for CAPD peritonitis. Perit Dial Int 1995; 15:269-271.
142. Goldberg L, Clemenger M, Azadian B, Brown EA: Initial treatment of peritoneal dialysis peritonitis without vancomycin with a once-daily cefazolin-based regimen. Am J Kidney Dis 2001; 37:49-55.
143. Vas S, Bargman J, Oreopoulos DG: Treatment in PD patients of peritonitis caused by gram positive organisms with single daily dose of antibiotics. Perit Dial Int 1997; 17:91-94.
144. Mulhern JG, Braden GL, O'Shea MH, et al: Trough serum vancomycin levels predict the relapse of gram-positive peritonitis in peritoneal dialysis patients. Am J Kidney Dis 1995; 25: 611-615.
145. Read RR, Eberwein P, Dasgupta MK, et al: Peritonitis in peritoneal dialysis: Bacterial colonization by biofilm spread along the catheter surface. Kidney Int 1989; 35:614-621.
146. Swartz R, Messana J, Reynolds J, Ranjit U: Simultaneous catheter replacement and removal in refractory peritoneal dialysis infections. Kidney Int 1991; 40:1160-1165.
147. Majkowski NL, Mendley SR: Simultaneous removal and replacement of infected peritoneal dialysis catheters. Am J Kidney Dis 1997; 29:706-711.
148. Fredensborg BB, Meyer HW, Joffe P, Fugleberg S: Reinsertion of PD catheters during PD-related infections performed either simultaneously or after an intervening period. Perit Dial Int 1995; 15:374-378.
149. Innes A, Burden RP, Finch RG, Morgan AG: Treatment of resistant peritonitis in continuous ambulatory peritoneal dialysis with intraperitoneal urokinase: A double-blind clinical trial. Nephrol Dial Transplant 1994; 9:797-799.
150. Williams AJ, Boletis I, Johnson BF, et al: Tenckhoff catheter replacement or intraperitoneal urokinase: A randomised trial in the management of recurrent continuous ambulatory peritoneal dialysis (CAPD) peritonitis. Perit Dial Int 1989; 9:65-67.
151. Nankivell BJ, Lake N, Gillies A: Intracatheter streptokinase for recurrent peritonitis in CAPD. Clin Nephrol 1991; 35:20-23.
152. Norris KC, Shinaberger JH, Reyes GD, Kraut JA: The use of intracatheter instillation of streptokinase in the treatment of recurrent bacterial peritonitis in continuous ambulatory peritoneal dialysis. Am J Kidney Dis 1987; 10:62-65.
153. Bernardini J, Holley JL, Johnston JR, et al: An analysis of ten-year trends in infections in adults on continuous ambulatory peritoneal dialysis (CAPD). Clin Nephrol 1991; 36:29-34.
154. Piraino B, Perlmutter JA, Holley JL, Bernardini J: Staphylococcus aureus peritonitis is associated with Staphylococcus aureus nasal carriage in peritoneal dialysis patients. Perit Dial Int 1993; 13(suppl 2):S332-S334.
155. Sesso R, Draibe S, Castelo A, et al: Staphylococcus aureus skin carriage and development of peritonitis in patients on continuous ambulatory peritoneal dialysis. Clin Nephrol 1989; 31: 264-268.
156. Oxton LL, Zimmerman SW, Roecker EB, Wakeen M: Risk factors for peritoneal dialysis-related infections. Perit Dial Int 1994; 14:137-144.
157. Pignatari A, Pfaller M, Hollis R, et al: Staphylococcus aureus colonization and infection in patients on continuous ambulatory peritoneal dialysis. J Clin Microbiol 1990; 28:1898-1902.
158. Davies SJ, Ogg CS, Cameron JS, et al: Staphylococcus aureus nasal carriage, exit-site infection and catheter loss in patients treated with continuous ambulatory peritoneal dialysis (CAPD). Perit Dial Int 1989; 9:61-64.
159. Swartz R, Messana J, Starmann B, et al: Preventing Staphylococcus aureus infection during chronic peritoneal dialysis. J Am Soc Nephrol 1991; 2:1085-1091.
160. Wanten GJ, van Oost P, Schneeberger PM, Koolen MI: Nasal carriage and peritonitis by Staphylococcus aureus in patients on continuous ambulatory peritoneal dialysis: A prospective study. Perit Dial Int 1996; 16:352-356.
161. Lye WC, Leong SO, Lee EJ: Methicillin-resistant Staphylococcus aureus nasal carriage and infections in CAPD. Kidney Int 1993; 43:1357-1362.
162. Peacock SJ, Howe PA, Day NP, et al: Outcome following staphylococcal peritonitis. Perit Dial Int 2000; 20:215-219.
163. Munoz de Bustillo E, Aguilera A, Jimenez C, et al: Streptococcal versus Staphylococcus epidermidis peritonitis in CAPD. A comparative study. Perit Dial Int 1997; 17:392-395.
164. Yinnon AM, Jain V, Magnussen CR: Group B streptococcus (agalactia) peritonitis and bacteremia associated with CAPD. Perit Dial Int 1993; 13:241.
165. Borra SI, Chandarana J, Kleinfeld M: Fatal peritonitis due to group B beta-hemolytic streptococcus in a patient receiving chronic ambulatory peritoneal dialysis. Am J Kidney Dis 1992; 19:375-377.
166. Winchester JF, Rakowski TA: Group A streptococcal peritonitis associated with continuous ambulatory peritoneal dialysis. Am J Med 1989; 87:487.
167. Cavalieri SJ, Allais JM, Schlievert PM, et al: Group A streptococcal peritonitis in a patient undergoing continuous ambulatory peritoneal dialysis. Am J Med 1989; 86:249-250.
168. Troidle L, Kliger AS, Gorban-Brennan N, et al: Nine episodes of CPD-associated peritonitis with vancomycin resistant enterococci. Kidney Int 1996; 50:1368-1372.
169. Leblanc M: Oral ciprofloxacin to treat bacterial peritonitis associated with peritoneal dialysis. Clin Nephrol 1997; 47:350-354.

170. Shemin D, Maaz D: Gram-negative peritonitis in peritoneal dialysis: Improved outcome with intraperitoneal ceftazidime. Perit Dial Int 1996; 16:638-641.
171. Szeto CC, Chow KM, Leung CB, et al: Clinical course of peritonitis due to Pseudomonas species complicating peritoneal dialysis: A review of 104 cases. Kidney Int 2001; 59:2309-2315.
172. Bunke M, Brier ME, Golper TA: Pseudomonas peritonitis in peritoneal dialysis patients: The Network 9 Peritonitis Study. Am J Kidney Dis 1995; 25:769-774.
173. Tebben JA, Rigsby MO, Selwyn PA, et al: Outcome of HIV infected patients on continuous ambulatory peritoneal dialysis. Kidney Int 1993; 44:191-198.
174. Szeto CC, Li PK, Leung CB, et al: Xanthomonas maltophilia peritonitis in uremic patients receiving continuous ambulatory peritoneal dialysis. Am J Kidney Dis 1997; 29:91-95.
175. Galvao C, Swartz R, Rocher L, et al: Acinetobacter peritonitis during chronic peritoneal dialysis. Am J Kidney Dis 1989; 14:101-104.
176. Lye WC, Lee EJ, Leong SO, Kumarasinghe G: Clinical characteristics and outcome of Acinetobacter infections in CAPD patients. Perit Dial Int 1994; 14:174-177.
177. Grefberg N, Danielson BG, Nilsson P: Peritonitis in patients on continuous ambulatory peritoneal dialysis. A changing scene. Scand J Infect Dis 1984; 16:187-194.
178. Boroujerdi-Rad H, Juergensen P, Mansourian V, et al: Abdominal abscesses complicating peritonitis in continuous ambulatory peritoneal dialysis patients. Am J Kidney Dis 1994; 23:717-721.
179. Johnson RJ, Ramsey PG, Gallagher N, Ahmad S: Fungal peritonitis in patients on peritoneal dialysis: Incidence, clinical features and prognosis. Am J Nephrol 1985; 5:169-175.
180. Goldie SJ, Kiernan-Tridle L, Torres C, et al: Fungal peritonitis in a large chronic peritoneal dialysis population: A report of 55 episodes. Am J Kidney Dis 1996; 28:86-91.
181. Bibashi E, Memmos D, Kokolina E, et al: Fungal peritonitis complicating peritoneal dialysis during an 11-year period: Report of 46 cases. Clin Infect Dis 2003; 36:927-931.
182. Warady BA, Bashir M, Donaldson LA: Fungal peritonitis in children receiving peritoneal dialysis: A report of the NAPRTCS. Kidney Int 2000; 58:384-389.
183. Wang AY, Yu AW, Li PK, et al: Factors predicting outcome of fungal peritonitis in peritoneal dialysis: Analysis of a 9-year experience of fungal peritonitis in a single center. Am J Kidney Dis 2000; 36:1183-1192.
184. Michel C, Courdavault L, al Khayat R, et al: Fungal peritonitis in patients on peritoneal dialysis. Am J Nephrol 1994; 14:113-120.
185. Andersen K, Olsen H: Candida peritonitis in a patient receiving chronic intermittent peritoneal dialysis. Scand J Infect Dis 1978; 10:91-92.
186. Holdsworth SR, Atkins RC, Scott DF, Jackson R: Management of Candida peritonitis by prolonged peritoneal lavage containing 5-fluorocytosine. Clin Nephrol 1975; 4:157-159.
187. Montenegro J, Aguirre R, Gonzalez O, et al: Fluconazole treatment of candida peritonitis with delayed removal of the peritoneal dialysis catheter. Clin Nephrol 1995; 44:60-63.
188. Lui SL, Lo CY, Choy BY, et al: Optimal treatment and long-term outcome of tuberculous peritonitis complicating continuous ambulatory peritoneal dialysis. Am J Kidney Dis 1996; 28:747-751.
189. Chow KM, Chow VC, Hung LC, et al: Tuberculous peritonitis? associated mortality is high among patients waiting for the results of mycobacterial cultures of ascitic fluid samples. Clin Infect Dis 2002; 35:409-413.
190. Mallat SF, Brensilver JM: Tuberculous peritonitis in a CAPD patient cured without catheter removal: Case report, review of the literature, and guidelines for treatment and diagnosis. Am J Kidney Dis 1989; 13:154-157.
191. Szeto CC, Wong TY, Chow KM, et al: The clinical course of culture-negative peritonitis complicating peritoneal dialysis. Am J Kidney Dis 2003; 42:567-574.
192. de Fijter CW, Oe LP, Nauta JJ, et al: Clinical efficacy and morbidity associated with continuous cyclic compared with continuous ambulatory peritoneal dialysis. Ann Intern Med 1994; 120: 264-271.
193. Holley JL, Bernardini J, Piraino B: Continuous cycling peritoneal dialysis is associated with lower rates of catheter infections than continuous ambulatory peritoneal dialysis. Am J Kidney Dis 1990; 16:133-136.
194. de Fijter CW, Verbrugh HA, Oe LP, et al: Peritoneal defense in continuous ambulatory versus continuous cyclic peritoneal dialysis. Kidney Int 1992; 42:947-950.
195. Wrenger E, Baumann C, Behrend M, et al: Peritoneal mononuclear cell differentiation and cytokine production in intermittent and continuous automated peritoneal dialysis. Am J Kidney Dis 1998; 31:234-241.
196. Manley HJ, Bailie GR, Frye R, et al: Pharmacokinetics of intermittent intravenous cefazolin and tobramycin in patients treated with automated peritoneal dialysis. J Am Soc Nephrol 2000; 11:1310-1316.
197. Troidle L, Gorban-Brennan N, Kliger A, Finkelstein F: Once-daily intraperitoneal cefazolin and oral ciprofloxacin as empiric therapy for the treatment of peritonitis. Adv Perit Dial 1999; 15: 213-216.
198. Liberek T, Topley N, Jorres A, et al: Peritoneal dialysis fluid inhibition of phagocyte function: Effects of osmolality and glucose concentration. J Am Soc Nephrol 1993; 3:1508-1515.
199. Ejlersen E, Brandi L, Lokkegaard H, et al: Is initial (24 hours) lavage necessary in treatment of CAPD peritonitis? Perit Dial Int 1991; 11:38-42.
200. Pannekeet MM, Zemel D, Koomen GC, et al: Dialysate markers of peritoneal tissue during peritonitis and in stable CAPD. Perit Dial Int 1995; 15:217-225.
201. Peers E, Gokal R: Icodextrin: Overview of clinical experience. Perit Dial Int 1997; 17:22-26.
202. Szeto CC, Chow KM, Wong TY, et al: Feasibility of resuming peritoneal dialysis after severe peritonitis and Tenckhoff catheter removal. J Am Soc Nephrol 2002; 13:1040-1045.
203. Swartz RD, Messana JM: Simultaneous catheter removal and replacement in peritoneal dialysis infections: Update and current recommendations. Adv Perit Dial 1999; 15:205-208.
204. Posthuma N, Borgstein PJ, Eijsbouts Q, ter Wee PM: Simultaneous peritoneal dialysis catheter insertion and removal in catheter-related infections without interruption of peritoneal dialysis. Nephrol Dial Transplant 1998; 13:700-703.
205. Mayo RR, Messana JM, Boyer CJ Jr, Swartz RD: Pseudomonas peritonitis treated with simultaneous catheter replacement and removal. Perit Dial Int 1995; 15:389-390.
206. Paterson AD, Bishop MC, Morgan AG, Burden RP: Removal and replacement of Tenckhoff catheter at a single operation: Successful treatment of resistant peritonitis in continuous ambulatory peritoneal dialysis. Lancet 1986; 2:1245-1247.
207. Lui SL, Li FK, Lo CY, Lo WK: Simultaneous removal and reinsertion of Tenckhoff catheters for the treatment of refractory exit-site infection. Adv Perit Dial 2000; 16:195-197.
208. Blumenkrantz MJ, Gahl GM, Kopple JD, et al: Protein losses during peritoneal dialysis. Kidney Int 1981; 19:593-602.
209. Rubin J, Ray R, Barnes T, Bower J: Peritoneal abnormalities during infectious episodes of continuous ambulatory peritoneal dialysis. Nephron 1981; 29:124-127.
210. Jones MR: Etiology of severe malnutrition: Results of an international cross-sectional study in continuous ambulatory peritoneal dialysis patients. Am J Kidney Dis 1994; 23:412-420.
211. Sennesael JJ, De Smedt GC, Van der Niepen P, Verbeelen DL: The impact of peritonitis on peritoneal and systemic acid-base status of patients on continuous ambulatory peritoneal dialysis. Perit Dial Int 1994; 14:61-65.
212. Dobbie JW: Pathogenesis of peritoneal fibrosing syndromes (sclerosing peritonitis) in peritoneal dialysis. Perit Dial Int 1992; 12:14-27.

213. Hendriks PM, Ho-dac-Pannekeet MM, van Gulik TM, et al: Peritoneal sclerosis in chronic peritoneal dialysis patients: Analysis of clinical presentation, risk factors, and peritoneal transport kinetics. Perit Dial Int 1997; 17:136-143.
214. Davies SJ, Bryan J, Phillips L, Russell GI: Longitudinal changes in peritoneal kinetics: The effects of peritoneal dialysis and peritonitis. Nephrol Dial Transplant 1996; 11:498-506.
215. Selgas R, Fernandez-Reyes MJ, Bosque E, et al: Functional longevity of the human peritoneum: How long is continuous peritoneal dialysis possible? Results of a prospective medium long-term study. Am J Kidney Dis 1994; 23:64-73.
216. Nomoto Y, Kawaguchi Y, Kubo H, et al: Sclerosing encapsulating peritonitis in patients undergoing continuous ambulatory peritoneal dialysis: A report of the Japanese Sclerosing Encapsulating Peritonitis Study Group. Am J Kidney Dis 1996; 28:420-427.
217. Lindblad AS, Noval JW, Nolph KD (eds): Continuous Ambulatory Peritoneal Dialysis in the USA: Final Report of the National CAPD Registry 1981–1988. Dordrecht, The Netherlands, Kluwer Academic Publishers, 1989.
218. Scalamogna A, Castelnovo C, De Vecchi A, Ponticelli C: Exit-site and tunnel infections in continuous ambulatory peritoneal dialysis patients. Am J Kidney Dis 1991; 18:674-677.
219. Lye WC, Wong PL, Leong SO, Lee EJ: A prospective study of peritoneal dialysis-related infections in CAPD patients with diabetes mellitus. Adv Perit Dial 1993; 9:195-197.
220. Pierratos A: Peritoneal dialysis glossary. Perit Dial Bull 1984; 1:2-3.
221. Gloor HJ, Nichols WK, Sorkin MI, et al: Peritoneal access and related complications in continuous ambulatory peritoneal dialysis. Am J Med 1983; 74:593-598.
222. Flanigan MJ, Hochstetler LA, Langholdt D, Lim VS: Continuous ambulatory peritoneal dialysis catheter infections: Diagnosis and management. Perit Dial Int 1994; 14:248-254.
223. Twardowski ZJ, Prowant BF: Classification of normal and diseased exit sites. Perit Dial Int 1996; 16(suppl 3):S32-S50.
224. Gokal R, Alexander S, Ash S, et al: Peritoneal catheters and exit-site practices toward optimum peritoneal access: 1998 update. Perit Dial Int 1998; 18:11-33.
225. Holley JL, Foulks CJ, Moss AH, Willard D: Ultrasound as a tool in the diagnosis and management of exit site infections in patients undergoing continuous ambulatory peritoneal dialysis. Am J Kidney Dis 1989; 14:211-216.
226. Vychytil A, Lorenz M, Schneider B, et al: New criteria for management of catheter infections in peritoneal dialysis patients using ultrasonography. J Am Soc Nephrol 1998; 9:290-296.
227. Korzets Z, Erdberg A, Golan E, et al: Frequent involvement of the internal cuff segment in CAPD peritonitis and exit-site infection: An ultrasound study. Nephrol Dial Transplant 1996; 11:336-339.
228. Twardowski ZJ, Dobbie JW, Moore HL, et al: Morphology of peritoneal dialysis catheter tunnel: Macroscopy and light microscopy. Perit Dial Int 1991; 11:237-251.
229. Luzar MA, Coles GA, Faller B, et al: Staphylococcus aureus nasal carriage and infection in patients on continuous ambulatory peritoneal dialysis. N Engl J Med 1990; 322:505-509.
230. Zimakoff J, Bangsgaard Pedersen F, Bergen L, et al: Staphylococcus aureus carriage and infections among patients in four haemo- and peritoneal-dialysis centres in Denmark. The Danish Study Group of Peritonitis in Dialysis (DASPID). J Hosp Infect 1996; 33:289-300.
231. Lye WC, Leong SO, van der Straaten J, Lee EJ: Staphylococcus aureus CAPD-related infections are associated with nasal carriage. Adv Perit Dial 1994; 10:163-165.
232. Holley JL, Bernardini J, Piraino B: Risk factors for tunnel infections in continuous peritoneal dialysis. Am J Kidney Dis 1991; 18:344-348.
233. Vychytil A, Lorenz M, Schneider B, et al: New strategies to prevent Staphylococcus aureus infections in peritoneal dialysis patients. J Am Soc Nephrol 1998; 9:669-676.
234. Gokal R, Ash SR, Helfrich GB, et al: Peritoneal catheters and exit-site practices: Toward optimum peritoneal access. Perit Dial Int 1993; 13:29-39.
235. Sherman RA: Ophthalmic antibiotic solutions for equivocal exit sites. Semin Dial 1993; 6:327.
236. Wadhwa NK, Cabralda T, Suh H, et al: Exit-site/tunnel infection and catheter outcome in peritoneal dialysis patients. Adv Perit Dial 1992; 8:325-327.
237. Peng SJ, Yang CS, Ferng SH: The clinical experience and natural course of peritoneal catheter exit site infection among continuous ambulatory peritoneal dialysis patients. Dial Transplant 1998; 27:71-78.
238. Nichols WK, Nolph KD: A technique for managing exit site and cuff infection in Tenckhoff catheters. Perit Dial Bull 1983; 3(suppl 1):S4-S5.
239. Scalamogna A, De Vecchi A, Maccario M, et al: Cuff-shaving procedure. A rescue treatment for exit-site infection unresponsive to medical therapy. Nephrol Dial Transplant 1995; 10: 2325-2327.
240. Bazzato G: CAPD by means of double-bag, closed drainage infusion system. CAPD Proc Int Symp, Paris, 1979. Amsterdam, Excerpta Medica, 1980, pp 171-173.
241. Scalamogna A, De Vecchi A, Castelnovo C, et al: Long-term incidence of peritonitis in CAPD patients treated with the Y set technique: Experience in a single center. Nephron 1990; 55:24-27.
242. Burkart JM, Hylander B, Durnell-Figel T, Roberts D: Comparison of peritonitis rates during long-term use of standard spike versus ultraset in continuous ambulatory peritoneal dialysis. Perit Dial Int 1990; 10:41-43.
243. Prowant BF: Nursing interventions related to peritonitis. Adv Ren Replace Ther 1996; 3:237-239.
244. Dryden MS, Ludlam HA, Wing AJ, Phillips I: Active intervention dramatically reduces CAPD-associated infection. Adv Perit Dial 1991; 7:125-128.
245. Andrews PA, Warr KJ, Hicks JA, Cameron JS: Impaired outcome of continuous ambulatory peritoneal dialysis in immunosuppressed patients. Nephrol Dial Transplant 1996; 11:1104-1108.
246. Bernardini J, Piraino B, Holley J, et al: A randomized trial of Staphylococcus aureus prophylaxis in peritoneal dialysis patients: Mupirocin calcium ointment 2% applied to the exit site versus cyclic oral rifampin. Am J Kidney Dis 1996; 27: 695-700.
247. Mupirocin Study Group. Nasal mupirocin prevents Staphylococcus aureus exit-site infection during peritoneal dialysis. J Am Soc Nephrol 1996; 7:2403-2408.
248. Perez-Fontan M, Rosales M, Rodriguez-Carmona A, et al: Treatment of Staphylococcus aureus nasal carriers in CAPD with mupirocin. Adv Perit Dial 1992; 8:242-245.
249. Perez-Fontan M, Garcia-Falcon T, Rosales M, et al: Treatment of Staphylococcus aureus nasal carriers in continuous ambulatory peritoneal dialysis with mupirocin: Long-term results. Am J Kidney Dis 1993; 22:708-712.
250. Zimmerman SW, Ahrens E, Johnson CA, et al: Randomized controlled trial of prophylactic rifampin for peritoneal dialysis-related infections. Am J Kidney Dis 1991; 18:225-231.
251. Holley JL, Bernardini J, Piraino B: Infecting organisms in continuous ambulatory peritoneal dialysis patients on the Y-set. Am J Kidney Dis 1994; 23:569-573.
252. Scalamogna A, Castelnovo C, De Vecchi A, et al: Staphylococcus aureus exit-site and tunnel infection in CAPD. Adv Perit Dial 1990; 6:130-132.
253. Gadallah MF, Ramdeen G, Mignone J, et al: Role of preoperative antibiotic prophylaxis in preventing postoperative peritonitis in newly placed peritoneal dialysis catheters. Am J Kidney Dis 2000; 36:1014-1019.
254. Waite NM, Webster N, Laurel M, et al: The efficacy of exit site povidone-iodine ointment in the prevention of early peritoneal dialysis-related infections. Am J Kidney Dis 1997; 29:763-768.

255. Copley JB, Smith BJ, Koger DM: Prevention of postoperative peritoneal dialysis catheter related infections. Perit Dial Int 1988; 8:195-197.
256. Danielsson A, Blohme L, Tranaeus A, Hylander B: A prospective randomized study of the effect of a subcutaneously buried peritoneal dialysis catheter technique versus standard technique on the incidence of peritonitis and exit-site infection. Perit Dial Int 2002; 22:211-219.
257. Patel UD, Mottes TA, Flynn JT: Delayed compared with immediate use of peritoneal catheter in pediatric peritoneal dialysis. Adv Perit Dial 2001; 17:253-259.
258. Crabtree JH, Burchette RJ, Siddiqi RA, et al: The efficacy of silver-ion implanted catheters in reducing peritoneal dialysis-related infections. Perit Dial Int 2003; 23:368-374.
259. Wadhwa NK, Suh H, Cabralda T: Antifungal prophylaxis for secondary fungal peritonitis in peritoneal dialysis patients. Adv Perit Dial 1996; 12:189-191.
260. Robitaille P, Merouani A, Clermont MJ, Hebert E: Successful antifungal prophylaxis in chronic peritoneal dialysis: A pediatric experience. Perit Dial Int 1995; 15:77-79.
261. Lo WK, Chan CY, Cheng SW, et al: A prospective randomized control study of oral nystatin prophylaxis for Candida peritonitis complicating continuous ambulatory peritoneal dialysis. Am J Kidney Dis 1996; 28:549-552.
262. Zaruba K, Peters J, Jungbluth H: Successful prophylaxis for fungal peritonitis in patients on continuous ambulatory peritoneal dialysis: Six years' experience. Am J Kidney Dis 1991; 17: 43-46.
263. Li PK, Chow KM: How to have a successful PD programme. Perit Dial Int (In press).
264. Li PKT, Chow KM: How to have a successful PD programme? Perit Dial Int 2003; 23: S183-S187.

Metabolic and Noninfectious Complications of Peritoneal Dialysis

Sarah Prichard, M.D., F.R.C.P.C. • Joanne M. Bargman, M.D., F.R.C.P.C.

METABOLIC COMPLICATION OF PERITONEAL DIALYSIS

All renal failure patients face a number of metabolic disturbances that are the result of the uremic condition. These include acid-based abnormalities, disturbances of mineral metabolism, electrolyte imbalances, and nutritional disorders. This chapter focuses on the common systemic metabolic problems that are related specifically to the modality of peritoneal dialysis (PD).

Systemic Metabolic Effects of Glucose Dialysate

Glucose has served as the osmotic agent added to standard peritoneal dialysate since its inception. It has proven to be generally safe, inexpensive, and stable.[1] More recently there have been concerns about its local effect on the peritoneum.[2] Glucose and its degradation products have been implicated in the long-term changes that are seen in the structure and function of the peritoneum in long-standing peritoneal dialysis patients. There has been a search for an alternative to glucose as an osmotic agent since PD was introduced as a chronic therapy. Today amino acids and icodextrin, a glucose polymer, are used in many parts of the world as a glucose alternative in one exchange per day. However, glucose remains the standard osmotic agent in PD fluids in the majority of patients for the majority of their exchanges. Glucose has systemic metabolic effects that need to be understood and treated.[3,4]

Glucose Absorption

Glucose has a molecular weight of 180 and is easily transferred across the peritoneum by diffusion. Given that the normal blood sugar is approximately 5 mmol/L and that the 1.5%, 2.5%, and 4.25% glucose concentrations in PD fluids are approximately 80 mmol/L, 130 mmol/L, and 230 mmol/L, respectively, there is rapid absorption of glucose into the patient.[5] There is variability from patient to patient as to how much of the glucose is absorbed.[6] Based on the standard peritoneal equilibrium test (PET), at 4 hours, the concentration of glucose in the dialysate will have decreased by 20% to 80%.[7] This is usually expressed as a ratio of the concentration of dialysate glucose at the time of drainage (G_4) over its concentration at the time of infusion (G_0) and, together with the dialysate creatinine, serves to characterize a patient as being a rapid or slow transporter. Those who are rapid transporters will be subject to the greatest glucose loading with its positive and negative effects.[8]

The positive aspect of the glucose absorption is its contribution to the nutritional needs of the patients. Each gram of glucose absorbed contributes 4 calories. Thus, if a patient absorbs 50% of the glucose from a 1.5% 2-L bag, he or she will have absorbed 15 g of glucose and 60 calories. Because most patients use a prescription with variable glucose concentrations and, on average, approximately 60% of dialysate glucose is absorbed regardless of the bag used, the caloric intake from the dialysis alone can range from 300 to 800 calories per day. Current recommendations are that PD patients take in 35 calories/kg of body weight per day.[9] Yet many PD patients remain malnourished for a variety of reasons ranging from gastric motility disorders to depression. This dialysate glucose absorption makes an important contribution toward reaching the nutritional goal with respect to caloric intake.

Adverse Effects of Glucose Absorption

Hyperinsulinemia has been implicated as an important risk factor for the development of atherosclerosis.[10] Most all renal failure patients have insulin resistance.[11] Inevitably, insulin levels rise as glucose loading takes place during a PD exchange. Hyperinsulinemia has been suggested as one of the particular risk factors attributable to the renal failure population, who have such a high incidence of cardiovascular morbidity and mortality. Just how important this is as a cardiovascular risk factor remains uncertain. Rosiglitazone appears to improve insulin resistance and to decrease insulin levels in nondiabetic PD patients.[12]

Weight gain is common when patients start peritoneal dialysis.[13,14] Although part of this is attributable to the relief of uremic symptoms and overall improvement in nutritional status, at least part of the weight gain must be attributed to the caloric loading from the dialysate. In PD patients, the weight gain results in significant fat accumulation,[15–17] particularly an accumulation of abdominal fat.[18,19] This fat distribution is implicated as a risk factor for cardiovascular disease and is part of the metabolic syndrome characterized by abdominal obesity, insulin resistance, hyperlipidemia, and endothelial dysfunction. Type II diabetes remains the most common cause of renal failure in most parts of the world, and most of these patients already have the abnormalities associated with the metabolic syndrome. Thus, PD can further exaggerate these metabolic disturbances.[20,21] Recent studies have shown that low carbohydrate diets facilitate weight loss.[22,23] PD patients will always have carbohydrate loading through the dialysate and, therefore, this may impair weight loss as well as contribute to weight gain.

High transporters have been reported to have a worse outcome on PD.[24] These patients will have higher glucose absorption as well as greater protein losses across the peritoneum. Whether the high transporter status simply reflects an underlying higher comorbidity burden, an inflammatory state, or a predisposition to chronic fluid overload, is unknown.[25] A role for the glucose loading in contributing to that worse outcome cannot be excluded.

Studies have repeatedly demonstrated that a high body weight is associated with better, or is neutral with regard to, outcomes for dialysis patients.[13,26–30] This is the opposite to the general population.[31] The explanation for the protective effect of obesity in uremia remains uncertain. It could be that it is simply a marker for good nutrition. Interestingly, there are now studies that show obesity is associated with inflammation and worse outcomes in PD patients.[32,33] Therefore, obesity in PD patients, which, as noted, is abdominal obesity, may predispose them to metabolic changes that increase their risk for cardiovascular events. This remains speculative and is being further investigated.

Some patients who have no history of glucose intolerance will develop hyperglycemia following the initiation of PD. Tight glucose control has been found to reduce diabetic complications and may help to preserve residual renal function. Poor glycemic control at the initiation of dialysis is associated with worse outcomes.[34] Therefore, every effort should be made to keep patients euglycemic. Hyperglycemia needs to be corrected through judicious use of hypertonic PD solutions, diet, and medication. New insulin receptor sensitizing agents have proven to be effective in this regard and significantly reduce the insulin resistance.[12] Some patients require the initiation of hypoglycemic drugs and insulin. Current recommendations are to keep the hemoglobin A1C at less than 7.2% for patients on PD. Insulin therapy, when required, can be administered via a subcutaneous or intraperitoneal route, and some patients use a combination of administration of both routes.[35] Either strategy can result in good glucose control.[36]

PD patients with hyperglycemia are at particular risk for the development of hyperosmolar states. Since the peritoneum allows for sodium sieving, that is, the movement of water in excess of solute into the peritoneal cavity, PD patients will continue to lose water from the extracellular space in spite of hyperosmolality. In this regard, PD patients have the equivalent of an osmotic diuresis even in the absence of renal function. At the same time, their impaired renal function makes them incapable of conserving water. Furthermore, they drink fluids in response to the thirst stimulated by the hyperglycemia, which PD patients then try to remove by using more hypertonic PD solutions, causing more glucose loading, and a vicious cycle follows. It is, therefore, imperative that blood glucose levels be normalized.

All of these negative effects of glucose-based PD solutions have led investigators and clinicians to adopt a glucose sparing strategy in prescribing peritoneal dialysis[37] for patients who are at high risk for the adverse effects of glucose.[38,39] This includes the use of amino acid-based solutions, icodextrin, and minimizing the use of hypertonic glucose exchanges. There is evidence that the lipid profile of patients can be improved when daily amino acid and icodextrin exchanges are used to replace glucose-based exchanges. Insulin levels fall with the use of icodextrin.[40] However, detailed studies on the metabolic advantage of glucose sparing strategies in PD are not yet available.

DYSLIPIDEMIA IN PERITONEAL DIALYSIS

A great deal has been written about the lipid abnormalities found in patients with chronic kidney disease, including those requiring renal replacement therapy.[41,42] This keen interest in the lipid abnormalities arises from the search for treatable risk factors for cardiovascular disease in this population, in whom the rates of cardiovascular death are staggeringly high.

Patients on peritoneal dialysis have a variety of lipid abnormalities.[43–49] Typically, they have high total and low-density lipoprotein (LDL) cholesterol, high triglycerides, low high-density lipoprotein (HDL) cholesterol, high apolipoprotein B (apoB), low apoA-I, and high lipoprotein(a) [Lp(a)] levels. The apolipoprotein E genotype 2/3 is associated with high cholesterol and TG levels in PD patients.[50] Compared with hemodialysis patients, the most striking differences are the high apoB protein and LDL cholesterol levels, which are usually normal in hemodialysis patients.[51] Levels of oxidized LDL and antibodies to oxidized LDL are elevated in end-stage renal disease (ESRD) patients on both PD and hemodialysis.[52]

Intermediate density lipoprotein (IDL) levels are also elevated. These are the lipoprotein particles that are intermediate in size between VLDL and LDL, and an increase in their levels represents the delay in removal of the triglyceride component of the VLDL as it is transformed into the cholesterol ester rich LDL. These abnormalities are summarized in Table 30–1.

This lipid/lipoprotein profile of peritoneal dialysis is markedly atherogenic. The LDL particles are small and dense, indicated by the high apoB protein levels with modest elevations of LDL cholesterol.[47,53] Small, dense LDL particles are particularly atherogenic in that they cross the endothelium with greater ease and are oxidized more readily than larger LDL particles.

The pathogenesis of the overproduction of LDL particles in peritoneal dialysis remains obscure. Hypoalbuminemia secondary to peritoneal protein loss may partly contribute to the abnormality. In this regard, PD patients can be considered similar to patients with nephrotic syndrome. Studies using HepG2 cells, a cell line derived from hepatomas, suggest that low amino acid levels might also contribute to overproduction of the apolipoprotein B hepatic derived VLDL, which

Table 30–1 Lipid Abnormalities in End-Stage Renal Disease

Factor	PD	HD	
Total cholesterol		↑	normal
LDL cholesterol		↑	normal
HDL cholesterol	↓	↓	
Triglycerides	↑↑	↑	
Apo A1 protein	↓	↓	
Apo B protein	↑↑		normal
Lp(a)	↑↑	↑↑	
LDL oxidation	↑	↑	

PD, peritoneal dialysis; *HD,* hemodialysis; *LDL,* low-density lipoprotein; *HDL,* high-density lipoprotein; *Lp(a),* lipoprotein(a).

would account for the high LDL levels because LDL is derived from VLDL.[54,55] However, a randomized, controlled trial using a single daily amino acid exchange did not improve the lipid profile.[56] More recently, the use of an icodextrin to substitute for a glucose-based exchange did result in an improved lipid profile.[39] This implies that glucose loading may contribute to the dyslipidemia. Glucose can exacerbate hypertriglyceridemia in glucose intolerant patients. One study has reported that the use of amino acid dialysate increased homocysteine levels.[57] Therefore, the use of the new nonglucose-based solutions to modify the cardiovascular risk profile of patients cannot yet be strongly advocated.[58]

The high level of IDL is attributed to the overproduction of VLDL and to defective function of lipoprotein lipase. The low HDL levels seen in PD patients is also poorly understood, but the loss of HDL across the peritoneum may be a contributing factor.[59] High Lp(a) levels have been associated with malnutrition and inflammatory states and may simply be part of the overall inflammatory response, similar to the other observed elevations of acute phase reactants.

The hypertriglyceridemia (hyperTg) seen in peritoneal dialysis results from the overproduction of VLDLs and a deficiency in lipoprotein lipase. There may also be a partial deficiency of hepatic lipase. The pathogenesis of these abnormalities is not understood, but the use of glucose-based peritoneal dialysis solutions and a variety of drugs, such as β-blockers, aggravate the problem. The usual level of triglycerides seen in peritoneal dialysis patients is 220 to 400 mg/dL (2.5–4.5 mmol/ L), but levels greater than 530 mg/dL (6 mmol/L) are not unusual.

Compared with hemodialysis patients, PD patients have a more obviously atherogenic lipid profile. The importance of these abnormalities as a cardiovascular risk factor in renal failure patients remains uncertain. There are no clinical studies to demonstrate the efficacy of treating dyslipidemias in dialysis patients with respect to improving cardiovascular outcomes in PD patients. Furthermore, in many studies that have analyzed risk factors for cardiovascular disease in dialysis patients, lipids have often not been shown to confer significant risk in this population. The explanation for this difference in the role of lipids as a risk factor in renal failure patients compared to the general population in whom it is a very powerful risk factor, remains unclear. Perhaps other factors, such as inflammatory states,[60–64] abnormalities of mineral metabolism, and preexisting comorbidities, have such a powerful impact on outcome that the lipid profiles fail to emerge as significant. At least one study has linked coronary artery calcification with abnormal lipid profiles.[65] This implies that there could be an interaction or facilitation for calcification when dyslipidemia exists. Alternatively, since almost all dialysis patients have lipid abnormalities, it may not be a discriminating risk factor in this population.

In spite of this lack of data, guidelines from the International Society for Peritoneal Dialysis[66] and from the National Kidney Foundation Dialysis Outcomes Quality Initiative[67] (K/DOQI) recommend treating lipid abnormalities in all renal failure patients. The recommendations for treatment follow the same targets for therapy that are currently applied to patients in the general population who have known coronary artery disease. Thus, it has been the best judgment of experts that, notwithstanding a lack of clear evidence, and given the extraordinarily high rate of cardiovascular morbidity and mortality in renal failure patients, this patient population be regarded as having equivalent risk to someone with established coronary artery disease.

Treatment for PD patients with lipid abnormalities is usually successful in reaching the set targets for therapy. Although dietary and weight management is a strategy that can be applied to all patients, it has limitations in PD patients. Achieving adequate nutrition can be a challenge for all PD patients, and adding dietary restrictions for purposes of lipid management may compromise the patient's ability to achieve the daily nutritional goals that are recommended. Daily exercise and achieving optimal body weight might be desirable, but the patient's general condition can preclude an active exercise program, and weight loss plans could compromise the patient's nutritional status. Therefore, medications are the mainstay of lipid management in the PD population. Specifically, HMG Co-A reductase inhibitors (statins) are recommended as first-line drugs.[67] They have proven to be both safe and effective in studies of dialysis patients, including PD patients.[68] As in the general population, the most common side effects are muscle pain, elevations of creatine kinase, and, rarely, abnormalities of liver enzymes. Severe rhabdomyolysis is a rare but serious complication. It is recommended that the relevant muscle and liver enzymes be followed after a patient is started on a statin. However, only a small percentage of patients have enzyme abnormalities severe enough to warrant discontinuing the drug.

Fibrates as a class of drugs should be used with caution in renal failure.[67] They are excreted by the kidneys and dose adjustment is required. The combination of a statin and a fibrate is not recommended in dialysis patients.

Ezetimibe is the first of a new class of drug that blocks the absorption of cholesterol in the small intestine.[69] It usually lowers LDL cholesterol levels by approximately 20%. The drug has been reported to be safe in renal failure patients and might be a good option for patients who are intolerant of statins or for those who are unsuccessful in achieving the therapeutic target with statins alone.

Sevelamer, a noncalcium-based phosphate binder, has also been shown to reduce LDL and total cholesterol levels in hemodialysis patients by 20% on average.[70,71] Although no recommendation has been made to use sevelamer for the purpose of managing the lipid abnormalities found in dialysis patients, its lipid-lowering effect is a side effect of the drug that helps patients to achieve the therapeutic goal for their cholesterol.

Finally, with regard to the dialysis itself, the use of nonglucose-based dialysate has been shown to improve the lipid profile. Icodextrin, in particular, may have an advantage in this regard.[39]

PROTEIN LOSS

PD patients have lower serum albumin and total protein levels than hemodialysis patients, with typical values being 3.3 to 3.6 g/dL in PD patients. This is, at least in part, related to significant loss of protein across the peritoneum.[72] The loss is about 0.5 g/L of dialysate protien but can be higher and account for as much as 10 to 20 g/day in patients who are high transporters.[73–75] The major component of the protein losses is albumin, but immunoglobulin G (IgG) accounts for up to 15%.

Protein losses are greatest in high and high-average transporters. Amino acid losses of approximately 3 to 4 g/day also occur. Acute peritoneal inflammation, as seen in peritonitis, is associated with substantially greater protein losses, and a rapid reduction in serum albumin is common during episodes of peritonitis. Unresolving peritonitis is associated with protracted and exaggerated protein losses causing protein malnutrition. The protein loss itself sometimes becomes an indication to terminate peritoneal dialysis temporarily or, on occasion, permanently. In addition, inasmuch as peritoneal dialysis may help preserve residual renal function,[76] in patients with nephrotic syndrome, this preserved renal function may be at the cost of ongoing protein losses. Therefore, measurements of both peritoneal and urinary protein losses need to be evaluated in peritoneal dialysis patients, and appropriate dietary adjustments should be made.

Low serum albumin levels should not be attributed solely to protein loss in the dialysate and urine. Poor nutrition can occur because of persistent uremic symptoms due to under dialysis, gastroparesis, or other gastrointestinal pathologies,[77] depression, side effects of medications, and even limited financial resources to buy appropriate food.[78] Additionally, inflammatory states of known or unknown etiology are associated with low serum albumin levels.[79,80] Thus, a thorough evaluation of all PD patients is needed to appropriately assess the cause of low total serum protein and albumin levels.

Overall prognosis for PD patients is linked to hypoalbuminemia.[81] But the linkage between inflammatory conditions, as reflected by high C-reactive protein and Il-6 levels and hypoalbuminemia can make it difficult to ascertain how much of the low albumin level is actually due to the peritoneal losses.[82–84] There is also a linkage of markers of malnutrition to elevated homocysteine levels Lp(a) and other risk factors for cardiovascular disease.[85,86]

Amino acid dialysate was developed to serve as a nutritional supplement in response to the known protein losses of PD.[87–90] A 1.1% amino acid dialysate contains 22 g of amino acids and has an osmolality of 345 mmol/L, which is similar to a 1.5% glucose bag. It has proven to be safe and stable. Between 70% and 90% of the amino acids are absorbed in a 6-hour dwell. In a study of 20 patients, an average of 17.6 g of amino acids were absorbed with each 2-L exchange of 1.1% amino acid dialysate.[87] These patients went into positive nitrogen balance, but markers of improved nutritional status, such as serum albumin levels, did not significantly improve. Subsequent studies have failed to give convincing data to support the efficacy of amino acid based dialysate as an effective therapy for malnutrition in PD patients.[91] Amino acid dialysate has been found to reduce leptin levels, but the clinical significance of this is unclear.[92] New interest in amino acid solutions is now focused on its glucose sparing effect.

Patients with advanced liver disease and ascites have particularly large protein losses on PD. In spite of this concern, there are several series of such patients that report very successful use of PD as renal replacement therapy.[93] The dietary counseling of these patients should include consideration for the extra protein losses, but this should not preclude the use of PD, if the patient is otherwise suitable for PD. The caloric loading of glucose from the dialysate may be of special benefit to these challenging patients with advanced liver disease.

HYPONATREMIA/HYPERNATREMIA

Standard peritoneal dialysis solutions contain 132 mmol/L of sodium. Most patients maintain a normal serum sodium on peritoneal dialysis. With a better understanding of peritoneal physiology, we can now better account for observed changes in serum sodium in certain situations.[94–99] During an exchange, the dialysate sodium concentration falls early in the exchange as water moves across the endothelial aquaporin channels.[100] Sodium then moves into the peritoneum across the small pores, by diffusion. This dissociation of water and sodium movement across the peritoneal membrane accounts for the sodium sieving that has been observed since PD was started as a therapy.[101]

Hyponatremia

Patients who are excessive water drinkers can get a dilutional hyponatremia if the water intake exceeds the total water loss. The water losses in PD patients will be the sum of insensible losses, urinary free water clearance, and dialysate water losses. Insensible losses will vary according to the patient's losses through sweating, changes in body temperature, and respiratory losses. In this regard, PD patients are no different from the general population. In contrast, with loss of renal function, the ability to generate significant urinary free water loss is usually lost. The urine of patients with advanced renal failure is usually close to that of plasma. The water loss from dialysate occurs through the water channels and will increase with more hypertonic exchanges because the hypertonicity stimulates aquaporin function. But this water loss is a function of the peritoneal water channels and does not vary with water loading from diet. Therefore, even with the usual ongoing water losses, PD patients can become hyponatremic, if water intake is too large.

The use of icodextrin is associated with a small reduction in serum sodium levels.[102,103] In patients with marked hyperglycemia, hyponatremia can be seen as a result of water shifting into the extracellular fluid. Typically, the serum sodium falls about 1.3 mmol/L for each 100 mg/dL (5.6 mmol/L) rise in blood glucose. Finally, severe hyper Tg can also give hyponatremia, which is classified as factitious because it is caused by a reduction in the amount of water per liter of plasma rather than a true reduction of sodium per unit of plasma water.

Hypernatremia

With rapid ultrafiltration using hypertonic solutions, hypernatremia may occur due to the sieving effect of the peritoneal membrane on sodium. This is most pronounced in slower transporters, in whom the transfer of water across the ultrasmall pores, or aquaporin channels, remains in tact but the diffusion of sodium across the small and larger pores is relatively slow due to a reduction in the effective peritoneal surface area. Therefore, patients on frequent, short, hypertonic exchanges can become hypernatremic. Some authors have advocated a lower dialysate sodium concentration in hypertonic (4.25%) bags to enhance sodium removal by diffusion.

This same phenomenon accounts for the observation that some patients who change from CAPD to APD have a significant reduction in sodium removal across the peritoneum in spite of adequate fluid removal.[104] These patients maintain a good ultrafiltration volume, but because of the sodium sieving, the ultrafiltrate will be relatively hypotonic.

Correcting this problem requires that the exchanges be lengthened to allow sufficient time for sodium diffusion to take place.

HYPOKALEMIA/HYPERKALEMIA

Standard peritoneal dialysis solution contains no potassium. Potassium is removed during peritoneal dialysis by diffusion and convection; after a 4- to 6-hour exchange, the dialysate potassium level is slightly lower than plasma. As ultrafiltration increases, so will the removal of potassium. Total potassium losses through dialysis closely relate to total sodium losses.[105] For patients draining 10 L of dialysate daily, potassium loss through the dialysis would be 35 to 50 mmol/day, depending on the serum potassium level. Residual renal function may allow the further output of 10 to 30 mmol of potassium per day. These renal and peritoneal outputs of potassium are insufficient to account for the usual 80 mmol of potassium intake in most patients. Yet most patients maintain a normal serum potassium.[106] It is concluded, therefore, that in renal failure, gastrointestinal secretion of potassium is enhanced.[107]

Usually, only patients who are noncompliant in performing their dialysis exchanges or who have excessive potassium intake have ongoing problems with hyperkalemia. Medications, such as β-blockers and ACE inhibitors, may exaggerate the problem. Treatment of hyperkalemia in a PD patient is similar to HD and includes dietary counseling, increased dialysis, medication changes, and, occasionally, the addition of potassium binders. In acute renal failure treated with PD, hyperkalemia has been reported.[108]

Hypokalemia is reported in 10% to 30% of CAPD patients.[109] Occasionally, it is profound when associated with vomiting and diarrhea.[110] However, most cases are associated with poor nutritional intake, and most can be managed by liberalizing the diet. Increased bowel losses and the intracellular shift of potassium may also play a role. The high intracellular muscle content of potassium observed in PD patients supports this latter mechanism.[111]

The abnormal potassium metabolism of end-stage renal disease has been implicated in the high level of cardiac morbidity and mortality, and treatment is recommended.[112] Persistent levels lower than 3 mmol/L should be managed with potassium supplementation. For patients on digoxin, potassium levels are recommended to be kept above 3.5 mmol/L. Potassium chloride can be added to the dialysate, if necessary, but the risk of errors and infection make this option less attractive than oral supplementation for patients at home. Patients in a hospital setting, in whom intensive PD is being prescribed and oral intake is reduced, may benefit from adding the KCl to the dialysate, usually 2 to 4 mmol/L, but higher levels can be used when appropriate. In a case report, 20 mmol/L of KCl was added and the rate of increase in the serum potassium was 0.44 mmol/L over 2 to 3 hours.[113] The toxicity of high intraperitoneal potassium levels is unknown, and its use should be reserved for the short-term treatment of an urgent situation.

HYPOCALCEMIA/HYPERCALCEMIA

Peritoneal dialysis solutions are available with 2.5 mEq/L (1.25 mmol/L) or 3.5 mEq/L (1.75 mmol/L) calcium.[114–116] The standard solution is now considered to be the 2.5 mmol/L calcium solution.

Calcium balance with regard to the dialysis itself depends on the patient's serum calcium level, the dialysate calcium concentration, and the rate of ultrafiltration.[117–125] At the end of a 6-hour exchange, the dialysate calcium concentration is close to that of plasma. Given that the normal serum ultrafiltrable calcium is 1.12 to 1.33 mmol/L, when a 1.75 mmol/L bag is used, there will be a net gain of calcium by the patient. In the absence of ultrafiltration, the patient gains approximately 30 mg of calcium. With a large ultrafiltration, there can be a negative balance for calcium. However, over the course of a day, most patients will use a mix of hypertonic and less hypertonic exchanges, and the total calcium balance with respect to the dialysis, using the 1.75 mmol/L dialysate, will be positive. When this is added to the calcium absorbed from calcium-based phosphate binders, the net calcium balance can be positive by as much as 400 to 700 mg/day.[126] In contrast, the 1.25 mmol/L calcium solution will give neutral calcium balance in the absence of ultrafiltration. The larger the volume of drainage, the greater the output of calcium through the dialysis.[127,128] The net effect is that, on most exchanges with any degree of ultrafiltration, the 1.25 mmol/L calcium solution will put the patients in slightly negative balance for calcium with respect to the dialysis itself.[90] There are increases in serum PTH levels reported with the use of the low calcium solutions, which may be beneficial to patients with low turnover bone disease.[129,130] However, most patients remain in neutral or positive balance overall for calcium, using the 1.25 mmol/L calcium dialysate because of the high oral intake of calcium from diet and calcium-based phosphate binders. As concerns increase with regard to the risks of hyperphosphatemia,[131] phosphate binders, most commonly calcium-based phosphate binders, are prescribed in almost all dialysis patients. This likely accounts for the observation that hypercalcemia is frequent in PD and that the most common form of bone disease seen in PD patients is low turnover bone disease, with low PTH levels, which is unrelated to aluminum toxicity.[132]

Currently, there are concerns about widespread vascular and valvular calcification in dialysis patients, including PD patients.[133–137] This is often associated with other markers of inflammation and lipid abnormalities, although it is unclear whether the calcification is causal or secondary to the inflammation.[65] Because of these issues, the K/DOQI guidelines for bone metabolism and disease recommend the use of the physiologic 1.25 mmol/L calcium PD dialysate as the appropriate first-line solution for almost all PD patients.[138] Although sevelamer has not been studied in PD patients, its effect to reduce the progression of vascular calcification in hemodialysis patients has also led to its use in the PD population.[70] When noncalcium-based phosphate binders are not used in a PD patient, and the 1.25 mmol/L dialysate is used, the patients will often be in negative calcium balance, depending on the dietary intake of calcium. PTH rises when sevelamer replaces calcium-based binders in PD patients with low turnover bone disease.[139]

Hypocalcemia

Hypocalcemia is not common in patients initiating dialysis treatment because of the widespread use of calcium-based phosphate binders and vitamin D. When it does occur, it can be managed with calcium and vitamin D supplements and, when necessary, the use of 1.75 mmol/L calcium dialysate. This high-calcium dialysate brings about a net positive transfer of calcium to all patients except those with continuous high ultrafiltration. Patients using the higher calcium dialysate should be monitored for hypercalcemia and decreasing PTH levels. If either occur, they should be switched to the lower 1.25 mmol/L calcium solution.

There are a few case reports of hypocalcemia post parathyroidectomy, which were managed by the addition of calcium to the peritoneal dialysate.[140]

Hypercalcemia

Hypercalcemia is common in peritoneal dialysis patients, which, together with low PTH levels and low turnover bone disease, requires a strategy to correct the problem. It is usually the result of large doses of calcium supplements being used as phosphate binders and/or from inappropriate use of vitamin D and/or dialysis using the higher calcium dialysate. The use of the lower calcium dialysate, noncalcium-based phosphate binders, and the discontinuation of vitamin D supplementation are required in this situation. Recommendations in this regard are reviewed in the K/DOQI guidelines on bone disease, calcium, and phosphate.[138]

Peritoneal dialysis has occasionally been used in the treatment of severe hypercalcemia, using either the commercially available 1.25 mmol/L solution or a locally prepared calcium-free dialysate.[141–144]

ELEVATED SERUM LACTATE

The usual base in peritoneal dialysis solutions is lactate. The lactate is metabolized by the liver to bicarbonate. Under most circumstances, the liver's ability to metabolize lactate easily exceeds the daily delivery of lactate. However, patients on oral hypoglycemic agents (metformin and related compounds), with advanced liver disease, and with thiamine deficiency may not have sufficient reserve to handle the lactate load of peritoneal dialysis, and a lactic acidosis may ensue. In patients with ongoing lactic acidosis, as in patients with acute hepatic failure or other conditions seen in the intensive care setting, the addition of lactate-containing peritoneal dialysis solutions may exacerbate the problem. In such cases, bicarbonate-based solutions should be used. These are commercially available in many countries but may be locally prepared if necessary. See the chapter on PD solutions for a full discussion on the use of bicarbonate-based solutions.

NONINFECTIOUS COMPLICATIONS OF PERITONEAL DIALYSIS

Peritoneal dialysis is a home-based therapy that lends the patient autonomy to manage most aspects of treatment. It is evident to those who care for these patients that this modality of dialysis is underappreciated and underused in many parts of the world. There are many reasons for this, but part of the problem may be unfamiliarity or even discomfort with the unique complications that can occur in association with peritoneal dialysis.

The purpose of this chapter is to discuss some problems that can be encountered with the use of peritoneal dialysis. Some, like hernias, are common and not usually serious; others, like encapsulating peritoneal sclerosis, are very rare but result in marked morbidity and mortality for the patient. It is crucial that those who look after patients on peritoneal dialysis be familiar with the diagnosis and management of these noninfectious complications.

Hemoperitoneum

Bloody peritoneal dialysate, or hemoperitoneum, is an occasional complication of peritoneal dialysis that can be very distressing to the patient. Many of the causes of intraperitoneal bleeding occur also in individuals not on PD but remain clinically unnoticed. However, since peritoneal dialysis offers a "window" into the peritoneal cavity, the bleeding is detectable because it appears as a bloody effluent. So, for example, the intraperitoneal bleeding associated with menstruation probably occurs very frequently but is routinely seen only in the menstruating woman on peritoneal dialysis.

Causes of hemoperitoneum can be divided into those that likely occur routinely but remain undetected, such as menstruation, and those related to the peritoneal dialysis procedure itself and would not otherwise occur if the patient were not on PD. An example of the latter cause would be the traumatic laceration of an intraperitoneal blood vessel by the peritoneal dialysis catheter. Another way of subdividing the causes of hemoperitoneum is the benign versus more sinister causes of bleeding.

A recent review of recurrent hemoperitoneum reported that 46 of 549 (8.4%) of PD patients had at least one episode of hemoperitoneum during their time on PD, and half of these patients had recurrent episodes.[145] An earlier study found a similar incidence: 26 of 424 (6.1%) patients on peritoneal dialysis had one or more episodes of this complication.[146] Looked at another way, hemoperitoneum was temporally associated with the menses in over half of menstruating women on peritoneal dialysis.[147,148]

The majority of episodes of bloody dialysis effluent are indeed the result of menstruation.[145,146] There are two ways that menses can lead to blood in the peritoneal cavity. In the case of retrograde menstruation, the uterine blood is expelled not only through the cervix, but also with uterine contraction, retrogradely through the Fallopian tubes, which open into the peritoneal cavity. Therefore, intraperitoneal bleeding may occur regularly in this way and becomes obvious in the patient routinely draining intraperitoneal fluid as part of dialysis. Another possible cause for hemoperitoneum is studding of the intraperitoneal cavity, a known site for endometriosis, with ectopic endometrial tissue. The endometrial tissue sheds at the same time, under the same hormonal influence, as the intrauterine endometrium as part of the menstrual cycle. This could be a situation analogous to the cyclic pulmonary bleeding seen when ectopic endometrium is deposited in the lungs or pleura.[149]

Although the majority of episodes of hemoperitoneum are associated with menstruation, there are many other causes reported in the literature (see Table 30–2). It is clear that in the nonmenstruating individual other causes should be sought, and some of these may be serious.

Although there seems to be little in the way of long-term sequelae to hemoperitoneum, a more immediate worry is that the intraperitoneal blood may coagulate in and around the intraperitoneal portion of the dialysis catheter and lead to its obstruction. Although this appears to be an uncommon complication, it is recommended that heparin be instilled in the peritoneal fluid for as long as blood or fibrin is visible. The administration of anticoagulation in the setting of bleeding may sound counterintuitive, but the heparin does not exacerbate the bleeding of the most common causes, menstruation and ovulation. With other causes, the risk of heparinization worsening the bleeding would have to be weighed against the risk of the blood clotting inside the PD catheter, jeopardizing the whole PD process. In addition, since a negligible amount of heparin administered by this route is absorbed systemically, it is safe to give in patients in whom systemic anticoagulation is contraindicated. However, little is known about the use of intraperitoneal heparin in a patient with heparin-induced thrombocytopenia (HIT). In the absence of any evidence, it is best to avoid heparin in these patients because of the possibility that IP heparin may serve as an antigenic stimulus and a source of ongoing production of antibodies directed against that protein.

At the first appearance of bloody effluent, the patient should undertake a flush of the peritoneal cavity, which may be helpful in some instances to clear the blood and blood products. If it is not uncomfortable, the patient could also try infusing unwarmed dialysate, at room temperature. Because the temperature of the dialysis fluid is cooler than core body temperature, the consequent vasospasm may stop the source of the bleeding.[169] This maneuver would be particularly helpful in cases of hemoperitoneum from trauma induced by the PD catheter. This is analogous to patients who have blood in the peritoneal cavity at the end of PD catheter insertion, where flushing may be important to ensure the patency of the catheter.[159]

It is important to warn females of menstrual age that they may see bloody effluent at the time of ovulation or menstruation. The amount of blood loss is usually insignificant, but it can make the liters of fluid in the drain bag appear overtly bloody, falsely magnifying the amount of blood loss.

The diagnostic approach to the patient who presents with hemoperitoneum depends on the clinical setting. In a menstruating female, there is no need to undertake an extensive investigation, if the patient is otherwise well. However, if the bloody effluent is unassociated with menses, then investigation should include at least an abdominal ultrasound, which can screen for pathology of several of the implicated organs, including liver, spleen, and kidneys. The coagulation profile should be checked, along with the hemoglobin concentration, although hemoperitoneum infrequently leads to serious blood loss. As shown in the table, hemoperitoneum may be the first presentation of encapsulating peritoneal sclerosis, and this should be kept in mind, if bleeding occurs with no other explanation in the long-term PD patient.

Follow-up studies in patients who have experienced one or many episodes of hemoperitoneum suggest that the presence of the blood does not act as a growth medium for bacteria, leading to peritonitis.[145] Furthermore, the blood itself does not appear to compromise the integrity of the peritoneum or the ability to continue peritoneal dialysis.[145,170]

Table 30–2 Causes of Hemoperitoneum other than Menstruation

Cause or Disease	Reference
Rupture of the liver	150
Rupture of the spleen	151–153
Hepatocellular carcinoma and other liver tumors	154–157
Insertion of the PD catheter	158, 159
Acute systemic cytomegalovirus (CMV) infection	160
Bleeding diathesis/systemic anticoagulation	153
Colonic perforation as presentation of dialysis-associated amyloidosis	161
Retroperitoneal hematoma	162
Post-pericardiocentesis	163
Polycystic kidney or liver disease	164
Renal cell carcinoma	164
Ruptured ovarian cysts	166
Ovulation	147
Encapsulating peritoneal sclerosis (sclerosing peritonitis)	148
Spontaneous hematoma of iliopsoas muscle	167
Collagen vascular disease	160
Tuberous sclerosis	168

ENCAPSULATING PERITONEAL SCLEROSIS

Encapsulating peritoneal sclerosis (EPS) is one of the most dreaded complications of peritoneal dialysis. It was previously referred to as sclerosing encapsulating peritonitis (SEP), but given its chronic, noninflammatory characteristics, it less resembles "peritonitis" than a progressive sclerosing condition.

Literature on this condition is difficult to reconcile, given the inherent rarity of this complication, the differing rates of incidence in different countries, and a lack of uniformity in defining what constitutes the EPS syndrome.

The "classic" syndrome occurs in a long-term peritoneal dialysis patient and may be temporally associated with a severe case of bacterial peritonitis, especially if this has necessitated PD catheter removal and transfer to hemodialysis. In this classic scenario, some time afterward, the patient develops nonspecific complaints of anorexia and abdominal discomfort, which then progresses to malnutrition and recurrent episodes of small bowel or, less commonly, large bowel obstruction. Radiographic imaging typically shows thickened peritoneal membrane binding down or encapsulating loops of bowel. If laparotomy is undertaken, a thick cocoon of fibrous tissue can often be seen overlying and binding down underlying bowel.

In the case of the syndrome outlined previously, the diagnosis is straightforward, although if the patient has been changed to hemodialysis for awhile, the connection of symptoms to a complication of peritoneal dialysis may not be obvious. The patient may develop hemoperitoneum as in the case of the PD patient, but this would not be detected unless paracentesis is undertaken.[171] It is possible, therefore, that the incidence of EPS is underestimated, if the diagnosis is not considered in former PD patients who have been transplanted or transferred to hemodialysis. On the other hand, this condition can also be overestimated. For example, a thickened or even calcified peritoneal membrane[172,173] does not in itself constitute a diagnosis of EPS. Labeling long-term PD patients with anatomic changes in the peritoneal membrane as suffering from EPS will necessarily overestimate the incidence. These uncertainties must be kept in mind when discussing this condition.

Much of the literature on EPS comes from Japan, where, as a result of the low rate of renal transplantation, patients who undertake peritoneal dialysis tend to stay on this modality for a long time. A recent analysis from Japan[174] has shown that the incidence of EPS in patients on PD for less than 5 years is 0.3%, for 5 to 10 years is 4.5%, and rises to 7.1% in those who have been on this dialysis modality for more than 10 years. Similar values have been reported from Australia.[175] Given that patients in other countries tend to not stay on PD for as long as they do in Japan, these results are consistent with reports of a 0.5% to 1.5% prevalence elsewhere.[176–179]

Identified risk factors for the development of EPS include long duration of PD, an initial rapid transporter state, the use of more hypertonic glucose dialysate (which could be consequent to the rapid transporter status and unrelated to the development of EPS), and severe or recurrent episodes of peritonitis.[171] When this syndrome was first described, putative risk factors also included the use of acetate, instead of lactate, as the buffer in dialysis fluid, and spraying the catheter connection device with antiseptics such as chlorhexidine.[180,181] However, even though both of these practices have been discontinued, EPS continues to complicate peritoneal dialysis. Since the β-blocker practolol was withdrawn from patient use because of the development of retroperitoneal fibrosis,[182] inquiry has been made into a possible association between the use of β-blockers in general and the development of EPS.[183] Once again, however, given the rarity of this complication, it is difficult to pinpoint epidemiologic links. The observation that high transporters may be more prone to develop EPS suggests that subclinical inflammation may predispose to this complication. Interestingly, in one large center, the only two patients who developed EPS both had active systemic lupus erythematosus, which can lead to peritoneal inflammation as part of the polyserositis seen in this condition.[177] Perhaps EPS is the result of a "two hit" model, where the peritoneum is primed by one risk factor (such as long-term PD, serositis, β-blockade), but the disease is set off by another factor, such as an episode of peritonitis.

The clinical presentation of established disease has been outlined earlier. Certainly the onset of recurrent bowel obstruction in a patient on PD, or formerly on PD, should suggest the possibility of EPS. Investigators in Japan have suggested that there may be an earlier, more inflammatory stage, where there is a window of opportunity to better treat and, perhaps, reverse this complication. The earlier inflammatory stage is reported to be characterized by fever, increased C-reactive protein levels, and episodes of abdominal ileus.[184] If the patient is no longer on peritoneal dialysis, abdominal ascites may be noted.[183,171] It had been suggested previously that the acquisition of a "slow transporter" state coincident with poor ultrafiltration (type II ultrafiltration failure) may herald this complication, but this has not been a general observation.

Computer tomographic (CT) images of the abdomen reveal a thickened, dense peritoneal membrane that binds down loops of bowel. There may be air-fluid levels consistent with associated bowel obstruction.[185,186] The presence of intraperitoneal fluid in a patient no longer on PD may also be consistent with this diagnosis but is not the same condition as the poorly-understood "post peritoneal dialysis ascites" syndrome, which is usually not associated with disturbances of bowel motility and gradually resolves without specific treatment. It is important to note that the isolated finding of a thickened or calcified peritoneal membrane, in the absence of symptoms, also does not make a diagnosis of EPS. Many long-term PD patients will have these anatomic changes in the peritoneal membrane without any sequelae. Some reports suggest that on ultrasound there is a distinct trilaminar appearance to the membrane, with a lucent zone sandwiched between two more dense layers.[185]

Pathologic findings are perhaps what would be expected from the description earlier. The peritoneal membrane is densely fibrotic, with little in the way of active inflammation.[187] The fibrosis may encroach into the bowel wall itself[188] or extend transmurally.[189] Foci of calcification, and even ossification may be found.[188]

Treatment is difficult, and there is a high mortality rate. In the early inflammatory state, if it is recognized, pulse corticosteroids have been recommended.[184] This may be a difficult decision to make in the subclinical stage, because high dose corticosteroid therapy is not without risk. Further, it isn't clear which patient is going to proceed to the more established syndrome.

In established disease, therapy is based on three approaches, alone or in combination:

- Nutritional support, including parenteral feeding
- Anti-inflammatory and antifibrotic medication
- Emergent or planned surgical intervention

Much of the high mortality rate is the result of progressive malnutrition. Therefore, careful attention has to be paid to nutritional supplementation through the use of pureed feeds or other easily digested supplements. In those patients in whom enteral nutrition has become impossible, total parenteral nutrition is another option. Frequently, these patients have been converted already to hemodialysis, and therefore have vascular access. Intrahemodialytic parenteral nutrition can be administered, although a regimen of 4 hours thrice weekly may be too intermittent to effect a significant improvement in nutritional status,[190] and the patient may need ongoing total parenteral nutrition.[184,191] There has been a long-standing interest in the use of anti-inflammatory or immunosuppressive medications, such as corticosteroids and azathioprine, for treatment of this disorder.[192–194] Reports of treatment remain anecdotal, however. It is reasonable to conclude that corticosteroids are likely more effective in any earlier, inflammatory stage of the disease, rather than when the sclerosis and fibrosis are well established. In the latter case, there are reports of the use of antifibrotic medications. Tamoxifen, better known for its role in treating breast cancer, has antifibrotic properties. There are case reports of the use of tamoxifen in EPS[195] with benefit. The antifibrotic and immunosuppressive agent colchicine has also been reported to be helpful in one patient.[196] The antirejection drug sirolimus also has antifibrotic properties and has been advocated as a treatment for EPS[197] but, again, the rarity of this condition, and the variation in definition and outcome parameters make these claims difficult to assess.

Surgical intervention in the emergent setting is usually done for unremitting obstruction or secondary bowel perforation. The mortality rate is extremely high when surgery is done for these reasons. More attention, however, is being paid to planned surgical intervention with careful adhesiolysis and enterolysis. Careful release of intestinal loops, reexposing peritoneal surface area (neoperitonization), and avoiding primary anastomosis in the case of enterectomy, appears to be associated with a good outcome in a subset of patients.[184,198,199] Bowel perforation must be avoided at all costs, as it is associated with an early septic death.[184]

A basic question, which remains unanswered, is whether the patient, when first diagnosed, should be intentionally left on peritoneal dialysis to keep the loops of bowel "afloat," or whether it is best to change the patient to hemodialysis. Clearly, if the peritoneal dialysis is not working, then the patient must necessarily change to hemodialysis, although one could keep the peritoneal catheter in situ to periodically flush out the peritoneal cavity. On the other hand, change to hemodialysis and keeping the peritoneal membrane empty of fluid will allow the (inflamed?) loops of bowel to be in close contact with each other, and perhaps that is how a cocoon of fibrosis is able to encapsulate the loops of bowel. There are reports of good outcome in changing patients with EPS to hemodialysis,[199] but the decision must be weighed against the risk of accelerating the process with a dry abdomen.

COMPLICATIONS OF PD-RELATED INCREASED INTRA-ABDOMINAL PRESSURE

The instillation of dialysis fluid into the peritoneal cavity leads to increased pressure within this cavity. Patients new to PD will often comment on this sensation of tightness and raised intra-abdominal pressure. The pressure effects have been studied by introducing a pressure transducer into the peritoneal dialysis system.[200,201] Factors that increase the intra-abdominal pressure include increasing volume of dialysis fluid, increased body mass index, and the sitting and standing position compared to the supine position. Furthermore, coughing, straining at stool, and lifting weights are all associated with increases in the pressure. Indeed, coughing and straining at stool are associated with very high pressures for the duration of those activities.[200] These observations are important in managing complications in PD related to raised intra-abdominal pressure. These pressures can be reduced by having the patient assume the supine position during dialysis and by the use of smaller dwell volumes.

Hydrothorax in Peritoneal Dialysis

An interesting, but uncommon, complication of peritoneal dialysis is movement of dialysate from the peritoneal to the pleural cavity resulting in a pleural effusion composed of peritoneal dialysis fluid. This complication is referred to as *hydrothorax.* It shares much in common with "hepatic hydrothorax," where ascitic fluid migrates across the hemidiaphragm into the pleural space.

A recent review of 10 major series reporting hydrothorax between 1978 and 2002 found that the incidence of this complication ranged between 1.0% and 5.1%, with an average of 1.9%.[202] It is possible that some patients have a chronic mild hydrothorax that does not come to clinical attention, and so the incidence may be even higher.

The commonest presentation is shortness of breath, commensurate with a large pleural effusion. Rarely, we have seen patients complain of some chest discomfort. In the asymptomatic patients, the pleural effusion may be found incidentally during radiography or CT scanning done for some other reason. Other causes of pleural effusion, such as pulmonary embolism, tuberculosis, or congestive heart failure, need to be considered. However, since hydrothorax usually occurs soon after commencing peritoneal dialysis, the clinical presentation should suggest itself. Since many dialysis patients who are short of breath have fluid overload and congestive heart failure, the inclination may be to use more hypertonic dialysate to increase ultrafiltration. However, in the case of hydrothorax, increased ultrafiltration will increase intraperitoneal volume and pressure. This may encourage even more dialysis fluid to migrate across the hemidiaphragm, worsening, rather than improving, the symptoms. Therefore, the worsening of breathlessness with the use of hypertonic dialysate should suggest the possibility of dialysis-associated hydrothorax.

Sometimes hydrothorax does not occur at the beginning of peritoneal dialysis, but months to years later. It has been observed that hydrothorax can develop at the time of peritonitis, suggesting that defects in the diaphragm may somehow be exacerbated by the intraperitoneal infection.[203,204] A transient increase in intra-abdominal pressure can also predispose to acute hydrothorax. This phenomenon has been reported after a fit of coughing[205] or with the use of abdominal corsets.[206] A patient on peritoneal dialysis who fell and broke two left ribs developed hydrothorax on the left side, wherein it was postulated that the flail ribs tore diaphragmatic muscle fibers, allowing a conduit for the dialysate to enter the pleural space.[207] Patients with polycystic kidney disease may also be more at risk for hydrothorax.[208] One explanation is that the large kidneys occupy more space in the abdominal cavity, thereby leading to increased intra-abdominal pressure. Another possibility is that defects in the hemidiaphragm are more examples of the multiple defects in connective tissue seen in this disorder.

Interestingly, most series report a female predominance with hydrothorax.[208–213] The exception is reported from a large collaborative study in Japan, where the majority (54%) of the 50 patients with hydrothorax were male. However, the sex distribution of the PD population as a whole was not given, so that the 46% who were female may have still been a relative overrepresentation.[214] The reason for the predominance of females is unexplained, although stretching of the diaphragm as a result of previous pregnancy has been suggested.[203]

The dialysis fluid must traverse the hemidiaphragm to enter the pleural cavity. The pathway is felt to consist of congenital or acquired defects in the structure of the diaphragm. During development, pleuroperitoneal membranes form to separate the thoracic from the abdominal cavity, and myoblasts populate the membranes to form the muscular component of the diaphragm. Defects in this process, perhaps combined with raised abdominal pressure, can lead to gaps and herniations of this structure.[215] Autopsy studies have demonstrated discontinuities in the tendinous portions of the hemidiaphragms, and absence of the normal muscle fibers, which have been replaced by a disordered collagen network.[203,216] In some instances the weaker diaphragmatic tissue balloons into the pleural space, resulting in "blebs" that can be detected on inspection at surgery or thoracoscopy. In other instances these blebs have appeared to broken open completely, leaving a pathway of free communication across the hemidiaphragm between the peritoneal and pleural space.[216] Because of the higher intraperitoneal pressure, fluid will move along the pressure gradient from the intraperitoneal to intrapleural space, but a valve effect may stop the fluid from moving in the opposite direction. Others have suggested that the movement of fluid and particulate matter from the peritoneal to pleural space may occur through diaphragmatic lymphatics rather than discrete interruptions in the hemidiaphragm.[217] If the lymphatics contribute to this complication, however, it is likely in only a minority of cases.

Another interesting feature of the hydrothorax associated with peritoneal dialysis is that it is almost always on the right side. This is also seen in hepatic hydrothorax[215] and in ectopic endometriosis syndromes. Indeed, a review of thoracic endometriosis demonstrated that the pulmonary complications occurred in the right lung in more than 90% of cases.[149] Explanations include the observation that the right hemidiaphragm is more vulnerable to embryologic variation; that the heart and pericardium cover much of the left hemidiaphragm and so protect against the development of free communication between the peritoneal and pleural cavities; and that the solid fixed liver acts as a piston across the right side, whereas the increased mobility of the left subphrenic organs minimize spikes in pressure on that side.[218] Peritoneal dialysate has also been found in the pericardial space under extraordinary circumstances. In one case the patient had an indwelling pigtail catheter in the pericardial space for drainage of a pericardial effusion presumed secondary to uremic pericarditis. Pericardial fluid reaccumulated with the characteristics of PD fluid, and it was felt that the catheter had been the connection between the peritoneal and pericardial spaces.[219] In another patient whose pericardium had been disrupted for aortic valve surgery, massive pericardial effusion, composed of dialysate, developed.[220]

The diagnosis is straightforward when the patient, usually female, presents with sudden onset of shortness of breath at the initiation of peritoneal dialysis and chest X-ray shows a right-sided pleural effusion. As mentioned earlier, other causes of pleural effusion should be considered, especially if it is left-sided or in a clinical setting different from the one described. Hydrothorax from peritoneal dialysate can be usually confirmed by thoracentesis or imaging studies.

Thoracentesis is not only helpful for diagnosis but can be very effective to rapidly improve the dyspnea. The withdrawn fluid should have the characteristics of the dialysis fluid and so should be transudative. The LDH levels and white blood cell count are low. Because the glucose concentration in conventional peritoneal dialysis fluid is very high, in most instances the pleural fluid in the hydrothorax will be similarly elevated. Therefore, the finding of markedly elevated glucose concentration above blood glucose is virtually diagnostic of dialysate hydrothorax and obviates the need for further diagnostic study. However, if the fluid has been left in the pleural cavity for many hours, it is possible that the glucose can diffuse out of the pleural cavity along its concentration gradient, in which case the fluid may have a falsely normal glucose concentration. In other words, a very high glucose rules in the diagnosis of hydrothorax, but a normal glucose concentration does not rule it out. A recent study has suggested that if the pleural fluid glucose concentration is at least 50 mg/dL (2.8 mmol/L) higher than simultaneous blood glucose, then the pleural fluid is composed of peritoneal dialysate.[212] However, there have been subsequent reports where the glucose gradient was less than 50 mg/dL.[213]

Diagnostic and therapeutic thoracentesis is perhaps the most efficient way to confirm dialysis hydrothorax and relieve symptoms with one maneuver. In some instances, however, it may not be feasible to perform thoracentesis. Examples include an anticoagulated patient, a small pleural effusion that may not be amenable to drainage, or multiple comorbid conditions. In the case that thoracentesis is not done, there are other studies, which can document movement of dialysate from peritoneal to pleural cavity.

It has been previously recommended to instill a dye, such as methylene blue, into the peritoneal cavity, and then subsequently sample the pleural fluid to detect a blue coloration.[221] This technique should be used with caution. First, methylene blue can act as a chemical irritant to the peritoneum, causing additional discomfort to what is already a source of distress to the patient.[222,223] Second, there are many false negatives with this procedure, where, despite a leak, no obvious blue color appears in the pleural fluid.[213,224]

Peritoneal scintigraphy involves the instillation of radiolabel along with dialysate into the peritoneum. Examples of radiolabel include Technetium-99m macroaggregated human albumin,[225] and Technetium-99m sulphur colloid.[226–229] The macroaggregated albumin is larger than sulphur colloid and, theoretically, may more easily demonstrate the large defects felt to be responsible for the leakage across the diaphragm. However, one form has not been found to be uniformly superior to the other. Doses of radioisotope have ranged from 0.5 to 10 mCi. Subsequent scanning with a gamma camera can then locate radioactivity extending above the diaphragm, thereby demonstrating the peritoneal-pleural communication. There appears to be variability in the time it takes for the radioligand to cross the diaphragm, likely related to the size and patency of the diaphragmatic defect. It is recommended that the patient ambulate after instillation of the dialysate and label to increase the intra-abdominal pressure and facilitate the efflux of the dialysate from the peritoneal cavity.

Magnetic resonance imaging can be used to detect abnormal movement of dialysate. It has been used without gadolinium to detect dialysate leaks.[230] It has been used in hepatic hydrothorax where the diaphragmatic defect was detected as a hypodense jet flow across the diaphragm.[231]

If there is significant dyspnea and no contraindication to the procedure, thoracentesis should be done for relief of symptoms and for pleural fluid analysis. As mentioned above, a high glucose concentration in the pleural fluid may obviate the need for further investigation. The peritoneal dialysis should be discontinued immediately. If the patient has just started on dialysis and has significant residual renal function, there may be no need for urgent initiation of hemodialysis, and management of the hydrothorax can be undertaken.

There are a number of approaches to management of hydrothorax. Generally, the prevention of recurrence mandates either specific closure of the defects in the hemidiaphragm, which are allowing the movement of the dialysate into the pleural space, obliteration of the pleural space itself (pleurodesis), or dialysis under conditions of low intra-abdominal pressure so that there is not enough of a transdiaphragmatic pressure gradient to promote the flux of dialysate out of the peritoneal cavity.

Sometimes a rechallenge of the peritoneal dialysis, after a temporary hiatus from PD, can be done without recurrence.[232,233] The interruption of PD should be for at least 2 weeks, ideally even longer. The absence of recurrence may be the result of sclerosis of any defects as a result of the effect of the hyperosmolar, acidic dialysate on the pleural lining. A recent review of outcome studies of hydrothorax suggested that more than half of patients with hydrothorax have been able to resume PD successfully after a period of temporary discontinuation and rechallenge.[202] This seems somewhat high, but it does speak to the value of a trial of temporary discontinuation and subsequent rechallenge of PD as a first step in the management algorithm.

Because increased intra-abdominal pressure plays a role in movement of the dialysate from peritoneal to pleural cavity, sometimes dialysis under conditions of lower intra-abdominal pressure can be carried out without recurrence.[234] Lower intra-abdominal pressure can be attained by the use of a smaller dwell volume of dialysate with the patient in the supine position, such as in automated peritoneal dialysis.

The use of more aggressive interventions depends, of course, on how intent the patient is to pursue PD, and/or the availability of hemodialysis as an alternative option for renal replacement therapy. Conventional pleurodesis agents have been used successfully to effect pleurodesis for dialysis-related hydrothorax. These include talc,[213,235,236] autologous blood,[237–240] mechanical rubbing of the pleura,[234] bleomycin, tetracycline,[209,210] and, less frequently, fibrin glue,[241,242] N-CWS (*Nocardia rubra* cell wall skeleton),[214] and the hemolytic streptococcal preparation OK-432.[214] The effectiveness of one agent over the other is not clear. Autologous blood appears to be less painful than, for example, talc or tetracycline, but may require more than one instillation to effect pleurodesis. Some studies use thoracoscopy, either video-assisted (VATS) or conventional, to perform the pleurodesis. It is best to seek consultation from a thoracic surgeon who has experience in pleurodesis, and use the agent with which the surgeon feels most comfortable. In review of the literature, a closed chemical pleurodesis is not as effective as one with a chest drain and pleural visualization.[202] There have been no reported cases of pleurodesis agents leaking from pleural to peritoneal cavity and leading to, for example, peritoneal sclerosis.

Another option is surgical or VATS intervention to visualize the defects in the hemidiaphragm and close them directly. These can be closed by clipping,[243,244] suturing[242] and reinforcement with Teflon patches,[245,246] surgical stapling, and spraying of the surface with fibrin glue.[247]

It is important, in anticipation of a surgical or VATS intervention, to warn the surgeon or VATS operator that methylene blue is irritating to the peritoneum, and so should be avoided as a method to try to visualize the diaphragmatic blebs or locate the source of leak across the diaphragm. If a dye is to be used, indocyanine green is reported to be less irritating than methylene blue. Also, any dye instilled with dialysate into the peritoneal cavity can become too diluted to be detected, and so produce a "false negative" test for visual detection of a leak.[213]

It is unclear what the success rate is for the interventional procedures, because there is likely a bias to report successful results. Overall, there is roughly a 50% success rate. A review of the outcome studies in the literature concluded that results were even better in males, in those with a diagnosis other than polycystic kidney disease, and in late leaks (>30 days after catheter insertion).[202] The rate of successful return to PD will also be dictated by the necessity to perform peritoneal dialysis and the availability of hemodialysis as an alternative.

Hernias

The increased intra-abdominal pressure, which results from the instillation of dialysis fluid into the peritoneal cavity, can lead to new defects or unmasking of occult defects in the supporting structures of the abdominal wall. One consequence is the development of hernias.

Most studies suggest that between 10% and 20% of PD patients will develop a hernia some time on that modality,[248–250] although a recent study found that 25% of patients developed a hernia, for an incidence rate of 0.08/patient/year.[251] The detection rate may be affected by how vigorously the diagnosis is pursued with the use of radiography and other investigations.

Many different kinds and locations of hernias have been described in PD patients. The most common type of hernia is umbilical. Herniation can occur through the inguinal canal, where both direct and indirect hernias can occur. Other hernias described include ventral hernias, those at the catheter insertion site, or at the incision from some previous surgery (Figure 30–1). Less commonly-encountered hernias include epigastric hernias, cystocele or rectocele,[252] Spigelian,[253] paraesophageal hernia presenting as a mediastinal mass,[254] and herniation through the foramen of Morgagni.[255]

The most common presentation is of a lump or a bulge at the site in question. The PD patient will usually bring this to clinical attention. The relationship to the increased intra-abdominal pressure is highlighted by the observation that many of these patients will notice a lump or a swelling on the abdomen after a bout of physical exertion or coughing. Less frequently, and particularly in an obese patient, the lump or bulge may not be clinically obvious, but the patient may report a vague discomfort in the area.

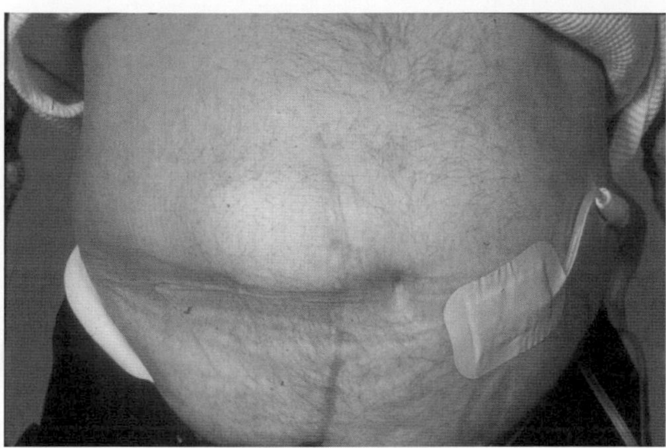

Figure 30-1 Ventral abdominal hernia.

Because a hernia can be associated with a defect in the integrity of the peritoneum, it may be associated with leak of dialysis fluid into the anterior abdominal wall. Therefore, the patient can present with abdominal wall edema (discussed later) or diminished dialysis effluent return, in association with a clinically occult hernia. Finally, a hernia can be a site of bowel incarceration and strangulation, with the strangulated bowel serving as a source of peritonitis, particularly with multiple enteric organisms. Rarely then, the first presentation of a hernia can be with this kind of peritonitis as a result of an undiagnosed hernia, which has incarcerated and then strangulated the involved bowel.[256]

It was originally observed that patients who are at risk for hernias include those with higher body mass index, because these patients will have higher intra-abdominal pressure for a given dwell volume.[200] Other studies have found the opposite result, namely that it is smaller patients who have the greater risk for hernias, when the height and weight are adjusted for sex.[250,257]

The relationship of dwell volume to the size of the patient may be a factor, and small patients may be more malnourished with less tissue strength, which may predispose to hernia. The insertion of the PD catheter through a midline abdominal incision is associated with risk of hernia development[258] because this is an area lacking in anatomic support. This practice has been avoided for many years and a paramedian approach is recommended.[259] Other risk factors for hernia development include older age, multiparity, and previous laparotomy or hernia repair.[260] Given the reduction in intra-abdominal pressure in the supine position, it is not surprising that patients ambulatory with CAPD are more at risk for this complication than those supine on cycler dialysis.[261]

Polycystic kidney disease (PKD) is also a risk for the development of hernias through multiple mechanisms. First, indirect inguinal hernias as a result of patent processus vaginalis has been encountered frequently in PKD males on PD, and it has been suggested that patent processus vaginalis may be another complication of this condition.[262] If the kidneys are massively enlarged, they may encroach upon the peritoneal space, so that a given volume of dialysate has less room to dwell and increases the pressure therein. A recent review of abdominal wall complications in PD patients found that PKD was the only factor significantly associated with the development of hernias,[251] although this finding has not been universal.[257,263]

One of the ways to increase clearance on PD is through the use of larger dwell volumes. There has been concern that the routine use of larger volumes may be associated with an increased risk of hernia. Although this concern has not been borne out in the literature,[249,257,261] there is a relationship between higher volumes and intra-abdominal pressure. This relationship should be kept in mind when prescribing dwell volumes, and the size of the patient should be taken into consideration. The volume-pressure curve is blunted by assuming the supine posture, so this is less of a problem in the APD patient (at least for the supine dwells at night), then in a patient who is on CAPD. In a patient who is at risk for hernia, or who perhaps has had a recent hernia repair, an optimum regimen might include night cycler with more normal volumes, but the use of smaller dwell volumes during the day, when activities will lead to an increase in pressure in the abdomen. Furthermore, if patients are anticipating an activity that could increase the pressure, such as an exercise class, they should be instructed to use a minimal volume of dialysate, or no dialysate at all, for the duration of the strenuous activity.

The diagnosis of hernia is usually straightforward. For example, a patient who reports being active and then feeling a "pop" in the groin and now has an inguinal mass is very consistent with an inguinal hernia. However, particularly in the obese patient, the diagnosis may not be as obvious. Further, a lump around the catheter exit site or tunnel could be a hernia, a collection of dialysis fluid from a leak, or infection. Therefore, there are ancillary tests to diagnose or confirm the hernia.

CT scanning can be helpful. The diagnostic utility is improved by the use of intraperitoneal dye. Depending on the volume of dialysate used, 100 to 150 mL of dye should be instilled into the peritoneal fluid and this fluid infused into the peritoneal cavity.[264–267] It is important that after this infusion the patient be ambulatory for some time (30 to 60 minutes) before going for CT examination. This ambulatory time will allow for the dye to distribute within the peritoneal fluid and, under the increased intra-abdominal pressure associated with being ambulatory, should allow the dye-labeled dialysate to enter the hernia sac and any potential area of leak. Placing the patient in the prone position for scanning is another way to increase the abdominal pressure.[268] It is also of benefit to speak to the radiologist about this study. In a center with a small PD population, this kind of study is uncommon, and so the radiologist may not be familiar with the dialysate and what exactly is happening with the patient. Most of the instilled dye will be removed from the patient when the dialysis fluid is drained, but a small amount may be absorbed systemically because sometimes a slight nephrogram effect will be reported.

A similar study can be done without dye. Radionuclide imaging using technetium-labelled tin or sulphur colloid, is an alternative method to investigate hernias and leaks. Subsequent scanning by gamma camera can then track the movement of dialysate, such as through the inguinal canal as a result of indirect inguinal hernia.[269–274] As with the CT studies, it is important for the patients to raise the intra-abdominal pressure for the labeled dialysate to move into the hernia sac. In suspected indirect inguinal hernia, the patient may be instructed to lean forward in the sitting position to increase the pressure in the abdomen.

Patients on peritoneal dialysis who develop a hernia should undergo laparoscopic or operative repair. Most patients find hernias to be unsightly and request that they be repaired. In addition to cosmetic considerations, hernias pose a risk for bowel incarceration and strangulation. As mentioned earlier, this can be the first presentation of a previously-undiagnosed hernia. It is the smaller hernias, with smaller orifices, in which bowel can get caught, that pose the greater risk of incarceration, compared with large ventral hernias. Given their prevalence and size, umbilical hernias are most frequently associated with these bowel complications.[248] A patient with a hernia awaiting repair should be reminded that they should always be able to manually reduce the hernia. If the hernia becomes irreducible, and especially if it becomes tender, the patient should report to the hospital as soon as possible. The third problem with hernias is that they represent a break in the integrity of the peritoneal membrane and, therefore, pose a source for dialysate leak, as discussed later. For these three reasons, most PD patients with hernias should undergo repair.

The repair is undertaken by conventional surgical techniques. The patient should be drained of dialysate before the surgery. The management of dialysis requirements around the surgery depends on the residual renal function. If the patient has about 3 mL/min residual glomerular filtration rate (the mean of a 24-hr urine urea and creatinine clearance) or more and is without significant comorbidity, such as a Grade IV left ventricle, then the patient can carry out the usual dialysis up until the day of surgery. Postoperatively, the patient should not recommence PD for at least 1 or 2 days.[275] The use of a mesh repair may allow for the faster return to PD.[275–277] Again, depending on the residual kidney function, the patient may need additional diuretics or dietary salt and potassium restriction during the time without dialysis, although oral intake during this postoperative time is usually not so much in any case. Dialysis should be gradually restarted under conditions of low intra-abdominal pressure, that is, small volumes and performed in the supine position. This is done so that a sudden increase in abdominal pressure does not threaten the repair. If the patient uses a home cycler, dialysis can be performed with small volume exchanges overnight, leaving the patient dry during the day. If the patient uses CAPD, 1 L exchanges can be used four or five times daily. While this is less than the usually accepted dose of dialysis, it should have little consequence in the face of residual renal function and for a short period of time. It is well to remember that the risk of "under-dialysis" has to be weighed against the risk of insertion of a temporary hemodialysis line and the hemodialysis procedure itself. On the other hand, if the patient is anuric and has multiple comorbid conditions, recommencing suboptimal dialysis could have deleterious consequences. Caution has to be taken about reducing the dialysis, especially the ultrafiltration, for any length of time. In this case, consideration may have to be given to a transient move to hemodialysis until the repair is healed. If the patient has significant comorbidity, another option is to forego the hernia repair altogether. In this instance, the patient should be warned about incarceration, but the hernia itself could just be observed, if it is not a source of leak.

Abdominal Wall and Genital Leaks

Under the influence of increased intra-abdominal pressure, dialysis fluid can leak out of the peritoneal cavity into other sites. Movement of dialysis fluid across the hemidiaphragm, leading to PD hydrothorax, has been discussed elsewhere in this chapter. Dialysate can also move into the abdominal wall, leading to abdominal wall edema, and into the genitalia.

In order to facilitate movement of the dialysate, there needs to be some pathway of low resistance through which the dialysate moves. In the case of the abdominal wall, the defects include the incisional site for the insertion of the PD catheter, at least until that has healed, the catheter tunnel and exit site, and other congenital or acquired defects, including hernias.

Genital edema can occur in two ways. The processus vaginalis is a connection from the peritoneal cavity into the scrotum or labia. It is through the processus vaginalis that the testes migrate into the scrotal sac. Normally, but not inevitably, the canal then obliterates. If the processus vaginalis remains patent, it can serve as a conduit between the peritoneal cavity and the scrotum or labia. If bowel or omentum migrates along the patent processus vaginalis, an indirect inguinal hernia can result. If fluid moves along the same path, the result is a hydrocele. Therefore, in the face of a patent processus vaginalis, dialysis fluid, under increased intra-abdominal pressure, can move into the scrotum or labia[278] leading to genital edema. This may or may not be accompanied by an indirect inguinal hernia.

The other defect that can result in genital edema is in the abdominal wall. If sufficient fluid traverses the defect, the dialysate can then migrate caudally by gravity and collect along the mons pubis or penis.

The patient is usually the first to notice abdominal wall or genital edema and will seek attention for it. Sometimes a patient may notice only that the abdomen has become more protuberant or asymmetric. Even less often, the presenting complaint is that of diminished effluent return and weight gain. In this instance, it is not the result of ultrafiltration problems, but rather that the fluid is moving into another compartment and so is not available for drainage through the PD catheter.

In the case of scrotal or labial edema, the diagnosis should be apparent. Local processes should be considered, such as epididymitis, but the scrotal swelling from leak is usually not as tender as that associated with acute local inflammation. On examination, an associated indirect inguinal hernia should be looked for, although it may be better discerned by CT scanning (see later text). In the case of abdominal wall edema or complaint of a protuberant abdomen, careful examination should be made with the patient standing. In the standing position, it is easier to see any obvious asymmetry, such as a bulging flank or a protuberance on the abdomen. In the supine position, the abdomen should be palpated for any fascial defects that may be allowing the passage of dialysate out of the peritoneal cavity. The abdominal wall often has a distinctive appearance when it is edematous. It truly looks somewhat "puffy," and the usual indentations made by the waistband of underpants or the catheter itself lying across the wall look deeper than normal.

A less common site of leakage is through the vagina. The peritoneal cavity reflects over the vaginal vault, and a defect in that location can leak to movement of dialysate through the vagina itself. Thankfully this is an uncommon event.[279–281] A pathway for communication should be suspected not only if there is a new complaint of clear vaginal "discharge," but also if there is peritonitis with a vaginal organism, such as *lactobacillus.*

Radionuclide scanning and CT scans are very helpful in the diagnosis. In the case of scrotal or labial edema, 3 to 10 mCi of technetium-labeled ligand or 100 to 150 mL of CT dye can be infused into the peritoneal cavity with the usual volume of dialysate. The patient should be instructed to move around to raise the intra-abdominal pressure. The subsequent scanning, if positive, will demonstrate movement of dialysate through a patent processus vaginalis into the scrotum or labia.[282] On CT scanning sometimes contents of a hernia are also seen in the processus vaginalis.[283] This information can be helpful if surgical intervention is being planned.

The same studies can be used for abdominal wall edema. There is experience with CT scanning[264,267,268,284] and isotopic scanning[269,272–274,285] for this condition. In this case the study can confirm that the edema is indeed the result of leakage of dialysate (now labeled with dye) and sometimes even demonstrate the site of the leak, such as a fascial defect or occult hernia. There is recent experience with magnetic resonance (MR) scanning, with and without[230] the use of gadolinium. Interestingly, one report on the use of MR scanning, using the dialysate as its own "tracer," demonstrated more extensive spread of dialysate through the surrounding tissue than what is usually detected with conventional CT peritoneography.[230] Ultrasound examination of the anterior abdominal wall can sometimes detect a fluid collection and may serve as a reasonable initial test.[286]

Since both abdominal wall and genital leaks are the result of some combination of increased intra-abdominal pressure and a low-resistance pathway for movement of peritoneal dialysate, the approach to management should address both these risk factors. First, if there is sufficient residual renal function, it is not automatic that the patient has to immediately be managed by hemodialysis. Often these leaks occur early on, and there is adequate renal function so that the dialysis dose can be adjusted and manipulated without worry of under-dialysis. The patient should be dialyzed under conditions of lower intra-abdominal pressure. This can be effected by having most, if not all, of the dialysis done while the patient is in the supine position by cycler dialysis. For example, the patient can be converted to nocturnal intermittent peritoneal dialysis (NIPD) with 1.5 or 2.0 L exchanges and be without dialysate during the daytime. This dialysis regimen is satisfactory in the face of kidney function but is not really a good long-term solution, because NIPD is not an ideal form of peritoneal dialysis when the patient eventually loses renal function. Sometimes a small day volume can be used without recurrence of edema, such as 1 L after coming off the cycler, and then a 1 L mid-day exchange. The CAPD patient can have smaller dwell volumes compensated for by more frequent exchanges. A suggested regimen is 1.5 L, five times a day. Again, this is not a satisfactory long-term solution, but it keeps the intra-abdominal pressure low and minimizes the recurrence of edema while other strategies to address the potential anatomic defect are considered.

Sometimes leak is the result of some abdominal tear, which can heal spontaneously. In this scenario NIPD for 2 weeks can be associated with spontaneous resolution of the leak without any other kind of intervention.[264,284,287] This conservative approach works better for early leaks, which may be related to incomplete healing of the surgery for catheter insertion.[287] There are a few reports of infiltration of a leak around the PD catheter with fibrin glue.[288] In the case of established hernias or patent processus vaginalis, it is likely that the leaks will recur unless more definitive surgical correction is undertaken. In the case of leak through the catheter exit site, a trial of NIPD is worthwhile, but if the leak recurs catheter replacement may be necessary.[289] It is important to discuss any leaks with the surgeon or laparoscopist to ensure that the peritoneal entry site is well-sealed with purse-string sutures to minimize leak.

There is a risk of developing peritonitis, if the leak occurs to the external surface. It has been recommended that prophylactic antibiotics be given for the duration of the leak[146] to minimize this risk.

In the case of surgical repair of leak secondary to hernia or patent processus vaginalis, the same postoperative principles apply as to repair of hernias, discussed earlier. If there is residual renal function (GFR >3 mL/min), the patient can usually miss dialysis for 2 to 3 days postoperatively and then recommence PD under conditions of lower intra-abdominal pressure, that is, smaller dwell volumes and the use of the supine position. In the case of the CAPD patient, 1 L exchanges can be done four or five times daily. Although this will transiently cause the patient to be relatively under-dialyzed and lead to increase in the concentration of creatinine and other dialyzable solutes, the long-term sequelae are likely unimportant and must be balanced against the risk of insertion of a temporary hemodialysis catheter. However, if the patient is likely to have a prolonged healing time (elderly patient or prolonged use of corticosteroids, as in the case of past renal transplant) and has borderline or no renal function, temporary hemodialysis may be required.

MALFUNCTION OF THE PERITONEAL DIALYSIS CATHETER

Malfunction of the peritoneal dialysis catheter, which usually occurs soon after the insertion of the catheter, remains one of the most dissatisfying aspects of starting a patient on PD. Oftentimes the patient has only recently learned that he or she has kidney failure, chooses home dialysis, undertakes the insertion of the catheter, only to find out that the catheter is not draining well. This complication will delay the instruction in home dialysis and is the source of much frustration. Further, unless the personnel involved have experience with sorting out the catheter complications, the easier option is to "default" to hemodialysis.

Catheter drainage problems include:

- "Two-way obstruction," that is, poor inflow and poor outflow
- "One-way obstruction," usually satisfactory inflow but poor outflow
- Pain associated with either inflow or outflow

The combination of poor inflow and poor outflow is not as common as poor outflow alone. The "two-way obstruction" is usually the result of some obstruction in the lumen of the catheter or a kink in the catheter that similarly will obstruct flow bidirectionally.[291] Material that has caused intraluminal obstruction includes blood clots, fibrin strands,[292] and, more rarely, fungus balls, stones, and cryoglobulins.[293] Very rarely, the ovarian fimbriae and related structures have been reported to block the intraperitoneal portion of the catheter.[294–297] If two-way obstruction is found, particularly soon after implantation of the PD catheter, the catheter should be flushed under high pressure with a syringe of heparinized saline.[298] Both vigorous flushing and aspiration should be attempted.[299] A brush to clean the lumen has also been used.[300,301] If that maneuver is unsuccessful, the catheter lumen can be filled with more heparinized saline, urokinase,[302–304] or tissue plasminogen activator (tPA) for a couple of hours, to try to effect thrombolysis of the occluding material.[305,306] If the catheter is still obstructed, consideration should be given to instilling dye through the catheter to determine whether there is indeed an intraluminal occlusion or whether the catheter itself is kinked. At the same radiologic sitting, the occlusion or kink can be treated by the intraluminal insertion of a rigid trochar, to either dislodge the occluding material or to attempt to straighten out the kink.

In the case of satisfactory inflow but poor outflow, the usual cause is obstruction around the holes in the intraperitoneal portion of the dialysis catheter. With inflow, the flow pressure pushes the obstruction away from these holes, so inflow proceeds normally, or perhaps just a little more slowly than normal. However, with the suction effect of the outflow, the obstructing material is sucked closer to the catheter, impeding the outflow of the effluent from the peritoneal cavity into the catheter. Causes of this kind of obstruction include constipation, with stool-filled colon taking up much intraperitoneal space and impinging on the catheter surface; wrapping of omentum and *appendices epiploicae* around the intraluminal portion of the catheter[307]; or catheter migration into the upper quadrants, where the draining holes may be out of contact with the effluent, which may be pooling caudally, particularly if the patient dialyzes in the sitting position.

Since constipation is such a common cause of early one-way dysfunction, it is strongly recommended that careful attention be paid to bowel movements, starting before the catheter insertion. The patient should receive regular treatment with docusate or sennosides to ensure that constipation does not supervene.[308] If the patient is on oral iron or calcium supplements, consideration should be given to temporarily holding these around the catheter insertion, because they can be constipating for many patients. In the postoperative period, the patient may need cathartics or enemas. Importantly, one bowel movement does not mean that the constipation has been relieved. We have seen patients with one-way obstruction after catheter insertion, who had large bowel movements with enemas, but whose flat plate radiographs of the abdomen still demonstrated copious amounts of stool in the colon. Interestingly, one of our patients had poor catheter function until he underwent a bowel preparation for an unrelated colonoscopy, at which point his catheter started to function perfectly.

In the case of catheter migration or omental wrapping, once again a semirigid wire can be inserted, under aseptic conditions, through the catheter. In the case of migration, the catheter can be gently brought down from the upper quadrant into the pelvis.[309–315] This procedure is associated with variable rates of success.[298] It must be done gently, because there is a risk of bowel tearing or perforation.[316] With omental wrapping, the catheter can be gently tugged free from the omentum in the successful instances. There are reports of manipulation with a Fogarty catheter instead of semirigid wire.[302,317]

In recent years laparoscopy has become very valuable, both to place the catheter[318–321] and to treat catheter malfunction.[315,322–325] Laparoscopy can be used to reposition a catheter that has migrated and even secure it in place with a suture.[326–329] The laparoscope can also be used to remove[330,331] or secure the omentum and associated *appendices epiploicae* so that they do not block the catheter holes.[332–334] This procedure can be done prophylactically at the time of catheter insertion or as needed to treat drainage problems.[335] Laparoscopy has even been used to free up the PD catheter from the fimbriae of the Fallopian tubes.[336]

References

1. Oreopoulos DG, Khanna R, Williams P, Vas SI: Continuous ambulatory peritoneal dialysis 1981. Nephron 1982; 30(4): 293-303.
2. Krediet RT, Lindholm B, Rippe B: Pathophysiology of peritoneal membrane failure. Perit Dial Int 2000; 20(S4):S22-S42.
3. Delarue J, Maingourd C: Acute metabolic effects of dialysis fluids during CAPD. Am J Kidney Dis 2001; 37(1 suppl 2):S103-S107.
4. Davies SJ, Russell L, Bryan J, et al: Impact of peritoneal absorption of glucose on appetite, protein catabolism and survival in CAPD patients. Clin Nephrol 1996; 45(3):194-198.
5. Grodstein GP, Blumenkrantz MJ, Kopple JD, et al: Glucose absorption during continuous ambulatory peritoneal dialysis. Kidney Int 1981; 19(4):564-567.
6. Bodnar DM, Busch S, Fuchs J, et al: Estimating glucose absorption in peritoneal dialysis using peritoneal equilibration tests. Adv Perit Dial 1993; 9:114-118.
7. Twardowski ZJ, Nolph KD, Khanna R, et al: Peritoneal equilibration test. Perit Dial Bull 1987; 7:138-147.
8. Krediet RT, Boeschoten EW, Zuyderhoudt FM, Arisz L: The relationship between peritoneal glucose absorption and body fluid loss by ultrafiltration during continuous ambulatory peritoneal dialysis. Clin Nephrol 1987; 27(2):51-55.
9. Lindholm B, Bergstrom J: Nutritional management of patients undergoing peritoneal dialysis. *In* Nolph KD (ed): Peritoneal Dialysis. Dordrecht, Kluwer Academic Publishers, 1988, pp 230-260.
10. Zavaroni A, Bonora E, Pagliara M, et al: Risk factor for coronary artery disease in healthy persons with hyperinsulinemia and normal glucose tolerance. N Engl J Med 1989; 320:702-706.
11. DeFronzo RA, Tobin JD, Rowe JW, Andres R: Glucose intolerance in uremia. Quantification of pancreatic beta cell sensitivity to glucose and tissue sensitivity to insulin. J Clin Invest 1978; 62(2): 425-435.
12. Lin SH, Lin YF, Kuo SW, et al: Rosiglitazone improves glucose metabolism in nondiabetic uremic patients on CAPD. Am J Kidney Dis 2003; 42(4):774-780.
13. Aslam N, Bernardini J, Fried L, Piraino B: Large body mass index does not predict short-term survival in peritoneal dialysis patients. Perit Dial Int 2002; 22(2):191-196.
14. Boeschoten EW, Zuyderhoudt FMJ, Krediet RT, Arisz L: Changes in weight and lipid concentrations during CAPD treatment. Perit Dial Int 1988; 8:19-24.
15. Soreide R, Dracup B, Svarstad E, Iversen BM: Increased total body fat during PD treatment. Adv Perit Dial 1992; 8:173-176.
16. Soreide R, Dracup B, Svarstad E, Iversen BM: Increased total body fat during PD treatment. Adv Perit Dial 1992; 8:173-176.16.
17. Bergia R, Bellini ME, Valenti M, et al: Longitudinal assessment of body composition in continuous ambulatory peritoneal dialysis

patients using bioelectric impedance and anthropometric measurements. Perit Dial Int 1993; 13(S2):512-514.
18. Nordfors L, Heimburger O, Lonnqvist F, et al: Fat tissue accumulation during peritoneal dialysis is associated with a polymorphism in uncoupling protein 2. Kidney Int 2000; 57(4): 1713-1719.
19. Fernstrom A, Hylander B, Moritz A, et al: Increase of intra-abdominal fat in patients treated with continuous ambulatory peritoneal dialysis. Perit Dial Int 1998; 18(2):166-171.
20. Lee P, O'Neal D, Murphy B, Best J: The role of abdominal adiposity and insulin resistance in dyslipidemia of chronic renal failure. Am J Kidney Dis 1997; 29(1):54-65.
21. Henriquez MA, Gonzalez A, Bemis JA, Esquivel J: Body composition and lipid abnormalities in Hispanic and black patients on continuous ambulatory peritoneal dialysis. Perit Dial Int 1993; 13(S2):S424-S427.
22. Samaha FF, Iqbal N, Seshadri P, et al: A low-carbohydrate as compared with a low-fat diet in severe obesity. N Engl J Med 2003; 348(21):2074-2081.
23. Foster GD, Wyatt HR, Hill JO, et al: A randomized trial of a low-carbohydrate diet for obesity. N Engl J Med 2003; 348(21): 2082-2090.
24. Churchill DN, Thorpe KE, Nolph KD, et al: Increased peritoneal membrane transport is associated with decreased patient and technique survival for continuous peritoneal dialysis patients. The Canada-USA (CANUSA) Peritoneal Dialysis Study Group. J Am Soc Nephrol 1998; 9(7):1285-1292.
25. Szeto CC, Law MC, Wong TY, et al: Peritoneal transport status correlates with morbidity but not longitudinal change of nutritional status of continuous ambulatory peritoneal dialysis patients: A 2-year prospective study. Am J Kidney Dis 2001; 37(2):329-336.
26. Abbott KC, Glanton CW, Trespalacios FC, et al: Body mass index, dialysis modality, and survival: Analysis of the United States. Renal Data System Dialysis Morbidity and Mortality Wave II Study. Kidney Int 2004; 65(2):597-605.
27. Johnson DW, Herzig KA, Purdie DM, et al: Is obesity a favorable prognostic factor in peritoneal dialysis patients? Perit Dial Int 2000; 20(6):715-721.
28. Hakim RM, Lowrie E: Obesity and mortality in ESRD: Is it good to be fat? Kidney Int 1999; 55(4):1580-1581.
29. Fried L, Bernardini J, Piraino B: Neither size nor weight predicts survival in peritoneal dialysis patients. Perit Dial Int 1996; 16(4): 357-361.
30. Salahudeen AK: Obesity and survival on dialysis. Am J Kidney Dis 2003; 41(5):925-932. 30.
31. Byers T: Body weight and mortality. N Engl J Med 1995; 333(11): 723-724.
32. McDonald SP, Collins JF, Johnson DW: Obesity is associated with worse peritoneal dialysis outcomes in the Australia and New Zealand patient populations. J Am Soc Nephrol 2003; 14(11): 2894-2901.
33. Stompor T, Sulowicz W, Dembinska-Kiec A, et al: An association between body mass index and markers of inflammation: Is obesity the proinflammatory state in patients on peritoneal dialysis? Perit Dial Int 2003; 23(1):79-83.
34. Wu MS, Yu CC, Wu CH, et al: Pre-dialysis glycemic control is an independent predictor of mortality in type II diabetic patients on continuous ambulatory peritoneal dialysis. Perit Dial Int 1999; 19(S2):S179-S183.
35. Diaz-Buxo JA: Peritoneal dialysis prescriptions for diabetic patients. Adv Perit Dial 1999; 15:91-95.
36. Marshall J, Jennings P, Scott A, et al: Glycemic control in diabetic CAPD patients assessed by continuous glucose monitoring system (CGMS). Kidney Int 2003; 64:1480-1486.
37. Holmes CJ, Shockley TR: Strategies to reduce glucose exposure in peritoneal dialysis patients. Perit Dial Int 2000; 20(S2):S37-S41.
38. Renzo S, Beatrice D, Giuseppe I: CAPD in diabetics: Use of amino acids. Adv Perit Dial 1990; 6:53-55.
39. Bredie SJ, Bosch FH, Demacker PN, et al: Effects of peritoneal dialysis with an overnight icodextrin dwell on parameters of glucose and lipid metabolism. Perit Dial Int 2001; 21(3):275-281.
40. Amici G, Orrasch M, Da Rin G, Bocci C: Hyperinsulinism reduction associated with icodextrin treatment in continuous ambulatory peritoneal dialysis patients. Adv Perit Dial 2001; 17:80-83.
41. Oda H, Keane WF: Lipid abnormalities in end stage renal disease. Nephrol Dial Transplant 1998; 13(S1):45-49.
42. Prichard SS: Impact of dyslipidemia in end-stage renal disease. J Am Soc Nephrol 2003; 14:S315-S320.
43. Prichard S: Major and minor risk factors for cardiovascular disease in peritoneal dialysis. Perit Dial Int 2000; 20(S2):S154-S159.
44. O'Riordan E, O'Donoghue DJ, Kalra PA, et al: Changes in lipid profiles in nondiabetic, nonnephrotic patients commencing continuous ambulatory peritoneal dialysis. Adv Perit Dial 2000; 16:313-316.
45. Little J, Phillips L, Russell L, et al: Longitudinal lipid profiles on CAPD: Their relationship to weight gain, comorbidity, and dialysis factors. J Am Soc Nephrol 1998; 9(10):1931-1939.
46. Sniderman A, Cianflone K, Kwiterovich PO Jr, et al: Hyperapobetalipoproteinemia: The major dyslipoproteinemia in patients with chronic renal failure treated with chronic ambulatory peritoneal dialysis. Atherosclerosis 1987; 65(3):257-264.
47. Moberly JB, Attman PO, Samuelsson O, et al: Alterations in lipoprotein composition in peritoneal dialysis patients. Perit Dial Int 2002; 22(2):220-228. 47.
48. Lameire N, Matthys D, Matthys E, Beheydt R: Effects of long-term CAPD on carbohydrate and lipid metabolism. Clin Nephrol 1988; 30(S1):S53-S58.
49. Wheeler DC: Abnormalities of lipoprotein metabolism in CAPD patients. Kidney Int 1998; 54(S1):45-49.
50. Choi KH, Song HY, Shin SK, et al: Influence of apolipoprotein E genotype on lipid and lipoprotein levels in continuous ambulatory peritoneal dialysis patients. Adv Perit Dial 1999; 15:243-246.
51. Attman PO, Samuelsson OG, Moberly J, et al: Apolipoprotein B-containing lipoproteins in renal failure: The relation to mode of dialysis. Kidney Int 1999; 55(4):1536-1542.
52. Salomon RG, Kaur K, Podrez E, et al: HNE-derived 2-pentylpyrroles are generated during oxidation of LDL, are more prevalent in blood plasma from patients with renal disease or atherosclerosis, and are present in atherosclerotic plaques. Chem Res Toxicol 2000; 13(7):557-564.
53. O'Neal D, Lee P, Murphy B, Best J: Low-density lipoprotein particle size distribution in end-stage renal disease treated with hemodialysis or peritoneal dialysis. Am J Kidney Dis 1996; 27(1): 84-91.
54. Sniderman A, Cianflone K, Kwiterovich PO Jr, et al: Hyperapobetalipoproteinemia: The major dyslipoproteinemia in patients with chronic renal failure treated with chronic ambulatory peritoneal dialysis. Atherosclerosis 1987; 65(3):257-264.
55. Prichard S, Cianflone K, Sniderman A: The role of the liver in the pathogenesis of hyperlipidemia in patients with end-stage renal disease treated with continuous ambulatory peritoneal dialysis. Perit Dial Int 1996; 16(Sl):S207-S210.
56. Misra M, Reaveley DA, Ashworth J, et al: Six-month prospective cross-over study to determine the effects of 1.1% amino acid dialysate on lipid metabolism in patients on continuous ambulatory peritoneal dialysis. Perit Dial Int 1997; 17(3):279-286.
57. Chang JM, Chen HC, Hwang SJ, et al: Does amino acid-based peritoneal dialysate change homocysteine metabolism in continuous ambulatory peritoneal dialysis patients? Perit Dial Int 2003; 23(S2):S48-S51.
58. Brulez HF, van Guldener C, Donker AJ, ter Wee PM: The impact of an amino acid-based peritoneal dialysis fluid on plasma total homocysteine levels, lipid profile and body fat mass. Nephrol Dial Transplant 1999; 14(1):154-159.

59. Kagan A, Bar-Khayim Y, Schafer Z, Fainaru M: Heterogeneity in peritoneal transport during continuous ambulatory peritoneal dialysis and its impact on ultrafiltration, loss of macromolecules and plasma level of proteins, lipids and lipoproteins. Nephron 1993; 63(1):32-42.
60. Stenvinkel P, Pecoits-Filho R, Lindholm B: Coronary artery disease in end-stage renal disease: No longer a simple plumbing problem. J Am Soc Nephrol 2003; 14(7):1927-1939.
61. Arici M, Walls J: End-stage renal disease, atherosclerosis, and cardiovascular mortality: Is C-reactive protein the missing link? Kidney Int 2001; 59(2):407-414.
62. Ducloux D, Bresson-Vautrin C, Kribs M, et al: C-reactive protein and cardiovascular disease in peritoneal dialysis patients. Kidney Int 2002; 62(4):1417-1422.
63. Kim SB, Min WK, Lee SK, et al: Persistent elevation of C-reactive protein and ischemic heart disease in patients with continuous ambulatory peritoneal dialysis. Am J Kidney Dis 2002; 39(2): 342-346.
64. Stenvinkel P, Chung SH, Heimburger O, Lindholm B: Malnutrition, inflammation, and atherosclerosis in peritoneal dialysis patients. Perit Dial Int 2001; 21(S3):S157-S162.
65. Stompor T, Pasowicz M, Sullowicz W, et al: An association between coronary artery calcification score, lipid profile, and selected markers of chronic inflammation in ESRD patients treated with peritoneal dialysis. Am J Kidney Dis 2003; 41(1): 203-211.
66. Fried L, Hutchison A, Stegmayr B, et al: Recommendations for the treatment of lipid disorders in patients on peritoneal dialysis. ISPD guidelines/recommendations. International Society for Peritoneal Dialysis. Perit Dial Int 1999; 19(1):7-16.
67. National Kidney Foundation. K/DOQI clinical practice guidelines for managing dyslipidemias in chronic kidney disease. Am J Kidney Dis 2003; 41:S1-S91.
68. Li PK, Mak TW, Lam CW, Lai KN: Lovastatin treatment of dyslipoproteinemia in patients on continuous ambulatory peritoneal dialysis. Perit Dial Int 1993; 13(S2):S428-S430.
69. Nutescu EA, Shapiro NL: Ezetimibe: A selective cholesterol absorption inhibitor. Pharmacotherapy 2003; 23(11):1463-1474.
70. Chertow GM, Burke SK, Raggi P: Treat to Goal Working Group. Sevelamer attenuates the progression of coronary and aortic calcification in hemodialysis patients. Kidney Int 2002; 62(1):245-252.
71. Chertow GM, Burke SK, Dillon MA, Slatopolsky E: Long-term effects of sevelamer hydrochloride on the calcium X phosphate product and lipid profile of haemodialysis patients. Nephrol Dial Transplant 1999; 14:2907-2914.
72. Nakamoto H, Imai H, Kawanishi H, et al: Low serum albumin in elderly continuous ambulatory peritoneal dialysis patients is attributable to high permeability of peritoneum. Adv Perit Dial 2001; 17:238-243.
73. Cooper S, Iliescu EA, Morton AR: The relationship between dialysate protein loss and membrane transport status in peritoneal dialysis patients. Adv Perit Dial 2001; 17:244-247.
74. Coronel F, Tornero F, Macia M, et al: Peritoneal clearances, protein losses and ultrafiltration in diabetic patients after four years on CAPD. Adv Perit Dial 1991; 7:35-38.
75. Spaia S, Christidou F, Pangidis P, et al: Variability of peritoneal protein loss in diabetic and nondiabetic patients on continuous ambulatory peritoneal dialysis. Perit Dial Int 1993; 13(S2):S242-S244. 75.
76. Moist LM, Port FK, Orzol SM, et al: Predictors of loss of residual renal function among new dialysis patients. J Am Soc Nephrol 2000; 11(3):556-564.
77. Ross EA, Koo LC: Improved nutrition after the detection and treatment of occult gastroparesis in nondiabetic dialysis patients. Am J Kidney Dis 1998; 31(1):62-66.
78. Wright M, Woodrow G, O'Brien S, et al: Disturbed appetite patterns and nutrient intake in peritoneal dialysis patients. Perit Dial Int 2003; 23(6):550-556.
79. Yeun JY, Kaysen GA: Acute phase proteins and peritoneal dialysate albumin loss are the main determinants of serum albumin in peritoneal dialysis patients. Am J Kidney Dis 1997; 30(6):923-927.
80. Stenvinkel P, Heimburger O, Lindholm B, et al: Are there two types of malnutrition in chronic renal failure? Evidence for relationships between malnutrition, inflammation and atherosclerosis (MIA syndrome). Nephrol Dial Transplant 2000; 15(7):953-960.
81. Leavey SF, Strawderman RL, Jones CA, et al: Simple nutritional indicators as independent predictors of mortality in hemodialysis patients. Am J Kidney Dis 1998; 31(6):997-1006.
82. Herzig KA, Purdie DM, Chang W, et al: Is C-reactive protein a useful predictor of outcome in peritoneal dialysis patients? J Am Soc Nephrol 2001; 12(4):814-821.
83. Iseki K, Tozawa M, Yoshi S, Fukiyama K: Serum C-reactive protein (CRP) and risk of death in chronic dialysis patients. Nephrol Dial Transplant 1999; 14(8):1956-1960.
84. Noh H, Lee SW, Kang SW, et al: Serum C-reactive protein: A predictor of mortality in continuous ambulatory peritoneal dialysis patients. Perit Dial Int 1998; 18(4):387-394.
85. Suliman ME, Qureshi AR, Barany P, et al: Hyperhomocysteinemia, nutritional status, and cardiovascular disease in hemodialysis patients. Kidney Int 2000; 57(4): 1727-1735.
86. Ducloux D, Heuze-Lecornu L, Gibey R, et al: Dialysis adequacy and homocyst(e)ine concentrations in peritoneal dialysis patients. Nephrol Dial Transplant 1999; 14(3):728-731.
87. Jones M, Hagen T, Boyle CA, et al: Treatment of malnutrition with 1.1% amino acid peritoneal dialysis solution: Results of a multicenter outpatient study. Am J Kidney Dis 1998; 32(5): 761-769.
88. Bruno M, Gabella P, Ramello A: Use of amino acids in peritoneal dialysis solutions. Perit Dial Int 2000; 20(S2):S166-S171.
89. Oreopoulous DR, Marliss E, Anderson GH, et al: Nutritional aspects of CAPD and the potential use of amino acid containing dialysis solutions. Perit Dial Bull 1983; 3:S10-S12.
90. Hutchison AJ, Gokal R: Improved solutions for peritoneal dialysis: Physiological calcium solutions, osmotic agents and buffers. Kidney Int 1992; 42(S38):S153-S159.
91. Li FK, Chan LY, Woo JC, et al: A 3-year, prospective, randomized, controlled study on amino acid dialysate in patients on CAPD. Am J Kidney Dis 2003; 42(1):173-183.
92. Grzegorzewska AE, Wiecek A, Mariak I, Kokot F: Amino-acid-based dialysis solution changes leptinemia and leptin peritoneal clearance. Adv Perit Dial 2000; 16:7-14.
93. Swartz RD: The use of peritoneal dialysis in special situations. Adv Perit Dial 1999; 15:160-166.
94. Heimburger O, Waniewski J, Werynski A, Lindholm B: A quantitative description of solute and fluid transport during peritoneal dialysis. Kidney Int 1992; 41(5):1320-1332.
95. Khandelwal M, Kothari J, Krishnan M, et al: Volume expansion and sodium balance in peritoneal dialysis patients. Part I: Recent concepts in pathogenesis. Adv Perit Dial 2003; 19:36-43.
96. Khandelwal M, Kothari J, Krishnan M, et al: Volume expansion and sodium balance in peritoneal dialysis patients. Part II: Newer insights in management. Adv Perit Dial 2003; 19:44-52.
97. Struijk DG, Krediet RT: Sodium balance in automated peritoneal dialysis. Perit Dial Int 2000; 20(S2):S101-S105.
98. Waniewski J, Werynski A, Heimburger O, Lindholm B: Simple membrane models for peritoneal dialysis. Evaluation of diffusive and convective solute transport. ASAIO J 1992; 38(4):788-796.
99. Waniewski J, Heimburger O, Werynski A, Lindholm B: Aqueous solute concentrations and evaluation of mass transport coefficients in peritoneal dialysis. Nephrol Dial Transplant 1992; 7(1):50-56.
100. Rippe B, Carlsson O: Role of transcellular water channels in peritoneal dialysis. Perit Dial Int 1999; 19(S2):S95-S101.

101. Ahearn DJ, Nolph KD: Controlled sodium removal with peritoneal dialysis. Trans Am Soc Artif Organs 1972; 18:423-428.
102. Grzegorzewska AE, Antczak-Jedrzejczak D, Leander M, Mariak I: Polyglucose dialysis solution induces changes in blood chemistry. Adv Perit Dial 2001; 17:101-108.
103. Gokal R, Moberly J, Lindholm B, Mujais S: Metabolic and laboratory effects of icodextrin. Kidney Int 2002; 62(S81):S62-S71.
104. Rodriguez-Carmona A, Fontan MP: Sodium removal in patients undergoing CAPD and automated peritoneal dialysis. Perit Dial Int 2002; 22(6):705-713.
105. Nolph KD, Sorkin MI, Moore H: Autoregulation of sodium and potassium removal during continuous ambulatory peritoneal dialysis. Trans Am Soc Artif Intern Organs 1980; 26:334-338.
106. Bargman J, Jamison R: Disorders of potassium homeostasis. *In* Sutton R, Dirks J (eds): Diuretics: Physiology, Pharmacology and Clinical Use. Philadelphia, PA, W.B. Saunders, 1986, pp 296-319.
107. Sandle GI, Gaiger E, Tapster S, Goodship TH: Evidence for large intestinal control of potassium homeostasis in uraemic patients undergoing long-term dialysis. Clin Sci (Lond) 1987; 73(3): 247-252.
108. Vaamonde CA, Michael UF, Metzger RA, Carroll KE Jr: Complications of acute peritoneal dialysis. J Chronic Dis 1975; 28(11-12):637-659.
109. Khan AN, Bernardini J, Johnston JR, Piraino B: Hypokalemia in peritoneal dialysis patients. Perit Dial Int 1996; 16(6):652.
110. Rostand SG: Profound hypokalemia in continuous ambulatory peritoneal dialysis. Arch Intern Med 1983; 143(2):377-378.
111. Lindholm B, Alvestrand A, Hultman E, Bergstrom J: Muscle water and electrolytes in patients undergoing continuous ambulatory peritoneal dialysis. Acta Med Scand 1986; 219(3):323-330.
112. Dolson GM: Do potassium deficient diets and K+ removal by dialysis contribute to the cardiovascular morbidity and mortality of patients with end stage renal disease? Int J Artif Organs 1997; 20(3):134-135.
113. Spital A, Sterns RH: Potassium supplementation via the dialysate in continuous ambulatory peritoneal dialysis. Am J Kidney Dis 1985; 6(3):173-176.
114. Hutchison AJ, Freemont AJ, Boulton HF, Gokal R: Low-calcium dialysis fluid and oral calcium carbonate in CAPD. A method of controlling hyperphosphataemia whilst minimizing aluminum exposure and hypercalcaemia. Nephrol Dial Transplant 1992; 7(12):1219-1225.
115. Hutchison AJ, Gokal R: Towards tailored dialysis fluids in CAPD: The role of reduced calcium and magnesium in dialysis fluids. Perit Dial Int 1992; 12(2):199-203.
116. Honkanen E, Kala AR, Gronhagen-Riska C, Ikaheimo R: CAPD with low calcium dialysate and calcium carbonate: Results of a 24-week study. Adv Perit Dial 1992; 8:356-361.
117. Kurz P, Tsobanelis T, Roth P, et al: Differences in calcium kinetic pattern between CAPD and HD patients. Clin Nephrol 1995; 44(4):255-261.
118. Bender FH, Bernardini J, Piraino B: Calcium mass transfer with dialysate containing 1.25 and 1.75 mmol/L calcium in peritoneal dialysis patients. Am J Kidney Dis 1992; 20(4):367-371.
119. Prichard S, Fried L: Hypercalcemia in a peritoneal dialysis patient. Perit Dial Int 2001; 21(4):420-427.
120. Parker A, Nolph KD: Magnesium and calcium mass transfer during continuous ambulatory peritoneal dialysis. Trans Am Soc Artif Intern Organs 1980; 26:194-196.
121. Banalagay EE, Bernardini J, Piraino B: Calcium mass transfer with 10-hour dwell time using 1.25 versus 1.75 mmol/L calcium dialysate. Adv Perit Dial 1993; 9:271-273.
122. Malberti F, Corradi B, Imbasciati E: Calcium mass transfer and kinetics in CAPD using calcium-free solutions. Adv Perit Dial 1993; 9:274-279.
123. Piraino B, Bernardini J, Holley J, et al: Calcium mass transfer in peritoneal dialysis patients using 2.5 mEq/L calcium dialysate. Clin Nephrol 1992; 37(1):48-51.
124. Banalagay E, Bernardini J, Holley J, et al: A randomized trial comparing 2.5 mEq/L calcium dialysate and calcitriol to 3.5 mEq/L calcium dialysate in patients on peritoneal dialysis. Adv Perit Dial 1993; 9:280-283.
125. Kwong M, Lee J, Chan M: Transperitoneal calcium and magnesium transfer during an eight-hour dialysis. Perit Dial Bull 1987; 7:85-89.
126. Martis L, Serkes KD, Nolph KD: Calcium carbonate as a phosphate binder: Is there a need to adjust peritoneal dialysate calcium concentrations for patients using CaCO3? Perit Dial Int 1989; 9(4):325-328.
127. Piraino B, Perlmutter JA, Holley JL, et al: The use of dialysate containing 2.5 mEq/L calcium in peritoneal dialysis patients. Perit Dial Int 1992; 12(1):75-76.
128. Pagliari B, Baretta A, De Cristofaro V, et al: Short-term effects of low-calcium dialysis solutions on calcium mass transfer, ionized calcium, and parathyroid hormone in CAPD patients. Perit Dial Int 1991; 11(4):326-329.
129. Montenegro J, Saracho R, Gonzalez O, et al: Reversibility of parathyroid gland suppression in CAPD patients with low i-PTH levels. Clin Nephrol 1997; 48(6):359-363.
130. Shigematsu T, Kawaguchi Y, Kubo H, et al: Low calcium (1.25 mmol/L) dialysate can normalize relative hypoparathyroidism in CAPD patients with low bone turnover. Adv Perit Dial 1996; 12:250-256.
131. Levin NW, Hoenich NA: Consequences of hyperphosphatemia and elevated levels of the calcium-phosphorus product in dialysis patients. Curr Opin Nephrol Hypertens 2001; 10(5):563-568.
132. Malberti F, Corradi B, Imbasciati E: Effect of CAPD and hemodialysis on parathyroid function. Adv Perit Dial 1996; 12:239-244.
133. Moe SM, O'Neill KD, Fineberg N, et al: Assessment of vascular calcification in ESRD patients using spiral CT. Nephrol Dial Transplant 2003; 18(6):1152-1158.
134. Wang AY, Wang M, Woo J, et al: Cardiac valve calcification as an important predictor for all-cause mortality and cardiovascular mortality in long-term peritoneal dialysis patients: A prospective study. J Am Soc Nephrol 2003; 14(1):159-168.
135. Wang AY, Woo J, Wang M, et al: Association of inflammation and malnutrition with cardiac valve calcification in continuous ambulatory peritoneal dialysis patients. J Am Soc Nephrol 2001; 12(9):1927-1936.
136. London GM, Guérin AP, Marchais SJ, et al: Arterial media calcification in end-stage renal disease: Impact on all-cause and cardiovascular mortality. Nephrol Dial Transplant 2003; 18:1731-1740.
137. Goodman WG, Goldin J, Kuizon BD, et al: Coronary-artery calcification in young adults with end-stage renal disease who are undergoing dialysis. N Engl J Med 2000; 342(20):1478-1483.
138. National Kidney Foundation. K/DOQI clinical practice guidelines for bone metabolic and disease in chronic kidney disease. Am J Kidney Dis 2003; 42:S1-S201.
139. Moe SM, Peterson JM, Murphy CL, et al: Sevelamer HCL improves parathyroid hormone (PTH) and bone function in peritoneal dialysis (PD) patients with probable low turnover bone disease. Am J Kidney Dis 2001; 37:A25.
140. Thompson TJ, Neale TI: Intraperitoneal calcium for resistant symptomatic hypocalcaemia after parathyroidectomy in chronic renal failure. Br Med J 1988; 296:896-897.
141. Heyburn PJ, Selby PL, Peacock M, et al: Peritoneal dialysis in the management of severe hypercalcaemia. Br Med J 1980; 280: 525-526.
142. Mars RL: Successful use of zero calcium dialysate to treat hypercalcemia in a postsurgical peritoneal dialysis patient. Adv Perit Dial 1993; 9:284-287.
143. Hamilton JW, Lasrich M, Hirszel P: Peritoneal dialysis in the treatment of severe hypercalcemia. J Dial 1980; 4(2-3):129-138.
144. Querfelf U, Salusky IB, Fine RN: Treatment of severe hypercalcemia with peritoneal dialysis in an infant with end-stage renal disease. Pediatr Nephrol 1988; 2:323-325.

145. Tse K, Yip P, Lam M, et al: Recurrent hemoperitoneum complicating continuous ambulatory peritoneal dialysis. Perit Dial Int 2002; 22:488-491.
146. Greenberg A, Bernardini J, Piraino BM, et al: Hemoperitoneum complicating chronic peritoneal dialysis: Single-center experience and literature review. Am J Kidney Dis 1992; 19:252-256.
147. Harnett J, Gill D, Corbett L, et al: Recurrent hemoperitoneum in women receiving continuous peritoneal dialysis. Ann Intern Med 1987; 107:341-343.
148. Holley J, Schiff M, Schmidt R, et al: Hemoperitoneum occurs in over half of menstruating women on peritoneal dialysis (Letter). Perit Dial Int 1996; 16:650.
149. Joseph J, Sahn S: Thoracic endometriosis syndrome: New observations from an analysis of 110 cases. Am J Med 1996; 100: 164-170.
150. Colucci P, Fortis D, Nicolini A, et al: Severe hemoperitoneum caused by spontaneous liver rupture: A case report. Perit Dial Int 2002; 22:417-419.
151. Dedi R, Bhandari S, Sagar PM, Turney JH: Delayed splenic rupture as a cause of haemoperitoneum in a CAPD patient with amyloidosis. Nephrol Dial Transplant 2001; 16:2446.
152. Kanagasundaram NS, Macdougall IC, Turney JH: Massive haemoperitoneum due to rupture of splenic infarct during CAPD. Nephrol Dial Transplant 1998; 13:2380-2381.
153. Wang JY, Lin YF, Lin SC, Tsao TY: Hemoperitoneum due to splenic rupture in a CAPD patient with chronic myelogenous leukemia. Perit Dial Int 1998; 18:334-337.
154. Peng S-J, Yang C-S: Hemoperitoneum in CAPD patients with hepatic tumors. Perit Dial Int 1996; 16:84-86.
155. Fine A, Novak C: Hemoperitoneum due to carcinomatosis in the liver of a CAPD patient. Perit Dial Int 1996; 16:181-183.
156. Dozio B, Scanziani R, Rovere G, et al: Hemoperitoneum in a continuous ambulatory peritoneal dialysis patient caused by a hepatocarcinoma treated with percutaneous embolization. Am J Kidney Dis 2001; 38:E11.
157. Posthuma N, van Eps RS, ter Wee PM: Hemoperitoneum due to (hepatocellular) adenoma. Perit Dial Int 1998; 18:446-447.
158. Miller R, Denman R, Saltissi D, et al: Erosion of a mesenteric vessel by a Tenckhoff catheter. Perit Dial Int 1996; 16:528-529.
159. Gadallah MF, Torres-Rivera C, Ramdeen G, et al: Relationship between intraperitoneal bleeding, adhesions, and peritoneal dialysis catheter failure: A method of prevention. Adv Perit Dial 2001; 17:127-129.
160. Ohtani H, Imai H, Komatsuda A, et al: Hemoperitoneum due to acute cytomegalovirus infection in a patient receiving peritoneal dialysis. Am J Kidney Dis 2000; 36:E33.
161. Min CH, Park JH, Ahn JH, et al: Dialysis-related amyloidosis (DRA) in a patient on CAPD presenting as haemoperitoneum with colon perforation. Nephrol Dial Transplant 1997; 12: 2761-2763.
162. Fernandez Giron F, Hermosilla Sanchez F, Paralle Alcalde M, Gonzalez Martinez J: Hemoperitoneum in peritoneal dialysis secondary to retroperitoneal hematoma (Letter). Perit Dial Int 1996; 16:644.
163. Bender F: Hemoperitoneum after pericardiocentesis in a CAPD patient (Letter). Perit Dial Int 1996; 16:330.
164. Rutecki G, Asfoura J, Whittier F: Autosomal dominant polycystic liver disease as an etiology for hemoperitoneum during CCPD. Perit Dial Int 1995; 15:367-368.
165. Twardowski ZJ, Schreiber M: A 55-year-old man with hematuria and blood-tinged dialysate (Peritoneal Dialysis Case Forum). Perit Dial Int 1992; 12:61-66.
166. Fraley D, Johnston JR, Bruns F, et al: Rupture of ovarian cyst: Massive hemoperitoneum in continuous ambulatory peritoneal dialysis patients: Diagnosis and treatment. Am J Kidney Dis 1988; 12:69-71.
167. Campisi S, Cavatorta F, De Lucia E: Iliopsoas spontaneous hematoma: An unusual cause of hemoperitoneum in CAPD patients (Letter). Perit Dial Int 1992; 12:78.
168. Ramon G, Miguel A, Caridad A, Colomer B: Bloody peritoneal fluid in a patient with tuberous sclerosis in a CAPD program (Letter). Perit Dial Int 1989; 9:353.
169. Goodkin D, Benning M: An outpatient maneuver to treat bloody effluent during continuous ambulatory peritoneal dialysis (CAPD). Perit Dial Int 1990; 10:227-229.
170. Vazelov E: Prolonged periodic intra-abdominal bleeding without serious consequences in a female patient on CAPD. Perit Dial Int 2000; 20:807.
171. Pollock CA: Bloody ascites in a patient after transfer from peritoneal dialysis to hemodialysis. Semin Dial 2003; 16:406-410.
172. Wakabayashi Y, Kawaguchi Y, Shigematsu T, et al: Extensive peritoneal calcification as a complication of long-term CAPD. Perit Dial Int 1995; 15:369-371.
173. Church C, Junor B: Images in clinical medicine. Sclerosing peritonitis during continuous ambulatory peritoneal dialysis. N Engl J Med 2002; 347:737.
174. Kawanishi H: Personal communication. 2003.
175. Rigby RJ, Hawley CM: Sclerosing peritonitis: The experience in Australia. Nephrol Dial Transplant 1998; 13:154-159.
176. Afthentopoulos IE, Passadakis P, Oreopoulos DG, Bargman J: Sclerosing peritonitis in continuous ambulatory peritoneal dialysis patients: One center's experience and review of the literature. Adv Ren Replace Ther 1998; 5:157-167.
177. Odama UO, Shih DJ, Korbet SM: Sclerosing peritonitis and systemic lupus erythematosus: A report of two cases. Perit Dial Int 1999; 19:160-164.
178. Mactier RA: The spectrum of peritoneal fibrosing syndromes in peritoneal dialysis. Adv Perit Dial 2000; 16:223-228.
179. Jenkins SB, Leng BL, Shortland JR, et al: Sclerosing encapsulating peritonitis: A case series from a single U.K. center during a 10-year period. Adv Perit Dial 2001; 17:191-195.
180. Junor B, Briggs J, Forwell M, et al: Sclerosing peritonitis: The contribution of chlorhexidine in alcohol. Perit Dial Bull 1985; 4:101-104.
181. Lo WK, Chan KT, Leung AC, et al: Sclerosing peritonitis complicating prolonged use of chlorhexidine in alcohol in the connection procedure for continuous ambulatory peritoneal dialysis. Perit Dial Int 1991; 11:166-172.
182. Marshall A, Baddeley H, Barritt D: Practolol peritonitis. Q J Med 1977; 46:135-149.
183. Harty R: Sclerosing peritonitis and propranolol. Arch Intern Med 1978; 138:1424-1426.
184. Kawanishi H, Harada Y, Noriyuki T, et al: Treatment options for encapsulating peritoneal sclerosis based on progressive stage. Adv Perit Dial 2001; 17:200-204.
185. Campbell S, Clarke P, Hawley C, et al: Sclerosing peritonitis: Identification of diagnostic, clinical, and radiological features. Am J Kidney Dis 1994; 24:819-825.
186. Stafford-Johnson DB, Wilson TE, Francis IR, Swartz R: CT appearance of sclerosing peritonitis in patients on chronic ambulatory peritoneal dialysis. J Comput Assist Tomogr 1998; 22:295-299.
187. Dobbie JW: Pathogenesis of peritoneal fibrosing syndromes (sclerosing peritonitis) in peritoneal dialysis. Perit Dial Int 1992; 12:14-27.
188. Okada K, Onishi Y, Oinuma T, et al: Sclerosing encapsulating peritonitis: Regional changes of peritoneum. Nephron 2002; 92:481-483.
189. Hauglustaine D, van Meerbeek J, Monballyu J, et al: Sclerosing peritonitis with mural bowel fibrosis in a patient on long-term CAPD. Clin Nephrol 1984; 22:158-162.
190. Kopple J: Therapeutic approaches to malnutrition in chronic dialysis patients: The different modalities of nutritional support. Am J Kidney Dis 1999; 33:180-185.
191. Pearson S, Jackson MA, Rylance PB: Sclerosing peritonitis complicating continuous ambulatory peritoneal dialysis managed by hemodialysis and home parenteral nutrition. Clin Nephrol 2002; 58:244-246.

192. Junor BJ, McMillan MA: Immunosuppression in sclerosing peritonitis. Adv Perit Dial 1993; 9:187-189.
193. Bhandari S, Wilkinson A, Sellars L: Sclerosing peritonitis: Value of immunosuppression prior to surgery. Nephrol Dial Transplant 1994; 9:436-437.
194. Mori Y, Matsuo S, Sutoh H, et al: A case of a dialysis patient with sclerosing peritonitis successfully treated with corticosteroid therapy alone. Am J Kidney Dis 1997; 30:275-278.
195. Allaria PM, Giangrande A, Gandini E, Pisoni IB: Continuous ambulatory peritoneal dialysis and sclerosing encapsulating peritonitis: Tamoxifen as a new therapeutic agent? J Nephrol 1999; 12:395-397.
196. Fagugli RM, Selvi A, Quintaliani G, et al: Immunosuppressive treatment for sclerosing peritonitis. Nephrol Dial Transplant 1999; 14:1343-1345.
197. Rajani R, Smyth J, Koffman CG, et al: Differential effect of sirolimus vs prednisolone in the treatment of sclerosing encapsulating peritonitis. Nephrol Dial Transplant 2002; 17:2278-2280.
198. Kawanishi H, Harada Y, Sakikubo E, et al: Surgical treatment for sclerosing encapsulating peritonitis. Adv Perit Dial 2000; 16: 252-256.
199. Klimopoulos S, Katsoulis IE, Margellos V, Nikolopoulou N: Sclerosing encapsulating peritonitis secondary to CAPD: The effect of fibrotic debridement on further dialysis. J R Coll Surg Edinb 2002; 47:485-490.
200. Twardowski ZJ, Khanna R, Nolph KD, et al: Intraabdominal pressures during natural activities in patients treated with continuous ambulatory peritoneal dialysis. Nephron 1986; 44:129-135.
201. Durand PY, Chanliau J, Gamberoni J, et al: Measurement of hydrostatic intraperitoneal pressure: A necessary routine test in peritoneal dialysis. Perit Dial Int 1996; 16(suppl 1):S84-S87.
202. Chow KM, Szeto CC, Li PK: Management options for hydrothorax complicating peritoneal dialysis. Semin Dial 2003; 16:389-394.
203. Boeschoten EW, Krediet RT, Roos CM, et al: Leakage of dialysate across the diaphragm: An important complication of continuous ambulatory peritoneal dialysis. Neth J Med 1986; 29:242-246.
204. Shemin D, Clarke D, Chazan J: Unexplained pleural effusions in the peritoneal dialysis population. Perit Dial Int 1989; 9:143.
205. Bundy JT, Pontier PJ: Cough-induced hydrothorax in peritoneal dialysis. Perit Dial Int 1994; 14:293.
206. Caravaca F, Arrobas M, Cubero JJ, et al: Tight corsets and hydrothorax on CAPD. Perit Dial Int 1991; 11:87-88.
207. Hausmann MJ, Basok A, Vorobiov M, Rogachev B: Traumatic pleural leak in peritoneal dialysis. Nephrol Dial Transplant 2001; 16:1526.
208. Fletcher S, Turney JH, Brownjohn AM: Increased incidence of hydrothorax complicating peritoneal dialysis in patients with adult polycystic kidney disease. Nephrol Dial Transplant 1994; 9:832-833.
209. Benz RL, Schleifer CR: Hydrothorax in continuous ambulatory peritoneal dialysis: Successful treatment with intrapleural tetracycline and a review of the literature. Am J Kidney Dis 1985; 5:136-140.
210. Green A, Logan M, Medawar W, et al: The management of hydrothorax in continuous ambulatory peritoneal dialysis (CAPD). Perit Dial Int 1990; 10:271-274.
211. Simmons LE, Mir AR: A review of management of pleuroperitoneal communication in five CAPD patients. Adv Perit Dial 1989; 5:81-83.
212. Chow KM, Szeto CC, Wong TY, Li PK: Hydrothorax complicating peritoneal dialysis: Diagnostic value of glucose concentration in pleural fluid aspirate. Perit Dial Int 2002; 22: 525-528.
213. Tang S, Chui WH, Tang AW, et al: Video-assisted thoracoscopic talc pleurodesis is effective for maintenance of peritoneal dialysis in acute hydrothorax complicating peritoneal dialysis. Nephrol Dial Transplant 2003; 18:804-808.
214. Nomoto Y, Suga T, Nakajima K, et al: Acute hydrothorax in continuous ambulatory peritoneal dialysis: A collaborative study of 161 centers. Am J Nephrol 1989; 9:363-367.
215. Lazaridis KN, Frank JW, Krowka MJ, Kamath PS: Hepatic hydrothorax: Pathogenesis, diagnosis, and management. Am J Med 1999; 107:262-267.
216. Lieberman F, Hidemura R, Peters R, Reynolds T: Pathogenesis and treatment of hydrothorax complicating cirrhosis with ascites. Ann Intern Med 1966; 64:341-351.
217. Johnston RF, Loo RV: Hepatic hydrothorax. Studies to determine the source of the fluid and a report of thirteen cases. Ann Intern Med 1964; 61:385-401.
218. Kirschner PA: Catamenial pneumothorax: An example of porous diaphragm syndromes. Chest 2000; 118:1519-1520.
219. Hou C-H, Tsai T-J, Hsu K-L: Peritoneopericardial communication after pericardiocentesis in a patient on continuous ambulatory peritoneal dialysis with dialysis pericarditis. Nephron 1994; 68:125-127.
220. Nather S, Anger H, Koall W, et al: Peritoneal leak and chronic pericardial effusion in a CAPD patient. Nephrol Dial Transplant 1996; 11:1155-1158.
221. Scheldewaert R, Bogaerts Y, Pauwels R, et al: Management of a massive hydrothorax in a CAPD patient: A case report and a review of the literature. Perit Dial Bull 1982; 2:69-72.
222. Kennedy J: Procedures used to demonstrate a pleuroperitoneal communication: A review. Perit Dial Bull 1982; 2:168-170.
223. Macia M, Gallego E, Garcia-Cobaleda I, et al: Methylene blue as a cause of chemical peritonitis in a patient on peritoneal dialysis (Letter). Clin Nephrol 1995; 43:136-137.
224. Singh S, Vaidya P, Dale A, Morgan B: Massive hydrothorax complicating continuous ambulatory peritoneal dialysis. Nephron 1983; 34:168-172.
225. Huang JJ, Wu JS, Chi WC, et al: Hydrothorax in continuous ambulatory peritoneal dialysis: Therapeutic implications of Tc-99m MAA peritoneal scintigraphy. Nephrol Dial Transplant 1999; 14:992-997.
226. Adam WR, Arkles LB, Gill G, et al: Hydrothorax with peritoneal dialysis: Radionuclide detection of a pleuro-peritoneal connection. Aust N Z J Med 1980; 10:330-332.
227. Gibbons GD, Baumert J: Unilateral hydrothorax complicating peritoneal dialysis. Use of radionuclide imaging. Clin Nucl Med 1983; 8:83-84.
228. Lepage S, Bisson G, Verreault J, Plante GE: Massive hydrothorax complicating peritoneal dialysis. Isotopic investigation (peritoneopleural scintigraphy). Clin Nucl Med 1993; 18: 498-501.
229. Mestas D, Wauquier JP, Escande G, et al: Diagnosis of hydrothorax complicating CAPD and demonstration of successful therapy by scintigraphy. Perit Dial Int 1991; 11:283-284.
230. Prischl FC, Muhr T, Seiringer EM, et al: Magnetic resonance imaging of the peritoneal cavity among peritoneal dialysis patients, using the dialysate as "contrast medium." J Am Soc Nephrol 2002; 13:197-203.
231. Zenda T, Miyamoto S, Murata S, Mabuchi H: Detection of diaphragmatic defect as the cause of severe hepatic hydrothorax with magnetic resonance imaging. Am J Gastroenterol 1998; 93:2288-2289.
232. Vezina D, Winchester JF, Rakowski TA: Spontaneous Resolution of Massive Hydrothorax in a CAPD Patient (Letter). Perit Dial Bull 1987; 7:212-213.
233. Ing A, Rutland J, Kalowski S: Spontaneous resolution of hydrothorax in continuous ambulatory peritoneal dialysis. Nephron 1992; 61:247-248.
234. Mak SK, Nyunt K, Wong PN, et al: Long-term follow-up of thoracoscopic pleurodesis for hydrothorax complicating peritoneal dialysis. Ann Thorac Surg 2002; 74:218-221.
235. Jagasia MH, Cole FH, Stegman MH, et al: Video-assisted talc pleurodesis in the management of pleural effusion secondary to

continuous ambulatory peritoneal dialysis: A report of three cases. Am J Kidney Dis 1996; 28:772-774.
236. Kanaan N, Pieters T, Jamar F, Goffin E: Hydrothorax complicating continuous ambulatory peritoneal dialysis: Successful management with talc pleurodesis under thoracoscopy. Nephrol Dial Transplant 1999; 14:1590-1592.
237. Hidai H, Takatsu S, Chiba T: Intrathoracic instillation of autologous blood in treating massive hydrothorax following CAPD. Perit Dial Int 1989; 9:221-223.
238. Catizone L, Zuchelli A, Zucchelli P: Hydrothorax in a PD patient: Successful treatment with intrapleural autologous blood instillation. Adv Perit Dial 1991; 7:86-90.
239. Okada K, Takahashi S, Kinoshita Y: Effect of pleurodesis with autoblood on hydrothorax due to continuous ambulatory peritoneal dialysis-induced diaphragmatic communication. Nephron 1993; 65:163-164.
240. Scarpioni R: Acute hydrothorax in a peritoneal dialysis patient: Long-term efficacy of autologous blood cell pleurodesis associated with small-volume peritoneal exchanges. Nephrol Dial Transplant 2003; 18:2200-2201.
241. Vlachojannis J, Boettcher I, Brandt L, Schoeppe W: A new treatment for unilateral recurrent hydrothorax during CAPD. Perit Dial Bull 1985; 5:180-181.
242. Di Bisceglie M, Paladini P, Voltolini L, et al: Videothoracoscopic obliteration of pleuroperitoneal fistula in continuous peritoneal dialysis. Ann Thorac Surg 1996; 62:1509-1510.
243. Tsunezuka Y, Hatakeyama S, Iwase T, Watanabe G: Video-assisted thoracoscopic treatment for pleuroperitoneal communication in peritoneal dialysis. Eur J Cardiothorac Surg 2001; 20:205-207.
244. Halstead JC, Lim E, Ritchie AJ: Acute hydrothorax in CAPD. Early thoracoscopic (VATS) intervention allows return to peritoneal dialysis. Nephron 2002; 92:725-727.
245. Pattison CW, Rodger RS, Adu D, Michael J, et al: Surgical treatment of hydrothorax complicating continuous ambulatory peritoneal dialysis. Clin Nephrol 1984; 21:191-193.
246. Allen SM, Matthews HR: Surgical treatment of massive hydrothorax complicating continuous ambulatory peritoneal dialysis. Clin Nephrol 1991; 36:299-301.
247. Okada H, Ryuzaki M, Kotaki S, et al: Thoracoscopic surgery and pleurodesis for pleuroperitoneal communication in patients on continuous ambulatory peritoneal dialysis. Am J Kidney Dis 1999; 34:170-172.
248. Suh H, Wadhwa NK, Cabralda T, et al: Abdominal wall hernias in ESRD patients receiving peritoneal dialysis. Adv Perit Dial 1994; 10:85-88.
249. Bleyer AJ, Casey MJ, Russell GB, et al: Peritoneal dialysate fill-volumes and hernia development in a cohort of peritoneal dialysis patients. Adv Perit Dial 1998; 14:102-104.
250. Tokgoz B, Dogukan A, Guven M, et al: Relationship between different body size indicators and hernia development in CAPD patients. Clin Nephrol 2003; 60:183-186.
251. Del Peso G, Bajo MA, Costero O, et al: Risk factors for abdominal wall complications in peritoneal dialysis patients. Perit Dial Int 2003; 23:249-254.
252. Nassberger L: Enterocele due to continuous ambulatory peritoneal dialysis (CAPD). Acta Obstet Gynecol Scand 1984; 63:283.
253. Francis D, Schofield I, Veitch PS: Abdominal hernias in patients treated with continuous ambulatory peritoneal dialysis. Br J Surg 1982; 69:409.
254. Hughes GC, Ketchersid TL, Lenzen JM, Lowe JE: Thoracic complications of peritoneal dialysis. Ann Thorac Surg 1999; 67:1518-1522.
255. Polk D, Madden R, Lipkowitz G, et al: Use of computerized tomography in the evaluation of a CAPD patient with a foramen of Morgagni hernia: A case report. Perit Dial Int 1996; 16:318-320.
256. Shohat J, Shapira Z, Shmuel iD, Boner GI: Intestinal incarceration in occult abdominal wall herniae in continuous ambulatory peritoneal dialysis. Israel J Med Sci 1985; 21:985-987.
257. Afthentopoulos IE, Panduranga Rao S, Mathews R, Oreopoulos DG: Hernia development in CAPD patients and the effect of 2.5 l dialysate volume in selected patients. Clin Nephrol 1998; 49:251-257.
258. Apostolidis NS, Tzardis PJ, Manouras AJ, et al: The incidence of postoperative hernia as related to the site of insertion of permanent peritoneal catheter. Am Surg 1988; 54:318-319.
259. Spence P, Mathews R, Khanna R, Oreopoulos DG: Improved results with a paramedian technique for the insertion of peritoneal dialysis catheters. Surg Gynecol Obstet 1985; 161(6):585-587.
260. O'Connor JP, Rigby RJ, Hardie IR, et al: Abdominal hernias complicating continuous ambulatory peritoneal dialysis. Am J Nephrol 1986; 6:271-274.
261. Hussain SI, Bernardini J, Piraino B: The risk of hernia with large exchange volumes. Adv Perit Dial 1998; 14:105-107.
262. Modi K, Grant A, Garret A, Rodger RS: Indirect inguinal hernia in CAPD patients with polycystic kidney disease. Adv Perit Dial 1989; 5:84-86.
263. Hadimeri H, Johansson AC, Haraldsson B, Nyberg G: CAPD in patients with autosomal dominant polycystic kidney disease. Perit Dial Int 1998; 18:429-432.
264. Twardowski ZJ, Tully RJ, Ersoy FF, Dedhia NM: Computerized tomography with and without intraperitoneal contrast for determination of intraabdominal fluid distribution and diagnosis of complications in peritoneal dialysis patients. ASAIO Trans 1990; 36:95-103.
265. Scanziani R, Dozio B, Caimi F, et al: Peritoneography and peritoneal computerized tomography: A new approach to non-infectious complications of CAPD. Nephrol Dial Transplant 1992; 7:1035-1038.
266. Hollett MD, Marn CS, Ellis JH, et al: Complications of continuous ambulatory peritoneal dialysis: Evaluation with CT peritoneography. Am J Roentgenol 1992; 159:983-989.
267. Camsari T, Celik A, Ozaksoy D, et al: Non-infectious complications of continuous ambulatory peritoneal dialysis: Evaluation with peritoneal computed tomography. Scand J Urol Nephrol 1997; 31:377-380.
268. Hawkins SP, Homer JA, Murray BB, et al: Modified computed tomography peritoneography: Clinical utility in continuous ambulatory peritoneal dialysis patients. Australas Radiol 2000; 44:398-403.
269. Johnson BF, Segasby CA, Holroyd AM, et al: A method for demonstrating subclinical inguinal herniae in patients undergoing peritoneal dialysis: The isotope "peritoneoscrotogram." Nephrol Dial Transplant 1987; 2:254-257.
270. Berman C, Velchik MG, Shusterman N, Alavi A: The clinical utility of the Tc-99m SC intraperitoneal scan in CAPD patients. Clin Nucl Med 1989; 14:405-409.
271. Johnson J, Baum S, Smink RD Jr: Radionuclide imaging in the diagnosis of hernias related to peritoneal dialysis. Arch Surg 1987; 122:952-954.
272. Sissons GR, Jones SM, Evans C, Richards AR: Scintigraphic detection of abdominal hernias associated with continuous ambulatory peritoneal dialysis. Br J Radiol 1991; 64:1158-1161.
273. Juergensen PH, Rizvi H, Caride VJ, et al: Value of scintigraphy in chronic peritoneal dialysis patients. Kidney Int 1999; 55:1111-1119.
274. Rajnish A, Ahmad M, Kumar P: Peritoneal scintigraphy in the diagnosis of complications associated with continuous ambulatory peritoneal dialysis. Clin Nucl Med 2003; 28:70-71.
275. Mettang T, Stoeltzing H, Alscher DM, et al: Sustaining continuous ambulatory peritoneal dialysis after herniotomy. Adv Perit Dial 2001; 17:84-87.
276. Lewis DM, Bingham C, Beaman M, et al: Polypropylene mesh hernia repair: An alternative permitting rapid return to peritoneal dialysis. Nephrol Dial Transplant 1998; 13:2488-2489.
277. Imvrios G, Tsakiris D, Gakis D, et al: Prosthetic mesh repair of multiple recurrent and large abdominal hernias in continuous

ambulatory peritoneal dialysis patients. Perit Dial Int 1994; 14:338-343.

278. Kopecky RT, Funk M, Kreitzer P: Localized genital edema in patients undergoing continuous ambulatory peritoneal dialysis. J Urol 1985; 134:880-884.

279. Diaz-Buxo J, Burgess P, Walker J: Peritoneovaginal fistula: Unusual complication of peritoneal dialysis. Perit Dial Bull 1983; 13:142-143.

280. Ogunc G, Oygur N: Vaginal fistula: A new complication in CAPD (Letter). Perit Dial Int 1995; 15:84-85.

281. Bradley AJ, Mamtora H, Pritchard N: Transvaginal leak of peritoneal dialysate demonstrated by CT peritoneography. Br J Radiol 1997; 70:652-653.

282. Mandel P, Faegenburg D, Imbriano LJ: The use of technetium-99m sulfur colloid in the detection of patent processus vaginalis in patients on continuous ambulatory peritoneal dialysis. Clin Nucl Med 1985; 10:553-555.

283. Capelouto CC, DeWolf WC: Genital swelling secondary to leakage from continuous ambulatory peritoneal dialysis: Computerized tomography diagnosis. J Urol 1993; 150:196-198.

284. Litherland J, Lupton E, Ackrill P, et al: Computed tomographic peritoneography: CT manifestations in the investigation of leaks and abnormal collections in patients on CAPD. Nephrol Dial Transplant 1994; 9:1449-1452.

285. Walker JV, Fish MB: Scintigraphic detection of abdominal wall and diaphragmatic peritoneal leaks in patients on continuous ambulatory peritoneal dialysis. J Nucl Med 1988; 29:1596-1602.

286. Portoles J, Coronel F, Ganado T: Abdominal wall leakage on CAPD: Usefulness of ultrasonography. Nephron 1995; 69:348-349.

287. Tzamaloukas AH, Gibel LJ, Eisenberg B, et al: Early and late peritoneal dialysate leaks in patients on CAPD. Adv Perit Dial 1990; 6:64-71.

288. Joffe P: Peritoneal dialysis catheter leakage treated with fibrin glue. Nephrol Dial Transplant 1993; 8:474-476.

289. Hirsch D, Jindal K: Late leaks in peritoneal dialysis patients. Nephrol Dial Transplant 1990; 6:670-671.

290. Holley J, Bernardini J, Piraino B: Characteristics and outcome of peritoneal dialysate leaks and associated infections. Adv Perit Dial 1993; 9:240-243.

291. Cacho CP, Tessman MJ, Newman LN, Friedlander MA: Inflow obstruction due to kinking of coiled catheters during placement. Perit Dial Int 1995; 15:276-278.

292. Guiserix J, Ramdane M, Rajaonarivelo P, Finielz P: Obstructive fibrin clot in the peritoneal catheter. Perit Dial Int 1996; 16:93.

293. De Vecchi AF, Cresseri D, Scalamogna A: Obstruction of the peritoneal catheter caused by cryoglobulin precipitation. Perit Dial Int 2002; 22:276-277.

294. Abidin MR, Spector DA, Kittur DS: Peritoneal dialysis catheter outflow obstruction due to oviductal fimbriae: A case report. Am J Kidney Dis 1990; 16:256-258.

295. Abouljoud MS, Cruz C: Obstruction of PD catheters by fallopian tubes. Perit Dial Int 1994; 14:90.

296. Borghol M, Alrabeeah A: Entrapment of the appendix and the fallopian tube in peritoneal dialysis catheters in two children. J Pediatr Surg 1996; 31:427-429.

297. Macallister RJ, Morgan SH: Fallopian tube capture of chronic peritoneal dialysis catheters. Perit Dial Int 1993; 13:74-76.

298. Diaz-Buxo JA: Management of peritoneal catheter malfunction. Perit Dial Int 1998; 18:256-259.

299. Hashimoto Y, Yano S, Nakanishi Y, et al: A simple method for opening an obstructed peritoneal catheter using an infusion accelerator. Adv Perit Dial 1996; 12:227-230.

300. Kumwenda MJ, Wright FK: The use of a channel-cleaning brush for malfunctioning Tenckhoff catheters. Nephrol Dial Transplant 1999; 14:1254-1257.

301. Tranter SA: Re-establishment of flow in peritoneal dialysis catheters using the endoluminal FAS brush. Perit Dial Int 2002; 22:275-276.

302. Stringel G, Olsen S, Cascio C: Unblocking peritoneal dialysis catheters with a combination of urokinase and Fogarty catheter manipulation. Adv Perit Dial 1995; 11:200-201.

303. Majors DS: Thrombolytic therapy with urokinase. Anna J 1996; 23:627-629.

304. Stadermann MB, Rusthoven E, van de Kar NC, et al: Local fibrinolytic therapy with urokinase for peritoneal dialysis catheter obstruction in children. Perit Dial Int 2002; 22:84-86.

305. Sakarcan A, Stallworth JR: Tissue plasminogen activator for occluded peritoneal dialysis catheter. Pediatr Nephrol 2002; 17:155-156.

306. Shea M, Hmiel SP, Beck AM: Use of tissue plasminogen activator for thrombolysis in occluded peritoneal dialysis catheters in children. Adv Perit Dial 2001; 17:249-252.

307. Maccario M, De Vecchi A, Scalamogna A, et al: Reversible catheter obstruction by omental wrapping in a CAPD patient. Perit Dial Int 1995; 15:278-279.

308. Garcia Ramon R, Carrasco SM, Ballester Sapina B: Correction of outflow obstruction with the use of sennosides in CAPD patients. Perit Dial Int 1996; 16:642-643.

309. Diaz-Buxo JA, Turner MW, Nelms M: Fluoroscopic manipulation of Tenckhoff catheters: Outcome analysis. Clin Nephrol 1997; 47:384-388.

310. Dobrashian RD, Conway B, Hutchison A, et al: The repositioning of migrated Tenckhoff continuous ambulatory peritoneal dialysis catheters under fluoroscopic control. Br J Radiol 1999; 72:452-456.

311. Kappel JE, Ferguson GM, Kudel RM, et al: Stiff wire manipulation of peritoneal dialysis catheters. Adv Perit Dial 1995; 11:202-207.

312. Jones B, McLaughlin K, Mactier RA, Porteous C: Tenckhoff catheter salvage by closed stiff-wire manipulation without fluoroscopic control. Perit Dial Int 1998; 18:415-418.

313. Simons ME, Pron G, Voros M, et al: Fluoroscopically-guided manipulation of malfunctioning peritoneal dialysis catheters. Perit Dial Int 1999; 19:544-549.

314. McLaughlin K, Jardine AG: Closed stiff-wire manipulation of malpositioned Tenckhoff catheters offers a safe and effective way of prolonging peritoneal dialysis. Int J Artif Organs 2000; 23:219-220.

315. Kim HJ, Lee TW, Ihm CG, Kim MJ: Use of fluoroscopy-guided wire manipulation and/or laparoscopic surgery in the repair of malfunctioning peritoneal dialysis catheters. Am J Nephrol 2002; 22:532-538.

316. Asif A, Byers P, Vieira CF, et al: Peritoneoscopic placement of peritoneal dialysis catheter and bowel perforation: Experience of an interventional nephrology program. Am J Kidney Dis 2003; 42:1270-1274.

317. Gadallah MF, Arora N, Arumugam R, Moles K: Role of Fogarty catheter manipulation in management of migrated, nonfunctional peritoneal dialysis catheters. Am J Kidney Dis 2000; 35:301-305.

318. Barone GW, Lightfoot ML, Ketel BL: Technique for laparoscopy-assisted complicated peritoneal dialysis catheter placement. J Laparoendosc Adv Surg Tech A 2002; 12:53-55.

319. Batey CA, Crane JJ, Jenkins MA, et al: Mini-laparoscopy-assisted placement of Tenckhoff catheters: An improved technique to facilitate peritoneal dialysis. J Endourol 2002; 16: 681-684.

320. Hodgson D, Rowbotham C, Peters JL, Nathan S: A novel method for laparoscopic placement of Tenckhoff peritoneal dialysis catheters. BJU Int 2003; 91:885-886.

321. Lu CT, Watson DI, Elias TJ, et al: Laparoscopic placement of peritoneal dialysis catheters: 7 years experience. ANZ J Surg 2003; 73:109-111.

322. Amerling R, Maele DV, Spivak H, et al: Laparoscopic salvage of malfunctioning peritoneal catheters. Surg Endosc 1997; 11: 249-252.

323. Brandt CP, Ricanati ES: Use of laparoscopy in the management of malfunctioning peritoneal dialysis catheters. Adv Perit Dial 1996; 12:223-226.

324. Zadrozny D, Lichodziejewska-Niemierko M, Draczkowski T, et al: Laparoscopic approach for dysfunctional Tenckhoff catheters. Perit Dial Int 1999; 19:170-171.
325. Ogunc G: Malfunctioning peritoneal dialysis catheter and accompanying surgical pathology repaired by laparoscopic surgery. Perit Dial Int 2002; 22:454-462.
326. Chao SH, Tsai TJ: Laparoscopic rescue of dysfunctional Tenckhoff catheters in continuous ambulatory peritoneal dialysis patients. Nephron 1993; 65:157-158.
327. Fukui M, Maeda K, Sakamoto K, et al: Laparoscopic manipulation for outflow failure of peritoneal dialysis catheter. Nephron 1999; 83:369.
328. Jonler M, Lund L, Kyrval H: Laparoscopic correction and fixation of displaced peritoneal dialysis catheters. Int Urol Nephrol 2003; 35:85-86.
329. Quiroga I, Reddy SP, Bhattacharjya S, Darby CR: Tenckhoff catheters:The pull technique. Nephrol Dial Transplant 2003; 18:1682.
330. Campisi S, Cavatorta F, Ramo E, Varano P: Videolaparoscopy with partial omentectomy in patients on peritoneal dialysis. Perit Dial Int 1997; 17:211-212.
331. Lee M, Donovan JF: Laparoscopic omentectomy for salvage of peritoneal dialysis catheters. J Endourol 2002; 16:241-244.
332. Crabtree JH, Fishman A: Laparoscopic epiplopexy of the greater omentum and epiploic appendices in the salvaging of dysfunctional peritoneal dialysis catheters. Surg Laparosc Endosc 1996; 6:176-180.
333. Ogunc G: Videolaparoscopy with omentopexy: A new technique to allow placement of a catheter for continuous ambulatory peritoneal dialysis. Surg Today 2001; 31:942-944.
334. Crabtree JH, Fishman A: Selective performance of prophylactic omentopexy during laparoscopic implantation of peritoneal dialysis catheters. Surg Laparosc Endosc Percutan Tech 2003; 13:180-184.
335. Giannattasio M, La Rosa R, Balestrazzi A: How can videolaparoscopy be used in a peritoneal dialysis programme? Nephrol Dial Transplant 1999; 14:409-411.
336. Klein Z, Magen E, Fishman A, Korzets Z: Laparoscopic salpingectomy: The definitive treatment for peritoneal dialysis catheter outflow obstruction caused by oviductal fimbriae. J Laparoendosc Adv Surg Tech A 2003; 13:65-68.

SECTION E

Transplantation

Chapter 31

Transplantation Immunobiology

Nader Najafian, M.D. • Alan M. Krensky, M.D. • Mohamed H. Sayegh, M.D.

When an organ or tissue from one member of a species is transplanted into a nonidentical member of the same species, an immune response ensues. This response is termed the *alloimmune response.* The alloimmune response is primarily orchestrated by initial T cell recognition of alloantigens (allorecognition) followed by a series of cellular and molecular events leading to the effector mechanisms of allograft destruction. The first and major component of this chapter reviews the mechanisms of the alloimmune response and how it leads to allograft rejection. Last but not least, the ultimate goal in clinical transplantation is to induce a state of donor-specific immunologic tolerance, where recipients can accept organs without the need of exogenous immunosuppression. Greater understanding of the interplay of the various costimulatory and inhibitory signals has led to important insights into how lymphocytes differentiation is specified, how effector cells are regulated, how memory is generated, and how tolerance is maintained. The second part of this chapter will review these concepts.

THE ALLOIMMUNE RESPONSE

Transplantation Antigens

Major Histocompatibility Complex

The major histocompatibility complex (MHC) antigens are the strongest transplantation antigens and can stimulate a primary immune response without priming. The alloimmune response arises as a direct result of the normal function of MHC molecules. T lymphocytes recognize foreign (nonself) antigens in the context of self cell-surface molecules encoded in the MHC.[1] In humans, this genetic region is located in a 3.5-million base-pair region on the short arm of chromosome 6. This locus is further subdivided into three clusters based on the structure and function of the proteins encoded by the genes. Human MHC molecules are called *human leukocyte antigens* (HLAs), and the three regions have been designated HLA class I, class II, and class III (Figure 31–1).

HLA class I molecules (classic HLA-A, -B, and -C and other nonclassic molecules) are composed of a 44-kD heavy chain and a 12-kD light chain (Figure 31–2*A*; see Color Figure).[1,2] The amino terminus portion of the heavy chain that extends into the extracellular space is composed of three domains: $\alpha1$, $\alpha2$, and $\alpha3$. The $\alpha1$ and $\alpha2$ domains interact to form the sides of a cleft (or groove). The cleft is the site where foreign proteins bind to MHC molecules for presentation to T cells. The highly variable amino acid residues located in the groove determine the specificity of peptide binding and T-cell antigen recognition. The light chain, β_2-microglobulin, stabilizes the heavy chain, such that displacement of β_2-microglobulin from the class I molecule causes a loss of heavy chain native structure. The function of intact class I molecules is to present antigenic peptides as protein fragments (peptides) in the context of self to T lymphocytes. HLA class I molecules are highly polymorphic. This polymorphism aids in maximizing the potential for peptide binding by the species. Peptides bind within the HLA class I groove (Figure 31–3*A*; see Color Figure) based on the sequence of amino acids in the peptide-binding region.[3] HLA class I molecules tend to bind peptides of 9 to 10 amino acids in length. These peptides fit tightly into the groove and do not extend out of the ends of the molecule.

MHC class I molecules generally present endogenous proteins (Figure 31–4). These proteins, such as viruses and normal self proteins, are degraded in the cytoplasm in proteosomes. Short peptide sequences are then moved to the endoplasmic reticulum through specific transporters associated with antigen presentation (TAP transporters). In the endoplasmic reticulum, these peptides associate with class I heavy chain and β_2-microglobulin, and the mature complex is transported to the cell surface, where it can be recognized by T lymphocytes. Peptides sit in the middle of the groove and run the length of the cleft. The rules for peptide binding are restricted to certain "motifs" based on the polymorphisms described earlier but are lax enough to permit the binding of many different peptides to a single HLA type (allele). Antigens associated with class I molecules are recognized by cytotoxic CD8+ T lymphocytes.

The second major region of the MHC is called the *class II locus* (see Figure 31–1).[1] HLA class II molecules, HLA-DP, DQ, and DR, are composed of heavy (α) and light (β) chains of about 35 and 31 kD, respectively. These two chains associate to form a peptide-binding region, but unlike class I molecules, determinants of the peptide-binding region are contributed by both

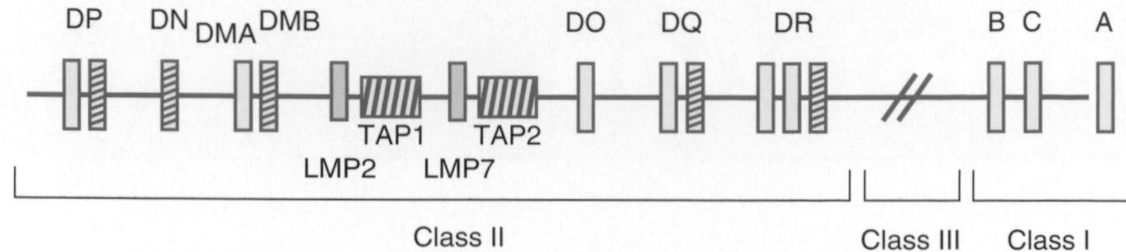

Figure 31–1 Genomic organization of the human major histocompatibility complex (MHC). See text for explanation. (From Noessner E, Krensky AM: HLA and antigen presentation. *In* Tilney NL, Strom TB, Paul LC [eds]: Transplantation Biology: Cellular and Molecular Aspects. New York, Lippincott-Raven, 1996, p 31.1.)

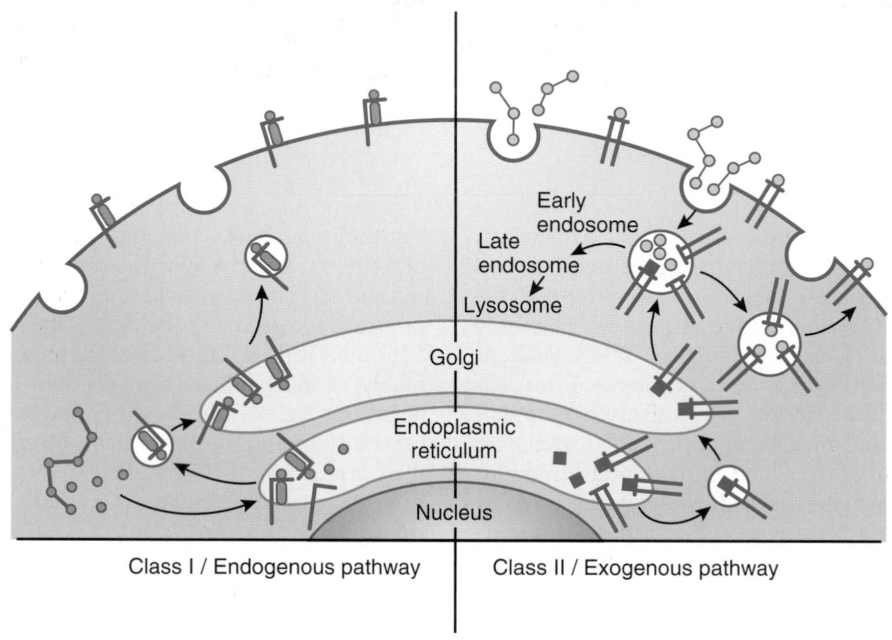

Figure 31–4 Antigen processing and presentation. In the endogenous pathway *(left),* HLA class I molecules bind to peptides from endogenous antigens. The proteosome breaks up cytoplasmic proteins into peptides that enter the endoplasmic reticulum via specific transporters. In the endoplasmic reticulum, peptides associate with HLA class I molecules and from the mature complex which is exported through the Golgi apparatus to the plasma membrane. In the exogenous pathway *(right),* HLA class II molecules bind peptides from exogenous antigens. Exogenous proteins enter the cell by endocytosis and are degraded to peptides in endosomes and lysosomes. Class II molecules bind peptides in the "compartment for peptide loading" and are transported to the plasma membrane. (From Krensky AM: Transplantation Immunobiology. *In* Jamison R, Wilkinson R [eds]: Nephrology. London, Chapman and Hall, 1997, p 1051. Reprinted by permission of Hodder Arnold.)

chains (see Figure 31–2*B*).[2] MHC class II molecules bind longer peptides, typically of 12 to 28 amino acids. In contrast to class I, MHC class II molecules have binding grooves that are open at the ends, permitting peptides of greater length to extend beyond the groove (see Figure 31–3*B*).[4] Class II molecules tend to bind antigens derived from the exogenous pathway (see Figure 31–4). MHC class II α and β chains associate in the endoplasmic reticulum with an invariant chain, a portion of which binds in the antigen-binding groove. This invariant chain appears to both protect the groove from peptide binding and permit proper folding of the class II complex. A nonameric form exits the endoplasmic reticulum and moves through the Golgi apparatus and into an endosomal compartment. Within the endosome, the invariant chain is degraded, leaving a shorter class II–associated invariant chain peptide (CLIP) fragment in the groove. Peptides from the extracellular space are taken up into endosomes by endocytosis and targeted to the "compartment for peptide loading." Within this specialized intercellular compartment, exogenous peptides displace CLIP, and the mature heterotrimeric complex (α, β, and peptide) is transported to the cell surface, where it can be recognized by T lymphocytes.

In addition to the classic class II antigens, the MHC class II region encodes proteins that make up the proteasome (low-molecular-weight proteins, LMP-2 and LMP-7) and the TAP transporters (TAP-1 and TAP-2) (see Figure 31–1). Polymorphisms associated with these structures also contribute probably to the specificity and diversity of peptide binding and antigen presentation.

The class III region encodes a variety of proteins of immunologic relevance (see Figure 31–1). These include tumor necrosis factor (TNF) and complement proteins, factor B, and C4.

The alloimmune response is strong and does not require priming.[5] At least part of the basis for the greater magnitude

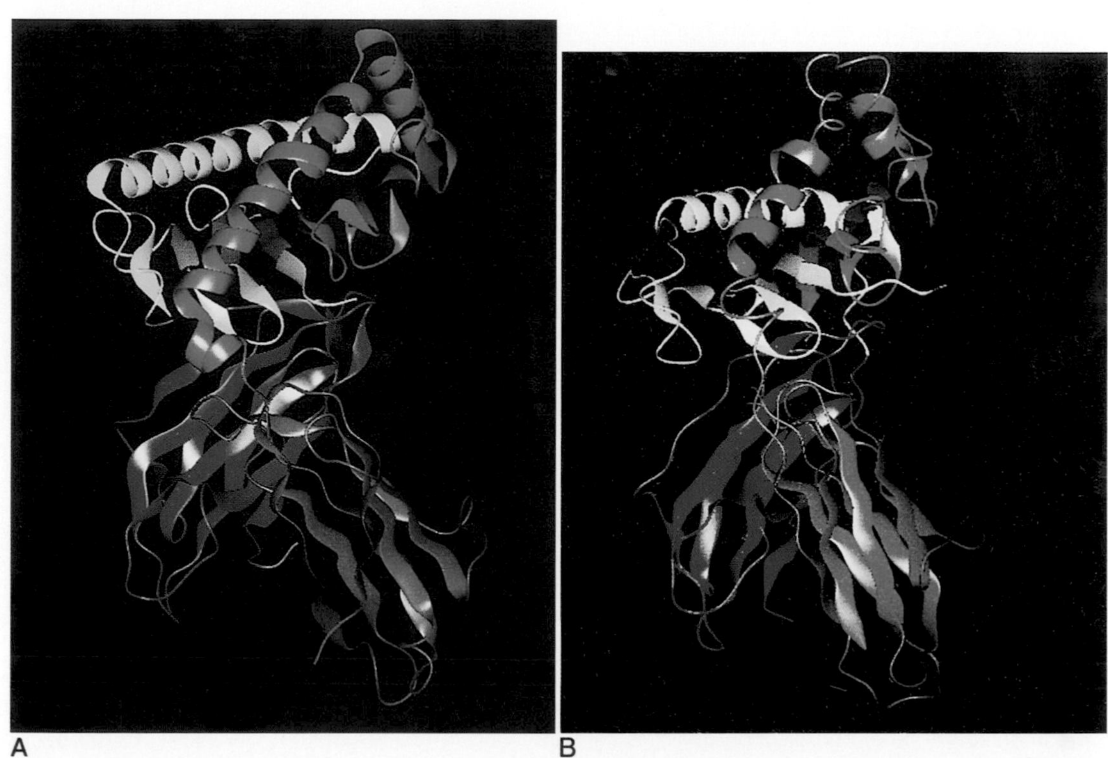

Figure 31–2 **(A)** Computer model of HLA class I (HLA-B27) and **(B)** class II (HLA-DR1) structures. The peptide-binding region, made up of two a helices supported by a floor of b strands, is at the top of both views. For HLA-B27, a_1 domain is yellow, a_2 domain is red, b_1 domain is blue, and b_2 domain is green. The colors are the same for homologous domains in the two proteins. (From Germain R: MHC-dependent antigen processing and peptide presentation: Providing ligands for T lymphocyte activation. Cell 1994; 76:288.)

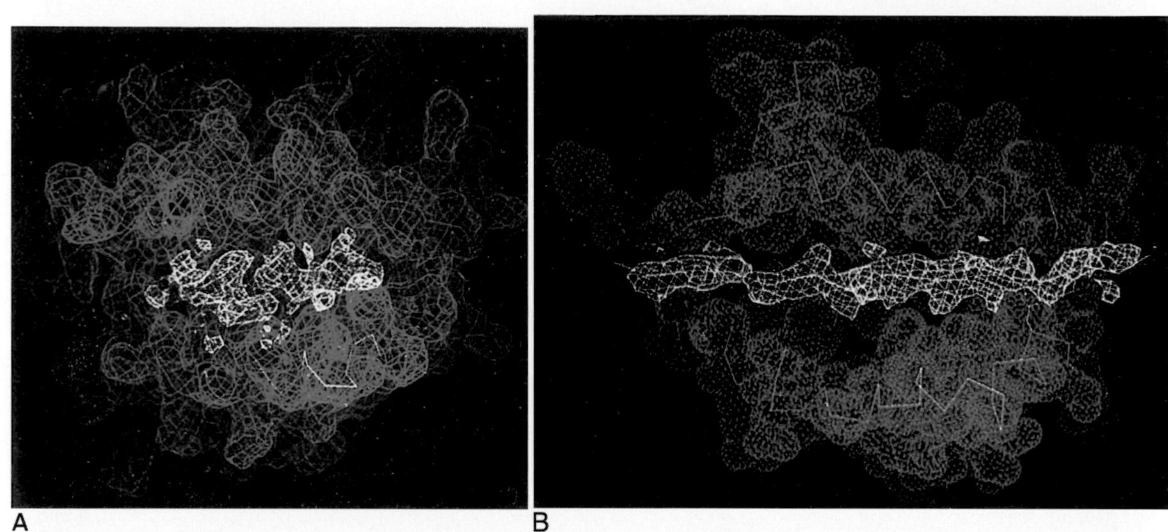

Figure 31–3 **(A)** Peptide binding to HLA class I (HLA-A2) and **(B)** class II (HLA-DR1). The view is looking down on the molecule as a T lymphocyte might "see" it. The two α helices forming the rim of the peptide binding site are blue, and electron densities corresponding to bound peptides are shown in red. (*A* from Bjorkman PJ, Saper MA, Samraoui B, et al: Structure of the human class I histocompatibility antigen, HLA-A2. Nature 1987; 329:506; *B* from Brown JH, Jardetzky TS, Gorga JC, et al: Three-dimensional structure of the human class II histocompatibility antigen HLA-DR1. Nature 1994; 364:35.)

of the allogeneic response is the relatively high frequency of T cell precursors capable of responding to a foreign MHC antigen. For example, the frequency of specific T cells to conventional antigens is approximately 1 in 10^4 to 10^5, whereas the frequency responding during allogeneic stimulation can be as high as 1 in 10^1 to 10^2. The concept of positive and negative selection in the thymus (see Mechanisms of Self Tolerance) also helps to explain the strength of the alloimmune response.[6] During development, T cells with receptors of too high affinity are deleted (negative selection), whereas those with too low affinity are not selected. The end result of this selection is that TCRs of intermediate affinity exit the thymus and enter the periphery. Within an individual, clonal deletion occurs early in development. Potentially, autoreactive clones (with too high affinity for self) are deleted; failure of deletion of some clones may lead to autoimmunity. In the case of transplantation across an allelic difference, however, the recipient's T cells do not contact allo-MHC molecules during development in the thymus and thus escape the deletion (negative selection) imposed by interaction with self-MHC. Thus, the end result is the large number of donor MHC/peptide complexes on the graft to which a potential recipient has not been tolerized during ontogeny. Moreover, the relatively low affinity of any given TCR for its ligand suggests that each T cell could potentially recognize more than one MHC/peptide complex.[7] The high density of alloantigens on the surface of an allograft contributes additionally to the strong T-cell response. In addition, because recipient T cells recognize intact allogeneic MHC molecules directly (see following text), they are stimulated maximally by the high density of MHC on the surfaces of transplanted cells.

Minor Transplantation Antigens

Studies involving MHC identical grafts in mice indicate that minor histocompatibility antigens can also mediate rejection. Recipient T cells can be directly primed to minor histocompatibility antigens. A minor histocompatibility antigen is molecularly defined as a donor-derived peptide presented on a donor cell by an MHC molecule shared by donor and recipient. Note that donor and recipient express the same MHC molecules. Donor DCs directly prime CD8+ T cells to become effector cells without the need for further antigen processing by recipient APCs. As one illustration, CD8+ T cells from female C57BL/6 mice specific for male-derived H-Y Uty peptide + MHC class I mediate rejection of syngeneic C57/BL6 male skin.[8] In humans, it has been appreciated for several years that minor histocompatibility antigens can be immunogenic, from observations based on organ graft rejections and bone marrow graft-versus-host reactions in cases of genetically matched HLA antigens. A few cases of donor-directed, HLA class I–restricted, cytotoxic T-cell responses have been demonstrated in such cases.[9,10] Two general families of such antigens have been identified:

1. H-Y antigens are proteins encoded on the Y chromosome. Females of the species may mount an immune response against these proteins.
2. T cells recognize peptidic antigens corresponding to polymorphisms among autosomal proteins expressed by individuals of the species. Examples include mitochondrial proteins and enzymes.

In the presence of both major and minor incompatibilities, it is clear that the alloimmune response targeted against the MHC molecules predominates.

ABO Blood Group Antigens

The A and B groups are glycosylated differentially, whereas group O lacks the enzymes necessary for glycosylation. The antigens are readily recognized by natural antibodies, termed *hemagglutinins* because they cause red cell agglutination. They are relevant to transplantation because they are expressed on other cell types, including the endothelium. Thus, they cause hyperacute rejection of vascular allografts due to preformed natural antibodies. Allograft rejection due to red blood cell type mismatching can be readily prevented by routine blood typing before transplantation. The rhesus (Rh) factor and other red cell antigens are of little concern because they are not expressed on endothelial cells.

Monocyte and Endothelial Cell Antigens

Occasionally, allografts undergo hyperacute rejection, despite appropriate ABO matching. Some of these rejection episodes have been attributed to additional non-ABO antigens expressed on endothelial cells and monocytes[11]; however, these antigen systems remain poorly understood. Pretransplant tissue typing does not currently evaluate the endothelial/monocyte antigens, owing to the apparent rarity of such antibodies and the lack of accurate reagents for typing.

CELLULAR EVENTS LEADING TO ALLOGRAFT REJECTION

In the context of allograft rejection, T cells play a central role in orchestrating the immune response as they recognize alloantigens through two distinct non-mutually exclusive pathways (see later text). Once activated, they secrete cytokines and chemokines to activate and attract various effector cells, such as CD8+ T cells and macrophages into the allograft. They are also able to interact with B cells that will secrete highly specific alloreactive antibodies. These cells in turn mediate the effector mechanisms of allograft destruction (see later text). Table 31–1 summarizes the steps leading to allograft rejection.

Allorecognition Pathways

The first step in an alloimmune response is the recognition of alloantigens by T cells (priming of alloreactive T cells). In the setting of a transplant, there is the potential for two different cellular mechanisms of allorecognition; these have been called the *direct* and *indirect* pathways of allorecognition (Figure 31–5).[12-14]

Direct refers to cell recognition of a whole intact foreign MHC molecule on the surface of donor cells. Although the specific peptide (typically derived from endogenous proteins, including MHC antigens) bound in the groove of the MHC molecule may be important in this recognition process, it does not restrict this response. The graft, which includes donor bone marrow-derived APCs, usually expresses several class I and class II MHC molecules that

Table 31–1 Steps in Allograft Rejection

1. Recognition of the alloantigen (direct and indirect pathways)
2. T-cell and B-cell activation, differentiation and expansion
3. Effector functions
4. Resolution of the response with residual memory

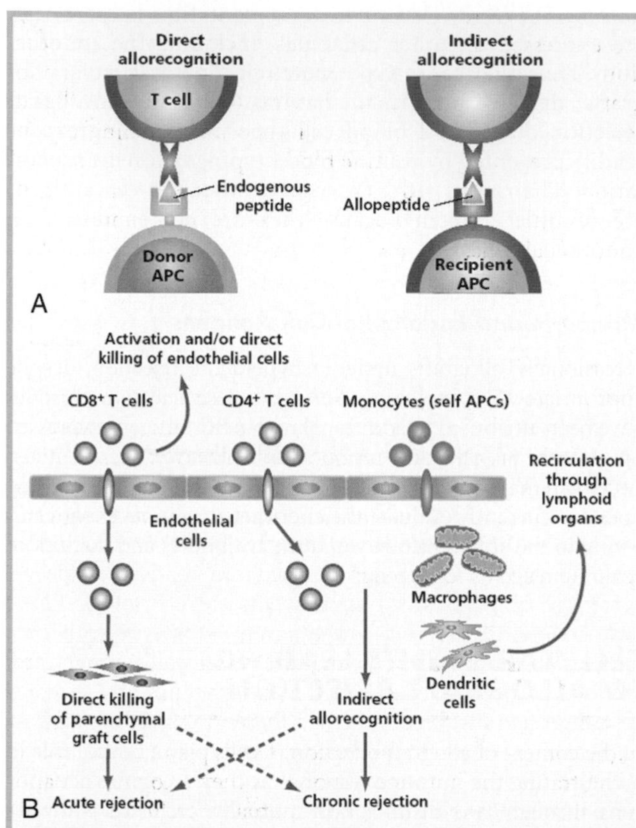

Figure 31–5 Allorecognition pathways and graft rejection. ***A,*** Graft rejection is initiated by CD4+ T cells, which recognize alloantigens. In the "direct" pathway of allorecognition, the T cell binds to a major histocompatibility complex (MHC) molecule on donor antigen-presenting cells *(left)*. In the "indirect" pathway, the foreign MHC molecule is processed into allopeptides, which are presented to the T cell by self antigen–presenting cells *(right)*. Activated CD4+ T cells proliferate and secrete a variety of cytokines that act as growth and activation factors for CD8+ cytotoxic T cells, B cells, and macrophages. ***B,*** Interactions among endothelial cells, T cells, and recipient antigen-presenting cells in allograft rejection. Recipient monocytes are recruited by endothelial cells to the graft tissue. They are also transformed to become highly efficient antigen-presenting dendritic cells that may need to recirculate to peripheral lymphoid organs for maturation. The dendritic cells and intragraft macrophages present donor peptides via the indirect pathway to recruited CD4+ T cells. CD8+ T cells, on the other hand, are activated by donor endothelial cells and can either directly kill endothelial cells or traverse the endothelium and kill parenchymal graft. (Adapted from Briscoe DM, Sayegh MH: A rendezvous before rejection: Where do T cells meet transplant antigens? Nature Med 2002; 8[3]:220-222.)

differ from the recipient's MHC molecules and can directly stimulate recipient T cells. In sum, donor APCs prime CD4+ and CD8+ T cells through the direct pathway. However, as these donor APCs are destroyed during the priming process, direct T-cell priming is likely to be time-limited. Thus, direct allorecognition may account for early acute cellular rejection. Consistent with this idea, direct alloreactivity was not detectable in the peripheral blood of a cohort of renal allograft recipients with chronic allograft dysfunction several years after transplantation.[15,16] In contrast, *indirect* refers to T cell recognition of nonself MHC-derived peptides (allopeptides) in the context of self MHC molecules expressed on recipient antigen-presenting cells (APCs). In this case, similar to the physiologic pathway of antigen recognition, the peptide sequence determines the response. Indirect presentation could occur through a number of mechanisms: soluble donor MHC molecules are shed from the graft and drain through the bloodstream/lymphatics to the recipient secondary lymphoid organs, where they would be processed/presented by recipient APCs to recipient T cells. Alternatively, donor graft cells that migrate to recipient secondary lymphoid organs could be endocytosed by recipient APCs. Third, recipient monocyte/macrophages entering the donor graft could endocytose donor antigens and present the peptides to recipient T cells. Other allopeptides may be derived from minor histocompatibility antigens or tissue-specific antigens. Because recipient monocytes migrating through the allograft can constantly endocytose donor antigen, priming through the indirect pathway could occur for as long as the graft is present in the host. Thus, while indirect alloreactive T cells may participate in acute rejection, they may play a predominant role in chronic rejection.[17] Consistent with this concept, several groups have now provided data correlating the indirect alloreactive T cells with the presence of chronic allograft dysfunction.[18-20] Interestingly, recent emerging data demonstrate that not only CD4+ T cells, as traditionally thought, but also CD8+ T cells can be primed through the indirect pathway of allorecognition and contribute to graft destruction.[21]

Endothelial cells of donor origin are located at the interface between the recipient's blood and the allograft and have been implicated in graft rejection (Figure 31–5).[13] Graft endothelial cells express MHC class I and class II molecules and have been shown recently to promote direct allorecognition by serving as antigen-presenting cells and as targets for T cell–mediated cytotoxicity. In addition, endothelial cells may promote indirect allorecognition by a crosstalk mechanism, which involves the recruitment and transformation of recipient monocytes by endothelial cells into highly efficient antigen presenting dendritic cells.[13]

Finally, there has been recent interest in studying where T cells meet the transplant antigens. The site of alloantigen recognition had until recently been believed to be in the allograft itself, but recent data seem to indicate that peripheral lymphoid organs are required for allograft rejection.[22] Whether unprimed T cells encounter antigens first outside of the allograft in peripheral lymphoid tissue or they migrate to secondary lymphoid organs after they encounter the alloantigens in the graft for further maturation and differentiation remains controversial. Interestingly, primed/ effector/memory cells appear to mediate graft rejection independent of peripheral lymphoid organs, suggesting that they do get activated by alloantigens in the graft itself.[22]

T-Cell Activation

Allograft rejection is a T cell–dependent process; animals that lack T cells do not reject an allograft. In particular, CD4+ helper T cells appear to be essential orchestrators of the alloimmune response leading to allograft rejection.[23] T lymphocytes initiate the immune response, which ultimately results in graft rejection. In addition, they can function as regulators and effectors in the immune response (see later text). As discussed earlier, allorecognition is the essential initial step for initiation of the cascade of events that results in rejection of the graft (Table 31–1). The essential cell-cell interactions between T cells and APCs (donor or self) may involve five classes of receptors: the antigen-specific TCR, the CD4 or CD8 coreceptor, costimulatory molecules, accessory or adhesion molecules, and lymphokine receptors. Members of each class of receptors may present suitable targets for therapeutic and experimental manipulation and are thus discussed in the following text.

T Cell Receptor-CD3 Complex

T-cell recognition of alloantigens on APCs is the central event that initiates allograft rejection.[12,14,24] The interaction between T lymphocytes and APCs involves multiple T-cell surface molecules and their counter-receptors expressed by APCs. Antigen specificity is determined by the TCR, which recognizes processed antigen in the form of short peptides bound to an MHC molecule. Clonally restricted TCRs are made up of two chains. The major TCR is an α, β heterodimer; a less commonly expressed TCR consists of γ and δ chains. The TCR consists of constant and variable portions involved in binding to HLA and recognition of the specific alloantigenic targets. Although the TCR allows T cells to recognize antigen-MHC complexes, the cell-surface expression of TCR molecules and the initiation of intracellular signaling depend on a complex of additional peptides known as the CD3 complex. After a given TCR is engaged by alloantigen, the T cell is activated, and a signal (signal 1) is transduced through the TCR–CD3 complex. As we will discuss further in later text, full activation of T cells requires two synergistic signals (see "Costimulatory Molecules" section).

The OKT3 monoclonal antibody binds to the CD3 complex. There are at least two components to the mechanism of immunosuppression by OKT3.[25] Within hours after administration, OKT3 causes profound depletion of peripheral T cells. Because OKT3 is not cytotoxic, the depletion is attributed to sequestration of the T cells. In addition, T cells downmodulate the expression of the TCR complex. Thus, after a few days of treatment, by flow cytometry circulating CD4+ and CD8+ cells can be shown to lack detectable TCR. It is thought that the TCR is internalized by endocytosis or shedding. The modulation of TCR expression is reversible, and, after elimination of OKT3, the TCR-CD3 complex is again expressed on the cell surface. Recently, a new generation of anti-CD3 monoclonal antibodies has been generated and is currently being tested in the clinic.[26-28] These antibodies are humanized (OKT3 is a mouse antibody) and nonmitogenic, and thus may prove to be promising in minimizing some of the side effects of OKT3 mediated by its mitogenic properties.

CD4 and CD8 TCR Coreceptors

The two major subsets of T cells, cytotoxic CD8+ T cells and helper CD4+ T cells, recognize processed antigen on MHC class I and class II molecules, respectively. CD4 and CD8 molecules enhance the interaction between the TCR and APCs through the MHC. By binding class II MHC molecules, the CD4 molecule facilitates TCR-CD3 complex-mediated signal transduction and assists the actions of class II MHC-restricted T cells. Similarly, the CD8 molecule binds to class I MHC molecules and stabilizes the interaction of the class I MHC-restricted T cell with a target cell-mediating signal transduction. Thus, CD4/CD8+TCR-CD3 complex proteins function together in initiating the signals for T-cell activation. Monoclonal antibodies against CD4 or CD8 molecules inhibit T-cell activation and may be important targets for immunosuppression.

Adhesion Molecules

Immune cells gain access to the site of inflammation in the graft from nearby lymph nodes and the bloodstream. Associated with transplantation, alloantigens enter local lymph nodes. APCs, such as dendritic cells and tissue macrophages, take up foreign HLA (indirect allorecognition), or foreign HLA on donor APCs is recognized directly (direct allorecognition). Antigen-specific T cells are activated, differentiate, divide, and enter the bloodstream. Immune cells move from the bloodstream into the site of inflammation by a three-step process.

First, immune cells roll along the vessel wall through interactions between selectins on the endothelium and receptors on immune cells. Second, they adhere to vessel endothelium. Third, chemoattractant cytokines (chemokines) are released (Figure 31–6). Adhesion molecules and chemokines are important regulators of rejection and appear to be targets for immunotherapy. Adhesion molecules (integrins) are well known for their ability to facilitate adhesion between cells and between cells and the extracellular matrix. Integrins on T cells include lymphocyte function–associated antigen-1 (LFA-1), which interacts with intercellular adhesion molecules (ICAM-1 and ICAM-2); CD2, which interacts with CD58 (leukocyte function-associated antigen-3 [LFA-3]); and very-late-appearing antigen (VLA-4) (CDw49d, CD29), which interacts with vascular cell adhesion molecule (VCAM-1, CD106).These receptors are of two large structural families. The integrins, including LFA-1 and VLA-4, are made up of α, β heterodimers, whereas members of the immunoglobulin superfamily, including CD2, LFA-3, VCAM-1, and the ICAMs, are made up of disulfide-linked "receptor" domains. The inhibition of adhesion cell function has been shown to be immunosuppressive. Previous studies in murine and primate models showed increased graft survival with anti-ICAM-1 monoclonal antibodies; however, in a recent randomized multicenter trial, short-term use of the anti-ICAM-1 monoclonal antibody enlimomab for induction therapy after renal transplantation did not reduce the rate of acute rejection or delayed graft function.[29] Blockade of LFA-1 as induction treatment, on the other hand, is being studied in the context of preventing delayed graft function after transplantation.[30] Recently,

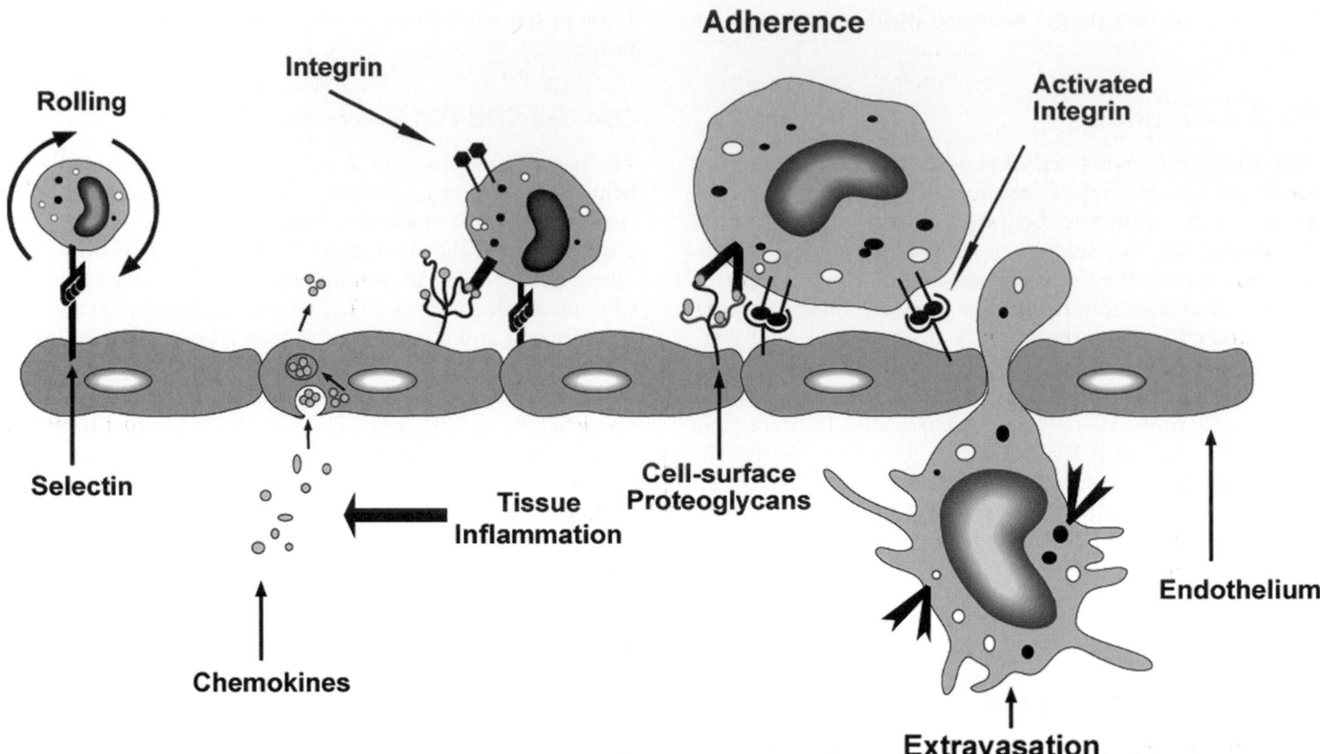

Figure 31–6 Three-step model of inflammatory cell migration from the bloodstream into the site of rejection. Rolling of monocytes and T lymphocytes along the vascular endothelium is mediated by selectins. Chemokines may be synthesized by the endothelial cell or produced by tissue cells and subsequently transported across the endothelium. Then they bind to glycosoaminoglycans on the endothelial cell surface, where they can activate leukocyte chemokine receptors causing integrin activation, flow arrest, and movement across the endothelial cell barrier into the tissues following the chemoattractant gradient. (From Dong VM, McDermott DH, Abdi R: Chemokines and diseases. Eur J Dermatology 2003; 13[3]:224-230.)

efalizumab, a humanized anti-LFA-1 monoclonal antibody, was shown to be well tolerated and effective at reducing the severity of the disease in patients with psoriasis. Initial results in renal transplant patients are also promising.[31]

Costimulatory Molecules

T cells require two signals for full activation (Figure 31–7). One signal is provided by the interaction of the TCR with the MHC–peptide complex; the second costimulatory signal depends on one or more additional receptor-ligand interactions between T cells and APCs.[26-28] The two-signal model has gained enormous support in recent years, defining several costimulatory pathways and is now widely accepted (Figure 31–8).[32,33] The CD28-B7 and CD154-CD40 pathways have been described as the critical costimulatory pathways for T-cell activation. Blockade of these pathways has been reported to regulate both autoimmune and alloimmune responses in experimental models and in human disease. However, studies have indicated that inhibition of these pathways is insufficient to reproducibly induce long-lasting immunologic tolerance in some experimental autoimmunity and transplantation models, indicating a role for other costimulatory pathways. The recent discovery of new members of the B7-CD28 family,[32,33] inducible costimulator (ICOS), its ligand B7h, as well as programmed death-1 (PD-1) and its ligands, PD-L1 and PD-L2, have therefore been of major interest. Other molecules belonging to the tumor necrosis factor (TNF) superfamily and their receptors (TNF-R), including 4-1BB, CD30, CD134 (OX40) and CD27, and their respective ligands, 4-1BBL, CD30L, CD134L and CD70, also act as efficient costimulatory molecules for T cells.[32,33] The role of these novel costimulatory molecules is currently under intense investigation, and their role in autoimmunity and transplantation is just beginning to emerge. Thus, we will review later the role of the CD28-B7 and CD154-CD40 pathways in transplantation.

The CD28/CTLA4-B7 Pathway

Many T-cell molecules may serve as receptors for costimulatory signals; the CD28 molecule is the best characterized of these molecules (see Figure 31–8). According to recent gene expression studies, CD28 costimulation can lead to significant augmentation of expressions of genes induced by TCR signaling alone. These findings are consistent with a model of costimulation in which CD28 signaling lowers TCR thresholds for activation of cells.[34,35] CD28 has two known ligands, B7-1 (CD80) and B7-2 (CD86), both of which are expressed primarily on activated professional bone marrow-derived APCs. T cells also express CTLA-4, a molecule that is highly homol-

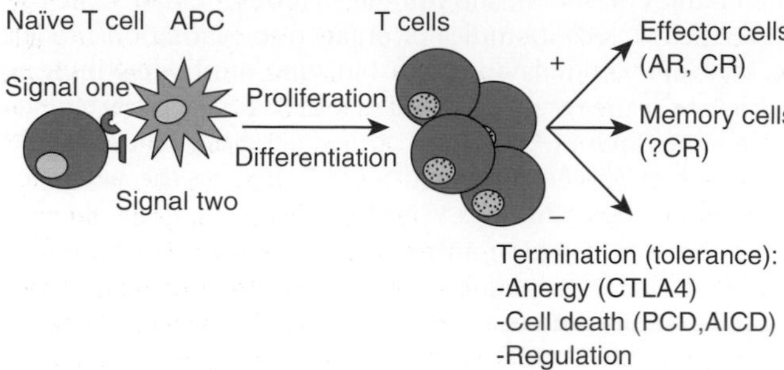

Figure 31–7 Stimulation of T cells through binding of a peptide-MHC complex to the T cell receptor (signal 1) in the presence of a costimulatory signal (signal two) leads to proliferation and differentiation of these cells. Apoptosis, cell cycle arrest, and active suppression are known regulators of this immune response. A few antigen-specific cells are spared and become memory cells. (From Najafian N, Khoury SJ, Sayegh MH: T cell costimulatory blockade as a novel immune intervention in auoimmune diseases. Clin Dermatol 2001; 19[5]:586-591.)

ogous to CD28 that also binds CD80 and CD86.[36] However, unlike CD28, CTLA-4 transmits an inhibitory signal that serves to terminate the immune response. Whereas CD28 is expressed by both resting and activated T cells, CTLA-4 is expressed on activated T cells only. Because CTLA-4 binds B7 molecules with a higher affinity than does CD28, its inhibitory interaction eventually predominates, leading to the termination of the immune response. The importance of CTLA-4 as a negative regulatory T-cell costimulatory molecule in the physiologic termination of T cell responses is highlighted by the observation that CTLA-4 gene knockout mice develop massive lymphoproliferation and early death. One point that needs to be emphasized is the critical role of costimulation in T-cell responses. In the absence of costimulatory signals, sometimes the T cell simply ignores the peptide-MHC-complex presented to it. At other times, the T cell undergoes apoptotic death[37,38] or is rendered anergic for up to several weeks[37]; that is, the T cell is unable to respond to antigens, even when it is presented by APCs that express a costimulatory molecule. Precisely what determines the outcome of the stimulation of T-cell antigen receptors in the absence of costimulation (ignorance, apoptosis, or anergy) is not known. This process is considered one important factor in induction of peripheral tolerance. Thus, manipulation of CD28/B7 pathway has been envisioned as a potential strategy for achieving therapeutically useful immunosuppression or tolerance. T-cell costimulatory blockade, in the form of CTLA4Ig (LEA29Y), which blocks CD28 interaction with B7, is currently being studied as a means of immunosuppression.[36]

The CD154-CD40 Pathway

The CD154-CD40 pathway, initially described as having a role in B-cell activation, has been recognized as a key pathway for T-cell activation as well (see Figure 31–8). CD40 is expressed on APCs, such as B cells, macrophages, and dendritic cells, as well as other cell types such as endothelial cells. The ligand for CD40 (originally called CD40L and recently named CD154) is expressed on activated CD4 T cells. CD154 was later found on stimulated mast cells and basophils and, most recently, on activated platelets in vitro and in vivo and also in vivo on platelets in the process of the thrombus formation. Stimulation of CD40 provides important signals for antibody production by B cells and strongly induces B7 expression on all APCs.[39] In this manner, the CD154-CD40 system may have an important role in T-cell costimulation. Activation of APCs through CD40 also induces the expression of adhesion molecules and inflammatory cytokines that participate in T-cell activation. Therefore, CD154 may act in T-cell costimulation by directly providing costimulation, by inducing B7, or by inducing other costimulatory ligands. CD154-CD40 blockade has been shown to be efficient in preventing acute graft rejection in several small animal models. When anti-CD154 monoclonal

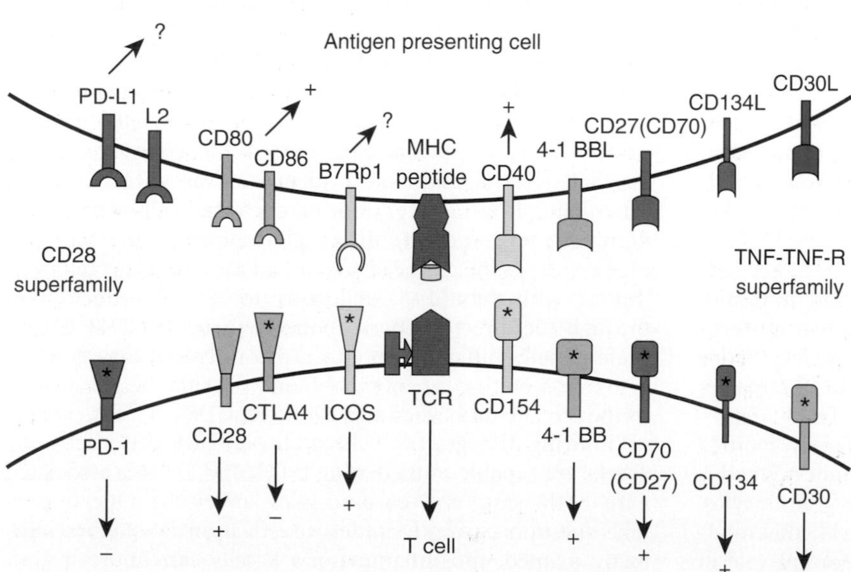

Figure 31–8 Overview of the main costimulatory molecules belonging to the CD28-B7 and TNF-TNF-R super families. Following ligation of the receptor-ligand pairs, the signal transduced results in a net stimulatory (+) or inhibitory (–) response. (From Salama AD, Salama AD, Sayegh MH: Alternative T-cell costimulatory pathways in transplant rejection and tolerance induction: Hierarchy or redundancy? Am J Transplantation 2003; 3:509-511.)

antibody was used as part of a strategy to induce mixed allogeneic chimerism in a renal transplant model, the primates developed donor-specific tolerance. However, some recipients developed thromboembolic complications. Such a complication was also observed in some humans entered in the phase I and phase II transplant trial with the humanized anti-CD154 (Biogen Inc., Cambridge, MA) monoclonal antibody, resulting in premature termination of trial. Thus, the plans for future development of this agent in transplantation remain unclear.

In summary, there are complex interactions between the various costimulatory pathways that influence their actions. These interactions ultimately determine the fate of the alloimmune response in vivo. A major focus of future research is thus directed at dissecting these functions to provide the rationale for developing novel therapeutic targets and strategies for induction of robust and durable transplantation tolerance.

Cytokines/Chemokines

In addition to cell–cell interactions, cell function can be directed through proteins produced by a variety of cell types. These cytokines can function as chemoattractant (chemokines, see later text), as well as growth, activation, and differentiation factors. After antigenic stimulation, CD4+ T cells differentiate into two distinct populations, each producing its own set of cytokines and mediating separate effector functions.[40,41] *Type 1* helper T cells (Th1 cells) produce interleukin-2 (IL-2) and interferon-γ (IFN-γ) and mediate activation of macrophages and induction of delayed-type hypersensitivity (DTH) responses (see later text). *Type 2* helper cells (Th2 cells) produce IL-4, IL-5, IL-10, and IL-13, which provide help for B-cell function. However, the functional segregation between the Th1 and Th2 subsets remains incompletely understood. Studies with specific Th1 or Th2 cytokine gene-knockout animals indicate the complexity of the Th1-Th2 paradigm in graft rejection and tolerance.[40-42] Data from animal and human studies showed that Th2 clones propagated from patients with stable renal transplant function, or animals tolerant to kidney transplants can regulate a proliferative response from Th1 clones isolated from patients or animals undergoing active rejection.[43,44] Except for blockade of the IL-2R, therapeutic strategies that specifically modulate lymphokines have not proved highly effective. Therefore, although manipulation of lymphokine functions may hold promise as a therapeutic modality, we will have to better understand the role of lymphokines in graft rejection and tolerance under physiologic conditions, if we are to develop effective treatments.

Chemokines are *chemoattractant cytokines.*[45] They are structurally related by amino acid homologies and, in particular, by the placement of cysteines. The nomenclature of chemokines is becoming increasingly complex. Four chemokine families are now recognized, of which the majority of members belong to the C-C chemokine family, represented by RANTES, or the C-X-C chemokine family, typified by IL-8. In general, C-C chemokines attract monocytes and T lymphocytes, and C-X-C chemokines attract granulocytes. Detection of altered chemokine mRNA in experimental models of rejection suggests that they play an important role in this process; however, because of redundancy and differences between the function of chemokines in rodents and in humans, for the most part, the exact role that individual chemokines play in an alloimmune response remains unclear. Nevertheless, recent studies in organ transplantation models in knockout animals and with blocking antibodies indicate key roles for the receptors CXCR3 and CCR5 and selected targeting chemokines.[46,47] Mean cardiac allograft survival of 58 days in CXCR3–/– compared with 7 days in the wild-type underlines these findings. Similar effects on graft survival were obtained using an anti-CXCR3 antibody in CXCR3+/+ recipients. MHC disparate cardiac allografts transplanted into CCR5–/– mice show a tripling of graft survival. Whereas chemokine expression in the heart is primarily by EC or infiltrating mononuclear cells, kidneys have a heterogeneous population of resident cells, which express inflammatory chemokines when stimulated. Further studies of these knockout mice in studies on renal transplantation will help prove the applicability of these data to renal transplantation.

Effector Mechanisms of Allograft Rejection

Transplant rejection has both cellular (DTH responses, cell-mediated cytotoxicity) and humoral components. Once fully activated via the direct or indirect pathway (see earlier text), T cells produce cytokines and chemokines that orchestrate various effector arms of the alloimmune response. Primed CD4+ T cells can provide help for production of alloantibody and can also provide helper signals required for the induction of CD8+ CTLs,[14,23] both of which can subsequently mediate graft injury. Moreover, CD4+ T cells capable of recognizing donor antigen on donor cells can directly mediate acute graft rejection,[48] but there is some evidence that this outcome is frequency-dependent.[49] Below a certain frequency threshold, primed T cells may not reject the transplanted organ but may alternatively be capable of inducing chronic injury that results in fibrosis and vasculopathy, characteristic of chronic allograft dysfunction.[50] Furthermore, directly primed Th1 cells and macrophages can mediate delayed-type hypersensitivity (DTH) reactions and contribute to the destruction of the graft. In this setting, it is hypothesized that some of the cytokines produced by T cells and macrophages (TNF-α) may mediate apoptosis of graft cells. The pathology of a transplanted organ may also be dependent on the specific graft cell with which the primed T cells interact. It is tempting to speculate that direct recognition of donor endothelial cells by primed CD8+ T cells may participate in those acute rejections associated with pathologic evidence of vasculitis.[51] On the other hand, if intragraft donor parenchymal cells are the predominant targets of the direct alloresponse, acute rejection may appear as the classically described mononuclear cell infiltration with tubulitis. Analogous to T cells functioning through the direct pathway, indirectly primed CD4+ T cells preferentially differentiate into a pro-inflammatory type –1 cytokine-secreting phenotype[52] and provide helper signals to induce alloantibodies and cytotoxic CD8+ T cells capable of injuring the graft.[53-55] In addition, indirectly activated T cells are capable of mediating DTH, and DTH is associated with both acute and chronic graft injury.[56,57] One important question currently under investigation is whether indirectly primed, pro-inflammatory T cells can injure a graft even though they cannot interact with any antigen expressed on the graft cells. At least in skin graft models, it is possible that recipient-derived vascular endothelial cells found on vessels feeding the graft may act as a target of the indirectly primed immune response.[58] The frequency of activated cells may also influence the eventual outcome. Higher frequencies of indirectly primed CD4+ T cells seem to be associated with acute rejection, whereas lower frequencies may mediate fibrosis and vasculopathy.[48]

In summary, the pattern of transplant rejection is not only influenced by the T-cell recognition pathway, but also by the frequency, the induced effector functions, and the specific cellular targets of the alloreactive T cells.

B lymphocytes express clonally restricted antigen-specific cell-surface receptors, called *immunoglobulins*.[59] When cell-surface immunoglobulin binds specific antigen in the context of soluble helper factors (such as IL-4, IL-6, and IL-8), B cells are activated. They differentiate, divide, and become plasma cells, which secrete soluble forms of antigen-specific antibodies displayed on their cell surface. These antibodies, in turn, can bind allogeneic target antigens and induce graft damage by binding complement or by directing antibody-dependent cellular cytotoxicity. Both immunoglobulin M (IgM) and IgG alloantibodies can be detected in the serum as well as in the graft of animals and humans undergoing allograft rejection. Preformed anti-HLA class I antibodies and, occasionally, anti-endothelial antibodies play an important role in the hyperacute rejection and accelerated vascular rejection seen in previously sensitized transplant recipients. In the case of xenotransplantation, naturally occurring xenoreactive antibodies play a critical role in the hyperacute rejection of xenografts (see Chapter 37). Finally, alloantibodies, particularly IgG, play an important pathogenetic role in the development of chronic rejection and graft arteriosclerosis.

Other soluble factors induce additional effector mechanisms, including phagocytosis by granulocytes and macrophages, and cell death by natural killer (NK) cells. NK cells express cell-surface receptors called "killer-inhibitory receptors" (KIR) that recognize HLA class I molecules.[60] When self HLA is recognized, NK cells are prevented from killing. If the killer-inhibitory receptors do not bind to a self HLA molecule, as in certain tumors or viral infections, the target cell is lysed. In addition, NK cells can lyse certain targets expressing non-self HLA (alloantigens). Although the role of NK cell–mediated cytotoxicity in allograft rejection remains controversial, NK cells appear to play a key role in mediating delayed xenograft rejection (see Chapter 37).

Resolution and Memory

Apoptosis, cell cycle arrest, and active suppression are known regulators leading to a dampening of the induced immune response (see "Tolerance" section).[61] Nevertheless, a few antigen-specific cells are spared and these become memory cells (see Figure 31–7). Memory cells have a lower activation threshold than do naïve cells and can respond rapidly to previously encountered antigens. Memory T cells not only endanger allograft survival by causing both acute and chronic rejection, but recent studies suggest that they impede the induction of transplantation tolerance.[62] Evidence that memory T cells impede tolerance induction derives from studies using costimulation blockade and mixed allogeneic chimerism strategies.

TOLERANCE

Immunologic tolerance to an allograft can be defined as normal graft function and histology in the absence of immunosuppression, associated with absence of a destructive specific alloimmune response to the graft, but with an otherwise fully functional immune system.[32] Renal transplantation has been made possible by the development of powerful immunosuppressive drugs that can prevent the rejection process but usually require lifelong administration, patient compliance, and the risk for a wide range of unwanted side effects. Although there has been great success in improving short-term allograft survival in recent years, chronic allograft nephropathy (CAN) remains the principal cause of late renal allograft failure and may even be accelerated by some immunosuppressive drugs. Immunologic tolerance would ideally prevent the side effects of immunosuppression and would hopefully prevent chronic rejection, as demonstrated in several animal models.[63] An individual is usually tolerant to self antigens. Understanding mechanisms of self tolerance has yielded important information regarding the mechanisms of immune responses and has provided the rationale to develop strategies for induction of acquired tolerance. As discussed previously, the T-cell repertoire is modified through negative and positive selection processes in the thymus to delete potentially self-reactive T-cell clones. Self tolerance is partially mediated by "negative selection" through deletion of autoreactive T-cell clones in thymus (central tolerance). On the other hand, potentially autoreactive T cells that had escaped deletion during intrathymic ontogeny are kept under control by mechanisms of peripheral tolerance. Clonal deletion through apoptosis, anergy, and immunoregulation have all been suggested as nonmutually exclusive and probably complementary mechanisms of peripheral tolerance.[61] Stimulation of lymphocytes through the antigen receptor in the absence of costimulation is not a neutral event and mediates specific inactivation through anergy, a further safeguard against self-reactivity. Thus, it has been suggested that the absence of costimulation on resting tissue APCs could serve to induce and maintain T-cell tolerance to self-antigens, and that aberrant expression of costimulatory molecules on nonprofessional APCs could activate self-reactive T cells, resulting in autoimmunity. Recent findings suggest that an additional level of regulation may be achieved by the expression of novel inhibitory molecules (CTLA4 and PD1) on T cells that can provide negative signals to terminate immune responses.[33]

Similar to self tolerance, the mechanisms of acquired tolerance are listed in Table 31–2. There are two types of acquired tolerance:

1. *Central tolerance* involves thymic deletional mechanisms analogous to self tolerance.
2. *Peripheral tolerance* is mediated by T-cell anergy and deletion, by regulatory/suppressor cells, and/or by suppressive cytokines.

The occurrence of natural tolerance was first described by Owen,[64] who showed that dizygotic twin cattle that shared a common placenta in utero would continue to have circulating blood cells of their twin specificity after birth. The resultant animals were said to be *chimeric*, and they could not reject skin grafts of the other twin in adult life. This was followed by studies by Billingham, Brent, and Medawar,[65] who

Table 31-2 Mechanisms of Transplantation Tolerance

- Central tolerance
- Peripheral tolerance
  - Anergy
  - Apoptosis
  - Regulation (regulatory cells, suppressive cytokines)

demonstrated that it was possible to induce mice to accept skin grafts from a different genetic background, if the recipient mice were injected while still in utero (or neonatally) with hematopoietic cells of donor origin. This was the first description of acquired tolerance. Neonatal tolerance is thought to be due largely to clonal deletion, whereby T cells reactive with alloantigen are deleted in the thymus, presumably by the same mechanisms that delete self reactive T cells. Other mechanisms (e.g., immune deviation to Th2 cells), however, have been described as possible mediators of neonatal tolerance.

Anergy is a state of functional inactivation in which antigen-specific T lymphocytes are present but are unable to respond (by proliferating or producing cytokines) to rechallenge with antigen. Anergy is typically induced when T cells do not receive a positive costimulatory signal, when positive costimulatory signals are blocked, or when they receive a negative costimulatory signal. Anergy can sometimes be reversed by IL-2 and thus may not be a desirable clinical approach to induce tolerance because infections may activate the immune system and reverse anergy.

Another mechanism of peripheral tolerance is through the function of antigen-specific regulatory or suppressor cells. Such cells have been demonstrated by *in vitro* assays and by adoptive transfer experiments *in vivo*. *Infectious tolerance*, whereby T cells from a tolerant animal can actively transfer specific tolerance to a naïve animal, indicates the presence of regulatory cells. Indeed, the existence of CD4+CD25+ regulatory T cells in the blood of healthy adult volunteers have been previously reported.[66] A recent study provided the first evidence that such regulatory cells appear and persist in renal transplant patients and account for indirect pathway hyporeactivity in a proportion of renal transplant patients with stable allograft function.[67] Therefore, while T-cell anergy and death are most likely the main regulatory mechanisms contributing to direct pathway hyporesponsiveness,[68] regulatory CD4+CD25+ T cells appear to play a role in regulation of indirect antidonor alloresponse in stable renal transplant patients.[67] Besides CD4+CD25+ regulatory cells, it has been recognized that CD4+ helper T cells can be subdivided into Th1 and Th2 subsets. Th2 cytokines are expressed in tolerant grafts.[69] This state of immune deviation toward predominantly Th2 cell function has been associated with tolerance in experimental models of autoimmunity and transplantation. In the case of transplantation, however, a causal relation has not been proved. Data indicating that IL-2 or IFN-γ knockout animals are capable of rejecting allografts and that IL-4 knockout animals can be "tolerized" may question the validity of the Th1 and Th2 paradigm in allograft rejection and tolerance.[41] Recently, NK1.1+ T cells have been shown to act as natural suppressor cells preventing graft versus host disease after bone marrow transplantation.[70,71] In the setting of transplantation tolerance, NKT cells also seem to be required for the induction of cardiac transplant tolerance by costimulation. Furthermore, CD8+CD28-T cells that are capable of suppressing CD4+ T cells with allospecificity or xenospecificity could be generated by repetitive allostimulation or xenostimulation in vitro.

Novel approaches to induce transplantation tolerance in humans include T cell non-myeloablative therapy with donor bone marrow transplantation plus a solid organ transplant. One recent paper demonstrated that this is feasible in a patient with myeloma and renal failure.[72] Other strategies that may be explored in the future include T-cell costimulatory blockade, T-cell depletion protocols (thymoglobulin, Campath-1, anti-CD2, and nonmitogenic anti-CD3), and mixed allogeneic chimerism in haploidentical transplant recipients in the absence of hematologic malignancies.[32]

Finally, although the induction of immunologic tolerance remains an important clinical goal in transplantation, there are several immunologic hurdles that has made it difficult to translate animal studies to humans; these barriers include the large repertoire of alloreactive T cells in the case of transplantation, the limitations of peripheral immune regulatory mechanisms that are commonly exploited to induce tolerance (T-cell deletion, anergy, and suppression), and last, but not least, the difficult task of "tolerizing" memory T cells.[32,62]

SUMMARY

In this chapter, we have highlighted our current understanding of the cellular and molecular mechanisms involved in transplant rejection and acceptance. This information has been important in the design of current therapies and may help usher in a new generation of approaches that will result in immunologic tolerance, the ultimate goal of transplantation biologists.

References

1. Lamm LU, Friedrich U, Petersen CB, et al: Assignment of the major histocompatibility complex to chromosome no. 6 in a family with a pericentric inversion. Hum Hered 1974; 24(3): 273-284.
2. Germain RN: MHC-dependent antigen processing and peptide presentation: Providing ligands for T lymphocyte activation. Cell 1994; 76(2):287-299.
3. Bjorkman PJ, Saper MA, Samraoui B, et al: Structure of the human class I histocompatibility antigen, HLA-A2. Nature 1987; 329(6139):506-512.
4. Brown JH, Jardetzky TS, Gorga JC, et al: Three-dimensional structure of the human class II histocompatibility antigen HLA-DR1. Nature 1993; 364(6432):33-39.
5. Garcia KC, Teyton L, Wilson IA: Structural basis of T cell recognition. Annu Rev Immunol 1999; 17:369-397.
6. Jameson SC, Hogquist KA, Bevan MJ: Positive selection of thymocytes. Annu Rev Immunol 1995; 13:93-126.
7. Brock R, Wiesmuller KH, Jung G, Walden P: Molecular basis for the recognition of two structurally different major histocompatibility complex/peptide complexes by a single T-cell receptor. Proc Natl Acad Sci U S A 1996; 93(23):13108-13113.
8. Scott DM, Ehrmann IE, Ellis PS, et al: Why do some females reject males? The molecular basis for male-specific graft rejection. J Mol Med 1997; 75(2):103-114.
9. Garovoy MR, Franco V, Zschaeck D, et al: Direct lymphocyte-mediated cytotoxicity as an assay of presensitisation. Lancet 1973; 1(7803):573-576.

10. Pfeffer PF, Thorsby E: HLA-restricted cytotoxicity against male-specific (H-Y) antigen after acute rejection of an HLA-identical sibling kidney: Clonal distribution of the cytotoxic cells. Transplantation 1982; 33(1):52-56.
11. Lucchiari N, Panajotopoulos N, Xu C, et al: Antibodies eluted from acutely rejected renal allografts bind to and activate human endothelial cells. Hum Immunol 2000; 61(5):518-527.
12. Sayegh MH: Why do we reject a graft? Role of indirect allorecognition in graft rejection. Kidney Int 1999; 56(5):1967-1979.
13. Briscoe DM, Sayegh MH: A rendezvous before rejection: Where do T cells meet transplant antigens? Nat Med 2002; 8(3): 220-222.
14. Heeger PS: T-cell allorecognition and transplant rejection: A summary and update. Am J Transplant 2003; 3(5):525-533.
15. Baker RJ, Hernandez-Fuentes MP, Brookes PA, et al: Loss of direct and maintenance of indirect alloresponses in renal allograft recipients: Implications for the pathogenesis of chronic allograft nephropathy. J Immunol 2001; 167(12):7199-7206.
16. Baker RJ, Hernandez-Fuentes MP, Brookes PA, et al: The role of the allograft in the induction of donor-specific T cell hyporesponsiveness. Transplantation 2001; 72(3):480-485.
17. Womer KL, Vella JP, Sayegh MH: Chronic allograft dysfunction: Mechanisms and new approaches to therapy. Semin Nephrol 2000; 20(2):126-147.
18. Najafian N, Salama AD, Fedoseyeva EV, et al: Enzyme-linked immunosorbent spot assay analysis of peripheral blood lymphocyte reactivity to donor HLA-DR peptides: Potential novel assay for prediction of outcomes for renal transplant recipients. J Am Soc Nephrol 2002; 13(1):252-259.
19. Vella JP, Vos L, Carpenter CB, Sayegh MH: Role of indirect allorecognition in experimental late acute rejection. Transplantation 1997; 64(12):1823-1828.
20. Vella JP, Spadafora-Ferreira M, Murphy B, et al: Indirect allorecognition of major histocompatibility complex allopeptides in human renal transplant recipients with chronic graft dysfunction. Transplantation 1997; 64(6):795-800.
21. Yewdell JW, Bennink JR: Immunodominance in major histocompatibility complex class I-restricted T lymphocyte responses. Annu Rev Immunol 1999; 17:51-88.
22. Lakkis FG, Arakelov A, Konieczny BT, Inoue Y: Immunologic "ignorance" of vascularized organ transplants in the absence of secondary lymphoid tissue. Nat Med 2000; 6(6):686-688.
23. Krieger NR, Yin DP, Fathman CG: CD4+ but not CD8+ cells are essential for allorejection. J Exp Med 1996; 184(5):2013-2018.
24. Sayegh MH, Turka LA: The role of T-cell costimulatory activation pathways in transplant rejection. N Engl J Med 1998; 338(25):1813-1821.
25. Denton MD, Magee CC, Sayegh MH: Immunosuppressive strategies in transplantation. Lancet 1999; 353(9158):1083-1091.
26. Hubbard WJ, Moore JK, Contreras JL, et al: Phenotypic and functional analysis of T-cell recovery after anti-CD3 immunotoxin treatment for tolerance induction in rhesus macaques. Hum Immunol 2001; 62(5):479-487.
27. Knechtle SJ: Treatment with immunotoxin. Philos Trans R Soc London [Biol] 2001; 356(1409):681-689.
28. Weetall M, Digan ME, Hugo R, et al: T-cell depletion and graft survival induced by anti-human CD3 immunotoxins in human CD3epsilon transgenic mice. Transplantation 2002; 73(10):1658-1666.
29. Salmela K, Wramner L, Ekberg H, et al: A randomized multicenter trial of the anti-ICAM-1 monoclonal antibody (enlimomab) for the prevention of acute rejection and delayed onset of graft function in cadaveric renal transplantation: A report of the European Anti-ICAM-1 Renal Transplant Study Group. Transplantation 1999; 67(5):729-736.
30. Hourmant M, Bedrossian J, Durand D, et al: A randomized multicenter trial comparing leukocyte function-associated antigen-1 monoclonal antibody with rabbit antithymocyte globulin as induction treatment in first kidney transplantations. Transplantation 1996; 62(11):1565-1570.
31. Dedrick RL, Walicke P, Garovoy M: Anti-adhesion antibodies efalizumab, a humanized anti-CD11a monoclonal antibody. Transpl Immunol 2002; 9(2-4):181-186.
32. Salama AD, Remuzzi G, Harmon WE, Sayegh MH: Challenges to achieving clinical transplantation tolerance. J Clin Invest 2001; 108(7):943-948.
33. Rothstein DM, Sayegh MH: T-cell costimulatory pathways in allograft rejection and tolerance. Immunol Rev 2003; 196: 85-108.
34. Diehn M, Alizadeh AA, Rando OJ, et al: Genomic expression programs and the integration of the CD28 costimulatory signal in T cell activation. Proc Natl Acad Sci U S A 2002; 99(18):11796-11801.
35. Riley JL, Mao M, Kobayashi S, et al: Modulation of TCR-induced transcriptional profiles by ligation of CD28, ICOS, and CTLA-4 receptors. Proc Natl Acad Sci U S A 2002; 99(18):11790-11795.
36. Najafian N, Sayegh MH: CTLA4-Ig: A novel immunosuppressive agent. Expert Opin Investig Drugs 2000; 9(9):2147-2157.
37. Gimmi CD, Freeman GJ, Gribben JG, et al: Human T-cell clonal anergy is induced by antigen presentation in the absence of B7 costimulation. Proc Natl Acad Sci U S A 1993; 90(14):6586-6590.
38. Noel PJ, Boise LH, Green JM, Thompson CB: CD28 costimulation prevents cell death during primary T cell activation. J Immunol 1996; 157(2):636-642.
39. Yamada A, Salama AD, Sayegh MH: The role of novel T cell costimulatory pathways in autoimmunity and transplantation. J Am Soc Nephrol 2002; 13(2):559-575.
40. Nickerson P, Steurer W, Steiger J, et al: Cytokines and the Th1/Th2 paradigm in transplantation. Curr Opin Immunol 1994; 6(5):757-764.
41. Lakkis FG: Role of cytokines in transplantation tolerance: Lessons learned from gene-knockout mice. J Am Soc Nephrol 1998; 9(12):2361-2367.
42. Dai Z, Konieczny BT, Baddoura FK, Lakkis FG: Impaired alloantigen-mediated T cell apoptosis and failure to induce long-term allograft survival in IL-2-deficient mice. J Immunol 1998; 161(4):1659-1663.
43. Kist-van Holthe JE, Gasser M, Womer K, et al: Regulatory functions of alloreactive Th2 clones in human renal transplant recipients. Kidney Int 2002; 62(2):627-631.
44. Waaga AM, Gasser M, Kist-van Holthe JE, et al: Regulatory functions of self-restricted MHC class II allopeptide-specific Th2 clones in vivo. J Clin Invest 2001; 107(7):909-916.
45. Hancock WW, Gao W, Faia KL, Csizmadia V: Chemokines and their receptors in allograft rejection. Curr Opin Immunol 2000; 12(5):511-516.
46. Nelson PJ, Krensky AM: Chemokines and allograft rejection: Narrowing the list of suspects. Transplantation 2001; 72(7):1195-1197.
47. Nelson PJ, Krensky AM: Chemokines, chemokine receptors, and allograft rejection. Immunity 2001; 14(4):377-386.
48. Pietra BA, Wiseman A, Bolwerk A, et al: CD4 T cell-mediated cardiac allograft rejection requires donor but not host MHC class II. J Clin Invest 2000; 106(8):1003-1010.
49. Jones ND, Turvey SE, Van Maurik A, et al: Differential susceptibility of heart, skin, and islet allografts to T cell-mediated rejection. J Immunol 2001; 166(4):2824-2830.
50. Ardehali A, Fischbein MP, Yun J, et al: Indirect alloreactivity and chronic rejection. Transplantation 2002; 73(11):1805-1807.
51. Kreisel D, Krupnick AS, Gelman AE, et al: Non-hematopoietic allograft cells directly activate CD8+ T cells and trigger acute rejection: An alternative mechanism of allorecognition. Nat Med 2002; 8(3):233-239.
52. Benichou G, Valujskikh A, Heeger PS: Contributions of direct and indirect T cell alloreactivity during allograft rejection in mice. J Immunol 1999; 162(1):352-358.

53. Auchincloss H Jr, Lee R, Shea S, et al: The role of "indirect" recognition in initiating rejection of skin grafts from major histocompatibility complex class II-deficient mice. Proc Natl Acad Sci U S A 1993; 90(8):3373-3377.
54. Lee RS, Grusby MJ, Glimcher LH, et al: Indirect recognition by helper cells can induce donor-specific cytotoxic T lymphocytes in vivo. J Exp Med 1994; 179(3):865-872.
55. Steele DJ, Laufer TM, Smiley ST, et al: Two levels of help for B cell alloantibody production. J Exp Med 1996; 183(2):699-703.
56. Sirak J, Orosz CG, Wakely E, VanBuskirk AM: Alloreactive delayed-type hypersensitivity in graft recipients: Complexity of responses and divergence from acute rejection. Transplantation 1997; 63(9):1300-1307.
57. Carrodeguas L, Orosz CG, Waldman WJ, et al: Trans vivo analysis of human delayed-type hypersensitivity reactivity. Hum Immunol 1999; 60(8):640-651.
58. Valujskikh A, Lantz O, Celli S, et al: Cross-primed CD8(+) T cells mediate graft rejection via a distinct effector pathway. Nat Immunol 2002; 3(9):844-851.
59. Krensky AM, Weiss A, Crabtree G, et al: T-lymphocyte-antigen interactions in transplant rejection. N Engl J Med 1990; 322(8):510-517.
60. Young NT, Bunce M, Morris PJ, Welsh KI: Killer cell inhibitory receptor interactions with HLA class I molecules: Implications for alloreactivity and transplantation. Hum Immunol 1997; 52(1):1-11.
61. van Parijs L, Perez VL, Abbas AK: Mechanisms of peripheral T cell tolerance. Novartis Found Symp 1998; 215:5-14; discussion 14-20, 33-40.
62. Lakkis FG, Sayegh MH: Memory T cells: A hurdle to immunologic tolerance. J Am Soc Nephrol 2003; 14(9):2402-2410.
63. Sayegh MH, Carpenter CB: Tolerance and chronic rejection. Kidney Int Suppl 1997; 58:S11-S14.
64. Owen: Immunogenetic consequences of vascular anastomosis between bovine twins. Science 1945; 102:400.
65. Billingham RE, Brent L, Medawar PB: Activity acquired tolerance of foreign cells. Nature 1953; 172(4379):603-606.
66. Ng WF, Duggan PJ, Ponchel F, et al: Human CD4(+)CD25(+) cells: A naturally occurring population of regulatory T cells. Blood 2001; 98(9):2736-2744.
67. Salama AD, Najafian N, Clarkson MR, et al: Regulatory CD25+ T cells in human kidney transplant recipients. J Am Soc Nephrol 2003; 14(6):1643-1651.
68. Lechler RI, Garden OA, Turka LA: The complementary roles of deletion and regulation in transplantation tolerance. Nat Rev Immunol 2003; 3(2):147-158.
69. Sayegh MH, Akalin E, Hancock WW, et al: CD28-B7 blockade after alloantigenic challenge in vivo inhibits Th1 cytokines but spares Th2. J Exp Med 1995; 181(5):1869-1874.
70. Seino KI, Fukao K, Muramoto K, et al: Requirement for natural killer T (NKT) cells in the induction of allograft tolerance. Proc Natl Acad Sci U S A 2001; 98(5):2577-2581.
71. Zeng D, Lewis D, Dejbakhsh-Jones S, et al: Bone marrow NK1.1(−) and NK1.1(+) T cells reciprocally regulate acute graft versus host disease. J Exp Med 1999; 189(7):1073-1081.
72. Spitzer TR, Sykes M: Treatment of renal-cell cancer by transplantation of allogeneic stem cells. N Engl J Med 2001; 344(2):137-138.

Chapter 32

Evaluation of Donors and Recipients

Colm C. Magee, M.D., M.P.H.

EVALUATION OF THE LIVING DONOR

Live kidney donation is increasingly common in the United States and in other countries. This reflects many factors, including the ongoing shortage of suitable deceased donors, the excellent results achieved with live kidney donation (even between unrelated donors and recipients), and greater physician and public awareness of its benefits. These potential benefits are summarized in Table 32–1. The number of living related and unrelated donors has increased by 68% and 100%, respectively, in the United States over the last decade.[1] In fact, the number of living donors surpassed that of cadaveric donors in 2001.

One major advantage is that preemptive transplantation (before the need for dialysis) is often feasible. Not only does this avoid complications associated with dialysis itself, but recent studies show it is associated with less acute rejection and better allograft survival.[2] This intriguing finding may reflect the avoidance of pro-inflammatory effects of advanced uremia or dialysis itself. Despite the poor matching for HLA antigens associated with unrelated donation, outcomes are excellent.[3] This emphasizes the benefits of transplanting a "healthy" kidney with minimum perioperative ischemia and reperfusion injury.

DONOR NEPHRECTOMY TECHNIQUES

Open nephrectomy is the traditional method. The advantages and disadvantages of this technique are summarized in Table 32–2. For reasons that include patient preference, surgeon preference and marketing strategy, laparoscopic nephrectomy is becoming the donor nephrectomy method of choice in the larger U.S. transplant centers.[4] This can be done as a full or hand-assisted laparoscopic procedure. The advantages and disadvantages of this technique are shown in Table 32–3. There is some evidence that the perceived advantages of laparoscopic nephrectomy have contributed to the increase in donation rates.[5] However, rates of early graft dysfunction may be higher with this technique for the following reasons: higher intra-abdominal pressures required during the procedure, longer warm ischemia times, less experience with the technique—entailing a learning curve—and more manipulation of the renal vessels.[6] One randomized trial found better donor and equivalent recipient outcomes with hand-assisted as opposed to open live donor nephrectomy.[7] It is quite likely, however, that there is a publication bias favoring the laparoscopic method. Adverse outcomes associated with this newer technique are unlikely to be submitted for publication!

CHOOSING THE POTENTIAL DONOR

The general schema for evaluation of a possible donor is shown in Figure 32–1. In general, biologically related donors are preferable to unrelated ones. ABO blood group testing is performed before HLA typing and cross-matching because ABO incompatibility traditionally precludes transplant (a limited number of ABO incompatible transplants are now being performed). When more than one family member is interested in, and suitable for, donation, the best matched donor is preferable. A two haplotype matched sibing is of course the ideal. However, older donors, such as parents, are sometimes preferred in case a subsequent transplant might be required.

Age

There is no absolute age above which donation is contraindicated; more important is whether or not there are medical contraindications (the prevalence of hypertension and type 2 diabetes mellitus, for example, increases with age). A different situation applies in the young where there are major concerns about minors' rights, the ability to freely give informed consent, and the fact that the donor will be exposed to many years of the "single kidney" state. The majority of centers do not allow donation by those less than 18 years (exceptions are sometimes made for identical twins); some centers have higher thresholds, such as 25 years. Unfortunately, there is some evidence that inappropriate donation by minors is occurring.[8]

Safety of Donation: Risks to the Donor

An important issue in the evaluation of persons for living kidney donation is balancing the professional goal of alleviating the recipient's illness with the philosophy of "first, do no harm." Four conditions must be satisfied before living donation can proceed: (1) The risk to the donor must be low, (2) the donor must be fully informed, (3) the decision to donate must be independent and voluntary, and (4) there must be a good chance of a successful recipient outcome.[9]

The risks are most easily explained to the donor as short- and long-term risks. The short-term risks are those associated with the major surgery itself, including death, thromboembolism, myocardial infarction, and wound infection. Because donors are carefully selected and the surgery is elective, major complications are rare. Of more concern to the physician evaluating the donor is the long-term risk, particularly of hypertension and kidney disease. The majority of data regarding mortality in subjects who have undergone unilateral

Table 32–1 Advantages and Disadvantages of Living Donor Kidney Transplantation

Advantages
Potential for minimum waiting time on dialysis and for pre-emptive transplantation
Close HLA matching often feasible
Expansion of total donor pool
Elective surgery
Minimal ischemic damage to allograft
Potential for less aggressive immunosuppression
Excellent graft survival and recipient survival
Psychosocial benefits to donor
Disadvantages
Psychological stress on donor and family
Perioperative donor morbidity (wound infection, thrombosis, etc.)
Perioperative donor mortality (rare)
Potential to excacerbate donor hypertension, proteinuria or kidney disease over the long term

Table 32–2 Advantages and Disadvantages of Open Nephrectomy

Advantages
Tried-and-trusted technique; long-term outcomes excellent
Risk of perioperative ischemic damage very low
Retroperitoneal approach minimizes bowel and other abdominal complications
Disadvantages
Relatively invasive surgery
Large scar with risk of hernia

Table 32–3 Advantages and Disadvantages of Laparoscopic Nephrectomy

Advantages
Less invasive surgery; postoperative recovery faster
Smaller scar
Shorter hospital stay
More acceptable to many donors
Disadvantages
Long-term outcomes not available
Learning curve
Potential for more perioperative ischemic damage and delayed graft function

nephrectomy (for reasons including trauma, neoplasia, or donation) are very reassuring. In fact, a well-performed follow-up study of donors in Sweden found that survival was better in donors compared to that in the general population.[10] Low-grade microalbuminuria or proteinuria has been observed in up to 30% of donors; this is very rarely progressive. The majority of the evidence suggests that nephrectomy is associated with a slight increase in blood pressure. How much this reflects the natural history in a given donor is unclear; when donors were compared to siblings, a similarly high incidence was found in both.[11] Although limited data suggest that long-term renal function remains adequate in the majority of donors, there is growing concern that not enough is known about their long-

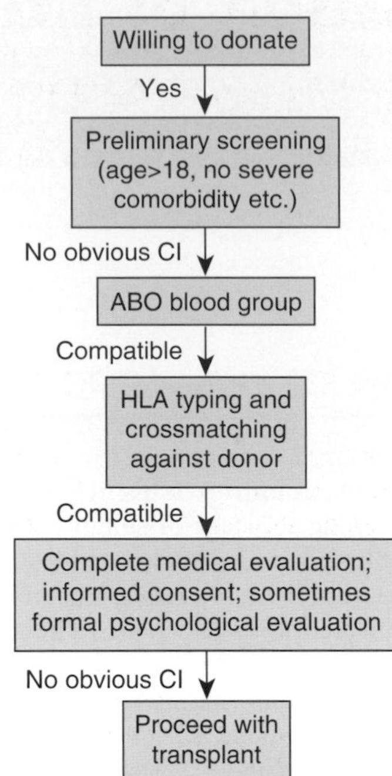

Figure 32–1 Typical steps in the evaluation of a patient for live kidney donation. *CI*, contraindication.

term outcomes.[12] Ideally, a national registry of donors would be established to allow more rigorous long-term follow-up; this has yet to be done in the United States. One recent study of the OPTN database found that 56 previous living donors had been listed for transplantation; the number of patients with less severe kidney disease could, of course, be much greater.[12]

Clinical Assessment of the Donor

To avoid conflict of interest, the proposed donor should be meticulously evaluated by a physician not involved in care of the proposed recipient. The physician must confirm that the patient's wish to donate is voluntary. This is more of a concern with nonrelated donors. The physician must also fully explain the short- and long-term consequences of donation.

The history and examination and tests (Table 32–4) should focus on excluding contraindications to donation. Many of these contraindications are shown in Table 32–5. Not all of these listed are absolute contraindications, but in general it is better to err on the side of minimizing damage to the donor. Occasionally, disagreements will arise wherein the evaluating physician will advise against donation and the patient will still want to donate, "whatever the risk." A second opinion is often of use in such cases.

Family History of Type 2 Diabetes Mellitus

Type 2 diabetes mellitus is an increasingly common cause of ESRD. Not surprisingly, when the recipient has these diseases, the risk of related donors developing diabetes later in life is a major concern. Although little is known as to whether single-kidney status would accelerate the progression of diabetic nephropathy, it seems prudent to avoid donation in those

Table 32–4 Initial Tests for Potential Live Kidney Donors*

CBC, PT, PTT
Plasma creatinine, calcium, urea, electrolytes
Fasting plasma glucose (and glucose tolerance test if patient obese or if family history of type 2 diabetes mellitus)
Chest X-Ray, EKG
Estimate of GFR (creatinine clearance or isotope)
Spot urine albumin:creatinine ratio (twice)
Urinalysis and urine culture
Tests for HIV, hepatitis B, hepatitis C, cytomegalovirus, Epstein-Barr virus

*This assumes no ABO-blood group or HLA antigen incompatibilities. Imaging studies of the renal vasculature are usually performed later.

Table 32–5 Relative or Absolute Contraindications to Live Kidney Donation

Age <18-25 or >70-75 years
Hypertension (BP >140/90 or on antihypertensive medication)
BMI >30-35 kg/m^2
Diabetes mellitus or abnormal glucose tolerance test
History of gestational type 2 diabetes mellitus
Strong family history of diabetes mellitus
Malignancy
Significant comorbidity
Microalbuminuria or overt proteinuria
Recurrent kidney stone disease
Other kidney disease
Low GFR (<70-80 ml/min)
Transmissable serious infection (e.g., HIV, hepatitis B, hepatitis C)

thought to be at high risk of developing type 2 diabetes mellitus later in life. In addition to family history (especially first-degree relative) of type 2 diabetes mellitus, the following factors increase risk: obesity, increasing age, non-white ethnicity and history of gestational diabetes. All patients with a family history of type 2 diabetes mellitus should have a glucose tolerance test; if this is abnormal, donation is prohibited due to the very high risk of developing diabetes. If the glucose tolerance test is normal and there are no other risk factors, it is reasonable to allow donation. More difficult is where the test is normal but the patient has one or both of the additonal factors mentioned. The protocol in our institution is to advise lifestyle modification for 3 to 6 months, then further review and discuss with the donor. It is sobering to note that the estimated lifetime probability of developing diabetes mellitus in the United States is now about 1 in 3.[13]

Hereditary Kidney Disease

When kidney disease in the recipient is due to an inherited disease, it is essential that the disease is excluded in related donors. This will sometimes require close consultation with a geneticist. The most common scenario is a family history of autosomal dominant polycystic kidney disease (ADPKD). If the potential donor is over age 30, the absence of cysts on a carefully performed ultrasound virtually excludes the diagnosis. If the donor is 20 to 30 years old, however, a negative ultrasound does not exclude ADPKD type II (a negative ultrasound or CT are probably adequate to exclude ADPKD type I) and genetic testing such as linkage analysis may be helpful.[14]

Alport's syndrome is a genetically heterogeneous disease with X-linked, autosomal recessive, and autosomal dominant variants. The majority of cases are X-linked. Screening of donors involves urinalysis, tests of GFR, and specialized eye and ear testing. Male siblings greater than 20 years of age are very unlikely to have the disease if hematuria is absent. Sisters of affected male recipients with X-linked diseases have a 50% chance of being carriers; a small percent of such females carrying the abnormal gene do develop renal failure. Thus, female heterozygotes (identified as having hematuria but normal renal function) should only be allowed to donate after detailed consultation with a nephrologist and geneticist.

Donor with Asymptomatic Microhematuria

Urine dipstick testing—in the absence of fever, trauma, menstruation, or vigorous exercise—should be repeated twice to confirm the presence of microhematuria. Urinary tract infection must be excluded. Urine microscopy should be performed to confirm the presence of red blood cells and to determine whether red blood cell casts are present. The presence of unexplained microhematuria at this stage does not exclude donation, but the donor must be informed that further invasive testing is required before he or she can be deemed fit to donate. The following tests may all be required: cystoscopy, imaging of kidneys and of urinary tract, and kidney biopsy. Only if these tests are normal should the hematuria be considered benign and donation be allowed.

Renal Stone Disease

A history of urinary tract stones is at least a relative contraindication to donation because stones tend to recur and obstruction of a solitary kidney could of course be catastrophic. Some centers will consider donation where all of the following apply: passage of only one stone and that at least 10 years prior to donation, no evidence of a metabolic cause (such as hypercalciuria) of stone formation, and current imaging studies showing no urinary tract stones.[15] Any such donors should be advised to continue lifelong high fluid intake.

Conclusion

Live kidney donation is likely to increase further in the United States and in other countries. It is imperative that donors are carefully selected and that the short- and long-term risks of donation are minimized. Ideally, long-term follow-up of donors will be improved; a national donor registry in the United States would be very helpful in this regard.

EVALUATION OF THE RECIPIENT

Evaluation of the patient with chronic kidney disease for transplantation should begin before initiation of dialysis. This allows preemptive (before dialysis) transplantation if a living donor is available. Even if living donation is not an option, completion of the evaluation and testing means that the patient can be listed for cadaveric kidney transplantation as soon as dialysis is started. The initial evaluation must be thorough (Figure 32–2). Not only must the patient be extensively educated as to the risks and benefits of transplantation, but contraindications to transplant must be excluded. In addition to a thorough history and examination, a number of routine tests are required (Table 32–6). General contraindications to transplant are discussed in the following paragraph and shown in Table 32–7.

Contraindications to Transplantation

Cancer

At least 2 years disease-free status is required for almost all cancers; many programs require 5 years for breast cancer and melanoma. Close consultation with oncology colleagues is essential. Active cancer is a contraindication to transplant for at least two reasons. First, immunosuppression could accelerate progression of cancer. Second, early recurrence with associated morbidity and mortality would "waste" the transplanted organ.

Acute or Chronic Infections

Whenever possible, acute or chronic infections should be eliminated before transplant. In certain situations, complete cure is not possible and the risks and benefits of transplantation and associated immunosuppression must be very carefully considered, for instance, hepatitis C infection (response to antiviral therapy is often incomplete) or HIV infection.

Hepatitis C.

Immunosuppression can accelerate the progression of this systemic disease. This does not mean that HCV-infected patients should forego transplantation. In fact, although HCV-positive dialysis and transplant patients had poorer survival compared to HCV-positive, transplantation still conferred a survival benefit over dialysis in those with HCV infection.[16] The management of the pretransplant HCV-positive patient has not been standardized. However, most experts recommend liver biopsy in all transplant candidates to guide prognosis and therapy.[17] The goal—not always achievable—is to eliminate viral replication or, at least, slow progression to cirrhosis. An algorithm for management of the HCV-positive pretransplant patient is shown in Figure 32–3. Interestingly, the response rates to interferon-α monotherapy are probably higher in dialysis than in nondialysis patients. However, ribavirin is contraindicated in the former group because of its accumulation in renal failure and associated risk of severe anemia.

HIV.

Until recently, HIV infection was considered an absolute contraindication to renal transplantation in most centers. This reflected fears that immunosuppression would facilitate progression of infection and that the short survival of

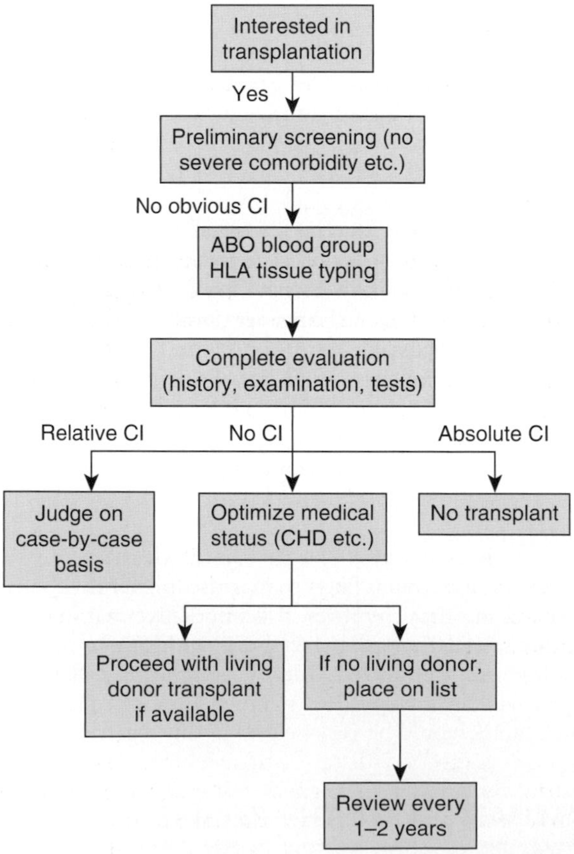

Interested in transplantation
Yes
Preliminary screening (no severe comorbidity etc.)
No obvious CI
ABO blood group HLA tissue typing
Complete evaluation (history, examination, tests)
Relative CI | No CI | Absolute CI
Judge on case-by-case basis
Optimize medical status (CHD etc.)
No transplant
Proceed with living donor transplant if available
If no living donor, place on list
Review every 1–2 years

Figure 32–2 Typical steps in the evaluation of a patient for kidney transplantation. *CI,* contraindication; *CHD,* coronary heart disease.

Table 32–6 Routine Tests for Potential Kidney Transplant Recipients

ABO blood typing and HLA tissue typing
CBC, PT, PTT
Plasma creatinine, urea, electrolytes, calcium, glucose, PTH
Chest X-Ray, EKG
Urinalysis and urine culture
Tests for HIV, hepatitis B, hepatitis C, cytomegalovirus, Epstein-Barr virus, syphilis
If >50 yrs: stool occult blood testing +/− colonoscopy
Women: Pap smear; mammogram if >40 yrs
Men: PSA if >50 yrs

Table 32–7 Contraindications to Kidney Transplantation

Active cancer
Active infection
Active psychiatric illness
Ongoing non-compliance with dialysis or medicine regimen
Major morbidity which would be worsened by transplant or would lead to very short posttransplant survival
High operative risk
ABO-incompatibility*
Positive T-cell crossmatch*
Severe obesity eg BMI >35 kg/m^2

*Protocols are available to facilitate transplantation across these barriers.

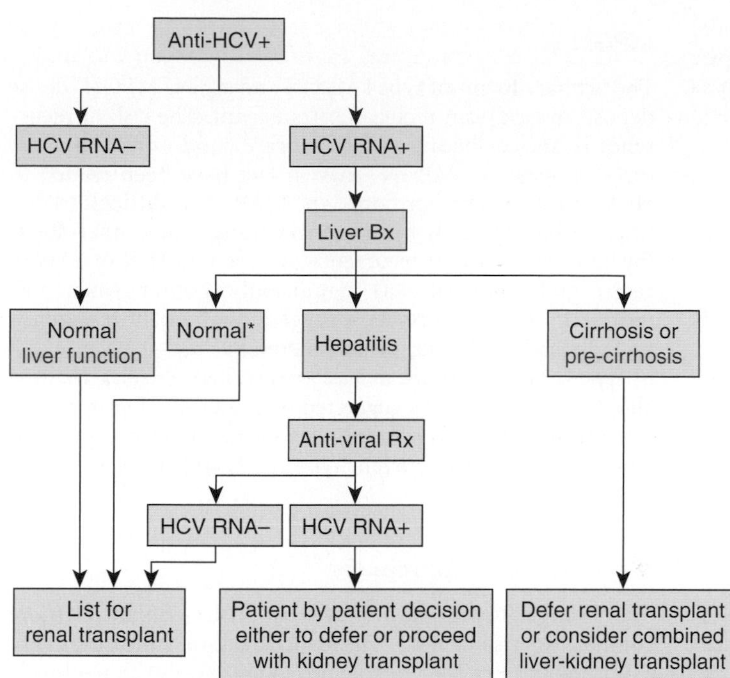

Figure 32–3 Management of the anti-HCV antibody positive ESRD patient being considered for kidney transplant. *Some centers might try course of anti-viral therapy, before transplant.

HIV–positive transplanted patients would waste valuable allografts. With dramatic improvements in the survival of HIV-positive patients, these premises are being reexamined.[18] These patients should be referred to centers specializing in the management of transplanted HIV-positive patients as their management is complex. One difficulty is the potential for interactions between the multiple antiviral medicines, some of which inhibit and some of which induce the cytochrome P450 system.

Tuberculosis.

Active tuberculosis, of course, requires full treatment and cure before transplant. Transplant candidates who are PPD positive and who have no clinical or radiologic evidence of active disease should receive a course of antituberculosis prophylaxis if this has not been administered before. Typically, isoniazid is prescribed for 9 months. The major adverse effect of this drug is hepatotoxicity, and monitoring of LFTs is mandatory. Ideally, the complete course of isoniazid is given pretransplant but posttransplant administration is acceptable.

Ongoing Psychiatric Illness

Psychiatric illness is only a contraindication if severe enough to impair understanding of the risks and benefits of transplantation and if severe enough to prevent normal posttransplant follow-up and compliance. Addiction to alcohol or other drugs should be successfully treated before transplantation. Mental retardation of itself is not a contraindication if adequate posttransplant support is available. The issue of informed consent for surgery can be difficult, however.

Specific Renal or Systemic Diseases that Can Recur Posttransplant

Certain renal and systemic diseases recur posttransplant and, in such cases, the recipient must be informed of this risk. Usually transplantation is not contraindicated but a waiting period, until the disease becomes quiescent, is sometimes required.

Primary Focal Segmental Glomerulosclerosis (FSGS)

Primary FSGS has a reported recurrence rate of 20% to 40% and causes graft loss in approximately 50% of recurrent cases.[19] Risk factors for graft loss from recurrence (by analysis of registry data) include white recipient, black donor, younger recipient, and treatment for rejection.[19] Other factors thought to predict recurrence and/or graft loss are rapidly progressive FSGS in the recipient's native kidneys and recurrence of disease in a previous allograft. Treatment options include plasmapheresis or immunoadsorption, high dose glucocorticoids, high dose CNIs and cyclophosphamide but controlled studies are lacking. Those at very high risk of recurrence should be offered cadaveric rather than living donor kidneys.

Anti-GBM Disease

Before transplantation, patients with ESRD due to anti-GBM disease should be on dialysis for at least 6 months and have negative anti-GBM serology. If these criteria are fulfilled, posttransplant recurrence is very rare.

De Novo Anti-GBM Disease

De novo anti-GBM disease occasionally arises in the early posttransplant period in grafts transplanted into recipients with Alport's syndrome. Here the recipient with abnormal type IV collagen α chains produces antibodies against the previously "unseen" normal α chain in the basement membrane of the transplanted kidney. Patients with graft dysfunction should be treated with plasmapheresis and cyclophosphamide.

Those with only immunofluorescence evidence of recurrence (i.e., linear staining of GBMs by IgG) do not require therapy. Graft failure due to anti-GBM disease is more common in retransplants.

HUS/TTP

Recurrence of classical (diarrhoea associated) HUS/TTP is uncommon. In contrast, recurrence of atypical (nondiarrhoea associated) HUS/TTP, particularly if inherited, is common. In one series of patients with an autosomal recessive form of HUS/TTP, there was recurrence in six of seven cases.[20] In general, the prognosis for the graft is poor if there is recurrence. Even when ESRD is due to the classical form, transplantation should be deferred until the disease is quiescent for at least 6 months.

IgA Glomerulonephritis

Studies with longer follow-up have shown that histologic recurrence of this condition is common; in one recent series it was at least 35%.[21] On multivariable analysis, recurrence was not associated with greater risk of graft failure. IgA glomerulonephritis is not a contraindication to transplant, although it would seem prudent in very aggressive forms of this condition to allow a period of 6 to 12 months before transplant.

SLE Nephritis

Graft and patient survival overall are similar in patients with ESRD secondary to lupus nephritis compared to those with ESRD from other causes.[22] Recurrence of severe SLE, systemically or within the graft, is uncommon after transplant. This probably reflects the following: patient selection, disease activity "burning out" on chronic dialysis, and the effects of powerful posttransplant immunosuppression. After starting dialysis, patients should have clinically quiescent disease for 3 to 6 months before undergoing transplantation. Clinical criteria are a better guide to suitability for transplant than serologic criteria alone. SLE patients with anti-phospholipid antibody syndrome probably have poorer graft and patient survival because of recurrent APS after transplant. These patients should resume full anticoagulation immediately after surgery.

Wegener's Granulomatosis and Microscopic Polyangiitis

Renal and extrarenal recurrence of Wegener's granulomatosis and polyangiitis have been described after renal transplantation. It is not yet known whether current regimens incorporating MMF or tacrolimus reduce that risk. In the largest reported series, with a mean follow-up time of 44 months, ANCA associated small vessel vasculitis recurred in 17% of cases; renal involvement recurred in 10% of cases; the recurrence rate was not lower with CsA therapy.[23] This and other studies have found that positive ANCA serology at the time of transplant does not predict later relapse. Of course, patients with ESRD secondary to ANCA vasculitis should not be transplanted until the disease is clinically in remission. Relapses usually respond to cyclophosphamide.

MPGN

The primary forms of type I MPGN and type II MPGN (dense deposit disease) can recur after transplant. The risk of recurrence is unclear because these are rare conditions and some cases of "primary MPGN" may in fact have been related to HCV infection. Furthermore, type I MPGN is difficult to distinguish histologically from primary transplant glomerulopathy. One series found recurrence of type I MPGN in 33% of cases; graft survival was significantly poorer when this recurred.[24] Case reports have suggested a benefit of steroids, cyclophosphamide, and plasmapheresis.

Type II MPGN recurs, at least by histologic criteria, in most allografts. Early reports suggested that associated graft failure was unusual. However, more recent series have documented allograft loss from recurrent type II MPGN in over 20% of cases.[25]

Membranous Nephropathy

Membranous nephropathy may recur posttransplant, or more commonly, arise *de novo*. The associated clinical features vary from nonexistent (i.e., histologic evidence only) to nephrotic syndrome. In one series of 30 patients, the actuarial risk of recurrence at 3 years was 29% and recurrence was associated with poor graft survival.[26] *De novo* membranous nephropathy is often associated with chronic allograft nephropathy. As with native kidney disease, HCV infection and other causes of this glomerulopathy should be excluded.

Primary Hyperoxaluria

Primary hyperoxaluria is a rare inherited metabolic disorder characterized by hyperproduction of oxalate with resultant massive deposition in the kidney and urinary tract. Deposition can recur immediately posttransplant, leading to early graft loss. The treatment for choice is therefore often combined liver-kidney transplantation as the hepatic allograft corrects the enzyme defect.

Sickle Cell Disease

Many centers consider sickle cell disease a contraindication to transplant. Sickling may actually worsen posttransplant because of the higher blood hemoglobin. Nevertheless, some patients may be candidates for transplantation, if the disease is well controlled and if expert hematologic input (for therapies such as exchange blood transfusion) is available in the perioperative period.

Diabetes Mellitus

It is important to note that diabetics, in particular, gain a significant survival advantage with transplantation as compared to those diabetics remaining on dialysis on the waiting list.[27] Recurrence of diabetic nephropathy in the allograft has not been well studied. This reflects the poor long-term survival of diabetic transplant recipients; the duration of exposure to the diabetic milieu is often insufficient to allow development of severe diabetic nephropathy. Kim and Cheigh[28] performed a case control study of 78 patients with ESRD due to type I DM. Overall graft survival was poorer in the diabetic group; if death were excluded as a cause of graft failure, however, graft survival would be little different. Six of 16 patients who were biopsied had histologic evidence of recurrence, but this resulted in graft loss in only one case. It is likely that with better management of risk factors for cardiovascular disease, overall survival for diabetics will improve. Thus, recurrence of clinically significant diabetic nephropathy will probably become more common.

Other Conditions that Complicate Transplantation

High Sensitization to HLA Antigens

ESRD patients can develop antibodies against HLA antigens after exposure to these antigens in previous allografts, blood products, or pregnancy. Obtaining a suitable allograft for highly sensitized patients has traditionally proved difficult—such patients may wait many years for a compatible kidney. Furthermore, rejection tends to be more common and severe. Two protocols are evolving for the "desensitization" of such patients. One involves intermittent infusions of very high dose IgG; the IgG probably has multiple immune effects. Another protocol involves pretransplant plasmapheresis, lower dose IgG, MMF, tacrolimus, and steroids. In each case, transplant is done if and when the donor-recipient cross-match turns negative. Short-term results have been very encouraging.[29,30] Longer-term results of these approaches are awaited but desensitization will likely be increasingly offered to highly sensitized patients otherwise precluded from transplantation.

Age

There is no absolute age above which transplantation is contraindicated; biologic age is more important than chronological age. Each case should be assessed on its merits. A reasonable criterion is that the patient would be expected to live for at least 5 years after transplant. Of course, many elderly patients will still need to wait several years before obtaining a cadaveric transplant. Where available, additional listing for marginal kidney transplants should be discussed.

Obesity

Obesity is associated with more transplant surgery-related complications, more DGF, higher mortality (related to cardiovascular complications), and poorer graft survival.[31,32] Poorer long-term graft survival probably reflects the effects of DGF, nephron overwork, and more difficult dosing of immunosuppressive drugs. Nevertheless, there are some data suggesting that transplantation provides a survival benefit over remaining on the waiting list (on dialysis); no benefit was noted in those with BMI greater than or equal to 41 kg/m^2.

The question is: At what BMI are the risks of transplantation excessive? A reasonable approach is to enter all prospective recipients with BMI greater than 30 kg/m^2 into weight loss programs and, of course, to rigorously exclude/treat any cardiac disease. In those with persistent BMI greater than 30 kg/m^2 but without cardiac contraindications to surgery, eligibility for transplantation should be judged on a case-by-case basis.

Liver Disease

Hepatitis C has been discussed previously. General principles related to liver disease (of any sort) are that transplantation should not be performed where there is active hepatitis or advanced cirrhosis. Less severe forms of liver disease may not preclude transplantation, but wherever possible, treatment should be completed pretransplant.

Transplantation and immunosuppression can undoubtedly worsen hepatitis B. A generally accepted strategy for the assessment of the ESRD patient chronically infected with HBV (i.e., chronically HBV surface antigen positive) is shown in Figure 32–4. Current guidelines are that all HBV surface antigen positive patients who do receive a kidney transplant should receive

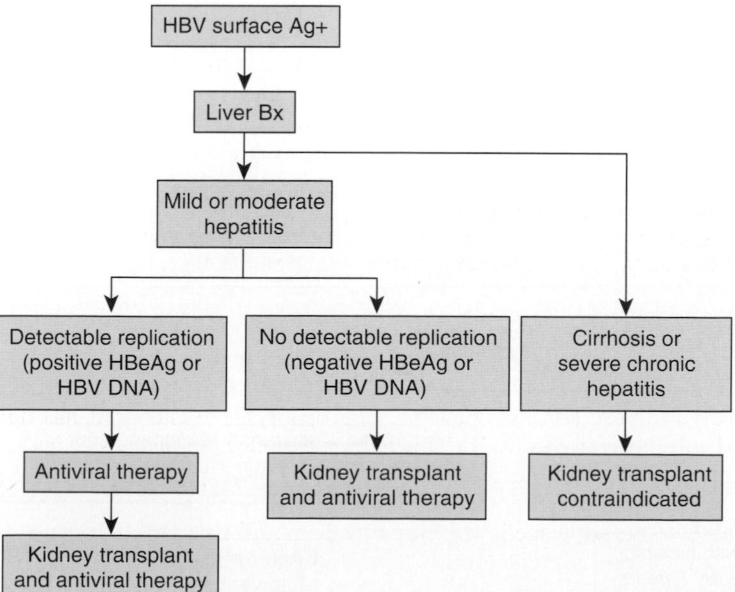

Figure 32–4 Management of the HBV surface antigen positive ESRD patient being considered for kidney transplant.

lamivudine for the following 18 to 24 months.[33] Lamivudine has the major advantage over interferon-α of not promoting allograft rejection.

Cardiac Disease

The high prevalence of cardiovascular disease in ESRD patients is well known. It is very important to optimize the cardiovascular status of the transplant candidate before surgery for the following reasons: (1) The stress of surgery and anesthesia can precipitate serious cardiac events such as myocardial infarction; (2) perioperative cardiac events can contribute to delayed graft function; and (3) performing major interventions such as coronary angioplasty/stenting or coronary artery bypass grafting posttransplant could damage the allograft (whereas renal damage is not a concern in those on dialysis). Thus, all patients require careful evaluation for clinically significant coronary heart disease. A suggested schema is shown in Figure 32–5. Protocols differ substantially between centers; in some, for example, all diabetic patients undergo diagnostic cardiac catheterization. Obviously, close consultation with the candidate's cardiologist is important. The type of noninvasive test used to screen for coronary heart disease depends on center expertise and availability. In general, an exercise-based (treadmill) test is most desirable, as it best simulates the "stress" of surgery. However, many ESRD patients are not robust enough to achieve adequate heart rates or workloads on the treadmill; in such cases, pharmacologic agents can be combined with echocardiography or scintigraphy. Unless contraindicated, ESRD patients known to have coronary heart disease should receive perioperative aspirin and β-blockade.

Diseases of the Gastrointestinal Tract

These are rarely contraindications to renal transplant. Obviously, acute exacerbations of peptic ulcer disease, diverticulitis, and so forth, should be treated before transplant. Those with a history of acute cholecystitis should probably undergo cholecystectomy. Some centers perform cholecystectomy in diabetic transplant candidates with asymptomatic cholelithiasis. Sometimes partial colectomy is performed in transplant candidates with recurrent diverticulitis—the rationale again being that recurrence of the disease posttransplant would be more harmful.

Seizure Disorders

Many antiseizure medications upregulate activity of hepatic cytochrome P450 enzymes. Continuation of such medications after transplant may thus lead to difficulty obtaining therapeutic blood concentrations of the calcineurin inhibitors (and presumably other medications metabolized by this enzyme system).Transplant candidates taking antiseizure medications should be assessed as to whether such medications can be stopped or changed to less enzyme-inducing alternatives (for example, carbamazepine is less inducing than phenytoin).

MANAGING PATIENTS ON THE WAITING LIST

Waiting times in the United States and elsewhere for cadaveric grafts are increasing and are typically several years. Some patients wait more than 5 to 10 years. Thus, dialysis patients are at relatively high risk of developing new complications, particularly cardiovascular disease, while waiting for a cadaveric kidney. Ideally, all patients on the list, or at least those at highest risk of developing new complications (e.g., elderly, diabetics), should be reassessed every 1 to 2 years. This requires a lot of work! Close communication with the patient's outside nephrologist is essential.

CONCLUSION

Thorough evaluation of the candidate transplant recipient is essential. The risks and benefits of transplantation must be carefully assessed for each individual patient. As the waiting list grows longer, more attention must be paid to those on the list to ensure that they remain optimally prepared for their transplant.

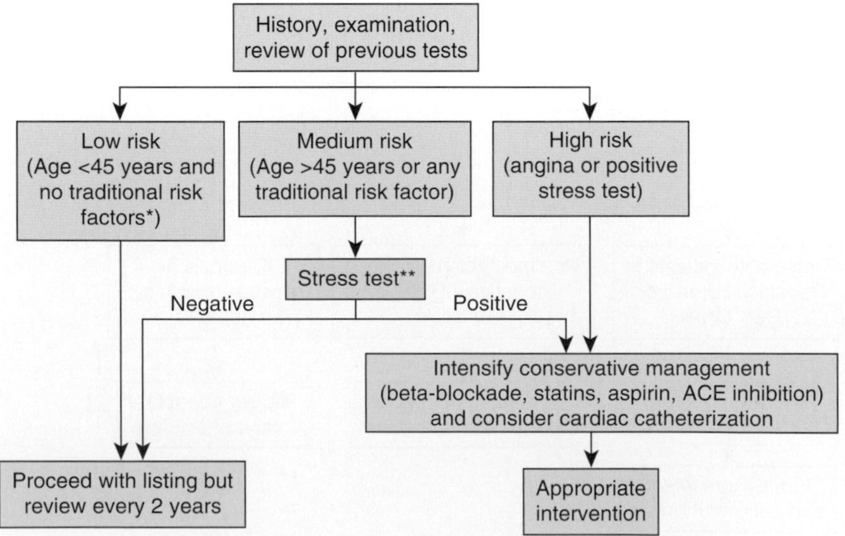

Figure 32–5 Suggested evaluation for coronary heart disease pretransplant. *Hypertension, hyperlipidemia, diabetes mellitus, smoking. **Specific test will depend on patients's ability to exercise and on local expertise.

References

1. United States Renal Data System: 2002 Annual Data Report: Atlas of end stage renal disease in the United States. Accessed on-line at www.usrds.org, USRDS, 2003.
2. Mange KC, Joffe MM, Feldman HI: Effect of the use or nonuse of long-term dialysis on the subsequent survival of renal transplants from living donors. N Engl J Med 2001; 344:726-731.
3. Gjertson DW, Cecka JM: Living unrelated donor kidney transplantation. Kidney Int 2000; 58:491-499.
4. Finelli FC, Gongora E, Sasaki TM, Light JA: A survey: The prevalence of laparoscopic donor nephrectomy at large U.S. transplant centers. Transplantation 2001; 71:1862-1864.
5. Schweitzer EJ, Wilson J, Jacobs S, et al: Increased rates of donation with laparoscopic donor nephrectomy. Ann Surg 2000; 232: 392-400.
6. Novick AC: Laparoscopic live donor nephrectomy: Con. Urology 1999; 53:668-670.
7. Wolf JS Jr, Merion RM, Leichtman AB, et al: Randomized controlled trial of hand-assisted laparoscopic versus open surgical live donor nephrectomy. Transplantation 2001; 72:284-290.
8. Delmonico FL, Harmon WE: The use of a minor as a live kidney donor. Am J Transplant 2002; 2:333-336.
9. Anonymous: Ethical issues. UK guidelines for living donor kidney donation. BTS 2000:9-14.
10. Fehrman-Ekholm I, Elinder CG, Stenbeck M, et al: Kidney donors live longer. Transplantation 1997; 64:976-978.
11. Najarian JS, Chavers BM, McHugh LE, Matas AJ: 20 years or more of follow-up of living kidney donors. Lancet 1992; 340: 807-810.
12. Ellison MD, McBride MA, Taranto SE, et al: Living kidney donors in need of kidney transplants: A report from the organ procurement and transplantation network. Transplantation 2002; 74:1349-1351.
13. Narayan KM, Boyle JP, Thompson TJ, et al: Lifetime risk for diabetes mellitus in the United States. JAMA 2003; 290:1884-1890.
14. Nicolau C, Torra R, Badenas C, et al: Autosomal dominant polycystic kidney disease types I and II: Assessment of U.S. sensitivity for diagnosis. Radiology 1999; 213:273-276.
15. Kasiske BL, Ravenscraft M, Ramos EL, et al: The evaluation of living renal transplant donors: Clinical practice guidelines. Ad Hoc Clinical Practice Guidelines Subcommittee of the Patient Care and Education Committee of the American Society of Transplant Physicians. J Am Soc Nephrol 1996; 7:2288-2313.
16. Pereira BJ, Natov SN, Bouthot BA, et al: Effects of hepatitis C infection and renal transplantation on survival in end-stage renal disease. The New England Organ Bank Hepatitis C Study Group. Kidney Int 1998; 53:1374-1381.
17. Morales JM, Campistol JM: Transplantation in the patient with hepatitis C. J Am Soc Nephrol 2000; 11:1343-1353.
18. Halpern SD, Ubel PA, Caplan AL: Solid-organ transplantation in HIV-infected patients. N Engl J Med 2002; 347:284-287.
19. Abbott KC, Sawyers ES, Oliver JD III, et al: Graft loss due to recurrent focal segmental glomerulosclerosis in renal transplant recipients in the United States. Am J Kidney Dis 2001; 37:366-373.
20. Kaplan BS, Papadimitriou M, Brezin JH, et al: Renal transplantation in adults with autosomal recessive inheritance of hemolytic uremic syndrome. Am J Kidney Dis 1997; 30:760-765.
21. Ponticelli C, Traversi L, Feliciani A, et al: Kidney transplantation in patients with IgA mesangial glomerulonephritis. Kidney Int 2001; 60:1948-1954.
22. Ward MM: Outcomes of renal transplantation among patients with end-stage renal disease caused by lupus nephritis. Kidney Int 2000; 57:2136-2143.
23. Nachman PH, Segelmark M, Westman K, et al: Recurrent ANCA-associated small vessel vasculitis after transplantation: A pooled analysis. Kidney Int 1999; 56:1544-1550.
24. Andresdottir MB, Assmann KJ, Hoitsma AJ, et al: Recurrence of type I membranoproliferative glomerulonephritis after renal transplantation: Analysis of the incidence, risk factors, and impact on graft survival. Transplantation 1997; 63:1628-1633.
25. Andresdottir MB, Assmann KJ, Hoitsma AJ, et al: Renal transplantation in patients with dense deposit disease: Morphological characteristics of recurrent disease and clinical outcome. Nephrol Dial Transplant 1999; 14:1723-1731.
26. Cosyns JP, Couchoud C, Pouteil-Noble C, et al: Recurrence of membranous nephropathy after renal transplantation: Probability, outcome and risk factors. Clin Nephrol 1998; 50:144-153.
27. Wolfe RA, Ashby VB, Milford EL, et al: Comparison of mortality in all patients on dialysis, patients on dialysis awaiting transplantation, and recipients of a first cadaveric transplant. N Engl J Med 1999; 341:1725-1730.
28. Kim H, Cheigh JS: Kidney transplantation in patients with type I diabetes mellitus: Long-term prognosis for patients and grafts. Korean J Intern Med 2001; 16:98-104.
29. Schweitzer EJ, Wilson JS, Fernandez-Vina M, et al: A high panel-reactive antibody rescue protocol for cross-match-positive live donor kidney transplants. Transplantation 2000; 70:1531-1536.
30. Montgomery R, Zachary A, Racusen L, et al: Plasmapheresis and intravenous immune globulin provides effective rescue therapy for refractory humoral rejection and allows kidneys to be successfully transplanted into cross-match-positive recipients. Transplantation 2000; 70:887-895.
31. Pischon T, Sharma AM: Obesity as a risk factor in renal transplant patients. Nephrol Dial Transplant 2001; 16:14-17.
32. Meier-Kriesche HU, Arndorfer JA, Kaplan B: The impact of body mass index on renal transplant outcomes: A significant independent risk factor for graft failure and patient death. Transplantation 2002; 73:70-74.
33. Kasiske BL, Vazquez MA, Harmon WE, et al: Recommendations for the outpatient surveillance of renal transplant recipients. American Society of Transplantation. J Am Soc Nephrol 2000; 11:S1-S86.

Surgical Aspects of Renal Transplantation

Nahel Elias, M.D. • Francis L. Delmonico, M.D. • Dicken S.C. Ko, M.D., F.R.C.S.C.

HISTORIC ASPECTS

The early development of renal transplantation has much of its history rooted in Boston at the Peter Bent Brigham Hospital.[1] As the chief of the Department of Surgery during those formative years, Francis D. Moore created an environment filled with energy and resources, enabling significant innovation. The careful and logical progression of the Brigham's investigative work in transplantation eventually captured the Nobel Prize, which was awarded to Joseph Murray in 1990.

Some transplant physicians may not be aware of the depth of the Brigham research that preceded Murray's accomplishments. Prior to the first successful kidney transplant between identical twins performed by Murray in 1954, a series of nine recipients of cadaveric renal allografts was published by David Hume and colleagues,[2] who were also working in Moore's department. One of Hume's patients experienced adequate renal function for nearly 6 months following transplantation. This recipient eventually suffered a rejection of the "homograft," a fate that the Brigham group had observed previously in numerous renal transplants in dogs. Hume's technique for human renal transplantation was, in retrospect, primitive; the renal allograft was placed in the thigh and a cutaneous ureterostomy was established for urinary tract drainage.[2] The patient, who enjoyed several months of renal function, wore a leg bag to collect the allograft urine, and he was able to manage the stoma without difficulty, traveling by public transportation to the hospital for follow-up on many occasions (Joseph Murray, M.D., personal communication, 1998). A total of 13 such renal transplantations were performed by the Brigham team using the upper thigh vessels for vascular anastomoses and the skin ureterostomy for drainage.[3]

Hume[4] made other contributions to transplantation that we are familiar with today, including the development of tissue typing and a network of organ sharing. His vision of an organ bank led to the formation of the Southeast Organ Procurement Foundation, the forerunner of the United Network for Organ Sharing (UNOS). The concept of removing human kidneys from cadavers was first undertaken by Hume in 1947, as he and Charles Hufnagle resolved the postpartum renal failure of a young woman by suturing the renal artery and vein of a cadaver kidney to the brachial vessels of this patient (Francis D. Moore, M.D., personal communication, 1998). The cadaver kidney provided a method of dialysis until the recovery of this patient's native kidney function permitted her survival.[4]

Had it not been for the untimely death of Hume[1] in 1973, he likely would have shared the Nobel Prize with Murray. It should be noted, however, that more than a decade before Hume's pioneering work, a Russian surgeon named Voronoy[5] attempted a renal transplantation from a cadaver (6 hours after the patient's death) (Figs. 33–1 and 33–2). Although this transplant was unsuccessful in producing urine, Hume and colleagues[2] acknowledged Voronoy in their original report of the Boston series. An informative review of the Voronoy procedure was published by Hamilton and Reid[6] in 1984.

Starzl[5] has recorded that the extraperitoneal site of renal transplantation was first considered by French surgeons prior to Murray's successful transplantation. Nevertheless, this retroperitoneal pelvic location was later chosen for the identical twin renal transplantation by Murray and colleagues[3] because it enabled implantation of a short segment of ureter into the bladder. An insufficient length of the transplanted ureter was the principal reason not to use the native renal fossa. However, performing a simultaneous nephrectomy was also viewed as an impediment. Other advantages of the heterotopic location included the following[3]:

- The kidney was placed in a "more natural environment" (versus the thigh).
- Normal physiologic conditions would be re-created by gravity drainage of the renal pelvis.

In 1954, a 24-year-old patient with malignant hypertension and a blood urea nitrogen (BUN) value of 185 mg/dL was referred to Dr. John Merrill and his colleagues at the Peter Bent Brigham Hospital.[7] The patient was disoriented and was experiencing generalized seizures. It was subsequently determined that the patient had a healthy twin brother. To confirm the genetic identity of these siblings, skin grafts were exchanged between the twins. (This approach still has a contemporary application, in the rare instances in which immunosuppression is to be withdrawn after the transplantation of a renal allograft from a sibling thought to be an identical twin.) At the time of the first transplant, no immunosuppression was available. Nevertheless, Murray concluded correctly that the kidney would not be rejected because of the genetic identity. He also anticipated that the kidney would function normally because he had established that a renal autograft had an indefinite period of normal physiologic status in experimental animals. A left donor nephrectomy was performed and the right ilia fossa was used for the recipient site of transplantation. The donor renal artery was anastomosed to the recipient's hypogastric artery in an end-to-end fashion, and the end of the renal vein was sewn to a venotomy in the side of the common iliac vein. The total ischemia time was 1 hour 22 minutes; nevertheless, the kidney made urine immediately. The ureter was tunneled through the submucosa of the bladder, and an anastomosis between mucosa of the donor ureter with mucosa of the recipient bladder was then performed.

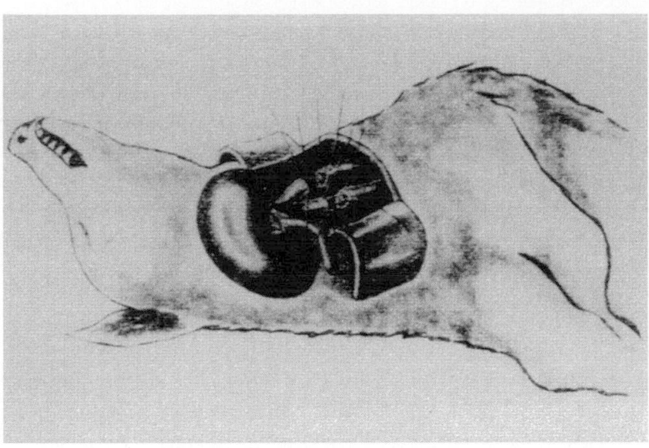

Figure 33–1 Y. Y. Voronoy experimented with dog allografts before carrying out the first human kidney allograft in 1933 at Kherson in Ukraine. His experimental animal model is shown here. (From Hamilton D: Kidney transplantation: A history. *In* Morris PJ [ed]: Kidney Transplantation: Principles and Practice, 4th ed. Philadelphia, WB Saunders, 1994, p 4.)

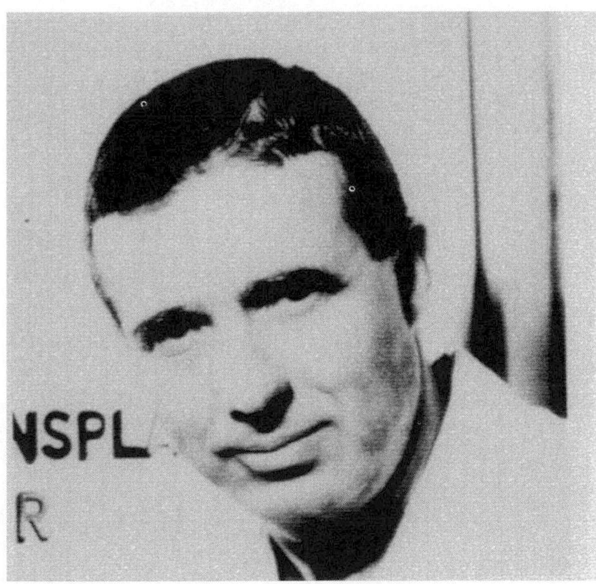

Figure 33–2 David M. Hume (1917–1973) pioneered human kidney transplantation at the Peter Bent Brigham Hospital, Boston, and the Medical College of Virginia. (From Hamilton D: Kidney transplantation: A history. *In* Morris PJ [ed]: Kidney Transplantation: Principles and Practice, 4th ed. Philadelphia, WB Saunders, 1994, p 4.)

The recipient's native kidneys were subsequently removed separately at 3 and 5 months after transplantation because of (1) concern that either kidney might become the source of infection and (2) recurrent hypertension.

In awarding Joseph Murray the Nobel Prize, the committee recognized not only the first successful transplantation in 1954 but also two of his other significant accomplishments: the first successful transplantation of a renal allograft between two fraternal (nonidentical) twins in 1959 using total body irradiation as immunosuppression and, 4 years later, one of the first successful transplantations from a nontwin donor using azathioprine for immunosuppression. Although the focus of this chapter is to recount the surgical aspects of renal transplantation, the contributions of Calne[1] as a Brigham colleague of Murray's should not be overlooked. The routine use of immunosuppression for cadaver donor renal transplants soon thereafter became broadly applied by Hume, Starzl, Russell, Hamburger, and Najarian.

PREOPERATIVE EVALUATION OF RENAL TRANSPLANT RECIPIENTS

The renal disease most commonly associated today with end-stage renal disease (ESRD) is glomerulonephropathy, usually the result of diabetes mellitus. However, individuals who have lost their primary renal transplants because of rejection now constitute the next largest group of patients with renal failure being listed for transplantation. More recently, ESRD combined with another end-stage organ dysfunction necessitating double organ transplants, such as combined kidney-liver and kidney-heart, are on the increase. When there are instances in which the cause of renal failure is unknown, it remains very important to clearly establish its irreversibility before proceeding to renal transplantation.

The success of renal transplantation since the 1960s has been so favorable that it is clearly the optimal therapy for end-stage renal disease. Nevertheless, we have become victims of our own success because the number of potential recipients now far exceeds the number of donors. Thus, prospective patients must be carefully considered for renal transplantation to ensure that they are appropriate candidates for such a scarce resource. An efficient format for evaluating candidates for transplantation is to assemble a meeting of multidisciplinary representatives to assess each patient with the family in attendance. All of the pertinent medical history, laboratory data, and social information should be reviewed by the team at this family meeting to reach a clinically sound recommendation. Psychiatric assessment of a patient's compliance with the medical regimen must be determined before the patient is accepted for transplantation.

Although older age is associated with a higher incidence of other medical illnesses that may lead to a decreased life expectancy, the age of the individual is not an absolute restriction to renal transplantation. Cadaveric renal transplantation can be considered for patients older than 70 years who are otherwise in satisfactory condition for an operative procedure and who may still have a good life expectancy and, therefore, will benefit from a renal allograft.

The overall medical condition of the patient with extrarenal comorbid factors, such as cardiovascular (coronary, valvular, or peripheral vascular), pulmonary disease, hepatitis, and malignancy, also influences patient suitability. This is discussed more in Chapter 32. From a surgical perspective, assessment of arteriosclerotic peripheral vascular disease and its extent is essential. Aortoiliac disease proximal to the transplant may compromise circulation to the allograft and iliofemoral disease distally may result in steal of the lower extremity circulation by the allograft.[8] Assessment of the urinary tract is very important. In males, bladder outlet obstruction secondary to benign prostatic hypertrophy, bladder neck contracture, or urethral strictures must be evaluated before transplant surgery. Although the presence of structural abnormalities of the urinary tract has previously precluded renal transplantation, anatomic reconstructions of the urinary tract, including continent urinary diversion, now permit affected patients to be considered for transplant. In the cases where the storage capacity of the bladder is insufficient for normal function, these bladders may be amenable to cyclic hydrodistention, augmentation cystoplasty, continent urinary diversion, or ileal conduit construction in preparation for transplant.

Ultrasonography may be useful to determine structural of the native kidneys prior to transplantation. Patients with renal failure secondary to chronic pyelonephritis are at risk for persistent urinary tract infection following transplantation; thus, a native nephrectomy prior to or at the time of transplantation may be indicated. Polycystic kidneys may also require nephrectomy prior to transplantation because of bleeding, infection, nephrolithiasis, or mass effect (compromising the space for the allograft). Renal cysts that develop in patients undergoing long-term hemodialysis are a risk factor for renal cell carcinoma.[9–11] If an abnormal mass is identified in the renal parenchyma, further anatomic definition by computed tomography (CT) is required. A native nephrectomy may be indicated to diagnose and to treat renal malignancies prior to transplantation. A renal cell carcinoma is not an absolute contraindication to transplantation, but Penn[12] has advised that an extended period of observation is necessary to rule out development of metastasis before immunosuppression is instituted.

If the patient is anuric or if obstructive/reflux uropathy is a cause of ESRD, a voiding cystourethrogram (VCUG) is often performed preoperatively. Urinary reflux and potential stagnation in a large tortuous upper tract that empties poorly may predispose to further urosepsis after transplantation. A VCUG is also useful to assess the bladder volume of patients with a history of bladder dysfunction.[13] In a large retrospective series, however, routine VCUG evaluation prior to renal transplantation found only 2.5% of 517 patients to have abnormalities.[14] A VCUG presents the potential risk of introducing infection into an otherwise sterile compartment or of causing trauma to the lower urinary tract. In the series just cited, patients with reflux alone (3 of 517) did not require intervention before transplantation.[14] Moreover, a VCUG may not distinguish reflux from a normal urinary tract in approximately 22% of patients when two consecutive VCUGs are performed successively in the same patient. The diagnostic value of a VCUG must be balanced with its risks and costs, thus making its routine use inadvisable.[13]

LIVE KIDNEY DONATION

The notion of removing an organ for transplantation is unique among major surgical procedures because it exposes the healthy donor to the risks of surgery solely for the benefit of another individual. Despite the compelling reasons for using live kidney donors, the procedure could not be justified if unacceptable morbidity or mortality were to be incurred. This concept has been critically evaluated to ensure short-term and long-term safety for the altruistic donor. In the last 50 years, live donor renal transplantation has clearly become an accepted medical procedure using related or unrelated volunteers. Evaluation of candidate donors is discussed in detail in Chapter 32.

OPERATIVE TECHNIQUES

Open Donor Nephrectomy

The techniques of donor nephrectomy can vary among different centers; some favor a posterior rib spreading approach, whereas most now employ a mini-incision anterior flank incision. Regardless of the type of open surgical approach, there are a number of fundamental surgical principles that are of importance. One must have adequate exposure to visualize the important anatomic structures during dissection. The tissues around the renal arteries must be carefully handled to minimize vascular spasm. The vasculature to the ureter must be maintained and meticulously preserved to limit the possibility of subsequent ureteral ischemia. It is also important to maintain an active diuresis so that there will be brisk resumption of renal function after transplantation into the recipient.

Most often, the living donor patient is placed in an extended flank position so that either a supra-11th or supra-12th rib incision can be performed through the latissimus dorsi muscle posteriorly and external oblique muscle anteriorly. The internal oblique and transverse abdominis muscles are then divided with the underlying transversalis fascia to provide full retroperitoneal exposure of the kidney. The paranephric fat and Gerota's fascia, lying in the central part of the wound, are entered. The renal vein is dissected to its junction with the vena cava, the adrenal and gonadal tributaries being ligated and divided. The renal artery is skeletonized at its origin from the aorta after lifting the kidney from its bed and rotating it anteriorly. The ureter is freed, with its investing vessels and fat, down to or below the pelvic brim and then transected. Once urinary output from the skeletonized kidney is assured, the renal artery and vein are clamped and divided, taking care to leave a sufficient cuff of the retained donor vessel to allow secure repair.

The left kidney is usually preferred for transplantation because of the anatomic advantage of a longer renal vein. The left renal vein is transected just proximal to the origins of the adrenal and gonadal veins, providing sufficient length of the vein. If the right kidney is selected, the right renal vein is transected at its origin at the inferior vena cava. The excised kidney is perfused with a chilled, heparinized electrolyte solution. Increasing the osmolarity of the perfusate with mannitol is believed by some to further protect the kidney from ischemic damage. The use of more complex and thus more expensive preservation solutions is not required for living donor kidneys, which will typically be reimplanted with only a brief cold ischemic interval. The wound is closed without drains, and the patient is returned to the recovery room where a chest radiograph is obtained to exclude the possibility of pneumothorax.

Laparoscopic Nephrectomy

Minimally invasive techniques using laparoscopy have made remarkable changes in the field for surgery in the last decade.

A variation of the laparoscopic living donor nephrectomy approach using retroperitoneal endoscopy with special retractors was first reported in 1995[90]; however, the first reported case of a successful laparoscopic nephrectomy in a living donor was performed by Ratner and colleagues[91] at Johns Hopkins University. A subsequent report of 10 consecutive successful laparoscopic living donor nephrectomies performed at the same institution was evaluated against a historic control group of open nephrectomies. The renal allograft warm ischemic time was 4.2 ± 1.3 minutes during the retrieval process through a small (4 to 5 cm) infraumbilical incision. All laparoscopically procured kidneys immediately functioned upon revascularization in the recipients. Compared with the open approach, the laparoscopic procedure was associated with the following advantages[92]:

- Significantly decreased postoperative use of analgesics
- Reduced estimated blood loss
- Earlier resumption of normal diet
- Shorter hospitalization

A later study from the University of Maryland, involving 70 cases of attempted laparoscopic living donor nephrectomy, demonstrated a success rate in 94% of cases. Renal allograft survival rates were 97% in the laparoscopic nephrectomy group and 98% in the open surgery group. Similar to prior reports, this study found that narcotic requirements, length of stay, blood loss, and interval until return to normal activity were significantly less in the laparoscopic donor group.[93] These initial successes in laparoscopic living donor nephrectomies have led to further series that have demonstrated long-term safety and cost-effectiveness associated with the inherent advantages of the procedure.

Some of the initial concerns about laparoscopic donor nephrectomy included warm ischemic injury and prolonged surgical times compared to open donor nephrectomy. With the advent of many ingenious minimally invasive products over the last few years, the incorporation of endocatch and hand-assisted (Handport, LapDisc, or Pneumosleeve) devices enables shortening of ischemic times to intervals comparable to those of open donor nephrectomies. Accordingly, the results for laparoscopically removed kidneys are now quite comparable to those achieved following transplantation of organs procured via the classic open incision.[92]

Many potential live kidney donors continue to be concerned about the potential complications of open surgical approach and the resultant cosmetic appearance of a flank incision. Historically, open donor nephrectomy has been reported to have less than 1% significant morbidity.[86–89] Nevertheless, the issues of postoperative pain, hospitalization, and convalescence requiring an extended period of absence from employment have deterred potential candidates. The availability of the minimally invasive nephrectomy techniques offers a more "patient friendly" option.

Cadaveric Donor Nephrectomy

Viable organs for transplantation are also retrieved from brain dead "heart-beating" patients who are maintained in stable physiologic balance by artificial support. These donors are brought to the operating room, where organ procurement is undertaken under semi-elective conditions employing the usual sterile precautions of any aseptic surgical procedure.

There are situations in which the criteria for brain death have been fulfilled but the concept of heart-beating donation has not been culturally accepted, and in which there is irreversible brain injury but not fulfilling the criteria of brain death, these patients may be candidates for "non-heart beating" (NHBD) or donation after cardiac death (DCD). In NHBD/DCD donors, respiratory support is discontinued. After cardiac function ceases, the donor is declared dead by an independent medical professional and the surgical procurement procedure is expeditiously undertaken. The kidneys must be cooled and removed more rapidly than in the heart-beating donation procedure to minimize warm ischemic injury to the retrieved organs. The goal is to limit the warm ischemic period to, whenever possible, less than 30 minutes. To further increase the number of kidneys available for transplantation, interest has also been revived in the possible procurement of organs from donors who are dead on arrival or who die following unsuccessful cardiorespiratory resuscitation ("uncontrolled" NHBD). Several studies have confirmed that significant numbers of patients succumb either in emergency rooms or intensive care units without brain death being declared.

If only the kidneys are to be removed, bilateral nephrectomy is accomplished through a long midline incision. The peritoneum is incised around the right colon so that the bowel can be retracted upward and to the left. The proximal aorta is freed to above the celiac axis, dividing and ligating the superior mesenteric artery, tapes, or large silk sutures are passed around the distal aorta and vena cava just above the iliac bifurcations. After achieving proximal aortic, distal aortic, and distal caval occlusion, preservation of the kidneys *in situ* is begun by perfusion either with chilled University of Wisconsin (UW) solution, Euro-Collin's solution, or Ringer's lactate solution containing mannitol (18 g/L) and heparin (20,000 units/L) infused through sterile intravenous tubing that has been placed directly into the distal infrarenal aorta. The objective is to take both kidneys with the full length of the renal artery and vein, preferably on aortic and vena–caval cuffs. This approach limits the possibility of injuring accessory vessels, which are present in 12% to 15% of normal kidneys. The technique we prefer entails *en bloc* removal of both kidneys with an intact segment of aorta and inferior vena cava to allow early *in situ* cooling of the kidneys. This approach also reduces the time required for the nephrectomies, because the fine dissection necessary for identification and isolation of the artery and vein can be performed after the kidneys are removed. With this technique, the risk of damaging accessory vessels is essentially eliminated. The final mobilization of the kidneys is undertaken within the plane of Gerota's fascia in a more leisurely manner. Care is taken to free and section the ureters as far down toward the bladder as possible and to avoid dissection within the renal hilus. The distal aorta and vena cava are divided, and the entire block is lifted anteriorly to expose the lumbar vessels posteriorly. Once the proximal aorta and vena cava have been divided, the block consisting of both kidneys and ureters, aorta, and inferior vena cava can be lifted out of the abdomen and placed immediately into a basin of cooled perfusion solution.

The more typical situation involves multiple-organ procurement from the same donor. Although the details will differ, depending on the combination of organs to be removed, certain common principles prevail. These include wide exposure, dissection of each organ to its vascular connection while the heart is still beating, and placement of cannulas for *in situ* cooling and removal of organs while perfusion continues, usually in the order of heart, lungs, liver, pancreas, and then kidneys. The aortic perfusion cannula is placed in the infrarenal aorta as described previously, then the aorta is cross-clamped at the diaphragm and the aortic flush is begun for rapid cooling of the abdominal organs. Precise coordination among the retrieval teams is required at this critical stage. The thoracic organs are removed first; the liver is next, followed by the pancreas and kidneys. The kidneys are mobilized and removed in the same process described for kidney only retrieval.

RECIPIENT OPERATION

Vascular Anastomosis

The natural orientation of the renal vein, renal artery, and ureter is the anatomic basis for transposing the kidney to the contralateral iliac fossa. The left kidney of the donor is usually transplanted to the right iliac fossa of the recipient, and vice versa. However, the donor kidney can be placed on the ipsilateral side without technical hazard. Iliac vessel anastomoses are performed through an extraperitoneal approach.

In the recipient, a modified Gibson's incision can be made in either the left or right lower quadrant of the abdomen. The curvilinear incision allows dissection through the anterior abdominal wall and medial mobilization of the peritoneum. This approach facilitates full exposure of the retroperitoneal iliac fossa, the iliac vessels, and the bladder in preparation for implantation of the renal allograft. If a ureteropyelostomy is indicated as the method of urinary reconstruction, the Gibson's incision can be extended to the tip of the twelfth rib. This enables exposure of the inferior aspects of the Gerota's fascia and permits dissection to perform a standard simple nephrectomy.

The donor renal artery can be anastomosed to the recipient's common, internal, or external iliac artery. The location of the recipient arteriotomy is influenced by the length of the donor artery, the length of the donor ureter, and the presence of atherosclerotic plaques. Although historically either the internal iliac or hypogastric artery was preferentially selected for an end-to-end anastomosis to the donor renal artery (theoretically because of better flow dynamics for the allograft), it has not been shown to be superior to an end-to-side anastomosis of the renal artery to the common or the external iliac artery. Thus, the most common anastomosis performed today is between the end of the donor renal artery and the side of the recipient external iliac artery. This position allows use of the shortest segment of donor artery. Moreover, the proximity of these vessel anastomoses to the bladder also facilitates the creation of the ureteroneocystostomy without compromising the distal ureteric blood supply (Figure 33–3).

The hypogastric artery is now reserved as a last alternative to be used when the other vessels are deemed unsuitable. If the internal iliac artery is to be used, it is divided at the origin of the superior gluteal artery. However, transection of the hypogastric artery may contribute to vasculogenic impotence in males if there is significant occlusive disease of the iliac vessels.[15,16]

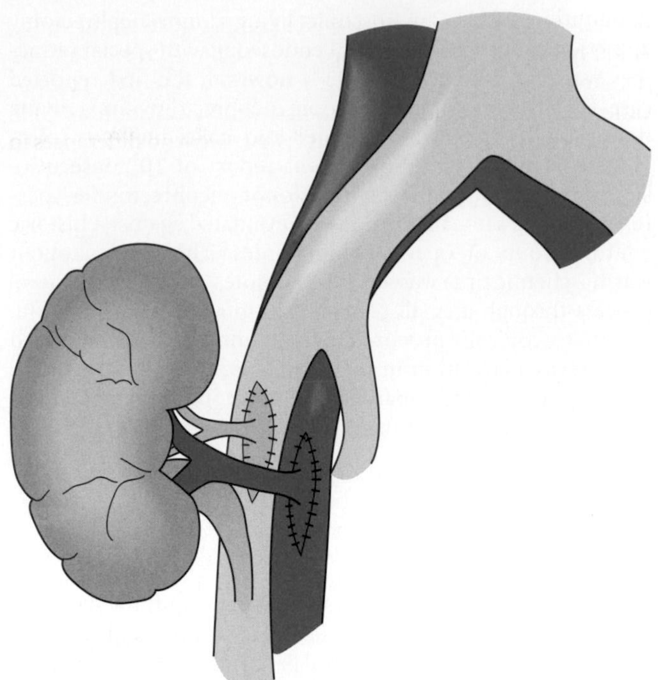

Figure 33–3 Use of Carrel patch on donor artery and vein end-to-side to external iliac artery and vein. (From Salvatierra O Jr: Renal transplantation. *In* Glenn JF [ed]: Urologic Surgery. Philadelphia, JB Lippincott, 1983, p 364.)

The existence of multiple donor renal arteries can be challenging for the transplant surgeon.[17] The loss of a polar vessel results in segmental infarction of the allograft. The lower pole vessel often provides blood supply to the ureter, so compromise of this artery may result in ureteral complications. Thus, during donor organ procurement, the surgical team must be cognizant of multiple renal arteries supplying either kidney. For example, the lower pole artery to the right kidney may course anterior to the vena cava, affecting the cannulation site of the vena cava during a multiorgan procurement from a cadaver donor. When a polar vessel is visualized, it can be traced to the origin of the aorta and salvaged on a Carrel patch of the aorta. Polar vessels can also be anastomosed to the main renal artery in an end-to-side manner to accommodate a single large-vessel anastomosis to the iliac arterial supply. However, very small arterial vessels may supply less than 10% of the kidney; therefore, ligation may be preferable because revascularization may not be feasible.

The placement of the renal vein anastomosis depends on the chosen site for the artery. If the external artery is selected, the renal vein is usually positioned anterior to the artery and is sewn on-end to the side of the external iliac vein. If the common iliac artery is used, the renal vein may be anastomosed to the common iliac vein posterior to the iliac artery. The posterior positioning of the renal vein on the common iliac vein prevents the possibility of poor flow when the patient is supine.

In cadaveric renal transplantation, the use of the donor vena cava to extend the short right renal vein is controversial.[18] Extension of the right renal vein enables an easier technical anastomosis and, possibly, better positioning of the kidney. However, this arrangement may theoretically cause low-flow hemodynamics because of possible kinking of the long vessel. A study examining 305 transplanted right cadaveric kidneys demonstrated no higher rate of technical vascular complications in the 76 kidneys that had venous extensions than in those without venous extension[18]; there were no differences in 1- and 2-year graft survivals between those with and those without an extension. Some researchers have recommended that the donor procurement team provide the right kidney with the vena cava attached routinely, thus allowing the recipient surgical team to determine whether an extension is appropriate for the particular recipient's pelvic anatomy.

Urinary Drainage Reconstruction Techniques

Several strategies are employed for urinary tract reconstruction in renal transplantation. Although Hume and colleagues[2] experimented with a cutaneous ureterostomy in their pioneering series, the likely high rate of surgical complication discouraged this method of urinary drainage from gaining further acceptance. Instead, using either the bladder or ureter of the recipient offered the obvious advantage of enabling the recipient to void naturally.

Ureteroneocystostomy

The technique of ureteroneocystostomy, that is, the implantation of the donor ureter into the recipient bladder, can be classified as either an intravesical, extravesical, or combined intravesical and extravesical repair. Ureteroneocystostomy was first used for the correction of ureteral reflux in children more than 100 years ago by Witzel.[19] Intravesical repair of ureterovesical reflux gained favor in the 1940s with the Hess procedure,[20] which was designed to resolve distal ureteral stricture following reimplantation.

Historically, the most widely practiced intravesical ureteroneocystostomy was the Leadbetter-Politano technique.[21] This approach was used by Leadbetter in the early era of renal transplantation as the method of choice for urinary tract reconstruction. It involved a suprahiatal repair suitable for renal transplantation because the donor ureter was not advanced into the bladder trigone. The advantages of this procedure were (1) the elimination of ureteric kinking at the new muscular hiatus and (2) the hooking of the donor ureter by lateral placement in an expandable bladder. Nevertheless, the disadvantages of a formal cystostomy, enabling intravesical exposure and thereby necessitating prolonged bladder drainage, subsequently made the Leadbetter ureteroneocystostomy obsolete.

Extravesical ureteroneocystostomy creates an extravesical submucosal tunnel by defining a segment of detrusor bladder muscle under which the ureter passes. The most commonly used methods have been those popularized by Lich and Gregoir and by Barry.[22] Interestingly, Lich and Gregoir independently developed this technique simultaneously in the early 1960s (Figure 33–4). Gregoir's approach received much acclaim for its success in the repair of reflux in children in Europe. However, the negative experience as described by Hendren, with high reflux recurrence rates, adversely influenced its use in North America. Nevertheless, later series demonstrated its merits, which were excellent long-term results and few technical complications.[23,24] The Lich-Gregoir method of extravesical urinary reconstruction is favored in transplantation because of its simplicity. The need for minimal bladder dissection and the avoidance of complications of a formal cystostomy contribute to its effectiveness.

The concept of the Barry repair is similar to that of the Lich-Gregoir method, but the difference resides in the method of developing a submucosal tunnel. The Barry method utilizes a parallel incision in the detrusor muscle, which is followed by tunneling of the ureter submucosally between the incisions.[25] This procedure has a low complication rate, requiring reoperation in 2.1% of 1000 transplants reported.[26] Depending on the specific preferences of the treatment center and the experiences of the transplant surgeons, both methods are acceptable techniques for ureteroneocystostomy in renal transplantation.

The extravesical single-stitch technique was reviewed and compared with the Leadbetter-Politano and Lich-Gregoir

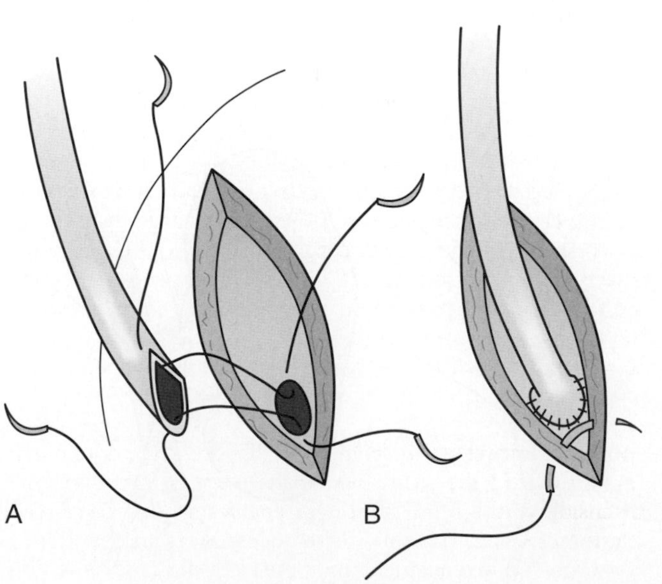

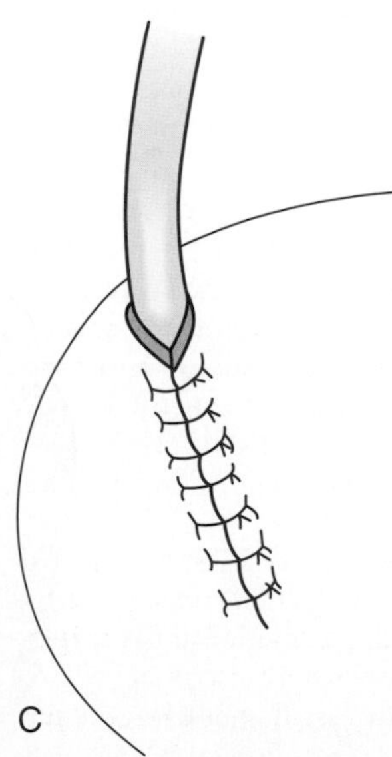

Figure 33–4 Lich-Howerton-Gregoir extravesical technique, which may be used as an alternative to the Leadbetter-Politano tunnel. ***A,*** Extravesical dissection of bladder seromuscular layer and opening into bladder lumen at inferior aspect. ***B,*** Ureter is anastomosed to bladder mucosa, and then seromuscular layer is closed over ureter. ***C,*** Completed ureteral anastomosis. (From Sagalowsky AI: Renal transplantation. *In* Gillenwater JY [ed]: Adult and Pediatric Urology. St. Louis, Mosby-Year Book, 1987, p 847.)

techniques at the University of Minnesota Hospital over an 8-year period in 1183 consecutive renal transplantations.[27] Overall, urologic complications occurred in 81 patients (6.8%); 68 (5.7%) of these complications occurred within 4 months of transplantation, and 13 (1.1%) were late. The complication rates for Politano-Leadbetter, Lich-Gregoir, and single-stitch techniques were 7.8%, 5.8%, and 6.7%, respectively. There was no difference among the techniques in rates of early and late complications of leakage, stricture, and hematuria in either cadaveric or living donor transplant recipients. Each technique has its inherent advantages, and every surgeon should become familiar with the different procedures to facilitate their use as dictated by individual circumstances.

Ureteropyelostomy

Leadbetter first described the technique of ureteropyelostomy for urinary tract reconstruction in renal transplantation 30 years ago. Updated revisions have subsequently been reported by Whelchel, Jaffers and colleagues,[28] and Hughes and colleagues[29] (Figure 33–5). The technique of ureteropyelostomy used in transplantation today employs the same surgical principles used by Foley in 1937 and by Anderson and Hynes in 1949, who earlier devised the method, that is, suturing a spatulated recipient ureter to the lowest portion of the donor renal pelvis. A ureteropyelostomy is usually accomplished after an ipsilateral native nephrectomy in which the recipient ureter is retained as a freestanding structure.

Ureteropyelostomy has distinct advantages, which include:

- Avoiding a cystostomy
- Shortening the duration of urethral catheterization
- Minimizing the complications of distal ureteral obstruction and stenosis
- Eliminating reflux in an otherwise predetermined normal ureter

In addition, a ureteropyelostomy theoretically preserves blood supply to the donor renal pelvis because the arterial supply to the native ureter is undisrupted. These technical features minimize the possibility of a poorly perfused donor distal ureter, especially after an episode of rejection. Rejection may affect ureteral blood flow and thus may contribute to the development of early ureteric leaks or late ureteric strictures.

Despite these attractive aspects, the popularity of ureteropyelostomy has been hindered historically by a high rate of urinary leaks, mainly related to the suture materials used to perform the anastomosis. With the advent of superior absorbable sutures (characterized by short duration of dissolution with good handling characteristics and appropriate needle configuration), the leak rate has become negligible. The long-term benefits of ureteropyelostomy have subsequently become more prominent compared with the uretero-

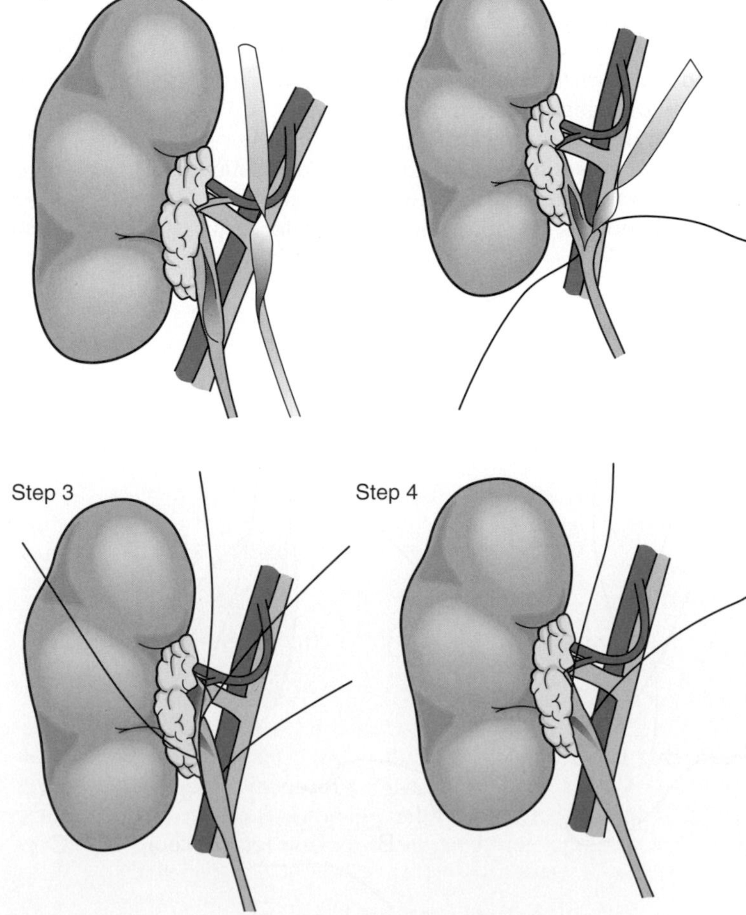

Figure 33–5 Technique of ureteropyelostomy. *Step 1*, Alignment of ureteral segments after partial transection and spatulation of the ureters. *Step 2*, Transection of the distal donor ureter after ligation of the apex stitch. Initiation of the anastomosis with direct visualization of the recipient ureter. *Step 3*, Ligation of the second corner suture with completion of the lateral suture. *Step 4*, Completion of the medial anastomosis. (From Jaffers GJ: Experience with pyeloureterostomy in renal transplantation. Ann Surg 1982; 196:588.)

neocystostomy method. The ureteropyelostomy does add time to the renal transplant procedure because the use of the ipsilateral ureter necessitates a concurrent native nephrectomy. An incidental—but important—advantage of concurrent native nephrectomy (with subsequent pathologic analysis) is that the original cause of the recipient's kidney disease can sometimes be better determined.

Ureteric Stents in Transplantation

Whether performed by ureteroneocystostomy or ureteropyelostomy, the major technical hazard of renal allograft transplantation is the reconstruction of the urinary tract. The rates of urinary leaks and obstructions in the immediate post-transplantation period range from 6% to 12%.[30] A ureteral stent can theoretically protect the urinary reconstruction through the creation of a conduit that drains the renal pelvis without exerting pressure on a healing anastomosis.

The use of ureteric stents is still controversial because of several disadvantages related to an indwelling foreign body in the immunosuppressed recipient of an allograft.[31] For example, a blood clot from the fresh anastomosis can easily obstruct the lumen of the stent. Ureteric stents may become structurally defective after urinary infection, resulting in stent breakage at the time of their removal via cystoscope. The peristaltic action of the ureter can dislodge the stent from its functional position. As a foreign body, the stent is a nidus for calculus formation, especially in a patient population predisposed to hypercalciuria because of secondary hyperparathyroidism. The distal portion of the stent may irritate the trigone of the bladder to give symptoms of irritative voiding, which is unacceptable for many patients. Because most patients undergo a meticulous urinary tract reconstruction without an increased risk of urinary leak, the use of a ureteric stent is recommended only in those circumstances in which there is a known technical hazard.[32] Such circumstances are:

1. Thin bladder secondary to disuse atrophy from chronic renal failure.
2. Anatomic outflow restriction, which may transmit elevated intravesical pressures directly onto the ureteroneocystostomy.
3. Neurogenic bladders compromised by uninhibited contractions.
4. Pediatric en bloc kidneys.[33]
5. Ureteric anastomosis into intestinal segments, such as ileal conduits or augmentation ileocystoplasties.

If a ureteric stent is required, the stent should be removed by 2 months after transplantation.

Abnormal Lower Urinary Tract

Renal failure can arise from functional abnormalities of the bladder that create high intravesical pressures leading to ureterovesical reflux. A dysfunctional bladder is associated with spinal dysraphisms and spinal cord injuries.[34,35] Such neurogenic bladders have difficulties with the storage and emptying of urine and, thus, have a propensity for urinary tract infections.[36] Patients with these conditions often require intermittent catheterization because they have lost the coordinated control of bladder function.[37] Autonomic dysreflexia associated with neurogenic bladder can cause uninhibited bladder spasms, which may be resolved by urinary sphincterotomy and condom catheter drainage.[38] Even the most successful sphincterotomies subsequently scar and cause bladder outlet obstruction. Thus, an ileal conduit is the preferred choice of long-term urologic management for patients with dysfunctional bladder, despite the necessity of an external drainage appliance.[39,40]

The bladder with low compliance may be inadequate to perform the intended storage function. This form of bladder function predisposes to frequency and urinary incontinence. A small contracted bladder may warrant an augmentation to reconstruct the urinary tract[41–44] (Figure 33–6). This procedure provides a larger reservoir that, in combination with intermittent catheterization, may overcome the neurogenic component and allow for preservation of the native bladder.[45, 46]

Nevertheless, there are several potential problems with the ileocystoplasty. First, the intestinal mucosa is secretive in nature; thus, the presence of oliguria or anuria predisposes to accumulation of secretions, leading to outflow obstruction and subsequent bladder distention. Ileocystoplasty can be considered only in an individual with a small contracted bladder who still has satisfactory daily urine output. Second, the compliances of the ileum and bladder are dissimilar; therefore, when an ileocystoplasty is distended following successful renal transplantation, it is prone to disruption at the bladder-ileum anastomosis.[47,48] Reconstructive bladder surgery should be planned well in advance of the renal transplantation to allow for healing and appropriate maturation of the storage reservoir.[49] Third, many patients who have undergone augmentation ileocystoplasty do not void adequately and require continued intermittent catheterization. The overall problems with intermittent catheterization result in a symptomatic urinary tract infection rate of more than 40% in a nonimmunosuppressed host.[50] The development of urosepsis after transplantation may be detrimental to both patient and allograft survival.[39]

For the foregoing reasons, an ileal conduit is still the preferred treatment of choice for managing a poorly functioning lower urinary tract to reduce the potential complications associated with an abnormal lower urinary tract.

COMPLICATIONS OF RENAL TRANSPLANTATION

Vascular Complications

Thrombosis of a renal allograft can occur following hyperacute rejection; however, in the majority of cases, the cause of thrombosis remains obscure.[52–54] The associated risk factors for graft thrombosis without evidence of rejection have not been clearly established. Bakir and colleagues[55] reported the occurrence of 34 graft thromboses without pathologic evidence of rejection in 558 consecutive cadaveric kidney transplantations performed in a single center. The incidence of primary renal graft thrombosis was 6% (1.9% arterial, 3.4% venous, and 0.7% both), and this complication accounted for 45% of early (90 days) and 37% of 1-year graft losses. The multivariate analysis identified five independent risk factors for primary renal graft thrombosis:

- Use of donor's right kidney
- History of venous thrombosis (renal or extrarenal)

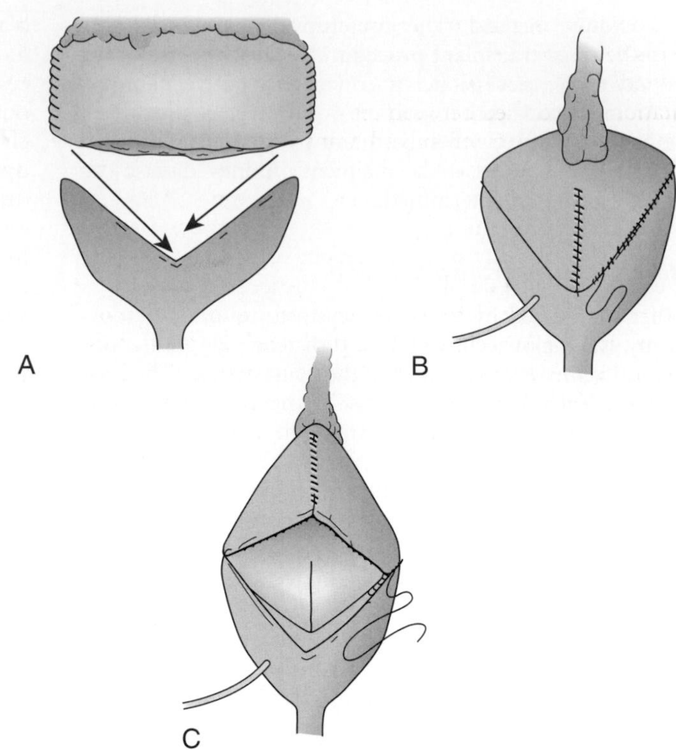

Figure 33–6 "Clam cystoplasty" with "cup patch" of bowel. ***A,*** The bladder is opened in a sagittal plane almost from anterior bladder neck to trigone. ***B,*** The bowel patch is reshaped to match the size of the opened bladder. ***C,*** Note that bowel is closed beginning at open ends, effectively disrupting peristalsis. (From Mitchell ME: Use of bowel in undiversion. Urol Clin North Am 1986; 13:352.)

- Diabetic nephropathy in the recipient
- Technical complications
- Recipient's perioperative and early postoperative hemodynamic status

There was no association between (1) primary renal graft thrombosis and recipient's age or sex; (2) number of previous transplants; (3) type of dialysis; (4) pretransplantation treatment with erythropoietin, antiplatelet agents, or oral anticoagulants; (5) donor's age or sex; (6) number of graft vessels; (7) warm and cold ischemia times; (8) site of transplantation (right or left iliac fossa); or (9) type of immunosuppressive agent used for induction.

In another series of 6153 consecutive renal transplantations, 134 index cases of graft loss from renal allograft thrombosis were reported to the Australian and New Zealand Dialysis and Transplant Registry between 1980 and 1992.[56] Renal allograft thrombosis was not associated with recipient age or sex, primary renal disease, type of dialysis, treatment with cyclosporine, extent of HLA antigen mismatch, panel-reactive antibody levels, perfusion solution and perfusion technique, or immunosuppressive therapy. However, there was a significantly higher incidence of renal allograft thrombosis in association with[56]:

- Both extremes of donor age
- Female donors
- Prolonged total ischemic time

Hematologic evaluation for hypercoagulable states is often negative in most of the patients seen for primary renal graft thrombosis. Not infrequently, the need for an anticoagulation regimen is difficult to assess because high-risk patients are not often identified preoperatively. Strategies have been developed to allow for early detection of anatomic or functional complications of renal transplantation. Color flow Doppler imaging and radionucleotide scanning have been used to assess vascular integrity of renal allografts in the post-transplantation period.[57–59] When both tests are used together, they effectively differentiate delayed graft function due to acute tubular necrosis from renal allograft thrombosis.

The report from the North American Pediatric Renal Transplant Cooperative Study examined the incidence of graft thrombosis in pediatric renal transplant recipients.[60] Of 213 pediatric renal transplant failures, 27 (2.6%) were a result of thrombosis. Among recipients of living donor kidneys, the majority of graft failures occurred in patients less than 6 years old. The recipient age was not identified as a factor in cadaveric kidneys transplanted into pediatric patients. In addition, recipients of pediatric cadaveric kidneys with long cold ischemic times were observed to have a greater risk of thrombosis.

The use of kidney allografts with multiple renal arteries has been evaluated to determine its effects on survival of both renal allografts and patients. In the early experience, kidney allografts with multiple renal arteries have been associated with a higher incidence of early vascular complications. Benedetti and colleagues[17] analyzed 998 adult kidney transplantations performed between December 1, 1985, and June 30, 1993, to evaluate the complications of multiple renal arteries in donor allografts. The rate of early vascular complications in kidneys with multiple arteries was not different from that in kidneys with single arteries; however, the rate of the late complication renal artery stenosis was found to be slightly higher in kidneys with multiple arteries. Nevertheless, the overall results for kidney transplantation using allografts with multiple and single arteries are similar. The findings further suggested no significant differences in rates of posttransplantation hypertension, acute tubular necrosis, acute rejection, or creatinine levels.[17]

The outcome of renal transplantation with an arterial anastomosis to an aortofemoral vascular prosthesis was evaluated in a series of 13 cases (0.2%) from 5791 cadaveric renal transplantations performed between 1978 and 1994.[61] In six cases, the vascular reconstruction and transplant operation were performed simultaneously. In the remaining seven cases, the procedures were performed separately with a mean interval of 3.5 years. The indications for vascular reconstruction were aneurysmal disease in four cases and occlusive disease in nine. The early vascular complications of these procedures were hemorrhage (four patients) and renal vein thrombosis (one patient). Two of 13 recipients had graft loss with a mortality rate of 15%. The graft and patient survival rates were 68% and 83%, respectively, after 1 year, and 17% and 37%, respectively, after 5 years. Not unexpectedly, late mortality was mainly due to cardiovascular disease. Renal transplantation that involves an arterial anastomosis to an aortofemoral vascular prosthesis is a high-risk procedure with relatively poor short-term and long-term results. These observations should be considered in the evaluation of renal replacement therapy in this special patient population.

Urologic Complications

In our experience with the ureteropyelostomy technique of urinary tract reconstruction at the Massachusetts General Hospital, the rate of complication has been less than 2% over the past decade.

Most initial urinary tract complications after transplantation manifest as either a leak or an obstruction. For example, in the first 1000 consecutive renal transplantations performed at Oxford University, in which the Leadbetter-Politano technique was employed for all but three cases, there were 71 primary complications in 68 patients (7.1%).[62] The complications included 36 ureteral obstructions, 25 ureteral or bladder leaks, 7 bladder outflow obstructions, 2 ureteral stones, and 1 case of symptomatic vesicoureteral reflux. Although no grafts were lost as a result of urologic complications, two patients died, following septic and hemorrhagic complications despite therapeutic interventions. Induction with high-dose steroids in the early period of renal transplantation was associated with urologic complication rate of 10%. However, with later administration of low-dose steroids combined with azathioprine and cyclosporine, the incidence of complications decreased to 4%.

Urinary leaks may be the result of ischemic injury to the distal donor ureter at the site of bladder implantation. The cut end of the donor ureter must bleed sufficiently to indicate its viability prior its anastomosis to the bladder. Rejection may also cause ureteral necrosis because of renal allograft swelling and compromise of the ureteral blood supply.[63] Children are especially susceptible. If the native ureter is available, it may be used to resolve the obstruction or leak associated with distal ureteral necrosis at the site of bladder implantation. The donor ureter can be resected, and a ureteropyelostomy may be performed.

Urinary obstruction may be noted immediately after transplantation because the tunnel may compress the ureter and block its peristalsis. Placement of a stent or a revision of the ureteroneocystostomy may be indicated. If the donor ureteral blood supply is not compromised, a urinary leak of either the ureteropyelostomy or the ureteroneocystostomy can be treated by either direct operative or endoscopic placement of a stent. Percutaneous nephrostomy, with or without stenting, is not commonly used today.

Lymphatic Complications

Lymphoceles may develop following renal transplantation because (1) lymphatic channels are transected during the iliac dissection of the transplant procedure or (2) from open-ended lymphatic vessels following donor nephrectomy. Allografts undergoing rejection, which become swollen with infiltration inflammatory cells, are prone to releasing lymphatic fluid. Lymphoceles may also be associated with ureteral obstruction, venous obstruction, venous thrombosis, and infection. In a study by Khauli and colleagues,[64] univariate analysis showed a significant risk for the development of lymphoceles in transplants with acute tubular necrosis and delayed graft function, rejection, and high-dose steroids. However, multivariate analyses showed that only rejection was associated with a significant risk for lymphoceles.

The incidence of lymphoceles may be as high as 20%, but only 1 in 20 patients noted to have lymphoceles with a diameter of 5 cm or greater has symptoms that require drainage.[64] The interval for development of symptomatic lymphoceles ranges from 1 week to 3.7 years with a median of 10 months. The size and pressure of the lymphocele may cause discomfort or urinary tract obstruction or may compromise the circulation to the allograft.

Simple needle aspiration or external drainage with sclerotherapy of lymphoceles is associated with an unacceptably high incidence of recurrence and complications. Moreover, many lymphocele collections are multiloculated, thus limiting the value of percutaneous catheter drainage. The treatment of choice is a surgical approach via the retroperitoneal transplant incision or transperitoneally through an abdominal incision.

In the era of minimally invasive surgery, achieving internal drainage by laparoscopically deroofing the lymphocele and creating a peritoneal fenestration has evolved to become an alternative method of management.[65] In an early series reporting on nine patients so treated, the postoperative course was uneventful and hospitalization did not exceed 7 days; moreover, evaluation using CT scanning or ultrasonography did not demonstrate recurrence in any of the patients after a mean follow-up period of 11 months.[66] Further reports in four patients with symptomatic lymphoceles operated on laparoscopically by Boeckmann and colleagues[67] effectively demonstrated that lymphocele drainage can be achieved in 40 to 70 minutes. Most surgeons who have had extensive experience with this minimally invasive technique believe that symptomatic posttransplantation lymphocele represents an ideal indication for laparoscopic drainage.[65,67]

RETRANSPLANTATION

The number of renal allografts necessitating transplant nephrectomy because of rejection failure has declined.[68,69] The current indications for transplant nephrectomy are:

- Primary nonfunction
- Acute hemorrhage
- Uncontrolled hypertension
- Allograft infection

Otherwise, retaining the transplant kidney with low-dose immunosuppression may prevent the development of alloantibodies.[70]

Removing a failed allograft is a more challenging procedure than native nephrectomy.[71] The early removal of a nonfunctioning kidney does not pose any additional difficulty because the tissue planes from the recent procedure are preserved; they can be dissected out to expose the necessary structure for ligation and subsequent removal of the kidney.[72] The kidney being removed because of chronic rejection, however, often has significant surrounding scar tissue, thus making dissection of the kidney more difficult. The intracapsular approach was devised so that the allograft capsule is not resected and only the renal parenchyma are removed. This approach allows exposure and ligation of the main renal vessels so that the nephrectomy can be performed safely.

The choice of allograft placement for the second kidney transplant is the side contralateral from the previous allograft. When the kidney has to be placed on the same side as the previous transplant for technical reasons, an allograft nephrectomy should be performed. It is also important to exclude the possibility of an arteriovenous fistula resulting from ligated renal vessels of the previous allograft. Moreover, the new vessel anastomoses should be placed in new segments of the iliac artery and vein. If there was a previous bladder anastomosis, the use of the native ureter to perform a ureteropyelostomy should be the preferred procedure. Alternatively, if a primary ureteropyelostomy was previously performed, then a ureteroneocystostomy is indicated.

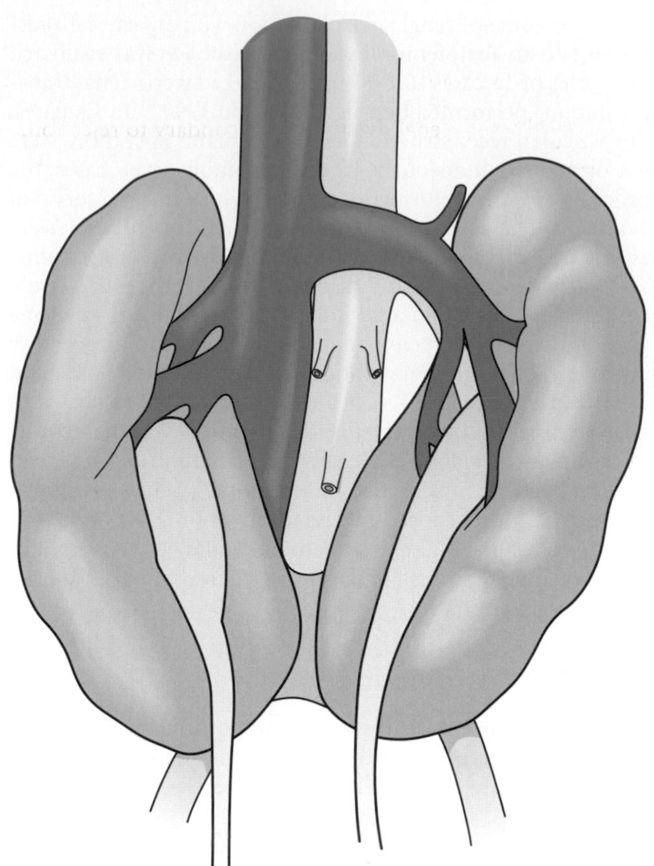

Figure 33–7 Classic features of horseshoe kidney. Fusion of lower poles produces an isthmus and shifts the axis of the kidneys toward the lumbosacral vertebrae. (From Koff SA: Anomalies of the kidney. *In* Gillenwater JY [ed]: Adult and Pediatric Urology. St. Louis, Mosby-Year Book, 1987, p 1820.)

UNIQUE CONFIGURATIONS AND SPECIAL CONSIDERATIONS

Horseshoe Kidneys

Horseshoe kidneys develop after the embryologic fusion of a portion of the renal blastema across the midline at 4 to 8 weeks of gestation (Figure 33–7). The normal medial rotation and upward migration of the kidney to an anatomic location cephalad to the inferior mesenteric artery is prevented by the isthmus of the fused kidney. Horseshoe kidneys are considered to be at high risk for complication after transplantation.[73] Most transplant surgeons are reluctant to utilize horseshoe kidneys because of their unpredictable arterial and venous anatomy. In addition, other congenital anomalies may be associated with this abnormality, including ureteral duplications, ureteropelvic junction obstructions, and vesicoureteral reflux.

Nevertheless, horseshoe kidneys have been used for transplantation either as an en bloc engraftment into a single recipient[74] or following an isthmectomy that divides the kidneys for transplantation into two recipients.[75–81] Although isthmectomy may theoretically lead to urinary fistula formation and parenchymal hemorrhage, these complications have not been reported thus far in the literature. The use of horseshoe kidneys is driven by the shortage of cadaveric donor organs and by the fact that the fused kidneys are histologically normal. Thus, if the isthmectomy is performed successfully and if other anatomic considerations, such as ureteropelvic junction obstruction, can be overcome by a ureteropyelostomy for urinary tract reconstruction, horseshoe kidneys may be appropriate for transplantation.

Pediatric En Bloc Kidney Transplantation

Pediatric kidneys are an important source of cadaveric renal allografts for transplantation.[82–84] Sustained and significant hypertrophy of such a single kidney does occur. The decision whether to retain kidneys recovered from a pediatric donor is influenced by the donor's age and body weight and the cortical dimensions of the kidneys. If the donor is older than 3 years and weighs more than 15 kg (30 lb), and if the polar length of the donor kidneys exceeds 8 cm, the kidneys can safely be divided and transplanted even to two adult recipients because they provide enough nephron mass to maintain normal renal function.

The reported surgical complication rate (~5%) is not sufficient to discard pediatric kidneys because of vascular thromboses; however, these pediatric allografts are also susceptible to failure because of rejection.[83,84] Nevertheless, there is no statistical difference in allograft survival between single pediatric kidneys and cadaveric kidneys from donors older than 50 years.

The use of en bloc cadaveric kidneys from younger pediatric donors (<3 years) is more controversial. The overall long-term results have not paralleled those of kidneys from

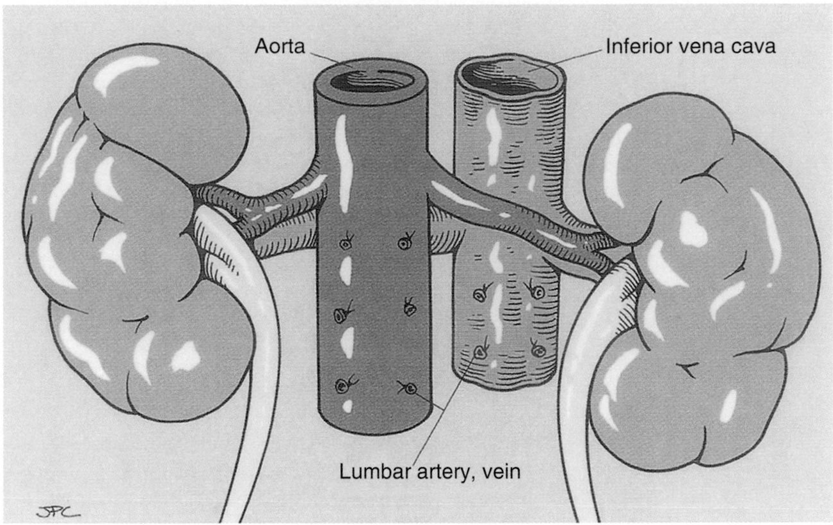

Figure 33–8 Pediatric en bloc kidneys. (From Shapiro R: Renal transplantation. *In* Starzl TE [ed]: Atlas of Organ Transplantation. Philadelphia, JB Lippincott, 1992, p 4.11.)

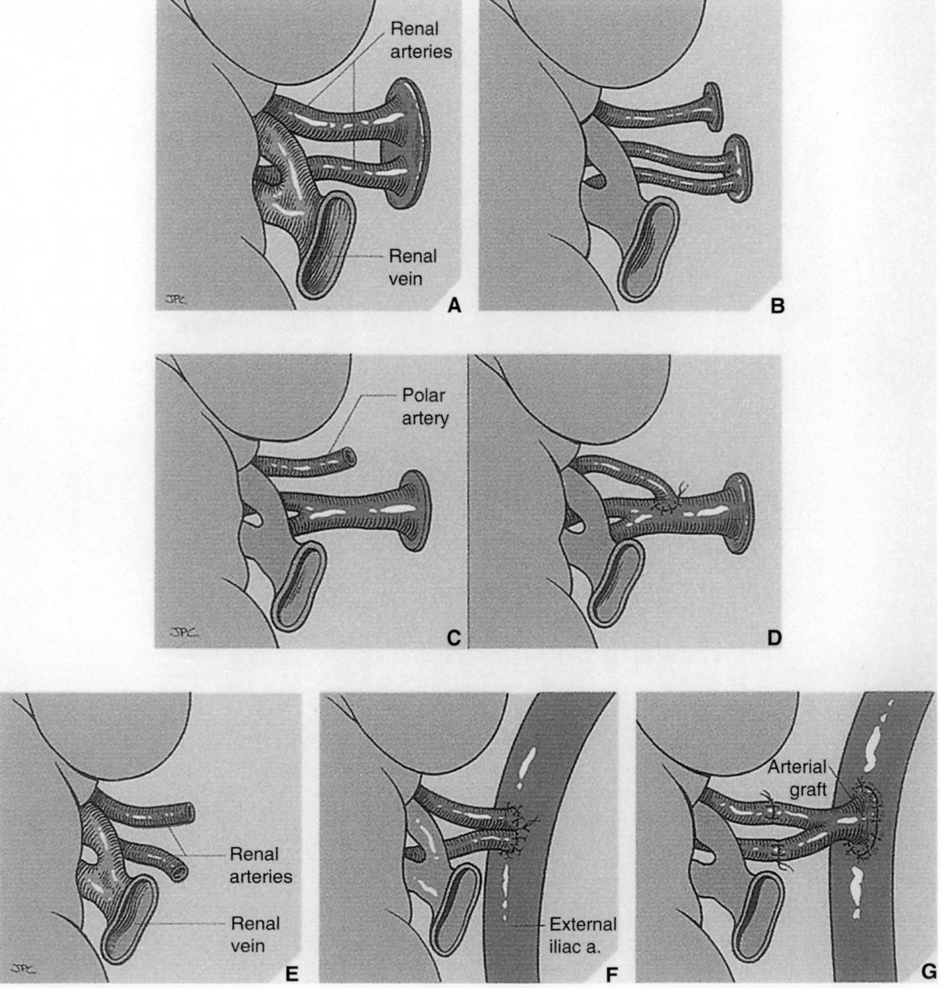

Figure 33–9 Multiple renal artery and reconstruction. (From Shapiro R: Renal transplantation. *In* Starzl TE (ed): Atlas of Organ Transplantation. Philadelphia, JB Lippincott, 1992, p 4.7.)

adult donors. The factors that have been implicated in failure of kidneys from younger pediatric donors include:

1. Reported higher incidences of technical complications.
2. Observed severe renal dysfunction secondary to rejection.
3. The inadequate nephron mass provided to adult recipients, despite the en bloc preparation.

Several technical alternatives have been developed for en bloc transplantation of pediatric kidneys.[85] All of the options are designed to overcome the anatomic impediments of small renal vessels and short double ureters (Figure 33–8; see Color Figure). Most surgeons place the kidneys in a retroperitoneal position using iliac sites of arterial and venous anastomoses that allow the shorter pediatric ureters to reach the recipient bladder. The superior cut ends of the donor aorta and the vena cava above the renal vessels are oversewn, and the inferior aorta and vena cava complete the vascular reconstruction.

Our preferred procedure for ureteric implantation of en bloc pediatric allografts is to create separate tunnels for two cystostomy sites, anastomosing each ureter extravesically by the Lich-Gregoir technique. This approach avoids a formal Leadbetter-Politano cystostomy and implantation. The major advantage of a double cystostomy site is the preservation of renal function of the contralateral renal unit if a complication does occur with one of the ureteroneocystostomies. Alternatively, others have favored joining the ureters together distally and constructing a single ureteroneocystostomy, reducing the potential for a complication by another ureteric anastomosis. Because ureteral leaks can result in a technical failure and loss of both kidneys, stents may be advisable.

We have performed renal transplantations using an en bloc pediatric preparation since 1993 without technical complications. All of our recipients continue to display normal renal function. Thus, en bloc pediatric transplants are a suitable source of kidneys.

Multiple Renal Arteries

Multiple renal arteries can be challenging because they present a diverse arterial supply that must be restored.[17] The loss of an accessory polar artery results in a segmental infarction of the kidney. The donor surgical team must search for the aberrant distribution of additional renal arteries. For example, the lower pole artery to the right kidney usually crosses anterior to the inferior vena cava. The presence of urologic anomalies, such as double ureters, may alert the donor surgeon to the possibility of additional renal vessels.

Polar vessels are preserved by dissecting each artery to its aortic origins (Figure 33–9; see Color Figure). The accessory artery may be in close proximity to the main renal artery, thus allowing for a single Carrel patch to be used for the recipient vascular anastomosis. The polar circulation can also be restored by anastomosing the accessory artery to the side of the main renal artery. Rarely, the inferior epigastric artery may be used for separate anastomosis to the accessory renal artery, if there is significant atherosclerotic plaque in the donor renal artery that precludes a satisfactory vascular reconstruction. However, when the accessory renal artery supplies less than 10% of a kidney, revascularization may not be feasible, given the small caliber of the artery.

Two-for-One Kidney Transplantation from Older Donors

The shortage of cadaver organ donors has prompted organ procurement organizations, such as the New England Organ Bank (NEOB), to expand the pool of acceptable cadaver donors by recovering organs from cadavers of ever-increasing age.[94] The data from the NEOB reveal a significant change in the characteristics of the donor pool.[95] Less than 40% of the NEOB donor population are trauma victims, and the largest category now represents individuals dying of cerebral vascular accidents (55%). These patients are much older and frequently have additional medical complications. The rate of survival for renal allografts obtained from older donors is not as good as that for kidneys procured from younger donors.[96] In an effort to provide a better estimate of immediate and long-term function of an allograft procured from an older donor, the NEOB has performed routine postrecovery biopsies on all such kidneys. The decreased survival of kidneys transplanted from older donors may be a result of an insufficient renal mass to support the recipient.[97] Thus, when a single kidney from an older donor is transplanted, and the kidney has a smaller number of functioning nephrons as a result of obsolescence, the kidney may suffer chronic dysfunction.

One approach to improve utilization of a source of allografts that otherwise might be discarded is to offer two allografts from an older age donor to a single recipient (a two-for-one approach). The reason for allocating both kidneys from an older donor to a single recipient is that the literature suggests that offering only one obsolescent allograft is not likely to provide a sufficient nephron mass to enable normal long-term renal function in the recipient.[98–104] This clinical concern is the principal reason that treatment centers have declined single kidneys from such older donors. The donor inclusion criteria to establish an automatic two-for-one allocation are:

- Age 60 or greater
- Creatinine clearance less than 65 mL/min
- 20% or greater glomerulosclerosis of both kidneys as determined by frozen-section biopsy

Most of the experience with the two-for-one approach has been reported by the University of Maryland and Stanford University Medical Centers.[105] This allocation scheme was established only after all UNOS (United Network of Organ Sharing) centers throughout the country had declined the kidneys offered singly. The NEOB procedure mandates a two-for-one allocation if the donor inclusion criteria are met. To delay and permit centers to consider transplanting only one of these kidneys before considering transplanting two would increase the ischemic time for these allografts, thereby compromising their function.[96]

A 1998 review of the NEOB experience regarding the transplantation of a single older donor kidney reveals the following data:

1. The preservation time for kidneys transplanted from 60-year-old donors was 23.4 ± 11 hours, versus 20.2 ± 10 for kidneys transplanted from donors younger than 60 years ($P < .01$).
2. A reduction in the duration of preservation was associated with immediate allograft function from all NEOB donors.

For kidneys from 60-year-old donors that had immediate function, the preservation time was 22.2 ± 9 hours (for those with delayed function, preservation time 25.4 ± 13 hours; $P = .1$ NS); for kidneys from donors younger than 60 years of age that had immediate function, the preservation time was 18.8 ± 9 hours (for those with delayed function, preservation time 24.9 ± 11 hours; $P < .01$).

3. A preservation time of less than 12 hours was associated with a reduction in the dysfunction rate of the kidneys from the 60-year-old donors (<12 hours, 23.1%; >12 hours, 43.5%; $P = .19$). Thus, centers appear to delay in deciding whether to accept a single older kidney. This increase in preservation time may influence immediate function of the allograft.

The two-for-one concept does not suggest that two kidneys will immediately function better than one. The risk factors that might influence immediate allograft dysfunction must be considered; these factors include maintaining the hemodynamic stability of the donor (especially in older donors, maintaining normovolemia and good urine output) and minimizing the preservation time.

The NEOB has developed a separate recipient selection list to reduce the ischemic time while we identify potential recipients. The patients on this list give informed consent to accept two-for-one kidneys well in advance of the potential allocation. The informed consent procedure is needed because of ethical concerns not only regarding acceptance of the marginal kidneys but also because the operating time, as well as the risk of technical complications, may be doubled.

References

1. Moore FD: A Nobel Award to Joseph E. Murray, MD: Some historical perspectives. Arch Surg 1992; 127:627.
2. Hume DM, Merrill JP, Miller BF, Thorn GW: Experiences with renal homotransplantation in the human: Report of nine cases. J Clin Invest 1955; 34:327.
3. Murray JE, Merrill JP, Harrison JH: Renal homotransplantation in identical twins. Surg Forum 1955; 6:432.
4. Diethelm AG: Ethical decisions in the history of organ transplantation. Ann Surg 1990; 211:505.
5. Starzl TE: The development of clinical renal transplantation. Am J Kidney Dis 1990; 16:548.
6. Hamilton DN, Reid WA: Yu Yu Voronoy and the first human kidney allograft. Surg Gynecol Obstet 1984; 159:289.
7. Merrill JP, Murray JE, Harrison JH, Guild WR: Successful homotransplantation of the human kidney between identical twins. JAMA 1956; 160:277.
8. Lemmers MJ, Barry JM: Major role for arterial disease in morbidity and mortality after kidney transplantation in diabetic recipients. Diabetes Care 1991; 14:295.
9. Doublet JD, Peraldi MN, Gattegno B, et al: Renal cell carcinoma of native kidneys: Prospective study of 129 renal transplant patients. J Urol 1997; 158:42.
10. Levine E: Acquired cystic kidney disease. Radiol Clin North Am 1996; 34:947.
11. Mattoo TK, Greifer I, Geva P, Spitzer A: Acquired renal cystic disease in children and young adults on maintenance dialysis. Pediatr Nephrol 1997; 11:447.
12. Penn I: Kidney transplantation in patients previously treated for renal carcinomas (Comment). Transpl Int 1993; 6:350.
13. Shandera KC, Rozanski TA, Jaffers G: The necessity of voiding cystourethrogram in the pretransplant urologic evaluation. Urology 1996; 47:198.
14. Glazier DB, Whang MI, Geffner SR, et al: Evaluation of voiding cystourethrography prior to renal transplantation. Transplantation 1996; 62:1762.
15. Burns JR, Houttuin E, Gregory JG, et al: Vascular-induced erectile impotence in renal transplant recipients. J Urol 1979; 121: 721.
16. Taylor RM: Impotence and the use of the internal iliac artery in renal transplantation: A survey of surgeons' attitudes in the United Kingdom and Ireland. Transplantation 1998; 65:745.
17. Benedetti E, Troppmann C, Gillingham K, et al: Short- and long-term outcomes of kidney transplants with multiple renal arteries. Ann Surg 1995; 221:406.
18. Benedetti E, Fryer J, Matas AJ, et al: Kidney transplant outcome with and without right renal vein extension. Clin Transplant 1994; 8:416.
19. Payne RL: Ureteral-vesical implantation: A new method of anastomosis. JAMA 1908; 51:1321.
20. Hess E: Intracystic reimplantation of the ureter: A new operative technique. J Urol 1941; 46:866.
21. Politano VA, Leadbetter WF: An operative technique for the correction of vesicoureteral reflux. J Urol 1958; 79:932.
22. Caparros J, Regalado RI, Sanchez-Martin F, Villavicencio H: A simplified technique for ureteroneocystostomy in renal transplantation. World J Urol 1996; 14:236.
23. Marberger M, Altwein JE, Straub E, et al: The Lich-Gregoir antireflux plasty: Experiences with 371 children. J Urol 1978; 120: 216.
24. Santiago-Delpin EA, Baquero A, Gonzalez Z: Low incidence of urologic complications after renal transplantation. Am J Surg 1986; 151:374.
25. Barry JM, Hatch DA: Parallel incision, unstented extravesical ureteroneocystostomy: Follow-up of 203 kidney transplants. J Urol 1985; 134:249.
26. Gibbons WS, Barry JM, Hefty TR: Complications following unstented parallel incision extravesical ureteroneocystostomy in 1000 kidney transplants. J Urol 1992; 148:38.
27. Hakim NS, Benedetti E, Pirenne J, et al: Complications of ureterovesical anastomosis in kidney transplant patients: The Minnesota experience. Clin Transplant 1994; 8:504.
28. Jaffers GJ, Cosimi AB, Delmonico FL, et al: Experience with pyeloureterostomy in renal transplantation. Ann Surg 1982; 196:588.
29. Hughes JD, Delmonico FL, Auchincloss H Jr, Cosimi AB: Ureteropyelostomy with a monofilament absorbable suture. Transplantation 1987; 44:459.
30. Benoit G, Blanchet P, Eschwege P, et al: Insertion of a double pigtail ureteral stent for the prevention of urological complications in renal transplantation: A prospective randomized study. J Urol 1996; 156:881.
31. Eschwege P, Blanchet P, Alexandre L, et al: Infectious complications after the use of double J ureteral stents. Transplant Proc 1996; 28:2833.
32. Barry JM: Unstented extravesical ureteroneocystostomy in kidney transplantation. J Urol 1983; 129:918.
33. Bergmeijer JH, Nijman R, Kalkman E, et al: Stenting of the ureterovesical anastomosis in pediatric renal transplantation. Transpl Int 1990; 3:146.
34. Selzman AA, Elder JS, Mapstone TB: Urologic consequences of myelodysplasia and other congenital abnormalities of the spinal cord. Urol Clin North Am 1993; 20:485.
35. Hollander JB, Diokno AC: Urinary diversion and reconstruction in the patient with spinal cord injury. Urol Clin North Am 1993; 20:465.
36. Kotkin L, Milam DF: Evaluation and management of the urologic consequences of neurologic disease. Tech Urol 1996; 2:210.
37. Perkash I: Long-term urologic management of the patient with spinal cord injury. Urol Clin North Am 1993; 20:423.
38. Kursh ED, Freehafer A, Persky L: Complications of autonomic dysreflexia. J Urol 1977; 118:70.

39. Hatch DA, Belitsky P, Barry JM, et al: Fate of renal allografts transplanted in patients with urinary diversion. Transplantation 1993; 56:838.
40. Hatch DA: Kidney transplantation in patients with an abnormal lower urinary tract. Urol Clin North Am 1994; 21:311.
41. Sidi AA, Becher EF, Reddy PK, Dykstra DD: Augmentation enterocystoplasty for the management of voiding dysfunction in spinal cord injury patients. J Urol 1990; 143:83.
42. Serrano DP, Flechner SM, Modlin CS, et al: Transplantation into the long-term defunctionalized bladder. J Urol 1996; 156:885.
43. Hendren WH, Hendren RB: Bladder augmentation: Experience with 129 children and young adults. J Urol 1990; 144:445.
44. McInerney PD, Picramenos D, Koffman CG, Mundy AR: Is cystoplasty a safe alternative to urinary diversion in patients requiring renal transplantation? Eur Urol 1995; 27:117.
45. Thomalla JV: Augmentation of the bladder in preparation for renal transplantation. Surg Gynecol Obstet 1990; 170:349.
46. Hatch DA: A review of renal transplantation into bowel segments for conduit and continent urinary diversions: Techniques and complications. Semin Urol 1994; 12:108.
47. Bauer SB, Hendren WH, Kozakewich H, et al: Perforation of the augmented bladder. J Urol 1992; 148:699.
48. Couillard DR, Vapnek JM, Rentzepis MJ, Stone AR: Fatal perforation of augmentation cystoplasty in an adult. Urology 1993; 42:585.
49. Zaragoza MR, Ritchey ML, Bloom DA, McGuire EJ: Enterocystoplasty in renal transplantation candidates: Urodynamic evaluation and outcome. J Urol 1993; 150:1463.
50. Shneidman RJ, Pulliam JP, Barry JM: Clean, intermittent self-catheterization in renal transplant recipients. Transplantation 1984; 38:312.
51. Middleton AW Jr, Hendren WH: Ileal conduits in children at the Massachusetts General Hospital from 1955 to 1970. J Urol 1976; 115:591.
52. Benoit G, Jaber N, Moukarzel M, et al: Incidence of vascular complications in kidney transplantation: Is there any interference with the nature of the perfusion solution? Clin Transplant 1994; 8:485.
53. Benoit G, Jaber N, Moukarzel M, et al: Incidence of arterial and venous complications in kidney transplantation: Role of the kidney preservation solution. Transplant Proc 1994; 26:295.
54. Bolander JE II, Carter CB: Cholesterol embolization in renal allografts. J Am Soc Nephrol 1996; 7:18.
55. Bakir N, Sluiter WJ, Ploeg RJ, et al: Primary renal graft thrombosis. Nephrol Dial Transplant 1996; 11:140.
56. Penny MJ, Nankivell BJ, Disney AP, et al: Renal graft thrombosis: A survey of 134 consecutive cases. Transplantation 1994; 58:565.
57. Blane CE, Gagnadoux MF, Brunelle F, et al: Doppler ultrasonography in the early postoperative evaluation of renal transplants in children. Can Assoc Radiol J 1993; 44:176.
58. Chung SY, Bae MO, Choi SJ, et al: Evaluation of renal allografts with duplex ultrasonography. Transplant Proc 1996; 28:1531.
59. Turetschek K, Nasel C, Wunderbaldinger P, et al: Power Doppler versus color Doppler imaging in renal allograft evaluation. J Ultrasound Med 1996; 15:517.
60. Harmon WE, Stablein D, Alexander SR, Tejani A: Graft thrombosis in pediatric renal transplant recipients: A report of the North American Pediatric Renal Transplant Cooperative Study. Transplantation 1991; 51:406.
61. van der Vliet JA, Naafs DB, van Bockel JH, et al: Fate of renal allografts connected to vascular prostheses. Clin Transplant 1996; 10:199.
62. Shoskes DA, Hanbury D, Cranston D, Morris PJ: Urological complications in 1000 consecutive renal transplant recipients.J Urol 1995; 153:18.
63. Maier U, Madersbacher S, Banyai-Falger S, et al: Late ureteral obstruction after kidney transplantation: Fibrotic answer to previous rejection? Transpl Int 1997; 10:65.
64. Khauli RB, Stoff JS, Lovewell T, et al: Post-transplant lymphoceles: A critical look into the risk factors, pathophysiology and management. J Urol 1993; 150:22.
65. Thurlow JP, Gelpi J, Schwaitzberg SD, Rohrer RJ: Laparoscopic peritoneal fenestration and internal drainage of lymphoceles after renal transplantation. Surg Laparosc Endosc 1996; 6:290.
66. Fahlenkamp D, Raatz D, Schonberger B, Loening SA: Laparoscopic lymphocele drainage after renal transplantation. J Urol 1993; 150:316.
67. Boeckmann W, Brauers A, Wolff JM, et al: Laparoscopical marsupialization of symptomatic post-transplant lymphoceles. Scand J Urol Nephrol 1996; 30:277.
68. Roberts CS, LaFond J, Fitts CT, et al: New patterns of transplant nephrectomy in the cyclosporine era. J Am Coll Surg 1994; 178:59.
69. Madore F, Hebert MJ, Leblanc M, et al: Determinants of late allograft nephrectomy. Clin Nephrol 1995; 44:284.
70. McCarty GA, King LB, Sanfilippo F: Autoantibodies to nuclear, cytoplasmic, and cytoskeletal antigens in renal allograft rejection. Transplantation 1984; 37:446.
71. O'Sullivan DC, Murphy DM, McLean P, Donovan MG: Transplant nephrectomy over 20 years: Factors involved in associated morbidity and mortality. J Urol 1994; 151:855.
72. Rosenthal JT, Peaster ML, Laub D: The challenge of kidney transplant nephrectomy. J Urol 1993; 149:1395.
73. Ratner LE, Kraus E, Magnuson T, Bender JS: Transplantation of kidneys from expanded criteria donors. Surgery 1996; 119:372.
74. Lowell JA, Taylor RJ, Cattral M, et al: En bloc transplantation of a horseshoe kidney from a high risk multi-organ donor: Case report and review of the literature. J Urol 1994; 152:468.
75. Brandina L, Mocelin AJ, Fraga AM, Lacerda G: Transplantation of a horseshoe kidney. Br J Urol 1978; 50:284.
76. Majeski JA, Alexander JW, First R, et al: Transplantation of a horseshoe kidney. JAMA 1979; 242:1066.
77. Barry JM, Fincher RD: Transplantation of a horseshoe kidney into 2 recipients. J Urol 1984; 131:1162.
78. Brandina L, Fraga AM, Bergonse MR, et al: Kidney transplantation: The use of abnormal kidneys. Nephron 1983; 35:78.
79. Kim SM, Intenzo CM, Park CH: Renal transplantation of a horseshoe kidney. Clin Nucl Med 1993; 18:1004.
80. Ratner LE, Zibari G: Strategies for the successful transplantation of the horseshoe kidney. J Urol 1993; 150:958.
81. Botta GC, Capocasale E, Mazzoni MP: Transplantation of horseshoe kidneys: A report of four cases. Br J Urol 1996; 78:181.
82. Gourlay W, Stothers L, McLoughlin MG, et al: Transplantation of pediatric cadaver kidneys into adult recipients. J Urol 1995; 153:322.
83. Wright FH Jr, Banowsky LH, Floyd M, et al: Single pediatric donor kidneys for adult recipients: The San Antonio experience. Clin Transpl 1995:233.
84. Salvatierra O, Alfrey E, Tanney DC, et al: Superior outcomes in pediatric renal transplantation. Arch Surg 1997; 132:842.
85. Amante AJ, Kahan BD: En bloc transplantation of kidneys from pediatric donors. J Urol 1996; 155:852.
86. Ottelin MC, Bueschen AJ, Lloyd LK, et al: Review of 333 living donor nephrectomies. South Med J 1994; 87:61.
87. Yasumura T, Nakai I, Oka T, et al: Experience with 247 living related donor nephrectomy cases at a single institution in Japan. Jpn J Surg 1988; 18:252.
88. Weinstein SH, Navarre RJ Jr, Loening SA, Corry RJ: Experience with live donor nephrectomy. J Urol 1980; 12:321.
89. DeMarco T, Amin M, Harty JI: Living donor nephrectomy: Factors influencing morbidity. J Urol 1982; 127:1082.
90. Yang SC, Park DS, Lee DH, et al: Retroperitoneal endoscopic live donor nephrectomy: Report of 3 cases. J Urol 1995; 153:1884.
91. Ratner LE, Ciseck LJ, Moore RG, et al: Laparoscopic live donor nephrectomy. Transplantation 1995; 60:1047.

92. Ratner LE, Kavoussi LR, Sroka M, et al: Laparoscopic assisted live donor nephrectomy—a comparison with the open approach. Transplantation 1997; 63:229.
93. Flowers JL, Jacobs S, Cho E, et al: Comparison of open and laparoscopic live donor nephrectomy. Ann Surg 1997; 226:483.
94. Alexander JW, Zola JC: Expanding the donor pool: Use of marginal donors for solid organ transplantation. Clin Transplant 1996; 10:1.
95. Delmonico FL: Discarding the older age kidney: Establishing the need for innovative utilization. Transplant Proc 1997.
96. Cecka JM, Terasaki PI: The UNOS scientific renal transplant registry: United Network for Organ Sharing. Clin Transpl 1995; 1.
97. Brenner BM, Cohen RA, Milford EL: In renal transplantation, one size may not fit all. J Am Soc Nephrol 1992; 3:162. (Erratum in J Am Soc Nephrol 1992; 3:1038.)
98. Heemann UW, Tullius SG, Azuma H, et al: Evidence for a beneficial effect of increased functional kidney mass upon chronic kidney rejection in rats. Transplant Proc 1994; 26:2047.
99. Hostetter TH, Olson JL, Rennke HG, et al: Hyperfiltration in remnant nephrons: A potentially adverse response to renal ablation. Am J Physiol 1981; 241:F85.
100. Modena FM, Hostetter TH, Salahudeen AK, et al: Progression of kidney disease in chronic renal transplant rejection. Transplantation 1991; 52:239.
101. Morrison AB: Experimentally induced chronic renal insufficiency in the rat. Lab Invest 1962; 11:321.
102. Shimamura T, Morrison AB: A progressive glomerulosclerosis occurring in partial five-sixths nephrectomized rats. Am J Pathol 1975; 79:95.
103. Terasaki PI, Koyama H, Cecka JM, Gjertson DW: The hyperfiltration hypothesis in human renal transplantation [Comments]. Transplantation 1994; 57:1450.
104. Terasaki PI, Gjertson DW, Cecka JM, Takemoto S: Fit and match hypothesis for kidney transplantation. Transplantation 1996; 62:441.
105. Johnson LB, Kuo PC, Dafoe DC, et al: The use of bilateral adult renal allografts—a method to optimize function from donor kidneys with suboptimal nephron mass. Transplantation 1996; 61:1261.

Induction Therapy in Kidney Transplantation

Flavio Vincenti, M.D.

Induction therapy with polyclonal and monoclonal antibodies (MAbs) has been an important component of immunosuppression dating back to the 1960s as demonstrated by Starzl and colleagues in 1967 on the beneficial effect of antilymphocyte globulin (ALG) in the prophylaxis of rejection in renal transplant recipients. Over the past 40 years, several polyclonal antilymphocyte preparations have been used in renal transplantation; however, only two preparations are currently FDA approved, Atgam and Thymoglobulin.[2-4] Another important milestone in biologic therapy was the development of monoclonal antibodies (MAbs) and the introduction of the murine anti CD3 MAb, OKT3 for the treatment of acute rejection.[5] Table 34–1 lists the currently used biologic agents in renal transplantation. Horse antithymocyte globulin (Atgam) and OKT3 (Orthoclone OKT3) were introduced in the 1980s and rabbit antithymocyte globulin (Thymoglobulin) was approved in the United States for use in the late 1990s. While the registered indication of these three biologic agents is to treat acute rejection or steroid resistant acute rejection, they have been used extensively as induction agents in the prophylaxis of rejection.[6] The anti-interleukin-2 receptor (IL-2R) MAbs (frequently referred to as anti-CD25) were the first biologics that were proved to be effective as induction agents in pivotal randomized double-blind prospective trials.[7-10] Over the past 7 years, the use of biologic agents for induction therapy in the prophylaxis of rejection has increased (Fig. 34–1). The popularity of induction therapy has been propelled by several factors, including the introduction of the anti IL-2R antibodies, the emergence of Thymoglobulin as a safer and more effective alternative than Atgam or OKT3 and the increased popularity of drug minimization regimens that spare calcineurin inhibitors or steroids but require coverage with biologic induction.[11]

Biologics for induction can be divided into two groups: the depleting agents and the immune modulators. The depleting agents consist of Atgam, Thymoglobulin, and OKT3 (the latter also produces immune modulation); their efficacy is derived from depleting the recipients of CD3 positive cells at the time of transplantation. The second group of biologic agents, the anti IL-2R MAbs do not result in depletion but block IL-2 mediated T-cell activation by binding to the α chain of IL-2R.

The benefits of induction therapy with the anti IL-2R MAbs were conclusively demonstrated in phase III clinical trials that showed that therapy with either daclizumab (humanized anti-IL2R) or basiliximab (chimeric anti-IL2R) resulted in significantly lower rejection rates than placebo.[7-10]

The decision to use induction therapy is often based on the clinical evaluation of the immunologic risks of transplant recipients. Although all patients can benefit from induction therapy, cost considerations tend to limit induction to the following category of patients:

1. Patients at high immunologic risk of rejection (i.e. blacks, sensitized patients, patients with delayed graft function, retransplant patients)
2. Patients that require or are being considered for calcineurin inhibitor sparing regimens
3. Patients in whom corticosteroids are completely avoided or withdrawn within days after transplantation.

The next important decision in induction therapy is the selection of the desired type of biologic agent, depleting antibody (Thymoglobulin, Atgam, or OKT3) or a nondepleting anti-IL2R. The regimens, benefits, and side effects of these two groups of biologic agents are shown in Tables 34–2 and 34–3. The choice of the specific antibody within each class is often arbitrary but may be based on a number of factors.

Thymoglobulin has displaced both Atgam (because of efficacy) and OKT3 (because of the cytokine release syndrome and excessive toxicity) as the depleting antibody of choice. The anti-IL-2R antibodies, daclizumab and basiliximab, are used interchangeably, although differences can exist between these two agents. Basiliximab is a chimeric antibody and thus could potentially elicit more side effects than daclizumab. Because basiliximab retains the variable domains from the parent murine antibody it has higher affinity to the IL-2Rα than the fully humanized daclizumab. The dose and regimen of basiliximab is fixed at 20 mg at day 0 and day 4 after transplantation. Daclizumab is approved for use in a prolonged five-dose regimen of 1 mg/kg administered at 2 weekly intervals after transplantation. However, increasingly daclizumab is being used in a two-dose regimen similar to basiliximab.[12]

POLYCLONAL ANTILYMPHOCYTE SERA

Polyclonal antilymphocyte agents are produced by immunizing animals with human lymphoid cells. The most frequent immunogen is a thymocyte. The sera from immunized animals are harvested and processed to obtain purified globulin. The final product, however, contains many antibodies that react against a variety of other targets, including red blood cells, neutrophils, and platelets. Within hours of administration polyclonal agents result in lymphocyte depletion secondary to a number of mechanisms, including complement dependent and Fc-dependent opsonization and lysis. The polyclonal agents also contain antibodies to a wide variety of cell surface antigens, including the IL-2R adhesion molecules and costimulatory molecules. The role of these targets in the overall effectiveness of the polyclonal agents is supported by the findings of a recent study showing that administration of Thymoglobulin intraoperatively as opposed to postoperatively resulted in a decrease of delayed graft function presumably by preventing ischemia reperfusion injury.[13]

Table 34–1 Antibodies in Current Use in Renal Transplantation

- **Polyclonal Antibodies**
  Atgam (horse derived globulin)
  Thymoglobulin (rabbit derived globulin)
- **Monoclonal Antibodies**
  OKT3 (murine anti CD3)
  Basiliximab (chimeric anti-IL-2R)
  Daclizumab (humanized anti-IL-2R)

Polyclonal agents are xenogeneic proteins and therefore elicit a number of side effects including fever and chills. Less commonly they can also induce a serum sickness-like syndrome and rarely ARDS. Anaphylaxis is extremely rare even upon reexposure.

Table 34–3 The Dose and Regimen of Currently Available Induction Agents

- Thymoglobulin
  1-2 mg/kg IV up to 14 doses or until renal function improves
- Atgam
  10-20 mg/kg IV up to 14 doses or until renal function improves
- OKT3
  5 mg IV 7-14 days
- Basiliximab
  20 mg IV at days 0 and 4 after transplantation
- Daclizumab

Phase III regimen: five doses of 1 mg/kg at day 0 and every 2 weeks thereafter transplantation. Increasingly used regimen: one (2 mg/kg) or two doses (second dose 1 mg/kg)

ANTI-CD3 MONOCLONAL ANTIBODIES

OKT3 was approved in 1986 for the treatment of acute rejections. OKT3 is a murine IgG2 monoclonal antibody targeting the CD3 complex adjacent to the T cell receptor. Soon after the injection of OKT3, T cells disappear from circulation as a result of opsonization and their removal from circulation by mononuclear cells in the liver and spleen. In addition, initially OKT3 can activate T cells and result in release of several cytokines including IL-2, interferon γ, IL-6, and TNF.[14] These cytokines cause a syndrome that has been referred to as the cytokine release syndrome and consists of fever, chills, headache, gastrointestinal complaints and, less commonly, ARDS, aseptic meningitis, and encephalopathy. The availability of other induction agents and the severity of the side effects associated with the cytokine release syndrome have resulted in a marked reduction in the use of OKT3 in the past several years. Furthermore, OKT3 is immunogenic in humans, and approximately 50% of patients will make antibodies to it following a course of treatment.[15] Many of these patients will develop high titer anti-mouse antibodies that preclude retreatment with OKT3.

There are several humanized nonactivating anti-CD3 MAbs that offer clear-cut advantages over the murine OKT3 but have yet to be developed for use in renal transplantation.

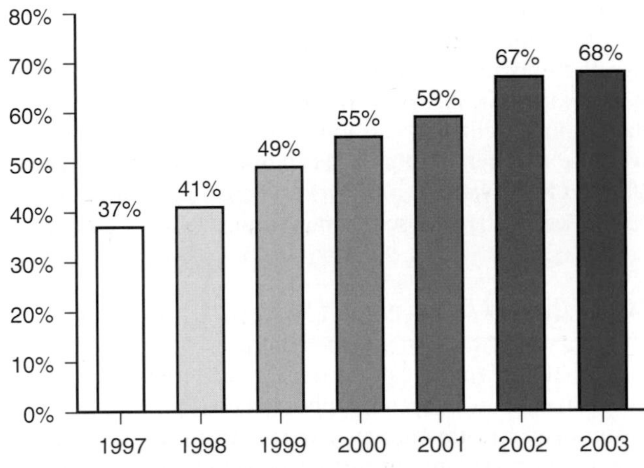

Figure 34–1 Percent of de novo patients receiving induction therapy (1997–2003).

ANTI IL-2R MONOCLONAL ANTIBODIES

The successful introduction of two monoclonal antibodies (MAb), daclizumab (Zenapax, Roche Laboratories) and basiliximab (Simulect, Novartis Pharmaceuticals Inc.), targeting the α chain of the IL-2R, can be attributed to the extensive investigative efforts performed on the IL-2R in the early 1980s.[16] The α chain was the first of the three IL-2R subchains to be fully characterized and was initially identified as Tac (for T-cell activation) protein. The IL-2R β and γ chains are required to transduce the IL-2 signal inside the cell, while the addition of the α chain leads to the expression of the high-affinity IL-2R. A MAb with the ability to block the interaction

Table 34–2 The Pros and Cons of Depleting and Nondepleting (Anti IL-2Ra MAbs) Biologics

Depleting Antibodies	Nondepleting Antibodies
• Rejection rare during use • Calcineurin inhibitors can be used sequentially (i.e., delayed) • Acute side effects with administration • Associated with increased infections and malignancies	• Rejection occurs during use • Calcineurin inhibitors should not be delayed • No acute side effects • Very safe and not associated with complications of over-immunosuppression

between IL-2 and the α chain of the high-affinity IL-2R αβγ has the potential to block the amplification of the immune response and the prevention of rejection. Promising clinical trials of murine or rat anti IL-2R MAbs followed soon thereafter and were published in the late 1980s and early 1990s.[17,18] The chimerization and humanization of rodent antibodies resulted in more humanized constructs that had prolonged half-life and lacked immunogenicity. The phase III trials with daclizumab and basiliximab provided convincing and conclusive proof that blockade of the IL-2 pathway can result in significant reduction in acute rejection.[7-10]

The exact mechanism of action of the anti-CD25 MAbs is not completely understood. There is no evidence that long-term tolerance occurs with therapy with anti-CD25 MAb. Significant depletion of T cells does not appear to play a major role in the mechanism of action of these MAbs. Studies with the anti-IL-2R MAbs suggest that the main mechanism of action of these antibodies is through saturation and blockade of the IL-2Rα.[7,19] However, other mechanisms of actions may mediate the effect of these antibodies. In a study of daclizumab-treated patients, there is approximately a 50% decrease in circulating lymphocytes staining with 7G7, a fluorescein-conjugated antibody that binds on the α chain to an epitope distinct from the epitope that is recognized and bound by daclizumab.[7] Similar results were obtained by Amlot and colleagues[19] in studies with basiliximab. These findings indicate that therapy with the anti-IL-2R MAbs results in a relative decrease of the expression of the α-chain either from depletion of coated lymphocytes and/or modulation of the α-chain secondary to decreased expression or increased shedding. There is also recent evidence that the β-chain may be downregulated by the anti-CD25 antibody.

CLINICAL ADMINISTRATION AND MONITORING IN TRANSPLANTATION

There are two anti-IL-2R preparations for use in clinical transplantation. Daclizumab was approved by the FDA in December of 1997, and basiliximab was approved in May of 1998. Daclizumab was administered in the phase III trials in five doses starting immediately preoperatively, and subsequently at biweekly intervals.[7,8] The dose of daclizumab used was 1 mg/kg given intravenously over 15 minutes in 50 to 100 cc solution of normal saline. This regimen was shown to result in saturation of the IL-2R α on circulating lymphocytes for up to 120 days after transplantation. The half-life of daclizumab was 20 days. Daclizumab blood concentrations of about 5μg/mL persisted in circulation for up to 70 days after transplantation. A higher concentration of daclizumab is required to block IL-2-mediated biologic responses than just to saturate IL-2R. While 1μg/mL of daclizumab saturates the IL-2R on circulating lymphocytes, concentrations of about 5μg/mL are required to block IL-2–mediated biologic responses.[12] In the phase III trials, daclizumab was used with a maintenance immunosuppression regimen that consisted of cyclosporine, azathioprine and steroids, or double-therapy, cyclosporine and steroids. Subsequently, daclizumab was successfully used with a maintenance triple-therapy regimens either with cyclosporine or tacrolimus, steroids and mycophenolate mofetil (MMF) substituting for azathioprine.[20,21]

In the phase III trials, basiliximab was administered in a fixed dose of 20 mg preoperatively and on day 4 after transplantation.[9,10] This regimen of basiliximab was shown to result in a concentration of greater than or equal to 0.2 μg/mL, sufficient to saturate IL-2R on circulating lymphocytes, for 25 to 35 days after transplantation. Concentrations of basiliximab required to block IL-2-mediated biologic responses are about 1μg/mL. The half-life of basiliximab was 7 days. In the phase III trials, basiliximab was used with a maintenance regimen consisting of cyclosporine and prednisone. In a recently reported randomized trial, basiliximab was shown to be safe and effective when used in a maintenance regimen consisting of cyclosporine, MMF, and prednisone.[22]

At present, there is no marker or test to monitor the effectiveness of anti-IL-2R therapy. Saturation of α chain on circulating lymphocytes, although important as a determinant of minimal blood concentrations, is not predictive of rejection that occurs during anti-IL-2R MAb therapy. Kovarik and colleagues[23] analyzed the influence and duration of IL-2R blockade on the incidence of acute rejection episodes in patients who participated in the phase III basiliximab trials and who had detailed disposition analysis of basiliximab.[23] Duration of receptor blockade was similar in patients with rejection and without rejection (34 ± 14 days vs. 37 ± 14 days, mean + SD). In another daclizumab trial, patients with acute rejection were found to have circulating as well as intragraft lymphocytes with saturated IL-2R.[24] A possible explanation is that those patients who reject on anti-IL-2R blockade do so through a mechanism that bypasses the IL-2 pathway due to cytokine–cytokine receptor redundancy (i.e., IL7, IL15).

THE CHOICE OF INDUCTION: DEPLETING VERSUS ANTI-IL2R MABS

Several studies have compared the effectiveness and safety of Thymoglobulin to the anti-IL-2R MAbs antibodies.[25,26] The first study is an open label randomized multicenter French trial comparing the efficacy and tolerability of Thymoglobulin versus basiliximab.[25] The protocol compared basiliximab plus immediate (within the first 24-hours post transplantation) cyclosporine therapy versus Thymoglobulin plus delayed (initiated when the serum creatinine is less than 2.8mg/dL) cyclosporine therapy. All patients also received corticosteroids and MMF at standard doses beginning on the day of transplantation. Fifty predominantly low immunologic risk patients were randomized to each treatment group. The incidence of acute rejection and overall outcome was similar between the two treatment groups, but patients in the Thymoglobulin arm had a higher incidence of side effects (Table 34–4). In contrast, Brennan and colleagues[26] performed a prospective, randomized, multicenter study of Thymoglobulin compared with basiliximab for induction immunosuppression in high immunologic risk patients. High immunologic risk patients were defined as recipients of kidneys likely to have delayed graft function, retransplants, patients with high levels of panel reactive antibodies (PRA) greater than 20%, six antigen mismatch and patients of African descent. Maintenance immunosuppression consisted of cyclosporine, MMF, and prednisone. Table 34–5 shows that patients treated with Thymoglobulin as compared with basiliximab had significantly lower composite endpoints as well as

Table 34–4 Outcomes During the 6-Month Posttransplantation Period (Intention-To-Treat Analysis)

Variable	Basiliximab (n=50)	Thymoglobulin (n=50)
First biopsy-confirmed rejection episode	4 (8%)	4 (8%)
First acute rejection episode treated with antibody therapy	0	1 (2%)
First acute rejection episode treated with tacrolimus	1 (2%)	0
Graft loss*	2 (4%)	0
Death	1 (2%)	0
Treatment failure†	7 (14%)	4 (2%)

*Need for regular postoperative dialysis or nephrectomy or retransplantation.
†Acute rejection, graft loss, or death ? whichever occurred first.

biopsy proven rejection. Taken together these two studies suggest that for lower immunologic risk patients the anti-IL2 MAbs may be the safer choice while for the higher immunologic risk patients, the depleting antibodies such as Thymoglobulin are likely to be the more effective therapy.

BIOLOGIC AGENTS IN DRUG MINIMIZATION TRIALS

As mentioned earlier, induction with biologic agents has been used predominately to enhance the effectiveness of immunosuppression at the time of antigen presentation and increased antigen load. Recently, however, induction therapy has been utilized to leverage drug minimization protocols, especially steroid avoidance or very rapid steroid discontinuation strategies. Table 34–6 details the various steroid-sparing regimens that have utilized different induction regimens to either completely eliminate corticosteroids or withdraw them very rapidly after transplantation. In a single center open label trial at Stanford University, 43 pediatric patients were treated with an extended regimen of daclizumab (6 months) after transplantation as a replacement for corticosteroids with patients maintained on tacrolimus and MMF.[27] With a mean follow-up of 16 ± 9 months, acute rejection occurred in approximately 5% of patients. In a Canadian multicenter, single arm open label trial, patients were also treated with cyclosporine, MMF, and a corticosteroid avoidance protocol but with a shorter course of daclizumab (the conventional five doses, given 1 mg/kg every 2 weeks). The acute rejection rate at 1 year was 25% with the majority of rejections being mild.[28] The other three studies (Table 34–6) utilized steroids only during the perioperative period followed by early discontinuation with induction therapy with either an anti IL-2R MAb or Thymoglobulin and were associated with low acute rejection rates. However, longer-term follow-up will still be required to determine whether this approach is, in fact, safe and beneficial.

INDUCTION THERAPY IN CALCINEURIN INHIBITORS (CNI) SPARING REGIMENS

Induction therapy is also being utilized to facilitate a CNI free regimen combining the two anti-proliferative agents, sirolimus, and MMF in conjunction with steroids. Flechner and colleagues[32] treated 61 patients randomized to either cyclosporine or sirolimus with induction therapy with basiliximab. All patient were treated with MMF and steroids. At 1 year, patient and graft survival were not significantly different between the two treatment groups. The sirolimus-treated patients had a rejection rate of 6.4% compared with 16% in the cyclosporine treatment group. At 12 months following transplantation, the sirolimus treated patients had a significantly lower mean serum creatinine than the cyclosporine treated patients (1.3 mg/dL vs. 1.78 mg/dL, p=.004). These results were appreciably better than those obtained by Kreis and colleagues[33] in a multicenter European study in patients treated with the same maintenance regimen but without biologic induction. The incidence of biopsy-proven acute rejection was 27% with the majority of rejection being moderate in severity. Thus, the superior results obtained by Flechner and colleagues are likely due to the addition of induction therapy to their maintenance regimen. Larson and colleagues[11] treated a randomized group of patients with Thymoglobulin induction and maintenance with either sirolimus, MMF, and prednisone; or tacrolimus, MMF, and prednisone. At 6 months the overall rejection rate in the CNI free treatment arm was 17% with the majority of rejections being subclinical and mild. In

Table 34–5 Efficacy Results: Interim Analysis

	Interim Patients Analyzed (n=212)		
	Thymoglobulin (n=106)	Basiliximab (n=106)	*P* value
Composite (AR/GL/death)	10.4%	23.6%	.017
BPAR	7.6%	18.9%	.023
Graft loss	5.7%	7.6%	P = NS
Death	2.8%	2.8%	P = NS

AR, acute rejection; *BPAR,* biopsy-proven acute rejection; *GL,* graft loss.

Table 34–6 Design and Outcome of Induction Therapy with Corticosteroid Sparing Trials

Design	Immunosuppression	Corticosteroid Regimens	Outcome	Ref
Canadian single arm open label multicenter trial (n=57)	Daclizumab induction MMF-CsA	None	AR at 1 year 25%	26
The "Stanford" protocol single center pediatric trial (n=43)	Prolonged daclizumab induction (for 6 months) MMF-tacrolimus	None	AR 5% at a mean follow-up of 16±9 months	27
Open label randomized multicenter trial (n=83)	Basiliximab induction MMF-CsA	Standard steroids (dosage, mg: 500-250-125-65-30 then gradually taper to 5-10)	AR at 1 year 19%	28
		5 days of steroids (dosage, mg: 500-250-125-65-30)	AR at 1 year 20%	
Open label single center trial in living donor kidney transplantation (n=51)	Thymoglobulin induction MMF-CsA	6 days of steroids (dosage: 500 mg, 1 mg/kg, 0.5 g/kgx2 days, 0.25 mg/kgx2 days)	AR at 1 year 13%	29
Open label single arm multicenter trial (n=80)	Basiliximab induction SRL-tacrolimus	5 days of steroids (dosage, mg: 250-250-125-65-30)	AR at 6 months 8.5%	30

AR, acute rejection; *CsA*, cyclosporine; *MMF*, mycophenolate mofetil; *SRL*, sirolimus.

summary, induction therapy appears to be useful both in corticosteroid sparing as well as in CNI sparing regimens.

EMERGING BIOLOGIC INDUCTION REGIMENS

Two additional biologic agents are being used in novel immunosuppressive regimens to achieve drug minimization. The first agent is CAMPATH 1H, a humanized anti-CD52 monoclonal antibody approved for use for chronic lymphocytic leukemia. A single dose of anti-CD52 results in prolonged depletion of lymphocytes (6 months or greater) and has been used in several trials to eliminate CNI, steroids or both.[34,35] These trials have been investigator-initiated and at the present time no pivotal study is planned with anti-CD52. The long-term safety of prolonged lymphocyte depletion remains unresolved, although early and intermediate follow-up has not witnessed the emergence of PTLD or opportunistic infections.

The most promising area for biologic induction is blockade of the costimulatory pathway in an attempt to induce tolerance or the very least, graft acceptance with minimal maintenance immunosuppression. This represents a new paradigm in terms of biologic induction as these agents are being developed to be used chronically, intermittently, and indefinitely. The prototype is LEA29Y, a second generation CTL4Ig, which binds with enhanced affinity to CD80 and CD86, thus preventing their binding to CD28 and the subsequent necessary signaling for T-cell activation. In a large multicenter, prospective randomized study, costimulatory blockade is being tested for its efficacy and safety in a regimen consisting of intermittent LEA29Y intravenous therapy (initially every 2 weeks, then either every 4 or 8 weeks) and maintenance immunosuppression consisting of MMF and prednisone versus a standard regimen of cyclosporine, MMF, and prednisone.[36] While the results of these trials are yet to be reported, in a recently published study in nonhuman primates, a regimen of LEA29Y and sirolimus was successful in producing prolonged engraftment of islet cells without the use of CNI or corticosteroids.[37]

SUMMARY

Biologic induction therapy is currently an important component of immunosuppression therapy, and, in the future, it is more likely to replace rather than be replaced by maintenance oral immunosuppressive drugs.

References

1. Starzl TE, Marchioro TL, Hutchinson DE, et al: The clinical use of antilymphocyte globulin in renal homotransplantations. Transplantation 1967; 5:1100-1105.
2. Howard RJ, Condie RM, Sutherland DE, et al: The use of antilymphoblast globulin in the treatment of renal allograft rejection: A double-blind, randomized study. Transplantation 1997; 24:419-423.
3. Gaber AO, First MR, Tesi RJ, et al: Results of the double-blind, randomized, multicenter, phase III clinical trial of thymoglobulin versus Atgam in the treatment of acute graft rejection episodes after renal transplantation. Transplantation 1998; 66:29-37.
4. Monaco AP: A new look at polyclonal antilymphocyte antibodies in clinical transplantation. Graft 1999; 2:S2-S5.
5. Ortho Multicenter Transplant Study Group: A randomized clinical trial of OKT3 monoclonal antibody for acute rejection of cadaveric renal transplants. N Engl J Med 1985; 313:337-342.
6. Szczech LA, Berlin JA, Aradhye S, et at: Effect of anti-lymphocyte induction therapy on renal allograft survival: A meta-analysis. J Am Soc Nephrol 1997; 8:1771-1777.
7. Vincenti F, Kirkman R, Light S, et al: Interleukin-2-receptor blockade with daclizumab to prevent acute rejection in renal transplantation. New Engl J Med 1998; 338:161-165.

8. Nashan B, Light S, Hardie IR, et al: Reduction of acute renal allograft rejection by daclizumab. Daclizumab Double Therapy Study Group. Transplantation 1999; 67:110-115.
9. Nashan B, Moore R, Amlot P, et al: Randomized trial of basiliximab versus placebo for control of acute cellular rejection in renal allograft recipients. CHIB 201 International Study Group. Lancet 1997; 350:1193-1198.
10. Kahan BD, Rajagopalan PR, Hall M: Reduction of the occurrence of acute cellular rejection among renal allograft recipients treated with basiliximab, a chimeric anti-interleukin-2-receptor monoclonal antibody. United States Simulect Renal Study Group. Transplantation 1999; 67:276-284.
11. Vincenti F: Immunosuppression Minimization: Current and future trends in transplant immunosuppression. J Am Soc Nephrol 2003; 14:1940-1948.
12. Vincenti F, Pace D, Birnbaum J, Lantz M: Pharmacokinetic and pharmacodynamic studies of one or two doses of daclizumab in renal transplantation. Am J Transplant 2003; 3:50-52.
13. Goggins WC, Pascual MA, Powelson JA, et al: A prospective, randomized, clinical trial of intraoperative versus postoperative Thymoglobulin in adult cadaveric renal transplant recipients. Transplantation 2003; 76:798-802.
14. Sgro C: Side effects of a monoclonal antibody, muromonab CD3/orthoclone OKT3: Bibliographic review. Toxicology 1995; 105:23-29.
15. Kimball JA, Norman DJ, Shield CF, et al: The OKT3 Antibody Response Study: A multicenter study of human anti-mouse antibody (HAMA) production following OKT3 use in solid organ transplantation. Transpl Immunol 1995; 3:212-221.
16. Waldmann TA, Goldman CK: The multichain interleukin-2 receptor: A target for immunotherapy of patients receiving allografts. Am J Kidney Dis 1989; 14(suppl 2):45-53.
17. Kirkman R, Barrett L, Carpenter C, et al: A randomized trial of anti-Tac monoclonal antibody in human renal transplantation. Transplantation 1991; 51:107-113.
18. Soulillou JP, Cantarovich D, Le Mauff B, et al: Randomized controlled trial of a monoclonal antibody against the interleukin-2 receptor (33B3.1) as compared with rabbit antithymocyte globulin for prophylaxis against rejection of renal allografts. N Engl J Med 1990; 322:1175-1182.
19. Amlot PL, Rawlings E, Fernando ON, et al: Prolonged action of chimeric interleukin-2 receptor (CD25) monoclonal antibody used in cadaveric renal transplantation. Transplantation 1995; 60:748-756.
20. Ciancio G, Burke GW, Suzart K, et al: Efficacy and safety of daclizumab induction for primary kidney transplant recipients in combination with tacrolimus, mycophenolate mofetil, and steroids as maintenance immunosuppression. Transplant Proc 2003; 35: 873-874.
21. Pescovitz MD, Bumgardner GL, Gaston RS, et al: Addition of daclizumab to mycophenolate mofetil, cyclosporine, and steroids in renal transplantation: Pharmacokinetics, safety, and efficacy. Clin Transpl 2003 (in press).
22. Lawen J, Davies E, Morad F, et al: Basiliximab (Simulect) is safe and effective in combination with triple therapy of Neoral, steroids and CellCept in renal transplant recipients. Transplantation 2000; 69:S260.
23. Kovarik JM, Kahan BD, Rajagopalan PR, et al: Population pharmacokinetics and exposure-response relationships for basiliximab in kidney transplantation. The US Simulect Renal Transplant Study Group. Transplantation 1999; 68:1288-1294.
24. Vincenti F, Ramos E, Brattstrom C, et al: Multicenter trial exploring calcineurin inhibitors avoidance in renal transplantation. Transplantation 2001; 71:1282-1287.
25. Lebranchu Y, Bridoux F, Buchler M, et al: Immunoprophylaxis with basiliximab compared with antithymocyte globulin in renal transplant patients receiving MMF-containing triple therapy. Am J Transpl 2002; 2:48-56.
26. Brennan DC: The Thymoglobulin Induction Study Group. A prospective, randomized, multi-center study of Thymoglobulin compared to basiliximab for induction immunosuppression: Preliminary results (Abstract 398). Am J Transpl 2002; 2:238.
27. Cole E, Landsberg D, Russell D, et al: A pilot study of steroid-free immunosuppression in the prevention of acute rejection in renal allograft recipients. Transplantation 2001; 72:845-850.
28. Sarwal MM, Yorgin PD, Alexander S, et al: Promising early outcomes with a novel, complete steroid avoidance immunosuppression protocol in pediatric renal transplantation. Transplantation 2001; 72:13-21.
29. Vincenti F, Monaco A, Grinyo J, et al: Multicenter randomized prospective trial of steroid withdrawal in renal transplant recipients receiving basiliximab, cyclosporine microemulsion and mycophenolate mofetil. Am J Transpl 2003; 3:306-311.
30. Matas AJ, Ramcharan T, Paraskevas S, et al: Rapid discontinuation of steroids in living donor kidney transplantation: A pilot study. Am J Transpl 2001; 1:278.
31. Woodle S, Vincenti F, Lorber M, et al: A multicenter, open label pilot study of early (5 day) corticosteroid cessation in de novo renal transplant recipients under Simulect, tacrolimus, and sirolimus therapy: Interim analysis (Abstract #1128). Am J Transpl 2003; 3(suppl 5):440.
32. Flechner M, Goldfarb D, Modlin C, et al: Kidney transplantation without calcineurin inhibitor drugs: A prospective, randomized trial of sirolimus versus cyclosporine. Transplantation 2002; 74:1070-1076.
33. Kreis H, Cisterne J-M, Land W, et al: Sirolimus European Renal Transplant Study Group. Sirolimus in association with mycophenolate mofetil induction for the prevention of acute graft rejection in renal allograft recipients. Transplantation 2000; 69:1252-1260.
34. Knechtle SJ, Pirsch JD, Fechner JH, et al: Campath-1H induction plus Rapamycin monotherapy for renal transplantation: Results of a pilot study. Am J Transpl 2003; 3:722-730.
35. Kirk AD, Hale DA, Mannon RB, et al: Results from a human renal allograft tolerance trial evaluating the humanized CD52-specific monoclonal antibody alemtuzumab (campath-1H). Transplantation 2003; 76:120-129.
36. Vincenti F, Durrbach A, Larsen C, et al: Study design and baseline characteristics of a multiple dose, randomized, controlled open-label study comparing a costimulation blocker based regimen of BMS224818 (LEA29Y) vs. cyclosporine in renal transplant (Abstract A1253). Am J Transpl 2003; 3(suppl 5):473.
37. Adams AB, Shirasugi N, Durham MM, et al: Calcineurin inhibitor-free CD28 blockade-based protocol protects allogeneic islets in nonhuman primates. Diabetes 2002; 51:265-270.

Current and Emerging Maintenance Immunosuppressive Therapy

Simin Goral, M.D. • J. Harold Helderman, M.D.

This chapter reviews current immunosuppressive management in kidney transplantation while emphasizing the emerging features that have led to a more individualized approach to each patient.

The dictum of accommodation between host and graft drives the construction of renal transplantation immunosuppressive management strategies. It has been observed that the technical, drug toxicity-related, and immunologic graft loss rates are highest within the first several months after engraftment. Certainly, after 1 year of allograft survival, loss rates become nearly linear over time, permitting construction of graft half-life survival curves with high confidence.[1] Corollary to the law of graft half-life accommodation is the rule that heightened immunosuppression is required early, with progressive reduction in the amount and stringency over time. Until highly allospecific immunity or even alloantigenic tolerance can be achieved, this strategy of "more early and less late" will continue to define the role of immunosuppression, regardless of the agents employed.

Pursuant to the dictum of accommodation, three distinct periods of transplantation immunosuppression have been defined:

1. The perioperative *induction* period
2. *Early maintenance,* characterized by progressive taper of the individual drugs in the regimen
3. *Chronic maintenance,* characterized by a relatively fixed package of agents used at the lowest, effective doses until an intervening event occurs, such as late acute rejection, infection, or neoplasm

In this chapter, induction therapy will be discussed briefly, followed by the agents used in the early and late maintenance phases of immunosuppression. Since they are similar, they are discussed together.

INDUCTION IMMUNOSUPPRESSION

In the perioperative period, steroids are given initially at high doses; rapid tapering is then instituted to achieve the levels used in the early maintenance phase. The rapidity of the tapering varies from center to center. Usually, the patient receives a 250-mg to 500-mg pulse of IV methylprednisolone during surgery. Cytotoxic drugs such as azathioprine or mycophenolate mofetil (MMF) are frequently used. Azathioprine is typically given as an intravenous dose of 3 to 5 mg/kg, followed by a rapid taper to the induction dose of 150 mg/day for 5 days, and leading into the early maintenance dose of 100 mg/day or 2 mg/kg/day, whichever is lower, adjusted by marrow toxicity. Initial doses of MMF are typically 2 to 3 g/day in divided doses.

The greatest differences in induction strategies involve the decisions: (1) whether or not to use a calcineurin inhibitor (CI) such as cyclosporine or tacrolimus or (2) whether or not to provide a T cell–directed polyclonal or monoclonal antibody for a defined period before introducing the calcineurin inhibitor to enter the early maintenance phase of immunosuppression. The development of the *antibody-induction approach* stemmed from the recognition that cyclosporine and tacrolimus are nephrotoxic, thus potentially compromising early graft function.

A sequential induction approach, which was developed to avoid early cyclosporine use, employs anti–T cell antibodies that are extraordinarily effective at forestalling acute rejection when used early.[2] A short overlap period follows, during which cyclosporine or tacrolimus is introduced. The achievement of target blood levels of calcineurin inhibitor is determined empirically at rejection prophylaxis.[3] When these target levels are achieved, the antibody is discontinued, the induction phase is considered complete, and the recipient enters the early maintenance phase of immunosuppression.

Testing the role of antibody induction requires carefully constructed, large trials (which have been rare) or an approach to the data that employs statistical tools of meta-analysis. A combined group of investigators from the Vanderbilt Transplant Center and the Brigham and Women's program in Boston performed a meta-analysis of data in the published literature.[4] When taken together, statistically significant graft survival outcomes in the United States improved in cases in which polyclonal or monoclonal antibodies were used. More recently, Shield and colleagues[5] analyzed the large United Network for Organ Sharing (UNOS) database and reached the same conclusion. In another study, Szczech and colleagues[6] looked at the combined individual patient-level data from published trials to examine the effect of induction therapy on allograft survival. They showed a benefit of induction therapy at 2 years, particularly among presensitized patients. Although the benefit of this therapy subsequently waned, presensitized patients continued to have benefit at 5 years. Induction antibodies are discussed in more detail in Chapter 34.

MAINTENANCE PHASE

Therapeutic Approach

Following the accommodation dictum, the transplant recipient enters early and then late maintenance with progressive graft survival. In the next part of this chapter, we review each agent available for use for immunosuppressive maintenance individually, with a focus on newer approaches. It is appropriate to first provide a general framework for the therapeutic approach in these next two immunosuppressive periods.

The bedrock of maintenance immunosuppression since the early 1980s has been a calcineurin inhibitor with some form of adjunctive immunosuppression. In most programs, steroids were added as a second immunosuppressive drug ("double therapy"), or a cytotoxic agent was also used ("triple therapy"). Azathioprine was the predominant cytotoxic agent used until the early 1990s, when it was superseded in most programs by mycophenolate mofetil (MMF), based on evidence from three large randomized, prospective, blinded cooperative treatment trials conducted worldwide.[8] No clear graft survival advantage has been shown with azathioprine-based triple therapy over double therapy.[9,10] The important reduction in early acute rejection rates with MMF-based triple therapy drives the popularity of that regimen.

Immunosuppressive Agents

Steroids

Although not an emerging maintenance therapeutic agent, steroids remain a basic element in almost all protocols; thus, a brief discussion of standard uses and attempts at steroid withdrawal is in order. Corticosteroids have been used for prevention as well as for treatment of acute allograft rejection since the early 1960s. They block the expression of several cytokine genes and the synthesis and action of several chemoattractants and vasodilators as part of their anti-inflammatory properties. In some transplantation centers, steroids are administered in the perioperative period as part of induction therapy (e.g., methylprednisolone, 250–500 mg, given intravenously), followed by prednisone, 30 mg/day in two or three separate doses. The dose is gradually tapered over 3 months to a maintenance dose of 5 to 10 mg, or to lower doses in some centers.

The long-term use of steroids causes numerous and diverse complications, including growth retardation in children, osteoporosis, avascular necrosis, hyperlipidemia, hypertension, cataracts, and diabetes. To minimize or eliminate the occurrence of these complications, studies have been undertaken and are in progress at a number of transplantation centers. The potential benefits of eliminating steroids from the immunosuppressive regimens must be weighed against the risk of acute or chronic rejection and eventually early loss of the allograft. A meta-analysis by Hricik and colleagues[11] suggested that the elimination of steroids is associated with an increased short-term risk of acute rejection, with no statistically significant adverse effect on long-term patient or allograft survival. These studies, however, had a great deal of heterogeneity in their designs and outcomes as well as short follow-up periods. Moreover, the experience of the Canadian Multicentre Transplant Study Group[12] with steroid withdrawal revealed that statistically significant differences in outcomes can be seen only after prolonged follow-up (more than 3 years), raising caution and potentially explaining the results of the Hricik study. Two randomized trials studied the potential risks and the benefits of late steroid withdrawal (3 months after transplantation) while patients are on cyclosporine and MMF.[13,14] The investigators concluded that for recipients on cyclosporine, mycophenolate mofetil, prednisone with no acute rejection at 90 days, the chance of developing subsequent acute rejection is small. When prednisone was tapered and withdrawn, the risk of acute rejection increased but withdrawal patients had a lower cholesterol level, less need for antihypertensives, and increased lumbar spine bone density. Of note, acute rejection risk was higher in blacks (39.6%) versus non-blacks (16%). There have been recent studies favoring immunosuppressive regimens in which steroids are withdrawn very early (usually in the 1st week) after transplantation or completely avoided.[15,16] Although there are many benefits of withdrawing steroids from the maintenance immunosuppressive regimens, we believe that clinicians should be cautious when considering steroid minimization because of the unresolved issues such as the timing of steroid discontinuation, concerns over the lack of long-term follow-up, infrequent use of controls in most of the trials, and the other immunosuppressive drugs included in the protocol, allowing the safest steroid minimization protocol.

Randomized, controlled studies are in progress to assess the risk of rejection and graft loss with the newer immunosuppressive agents, including MMF and rapamycin, which may facilitate withdrawal of steroids in the future.

Cyclosporine

Before the discovery of the antirejection properties of cyclosporine, the graft and patient survival rates after kidney transplantation were barely acceptable, and transplantation of other solid organs remained highly experimental. The introduction of cyclosporin A into the clinical arena of transplantation in 1978 revolutionized medical management after transplantation and improved early graft survival significantly. Because of its profound impact on transplantation, a cyclosporine-based immunosuppressive regimen had become the gold standard of medical maintenance immunosuppression.

Cyclosporine is a small polypeptide of fungal origin. It binds to cyclophilin, a cytoplasmic receptor protein and creates an active complex. By binding to calcineurin, a calcium-regulated enzyme, the cyclosporine-cyclophilin complex inhibits the expression of several critical T-cell activation gene transcription factors, thus forestalling the activation and proliferation of lymphocytes (Figure 35–1). The form of this drug initially available, Sandimmune, has pharmacokinetic properties that have made it difficult to use. There is a great deal of interpatient and intrapatient variability in exposure to drug with standard dosing, whereas 12-hour trough blood levels are poorly reflective of drug exposure. Both gut motility and bile are required for adequate gastrointestinal absorption. Certain groups of patients (e.g., children, African-Americans, and diabetic patients) absorb drugs poorly and are thus vulnerable to rejection.

A microemulsion formulation of cyclosporine (Neoral) entered the clinical arena of transplantation in 1995. This formulation is a preconcentrate that, on contact with gastrointestinal fluids, rapidly forms a microemulsion, resulting in increased absorption of cyclosporine that is unaffected by food intake or the presence of bile. Neoral has shown increased bioavailability and decreased intrapatient and interpatient variability. Area under the curve (AUC) 0 to 4 hours represents the period of greatest variability among transplant recipients. Adequate absorption is very important for effective rejection prophylaxis. It has been shown previously that although the correlation between cyclosporine trough blood concentrations and total systemic exposure measured by the AUC is improved with Neoral, C0 trough level does not correlate well with AUC.[17,18] Recent studies indicated that 2-hour

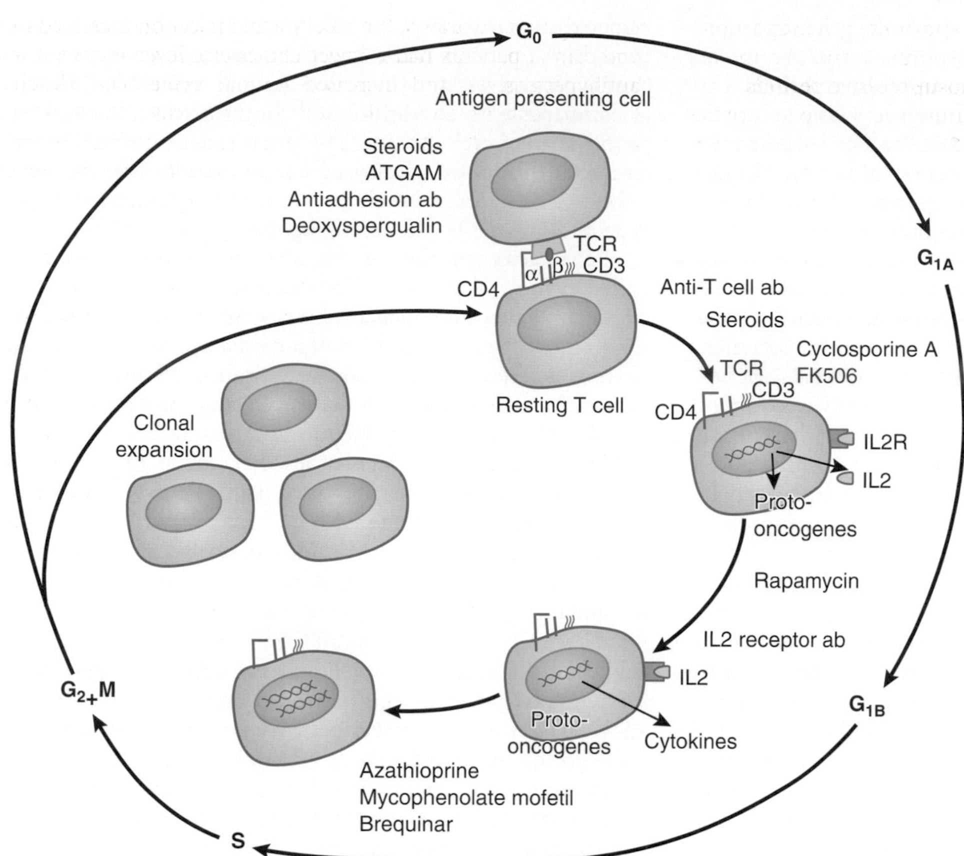

Figure 35–1 Lymphocyte activation cascade, with mechanism of actions of various immunosuppressive agents. *ab,* Antibody; *ATGAM,* antithymocyte globulin; *IL2,* interleukin-2; *TCR,* T-cell receptor.

post dose sample, C2, is the best single time-point predictor of AUC 0 to 4 in all solid organ transplants.[19, 20] Dose reduction depending on C2 levels in many overexposed patients may lead to improvements in renal function and blood pressure and a decrease in the incidence of chronic allograft nephropathy as well. Further studies are required to confirm the long-term benefits of this strategy. Replication of these studies in patient groups with different absorptive characteristics such as children and diabetics with gastroparesis would also be necessary.

No significant difference has been demonstrated in safety and tolerability between the standard oil-based cyclosporine (Sandimmune) and the new formulation.[21] The absorption of cyclosporine has been markedly improved by conversion of even stable patients from Sandimmune to Neoral, especially poor absorbers, such as diabetic recipients of simultaneous kidney and pancreas allografts.[22] Indeed, a meta-analysis of a global database of worldwide studies of conversion showed the most dramatic improvement in the worst absorbers.[23] Finally, Kahan and colleagues[24] revealed an association between variable oral bioavailability of cyclosporine and risk of chronic rejection, which theoretically can be reduced by switching patients from Sandimmune to Neoral.

New patients are started on Neoral at a dose similar to that of Sandimmune, with adjustments in dosing made to achieve the same target blood levels. In several studies, 1:1 dosage conversion from Sandimmune to Neoral was safe for most stable patients.[25,26] However, it is strongly recommended that serum creatinine and cyclosporine blood levels be closely monitored, with the first time point at 7 days after conversion, to capture any cyclosporine-related toxic events because a 10% to 20% dose reduction is frequently required. Neoral is available in the same oral dosage strengths and forms as Sandimmune (25 and 100 mg, capsules, and 100 mg/mL, oral solution).

Table 35–1 reviews the toxicity profile of cyclosporine. Similar adverse effects have been reported with Neoral. Long-term studies should help determine whether the improved bioavailability and higher peak concentrations of Neoral will lead to reduced chronic rejection and longer graft survival or to increased chronic nephrotoxicity.

Another major development in transplantation therapeutics involving the cyclosporine molecule is the advent of generic formulations for study; these have already triggered discussion,

Table 35–1 Potential Adverse Effects of Cyclosporine

Nephrotoxicity
Hypertension
Hyperkalemia
Hypomagnesemia
Hyperuricemia
Thromboembolic events
Hepatotoxicity
Thrombotic microangiopathy
Hypertrichosis
Gingival hyperplasia
Hyperlipidemia
Glucose intolerance
Neurotoxicity
Chronic renal interstitial fibrosis
BK virus nephropathy

even before market availability. The type of the generic formulations (the old formulation of cyclosporine versus the newer microemulsion), their success in clinical trials, and their cost will have a major impact on their future use. Using an open-label, three-period design, Roza and colleagues[27] studied 50 renal transplant recipients taking stable doses of Neoral. Subjects switched from Neoral on a milligram-for-milligram basis to Gengraf. The pharmacokinetics of Gengraf were equivalent and indistinguishable from those of Neoral. Gengraf was well tolerated and interchangeable with Neoral in these stable renal transplant recipients. To gain wide acceptance in the transplantation community, the generic cyclosporine formulations must be held to a higher standard than is usually applied by the U.S. Food and Drug Administration (FDA) censure of generic drugs. In this medical arena, in which survival of the organ transplant is at stake, mere bioequivalence (within 30%) after single-dose comparisons in young healthy volunteers is an inadequate criterion for acceptance. In the least, especially because this molecule has a complex pharmacokinetic profile, different patient populations and perhaps even efficacy data should be the standards on which approval is based.

Because of the significant long-term side effects of calcineurin inhibitors including nephrotoxicity, cardiovascular diseases and malignancy, there are new trials on the way to minimize the use these agents. The introduction of newer and potent agents in the recent years has prompted interest in CI-sparing (the initial use of a standard or low dose CI with subsequent withdrawal) and CI-avoidance (completely avoiding the use of CI) protocols. The physicians should be aware that these strategies are not safe for all patients. The studies are in progress.

Tacrolimus

Tacrolimus (FK-506; Prograf) is an immunosuppressive agent that was approved by the FDA in 1994 for use in liver transplant recipients and in 1997 for use in kidney transplant recipients based on trials in which FK-506 was used either as the primary immunosuppressive agent or as rescue therapy in steroid-resistant rejection.[28,29] Tacrolimus is a macrolide antibiotic that was isolated in 1985 from a soil actinomycete. It blocks T-cell activation genes by a mechanism similar to that of cyclosporine (see Figure 35–1). By binding to a ubiquitous, highly conserved cytosolic protein (FK-506–binding protein [FKBP]), the class of which has been labeled the *immunophilins*, FK-506 blocks the activation of calcineurin, a calcium-activated serine-threonine phosphatase, and inhibits the calcium-dependent signal transduction pathway in T lymphocyte activation. In open-label phase III studies, acute early transplant rejection rates, antirejection medication use, and the histologic severity of rejection were all reduced by FK-506, as compared with Sandimmune.[30] In these trials, the toxicity profile favored cyclosporine. The target range of trough blood level that optimizes efficacy and minimizes toxicity appears to be 5 to 15 ng/mL. The corresponding recommended initial dose of FK-506 is 0.1 to 0.2 mg/kg/day.

Table 35–2 Potential Adverse Effects of FK-506

Nephrotoxicity
Neurotoxicity
Gastrointestinal disturbances
Diabetes
Thrombotic microangiopathy
Alopecia
Hypertension
BK virus nephropathy
Chronic renal interstitial fibrosis
Hyperkalemia
Hypomagnesemia

The toxicity profile of FK-506 is similar to that of cyclosporine (Table 35–2). The characteristics of nephrotoxicity include new arteriolar hyalinosis, degeneration or necrosis of smooth muscle cells of the media of the afferent and efferent arteriolar walls, and vacuolization of the proximal tubule. Neurotoxicity and diabetes occur more frequently with FK-506 than with cyclosporine.

Although the pathogenesis of diabetes due to FK-506 is not well understood, it has been reported that FK-506 decreases glucose-induced insulin release at high concentrations in animal and human pancreatic cells. Obesity, a family history of diabetes, a history of glucose intolerance, positive hepatitis C status, and the use of high steroid doses are some of the risk factors for diabetes in patients taking FK-506. A recent retrospective study by First and colleagues[31] showed that the incidence of post-transplant diabetes mellitus (PTDM) was 4.9% in tacrolimus-treated patients compared to 3.3% in cyclosporine-treated patients (p=.453). In this particular study, the absence of an antiproliferative agent correlated with the development of PTDM. In another study, using data from the United States Renal Data System, Kasiske and colleagues[32] identified 11,659 Medicare beneficiaries who received their first kidney transplant from 1996 to 2000. The cumulative incidence of PTDM was 9.1%, 16.0%, and 24.0% at 3, 12, and 36 months posttransplant, respectively. Using Cox's proportional hazards analysis, they demonstrated that risk factors for PTDM included age, African-American race, Hispanic ethnicity, male donor, increasing HLA mismatches, hepatitis C infection, body mass index greater or equal to 30 kg/m^2, and the use of tacrolimus as the initial maintenance immunosuppressive medication. Tremors, headache, seizures, and insomnia are also reported with use of this drug. Diarrhea, nausea, and anorexia are relatively common in patients receiving FK-506. The incidence of hyperlipidemia as well as hypertension is lower with FK-506 than with cyclosporine. Gloor and colleagues[33] also demonstrated that subclinical rejection episodes were much lower in patients treated with tacrolimus, MMF, and steroids (2.6%) compared to historic controls treated with cyclosporine (30%).

There is tantalizing evidence that FK-506 is a potent and useful immunosuppressive agent for the prevention of acute rejection and reversal of steroid-resistant rejection. Recently, in a 5-year follow-up study, Vincenti and colleagues[34] demonstrated that tacrolimus-based therapy resulted in significantly reduced risk of graft failure, without an increase in the incidence of adverse events associated with long-term immunosuppression.

Prospective, randomized studies are underway looking at the incidence of chronic allograft nephropathy, long-term renal function, steroid withdrawal, and cardiovascular risk factors comparing cyclosporine and tacrolimus, as well as testing the long-acting FK-506 molecule.

Azathioprine

Azathioprine is a purine analogue with a complex mechanism of action. It is metabolized in the liver to 6-mercaptopurine and 6-thioinosinic acid. Azathioprine can inhibit both deoxyribonucleic acid (DNA) and ribonucleic acid (RNA) synthesis by preventing interconversion among the precursors of purine synthesis and by inhibiting the initial steps of the de novo purine synthesis pathway through suppression of the enzyme glutamine phosphoribosyl pyrophosphate aminotransferase. It was widely used with steroids for maintenance immunosuppression before the introduction of cyclosporine to clinical transplantation.

The usual maintenance dose of azathioprine is 1 to 3 mg/kg/day as a single oral dose. One can adjust the dosage by monitoring the hematologic side effects, not by assessing blood level measurements. The most important side effect of azathioprine is bone marrow suppression, which can usually be reversed by decreasing the dose or temporarily discontinuing the drug. Hepatitis, pancreatitis, and hair loss have also been reported. There is an important drug interaction with allopurinol, which by inhibiting the enzyme xanthine oxidase, can increase the toxicity of azathioprine. Therefore, simultaneous administration of azathioprine and allopurinol should be followed closely, and the dose of allopurinol may need to be reduced to 25% to 50% of the usual dose.

In two separate meta-analyses of triple therapy (cyclosporine, prednisone, azathioprine) versus double therapy (cyclosporine, prednisone) no graft outcome advantage could be statistically discerned for azathioprine in cyclosporine-based maintenance regimens.[9,10] The new immunosuppressive agent MMF, which has decreased marrow toxicity, has entered the clinical arena of transplantation and gained popularity as part of the triple-drug regimen (cyclosporine or tacrolimus, MMF, and1 steroids). In one way, MMF has reduced acute rejection episodes by half compared with triple-therapy regimens that include azathioprine; however, the molecule is much more expensive.

Mycophenolate Mofetil

MMF is a semisynthetic derivative of mycophenolic acid produced by the fungus *Penicillium.* It was approved by the FDA in 1995 for use in rejection prophylaxis in kidney transplantation and has already replaced azathioprine in many centers around the world. Mycophenolic acid is poorly absorbed after oral administration; the use of MMF, the pro-drug, improves the drug's bioavailability. After oral administration, MMF is rapidly and completely converted to mycophenolic acid, which functions as a noncompetitive inhibitor of the rate-limiting enzyme inosine monophosphate dehydrogenase in the de novo purine biosynthesis pathway (Figure 35–2). Because lymphocytes are highly dependent on the de novo pathway of purine synthesis and cannot efficiently use the salvage pathway, MMF, in theory, selectively inhibits the proliferation of T and B lymphocytes. A second action to inhibit intracellular glycosylation of peptides may prove equally important because many growth factors and their receptors require the addition of glycosyl residues to traffic from the endoplasmic reticulum to the cell surface.

The efficacy and safety of MMF in renal transplantation have been evaluated in three large multicenter studies.[35-37] These studies indicated that MMF reduces the incidence of acute rejection significantly compared with azathioprine or placebo when combined with cyclosporine and steroids. Side effects were greater in patients who received 3 g/day of MMF in all studies and included diarrhea, esophagitis, gastritis, leukopenia, and anemia. Nephrotoxicity, neurotoxicity, and hepatotoxicity have not been reported with MMF (Table 35–3).

Although MMF is a promising agent for both induction and maintenance therapy, it has also been used successfully as rescue therapy for biopsy-proven rejection refractory to treatment with high-dose steroids, OKT3, or both.[38] Its long-term graft survival advantage as well as effects on decreasing the

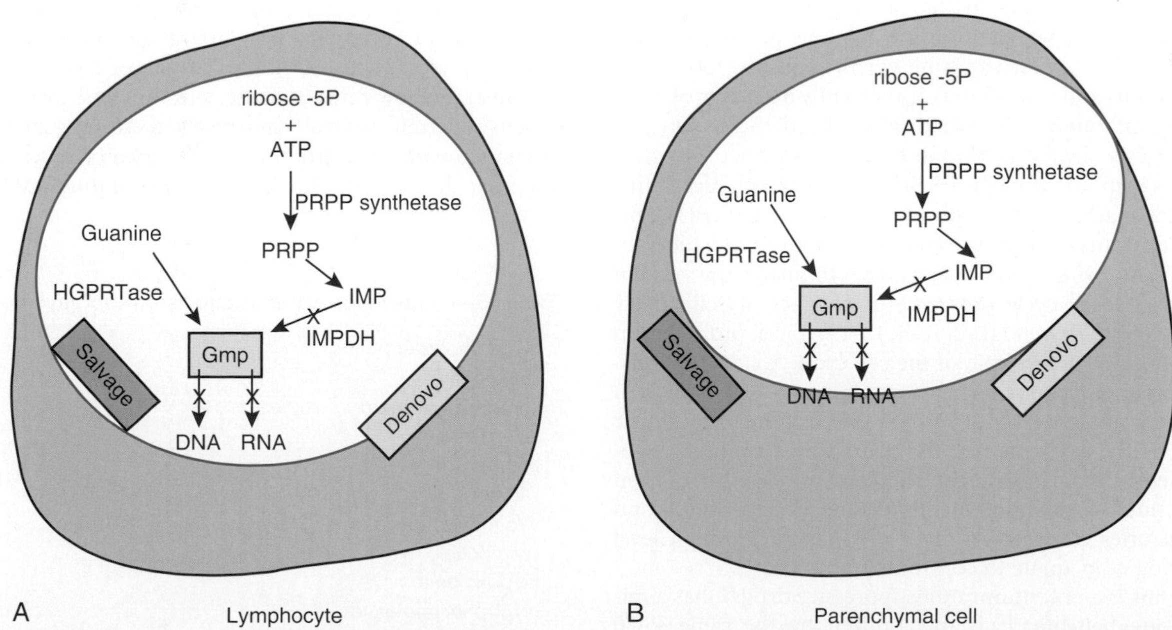

Figure 35–2 The mechanism of action of mycophenolate mofetil. ***A,*** Purine metabolism in the lymphocyte. ***B,*** Purine metabolism in the parenchymal cells. *Gmp,* Guanosine monophosphate; *HGPRTase,* hypoxanthine guanine phosphoribosyl transferase; *IMP,* inosine monophosphate; *IMPDH,* inosine monophosphate dehydrogenase; *PRPP,* 5-phosphoribosyl-1-phosphate; *DNA,* deoxyribonucleic acid; *RNA,* ribonucleic acid; *ATP,* adenosine triphosphate.

Table 35–3 Potential Adverse Effects of Mycophenolate Mofetil

Nausea
Anorexia
Diarrhea
Gastritis
Leukopenia
Anemia

risk of late acute rejection over azathioprine have also been shown in several recent studies.[39,40]

In addition, experimental animal data suggest that MMF may directly inhibit many mechanisms thought to be involved in chronic rejection. Although many authorities believe that MMF is an important adjunct to steroids and to some IL-2–blocking agents for early maintenance therapy, the duration of treatment with this relatively expensive agent is unclear. Trials to address this issue, especially in light of the impact on preventing rather than reversing chronic rejection, are being initiated. Ongoing trials are also looking at steroid withdrawal in patients taking MMF and at the use of MMF in combination with rapamycin and steroids in patients receiving marginal donor kidneys. Use of enteric-coated formulation of MMF allowing more therapeutic mycophenolic acid exposure is also underway.

Sirolimus

Sirolimus (rapamycin) is a macrolide antibiotic produced by *Streptomyces hygroscopicus* that has demonstrated potent immunosuppressive activity in a number of studies in both animals and humans. It has been approved in 1999 by the FDA for prophylaxis of acute rejection in renal transplant recipients after a series of clinical trials from Europe and United States demonstrated that, when used in combination with cyclosporine and steroids, it decreased the incidence of acute rejection episodes in the early posttransplant period, compared with either azathioprine or placebo. Another indication to withdraw cyclosporine when used in combination with sirolimus and steroids has also recently been approved by the FDA. Although it is structurally related to FK-506 and binds to FKBP, sirolimus has a distinct mechanism of action.[32] It forms a complex with the FKBP that binds with high affinity to the mammalian target of rapamycin (mTOR). This interaction causes dephosphorylation and inactivation of p70S6 kinase, which, when activated, stimulates the protein synthesis and cell cycle progression. This activity effectively blocks cytokine-driven (IL-2, IL-4, IL-15) T-cell proliferation by inhibiting G1 to S phase of the cell cycle. A clear synergistic effect with cyclosporine has been shown.

Although antagonistic to FK-506 in vitro, the intracellular pool of FKBP is so large that the two agents have been effectively used in renal transplant recipients *in vivo.* It has been demonstrated that simultaneous dosing of tacrolimus and sirolimus after transplantation is safe and that trough level monitoring is adequate to control therapy.

Sirolimus is a potent immunosuppressive drug. It has a relatively long half-life. It is metabolized by the same P450 enzyme system involved in the metabolism of CIs. It can be used both with and without a CI. Recent trials using sirolimus in combination with MMF and steroids demonstrated that sirolimus may be safely and effectively used as primary therapy for the prevention of acute rejection in kidney transplantation.[42] In another study, Oberbauer and colleagues[43] showed that early cyclosporine withdrawal followed by a sirolimus-steroids maintenance regimen resulted in long-term improvement in both renal function and blood pressure, without increased risk of graft loss or late acute rejection.

The drug is relatively safe and well tolerated.[44] Reported side effects include headache, leukopenia, thrombocytopenia, hyperlipidemia, diarrhea, delayed wound healing, and lymphocele (Table 35–4). Nephrotoxicity does not occur when the drug is used without a CI but it can exacerbate CI nephrotoxicity. Animal studies showed that rapamycin also inhibits smooth muscle cell proliferation and migration as well as chronic graft vessel disease in rat transplant models of chronic rejection, which raises hope that this agent may have a role in the prevention of clinical chronic rejection as well.[45]

Interestingly, in a recent study, Morice and colleagues[46] showed that a rapamycin-eluting coronary stent compared to a standard stent showed considerable promise for the prevention of neointimal proliferation, restenosis and associated cardiac events in patients with coronary artery disease.

There is also evidence from animal studies that sirolimus can block regional tumor growth and metastatic progression of the tumor by showing an antiangiogenic effect linked to a decrease in production of vascular endothelial growth factor (VEGF) and to markedly inhibited response of vascular endothelial cells to stimulation by VEGF, as well as increasing the expression of E-cadherin.[47,48] In another animal model, sirolimus inhibited the growth of EBV-associated B-cell lymphomas.[49] Thus, the use of sirolimus may be of value for the management of posttransplant malignancy. Future trials as well as the long-term results of current trials with sirolimus can shed light to this issue.

Since it probably has no adverse effects on renal function (when used without a CI), sirolimus has been used in patients with delayed graft function. By using a CI-free protocol of antibody induction, sirolimus, mycophenolate mofetil, and prednisone in recipients with marginal donor kidneys or delayed graft function, Shaffer and colleagues[50] recently demonstrated low rates of acute rejection and excellent early patient and graft survival. Conversely, there are concerns that, when used with a CI, sirolimus could exacerbate delayed graft function; this requires further study. Sirolimus use has also

Table 35–4 Potential Adverse Effects of Rapamycin

Hypercholesterolemia
Leukopenia
Thrombocytopenia
Anemia
Arthralgias
Diarrhea
Wound complications
Lymphocele
Hypokalemia
Hypophosphatemia
Eyelid edema
Interstitial pneumonitis
Worsening of delayed graft function (DGF)

been reported in hemolytic-uremic syndrome, in steroid-free regimens, as a rescue agent in severe acute rejection, and as a substitute for CI in patients with chronic rejection.

Everolimus or SDZ RAD is a derivative of sirolimus. Its half-life is shorter than that of sirolimus. Trials are in progress in which it is being tested in combination with calcineurin inhibitors in renal transplant recipients.

Leflunomide

Leflunomide is a synthetic isoxazole derivative with anti-inflammatory and antiviral properties, which inhibits pyrimidine nucleotide synthesis with secondary effects on IL-2, transforming growth factor alpha and antibody production. It has been reported to prevent acute rejection and delay progression of chronic allograft nephropathy as well as prolong graft survival in different animal models. Interestingly, it has inhibitory effects on herpes virus replication. Side effects include anemia, gastrointestinal toxicity, elevated liver enzymes, and weight loss. Studies using leflunomide and its analogue, FK778, are being tested in phase II trials.

SUMMARY

For many years, the mainstay of immunosuppressive therapy in kidney transplantation has been the combination of Sandimmune, azathioprine, and prednisone. In recent years, the introduction of cyclosporine microemulsion, tacrolimus, mycophenolate mofetil, sirolimus, and leflunomide for maintenance therapy has provided transplant physicians with a wide variety of choices in order to be able to pick and choose the best individual immunosuppressive regimen for the individual patient.

Numerous potent immunosuppressive agents are in the design stage or undergoing trial. The questions such as whether these new agents are providing more specific immunosuppression, or what would be the best combination to achieve maximum efficacy and minimum harm, or whether these agents would prevent chronic rejection and improve long-term graft survival, and, finally, whether these agents affect tolerance induction still remain unanswered.

ACKNOWLEDGMENT

A special note of appreciation is due Mrs. Nadine Cline, whose patience in dealing with cross-country manuscript preparation was most important for completion of this project.

References

1. Cecka JM: The UNOS Scientific Renal Transplant Registry. *In* Cecka JM, Terasaki PI (eds): Clinical Transplants 1996. Los Angeles, UCLA Tissue Typing Laboratory, 1995, pp 1–14.
2. Wechter WJ, Brodie JA, Morrell RM, et al: Antithymocyte globulin (ATGAM) in renal allograft recipients: Multicenter trials using a 14-dose regimen. Transplantation 1979; 28(4):294–302.
3. Sommer BG, Henry M, Ferguson RM: Sequential antilymphoblast globulin and cyclosporine for renal transplantation. Transplantation 1987; 43:85–90.
4. Murphy B, Goral S, Sayegh MH, et al: The role of anti-lymphocyte induction therapy in renal transplantation. Chicago, 14th Annual Meeting of the American Society of Transplant Physicians, May 14–16, 1995.
5. Shield CF, Edwards EB, Davies DB, et al: Antilymphocyte induction therapy in cadaver renal transplantation: A retrospective, multicenter United Network for Organ Sharing Study. Transplantation 1997; 63(9):1257–1263.
6. Szczech LA, Berlin JA, Feldman HI: The effect of antilymphocyte induction therapy on renal allograft survival. A meta-analysis of individual patient-level data. Anti-Lymphocyte Antibody Induction Therapy Study Group. Ann Intern Med 1998; 128(10): 817-826.
7. Adu D, Cockwell P, Ives NJ, et al: Interleukin-2 receptor monoclonal antibodies in renal transplantation: Meta-analysis of randomized trials. BMJ 2003; 326(7393):789-793.
8. Halloran P, Mathew T, Tomlanovich S, et al: International Mycophenolate Mofetil Renal Transplant Study Groups: Mycophenolate mofetil in renal allograft recipients: A pooled efficacy analysis of three randomized, double-blind, clinical studies in prevention of rejection. Transplantation 1997; 63(1):39–47.
9. Helderman JH, Van Buren DH, Amend WJ Jr, et al: Chronic immunosuppression of the renal transplant patient. J Am Soc Nephrol 1994; 4(suppl 8):S2–S9.
10. Kunz R, Neumayer HH: Maintenance therapy with triple versus double immunosuppressive regimen in renal transplantation: A meta-analysis. Transplantation 1997; 63(3):386–392.
11. Hricik DE, O'Toole MA, Schulak JA, et al: Steroid-free immunosuppression in cyclosporine-treated renal transplant recipients: A meta-analysis. J Am Soc Nephrol 1993; 4:1300–1305.
12. Sinclair NR: Canadian Multicentre Transplant Study Group: Low-dose steroid therapy in cyclosporine-treated renal transplant recipients with well-functioning grafts. Can Med Assoc J 1992; 147(5):645–657.
13. Ahsan N, Hricik D, Matas A, et al: Prednisone withdrawal in kidney transplant recipients on cyclosporine and mycophenolate mofetil: A prospective randomized study. Steroid Withdrawal Study Group. Transplantation 1999; 68(12):1865-1874.
14. Vanrenterghem Y, Lebranchu Y, Hene R, et al: Double-blind comparison of two corticosteroid regimens plus mycophenolate mofetil and cyclosporine for prevention of acute renal allograft rejection. Transplantation 2000; 70(9):1352-1359.
15. Sarwal MM, Yorgin PD, Alexander S, et al: Promising early outcomes with a novel, complete steroid avoidance protocol in pediatric renal transplantation. Transplantation 2001; 72(1): 13-21.
16. Matas AJ, Ramcharan T, Paraskevas S, et al: Rapid discontinuation of steroids in living donor kidney transplantation: A pilot study. Am J Transplant 2001; 1(3):278-283.
17. Feutren G, Wong R, Jin J, et al: Safety and tolerability of Neoral in transplant recipients. Transplant Proc 1996; 28(4):2177–2182.
18. Mueller EA, Kovarik JM, Van Bree JB, et al: Pharmacokinetics and tolerability of a microemulsion formulation of cyclosporine in renal allograft recipients: A concentration-controlled comparison with the commercial formulation. Transplantation 1994; 57:1178–1182.
19. Kazancioglu R, Goral S, Shockley SL, et al: A systematic examination of estimates of cyclosporine area under the curve in renal transplant recipients. Transplantation 2002; 73(2):301-302.
20. Levy G, Thervet E, Lake J, et al: Patient management by Neoral C2 monitoring: An international consensus statement. Transplantation 2002; 73(9):S12-S18.
21. Pescovitz MD, Barone G, Choc MG Jr, et al: Safety and tolerability of cyclosporine microemulsion versus cyclosporine: Two-year data in primary renal allograft recipients. A report of the Neoral Study Group. Transplantation 1997; 63(5):778–780.
22. Chapman JR, O'Connell PJ, Bovington KJ, et al: Reversal of cyclosporine malabsorption in diabetic recipients of simultaneous

pancreas and kidney transplant using a microemulsion formulation. Transplantation 1996; 61(12):1699–1704.

23. Helderman JH: Lessons from the Neoral global database for renal transplantation. Transplant Proc 1999; 31(3):1659-1663.
24. Kahan BD, Welsh M, Schoenberg L, et al: Variable oral absorption of cyclosporine: A biopharmaceutical risk factor for chronic renal allograft rejection. Transplantation 1996; 62(5): 599–606.
25. The Canadian Neoral Renal Transplantation Group: A randomized, prospective multicenter pharmacoepidemiologic study of cyclosporine microemulsion in stable renal graft recipients. Transplantation 1996; 62(12):1744–1752.
26. Neumayer HH, Budde K, Farber L, et al: Conversion to microemulsion cyclosporine in stable renal transplant patients: Results after one year. Clin Nephrol 1996; 45(5):326–331.
27. Roza A, Tomlanovich S, Merion R, et al: Conversion of stable renal allograft recipients to a bioequivalent cyclosporine formulation. Transplantation 2002; 74(7):1013-1017.
28. Woodle ES, Thistlethwaite R, Gordon JH, et al: A multicenter trial of FK506 (tacrolimus) therapy in refractory acute allograft rejection. Transplantation 1996; 62(5):594–599.
29. Laskow DA, Vincenti F, Neylan JF, et al: An open-label, concentration-ranging trial of FK506 in primary kidney transplantation. Transplantation 1996; 62(7):900–905.
30. Pirsch JD, Miller J, Deierhoi MH, et al: Comparison of tacrolimus (FK506) and cyclosporine for immunosuppression after cadaveric renal transplantation. Transplantation 1997; 63(7):977–983.
31. First MR, Gerber DA, Hariharan S, et al: Posttransplant diabetes mellitus in kidney allograft recipients: Incidence, risk factors, and management. Transplantation 2002; 73(3):379-386.
32. Kasiske BL, Snyder JJ, Gilbertson D, et al: Diabetes mellitus after kidney transplantation in the United States. Am J Transplant 2003; 3(2):178-185.
33. Gloor JM, Cohen AJ, Lager DJ, et al: Subclinical rejection in tacrolimus-treated renal transplant recipients. Transplantation 2002; 73(12):1965-1968.
34. Vincent F, Jensik SC, Filo RS, et al: A long-term comparison of tacrolimus (FK506) and cyclosporine in kidney transplantation: Evidence for improved allograft survival at five years. Transplantation 2002; 73(5):775-782.
35. European Mycophenolate Mofetil Cooperative Study Group: Placebo-controlled study of mycophenolate mofetil combined with cyclosporine and corticosteroids for prevention of acute rejection. Lancet 1995; 345(8961):1321–1325.
36. The Tricontinental Mycophenolate Mofetil Renal Transplantation Study Group: A blinded, randomized clinical trial of mycophenolate mofetil for the prevention of acute rejection in cadaveric renal transplantation. Transplantation 1996; 61(7): 1029–1037.
37. Sollinger HW: U.S. Renal Transplant Mycophenolate Study Group: Mycophenolate mofetil for the prevention of acute rejection in primary cadaveric renal allograft recipients. Transplantation 1995; 60(3):225–232.
38. The Mycophenolate Mofetil Renal Refractory Rejection Study Group: Mycophenolate mofetil for the treatment of refractory, acute, cellular renal transplant rejection. Transplantation 1996; 61(5):722–729.
39. Ojo AO, Meier-Kriesche HU, Hanson JA, et al: Mycophenolate mofetil reduces late renal allograft loss independent of acute rejection. Transplantation 2000; 69(11):2405-2409.
40. Meier-Kriesche HU, Steffen BJ, Hochberg AM, et al: Mycophenolate mofetil versus azathioprine therapy is associated with a significant protection against long-term renal allograft function deterioration. Transplantation 2003; 75(8):1341-1346.
41. Molnar-Kimber KL: Mechanism of action of rapamycin (sirolimus, Rapamune). Transplant Proc 1996; 28(2):964–969.
42. Kreis H, Cisterne JM, Land W, et al: Sirolimus in association with mycophenolate mofetil induction for the prevention of acute graft rejection in renal allograft recipients. Transplantation 2000; 69(7):1252-1260.
43. Oberbauer R, Kreis H, Johnson RW, et al: Long-term improvement in renal function with sirolimus after early cyclosporine withdrawal in renal transplant recipients: 2-year results of the Rapamune Maintenance Regimen Study. Transplantation 2003; 76(2):364-370.
44. Brattstrom C, Tyden G, Sawe J, et al: A randomized, double-blind, placebo-controlled study to determine safety, tolerance, and preliminary pharmacokinetics of ascending single doses of orally administered sirolimus (rapamycin) in stable renal transplant recipients. Transplant Proc 1996; 28(2):985–986.
45. Schmid C, Heeman U, Azuma H, et al: Comparison of rapamycin, RS 61443, cyclosporine, and low-dose heparin as treatment for transplant vasculopathy in a rat model of chronic allograft rejection. Transplant Proc 1995; 27:438–439.
46. Morice MC, Serruys PW, Sousa JE, et al: A randomized comparison of a sirolimus-eluting stent with a standard stent for coronary revascularization. N Engl J Med 2002; 346(23):1773-1780.
47. Luan FL, Hojo M, Maluccio M, et al: Rapamycin blocks tumor progression: Unlinking immunosuppression from antitumor efficacy. Transplantation 2002; 73(10):1565-1572.
48. Guba M, von Breitenbuch P, Steinbauer M, et al: Rapamycin inhibits primary and metastatic tumor growth by antiangiogenesis: Involvement of vascular endothelial growth factor. Nat Med 2002; 8(2):128-135.
49. Nepomuceno RR, Balatoni CE, Natkunam Y, et al: Rapamycin inhibits the interleukin 10 signal transduction pathway and the growth of Epstein Barr virus B-cell lymphomas. Cancer Res 2003; 63(15):4472-4480.
50. Shaffer D, Langone A, Nylander WA, et al: A pilot protocol of a calcineurin-inhibitor free regimen for kidney transplant recipients of marginal donor kidneys or with delayed graft function. Clin Transpl 2003; l17(S9):31-34.

Chapter 36

Diagnosis and Therapy of Graft Dysfunction

Phuong-Thu T. Pham, M.D. • Cynthia Nast, M.D. •
Phuong-Chi T. Pham, M.D. • Gabriel M. Danovitch, M.D.

Important advances in immunosuppressive therapy and refinement in surgical techniques have allowed renal transplantation to become the preferred treatment modality for virtually all suitable candidates with end-stage renal disease. Ideally, a renal allograft recipient receives a high quality donor kidney, undergoes a smooth surgical grafting, develops an immediate post-transplantation diuresis with a steady improvement in renal function, and achieves excellent renal function with long-term stability. Although such idealized course is realized for many patients, graft dysfunction is an incessant threat throughout the graft lifetime for many others. The etiology and management of graft dysfunction vary over time. In this chapter, graft dysfunction will be discussed in three arbitrarily defined phases:

1. *Delayed graft function* (DGF), occurring in the immediate post-transplantation period
2. *Early graft dysfunction,* occurring in the first 2 to 3 months post-transplantation months
3. *Late graft dysfunction,* occurring thereafter

DELAYED GRAFT FUNCTION

Definition

Despite the exponential growth in renal transplantation, no universally defined criteria for delayed graft function have been established. Nevertheless, various indices, including urine volume, dialysis requirement, and serum creatinine, have been used by transplant nephrologists to diagnose "delayed graft function."

In general, a urine output greater than 20 mL/kg/day in the immediate postoperative period is a good clinical indicator of adequate renal function. Using urine output as an indication for early allograft function, however, is limited in cases where large urine volume is still being produced by the native kidneys. A large urine output from the native kidneys in the immediate postoperative period may be mistaken for an early functioning allograft. Similarly, in these same patients, no increase in urine output postoperatively does not necessarily indicate delayed graft function.

In studies evaluating the causes and management of DGF, a modified definition of "the need for more than one dialysis" is sometimes applied to take into account the need for a single postoperative dialysis for the management of hyperkalemia or fluid overload or the safe administration of blood products.[1] Using the need for dialysis alone to define DGF, however, may lead to underdiagnosis, particularly if there is some residual native kidney function. It has been proposed that an elevated serum creatinine concentration (>400 mmol/L) 1 week after transplantation should be used as a more sensitive and specific measure of DGF.[2]

Differential Diagnosis

The differential diagnosis of DGF is shown in Table 36–1. Although most cadaveric kidneys with DGF are afflicted with the clinicopathologic entity of acute tubular necrosis (ATN), it is important to not use the term loosely lest other causes of DGF not be considered. Post-transplantation ATN, like ATN in the nontransplant setting, is essentially a diagnosis of exclusion, and the diagnostic algorithms in the transplant and nontransplant settings have much in common. A systematic approach to the evaluation of DGF may be divided into prerenal (or preglomerular type), intrinsic, and postrenal. Although uncommon, vascular causes of DGF must be excluded, particularly in the early postoperative period (see Table 36–1). The term *primary nonfunction* should best be applied to kidneys that never function, and allograft nephrectomy is usually indicated.

Prerenal Causes of DGF

Severe intravascular volume depletion or significant fall in blood pressures is usually suggested by a careful review of patients' preoperative history and intraoperative report. Knowing patients' dialysis dry weight and their preoperative weight may be invaluable in the assessment of their volume status in the immediate postoperative period. Intraoperative Swan-Ganz placement for continuous monitoring of central venous or pulmonary artery wedge pressure may be useful in assessing the volume status of patients with cardiomyopathy and/or coronary artery disease.

Both calcineurin inhibitors (CNI) cyclosporine and, to a lesser extent, tacrolimus have been shown to cause a dose-related reversible afferent arteriolar vasoconstriction and "preglomerular type" allograft dysfunction that manifests clinically as delayed recovery of allograft function. Angiotensin-converting enzyme inhibitors or angiotensin receptor blockers, Amphotericin B, nonsteroidal anti-inflammatory drugs (NSAIDs), and radiocontrast dye are commonly used drugs that may potentially precipitate or exacerbate acute preglomerular type allograft dysfunction. A thorough chart review should focus on the recent use of nephrotoxic medications and perioperative blood pressure curves.

Intrinsic Renal Causes of DGF

Intrinsic renal causes of DGF typically include acute tubular necrosis (ATN), acute rejection, infection, thrombotic

Table 36–1 Differential Diagnosis of Delayed Graft Function (DGF)

Prerenal (or Preglomerular Type)
Volume contraction
Nephrotoxic drugs (see text)
Vascular Complications
Arterial or venous thrombosis
Renal artery stenosis
Intrinsic Renal
Acute tubular necrosis
Accelerated acute or acute rejection
Thrombotic microangiopathy
Recurrence of primary glomerular disease (particularly FSGS)
Postrenal
Catheter obstruction
Perinephric fluid collection (lymphocele, urine leak, hematoma)
Ureteral obstruction:
Intrinsic (blood clots, poor reimplantation, ureteral slough)
Extrinsic (ureteral kinking)
Neurogenic bladder
Benign prostatic hypertrophy

(Adapted from Pham PT, Pham PC, Wilkinson AH: Management of the transplant recipient in the early postoperative period. *In* Davidson (ed): Oxford Textbook of Clinical Nephrology, 3rd ed. New York, Oxford University Press [In press]).

microangiopathy, or recurrence of glomerular disease affecting the native kidneys.

Acute Tubular Necrosis

Post-transplant acute tubular necrosis is the most common cause of DGF. The two terms are often used interchangeably, although not all cases of DGF are caused by ATN. Its incidence varies widely among centers and has been reported to occur in 20% to 25% of patients (range 10% to 60%).[3–8] The difference in the incidence reported may, in part, be due to the more liberal use of organs from marginal donors by some centers but not by others and/or the difference in the criteria used to define DGF. Unless an allograft biopsy is performed, post-transplant ATN should be a diagnosis of exclusion. Both donor and/or recipient factors are important determinant(s) of early allograft dysfunction (Table 36–2).

Pathogenic Mechanisms

ATN found in the post-transplant setting is essentially an ischemic injury that may be synergistically exaggerated by both immunologic and nephrotoxic insults.[1] All transplanted kidneys are subject to injury at various steps in the transplantation process—from donor death to organ procurement, surgical reanastomosis, and postoperative course. Understanding, identifying, and addressing the potential for injury at every step of this complex process are critical to the prevention of post-transplant ATN. Some degree of ischemic injury is invariably unavoidable in cadaveric renal transplantation.

Table 36–2 Risk Factors for Delayed Graft Function (DGF) Due to Acute Tubular Necrosis (ATN) in Cadaveric Renal Transplantation

Donor Factors	Recipient Factors
Premorbid Factors	**Premorbid Factors**
Age (<10 or >50)	African American (compared to Caucasians)
Donor hypertension	Peripheral vascular disease
Donor macrovascular or microvascular disease	Presensitization (PRA>50)
Cause of death (cerebrovascular vs. traumatic)	Reallograft transplantation
Preoperative Donor Characteristics	**Perioperative and Postoperative Factors**
Brain–death stress	Recipient volume contraction
Hypotension, shock	Early high dose calcineurin inhibitors
Prolonged use of vasopressors	+/– Early use of OKT3
Preprocurement ATN	
Non–heart beating donor	
Nephrotoxic agents	
Organ Procurement Surgery	
Hypotension prior to cross-clamping of aorta	
Traction on renal vasculatures	
Cold storage flushing solutions	
Kidney Preservation	
Prolonged warm ischemia time (+/– contraindication to donation)	
Prolonged cold ischemia time	
Cold storage vs. machine perfusion	
Intraoperative Factors	
Intraoperative hemodynamic instability	
Prolonged rewarm time (anastomotic time)	

(Adapted from Pham PT, Pham PC, Wilkinson AH: Management of the transplant recipient in the early postoperative period. *In* Davidson (ed): Oxford Textbook of Clinical Nephrology, 3rd ed. New York, Oxford University Press [In press]).

Much can be inferred about the cellular and molecular mechanisms of post-transplant ATN from observations in nontransplant animal models and ATN in native kidneys. Readers are referred to extensive reviews of this topic.[9–13] In essence, during ischemia, cellular metabolism continues and the resulting shift to anaerobic metabolism leads to accumulation of lactic acid, failure of sodium-potassium-ATPase pumps, loss of cell polarization, cell swelling, and subsequent lysis with release of cytotoxic oxygen-free radicals.

Because of the unique sequence of events leading to organ transplantation, the transplanted kidney is particularly susceptible to reperfusion injury. The reintroduction of oxygen into tissues with a high concentration of oxygen-free radicals leads to the production of superoxide anion and hydrogen peroxide leading to lipid peroxidation of cell membranes. This process may be responsible for the commonly occurring clinical sequence, where an early post-transplantation diuresis is followed by oliguria within hours.

Damage to the vascular epithelium leads to the release of vasoactive molecules that may be responsible for the hemodynamic changes typical of ATN.[11] The term *vasomotor nephropathy* may be more appropriate than ATN because it describes a physiologically altered state that may not be necessarily accompanied by tubular necrosis histologically.[12] As a result of increased renovascular resistance and decreased glomerular permeability, the glomerular filtration rate (GFR) falls. In ATN, tubules obstructed with cellular debris further reduce the GFR and the increased intrarenal pressure due to edema further reduces blood flow.[13] Although blood flow to the renal cortex is reduced, there is a relatively greater reduction in GFR and tubular function, which accounts for the common findings of "good flow and poor excretion" on scintigraphic studies.[14] The alterations in vascular resistance and increased intracapsular pressure result in the increased resistive index and reduced or reversed diastolic blood flow observed on Doppler ultrasound.

Although ischemic injury has been regarded as a major risk factor for the development of post-transplant ATN, several lines of evidence suggest that immunologic factors may be equally important. The former is suggested by the observation that the incidence of DGF was significantly higher among recipients of cadaveric kidneys than for living-donor transplants and the latter by the observation that DGF is more prevalent in recipients of re-allograft transplants compared to those of primary transplant, particularly if they have high levels of preformed panel-reactive antibodies.[3,15] A positive flow cytometry cross-match in the absence of a positive standard complement-dependent cytotoxicity cross-match has also been shown to be associated with a greater incidence of ATN and delayed lowering of the post-transplant plasma serum creatinine level.[16] Presumably, the immunologic factors make the newly transplanted kidney more susceptible to ischemic injury.

The Effect of ATN on Host Immunogenicity

Some but not all evidence suggest that ATN may contribute to the upregulation and exposure of histocompatibility antigens and increase the immunogenicity of the transplanted kidney, hence enhance its susceptibility to both acute and chronic rejections.[17–18] The stress of brain death itself likely has a similar effect. In a rat study, explosive brain death has been shown to be associated with upregulation of macrophage (IL-1, IL-6, and TNFα) and T-cell–associated products (IL-2 and IF-α) in the peripheral organs, rendering them more susceptible to subsequent host inflammatory and immunologic responses.[19] Nitric oxide produced by the inducible nitric oxide synthase (iNOS) enzymes in response to ischemic cell injury has been suggested to a play a key role in the link between ischemic reperfusion injury and graft rejection.[20] Renal epithelial regeneration after ischemic damage is mediated by growth factors and cytokines, such as epidermal growth factors (EGF) and transforming growth factor β (TGF-β), which may facilitate the development of the low-grade inflammation and fibrosis that occurs in chronic rejection.[21] Injury, in the form of ATN, leads to inflammation, which, in turn, facilitates an immune response that causes further injury.[15,17] A number of studies have shown that in the long-term, ATN kidneys that do not develop rejection do as well as non-ATN kidneys that do not develop rejection, lending support to the theory that it is the immunologic consequences of ATN that are responsible for its prognostic significance.[22] Yet studies on the impact of DGF (presumably due to ATN) with or without early acute rejection on long-term graft survival have yielded conflicting results (discussed in a later section).

Histology

ATN in the allograft is similar to that in the native kidney. Tubular epithelial cells show necrosis, often with sloughed, degenerated, or apoptotic epithelial cells in the tubular lumina, a feature more prominent in ATN involving transplanted kidneys.[23] Proximal cell brush border staining is focally absent with flattening of tubular cells, and there may be regeneration in the form of mitotic figures (Figure 36–1).[24] The interstitium is variably edematous, with a minimal or patchy interstitial lymphocytic infiltrate; however, there is no associated inflammation in the walls of tubules. No specific changes of glomeruli or the vasculature are found in ATN.

Prediction and Prevention

Kidneys from living, related, or biologically unrelated donors rarely suffer from DGF, whereas the incidence of DGF in recipients of cadaveric transplants varies from 10% to 60%.[3–8] Living donors undergo an extensive evaluation process to ensure their health and that of their kidneys, and the circumstances of live donor organ harvesting permit minimalization of ischemic damage to the organ. On the contrary, the circumstances of sudden death are always, in varying degrees, detrimental to renal function, and some degree of ischemic damage is inevitable, considering the complexities of the cadaveric organ procurement process.

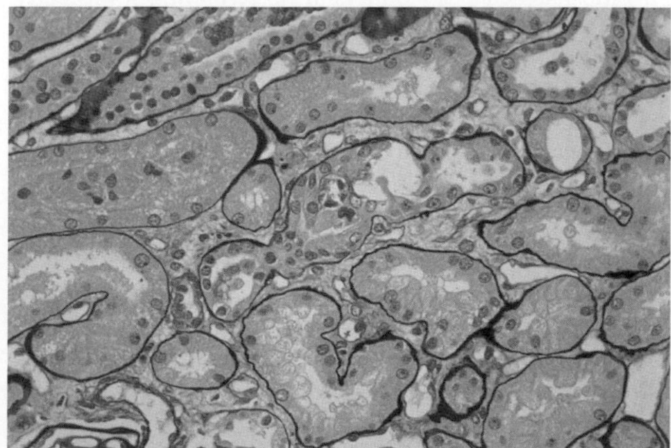

Figure 36–1 Acute tubular necrosis. Tubular cells show flattening and necrosis and focally are desquamated into the tubular lumina. The central tubule contains calcium oxalate in the lumen, a product of cellular debris. (Jones methenamine silver × 250)

Donor factors before the procurement of cadaveric organs are important predictors of early and late graft function. Kidneys from older donors have a higher incidence of ATN,[25] a finding that is reminiscent of the clinical observation that older patients in the nontransplantation setting are also more susceptible to ATN when faced with ischemic or nephrotoxic insult.[26] The common factor linking older age to ATN is probably diminished capacity of the aging vasculature to vasodilate adequately to protect the transplant from anoxic damage.

In this respect, donor death from traumatic injury is less likely to be associated with ATN than death from cerebrovascular causes because the trauma victim is more likely to have been younger and healthier than a stroke victim.[27] Even the "ideal" trauma victim is likely to have experienced an episode of hypotension, and a history of fluctuating or deteriorating renal function is not uncommon. Kidneys from young donors typically recover from pre-transplantation injury, whereas the prognosis for kidneys from older donors with pre-transplantation impairment of function is often poor, and it has previously been suggested that such kidneys should not be routinely transplanted.[28] However, with the ever-increasing disparity between supply and demand for cadaveric donor kidneys, expanded criteria donor kidneys (ECD) have been increasingly used by some centers. These kidneys are defined by donor characteristics that are associated with a 70% greater risk of kidney graft failure when compared to a reference group of nonhypertensive donors of ages 10 through 39 years whose cause of death was not cerebrovascular accident (CVA) and whose terminal creatinine was less than or equal to 1.5 mg/dL. The donor factors associated with this increased relative rate of graft failure include age 60 or older, or ages 50 to 59, with at least 2 comorbid factor. The latter may include CVA as a cause of death, hypertension, and/or terminal creatinine greater than 1.5 mg/dL (Table 36–3). To optimize allograft outcome using these "marginal" kidneys, the United Network of Organ Sharing (UNOS) has implemented a system to minimize cold ischemia time and to expedite ECD kidney placement. Currently, the allocation of ECD kidneys is based on prior identification of and consent by ECD wait-listed candidates, pre-procurement tissue typing of ECD kidneys, and abbreviated time period (2 hours) for placement of zero mismatched ECD kidneys. If no zero antigen mismatch transplant candidate is identified, the ECD kidney will be allocated to all other "pre-identified" candidates by waiting time alone, first locally, then regionally, and then nationally.

Despite the efforts to decrease cold ischemia time, the use of ECD kidneys inevitably increases the incidence of post-transplantation ATN. Similarly, attempts to bolster the cadaveric donor supply by the use of non–heart-beating donors (NHB) that are, by definition, susceptible to warm ischemia resulted in an elevated DGF rates.[28] Analysis of the U.S. Renal Data System database revealed that recipients of NHB donor organs experienced nearly twice the incidence of DGF compared with heart-beating donors (42.4% vs. 23.3%, respectively). Nonetheless, NHB donor transplants experienced comparable allograft survival when compared with cadaveric transplant at 6-year follow up (73.2% vs. 72.5%, respectively: P=NS). Interestingly, patient survival was greater at 6 years for NHB compared with cadaveric renal transplant recipients, although this did not reach statistical significance. Significant factors for allograft loss for NHB donor organ recipients include repeat transplant, DGF, donor age older than 35 years, and head trauma as a cause of initial injury.[29] Acknowledging these risk factors may maximize the use of cadaveric donor organs while minimizing the risk of accepting kidneys with primary nonfunction.

Table 36–3 Factors that Determine Expanded Criteria Donors (Adapted from UNOS)

Donor Condition	Donor Age Categories 50–59	≥60
CVA + HTN + Creat >1.5	X	X
CVA + HTN	X	X
CVA + Creat >1.5	X	X
HTN + Creat >1.5	X	X
CVA		X
HTN		X
Creat >1.5		X
None of the above		X

X, expanded criteria donor; *CVA*, cerebrovascular accident (as the cause of death); *HTN*, hypertension; *Creat*, creatinine.

In selected cases, dual transplant of ECD kidneys have been offered to older recipients with excellent short-term allograft outcome, comparable to that of recipients of single non-ECD control kidneys.[30] It has been suggested that the salutary effect of dual kidney transplant is due to increasing viable nephron mass. Experimental studies in rats have shown that increasing the number of viable nephron mass by dual kidney transplantation prevented the progressive deterioration in renal function that occurred in control rats receiving single kidney.[31] Studies on long-term graft function and survival in human recipients of ECD kidneys are currently limited. In a single center retrospective study consisting of 10 dual renal transplant recipients and 10 age matched single cadaver kidney recipients, allograft function and the incidence of graft loss at 4-year follow-up were comparable between the two groups.[32]

Organ Procurement and Preservation

Early ischemic injury adversely affects both short- and long-term allograft function and/or survival. In cadaveric kidneys the earliest injury begins with organ procurement and preservation. The technical aspect of donor management and organ procurement in the era of multiorgan harvesting are beyond the scope of this chapter. The purpose of donor management is to maintain adequate organ perfusion before rapid cooling and flushing of the kidneys to minimize warm ischemia. The warm ischemia time refers to the period between circulatory arrest and the commencement of cold storage.[33] Ischemia at body temperature can be tolerated for only a few minutes, after which irreversible cellular injury begins to occur such that within about 30 minutes, the organ becomes nonviable. The cold ischemia time refers to the period of cold storage or machine perfusion. Fortunately, for the purposes of transplantation, anaerobic metabolism can maintain renal cellular energy requirements for up to 48 hours, provided the organ is cooled to about 4°C with an appropriate preservation solution.[34] Increasing both the warm and cold ischemia times leads to a progressive decline in graft survival rates and an increase in the incidence of DGF.[33] Ideally, kidneys are transplanted without significant warm ischemia and with cold ischemia time of less than 24 hours, although longer cold ischemia may be acceptable.

Organ Preservation: Collins Solution versus University of Wisconsin Solution

Although the method of kidney preservation differs between centers, simple cold storage is currently the most widely used technique. The goal of preservation is to maximize ischemic tolerance during anaerobic metabolism and to minimize ischemic reperfusion injury. Collins solution was used for many years for flushing and for organ preservation until the 1990s, when University of Wisconsin solution started to gain popularity. University of Wisconsin solution has been shown to be superior to Collins solution in reducing the rate of DGF and in extending cold ischemia time.[8,35] Both solutions have high potassium content and are hyperosmolar. UW solution contains lactobionate, raffinose, and hydroxyethyl starch as osmotic component, whereas Collins solution contains glucose. UW solution also contains glutathione, adenosine, and the free-radical scavenger allopurinol, and it has a higher viscosity than that of Collins solution. Although the higher viscosity of Wisconsin solution may impede a sufficient initial flush, glutathione content in UW solution may serve to facilitate regeneration of cellular adenosine triphosphate (ATP) and to maintain membrane integrity, whereas during reperfusion, adenosine may provide the substrate for regeneration of ATP. Newer solutions with increasing chemical stability, lower potassium content, and lower viscosity are currently in the investigational stages. Although controversies remain regarding the relative benefits of cold storage versus pulsatile perfusion of the newly procured organ during the period of cold ischemia, pulsatile preservation is preferred by some centers.[36] A number of studies have shown that pulsatile perfusion is associated with a lower incidence of DGF and an improvement in early and long-term allograft function.[36,37] Pulsatile perfusion may also permit identification of kidney(s) that will likely result in primary nonfunction, hence sparing a recipient of the morbidity associated with the transplant operation and of the potential for the development of allosensitization.[36] In this respect, pulsatile perfusion of kidneys may aid in optimizing the use of marginal kidneys.

Rewarm time refers to the period between the removal of the kidney from cold storage and the completion of the vascular anastomosis.[33] The length of this period is strongly correlated to the incidence of DGF. Minimalization of this time period is, to a large extent, a reflection of surgical technical expertise. Ischemic damage can be minimized, if the kidney is kept cool with cold packs during this period. Before, during, and after recipient surgery, compulsive attention to the volume status helps minimize post-transplant dysfunction. If recipients require dialysis preoperatively, care should be taken to ensure that at the completion of the dialysis, the patient is at or above, but not below, his or her "dry weight" en route to the operating room. During the surgery, a state of mild volume expansion should be maintained, as permitted by the cardiovascular status of the patient. Central venous pressure should be maintained at about 10 mmHg with the use of isotonic saline and albumin infusions, and systolic blood pressure should be kept above 120 mmHg.[38]

Prevention Using Drug Therapy

Various pharmaceutical agents and protocol modifications have been made to encourage postoperative diuresis and to reduce the incidence or severity of ATN.[39] The use of diuretics is discussed in the section on management. Some immunosuppressive protocols do not permit the use of intravenous cyclosporine in the early postoperative period. Some programs use routine induction therapy with antilymphocytic agents in all patients, thereby obviating the vasoconstrictive effect of both cyclosporine and tacrolimus. More commonly, however, induction therapy is used selectively in patients with anticipated or established DGF. As ATN may render the allograft more susceptible to immunologic injury, the use of antilymphocyte antibodies in this setting may also be beneficial due to their potent immunosuppressive effect. Dopamine infusions at renal dose levels of 1 to 5 mcg/kg/min are used routinely at some centers to promote renal blood flow and to counteract cyclosporine-induced renal vasoconstriction.[39] The benefits of dopamine have not been proved in randomized trials, although its use has become institutionalized. Fenoldopam, a selective agonist of dopamine-1 receptors with both systemic and renal vasodilator properties, has been shown to reverse cyclosporine-mediated renal vasoconstriction in stable renal transplant recipients.[40] However, its role in reducing the incidence or severity of post-transplant DGF remains to be determined. Administration of calcium channel blockers to the donor or recipient, or at the time of the vascular anastomosis, has become routine in many transplant centers largely as a result of randomized clinical trials showing improved initial function with their use.[41] The presumed mechanism of action is by virtue of a direct vasodilatory effect. The kidney is often observed to "pink-up" when verapamil is injected into the renal artery during surgery.[38]

Randomized trials of allopurinol and other oxygen-free radical scavengers have not shown convincing benefit in graft function.[42] Although prostaglandins have been shown in animal models to minimize ischemic injury,[43] no benefit was found in a blinded trial of the prostaglandin E analogue enisoprost.[44] Similarly, although pretreatment with an antibody preparation against the intercellular adhesion molecule 1 (anti-ICAM-1) has been shown in experimental rat models to alleviate ischemic reperfusion injury, no benefit was found in a randomized multicenter trial of the anti-ICAM-1 monoclonal antibody enlimonab.[45] Blinded trials of atrial natriuretic factor administration have shown only marginal benefit in native kidney ATN,[46] and it is unlikely that this agent will find a place in the transplantation setting. In renal transplant recipients with DGF, it has been shown that neither renal vasoconstriction nor hypofiltration is alleviated by a progressive elevation of endogenous plasma atrial natriuretic peptide levels.[47]

Management of Delayed Graft Function

The differential diagnosis of DGF (see Table 36–1) must be considered before a patient is labeled with the most likely explanation—post-transplantation ATN. Most patients with DGF are oliguric or anuric. Knowledge of the patient's native urine output is critical to assess the origin of the early post-transplantation urine output. From the previous discussion on the etiology of DGF, it is clear that information about the donor kidney itself is critical. When the transplant is from a living donor, postoperative oliguria is rare because of the short ischemia time, and if it occurs, it must raise immediate concern regarding the vascularization of the graft. However, when a patient receives a cadaveric kidney from a nonideal donor, DGF may be anticipated. The mate kidney from a cadaveric donor often behaves in a similar manner, and information on its function can be useful.[1]

Anuria is easy to define. Oliguria in the peri-transplantation and early post-transplantation period usually refers to a urine output of less than about 50 mL/hr. Before the low urine output is therapeutically and diagnostically addressed, the patient's volume status and fluid balance must be assessed and the Foley catheter irrigated to ensure patency. If clots are present, the catheter should be removed while gentle suction is applied in an attempt to capture the offending clot. Thereafter, a large catheter may be required. If the Foley catheter is patent and the patient is clearly hypervolemic, up to 200 mg of furosemide should be given intravenously. If the patient is judged to be hypovolemic or if a confident clinical assessment cannot be made, a judicious isotonic saline should be given, followed by a large dose of furosemide. A suggested algorithmic approach to postoperative fluid management in an oliguric patient is shown in Figure 36–2.

Indications for dialysis in the transplant recipient with DGF are essentially the same as in any patient with postoperative renal dysfunction. Hyperkalemia is a persistent danger and must be monitored repeatedly and treated aggressively. It is usually safest to dialyze patients once the potassium level reaches the "high fives." Other treatment modalities, such as intravenous calcium, and glucose with insulin, are valuable temporizing measures but do not obviate the need for dialysis. Sodium polystyrene sulfonate (Kayexalate) should not be administered rectally in the early post-transplant period because it may induce colonic dilatation and predispose to perforation.[48]

Patients with DGF often become volume overloaded in the early post-transplantation period because they are frequently subjected to repeated volume challenges. It is not infrequent for such patients to be several kilograms over their dialysis dry weight, and this fluid gain may not be always clinically obvious. Ultrafiltration with or without dialysis may be required. When dialyzing post-transplantation patients who have DGF, one must take particular care to avoid hypotension, which may perpetuate the graft dysfunction. A bicarbonate bath and a biocompatible dialyzer should be used. In patients with established DGF, the dialysis requirement should be assessed daily until graft function improves.[1]

Diagnostic Studies in Persistent Oliguria or Anuria

Failure to respond to volume challenge and furosemide administration warrants further evaluation with diagnostic imaging studies to determine the cause of the early post-transplant oliguric state. The urgency of this evaluation partially depends on the clinical circumstances. If diuresis is anticipated, such as after a living donor kidney transplantation, diagnostic studies should be performed immediately—in the recovery room if necessary. If oliguria is anticipated, studies can usually be safely delayed by several hours.

Diagnostic studies are used to confirm the presence of blood flow to the graft and the absence of a urine leak or obstruction. Blood flow studies are performed scintigraphically or by Doppler ultrasound.[49] The typical scintigraphic finding in ATN is relatively good flow to the graft compared with poor excretion. If the flow study reveals no demonstrable blood flow, a prompt surgical reexploration is necessary to attempt to repair any vascular technical problem and diagnose hyperacute rejection. These kidneys are usually lost, however, and are removed during the second surgery. If adequate blood flow is visible with the scintiscan or Doppler studies, the possibility of ureteral obstruction or urinary leak needs to be considered and can be evaluated by the same imaging studies. In the first 24 hours after transplantation, as long as the Foley catheter has been providing good bladder drainage, the obstruction or leak is almost always at the ureterovesical junction and represents a technical problem that needs surgical correction.[38]

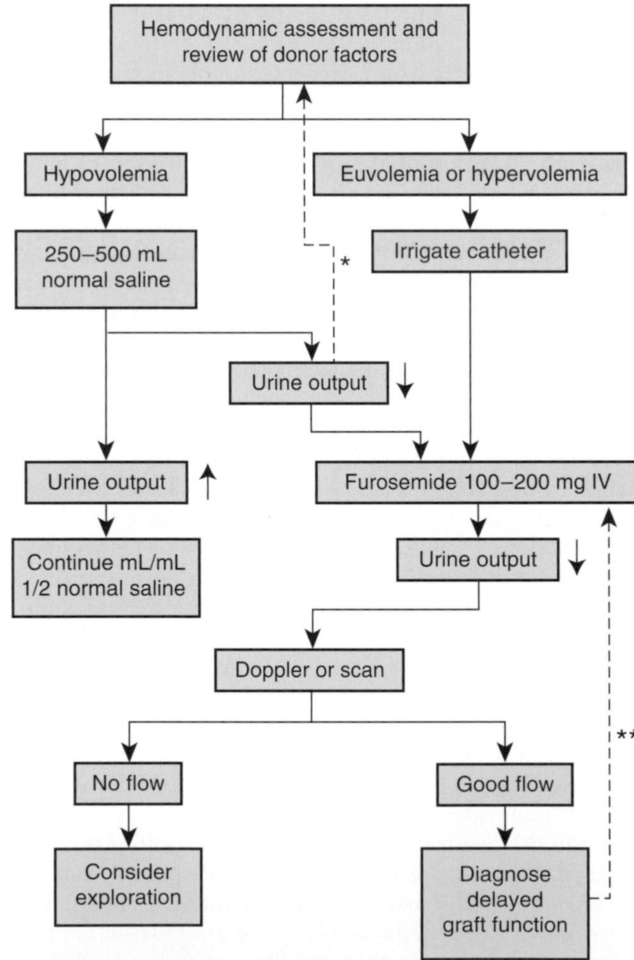

Figure 36–2 Algorithmic approach to post-transplant oliguria. *The volume challenge can be repeated, but only after careful reassessment of the volume status and fluid balance. **Repeated doses of intravenous furosemide or furosemide "drips" may be valuable in patients whose urine output fluctuates. Persistent oliguria will usually not respond to a repeat dose. (From Amend WJ, Vincenti I, Tomlanovich SJ: The first two post-transplant months. *In* Danovitch GM [ed]: Handbook of Kidney Transplantation. Boston, Little, Brown & Co, 2001, p 167.)

Other Causes of Graft Dysfunction During the First Week After Transplantation

Early Acute Rejection

Hyperacute Rejection

Rejection occurring immediately after transplantation or hyperacute rejection is due to presensitization and is mediated by antibodies to donor human leukocyte antigens (HLA). The rejection occurs after an anamnestic response, and a critical level of antibodies is produced that results in an irreversible vascular rejection. Hyperacute rejection may be evident before wound closure or it may be "hidden" and manifest itself as primary nonfunction of the kidney allograft.[50] Patients are usually anuric or oliguric and often have fever and graft tenderness. The renal scan shows little or no uptake, a finding that differentiates this cause of graft dysfunction from the much more frequent ATN. There may be evidence of intravascular coagulation. Prompt surgical exploration of the allograft is often indicated, and when in doubt, an intraoperative biopsy is performed to determine viability. Because of assiduous attention to the pretransplantation cross-match, it occurs rarely in modern transplantation practice.

Because hyperacute rejection is due to preformed antibodies, it is characterized morphologically by arterial and glomerular thrombi, which often contain neutrophils or may have accumulation of intravascular neutrophils as the initial event. The interstitium is edematous and variable parenchymal necrosis or infarction is observed, depending on the length of time from thrombosis to nephrectomy. There is no significant vascular or tubulointerstitial inflammation. Immunofluorescence microscopy reveals fibrin within the intravascular thrombi, and immunoglobulin M (IgM), IgG, C3, and fibrin may be found lining portions of the arterial and capillary lumens. In this setting, most allografts need to be removed.[51]

Accelerated Acute Rejection

Accelerated acute rejection or delayed hyperacute rejection occurs within 24 hours to a few days after transplantation and may involve both humoral and cellular immune mechanisms. Accelerated acute rejection probably represents a delayed amnestic response to prior sensitization and may be seen after donor-specific transfusions in recipients of living-donor transplant due to a primed T-cell response.[52] HLA allosensitization through repeat transplants, multiple pregnancies, or multiple transfusions are well-substantiated risk factors for hyperacute or accelerated acute rejection. However, with the current sensitive cross-matching techniques, such as flow cytometry or antihuman globulin augmentation tests, hyperacute rejection has virtually been nonexistent.

Early Cell-Mediated Acute Rejection

Early cell-mediated rejection, with a typical interstitial infiltrate or vasculitis, can also be detected in the latter part of the first week after transplantation, although it typically occurs somewhat later. It may develop in an allograft already suffering from ATN and may be difficult to recognize clinically because the patient is anuric or oliguric. An allograft with DGF, presumably due to ATN, should undergo serial biopsies at intervals of about 10 days to detect the covert development of rejection. The prognosis for long-term function of these grafts is poor, although adequate function may be achieved, if the ATN reverses and the rejection responds to intensification of immunosuppression (see Chapters 29 and 30).

Nonimmunologic Causes

Nonimmunologic causes of DGF (other than ATN) of various etiologies may occur in the first post-transplant week or any time thereafter and are discussed under graft dysfunction in the early post-transplant period.

Long-Term Impact of Delayed Graft Function

Studies on the impact of DGF on long-term graft function have yielded conflicting results.[3,4,6,7,53] Data from the UNOS Scientific Renal Transplant Registry revealed that DGF reduced 1-year graft survival from 91% to 75% ($p <.0001$) and graft half-life from 12.9 to 8.0 years, independent of early acute rejection. The deleterious effect of DGF with or without acute rejection on graft half-life remained significant after adjusting for discharge serum creatinine of less than 2.5 mg/dL. Interestingly, in the presence of DGF with or without acute rejection, the survival advantage of well-matched kidneys (0–1 mismatch) over those of poorly matched (5–6 mismatch) kidneys was no longer seen.[54] Some group of investigators showed that DGF, when combined with rejection had an additive adverse effect on allograft survival, whereas others suggested that DGF is deleterious to graft outcome only when associated with reduced renal mass and hyperfiltration injury.[53,55] The harmful effect of DGF may also be more pronounced when marginal donor kidneys are used. It should be noted that in most studies reported transplant biopsies were not performed and DGF was presumed to be due to ATN. This, along with the difference in the criteria used to define DGF may explain, in part, the conflicting results between various studies.

GRAFT DYSFUNCTION IN THE EARLY POST-TRANSPLANT PERIOD

The early post-transplantation period usually refers to the time span following discharge from the hospital until the second or third month, at which time most patients have achieved stable graft function and a stable immunosuppressive regimen. Although the differentiation, at this stage, between the early and late post-transplantation is clearly somewhat arbitrary, it is based on the finding that most acute rejection episodes occur within the first few months. In randomized trials that have used episodes of acute rejection as their end points, more than 90% of acute rejection episodes occur during the first year.[56,57] Similarly, most episodes of cyclosporine or tacrolimus toxicity occur during this period, as do most cases of surgery-related graft dysfunction.

By the second week, graft function of most patients with DGF due to ATN begins to improve, although some patients remain oliguric for several weeks. In all patients who have become independent of dialysis, measurement of the serum creatinine (SCr) concentration is a simple yet invaluable marker of kidney transplant function, and the universal availability of this test greatly facilitates post-transplantation management. In clinical transplantation management, it is generally not necessary to measure renal function by more accurate and sophisticated techniques, such as creatinine clearance and isotope filtration rates, although these techniques may be valuable in assessing the significances of changes in SCr with time and in providing a more accurate baseline value for follow-up. The level of SCr reached by the second week is an important determinant of long-term graft function, and any baseline level greater than the "low twos" is a source of concern necessitating evaluation. The relationship between SCr and adverse outcome in renal transplantation remains the most robust predictor of graft survival at all time points.[2] Recent analysis of the UNOS database involving 105,742 adult renal transplant recipients performed in the United States between 1988 and 1998 revealed that post-transplant serum creatinine greater than 1.5 mg/dL at 1 year significantly decreased graft half-life regardless of whether or not patients had an episode of acute rejection[58] (discussed in further details under graft dysfunction during long-term follow up).

Elevations in SCr of greater than 25% from baseline almost always indicate a significant, potentially graft-endangering event. Smaller elevations may represent laboratory variability, and if there is any question regarding a small asymptomatic rise in SCr, the test should be repeated within 48 hours. The clinical algorithm in approaching SCr elevations (or failure to reach a low baseline value) is similar, in principle, to that used in the nontransplant setting in that "prerenal," "renal," and "postrenal" causes need to be considered. In the early post-transplantation period, acute rejection and nephrotoxicity are constant threats to graft function; anatomic or surgical problems must be considered, however, before medical diagnoses are made to explain deteriorating graft function.

Acute Rejection

Clinical Presentation

Acute rejection is the term conventionally used to describe the cellular immune response to the transplant that produces enough inflammation and destruction to cause recognizable graft dysfunction, as measured by an elevation of the SCr. More recently it has been suggested that humoral immune response or more specifically, donor specific anti-HLA antibodies can also cause direct graft injury and acute allograft dysfunction. Although using the SCr to define the occurrence of rejection is highly convenient it is insensitive in detecting subclinical pathogenic allograft inflammation or "subclinical rejection." Up to 30% to 80% of protocol biopsies performed in the first 3 months post-transplantation in patients with stable allograft function have been shown to meet Banff criteria for type I rejection.[59] More importantly, untreated subclinical rejection has been suggested to be a precursor to chronic rejection and chronic allograft nephropathy.[59,60] Conversely, treatment of subclinical rejection in the first 3 months post-transplantation has been shown to prevent both late clinical rejections and the development of chronic rejection.[61,62]

The classic symptoms and signs of acute rejection are fever, malaise, graft tenderness, and oliguria. Acute rejection can present with a seemingly innocuous influenza-like illness, and transplant recipients should be warned of the potential significance of these symptoms. These symptoms consistently and rapidly resolve when the rejecting patient receives pulse steroids, presumably as a result of the blockade of interleukin-1 by corticosteroids.[63] Since the advent of cyclosporine and of potent immunosuppressive agents in general, these findings are seen less frequently, and many rejections present as asymptomatic elevations of the SCr. In the presence of fever, graft tenderness, and/or oliguria, a search for alternative causes of graft dysfunction is warranted.

Fever may indicate either rejection or infection and should never be presumed to be due to the former without considering the latter. Infection during the first few weeks usually results from bacterial pathogens in the wound, urinary tract, or respiratory tract and may be associated with an elevated SCr level as a result of vasodilatation or volume contraction.[64] A thorough history, physical exam, standard laboratory tests, and a chest radiograph must, therefore, precede the diagnosis and treatment of rejection. An elevated white blood cell count is frequently seen in the post-transplantation period, particularly in patients still receiving high baseline doses of corticosteroids, and is often unhelpful in the differential diagnosis. Fever due to infection with opportunistic organisms usually does not occur in renal transplant recipients until several weeks after transplantation. Cytomegalovirus (CMV) infection may mimic acute rejection, and its possible presence always needs to be considered, particularly in CMV-negative recipients of kidneys from CMV-positive donors.[64]

Many patients comment on incisional tenderness in the first few days and can be reassured that this is of little clinical significance. The new onset of graft tenderness in a previously pain-free patient, however, is a significant symptom that needs to be evaluated. A tender, swollen graft in a patient with a rising SCr concentration and fever usually indicates rejection, although the possibility of acute pyelonephritis must also be considered.[64] Cyclosporine and tacrolimus toxicity and CMV infection do not produce graft tenderness. Excruciating localized perinephric pain is usually a result of a urine leak.[65]

Both rejection and cyclosporine toxicity may produce weight gain and edema as a result of impaired graft function and avid tubular sodium reabsorption. Mild peripheral edema is common in stable patients receiving cyclosporine. Acute rejection, cyclosporine toxicity, and tacrolimus toxicity can all produce graft dysfunction in the absence of oliguria. Oliguria is common in severe acute rejection; its occurrence makes a diagnosis of drug toxicity less likely and makes the necessity to exclude an anatomic cause all the more critical.

Imaging Studies

The morphologic findings in acute rejection are nonspecific and somewhat subjective, and imaging studies are performed to exclude alternative causes of graft dysfunction. In mild acute rejection episodes, ultrasonographic and nuclear medicine study results may be normal.[14,49] Ultrasonographic abnormalities include graft enlargement, obscured corticomedullary definition, prominent hypoechoic medullary pyramids, decreased echogenicity of the renal sinus, thickened uroepithelium, and scattered heterogenous areas of increased echogenicity. The resistive index is also elevated as it is in other causes of graft dysfunction that produce increased vascular resistance to the kidney.[14]

Acute rejection may appear on nuclear medicine technetium 99m DTPA and MAG-3 scans as delayed visualization (decreased perfusion) of the transplant in the first-pass renal scintiangiogram.[49] Poor parenchymal uptake with high background activity (poor kidney function and clearance) may be seen in the second and third phases of the three-phases imaging study. However, it should be noted that neither renal Doppler ultrasound nor radioisotope flow scan is sufficiently sensitive or specific in the diagnosis of acute rejection. Although invasive, tissue diagnosis remains the most accurate means of differentiating acute rejection from other causes of acute deterioration of allograft function.

Histopathologic Diagnosis

Percutaneous renal biopsy is the gold standard diagnostic tool for acute rejection. Although readily accessible and less invasive, allograft fine needle aspiration has significant diagnostic limitations, and its use has lost popularity. The timing and frequency of kidney biopsies vary among centers. One clinical approach to graft dysfunction is to base a therapeutic intervention empirically on the clinical presentation and laboratory values. A favorable response confirms the diagnosis, but a lack of response requires tissue diagnosis. It is probably wise to obtain tissue diagnosis of rejection before embarking on a course of OKT3 or polyclonal antibodies because occasionally CMV infection may present as fever and graft dysfunction,[64] in which case potent immunosuppressive therapy could be catastrophic. A more aggressive approach to graft dysfunction is to perform a kidney biopsy whenever the SCr level rises 25% over the baseline value. Therapy is then based on the morphologic findings.

Types of Acute Rejection

Acute rejections occur, most typically, between the first week and the first 3 months after transplantation. In unsensitized patients with low levels of preformed antibodies, acute rejections rarely occur in the first week, while very early rejections (or accelerated acute rejection) may occur in sensitized patients (as previously described). On the basis of the underlying immunopathogenic mechanisms, acute rejection can be divided into cell-mediated and humoral immunity. Approximately 90% of the episodes of acute rejection are predominantly cell-mediated, whereas 20% to 30% of all acute rejection episodes have a humoral component.[66] The histologic diagnostic criteria are different for these two types of rejection and are discussed separately. It should be noted, however, that the histopathologic findings of acute cellular rejection can be seen in allograft biopsies with acute humoral rejection or vice versa.

Acute Cellular Rejection

Acute cellular rejection generally occurs after the first posttransplant week and most commonly occurs within 3 months after transplantation. It has been suggested that CD4+ T cells play an important role in the initiation of rejection, whereas CD8+ T cells are critical at a later stage.[52] There has been accumulating evidence indicating that the effector pathway of cytotoxicity T lymphocytes killing (CTL) leading to acute renal allograft rejection involves the perforin/granzyme degranulation pathway.[67] Urinary perforin mRNA and granzyme B have been shown to be elevated in acute allograft rejection. It has been suggested that measurement of urine perforin mRNA and granzyme B messenger RNA may offer a noninvasive means of diagnosing acute renal allograft rejection with a sensitivity of 79% to 83% and a specificity of 77% to 83%.[68] Nonetheless, whether measurement of these cytotoxic proteins may be beneficial in monitoring or in the diagnosis of acute cellular rejection awaits further studies.

Acute Humoral Rejection

Acute humoral rejection generally occurs within the first 1 to 3 weeks after transplantation.[69] Its incidence has been difficult to determine in part due to the lack of well-defined diagnostic criteria. Although the detection of the complement degradation product C4d deposition in peritubular capillaries (PTC) of renal allograft biopsies has been regarded as a footprint of a humoral response, focal PTC C4d staining has also been found to be present in ischemic injury. More recently, Mauiyyedi and associates[69] suggested that a definitive diagnosis of AHR requires demonstration of circulating donor specific antibodies (DSA). Yet other investigators speculated that non-HLA, anti-endothelial antibodies or subthreshold levels of DSA may account for the C4d(+) DSA(−) cases of AHR? hyperacute rejection as a result of antibodies to endothelial cells has been reported.[69,70] The currently suggested histologic and immunopathologic criteria for AHR is shown in Table 36–4.

Core Biopsy

Biopsy evaluation for acute changes should be performed in unscarred portions of the renal cortex. Cell-mediated acute rejection occurs in two forms, including the tubulointerstitial and vascular types. Tubulointerstitial acute rejection is characterized by lymphocytes in the walls of tubules (tubulitis) with associated interstitial edema and inflammation, including lymphocytes, activated lymphocytes, monocytes, and occasional scattered eosinophils or plasma cells. Variable degrees of tubular cell flattening, necrosis, and regenerative

Table 36–4 Pathologic Criteria for Acute Humoral Rejection*

- C4d deposition in peritubular capillaries†
- At least one of the following‡:
  - Neutrophils in peritubular capillaries
  - Arterial fibrinoid necrosis
  - Acute tubular injury
- Circulating donor-specific antibodies

*Cases that also meet the criteria of type I or II acute cellular rejection (Banff) are considered to have both processes.
†Bright and diffusely positive staining (at least 2/4+ by immunofluorescence) for C4d in peritubular capillaries (PTCs).
‡Neutrophils in PTCs, on average, two or more neutrophils per high power field, in PTC, in 10 consecutive 40 × (500 μm diameter) fields; fibrinoid necrosis in an artery larger than an arteriole; acute tubular injury, loss of brush borders, flattened epithelium, apoptosis. If only two of the three numbered criteria are present, the term "suspicious for acute humoral rejection" is recommended (for example, when donor-specific antibodies are not tested). (Adapted from Racusen LC, Colvin RB, Solez K, et al: Antibody-mediated rejection criteria: An addition to the Banff '97 classification of renal allograft rejection. Am J Transplant 2003; 3:708-714.).

change are also present (Figure 36–3). Vascular cell-mediated rejection is characterized by lymphocytes, monocytes, or both extending under the endothelial lining into the intima (endothelialitis), with endothelial cells appearing swollen and often detached from the vascular wall (Figure 36–4). Infrequently in severe cases, the inflammatory cells are found in the arterial media and may be associated with smooth muscle cell necrosis.[71] This process involves small and medium-sized intrarenal arteries and tends to be present focally, so it may be missed on biopsy. Therefore, a minimum of two arteries within the biopsy and at least 12 sections of the tissue are required for an adequate assessment of vascular rejection. Vascular rejection is usually accompanied by the tubulointerstitial form and may be associated with interstitial hemorrhage due to increased permeability of peritubular capillaries. The finding of interstitial hemorrhage suggests the presence of vascular rejection even in the absence of diagnostic arteries, if other causes of hemorrhage, such as prior biopsy site and infarction, have been excluded.[72] Glomeruli may display a form of capillary rejection termed *acute transplant glomerulopathy*, in which capillary lumens contain mononuclear leukocytes.[73]

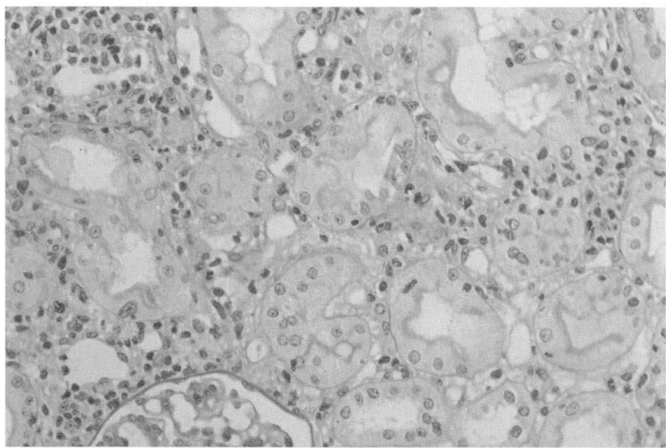

Figure 36–3 Acute cell-mediated tubulointerstitial rejection. There are interstitial edema and lymphocytes with lymphocytes in the walls of most tubules. (Periodic acid-Schiff × 250)

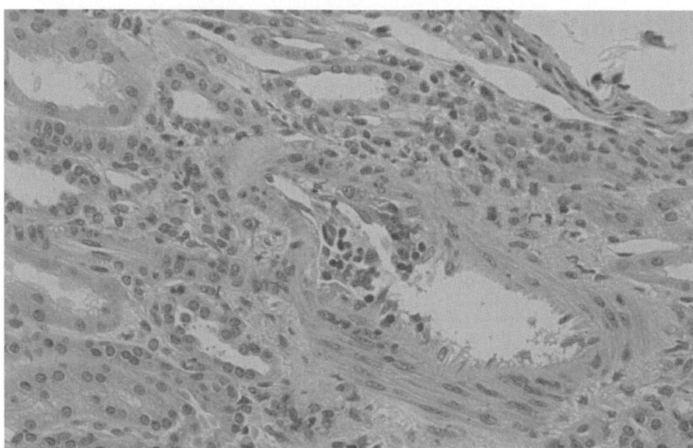

Figure 36–4 Acute cell-mediated vascular rejection. The artery contains swollen endothelial cells that are focally detached from the artery wall with undermining lymphocytes. The adjacent interstitium has edema and a lymphocytic infiltrate. (Hematoxylin and eosin × 250)

Humoral antibody-mediated rejection in its classic form is a vascular process wherein neutrophils infiltrate artery walls, with fibrin deposition inducing fibrinoid necrosis, often accompanied by mononuclear leukocytes.[70] There may be associated intravascular thrombosis, glomerular inflammation, and foci of renal parenchymal necrosis or infarction. Another type of antibody-mediated rejection is associated with C4d deposition around PTC, best demonstrated by immunofluorescence microscopy (Figure 36–5).[74] This may be associated with only minor tubular cell necrosis, with neutrophil infiltrates or in the setting of arterial fibrinoid necrosis. The currently suggested histologic and immunopathologic criteria for AHR are shown in Table 36–4.

Attempts are underway to provide standardized morphologic definitions of acute rejection. The Banff '97 working classification[75] includes separate categories for cell-mediated and antibody-mediated rejection. The former requires as a minimum greater than 25% of the interstitium to contain inflammation and greater than four mononuclear leukocytes in a tubule, and the category is subdivided into tubulointerstitial and vascular forms of rejection. The antibody-mediated rejection category was recently revised[76] and now is reflected in Table 36–4. More than one form of rejection may be present simultaneously. The borderline category, characterized by inflammation less than that required for a diagnosis of cell-mediated acute rejection, remains controversial as to its immunologic significance. Further study is required, possibly with the application of cytokine analysis, to determine accurately the meaning of low grade inflammation within the allograft.

Cyclosporine and Tacrolimus Toxicity

Although biochemically distinct, cyclosporine and tacrolimus are two potent immunosuppressive agents with similar mechanism of action as well as clinical and pathologic patterns of nephrotoxicity. Their potential for impairment of graft function, particularly in the early post-transplant period should be included in the differential diagnosis of the elevated serum creatinine level. It is important to note that there are various

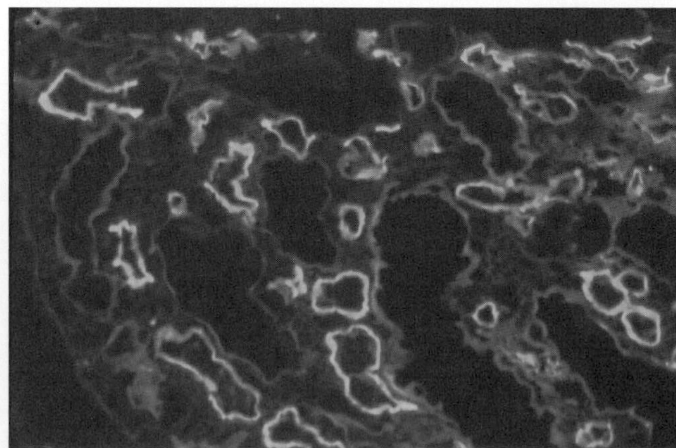

Figure 36–5 Acute antibody-mediated (humoral) rejection. There is bright staining of peritubular capillaries for C4d in a linear pattern. (C4d immunofluorescence × 500)

clinical and histologic manifestations of cyclosporine and tacrolimus toxicity; in the early post-transplant period, the most important are the frequently occurring functional decrease in renal blood flow and GFR and the infrequently occurring thrombotic microangiopathy.

Functional Decrease in Renal Blood Flow and Filtration Rate

Cyclosporine and tacrolimus produce a dose-related, reversible, renal vasoconstriction that particularly affects the afferent arteriole.[39] The glomerular capillary ultrafiltration coefficient (Kf) also falls, possibly because of increased mesangial cell contractility. Clinically, this condition is reminiscent of prerenal dysfunction, and in the acute phase, tubular function is intact. The mechanism of the vasoconstriction is discussed in Chapter 38. Cyclosporine- and tacrolimus-induced renal vasoconstriction may manifest clinically as delayed recovery from ATN and as transient, reversible, dose-dependent and blood level-dependent elevation in SCr concentration that may be difficult to distinguish from other causes of graft dysfunction.

Cyclosporine and Tacrolimus Blood Levels

The use of blood levels of cyclosporine and tacrolimus in clinical immunosuppressive management is discussed in Chapter 38. High blood levels of cyclosporine and tacrolimus do not preclude a diagnosis of rejection, although they may make it less likely, particularly in the case of tacrolimus.[57] Nephrotoxicity may develop at apparently low levels of both drugs, and some degree of toxicity may be intrinsic to their use.[77] Nephrotoxicity and rejection may coexist. In clinical practice, particularly when SCr elevation is modest, it is fair to initially presume that a patient with a very high cyclosporine or tacrolimus level is probably suffering from nephrotoxicity and that a patient with deteriorating graft function and very low drug level is probably undergoing rejection. If the appropriate clinical therapeutic response does not have a salutary effect on graft function, the clinical premise needs to be reconsidered. Cyclosporine toxicity usually resolves within 24 to 48 hours of a dose reduction, whereas tacrolimus toxicity may take longer to resolve. Progressive elevation of the plasma creatinine level, even in the face of persistently high drug levels, suggests rejection.

Patients may detect somatic manifestations of toxicity, and these symptoms may suggest the diagnosis. Tremor and headache are produced by both drugs but are particularly marked with tacrolimus.[77] Compared to Sandimmune, the Neoral formulation of cyclosporine produces higher peak levels and a more consistent pharmacokinetic profile with a magnified area under the curve (AUC) in some patients.[78] The high peak level may be detected by patients as headache and flushing, whereas the magnified AUC may predispose to nephrotoxicity at a time that trough levels are deemed not elevated. More recently, Neoral cyclosporine monitoring using the 2-hour postdose (C2) has been suggested to correlate better with the risk for acute rejection and cyclosporine-induced nephrotoxicity compared with trough (C0) monitoring.[79] We are currently conducting a pilot study to assess whether improved renal function can be achieved at 6 and 12 months post-transplant in de novo renal transplant recipients receiving Neoral using C2 for dosing determination as compared to historical controls using trough monitoring. Adoption of C2 monitoring as a new tool to monitor Neoral dose adjustment awaits further studies. Prospective randomized trials are needed.

Drug Interactions

Well-substantiated potentiation of renal impairment has been described when amphotericin, aminoglycosides, nonsteroidal anti-inflammatory drugs, angiotensin-converting enzyme inhibitors, and/or angiotensin receptor antagonists are used in patients receiving calcineurin inhibitor therapy. More recently, exacerbation of nephrotoxicity has been observed in renal transplant recipients receiving the newer immunosuppressant sirolimus and cyclosporine combination therapy.[80,81]

Sirolimus is a potent immunosuppressant with a mechanism of action and a side effect profile distinct from that of the calcineurin inhibitors. When used as base therapy without a calcineurin inhibitor sirolimus has been shown to be devoid of nephrotoxicity.[82,83] However, in two phase III clinical trials (The Global and U.S. Rapamune Study Group) concomitant administration of cyclosporine and sirolimus has been shown to potentiate cyclosporine-induced nephrotoxicity.[80,81] There has been substantial evidence suggesting that cyclosporine exposure is increased by a pharmacokinetic interaction with sirolimus. In rat animal models sirolimus has also been shown to increase partitioning into renal tissue to a greater extent than it increases whole blood concentrations.[84] When combination therapy is used, a reduction in therapeutic cyclosporine level is desirable, particularly when there is an unexplained rise in SCr level. The pharmacologic interaction between sirolimus and tacrolimus has been less rigorously studied. Co-administration of tacrolimus and sirolimus has been shown to result in reduced exposure to tacrolimus at sirolimus doses of greater than or equal to 2 mg/day.[85] However, cases of acute allograft failure following sirolimus-tacrolimus therapy have been reported.[86] Caution should be exercised when combination immunosuppressive agents are used.

Thrombotic Microangiopathy (TMA)

Use of both cyclosporine and tacrolimus may be associated with drug-induced thrombotic microangiopathy. Although the exact pathogenic mechanism of cyclosporine-induced TMA remains speculative, multiple prothrombotic effects of cyclosporine have been implicated in the pathogenesis of cyclosporine-associated TMA. These include a direct cytotoxic effect on endothelial cells, a reduction of prostacyclin synthesis, and alterations in the thromboxane A2 to prostacyclin ratio, leading to vasoconstriction, platelet aggregation, and thrombus formation.[87] Cyclosporine has also been found to reduce the generation of activated protein C from endothelial cells and to increase thromboplastin expression from mononuclear and endothelial cells. More recently, deficiency in the activity of von Willebrand factor cleaving metalloprotease ADAMTS13 and the presence of its inhibitory antibodies has been reported to cause TMA in a renal allograft transplant recipient receiving cyclosporine-based immunosuppression. However, whether cyclosporine or calcineurin inhibitor plays a role in the formation of autoantibodies to ADAMTS13 remains to be determined.[88] As is the case with cyclosporine, it is suggested that endothelial cell damage may be the inciting event in tacrolimus-induced TMA. However, tacrolimus has mixed effects on the synthesis of prostaglandins.

TMA may develop as early as 4 days postoperative to as late as 6 years post-transplantation. It may be evident clinically by virtue of the typical laboratory findings of intravascular coagulation (e.g., thrombocytopenia, distorted erythrocytes, elevated lactate dehydrogenase levels) accompanied by an arteriolopathy and intravascular thrombi on transplant biopsy. Unlike the primary form of thrombotic thrombocytopenic purpura or hemolytic-uremic syndrome, however, cyclosporine- or tacrolimus-associated TMA may be covert, and the laboratory findings may be inconsistent. In recipients of renal allograft, renal dysfunction is the most common manifestation. Thrombocytopenia and microangiopathic hemolysis are often mild or absent and the diagnosis is often made on graft biopsies performed to determine the cause of DGF or to rule out acute rejection.[87] Although there have been no controlled trials comparing the different treatment modalities of this condition, dose reduction or discontinuation of the offending agent appears to be pivotal to management. Adjunctive plasmapheresis with fresh frozen plasma replacement may offer survival advantages. In transplant recipients with cyclosporine-associated TMA, successful use of tacrolimus immunosuppression has been reported. However, recurrence of TMA in renal transplant recipients treated sequentially with cyclosporine and tacrolimus has been described, and clinicians must remain vigilant for signs and symptoms of recurrence of TMA in patients who are switched from cyclosporine to tacrolimus or vice versa.[87] There have been anecdotal reports of the successful use of sirolimus and/or mycophenolate mofetil in transplant recipients with calcineurin inhibitor associated TMA.[89,90] However, recently sirolimus has also been reported to cause TMA in recipients of renal allografts.[91] The use of the monoclonal antibody muromonab-CD3 OKT3 has also been associated with the development of post-transplant TMA, although infrequently.

Other potential causative factors of post-transplant-associated TMA include the presence of lupus anticoagulant and/or anticardiolipin antibody, cytomegalovirus infection, and, less frequently, systemic viral infection with parvovirus B19 or influenza A virus.[92] An increased incidence of TMA has also been described in a subset of renal allograft recipients with concurrent hepatitis C virus infection and anticardiolipin antibody positivity.[93]

Histologic Features

Cyclosporine and tacrolimus nephrotoxicity have similar appearances in renal allografts. The most common form of acute toxicity is a variant of ATN, with scattered individual necrotic tubular cells, considerable dilatation of tubular lumina and epithelial cell flattening without extensive loss of brush border staining.[94] The characteristic feature, often not present, is isometric vacuolization of proximal tubular cell cytoplasm, which tends to involve all tubular cells in few tubular profiles (Figure 36–6).[95] There is mild interstitial edema without significant inflammation or with focal aggregates of inactive lymphocytes often in perivenous locations; tubulitis is absent. There are no specific glomerular abnormalities, but arterioles have muscular hypertrophy and may contain rounded plasma protein collections (insudates) in the outer aspect of the muscular walls and individual smooth muscle cell necrosis. The juxtaglomerular apparatus is enlarged.

Thrombotic microangiopathy has an identical morphologic appearance regardless of the underlaying pathogenetic cause. Therefore, TMA associated with the calcineurin inhibitors has the usual features, including glomerular capillary, arteriolar, and occasionally arterial thrombosis (Figure 36–7).[96] Vascular walls have muscular hypertrophy, loose mucoid intimal thickening, and fibrin deposition with luminal narrowing. This process may be patchy and subtle or widespread and associated with cortical infarction. The histologic features of chronic cyclosporine and tacrolimus toxicity are discussed in the section on chronic rejection and chronic allograft toxicity.

Infection

The most common infections in the early post-transplantation period that are associated with graft dysfunction are uri-

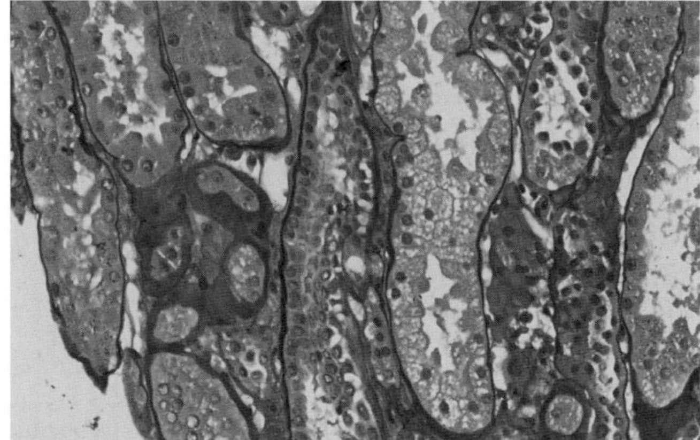

Figure 36–6 Acute calcineurin-inhibitor nephrotoxicity. Isometric vacuoles are in the cytoplasm of all epithelial cells in the center proximal tubular profile. (Jones methenamine silver × 300)

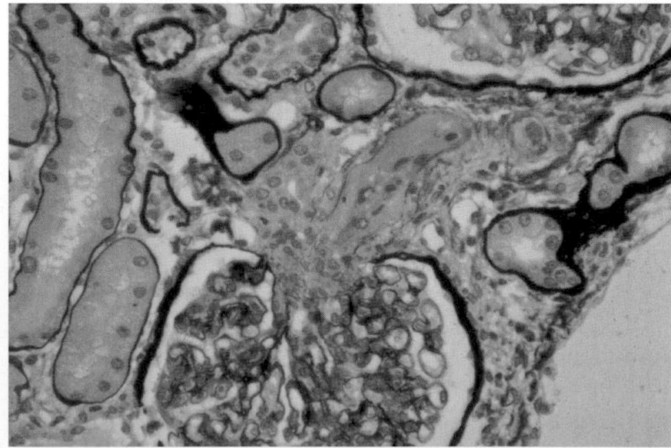

Figure 36–7 Thrombotic microangiopathic form of acute calcineurin-inhibitor nephrotoxicity. The arteriole has swollen endothelial cells and nuclear fragments entrapped in a luminal thrombus. The adjacent juxtaglomerular apparatus is enlarged. (Jones methenamine silver × 250)

nary tract and CMV infections. Uncomplicated urinary tract infections do not usually lead to graft dysfunction, unless they are complicated by pyelonephritis or urosepsis. Clinical CMV infection may mimic acute rejection and is discussed in Chapter 40.

Vascular Complications: Renal Artery Stenosis

Transplant renal artery stenosis may occur as early as the first week but is usually a late complication and is discussed under allograft dysfunction during long-term follow-up. Arterial or venous thrombosis generally occurs within the first 2 to 3 postoperative days but may occur as long as 2 months post-transplant. In most series reported, the incidence of graft thrombosis ranges from 0.5% to as high as 8% with arterial accounting for one third and venous thrombosis for two thirds of cases.[38,97] Thrombosis occurring early after transplantation is most often due to technical surgical complications, whereas the later onset is generally due to acute rejection.[38] In patients with initial good allograft function, thrombosis is generally heralded by the acute onset of oliguria or anuria associated with deterioration of allograft function. Abnormal laboratory findings may include thrombocytopenia, hyperkalemia, and a rising lactate dehydrogenase level. Clinically, the patient may present with graft swelling or tenderness, and/or gross hematuria. In patients with DGF and good residual urine output from the native kidneys there may be no overt signs or symptoms, and the diagnosis rests on clinical suspicion and prompt imaging studies. The diagnosis is usually made by Doppler ultrasound or isotope flow scan. Confirmed arterial or venous thrombosis typically necessitates allograft nephrectomy. In recipients of kidneys with multiple arteries, thrombosis may occur in a single branch, and depending on the extent of renal parenchymal supplied, adequate functioning tissue may remain.

Suggested predisposing factors for vascular thrombosis include arteriosclerotic involvement of the donor or recipient vessels, intimal injury of graft vessels, kidney with multiple arteries, history of recurrent thrombosis, thrombocytosis, younger recipient and/or donor age, and the presence of antiphospholipid antibody (anticardiolipin antibody and/or lupus anticoagulant).[92] There has been no consensus on the optimal management of recipients with abnormal hypercoagulability profile, such as abnormal activated protein C resistance ratio or factor V Leiden mutation, antiphospholipid antibody positivity, protein C, or protein S deficiency or antithrombin III deficiency. However, unless contraindicated, perioperative and/or postoperative prophylactic anticoagulation should be considered, particularly in patients with a prior history of recurrent thrombotic events. Transplant of pediatric en bloc kidneys into adult recipient with a history of thrombosis should probably be avoided. The duration of anticoagulation has not been well defined, but lifelong anticoagulation should be considered in high-risk candidates.[92]

Ureteral Obstruction

Ureteral obstruction occurs in 2% to 10% of renal transplants[98] and is usually manifested by painless impairment of graft function due to the lack of innervation of the engrafted kidney. Hydronephrosis may be minimal or absent in early obstruction, whereas low-grade dilatation of the collecting system secondary to edema at the ureterovesical anastomosis may be seen early post-transplantation and does not necessarily indicate obstruction. A full bladder may also cause mild calyceal dilatation due to ureteral reflux, and repeat ultrasound with an empty bladder should be carried out. Persistent or increasing hydronephrosis on repeat ultrasound examinations is highly suggestive of obstruction. Renal scan with furosemide washout may help support the diagnosis, but it does not provide clear anatomic detail.[14,99] Although invasive, percutaneous nephrostomy tube placement with antegrade nephrostogram is the most effective way to visualize the collecting system and can be of both diagnostic and therapeutic value.

Blood clots, a technically poor reimplant, and ureteral slough are the common causes of early acute obstruction after transplantation.[38,65,92] Ureteral fibrosis secondary to either ischemia or rejection can cause an intrinsic obstruction. The distal ureter close to the ureterovesical junction is particularly vulnerable to ischemic damage due to its remote location from the renal artery and hence its compromised blood supply. Ureteral fibrosis associated with polyoma BK virus is a newly recognized cause of ureteral obstruction in the setting of renal transplantation.[100] Ureteral kinking, lymphocele, pelvic hematoma or abscess, and malignancy are potential causes of extrinsic obstruction. Calculi are uncommon causes of transplant ureteral obstruction.[38]

Definitive treatment of ureteral obstruction due to ureteral strictures consists of either endourologic techniques or open surgery. Intrinsic ureteral scars can be treated effectively by endourologic techniques in an antegrade or retrograde approach. A stent is left indwelling to bypass the ureteral obstruction and can be removed cystoscopically after 2 to 6 weeks.[38] Routine ureteral stent placement at the time of transplantation has been suggested to be associated with a lower incidence of early postoperative obstruction.[101] Extrinsic strictures or strictures that are longer than 2 cm are less likely to be amenable to percutaneous techniques and are more likely to require surgical treatment, as do strictures that fail endourologic incision.[38] Obstructing calculi can be managed by endourologic techniques or by extracorporeal shock wave lithotripsy.

Perinephric Fluid Collections

Symptomatic perinephric fluid collections in the early postoperative period can be due to lymphoceles, hematoma, urinoma, or abscesses. Lymphoceles are collections of lymph caused by leakage from severed lymphatics. They typically develop within weeks after transplantation. Most lymphoceles are small and asymptomatic. Generally, the larger the lymphocele, the more likely it is to produce symptoms and to require treatment, although very small but strategically placed lymphoceles can result in ureteral obstruction. Lymphoceles may also compress the iliac vein, leading to ipsilateral leg swelling or deep vein thrombosis, or they may occasionally produce urinary incontinence due to bladder compression.[38]

Lymphoceles are usually detected by ultrasound either as an incidental finding or during evaluation of allograft dysfunction. They appear as a roundish, sonolucent, septated mass.[49] Hydronephrosis may be present, and the ureter may be seen adjacent to and compressed by presentation, and ultrasound appearance distinguish a lymphocele from other types of perinephric fluid collections, such as a hematoma or urine leak. Needle aspiration reveals a clear fluid with a creatinine concentration equal to that of the serum.

No therapy is necessary for the common, small, asymptomatic lymphocele. Percutaneous aspiration should be performed if a ureteral leak, obstruction, or infection is suspected. The most common indication for treatment is ureteral obstruction. If the cause of the obstruction is simple compression resulting from the mass effect of the lymphocele, percutaneous drainage alone usually resolves the problem. The ureter is often narrowed and may need to be reimplanted because of its involvement in the inflammatory reaction in the wall of the lymphocele. Repeated percutaneous aspirations are not advised because they seldom lead to dissolution of the lymphocele and often result in infection. Infected or obstructing lymphoceles can be drained externally. Sclerosing agents, such as povidone-iodine, tetracycline, or fibrin-glue, can be instilled into the cavity with variable results.[38] Lymphoceles can also be marsupialized into the peritoneal cavity, where the fluid is reabsorbed.

An obstructed hematoma is best managed by surgical evacuation. Urinoma or evidence of a urine leak should be treated without delay. A small leak can be managed expectantly with insertion of a Foley catheter to reduce intravesical pressure. This maneuver may occasionally reduce or stop the leak altogether. Persistent allograft dysfunction, particularly in a symptomatic patient, often necessitates early surgical exploration and repair. Infected perinephric fluid collections should be treated by external drainage or open surgery in conjunction with systemic antibiotics.

GRAFT DYSFUNCTION DURING LONG-TERM FOLLOW-UP

The causes of graft loss after the first year are listed in Table 36–5. Both immunologic and nonimmunologic factors have been suggested to play an interactive role in the development of chronic allograft dysfunction. Hence, the term "chronic rejection" has been replaced by the less specific but more accurate term *chronic allograft nephropathy.* Graft loss from recurrent diseases is discussed in Chapter 35.

Table 36–5 Causes of Chronic Allograft Failure

Alloantigen-Dependent	Alloantigen-Independent
Acute rejection	Delayed graft function
Poor HLA matching	Nephron "dose"
Prior sensitization	Donor age
Inadequate immunosuppression	Ischemia-reperfusion injury
Poor adherence to medications	Hypertension
	Hyperlipidemia
	Calcineurin inhibitor nephrotoxicity
	Cyto-megalovirus infection

HLA, human leukocyte antigen.

Chronic Rejection and Chronic Allograft Nephropathy

Chronic allograft nephropathy (CAN) usually occurs months or years after transplantation and can be loosely defined as progressive deterioration of graft function in the absence of any other causes, such as rejection, recurrent or de novo glomerular diseases, or structural abnormalities. Similar to chronic kidney disease of the native kidneys, CAN may be accompanied by hypertension and/or proteinuria. The characteristic histopathologic changes of CAN are provided in detail below. The development of CAN is multifactorial in etiologies and include both alloantigen-dependent and alloantigen-independent factors.

Alloantigen-Dependent Factors

Acute rejection episodes, poor HLA matching, prior sensitization, inadequate immunosuppression, and noncompliance have all been implicated in the development of CAN.

Acute Rejection Episodes

Numerous retrospective studies have shown that the most significant predictive factor for the development of CAN and late graft loss is the incidence of acute rejection episodes.[102–105] In some studies, even a single episode occurring within the first 2 months has a negative predictive effect, although multiple episodes and late episodes are more powerful predictors. It should also be noted that treatment of acute rejection episodes after the first year is often followed by incomplete recovery of graft function and expedited graft loss. It has been estimated that the half-life of allografts with no rejection episodes is 13 years, compared with 6 years for allografts with more than one episode.[104]

In addition to the frequency and timing of occurrence, the severity and histopathologic type of rejection have also been shown to be predictive of subsequent development of CAN. In this respect, early cell-mediated vascular rejections are more likely than tubulointerstitial rejections to herald CAN.[106] Interestingly, however, untreated subclinical rejections have also been suggested to result in the early appearance of chronic graft pathology and impaired graft function at long-term follow-up.[59, 61]

More recently, humoral immune mechanisms have also been suggested to have an important role in the pathogenesis of CAN.[107] In a retrospective study consisting of 152 renal allograft biopsies performed for evaluation of chronic allograft nephropathy, 23 of 38 (61%) of chronic rejection cases had peritubular capillaries staining for C4d, compared with 1 of 46 (2%) of controls (the former include allograft biopsies showing either glomerular basement membrane duplication in the absence of de novo or recurrent glomerulonephritis or arterial intimal fibrosis with intimal mononuclear cell infiltration, and the latter include allograft biopsies that showed chronic cyclosporine toxicity or nonspecific interstitial fibrosis, and native kidneys with end-stage renal disease). It was further demonstrated that circulating anti-donor HLA antibody was present in the majority of C4d-positive chronic rejection cases, whereas it was absent in C4d-negative chronic rejection cases (antidonor HLA positivity: 88% vs. 0% $p < .0002$, respectively). Whether complement C4d deposits in peritubular capillaries found on biopsy samples from patients with CAN represents an ongoing immunologic process and merits intervention remains to be determined.

Histocompatibility

Well-matched kidneys tend to last longer than less well-matched kidneys. This observation is true for both living donor and cadaveric transplants.[108] Among living donor transplants, the half-life for two-haplotype–matched transplants has been estimated to be 22.7 years compared with 13.1 years for one-haplotype–matched transplants, which, in turn, tend to function longer than zero-haplotype–matched and transplants from living, unrelated donors.[27,109] The importance of matching is particularly evident for cadaveric transplants: six-antigen–matched or zero-mismatched cadaveric transplants have a 5-year survival rate approaching 80% and a half-life approaching 13 years, compared with about 50% and 8 years, respectively, for completely mismatched transplants.[110] For many years, the improved long-term prognosis of living, related donor transplant over cadaveric donor transplants was presumed to be due largely to better histocompatibility matching. Although matching is important, the excellent short-term and long-term results of living, unrelated transplants suggest that the condition of the kidney at the time of transplantation is a critical, nonalloantigen-dependent factor.[109]

Noncompliance and Suboptimal Immunosuppression

The importance of alloantigen-dependent factors is clearly illustrated by the ongoing necessity to maintain adequate immunosuppression for the life span of the graft[111]; the definition of "adequate immunosuppression," however, remains controversial, and long-term prospective randomized trials comparing immunosuppressive regimens of varying intensity have not been performed. The discontinuation of corticosteroid in patients receiving triple therapy with cyclosporine, azathioprine, and prednisone has variably been shown to result in an unacceptable increased risk of acute and chronic rejection.[63,112,113] An increased incidence of rejection following steroid withdrawal was also seen in recipients receiving triple therapy with cyclosporine, prednisone, and mycophenolate mofetil, even among recipients who had been rejection free prior to steroid cessation.[114] More recent studies have shown that adequate immunosuppression can be achieved with regimens consisting of tacrolimus and mycophenolate mofetil or sirolimus (with or without antibody induction), hence allowing safer discontinuation of corticosteroids.[115,116] However, long-term follow-up data is currently lacking.

Noncompliance is a potent cause of late graft loss, and although occasional long-term, stable patients may "get away" with discontinuation of immunosuppression, such a policy is fraught with danger and should be discouraged, unless there is specific overriding indication, such as malignancy. The development of an acute rejection episode in a previously stable patient should prompt suspicion of noncompliance or inadequacy of the immunosuppressive regimen.

Alloantigen-Independent Factors

Nephron Dose and Hyperfiltration

The concept of nephron dose is based on the presumption that circumstances associated with an unfavorable ratio between the supply of functioning nephrons transplanted and the demands of the recipient make the allograft more susceptible to chronic loss of function.[117] The supply of functioning nephrons may be an absolute feature of the allograft (young or old age, female sex, African-American race, all of which are associated with a reduced nephron supply) or a feature of perioperative events, such as prolonged ischemia times and ATN. Limited data have shown that dual transplant of marginal kidneys have resulted in excellent short- and long-term allograft outcome, presumably due to increased viable nephron mass.[30] In a rat model of chronic rejection, the transplanted kidney appeared to be protected from progressive damage by the presence of a retained, functioning, recipient native kidney.[118] This finding supports the hypothesis that hyperfiltration in the remaining nephrons makes them susceptible to chronic damage in a manner similar to that proposed to explain the inexorable loss of function of the diseased nephrons of patients with chronic kidney disease. Interestingly, in a single center retrospective study, baseline glomerular hypertrophy (identified on intraoperative biopsies after vascular anastomosis) was shown to be an important determinant of late allograft dysfunction.[119] In addition to nephron "dose," perioperative damage to the allograft may also contribute to nonspecific tissue injury, cytokine release, upregulation of cell-surface markers and adhesion molecules, and chemoattraction of neutrophils, with further cycles of injury and repair.[120]

Recently, renal function in the first post-transplant year has been shown to serve as a predictor of renal allograft survival regardless of whether or not patients had prior episodes of acute rejection. For recipients of cadaveric renal allografts who had no clinical evidence of acute rejection within 1 year post-transplantation and who had a serum creatinine of less than 1.5 mg/dL at 1 year and a change in serum creatinine of less than 0.3 mg/dL between 6 months and 1 year post-transplant, the estimated median graft half-life is 17 years compared with 5 to 6 years for those who had no acute rejection episodes within 1 year but who had a serum creatinine at 1 year post-transplant of greater than 1.5 mg/dL and a change in SCr of greater than 0.3 mg/dL between 6 months and 1 year post-transplant.[58]

Other Factors

Systemic hypertension may exaggerate and perpetuate the vascular injury associated with allograft nephropathy, which has pathologic features in common with hypertensive nephrosclerosis.[106] One mechanism by which hypertension could lead to progressive renal allograft dysfunction is by increasing shear stress in renal vessels. It has been suggested that shear stress could promote atherosclerosis and hypertension by causing an upregulation of endothelin-1, PDGF, and other growth factors within the endothelium and by reducing NO secretion.[121] In rat orthotopic renal transplant models, it has been shown that hypertension increases the expression of growth factors and MHC class II.[122] In essence, hypertension may act in concert with or synergistically with immunologic factors to cause progressive graft dysfunction. Dyslipidemia, calcineurin inhibitor nephrotoxicity, number of transplants, proteinuria, CMV infection, and donor age and gender are other suggested risk factors for chronic allograft dysfunction. In a recent retrospective study consisting of 40,289 primary solitary Caucasian adult renal transplants, older donor and recipient age were shown to have an independent, yet equally detrimental effect on renal allograft survival.[123]

Histopathologic Features

The term *chronic allograft nephropathy* is used when it is uncertain which immunologic and nonimmunologic factors have contributed to the chronic changes, although it may be used synonymously with chronic transplant rejection.[124] CAN has characteristic morphologic features, including focal tubular atrophy and/or tubular dropout with interstitial fibrosis and variable degrees of associated mononuclear inflammation. When chronic transplant rejection is present there is intimal fibrosis of arteries with entrapped mononuclear leukocytes in the thickened vascular wall, disruption of the internal elastic lamina, and narrowing of the lumens.[125] Lymphocytes are frequently present in the scarred interstitium and in atrophic tubules. Glomeruli may be normal or ischemic or may show chronic transplant glomerulopathy, a lesion consisting of capillary wall double contours, mesangial widening with mild hypercellularity, mesangiolysis and leukocytes in capillary lumens; segmental glomerulosclerosis may also be present (Figure 36–8).[6] These glomeruli have variable deposition of IgM, complement, and fibrin focally in capillary walls identified by immunofluorescence. Ultrastructurally, mesangial migration and interposition, and subendothelial flocculent material are present, whereas peritubular capillaries have been reported to contain multilayered basement membranes.[127] Chronic transplant glomerulopathy confirms that chronic rejection is present, even in the absence of a diagnostic artery. The arterial and glomerular lesions, although diagnostic, tend to be focal and may not be present in a biopsy specimen. In this event, it may be difficult to differentiate between nephrosclerosis, chronic cyclosporine and tacrolimus nephrotoxicity, and chronic rejection, and the term *chronic allograft nephropathy* should be used. Active cell mediated and/or antibody-mediated acute rejection may occur simultaneously with CAN.

Chronic cyclosporine and tacrolimus toxicity is characterized by focal "striped" interstitial fibrosis, thought to be cortical medullary rays,[128] with associated tubular atrophy and little inflammation.[129] Arteries are normal, but arterioles may show muscular hypertrophy and rounded insudates in the walls, particularly the outer portion (Figure 36–9). The glomeruli are unremarkable or show mild ischemic change. The chronic toxicity of cyclosporine and tacrolimus cannot be differentiated histologically.[129,130]

Clinical Course

Chronic rejection typically occurs in patients who have suffered episodes of acute rejection, particularly when these episodes are multiple or late or when recovery of graft function, as judged by the return of the serum creatinine level to baseline is incomplete.[131] It presents clinically as deterioration of graft function, typically with proteinuria of varying degrees and hypertension. The time course to allograft failure is extremely variable, ranging from months to years. In most cases, the loss of graft function is inexorable, although spontaneous reduction and arrest of the rate of decline may occur. Proteinuria is usually moderate (1 to 3 g/day), but nephrotic-range proteinuria may occur. Chronic rejection is the most common cause of transplant nephrotic syndrome.[132,133]

Renal function in chronic rejection is typically monitored by the rise of the serum creatinine. The creatinine clearance, however, may overestimate the true GFR in the presence of chronic renal failure and proteinuria. As a result, the early stages of graft dysfunction may be associated with apparently minor rises in the SCr level, whereas small changes in GFR produces big changes in creatinine levels as the graft approaches end-stage failure.[134]

Differential Diagnosis

Chronic rejection needs to be differentiated from other causes of late graft dysfunction. The absence of a history of rejection, hypertension, and proteinuria should arouse diagnostic skepticism.[132,133] A renal ultrasound should be performed at least once to exclude obstructive causes of graft dysfunction, and the possibility of renal artery stenosis should be considered, particularly if hypertension is severe or the hemoglobin/hematocrit is high. Kidney biopsy provides a definitive diagnosis and may allow an estimate of the severity of the lesion

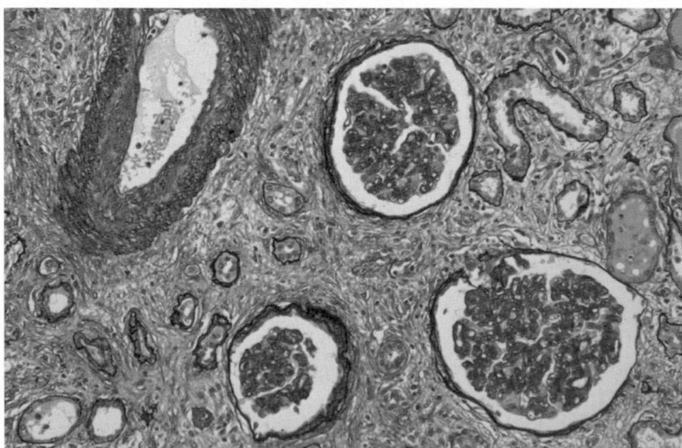

Figure 36–8 Chronic rejection. Arterial intimal fibrosis, tubular atrophy with interstitial fibrosis, interstitial lymphocytes and chronic transplant glomerulopathy are present. (Jones methenamine silver × 125)

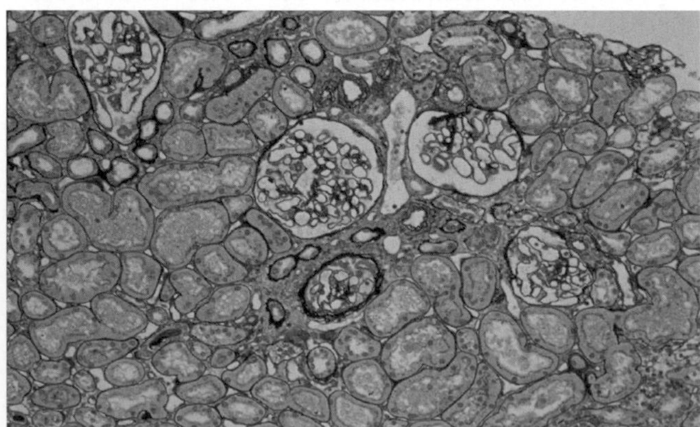

Figure 36–9 Chronic calcineurin-inhibitor nephrotoxicity. There is "striped" tubular atrophy with interstitial fibrosis without a significant lymphocytic infiltrate. The intervening tubules are unremarkable as are the majority of glomeruli. The small glomerulus has mild ischemic features. (Jones methenamine silver × 125)

and show the presence of coexisting acute rejection or de novo or recurrent glomerular lesions.

Treatment

The optimal management of immunosuppression for the chronically failing allograft has yet to be defined. If an element of acute rejection is suspected, a steroid pulse should be given, but this therapy should not be repeated if it is ineffective. Monoclonal and polyclonal antibodies should not be given in the presence of chronic rejection. Intensification of calcineurin inhibitor therapy often merely exaggerates nephrotoxicity. In contrast, a reduction or cessation of CNI in conjunction with either the addition, continuation, or increase in the dose of mycophenolate mofetil may slow the rate of decline of renal function in patients with biopsy-proven CAN and deteriorating allograft function.[135,136] There has been some evidence suggesting that Neoral C2 monitoring is superior to trough monitoring in detecting cyclosporine underexposure or overexposure.[137] In the latter dose reduction has been reported to result in stabilization or improvement of allograft function. More recently, conversion from cyclosporine or tacrolimus to sirolimus has been shown to preserve graft function in patients with biopsy-confirmed CAN.[138] Although a number of studies have demonstrated that CNI dose reduction or withdrawal in conjunction with MMF or sirolimus treatment may improve or slow the progression of CAN, manipulation of immunosuppressive therapy may be of little beneficial effect when SCr is 3.0 to 3.5 mg/dL or higher at the time of therapeutic intervention (unpublished observation).

The relative contribution of nonimmune mechanism(s) to the development of progressive allograft dysfunction is difficult to define, and the management of CAN should be targeted at risk factor modification. Blood pressure control and aggressive management of dyslipidemia are mandatory. The use of angiotensin converting enzyme inhibitor (ACEI) and/or angiotensin receptor blocker (ARB) has also been advocated due to its well-established antiproteinuric and cardioprotective effects. However, these drugs should be used with care because of their potential to cause or exacerbate anemia, hyperkalemia, and renal dysfunction. A rising serum creatinine should alert clinicians to the possibility of renal artery stenosis.

References

1. Shokes DA, Halloran PF: Delayed graft function in renal transplantation: Etiology, management, and long-term significance. J Urol 1996; 155:1831-1840.
2. Homik J, Huiziga RB, Cockfield SM, et al: Elevated serum creatinine: A valuable objective measure of delayed graft function in renal transplant (Abstract). Am Soc Transplant Phys 1997;156.
3. Shokes DA, Cecka JM: Effect of delayed graft function on short- and long-term kidney graft survival. *In* Cecka JM and Terasaki PI (eds): Clinical Transplants. Los Angeles, CA, UCLA Tissue Typing Laboratory, 1997, pp 297-303.
4. Lehtonen SRK, Isoniemi HM, Salmela KT, et al: Long-term graft outcome is not necessarily affected by delayed onset of graft function and early acute rejection. Transplantation 1997; 64:103-107.
5. Paff WW, Howard RJ, Patton HP, et al: Delayed graft function after renal transplantation. Transplantation 1998; 65:219-223.
6. Ojo AO, Wolfe RA, Held WP, et al: Delayed graft function: Risk factors and implication for renal allograft survival. Transplantation 1997; 63:968-974.
7. Marcen R, Orofino L, Pascual J, et al: Delayed graft function does not reduce the survival of renal transplant allografts. Transplantation 1998; 66:461-466.
8. Ploeg RJ, van Bockel JH, Langendijk PT, et al: European Multicentre Study Group: Effect of preservation solution on results of cadaveric kidney transplantation. Lancet 1992; 340: 129-137.
9. Edelstein CL, Ling H, Schrier RW: The nature of renal injury. Kidney Int 1997; 51:134-151.
10. Alkhaunaizi AM, Schrier RW: Management of acute renal failure: New perspectives. Am J Kidney Dis 1996; 28:315-328.
11. Paller MS: Free radical-mediated postischemic injury in renal transplantation. Ren Fail 1992; 14:257-260.
12. Oken DE: Acute renal failure (vasomotor nephropathy): Micropuncture studies of the pathogenic mechanisms. Annu Rev Med 1975; 26:307-319.
13. Humes HD: Acute renal failure: The promise of new therapies. N Engl J Med 1997; 336:870-871.
14. Zimmerman P, Ragavendra N, Hoh CK, Barbaric LB: Diagnostic imaging in kidney transplantation. *In* Danovitch GM (ed): Handbook of Kidney Transplantation. Boston, Little, Brown, 2001, pp 272-289.
15. Shoskes DA, Churchill BM, McLorie GA, et al: The impact of ischemic and immunologic factors on early graft function in pediatric renal transplantation. Transplantation 1990; 50:877-881.
16. Utzig MJ, Blumke M, Wolff-Vorbeck G, et al: Flow cytometry crossmatch: A method for predicting graft rejection. Transplantation 1997; 63:551-554.
17. Lu CY: Ischemia, injury and renal allograft rejection. Curr Opin Nephrol Hypertens 1996; 5:107-110.
18. Nast CC, Zuo X, Prehn J, et al: Gamma-interferon gene expression in human renal allograft fine needle aspirates. Transplantation 1994; 57:498-502.
19. Takada M, Nadeau KC, Hancock WW, et al: Effects of explosive brain death on cytokine activation of peripheral organs in the rat. Transplantation 1998; 65:1533-1542.
20. Shoskes DA, Xie Y, Gonzalez Cadavid NF: Nitric oxide synthase activity in renal ischemia-reperfusion injury in the rat. Transplantation 1997; 63:495-500.
21. Tobak FG: Regeneration after acute tubular necrosis. Kidney Int 1992; 41:226-246.
22. Shoskes DA, Hodge EE, Goormastic M, et al: HLA matching determines susceptibility to harmful effects of delayed graft function in renal transplant recipients. Transplant Proc 1995; 27: 1068-1069.
23. Marcusen N, Lai R, Olson TS, et al: Morphometric and immunohistochemical investigation of renal biopsies from patients with transplant ATN, native ATN, or acute graft rejection. Transplant Proc 1996; 28:479.
24. Solez K, Racusen LC, Marcussen N, et al: Morphology of ischemic acute renal failure, normal function, and cyclosporine toxicity in cyclosporine-treated renal allograft recipients. Kidney Int 1993; 43:1058.
25. Cecka JM, Cho YW, Terasaki PI: Analysis of the UNOS Scientific Renal Transplant Registry at three years: Early events affecting transplant success. Transplantation 1992; 53:59-64.
26. Thadhani R, Pascual M, Bonventr JV: Acute renal failure. N Engl J Med 1996; 334:1448-1460.
27. Cecka JM, Terasaki PI: The UNOS Scientific Renal Transplant Registry. Clin Transpl 1996; 95:1.
28. Wijnen RM, Booster MH, Stubenitsky BM, et al: Outcome of transplantation of non-heart-beating donor kidneys. Lancet 1995; 345:1067-1070.
29. Rudich SM, Kaplan B, Magee JC, et al: Renal transplantations performed using non-heart-beating organ donors: Going back to the future? Transplantation 2002; 74:1715-1720.

30. Lu AD, Carter JT, Weinstein RJ, et al: Excellent outcome in recipients of dual kidney transplants. Arch Surg 1999; 134: 971-976.
31. MacKenzie HS, Azuma H, Rennke HG, et al: Renal mass as a determinant of late allograft outcome: Insights from experimental studies in rats. Kidney Int 1995; 52:S38-S42.
32. Lee RS, Miller E, Marsh CL, et al: Intermediate outcomes of dual renal allografts: The University of Washington experience. J Urol 2003; 169:855-858.
33. Gritsch HA, Rosenthal JT, Danovitch GM: Living and cadaveric kidney donation. *In* Danovitch GM (ed): Handbook of Kidney Transplantation. Boston, Little, Brown, 2001, pp 111-129.
34. Belzer FO, Southard JH: Principles of solid organ preservation by cold storage. Transplantation 1988; 45:673-676.
35. Ploeg RJ: Kidney preservation with UW and Euro-Collins solutions. A preliminary report of a clinical comparison. Transplantation 1990; 49:281-284.
36. Sellers MT, Gallichio MH, Hudson SL, et al: Improved outcomes in cadaveric renal allografts with pulsatile preservation. Clin Transpl 2000; 14:543-549.
37. Polyak MM, Arrington BO, Stubenbord WT, et al: The influence of pulsatile preservation on renal transplantation in the 1990s. Transplantation 2000; 69:249-258.
38. Gritsch HA, Rosenthal JT: The transplant operation and its surgical complications. *In* Danovitch GM (ed): Handbook of Kidney Transplantation. Boston, Little, Brown, 2001, pp 146-162.
39. Danovitch GM: Immunosuppressive medications and protocols for kidney transplantation. *In* Danovitch GM (ed): Handbook of Kidney Transplantation. Boston, Little, Brown, 2001, pp 62-110.
40. Jorkasky DK, Audet P, Shusterman N, et al: Fenoldopam reverses cyclosporine-induced renal vasoconstriction in kidney transplant recipients. Am J Kidney Dis 1992; 19:567-572.
41. Ferguson CJ, Hillis AN, Williams JD, et al: Calcium-channel blockers and other factors influencing delayed function in renal allografts. Nephrol Dial Transplant 1990; 5:816-820.
42. Pollack R, Andrisevic JH, Maddux MS, et al: A randomized double-blind trial of the use of human recombinant superoxide dismutase in renal transplantation. Transplantation 1993; 55: 57-60.
43. Finn WF, Hak LJ, Grossman SH: Protective effect of prostacyclin on postischemic acute renal failure in the rat. Kidney Int 1987; 32:479-487.
44. Adams MB: Enisoprost Renal Transplant Study Group: Enisoprost in renal transplantation. Transplantation 1992; 53: 338-345.
45. Kaija S, Lars W, Henrick E, et al: A randomized multicenter trial of the anti-ICAM-1 monoclonal antibody (enlimonab) for the prevention of acute rejection and delayed onset of graft function in cadaveric renal transplantation: A report of the European Anti-ICAM-1 Renal Transplant Study Group. Transplantation 1999; 67(5):729-736.
46. Allgren RL, Marbury TC, Rahman SN, et al: Anaritide in acute tubular necrosis. N Engl J Med 1997; 336:828-834.
47. Vinot O, Bialek J, Canaan-Kuhl S, et al: Endogenous ANP in postischemic acute renal allograft failure. Am J Physiol 1995; 269:F125-F133.
48. Pirenne J, Lled-Garcia E, Benedetti E: Colonic perforation after renal transplantation. Clin Transpl 1997; 11:88-93.
49. Phillips AO, Deanne C, O'Donnell P, et al: Evaluation of Doppler ultrasound in primary non-function of renal transplants. Clin Transpl 1994; 8:83-86.
50. Terasaki PI: Humoral theory of transplantation. Am J Transplant 2003; 3:665-673.
51. Nast CC, Cohen AH: Pathology of kidney transplantation. *In* Danovitch GM (ed): Handbook of Kidney Transplantation. Boston, Little, Brown, 2001, pp 290-312.
52. Helderman JH, Goral S: Transplantation immunobiology. *In* Danovitch GM (ed): Handbook of Kidney Transplantation. Boston, Little, Brown, 2001, pp 17-38.
53. Troppmann C, Gillingham KJ, Gruessner RW, et al: Delayed graft function in the absence of rejection has no long-term impact. Transplantation 1996; 61:1331-1337.
54. Shoskes DA, Cecka JM: Deleterious effects of delayed graft function in cadaveric renal transplant recipients independent of acute rejection. Transplantation 1998; 66:1697-1701.
55. Barrientos A, Portoles J, Herrero JA, et al: Glomerular hyperfiltration as a nonimmunologic mechanism of progression of chronic renal rejection. Transplantation 1994; 57:753-756.
56. Sollinger HW: U.S. Renal Transplant Mycophenolate Study Group: Mycophenolate mofetil for the prevention of acute rejection in primary cadaveric renal allograft recipients. Transplantation 1995; 60:225.
57. Vicente FK, Laskow DA, Neylan J, et al: One-year follow-up of an open-label trial of FK506 for primary kidney transplantation. Transplantation 1996; 61:1576-1581.
58. Hariharan S, McBride MA, Cherikh WS, et al: Post-transplant renal function in the first year predicts long-term kidney transplant survival. Kidney Int 2002; 62:311-318.
59. Rush DN, Karpinski ME, Nickerson P, et al: Does subclinical rejection contribute to chronic rejection in renal transplant patients? Clin Transpl 1999; 13:441-446.
60. Legendre C, Thervet E, Skhiri H, et al: Histologic features of chronic allograft nephropathy revealed by protocol biopsies in kidney transplant recipients. Transplantation 1998; 65:1506-1509.
61. Rush DN, Nickerson P, Gough J, et al: Beneficial effects of treatment of early subclinical rejection: A randomized study. J Am Soc Nephrol 1998; 9:2129-2134.
62. Nickerson P, Jeffery JR, Gough J, et al: Effect of increasing baseline immunosuppression on the prevalence of clinical and subclinical rejection: A pilot study. J Am Soc Nephrol 1999; 10:1801-1805.
63. Hricik DE, Almawi W, Strom B: Trends in the use of glucocorticoids in renal transplantation. Transplantation 1994; 57:979-989.
64. Kubak BM, Pegues DA, Holt CD: Infectious complications of kidney transplantation and their management. *In* Danovitch GM (ed): Handbook of Kidney Transplantation. Boston, Little, Brown, 2001, pp 221-262.
65. Nargund VH, Cranston D: Urologic complications after renal transplantation. Transplant Rev 1996; 10:24.
66. Watschinger B, Pascual M: Capillary C4d deposition as a marker of humoral immunity in renal allograft rejection. J Am Soc Nephrol 2002; 13:2420-2423.
67. Olive C, Cheung C, Falk MC: Apoptosis and expression of cytotoxic T lymphocyte effector molecules in renal allografts. Transpl Immunol 1999; 7:27-36.
68. Li B, Hartono C, Ding R, et al: Noninvasive diagnosis of renal allograft rejection by measurement of messenger RNA for perforin and granzyme B in urine. N Engl J Med 2001; 344: 947-954.
69. Mauiyyedi S, Covin RB: Humoral rejection in kidney transplantation: New concepts in diagnosis and treatment. Curr Opin Nephrol Hypertens 2002; 11:609-618.
70. Mauiyyedi S, Crespo M, Collins AB, et al: Acute humoral rejection in kidney transplantation: II. Morphology, immunology, and pathologic classification. J Am Soc Nephrol 2002; 13: 779-787.
71. Colvin RB: Renal transplant pathology. *In* Jennette JC, Olson JL, Schwartz MM, Silva FG (eds): Heptinstall's Pathology of the Kidney. Philadelphia, Lippincott-Raven, 1998, p 1409.
72. Leszczynski D, Laszczynska M, Halttunen J, et al: Renal target structures in acute allograft rejection: A histochemical study. Kidney Int 1987; 31:1311.
73. Olsen S, Spencer E, Cockfield S, et al: Endocapillary glomerulitis in the renal allograft. Transplantation 1995; 59:1421.
74. Feucht HE: Complement C4d in graft capillaries: The missing link in the recognition of humoral alloreactivity. Am J Transplant 2003; 3:646.

75. Racusen L, Solez K, Colvin RB, et al: The Banff 97 working classification of renal allograft pathology. Kidney Int 1999; 55: 713.
76. Racusen LC, Colvin RB, Solez K, et al: Antibody-mediated rejection criteria: An addition to the Banff '97 classification of renal allograft rejection. Am J Transplant 2003; 3:708-714.
77. Danovitch GM: Cyclosporine and tacrolimus: Which agent to choose? Nephrol Dial Transplant 1997; 12:1566-1568.
78. Kahan BD, Dunn J, Fitts C, et al: The neoral formulation: Improved correlation between cyclosporine trough levels and exposure in stable renal transplant recipients. Transplant Proc 1994; 26:2940-2943.
79. Mahalati K, Belitski P, Sketris I, et al: Neoral monitoring by simplified sparse sampling area under the concentration-time curve: Its relationship to acute rejection and cyclosporine nephrotoxicity early after kidney transplantation. Transplantation 1999; 68: 55-62.
80. Kahan BD: The Rapamune U.S. Study Group: Efficacy of sirolimus compared with azathioprine for reduction of acute renal allograft rejection: A randomized multicentre study. Lancet 2000; 356:194-202.
81. MacDonald AS: The Rapamune Global Study Group: A worldwide, phase III, randomized, controlled, safety and efficacy study of a sirolimus/cyclosporine regimen for prevention of acute rejection in recipients of primary mismatched renal allografts. Transplantation 2001; 71:271-280.
82. Groth CG, Backman L, Morales J-M, et al: The Sirolimus European Renal Transplant Study Group: Sirolimus (rapamycin)-based therapy in human renal transplantation. Transplantation 1999; 67:1036-1042.
83. Kreis H, Cisterne J-M, Land W, et al: The Sirolimus European Renal Transplant Study Group: Sirolimus in association with mycophenolate mofetil induction for the prevention of acute graft rejection in renal allograft recipients. Transplantation 2000; 69:1252-1260.
84. Podder H, Stepkowski SM, Napoli KL, et al: Pharmacokinetic interactions augment toxicities of sirolimus/cyclosporine combinations. J Am Soc Nephrol 2001; 12:1059-1071.
85. Undre NA: Pharmacokinetics of tacrolimus-based combination therapies. Nephrol Dial Transplant 2003; 18:S12-S15.
86. Lawsin L, Light JA: Severe acute renal failure after exposure to sirolimus-tacrolimus in two living donor kidney recipients. Transplantation 2003; 75:157-160.
87. Pham PT, Peng A, Wilkinson AH, et al: Cyclosporine and tacrolimus-associated thrombotic microangiopathy. Am J Kidney Dis 2000; 36:844-850.
88. Pham PT, Danovitch GM, Wilkinson AH, et al: Inhibitors of ADAMTS13: A potential factor in the etiology of thrombotic microangiopathy in a renal allograft recipient. Transplantation 2002; 74:1077-1080.
89. Edwards C, House A, Shahinian V, et al: Sirolimus-based immunosuppression for transplant-associated thrombotic microangiopathy. Nephrol Dial Transplant 2002; 17:1254-1256.
90. Franco A, Hernandez D, Capdevilla L, et al: De novo hemolytic-uremic syndrome/thrombotic microangiopathy in renal transplant patients receiving calcineurin inhibitors: Role of sirolimus. Transplant Proc 2003; 35:1764-1766.
91. Barone GW, Gurley BJ, Abul-Ezz SR, et al: Sirolimus-induced thrombotic microangiopathy in a renal transplant recipient. Am J Kidney Dis 2003; 42:202-206.
92. Pham PT, Pham PC, Wilkinson AH: Management of the transplant recipient in the early postoperative period. *In* Davidson (ed): Oxford Textbook of Clinical Nephrology, 3rd ed. New York, Oxford University Press (In press).
93. Baid S, Pascual M, Williams WW, et al: Renal thrombotic microangiopathy associated with anti-cardiolipin antibodies in hepatitis C-positive renal allograft recipients. J Am Soc Nephrol 1999; 10:146-153.
94. Bergstrand A, Bohman SO, Farnsworth A, et al: Renal histopathology in kidney transplant recipients immunosuppressed with cyclosporin A: Results of an international workshop. Clin Nephrol 1985; 24:107.
95. Mihatsch MJ, Thiel G, Ryffel G: Cyclosporine nephrotoxicity. Adv Nephrol 1988; 17:303.
96. Young BA, Marsh CL, Alpers CE, Davis CL: Cyclosporine-associated thrombotic microangiopathy/hemolytic uremic syndrome following kidney and kidney-pancreas transplantation. Am J Kidney Dis 1996; 28:561.
97. Fotiadis CN, Govani MV, Helderman JH: Renal allograft dysfunction. *In* Massary SG, Glassock RJ (eds): Textbook of Nephrology. Philadelphia, Lippincott, Williams & Wilkins, 2001, pp 1617-1635.
98. Berger PM, Diamond JR: Ureteral obstruction as complication of renal transplantation: A review. J Nephrol 1998; 11:20-23.
99. Zimmerman P, Ragavendra N, Hoh C, et al: Radiology of kidney transplantation. *In* Danovitch GM (ed): Handbook of Kidney Transplantation. Boston, Little, Brown, 1996, pp 214-231.
100. Mylonakis E, Goes N, Rubin RH, et al: BK virus in solid organ transplant recipients: An emerging syndrome. Transplantation 2002; 72:1587-1592.
101. Nicol DL, P'ng K, Nardic DR, et al: Routine use of indwelling ureteral stents in renal transplantation: A review. J Nephrol 1998; 11:20-23.
102. Almond PS, Matas A, Gillingham K, et al: Risk factors for chronic rejection in renal allograft recipients. Transplantation 1993; 55:752-757.
103. Kahan BD: Toward a rational design of clinical trials of immunosuppressive agents in transplantation. Immunol Rev 1993; 136:29-49.
104. Cecka JM, Cho YW, Terasaki PI: Analysis of the UNOS Scientific Renal Transplant Registry at three years: Early events affecting transplant success. Transplantation 1992; 53:59-64.
105. Brazy PC, Pirsch JD, Belzer FO: Factors affecting renal allograft function in long-term recipients. Am J Kidney Dis 1992; 19:558-566.
106. Van Saase JL, Van der Woude FJ, Thorogood J, et al: The relation between acute vascular and interstitial renal allograft rejection and subsequent chronic rejection. Transplantation 1995; 59:1280-1285.
107. Mauiyyedi S, Pelle PD, Saidman S, et al: Chronic humoral rejection: Identification of antibody-mediated chronic renal allograft rejection by C4d deposits in peritubular capillaries. J Am Soc Nephrol 2001; 12:574-582.
108. Katznelson S, Terasaki PI, Danovitch GM: Histocompatibility testing, crossmatching, and allocation of cadaveric kidney transplants. *In* Danovitch GM (ed): Handbook of Kidney Transplantation. Boston, Little, Brown, 1996, pp 32-54.
109. Terasaki PI, Cecka JM, Gjerson DW, et al: High survival rates of kidney transplants from spousal and living unrelated donors. N Engl J Med 1995; 333:333-336.
110. Opelz G, Mytilineos J, Scherer S, et al: Analysis of HLA-DR matching in DNA-typed cadaver kidney transplants. Transplantation 1993; 55:782-785.
111. Burke JF, Pirsch JD, Ramos EL, et al: Long term efficacy and safety of cyclosporine in renal transplant recipients. N Engl J Med 1994; 331:358-363.
112. Dunn TB, Asolati M, Holman DM, et al: Long-term outcome of a prospective trial of steroid withdrawal after kidney transplantation. Surgery 1999; 125:155-159.
113. Ratcliffe PJ, Dudley CRK, Higgins RM, et al: Randomised controlled trial of steroid withdrawal in renal transplant recipients receiving triple immunosuppression. Lancet 1996; 348:643-648.
114. Ahsan N, Hricik D, Matas A, et al: Prednisone withdrawal in kidney transplant recipients on cyclosporine and mycophenolate mofetil: A prospective randomized study. Transplantation 1999; 68:1865-1874.

115. Kuypers DR, Evenepoel P, Maes B, et al: The use of an anti-CD25 monoclonal antibody and mycophenolate mofetil enables the use of low-dose tacrolimus and early withdrawal of steroids in renal transplant recipients. Clin Transpl 2003; 17: 234-241.
116. Hricik DE, Knauss TC, Bodziak KA, et al: Withdrawal of steroid therapy in African American kidney transplant recipients receiving sirolimus and tacrolimus. Transplantation 2003; 76: 938-942.
117. Brenner BM, Cohen RA, Milford EL: In renal transplantation one size may not fit all. J Am Soc Nephrol 1992; 3:162-169.
118. Tullius SG, Hancock WW, Heeman UW, et al: Reversibility of chronic renal allograft rejection: Critical effect of time after transplantation suggests both host immune dependent and independent phases of progressive injury. Transplantation 1999; 58:93.
119. Mingxi L, Nicholls KM, Becker GJ, et al: Risk factors for late allograft dysfunction: Effects of baseline glomerular size. J Nephrol 2002; 15:620-625.
120. Hayry P: Aspects of allograft rejection: Molecular pathology of acute and chronic rejection. Transplant Rev 1995; 9:113.
121. Fellstrom B: Nonimmune risk factors for chronic renal allograft dysfunction. Transplantation 2001; 11:SS10-SS16.
122. Schindler R, Tullius SG, Tanriver Y, et al: Hypertension increases expression of growth factors and MHC II in chronic allograft nephropathy. Kidney Int 2003; 63:2302-2308.
123. Meir-Kriesche H-U, Cibrick DM, Ojo AO, et al: Interaction between donor and recipient age in determining the risk of chronic renal allograft failure. J Am Geriatr Soc 2002; 50:14-17.
124. Racusen L, Solez K, Colvin RB: Fibrosis and atrophy in the renal allograft: Interim report and new directions. Am J Transplant 2002; 2:203.
125. Sibley RK: Morphologic features of chronic rejection in kidney and less commonly transplanted organs. Clin Transpl 1994; 8:293.
126. Maryniak RK, Weiss MA, First MR: Transplant glomerulopathy: Evolution of morphologically distinct changes. Kidney Int 1985; 27:799.
127. Gough J, Yilmaz A, Miskulin D, et al: Peritubular capillary basement membrane reduplication in allografts and native kidney disease: A clinicopathologic study of 278 consecutive renal specimens. Transplantation 2001; 71:1390.
128. Rosen S, Greenfeld Z, Brezis M: Chronic cyclosporine-induced nephropathy in the rat. Transplantation 1990; 49:445.
129. Nast CC, Cohen AH: Pathology of kidney transplantation. *In* Danovitch GM (ed): Handbook of Kidney Transplantation. Boston, Little, Brown, 1996, p 232.
130. Palestine AG, Austin HA, Balow JE, et al: Renal histopathologic alterations in patients with cyclosporine for uveitis. N Engl J Med 1986; 314:1293.
131. Matas A: Chronic rejection in renal transplant recipients: Risk factor and correlates. Clin Transpl 1994; 8:332-335.
132. Meyer MM, Norman DJ, Danovitch GM: Long-term posttransplant management and complications. *In* Danovitch GM (ed): Handbook of Kidney Transplantation. Boston, Little, Brown, 1996, pp 154-186.
133. Kasiske BL: Long-term posttransplantation management and complications. *In* Danovitch GM (ed): Handbook of Kidney Transplantation. Boston, Little, Brown, 2001, pp 182-220.
134. Ross E, Wilkinson A, Hawkins R, et al: The plasma creatinine concentration is not an accurate reflection of the glomerular filtration rate in stable renal transplant patients receiving cyclosporine. Am J Kidney Dis 1987; 10:113-117.
135. Weir M, Ward MT, Blahut SA: Long-term impact of discontinued or reduced calcineurin inhibitor in patients with chronic allograft nephropathy. Kidney Int 2001; 59:1567-1573.
136. Ducloux D, Motte G, Billerey C, et al: Cyclosporin withdrawal with concomitant conversion from azathioprine to mycophenolate mofetil in renal transplant recipients with chronic allograft nephropathy: A 2-year follow-up. Transplant Int 2002; 15:387-392.
137. Cole E, Maham N, Cardella C, et al: Clinical benefits of C2 monitoring in the long-term management of renal transplant recipients. Transplantation 2003; 75:2086-2090.
138. Egidi MF, Cowan PA, Naseer A, et al: Conversion to sirolimus in solid organ transplantation: A single center experience. Transplant Proc 2003; 35:131S-137S.

Chapter 37

Infection in Renal Transplant Recipients

Jay A. Fishman, M.D. • Emilio Ramos, M.D.

Successful management of infections in the immunocompromised renal transplant recipient is complicated by a variety of factors.[1] These include increased susceptibility to a broad spectrum of infectious pathogens and the difficulty in making a diagnosis of infection in the face of diminished signs and symptoms of infection, an array of noninfectious etiologies of fever (e.g., graft rejection, drug toxicity), and the possibility that multiple processes are present simultaneously. Further, because immunocompromised patients tolerate invasive and established infection poorly with high morbidity and mortality, the urgency for an early and specific diagnosis to guide antimicrobial therapy is increased. Given the primacy of T-lymphocyte dysfunction in transplantation, viral infections in particular are increased and contribute to graft dysfunction, systemic illness, graft rejection, and enhancing the risk for other opportunistic infections (e.g., *Pneumocystis* and *Aspergillus* species) and for virally-mediated cancers.

RISK OF INFECTION

The risk of infection in the renal transplant recipient is determined by the interaction of two factors:

1. The epidemiologic exposures of the patient, including those unrecognized by the patient or distant in time (Table 37–1).
2. The patient's net state of immunosuppression, including all of the factors contributing to the risk for infection in the transplant recipient (Table 37–2).

Epidemiologic Exposures

The prevention and treatment of infection is central to the optimal management of transplant recipients, given the adverse impact of infections on quality of life. Consideration of the epidemiology of infection allows the clinician to establish a differential diagnosis for a given "infectious" presentation and to design the optimal preventive strategy for each patient. Donor and recipient screening are critical components to the post-transplant health maintenance of the patient (Table 37–3). Of these, consideration should be given to empiric therapy for purified protein derivative (PPD) positive patients, for *Strongyloides stercoralis* in patients from endemic regions, and for patients known to have received organs from donors with acute bacterial and fungal infections. Specific antiviral strategies stratified according to individual risk should be considered for all kidney recipients.

Exposures of importance can be divided into four overlapping categories: donor- or recipient-derived infections, and community- or nosocomial-acquired exposures.

Donor-Derived Infections

Infections that are derived from the donor tissues and activated in the recipient are among the most important exposures in transplantation. Some of these are latent while others are the result of bad timing—active infection transmitted at the time of transplantation. All of the known types of infections have been recognized in transplant recipients. The activation of these infections may reflect the intensity of immune suppression or result from the allogeneic response (graft rejection), which activates latent viral pathogens. Three types of infection merit special attention. First, in donors who are bacteremic or fungemic at the time of donation, these infections—staphylococci, pneumococcus, *Candida* species, *Salmonella, E. coli*—tend to "stick" to anastamotic sites (vascular, urinary) and may produce leaks or mycotic aneurysms. Second, viral infections, including cytomegalovirus (CMV) and Epstein-Barr virus (EBV), are associated with particular syndromes and morbidity in the immunocompromised population (discussed later in text). The greatest risk of such infections is in recipients who are seronegative (immunologically naïve) and receive infected grafts from seropositive donors (latent viral infection). Third, late, latent infections, including tuberculosis, may activate many years after the initial exposure. Disseminated mycobacterial infection is often difficult to treat once established due largely to interactions between the antimicrobial agents used to treat infection (e.g., rifampin, streptomycin, isoniazid) and the agents used in immune suppressive therapy.

Given the risk of transmission of infection from the organ donor to the recipient, certain infections should be considered relative contraindications to organ donation. Given that renal transplantation is, in general, elective surgery, it is reasonable to avoid donation from individuals with unexplained fever, rash, or infectious syndromes. Some of the common criteria for exclusion of organ donors are listed in Table 37–4.

Recipient-Derived Exposures

Infections in this category are generally latent infections activated in the setting of immune suppression. It is necessary to obtain a careful history of travel and exposures to guide preventive strategies and empiric therapies. Notable among these infections are tuberculosis, strongyloidiasis, viral infections (herpes simplex and Varicella zoster or shingles), histoplasmosis, coccidioidomycosis, hepatitis B or C, and human immunodeficiency virus (HIV). Vaccination status should be evaluated (tetanus, hepatitis B, childhood vaccines, influenza, pneumococcal vaccine). Dietary habits should also be considered, including the use of well water (*Cryptosporidia*), uncooked meats (*Salmonella, Listeria*), and unpasteurized dairy products (*Listeria*).

Table 37–1 Significant Epidemiologic Exposures Relevant to Transplantation

Donor-Derived

Viral

- Herpes group (cytomegalovirus, Epstein-Barr virus, human herpes viruses 6, 7, 8, herpes simplex)
- Hepatitis viruses (notably B and C)
- Retroviruses (HIV, HTLV-1 and -2)
- Others

Bacteria

- Gram-positive and gram-negative bacteria (*Staphylococcus* species, *Pseudomonas spp.*, Enterobacteriaceae)
- Mycobacteria (tuberculosis and nontuberculous)
- Nocardia asteroides

Fungi

- *Candida* species
- *Aspergillus* species
- Endemic fungi (*Cryptococcus neoformans*)
- Geographic fungi (histoplasma capsulatum, *Coccidioides immitis*, blastomyces)

Parasites

- *Toxoplasma gondii*
- *Trypanosoma cruzi*

Nosocomial Exposures

Methicillin-resistant staphylococci
Vancomycin-resistant enterococci (also linezolid and quinupristin-dalfopristin resistance)
Aspergillus species
Candida non-albicans strains

Community Exposures

Food and water-borne (*Listeria monocytogenes, Salmonella spp., Cryptosporidium spp.*, hepatitis A, *Campylobacter spp.*)
Respiratory viruses (RSV, Influenza, parainfluenza, adenovirus, metapneumovirus)
Common viruses: often with exposure to children (Coxsackie, parvovirus, polyomavirus, papilloma virus)
Atypical respiratory pathogens (*Legionella spp., Mycoplasma spp., Chlamydia*)
Geographic fungi and *Cryptococcus, Pneumocystis jiroveci*
Parasites (often distant)

- *Strongyloides stercoralis*
- *Leishmania* species
- *Toxoplasma gondii*
- *Trypanosoma cruzi*
- *Naeglaeria spp.*

Table 37–2 Factors Contributing to the "Net State of Immunosuppression"

Immunosuppressive Therapy: Type, Temporal Sequence, Intensity

Prior therapies (chemotherapy or antimicrobials)
Mucocutaneous barrier integrity (catheters, lines, drains)
Neutropenia, lymphopenia (often drug-induced)
Underlying immune deficiency

- Hypogammaglobulinemia from proteinuria
- Systemic lupus, complement deficiencies

Metabolic Conditions: Uremia, Malnutrition, Diabetes, Alcoholism/Cirrhosis

Viral infection (CMV, hepatitis B and C, RSV)
Immune suppression
Graft rejection
Cancer/cellular proliferation

Community Exposures

Common exposures in the community are often related to contaminated food and water ingestion, exposure to infected children or coworkers, or exposures due to hobbies (gardening), travel, or work. Respiratory virus infection due to influenza, respiratory syncytial virus, and adenoviruses and more atypical pathogens (Herpes simplex virus, Herpes zoster virus) carries the risk for viral pneumonia but increased risk for bacterial superinfection. Community (social or transfusion-associated) exposure to CMV and EBV may produce severe primary infection in the nonimmune host. Recent and remote exposures to endemic, geographically restricted systemic mycoses (*Blastomyces dermatitidis, Coccidioides immitis,* and *Histoplasma capsulatum*) and *Mycobacterium tuberculosis* can result in localized pulmonary, systemic, or metastatic infection. Asymptomatic *strongyloides stercoralis* infection may activate more than 30 years after initial exposure due to the effects of immunosuppressive therapy. Such reactivation can result in either a diarrheal illness and parasite migration with hyperinfestation syndrome (characterized by hemorrhagic enterocolitis, hemorrhagic pneumonia, or both) or disseminated infection with accompanying (usually) gram-negative bacteremia or meningitis. Gastroenteritis due to *Salmonella* species, *campylobacter jejuni,* and a variety of enteric viruses can result in persistent infection, more severe and prolonged diarrheal disease as well as an increased risk of bloodstream invasion and metastatic infection.

Nosocomial Exposures

Nosocomial infections are of increasing importance because organisms with significant antimicrobial resistance predominate in many centers. These include vancomycin, linezolid and quinupristin/dalfopristin-resistant enterococci, methicillin-resistant staphylococci, and fluconazole-resistant *Candida* species. A single case of nosocomial *Aspergillus* infection in a compromised host should be seen as an indication of the failure of infection control practices. Antimicrobial abuse has resulted in increased rates of *C. difficile* colitis. Outbreaks of infections due to *Legionella* species have been associated with hospital plumbing and contaminated water supplies or ventilation systems. Each nosocomial infection should be investigated to ascertain the source and prevent subsequent infections. Nosocomial spread of *P. jiroveci* between immunocompromised patients has also been suggested by a variety of case series. Respiratory viral infections may be acquired from medical staff and should be considered among the causes of fever and respiratory decompensation among hospitalized or institutionalized, immunocompromised individuals.

Table 37–3 The Pre-Transplant Evaluation of the Donor and Recipient (Consider the Following)

Laboratory Test	All Patients	Patients with Exposure to Endemic Area	Quantitative Viral Studies Available (PCR)
Serologies			
CMV	√		√
HSV	√		√
VZV	√		
EBV	√		√
HIV	√		√
HBV: HBsAg	√		√
anti-HBs	√		
HCV	√		√
Treponema pallidum	√		
Toxoplasma gondii	√		
Strongyloides stercoralis		√	
Leishmania spp.		√	
Trypanosoma cruzi		√	Blood smear
Histoplasma capsulatum		√	
Cryptococcus neoformans		√	Cryptococcal antigen
Coccidioides immitis		√	
Cultures, etc.			
Urinalysis and culture	√		
Skin test: PPD	√		
Chest x-ray (routine)	√		
Stool O&P (Strongyloides)		√	
Urine ova & parasites/cystoscopy		√(for kidneys)	(Schistosomiasis endemic areas)

Table 37–4 Common Infectious Exclusion Criteria for Organ Donors*

Active Infectious Disease
Unknown infection of central nervous system (encephalitis, meningitis)
Herpes simplex encephalitis or other encephalitis
H/o JC virus infection
West Nile virus infection
Cryptococcal infection of any site
Rabies
Creutzfelt-Jacob disease
Other fungal or viral encephalitis
Untreated bacterial meningitis (proof of cure)
Infection with HIV (serologic or molecular)
Active viremia: herpes, acute EBV (mononucleosis)
Serologic or molecular evidence of HTLV-I/II
Active hepatitis A, B
Infection by: *Trypanosoma cruzi, Leishmania, Strongyloides, Toxoplasmosis*
Active tuberculosis
SARS
Untreated pneumonia
Untreated bacterial or fungal sepsis (e.g., candidemia)
Untreated syphilis
Multisystem organ failure due to overwhelming sepsis, gangrenous bowel

*Must be considered in the context of the individual donor and recipient.

Net State of Immunosuppression

The net state of immunosuppression is a measure of all of the factors contributing to the patient's risk for infection (Table 37–2). Among these are:

1. The specific immunosuppressive therapy, including dose, duration, and sequence of agents.
2. Technical problems from the transplant procedure, resulting in leaks (blood, lymph, urine) and fluid collections, devitalized tissue, poor wound healing, and surgical drainage catheters for prolonged periods.
3. Prolonged airway intubation
4. Prolonged use of broad-spectrum antibiotics
5. Renal and/or hepatic dysfunction
6. Prolonged use of vascular access or dialysis catheters

Presence of infection with one of the immunomodulating viruses, including CMV, EBV, hepatitis B (HBV) or C (HCV), or HIV.

Specific immunosuppressive agents are associated with increased risk for certain infections (Table 37–5). Combinations of these agents may enhance this risk or cause toxicity (e.g., nephrotoxicity) and may further enhance risk.

TIMETABLE OF INFECTION

As immunosuppressive regimens have become more standardized, the specific infections that occur most often will vary in a predictable pattern depending on the time elapsed

Table 37–5 Specific Immunosuppressive Drugs and Infection

- Antilymphocyte globulins (lytic) and alloimmune response: Activation of latent (herpes)virus, fever, cytokine release
- Plasmapheresis: Encapsulated bacteria
- Co-stimulatory blockade: Unknown so far
- Corticosteroids: Bacteria, PCP, hepatitis B, C
- Azathioprine: Neutropenia, papilloma virus?
- Mycophenylate mofetil (MMF): Early bacterial infection, B-cells, late CMV?
- Calcineurin inhibitors (cyclosporine/tacrolimus): Enhanced viral replication (absence of immunity), gingival infection, intracellular pathogens
- Sirolimus: Excess infections in combination with current agents, idiosyncratic pneumonitis?

since transplantation (Figure 37–1). This is a reflection of the changing risk factors (surgery/hospitalization, immune suppression, acute and chronic rejection, emergence of latent infections, and exposures to novel community infections.[1] The pattern of infections will be changed with alterations in the immunosuppressive regimen (pulse dose steroids or intensification for graft rejection), intercurrent viral infection, neutropenia (drug toxicity), graft dysfunction, or significant epidemiologic exposures (travel or food).

The time line reflects three overlapping periods of risk for infection: (1) the perioperative period to approximately 4 weeks after transplantation; (2) the period 1 to 6 months after transplantation (depending on the rapidity of taper of immune suppression and the type and dosing of antilymphocyte "induction" that may persist); and (3) the period beyond the first year after transplantation. These periods reflect the changing major risk factors associated with infection: (1) surgery and technical complications; (2) intensive immune suppression with viral activation; and (3) community-acquired exposures with the return of normal activities.

The time line may be used in a variety of ways: (1) to establish a differential diagnosis for the transplant patient suspected of having infection; (2) as a clue to the presence of an excessive environmental hazard for the individual, either within the hospital or in the community; and (3) as a guide to the design of preventive antimicrobial strategies. Infections occurring outside the usual period or of unusual severity suggest either excessive epidemiologic hazard or excessive immunosuppression. The prevention of infection must be linked to the risk for infection at various times after transplantation. Routine preventive strategies from the Massachusetts General Hospital are outlined in Table 37–6. It should be noted that such strategies serve only to delay the onset of infection in the face of epidemiologic pressure. The use of antibiotic prophylaxis, vaccines, and behavioral modifications (e.g., routine hand washing or advice against digging in gardens without masks) may only result in a "shift to the

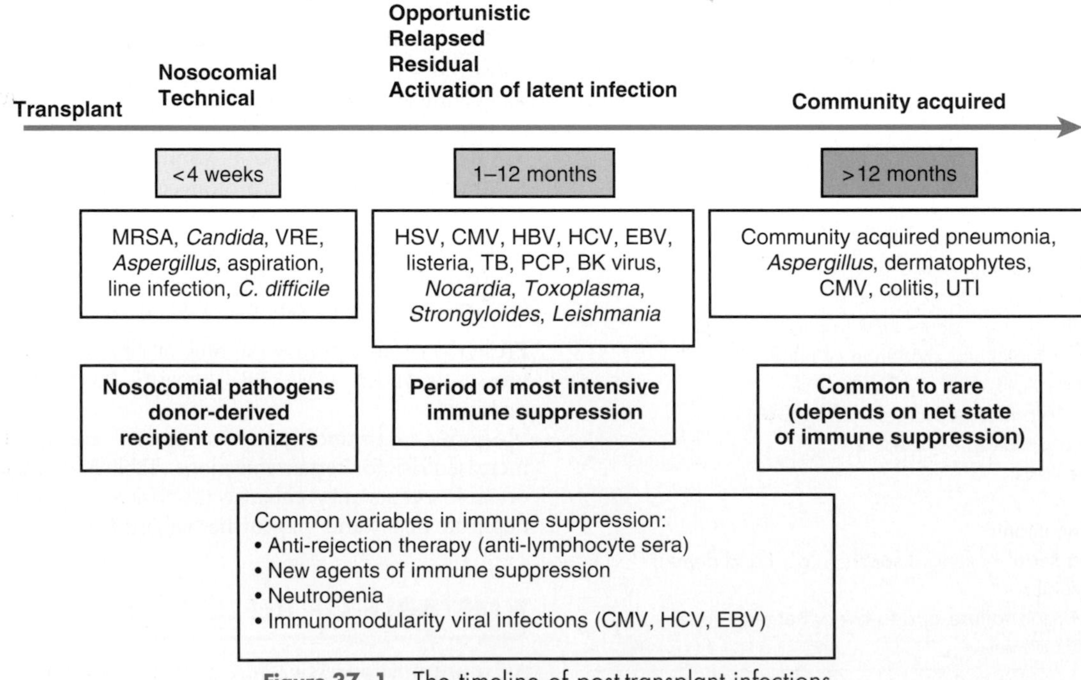

Figure 37–1 The timeline of post-transplant infections.

Table 37-6 Renal Transplantation Antimicrobial Protocols at the Massachusetts General Hospital, Boston, Massachusetts

A. Anti-*Pneumocystis* jiroveci Pneumonia (PCP) and General Antibacterial Prophylaxis

Background: Low dose trimethoprim-sulfamethoxazole prophylaxis (in adults: 1 single strength per day orally) is well tolerated and essentially eradicates *Pneumocystis* infection from this patient population. Lower doses (3 days per week) prevent PCP but may not prevent other infections such as urinary tract infection, nocardiosis and listeriosis, toxoplasmosis, and a variety of gastrointestinal and pulmonary infections.

Regimen: One single strength trimethoprim-sulfamethoxazole tablet (containing 80 mg trimethoprim, 400 mg sulfamethoxazole) po qhs for a minimum of 4–6 months post-transplant. Patients infected with CMV, with chronic rejection, or recurrent infections are maintained on lifelong prophylaxis.

Alternative Regimen: For those patients proven to not tolerate trimethoprim-sulfamethoxazole, alternative regimens include: (1) a combination of atovaquone 1500 mg po with meals once daily plus levofloxacin (or equivalent fluoroquinolone without anti-anaerobic spectrum) 250 mg once daily; (2) pentamidine (300 mg iv or inhaled q 3–4 weeks); and (3) Dapsone (100 mg po qd to biweekly) +/– pyrimethamine. Each of these agents has toxicities that must be considered, including hemolysis in G6PD-deficient hosts with dapsone. None of these alternative programs offer the same broad protection of TMP-SMX.

B. Herpes Group Virus Prevention

Background: The human herpes viruses (cytomegalovirus, CMV; herpes simplex viruses 1 and 2, HSV-1 and HSV-2; Epstein-Barr virus, EBV; varicella-zoster virus, VZV; human herpes virus-6, HHV-6; human herpes virus-7, HHV-7; and human herpes virus-8, HHV-8/Kaposi's sarcoma-associated herpes virus) are among the most important causes of infectious disease morbidity and mortality in the transplant recipient. Different regimens are determined by the clinical risk, the major determinants of which are the past experience of donor and recipient with the virus (as defined by the presence or absence of circulating antibody prior to transplant) and the nature of the immunosuppressive therapy.

1. Treatment of Symptomatic CMV Disease

a. Reduce immune suppression, if possible
b. Consider CMV hyperimmune globulin
c. The standard of care for treating symptomatic CMV disease is a minimum of 2 to 3 weeks of intravenous ganciclovir at a dose of 5 mg/kg twice daily (with dosage adjustment for renal dysfunction). It is not yet clear whether oral valganciclovir may be substituted for intravenous therapy. Regardless of the type of therapy, microbiologic and clinical responses must be demonstrated. The main side effect of ganciclovir is hematopoietic toxicity (some renal toxicity). Alternative agents (cidofovir with renal toxicity, foscarnet with renal, CNS and hepatic and hematopoietic toxicity) are also available and may be preferred in individual patients. The end point of intravenous therapy is the documented clearance of virus from the blood as demonstrated by a negative CMV antigenemia assay or quantitative PCR assay. In seropositive individuals, the risk of subsequent relapse can be essentially eliminated by following intravenous therapy with oral valganciclovir 450 mg PO qd (not FDA approved dose—check creatinine clearance) in renal transplant recipients (see following table) for 3 additional months. Such follow-up oral therapy is obligatory for individuals with primary CMV disease (donor seropositive, recipient seronegative [D+R–]), in whom the risk of relapse without oral therapy is high.
d. Dosing Nomogram for Ganciclovir Treatment of CMV Infections

Serum Creatinine (mg/dL)	Intravenous Dose (mg/kg)	Frequency
<2.0	5	Q12h
2–3	5	Daily
3–5	1.25*	Daily
>5.0	1.25*	QOD
Hemodialysis	5	Post-dialysis
Peritoneal dialysis	2.5*	Daily

*After loading dose of 5 mg/kg. All patients (prophylaxis or therapeutic) received: leukocyte or CMV-negative blood; CMV-hyperimmune globulin 150 mg/kg IV for first dose and 100 mg/kg × 4 at the discretion of the physician.
Data from Fishman JA, Doran MT, Volpicelli SA, et al: Dosing of intravenous ganciclovir for the prophylaxis and treatment of cytomegalovirus infection in solid organ transplant recipients. Transplantation 2000; 69:389-393.

Valganciclovir Conversions: With the availability of oral valganciclovir (full dose therapy as 900 mg po bid), many patients can be converted to oral therapy. It may be preferable to load intravenously and to document a clinical response before conversion. Gastrointestinal CMV requires prolonged therapy.

Valganciclovir Dose Modifications for Patients with Impaired Renal Function*

Serum Cr	CrCl (mL/min)	Treatment dose	Prophylaxis dose
≤ 1.5	≥ 60	900 mg bid	450 renal; 900 mg qd other
1.6–2.5	40–59	450 mg bid	450 mg qd
2.6–4.0	25–39	450 mg qd	450 mg qod
> 4.0	10–24	450 mg qod	450 mg twice weekly

*Formal measurement of creatinine clearance is preferred because measurements of serum creatinine may be misleading. Hemodialysis patients: There are no data on dosing for HD patients at present.

Continued

Table 37-6 Renal Transplantation Antimicrobial Protocols at the Massachusetts General Hospital, Boston, Massachusetts—cont'd

2. Guidelines for Prevention of Cytomegalovirus Infection

Prophylaxis of High-Risk Patients: Prophylaxis is achieved with 50% of the therapeutic dose of ganciclovir or valganciclovir (corrected for renal function). In some patients, intravenous immune globulin (IvIG or hyperimmune globulin) is used as an adjunctive therapy for prophylaxis.

Certain subgroups merit routine prophylaxis. These include:

- Solid organ transplant recipients who are naïve (seronegative) and receive an organ from a seropositive donor (D+/R–)
- Solid organ transplant recipients who are seropositive (R+) and receive antilymphocyte antibodies or other intensive immune suppression (e.g., for graft rejection)

Antiviral Prophylaxis Made Simple*

CMV Serologic Status +/– Antilymphocyte Antibody Therapy	Therapy	Screening (Antigenemia)
D+/R-	Intravenous ganciclovir 5mg/kg iv for loading dose then per renal function to discharge; then po valganciclovir (450 mg/d for renal transplants) × 3 mo	Monthly for 6 months after D/C of therapy+
D+ or R+ with antilymphocyte antibody therapy	Intravenous ganciclovir 5mg/kg iv for first dose then per renal function to discharge; D/C on po valganciclovir (450 mg/d renal) × 6 months	Monthly for 6 months after D/C of therapy+
D–/R+ (no antilymphocyte antibody therapy)	Oral valganciclovir (450 mg/d renal) × 3 months	Symptoms only
D–/R–	Oral famciclovir (Famvir) 500 mg po qd × 3–4 mo (or valacyclovir 500 bid or acyclovir 400 tid) Use of CMV-negative or leukocyte-filtered blood	Symptoms, fever/neutropenia
Status unknown with ALS	Intravenous ganciclovir 5mg/kg iv for first dose and QD (corrected for renal function) until sero-status determined.	

Neutropenia: The dose of antiviral and antibacterial therapies ARE NOT, in general, reduced for neutropenia. Consider other options first!

+ ALS: Antilymphocyte antibodies include any of the lytic, lymphocyte-depleting antisera

*Note: Not FDA approved at these doses

3. Anti-*Candida* Prophylaxis:

Prevention of mucocutaneous infection can be accomplished with oral clotrimazole (may increase CyA levels) or nystatin 2 to 3 times per day at times of steroid therapy or in the face of antibacterial therapy. Fluconazole, at a dose of 200–400 mg/day for 10–14 days is utilized in the treatment of prophylaxis failures. Routine prophylaxis with fluconazole is used for pancreas transplants.

right" of the infection time line, unless the intensity of immune suppression is reduced or immunity develops.

Phase One: 1 to 4 Weeks After Transplantation

During the first month after transplantation, three types of infection occur.

The first type of infection is that present in the recipient prior to transplantation, was inadequately treated, and now has emerged in the setting of surgery, anesthesia, and immunosuppression. Pre-transplantation pneumonia and vascular access infections are common examples of this type of infection. Colonization of the recipient with resistant organisms is also common (e.g., MRSA). The first rule of successful transplant infectious disease is the eradication of all infection possible prior to transplantation.

The second type of early infection was present in the donor before transplantation. This is often a nosocomial-acquired organism (resistant gram-negative bacilli and *S. aureus* or *Candida* species) due to (1) systemic infection in the donor (e.g., line infection) or (2) contamination during the organ procurement process. The end result is a high risk of infection of vascular suture lines with resultant mycotic aneurysm. Uncommonly, infections have been transmitted from donor to recipient, including tuberculosis or fungal (e.g., histoplasmosis) infection that may emerge earlier in the time line than would be predicted (i.e., in the first month).

The third type and the most common source of infections in this period are related to the complex surgical procedure of transplantation. These include surgical wound infections, pneumonia (aspiration), bacteremia due to vascular access or surgical drainage catheters, urinary tract infections, or infections of fluid collections—leaks of vascular or urinary anastamoses or of lymphoceles. These are nosocomial infections and, as such, are due to the same bacteria and *Candida* infections observed in nonimmunosuppressed patients undergoing comparable surgery. However, given the immune suppression, the signs of infection may be subtle and the severity or duration may be greater. The technical skill of the surgeons and meticulous postoperative care (i.e., wound care, endotracheal tubes, vascular access devices, and drainage catheters) are the determinants of risk for these infections. Also among the common infections is *C. difficile* colitis. Limited perioperative antibiotic prophylaxis (i.e., from a single dose to 24 hours of an antibiotic such as cefazolin) is usually adequate with additional coverage only for known risk factors (e.g., prior colonization with MRSA). For pancreas transplantation, perioperative prophylaxis against yeasts with fluconazole is used in addition, bearing in mind the interactions between azole antifungal agents and calcineurin inhibitors and sirolimus (levels may be increased significantly).

Notable by their absence in the 1st month after transplantation are opportunistic infections, even though the daily doses of immunosuppressive drugs are at their highest during this time. The implications of this observation are important: The net state of immunosuppression is not great enough to support the occurrence of opportunistic infections unless an exposure has been excessive; this observation suggests that it is not the daily dose of immunosuppressive drugs that is of importance but rather the sustained administration of these drugs, the "area under the curve," in determining the net state of immunosuppression. Thus, the occurrence of a single case of opportunistic infection in this period should trigger an epidemiologic investigation for an environmental hazard.

Phase Two: 1 to 6 Months After Transplantation

Infection in the transplant recipient 1 to 6 months after transplantation has one of three causes:

1. Lingering infection from the peri-surgical period, including relapsed *C. difficile* colitis, inadequately treated pneumonia, or infection related to a technical problem (e.g., urine leak, lymphocele, hematoma). Fluid collections require drainage.
2. Viral infections, including CMV, HSV, shingles (VZV), human herpesvirus 6 or 7, EBV, relapsed hepatitis (HBV, HCV), and HIV. This group of viruses is unique: lifelong infection; tissue-associated (often transmitted with the allograft from seropositive donors); immunomodulating—systemically immune suppressive and, potentially, predisposing to graft rejection. It is also notable that the herpesviruses are prominent due to the attenuated ability of T cells to control these infections. Among the other viral pathogens of this period must be included BK polyomavirus in association with allograft dysfunction and community-acquired respiratory viruses (adenovirus, influenza, parainfluenza, respiratory syncytial virus, metapneumovirus). The suppression of antibody production (e.g., using tacrolimus and mycophenylate mofetil or with lymphopenia) may predispose to other infections.
3. Opportunistic infection due to *P. jiroveci*, *Listeria monocytogenes*, *T. gondii*, *Nocardia* species, *Aspergillus* species, and other agents.

In this period, the stage is also set for the emergence of a subgroup of patients, the "chronic ne'er-do-wells"—individuals who require higher than average immune suppression to maintain graft function or who have prolonged untreated viral infections and other opportunistic infections, predicting long-term susceptibility to many other infections (third phase, discussed later). Such individuals may merit prolonged (lifelong) prophylaxis (antibacterial and/or antiviral) to prevent life-threatening infection.

The specific opportunistic infections that occur, reflect the specific immunosuppressive regimen used and the presence or absence of immunomodulating viral infection. Viral pathogens (and rejection) are responsible for the majority of febrile episodes that occur in this period. During this period, anti-CMV strategies and trimethoprim-sulfamethoxazole prophylaxis are effective in decreasing the risk of infection. Trimethoprim-sulfamethoxazole prophylaxis eliminates *P. jiroveci* pneumonia (PCP) and reduces the incidence of urinary tract infection and urosepsis, *L. monocytogenes* meningitis, *Nocardia* species infection, and *Toxoplasma gondii.*

Phase Three: More Than 6 to 12 Months After Transplantation

Transplant recipients who are more than 6 months past the procedure can be divided into three groups in terms of infection risk.

The first group consists of the majority of transplant recipients (70%–80%) who had a technically good procedure with satisfactory allograft function, reduced and maintenance immunosuppression, and absence of chronic viral infection. These patients resemble the general community in terms of infection risk, with community-acquired respiratory viruses constituting their major risk. Occasionally, such patients will develop primary CMV infection (socially acquired) or infections related to underlying diseases (e.g., skin infections in diabetes).

The second group (~10% of patients) suffers chronic viral infection, which, in the absence of effective therapy, will lead inexorably to one of three results:

- End organ damage (e.g., BK polyomavirus nephropathy, cryoglobulinemia, or cirrhosis from HCV—HBV being relatively well managed at present)
- Malignancy (post-transplantation lymphoproliferative disease [PTLD] due to EBV, skin, or anogenital cancer due to papilloma viruses)
- Acquired immunodeficiency syndrome (HIV/AIDS)

The third group of patients (~10% of all recipients) has less than satisfactory allograft function and requires excessive amounts of immunosuppressive therapy for recurrent graft rejection. This may be associated with chronic viral infection. This is the subgroup of transplant recipients, often termed the "chronic ne'er-do-wells," who are at highest risk for opportunistic infection with such pathogens as *P. jiroveci*, *L. monocytogenes*, *N. asteroides*, and *Cryptococcus neoformans.* It is our practice to give these patients lifetime maintenance trimethoprim-sulfamethoxazole prophylaxis and to consider the use of fluconazole prophylaxis. Also, this group is susceptible to organisms more often associated with immune dysfunction of AIDS (Bartonella, Rhodococcus, Cryptosporidium, and Microsporidium species) and invasive fungal pathogens

(*Aspergillus*, *Zygomycetes*, and the *Dematiaceae*, or pigmented, molds). Minimal signs or symptoms merit careful evaluation in this group of "high-risk" individuals.

ASSESSMENT OF INFECTIOUS DISEASE IN RECIPIENT AND POTENTIAL DONOR BEFORE TRANSPLANTATION

Guidelines for pre-transplant screening have been the subject of several recent publications including a consensus conference of the Immunocompromised Host Society (ICHS), the American Society for Transplantation (AST) Clinical Practice Guidelines on the evaluation of renal transplant candidates, and the ASTP Clinical Practice Guidelines on the evaluation of living renal transplant donors.[2–9]

The Transplant Donor

Deceased Donor Evaluation

The critical feature of screening for deceased donors is time limitation. A useful organ must be procured and implanted before some microbiologic assessments have been completed. Thus, major infections must be excluded and appropriate cultures and stored samples obtained for future reference. As a result, bacteremia or fungemia may not be detected until after the transplant has occurred. Such infections have not generally resulted in transmission of infection as long as the infection has been adequately treated, both in terms of use of antimicrobial agents to which the organism is susceptible and time. In recipients of tissues from 95 bacteremic donors, a mean of 3.8 days of effective therapy post-transplantation appeared adequate to prevent transmission; longer courses of therapy in the recipient are preferred, targeting known potential pathogens from the donor.[10] Bacterial meningitis must also be treated with antibiotics that penetrate the CSF before procurement. Similarly, due to the limited time for testing, certain acute infections (CMV, EBV, HIV, HBV, or HCV) may be undetected in the period prior to antibody formation, and viral DNA detection is preferred. As a result, the donor's clinical, social, and medical histories are essential to reducing the risk of such infections. However, in the presence of known infection, such infections must be treated prior to procurement, if possible. Major exclusion criteria are outlined in Table 37–4.

Living Donor Evaluation

The differences in screening of the living donor and the cadaver donor are largely based on the different time frames during which this screening takes place. The living donor procedure should be considered elective—and, thus, evaluation completed and infections treated prior to such procedures. An interim history must be taken at the time of surgery to assess the presence of new infections since the initial donor evaluation. Intercurrent infections (flu-like illness, headache, confusion, myalgia, cough) might be the harbinger of important infection (West Nile Virus, SARS, rabies, *Trypanosoma cruzi*). Live donors undergo a battery of serologic tests (Table 37–3) as well as PPD skin test and, if indicated, chest radiograph. The testing must be individualized based on unique risk factors (e.g., travel). Of particular importance to the renal transplant recipient is the exclusion of urinary tract infection. Whether focal infections in the donor outside the procured organs merit therapy remains unresolved.

Special Considerations in Procurement

Mycobacterium tuberculosis. This bacterium from the donor represented approximately 4% of reported post-transplant TB cases in a review of 511 patients by Singh and colleagues.[11] Active disease should be excluded in PPD positive donors, including chest radiograph, sputum cultures, and chest CT, if the chest radiograph is abnormal. Urine AFB cultures may be useful in the PPD-positive kidney donor. Isoniazid prophylaxis of the recipient should be considered for untreated, PPD-positive donors.[12] Factors mitigating towards prophylaxis include donor from endemic region, use of high-dose steroid regimen, or high-risk social environment.

Chagas' disease (T. cruzi). This parasitic disease has been transmitted by transplantation in endemic areas and recently in the United States. Schistosomiasis and infection by *Strongyloides stercoralis* are generally recipient-derived problems.

Viral Infections other than CMV

Epstein-Barr virus. The risk for post-transplant lymphoproliferative disease (PTLD) is greatest in the EBV seronegative recipient of an EBV seropositive allograft (i.e., D+/R–). This is most common in pediatric transplant recipients and in adults coinfected with CMV or on higher levels of immune suppression. Monitoring should be considered for at-risk individuals using a quantitative, molecular assay (e.g., PCR) for EBV.[13,14] EBV is also a cofactor for other lymphoid malignancies.

Varicella screening should be used to identify seronegative individuals (no history of chicken pox or shingles) for vaccination prior to transplantation. HSV screening is performed by most centers despite the use of antiviral prophylaxis during the post-transplant period. VZV serologic status is particularly important in children who may be exposed at school (for antiviral or varicella immune globulin prophylaxis) and in adults with atypical presentations of infection (pneumonia or GI disease). Other herpesviruses may reactivate with HHV-6 and HHV-7 serving as cofactors for CMV and fungal infections and in endemic regions, Kaposi's sarcoma-associated herpesvirus (HHV-8/KSHV) causing malignancies.

Hepatitis B virus (HBV). HBsAg and HBV core antibody (HBcAb) are used for screening purposes with HBsAb positivity indicating either vaccination or prior infection. HBcAb-IgM positivity suggests active HBV infection, whereas IgG positivity suggests a more remote or persistent infection. The HBsAg negative, HBcAb-IgG positive donor may have viral DNA in the liver but may be appropriate as a donor for HBV-infected renal recipients. Quantitative assays for HBV should be obtained to guide further therapy. The presence of HBsAg negative, HBcAb-IgG positive assays may be a false-positive or reflect true, latent HBV infection.

Hepatitis C virus (HCV) infection will generally progress more rapidly with immune suppression and with CMV coinfection. HCV seropositive renal transplant candidates are more likely to develop cirrhosis and complications of liver failure. There is no good therapy for HCV infection; management is by quantitative molecular viral assays.

HIV-infected donors have not been utilized. The progression of disease is rapid and outweighs the benefits of transplantation. Donors may be excluded based on historic evidence of "high-risk" behavior for HIV infection. Western blot testing and molecular assays (PCR) should be obtained prior to the use of tissues from any HIV-seropositive donor.

Human T-lymphotropic virus I (HTLV-I) is endemic in the Caribbean and parts of Asia (Japan) and can progress to HTLV-I-associated myelopathy/tropical spastic paraparesis (HAM/TSP) or to adult T cell leukemia/lymphoma (ATL). HTLV-II is similar to HTLV-I serologically but is less clearly associated with disease. Use of organs from such donors is generally avoided.[15,16]

West Nile virus (WNV) is a flavivirus associated with viral syndromes and meningoencephalitis and may be transmitted by blood transfusion and organ transplantation.[17,18] Routine screening of donors is not advocated other than in areas with endemic infection of the blood supply. Donors with unexplained changes in mental status or recent viral illness with neurologic signs should be avoided.

SARS (Severe Acute Respiratory Syndrome) is a recently described coronavirus, thought to be associated with exposure to civets or other animals common to the diet of certain regions of China. Tissue persistence is prolonged and infection of transplant recipients appears to be severe and often symptomatic. Organ procurement should exclude patients with recent acute illnesses meeting SARS criteria.

Recipient Screening

The pre-transplant period is useful for a thorough travel, animal, and environmental and exposure history; updating immunizations; and counseling of the recipient regarding travel, food, and other infection risks. Ongoing infection must be eradicated prior to transplantation. Two forms of infection pose a special risk:

1. Bloodstream infection: This is related to vascular access, including that for dialysis and pneumonia, which puts the patient at high risk for subsequent lung infection with nosocomial organisms. Infected ascites or peritoneal dialysis fluid must also be cleared prior to surgery. Urinary tract infection (UTI) must be eliminated prior to transplantation with antibiotics with or without nephrectomy. Similarly, skin disease that threatens the integrity of this primary defense against infection should be corrected before transplantation, even if doing so requires the initiation of immunosuppression prior to transplantation (e.g., the initiation of immune suppression to treat psoriasis or eczema). Finally, the history of more than one episode of diverticulitis should initiate an evaluation to determine whether sigmoid colectomy should be carried out prior to transplantation.
2. Tuberculosis: Both the incidence of active disease and the occurrence of disseminated infection due to *M. tuberculosis* are far higher in the transplant recipient than in the general population. Active tuberculous disease must be eradicated prior to transplantation. The major antituberculous drugs are potentially hepatotoxic, and significant drug interactions are common between the anti-TB agents and the agents of immune suppression. In patients with active infection, from endemic regions or with high risk exposures, TB therapy should be initiated in all PPD positive individuals prior to transplantation. Some judgment may be used as to the optimal timing of treatment in individuals without evidence of active or pleuropulmonary disease. Greater risk may include:

- Previously active tuberculosis or significant signs of old tuberculosis on chest radiograph
- Recent tuberculin reaction conversion
- Known exposure to active disease
- Protein-calorie malnutrition, cirrhosis, or other immune deficiency
- Living in a shelter or other group housing

AIDS

For those benefiting from HAART, AIDS has been converted from a progressively fatal disease to a chronic infection controlled by complex regimens of antiviral agents. HAART has been associated with reduced viral loads, improved CD4 lymphocyte counts, and reduced susceptibility to opportunistic infections. In the pre-HAART era, organ transplantation was generally associated with a rapid progression of AIDS. As a result, HIV-infected individuals have been excluded at most transplantation centers. However, prolonged disease-free survival with HAART has lead to a reconsideration of this policy. Renal transplantation in HIV has been associated with good outcomes in individuals with controlled HIV infection and in the absence of HCV co-infection.[19] Management requires some sophistication regarding both the immune suppressive agents and the various HAART regimens.

SELECTED INFECTIONS OF IMPORTANCE

General Considerations

The spectrum of infection in the immunocompromised host is quite broad. Given the toxicity of antimicrobial agents and the need for rapid interruption of infection, early, specific diagnosis is essential in this population. Advances in diagnostic modalities (CT or MRI scanning, molecular microbiologic techniques) may greatly assist in this process. However, the need for invasive diagnostic tools cannot be overemphasized. Given the diminished immune responses of the host and the frequency of multiple simultaneous processes, invasive diagnosis is often the only method for optimal care. The initial therapy will, by necessity, be broad with a rapid narrowing of the antimicrobial spectrum as data become available. *The first choice of therapy is to reduce the intensity of immune suppression.* The risk of such an approach is that of graft rejection. The selection of the specific reduction may depend upon the organisms isolated. Similarly, reversal of some immune deficits (neutropenia, hypogammaglobulinemia) may be possible with adjunctive therapies (colony stimulating factors or IgG). Co-infection with virus (CMV) is common and merits additional therapy.

Viral Pathogens

Cytomegalovirus (CMV)

CMV is the single most important pathogen in transplant recipients, having a variety of direct and indirect effects.[1,27] The direct effects include:

- Fever and neutropenia syndrome with features of infectious mononucleosis, including hepatitis, nephritis, leukopenia, and/or thrombocytopenia
- Pneumonia
- Gastrointestinal invasion with colitis, esophagitis, gastritis, ulcers, bleeding, or perforation
- Hepatitis, pancreatitis, chorioretinitis

With the exception of chorioretinitis, the direct clinical manifestations of CMV infection usually occur 1 to 4 months after transplantation; chorioretinitis usually does not begin until later in the transplant course.

Although CMV is the most common cause of clinical infectious disease syndromes, its "indirect effects" are often more important. CMV infection produces a profound suppression of a variety of host defenses, predisposing to secondary invasion by such pathogens as *P. jiroveci*, *Candida* and *Aspergillus* species, and some bacterial infections. CMV also contributes to the risk for graft rejection, PTLD, HHV6, and HHV7 infections. The mechanisms for this effect are complex, including altered T-cell subsets and MHC synthesis, and the elaboration of an array of pro-inflammatory cytokines, chemokines, and growth factors.

Patterns of Transmission

Transmission of CMV in the transplant recipient occurs in one of three patterns: primary infection, reactivation infection, and superinfection.[1]

Primary CMV infection

Primary infection occurs when seronegative individuals receive grafts from latently infected, seropositive donors (donor seropositive, recipient seronegative [D+R−]), with subsequent reactivation of the virus and systemic dissemination after transplantation. Between 40% and 50% of these patients experience direct infectious disease manifestations of CMV while the majority are viremic, often without symptoms. Primary CMV infection may also occur in seronegative individuals after transfusion or sexual contacts in the community. This disease may be severe.

Reactivation CMV infection

In reactivation infection, seropositive individuals reactivate endogenous virus after transplantation (donor seropositive or seronegative, recipient seropositive [D+R+ or D−R+]). When conventional immunosuppressive therapy is used (e.g., no antilymphocyte antibody treatment), approximately 10% to 15% experience direct infectious disease syndromes with a higher rate with the use of induction antilymphocyte therapy. Up to 50% of these individuals are viremic, often without symptoms.

CMV superinfection

Virus may be reactivated in the setting of an allograft from a seropositive donor transplanted into a seropositive recipient (D+R+).

Pathogenesis

Control of CMV infection is via MHC-restricted, virus-specific, cytotoxic T lymphocyte response (CD8+ cells) controlled by CD4+ lymphocytes. Seroconversion is a marker for the development of host immunity. Thus, the major effector for activation of virus is the nature of the immunosuppressive therapy being administered. The lytic antilymphocyte antibodies, both polyclonal and monoclonal, are direct activators of viral infection (mimicking the alloimmune response) and also provoke the elaboration of TNF and the other pro-inflammatory cytokines that enhance viral replication. Cyclosporine, tacrolimus, sirolimus, and prednisone (other than pulse doses) have limited ability to reactivate latent CMV while azathioprine, mycophenolate, and cyclophosphamide are moderately potent in terms of promoting viral reactivation. These agents perpetuate infection once established.

Allograft rejection is a major stimulus for CMV activation and vice versa. Thus, the CMV infection has been linked to a diminished outcome of renal and other allografts. As a result, Reinke and colleagues[27] showed that 17 of 21 patients for whom biopsy revealed evidence of "late acute rejection" demonstrated a response to antiviral therapy. Further, Lowance and colleagues[28] demonstrated that the prevention of CMV infection also resulted in a lower incidence of graft rejection.

Diagnosis

Clinical management of CMV, both prevention and treatment, is of great importance for the transplant recipient. It is based on a clear understanding of the causes of CMV activation and the variety of diagnostic techniques available. CMV cultures are generally too slow and insensitive for clinical utility. Further, a positive CMV culture (or shell vial culture) derived from respiratory secretions or urine is of little diagnostic value—many patients secrete CMV in the absence of invasive disease. Serologic tests are useful prior to transplantation to predict risk but are of little value after transplantation in defining clinical disease (this statement includes measurements of anti-CMV immunoglobulin M [IgM] levels). Should a patient seroconvert to CMV, this is evidence that the patient has been exposed to CMV and has developed some degree of immunity. However, seroconversion in transplantation is generally delayed and, thus, not useful for clinical diagnosis. The demonstration of CMV inclusions in tissues in the setting of a compatible clinical presentation is the "gold standard" for diagnosis.

Quantitation of the intensity of CMV infection has been linked to the risk for infection in transplant recipients.[29–33] Two types of quantitative assays have been developed: the molecular assays and the antigen detection assays. The antigenemia assay is a semiquantitative fluorescent assay in which circulating neutrophils are stained for CMV early antigen (pp65), which is taken up nonspecifically as a measure of the total viral burden in the body. The molecular assays (direct DNA PCR, hybrid capture, amplification assays) are highly specific and sensitive for the detection of viremia. Most commonly used assays include plasma-based PCR testing and the whole-blood hybrid capture assay, noting that whole blood and plasma-based assays cannot be directly compared. The highest viral loads are often associated with tissue-invasive disease with the lowest in asymptomatic CMV infection. Viral loads in the CMV syndrome are variable. Either assay can be used in management.

The advent of quantitative assays for the diagnosis and management of CMV infection has allowed noninvasive diagnosis in many patients with two important exceptions:

1. Neurologic disease, including chorioretinitis
2. Gastrointestinal disease, including invasive colitis and gastritis.

In these syndromes, the CMV assays are often *negative* and invasive (biopsy) diagnosis may be needed.

The central role of assays is illustrated by the approach to prevention and treatment of CMV (Table 37–6). The schedule for screening is linked to the risk for infection. Thus, in the high risk patient (D+/R– or R+ with antilymphocyte globulin) after the completion of prophylaxis, monthly screening is performed to assure the absence of infection for 3 to 6 months. In the patient being treated for CMV infection, the assays provide an end point (zero positivity) for therapy and the initiation of prophylaxis.

CMV Prevention

Prevention of CMV infection must be individualized for immunosuppressive regimens and the patient. Two strategies are commonly used for CMV prevention: (1) universal prophylaxis and (2) preemptive therapy. Universal prophylaxis involves giving antiviral therapy to all "at-risk" patients beginning at or immediately post-transplant for a defined time period. In preemptive therapy, quantitative assays are used to monitor patients at predefined intervals to detect early disease. Positive assays result in therapy. Preemptive therapy incurs extra costs for monitoring and coordination of outpatient care while reducing the cost of drugs and the inherent toxicities. Prophylaxis has the possible advantage of preventing not only CMV infection during the period of greatest risk, but also diminishing infections due to HHV6, HHV7, and EBV. Further, the indirect effects of CMV (i.e., graft rejection, opportunistic infection) may also be reduced by routine prophylaxis. In practice neither strategy is perfect. Both breakthrough disease and ganciclovir resistance have been observed in both approaches.

Given the risk for invasive infection, patients at risk for primary infection (CMV D+/R–) are generally given prophylaxis for 3 to 6 months after transplantation. We utilize 6 months of prophylaxis in patients receiving lytic antilymphocyte antibodies. Other groups are candidates for preemptive therapy *if* an appropriate monitoring system is in place and patient compliance is good.

Treatment

The standard of care for treating CMV disease is 2 to 3 weeks of intravenous ganciclovir (5 mg/kg twice daily, with dosage adjustments for renal dysfunction). In patients slow to respond to therapy and who are seronegative, the addition of 3 months of CMV hyperimmune globulin in seronegative individuals (150 mg/kg/dose iv) may be useful. Relapse does occur, primarily in those not treated beyond the achievement of a negative quantitative assay. Therefore, we treat intravenously until viremia has been cleared and following it with prophylaxis with 2 to 4 months of oral ganciclovir (1 g two or three times daily) or valganciclovir (based on creatinine clearance). This approach has resulted in rare symptomatic relapses and appears to prevent the emergence of antiviral resistance.

A number of issues remain. First, the role of oral valganciclovir in treatment has not been well studied. This agent provides good bioavailability but is not approved for this indication. Further, some relapses occur in GI disease because the assays used to follow disease are not reliable in this setting. Thus, repeat endoscopy should be considered to assure the clearance of infection. The optimum dosing of valganciclovir for prophylaxis in renal transplant recipients is also unclear. Many centers use 450 mg/day po (given reduced creatinine clearance) although the FDA approved dosing 900 mg/day. It is worth measuring the creatinine clearance to ensure appropriate dosing.

Alternative therapies are available in intravenous form only. These include foscarnet and cidofovir. Foscarnet has been used extensively for therapy of CMV in AIDS patients. It is active against most ganciclovir-resistant strains of CMV, although we prefer combination therapy (ganciclovir and foscarnet) for such individuals, given the toxicities of each agent and the antiviral synergy demonstrated. Cidofovir has been used in renal transplant recipients, often with nephrotoxicity. Both foscarnet and cidofovir may exhibit synergistic nephrotoxicity with calcineurin inhibitors. A newer class of agents (leflunamide) has been approved for immune suppression and treatment of rheumatologic diseases but also appears to have useful activity against CMV (and possibly BK polyomavirus).

Epstein-Barr Virus

EBV is a ubiquitous herpesvirus (the majority of adults are infected) that has B-lymphocytes as a primary target for infection. In immunosuppressed transplant recipients, primary EBV infection (and relapses in the absence of antiviral immunity) causes a mononucleosis-type syndrome, generally presenting as a lymphocytosis (B-cells) with or without lymphadenopathy or pharyngitis. Meningitis, hepatitis, and pancreatitis may also be observed. Remitting-relapsing EBV infection is common in children and may reflect the interplay between evolving antiviral immunity and immune suppression. This syndrome should suggest relative over-immune suppression.

EBV also plays a central role in the pathogenesis of post-transplant lymphoproliferative disorder or PTLD.[34–37] The most clearly defined risk factor for PTLD is primary EBV infection that increases the risk for PTLD by 10- to 76-fold. PTLD may occur, however, in the absence of EBV infection or in seropositive patients. Post-transplant non-Hodgkin's lymphoma (NHL) is a common complication of solid organ transplantation. Lymphomas comprise up to 15% of tumors among adult transplant recipients (51% in children) with mortality of 40% to 60%. Many deaths are associated with allograft failure after withdrawal of immune suppression during treatment of malignancy. Compared with the general population, PTLD has increased extranodal involvement, poor response to conventional therapies, and poor outcomes. The spectrum of disease ranges from benign polyclonal, B-cell infectious mononucleosis-like disease to malignant, monoclonal lymphoma.[38] The majority is of B-cell origin, although T-cell, NK-cell and null cell tumors are described. It should be noted that EBV-negative PTLD has been described and that T-cell PTLD has been demonstrated in allografts, confused with graft rejection or other viral infection. PTLD late (more than 1–2 years) after transplantation is more often EBV-negative in adults.

The clinical presentations of EBV-associated PTLD vary:

1. Unexplained fever (fever of unknown origin)
2. A mononucleosis-type syndrome, with fever, malaise, with or without pharyngitis or tonsillitis (often diagnosed incidentally in tonsillectomy specimens); often no lymphadenopathy is observed.
3. Gastrointestinal bleeding, obstruction, perforation
4. Abdominal mass lesions
5. Infiltrative disease of the allograft
6. Hepatocellular or pancreatic dysfunction
7. Central nervous system disease

Diagnosis

Serologic testing is not useful for the diagnosis of acute EBV infection or PTLD in transplantation. Thus, quantitative EBV viral load testing is required for the diagnosis and management of PTLD.[39–42] Serial assays are more useful in an individual patient than specific viral load measurements. These assays are not standardized and cannot be directly compared between centers. There are some data to suggest that assays using unfractionated whole blood are preferable to plasma samples for EBV viral load surveillance.

Management

Clinical management depends on the stage of disease. In the polyclonal form, particularly in children, reestablishment of immune function may suffice to cause PTLD to regress. At this stage, it is possible that antiviral therapy might have some utility given the viremia and role of EBV as an immune suppressive agent. With the progression of disease to extra-nodal and monoclonal malignant forms, reduction in immune suppression may be useful, but alternate therapies are often required. In renal transplantation, the failure to regress with significant reductions in immune suppression may suggest the need to sacrifice the allograft for patient survival. Combinations of anti-B-cell therapy (anti-CD20 rituximab), chemotherapy (CHOP), and/or adoptive immunotherapy with stimulated T cells have been utilized.[43–46]

Polyomaviruses

Polyomaviruses have been identified in transplant recipients in association with nephropathy and ureteral obstruction (BK virus) and in association with demyelinating disease of the brain (JC virus) similar to that in AIDS. Polyomaviruses are small nonenveloped viruses with covalently closed, circular, double-stranded DNA genomes. Adult levels of seroprevalence are 65% to 90%. BK virus appears to achieve latency in renal tubular epithelial cells. JC virus has also been isolated from renal tissues but appears to have preferred tropism for neural tissues. Reactivation occurs with immune deficiency and suppression and tissue injury (e.g., ischemia-reperfusion).

BK Polyomavirus Infection

BK virus is associated with a range of clinical syndromes in immunocompromised hosts: viruria and viremia, ureteral ulceration and stenosis, and hemorrhagic cystitis.[47–54] Active infection of renal allografts has been associated with progressive loss of graft function (BK nephropathy) in some individuals. This may be referred to as polyomavirus-associated nephropathy or PVAN. BK nephropathy is rarely recognized in recipients of nonrenal organs. The clinical presentation of disease is usually as sterile pyuria, reflecting shedding of infected tubular and ureteric epithelial cells. These cells contain sheets of virus and are detected by urine cytology as "decoy cells." In most cases, such cells are not detected and the patient presents with diminished renal allograft function or with ureteric stenosis and obstruction. In such patients, the etiologies of decreased renal function must be carefully evaluated (e.g., mechanical obstruction, drug toxicity, pyelonephritis, rejection, thrombosis, recurrent disease), and choices must be made between *increasing immune suppression* to treat suspected graft rejection and *reducing immune suppression* to allow the immune system to control infection. Patients with BK nephropathy treated with increased immune suppression have a high incidence of graft loss. Reduced immune suppression may stabilize renal allograft function but risks graft rejection. Polyoma-associated nephropathy manifested by characteristic histologic features and renal dysfunction is found in about 1% to 8% of renal transplant patients.

Risk factors for nephropathy are poorly defined. Nickeleit and colleagues[51,52] found that cellular rejection occurred more commonly in patients with BK nephropathy than in controls. Other studies have implicated high dose immunosuppression (particularly tacrolimus and mycophenolate mofetil), pulse dose steroids, severe ischemia-reperfusion injury, exposure to antilymphocyte antibody therapy, increased number of HLA mismatches between donor and recipient, cadaver renal transplants, and presence and degree of viremia in the pathogenesis of disease. The role of specific immunosuppressive agents has not been confirmed.

Diagnosis

The use of urine cytology to detect the presence of infected decoy cells in the urine has approximately 100% sensitivity for BK virus infection but a low (29%) predictive value.[53,54] It is, therefore, a useful screening tool but cannot establish a firm diagnosis. The use of molecular techniques to screen blood or urine has also been advocated but is more useful in management of established cases (viral clearance with therapy) than in specific diagnosis.[55–60] Hirsch and colleagues[53] showed that patients with BK nephropathy have a plasma viral load statistically significantly higher (>7700 BK virus copies per mL of plasma, $p<.001$, 50% positive predictive value, 100% negative predictive value) when compared to patients without such disease.[53]

Given the presence of viremia in renal allograft recipients, it is critical to reduce immune suppression when possible. However, the possible coexistence of rejection with BK infection makes renal biopsy essential for the management of such patients. Renal biopsies will demonstrate cytopathic changes in renal epithelial cells without cellular infiltration with the gradual evolution of cellular infiltration consistent with the diagnosis of interstitial nephritis. Fibrosis is often prominent occasionally with calcification. Immunostaining for cross reacting SV40 virus demonstrates patchy staining of viral particles within tubular cells.

Treatment

There is no accepted treatment for PVAN other than a marked reduction in the intensity of immune suppression. It is possible to monitor the response to such maneuvers using urine cytology (decoy cells) and viral load measures in blood and/or urine. The greatest incidence of BK nephropathy is at centers with the most intensive immune suppressive regimens. Thus, it is unclear whether reduction of calcineurin inhibitors or antimetabolites should be considered first. Given the toxicity of calcineurin inhibitors for tubular cells and the role of injury in the activation of BK virus, as well as the need for anti-BK T-cell activity, we have generally reduced these agents first. Other centers have selected reduction of the antimetabolite first. Regardless of the approach, renal function, drug levels, and viral loads must be monitored carefully.

Some centers advocate the use of cidofovir for BK nephropathy in low doses (0.25–1 mg/kg every 2 weeks).[61–64] Significant renal toxicity may be observed with this agent, especially in combination with the calcineurin inhibitors. Retransplantation has been achieved in such patients with failed allografts, possibly as a reflection of immunity developing subsequent to reduction in immune suppression.[65]

JC Virus

Infection of the central nervous system by JC polyomavirus has been observed uncommonly in renal allograft recipients as progressive multifocal encephalopathy. This infection generally presents with focal neurologic deficits or seizures and may progress to death following extensive demyelination. PML may be confused with calcineurin neurotoxicity; both may respond to a reduction in drug levels. It is thought that these are distinct entities, but further studies are underway.

Fungal Infections

In addition to the endemic mycoses, transplant recipients are at risk for opportunistic infection with a variety of fungal agents, the most important of which are *Candida* species, *Aspergillus* species, and *C. neoformans.*

Candida Species

The most common fungal pathogen in these patients is *Candida*, with *C. albicans* and *C. tropicalis* accounting for 90% of the infections and *C. glabrata* for most of the rest. Mucocutaneous candidal infection (e.g., oral thrush, esophageal infection, cutaneous infection at intertriginous sites, candidal vaginitis) occurs particularly when candidal overgrowth is promoted by the presence of high levels of glucose and glycogen in tissues and fluids (e.g., with poorly controlled diabetes, high-dose steroid therapy) and by broad-spectrum antibacterial therapy). These infections are usually treatable through correction of the underlying metabolic abnormality and topical therapy with clotrimazole or nystatin.

More difficult to manage is candidal infection occurring in association with the presence of foreign bodies that violate the mucocutaneous surfaces of the body (e.g., vascular access catheters, surgical drains, and bladder catheters). Optimal management of these infections requires removal of the foreign body and systemic antifungal therapy with either fluconazole or amphotericin.

A special problem in renal transplant recipients is candiduria, even if the patient is asymptomatic. Particularly in individuals with poor bladder function, obstructing fungal balls can develop at the ureteropelvic junction, resulting in obstructive uropathy, ascending pyelonephritis, and the possibility of systemic dissemination. A single positive culture result for *Candida* species from a blood specimen necessitates systemic antifungal therapy, because this finding carries a risk of visceral invasion of more than 50% in this population. Fluconazole (400-600 mg/day, with adjustment for renal dysfunction), because of its better safety profile, is usually used as initial therapy, unless the patient is critically ill or a fluconazole-resistant species (e.g., *C. glabrata* or *C. krusei*) is present. In these instances, therapy is with caspofungin or amphotericin B, usually in a lipid preparation. Flucytosine may be useful as an adjunctive therapy in resistant infections but must be guided by drug levels and attention to hematopoietic toxicity.

Aspergillus Species

Invasive aspergillosis is a medical emergency in the transplant recipient, with the portal of entry being the lungs and sinuses in more than 90% of patients and the skin in most of those remaining. Two species, *A. fumigatus* and *A. flavum*, account for most of these infections, although amphotericin-resistant isolates (*A. terreus*) are occasionally recognized. The pathologic hallmark of invasive aspergillosis is blood vessel invasion, which accounts for the three clinical characteristics of this infection: tissue infarction, hemorrhage, systemic dissemination with metastatic invasion. Early in the course of transplantation, central nervous system involment with fungal infection is most often due to *Aspergillus* species; more than 1 year after transplantation, other fungi (zygomycetes, dematiaceous fungi) are increasingly prominent.

The drug of choice for this infection is probably voriconazole, noting the intense interactions between this agent and the calcineurin inhibitors and sirolimus. Liposomal amphotericin is a reasonable alternative, and combination therapies are under study. Of note, surgical debridement is often essential for the successful clearance of such invasive infections.

Central Nervous System Infection and *Cryptococcus neoformans*

Central nervous system (CNS) infection in the transplant recipient is an important differential for the clinician. The spectrum of causative organisms is broad and must be considered in terms of the timeline for infection in this population. Many infections are metastatic to the CNS, often from the lungs. Thus, a "metastatic workup" is a component of evaluation of CNS lesions, including those due to *Aspergillus*, *Cryptococcus*, *Nocardia*, or *Strongyloides stercoralis.* Viral infections include cytomegalovirus (nodular angiitis), herpes simplex meningoencephalitis, JC virus (PML), and varicella zoster virus. Common bacterial infections include *Listeria monocytogenes*, mycobacteria, *Nocardia*, and occasionally *Salmonella* species. Brain abscess and epidural abscess may be observed with methicillin-resistant staphylococcus, penicillin resistant pneumococcus and quinolone-resistant streptococci problematic. Metastatic fungi include *Aspergillus* and *Cryptococcus* but also spread from sinuses (*Mucoraceae*), skin (*Dematiaceae*), and bloodstream (*Histoplasma* and *Pseudoallescheria/Scedosporium*, *Fusarium* species). Parasites include *Toxoplasma gondii* and *Strongyloides*. Given the spectrum of etiologies, precise diagnosis is essential. In particular, empiric therapy must "cover" *Listeria* (ampicillin), *Cryptococcus* (fluconazole or amphotericin), and herpes simplex virus (acyclovir) while awaiting data from lumbar puncture, blood cultures, and radiographic studies. Included in the differential diagnosis are noninfectious etiologies, including calcineurin inhibitor toxicity and lymphoma, as well as metastatic cancer. Biopsy is often needed for a firm diagnosis.

Cryptococcus neoformans

Cryptococcal infection is rarely seen in the transplant recipient until more than 6 months after transplantation. In the relatively intact transplant recipient, the most common presentation of cryptococcal infection is that of an asymptomatic pulmonary nodule, often with active organisms present. In the "chronic ne'er-do-well" patient, pneumonia and meningitis are common with skin involvement at sites of tissue injury (catheters) also being observed.

Cryptococcosis should be suspected in transplant recipients present with unexplained headaches (especially when accompanied by fevers), decreased state of consciousness, failure to thrive, or unexplained focal skin disease (which requires biopsy for culture and pathologic evaluation) more than 6 months after transplantation. Diagnosis is often achieved by serum cryptococcal antigen detection, but all such patients should have lumbar puncture for cell counts and cryptococcal antigen studies. Initial treatment is probably best with amphotericin and 5-flucytosine followed by high dose fluconazole until the cryptococcal antigen is cleared from blood and cerebrospinal fluid. Scarring and hydrocephalus may be observed.

Fever and Pneumonitis and *Pneumocystis* Infection

The spectrum of potential pathogens of the lungs in transplantation is too broad for this discussion. However, some general concepts are worth mentioning. As for all infections in transplantation, invasive diagnostic techniques are often necessary in these hosts. The depressed inflammatory response of the immunocompromised transplant patient may greatly modify or delay the appearance of a pulmonary lesion on radiograph. Focal or multifocal consolidation of acute onset will quite likely be caused by bacterial infection. Similar multifocal lesions with subacute to chronic progression are more likely secondary to fungi, tuberculosis, or nocardial infections. Large nodules are usually a sign of fungal or nocardial infection, particularly if they are subacute to chronic in onset. Subacute disease with diffuse abnormalities, either of the peribronchovascular type or miliary micronodules, are usually caused by viruses (especially CMV) or *Pneumocystis jiroveci*.[66,67] Additional clues can be found by examining pulmonary lesions for cavitation; cavitation suggests such necrotizing infections as those caused by fungi (*Aspergillus* or *Mucoraceae*), *Nocardia*, *Staphylococcus*, certain gram-negative bacilli, most commonly with *Klebsiella pneumoniae* and *Pseudomonas aeruginosa*.[68–70] CT of the chest is useful when the chest radiograph is negative or when the radiographic findings are subtle or nonspecific. CT is also essential to the definition of the extent of the disease process, the possibility of multiple simultaneous processes (superinfection), and to the selection of the optimal invasive technique to achieve microbiologic diagnosis.

Pneumocystis jiroveci Pneumonia

The risk of infection with *Pneumocystis* is greatest in the first 6 months after transplantation and during periods of increased immune suppression.[1,66,67] The natural reservoir of infection remains unknown. Aerosol transmission of infection has been demonstrated by a number of investigators in animal models, and clusters of infections have developed in clinical settings, including between HIV-infected persons and renal transplant recipients. Activation of latent infection remains a significant factor in the incidence of disease in immunocompromised hosts. In the solid organ transplant recipient, chronic immune suppression that includes corticosteroids is most often associated with pneumocystosis. Bolus corticosteroids, cyclosporine, or co-infection with CMV may also contribute to the risk for *Pneumocystis* pneumonia.

In patients not receiving trimethoprim-sulfamethoxazole (or alternative drugs) as prophylaxis, most transplant centers report an incidence of *Pneumocystis jiroveci* pneumonia of approximately 10% in the first 6 months post-transplant. There is a continued risk of infection in three overlapping groups of transplant recipients: (1) those who require higher than normal levels of immune suppression for prolonged periods of time due to poor allograft function or chronic rejection; (2) those with chronic cytomegalovirus infection; and (3) those undergoing treatments that increase the level of immune deficiency, such as cancer chemotherapy or neutropenia due to drug toxicity. The expected mortality due to *Pneumocystis* pneumonia is increased in patients on cyclosporine when compared to other immunocompromised hosts. The hallmark of infection due to *P. jiroveci* is the presence of marked hypoxemia, dyspnea, and cough with a paucity of physical or radiologic findings. In the transplant recipient, *Pneumocystis* pneumonia is generally acute to subacute in development. Atypical *Pneumocystis* infection (radiographically or clinically) may be seen in patients who have coexisting pulmonary infections or who develop disease while receiving prophylaxis with second choice agents (e.g., pentamidine or atovaquone). Patients outside the usual period of greatest risk for PCP may present with indolent disease confused with heart failure. In such patients, diagnosis often has to be made by invasive procedures. The role of sirolimus therapy in the clinical presentation is unknown. A number of patients have been identified with interstitial pneumonitis while receiving sirolimus; it is not known whether this syndrome is directly attributable to sirolimus or reflects concomitant infection.

Diagnosis

The characteristic hypoxemia of *Pneumocystis* pneumonia produces a broad alveolar-arterial PO_2 gradient. The level of serum lactic dehydrogenase (LDH) is elevated in most patients with *Pneumocystis* pneumonia (>300 international units [IU]/mL). However, many other diffuse pulmonary processes also raise serum LDH levels.

Like many of the "atypical" pneumonias (pulmonary infection without sputum production), no diagnostic pattern exists for *Pneumocystis* pneumonia on routine chest radiograph. The chest radiograph may be entirely normal or develop the classical pattern of perihilar and interstitial "ground glass" infiltrates. Microabscesses, nodules, small effusions, lymphadenopathy, asymmetry, and linear bands are common. Chest computerized tomography (CT-scans) will be more sensitive to the diffuse interstitial and nodular pattern than routine radiographs. The clinical and radiologic manifestations of *P. jiroveci* pneumonia are virtually identical to those of CMV. Indeed, the clinical challenge is to determine whether both pathogens are present. Significant extrapulmonary disease is uncommon in the transplant recipient.

Identification of *P. jiroveci* as a specific etiologic agent of pneumonia in an immunocompromised patient should lead to successful treatment. A distinction should be made between the diagnosis of *Pneumocystis* infection in AIDS and in non-AIDS patients. The burden of organisms in infected AIDS patients is generally greater than that of other immunocompromised hosts and noninvasive diagnosis (sputum induction) more often achieved. In general, noninvasive testing should be attempted to make the initial diagnosis, but invasive techniques should be used when clinically feasible. The diagnosis of *P. jiroveci* infection has been improved by the use of induced sputum samples and of immunofluorescent monoclonal antibodies to detect the organism in clinical specimens. These antibodies bind both cysts and trophozoites. The cyst wall can be displayed by a variety of staining techniques; of these, the Gomori's methenamine-silver nitrate method (which stains organisms brown or black) is most reliable, even though it is susceptible to artifacts. Sporozoites and trophozoites are stained by polychrome stains, particularly the Giemsa stain.

Therapy

Early therapy, preferably with trimethoprim-sulfamethoxazole (TMP-SMZ) is preferred; few renal transplant patients will tolerate full-dose TMP-SMZ for prolonged periods of time. This reflects both the elevation of creatinine due to trimethoprim (competing for secretion in the kidney) and the toxicity of sulfa agents for the renal allograft. Hydration and the gradual initiation of therapy may help. Alternate therapies are less desirable but have been used with success, including: intravenous pentamidine, atovaquone, clindamycin with primaquine or pyrimethamine, and trimetrexate. Although a reduction in the intensity of immune suppression is generally considered a part of anti-infective therapy in transplantation, the use of short courses of adjunctive steroids with a gradual taper is sometimes used in transplant recipients (as in AIDS patients) with severe respiratory distress associated with PCP.

The importance of preventing *Pneumocystis* infection cannot be overemphasized. Low dose trimethoprim-sulfamethoxazole is well tolerated and should be used in the absence of concrete data demonstrating true allergy. Alternative prophylactic strategies including dapsone, atovaquone, inhaled or intravenous pentamidine, are less effective than trimethoprim-sulfamethoxazole but useful in the patient with significant allergy to sulfa drugs. TMP-SMX is the most effective agent for prevention of infection due to *P. jiroveci.* The advantages of TMP-SMX include increased efficacy, lower cost, the availability of oral preparations, and possible protection against other organisms, including *Toxoplasma gondii*, *Isospora belli*, *Cyclospora cayetanensis*, *Nocardia asteroides*, and common urinary, respiratory, and gastrointestinal bacterial pathogens. It should be noted that alternative agents lack this spectrum of activity.

Table 37–7 Vaccinations to Consider Prior to Transplantation

Measles/mumps/rubella (MMR)
Diphtheria/tetanus/pertussis (DTP)
Poliovirus
Haemophilus influenzae type b
Hepatitis B
Pneumococcus
Influenza
Varicella

Vaccination

Due to concerns about the efficacy of vaccines following transplantation, patients should complete vaccinations at least 4 weeks beforehand to allow time for an optimal immune response and resolution of subclinical infection from live vaccines. Vaccinations should include pneumococcal vaccine (if not vaccinated in last 3–5 years), documentation of tetanus and MMR (measles, mumps, rubella) and polio status, as well as vaccines for hepatitis B and Varicella zoster (if no history of chickenpox or shingles) (see also Table 37–7). After transplant, influenza vaccination should be performed yearly or as per local guidelines. Recommended schedules and doses for routine vaccinations can be obtained from the United States Centers for Disease Control and Prevention (CDC) at www.immunize.org or the CDC Immunization Information Hotline, (800) 232-2522.

References

1. Fishman JA, Rubin RH: Infection in organ-transplant recipients. N Engl J Med 1998; 338:1741–1751.
2. Schaffner A: Pretransplant evaluation for infections in donors and recipients of solid organs. Clin Infect Dis 2001; 33(suppl 1):S9–S14.
3. Avery RK, Ljungman P: Prophylactic measures in the solid-organ recipient before transplantation. Clin Infect Dis 2001; 33(suppl 1):S15–S21.
4. Delmonico FL, Snydman DR: Organ donor screening for infectious diseases: Review of practice and implications for transplantation. Transplantation 1998; 65:603–610.
5. Delmonico FL: Cadaver donor screening for infectious agents in solid organ transplantation. Clin Infect Dis 2000; 31:781–786.
6. Avery RK: Recipient screening prior to solid-organ transplantation. Clin Infect Dis 2002; 35:1513–1519.

7. Kasiske BL, Cangro CB, Hariharan S, et al: American Society of Transplantation. The evaluation of renal transplant candidates: Clinical practice guidelines. Am J Transplant 2001; 2(suppl 1):5–95.
8. Kasiske BL, Ravenscraft M, Ramos EL, et al: The evaluation of living renal transplant donors: Clinical practice guidelines. Ad Hoc Clinical Practice Guidelines Subcommittee of the Patient Care and Education Committee of the American Society of Transplant Physicians. J Am Soc Nephrol 1996; 7:2288–2313.
9. Rosengard BR, Feng S, Alfrey EJ, et al: Report of the Crystal City meeting to maximize the use of organs recovered from the cadaver donor. Am J Transplant 2002; 2:701–711.
10. Freeman RB, Giatras I, Falagas ME, et al: Outcome of transplantation of organs procured from bacteremic donors. Transplantation 1999; 68:1107–1111.
11. Singh N, Paterson DL: Mycobacterium tuberculosis infection in solid-organ transplant recipients: Impact and implications for management. Clin Infect Dis 1998; 27:1266–1277.
12. Antony SJ, Ynares C, Dummer JS: Isoniazid hepatotoxicity in renal transplant recipients. Clin Transplant 1997; 11:34–37.
13. Preiksaitis JK, Keay S: Diagnosis and management of posttransplant lymphoproliferative disorder in solid-organ transplant recipients. Clin Infect Dis 2001; 33(suppl 1):S38–S46.
14. Green M, Cacciarelli TV, Mazariegos GV, et al: Serial measurement of Epstein-Barr viral load in peripheral blood in pediatric liver transplant recipients during treatment for posttransplant lymphoproliferative disease. Transplantation 1998; 66:1641–1644.
15. Guidelines for counseling persons infected with human T-lymphotropic virus type I (HTLV-I) and type II (HTLV-II). Centers for Disease Control and Prevention and the U.S.P.H.S. Working Group. Ann Intern Med 1993; 118:448–454.
16. Tanabe K, Kitani R, Takahashi K, et al: Long-term results in human T-cell leukemia virus type 1-positive renal transplant recipients. Transplant Proc 1998; 30:3168–3170.
17. Update: Investigations of West Nile virus infections in recipients of organ transplantation and blood transfusion. MMWR Morb Mortal Wkly Rep 2002; 51:833–836.
18. Update: Investigations of West Nile virus infections in recipients of organ transplantation and blood transfusion? Michigan, 2002. MMWR Morb Mortal Wkly Rep 2002; 51:879.
19. Fishman JA: Transplantation for patients infected with human immunodeficiency virus: no longer experimental, but not yet routine. J Infect Dis 2003; 188:1405–1411.
20. Aguado JM, Herrero JA, Gavalda J, et al: Clinical presentation and outcome of tuberculosis in kidney, liver and heart transplant recipients in Spain. Transplantation 1997; 63:1278–1286.
21. Delaney V, Sumrani N, Hong JH, Sommer B: Mycobacterial infections in renal allograft recipients. Transplant Proc 1993; 25:2288–2289.
22. Lichtenstein IH, MacGregor RR: Mycobacterial infections in renal transplant recipients: Report of five cases and review of the literature. Rev Infect Dis 1983; 5:216–226.
23. Lloveras J, Peterson PK, Simmons Rl, Najarian JS: Mycobacterial infections in renal transplant recipients: Seven cases and a review of the literature. Arch Intern Med 1982; 142:888–892.
24. Qunibi WY, Al-Sibai MB, Taher S, et al: Mycobacterial infections after renal transplantation: Report of fourteen cases and review of the literature. QJM 1990; 77:1039–1060.
25. Roy V, Weisdorf D: Typical and atypical mycobacterium. *In* Bowden RA, Ljungman P, Paya CV (eds): Transplant Infections. Philadelphia, Lippincott Raven, 1998.
26. Singh N, Paterson DL: Mycobacterium tuberculosis infection in solid-organ transplant recipients: Impact and implications for management. Clin Infect Dis 1998; 27:1266–1277.
27. Reinke P, Fietze E, Ode-Hakum S, et al: Late-acute renal allograft rejection and symptomless cytomegalovirus infection. Lancet 1994; 344:1737–1738.
28. Lowance D, Neumayer HH, Legendre CM, et al: Valacyclovir for the prevention of cytomegalovirus disease after renal transplantation. International Valacyclovir Cytomegalovirus Prophylaxis Transplantation Study Group. N Engl J Med 1999; 340:1462–1470.
29. Caliendo AM, St George K, Kao SY, et al: Comparison of quantitative cytomegalovirus (CMV) PCR in plasma and CMV antigenemia assay: Clinical utility of the prototype AMPLICOR CMV MONITOR test in transplant recipients. J Clin Microbiol 2000; 38:2122–2127.
30. Humar A, Kumar D, Boivin G, Caliendo AM: Cytomegalovirus (CMV) virus load kinetics to predict recurrent disease in solid-organ transplant patients with CMV disease. J Infect Dis 2002; 186:829–833.
31. Mazzulli T, Drew LW, Yen-Lieberman B, et al: Multicenter comparison of the digene hybrid capture CMV DNA assay (version 2.0), the pp65 antigenemia assay, and cell culture for detection of cytomegalovirus viremia. J Clin Microbiol 1999; 37:958–963.
32. Paya C: Prevention of cytomegalovirus disease in recipients of solid-organ transplants. Clin Infect Dis 2001; 32:596–603.
33. Sia IG, Patel R: New strategies for prevention and therapy of cytomegalovirus infection and disease in solid-organ transplant recipients. Clin Microbiol Rev 2000; 13:83-121; table of contents.
34. Opelz G, Henderson R: Incidence of non-Hodgkin lymphoma in kidney and heart transplant recipients. Lancet 1993; 342: 1514–1516.
35. Paya C, Fung JJ, Nalesnik MA, et al: Epstein-Barr virus-induced posttransplant lymphoproliferative disorders. Transplantation 1999; 68:1517–1525.
36. Nalesnik M: The diverse pathology of posttransplant lymphoproliferative disorders: Importance of a standardized approach. Transplant Infect Dis 2001; 3:88–96.
37. Preiksaitis JK, Keay S: Guidelines for the diagnosis and management of post transplant lymphoproliferative disorder in solid organ transplant recipients. Clin Infect Dis 2001; 33(suppl 1): S38–S46.
38. Harris NL, Swerdlow SH, Frizzera G, et al: Posttransplant lymphoproliferative disorders (PTLD) pathology and genetics: Tumours of haematopoietic and lymphoid tissues. *In* Jaffe ES, Harris NL, Stein H, Vardiman JW (eds): WHO Classification of Tumours. Lyons, France, IARC Press, 2001, pp 264–269.
39. Green M: Management of Epstein-Barr virus-induced post-transplant lymphoproliferative disease in recipients of solid organ transplantation. Am J Transplant 2001; 1:103–108.
40. Mutimer D, Kaur N, Tang H, et al: Quantitation of Epstein-Barr virus DNA in the blood of adult liver transplant recipients. Transplantation 2000; 69:954–959.
41. Gartner BC, Fischinger J, Schafer H, et al: Epstein-Barr viral load as a tool to diagnose and monitor post-transplant lymphoproliferative disease. Recent Results Cancer Res 2002; 159:49–54.
42. Rowe DT, Webber S, Schauer EM, et al: Epstein-Barr virus load monitoring: Its role in the prevention and management of PTLD. Transplant Infect Dis 2001; 3:79–87.
43. Straathof KCM, Savoldo B, Heslop H, et al: Immunotherapy for post-transplant lymphoproliferative disease. Br J Hematol 2002; 118:728–740.
44. Durandy A: Anti-B cell and anti-cytokine therapy for the treatment of PTLD: Past, present and future. Transplant Infect Dis 2001; 3:104–107.
45. Haque T, Wilkie GM, Taylor C, et al: Treatment of Epstein-Barr-virus-positive post-transplantation lymphoproliferative disease with partly HLA-matched allogeneic cytotoxic T cells. Lancet 2002; 360:436–442.
46. Davis CL: Interferon and cytotoxic chemotherapy for the treatment of post transplant lymphoproliferative disorder. Transplant Infect Dis 2001; 3:108–118.
47. Heritage J, Chesters PM, McCance DJ: The persistence of papovavirus BK DNA sequences in normal human renal tissue. J Med Virol 1981; 8:143–150.
48. Randhawa P, Vats A, Shapiro R, et al: BK virus: Discovery, epidemiology, and biology. Graft 2002; 5(suppl):S19–S27.

49. Mylonakis E, Goes N, Rubin RH, et al: BK virus in solid organ transplant recipients: An emerging syndrome. Transplantation 2001; 72:1587–1592.
50. Randhawa PS, Finkelstein S, Scantlebury V, et al: Human polyoma virus-associated interstitial nephritis in the allograft kidney. Transplantation 1999; 67:103–109.
51. Nickeleit V, Hirsch HH, Zeiler M, et al: BK-virus nephropathy in renal transplants-tubular necrosis, MHC-class II expression and rejection in a puzzling game. Nephrol Dial Transplant 2000; 15:324–332.
52. Nickeleit V, Hirsch HH, Binet IF, et al: Polyomavirus infection of renal allograft recipients: From latent infection to manifest disease. J Am Soc Nephrol 1999; 10:1080–1089.
53. Hirsch HH, Knowles W, Dickenmann M, et al: Prospective study of polyomavirus type BK replication and nephropathy in renal-transplant recipients. N Engl J Med 2002; 347:488–496.
54. Fishman JA: BK virus nephropathy? polyomavirus adding insult to injury. N Engl J Med 2002; 347:527–530.
55. Drachenberg RC, Drachenberg CB, Papadimitriou JC, et al: Morphological spectrum of polyoma virus disease in renal allografts: Diagnostic accuracy of urine cytology. Am J Transplant 2001; 1:373–381.
56. Gardner SD, Mackenzie EF, Smith C, Porter AA: Prospective study of the human polyomaviruses BK and JC and cytomegalovirus in renal transplant recipients. J Clin Pathol 1984; 37(5):578–586.
57. Ramos E, Drachenberg CB, Papadimitriou JC, et al: Clinical course of polyoma virus nephropathy in 67 renal transplant patients. J Am Soc Nephrol 2002; 13:2145–2151.
58. Purighalla R, Shapiro R, McCauley J, Randhawa P: BK virus infection in a kidney allograft diagnosed by needle biopsy. Am J Kidney Dis 1999; 67:918–922.
59. Haririan A, Hamze O, Drachenberg CB, et al: Polyomavirus reactivation in native kidneys of pancreas alone allograft recipients. Transplantation 2003; 75:1186–1190.
60. Ramos E, Drachenberg CB, Portocarrero M, et al: BK virus nephropathy diagnosis and treatment: Experience at the University of Maryland Renal Transplant Program. *In* Cecka JM, Terasaki PI (eds): Clinical Transplantation. Los Angeles, CA, UCLA Immunogenetics Center, 2003, pp 143–153.
61. Chapman C, Flower AJ, Durrant ST: The use of vidarabine in the treatment of human polyomavirus associated acute haemorrhagic cystitis. Bone Marrow Transplant 1991; 7:481–483.
62. Andrei G, Snoeck R, Vandeputte M, De Clercq E: Activities of various compounds against murine and primate polyomaviruses. Antimicrob Agents Chemother 1997; 41:587–593.
63. Cundy KC, Petty BG, Flaherty J, et al: Clinical pharmacokinetics of cidofovir in human immunodeficiency virus-infected patients. Antimicrob Agents Chemother 1995; 39:1247–1252.
64. Vats A, Shapiro R, Singh RP, et al: Quantitative viral load monitoring and cidofovir therapy for the management of BK virus-associated nephropathy in children and adults. Transplantation 2003; 75:105–112.
65. Poduval RD, Meehan SM, Woodle ES, et al: Successful retransplantation following renal allograft loss to polyoma virus interstitial nephritis. Transplantation 2002; 73:1166–1169.
66. Fishman JA: Prevention of infection caused by Pneumocystis carinii in transplant recipients. Clin Infect Dis 2001; 33: 1397–1405.
67. Fishman JA: Prevention of infection due to Pneumocystis carinii. Antimicrob Agents Chemother 1998; 42:995–1004.
68. Chapman SW, Wilson JP: Nocardiosis in transplant recipients. Semin Respir Infect 1990; 5:74–79.
69. King CT, Chapman SW, Butkes DE: Recurrent nocardiosis in a renal transplant recipient. South Med J 1993; 86:225–228.
70. Kontoyiannis DP, Jacobson KL, Whimbey EE, et al: Central venous catheter-associated Nocardia bacteremia: An unusual manifestation of nocardiosis. Clin Infect Dis 2000; 31:617–618.

Noninfectious Complications in Renal Transplant Recipients

Anil Chandraker, M.D. • Colm C. Magee, M.D.

The survival of cadaveric and living donor renal allografts continues to improve. This reflects many factors, including lower rates of acute rejection (mainly due to better immunosuppressive regimens), better antimicrobial prophylaxis, and probably improvements in general medical and surgical care. With recipients and allografts surviving longer, more attention is being focused on ways to reduce the relatively high burden of morbidity and mortality in renal transplant recipients. Patient death is actually the leading cause of allograft loss beyond the first post-transplant year, with cardiovascular disease, infection, and malignancy being the main causes of death. The management of these and other problems is reviewed in this chapter.

CARDIOVASCULAR DISEASE

Death from cardiovascular disease is the leading cause of late mortality in renal transplant recipients.[1,2] Data from USRDS suggest that death from cardiovascular disease in the first year post-transplant accounts for 40% of deaths with graft function. Other estimates place the figure anywhere between 17% and 51%.[2] Post-transplant heart disease can take the form of either coronary heart disease (CHD) or cardiomyopathy (left ventricular hypertrophy or congestive heart failure).[2] This division may be somewhat arbitrary because some degree of CHD and cardiomyopathy is usually present in patients with cardiovascular disease, and either condition can exacerbate the other. A high prevalence of cardiomyopathy (presenting clinically as congestive heart failure or as left ventricular enlargement on echocardiography) has been noted.[2,3] One retrospective analysis found that the development of congestive heart failure after transplant was as common as the development of coronary heart disease; furthermore, it was associated with the same risk of death.[3] The authors thus proposed the interesting concept that transplantation is a state of "accelerated heart failure." The effects of treating anemia and hypertension (which are very prevalent after transplant—see later text) on rates of development of cardiomyopathy require study.

Although there is no reason to believe that the cardiac risk factors present in patients with chronic kidney disease or ESRD are different in renal transplant recipients, studies of causes of cardiovascular disease in the renal transplant population are limited.[4] Kasike and associates[5] reported that risk factors associated with cardiovascular disease in the general population, namely hypertension, hyperlipidemia, and cigarette smoking, were also predictive of cardiac disease in renal transplant recipients. Two or more episodes of acute rejection within the first year of transplant were also associated with a greater risk.

PREEXISTING CARDIOVASCULAR DISEASE

The majority of renal transplant recipients have risk factors for cardiovascular disease prior to transplant. Patients with chronic and end-stage kidney disease have a very adverse cardiovascular risk profile with a 10- to 20-fold increased risk of cardiovascular disease compared with the general population.[4] Hypertension, hypervolemia, anemia, diabetes, hyperlipidemia, and physical inactivity are all more common than in the general population.[6]

Given the high incidence of preexisting disease in the ESRD population, screening for cardiac disease is an important part of renal transplant evaluation. This is discussed in Chapter 33. Any patient with symptomatic coronary artery disease or positive stress testing should receive intensified medical therapy and be considered for coronary angiography and pre-transplant; this has been shown to decrease cardiovascular events after transplantation when compared to medical treatment alone.[7] Following transplantation, risk factors for development of CHD and cardiomyopathy should be aggressively controlled, and patients at risk for CHD should be placed on standard prophylaxis, including aspirin.[5,8]

Hypertension

Hypertension is common in renal transplant recipients and can have many causes. These include: high renin output state from diseased native kidneys, immunosuppressive drugs, chronic allograft nephropathy, obesity, hypercalcemia, transplant renal artery stenosis, and donor kidney with a family history of hypertension.[9]

Cyclosporine is well known to cause hypertension, although the mechanisms responsible are not fully understood.[10] Cyclosporine causes vasoconstriction of the renal vasculature (perhaps mediated by endothelin) and sodium retention (and thus a volume dependent form of hypertension).[11] Evidence to support the latter comes from observations of cyclosporine-treated diabetic patients transplanted with simultaneous kidney and bladder draining pancreas grafts; these patients do not develop the same degree of hypertension when compared to kidney only transplant recipients, probably because of sodium wastage in the exocrine pancreatic excretion.[12] High plasma renin does not appear to be an important mechanism in the development of cyclosporine-induced hypertension because patients treated with the drug are less responsive to ACE-inhibitors than are those treated with azathioprine.

Data on whether tacrolimus has the same adverse effects on hypertension are mixed, but overall it is probably less hypertension-inducing. Long-term studies in liver allograft recipients suggest that cyclosporine and tacrolimus have similar effects on blood pressure (BP), and another study directly comparing the two calcineurin inhibitors showed no difference in mean blood pressures or incidence of hypertension.[13,14] However, by 5 years fewer patients treated with tacrolimus needed antihypertensive medications compared with cyclosporine treated patients.[15] Hypertension has also been shown to resolve when patients were switched from cyclosporine to tacrolimus and to increase again when switched to cyclosporine treatment.[16] In addition, normal subjects without renal disease are more likely to develop hypertension, if given cyclosporine rather than tacrolimus.[17]

It has been suggested that because of their vasodilatory action, calcium channel blockers should be more effective in counteracting calcineurin inhibitor-induced hypertension. However, studies have not resolved this issue.[18,19] Caution should be exercised when prescribing calcium channel blockers because of their potential adverse cardiovascular effects or because several calcium channel blockers can interfere with the metabolism of calcineurin inhibitors and raise their plasma concentrations.

Steroids also elevate blood pressure. The effects are dose related and the relatively low doses of steroids used after the first 6 to 12 months are thought to have a minimal effect on blood pressure, although patients with preexisting hypertension appear to be susceptible to this adverse effect of chronic steroid use.[20] Obesity is exacerbated by use of steroids, which is discussed later.

Chronic allograft nephropathy (CAN) is also associated with hypertension. Multiple immunologic and nonimmunologic factors are associated with development of this condition (see Chapter 37). Hypertension itself is also thought to accelerate development of CAN. Treatment is directed at preventing progression of CAN, including reduction/elimination of calcineurin inhibitors.

Transplant renal artery stenosis is a less common but important cause (in that it is potentially treatable) of hypertension in transplant recipients. It is thought to be more common in recipients of living kidneys where an end-to-side anastomosis of donor renal artery to iliac artery is made compared to recipients of cadaveric grafts, where an aortic cuff protecting the orifice of the renal artery can be harvested.[21] The true incidence of this condition is difficult to define; one recent study found significant lesions in 5.4% of renal transplant recipients with at least 1 year of follow-up.[22] Development of the lesion was associated with weight at time of transplant, male gender, discharge serum creatinine greater than 2 mg/dL, and donor age. The presence of significant transplant renal artery stenosis is suggested by a reversible rise in plasma creatinine after administration of an ACE-inhibitor or angiotensin receptor blocker.[23] Unlike native renal artery stenosis, Doppler studies can be highly sensitive but are operator dependent. MR imaging is a useful screening test, but arteriography remains the gold standard diagnostic test. If multiple lesions or kinking of the artery is not present, percutaneous balloon angioplasty is successful about 80% of the time in previously untreated stenoses, however, lesions recur in about 20% of patients, who should then be considered for placement of a stent.[21,24–26] It is likely that primary placement of stents will be increasingly used.

Finally, studies have shown that donor and recipient family histories of hypertension are important in determining the need for blood pressure medications post-transplant.[27,28] For example, kidneys from a donor with a family history of hypertension transplanted into a recipient without a family history of hypertension lead to an increased need for antihypertensive medications post-transplant.

With the lack of good studies to confirm specific treatments, the Ad Hoc Group for the Prevention of Post-Transplant Cardiovascular Disease defers to the recommendations of the National Kidney Foundation Task Force on Cardiovascular Disease, setting a blood pressure control of less than 135/85 mmHg.[8] For patients with any of the following: diabetes, proteinuria greater than 500 mg/24 hr, greater than normal risk factors for CVD, or evidence of end organ damage, the goal blood pressure target should be less than or equal to 125/75 mmHg. Guidelines for treatment of BP post-transplant should generally follow the recommendations set by the Joint National Committee on prevention, detection, evaluation, and treatment of high blood pressure.[8,29] Depending on the cause, more specific treatment for elevated blood pressure is possible, such as reversing renal artery stenosis. The minimization/elimination of cyclosporine (and probably tacrolimus) has been shown to be effective in reducing the need for blood pressure medications.[30,31] Table 38–1 summarizes drugs commonly used to treat post-transplant hypertension; in practice, more than one agent is often needed to achieve adequate control of hypertension.

Smoking

There is accumulating evidence that continued smoking after transplant is associated with poorer renal allograft survival, even after censoring for death.[32] The mechanisms by which this might occur are unknown but could include exacerbation of transplant renovascular disease or of chronic rejection. Smoking, of course, also increases the risk of many squamous cell cancers, which are more common in transplant recipients. Thus, all recipients should be strongly encouraged to stop smoking, both to prolong recipient and allograft survival.

Dyslipidemia

The prevalence of hypercholesterolemia and hypertriglyceridemia after transplantation has been estimated as 60% and 35%, respectively.[33] Dyslipidemia very likely contributes to the high risk of cardiovascular disease. A major contributor to the development of post-transplant dyslipidemia is the use of immunosuppressive drugs. Sirolimus, corticosteroids, and the calcineurin inhibitors are all known to cause elevated plasma lipids with sirolimus probably having the greatest effect.[34] One study found around 80% of patients treated with this drug had serum cholesterol levels greater than 240 mg/dL or serum triglyceride levels greater than 200 mg/dL at some point after transplantation.[35] In this study, high-dose sirolimus was used; others have shown that dose reduction appears to reduce the degree of lipid abnormality, as does the withdrawal of steroids.[20]

Tacrolimus appears to have a less adverse effect on the lipid profile than does cyclosporine, which, in turn, is better than sirolimus.[36] Interestingly, sirolimus-coated stents reduce rates of re-stenosis in coronary arteries, but whether sirolimus has any such effect when given orally is not known. Both animal

Table 38–1 Antihypertensive Drugs Commonly Used in Renal Transplant Recipients

Drug	Potential Advantages	Potential Disadvantages	Comment
Thiazides	Well proven to reduce the complications of hypertension in the general population; inexpensive	Increase plasma creatinine; exacerbate gout and glucose intolerance	Avoid in first 2–3 months because of effect on plasma creatinine; probably underused in RTRs
Loop diuretics	Effectively treat volume component of hypertension	Increase plasma creatinine	Avoid in first 2–3 months, if possible
β-Blockers	Cardioprotective effects useful in many recipients because of high prevalence of coronary heart disease	As for non-transplant patients	Indications are the same as those for non-transplant patients
Calcium channel blockers	May ameliorate toxicity of calcineurin inhibitors; some evidence that they improve graft outcomes	Verapamil and diltiazem inhibit metabolism of calcineurin inhibitors; nifedipine exacerbates gum enlargement	Often used in the early post-transplant period because no effect on plasma creatinine
ACE-inhibitors, angiotensin receptor blockers	Postulated to slow progression of allograft failure, as in native kidney disease	Increase plasma creatinine; exacerbate anemia	Avoid in first 2–3 months because of effect on creatinine; useful in treating plasma post-transplant erythrocytosis
α-Blockers	Usually well tolerated	Allhat study showed inferior outcomes with α-blockers	Use for resistant hypertension only

and clinical studies have suggested an association between hyperlipidemia and progression of chronic allograft nephropathy.[37] Although this does not prove causality, cardiac disease in the general population is accelerated by occurrence of the so-called dysmetabolic state known as syndrome X, consisting of atherogenic lipid profile, hypertension, diabetes mellitus, and a chronic prothrombotic state.[38] These factors are known to contribute to the progression of renal failure, which would include chronic allograft nephropathy.[4]

Because cardiovascular disease is so prevalent in renal transplant recipients, it is reasonable to consider the renal transplant state a "coronary heart disease risk equivalent" when applying guidelines.[8,39] This implies targeting plasma LDL cholesterol less than 100mg/dL (newer guidelines are now suggesting < 70 mg/dL in high-risk patients) via a combination of therapeutic lifestyle changes and drug therapy. Reduction in steroid dose and switching cyclosporine to tacrolimus will also aid treatment of dyslipidemia.

Statins are the cholesterol-lowering drug of choice in transplant recipients. A recently published trial of statin use in renal transplant recipients showed them to be safe and effective in lowering plasma LDL cholesterol concentrations.[40] Cardiac deaths and nonfatal myocardial infarcts—although not overall mortality—were reduced. Because metabolism of many statins is partly inhibited by the calcineurin inhibitors, blood and tissue concentrations of statins may be increased in transplant recipients, thereby increasing the risk of adverse effects, such as rhabdomyolysis. This interaction is further enhanced, if additional inhibitors of cytochrome P450, such as diltiazem, are administered. Measures to minimize the risk of statin toxicity include the following: (1) starting with low statin doses, (2) use of pravastatin or fluvastatin (which appear to have the least interaction with CNIs), (3) avoidance of other inhibitors of the cytochrome P450 system, (4) avoidance of fibrates, and (5) periodic checking of plasma creatine kinase and liver function tests.[41] Rarely, nonstatin drugs are used to lower plasma lipids in transplant patients. Bile acid sequestrants, if used, should be taken separately from calcineurin inhibitors as they impair absorption of these drugs. Fibrates should be prescribed with extreme caution to patients on statins and calcineurin inhibitors.

HYPERHOMOCYSTEINEMIA

As in the general population, hyperhomocysteinemia has been recognized as an independent risk factor for the development of cardiovascular disease.[42] The use of cyclosporine has also been associated with higher plasma levels of homocysteine.[43] Even though administration of folate and vitamins B_6 and B_{12} effectively lowers homocysteine levels in transplant patients, no effect on outcome of cardiovascular disease has yet been shown.[8]

Post-Transplant Diabetes Mellitus

A recent study examined the economic impact of developing new onset diabetes mellitus post-transplant.[44] The cost to Medicare 2 years post-transplant was estimated as $21,500 per incident case. The "cost" in terms of morbidity and mortality is obviously much greater. There is no reason to believe that the effects of post-transplant diabetes mellitus (PTDM) are any different from those encountered by other diabetic patients. As in other diabetics, development of PTDM is associated with an adverse cardiovascular profile, including higher cholesterol and triglyceride levels as well as increased systolic blood pressure.[45]

Although the incidence of PTDM was exceptionally high (40%–60%) in the early days of renal transplantation, this was associated with use of very large doses of steroids. The incidence had declined but appears to be increasing again. The incidence of PTDM varies widely in different centers and in different studies. This is partially due to a varying definition of PTDM/impaired glucose tolerance. One study of USRDS patients who received their first renal allograft between 1996 and 2000 estimated the incidence of PTDM at 36 months post-transplant to be as high as 24%.[46] Risk factors for development of PTDM included age, black or Hispanic ethnicity, male donor, increasing HLA mismatches, hepatitis C infection, body mass index greater than or equal to 30 kg/m^2, and the use of tacrolimus as initial maintenance immunosuppression. Not surprisingly PTDM was associated with a poorer outcome in terms of increased graft failure, death-censored graft failure, and mortality. Other studies have found that PTDM is associated with not just the use, but also the dose of calcineurin inhibitor, use of intravenous methylprednisolone for treatment of acute rejection, cadaveric allograft donor, family history of diabetes as well as older recipient age, CMV infection, and use of furosemide.[47–50]

The mechanisms responsible for the development of PTDM appear to be mixed. In early studies where development of PTDM was related to high doses of steroids and weight gain, the major mechanisms appeared to be related to insulin resistance, that is, decreased activity of glycogen synthase, decreased number and binding affinity of insulin receptors, malabsorption of glucose in peripheral organs, or activation of the glucose/fatty acid pathway. This appears still to be important in some patients, especially those who gain significant amounts of weight post-transplant.[51] The introduction of calcineurin inhibitors appears to have exacerbated the situation, however, through decreased insulin secretion.[52] Most studies indicate that tacrolimus has a greater effect than cyclosporine. Even though animal models have shown that both cyclosporine and tacrolimus inhibit the ability of cells to secrete insulin, the precise mechanisms by which these drugs exert their diabetogenic effects in humans may differ.

Although both insulin resistance and impaired insulin secretion appear to be responsible for the development of PTDM, recent data suggest that abnormal insulin secretion is the dominant mechanism responsible.[51,53] Patients on high dose tacrolimus or methylprednisone who are also hepatitis C positive have a higher likelihood of developing PTDM. This appears to be related to active viral replication because treatment with antiviral medication brought the glycemia under control.[54,55]

PTDM is a potentially treatable condition. Some studies have indicated that one third of patients initially diagnosed with PTDM can return to normal glucose tolerance.[49] This figure may well be higher, if patients with PTDM are aggressively treated with reduction of steroids and lowering of calcineurin inhibitor levels.[56] Once PTDM has developed, treatment should be aggressive and take into account the primary cause of PTDM in that individual, for example, emphasizing weight reduction in an overweight patient with insulin resistance. Most patients, however, will require a multipronged approach with lifestyle modification, reduction in steroids and calcineurin inhibitors (if safe), and use of oral hypoglycemics and/or insulin. Metformin has the advantages of causing weight loss and not causing hypoglycemia but should be used with caution in those with renal impairment. Tight control of blood sugar has been shown to slow the progression of end-organ damage in diabetes; similar benefits are likely in renal transplant patients.

Obesity

Transplantation can exacerbate obesity, probably because of the effects of steroids. Dietary intervention after transplant can limit weight gain and hyperlipidemia.[57,58] It is likely that pharmacologic treatment of obesity will be increasingly prescribed to transplant recipients. This subject has recently been reviewed.[59] Orlistat and similar compounds can reduce absorption of cyclosporine (and probably other immunosuppressives) and should be administered at least 2 hours separately; concentrations of cyclosporine and tacrolimus should be closely monitored.[59]

Post-Transplant Anemia

Post-transplant anemia (PTA) is common; causes are shown in Table 38–2. A drop in hematocrit is associated with the perioperative period, and one study reported that 76% of patients had a hematocrit of less than 36 at the time of transplantation; this figure decreased to 21% at 1 year and rose again to 36% at 4 years.[60] Lorenz and associates[61] found a 40% prevalence of anemia and a 20% prevalence of iron deficiency (as measured by ≥2.5% hypochromic peripheral red blood cells) in renal transplant recipients. A similar retrospective study found that 30% of patients were anemic at some point during the post-transplant period.[62] The cause of anemia in the early post-transplant period is likely to be related to blood loss at the time of transplant and the sudden loss of exogenous erythropoietin supplementation. Surprisingly, given its prevalence, anemia is often not corrected in the transplant recipients, and the causes and effects of anemia in this population have not been well studied.[60] The association of anemia with the new development of left ventricular hypertrophy has been discussed earlier.[2,3,63]

Although there is a correlation between anemia and renal function in transplant patients, the degree of anemia is more severe than one would expect from renal dysfunction alone. Medication is an important cause. Mycophenolate mofetil, azathioprine, sirolimus, (val)gancyclovir, and SMX-TMP are all associated with bone marrow suppression. ACE-inhibitors and angiotensin receptor blockers are used to treat post-transplant erythrocytosis and were long suspected to be a potential cause of post-transplant anemia; this effect has recently been confirmed in the TRESAM study.[64] The benefits of ACE-inhibitor therapy in patients with progressive renal dysfunction probably outweigh the small associated drop in hematocrit. Gastrointestinal bleeding—perhaps related to steroids—can also contribute to post-transplant anemia. Other causes are shown in Table 38–2.

A common finding in the previously mentioned studies is that the causes of anemia are not aggressively investigated. A "standard" anemia workup should be performed (e.g., careful history and examination, fecal occult blood testing, iron studies, plasma LDH). As with anemia in general, treatment should be directed at the cause. Adequate treatment of anemia often requires use of erythropoietin, however.

Studies looking at the use of erythropoetin in transplant patients have found a low use of this medication.[60,64] It is not clear why this is so. The majority of anemic renal transplant

Table 38–2 Causes of Anemia in Renal Transplant Recipients

Cause	Mediated By	Ultimate Effect
Allograft dysfunction	Impaired production of erythropoietin	Decreased bone marrow production of RBCs
Azathioprine, MMF, sirolimus, SMX-TMP, (val)ganciclovir	Direct suppression of bone marrow turnover (all cell lines)	Decreased bone marrow production of RBCs
Acute inflammatory state, hyperparathyroidism	Impaired production of, or resistance to, erythropoietin	Decreased bone marrow production of RBCs
ACE-inhibitors, angiotensin receptor blockers	Impaired production of, or resistance to, erythropoietin	Decreased bone marrow production of RBCs
Iron deficiency	Impaired synthesis of hemoglobin	Decreased bone marrow production of RBCs
Minor ABO incompatibility	Donor antibodies	RBC hemolysis
Post-transplant hemolytic uremic syndrome	Multiple factors, including genetic defects, viral infection, calcineurin inhibitors, antiphospholipid antibodies	RBC hemolysis
Gastrointestinal or other bleeding		RBC losses exceed production

RBC, red blood cell.
This table shows only the more common causes of anemia post-transplant. Frequently, more than one is present in the individual recipient.

patients may not have as profound a drop in their glomerular filtration rate as what occurs in non-transplanted patients because of the additive effect of marrow suppressing medications. Because the recommendations for treatment for anemia with chronic kidney disease is based on GFRs from non-transplanted patients, there may be difficulty prescribing or getting reimbursement for use of erythropoietin in some transplant patients. Regardless, erythropoetin appears to work well in this population, and, although there are no prospective studies showing that correction of anemia slows progression of left ventricular hypertrophy in renal transplant patients, it would appear reasonable that the findings from treatment of anemia in the chronic kidney disease population could be extrapolated to the renal transplant population.

Peripheral and Cerebrovascular Disease

Data on the prevalence and risk factors for the development of peripheral vascular and cerebrovascular disease in renal transplant recipients are scarce. Kasiske and associates[33] reported a 15% prevalence of peripheral vascular disease at 15 years post-transplant. Sung and associates[65] retrospectively studied 664 adult recipients and found a cumulative 5- and 10-year incidence of 4.2% and 5.9%, respectively; the presence of peripheral vascular disease was independently associated with poorer recipient survival. There is also some evidence from registry data that peripheral vascular disease is a risk factor for poorer graft outcome.[66] It therefore seems reasonable to aggressively treat patients with this condition with measures, such as aspirin, statins, cessation of smoking, and revascularization where appropriate.

The 15-year cumulative incidence of cerebrovascular disease has been estimated as 15%.[33] As with the non-transplant population the benefits of carotid endarterectomy in patients with asymptomatic disease have not been proven. Management should be similar to that recommended by expert groups for the general population.[67,68] Control of hypertension is, of course, vital to prevent stroke.

Cancer

Data from many tumor registries clearly demonstrate that the overall incidence of cancer in renal transplant recipients is greater than in dialysis patients and the general population.[69–71] This increase in incidence applies to many cancers but particularly to those of the skin, lymphoid tissue, or urogenital tract. Table 38–3 shows data from one of the most comprehensive registries. Note that cancers common in the general population (those of the breast, lung, large bowel, and prostate) are only slightly increased in incidence. Exposure to excess ultraviolet light is particularly common in Australia; the cumulative risk of nonmelanotic skin cancers 20 years post-transplant in Australia is greater than 50%.[70]

Table 38–3 Relative Risk of Cancer Following Primary Cadaveric Kidney Transplantation (n = 8881), Compared to an Age-Matched Australian Population, 1963–2002*

Cancer	RR	95% CI
Carcinoma or vulva or vagina	35.5	25.7–49.1
In situ carcinoma of uterine cervix	17.2	13.5–21.9
Non-Hodgkin's lymphoma	8.7	7.3–10.3
Liver	7.8	4.8–12.9
Kidney	6.7	5.3–8.4
Malignant melanoma	3.6	3.0–4.2
Invasive carcinoma of uterine cervix	3.0	1.8–5.0
Colon	2.6	2.1–3.2
Lung, trachea	2.1	1.7–2.6
Breast	1.2	0.9–1.5
Prostate	0.7	0.5–0.9
Total (includes others not shown)	3.0	2.9–3.2

*Nonmelanotic skin cancers are not included. (Adapted from Chapman J, Webster A: 2002 Report of the ANZDATA Registry. Chapter 10: Cancer report: Australia and New Zealand Dialysis and Transplant Registry [ANZDATA], 2002.)

The reported incidence of cancers in transplant recipients is increased for several reasons. First, immunosuppression allows relatively uncontrolled proliferation of oncogenic viruses and probably inhibits normal tumor surveillance mechanisms. There is also experimental evidence that calcineurin inhibitors may promote tumor growth via their effects on TGFβ production.[72] Second, recipient factors associated with the primary renal disease may also be associated with neoplasia. Thus, viral hepatitis can cause both kidney disease and liver cancer. Finally, ascertainment bias may occur due to more complete reporting of cancers in RTRs compared to the general population; this is not a major factor, however.

It is believed that the cumulative amount of immunosuppression is the most important factor increasing the cancer risk. Aggressive immunosuppression with any one drug, such as tacrolimus, cyclosporine, or OKT3, can suffice. For example, renal transplant recipients were randomized in one study at 1 year post-transplant to either a standard or low-dose cyclosporine regimen. After 66 months follow-up, rates of rejection were higher in the low-dose group, but allograft survival was similar.[73] The cumulative incidence of cancers in the low-dose group was 20%; in the high-dose group, it was significantly increased to 32% (the majority being skin cancers).

The single most important measure to prevent cancers is, therefore, to minimize excess immunosuppression. Of course, achieving the optimum balance between excess and inadequate immunosuppression is a matter of subjective clinical judgement with an individual patient. Current guidelines are to employ primary and secondary preventive strategies for breast, lung, bowel, and urogenital cancers similar to those recommended for the general population (i.e., mammography, smoking cessation, endoscopy, pelvic examination in females). Because of the particularly high prevalence of skin cancers in transplant recipients, preventive measures for these cancers should be more rigorous.[74] Thus, patients should be specifically counseled to minimize exposure to ultraviolet light, to wear protective clothing, and to apply sunscreen to exposed areas. Premalignant skin lesions should be treated with cryotherapy or surgical excision.[74]

In general, when cancer occurs, immunosuppression should be decreased. Obviously, this increases the risk of graft rejection and loss. Fortunately, loss of the renal allograft is not fatal (unlike the situation in cardiac and lung transplantation), because dialysis is an option. There is experimental evidence that sirolimus has antineoplastic effects,[75,76] but long-term data are not yet available as to whether this new immunosuppressive drug can reduce the incidence of post-transplant cancers. The long-term effects of newer, more intensive immunosuppression regimens (using drugs such as tacrolimus and MMF) on the risk of developing post-transplant cancers are unknown. Certainly, the recent rise in reported cases of polyoma virus infections is a warning that some of our patients are being over-immunosuppressed.

Post-Transplant Lymphoproliferative Disease

Post-transplant lymphoproliferative disease (PTLD) is one of the most serious complications of transplantation because of its high associated morbidity and mortality. The cumulative incidence in renal transplant recipients overall is 1% to 5%, with most cases arising in the first 24 months after transplant.[33] The majority are non-Hodgkin's lymphomas and of recipient B cell origin.[77] Risk factors include: (1) the combination of an EBV+ donor and EBV− recipient, (2) the combination of a CMV+ donor and CMV− recipient, (3) pediatric recipient (in part because children are more likely to be EBV−), and (4) more intensive immunosuppression.[78] In many cases of PTLD, the pathogenesis involves infection and transformation of B cells by EBV; transformed B cells then undergo proliferation, which is initially polyclonal, but a malignant clone may evolve. The clinical and pathologic spectrum and treatment of PTLD are quite variable, and readers are referred to recent reviews for more information.[79,80]

Treatment involves drastic reduction in immunosuppression (e.g., to low-dose steroids alone) and variable combinations of antiviral therapy, radiotherapy, chemotherapy, and surgery. The prognosis of severe forms of PTLD is poor but there is optimism it will improve. Techniques for monitoring EBV viral load after transplantation are being developed. These may allow earlier identification of transplant recipients who are at high risk of developing PTLD or who have early disease, thus allowing preemptive or early therapy of such patients. In addition, nontoxic immunotherapies have been developed or are already in clinical use. These include biologic immune-modifiers, such as interferon-α and IL-6, adoptive immunotherapy with virus-specific T cells, and, most promisingly to date, elimination of B cells by the anti-CD20 monoclonal antibody, rituximab.[80]

Electrolyte Disorders

Electrolyte disorders are common after kidney transplant but rarely severe. Hyperkalemia can be caused by poor graft function, calcineurin inhibitors, and other drugs, such as ACE-I or β-blockers. Treatment is similar to that of hyperkalemia in chronic (native) kidney disease: reduction in potassium intake, adjustment in medications, and so forth. Post-transplant hypercalcemia can be caused by tertiary hyperparathyroidism and by administration of calcium or vitamin D (these drugs are used to prevent loss of bone density) or by both. Severe tertiary hyperparathyroidism requires parathyroidectomy (see later text). Many patients have hypophosphatemia in the first 6 months after transplant. This is due to increased urinary excretion of phosphate (mainly secondary to persistence of hyperparathyroidism) and probably decreased intestinal absorption secondary to steroids. Post-transplant hypophosphatemia is usually asymptomatic but can rarely cause severe muscle weakness, including weakness of respiratory muscles. The benefits of phosphate supplementation in the setting of mild or moderate post-transplant hypophosphatemia have not been well studied. Phosphate supplementation should be prescribed for severe (e.g., plasma phosphate <1.2 mg/dL) or symptomatic cases.

Bone Disorders after Renal Transplantation

Bone disease in the dialysis patient is multifactorial, involving varying degrees of hyperparathyroidism, vitamin D deficiency, adynamic bone disease, aluminum intoxication, and amyloidosis. Successful renal transplantation can reverse or at least prevent further progression of these conditions. Unfortunately, bone disease continues to be a major problem after renal transplantation due to persistence of the previously mentioned conditions, suboptimal kidney function, and the superimposed effects of steroids on bone.

Osteoporosis

Reduction in bone mineral density is a common complication of all forms of solid organ transplantation; one recent review estimated an incidence of up to 60% in the first 18 months after renal transplant.[33] The main cause of post-transplant osteoporosis is steroids through multiple effects, including direct inhibition of osteoblastogenesis, induction of apoptosis in bone cells, inhibition of sex hormone production (in both men and women), decreased gut calcium absorption, and increased urinary calcium excretion.[81] Other factors that may contribute to post-transplant osteoporosis include persistent hyperparathyroidism, presence of type 1 diabetes, post-menopausal state, vitamin D deficiency/resistance, and phosphate depletion. Thus, the pathophysiology of osteoporosis often differs from that seen in the non-transplant population (see Table 38–4).

Whether low bone mineral density (as identified by dual energy X-ray absorptiometry [DEXA] correlates with risk of fracture in RTRs remains unclear.[82,83] Certainly, pathologic fractures are common after renal transplantation. The estimated total fracture rate in nondiabetics renal transplant recipients is 2% to 3% per year; in type I diabetics 5% per year; and in pancreas–kidney recipients up to 12% per year.[82,84]

Measures to minimize post-transplant bone loss are summarized in Table 38–4. It is important that these measures are instituted immediately post-transplant, because most bone loss occurs in the first 6 months, when steroid doses are highest. All transplant recipients should receive calcium (at least 1000 mg elemental calcium per day) and vitamin D (at least 800 IU/day; more if serum 25-vitamin D3 concentrations are low or low-normal) and should be encouraged to perform weight-bearing exercises, stop smoking, and avoid excess alcohol consumption. Several trials have shown a benefit with the post-transplant use of vitamin D analogues and calcium.[85,86]

The role of DEXA and bisphosphonates in the prevention and treatment of post-transplant bone disease requires further prospective study. There is evidence that bisphosphonates prevent post-transplant bone loss, but trials reported to date have not been adequately powered to detect reductions in post-transplant fracture rates.[87] There is still concern that these agents, by suppressing bone remodeling, could worsen the mechanical integrity of bone in conditions, such as osteomalacia or adynamic bone.[84,87] A reasonable approach is to obtain DEXA from three bone sites (lumbar spine, forearm, hip) at the time of transplant in all patients. In those considered to be at high risk of osteoporosis related fracture based on their clinical features and DEXA results, post-transplant administration of bisphosphonates and the use of minimal dose steroid protocols should be considered.

Hyperparathyroidism

Incomplete resolution of hyperparathyroidism is common after renal transplantation. This probably reflects multiple factors: inherent slow involution of parathyroid cells, suboptimal renal function, suboptimal production of 1,25 vitamin D3, and steroid-induced reduction in intestinal calcium absorption.[83] Two clinical characteristics identify those at risk of post-transplant hyperparathyroidism: duration of dialysis and degree of pre-transplant hyperparathyroidism.[83] Patients scheduled for transplant who have persistent elevated PTH greater than 300 pg/mL, despite medical therapy should be considered for pretransplant parathyroidectomy. The most important complications of post-transplant

Table 38–4 Comparison of Postmenopausal and Postrenal Transplant Osteoporosis

	Postmenopausal Osteoporosis	Post-Transplant Osteoporosis
Pathophysiology		
Deficiency of sex hormones	Yes	Sometimes
Increased activity of osteoclasts; accelerated breakdown of bone	Yes	Sometimes
Decreased activity of osteoblasts; reduced bone sythesis	No	Yes
Background of renal osteodystrophy	No	Yes
Associated renal dysfunction	No	Frequent
Clinical		
Fracture sites	Mainly axial skeleton	Mainly appendicular skeleton
Diagnosis		
DEXA predicts fracture risk	Yes	Unclear
Recommended prevention/treatment measures		
Weight-bearing exercise	Yes	Yes
Calcium	Yes	Yes
Vitamin D	Yes	Yes; use calcitriol if GFR< 50 mL/min
Hormone replacement therapy	Only if other indications	Only if other indications
Bisphosphonates	Yes	Unclear

hyperparathyroidism are hypercalcemia and exacerbation of bone loss. If hypercalcemia is severe and associated with complications, early parathyroidectomy is indicated. Less severe cases can be managed conservatively in the hope that overactivity of the gland resolves; late parathyroidectomy may ultimately be required, however.

Osteonecrosis

Osteonecrosis, or avascular necrosis of bone, has been reported to occur in 3% to 16% of renal transplant recipients.[82] Hip, knee, ankle, shoulder, or elbow joints can be involved. If severe, significant joint damage can occur. The principal cause is steroids. Fortunately, the incidence has declined because RTRs are now receiving lower cumulative doses of steroids (maintenance doses are lower, and fewer "pulses" are required because acute rejection is less common). The presenting symptom is joint pain. MRI, radionuclide bone scan, and plain films (in order of decreasing sensitivity) are used to confirm the diagnosis. Severe cases require surgery.

CONCLUSION

Although acute rejection and early graft loss have become relatively uncommon, late graft loss and premature death (mainly from cardiovascular disease) remain major problems. Morbidity from diabetes mellitus and bone disease is also substantial. More attention is therefore being paid toward preventing and treating these "medical complications" of transplantation. In many ways, renal transplant recipients need to be managed similarly to those with chronic kidney disease. More effective intervention at the pre-dialysis or dialysis stage is also needed to reduce the burden of morbidity in transplant patients. Finally, reduction in long-term immunosuppression should be strongly considered in all patients.

References

1. Dimeny EM, Sarnak MJ, Levey AS, Kasiske BL: Cardiovascular disease after renal transplantation. Kidney Int Suppl 2002; 35:78-84.
2. Rigatto C: Clinical epidemiology of cardiac disease in renal transplant recipients. Semin Dial 2003; 16:106-110.
3. Rigatto C, Parfrey P, Foley R, et al: Congestive heart failure in renal transplant recipients: Risk factors, outcomes, and relationship with ischemic heart disease. J Am Soc Nephrol 2002; 13: 1084-1090.
4. Sarnak M, Levey A: Cardiovascular disease and chronic renal disease: A new paradigm. Am J Kidney Dis 2000; 35:S117-S131.
5. Kasiske BL: Epidemiology of cardiovascular disease after renal transplantation. Transplantation 2001; 72:S5-S8.
6. Levey AS, Beto JA, Coronado BE, et al: Controlling the epidemic of cardiovascular disease in chronic renal disease: What do we know? What do we need to learn? Where do we go from here? National Kidney Foundation Task Force on Cardiovascular Disease. Am J Kidney Dis 1998; 32:853-906.
7. Manske CL, Thomas W, Wang Y, Wilson RF: Screening diabetic transplant candidates for coronary artery disease: Identification of a low risk subgroup. Kidney Int 1993; 44:617-621.
8. Bostom AD, Brown RS Jr, Chavers BM, et al: Prevention of post-transplant cardiovascular disease: Report and recommendations of an ad hoc group. Am J Transplant 2002; 2:491-500.
9. Luke RG: Pathophysiology and treatment of posttransplant hypertension. J Am Soc Nephrol 1991; 2:S37-S44.
10. Curtis JJ: Hypertensinogenic mechanism of the calcineurin inhibitors. Curr Hypertens Rep 2002; 4:377-380.
11. Curtis JJ, Luke RG, Jones P, Diethelm AG: Hypertension in cyclosporine-treated renal transplant recipients is sodium dependent. Am J Med 1988; 85:134-138.
12. Curtis JJ: Cyclosporine and posttransplant hypertension. J Am Soc Nephrol 1992; 2:S243-S245.
13. Pirsch JD, Miller J, Deierhoi MH, et al: A comparison of tacrolimus (FK506) and cyclosporine for immunosuppression after cadaveric renal transplantation. FK506 Kidney Transplant Study Group. Transplantation 1997; 63:977-983.
14. Randomised trial comparing tacrolimus (FK506) and cyclosporin in prevention of liver allograft rejection. European FK506 Multicentre Liver Study Group. Lancet 1994; 344:423-428.
15. Vincenti F, Jensik SC, Filo RS, et al: A long-term comparison of tacrolimus (FK506) and cyclosporine in kidney transplantation: Evidence for improved allograft survival at five years. Transplantation 2002; 73:775-782.
16. Ligtenberg G, Hene RJ, Blankestijn PJ, Koomans HA: Cardiovascular risk factors in renal transplant patients: Cyclosporin A versus tacrolimus. J Am Soc Nephrol 2001; 12: 368-373.
17. Klein IH, Abrahams A, van Ede T, et al: Different effects of tacrolimus and cyclosporine on renal hemodynamics and blood pressure in healthy subjects. Transplantation 2002; 73:732-736.
18. Midtvedt K, Hartmann A, Foss A, et al: Sustained improvement of renal graft function for two years in hypertensive renal transplant recipients treated with nifedipine as compared to lisinopril. Transplantation 2001; 72:1787-1792.
19. Mourad G, Ribstein J, Mimran A, et al: Converting-enzyme inhibitor versus calcium antagonist in cyclosporine-treated renal transplants: Sustained improvement of renal graft function for two years in hypertensive renal transplant recipients treated with nifedipine as compared to lisinopril. Kidney Int 1993; 43: 419-425.
20. Hricik DE, Bartucci MR, Mayes JT, Schulak JA: The effects of steroid withdrawal on the lipoprotein profiles of cyclosporine-treated kidney and kidney-pancreas transplant recipients. Transplantation 1992; 54:868-871.
21. Sankari BR, Geisinger M, Zelch M, et al: Post-transplant renal artery stenosis: Impact of therapy on long-term kidney function and blood pressure control. J Urol 1996; 155:1860-1864.
22. Becker BN, Odorico JS, Becker YT, et al: Peripheral vascular disease and renal transplant artery stenosis: A reappraisal of transplant renovascular disease. Clin Transplant 1999; 13:349-355.
23. Shamlou KK, Drane WE, Hawkins IF, Fennell RS III: Captopril renography and the hypertensive renal transplantation patient: A predictive test of therapeutic outcome. Radiology 1994; 190:153-159.
24. Ruggenenti P, Mosconi L, Bruno S, et al: Post-transplant renal artery stenosis: The hemodynamic response to revascularization: Treatment of recurrent transplant renal artery stenosis with metallic stents. Kidney Int 2001; 60:309-318.
25. Sierre SD, Raynaud AC, Carreres T, et al: Treatment of recurrent transplant renal artery stenosis with metallic stents. J Vasc Interv Radiol 1998; 9:639-644.
26. Fervenza FC, Lafayette RA, Alfrey EJ, Petersen J: Renal artery stenosis in kidney transplants. Am J Kidney Dis 1998; 31:142-148.
27. Guidi E, Cozzi MG, Minetti E, Bianchi G: Donor and recipient family histories of hypertension influence renal impairment and blood pressure during acute rejections. J Am Soc Nephrol 1998; 9:2102-2107.
28. Guidi E, Menghetti D, Milani S, et al: Hypertension may be transplanted with the kidney in humans: A long-term historical prospective follow-up of recipients grafted with kidneys coming from donors with or without hypertension in their families. J Am Soc Nephrol 1996; 7:1131-1138.
29. Chobanian AV, Bakris GL, Black HR, et al: The Seventh Report of the Joint National Committee on Prevention, Detection,

Evaluation, and Treatment of High Blood Pressure: The JNC 7 report. JAMA 2003; 289:2560-2572.
30. Tran HT, Acharya MK, McKay DB, et al: Avoidance of cyclosporine in renal transplantation: Effects of daclizumab, mycophenolate mofetil, and steroids. J Am Soc Nephrol 2000; 11: 1903-1909.
31. Johnson RW, Kreis H, Oberbauer R, et al: Sirolimus allows early cyclosporine withdrawal in renal transplantation resulting in improved renal function and lower blood pressure. Transplantation 2001; 72:777-786.
32. Sung RS, Althoen M, Howell TA, et al: Excess risk of renal allograft loss associated with cigarette smoking. Transplantation 2001; 71:1752-1757.
33. Kasiske BL, Vazquez MA, Harmon WE, et al: Recommendations for the outpatient surveillance of renal transplant recipients. American Society of Transplantation. J Am Soc Nephrol 2000; 11(suppl 15):S1-S86.
34. Groth CG, Backman L, Morales JM, et al: Sirolimus (rapamycin)-based therapy in human renal transplantation: Similar efficacy and different toxicity compared with cyclosporine. Sirolimus European Renal Transplant Study Group. Transplantation 1999; 67:1036-1042.
35. Chueh SC, Kahan BD: Dyslipidemia in renal transplant recipients treated with a sirolimus and cyclosporine-based immunosuppressive regimen: Incidence, risk factors, progression, and prognosis. Transplantation 2003; 76:375-382.
36. Satterthwaite R, Aswad S, Sunga V, et al: Incidence of new-onset hypercholesterolemia in renal transplant patients treated with FK506 or cyclosporine. Transplantation 1998; 65:446-449.
37. Massy ZA, Kasiske BL: Post-transplant hyperlipidemia: Mechanisms and management. J Am Soc Nephrol 1996; 7:971-977.
38. Nicholas SB: Syndrome X following renal transplantation. Curr Hypertens Rep 2001; 3:121-123.
39. National Heart LaBI: Detection, Evaluation, and Treatment of High Blood Cholesterol in Adults (Adult Treatment Panel III), 2001.
40. Holdaas H, Fellstrom B, Jardine A, et al: Effect of fluvastatin on cardiac outcomes in renal transplant recipients: A multicentre, randomised, placebo-controlled trial. Lancet 2003; 361:2024-2031.
41. Bae J, Jarcho JA, Denton MD, Magee CC: Statin specific toxicity in organ transplant recipients: Case report and review of the literature. J Nephrol 2002; 15:317-319.
42. Ducloux D, Motte G, Challier B, et al: Serum total homocysteine and cardiovascular disease occurrence in chronic, stable renal transplant recipients: A prospective study. J Am Soc Nephrol 2000; 11:134-137.
43. Arnadottir M, Hultberg B, Vladov V, et al: Hyperhomocysteinemia in cyclosporine-treated renal transplant recipients. Transplantation 1996; 61:509-512.
44. Woodward RS, Schnitzler MA, Baty J, et al: Incidence and cost of new onset diabetes mellitus among U.S. wait-listed and transplanted renal allograft recipients. Am J Transplant 2003; 3:590-598.
45. Cosio FG, Pesavento TE, Kim S, et al: Patient survival after renal transplantation: IV. Impact of post-transplant diabetes. Kidney Int 2002; 62:1440-1446.
46. Kasiske BL, Snyder JJ, Gilbertson D, Matas AJ: Diabetes mellitus after kidney transplantation in the United States. Am J Transplant 2003; 3:178-185.
47. Hjelmesaeth J, Hartmann A, Kofstad J, et al: Glucose intolerance after renal transplantation depends upon prednisolone dose and recipient age. Transplantation 1997; 64:979-983.
48. Hjelmesaeth J, Jenssen T, Hagen M, et al: Determinants of insulin secretion after renal transplantation. Metabolism 2003; 52: 573-578.
49. Hjelmesaeth J, Hartmann A, Kofstad J, et al: Tapering off prednisolone and cyclosporin the first year after renal transplantation: The effect on glucose tolerance. Nephrol Dial Transplant 2001; 16:829-835.
50. Filler G, Neuschulz I, Vollmer I, et al: Tacrolimus reversibly reduces insulin secretion in paediatric renal transplant recipients. Nephrol Dial Transplant 2000; 15:867-871.
51. Nam JH, Mun JI, Kim SI, et al: Beta-cell dysfunction rather than insulin resistance is the main contributing factor for the development of postrenal transplantation diabetes mellitus. Transplantation 2001; 71:1417-1423.
52. Ekstrand AV, Eriksson JG, Gronhagen-Riska C, et al: Insulin resistance and insulin deficiency in the pathogenesis of posttransplantation diabetes in man. Transplantation 1992; 53:563-569.
53. Hagen M, Hjelmesaeth J, Jenssen T, et al: A 6-year prospective study on new onset diabetes mellitus, insulin release and insulin sensitivity in renal transplant recipients. Nephrol Dial Transplant 2003; 18:2154-2159.
54. Baid S, Cosimi AB, Farrell ML, et al: Posttransplant diabetes mellitus in liver transplant recipients: Risk factors, temporal relationship with hepatitis C virus allograft hepatitis, and impact on mortality. Transplantation 2001; 72:1066-1072.
55. Bloom RD, Rao V, Weng F, et al: Association of hepatitis C with posttransplant diabetes in renal transplant patients on tacrolimus. J Am Soc Nephrol 2002; 13:1374-1380.
56. Hricik DE, Bartucci MR, Moir EJ, et al: Influence of corticosteroid withdrawal on posttransplant diabetes mellitus in cyclosporine-treated renal transplant recipients. Transplant Proc 1991; 23:1007-1008.
57. Patel MG: The effect of dietary intervention on weight gains after renal transplantation. J Ren Nutr 1998; 8:137-141.
58. Lopes IM, Martin M, Errasti P, Martinez JA: Benefits of a dietary intervention on weight loss, body composition, and lipid profile after renal transplantation. Nutrition 1999; 15:7-10.
59. Yanovski SZ, Yanovski JA: Obesity. N Engl J Med 2002; 346:591-602.
60. Mix TC, Kazmi W, Khan S, et al: Anemia: A continuing problem following kidney transplantation. Am J Transplant 2003; 3:1426-1433.
61. Lorenz M, Kletzmayr J, Perschl A, et al: Anemia and iron deficiencies among long-term renal transplant recipients. J Am Soc Nephrol 2002; 13:794-797.
62. Yorgin PD, Scandling JD, Belson A, et al: Late post-transplant anemia in adult renal transplant recipients. An under-recognized problem? Am J Transplant 2002; 2:429-435.
63. Rigatto C, Foley R, Jeffery J, et al: Electrocardiographic left ventricular hypertrophy in renal transplant recipients: Prognostic value and impact of blood pressure and anemia. J Am Soc Nephrol 2003; 14:462-468.
64. Vanrenterghem Y, Ponticelli C, Morales JM, et al: Prevalence and management of anemia in renal transplant recipients: A European survey. Am J Transplant 2003; 3:835-845.
65. Sung RS, Althoen M, Howell TA, Merion RM: Peripheral vascular occlusive disease in renal transplant recipients: Risk factors and impact on kidney allograft survival. Transplantation 2000; 70:1049-1054.
66. Cho YW, Terasaki PI: Impact of new variables reported to the UNOS registry. Clin Transpl 1997; 305-314.
67. Biller J, Feinberg WM, Castaldo JE, et al: Guidelines for carotid endarterectomy: A statement for healthcare professionals from a special writing group of the Stroke Council, American Heart Association. Stroke 1998; 29:554-562.
68. Bettmann MA, Katzen BT, Whisnant J, et al: Carotid stenting and angioplasty: A statement for healthcare professionals from the Councils on Cardiovascular Radiology, Stroke, Cardio-Thoracic and Vascular Surgery, Epidemiology and Prevention, and Clinical Cardiology, American Heart Association: Guidelines for carotid endarterectomy: A statement for healthcare professionals from a special writing group of the Stroke Council, American Heart Association. Stroke 1998; 29:336-338.

69. Penn I: Posttransplant malignancies. Transplant Proc 1999; 31: 1260-1262.
70. Chapman J, Webster A: 2002 Report of the ANZDATA Registry. Chapter 10: Cancer Report: Australia and New Zealand Dialysis and Transplant Registry (ANZDATA), 2002.
71. Birkeland SA, Lokkegaard H, Storm HH: Cancer risk in patients on dialysis and after renal transplantation. Lancet 2000; 355: 1886-1887.
72. Hojo M, Morimoto T, Maluccio M, et al: Cyclosporine induces cancer progression by a cell-autonomous mechanism. Nature 1999; 397:530-534.
73. Dantal J, Hourmant M, Cantarovich D, et al: Effect of long-term immunosuppression in kidney-graft recipients on cancer incidence: Randomised comparison of two cyclosporin regimens. Lancet 1998; 351:623-628.
74. Jemec GB, Holm EA: Nonmelanoma skin cancer in organ transplant patients. Transplantation 2003; 75:253-257.
75. Luan FL, Hojo M, Maluccio M, et al: Rapamycin blocks tumor progression: Unlinking immunosuppression from antitumor efficacy. Transplantation 2002; 73:1565-1572.
76. Guba M, von Breitenbuch P, Steinbauer M, et al: Rapamycin inhibits primary and metastatic tumor growth by antiangiogenesis: Involvement of vascular endothelial growth factor. Nat Med 2002; 8:128-135.
77. Penn I: Neoplastic complications of transplantation. Semin Respir Infect 1993; 8:233-239.
78. Dharnidharka VR, Sullivan EK, Stablein DM, et al: Risk factors for posttransplant lymphoproliferative disorder (PTLD) in pediatric kidney transplantation: A report of the North American Pediatric Renal Transplant Cooperative Study (NAPRTCS). Transplantation 2001; 71:1065-1068.
79. Meijer E, Dekker AW, Weersink AJ, et al: Prevention and treatment of Epstein-Barr virus-associated lymphoproliferative disorders in recipients of bone marrow and solid organ transplants. Br J Haematol 2002; 119:596-607.
80. Straathof KC, Savoldo B, Heslop HE, Rooney CM: Immunotherapy for post-transplant lymphoproliferative disease. Br J Haematol 2002; 118:728-740.
81. Delmas PD: Osteoporosis in patients with organ transplants: A neglected problem. Lancet 2001; 357:325-326.
82. Heaf JG: Bone disease after renal transplantation. Transplantation 2003; 75:315-325.
83. Torres A, Lorenzo V, Salido E: Calcium metabolism and skeletal problems after transplantation. J Am Soc Nephrol 2002; 13:551-558.
84. Weber TJ, Quarles LD: Preventing bone loss after renal transplantation with bisphosphonates: We can . . . but should we? Kidney Int 2000; 57:735-737.
85. El-Agroudy AE, El-Husseini AA, El-Sayed M, Ghoneim MA: Preventing bone loss in renal transplant recipients with vitamin D. J Am Soc Nephrol 2003; 14:2975-2979.
86. De Sevaux RG, Hoitsma AJ, Corstens FH, Wetzels JF: Treatment with vitamin D and calcium reduces bone loss after renal transplantation: A randomized study. J Am Soc Nephrol 2002; 13:1608-1614.
87. Coco M, Glicklich D, Faugere MC, et al: Prevention of bone loss in renal transplant recipients: A prospective, randomized trial of intravenous pamidronate. J Am Soc Nephrol 2003; 14:2669-2676.

Recurrent and De Novo Renal Disease in Kidney Transplantation

Denise Sadlier, M.B., M.R.C.P.I. • Yvonne M. O'Meara, M.D., F.R.C.P.I.

Recurrence of original disease following renal transplantation affects 10% to 20% of patients in most series and accounts for up to 8% of graft failures at 10 years post-transplant.[1–7] There is, however, wide variation in the reported rates of recurrence of different diseases and the ensuing rates of graft loss (Tables 39–1 and 39–2). Accurate estimation of the incidence of recurrence is difficult for a number of reasons. First, definitive diagnosis of recurrence requires histologic confirmation of the primary disease in the native kidney by renal biopsy. The latter is often omitted in patients presenting with renal dysfunction and small kidneys, and many patients are classified clinically with "chronic glomerulonephritis." Second, biopsy of the allograft is undertaken in many centers only upon occurrence of a clinical indication, such as deterioration in renal function or the development of proteinuria. Thus, asymptomatic histologic recurrence will be missed without a policy of routine renal biopsy. Third, a variety of pathologic processes, such as ischemia, nephrotoxicity, hypertension, and acute and chronic rejection, can induce morphologic changes that mimic primary glomerulopathies and that may be difficult to distinguish from true recurrence.[8] Fourth, glomerular lesions can occur de novo in the transplanted kidney. In the absence of histologic confirmation of the patient's original disease, these lesions may also be misclassified.

Multiple factors influence the likelihood of recurrence. These include the type and severity of the original disease, the age at onset of the disease, the source of the donor kidney, and the immunosuppressive regimen used to prevent allograft rejection. In general, disease recurrence in an allograft implies persistence of an extrarenal pathogenetic stimulus. In certain diseases, modification of the pathogenetic stimulus can prevent or delay recurrence of the disease in the allograft. For example, in Goodpasture's syndrome, the presence of circulating anti-GBM antibodies in high titer at the time of transplantation increases the risk of recurrence in the allograft.[4,10] Conversely, clinical recurrence is extremely rare, if the antibody is undetectable over a 6- to 12-month period prior to transplantation.[10] Diabetic nephropathy invariably recurs in the allograft. However, this process can be delayed or prevented by improved glycemic control achieved by simultaneous pancreatic transplantation.[11,12] Similarly, in primary hyperoxaluria, another disease that invariably recurs, the use of simultaneous liver transplantation to provide a source of the absent hepatic peroxisomal alanine glyoxylate aminotransferase prevents disease recurrence in the renal allograft.[13–15]

The severity of disease in the native kidney influences the incidence of recurrence of certain diseases. Focal and segmental glomerulosclerosis (FSGS) illustrates this point. A culminant presentation with a short interval (<3 years) between diagnosis and development of end-stage renal disease (ESRD) increases the risk of disease recurrence in the allograft.[1,16] With regard to age of onset, recurrence of FSGS is greatest in younger patients whose primary disease presents before the age of 16 years.[17] Conversely, in Henoch-Schönlein purpura (HSP) recurrence is greatest in patients who develop their disease after the age of 14 years.[18]

With respect to the source of the renal allograft, some studies have demonstrated higher rates of recurrent glomerulonephritis in living related donor allografts compared with cadaveric grafts.[4,6] This observation suggests that phenotypic characteristics shared by related donor-recipient pairs may render the kidney more susceptible to humoral pathogens. It should be emphasized, however, that many studies fail to demonstrate an increased tendency to disease recurrence in recipients of living related grafts.[7,19]

Turning finally to the immunosuppressive regimen, cyclosporine A (CsA) is a potent immunosuppressive agent that induces remission of nephrotic syndrome associated with minimal change disease, FSGS, and membranous nephropathy, among other glomerulopathies.[20] It was anticipated that the introduction of CsA would reduce the incidence of recurrent glomerulonephritis. However, studies involving large numbers of transplant patients have failed to confirm this prediction.[21] CsA has been reported, however, to modify the course of recurrent glomerulonephritis and slow the rate of graft loss in some patients.[21]

The most recent and comprehensive data on graft loss, as a result of recurrent glomerulonephritis, derive from an Australian study involving 1505 patients with biopsy-proven glomerulonephritis as a primary cause of ESRD.[5] Post-transplantation patients were followed over a period of 10 years when the incidence of graft loss from recurrent glomerulonephritis was 8%. The diseases with the highest rates of graft loss were focal segmental glomerulosclerosis (31%) and type I membranoproliferative glomerulonephritis (17%). Both male gender and high pre-transplant panel-reactive antibody levels were noted to be independent risk factors for graft loss from recurrent disease. Recurrent glomerulonephritis was the third most common cause of graft loss at 10 years post-transplant, and, as previously reported, the relative importance of recurrence as a cause of graft loss increases with time post-transplant.[5]

Table 39–1 Estimated Rates of Recurrence of Primary Glomerulopathies and Consequent Graft Loss

	Recurrence Rate	Graft Loss in Patients with Recurrent Disease
FSGS	~30%	~50%
MGN	3%–10%	~30%
IgA nephropathy	30%–60%	10%–30%
MPGN I	15%–30%	~33%
MPGN II	~80%	10%–20%
Anti-GBM disease	~10%	<5%

FSGS, focal segmental glomerulosclerosis; *MGN,* membranous nephropathy; *MPGN,* membranoproliferative glomerulonephritis. See text for further details.

Table 39–2 Estimated Rates of Recurrence of Secondary Glomerulopathies and Consequent Graft Loss

	Recurrence Rate	Graft Loss in Patients with Recurrent Disease
Diabetic nephropathy	~100%	<5%
SLE	<3%	<5%
ANCA-associated vasculitis	~25%	<5%
HSP	~50%	~10%
HUS	10%–41%	10%–40%
Scleroderma	20%–30%	?
Amyloidosis	8%–26%	~40%
LCCD	~50%	?
EMC	~50%	?
Multiple myeloma	~27%	<5%
Fibrillary GN	~50%	~50%

SLE, systemic lupus erythematosus; *ANCA,* anti-neutrophil cytoplasmic antibody; *HSP,* Henoch-Schönlein purpura; *HUS,* hemolytic uremic syndrome; *LCDD,* light chain deposition disease; *EMC,* essential mixed cryoglobulinemia. See text for further details.

PRIMARY GLOMERULOPATHIES

Focal Segmental Glomerulosclerosis

Recurrent Disease

Primary or idiopathic FSGS accounts for approximately 10% and 20% of cases of idiopathic nephrotic syndrome in children and adults, respectively, and the lesion progresses to ESRD in about 60% of patients.[22] Since the first description of recurrent FSGS in renal transplantation,[23] the reported rates of recurrence have ranged from 15% to 50%.[10,16,24] Most authors report a recurrence rate of approximately 30% for first allografts[6,10,19,24,25] and a higher incidence in children.[24,26] The rate of recurrence may be as high as 80% in patients who have previously lost a graft to recurrent FSGS.[1,2,27] Collapsing glomerulopathy, an aggressive subtype of FSGS characterized by severe visceral epithelial cell injury, can also recur following transplantation and trigger rapid loss of GFR in the face of massive proteinuria.[28,29] It must be stressed that secondary FSGS can complicate a plethora of renal insults rendering the diagnosis of true recurrence difficult in many instances.

Recurrent FSGS presents clinically with heavy proteinuria, often with full-blown nephrotic syndrome and its attendant risk of thromboembolic complications.[25] Recurrence may be evident within days of transplantation, particularly in children.[26,30] Most patients display evidence of recurrent disease at the end of the first month post-transplantation. Graft failure occurs in as many as 50% of adult patients and is more likely in the presence of nephrotic syndrome.[2,16,27,31,32] Graft loss may be even higher in children, as exemplified in a series by Muller and colleagues[33] in which five of six grafts with recurrent FSGS were lost. A history of accelerated primary graft loss from recurrence significantly increases the risk of loss of subsequent grafts.[19] Conversely, patients who have had prolonged function of their primary graft, despite recurrent FSGS, may expect a similar, more slowly progressive course in subsequent grafts.[33]

A number of risk factors for recurrence of FSGS have been identified: (1) diffuse mesangial proliferation in the native kidney[1,9,16,17,19]; (2) rapid deterioration of renal function in the native kidney (i.e., renal failure <3 years after diagnosis)[10,16,17,27]; and (3) younger age at diagnosis.[9,16,17,19] Other less well-established predictors of recurrence are acute tubular necrosis in the immediate post-transplant period[33] and racial background, a few studies indicating a lower incidence of recurrence in blacks than in whites.[9,27,30–32] The routine use of CsA has not reduced the incidence of recurrent FSGS,[19,21,27,33,34] although some authorities claim that high doses ameliorate the clinical course.[27,35] Whereas some studies have found an increased incidence of graft loss due to recurrence in recipients of living related kidneys, no such statistically significant difference was found in the large series by Briganti and colleagues.[5]

It has long been postulated that a circulating factor(s), possibly of T lymphocyte origin is responsible for the induction of glomerular damage in FSGS.[36] A number of observations on recurrent disease in the renal allograft support this theory.[37–40] Savin and colleagues[37] recently isolated a "factor" from sera of patients with FSGS, which increases glomerular permeability to albumin *in vitro.* In 33 patients who had recurrent FSGS post-transplantation, there was a direct correlation between the level of this factor and the tendency to disease recurrence. Plasmapheresis in six patients reduced the level of this factor and decreased urinary protein excretion from 8.2 to 0.9 g/24hr. Subsequent work by the same group has shown the permeability factor to be a protein of molecular weight between 30 and 50 kDa.[39] Dantal and colleagues[40] showed that immunoadsorption of sera from patients with recurrent FSGS on a protein A column transiently reduced proteinuria by an average of 82%. Furthermore, elute from the protein A column enhanced urinary albumin excretion when injected into rats. In aggregate, these observations suggest a central role for a circulating humoral mediator in the pathogenesis of FSGS.

Current treatment strategies for recurrent FSGS are designed to inhibit secretion of the putative lymphocyte-derived "factor" (CsA or FK506) and enhance removal by plasmapheresis. As noted above, CsA has been reported to reduce proteinuria by some but not all investigators.[27,35] Similarly, variable success has been reported for plasmapheresis.* The latter appears most

*References 2,16,19,27,38,39,41,42.

useful if instituted early in the course of disease before glomerulosclerosis has become established.[38,41] For example, in a study by Artero and colleagues,[38] six of nine patients with recurrent FSGS had a rapid reduction in proteinuria when plasmapheresis was instituted within 2 weeks after documentation of recurrent proteinuria, at which time only one of these patients displayed evidence of glomerular hyalinosis on renal biopsy. Post-plasmapheresis biopsies showed evidence of restoration of foot processes in four of these patients. In one study, the use of prophylactic plasma exchange in the week prior to transplantation led to a significant reduction in the rate of recurrence from 66% to 37%.[43] However, it is not clear from this report whether benefit was sustained in the long-term. Dall'Amico and colleagues[42] reported a benefit with plasmapheresis combined with cyclophosphamide in a study of 15 patients with recurrence in 18 grafts. Reversal of proteinuria occurred in 9 of 11 treated patients, and a persistent remission was obtained in 7 patients.[42]

Angiotensin-converting enzyme inhibitors (ACEIs) also reduce proteinuria in patients with recurrent FSGS. It is not established as yet whether they prolong allograft survival. In a representative study, administration of ACEIs to nine patients with recurrent disease reduced average proteinuria from 11.1 to 4.22 g/24 hr.[27] Remission or amelioration of nephrotic syndrome has been described in occasional patients with recurrent FSGS treated with nonsteroidal anti-inflammatory agents (NSAIDs).[44] Potential benefits of NSAIDs must be weighed against the risk of exacerbating CsA toxicity.

De Novo Disease

Whereas de novo FSGS may be a direct consequence of immune attack, emerging evidence suggests that the disease is, at least in part, triggered by hemodynamic stress in remnant nephrons following injury to the kidney by rejection, ischemia, and CsA.[45] In many instances de novo FSGS is felt to be a manifestation of chronic rejection.[25] Histologically, this lesion is characterized by occlusive vascular changes typical of chronic rejection, which primarily involve the glomeruli in the outer cortical region. This observation contrasts with recurrent FSGS, where the mild obliterative arteriopathy preferentially involves the juxtamedullary glomeruli. Clinically de novo FSGS presents with proteinuria and a less aggressive course than recurrent FSGS, but it is nonetheless a negative independent predictor of graft survival.[46] Collapsing GN, the aggressive subtype of FSGS, has also been described as a de novo lesion in the renal allograft.[28]

Membranous Nephropathy

Recurrent Disease

Membranous nephropathy is the most common cause of idiopathic nephrotic syndrome in adults and progresses to ESRD in 20% of cases.[22] Membranous nephropathy may recur in allografts or develop as a de novo lesion, 75% being in the latter category.[1,10] Most studies quote a recurrence rate of 3% to 10%,[1,2,47,48] though figures as high as 25% to 57% have been reported.[4,9,10]

Recurrent membranous nephropathy occurs earlier post-transplantation than de novo disease and runs a more aggressive course. The average time from transplantation to recurrence is 10 months,[47] though appearance as early as one week[49] and as late as 7 years post-transplantation has been reported.[4] Patients typically present with nephrotic-range proteinuria, and graft loss is in the order of 30%.[10,47,48,50] However, many grafts lost to recurrent membranous nephropathy have displayed evidence of other pathologic processes, such as rejection, and the relative contribution of each process to graft failure is not often clear.[48]

Some studies suggest that a high degree of HLA matching between donor–recipient pairs and the use of living related kidneys also increases the risk of recurrence.[47] Furthermore, recurrent disease may manifest earlier (in the first 3 months post-transplantation) in living-related than in cadaveric grafts.[47] The routine use of CsA has not reduced the rate of recurrence.[21,48,50] High-dose steroids have not been successful in reducing proteinuria,[47,51] and no effective therapeutic regimen has been identified. Re-transplantation should be considered in patients who lose their initial graft, although consecutive recurrent membranous glomerulonephritis has been described.[48]

De Novo Disease

De novo membranous nephropathy is the most frequent cause of post-transplant nephrotic syndrome after rejection-induced transplant glomerulopathy (vide infra).[47,51] The reported incidence varies from 0.3% to 6.7%[51,52] with a higher frequency reported in centers with a policy of routine renal biopsy for assessment of non–nephrotic-range proteinuria. In one study, de novo membranous nephropathy recurred in four of seven patients in a second transplant.[53] The incidence of de novo membranous nephropathy increases with time, and, as overall graft survival rates improve, it is being increasingly recognized as a late complication in otherwise functional grafts.[51] De novo disease presents later than recurrent disease and manifests with gradual development of proteinuria. However, almost one third of patients remain asymptomatic with low-grade proteinuria.[51] Graft loss may occur in as many as 50% of patients with persistent nephrotic-range proteinuria.[54,55] However, because membranous nephropathy and chronic rejection often coexist, it may be difficult to determine the relative contribution of each to graft failure, and, indeed, graft loss has been attributed to chronic rejection rather than to membranous nephropathy in many cases.[51,52] For example, 14 of 21 grafts with de novo membranous nephropathy in one series failed, but chronic rejection was felt to be responsible for 13 of these graft losses.[51]

De novo membranous nephropathy is often associated with some degree of vascular rejection[51,52] and cyclosporine-induced vasculopathy.[51] An association with chronic viral infection, most commonly, hepatitis C, has been demonstrated in up to a third of patients with de novo membranous nephropathy, suggesting a potential viral trigger for immune complex formation.[51,55] Cyclosporin A is not effective in preventing development of the lesion.[21] Similarly, pulse steroid therapy was not effective in reducing proteinuria in larger series,[74] although occasional successes have been claimed.[56]

IgA Nephropathy

Immunoglobulin A (IgA) nephropathy is the most common primary glomerular disease worldwide.[57] Histologic evidence of recurrence is reported in 30% to 60% of allografts.[4,10,58–62] IgA deposition alone is not clinically significant unless accompanied by the development of mesangioproliferative changes. A recent retrospective study of 106 patients with biopsy proven IgA nephropathy demonstrated a similar 10-year graft survival in patients with IgA nephropathy when compared to 212 patients without IgA nephropathy who were transplanted during the same period.[60] Occasionally, recurrent IgA nephropathy presents as aggressive crescentic disease.[63,64] Recurrent IgA nephropathy has generally been considered a benign condition that causes graft loss in less than 10% of cases.[1,2,60] Interestingly, recent data suggest that recurrent IgA nephropathy may carry a more adverse prognosis and become an increasingly important cause of graft loss as overall allograft survival improves.[59–61] In one study, 9 of 13 patients with histologically confirmed recurrent IgA deposition had evidence of mesangioproliferative glomerulonephritis.[59] Although 5-year allograft survival was similar in the presence or absence of recurrent IgA nephropathy, four of these nine patients subsequently lost their grafts to recurrent disease from 60 to 119 months post-transplantation. Similarly, Frohnert and colleagues[61] reported that recurrent IgA nephropathy led to significant loss of graft function in 10 of 14 patients with prolonged follow-up and was responsible for 3 of 4 late graft losses.[61]

A recent report described recurrence of crescentic IgA nephropathy in a patient who had both IgA and IgG antineutrophil cytoplasmic antibodies (ANCA), with specificity for myeloperoxidase (MPO), prior to onset of ESRD.[65] The patient developed acute nephrotic syndrome with rapidly progressive renal failure due to recurrent crescentic IgA nephropathy associated with a rise in titer of IgA anti-MPO antibodies. The authors proposed the existence of a subgroup of patients who have an overlap syndrome of IgA nephropathy and microscopic polyangiitis in which IgA and IgG ANCA coexist and who are at increased risk of developing recurrent crescentic glomerulonephritis.[65] It is suggested that the titer of IgA anti-MPO antibodies but not IgG anti-MPO antibodies correlates with disease activity and tendency to recur. Further studies will be necessary to confirm the prognostic value of detection of IgA ANCA prior to renal transplantation.

Some studies suggest that recurrent IgA nephropathy is more frequent in living related than in cadaveric grafts,[58,64] though this is not a universal finding.[5,60,61] For example, in one study the recurrence rate was 83% in living related transplants compared with 14% in cadaveric grafts.[58] It is possible that inherited susceptibility factors, such as HLA DR4 in the case of IgA nephropathy, confer an increased risk of recurrence in living related transplants when shared by donor and recipient.[66] Alternatively, recurrence in this setting may reflect the presence of subclinical IgA nephropathy in the donor, with resultant inadvertent transmission of IgA deposits in the donor allograft to the recipient.[64] Instances of transplantation of kidneys containing mesangial IgA deposits have been described, and the glomerular mesangial deposits have been documented to disappear with time.[67] It has been suggested that when considering living related transplantation for patients with IgA nephropathy, the donor family should be evaluated for subtle evidence of nephritis and that pre-transplant donor biopsy or cadaveric transplantation should be considered if familial clustering is demonstrated.[64] In the study by Ponticelli and colleagues,[60] younger age was found to be a risk factor for recurrence with patients under 30 years having a relative risk of 2.6.

Several therapeutic strategies have been proposed for patients with recurrent IgA nephropathy, including combinations of steroids, cyclophosphamide, azathioprine, CsA, or plasma exchange, but without compelling evidence to support their use. Although the incidence of mesangial deposition of IgA is not altered by CsA, the latter agent has been reported by some[19] to ameliorate the clinical course and to reduce the rate of graft loss. Consistent with the known renoprotective effects of ACEI in native kidney disease, these agents have recently been reported to have a beneficial effect in patients with proteinuria secondary to recurrent IgA nephropathy.[68,69]

Membranoproliferative Glomerulonephritis Type I

Recurrent Disease

MPGN type I is an immune-complex-mediated glomerulonephritis that frequently follows an indolent clinical course and progresses to ESRD in approximately 20% of patients.[22] It recurs in 15% to 30% of renal allografts and causes graft loss in one-third of these patients.[2,4,5,9,70,71] Accurate estimation of disease recurrence has proved difficult in the past because of the similarities between this lesion and transplant glomerulopathy (vide infra) on light microscopy.[72] Routine examination of biopsy specimens by immunofluorescence and electron microscopy usually distinguishes between the two entities—subendothelial Ig-containing deposits being characteristic of MPGN but absent in transplant glomerulopathy.[10,73]

Recurrent MPGN type I may be a renal-limited disease or present in association with systemic signs of cryoglobulinemia. However, the prevalence of cryoglobulins, hypocomplementemia, and rheumatoid factor positivity is less in transplant MPGN, perhaps due to concomitant pharmacologic immunosuppression.[74,75] Recurrent renal disease presents clinically with heavy proteinuria and microscopic hematuria and may be evident within 3 weeks of transplantation.[75] No definite predictors of disease recurrence have been established. Crescentic disease with a rapidly progressive course in the native kidneys has been associated by some authors with an increased tendency to recurrence.[70] The use of living related kidneys and loss of a previous graft to recurrent disease may also favor recurrence.[71] Hypocomplementemia persisting after renal transplantation does not appear to be associated with higher recurrence rates.[70]

There are isolated reports in the literature of successful treatment of recurrent disease with increased immunosuppression. One group used long-term plasmapheresis over a 16-month period to maintain renal function along with the administration of monthly pulsed intravenous cyclophosphamide.[76] Cahen and colleagues[75] successfully induced remission of recurrent disease with a combination of prednisolone, cyclophosphamide, and dipyridamole. Aspirin and dipyridamole have also been shown to stabilize renal function.[70]

*References 2,4,5,9,70,71.

De Novo Disease

MPGN accounts for about 33% of cases of de novo glomerulonephritis in renal allografts.[21,74,77,78] The most important etiologic factor appears to be chronic hepatitis C infection, which is present in up to 30% of patients with ESRD.[77,79] In a study of a cohort of 94 hepatitis C–positive transplant recipients, de novo MPGN was demonstrated in 6 of 9 patients undergoing renal biopsy for investigation of proteinuria of greater than 1.5 g/day.[78] Type II cryoglobulinemia, circulating immune complexes, and classic pathway complement activation were observed in all patients. In another study of 98 hepatitis C–positive recipients, de novo MPGN was demonstrated in 5 of 8 patients who underwent biopsy for the investigation of proteinuria of greater than 1 g/day.[74] Interestingly, cryoglobulinemia was not a prerequisite for the development of MPGN as has also been noted with primary glomerulonephritis in the native kidney.

Hepatitis C infection is associated with development of a variety of glomerular lesions in native kidneys including MPGN. A similar spectrum has been observed in renal transplant recipients. Hepatitis C–positive transplant recipients have an increased incidence of both de novo glomerulonephritis and transplant glomerulopathy compared to hepatitis C negative patients (13.7% in hepatitis C–positive recipients versus 4.2% in hepatitis C–negative patients).[80] Intriguingly, Gallay and colleagues[77] described two hepatitis C–positive transplant recipients who developed a hybrid lesion with ultrastructural features of both MPGN and transplant glomerulopathy, namely electron-dense immune complex deposits typical of MPGN along with subendothelial accumulation of electron-lucent material, typical of transplant glomerulopathy (vide infra). It is not clear why only some transplant recipients with chronic hepatitis C infection develop glomerular lesions and what dictates the morphology of the glomerular lesion. Differences in viral strains, viral titers, and individual T cell–mediated responses may account for some of the variation. The occurrence of hybrid lesions as described by Gallay and colleagues[77] may simply reflect the coexistence of hepatitis C induced glomerulonephritis and allograft rejection, or, alternatively, it may reflect modification of the morphology of hepatitis C–associated glomerulonephritis by immunosuppressive therapy.

The role of interferon-α in treatment of hepatitis C–associated MPGN in renal transplant recipients is controversial because of the risk of precipitating acute cellular rejection. Whereas successful treatment of viral infection and stabilization of renal function has been reported in occasional patients,[77] interferon-α has been observed to trigger acute rejection when used as prophylaxis for CMV[81] and as treatment for hepatitis C–associated liver disease.[82,83]

Membranoproliferative GN Type II

Recurrent Disease

MPGN type II, which is characterized pathologically by accumulation of dense deposits within the glomerular basement membrane, is less common than MPGN type I and accounts for half as many cases of ESRD.[22] Recurrence of MPGN type II is very common affecting up to 80% of allografts.[1,4,10,84] The rate of graft loss from recurrence is in the order of 10% to 20%,[1,10] although a 50% graft failure rate was reported in one series of 10 transplant recipients with recurrent disease.[84] Recurrence of disease in a second graft after loss of the first allograft to recurrence has been described.[1]

Recurrence is usually clinically evident or ascertained by examination of renal biopsy specimens within the first year post-transplantation. Despite the high rate of histologic recurrence, clinical manifestations are absent in 40% of patients. The remainder present with proteinuria and slow, progressive deterioration of renal function. It appears that graft loss is more likely in male patients who present with nephrotic-range proteinuria and rapidly progressive glomerulonephritis.[84]

Unlike patients with native disease, most patients with recurrence do not have circulating C3 nephritic factor, probably reflecting the presence of chronic immunosuppression.[1] The use of CsA has generally not been found to influence the rate of recurrent MPGN, apart from one study, which suggested a reduced incidence.[34] Treatment of recurrent dense deposit disease has generally been ineffective, as in native disease. One isolated report described clinical and pathologic improvement with the use of plasma exchange.[85]

Anti-glomerular Basement Membrane Disease

Anti-GBM nephritis accounts for less than 2% of glomerulonephritis causing ESRD.[22] Recurrence, as defined by the reappearance of linear IgG deposition along the glomerular capillary walls, has been reported to occur in up to 55% of patients.[1] However, only 25% of these patients have clinical manifestations of recurrent disease, and graft loss is rare.[1,2] A more recent report by Pirson and colleagues[86] noted recurrence of IgG deposition in only 1 of 10 patients. Even in this patient, serum creatinine was normal after 15 months of follow-up. Of note, this patient had been on dialysis for 28 months prior to transplantation and had no detectable circulating antibodies at the time of transplantation.[86] Given the compelling evidence that anti-GBM antibodies are pathogenic in this disease, it is standard practice to delay transplantation for a 6- to 12-month period after this serum marker is undetectable.[87]

De Novo Crescentic Glomerulonephritis

De novo crescentic glomerulonephritis is rare in renal allografts, the most common setting being anti-GBM nephritis developing in allografts of patients with Alport's syndrome. The autoantigen in anti-GBM nephritis is a 28 kDa component of the α3 chain of type IV collagen.[88] In X-linked Alport's syndrome, a mutation in the gene encoding the α5 chain of type IV collagen is associated with abnormal assembly of the α3 chain of type IV collagen.[89] Anti-GBM antibodies may develop when the immune system of Alport patients encounters the Goodpasture antigen in the allograft for the first time. Whereas asymptomatic linear deposition of anti-GBM antibody is most common, full-blown rapidly progressive glomerulonephritis and graft loss can occur, albeit rarely.[90–93]

In a review of renal transplantation in a series of 30 patients with Alport's syndrome, patient and graft survival rates were similar to those of an age-matched control group.[94] Five of 15 grafts examined histologically were positive for linear IgG deposition; however, crescentic nephritis was not seen. Two patients underwent repeat biopsies. Linear IgG deposition had disappeared in one after 12 months but persisted in the second patient 5 years later.[94] The survival of the IgG positive and negative grafts was similar, as was the level of renal function. A single case of recurrent crescentic glomerulonephritis in a second allograft in an Alport's patient who had already lost the first graft to anti-GBM disease has been described.[93] In this patient renal function stabilized following plasmapheresis and an increase in the dose of CsA.

Development of de novo crescentic glomerulonephritis is very rare in patients with ESRD due to diseases other than Alport's syndrome.[95,96] In one report, de novo crescentic glomerulonephritis developed early in association with glomerular basement membrane deposition of IgG.[95] The author proposed that exposure of the allograft to a circulating antibody, perhaps contained in antilymphocyte globulin may have contributed to the development of this lesion. Treatment of de novo crescentic glomerulonephritis is similar to that for disease in the native kidney. Success has been claimed with early use of cyclophosphamide, plasmapheresis, steroids, and dipyridamole[93,95,96]; however, others dispute the long-term effectiveness of treatment.[91]

SECONDARY GLOMERULOPATHIES

Diabetes Mellitus

Diabetic nephropathy is the leading cause of ESRD and accounts for approximately 20% of renal transplants performed annually in North America. Diabetic nephropathy invariably recurs in the renal allograft and progresses at a similar rate to disease in the native kidney.[1,97,98] Recurrent disease typically presents with proteinuria and slow deterioration of renal function over a period of 15 to 20 years. Renal biopsy may reveal glomerular basement membrane deposition of IgG as the sole abnormality in the early post-transplant period. However, the classic histologic changes of diabetic nephropathy, such as glomerular basement membrane thickening, mesangial expansion, and arteriolar hyaline deposition, are seen within 2 to 4 years.[11,97,98] Graft loss from recurrent disease is seen in less than 5% of cases, largely because grafts fail from chronic rejection or patients die from extrarenal complications before diabetic nephropathy reaches end-stage.[12]

As with primary disease, the degree of glycemic control is a critical determinant of the rate of progression of recurrent diabetic nephropathy. It is also advisable to treat recurrent disease with ACEI, given the compelling evidence that they slow progression of primary disease in experimental animals and humans.[99] In selected patients, normalization of glucose levels with combined pancreatic and renal transplantation cures diabetes and prevents the development of diabetic renal disease in the transplanted kidney.[11,97,100]

Systemic Lupus Erythematosus

Lupus nephritis accounts for about 1% of cases of ESRD. In the majority of patients, disease activity declines upon institution of maintenance dialysis and declines further after renal transplantation.[101,102] It is not clear whether this response represents the natural history of SLE or the immunomodulatory effects of uremia and immunosuppression. In general, lupus nephritis recurs in less than 3% of patients following transplantation and is rarely responsible for graft loss.[1,2,10,103–107] In series by Nossent and colleagues[103] and Goss and colleagues,[105] only 1 of 28 patients and 1 of 14 patients, respectively, suffered recurrence. In another series of 80 patients with ESRD due to lupus nephritis, two patients (2.5%) suffered recurrence, one of whom lost their allograft.[106] More recent studies have documented a higher rate of recurrence.[108,109] For example, Stone and colleagues[108] documented a recurrence rate of 10% in a group of 97 transplant recipients with SLE; however, recurrence was felt to contribute to graft loss in only 4 patients. In most cases the recurrent lesion is of the same histologic class, as observed in the native kidney,[104,110] with occasional exceptions.[111] Overall, mean patient and graft survival following renal transplantation for lupus nephritis compare favorably with transplantation for other causes of ESRD.[104,110]

Several authorities recommend a 3- to 6-month waiting period between initiation of dialysis and transplantation in patients with lupus nephritis.[102,109] This approach allows time for recovery of any reversible component of renal failure and facilitates disease quiescence prior to transplantation. Some authors advocate delay of transplantation until patients are seronegative on the basis that active serology at the time of transplantation is associated with a worse outcome.[105,110] This view is not universally supported, however.[112]

Index case studies report a 1.5% rate of occurrence of lupus in first degree relatives.[102] Accordingly, it is of paramount importance to screen prospective living donors for hematuria and proteinuria prior to transplantation. A small increased risk of recurrent lupus nephritis in recipients of living related kidneys was suggested by the review of Mojcik and colleagues[104] but was not confirmed in other reports.[108] Furthermore, the results with living related kidneys are better than with cadaveric in patients with lupus nephritis, presumably because of shorter ischemic times and better HLA matching.[106] As mentioned above, disease recurrence rarely produces significant renal dysfunction and usually responds to increased immunosuppression.[109,111] Success has been reported with higher dose corticosteroids,[107] chlorambucil,[111] and cyclophosphamide.[110,112]

ANCA-Associated Vasculitis

The ANCA-associated renal diseases comprise Wegener's granulomatosis, Churg-Strauss syndrome, microscopic polyangiitis, and renal-limited crescentic glomerulonephritis.[113] ESRD requiring dialysis or transplantation occurs in approximately 10% of cases.[113] The data on renal transplantation derive mostly from small series of patients with Wegener's granulomatosis. In this setting, vasculitis–glomerulonephritis recurs in approximately 25%, but ensuing graft loss is rare.[114–119] A lower incidence of recurrence of 9% was reported by Allen and colleagues, possibly reflecting their policy of a longer duration of immunosuppressive therapy for patients once they commence maintenance dialysis.[115] In a series of 20 patients reported by Schmitt and colleagues[120] (6 of whom had active disease at the time of transplantation), 5 patients had clinical relapses during a 4-year follow-up, all of which were extrarenal. Graft survival in these patients was similar to that in the group as a whole. In a small series, the outcome of transplantation for microscopic polyangiitis and Wegener's granulomatosis seems to be similar.[117,121] In a pooled analysis of 127 patients the relapse rates of microscopic polyangiitis or renal limited crescentic GN (n = 51) was similar to Wegener's granulomatosis (n = 54).[114] Renal recurrence of Wegener's has been documented as early as 5 days after transplantation,[122] and typically presents with hematuria and deteriorating renal function. An interesting report described a patient with recurrent Wegener's granulomatosis who presented with obstructive uropathy secondary to ureteric stenosis caused by the vasculitic process.[119]

The preoperative ANCA titer does not appear to correlate with the risk of recurrence, and ANCA positivity is not a contraindication to transplantation.[114] Of eight patients described by Rostaing and colleagues,[117] seven had positive ANCA titers at the time of transplantation. Positive titers persisted in five patients after transplantation, and only one patient developed recurrent disease. Similarly, the reappearance of ANCA or a rising ANCA titer following transplantation does not accurately predict disease recurrence.[117,120] There are no data that suggest different risks of recurrence in patients with proteinase-3-specific c-ANCA or MPO-specific p-ANCA.[114]

The optimal immunosuppressive regimen post-transplantation in patients with ANCA-associated renal diseases has not been determined. Control of systemic disease as well as recurrent renal disease has to be considered. Some centers include cyclophosphamide in the immunosuppressive regimen for these patients, on the basis that it reduces the risk of recurrent disease. For example, Clarke and colleagues[118] noted a higher recurrence rate of Wegener's granulomatosis in patients receiving CsA without azathioprine or cyclophosphamide. Recurrences involved the lungs or ear, nose and throat more frequently than the kidney. In agreement with these data, Schmitt and colleagues reported a lower recurrence rate with triple therapy combining CsA and steroids with either azathioprine or cyclophosphamide than with CsA and steroids alone.[120] In the pooled analysis by Nachman and colleagues there was no difference in the rates of recurrence in patients receiving CsA compared to those not receiving CsA.[114] Recurrent disease usually remits following treatment with pulsed intravenous methylprednisolone and cyclophosphamide.[114,115,117,118] This overall favorable response to cyclophosphamide has led some authors to conclude that cyclophosphamide be reserved for those with recurrent disease, rather than used prophylactically.[123]

Henoch-Schönlein Purpura

HSP is an immune-complex disorder characterized by skin, joint, abdominal, and renal involvement. The pathologic hallmark of the disease is deposition of IgA in the glomerular mesangium and blood vessels of the dermis and intestine. The incidence of histologic recurrence following renal transplantation is approximately 50%.[10,18,58] This incidence is similar to IgA nephropathy, a disease that may be a renal-limited form of HSP.[58] Recurrent HSP is usually benign, but active proliferative nephritis with or without extrarenal manifestations has been noted in up to 20% of patients.[18] Purpura is noted in up to 10%. Although graft loss is reported to occur in 9% of cases of recurrence,[3] it may approach 50% in a subgroup of patients with renal involvement accompanied by recurrent purpura.[10,124] The actuarial risk of recurrence and resultant graft loss in two of the larger series was estimated at 35% and 11%, respectively, 5 years after transplantation.[18]

Severe systemic activity, especially purpura, in the year prior to transplantation[1, 2] and rapid progression of the primary disease to renal failure[18] are risk factors for recurrence. For these reasons, a waiting period of 6 to 12 months after resolution of purpura is generally advised before proceeding with transplantation.[1,2,124] Recurrence may be observed even with these precautions, however, as illustrated in a series by Meulders and colleagues, where two patients with recurrence had been on dialysis for 22 and 37 months prior to transplantation.[18] Age of onset of original disease of greater than 14 years may also predict recurrence.[18] Some but not all investigators have noted an increased incidence of recurrence in recipients of living-related kidneys.[18] In general, CsA does not appear to alter the incidence of recurrent HSP,[18,59] and no effective therapeutic regimen has been described.

Hemolytic Uremic Syndrome–Thrombotic Thrombocytopenic Purpura (HUS-TTP)

Recurrent Disease

HUS-TTP is a spectrum of disease characterized by microangiopathic hemolytic anemia, thrombocytopenia, intravascular coagulation, and acute renal failure, which may culminate in ESRD. The reported recurrence rates of HUS after renal transplantation vary widely from as low as 9% to as high as 56%.* Graft loss attributable to HUS occurs in 10% to 40% of these patients.[10,125,127–130] In a meta-analysis of 10 studies comprising 159 grafts in 127 patients, 1-year graft survival in patients with recurrence was as low as 33.3%.[128] Recurrence is less likely in diarrhea-associated HUS than in non-diarrhea–associated HUS, which might explain the lower incidence of recurrence in children, where the disorder is more frequently Shiga toxin–associated.[127] For example, Broyer and colleagues,[7] in an analysis of EDTA registry data, reported that of 71 failures of 170 first grafts in children with HUS only 1 was due to recurrent disease. In a series of 18 children in Argentina there was no documented case or recurrent HUS.[131]

Acute vascular rejection or CsA alone induces endothelial cell injury, which can trigger a de novo thrombotic microangiopathy with features similar to classic HUS and may predispose patients with ESRD due to primary HUS to development of recurrent disease.[132,133] Indeed, higher recurrence rates in some series have been related to more frequent use of CsA,[128,134] albeit with dissenting views.[21,129] In a recent review of 114 patients with recurrent HUS, Agarwal[126] found that about two thirds were exposed to CsA, whereas one third did not receive CsA. Other immunosuppressive agents that may predispose to recurrence are antilymphocyte globulin (ALG)[125] or OKT3.[135] In the meta-analysis by Duclox and colleagues,[128] additional risk factors for recurrence were a shorter mean interval between HUS and transplantation, older age at onset of HUS, a shorter mean interval between HUS and ESRD, and the use of living related donors. In one report a much lower rate of recurrence was found in patients who had

*References 1,2,10,24,125–130.

undergone pre-transplant bilateral nephrectomies than in those whose native kidneys were in situ.[130]

With these observations in mind, a number of strategies are advocated to reduce the risk of recurrence. Transplantation should not be undertaken until the clinical features (anemia, thrombocytopenia, abnormal smear) of HUS have subsided. OKT3, ALG, and the oral contraceptive pill (all risk factors for primary HUS) should be avoided.[135] Some authors urge avoidance of CsA if a previous graft was lost to recurrent HUS while on CsA.[126] Low-dose salicylates and dipyridamole have been recommended to prevent recurrence,[125] although without compelling evidence to support their use.

Treatment of recurrent HUS is essentially the same as for primary disease and centers around plasma exchange and plasma infusions. Although controlled trials are lacking in this area, anecdotal reports describe successful outcomes with plasmapheresis.[128,133] In patients on CsA, it is prudent to reduce the dose by 50% or withdraw CsA and replace it with FK506 or other agent, if additional immunosuppression is deemed necessary.[136]

De Novo Disease

De novo HUS has been reported more frequently since the incorporation of CsA into immunosuppressive regimens.[128] There are also a growing number of reports implicating tacrolimus in the causation of de novo HUS.[137–139] A more recent review by Schwimmer and colleagues[139] documented de novo HUS in 21 of 742 transplant recipients. The causative agent was deemed to be tacrolimus in 10 patients and CsA in 9 patients. Thirteen patients had systemic features, whereas 8 had localized renal disease. Graft loss was higher in patients with systemic manifestations (38% vs. 0%), and renal function improved in the group with localized disease on reduction, conversion, or temporary discontinuation of calcineurin inhibitor.[139] A number of prothrombotic mechanisms whereby CsA may perturb endothelial function *in vitro* and *in vivo* and trigger thrombotic microangiopathy have been postulated.[140] Viral infections have also been implicated as triggers for de novo HUS, as exemplified by a recent case report of HUS-TTP in association with HIV infection.[141] Recent reports suggest an association between sirolimus and de novo and recurrent thrombotic microangiopathy.[143,144] In a recent review of USRDS data additional risk factors identified for de novo TMA included younger age of recipient, older donor age, female recipients, and use of sirolimus.[144] De novo HUS in patients on CsA carries a poor prognosis with a high incidence of graft loss, even after withdrawal of the drug.[142] Again, treatment of de novo HUS is based on regimens for disease in native kidneys.

Systemic Sclerosis

The literature on renal transplantation in systemic sclerosis is rather limited. Patient and graft survival is poorer in this condition than in other causes of ESRD.[146,147] It is estimated that renal disease recurs in 20% to 30% of patients; this may be an overestimate given the rarity of the condition and the similarity of the pathologic lesion of renal scleroderma to vascular rejection. The risk of recurrence appears greatest in patients with a history of aggressive primary disease, particularly where the time interval from onset of systemic sclerosis to transplantation is less than 1 year.[3]

Graft survival can be maximized by ensuring that the patient is free of active disease at the time of transplantation and by aggressive control of hypertension post-transplantation. Early reports suggested that bilateral nephrectomy at the time of transplantation improved outcome; however, with improvement in antihypertensive therapy, this procedure should no longer be deemed necessary.[3] Cyclosporine does not appear to influence the incidence of recurrence.[205]

GLOMERULAR DEPOSITION DISEASES

Amyloidosis

Amyloid deposits recur in 8% to 26% of allografts in patients with primary (AL) and secondary (AA) amyloidosis, who survive longer than 1 year.[2,3,148–150] In the two largest single-center series, recurrent amyloidosis was documented in 4 of 45 patients by Pasternak and colleagues[148] and in 6 of 54 patients by Hartmann and colleagues.[150] In a review by Harrison and colleagues,[149] recurrent renal amyloidosis was documented in 21% of patients with familial Mediterranean fever, 15% of patients with AA amyloidosis secondary to rheumatic and chronic infectious disease, and 27% of patients with AL amyloidosis. The rate of loss of grafts with recurrent amyloidosis appears to be about 40%.[148,150] In general, survival of patients with amyloidosis has been found to be significantly less than for patients with other causes of ESRD, as a result of the high incidence of cardiovascular and other extrarenal complications, and death of the patient with a functioning graft accounts for as many as 60% of graft failures.[148,150] However, much better patient and graft survival were reported with living-donor renal transplantation in 23 patients with amyloidosis (16 with familial Mediterranean fever and 7 with primary amyloidosis) when compared to 47 nonamyloidotic controls.[151] In this report, both the 5- and 10-year patient and graft survival rates were similar to the control group, and recurrence was documented in only one case.[151]

Recurrent amyloidosis presents clinically with proteinuria or nephrotic syndrome, however, histologic recurrence is not invariably accompanied by clinical manifestations. The deterioration in renal function is often more gradual than in native kidneys. Controlling the activity of the underlying inflammatory focus may reduce the risk of recurrence of AA-amyloidosis.[152] No specific therapeutic strategies have been identified. Despite the risk of recurrence and the relatively high mortality rate, patients with amyloidosis should nonetheless be considered for transplantation, as survival appears superior with renal transplantation than with maintenance dialysis.

Essential Mixed Cryoglobulinemia

The clinical and serologic activity of essential mixed cryoglobulinemia decreases after the onset of ESRD. Data on the outcome of this disease following renal transplantation are sparse. Reactivation has been estimated to occur in as many as 50% of renal allograft recipients.[153] In two cases described by Hiesse and colleagues,[153] renal recurrence was accompanied by extrarenal disease and by the reappearance of rheumatoid factor positivity, the presence of serum cryoglobulins, and depressed levels of C3 and C4 components of complement. Recurrent renal disease can be seen as early as 30 days after engraftment, is often aggressive, and may ultimately result in graft loss. The high risk of significant recurrent disease has led some investigators to suggest that cadaveric grafts should be used in preference to living related grafts for these patients.[153]

Monoclonal Gammopathies

Lymphoplasmacytic disorders may cause renal insufficiency via a variety of pathologic mechanisms. Chief among these are AL amyloidosis (vide supra), light chain deposition disease (LCDD), myeloma cast nephropathy, and fibrillary-immunotactoid GN (vide infra).[154] Rarer manifestations include Fanconi's syndrome and heavy chain deposition disease. It is difficult to make strong inferences about the outcome of transplantation in these disorders because the available information is limited to case reports.[155–160]

LCDD recurs in approximately 50% of allografts.[155–157,159,161] Recurrent LCDD can cause severe impairment and loss of graft function,[156,157] although renal function may be well maintained in some patients despite histologic evidence of recurrence.[155,161] De novo LCDD without evidence of malignancy has been reported in a renal allograft 16 years after successful renal transplantation.[163]

Of seven reported patients with myeloma cast nephropathy who underwent renal transplantation, recurrence was observed in two patients without adversely affecting graft function.[158,160,162,164,165] However, a number of patients died from recurrent extrarenal disease or sepsis illustrating the poor prognosis in this disease. A few case reports have also described the occurrence of de novo multiple myeloma in renal allograft recipients following transplantation.[166,167] In one of these patients the myeloma was associated with LCDD in the allograft.[167]

Fibrillary-Immunotactoid Glomerulopathy

Fibrillary-immunotactoid glomerulopathy is characterized by extracellular deposition of congo-red–negative, nonbranching microfibrils or microtubules within the glomerular mesangium and capillary walls in the absence of light chains or cryoglobulins.[168] Patients with fibrillary immunotactoid glomerulopathy frequently progress to ESRD (50% after 5 years). Experience with transplantation in these patients is limited. From the small number of cases reported, it appears that fibril deposition recurs in at least 50% of patients.[168–172] Despite the high recurrence rate, the decline in renal function in allografts is usually slower than in native kidneys, and many patients maintain satisfactory function for over 5 years. Indeed, three patients with recurrent disease reported by Pronovost and colleagues[169] continued to have functioning grafts between 6 and 11 years post-transplantation. Whether the slower rate of progression in allografts reflects a beneficial effect of immunosuppressive therapy or spontaneous attenuation of disease activity is unclear.

NONGLOMERULAR DISEASES

Oxalosis

Oxalosis, or primary hyperoxaluria type I, is an autosomal recessive disease, which results from deficiency of hepatic peroxisomal alanine glyoxylate aminotransferase. Absence of this enzyme causes oxalate overproduction and recurrent calcium oxalate nephrolithiasis and nephrocalcinosis. Oxalosis was originally considered a contraindication to transplantation because of universal recurrence of renal disease and graft loss.[1,171] More recently, combined liver and kidney transplantation has produced encouraging results.[13–15,173,174] In one report, 17 of 24 patients had functioning grafts 1 to 6 years post-transplantation.[13] Some authors advocate liver transplantation simultaneously with the first kidney transplant,[13] whereas others suggest it be deferred until the first allograft fails from disease recurrence.[175] Several measures have been recommended to maximize successful engraftment.[176] First, renal replacement therapy should be instituted early (once the GFR approaches 20 mL/min) to limit tissue oxalate deposition, which will be released into the circulation and deposited in the allograft post-transplant.[124,174,175] Aggressive preoperative dialysis is recommended to deplete the extrarenal tissue oxalate pool. It is essential to establish a brisk postoperative diuresis, because deposition of oxalate in the allograft seems to be accelerated during periods of primary nonfunction.[176] The use of a large living related allograft and avoidance of the immediate use of CsA can accomplish this goal. Administration of pyridoxine, a coenzyme that functions in the conversion of glyoxylate to glycine and thereby decreases the glyoxylate pool, has also been recommended to maintain graft function.[177,178]

Cystinosis

Cystinosis is an autosomal recessive disorder that results from defective transport of cystine from lysosome to cytosol. Lysosomal accumulation of cystine in the renal interstitium ultimately causes interstitial fibrosis, glomerular sclerosis, and renal failure. Renal transplantation is very successful and is the preferred mode of treatment for children with this condition.[171,179] Cystinosis and cystine-induced tubular cell dysfunction per se do not recur.[124] However, cystine-laden cells, probably host macrophages, can be found in the transplanted kidney.[180] Despite successful renal transplantation, the systemic effects of pre-transplantation cystine accumulation in other organs persists and accounts for ongoing morbidity.

Fabry's Disease

Fabry's disease is an X-linked recessive disorder due to deficiency of the enzyme α-galactosidase, which results in the accumulation of glycosphingolipids in most tissues of the body, including the kidneys. Early reports of renal transplantation in Fabry's disease suggested a very poor outcome, and many patients died of pulmonary hemorrhage, thrombosis, and sepsis.[171,181] More recent reports indicate a better outcome, with 3 years graft survival rates of up to 80%.[124,182]

Initial hopes that kidney transplantation would provide an adequate source of the missing enzyme have not been realized[183] and recurrence has been described.[184] Recurrence does not result in clinical sequelae, however, and patient survival of up to 11 years has been reported.[184] Consequently, renal transplantation is now considered a reasonable option in this condition.

Sickle Cell Disease

Approximately 4% of patients with sickle cell disease progress to ESRD.[185] Experience with transplantation is rather limited.[254–257] Despite reasonable graft survival in some reports,[186–188] allograft failure in the first year was reported in six of eight patients in a series by Barber and colleagues.[188] Four of these grafts were deemed lost to recurrent sickling.[188] Graft loss may result from an acute vaso-occlusive crisis or from the more indolent effect of recurrent sickling episodes. Secondary focal sclerosis has been described in transplanted kidneys presumably a consequence of nephron loss due to intrarenal sickling.[187] An increased incidence of sickling crises has been described following renal transplantation, possibly due to the increased hematocrit and blood viscosity that follow successful engraftment.[186,188] Crises appear to be more common following transplantation in homozygotes than in heterozygotes.[186] There is a suspicion that OKT3 induces sickling crises in some patients, and this agent should be used with caution in this setting.

TRANSPLANT GLOMERULOPATHY

The term *transplant glomerulopathy* has been used to define a constellation of histologic, ultrastructural, and immunofluorescence findings in the renal allograft.[72,189,190] It is characterized pathologically by diffuse endothelial cell swelling, mesangial cell proliferation, and glomerular basement membrane reduplication with mesangial cell interposition. Immunofluorescence studies are usually negative but may show scant deposition of IgM and fibrin. Electron microscopy reveals reduplication of the basement membrane and widening of the subendothelial space by a layer of electrolucent flocculent material. This lesion resembles membranoproliferative glomerulonephritis (MPGN) by light microscopy; however, electron microscopy reveals absence of electron dense deposits in the capillary walls, which are typical of MPGN.[70,190]

The usual clinical presentation is with nephrotic syndrome and progressive impairment of renal function,[72,73] but a significant number of patients remain asymptomatic.[190] A diagnosis of transplant glomerulopathy was made in 4.3% of patients in a large series of long-term transplant recipients.[72] In a study by Habib and colleagues,[190] transplant glomerulopathy was demonstrated in 38 of 540 allografts (7%) in whom adequate tissue was available for pathologic examination. Although, typically considered a late occurrence, in the latter study it was noted as early as 4 months post-transplantation. Heavy proteinuria occurred in 29 patients, 10 of whom developed nephrotic syndrome, but, of note, 9 patients had absent or minimal proteinuria even on prolonged follow-up. Graft loss ultimately occurred in 60% of these patients, but 35% still had functioning grafts at a mean follow-up of 11 years.[190]

Nankivell and colleagues[189] recently studied the natural history of transplant glomerulopathy by performing serial renal biopsies in 120 patients with ESRD from diabetes mellitus who received a combined kidney and pancreas transplant (n = 119) or kidney transplant alone (n = 1). The natural history consisted of two distinct phases: an initial phase of early tubulointerstitial damage, due to ischemic injury, prior severe rejection, and subclinical rejection; and a later phase characterized by microvascular and glomerular injury. Calcineurin inhibitors were associated with increasing glomerulosclerosis and further tubulointerstitial damage. Severe chronic allograft glomerulopathy was present in 58% of patients at 10 years.[189]

Although no effective treatment has been identified for transplant glomerulopathy,[73,190] current treatment strategies include reduction or withdrawal of calcineurin inhibitors and the substitution of mycophenolate mofetil (MMF). In a series of 118 patients with biopsy proven transplant glomerulopathy reduction or withdrawal of either CsA or FK506, combined with the introduction or continuation of MMF, was found to be safe, well tolerated, and to either slow the rate of progression or stabilize renal function.[191] Future directions may include the combination of MMF and rapamycin, which has shown to be promising in experimental models.[192]

References

1. Kotanko P, Pusey CD, Levy JB: Recurrent glomerulonephritis following renal transplantation. Transplantation 1997; 8: 1045-1052.
2. Denton MD, Singh AK: Recurrent and de novo glomerulonephritis in the renal allograft. Semin Nephrol 2000; 2:164-175.
3. Ramos EL, Tisher CC: Recurrent diseases in the kidney transplant. Am J Kidney Dis 1994; 24:142-154.
4. Morzycka M, Croker BP, Seigler HF, et al: Evaluation of recurrent glomerulonephritis in kidney allografts. Am J Med 1982; 72:588-598.
5. Briganti EM, Russ GR, McNeil JJ, et al: Risk of renal allograft loss from recurrent glomerulonephritis. N Engl J Med 2002; 2: 103-109.
6. O'Meara Y, Green A, Carmody M, et al: Recurrent glomerulonephritis in renal transplants: Fourteen years' experience. Nephrol Dial Transplant 1989; 4:730-734.
7. Broyer M, Selwood N, Brunner F: Recurrence of primary renal disease on kidney graft: A European pediatric experience. J Am Soc Nephrol 1992; 2:S255-S257.
8. Croker BP, Salomon DR: Pathology of the renal allograft. *In* Tisher CC, Brenner BM (eds): Renal Pathology with Clinical and Functional Correlations. Philadelphia, JB Lippincott, 1989, pp 1518-1554.
9. Floege J: Recurrent glomerulonephritis following renal transplantation: An update. Nephrol Dial Transplant 2003; 7:1260-1265.
10. Chadban S: Glomerulonephritis recurrence in the renal graft. J Am Soc Nephrol 2001; 2:394-402.
11. Bilous RW, Mauer SM, Sutherland DE, et al: The effects of pancreas transplantation on the glomerular structure of renal allografts in patients with insulin-dependent mellitus. N Engl J Med 1989; 321:80-85.
12. Najarian JS, Kaufman DB, Fryd DS, et al: Long-term survival following kidney transplantation in 100 type I diabetic patients. Transplantation 1990; 47:106-113.
13. Watts RWE, Danpure CJ, de Pauw L, et al: Combined liver-kidney and isolated liver transplantations for primary hyperoxaluria type I: the European experience. Nephrol Dial Transplant 1991; 6:502-511.
14. McDonald JC, Landreneau MD, Rohr MS, et al: Reversal by liver transplantation of the complications of primary hyperoxaluria as well as the metabolic defect. N Engl J Med 1989; 321:1100-1103.
15. De Pauw L, Gelin M, Danpure CJ, et al: Combined liver-kidney transplantation in primary hyperoxaluria type I. Transplantation 1990; 50:886-887.
16. Newstead CG: Recurrent disease in renal transplants. Nephrol Dial Transplant 2003; 18(suppl 6):vi68-vi74.

17. Cameron JS, Senguttuvan P, Hartley B, et al: Focal segmental glomerulosclerosis in fifty-nine renal allografts from a single center: Analysis of risk factors for recurrence. Transplant Proc 1989; 21:2117-2118.
18. Meulders Q, Pirson Y, Cosyns JP, et al: Course of Henoch-Schönlein nephritis after renal transplantation. Report of ten patients and review of the literature. Transplantation 1994; 58:1179-1186.
19. Senggutuvan P, Cameron JS, Hartley RB, et al: Recurrence of focal segmental glomerulosclerosis in transplanted kidneys: Analysis of incidence and risk factors in 59 allografts. Pediatr Nephrol 1990; 4:21-28.
20. Glassock RJ: Role of cyclosporine in glomerular diseases. Cleve Clin J Med 1994; 61:363-369.
21. Schwarz A, Krause P-H, Offermann G, et al: Recurrent and de novo renal disease after kidney transplantation with or without cyclosporine A. Am J Kidney Dis 1991; 17:524-531.
22. Glassock RJ, Cohen AH, Adler SG: Primary glomerular diseases. *In* Brenner BM (ed): The Kidney. Philadelphia, WB Saunders, 1996, pp 1392-1497.
23. Hoyer JR, Vernier RL, Najarian JS, et al: Recurrence of idiopathic nephrotic syndrome after renal transplantation. Lancet 1972; 2:343-348.
24. Muller T, Sikora P, Offner G, et al: Recurrence of renal disease after kidney transplantation in children: 24 years of experience in a single center. Clin Nephrol 1998; 49:82-90.
25. Biesenbach G, Janko O, Hubmann R, et al: The incidence of thrombovenous and thromboembolic complications in kidney transplant patients with recurrent glomerulonephritis is dependent on the occurrence of severe proteinuria. Clin Nephrol 2000; 5:382-387.
26. Baum MA, Ho M, Stablein DM: NAPRTCS: Outcome of renal transplantation in adolescents with focal segmental glomerulosclerosis. Pediatr Transplantation 2002; 6:488-492.
27. Artero M, Biava C, Amend W, et al: Recurrent focal glomerulosclerosis: Natural history and response to therapy. Am J Med 1992; 92:375-383.
28. Detwiler RK, Hogan SL, Falk RJ: Collapsing glomerulopathy in renal transplant patients: Recurrence and de novo occurrence (Abstract). J Am Soc Nephrol 1996; 7:1331.
29. Clarkson MR, O'Meara YM, Murphy B, et al: Collapsing glomerulopathy: Recurrence in a renal allograft. Nephrol Dial Transplant 1998; 13:503-506.
30. Tejani A, Stablein DH: Recurrence of focal segmental glomerulosclerosis posttransplantation. A special report of the North American Pediatric Renal Transplant Cooperative Study. J Am Soc Nephrol 1992; 2:S258-S263.
31. Abbott KC, Sawyers ES, Oliver JD III, et al: Graft loss due to recurrent focal segmental glomerulosclerosis in renal transplant recipients in the United States. Am J Kidney Dis 2001; 2:366-373.
32. Butani L, Polinsky MS, Kaiser BA: Predictive value of race in post-transplantation recurrence of focal segmental glomerulosclerosis in children. Nephrol Dial Transplant 1999; 1:166-168.
33. Stephanian E, Matas AJ, Mauer SM, et al: Recurrence of disease in patients retransplanted for focal segmental glomerulosclerosis. Transplantation 1992; 53:755-757.
34. Tomlanovich S, Vincenti F, Amend W, et al: Is cyclosporin effective in preventing recurrence of immune-mediated glomerular disease after renal transplantation? Transplant Proc 1988; 20: 285-288.
35. Ingulli E, Tejani A, Khalid MHB, et al: High-dose cyclosporine therapy in recurrent nephrotic syndrome following renal transplantation. Transplantation 1990; 49:219-221.
36. Shalhoub RJ: Pathogenesis of lipoid nephrosis: A disorder of T-cell function. Lancet 1974; 2:556-560.
37. Savin VJ, Artero M, Sharma R, et al: Circulating factor associated with increased glomerular permeability to albumin in recurrent focal segmental glomerulosclerosis. N Engl J Med 1996; 334:878-883.
38. Artero ML, Sharma R, Savin VJ, et al: Plasmapheresis reduces proteinuria and serum capacity to injure glomeruli in patients with recurrent focal glomerulosclerosis. Am J Kidney Dis 1994; 23:574-581.
39. Sharma M, Sharma R, McCarthy ET: The FSGS Factor: Enrichment and in vivo effect of activity from focal segmental glomerulosclerosis plasma. J Am Soc Nephrol 1999; 3:552-561.
40. Dantal J, Bigot E, Bogers W, et al: Effect of plasma protein adsorption on protein excretion in kidney-transplant recipients with recurrent nephrotic syndrome. N Engl J Med 1994; 330:7-14.
41. Andresdottir MB, Ajubi N, Croockewit S, et al: Recurrent focal glomerulosclerosis: Natural course and treatment with plasma exchange. Nephrol Dial Transplant 1999; 11:2650-2656.
42. Dall'Amico R, Ghiggeri GM, Carraro M: Prediction and treatment of recurrent focal segmental glomerulosclerosis after renal transplantation in children. Am J Kidney Dis 1999; 34: 1048 –1055.
43. Kawaguchi H, Hattori M, Ito K, et al: Recurrence of focal glomerulosclerosis in allografts in children: The efficacy of intensive plasma exchange therapy before and after renal transplantation. Transplant Proc 1994; 26:7-8.
44. Kooijmans-Coutinho MF, Tegzess AM, Bruijn JA, et al: Indomethacin treatment of recurrent nephrotic syndrome and focal segmental glomerulosclerosis after renal transplantation. Pediatr Nephrol 1993; 8:469-473.
45. Brenner BM, Meyer TW, Hostetter TH: Dietary protein intake and the progressive nature of kidney disease: The role of hemodynamically mediated glomerular injury in the pathogenesis of progressive glomerular sclerosis in aging, renal ablation, and intrinsic renal disease. N Engl J Med 1982; 307:652-659.
46. Cosio FG, Frankel WL, Pelletier RP, et al: Focal segmental glomerulosclerosis in renal allografts with chronic nephropathy: Implications for graft survival. Am J Kidney Dis 1999; 4: 731-738.
47. Berger BE, Vincenti F, Biava C, et al: De novo and recurrent membranous glomerulopathy following kidney transplantation. Transplantation 1983; 35:315-319.
48. Josephson MA, Spargo B, Hollandsworth D, et al: The recurrence of recurrent membranous glomerulopathy in a renal transplant recipient: Case report and literature review. Am J Kidney Dis 1994; 24:873-878.
49. Lieberthal W, Bernard DP, Donohoe JF, et al: Rapid recurrence of membranous nephropathy in a related renal allograft. Clin Nephrol 1979; 12:222-228.
50. Couchoud C, Pouteil-Noble C, Colon S, et al: Recurrence of membranous nephropathy after renal transplantation. Transplantation 1995; 59:1275-1279.
51. Schwarz A, Krause P-H, Offermann G, et al: Impact of de novo membranous glomerulonephritis on the clinical course after kidney transplantation. Transplantation 1994; 58:650-654.
52. Antignac C, Hinglais N, Gubler M-C, et al: De novo membranous glomerulonephritis in renal allografts in children. Clin Nephrol 1988; 30:1-7.
53. Heidet L, Gagnadoux MF, Beziau A, et al: Recurrence of de novo membranous glomerulonephritis on renal grafts. Clin Nephrol 1994; 41:314-318.
54. Truong L, Gelfand J, D'Agati V, et al: De novo membranous glomerulopathy in renal allografts: A report of 10 cases and review of the literature. Am J Kidney Dis 1989; 14:131-144.
55. Morales JM, Pascual-Capdevila J, Campistol JM, et al: Membranous glomerulonephritis associated with hepatitis C virus infection in renal transplant patients. Transplantation 1997; 63:1634-1639.
56. Johnston PA, Goode NP, Aparicio SR, et al: Membranous allograft nephropathy: Remission of nephrotic syndrome with pulsed methylprednisolone and high-dose alternate-day steroids. Transplantation 1993; 55:214-216.

57. Galla JH: IgA nephropathy. Kidney Int 1995; 47:377-387.
58. Bachman U, Biava C, Amend W, et al: The clinical course of IgA nephropathy and Henoch-Schönlein purpura following renal transplantation. Transplantation 1986; 42: 511-515.
59. Kessler M, Hiesse C, Hestin D, et al: Recurrence of immunoglobulin A nephropathy after renal transplantation in the cyclosporin era. Am J Kidney Dis 1996; 28:99-104.
60. Ponticelli C, Traversi L, Feliciani A, et al: Kidney transplantation in patients with IgA mesangial glomerulonephritis. Kidney Intl 2001; 60:1948-1954.
61. Frohnert PP, Donadio JV Jr, Velosa JA, et al: The fate of renal transplants in patients with IgA nephropathy. Clin Transplant 1997; 11:127-133.
62. Ohmacht C, Kliem V, Burg M, et al: Recurrent immunoglobulin A nephropathy after renal transplantation: Significant contributor to graft loss. Transplantation 1997; 64:1493-1496.
63. Robles NR, Gomez Campdera FJ, Anaya F, et al: IgA nephropathy with a rapidly progressive course after kidney transplantation. Nephron 1991; 58:487-488.
64. Brensilver JM, Mallat S, Scholes J, et al: Recurrent IgA nephropathy in living-related donor transplantation: Recurrence or transmission of familial disease. Am J Kidney Dis 1988; 12:147-151.
65. Martin SJ, Audrain M, Barangler T, et al: Recurrence of immunoglobulin A nephropathy with immunoglobulin A antineutrophil cytoplasmic antibodies following renal transplantation. Am J Kidney Dis 1997; 29:125-131.
66. Kashiwabara H, Shishido H, Tomura S, et al: Strong association between IgA nephropathy and HLA-DR4 antigen. Kidney Int 1982; 22:377-382.
67. Sanfilippo F, Croker BP, Bollinger RR: Fate of four cadaveric renal allografts with mesangial IgA deposits. Transplantation 1982; 33:370-376.
68. Oka K, Imai E, Moriyama T, et al: A clinicopathological study of IgA nephropathy in renal transplant recipients: Beneficial effect of angiotensin-converting enzyme inhibitor. Nephrol Dial Transplant 2000; 5: 689-695.
69. Jeong HJ, Kim YS, Kwon KW, et al: Segmental glomerulosclerosis in IgA nephropathy after renal transplantation: Relationship with proteinuria and therapeutic response to enalapril. Clin Transplant 2003; 2:108-113.
70. Glicklich D, Matas AJ, Sablay LB, et al: Recurrent membranoproliferative glomerulonephritis type I in successive renal transplants. Am J Nephrol 1987; 7:143-149.
71. Andresdottir MB, Assmann KJ, Hoitsma AJ, et al: Recurrence of type I membranoproliferative glomerulonephritis after renal transplantation: Analysis of the incidence, risk factors, and impact on graft survival. Transplantation 1997; 63:1628-1633.
72. Maryniak RK, First MR, Weiss MA: Transplant glomerulopathy: Evolution of morphologically distinct changes. Kidney Int 1985; 27:799-806.
73. Cheigh JS, Mouradian J, Susin M, et al: Kidney transplant nephrotic syndrome: Relationship between allograft histopathology and natural course. Kidney Int 1980; 18:358-365.
74. Roth D, Cirocco R, Zucker K, et al: De novo membrano-proliferative glomerulonephritis in hepatitis C virus-infected renal allograft recipients. Transplantation 1995; 59:1676-1682.
75. Cahen R, Trolliet P, Dijoud F, et al: Severe recurrence of type I membrano-proliferative glomerulonephritis after transplantation: Remission on steroids and cyclophosphamide. Transplant Proc 1995; 27:1746-1747.
76. Lien YH, Scott K: Long-term cyclophosphamide treatment for recurrent type I membranoproliferative glomerulonephritis after transplantation. Am J Kidney Dis 2000; 3:539-543.
77. Gallay BJ, Alpers CE, Davis CL, et al: Glomerulonephritis in renal allografts associated with hepatitis C infection: A possible relationship with transplant glomerulopathy in two cases. Am J Kidney Dis 1995; 26:662-667.
78. Cruzado JM, Gil-Vernet S, Ercilla G, et al: Hepatitis C virus-associated membranoproliferative glomerulonephritis in renal allografts. J Am Soc Nephrol 1996; 7:2469-2475.
79. Davis CL, Gretch DR, Carithers RL: Hepatitis C virus in renal disease. Curr Opin Nephrol Hypertens 1994; 3:164-173.
80. Cockfield SM, Prieksaitis JK: Infection with hepatitis C virus increases the risk of de novo glomerulonephritis in renal transplant recipients. J Am Soc Nephrol 1995; 6:1078.
81. Kovarik J, Mayer G, Pohanka E, et al: Adverse effect of low-dose prophylactic human recombinant leukocyte interferon-alpha treatment in renal transplant recipients. Cytomegalovirus infection prophylaxis leading to an increased incidence of irreversible rejections. Transplantation 1988; 45:402-405.
82. Ozgur O, Boyacioglu S, Teletar H, et al: Recombinant alpha-interferon in renal allograft recipients with chronic hepatitis C. Nephrol Dial Transplant 1995; 10:2104-2106.
83. Harihara Y, Kurooka Y, Yanagisawa T, et al: Interferon therapy in renal allograft recipients with chronic hepatitis C. Transplant Proc 1994; 26:2075.
84. Andresdottir MB, Assmann KJ, Hoitsma AJ, et al: Renal transplantation in patients with dense deposit disease: Morphological characteristics of recurrent disease and clinical outcome. Nephrol Dial Transplant 1999; 7:1723-1731.
85. Oberkircher OR, Enama M, West JC, et al: Regression of recurrent membranoproliferative glomerulonephritis type II in a transplanted kidney after plasmapheresis therapy. Transplant Proc 1988; 20:418-423.
86. Pirson Y, Goffin E, Squifflet JP, et al: Outcome of patients with anti-GBM nephritis after renal transplantation. J Am Soc Nephrol 1993; 4:955.
87. Beleil OM, Coburn JW, Shinaberger JH, et al: Recurrent glomerulonephritis due to anti-glomerular basement membrane antibody in two successive allografts. Clin Nephrol 1973; 1:377-380.
88. Saus J, Wieslander J, Langeveld JPM, et al: Identification of the Goodpasture antigen as the $\alpha3$(IV) chain of collagen IV. J Biol Chem 1988; 263:13374-13380.
89. Hudson BG, Kalluri R, Gunwar S, et al: The pathogenesis of Alport syndrome involves type IV collagen molecules containing the $\alpha3$ (IV) chain: Evidence from anti-GBM nephritis after renal transplantation. Kidney Int 1992; 42:179-187.
90. Milliner DS, Pierides AM, Holley KE: Renal transplantation in Alport's syndrome. Anti-glomerular basement membrane glomerulonephritis in the allograft. Mayo Clin Proc 1982; 57:35-43.
91. Shah B, First MR, Mendoza NC, et al: Alport's syndrome: Risk of recurrent glomerulonephritis induced by antiglomerular-basement-membrane antibody after renal transplantation. Nephron 1988; 50:34-38.
92. Gobel J, Olbricht CJ, Frei U, et al: Renal transplantation in patients with Alport's syndrome: Long-term follow-up (Abstract). J Am Soc Nephrol 1990; 1:758.
93. Rassoul Z, Khader AAA, Al-Sulaiman M, et al: Recurrent allograft antiglomerular basement membrane glomerulonephritis in a patient with Alport's syndrome. Am J Nephrol 1990; 10:73-76.
94. Peten E, Pirson Y, Cosyns J-P, et al: Outcome of thirty patients with Alport's syndrome after renal transplantation. Transplantation 1991; 52:823-826.
95. Jones B, Trevillian P, Hibberd A, et al: De novo crescentic glomerulonephritis in a renal transplant. Am J Kidney Dis 1990; 16:501-503.
96. Boyce N, Holdsworth S, Atkins R, et al: De novo anti-GBM-antibody-induced glomerulonephritis in a renal transplant. Clin Nephrol 1984; 148-151.
97. Bohman SO, Wilczek H, Tyden G, et al: Recurrent diabetic nephropathy in renal allografts placed in diabetic patients and protective effect of simultaneous transplantation. Transplant Proc 1987; 19:2290-2293.

98. Najarian JS, Sutherland DER, Simmons RL, et al: Ten year experience with renal transplantation in juvenile onset diabetics. Ann Surg 1979; 190:487-500.
99. Lewis EJ, Hunsicker LG, Bain RP, et al: The effect of angiotensin-converting-enzyme inhibition on diabetic nephropathy. N Engl J Med 1993; 329:1456-1462.
100. Sollinger HW, Knechtle SJ, Reed A, et al: Experience with 100 consecutive simultaneous kidney-pancreas transplant with bladder drainage. Ann Surg 1991; 214:703-711.
101. Cheigh JS, Kim H, Stenzel KH, et al: Systemic lupus erythematosus in patients with end-stage renal disease: A long-term follow-up on the prognosis of patients and the evolution of lupus activity. Am J Kidney Dis 1990; 16:189-195.
102. Cheigh JS, Stenzel KH: End-stage renal disease in systemic lupus erythematosus. Am J Kidney Dis 1993; 21:2-8.
103. Nossent HC, Swaak TJG, Berden JHM: Systemic lupus erythematosus after renal transplantation: Patient and graft survival and disease activity. Ann Intern Med 1991; 114:183-188.
104. Mojcik CF, Klippel JH: End-stage renal disease and systemic lupus erythematosus. Am J Med 1996; 101:100-106.
105. Goss JA, Cole BR, Jendrisak MD, et al: Renal transplantation for systemic lupus erythematosus and recurrent lupus nephritis. Transplantation 1991; 52:805-810.
106. Lochhead KM, Pirsch JD, D'Alessandro AM, et al: Risk factors for renal allograft loss in patients with systemic lupus erythematosus. Kidney Int 1996; 49:512-517.
107. Kumano K, Sakai T, Mashimo S, et al: A case of lupus nephritis after renal transplantation. Clin Nephrol 1987; 27:94-98.
108. Stone JH, Millward CL, Olson JL, et al: Frequency of recurrent lupus nephritis among ninety-seven renal transplant patients during the cyclosporine era. Arthritis Rheum 1998; 41:678-686.
109. Roth D, Fernandez J, Diaz A, et al: Recurrence of lupus nephritis following renal transplantation. J Am Soc Nephrol 1992; 3:878.
110. Ward LA, Jelveh Z, Feinfeld DA: Recurrent membranous lupus nephritis after renal transplantation. A case report and review of the literature. Am J Kidney Dis 1994; 23:326-329.
111. Amend WJ, Vincenti F, Feduska NJ: Recurrent systemic lupus erythematosus involving renal allografts. Ann Intern Med 1981; 94:444-448.
112. Zara CP, Lipkowitz GS, Perri N, et al: Renal transplantation and end-stage lupus nephropathy in the cyclosporin and pre-cyclosporin eras. Transplant Proc 1989; 21:1648-1651.
113. Jennette JC, Falk JR: Small-vessel vasculitis. N Engl J Med 1997; 337:1512-1523.
114. Nachman PH, Segelmark M, Westman K, et al: Recurrent ANCA-associated small vessel vasculitis after transplantation: A pooled analysis. Kidney Int 1999; 56:1544-1550.
115. Allen A, Pusey C, Gaskin G: Outcome of renal replacement therapy in antineutrophil cytoplasmic antibody-associated systemic vasculitis. J Am Soc Nephrol 1998; 9:1258-1263.
116. Elmedhem A, Adu D, Savage COS: Relapse rate and outcome of ANCA-associated small vessel vasculitis after transplantation. Nephrol Dial Transplant 2003; 18:1001-1004.
117. Rostaing MD, Modesto A, Oskman F, et al: Outcome of patients with antineutrophil cytoplasmic autoantibody-associated vasculitis following cadaveric kidney transplantation. Am J Kidney Dis 1997; 29:96-102.
118. Clarke AE, Bitton A, Eappen R, et al: Treatment of Wegener's granulomatosis after renal transplantation: Is cyclosporin the preferred treatment? Transplantation 1990; 50:1047-1051.
119. Rich LM, Piering WF: Ureteral stenosis due to recurrent Wegener's granulomatosis after kidney transplantation. J Am Soc Nephrol 1994; 4:1516-1521.
120. Schmitt WH, Haubitz M, Mistry N, et al: Renal transplantation in Wegener's granulomatosis (Letter). Lancet 1993; 342:860.
121. Montalbert C, Carvallo A, Broumand B, et al: Successful renal transplantation in poly-arteritis nodosa. Clin Nephrol 1980; 14:206-209.
122. Reaich D, Cooper N, Main J, et al: Rapid catastrophic onset of Wegener's granulomatosis in a renal transplant. Nephron 1994; 67:354-357.
123. Lowance DC, Vosatka K, Whelchel J, et al: Recurrent Wegener's granulomatosis. Am J Med 1992; 92:573-575.
124. Ramos EL: Recurrent diseases in the renal allograft. J Am Soc Nephrol 1991; 2:108-121.
125. Hebert D, Sibley RK, Mauer SM: Recurrence of hemolytic uremic syndrome in renal transplant recipients. Kidney Int 1986; 30:S51-S58.
126. Agarwal A, Mauer SM, Matas AJ, et al: Recurrent hemolytic uremic syndrome in an adult renal allograft recipient: Current concepts and management. J Am Soc Nephrol 1995; 6:1160-1169.
127. Ruggenenti P: Post-transplant hemolytic-uremic syndrome. Kidney Int 2002; 62:1093-1104.
128. Ducloux D, Rebibou JM, Semhoun-Ducloux S, et al: Recurrence of hemolytic-uremic syndrome in renal transplant recipients: A meta-analysis. Transplantation 1998; 10:1405-1407.
129. Quan A, Sullivan EK, Alexander SR: Recurrence of hemolytic uremic syndrome after renal transplantation in children: A report of the North American Pediatric Renal Transplant Cooperative Study. Transplantation 2001; 4:742-745.
130. Lahlou A, Lang P, Charpentier B, et al: Hemolytic uremic syndrome. Recurrence after renal transplantation. Groupe Cooperatif de l'Ile-de-France (GCIF). Medicine (Baltimore) 2000; 2:90-102.
131. Bassani CE, Ferraris J, Gianantonio CA, et al: Renal transplantation in patients with classical hemolytic-uraemic syndrome. Pediatr Nephrol 1991; 5:607-611.
132. Giroux L, Smeesters C, Corman J, et al: Hemolytic uremic syndrome in renal allografted patients treated with cyclosporin. Can J Physiol Pharmacol 1987; 65:1125-1131.
133. Grino JM, Caralps A, Carreras L, et al: Apparent recurrence of hemolytic uremic syndrome in azathioprine-treated allograft recipients. Nephron 1988; 49:301-304.
134. Leithner C, Sinziger H, Pohanka E, et al: Recurrence of hemolytic uraemic syndrome triggered by cyclosporin A after renal transplantation. Lancet 1982; 1:1470.
135. Doutrelepont J-M, Abramowicz D, Florquin S, et al: Early recurrence of hemolytic uremic syndrome in a renal transplant recipient during prophylactic OKT3 therapy. Transplantation 1992; 53:1378-1379.
136. Kaufman DB, Kaplan B, Kanwar YS, et al: The successful use of tacrolimus (FK506) in a pancreas/kidney transplant recipient with recurrent cyclosporine-associated hemolytic uremic syndrome. Transplantation 1995; 59:1737-1739.
137. Zarifian A, Meleg-Smith S, O'Donovan R, et al: Cyclosporine-associated thrombotic microangiopathy in renal allografts. Kidney Int 1999; 6:2457-2466.
138. Pham PT, Peng A, Wilkinson AH, et al: Cyclosporine and tacrolimus-associated thrombotic microangiopathy. Am J Kidney Dis 2000; 4:844-850.
139. Schwimmer J, Nadasdy TA, Spitalnik PF, et al: De novo thrombotic microangiopathy in renal transplant recipients: A comparison of hemolytic uremic syndrome with localized renal thrombotic microangiopathy. Am J Kidney Dis 2003; 41:471-479.
140. Remuzzi G, Bertani T: Renal vascular and thrombotic effects of cyclosporin. Am J Kidney Dis 1989; 13:261-272.
141. Frem GJ, Rennke HG, Sayegh MH: Late renal allograft failure secondary to thrombotic microangiopathy-human immunodeficiency virus nephropathy. J Am Soc Nephrol 1994; 4:1643-1648.
142. Guttmann RD: Recurrent and de novo glomerulonephritis post-renal transplantation. Transplant Proc 1996; 28:1168-1170.
143. Barone GW, Gurley BJ, Abul-Ezz SR, et al: Sirolimus-induced thrombotic microangiopathy in a renal transplant recipient. Am J Kidney Dis 2003; 42:202-206.
144. Reynolds JC, Agodoa LY, Yuan CM, et al: Thrombotic microangiopathy after renal transplantation in the United States. Am J Kidney Dis 2003; 42:1058-1068.

145. Paul M, Bear RA, Sugar C: Renal transplantation in scleroderma. J Rheumatol 1984; 11:406-408.
146. Chang YJ, Spiera H: Renal transplantation in scleroderma. Medicine (Baltimore) 1999; 78:382-386.
147. Bleyer AJ, Donaldson LA, McIntosh M, et al: Relationship between underlying renal disease and renal transplantation outcome. Am J Kidney Dis 2001; 37:1152-1161.
148. Pasternack A, Ahonen J, Kuhlbäck B: Renal transplantation in 45 patients with amyloidosis. Transplantation 1986; 42:598-601.
149. Harrison KL, Alpers CE, Davis CL: De novo amyloidosis in a renal allograft: A case report and review of the literature. Am J Kidney Dis 1993; 22:468-476.
150. Hartmann A, Holdaas H, Fauchald P, et al: Fifteen years' experience with renal transplantation in systemic amyloidosis. Transplant Int 1992; 5:15-18.
151. Sherif AM, Refaie AF, Sobh MA-K, et al: Long-term outcome of live donor kidney transplantation for renal amyloidosis. Am J Kidney Dis 2003; 42:370-375.
152. Helin H, Pasternak A, Falck H, et al: Recurrence of renal amyloid and de novo membranous glomerulonephritis after transplantation. Transplantation 1981; 32:6-9.
153. Hiesse C, Bastuji-Garin S, Santelli G, et al: Recurrent essential mixed cryoglobulinaemia in renal allografts. Am J Nephrol 1989; 9:150-154.
154. Fang LST: Light-chain nephropathy. Kidney Int 1985; 27:582-592.
155. Briefel GR, Spees EK, Humphrey RL, et al: Renal transplantation in a patient with multiple myeloma and light-chain nephropathy. Surgery 1983; 93:579-584.
156. Alpers CE, Manchioro TL, Johnson RJ: Monoclonal immunoglobulin deposition disease in a renal allograft. Probable recurrent disease in a patient without myeloma. Am J Kidney Dis 1989; 13:418-423.
157. Gerlag PGG, Koene RAP, Berden JHM: Renal transplantation in light-chain nephropathy: Case report and review of the literature. Clin Nephrol 1986; 25:101-104.
158. Walker F, Bear RA: Renal transplantation in light-chain multiple myeloma. Am J Nephrol 1983; 3:34-37.
159. David-Neto E, Ianhez LE, Chocair PR, et al: Renal transplantation in systemic light-chain deposition (SLCD): A 44-month follow-up without recurrence. Transplant Proc 1989; 21:2128-2129.
160. De Lima JJG, Kourilsky O, Morel-Maroger L, et al: Kidney transplantation in multiple myeloma. Transplantation 1981; 31:223-224.
161. Scully RE (ed): Case records of the Massachusetts General Hospital. Case 1. N Engl J Med 1981; 304:33-43.
162. Bumgardner GL, Matas AJ, Payne WD, et al: Renal transplantation in patients with paraproteinemias. Clin Transplant 1990; 4:399-405.
163. Ecder T, Abdelghani A, Braun WE, et al: De novo light-chain deposition disease in a cadaver renal allograft. Am J Kidney Dis 1996; 28:461-465.
164. Spence RK, Hill GS, Goldwein MI, et al: Renal transplantation for end-stage myeloma kidney. Arch Surg 1979; 114:950-952.
165. Cosio FG, Pence TV, Shapiro FL, et al: Severe renal failure in multiple myeloma. Clin Nephrol 1981; 15:206-210.
166. Aparicio M, de Precigout V, Reiffers J, et al: Multiple myeloma and AL amyloidosis in a renal transplant recipient. Nephron 1989; 53:373-375.
167. Howard AD, Moore J, Tomaszewski M-M: Occurrence of multiple myeloma three years after successful renal transplantation. Am J Kidney Dis 1987; 10:147-150.
168. Alpers CE, Rennke HG, Hopper J Jr, et al: Fibrillary glomerulonephritis. An entity with unusual immunofluorescence features. Kidney Int 1987; 31:781-789.
169. Pronovost PH, Brady HR, Gunning ME, et al: Clinical features, predictors of disease progression and results of renal transplantation in fibrillary/immunotactoid glomerulopathy. Nephrol Dial Transplant 1996; 11:837-842.
170. Brady HR: Fibrillary glomerulopathy. Kidney Int 1998; 53:1421-1429.
171. Barnes BA, Bergan JJ, Braun WE, et al: Renal transplantation in congenital and metabolic diseases. JAMA 1975; 232:148-153.
172. Samaniego M, Nadasdy GM, Laszik Z, et al: Outcome of renal transplantation in fibrillary glomerulonephritis. Clin Nephrol 2001; 2:159-166.
173. Jamieson N, Watts R, Evans D, et al: Liver and kidney transplantation. Symposium and poster abstracts. XIII International Congress of the Transplantation Society, 1990, p 148.
174. Watts RWE, Morgan SH, Danpure CJ, et al: Combined hepatic and renal transplantation in primary hyperoxaluria type I: Clinical report of nine cases. Am J Med 1991; 90:179-188.
175. Katz A, Kim Y, Scheinman J, et al: Long-term outcome of kidney transplantation in children with oxalosis. Transplant Proc 1989; 21:2033-2035.
176. Schienman JI: Primary hyperoxaluria: Therapeutic strategies for the 90s. Kidney Int 1991; 40:389-399.
177. Whelchel JD, Alison DV, Luke RG, et al: Successful renal transplantation in hyperoxaluria Transplantation 1983; 35:161-164.
178. Knols G, Leunissen KML, Spaapen LJM, et al: Recurrence of nephrocalcinosis after renal transplantation in an adult patient with primary hyperoxaluria type I. Nephrol Dial Transplant 1989; 4:137-139.
179. Schneider JA, Katz B, Melles RB: Cystinosis. AKF Nephrol Lett 1990; 7:22-31.
180. Spear GS, Gubler MC, Habib R, et al: Renal allografts in cystinosis and mesangial demography. Clin Nephrol 1989; 32: 256-261.
181. Maizel SE, Simmons RL, Kjellstrand C, et al: Ten-year experience in renal transplantation for Fabry's disease. Transplant Proc 1981; 13:57-59.
182. Donati D, Novario R, Gaitaldi L: Natural history and treatment of uremia secondary to Fabry's disease. A European experience. Nephron 1987; 46:353-359.
183. Spence MW, MacKinnon KE, Burgess JK, et al: Failure to correct the metabolic defect by renal allotransplantation in Fabry's disease. Ann Intern Med 1976; 84:13-16.
184. Mosnier JF, Degott C, Bedrossian J, et al: Recurrence of Fabry's disease in a renal allograft eleven years after successful renal transplantation. Transplantation 1991; 51:759-762.
185. Powars DR, Elliot-Mills DD, Chan L, et al: Chronic renal failure in sickle cell disease. Risk factors, clinical course, and mortality. Ann Intern Med 1991; 115:614-620.
186. Montgomery R, Zibari G, Hill GS, et al: Renal transplantation in patients with sickle cell nephropathy. Transplantation 1994; 58:618-620.
187. Chatterjee S: National study on natural history of renal allografts with sickle cell disease or trait. Nephron 1980; 25:199-201.
188. Barber WH, Deierhoi MH, Julian BA, et al: Renal transplantation in sickle cell anemia and sickle disease. Clin Transplant 1987; 1:169-175.
189. Nankivell BJ, Borrows RJ, Fung CL, et al: The natural history of chronic allograft nephropathy. N Engl J Med 2003; 24: 2326-2333.
190. Habib R, Broyer M: Clinical significance of allograft glomerulopathy. Kidney Int 1993; 44(S43):S95-S98.
191. Weir MR, Ward MT, Blahut SA, et al: Long-term impact of discontinued or reduced calcineurin inhibitor in patients with chronic allograft nephropathy. Kidney Int 2001; 4:1567-1573.
192. Jolicoeur EM, Qi S, Xu D, et al: Combination therapy of mycophenolate mofetil and rapamycin in prevention of chronic renal allograft rejection in the rat. Transplantation 2003; 1:54-59.

Pediatric Renal Transplantation

William E. Harmon, M.D.

ROLE OF TRANSPLANTATION

Chronic dialysis and renal transplantation are both excellent treatments for end-stage renal disease (ESRD). The majority of adults with ESRD are receiving dialysis rather than undergoing renal transplantation, although the number seeking renal transplantation is continuing to rise substantially.[1] There is a survival advantage of transplantation for virtually all candidates. Unfortunately, the lack of suitable donors has limited the number of people who can receive transplants. Renal transplantation was recognized as the better form of treatment for children with ESRD two decades ago.[2] Both peritoneal dialysis, delivered as CAPD or CCPD, and hemodialysis lead to a deceleration of growth. Data from the dialysis component of the North American Pediatric Renal Transplant Cooperative Study (NAPRTCS) registry[3] show that the overall height deficit of −1.8 S.D. became more negative reaching a value of −2.16 S.D. at 24 months after initiation of dialysis. Additionally, children do not tolerate being "dependent" on any modality and maintenance dialysis induces loss of self-esteem and emotional maladjustment in them.[4] Cognitive achievement testing may diminish with prolonged time on dialysis.[5] In contrast, the mobility and freedom from dietary restrictions afforded by a functioning renal transplant enable children to live nearly normal lives. Although renal transplantation has not lived up to the promise of normal growth for all children, dramatic short-term improvements in height can be seen in many, and final adult height is improving after transplantation.[6–9] Most important, successful transplantation permits the child to attend school and to develop normally. School function testing improves dramatically following transplantation.[10,11] Also important is that young children now have the best long-term outcomes of all ages of transplant recipients, verifying the utility of transplantation in this age group.[12] For all of these reasons, successful renal transplantation remains the primary goal of programs that care for children with ESRD.

Incidence and Frequency of Transplantation

NAPRTCS has registered about 500 pediatric kidney transplants each year since its inception in 1987, accounting for 75% of all those performed in North America, and that number has remained relatively constant. In 2002 there were about 14,700 kidney transplants performed in the United States, suggesting that pediatric patients comprise about 5% of all transplant recipients. Although the number of pediatric transplants performed each year has varied by no more then 10%, the donor origin has undergone substantial changes. The Scientific Registry of Transplant Recipients (SRTR) data show that living kidney donation has expanded substantially, and the number of living donors (LD) exceeded the number of cadaver donors (CAD) for the first time in 2001.[1] Living donation now accounts for 43% of all kidney transplants in the United States. In 1987 only 40% of all transplants performed in children were from an LD source; by 1991 the figure had risen to 53%, and, for the last 5 years LDs accounted for over 60% of all pediatric renal transplants (Table 40–1).[13] Parents comprise 82% of LDs. Mothers comprise the majority of parent donors; fathers account for 46%. Since there are more boys than girls who receive kidney transplants, it should not be surprising that fathers donate to sons 64% of the time and mothers to sons 60%. There is no outcome advantage to either parent, with the possible exception that infants less than 1 year of age seem to have fewer rejections if the mother is the donor.[14,15] Because children most often have siblings who are too young to donate (less than 18 years), the NAPRTCS registry has recorded only 305 transplants between siblings. Of these, 150 grafts were from donors less than 21 years of age. A review of the NAPRTCS registry identified only 12 living donors under 18 years of age, of which 11 were transplants between siblings and 1 was from parent to child. It is quite clear that most programs are very reluctant to use minor donors.[16,17] However, a review of UNOS data revealed that from approximately 40,000 LDs in the United States between 1987 and 2000, 60 were from donors less than 18 years of age.[18] Twenty-four of the recipients were children and 36 were adults; only 7 of the transplants were between identical twins. In recent years there has been a substantial interest in living-unrelated donation in adult transplant literature because the outcome of the grafts has been shown to be better than that of cadaver source kidneys.[19] NAPRTCS identified 123 instances of living-unrelated donation between 1987 and 2001. In a preliminary analysis of the first 38 living-unrelated recipients, 23 (61%) were male, 30 (79%) were Caucasian, 8 were younger than 6 years old, and 20 were older than 12 years.[20] This was the primary transplant for 29 of the 38 recipients. Of the 38 donors, 22 were nonbiologic parents, and a family friend was the donor in 10 of the cases.

Thus, the majority of cadaver kidneys for children are recovered from adult donors. In the 1980s there was a tendency to preferentially place kidneys recovered from infants into infant recipients, with disastrous consequences for patient and graft survival.[21] As a result of widespread dissemination of these data,[22,23] there has been a marked change in the practice (Table 40–1). From 1987 through 1990, the percentage of cadaver donors older than 10 years ranged from 59% to 68%. From 1991 through 1994, these percentages ranged from 78% to 88%. Prior to 1991, children younger than 2 years of age comprised 3.2% of cadaver donors. In 1991 no pediatric recipient received a kidney from a cadaver donor less than 2 years of age; and in 1995 and 1996, there were no such kidneys utilized in children.[24] Between 1991

Table 40–1 Characteristics of Pediatric Kidney Donors and Recipients

	1987	1989	1991	1993	1995	1997	1999	2001
% Living Donors	43	46	51	51	52	55	58	63
% Recipients < 6 yr	25	23	22	23	15	18	17	17
% CAD donors < 10 yr	35	33	19	16	15	10	10	10

Adapted from Seikaly M, Ho PL, Emmett L, Tejani A: The 12th Annual Report of the North American Pediatric Renal Transplant Cooperative Study: Renal transplantation from 1987 through 1998 (updated at www.naprtcs.org). Pediatr Transplant 2001; 5:215-231.

and 2002, less than 1% (23/2464) of cadaver donors for children were less than 2 years of age.[13] This change in allocation of kidneys from young donors led to improvement in graft survival.[21] Some specialized pediatric programs have reported good results with young donors,[25] but many programs reserve grafts from very young donors for en bloc transplantation into older recipients.[26]

Primary Diagnosis

Because of the large database of the NAPRTCS, it is now possible to determine the percentages of each disease category leading to ESRD by age at transplantation as well as by gender and race. ESRD in children is generally due to congenital or inherited diseases. In reviewing 7651 transplants, the most common congenital diagnoses are obstructive uropathy and aplastic/hypoplastic/dysplastic kidneys, each representing about 16% of the patients[13] (Table 40–2). Among glomerular disorders, focal segmental glomerulosclerosis (FSGS) is the most common; 873 children received a renal transplant for FSGS between 1987 and 2002. The primary diagnosis also varies with the race of the recipient. Overall in the NAPRTCS registry, Caucasian children account for 62% of all recipients; however, Caucasian children account for less than 50% of the children transplanted for FSGS. The data regarding the role of FSGS in leading to ESRD can be better appreciated by observations from the dialysis section of the registry, in which the two most common diagnoses are FSGS and aplastic/dysplastic kidneys at 14% each. Of 733 children with FSGS on dialysis, Caucasian children account for only 34%, with African-American and Hispanic children accounting for 62% of the patients. Twenty-four percent of African-American children on dialysis and 30% of those greater than 12 years old have FSGS. Table 40–2 shows the primary diagnoses by gender and race of 7651 children who have received a transplant as recorded by NAPRTCS since 1987, as well as the percentage of biopsy proven diagnoses. It is important to observe that the biopsy confirmation of the primary diagnosis was made in 94% of FSGS, in 93% of systemic immunologic diseases and in 90% of congenital nephrotic syndrome patients. The information regarding primary diagnosis is critical in predicting graft survival as well as recurrence of the original disease, as discussed later.

Age at Transplantation

Kidney transplantation prior to 6 months of age, or in a recipient who weighs less than 6 kg is exceptional. From 1987 to 2002, NAPRTCS recorded 81 transplants performed in children younger than 12 months.[13] Of these, 5 transplants were performed in children between 3 and 5 months, 21 were performed in children between 6 and 8 months, and 55 were performed in children between 9 and 11 months of age. Only 12 infants have been reported since 1996. In general, the number of kidney transplants performed in infants and young children seems to be declining (Table 40–1). Since infants and adolescents have different risk factors for both patient and graft survival, children frequently have been grouped into five age categories: 0 to 1 year; 2 to 5 years; 6 to 12 years; 13 to 17 years; and 18 to 21 years of age. In 1987, 25% of all pediatric transplants were performed in children 0 to 5 years of age,[27] whereas in 1995, the same age group accounted for 15%,[24] and it is currently 17%.[13] Whether the decreased number of transplants in this group is due to a perception of their vulnerability or to the development of more optimum dialysis has not been established. It is important to note that excellent results have been obtained in very young patients in some individual centers.[28,29] The concept of a heightened immune response in young recipients is currently controversial.[30–32] Thus, the unique problems associated with transplantation in young recipients may be related to infections, technical issues, and differences in pharmacokinetics[14,33–36] rather than their immune response. Recent reports of outstanding long-term graft survival rates for these young children seem to indicate that their specific problems can be overcome successfully.[12]

Indications for Transplantation

Because of the shortage of donors for kidney transplantation, the evaluation of potential recipients and the indications for transplantation have recently been reviewed.[37,38] Virtually all children reaching ESRD are considered to be candidates for a renal transplant. In some settings, the definition of ESRD is related to the need for chronic dialysis to sustain life. Currently in the United States, dialysis is rarely indicated in adults until the serum creatinine has exceeded 8 mg/dL. The definition of dialysis dependency is inadequate in pediatrics, however, because a significant number of children receive a preemptive kidney transplant without ever having been on dialysis.[39] In a review of 7053 primary kidney transplants in children transplanted from 1987 through 2002, the NAPRTCS noted that 1713 (24%) of the patients had never received maintenance dialysis.[13] In the past, growth failure was considered one indication for transplantation, but the success of recombinant human growth hormone in overcoming this complication of chronic kidney disease (CKD) in children[8,40] has virtually eliminated growth failure as an absolute indication. A very disturbing result from an analysis of UNOS data demonstrated that African-Americans in the United States are less likely to be waitlisted for transplantation at any time after their first dialysis treatment than Caucasians.[41] The point at

Table 40-2 Pediatric Kidney Gender and Race Distribution by Primary Diagnosis

	N	%	% Male	% White	% Biopsied
Total	**7651**	**100**	**60**	**62**	**56**
Diagnosis					
Obstructive uropathy	1237	16	86	66	32
Aplasic/hypoplastic/dysplastic kidney	1222	16	62	65	28
Focal segmental glomerulosclerosis	873	11	58	48	94
Reflux nephropathy	397	5	45	74	33
Chronic glomerulonephritis	279	4	42	47	75
Polycystic disease	213	3	52	75	56
Medullary cystic disease	212	3	50	83	66
Hemolytic uremic syndrome	206	3	56	80	53
Prune belly	201	3	99	61	38
Congenital nephrotic syndrome	192	3	51	66	90
Familial nephritis	177	2	82	58	72
Cystinosis	162	2	50	90	44
Idiopathic crescentic glomerulonephritis	151	2	35	53	95
Membranoproliferative glommerulonehritis—Type I	150	2	46	55	97
Pyelo/interstitial nephritis	146	2	47	71	75
SLE nephritis	124	2	19	27	96
Renal infarct	119	2	49	78	37
Henoch-Schonlein nephritis	101	1	41	67	85
Berger's (IgA) nephritis	100	1	57	63	93
Membranoproliferative glommerulonehritis—Type II	68	1	50	76	96
Wilms' tumor	43	1	49	79	91
Drash syndrome	43	1	63	65	93
Oxalosis	43	1	58	81	74
Wegener's granulomatosis	42	1	40	79	93
Membranous nephropathy	36	1	61	56	97
Other systemic immunologic disease	30	0.4	13	53	93
Sickle cell nephropathy	14	0.2	57	0	71
Diabetic glomerulonephritis	8	0.1	25	38	62
Other	596	8	54	63	65
Unknown	466	6	51	31	30

Adapted from Seikaly M, Ho PL, Emmett L, Tejani A: The 12th Annual Report of the North American Pediatric Renal Transplant Cooperative Study: Renal transplantation from 1987 through 1998 (updated at www.naprtcs.org). Pediatr Transplant 2001; 5:215-231.

which a child with chronic renal insufficiency (CRI) should be considered for renal transplantation remains controversial.

PREEMPTIVE TRANSPLANTATION

Since preemptive transplantation is an important modality for children, NAPRTCS conducted a special study to determine the frequency and outcome of this approach[39] and has updated it in the annual reports.[13] From 1987 through 1992, 26% of the patients were registered as having had preemptive transplantation. The study compared data of those recipients who had been on maintenance dialysis versus patients who had no previous dialysis. Of 2213 primary grafts during that time period, 1150 (52%) were from an LD source, whereas for the preemptive group 70% were recipients of an LD kidney. More recently, of 7053 primary transplants, 1713 (24%) were preemptive. Preemptive transplantation was more common in LD (33%) than in CAD (13%) and in males (27%) than in females (20%). The rate varies among age groups with 20%, 24%, 28%, 27%, and 20% for the 0 to 1, 2 to 5, 6 to 12, 13 to 17, and 18 to 20 age groups, respectively. It also varies across races with Caucasians, African-Americans, Hispanics, and other races, having rates of 30%, 14%, 16%, and 16%, respectively. As noted above, African-Americans were also less likely to be waitlisted than Caucasians following initiation of dialysis.[41] A proposed objection against preemptive transplants has been that without the rigors of prior dialysis, compliance with immunosuppression might be poor. To determine whether this hypothesis might be correct, graft survival was compared between the two groups and was determined to not be different at 1 or 4 years.[39] When causes for graft loss were analyzed, the preemptive group did not have a higher incidence due to noncompliance. The NAPRTCS also surveyed the motive for preemptive transplantation and determined that the primary reasons were parents' desire to avoid dialysis (34%) and the nephrologists' recommendation (18%). Desire for improved growth was considered a contributory factor in 50% of the patients.[39]

CONTRAINDICATIONS TO TRANSPLANTATION

There are few absolute contraindications to transplantation. The concern of further immunosuppressing an already compromised host made transplantation of HIV-positive children a perceived relative contraindication. Many children who developed HIV nephropathy succumb to the systemic ravages of the virus, either before or very shortly after reaching ESRD status.[42] However, marked advances of treatment of HIV-positive patients, especially with protease inhibitors and other antiretroviral therapies, makes consideration of kidney transplantation more likely.[43,44] Ironically, initial results from a few centers suggest that HIV-positive patients with reasonable CD4 cell counts may have more problems with rejection rather than infection post-transplantation.

Another relative contraindication is a preexisting malignancy. The NAPRTCS dialysis registry contains 70 children with Wilms' tumor or Drash syndrome.[45] Thirteen of these did not receive a transplant because of metastatic disease and all 13 died. The transplant registry contains 86 children who have these diagnoses and who have received a kidney transplant, and no recurrences have been reported in any of them. The outcome of those who received transplants was similar to non-Wilms'/Drash recipients. However, children with already existing metastatic disease are generally not considered transplant candidates. Also, children with devastating neurologic dysfunction may not be suitable transplant candidates, but the wishes of the parents, as well as the potential for long-term rehabilitation, must be considered in these circumstances. Potential for recurrence of the original renal disease is of major concern but has not generally precluded at least an initial transplant. Oxalosis, which once was considered an absolute contraindication due to a high incidence of recurrence, can be treated successfully with combined liver and kidney transplantation,[46,47] although the complication rate remains high.[29,48,49]

PRE-TRANSPLANT PREPARATION

Recipient Preparation

Before a child can undergo transplantation, the problems caused by CKD must be addressed and repaired, if possible. In those cases where ESRD is due to urologic abnormalities, corrective reconstructive surgery should be undertaken, especially to the lower urinary tract, prior to transplantation. Two of the major consequences of CKD are anemia and growth retardation, both of which should be addressed prior to transplantation. A recent report of final adult height in pediatric renal transplant recipients suggests that the current improvement in final adult height post-transplantation is more related to improving height deficits prior to transplant than to any net gains achieved after transplantation.[8,9] Uremia also leads to wasting and malnutrition in the child, and this can compromise the success of the procedure. For example, prophylactic native nephrectomy and reversal of protein wasting and malnutrition improves the outcome of transplantation in children with congenital nephrotic syndrome.[50–52] Careful preparation is particularly important in children undergoing preemptive transplants. Although there exist guidelines for the evaluation of the adult transplant recipient,[37,38] there are no similar published reports for pediatric patients. Nonetheless, Table 40–3 details typical preparation utilized prior to surgery for pediatric recipients.

Table 40–3 Standard Preparation of Pediatric Renal Transplant Candidates

History and Physical Examination
Laboratory Tests
Hematology (CBC, platelets, differential)
Coagulation (PT, PTT, TT)
Chemistry (serum electrolytes, BUN, creatinine, liver function, lipid profile, Ca, PO_4, PTH)
Urine volume, culture, and urinalysis
Blood Bank / Immunology (ABO blood type, HLA type, histocompatability testing, anti-HLA antibody screening, hepatitis profile, HIV screening)
Virology (CMV, EBV, MMR titers)
X-Ray (VCUG,* CXR, bone age)
Consults
Dentist
Social Worker
Nutritionist
Vaccines
DPT/Polio, MMR, HIB, HBV
Pneumococcal
Varivax
PPD

*For selected recipients.

UROLOGIC EVALUATION

Children with the diagnoses described in Table 40–4 require a thorough urologic evaluation prior to transplantation. In the NAPRTCS report 1878 of 7651 (25%) pediatric transplant recipients were identified as having lower urinary tract abnormalities.[13] For all such patients, a history of voiding pattern prior to development of renal failure is most helpful. Preliminary investigations consist of measurement of urinary flow rate and ultrasound estimation of the post micturition urine volume. Urinary flow rate should be at least 15 mL/sec,[53] and the residual volume should be less than 30 mL. Further investigations would consist of urethrocystoscopy in patients suspected of a urethral stricture, and a voiding cystometrogram is essential for complete assessment of bladder function.[54] This provides information about bladder capacity, pressure rise, and the efficiency of voiding. Still more information can be obtained by combining urodynamic studies with radioisotope imaging. Routine voiding cystourethrogram is not indicated in older patients with no symptoms related to the urinary tract.[55]

A bladder with a very small capacity may not be adequate for a functioning transplant. Occasionally, the small capacity bladder may develop in patients with prolonged oligoanuria. However, if the bladder is distensible and the bladder wall compliant, such a bladder may be used safely for kidney transplantation. Other criteria for a usable bladder are an end-filling pressure less than 30 cm of H_2O and a good flow rate. In patients with a poor flow rate, if urethral and bladder outlet obstructions are ruled out, the problem may be due to detrusor malfunction.[53] When a bladder fails to empty completely, infection and obstruction are potential complications that may shorten graft survival. Intermittent, clean, self-catheterization, which is widely used in urologic practice, can be safely used post-transplantation in patients where the primary abnormality is inefficient and uncoordinated detrusor function.

Table 40-4 Possible Lower Urinary Tract Abnormalities of Pediatric Renal Transplant Recipients

Bladder exstrophy
Neuropathic bladder (meningomyelocele, spinal cord trauma, neurological disease)
Posterior urethral valves
Prune belly syndrome
Vesicoureteral reflux

Most pediatric patients have a urinary bladder that will adapt to the new kidney. Although the bladder may not appear to have the capacity, especially in patients on long-term dialysis prior to transplantation, it will most often distend with usage.[46] However, in patients with a truly low capacity or high pressure, bladder augmentation may be necessary prior to transplantation.[56–58] Augmentation cystoplasty consists of adding bowel or gastric wall to the bladder, whereas substitution cystoplasty is performed when most of the bladder is excised and replaced with bowel. Gastric remnants have been popular for augmentation, however, they do tend to cause excessive loss of acid in the urine, leading to discomfort and metabolic alkalosis. Early attempts to reconstruct bladders with bioengineered material are ongoing. There are promising reports of "bioengineered" bladder material, although these have not yet been tried in transplant recipients.[59,60] In those patients in whom augmentation has been performed prior to transplantation, long-term antibiotic therapy and intermittent catheterization may have to be carried out to prevent urine stasis and infection. In a very small subset of patients, whose bladder is unusable and augmentation unsuccessful, some form of urinary diversion may be necessary.[46]

PRETRANSPLANT BLOOD TRANSFUSIONS

In the precyclosporine era blood transfusions were shown to have a beneficial effect on graft outcome,[61] but their effect subsequently diminished,[62] and they are currently rarely utilized. The early beneficial effect of pre-transplant transfusions in children was similar to what was seen in adults. In the past, donor-specific transfusions were also given to children. Early results from such studies suggested better graft survival; however, more prolonged follow-up with improved immunosuppression showed diminished benefit,[63] and the practice of donor-specific transfusions has now been largely abandoned in pediatric renal transplantation. The theoretic advantages of pre-transplant tolerance induction by antigen presentation remain intriguing.[64] Two recent reports of the beneficial effects of deliberate pre-transplant transfusions have reinstated interest in their use.[65,66]

The role of random pre-transplant transfusions in improving graft survival remains unclear. In 1992, the NAPRTCS, in a study of 1667 transplants of which 57% were of CAD origin, did not observe any beneficial or detrimental effect of pre-transplant blood transfusions.[27] However, subsequently, a deleterious effect associated with pre-transplant transfusion became apparent. For LD source transplants the use of five or more prior transfusions was associated with graft loss with a relative risk (RR) of 1.8.[22] By 1995, the use of prior transfusions was a risk factor for CAD source transplants as well, and the use of five or more transfusions was associated with graft loss with a relative risk of 1.3.[3] The 1996 NAPRTCS report, which analyzed 4714 transplants, shows that greater than five transfusions were associated with graft loss with a relative risk of 1.7 for LD and 1.3 for CAD graft failure.[24] A NAPRTCS special analysis indicated that multiple transfusions have a deleterious effect on graft survival, but fewer then five transfusions may be associated with a decreased incidence of acute rejection episodes.[67] Sixty-five percent of pediatric living donor renal transplant recipients and 56% of cadaver donor recipients now have no random transfusions prior to transplantation, and donor-specific transfusion is rarely performed.[13] Pre-transplant blood transfusions would be of only historical interest except for a renewed interest related to tolerance induction and the recent reports mentioned above.[65,66] Whether they will be utilized in the future for this indication is unknown.

Effect of the Age of the Cadaver Donor

For many years there was a tendency to use kidneys recovered from infants and young children for transplantation into young recipients.[21] Early studies showed that 25% of all cadaver transplants performed in children were recovered from children under 10 years.[27] A special study of the NAPRTCS[68] demonstrated that the preferential placement of small kidneys into infants and very young children had disastrous consequences for graft survival, and this was subsequently confirmed by a larger study.[69] As a result, CAD allocation policies for pediatric recipients were changed resulting in improved outcome.[21] More recent information shows that this practice has now undergone substantial change.[13] Since 1991, less than 1% of cadaver kidneys for pediatric recipients have come from donors younger than 2 years. And, during the same time, the percentage of kidneys recovered from donors over the age of 10 years increased from 78% to 88%. Importantly, the kidneys from young donors have not been discarded but have been utilized for transplantation via the en bloc technique into adult recipients.[26,69,70] Also, single centers have reported better success with young donors, utilizing carefully controlled protocols.[25] Advanced donor age is also associated with diminished long-term graft survival[71,72] and should likely be avoided for young recipients.[68,73,74]

HLA Matching Results in Children

For CAD transplants the NAPRTCS registry indicates that a 2-DR mismatched graft has a relative hazard (RH) of first rejection of 1.27 compared to a 0-DR mismatch, and an RH of graft failure of 1.21 ($p = .002$).[13] These outcomes are consistent with the relationship between histocompatibility matching and graft outcome in adults.[75,76] Unfortunately, since children have waiting-time preference on the CAD waiting list in the United States, HLA-matching for them is generally poorer than for adults.[12] Because most living donors of renal transplants for children are parents, these transplants are mismatched at one haplotype.

ABO BLOOD TYPE IN CHILDREN

NAPRTCS has recorded 27 confirmed kidney transplants across ABO blood group compatibility barriers. Of these, most are

O recipients of A donors. A NAPRTCS special study of 11 of these patients concluded that the procedure could be successful if done under carefully controlled conditions.[77] Evaluation of recipient isohemagglutinin levels may be helpful to identify suitable donor-recipient pairs. A more recent strategy for ABO mismatching entails "donor-swaps," either with a complementary donor-recipient pair or with a CAD waiting list.[78,79]

THE TRANSPLANT PROCEDURE

Technical Issues in Transplantation

The operative technique differs based on the weight of the child. For small children less than 15 kg, the transplant is frequently done through a midline incision and the larger vessels are utilized for anastomosis with the donor kidney (Figure 40–1).[46] After reflection of the cecum and the right colon, the anterior wall of the aorta and the inferior vena cava are exposed and dissected.[80] The aorta is mobilized from above the inferior mesenteric artery to the external iliac artery on the right side. After ligating and dividing the lumbar branches, the iliac arteries and the inferior mesenteric are encircled. Next, the inferior vena cava is mobilized from the left renal vein to the iliac veins. After ligating the lumber veins the iliac veins are encircled. The donor renal vein is anastomosed to the recipient vena cava in an end-to-side technique.[81] The donor renal artery is then anastomosed to the recipient aorta in an end-to-side fashion. Careful attention needs to be paid to the recipient hemodynamic response upon clamping and unclamping of the major vessels, and it is desirable to maintain a central venous pressure of 15 to 18 cm H_2O prior to unclamping.[46,80] The filling of the transplanted kidney may be slow because a large adult kidney will take up a significant portion of the normal pediatric blood volume. Recent hemodynamic studies suggest that the cardiac output of infants must double to perfuse the adult donor kidney adequately.[82] Thus, volume replacement is critical. The ureteral anastomosis is done by implanting the donor's ureter into the recipient's bladder using either a Leadbetter-Politano procedure or a modification of it. Many surgeons now prefer a nonrefluxing extravesical rather than transvesical approach for ureteroneocystostomy because it is faster, a separate cystotomy is not required, and less ureteral length is necessary, thus assuring a distal ureteral blood supply.[83–85]

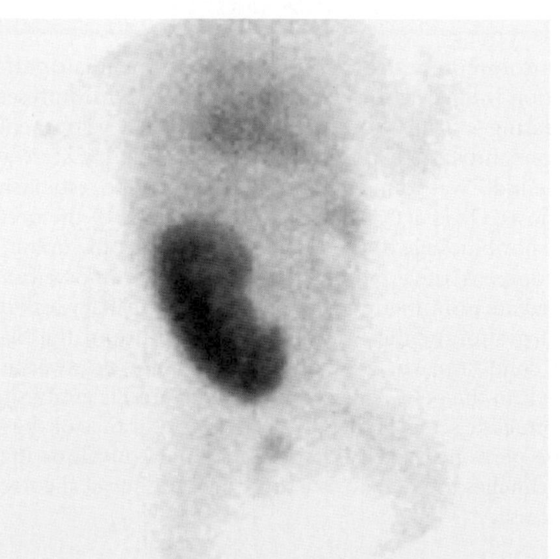

Figure 40–1 ^{99M}Tc-MAG3 radionuclide renal scan in a 9-month-old infant who received an LD renal transplant from his father. The graft is intraperitoneal and occupies most of the right side of the peritoneal space. Note the relative sizes of the graft and the heart.

The transplantation technique utilized in children with a body weight greater than 15 kg is similar to that employed in adults. Unlike the transperitoneal approach necessary in younger children, this transplant is extraperitoneal, with the renal vein anastomosed to the common iliac or to the external iliac vein.[80] The arterial anastomosis can be to either the common iliac or to the internal iliac artery. The ureterovesicular anastomosis is done using the techniques described earlier.

Evaluation of Graft Dysfunction

At the completion of the vascular anastomosis and release of the vascular clamps, immediate function of the transplanted kidney is demonstrated by the production of urine. Various causes, however, may prevent initial function, and evaluation of immediate nonfunction and the differential diagnosis of this condition is a critical component of the transplant physician's role.

ACUTE TUBULAR NECROSIS (ATN)

ATN represents the most frequent cause of immediate graft nonfunction. Data from the NAPRTCS 1996 Annual Report showed that ATN was observed in 5% of LD and 19% of CAD transplants.[24] Since the NAPRTCS definition for ATN is stringent, requiring dialysis in the first post-transplant week, these figures probably underrepresent the actual incidence of ATN. The risk of early ATN in LD kidneys is related to factors such as prior transplants and more than five transfusions. Similarly, the risk factors of ATN in CAD kidneys include prolonged cold ischemia, absence of prophylactic antibody therapy, and the use of more than five blood transfusions. The diagnosis is confirmed in most cases by the use of radionuclide scan (Figure 40–2). If recovery of graft function is delayed, however, a transplant biopsy may be necessary because other diagnostic tests cannot distinguish between ATN and rejection.[86,87] Importantly, early acute rejection can mimic ATN or coexist with it. The presence of ATN does not auger well for the transplant, particularly for those of cadaver source because graft failure and death are more common among patients with ATN.[48] The NAPRTCS data show that 71% of CAD grafts without ATN were functioning at 4 years compared to only 51% of those with ATN.[88]

GRAFT THROMBOSIS

Graft thrombosis is an important complication of pediatric transplantation. Although usually a major cause of immedi-

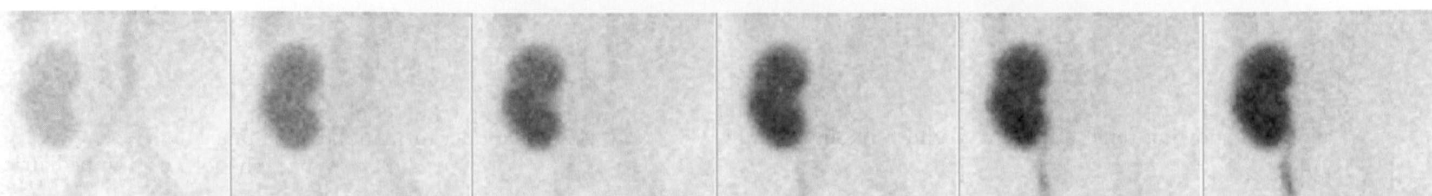

Figure 40–2 ^{99M}Tc-MAG3 radionuclide renal scan of a CAD renal transplant in a 15-year-old boy performed on the first post-op day. The cold ischemia time exceeded 24 hours, and the recipient experienced oliguric ATN. Note the good perfusion, followed by little excretion and "wash out" of the tracer from the graft.

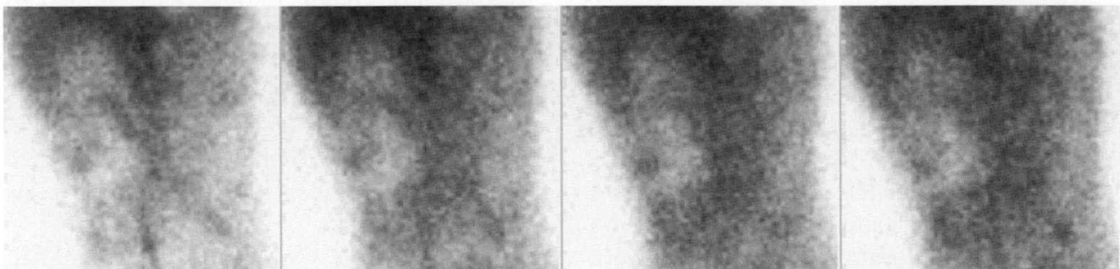

Figure 40–3 ^{99M}Tc-MAG3 radionuclide renal scan in a 6-year-old girl with FSGS who received an LD renal transplant, performed 16 hours post-operatively. Note the photopenic area in the right abdomen, indicating thrombosis of the graft with no perfusion.

ate graft nonfunction, it can be seen later in the course and has been recorded to occur as late as 15 days post-transplant following initial engraftment and function. Graft thrombosis has been the third most common cause of graft failure in pediatric renal transplantation[13] and may rise to second if acute rejection rates continue to fall.[89] The critical nature of this complication can be appreciated because it accounts for 11% of graft failure in index transplantation and 13% in repeat transplants in the NAPRTCS registry. A dreaded event, this condition is irreversible in most cases and necessitates removal of the graft. Graft thrombosis should be suspected in cases where there has been immediate function followed by the development of oligoanuria. The diagnosis is established by a radionuclide scan using diethylenetriamine pentaacetic acid (DTPA) or MAG3,[90] which reveals a photopenic defect with no uptake by the transplant kidney (Figure 40–3).

Because the outcome of graft thrombosis is uniformly dismal, numerous studies have been conducted in an attempt to understand and anticipate this complication. The etiology of graft thrombosis is multifactorial, but it is more commonly seen in young recipients.[91] In a special study of 2060 LD and 2334 CAD kidneys,[92] the NAPRTCS has shown that a history of prior transplantation increases the risk, whereas increasing recipient age has a protective effect for LD kidneys. The prophylactic use of antilymphocyte antibody also decreases the risk, and this may be particularly true for the monoclonal IL2r antibodies.[89] For cadaver source kidneys, a cold ischemia time longer than 24 hours increases the risk of thrombosis. The use of antibody induction therapy, the use of donors greater than 5 years of age, and increasing recipient age were factors that decreased the risk of thrombosis. A heightened thrombotic state has also been implicated.[90,93,94] One study showed that centers that performed fewer infant transplants had higher rates of graft thrombosis,[95] and another suggested that pre-transplant use of peritoneal dialysis increased the risk of thrombosis.[96,97] Some centers routinely administer anticoagulants to pediatric recipients at high risk of graft thrombosis, but no clinical studies of their effectiveness have been performed, and its use is not without complications.[98] This incidence of graft thrombosis has not changed over the past 15 years[13]; however, a preliminary report suggests that a new approach to induction therapy may have been associated with a decrease.[89]

OBSTRUCTION AND URINARY LEAK

An uncommon but correctable cause of immediate graft dysfunction is obstruction of the urinary flow, which presents as decreasing urine output and the development of hydronephrosis. An ultrasound or radionuclide scan with a furosemide washout enables the clinician to establish this diagnosis. Obstruction can be due to kinking of the ureter, to edema or blockage of the implantation site of the ureter, or to development of a lymphocele. A more ominous cause of immediate nonfunction is the rare case of urinary leak due to disintegration of the distal ureter or rupture of the bladder. This condition can be painful due to the extravasation of urine into the pelvis or peritoneal cavity and is established by radionuclide scan (Figure 40–4). The appearance of the tracer in the peritoneal cavity or in the scrotal, vulval, or inguinal area clinches the diagnosis and immediate surgical correction is necessary.

Induction Therapy

IL-2 Receptor Antibodies

There are two two high-affinity chimeric or humanized antibodies that act on the inducible α-chain of the interleukin-2

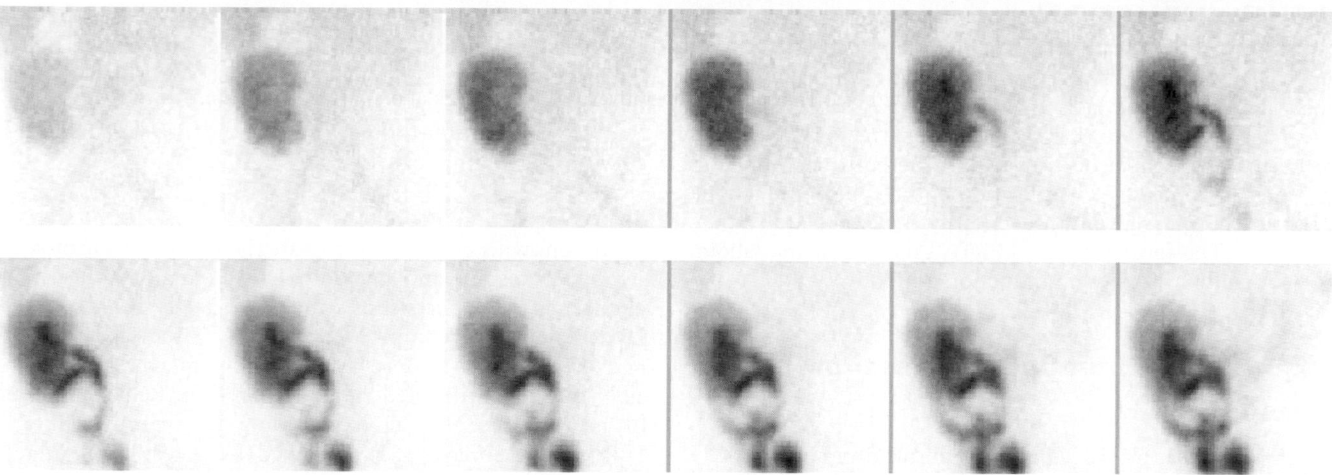

Figure 40–4 ^{99M}Tc-MAG3 radionuclide renal scan in an 8-year-old girl who received a CAD renal transplant, performed 12 hours post-operatively. Note the good perfusion of the graft and the rapid concentration and excretion from the kidney. Tracer, however, rapidly accumulates in the right lower quadrant, outside of the bladder. Investigation demonstrated a traumatic bladder rupture.

receptor (IL-2r) on the surface of the activated lymphocyte, basiliximab (Simulect, Novartis) and daclizumab (Zenapax, Roche). Basiliximab is generally given as two-dose regimen (generally 10 mg for children <40 kg and 20 mg for those >40 kg) on days 0 and 4 post-transplantation.[99] A pharmacologic study showed that basiliximab clearance in children is reduced by approximately half compared with adults and was independent of age, weight, or body surface area.[100] One study has noted that pediatric recipients receiving basiliximab may have significantly elevated levels of cyclosporine and may require reduced doses to avoid toxicity.[101] Daclizumab is generally given in a dose of 1 mg/kg intravenously on the day of transplantation and every 14 days thereafter for a total of five doses.[102] Higher doses may be required for saturation of IL-2 receptors in younger children.[6] Both antibodies are generally well tolerated without substantial side effects. Both antibodies have been studied extensively in children and have been shown to be safe and effective.[6,99,101,103–105] The precise mechanism of the antibodies is not known but is presumed to be saturation of the IL-2 receptor and subsequent competitive antagonism of IL-2-dependent proliferation. A novel 6-month dosing schedule of daclizumab has been reported as part of a steroid-avoidance pilot study and appears to be well tolerated.[6] There are no comparative studies between the two antibodies. Up to 65% of pediatric renal transplant recipients are now receiving an IL-2 receptor antibody as induction therapy.[13]

T-CELL ANTIBODIES

Retrospective data from the NAPRTCS do show a beneficial effect of prophylactic anti–T-cell antibody. In a review of LD transplants, 5-year graft survival was 81% in 1041 patients who received T-cell antibody therapy compared with 75% in 1399 patients who did not. Similar figures for CAD kidneys were 66% in 1423 T-cell antibody treated patients, compared to 56% in 1034 patients who did not receive T-cell antibody.[24] A major problem of these analyses is that several different types of T-cell antibody were used. In the early years a polyclonal antibody was used, the most common of which was prepared from horse serum and designated as MALG (Minnesota antilymphocyte globulin).[106] A monoclonal antibody directed at subsets of T cells, called OKT3, was subsequently employed.[107]

Two polyclonal antibodies currently available are Atgam (Upjohn), and Thymoglobulin (Sangstat). Atgam, because of the sclerosing nature of the preparation, is given intravenously through a central catheter for 10 to 15 days. The dose used is 15 mg/kg, and calcineurin inhibitors are generally withheld during the administration of the antibody. Thymoglobulin is provided through a peripheral vein at a dose of 1.5 to 2 mg/kg/dose. A recent report suggests daily monitoring of CD3+ subsets to guide therapy: the daily dose is given only when the CD3+ count exceeds 20 cells/mm^3.[108] Thymoglobulin has been studied in small groups of pediatric renal transplant recipients and was found to be effective.[109] Comparison of efficacy of removal of circulating T cells suggested that thymoglobulin may have some benefit over Atgam,[110] but no comparisons of clinical outcomes have been performed. The monoclonal antibody, OKT3, is administered as a bolus injection into a peripheral vein daily for 10 to 14 days at a dose of 5 mg for older children and 2.5 mg for children weighing less than 30 kg. Calcineurin inhibitors are also withheld during the use of OKT3. The major problem with these induction therapies include the "first-dose reaction"[111,112]; neurologic problems,[113] and the potential for the development of superimposed infections, such as cytomegalovirus (CMV) or Epstein-Barr virus (EBV) disease. Although retrospective analysis of pediatric kidney transplantation continues to show a clear benefit to the use of prophylactic induction antibody,[13] a recent prospective randomized trial of OKT3 induction showed no clear advantage.[114] Currently, less than 10% of pediatric renal transplant recipients receive an anti–T-cell antibody for induction therapy.[13] Depleting T-cell antibodies, such as Campath, have not yet been evaluated systematically in children.

OTHER INDUCTION

If T-cell antibody is not chosen for induction therapy, one of the calcineurin inhibitors may instead be used. Currently, there are two such drugs, cyclosporine and tacrolimus, which have similar mechanisms but act at different sites to inhibit calcineurin. A possible complication of this type of induction, particularly if it is given intravenously, is delayed graft function.[115,116] The most recent NAPRTCS data show that about 35% of children receive no induction antibody.[13]

Maintenance Immunosuppression

Cyclosporine

Cyclosporine was first used in renal transplantation by Calne[117] in 1978. The initial experience was followed by controlled trials in the United States, Canada, and Europe, all of which showed a significant improvement in graft survival over existing therapies. The drug was licensed in the United States in 1983 and has been used in all types of solid organ transplantation for over 20 years. There have been no controlled trials in children, but over the years of use a large body of information regarding its dosing and side effects has accumulated.[13]

Induction Dose

For induction purposes cyclosporine is given intravenously in a dose of 165 mg/m^2 daily for children under 6 years of age and 4.5 mg/kg daily in children over 6 years. The dose for younger children is calculated in square meter format because they metabolize the drug differently. The drug is preferably given in a continuous infusion over a 24-hour period starting intraoperatively. If practicality precludes a continuous infusion, the drug should be administered in three divided doses daily but over as long an interval as possible. If possible, induction therapy using cyclosporine should be continued for 48 hours only and then converted to oral cyclosporine. The recommended starting oral dose for children under the age of 6 years is 500 mg/m^2 daily, administered in three divided doses; for children over the age of 6 years, it is 15 mg/kg daily, administered in two divided doses. These doses are higher than those prescribed for adults because experience over the last 10 years has determined that the drug is metabolized more rapidly in children.[118] A calcium channel blocker is typically given with cyclosporine to reduce toxicity.[119]

Maintenance Dose

Because of its irregular absorption and inherent nephrotoxicity, dose adjustments of cyclosporine are constantly necessary.[120] Data from the NAPRTCS show that at 1 year post-transplant the mean cyclosporine dose can vary from 5.6 mg/kg to 8 mg/kg.[24] It has also been demonstrated that higher maintenance doses are associated with diminished chronic graft rejection.[118] Among cadaver kidney recipients the rate of rejection was 16% in those receiving doses higher than 8 mg/kg at 1 year post-transplant, compared to 24% in those receiving less than 6 mg/kg daily.[121] The difficulty of maintaining constant dosing has led to several methods of measuring cyclosporine blood levels.[116] Either high-pressure liquid chromatography (HPLC) or fluorescence polarization immunoassay (FPIA) techniques are used. Drug adequacy is considered to be a range of 100 to 200 ng/mL HPLC whole blood trough level or 200 to 450 ng/mL TDX whole blood levels for patients more than 3 months post-transplant. Higher levels are necessary in the first 3 months. Newer data suggest that measuring the level 2 hours after receiving the dose may lead to more accurate dosing, assessing the true area under the curve, and avoiding toxicity.[122–124]

Side Effects

Treatment with cyclosporine is associated with nephrotoxicity, hypertension, and hepatotoxicity. A major concern in children is the hypertrichosis and the facial dysmorphism.[125] Hyperkalemia is common in patients on cyclosporine[126] and also responds to dose reduction. The mechanism is possibly due to diminished tubular excretion. Renal handling of uric acid is also altered, leading to hyperuricemia.[127] Hypomagnesemia is also observed as a result of altered tubular function.[128] Tremors, convulsions, and parasthesias have been recorded in patients on cyclosporine.[129] These side effects may be multidrug induced rather than from cyclosporine alone; however, they are often seen with high blood levels. Both hypertension and hyperlipidemia are observed in patients on cyclosporine. A worrisome side effect in children is gingival hypertrophy,[130] seen more often with higher doses and in the presence of poor dental hygiene.[131] The most recent data from the NAPRTCS registry show that slightly less that 50% of renal transplant recipients are currently receiving cyclosporine as initial immunosuppression.[13]

Tacrolimus

Tacrolimus (Prograft, Fujisawa) was introduced as an immunosuppressant for kidney transplantation in the mid-1990s.[132–134] Recent data from the NAPRTCS show that slightly less than 50% of children are being maintained on tacrolimus at 31 days post-transplantation.[13]

Dosage

One method of initiation of tacrolimus is to provide 0.1 mg/kg/24 hr as a continuous infusion, with a switch to oral therapy within 2 to 3 days. However, because of the good absorption of the oral preparation and the concern about nephrotoxicity, many programs begin treatment via oral or NG tube very early post-transplant. Initial oral doses should not exceed 0.15 mg/kg twice daily and should be reduced to 0.1 mg/kg as maintenance dose. Blood monitoring is necessary as with cyclosporine, and target whole blood trough levels, measured by an enzyme linked immunosorbent assay (ELISA), should be maintained between 5 to 20 μGm/L. Diarrhea, which is common, particularly in infants, may lead to increased tacrolimus levels.[135]

Side Effects

Because of the similar mechanism of action, virtually all of the side effects of cyclosporine therapy are also seen with tacrolimus.[133] The nephrotoxic effect is similar.[136] The hypertrichosis and the dysmorphic features noted with cyclosporine are not seen with tacrolimus.[137] Neurologic side effects are common and may be seen more frequently than with cyclosporine.[138,139] A concern for the use of tacrolimus in pediatric renal transplantation was the development of post-transplant diabetes mellitus (PTDM), because in an early

Japanese renal study a third of the patients developed hyperglycemia requiring insulin therapy,[140] which has also been reported from other single center reports.[141,142] The mechanism may be related to a diminished insulin secretion in association with the insulin resistance related to steroid use.[143] The incidence of post-transplant lymphoproliferative disorder (PTLD) was much higher with the use of tacrolimus than with other immunosuppressants during early experience.[134,144] However, a more recent retrospective analysis showed that the use of tacrolimus was not a risk factor for development of PTLD, likely due to the lower doses currently utilized.[145]

Choice of Calcineurin Inhibitor

Calcineurin inhibitors have been mainstays of immunosuppression for pediatric transplantation for the past decade and likely account for the continuing improvement in graft survival rates.[12,146,147] The choice between the drugs has often been based on a center preference. An open-label randomized trial of the two drugs with steroids and azathioprine was recently completed.[148] Tacrolimus-treated patients had a lower rate of acute rejection (37%) than cyclosporine-treated patients (59%), although both rates were higher than current standards,[13] and not all episodes were biopsy-proven. One-year graft survival rates were similar, although the glomerular filtration rate (GFR) was higher in the tacrolimus group. Hypomagnesemia, diarrhea, and PTDM were higher in the tacrolimus group, and hypertrichosis and gum hyperplasia were higher in the cyclosporine group. In a retrospective analysis of NAPRTCS data of the two drugs given with MMF and steroids,[137] there was no difference in early rejection rate (29%), risk of rejection, or risk of graft loss. At 2 years, graft survival was not different (tacrolimus 91%, cyclosporine 95%). Tacrolimus-treated patients were less likely to require antihypertensives and had higher GFR at 2 years.

Azathioprine

For pediatric patients azathioprine is given in the dose of 1 to 2 mg/kg/day. Higher doses should be closely monitored for myelosuppression. In the early years of transplantation azathioprine was routinely used in all transplant recipients; when cyclosporine became available it was still widely used as an adjunct drug. In 1989 and 1990, 80% of pediatric patients in the NAPRTCS registry were receiving azathioprine, but as more familiarity is established with mycophenylate mofetil (MMF) the use of azathioprine has diminished substantially and is currently in less than 10% of patients.[13]

Mycophenylate Mofetil (MMF)

As of 1996 the NAPRTCS registry noted that only 6.5% of patients were being maintained on MMF,[24] but the most recent figures show that it is used in about two thirds of pediatric kidney transplant recipients.[13] There are mixed results concerning its advantages over azathioprine.[149–152] A well-controlled study, however, concluded that it was safe and effective for use in pediatric renal transplantation.[153] A major difficulty in widespread use of the drug in children has been the gastrointestinal disturbance, especially in young children.[154] Both nausea and vomiting are common, but in some patients the drug has to be withdrawn due to intolerable diarrhea. Current recommended dose of MMF for pediatric patients is 1200 mg/m²/day, divided into two, three, or four doses.[155] It is likely that therapeutic monitoring should be employed, but clear standards are not yet available to guide treatment.[156–161]

Corticosteroids

The NAPRTCS reports show that 96% of children with a functioning graft are maintained on prednisone.[24] The numerous mechanisms of action of steroids lead to side effects and toxicities. The important concern in children is growth retardation. Studies have shown that doses in excess of 8.5 mg/day will impair normal growth.[162] Other side effects include increased susceptibility to infection, impaired wound healing, aseptic necrosis of the bone, cataracts, glucose intolerance, hypertension, cushingoid facies, and acne.[163] The preparations commonly used are prednisolone, its 11-keto metabolite prednisone, and methylprednisone. Although the half-lives of these preparations are very short, they can be administered once daily because their effect on inhibition of lymphocyte production persists for 24 hours.[164] The dosage is usually high in the immediate post-transplant period, about 2 mg/kg/day, with a gradual reduction to approximately 0.2 to 0.3 mg/kg/day within a 6-month to 1-year period. Because of the multiple side effects of maintenance steroid therapy, attempts have been made to withdraw steroids altogether, reported both in adult and pediatric kidney transplantation.[165] Unfortunately, the majority of these attempts have failed because of the development of acute rejection episodes.[166–168] The use of alternate-day steroid therapy, which appears to reduce the growth inhibiting effect without unduly increasing rejection episodes,[169,170] seems reasonable, but only a minority of pediatric renal transplant recipients is receiving steroids in that manner.[13] Several ongoing studies are investigating the use of steroid avoidance or steroid withdrawal protocols, and it is likely that steroids will not be used for immunosuppression in the future.

Sirolimus

Sirolimus (Sirolimus, Rapamune [Wyeth]) is the newest immunosuppressive agent used for kidney transplantation. It is the product of a fungus that was discovered on Easter Island (Rapa Nui) in 1969. It was first investigated for antifungal properties, and its immunosuppressant properties were first discovered in 1988. It was approved by the FDA in 1999. A similar compound that may be an analogue, SDZ-RAD, is currently undergoing clinical trials. Rapamycin is classified as a TOR inhibitor. TOR is a cytosolic enzyme that regulates differentiation and proliferation of lymphocytes. Then TOR is activated as a result of the cascade of reactions in lymphocytes by the proliferation of cytokines, and it initiates production of messenger RNAs that trigger cell-cycle progression from G_1 to S phase. The TOR inhibitors bind to the immunophilin FKBP12 and inhibit the actions of TOR.[171–176] The TOR inhibitors may be particularly important in long-term immunosuppression because they stimulate T-cell apoptosis. TOR-inhibitors also inhibit mesenchymal proliferation, which may prove to be important in graft vascular disease.[177,178] Also, since the mechanism of action of sirolimus is different from other currently available immunosuppressants, it can be used in combination with all of them. Sirolimus has been found to be effective in combination with calcineurin inhibitors,[179–183] in a calcineurin-inhibitor sparing protocol,[184] and in a steroid-free protocol.[185] The role of sirolimus or SDZ-RAD in pediatric transplantation is undergoing study.[34,186,187]

Dosage

Sirolimus is available as an oral preparation, either as a solid or liquid. Sirolimus was shown to have a prolonged half-life in adults that allowed a single daily dose in adults.[181–183] However, pharmacokinetic studies in children have demonstrated a much shorter half-life, as short as 12 hours.[34,188] Thus, children may require twice-per-day schedules to maintain therapeutic levels. Retrospective analysis of early trials of sirolimus have suggested a relationship between blood levels and risk of rejection.[189] Current suggestions for therapeutic levels remain speculative and range between 25 ng/mL in the early post-transplant period without calcineurin inhibitors[34,184] and 5 to 10 ng/mL later in the course of transplantation.

Side Effects

Sirolimus's major side effects are hyperlipidemia, thrombocytopenia, leucopenia, and possibly delayed wound healing.[181] The former complications can respond to lipid lowering drugs or dose reduction. The latter complication may require suspension of the drug until the wound heals completely.

Maintenance Immunosuppression Combinations

Most pediatric renal transplant recipients are treated with triple immunosuppression.[13] When the number of drugs was limited, the number of possible combinations was small. However, there are at least 20 possible combinations of the 6 available drugs, and when the induction antibodies are added, there are over 60 possible reported protocols.[190] No "best" protocol for children has been established, although most clinical trials are currently directed at eliminating either steroids or calcineurin inhibitors, or both. Currently, most children are receiving prednisone, MMF, and cyclosporine or tacrolinus after kidney transplantation.[13]

There are many possible targets for immunosuppression strategies for children.[191] One promising new protocol of steroid avoidance has been recently reported.[6] This approach consists of 6 months of anti-IL2r antibody, tacrolimus, and MMF. Short-term patient and graft survival rates have been excellent, and growth rates have been very good. Major complications have included bone-marrow suppression and nephrotoxicity. Other protocols currently under investigation include calcineurin inhibitor avoidance or withdrawal and costimulation blockade with the eventual goal of avoiding both corticosteroids and calcineurin inhibitors.

ALLOGRAFT REJECTION

In the absence of tolerance the renal allograft is destined for loss by some form of rejection. Rejections are classified as hyperacute (occurring immediately upon grafting), accelerated acute (occurring within the first week after transplantation), acute (generally occurring within the first year of transplantation), late acute (occurring after the first year), and chronic, for which the time sequence is difficult to establish because it may occur as early as 3 months but generally occurs years later in the course of the transplant.

Hyperacute Rejection

Hyperacute rejection is the result of specific recurrent anti-donor antibodies against HLA, ABO, or other antigens.[192] Irreversible rapid destruction of the graft occurs. Histologically there is glomerular thrombosis, fibrinoid necrosis, and polymorphonuclear leukocyte infiltration. In the early years of transplantation, when the HLA matching techniques were not well developed, hyperacute rejection was more common. In most centers, it occurs very rarely. The latest data from the NAPRTCS show the incidence of hyperacute rejection to be less than 0.25% (17 cases) over the last 15 years. The only treatment is surgical removal of the allograft.

Acute Rejection

Information regarding the incidence and outcome of acute rejection in pediatric renal transplantation is available from the NAPRTCS data. Because NAPRTCS receives data from multiple sites that utilize many different diagnostic and treatment protocols, the definition of a rejection episode is based upon the circumstance of a patient having been treated with anti-rejection therapy, although biopsy confirmation is becoming more common. In a review of 8777 rejection episodes over a 15-year study, there were, on average, 0.89 rejection episodes for each LD transplant and 1.23 for each CAD transplant. A remarkable decrease in the incidence of acute rejection has occurred over the past 15 years (Table 40–5). In a study of two cohorts of pediatric renal transplant recipient (1469 in 1987–1989; 1189 in 1997–1999), the rejection ratios dropped from 1.6 to 0.7 per patient.[193] Sixty percent of the latter group were rejection-free compared to 29% of the former, and 1-year graft survival was 94% compared to 80%. Historically, over half of the patients experienced a rejection in the first post-transplant weeks, now the majority experiences a rejection-free first year. Risk factors for cadaver source transplants include the absence of prophylactic T-cell antibody therapy, donor age less than 5 years, black race, and no DR matches. Risk factors for living-related source transplants are the absence of T-cell antibody and one or two DR mismatches, black race, and ATN. In an earlier study the NAPRTCS noted that when reviewed by age groupings, rejection

Table 40–5 12-Month Probability (%) of First Rejection, by Transplant Year

Transplant Year	Living Donor %	Living Donor SE	Cadaver Donor %	Cadaver Donor SE
1987-1990	54.2	1.7	69.2	1.4
1991-1994	45.2	1.5	60.8	1.6
1995-1998	34.0	1.4	41.0	1.7
1999-2002	27.2	1.8	31.2	2.5

Adapted from Seikaly M, Ho PL, Emmett L, Tejani A: The 12th Annual Report of the North American Pediatric Renal Transplant Cooperative Study: Renal transplantation from 1987 through 1998 (updated at www.naprtcs.org). Pediatr Transplant 2001; 5:215-231.

ratios, time to first rejection, and the mean number of rejection episodes were not different; however, for the initial rejection episode, recipients less than 6 years of age had significantly increased irreversible rejections leading to graft loss.[23] There are conflicting data about whether infants and small children have a "heightened" immune response and an increased incidence of acute rejection episodes. Indirect evidence suggested a more vigorous immune response, especially in infants.[194] Also, data from the UNOS registry demonstrated a higher rate of acute rejections in young children after both living donor and cadaver donor transplantation, although adolescents were noted to have a higher rate of late acute rejections.[14] On the other hand, data from surveillance transplant biopsies suggest equivalent rejection responses in all groups.[31] Data from one large pediatric transplant program demonstrated that infants have a lower rate of acute rejection than older children.[33] A recent SRTR report demonstrated that infants and young children now have the best outcomes of all age groups.[12] Thus, either the proposed heightened immune response has been overcome by improved immunosuppression or the cause of previously poor outcome was related to other factors.

Diagnosis of Acute Rejection

Rejection is suspected when there is decreasing urinary outflow and a rising serum creatinine. In the past, classic signs of acute rejection included fever and graft tenderness. Under calcineurin inhibitors and prophylactic antibody therapy, however, these signs are rarely seen; thus, early evidence of graft dysfunction even without other signs, should initiate concern. The differential diagnosis consists of ureteral obstruction, renal artery stenosis, urinary leak, and an infectious process. When rejection is suspected, a urinalysis and urine culture should be performed to assess the possibility of infection. The urinalysis is also helpful if it suggests intragraft inflammation or an acute immune response as evidenced by proteinuria and the presence of leukocytes and other cells in the sediment. Blood or urinary cytokine analysis may also be useful for diagnosing rejection,[195,196] and examination of the sediment may be useful in detecting other reasons for graft dysfunction. An ultrasound is performed to rule out anatomic obstruction. Obstruction can be the result of perirenal fluid collection, a large lymphocele, hematoma, or rarely, an abscess. The ultrasound can also provide information about intragraft blood flow and pressure.[86] A radionuclide renal scan, using a tracer such as MAG 3, is a very helpful tool in establishing some diagnoses (Figures 40–2 to 40–4).[197] Rejection is suggested by rapid uptake of the tracer by the kidney but a delayed excretion. Unfortunately, radionuclide scans cannot distinguish among various causes of intragraft dysfunction, such as rejection, cyclosporine toxicity, and ATN. Thus, a definitive diagnosis of rejection requires a transplant biopsy.

Renal Transplant Biopsy

The renal transplant biopsy procedure is very easy and safe when conscious sedation and ultrasound guidance are utilized. Recent data evaluating over 150 pediatric renal transplant biopsies, including some in intraperitoneal kidneys and many perfomed during the first week post-transplantation, have demonstrated a very low risk.[87] One factor in reducing post-biopsy bleeding is the use of an automated biopsy "guns" using a small (18-gauge) rather than the standard (15-gauge) needle. Biopsies should be performed in pediatric renal transplant recipients whenever the diagnosis of rejection is in doubt.

Treatment of Acute Rejection

Standard treatment of an episode of acute rejection is intravenous methylprednisolone in a single daily dose of 20 to 25 mg/kg (maximum dose: 0.5 to 1 g), for 3 consecutive days. Most grades I and II rejections will respond to steroid therapy. Steroid resistant rejection episodes are treated with T-cell antibody, either the monoclonal OKT3 or the polyclonal antithymocyte globulin (Atgam or Thymoglobulin). OKT3 is administered in the dose of 2.5 mg for children with a body weight of 30 kg and 5 mg for children over 30 kg for 10 to 14 days. Atgam is given in the dose of 15 mg/kg, through a central venous catheter, for 10 to 14 days, depending upon the white cell and platelet count, because it will frequently deplete all formed elements in the blood system. It is advisable to maintain the white blood cell count above 2000/mm^3 and the platelet count above 20,000/mm^3. Thymoglobulin is given in a dose of 1.5 to 2 mg/kg/dose for a total of 10 to 14 days. It may be advisable to monitor CD3+ cells during treatment and restrict the frequency of dosing to days only when the count is greater than 20 cells/mm^3.[108] All antibodies have several side effects. Of concern are the first dose symptoms of OKT3 due to cytokine release.[111,112] This is clinically observed as fever with chills and, rarely, as pulmonary edema. Antipyretics, such as acetaminophen, should be given every 4 hours, and the administration of the antibody should be preceded by a bolus dose of 500 mg of methylprednisolone 1 hour prior to administration. Respiratory compromise, in the form of fluid extravasating into the pulmonary capillary bed, is seen only in patients with fluid overload. Fluid removal by dialysis should be considered prior to the administration of OKT3 in patients whose body weight exceeds 5% of their baseline. Precaution against the potential anaphylactic reaction related to polyclonal antibodies consists of using 500 mg of methylprednisone with the infusion of the antibody and administration of an antihistamine, such as diphenhydramine (Benadryl), 30 minutes prior to drug administration.

Reversibility of Acute Rejection

NAPRTCS data observe that among LD kidneys, 55% of rejection episodes are completely reversed, 40% are partially reversed, and 5% end in graft failure. Similar figures for CAD kidneys are 48%, 45%, and 7%, respectively.[24] When stratified by age, young transplant recipients have irreversible rejection episodes more frequently. Ten percent of acute rejections among infants receiving a LD kidney end in graft failure, compared to 4% for older children. For CAD kidneys the rate of graft failure in infants is 15%, compared to 7% for older children. Despite decreasing rejection frequency, complete reversal for pediatric living donor recipients seems to be improving in later cohort years. Molecular or genomic characterization of rejection biopsies may be helpful in describing different types of acute rejection.[195,196,198–200]

Rescue Therapy

In those patients in whom neither steroids nor antibody therapy have successfully reversed a rejection episode conversion to an alternative calcineurin inhibitor or to other immunosuppressants would appear to be warranted. There have been no controlled studies to document reversal of rejection with conversion to tacrolimus; however, anecdotal reports do suggest that in some cases conversion does help to stabilize graft function.[133,134,168]

Chronic Rejection

The gradation from acute to chronic rejection is gradual; however, many biopsies may show features of both, and some characteristic vascular changes of chronic rejection may be seen as early as 10 days post-transplant.[201] The clinical picture is that of gradually declining renal function together with varying degrees of proteinuria and hypertension. The clinical condition may also be referred to as *transplant glomerulopathy.* An ongoing controversy exists as to whether the changes seen in chronic rejection are immune mediated, ischemic in nature, or nonimmunologic injury due to hyperfiltration.[202,203] Data in children have shown clearly that acute rejection is a predictor of chronic rejection.[146] In a study of 1699 LD and 1795 CAD patients, the NAPRTCS noted that acute rejection was a relative risk (RR) factor for chronic rejection (RR = 3.1), and multiple acute rejections increased the RR to 4.3. Late acute rejections are also clinical correlates of chronic rejection.[204] Even if acute rejection is the most critical element in the genesis of chronic rejection, other immune mechanisms may mediate its progression. One possible explanation would be that in patients who go on to develop chronic rejection, the immune mediators of acute rejection, such as granzyme B, perforin and Fas ligand, are expressed in a more robust fashion and are quantitatively different from the responses of an acute rejection that does not lead to chronic rejection. Alternatively, the immune mediators of chronic rejection may be qualitatively different from those associated with an acute episode. For example, the multifunctional cytokine TGF-β1, which has fibrogenic properties, is present in biopsy tissue of patients with chronic rejection.[205] Identification of the mechanism of initiation or progression of chronic rejection will be vital to any attempts to control it.

Management of Chronic Rejection

Symptomatic therapy is currently the only available method of dealing with chronic rejection. Hypertension should be controlled, and the proteinuria may occasionally respond to ACE inhibitors; however, renal function will continue to decline. In children, chronic rejection produces an additional burden because decreased renal function will result in deceleration of growth.[206,207] It is in this context that prevention of chronic rejection by early aggressive therapy in patients who have had an episode of acute rejection may be rewarding. Because currently available immunosuppressive medications have been unsuccessful in preventing or slowing the progression of chronic rejection, the use of immunosuppressives, other than those currently approved, may be reasonable.

GRAFT SURVIVAL

Pediatric renal centers reporting graft survival show varying results. Because the number of patients at any one center is small, such data cannot represent the pediatric transplant population at large. Furthermore, multiple factors affect graft survival, such as donor and recipient age, histocompatibility matching, recipient race, and so forth. Thus, there cannot be accurate descriptions of graft survival rates without classification of the important variables. To obtain a proper population mix representing gender, age, and racial diversity, the NAPRTCS annual reports have been used.[13]

A total of 2201 graft failures occurred from 8399 (26%) transplants. Of index transplants 1924 of 7651 (23%) failed, whereas 277 of 748 (37%) subsequent transplants had graft failure. Of the failures, 1648 (75%) were returned to dialysis, and 132 (6%) were retransplanted at the time of failure. Table 40–6

Table 40–6 Cause of Graft Failure

	Index Graft Failures		Subsequent Graft Failures		All Graft Failures	
	N	%	N	%	N	%
Total	**1924**	**100**	**227**	**100**	**2201**	**100**
Death with functioning graft	183	9.5	21	7.6	204	9.3
Primary non-function	48	2.5	4	1.4	52	2.4
Vascular thrombosis	206	11.0	36	13.0	242	11.0
Other technical	29	1.5	4	1.4	33	1.5
Hyper-acute rejection < 24 hours	13	0.7	4	1.4	17	0.8
Accelerated acute rejection 2-7 days	32	1.7	8	2.9	40	1.8
Acute rejection	267	14.0	36	13.0	303	14.0
Chronic rejection	628	33.0	93	34.0	721	33.0
Recurrece of original disease	121	6.3	25	9.0	146	6.6
Renal atery stenosis	15	0.8	–	–	15	0.7
Bacterial / viral infection	39	2.0	40	1.4	43	2.0
Cyclosporine toxicity	10	0.5	–	–	10	0.5
De nova disease	6	0.3	2	0.7	8	0.4
Patient discontinued medication	93	4.8	8	2.9	101	4.6
Malignancy	27	1.4	101	4.6	28	1.3
Other / Unknown	99	5.1	16	5.8	115	5.2

Adapted from Seikaly M, Ho PL, Emmett L, Tejani A: The 12th Annual Report of the North American Pediatric Renal Transplant Cooperative Study: Renal transplantation from 1987 through 1998 (updated at www.naprtcs.org). Pediatr Transplant 2001; 5:215-231.

provides the distribution of causes of graft failure. With increased length of follow-up, chronic rejection continues to increase in importance. It is now the most common cause of graft failure. Overall, 47% of graft failures are caused by rejection with chronic rejection accounting for 33% and acute rejection accounting for 14%. Recurrence of original disease as a cause of graft failure was observed 146 times (focal segmental glomerulosclerosis, 66; membranoproliferative glomerulonephritis type II, 13; oxalosis, 10; hemolytic uremic syndrome, 16; chronic glomerulonephritis, 6; and others, 35). Vascular thrombosis remains a major cause of failure, and 204 graft failures were attributed to primary nonfunction, vascular thrombosis, or miscellaneous technical causes. These data show that such problems occur in 3.8% of pediatric transplants.[91–93,95–97,208]

Overall 5-year graft survival curves by donor source are shown in Figure 40–5. Current graft survival for index transplants at 1, 3, and 5 years for LD kidneys is 95%, 90%, and 83%, respectively, and for CAD kidneys it is 91%, 82%, and 73%, which are substantially better than previous results (Table 40–7). Table 40–8 shows relative hazards for graft failure for selected transplant characteristics for both LD and CAD kidneys. Five-year graft survival rates by selected variables for LD grafts are shown in Figure 40–6, and for CAD grafts survival rates are shown in Figure 40–7. An important trend in improved graft survival in pediatric LD and CAD renal transplant outcome has been reported,[12,121] and the most recent data are shown in Figures 40–8 and 40–9.

Registry based graft survival data can be used to establish risk factors. Relative risks of graft failure are derived using Cox proportional hazards regression models. For LD kidneys the risk factors for graft failure include blacks (RH = 1.88), more than five prior transfusions (RH = 1.41), and absence of HLA-B matches (RH = 1.39) (Table 40–8). No induction antibody is also a risk factor (1.13), as is transplant era (0.95).[13] A similar risk factor analysis for CAD kidneys has been reported,[13,24,209] and the most recent data are presented in Table 40–8. The risk factors are similar to those seen with LD grafts with additional hazards, such as young recipient age (RH = 1.80), young donor age, and prolonged cold ischemia time (RH = 1.20). Some factors that increase the relative risk of cadaver graft failure in children, such as recipient age, are integral to pediatrics. Other factors, such as recipient race, the degree of HLA matching, and prior transplantation, cannot be easily altered. Improvement in cadaver allograft survival rates, however, can be achieved by judicious choice of donors, pre-transplant management, changes of induction therapy, and optimal immunosuppressive therapy.[23]

Table 40–7 Percent Graft Survival by Source and Era

		Years Past Transplant		
		1	3	5
Living Donor	1995-2001	94.5%	90.0%	83.1%
	1987-1994	90.1%	83.5%	77.8%
Cadaver Donor	1995-2001	90.8%	81.9%	73.4%
	1987-1994	79.9%	69.6%	61.8%

Adapted from Seikaly M, Ho PL, Emmett L, Tejani A: The 12th Annual Report of the North American Pediatric Renal Transplant Cooperative Study: Renal transplantation from 1987 through 1998 (updated at *www.naprtcs.org*). Pediatr Transplant 2001; 5:215-231.

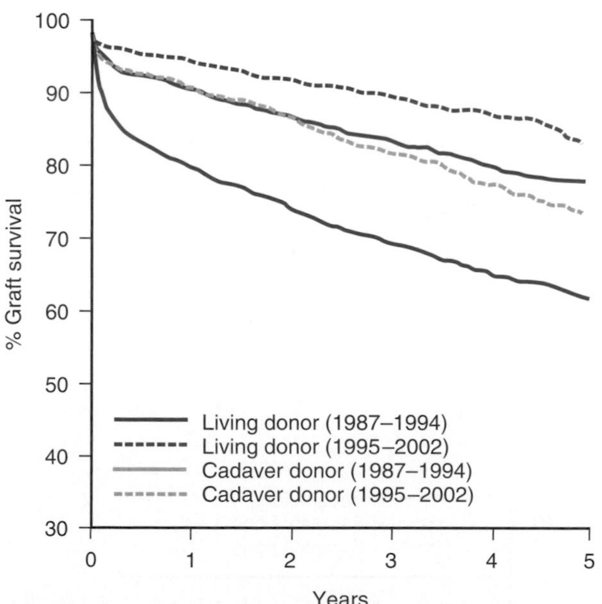

Figure 40–5 Five-year actuarial graft survival in children from LD and CAD renal transplantation. (Data adapted from Seikaly M, Ho PL, Emmett L, Tejani A: The 12th Annual Report of the North American Pediatric Renal Transplant Cooperative Study: Renal transplantation from 1987 through 1998 (updated at www.naprtcs.org). Pediatr Transplant 2001; 5:215-231, with permission.)

Another measure of long-term graft function is the calculation of graft half-life. A recent analysis of 8922 pediatric and 78,418 adult renal transplants demonstrated superior long-term graft function in young pediatric recipients.[14] Infants (ages 0–2) had the worst 1-year graft survival rates (71%) compared to children (ages 3–12) (83%), adolescents (ages 13–21) (85%), and adults (86%). However, for all grafts that survived at least 1 year, infants had the longest projected half-life (18 years), compared to children (11 years), adolescents (7 years), and adults (11 years). A similar analysis of UNOS data showed that young recipients who received adult donor kidneys and had immediate graft function had projected half-lives greater than 25 years, better than even HLA-identical adult donor-recipient pairs.[210]

The primary disease causing ESRD can have an effect on graft survival. Children with oxalosis used to have very bad outcomes, to the extent that the diagnosis was considered a contraindication to transplantation. However, improvements in outcome related to combined liver-kidney transplantation have been encouraging.[29,47–49] Similarly, infants with congenital nephrotic syndrome often had very poor outcomes,[48,211] but strategies designed to reduce the risk of thrombosis and to improve nutrition pre-transplantation have led to marked improvements.[50–52,94] Focal segmental glomerulosclerosis (FSGS) can be a devastating disease that recurs very quickly following renal transplantation, sometimes as early as the first post-transplant day.[211–215] Although recurrence is no more frequent in LD transplants, the graft survival advantage of LD transplantation is lost for children with FSGS.[216] Little is known about the pathophysiology of the disorder or the cause for recurrence.[217,218] There are sev-

Table 40–8 Relative Hazard Analysis for Graft Failure in Multivariate Proportional Hazards Model

	Living Donor		Cadaver Donor	
	RH	**P-Value**	**RH**	**P-Value**
Recipient Age (<2)	1.02	NS	1.80	<.0001
Prior Transplant	1.30	NS	1.41	<.0001
No Induction Antibody	1.13	.0090	1.14	.0430
>5 Lifetime Transfusions	1.41	.0003	1.32	<.0001
No HLA-B Matches	1.39	.0180	1.19	.0067
No HLA-DR Matches	1.09	NS	1.21	.0022
Black Race	1.88	<.0001	1.55	<.0001
Prior Dialysis	1.20	.0240	1.29	.0130
Cold Storage Time >24 Hours	—	—	1.20	.0060
Transplant Year	0.95	.0001	0.93	<.0001

Adapted from Seikaly M, Ho PL, Emmett L, Tejani A: The 12th Annual Report of the North American Pediatric Renal Transplant Cooperative Study: Renal transplantation from 1987 through 1998 (updated at *www.naprtcs.org*). Pediatr Transplant 2001; 5:215-231.

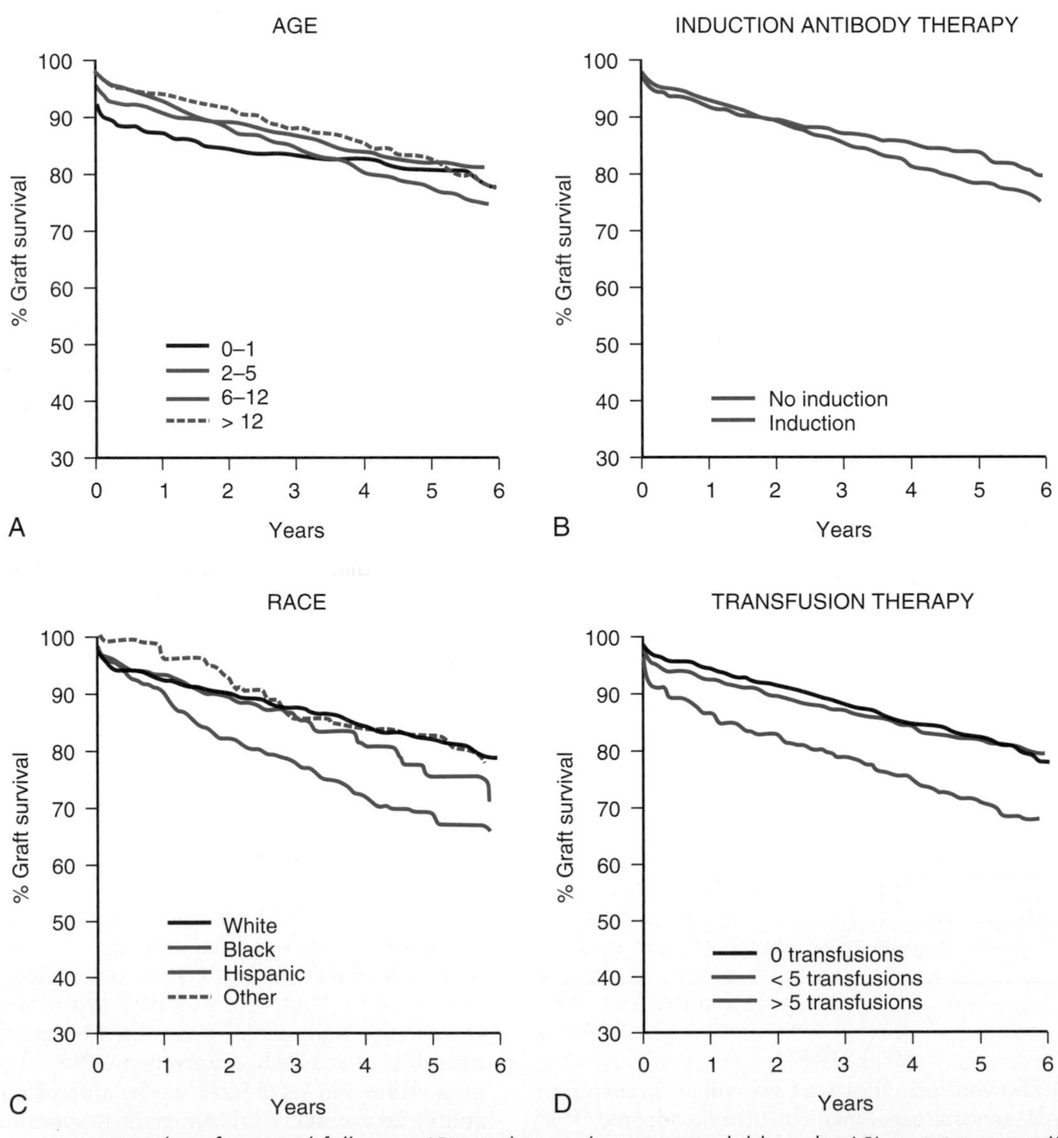

Figure 40–6 Five-year actuarial graft survival following LD renal transplantation in children, by (***A***) recipient age, (***B***) presence of antibody induction, (***C***) race, and (***D***) number of pre-transplant blood transfusions. (Data adapted from Seikaly M, Ho PL, Emmett L, Tejani A: The 12th Annual Report of the North American Pediatric Renal Transplant Cooperative Study: Renal transplantation from 1987 through 1998 [updated at www.naprtcs.org]. Pediatr Transplant 2001; 5:215-231, with permission.)

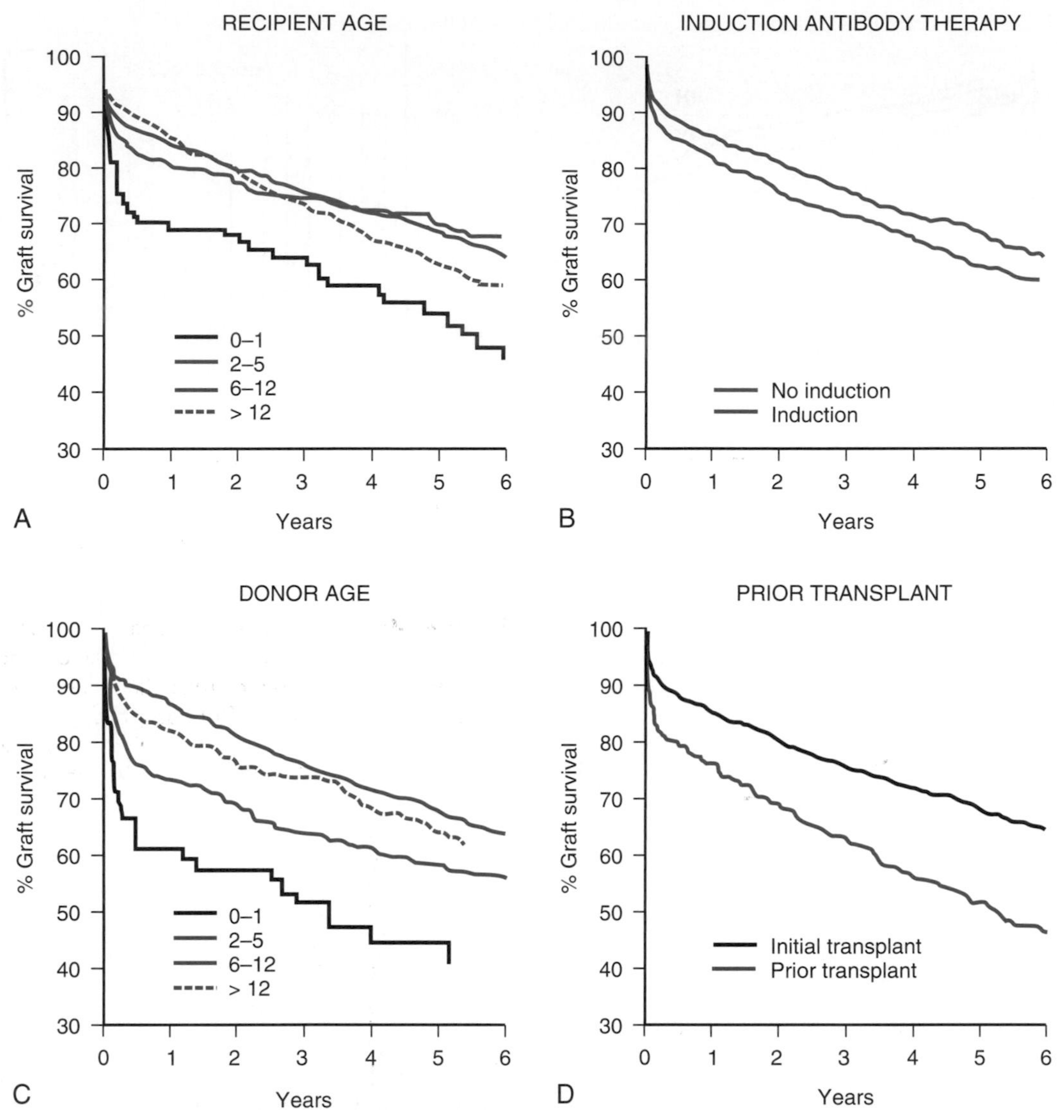

Figure 40–7 Five-year actuarial graft survival following CAD renal transplantation in children, by (***A***) recipient age, (***B***) presence of antibody induction, (***C***) donor age, and (***D***) prior transplant. (Data adapted from Seikaly M, Ho PL, Emmett L, Tejani A: The 12th Annual Report of the North American Pediatric Renal Transplant Cooperative Study: Renal transplantation from 1987 through 1998 [updated at www.naprtcs.org]. Pediatr Transplant 2001; 5:215-231, with permission.)

eral proposed approaches to preventing or treating recurrence, mostly involving enhanced immunosuppression with plasmapheresis.[215,219–224] Lupus nephritis surprisingly does not recur following renal transplantation to any great extent. Patients with lupus have similar outcomes compared to other patients,[225,226] except for a slight increase in mortality,[226] an increase in incidence of recurrent rejections, and a slight tendency to graft failure in those patients receiving CAD grafts following peritoneal dialysis.[225] Children with sickle cell disease and ESRD can receive kidney transplants successfully,[227] as can those with Down syndrome.[228,229] Hemolytic uremic syndrome (HUS) has been variably described as likely to recur or not.[211,230] After distinguishing the etiologic factors, epidemic shiga toxin-associated hemolytic syndrome is unlikely to recur following renal transplantation,[231,232] whereas atypical or familial HUS may recur with devastating and irreversible consequences.[232]

GROWTH FOLLOWING TRANSPLANTATION

A major distinguishing feature of pediatric from adult recipients is the need for children to grow. The growth failure commonly observed in children at the time of transplantation is multifactorial; however, the most important cause is the reduced response to endogenous growth hormone,[40] related to several mechanisms. Growth failure often begins insidiously early in the course of chronic renal insufficiency. In a NAPRTCS analysis of 1768 children with CKD (glomerular

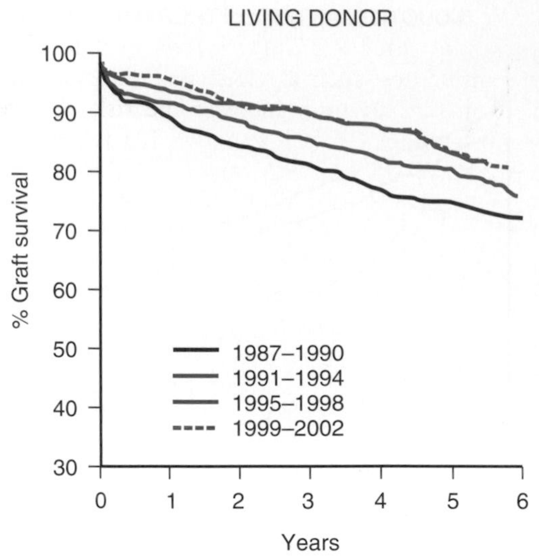

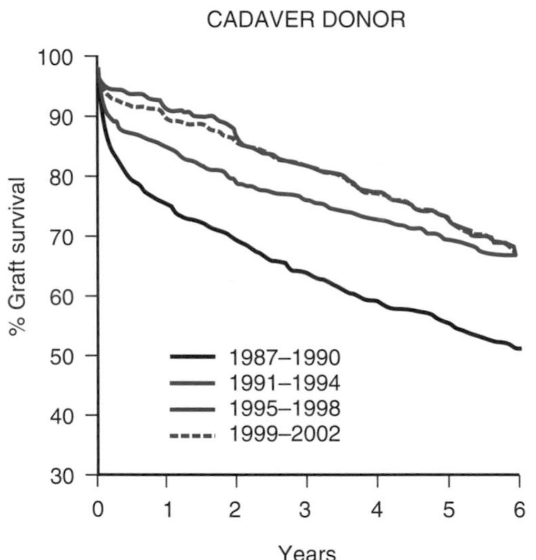

Figure 40–8 Actuarial graft survival CAD graft survival by year of renal transplantation. (Data adapted from Seikaly M, Ho PL, Emmett L, Tejani A: The 12th Annual Report of the North American Pediatric Renal Transplant Cooperative Study: Renal transplantation from 1987 through 1998 [updated at www.naprtcs.org]. Pediatr Transplant 2001; 5:215-231, with permission.)

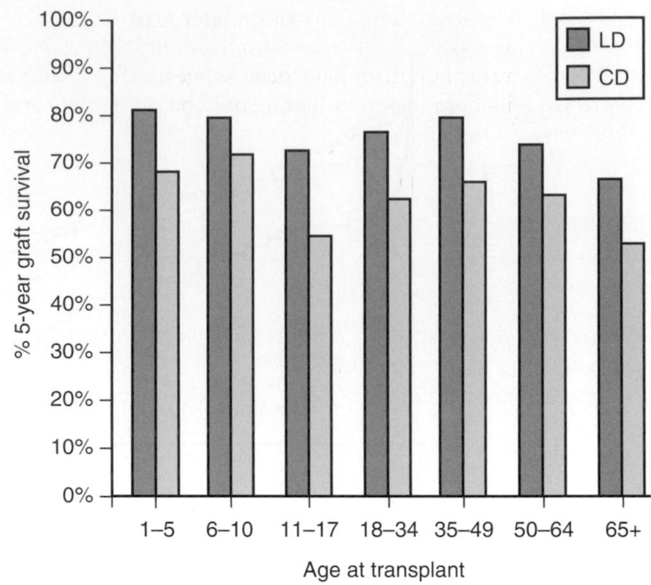

Figure 40–9 Five-rear actuarial patient survival following LD and CAD renal transplantation in children and adults by recipient age. Young children currently have the best long-term outcomes of all age groups. (Data adapted from Colombani PM, Dunn SP, Harmon WE, et al: Pediatric transplantation. Am J Transplant 2003; 3[suppl 4]:53-63, with permission.)

filtration rate <75/mL/min/m²), over one third had a height deficit of more than 2 SDS. It has been amply demonstrated that chronic renal insufficiency beginning in infancy leads to permanent reduction in growth potential.[233] Growth retardation continues in children on a dialysis regime, whether the mode of dialysis is peritoneal or hemodialysis. For several years it has been suggested that a functioning transplant would enable the child to achieve catch-up growth.[7] Unfortunately, long-term data from registry studies have shown a more disappointing outcome.

NAPRTCS data show that the mean height deficit at the time of transplantation is −1.88. Males (−1.92) and younger recipients have greater height deficits at the time of transplantation.[13] Younger children can show catch-up growth with complete inversion of Z-score up to 0.60 at 2 years for those less than 5 years of age at transplant. Older children may grow at a normal rate but rarely show catch-up growth. The Z-score for 19-year-olds is −1.5. Final adult height for children with ESRD is improving, but all of the improvements seem to be related to the gains achieved during treatment for CKD rather than after transplantation.[8]

These studies on long-term growth post-transplantation are disappointing; however, they do focus on mechanisms that prevent growth, despite a milieu with normal renal function. Individual center studies have adopted a variety of techniques, such as discontinuation of prednisone,[234,235] alternate-day steroid therapy,[169,170,236] steroid avoidance,[6] or the use of recombinant human growth hormone.[237] It has been known for several years that steroids used for immunosuppressive therapy will inhibit growth.[165] It has also been demonstrated that steroids affect growth hormone secretion.[206,238–240] Measurements of pulsatile and pharmacologically stimulated hormone release reveal that steroids play an inhibitory role.[165,241] Conversion of children to alternate-day steroid therapy has shown improvement in growth[169,170]; however, the best catch-up growth is seen in patients completely withdrawn from steroids.[6,134,166] Numerous uncontrolled studies have shown that steroids can be withdrawn from children post-transplantation[6,134,242]; however, acute rejection tends to occur shortly afterwards in many of these patients,[167] with marked detrimental long-term effects. An alternative method of attaining catch-up growth post-transplantation would be the use of growth hormone. Recombinant human growth hormone is not approved for use in children post-transplantation; however, numerous uncontrolled studies have shown its ability to accelerate growth in this setting.[243] Several complications of the use of rhGH post-transplantation have been suggested,[243–246] but a controlled trial demonstrated that it could be used safely and effectively.[247]

MORBIDITY

Hospitalization

The median duration of hospitalization at the time of transplantation in the most recent NAPRTCS report was 13 days, with longer stays required for young patients and for recipients of CAD transplants.[13] The mean hospital stay has fallen by about 8 days between 1987 and 2001. Most children require rehospitalization at least once after the initial discharge after renal transplantation. Fifty percent of LD recipients and 62% of CAD recipients are hospitalized during the first 6 post-transplant months. The hospitalization rate falls with increasing time after transplantation, but 16% require at least one hospital stay in the fourth post-transplant year.[24] The most common reason for hospitalization used to be for treatment of rejection. However, a recent analysis supports that treatment of viral and bacterial infections are the next most common reasons for hospitalization.[248] The most common bacterial infection in children less than or equal to 5 years of age is *Clostridium difficile* diarrhea and urinary tract infection for those greater than 5 years of age.[33] CMV appears to be the most common viral infection in older children. Treatment for hypertension is the cause for hospitalization in the first 6 months in 5% to 8% of recipients and falls to approximately 1% at 5 years after transplantation.[24]

Post-Transplant Lymphoproliferative Disease and Malignancy (PTLD)

Although PTLD has been reported as a complication of pediatric organ transplantation for many years,[249] the number of published reports seem to be increasing.[250] It is not clear whether this indicates that the incidence of this potentially lethal complication of immunosuppression is increasing or if it is just more readily recognized. If the incidence is increasing, it may be the unfortunate consequence of "improved" immunosuppression.[144] In a review of UNOS data, the most incidence of PTLD following pediatric renal transplantation is clearly increasing, and those who are less than 18 years of age, Caucasian, and male gender are significant risk factors.[251] Current incidence appears to be 1% to 2% of all pediatric renal transplants.

PTLD often presents within lymph nodes, but it can be extra-nodal, frequently occurring within the gastrointestinal tract,[252] proximate to or within the graft,[253] or distant from it.[254] Presentation of PTLD within the central nervous system is often devastating and rapidly fatal. PTLD is generally thought to emanate from EBV infection.[252,255,256] Thus, the pre-transplant EBV status of the donor and recipient may be an important determinant of the disease and may explain why the disease is more common in children than in adults.[257,258] In several reports, the incidence rate of PTLD for EBV-seronegative recipients was many times higher than that for EBV-seropositive recipients[259,260] and, in others, the source was the donor in most of the cases.[261] Concomitant primary infection with CMV may increase the risk of PTLD fivefold.[259] The intensity of immunosuppression may also predispose the child to PTLD.[262] Treatment with antilymphocyte antibodies, such as OKT3, as either induction or antirejection therapy, may increase the risk of developing PTLD substantially.[259,260,263] Although it has been reported following both cyclosporine and tacrolimus treatment, programs that have used both drugs have suggested that the incidence was higher in tacrolimus-treated recipients.[144,257,264] However, a recent registry report suggests that neither MMF nor tacrolimus were independent risk factors for PTLD; rather, the intensity of immunosuppression was most important.[145]

The diagnosis of PTLD has generally been made on the basis of characteristic pathologic findings, and the diagnosis cannot be made without biopsy material. Advances in detection of EBV DNA[265–269] and in the outgrowth of transformed lymphocytes[270,271] have permitted early detection of patients at high risk to develop PTLD. Surveillance of blood and prospective adjustment of immunosuppression has been proposed, but there are no universally-accepted standards in this area.[272] Similar tests have been used also to guide treatment,[265] but their absolute value for this function is not established.

The mainstay of treatment of PTLD is the reduction or discontinuation of immunosuppression.[261,273,274] Of interest, in many of these cases, the graft is not rejected despite the marked lowering or discontinuation of immunosuppressive medications. Interferon-α and intravenous γ-globulin,[275,276] ganciclovir,[277] and even chemotherapy have been suggested, but their efficacy has been variable. Prophylaxis of high-risk patients may be useful.[278] Recently, treatment with the monoclonal antibody rituximab has shown promising results.[279–283]

Other Infections

Immunosuppression renders the recipient susceptible to numerous viral and bacterial infections. Infections account for the majority of complications post-transplantation in children and are the principle cause of morbidity. Prophylactic therapy against the more common infections seen in the context of a renal transplantation is employed by most centers.

Cytomegalovirus (CMV)

CMV is an extremely important cause of infectious complications affecting transplant recipients. Unlike the situation seen in nonimmunocompromised individuals, cytomegalovirus infection in renal allograft recipients more often causes serious symptoms. CMV presents as a primary infection in seronegative patients; in seropositive patients the infection is secondary due to reactivation of the patient's own latent virus. Clinically, the two types cannot be distinguished although the former is generally more severe. Because of the high risk to the patient and renal allograft, prophylactic therapy is indicated for all seronegative patients who receive a seropositive kidney and for all patients who receive induction with a T-cell antibody. Prophylaxis can be carried out using either specific antiviral therapy or with high-titer CMV immunoglobulin, or both. The incidence of virologically confirmed CMV-associated syndromes was reduced from 60% in controls to 21% in recipients of CMV immune globulin. CMV immunoglobulin is generally given in the first 4 months post-transplantation. Both acyclovir[284] and ganciclovir[285] have been shown to be effective as prophylactic therapy; however, the latter should replace the former since the introduction of an oral preparation has been shown to be highly efficacious.[286,287] The dose of oral ganciclovir is 500 to 700 mg/m^2 every 8 hours.[288] There have been no controlled trials of CMV immunoglobulin versus ganciclovir, so the relative merits and indications of the two preparations are unknown, although the former seems to ameliorate the severity of CMV disease, whereas the latter decreases the frequency.

Pneumocystis Carinii Pneumonia (PCP)

Because of their defective cellular immunity, transplant patients are susceptible to respiratory infections by opportunistic organisms that are not of concern to normal children. Pneumonia is a common cause of morbidity in children with a renal allograft, and *Pneumocystis carinii* is the most important cause, occurring in about 3% of all renal transplant recipients.[289] Pneumocystis produces a diffuse pneumonia in which shortness of breath and hypoxemia are salient features. If diagnosed quickly it can be treated effectively; however, delay can be fatal and hence prophylaxis is standard therapy in most centers. The risk is highest in the first month and treatment with SMX-TMP in the dose of 10 mg/kg (trimethoprim component) three times per week should be given during the period of highest risk.

Varicella

Chickenpox is one of the constant worries of both the transplant physician and the patient's family, since exposure in the pediatric age range is extremely high.[33] The rash in an immunocompromised patient may become confluent, bullous, and hemorrhagic. If the disease becomes systemic, the fatality rate can be high.[290] Treatment of varicella in immunocompromised children generally consists of intravenous acyclovir at least until all lesions are crusted.[289,291] Prophylaxis, consisting of the administration of varicella zoster immunoglobulin (VZIG), is carried out routinely in all transplanted seronegative children upon exposure.[289] The administration of varicella vaccine (Varivax) prior to transplantation substantially reduces the frequency and severity of the disease post-transplant.[292] The use of varicella vaccine post-transplantation has been reported in only a small series,[293] but it is likely safe, although not uniformly successful.

Urinary Tract Infection (UTI)

UTI are extremely common during the first 3 months post-transplant and may be seen in as many as 50% of patients.[33,294] It appears that beyond the first 3 months episodes of asymptomatic bacteruria are more common. However, during the first 3 months UTI may be a common source of bacteremia.[295] Chemoprophylaxis, by the administration of SMX-TMP as described for *P. carinii*, should be provided in the first month in all patients and may be continued up to 1 year in patients whose original disease was urologic in origin.

Polyoma Virus

Polyoma BK virus infection may be an increasingly important cause of graft dysfunction and graft loss following renal transplantation,[296] but there has been little information about its frequency or severity in children. In one retrospective analysis of 100 pediatric renal transplants, 26 had BK virus detected in urine and 5 in blood.[297] Those with viremia had elevated serum creatinines and evidence of interstitial nephritis on graft biopsies. Screening of susceptible patients by urine analysis for BK messenger RNA has been proposed,[298] but proper therapeutic treatments in response to rising titers have not been identified.

Hypertension

The incidence of hypertension post-transplant is demonstrated in a NAPRTCS study wherein 70% of patients required antihypertensive medications at 1 month post-transplant; the incidence decreased to 59% at 24 months.[299] Hypertension may be detected more common if ambulatory blood pressure monitoring methods are used.[300,301] Hypertension post-transplant is primarily related to the side effects of drug therapy. The two most widely used immunosuppressives: calcineurin inhibitors and prednisone both exacerbate preexisting hypertension. Hypertension has been correlated with multiple complications of transplantation, including reduced graft survival and cardiovascular complications.[302–305]

Antihypertensive Therapy

With dose reduction of prednisone and calcineurin inhibitors almost all hypertensive patients can be managed, though multiple drug regimens may be necessary in some patients. An effective and safe drug to use is a calcium channel blocker, such as nifedipine, which also reduces cyclosporine toxicity (nifedipine may exacerbate gum enlargement, however).[119,306] Another drug particularly favored in adolescent patients due to concerns of noncompliance is clonidine, which is available in a transdermal patch. Clonidine may induce drowsiness, and sudden withdrawal tends to produce rebound hypertension. In patients who complain of palpitations due to drug-induced reflux tachycardia, prazosin is more effective because it induces the least amount of tachycardia. Minoxidil, an acute vasodilator, should only be used with severe hypertension and for only a limited duration because it causes hirsutism. ACE inhibitors should be used with caution because converting enzyme inhibition in a single kidney model leads to reduction in the glomerular filtration.[307,308]

Hyperlipidemia

Steroids, calcineurin inhibitors, and sirolimus induce hyperlipidemia. A fall in serum cholesterol levels on conversion from cyclosporine to azathioprine has been demonstrated.[309] The mechanism by which calcineurin inhibitors might increase plasma cholesterol is unclarified. The drugs are highly lipophylic and up to 80% is transported in plasma by binding to lipoproteins, particularly LDL. It is conceivable that the binding to LDL cholesterol results in impaired clearance of LDL from the circulation via cell-surface receptors.[310] Post-transplant hyperlipidemia in adults has an adverse effect on cardiovascular morbidity.[311,312] NAPRTCS reviewed post-transplant patients maintained under a rigid common protocol of immunosuppression and observed that at 1 year post-transplant they did exhibit significantly elevated levels of plasma cholesterol and VLDL cholesterol compared to normal controls; however, the elevated cholesterol levels (mean 213 mg/dL) were not high enough to require lipid lowering agents.[313] In cases with higher serum lipid levels (cholesterol 250 mg/dL or greater), 3-hydroxy-3 methylglutaryl (HMG) coenzyme (CoA) reductase inhibitors are particularly effective in reducing total cholesterol levels.[314,315] The use of sirolimus may increase the need for lipid-lowering agents in the future.

Post-Transplant Diabetes Mellitus

Hyperglycemia and post-transplant diabetes mellitus (PTDM) in children may be increasing in frequency.[142] Corticosteroids use leads to peripheral insulin insensitivity and hyperglycemia that is relatively insensitive to exogenous insulin. Steroid withdrawal has led to improvements in this condition.[316] A NAPRTCS study described an overall incidence of less than 3% of pediatric renal transplant recipients, with African-Americans at highest risk.[317] Tacrolimus use was identified as a significant risk factor, a finding confirmed by reports, some with incidence rates exceeding 50%.[133,140–142,318] Tacrolimus may diminish insulin secretion.[143] Treatment may be aided by reducing or eliminating corticosteroid or calcineurin inhibitor doses.[316,319]

Noncompliance

Noncompliance or nonadherence is often cited as a cause of long-term graft loss in pediatric renal transplant recipients, especially in adolescents. A major reason for noncompliance is thought to be the alteration in appearance that accompanies immunosuppressive medications, including the cushingoid facies and growth retardation related to long-term daily corticosteroid administration and the hirsutism and gingival hypertrophy associated with cyclosporine. However, the true incidence of noncompliance is unknown. Noncompliance rates of 22%,[320] 43%,[321] and as high as 64% in adolescents[322] have been reported. Some factors, such as young age, adolescence, poor socioeconomic status, and family stress have been associated with increased levels of noncompliance.[320,322–324] Importantly, however, health care workers are not able to identify a significant proportion of noncompliant patients.[325] Treatments, such as educational programs[321] and family-based therapy,[326] have been proposed, but these types of programs have not been universally succesful in changing motivation.

LONG-TERM OUTCOME

Rehabilitation

Organ transplantation typically results in dramatic improvement of all aspects of physical, emotional, and social functioning. Importantly, cognitive skills improve after successful renal transplantation,[11] suggesting stabilization of neurophysiologic functioning. Health related quality of life measures are generally good, especially in older children and adolescents, although all ages report some problems with usual activities.[327] Interestingly, the perceived emotional status of the children was actually better than controls, especially during and after adolescence.[327]

Long-term survival is generally excellent,[328] and measures of quality of life have demonstrated excellent rehabilitation in long-term survivors.[329,330] Over 90% have rated health as good or excellent, and most did not feel that health interfered with normal functioning. Most of them were full-time students or employed. The majority were below normal height, and up to a third were dissatisfied with their body appearance. In one report, only a small minority of long-term survivors were married,[331] but, in another, 50% were married and half of those had children.[330]

Mortality

Infection is generally the major cause of death, particularly in the first post-transplant years.[13] Other major causes include cancer/malignancy and cardiopulmonary causes. The best patient survival results are found in older pediatric recipients and in recipients of LD transplants.[48] Risk factors for excess mortality include young recipient age, graft dysfunction (ATN) at day 30 following transplant, and certain underlying renal diseases (oxalosis, congenital nephrotic syndrome, Drash syndrome).[48] Mortality after 10 years post-transplant seems to be related primarily to cardiovascular causes,[328] which may be linked to the hyperlipidemia and hypertension associated with chronic immunosuppression. The mortality rate of children, except for the very youngest, is very low and is generally better than what is found in adults.

References

1. Gaston RS, Alveranga DY, Becker BN, et al: Kidney and pancreas transplantation. Am J Transplant 2003; 3(suppl 4):64-77.
2. Fine RN: Renal transplantation for children: The only realistic choice. Kidney Int Suppl 1985; 17:S15-S17.
3. Warady BA, Hebert D, Sullivan EK, et al: Renal transplantation, chronic dialysis, and chronic renal insufficiency in children and adolescents. The 1995 Annual Report of the North American Pediatric Renal Transplant Cooperative Study. Pediatr Nephrol 1997; 11:49-64.
4. Trachtman H, Hackney P, Tejani A: Pediatric hemodialysis: A decade's (1974-1984) perspective. Kidney Int Suppl 1986; 19: S15-S22.
5. Brouhard BH, Donaldson LA, Lawry KW, et al: Cognitive functioning in children on dialysis and post-transplantation. Pediatr Transplant 2000; 4:261-267.
6. Sarwal MM, Yorgin PD, Alexander S, et al: Promising early outcomes with a novel, complete steroid avoidance immunosuppression protocol in pediatric renal transplantation. Transplantation 2001; 72:13-21.
7. Ingelfinger JR, Grupe WE, Harmon WE, et al: Growth acceleration following renal transplantation in children less than 7 years of age. Pediatrics 1981; 68:255-259.
8. Fine RN, Ho M, Tejani A: North American Pediatric Renal Transplant Cooperative Study. The contribution of renal transplantation to final adult height: A report of the North American Pediatric Renal Transplant Cooperative Study (NAPRTCS). Pediatr Nephrol 2001; 16:951-956.
9. Fine RN: Growth following solid-organ transplantation. Pediatr Transplant 2002; 6:47-52.
10. Mendley SR, Zelko FA: Improvement in specific aspects of neurocognitive performance in children after renal transplantation. Kidney Int 1999; 56:318-323.
11. Fennell EB, Fennell RS, Mings E, Morris MK: The effects of various modes of therapy for end stage renal disease on cognitive performance in a pediatric population: A preliminary report. Int J Pediatr Nephrol 1986; 7:107-112.

12. Colombani PM, Dunn SP, Harmon WE, et al: Pediatric transplantation. Am J Transplant 2003; 3(suppl 4):53-63.
13. Seikaly M, Ho PL, Emmett L, Tejani A: The 12th Annual Report of the North American Pediatric Renal Transplant Cooperative Study: Renal transplantation from 1987 through 1998 (updated at *www.naprtcs.org*). Pediatr Transplant 2001; 5:215-231.
14. Cecka JM, Gjertson DW, Terasaki PI: Pediatric renal transplantation: A review of the UNOS data. Pediatr Transplant 1997; 1:55-64.
15. Neu AM, Stablein DM, Zachary A, et al: Effect of parental donor sex on rejection in pediatric renal transplantation: A report of the North American Pediatric Renal Transplant Cooperative Study. Pediatr Transplant 1998; 2:309-312.
16. Spital A: Should children ever donate kidneys? Views of U.S. transplant centers. Transplantation 1997; 64:232-236.
17. Price DP: Minors as living donors: Ethics and law. Transplant Proc 1996; 28:3607-3608.
18. Delmonico FL, Harmon WE: The use of a minor as a live kidney donor (Comment). Am J Transplant 2002; 2:333-336.
19. Terasaki PI, Cecka JM, Gjertson DW, Takemoto S: High survival rates of kidney transplants from spousal and living unrelated donors (Comments). N Engl J Med 1995; 333:333-336.
20. Al-Uzri A, Sullivan EK, Fine RN, Harmon WE: Living-unrelated renal transplantation in children: a report of the North American Pediatric Renal Transplant Cooperative Study (NAPRTCS). Pediatr Transplant 1998; 2:139-144.
21. Davies DB, Breen TJ, Guo T, et al: Waiting times to pediatric transplantation: An assessment of the August 1990 change in renal allocation policy. Transplant Proc 1994; 26:30-31.
22. McEnery PT, Alexander SR, Sullivan K, Tejani A: Renal transplantation in children and adolescents: The 1992 annual report of the North American Pediatric Renal Transplant Cooperative Study. Pediatr Nephrol 1993; 7:711-720.
23. Tejani A, Stablein D, Alexander S, et al: Analysis of rejection outcomes and implications: A report of the North American Pediatric Renal Transplant Cooperative Study. Transplantation 1995; 59:500-504.
24. Feld LG, Stablein D, Fivush B, et al: Renal transplantation in children from 1987-1996: The 1996 Annual Report of the North American Pediatric Renal Transplant Cooperative Study. Pediatr Transplant 1997; 1:146-162.
25. Filler G, Lindeke A, Bohme K, et al: Renal transplantation from donors aged <6 years into children yields equal graft survival when compared to older donors. Pediatr Transplant 1997; 1:119-123.
26. Hiramoto JS, Freise CE, Randall HR, et al: Successful long-term outcomes using pediatric en bloc kidneys for transplantation. Am J Transplant 2002; 2:337-342.
27. McEnery PT, Stablein DM, Arbus G, Tejani A: Renal transplantation in children. A report of the North American Pediatric Renal Transplant Cooperative Study. N Engl J Med 1992; 326:1727-1732.
28. Briscoe DM, Kim MS, Lillehei C, et al: Outcome of renal transplantation in children less than two years of age. Kidney Int 1992; 42:657-662.
29. Najarian JS, Frey DJ, Matas AJ, et al: Renal transplantation in infants. Ann Surg 1990; 212:353-365.
30. Ingulli E, Matas AJ, Nevins TE, et al: Impact of age on renal graft survival in children after the first rejection episode. Pediatr Nephrol 1996; 10:474-478.
31. Strehlau J, Sharma VK, Pavalakis M, et al: Do children have a heightened immune response to acute allograft rejection? A preliminary comparative study of intragraft gene transcripts of immune activation markers in adult and pediatric graft rejection, 16th Annual Meeting of the American Society of Transplant Physicians (Abstract). Chicago, 1997.
32. Scomik JC, Cecka M: Clinical parameters of immune responsiveness in children and African American transplant patients, 16th Annual Meeting of the American Society of Transplant Physicians (Abstract). Chicago, 1997.
33. Chavers BM, Gillingham KJ, Matas AJ: Complications by age in primary pediatric renal transplant recipients. Pediatr Nephrol 1997; 11:399-403.
34. Schachter AD, Meyers KE, Spaneas LD, et al: Short sirolimus half-life in pediatric renal transplant recipients on a calcineurin inhibitor-free protocol. Pediatr Transplant 2004; 8:171-177.
35. Lemire J, Capparelli EV, Benador N, et al: Neoral pharmacokinetics in Latino and Caucasian pediatric renal transplant recipients. Pediatr Nephrol 2001; 16:311-314.
36. Hoppu K, Koskimies O, Holmberg C, Hirvisalo EL: Pharmacokinetically determined cyclosporine dosage in young children. Pediatr Nephrol 1991; 5:1-4.
37. Ramos EL, Kasiske BL, Alexander SR, et al: The evaluation of candidates for renal transplantation. The current practice of U.S. transplant centers. Transplantation 1994; 57:490-497.
38. Kasiske BL, Ramos EL, Gaston RS, et al: The evaluation of renal transplant candidates: Clinical practice guidelines. Patient Care and Education Committee of the American Society of Transplant Physicians (Review). J Am Soc Nephrol 1995; 6:1-34.
39. Fine RN, Tejani A, Sullivan EK: Pre-emptive renal transplantation in children: Report of the North American Pediatric Renal Transplant Cooperative Study (NAPRTCS). Clin Transplant 1994; 8:474-478.
40. Fine RN, Kohaut EC, Brown D, Perlman AJ: Growth after recombinant human growth hormone treatment in children with chronic renal failure: Report of a multicenter randomized double-blind placebo-controlled study. Genentech Cooperative Study Group. J Pediatr 1994; 124:374-382.
41. Furth SL, Garg PP, Neu AM, et al: Racial differences in access to the kidney transplant waiting list for children and adolescents with end-stage renal disease. Pediatrics 2000; 106:756-761.
42. Ingulli E, Tejani A, Fikrig S, et al: Nephrotic syndrome associated with acquired immunodeficiency syndrome in children. J Pediatr 1991; 119:710-716.
43. Roland ME, Stock PG: Review of solid-organ transplantation in HIV-infected patients. Transplantation 2003; 75:425-429.
44. Kuo PC, Stock PG: Transplantation in the HIV+ patient. Am J Transplant 2001; 1:13-17.
45. Kist-van Holthe JE, Ho PL, Harmon WE, Baum MA: Outcome of children after renal transplantation for Wilms' tumor and Drash syndrome: A report of the North American Pediatric Renal Transplant Cooperative Study. Am J Transplant 2003; 3:154.
46. Salvatierra O, Tanney D, Mak R, et al: Pediatric renal transplantation and its challenges. Transplant Rev 1997; 11:51-69.
47. Gagnadoux MF, Lacaille F, Niaudet P, et al: Long term results of liver-kidney transplantation in children with primary hyperoxaluria. Pediatr Nephrol 2001; 16:946-950.
48. Tejani A, Sullivan EK, Alexander S, et al: Posttransplant deaths and factors that influence the mortality rate in North American children. Transplantation 1994; 57:547-553.
49. Ellis SR, Hulton SA, McKiernan PJ, et al: Combined liver-kidney transplantation for primary hyperoxaluria type 1 in young children (Comment). Nephrol Dial Transplant 2001; 16:348-354.
50. Kim MS, Primack W, Harmon WE: Congenital nephrotic syndrome: Preemptive bilateral nephrectomy and dialysis before renal transplantation. J Am Soc Nephrol 1992; 3:260-263.
51. Fasola CG, Gillingham KJ, Troppmann C, et al: Kidney transplant or retransplant can effectively treat congenital nephrotic syndrome: A single-center experience. Transplant Proc 1994; 26:9.
52. Holmberg C, Jalanko H, Koskimies O, et al: Renal transplantation in small children with congenital nephrotic syndrome of the Finnish type. Transplant Proc 1991; 23:1378-1379.
53. Rudge CJ: Transplantation and the abnormal bladder. *In* Morris PJ (ed): Kidney Transplantation: Principles and Practice. Philadelphia, WB Saunders, 1994, pp 138-148.
54. Lopez Pereira P, Jaureguizar E, Martinez Urrutia MJ, et al: Does treatment of bladder dysfunction prior to renal transplant

improve outcome in patients with posterior urethral valves? Pediatr Transplant 2000; 4:118-122.

55. Ramirez SP, Lebowitz RL, Harmon WE, Somers MJ: Predictors for abnormal voiding cystourethrography in pediatric patients undergoing renal transplant evaluation (Comment). Pediatr Transplant 2001; 5:99-104.
56. Koo HP, Bunchman TE, Flynn JT, et al: Renal transplantation in children with severe lower urinary tract dysfunction (Comment). J Urol 1999; 161:240-245.
57. Power RE, O'Malley KJ, Khan MS, et al: Renal transplantation in patients with an augmentation cystoplasty. BJU Int 2000; 86:28-31.
58. Nahas WC, Mazzucchi E, Arap MA, et al: Augmentation cystoplasty in renal transplantation: A good and safe option? experience with 25 cases. Urology 2002; 60:770-774.
59. Atala A: Bladder regeneration by tissue engineering. BJU Int 2001; 88:765-770.
60. Atala A: Future trends in bladder reconstructive surgery. Semin Pediatr Surg 2002; 11:134-142.
61. Opelz G, Sengar DP, Mickey MR, Terasaki PI: Effect of blood transfusions on subsequent kidney transplants. Transplant Proc 1973; 5:253-259.
62. Opelz G: Improved kidney graft survival in nontransfused recipients. Transplant Proc 1987; 19:149-152.
63. Potter DE, Portale AA, Melzer JS, et al: Are blood transfusions beneficial in the cyclosporine era? Pediatr Nephrol 1991; 5:168-172.
64. Fedoseyeva EV, Tam RC, Popov IA, et al: Induction of T cell responses to a self-antigen following allotransplantation. Transplantation 1996; 61:679-683.
65. Niaudet P, Dudley J, Charbit M, et al: Pretransplant blood transfusions with cyclosporine in pediatric renal transplantation. Pediatr Nephrol 2000; 14:451-456.
66. Otsuka M, Yuzawa K, Takada Y, et al: Long-term results of donor-specific blood transfusion with cyclosporine in living related kidney transplantation (Comment). Nephron 2001; 88:144-148.
67. Chavers BM, Sullivan EK, Tejani A, Harmon WE: Pre-transplant blood transfusion and renal allograft outcome: A report of the North American Pediatric Renal Transplant Cooperative Study. Pediatr Transplant 1997; 1:22-28.
68. Harmon WE, Alexander SR, Tejani A, Stablein D: The effect of donor age on graft survival in pediatric cadaver renal transplant recipients: A report of the North American Pediatric Renal Transplant Cooperative Study. Transplantation 1992; 54:232-237.
69. Bresnahan BA, McBride MA, Cherikh WS, Hariharan S: Risk factors for renal allograft survival from pediatric cadaver donors: An analysis of united network for organ sharing data. Transplantation 2001; 72:256-261.
70. Ruff T, Reddy KS, Johnston TD, et al: Transplantation of pediatric en bloc cadaver kidneys into adult recipients: A single-center experience. Am Surg 2002; 68:857-859.
71. Takemoto S, Terasaki PI: Donor age and recipient age. Clin Transpl 1988; 345-356.
72. Terasaki PI, Gjertson DW, Cecka JM, et al: Significance of the donor age effect on kidney transplants. Clin Transplant 1997; 11:366-372.
73. Tejani AH, Stablein DM, Sullivan EK, et al: The impact of donor source, recipient age, pre-operative immunotherapy and induction therapy on early and late acute rejections in children: A report of the North American Pediatric Renal Transplant Cooperative Study (NAPRTCS). Pediatr Transplant 1998; 2:318-324.
74. Toma H, Tanabe K, Tokumoto T, et al: Time-dependent risk factors influencing the long-term outcome in living renal allografts: Donor age is a crucial risk factor for long-term graft survival more than 5 years after transplantation. Transplantation 2001; 72:940-947.
75. Cho YW, Cecka JM, Terasaki PI: HLA matching effect: Better survival rates and graft quality. Clin Transpl 1994; 435-449.
76. Terasaki PI, Cho Y, Takemoto S, et al: Twenty-year follow-up on the effect of HLA matching on kidney transplant survival and prediction of future twenty-year survival. Transplant Proc 1996; 28:1144-1145.
77. Osorio AV, Sullivan EK, Alexander SR, et al: ABO-mismatched renal transplantation in children: A report of the North American Pediatric Renal Transplant Cooperative Study (NAPRTCS) and the Midwest Organ Bank (MOB). Pediatr Transplant 1998; 2:26-29.
78. Ross LF, Rubin DT, Siegler M, et al: Ethics of a paired-kidney-exchange program (Comment). N Engl J Med 1997; 336:1752-1755.
79. Delmonico FL, Morrissey PE, Lipkowitz GS, et al: Donor kidney exchange for incompatible donors. Am J Transplant 2003; 3(suppl 5):550.
80. Jones JW, Matas AJ, Najarian JS: Surgical technique. *In* Tejani AH, Fine RN (eds): Pediatric Renal Transplantation. New York, Wiley-Liss, 1994, pp 187-200.
81. Lee HM: Surgical techniques of renal transplantation. *In* Morris PJ (ed): Kidney Transplantation: Principles and Practice. Philadelphia, WB Saunders, 1994, pp 127-137.
82. Salvatierra O, Singh T, Shifrin R, et al: Transplantation of adult-sized kidneys into infants induces major blood flow changes. Transplantation 1998; (In press).
83. French CG, Acott PD, Crocker JF, et al: Extravesical ureteroneocystostomy with and without internalized ureteric stents in pediatric renal transplantation. Pediatr Transplant 2001; 5:21-26.
84. Zaontz MR, Maizels M, Sugar EC, Firlit CF: Detrusorrhaphy: Extravesical ureteral advancement to correct vesicoureteral reflux in children. J Urol 1987; 138:947-949.
85. Wacksman J, Gilbert A, Sheldon CA: Results of the renewed extravesical reimplant for surgical correction of vesicoureteral reflux. J Urol 1992; 148:359-361.
86. Briscoe DM, Hoffer FA, Tu N, Harmon WE: Duplex Doppler examination of renal allografts in children: Correlation between renal blood flow and clinical findings. Pediatr Radiol 1993; 23: 365-368.
87. Benfield MR, Herrin J, Feld L, et al: Safety of kidney biopsy in pediatric transplantation: A report of the Controlled Clinical Trials in Pediatric Transplantation Trial of Induction Therapy Study Group. Transplantation 1999; 67:544-547.
88. Tejani A, Sullivan EK, Alexander SR, et al: Predictive factors for acute tubular necrosis (ATN) and its impact on renal graft survival in children, 16th Annual Meeting of the American Society of Transplant Physicians (Abstract). Chicago, 1997.
89. Smith JM, McDonald RA, Stablein D, et al: The impact of interleukin-2 receptor antibodies on renal allograft thrombosis: An analysis of the North American Pediatric Renal Transplant Cooperative Study. Am J Transplant 2003; 3(suppl 5):166.
90. Balachandra S, Tejani A: Recurrent vascular thrombosis in an adolescent transplant recipient (Review). J Am Soc Nephrol 1997; 8:1477-1481.
91. Harmon WE, Stablein D, Alexander SR, Tejani A: Graft thrombosis in pediatric renal transplant recipients. A report of the North American Pediatric Renal Transplant Cooperative Study. Transplantation 1991; 51:406-412.
92. Singh A, Stablein D, Tejani A: Risk factors for vascular thrombosis in pediatric renal transplantation: A special report of the North American Pediatric Renal Transplant Cooperative Study. Transplantation 1997; 63:1263-1267.
93. Wheeler MA, Taylor CM, Williams M, Moghal N: Factor V Leiden: A risk factor for renal vein thrombosis in renal transplantation. Pediatr Nephrol 2000; 14:525-526.
94. Kim MS, Stablein D, Harmon WE: Renal transplantation in children with congenital nephrotic syndrome: A report of the North American Pediatric Renal Transplant Cooperative Study (NAPRTCS). Pediatr Transplant 1998; 2:305-308.
95. Schurman SJ, Stablein DM, Perlman SA, Warady BA: Center volume effects in pediatric renal transplantation. A report of the North American Pediatric Renal Transplant Cooperative Study. Pediatr Nephrol 1999; 13:373-378.

96. Vats AN, Donaldson L, Fine RN, Chavers BM: Pretransplant dialysis status and outcome of renal transplantation in North American children: A NAPRTCS Study. North American Pediatric Renal Transplant Cooperative Study. Transplantation 2000; 69:1414-1419.
97. McDonald RA, Smith JM, Stablein D, Harmon WE: Pretransplant peritoneal dialysis and graft thrombosis following pediatric kidney transplantation: A NAPRTCS report. Pediatr Transplant 2003; 7:204-208.
98. Lundin C, Bersztel A, Wahlberg J, Wadstrom J: Low molecular weight heparin prophylaxis increases the incidence of lymphocele after kidney transplantation. Ups J Med Sci 2002; 107:9-15.
99. Offner G, Broyer M, Niaudet P, et al: A multicenter, open-label, pharmacokinetic/pharmacodynamic safety, and tolerability study of basiliximab (Simulect) in pediatric de novo renal transplant recipients. Transplantation 2002; 74:961-966.
100. Kovarik JM, Offner G, Broyer M, et al: A rational dosing algorithm for basiliximab (Simulect) in pediatric renal transplantation based on pharmacokinetic-dynamic evaluations. Transplantation 2002; 74:966-971.
101. Strehlau J, Pape L, Offner G, et al: Interleukin-2 receptor antibody-induced alterations of cyclosporin dose requirements in paediatric transplant recipients (Comment). Lancet 2000; 356:1327-1328.
102. Ciancio G, Burke GW, Suzart K, et al: Daclizumab induction, tacrolimus, mycophenolate mofetil and steroids as an immunosuppression regimen for primary kidney transplant recipients. Transplantation 2002; 73:1100-1106.
103. Swiatecka-Urban A, Garcia C, Feuerstein D, et al: Basiliximab induction improves the outcome of renal transplants in children and adolescents. Pediatr Nephrol 2001; 16:693-696.
104. Vester U, Kranz B, Testa G, et al: Efficacy and tolerability of interleukin-2 receptor blockade with basiliximab in pediatric renal transplant recipients. Pediatr Transplant 2001; 5:297-301.
105. Zamora I, Berbel O, Simon J, Sanahuja MJ: Anti-CD25 monoclonal antibody against polyclonal antibodies in pediatric renal transplantation. Nefrologia 2002; 22:66-70.
106. Simmons RL, Canafax DM, Fryd DS, et al: New immunosuppressive drug combinations for mismatched related and cadaveric renal transplantation. Transplant Proc 1986; 18:76-81.
107. Norman DJ: Mechanisms of action and overview of OKT3 (Review). Ther Drug Monit 1995; 17:615-620.
108. Peddi VR, Bryant M, Roy-Chaudhury P, et al: Safety, efficacy, and cost analysis of thymoglobulin induction therapy with intermittent dosing based on CD3+ lymphocyte counts in kidney and kidney-pancreas transplant recipients. Transplantation 2002; 73:1514-1518.
109. Ault BH, Honaker MR, Osama Gaber A, et al: Short-term outcomes of Thymoglobulin induction in pediatric renal transplant recipients. Pediatr Nephrol 2002; 17:815-818.
110. Brophy PD, Thomas SE, McBryde KD, Bunchman TE: Comparison of polyclonal induction agents in pediatric renal transplantation. Pediatr Transplant 2001; 5:174-178.
111. Norman DJ, Chatenoud L, Cohen D, et al: Consensus statement regarding OKT3-induced cytokine-release syndrome and human antimouse antibodies (Review). Transplant Proc 1993; 25:89-92.
112. Robinson ST, Barry JM, Norman DJ: The hemodynamic effects of intraoperative injection of muromonab CD3. Transplantation 1993; 56:356-358.
113. Shihab FS, Barry JM, Norman DJ: Encephalopathy following the use of OKT3 in renal allograft transplantation. Transplant Proc 1993; 25:31-34.
114. Tejani A, Harmon W, Benfield MR: A randomized, prospective, multicenter trial of T-cell antibody induction therapy in pediatric renal transplantation (Abstract). Transplantation 2000; 69:S111.
115. Jablonski P, Harrison C, Howden B, et al: Cyclosporine and the ischemic rat kidney. Transplantation 1986; 41:147-151.
116. Kahan BD: Cyclosporine (See comments). N Engl J Med 1989; 321:1725-1738.
117. Calne RY, Rolles K, White DJ, et al: Cyclosporin A initially as the only immunosuppressant in 34 recipients of cadaveric organs: 32 kidneys, 2 pancreases, and 2 livers. Lancet 1979; 2:1033-1036.
118. Harmon WE, Sullivan EK: Cyclosporine dosing and its relationship to outcome in pediatric renal transplantation. Kidney Int Suppl 1993; 43:S50-S55.
119. Suthanthiran M, Haschemeyer RH, Riggio RR, et al: Excellent outcome with a calcium channel blocker-supplemented immunosuppressive regimen in cadaveric renal transplantation. A potential strategy to avoid antibody induction protocols (See comments). Transplantation 1993; 55:1008-1013.
120. Tejani A, Sullivan EK: Higher maintenance cyclosporine dose decreases the risk of graft failure in North American children: A report of the North American Pediatric Renal Transplant Cooperative Study. J Am Soc Nephrol 1996; 7:550-555.
121. Tejani A, Sullivan EK, Fine RN, et al: Steady improvement in renal allograft survival among North American children: A five year appraisal by the North American Pediatric Renal Transplant Cooperative Study. Kidney Int 1995; 48:551-553.
122. David-Neto E, Araujo LP, Feres Alves C, et al: A strategy to calculate cyclosporin A area under the time-concentration curve in pediatric renal transplantation. Pediatr Transplant 2002; 6:313-318.
123. Belitsky P, Dunn S, Johnston A, Levy G: Impact of absorption profiling on efficacy and safety of cyclosporin therapy in transplant recipients. Clin Pharmacokinet 2000; 39:117-125.
124. Dunn SP: Neoral monitoring 2 hours post-dose and the pediatric transplant patient. Pediatr Transplant 2003; 7:25-30.
125. Crocker JF, Dempsey T, Schenk ME, Renton KW: Cyclosporin A toxicity in children. Transplant Rev 1993; 7:72.
126. Foley RJ, Hamner RW, Weinman EJ: Serum potassium concentrations in cyclosporine- and azathioprine-treated renal transplant patients. Nephron 1985; 40:280-285.
127. Chapman JR, Griffiths D, Harding NG, Morris PJ: Reversibility of cyclosporin nephrotoxicity after three months' treatment. Lancet 1985; 1:128-130.
128. Allen RD, Hunnisett AG, Morris PJ: Cyclosporin and magnesium (Letter). Lancet 1985; 1:1283-1284.
129. Beaman M, Parvin S, Veitch PS, Walls J: Convulsions associated with cyclosporin A in renal transplant recipients. Br Med J 1985; 290:139-140.
130. Thomas DW, Baboolal K, Subramanian N, Newcombe RG: Cyclosporin A-induced gingival overgrowth is unrelated to allograft function in renal transplant recipients. J Clin Periodontol 2001; 28:706-709.
131. Seymour RA, Jacobs DJ: Cyclosporin and the gingival tissues (Review). J Clin Periodontol 1992; 19:1-11.
132. Shapiro R, Jordan ML, Scantlebury VP, et al: The superiority of tacrolimus in renal transplant recipients? the Pittsburgh experience (Review). Clin Transpl 1995; 199-205.
133. McKee M, Segev D, Wise B, et al: Initial experience with FK506 (tacrolimus) in pediatric renal transplant recipients. J Pediatr Surg 1997; 32:688-690.
134. Ellis D: Clinical use of tacrolimus (FK-506) in infants and children with renal transplants (Review). Pediatr Nephrol 1995; 9: 487-494.
135. Eades SK, Boineau FG, Christensen ML: Increased tacrolimus levels in a pediatric renal transplant patient attributed to chronic diarrhea. Pediatr Transplant 2000; 4:63-66.
136. Shapiro R, Jordan M, Fung J, et al: Kidney transplantation under FK 506 immunosuppression. Transplant Proc 1991; 23:920-923.
137. Neu AM, Ho PL, Fine RN, et al: Tacrolimus vs. cyclosporine A as primary immunosuppression in pediatric renal transplantation: A NAPRTCS study. Pediatr Transplant 2003; 7:217-222.
138. Eidelman BH, Abu-Elmagd K, Wilson J, et al: Neurologic complications of FK 506. Transplant Proc 1991; 23:3175-3178.

139. Neu AM, Furth SL, Case BW, et al: Evaluation of neurotoxicity in pediatric renal transplant recipients treated with tacrolimus (FK506). Clin Transplant 1997; 11:412-414.
140. Japanese. FK506 Study Group. Morphological characteristics of renal allografts showing renal dysfunction under FK506 therapy: Is graft biopsy available to reveal the morphological findings corresponding with FK506 nephropathy? Transplant Proc 1993; 25:624.
141. Furth S, Neu A, Colombani P, et al: Diabetes as a complication of tacrolimus (FK506) in pediatric renal transplant patients. Pediatr Nephrol 1996; 10:64-66.
142. Greenspan LC, Gitelman SE, Leung MA, et al: Increased incidence in post-transplant diabetes mellitus in children: A case-control analysis. Pediatr Nephrol 2002; 17:1-5.
143. Filler G, Neuschulz I, Vollmer I, et al: Tacrolimus reversibly reduces insulin secretion in paediatric renal transplant recipients. Nephrol Dial Transplant 2000; 15:867-871.
144. Ciancio G, Siquijor AP, Burke GW, et al: Post-transplant lymphoproliferative disease in kidney transplant patients in the new immunosuppressive era. Clin Transplant 1997; 11:243-249.
145. Dharnidharka VR, Ho PL, Stablein DM, et al: Mycophenolate, tacrolimus and post-transplant lymphoproliferative disorder: A report of the North American Pediatric Renal Transplant Cooperative Study. Pediatr Transplant 2002; 6:396-399.
146. Tejani A, Ho PL, Emmett L, Stablein DM: North American Pediatric Renal Transplant Cooperative Study. Reduction in acute rejections decreases chronic rejection graft failure in children: A report of the North American Pediatric Renal Transplant Cooperative Study (NAPRTCS). Am J Transplant 2002; 2:142-147.
147. Tejani A, Stablein DM, Donaldson L, et al: Steady improvement in short-term graft survival of pediatric renal transplants: The NAPRTCS experience. Clin Transplant 1999; 95-110.
148. Trompeter R, Filler G, Webb NJ, et al: Randomized trial of tacrolimus versus cyclosporin microemulsion in renal transplantation. Pediatr Nephrol 2002; 17:141-149.
149. Benfield MR, Symons JM, Bynon S, et al: Mycophenolate mofetil in pediatric renal transplantation (Comment). Pediatr Transplant 1999; 3:33-37.
150. Butani L, Palmer J, Baluarte HJ, Polinsky MS: Adverse effects of mycophenolate mofetil in pediatric renal transplant recipients with presumed chronic rejection. Transplantation. 1999; 68:83-86.
151. Jungraithmayr T, Staskewitz A, Kirste G, et al: Pediatric renal transplantation with mycophenolate mofetil-based immunosuppression without induction: Results after three years. Transplantation 2003; 75:454-461.
152. Filler G, Gellermann J, Zimmering M, Mai I: Effect of adding mycophenolate mofetil in paediatric renal transplant recipients with chronical cyclosporine nephrotoxicity. Transplant Int 2000; 13:201-206.
153. Staskewitz A, Kirste G, Tonshoff B, et al: Mycophenolate mofetil in pediatric renal transplantation without induction therapy: Results after 12 months of treatment. German Pediatric Renal Transplantation Study Group. Transplantation 2001; 71: 638-644.
154. Bunchman T, Navarro M, Broyer M, et al: The use of mycophenolate mofetil suspension in pediatric renal allograft recipients. Pediatr Nephrol 2001; 16:978-984.
155. Ettenger R, Cohen A, Nast C, et al: Mycophenolate mofetil as maintenance immunosuppression in pediatric renal transplantation. Transplant Proc 1997; 29:340-341.
156. Oellerich M, Shipkova M, Schutz E, et al: Pharmacokinetic and metabolic investigations of mycophenolic acid in pediatric patients after renal transplantation: Implications for therapeutic drug monitoring. German Study Group on Mycophenolate Mofetil Therapy in Pediatric Renal Transplant Recipients. Ther Drug Monit 2000; 22:20-26.
157. Filler G, Feber J, Lepage N, et al: Universal approach to pharmacokinetic monitoring of immunosuppressive agents in children. Pediatr Transplant 2002; 6:411-418.
158. Shipkova M, Armstrong VW, Weber L, et al: Pharmacokinetics and protein adduct formation of the pharmacologically active acyl glucuronide metabolite of mycophenolic acid in pediatric renal transplant recipients. Ther Drug Monit 2002; 24:390-399.
159. Weber LT, Schutz E, Lamersdorf T, et al: Therapeutic drug monitoring of total and free mycophenolic acid (MPA) and limited sampling strategy for determination of MPA-AUC in paediatric renal transplant recipients. The German Study Group on Mycophenolate Mofetil (MMF) Therapy. Nephrol Dial Transplant 1999; 14:34-35.
160. Weber LT, Schutz E, Lamersdorf T, et al: Pharmacokinetics of mycophenolic acid (MPA) and free MPA in paediatric renal transplant recipients: A multicentre study. The German Study Group on Mycophenolate Mofetil (MMF) Therapy. Nephrol Dial Transplant 1999; 14:33-34.
161. Weber LT, Shipkova M, Armstrong VW, et al: The pharmacokinetic-pharmacodynamic relationship for total and free mycophenolic acid in pediatric renal transplant recipients: A report of the German Study Group on Mycophenolate Mofetil Therapy. J Am Soc Nephrol 2002; 13:759-768.
162. Potter D, Belzer FO, Rames L, et al: The treatment of chronic uremia in childhood. I. Transplantation. Pediatrics 1970; 45: 432-443.
163. Baqi N, Tejani A: Maintenance immunosuppression regimens. *In* Tejani AH, Fine RN (eds): Pediatric Renal Transplantation. New York, Wiley-Liss, 1994, pp 201-210.
164. Danovitch GB: Handbook of Kidney Transplantation. Boston, Little, Brown, 1996.
165. Ingulli E, Tejani A: Steroid withdrawal after renal transplantation. *In* Tejani AH, Fine RN (eds): Pediatric Renal Transplantation. New York, Wiley-Liss, 1994, pp 221-238.
166. Ingulli E, Sharma V, Singh A, et al: Steroid withdrawal, rejection and the mixed lymphocyte reaction in children after renal transplantation. Kidney Int Suppl 1993; 43:S36-S39.
167. Reisman L, Lieberman KV, Burrows L, Schanzer H: Follow-up of cyclosporine-treated pediatric renal allograft recipients after cessation of prednisone. Transplantation 1990; 49:76-80.
168. Hymes LC, Warshaw BL: Tacrolimus rescue therapy for children with acute renal transplant rejection. Pediatr Nephrol 2001; 16: 990-992.
169. Broyer M, Guest G, Gagnadoux MF: Growth rate in children receiving alternate-day corticosteroid treatment after kidney transplantation. J Pediatr 1992; 120:721-725.
170. Jabs K, Sullivan EK, Avner ED, Harmon WE: Alternate-day steroid dosing improves growth without adversely affecting graft survival or long-term graft function. A report of the North American Pediatric Renal Transplant Cooperative Study. Transplantation 1996; 61:31-36.
171. Sehgal SN, Molnar-Kimber K, Ocain TD, Weichman BM: Sirolimus: A novel immunosuppressive macrolide (Review). Med Res Rev 1994; 14:1-22.
172. Kim HS, Raskova J, Degiannis D, Raska K Jr: Effects of cyclosporine and sirolimus on immunoglobulin production by preactivated human B cells. Clin Exp Immunol 1994; 96: 508-512.
173. Ferraresso M, Tian L, Ghobrial R, et al: Sirolimus inhibits production of cytotoxic but not noncytotoxic antibodies and preferentially activates T helper 2 cells that mediate long-term survival of heart allografts in rats. J Immunol 1994; 153: 3307-3318.
174. Aagaard-Tillery KM, Jelinek DF: Inhibition of human B lymphocyte cell cycle progression and differentiation by sirolimus. Cell Immunol 1994; 156:493-507.
175. Dumont FJ, Staruch MJ, Koprak SL, et al: Distinct mechanisms of suppression of murine T cell activation by the related macrolides FK-506 and sirolimus. J Immunol 1990; 144:251-258.

176. Wood MA, Bierer BE: Sirolimus: Biologic and therapeutic effects, binding by immunophilins and molecular targets of action. Perspect Drug Discov Design 1994; 2:163-184.
177. Marx SO, Jayaraman T, Go LO, Marks AR: Sirolimus-FKBP inhibits cell cycle regulators of proliferation in vascular smooth muscle cells. Circ Res 1995; 76:412-417.
178. Cao W, Mohacsi P, Shorthouse R, et al: Effects of sirolimus on growth factor-stimulated vascular smooth muscle cell DNA synthesis. Inhibition of basic fibroblast growth factor and platelet-derived growth factor action and antagonism of sirolimus by FK506. Transplantation 1995; 59:390-395.
179. El-Sabrout R, Weiss R, Butt F, et al: Rejection-free protocol using sirolimus-tacrolimus combination for pediatric renal transplant recipients. Transplant Proc 2002; 34:1942-1943.
180. Montgomery SP, Mog SR, Xu H, et al: Efficacy and toxicity of a protocol using sirolimus, tacrolimus and daclizumab in a non-human primate renal allotransplant model. Am J Transplant 2002; 2:381-385.
181. Kahan BD, Camardo JS: Sirolimus: Clinical results and future opportunities. Transplantation 2001; 72:1181-1193.
182. Kahan BD, Julian BA, Pescovitz MD, et al: Sirolimus reduces the incidence of acute rejection episodes despite lower cyclosporine doses in Caucasian recipients of mismatched primary renal allografts: A phase II trial. Rapamune Study Group. Transplantation 1999; 68:1526-1532.
183. Kahan BD, Podbielski J, Napoli KL, et al: Immunosuppressive effects and safety of a sirolimus/cyclosporine combination regimen for renal transplantation. Transplantation 1998; 66:1040-1046.
184. Kreis H, Cisterne JM, Land W, et al: Sirolimus in association with mycophenolate mofetil induction for the prevention of acute graft rejection in renal allograft recipients. Transplantation 2000; 69:1252-1260.
185. Mital D, Podlasek W, Jensik SC: Sirolimus-based steroid-free maintenance immunosuppression. Transplant Proc 2002; 34:1709-1710.
186. Vester U, Kranz B, Wehr S, et al: Everolimus (Certican) in combination with neoral in pediatric renal transplant recipients: Interim analysis after 3 months. Transplant Proc 2002; 34:2209-2210.
187. Van Damme-Lombaerts R, Webb NA, Hoyer PF, et al: Single-dose pharmacokinetics and tolerability of everolimus in stable pediatric renal transplant patients. Pediatr Transplant 2002; 6:147-152.
188. Sindhi R, Webber S, Goyal R, et al: Pharmacodynamics of sirolimus in transplanted children receiving tacrolimus. Transplant Proc 2002; 34:1960.
189. MacDonald A, Scarola J, Burke JT, Zimmerman JJ: Clinical pharmacokinetics and therapeutic drug monitoring of sirolimus. Clin Ther 2000; 22:B101-B121.
190. Harmon WE, Stablein DM, Sayegh MH: Trends in immunosuppression strategies in pediatric kidney transplantation. Am J Transplant 2003; 3(suppl 5):285.
191. Sho M, Samsonov DV, Briscoe DM: Immunologic targets for currently available immunosuppressive agents: What is the optimal approach for children? Semin Nephrol 2001; 21:508-520.
192. Tilney NL: Early course of a patient. *In* Morris PJ (ed): Kidney Transplantation: Principles and Practice. Philadelphia, WB Saunders, 1988, pp 278-283.
193. McDonald R, Ho PL, Stablein DM, Tejani A: North American Pediatric Renal Transplant Cooperative Study. Rejection profile of recent pediatric renal transplant recipients compared with historical controls: A report of the North American Pediatric Renal Transplant Cooperative Study (NAPRTCS). Am J Transplant 2001; 1:55-60.
194. Ettenger RB, Blifeld C, Prince H, et al: The pediatric nephrologist's dilemma: Growth after renal transplantation and its interaction with age as a possible immunologic variable. J Pediatr 1987; 111:1022-1025.
195. Dadhania D, Muthukumar T, Ding R, et al: Molecular signatures of urinary cells distinguish acute rejection of renal allografts from urinary tract infection. Transplantation 2003; 75: 1752-1754.
196. Strehlau J, Pavlakis M, Lipman M, et al: Quantitative detection of immune activation transcripts as a diagnostic tool in kidney transplantation. Proc Natl Acad Sci U S A 1997; 94: 695-700.
197. Treves ST, Majd M, Kuruc A, et al: Kidneys. *In* Treves WT (ed): Pediatric Nuclear Medicine. New York, Springer-Verlag, 1995, pp 339-399.
198. Ding R, Li B, Muthukumar T, et al: CD103 mRNA levels in urinary cells predict acute rejection of renal allografts. Transplantation 2003; 75:1307-1312.
199. Li B, Hartono C, Ding R, et al: Noninvasive diagnosis of renal-allograft rejection by measurement of messenger RNA for perforin and granzyme B in urine (Comment). N Engl J Med 2001; 344:947-954.
200. Sarwal M, Chua MS, Kambham N, et al: Molecular heterogeneity in acute renal allograft rejection identified by DNA microarray profiling (Comment). N Engl J Med 2003; 349:125-138.
201. Dunnill MS: Histopathology of renal allograft rejection. *In* Morris PJ (ed): Kidney Transplantation: Principles and Practice. Philadelphia, WB Saunders, 1994, pp 266-285.
202. Feehally J, Harris KP, Bennett SE, Walls J: Is chronic renal transplant rejection a non-immunological phenomenon? Lancet 1986; 2:486-488.
203. Tilney NL, Guttmann RD: Effects of initial ischemia/reperfusion injury on the transplanted kidney (Review). Transplantation 1997; 64:945-947.
204. Tejani A, Cortes L, Stablein D: Clinical correlates of chronic rejection in pediatric renal transplantation. A report of the North American Pediatric Renal Transplant Cooperative Study. Transplantation 1996; 61:1054-1058.
205. Sharma VK, Bologa RM, Xu GP, et al: Intragraft TGF-beta 1 mRNA: A correlate of interstitial fibrosis and chronic allograft nephropathy. Kidney Int 1996; 49:1297-1303.
206. Jabs KL, Van Dop C, Harmon WE: Endocrinologic evaluation of children who grow poorly following renal transplantation. Transplantation 1990; 49:71-76.
207. Harmon WE, Jabs K: Factors affecting growth after renal transplantation (Review). J Am Soc Nephrol 1992; 2:S295-S303.
208. van Lieburg AF, de Jong MC, Hoitsma AJ, et al: Renal transplant thrombosis in children. J Pediatr Surg 1995; 30:615-619.
209. Tejani A, Fine RN: Cadaver renal transplantation in children. Incidence, immunosuppression, outcome, and risk factors (Review). Clin Pediatr 1993; 32:194-202.
210. Sarwal MM, Cecka JM, Millan MT, Salvatierra O Jr: Adult-size kidneys without acute tubular necrosis provide exceedingly superior long-term graft outcomes for infants and small children: A single center and UNOS analysis. United Network for Organ Sharing. Transplantation 2000; 70:1728-1736.
211. Kashtan CE, McEnery PT, Tejani A, Stablein DM: Renal allograft survival according to primary diagnosis: A report of the North American Pediatric Renal Transplant Cooperative Study. Pediatr Nephrol 1995; 9:679-684.
212. Tejani A, Stablein DH: Recurrence of focal segmental glomerulosclerosis posttransplantation: A special report of the North American Pediatric Renal Transplant Cooperative Study. J Am Soc Nephrol 1992; 2:S258-S263.
213. Baum MA, Ho M, Stablein D, Alexander SR: North American Pediatric Renal Transplant Cooperative Study. Outcome of renal transplantation in adolescents with focal segmental glomerulosclerosis. Pediatr Transplant 2002; 6:488-492.
214. Benfield MR, McDonald R, Sullivan EK, et al: The 1997 Annual Renal Transplantation in Children Report of the North American Pediatric Renal Transplant Cooperative Study (NAPRTCS). Pediatr Transplant 1999; 3:152-167.

215. Schachter AD, Harmon WE: Single-center analysis of early recurrence of nephrotic syndrome following renal transplantation in children. Pediatr Transplant 2001; 5:406-409.
216. Baum MA, Stablein DM, Panzarino VM, et al: Loss of living donor renal allograft survival advantage in children with focal segmental glomerulosclerosis. Kidney Int 2001; 59:328-333.
217. Schachter AD, Strehlau J, Zurakowski D, et al: Increased nuclear factor-kappaB and angiotensinogen gene expression in posttransplant recurrent focal segmental glomerulosclerosis. Transplantation 2000; 70:1107-1110.
218. Sharma M, Sharma R, McCarthy ET, Savin VJ: The FSGS factor: Enrichment and in vivo effect of activity from focal segmental glomerulosclerosis plasma. J Am Soc Nephrol 1999; 10:552-561.
219. Belson A, Yorgin PD, Al-Uzri AY, et al: Long-term plasmapheresis and protein A column treatment of recurrent FSGS. Pediatr Nephrol 2001; 16:985-989.
220. Dall' Amico R, Ghiggeri G, Carraro M, et al: Prediction and treatment of recurrent focal segmental glomerulosclerosis after renal transplantation in children. Am J Kidney Dis 1999; 34:1048-1055.
221. Greenstein SM, Delrio M, Ong E, et al: Plasmapheresis treatment for recurrent focal sclerosis in pediatric renal allografts. Pediatr Nephrol 2000; 14:1061-1065.
222. Ohta T, Kawaguchi H, Hattori M, et al: Effect of pre- and postoperative plasmapheresis on posttransplant recurrence of focal segmental glomerulosclerosis in children. Transplantation 2001; 71:628-633.
223. Raafat R, Travis LB, Kalia A, Diven S: Role of transplant induction therapy on recurrence rate of focal segmental glomerulosclerosis. Pediatr Nephrol 2000; 14:189-194.
224. Cochat P: Is there a need for a multicenter study to determine the optimal approach to recurrent nephrotic syndrome following renal transplantation? Pediatr Transplant 2001; 5:394-397.
225. Bartosh SM, Fine RN, Sullivan EK: Outcome after transplantation of young patients with systemic lupus erythematosus: A report of the North American pediatric renal transplant cooperative study. Transplantation 2001; 72:973-978.
226. Gipson DS, Ferris ME, Dooley MA, et al: Renal transplantation in children with lupus nephritis. Am J Kidney Dis 2003; 41:455-463.
227. Warady BA, Sullivan EK: Renal transplantation in children with sickle cell disease: A report of the North American Pediatric Renal Transplant Cooperative Study (NAPRTCS). Pediatr Transplant 1998; 2:130-133.
228. Edvardsson VO, Kaiser BA, Polinsky MS, Baluarte HJ: Successful living-related renal transplantation in an adolescent with Down syndrome (Comment). Pediatr Nephrol 1995; 9:398-399.
229. Baqi N, Tejani A, Sullivan EK: Renal transplantation in Down syndrome: A report of the North American Pediatric Renal Transplant Cooperative Study (Comment). Pediatr Transplant 1998; 2:211-215.
230. Broyer M, Selwood N, Brunner F: Recurrence of primary renal disease on kidney graft: A European pediatric experience. J Am Soc Nephrol 1992; 2:S255-S257.
231. Ferraris JR, Ramirez JA, Ruiz S, et al: Shiga toxin-associated hemolytic uremic syndrome: Absence of recurrence after renal transplantation. Pediatr Nephrol 2002; 17:809-814.
232. Quan A, Sullivan EK, Alexander SR: Recurrence of hemolytic uremic syndrome after renal transplantation in children: A report of the North American Pediatric Renal Transplant Cooperative Study. Transplantation 2001; 72:742-745.
233. Betts PR, Magrath G: Growth pattern and dietary intake of children with chronic renal insufficiency. Br Med J 1974; 2:189-193.
234. Tejani A, Ingulli E: Growth in children post-transplantation and methods to optimize post-transplant growth. Clin Transplant 1991; 5:214-218.
235. Shapiro R, Scantlebury VP, Jordan ML, et al: Pediatric renal transplantation under tacrolimus-based immunosuppression. Transplantation 1999; 67:299-303.
236. McEnery PT, Gonzalez LL, Martin LW, West CD: Growth and development of children with renal transplants. Use of alternate-day steroid therapy. J Pediatr 1973; 83:806-814.
237. Johansson G, Sietnieks A, Janssens F, et al: Recombinant human growth hormone treatment in short children with chronic renal disease, before transplantation or with functioning renal transplants: An interim report on five European studies. Acta Paediatr Scand Suppl 1990; 370:36-42.
238. Kaufmann S, Jones KL, Wehrenberg WB, Culler FL: Inhibition by prednisone of growth hormone (GH) response to GH-releasing hormone in normal men. J Clin Endocrinol Metab 1988; 67:1258-1261.
239. Rees L, Greene SA, Adlard P, et al: Growth and endocrine function after renal transplantation. Arch Dis Child 1988; 63: 1326-1332.
240. Wehrenberg WB, Janowski BA, Piering AW, et al: Glucocorticoids: Potent inhibitors and stimulators of growth hormone secretion. Endocrinology 1990; 126:3200-3203.
241. Schaefer F, Hamill G, Stanhope R, et al: Pulsatile growth hormone secretion in peripubertal patients with chronic renal failure. Cooperative Study Group on Pubertal Development in Chronic Renal Failure. J Pediatr 1991; 119:568-577.
242. Ghio L, Tarantino A, Edefonti A, et al: Advantages of cyclosporine as sole immunosuppressive agent in children with transplanted kidneys. Transplantation 1992; 54:834-838.
243. Ingulli E, Tejani A: An analytical review of growth hormone studies in children after renal transplantation (Review). Pediatr Nephrol 1995; 9:S61-S65.
244. Broyer M: Results and side-effects of treating children with growth hormone after kidney transplantation: A preliminary report. Pharmacia & Upjohn Study Group (See comments). Acta Paediatr Suppl 1996; 417:76-79.
245. Jabs K, Van Dop C, Harmon WE: Growth hormone treatment of growth failure among children with renal transplants. Kidney Int Suppl 1993; 43:S71-S75.
246. Chavers BM, Doherty L, Nevins TE, et al: Effects of growth hormone on kidney function in pediatric transplant recipients (Review). Pediatr Nephrol 1995; 9:176-181.
247. Fine RN, Stablein D, Cohen AH, et al: Recombinant human growth hormone post-renal transplantation in children: A randomized controlled study of the NAPRTCS. Kidney Int 2002; 62:688-696.
248. Dharnidharka VR, Stablein DM, Harmon WE: Post-transplant infections now exceed acute rejection as cause for hospitalization: a report of NAPRTCS. Am J Transplant 2004; 4:384-389.
249. Hanto DW, Frizzera G, Purtilo DT, et al: Clinical spectrum of lymphoproliferative disorders in renal transplant recipients and evidence for the role of Epstein-Barr virus. Cancer Res 1981; 41:4253-4261.
250. Nocera A, Ghio L, Dall'Amico R, et al: De novo cancers in paediatric renal transplant recipients: A multicentre analysis within the North Italy Transplant programme (NITp), Italy. Eur J Cancer 2000; 36:80-86.
251. Dharnidharka VR, Tejani AH, Ho PL, Harmon WE: Post-transplant lymphoproliferative disorder in the United States: Young Caucasian males are at highest risk. Am J Transplant 2002; 2:993-998.
252. Chang H, Wu JD, Cheng KK, Tseng HH: Epstein-Barr virus-associated lymphoproliferative disorders in oral cavity after heart transplantation: Report of a case. J Formos Med Assoc 1994; 93:332-336.
253. Renoult E, Aymard B, Gregoire MJ, et al: Epstein-Barr virus lymphoproliferative disease of donor origin after kidney transplantation: A case report. Am J Kidney Dis 1995; 26:84-87.
254. Gonthier DM, Hartman G, Holley JL: Posttransplant lymphoproliferative disorder presenting as an isolated skin lesion. Am J Kidney Dis 1992; 19:600-603.

255. Cen H, Williams PA, McWilliams HP, et al: Evidence for restricted Epstein-Barr virus latent gene expression and anti-EBNA antibody response in solid organ transplant recipients with posttransplant lymphoproliferative disorders. Blood 1993; 81:1393-1403.
256. Delecluse HJ, Kremmer E, Rouault JP, et al: The expression of Epstein-Barr virus latent proteins is related to the pathological features of post-transplant lymphoproliferative disorders. Am J Pathol 1995; 146:1113-1120.
257. Cox KL, Lawrence-Miyasaki LS, Garcia-Kennedy R, et al: An increased incidence of Epstein-Barr virus infection and lymphoproliferative disorder in young children on FK506 after liver transplantation. Transplantation 1995; 59:524-529.
258. Andrews W, Sommerauer J, Roden J, et al: 10 years of pediatric liver transplantation. J Pediatr Surg 1996; 31:619-624.
259. Walker RC, Marshall WF, Strickler JG, et al: Pretransplantation assessment of the risk of lymphoproliferative disorder. Clin Infect Dis 1995; 20:1346-1353.
260. Cockfield SM, Preiksaitis JK, Jewell LD, Parfrey NA: Post-transplant lymphoproliferative disorder in renal allograft recipients. Clinical experience and risk factor analysis in a single center. Transplantation 1993; 56:88-96.
261. Sokal EM, Caragiozoglou T, Lamy M, et al: Epstein-Barr virus serology and Epstein-Barr virus-associated lymphoproliferative disorders in pediatric liver transplant recipients (See comments). Transplantation 1993; 56:1394-1398.
262. Srivastava T, Zwick DL, Rothberg PG, Warady BA: Posttransplant lymphoproliferative disorder in pediatric renal transplantation. Pediatr Nephrol 1999; 13:748-754.
263. Swinnen LJ, Costanzo-Nordin MR, Fisher SG, et al: Increased incidence of lymphoproliferative disorder after immunosuppression with the monoclonal antibody OKT3 in cardiac-transplant recipients (See comments). N Engl J Med 1990; 323:1723-1728.
264. Ellis D, Shapiro R, Jordan ML, et al: Comparison of FK-506 and cyclosporine regimens in pediatric renal transplantation. Pediatr Nephrol 1994; 8:193-200.
265. Kenagy DN, Schlesinger Y, Weck K, et al: Epstein-Barr virus DNA in peripheral blood leukocytes of patients with posttransplant lymphoproliferative disease. Transplantation 1995; 60:547-554.
266. Campe H, Jaeger G, Abou-Ajram C, et al: Serial detection of Epstein-Barr virus DNA in sera and peripheral blood leukocyte samples of pediatric renal allograft recipients with persistent mononucleosis-like symptoms defines patients at risk to develop post-transplant lymphoproliferative disease. Pediatr Transplant 2003; 7:46-52.
267. Gupta M, Filler G, Kovesi T, et al: Quantitative tissue polymerase chain reaction for Epstein-Barr virus in pediatric solid organ recipients. Am J Kidney Dis 2003; 41:212-219.
268. Jabs WJ, Hennig H, Kittel M, et al: Normalized quantification by real-time PCR of Epstein-Barr virus load in patients at risk for posttransplant lymphoproliferative disorders. J Clin Microbiol 2001; 39:564-569.
269. Wagner HJ, Wessel M, Jabs W, et al: Patients at risk for development of posttransplant lymphoproliferative disorder: Plasma versus peripheral blood mononuclear cells as material for quantification of Epstein-Barr viral load by using real-time quantitative polymerase chain reaction. Transplantation 2001; 72:1012-1019.
270. Rooney CM, Loftin SK, Holladay MS, et al: Early identification of Epstein-Barr virus-associated post-transplantation lymphoproliferative disease. Br J Haematol 1995; 89:98-103.
271. Falco DA, Nepomuceno RR, Krams SM, et al: Identification of Epstein-Barr virus-specific CD8+ T lymphocytes in the circulation of pediatric transplant recipients. Transplantation 2002; 74:501-510.
272. Shroff R, Trompeter R, Cubitt D, et al: Epstein-Barr virus monitoring in paediatric renal transplant recipients. Pediatr Nephrol 2002; 17:770-775.
273. Harris KM, Schwartz ML, Slasky BS, et al: Posttransplantation cyclosporine-induced lymphoproliferative disorders: Clinical and radiologic manifestations. Radiology 1987; 162:697-700.
274. Chen JM, Barr ML, Chadburn A, et al: Management of lymphoproliferative disorders after cardiac transplantation. Ann Thorac Surg 1993; 56:527-538.
275. Taguchi Y, Purtilo DT, Okano M: The effect of intravenous immunoglobulin and interferon-alpha on Epstein-Barr virus-induced lymphoproliferative disorder in a liver transplant recipient. Transplantation 1994; 57:1813-1815.
276. Shapiro RS, Chauvenet A, McGuire W, et al: Treatment of B-cell lymphoproliferative disorders with interferon alfa and intravenous gamma globulin (Letter). N Engl J Med 1988; 318:1334.
277. Pirsch JD, Stratta RJ, Sollinger HW, et al: Treatment of severe Epstein-Barr virus-induced lymphoproliferative syndrome with ganciclovir: Two cases after solid organ transplantation. Am J Med 1989; 86:241-244.
278. Davis CL, Harrison KL, McVicar JP, et al: Antiviral prophylaxis and the Epstein Barr virus-related post-transplant lymphoproliferative disorder. Clin Transplant 1995; 9:53-59.
279. Herman J, Vandenberghe P, van den Heuvel I, et al: Successful treatment with rituximab of lymphoproliferative disorder in a child after cardiac transplantation. J Heart Lung Transplant 2002; 21:1304-1309.
280. Berney T, Delis S, Kato T, et al: Successful treatment of posttransplant lymphoproliferative disease with prolonged rituximab treatment in intestinal transplant recipients. Transplantation 2002; 74:1000-1006.
281. McGhee W, Mazariegos GV, Sindhi R, et al: Rituximab in the treatment of pediatric small bowel transplant patients with posttransplant lymphoproliferative disorder unresponsive to standard treatment. Transplantation Proc 2002; 34:955-956.
282. Serinet MO, Jacquemin E, Habes D, et al: Anti-CD20 monoclonal antibody (Rituximab) treatment for Epstein-Barr virus-associated, B-cell lymphoproliferative disease in pediatric liver transplant recipients (Comment). J Pediatr Gastroenterol Nutr 2002; 34:389-393.
283. Dotti G, Rambaldi A, Fiocchi R, et al: Anti-CD20 antibody (rituximab) administration in patients with late occurring lymphomas after solid organ transplant. Haematologica. 2001; 86: 618-623.
284. Balfour H Jr, Chace BA, Stapleton JT, et al: A randomized, placebo-controlled trial of oral acyclovir for the prevention of cytomegalovirus disease in recipients of renal allografts (See comments). N Engl J Med 1989; 320:1381-1387.
285. Schmidt GM, Horak DA, Niland JC, et al: A randomized, controlled trial of prophylactic ganciclovir for cytomegalovirus pulmonary infection in recipients of allogeneic bone marrow transplants. The City of Hope-Stanford-Syntex CMV Study Group (See comments). N Engl J Med 1991; 324:1005-1011.
286. Ahsan N, Holman MJ, Yang HC: Efficacy of oral ganciclovir in prevention of cytomegalovirus infection in post-kidney transplant patients. Clin Transplant 1997; 11:633-639.
287. Brennan DC, Garlock KA, Singer GG, et al: Prophylactic oral ganciclovir compared with deferred therapy for control of cytomegalovirus in renal transplant recipients. Transplantation 1997; 64:1843-1846.
288. Pescovitz MD, Brook B, Jindal RM, et al: Oral ganciclovir in pediatric transplant recipients: A pharmacokinetic study. Clin Transplant 1997; 11:613-617.
289. Harmon WE: Opportunistic infections in children following renal transplantation (Review). Pediatr Nephrol 1991; 5: 118-125.
290. Lynfield R, Herrin JT, Rubin RH: Varicella in pediatric renal transplant recipients. Pediatrics 1992; 90:216-220.
291. Kashtan CE, Cook M, Chavers BM, et al: Outcome of chickenpox in 66 pediatric renal transplant recipients. J Pediatr 1997; 131:874-877.

292. Broyer M, Tete MJ, Guest G, et al: Varicella and zoster in children after kidney transplantation: Long-term results of vaccination. Pediatrics 1997; 99:35-39.
293. Zamora I, Simon JM, Da Silva ME, Piqueras AI: Attenuated varicella virus vaccine in children with renal transplants. Pediatr Nephrol 1994; 8:190-192.
294. Prat V, Horcickova M, Matousovic K, et al: Urinary tract infection in renal transplant patients. Infection 1985; 13:207-210.
295. Peterson PK, Ferguson R, Fryd DS, et al: Infectious diseases in hospitalized renal transplant recipients: A prospective study of a complex and evolving problem. Medicine 1982; 61:360-372.
296. Drachenberg CB, Beskow CO, Cangro CB, et al: Human polyoma virus in renal allograft biopsies: Morphological findings and correlation with urine cytology. Hum Pathol 1999; 30:970-977.
297. Ginevri F, De Santis R, Comoli P, et al: Polyomavirus BK infection in pediatric kidney-allograft recipients: A single-center analysis of incidence, risk factors, and novel therapeutic approaches. Transplantation 2003; 75:1266-1270.
298. Ding R, Medeiros M, Dadhania D, et al: Noninvasive diagnosis of BK virus nephritis by measurement of messenger RNA for BK virus VP1 in urine. Transplantation 2002; 74:987-994.
299. Baluarte HJ, Gruskin AB, Ingelfinger JR, et al: Analysis of hypertension in children post renal transplantation: A report of the North American Pediatric Renal Transplant Cooperative Study (NAPRTCS). Pediatr Nephrol 1994; 8:570-573.
300. Morgan H, Khan I, Hashmi A, et al: Ambulatory blood pressure monitoring after renal transplantation in children. Pediatr Nephrol 2001; 16:843-847.
301. Sorof JM, Poffenbarger T, Portman R: Abnormal 24-hour blood pressure patterns in children after renal transplantation. Am J Kidney Dis 2000; 35:681-686.
302. Wigger M, Druckler E, Muscheites J, Stolpe HJ: Course of glomerular filtration rate after renal transplantation and the influence of hypertension. Clin Nephrol 2001; 56:S30-S34.
303. Mitsnefes MM, Schwartz SM, Daniels SR, et al: Changes in left ventricular mass index in children and adolescents after renal transplantation. Pediatr Transplant 2001; 5:279-284.
304. Mitsnefes MM, Omoloja A, McEnery PT: Short-term pediatric renal transplant survival: Blood pressure and allograft function. Pediatr Transplant 2001; 5:160-165.
305. Lilien MR, Stroes ES, Op't Roodt J, et al: Vascular function in children after renal transplantation. Am J Kidney Dis 2003; 41:684-691.
306. Shin GT, Cheigh JS, Riggio RR, et al: Effect of nifedipine on renal allograft function and survival beyond one year. Clin Nephrol 1997; 47:33-36.
307. Cohen LS, Friedman EA: Losartan-induced azotemia in a diabetic recipient of a kidney transplant (Letter). N Engl J Med 1996; 334:1271-1272.
308. Grekas D, Dioudis C, Kalevrosoglou I, et al: Renal hemodynamics in hypertensive renal allograft recipients: Effects of calcium antagonists and ACE inhibitors. Kidney Int Suppl 1996; 55:S97-S100.
309. Harris KP, Russell GI, Parvin SD, et al: Alterations in lipid and carbohydrate metabolism attributable to cyclosporin A in renal transplant recipients. Br Med J 1986; 292:16.
310. Raine AEG: Cardiovascular complications after renal transplantation. *In* Morris PJ (ed): Kidney Transplantation: Principles and Practice. Philadelphia, WB Saunders, 1994, pp 339-355.
311. Vathsala A, Weinberg RB, Schoenberg L, et al: Lipid abnormalities in cyclosporine-prednisone-treated renal transplant recipients. Transplantation 1989; 48:37-43.
312. Drueke TB, Abdulmassih Z, Lacour B, et al: Atherosclerosis and lipid disorders after renal transplantation (Review). Kidney Int Suppl 1991; 31:S24-S28.
313. Singh A, Tejani C, Benfield M, et al: Natural history of lipid abnormalities in children post-transplantation, 16th Annual Meeting of the American Society of Transplant Physicians (Abstract). Chicago, 1997.
314. Grundy SM: HMG-CoA reductase inhibitors for treatment of hypercholesterolemia (Review). N Engl J Med 1988; 319:24-33.
315. Silverstein DM: Indications and outcome of treatment of hyperlipidemia in pediatric allograft recipients (Comment). Pediatr Transplant 2003; 7:7-10.
316. Hricik DE, Bartucci MR, Moir EJ, et al: Effects of steroid withdrawal on posttransplant diabetes mellitus in cyclosporine-treated renal transplant recipients. Transplantation 1991; 51: 374-377.
317. Al-Uzri A, Stablein DM, A Cohn R: Posttransplant diabetes mellitus in pediatric renal transplant recipients: A report of the North American Pediatric Renal Transplant Cooperative Study (NAPRTCS). Transplantation 2001; 72:1020-1024.
318. Ferraresso M, Ghio L, Edefonti A, et al: Conversion from cyclosporine to tacrolimus in pediatric kidney transplant recipients. Pediatr Nephrol 2002; 17:664-667.
319. Butani L, Makker SP: Conversion from tacrolimus to neoral for postrenal transplant diabetes. Pediatr Nephrol 2000; 15:176-178.
320. Meyers KE, Weiland H, Thomson PD: Paediatric renal transplantation non-compliance. Pediatr Nephrol 1995; 9:189-192.
321. Beck DE, Fennell RS, Yost RL, et al: Evaluation of an educational program on compliance with medication regimens in pediatric patients with renal transplants. J Pediatr 1980; 96:1094-1097.
322. Ettenger RB, Rosenthal JT, Marik JL, et al: Improved cadaveric renal transplant outcome in children. Pediatr Nephrol 1991; 5:137-142.
323. Foulkes LM, Boggs SR, Fennell RS, Skibinski K: Social support, family variables, and compliance in renal transplant children. Pediatr Nephrol 1993; 7:185-188.
324. Bell F: Post-renal transplant compliance. J Child Health Care 2000; 4:5-9.
325. Blowey DL, Hebert D, Arbus GS, et al: Compliance with cyclosporine in adolescent renal transplant recipients. Pediatr Nephrol 1997; 11:547-551.
326. Fennell RS, Foulkes LM, Boggs SR: Family-based program to promote medication compliance in renal transplant children. Transplant Proc 1994; 26:102-103.
327. Apajasalo M, Rautonen J, Sintonen H, Holmberg C: Health-related quality of life after organ transplantation in childhood. Pediatr Transplant 1997; 1:130-137.
328. Kim MS, Jabs K, Harmon WE: Long-term patient survival in a pediatric renal transplantation program. Transplantation 1991; 51:413-416.
329. Morel P, Almond PS, Matas AJ, et al: Long-term quality of life after kidney transplantation in childhood. Transplantation 1991; 52:47-53.
330. Potter DE, Najarian J, Belzer F, et al: Long-term results of renal transplantation in children. Kidney Int 1991; 40:752-756.
331. Ehrich JH, Rizzoni G, Broyer M, et al: Rehabilitation of young adults during renal replacement therapy in Europe. II. Schooling, employment, and social situation. Nephrol Dial Transplant 1992; 7:579-586.

Emerging Strategies in Kidney Transplantation

Marilia Cascalho, M.D., Ph.D. • Brenda M. Ogle, Ph.D. • Jeffrey L. Platt, M.D.

No area of medicine has provoked so much excitement and so much frustration as transplantation. The excitement stems from the possibility that transplanting an organ such as a kidney into a desperately ill individual can change that individual's condition almost immediately to one of good health. The frustration stems from the fact that organs, such as the kidney, are not available for transplantation into all of those who need them[1] and from the fact that those who are fortunate enough to receive an organ transplant must also be treated for life with toxic immunosuppressive therapies to avoid rejection of the graft. New developments in medicine and biotechnology may add substantially to the excitement and frustration.

One new development that may change the demand for transplantation is molecular and genomic diagnosis. Advances in molecular diagnostics, genomics, and possibly proteomics may soon make it possible to predict the onset of disease long before the symptoms are manifest and to predict the course once disease has become apparent. With this information, the clinician may be tempted even more than before to carry out "preemptive" transplantation to spare the patient from adding the risks of organ failure or other diseases to the risks of transplantation.[2] For example, molecular diagnostics and genomics are approaching the levels of specificity and sensitivity that may make it possible to diagnose cancer before it can be localized by imaging. If new diagnostic tools make it possible to say with reasonable certainty that an individual has renal-cell or bladder cancer but that the cancer is too small to be localized by imaging, then it may be tempting to consider removing the kidneys or the bladder and replacing them with suitable substitutes. This type of preemptive transplant is sometimes carried out when an infant with ambiguous genitalia is found to have the Denys-Drash syndrome.[3,4] Extending preemptive transplantation to adults with high likelihood of tumor formation could add as many as 89,000 potential recipients per year to those awaiting kidney transplants. The circumstances are worse for the lung; preemptive transplantation would increase the demand for transplantation by 100-fold.

Another advance that could vastly increase the demand for kidney transplantation or renal cell transplantation comes from recent studies on the epidemiology of cardiovascular disease. Mann and associates[5] found that small decreases in glomerular filtration and the presence of microalbuminuria correlate with heightened risk of atherosclerosis, ischemic heart disease, and death.[6] Of course, this association between minor renal abnormalities and cardiovascular disease may simply mean that the kidney is a sentinel for diseases of the blood vessels and the heart. However, a more intriguing explanation for these findings is that the kidney may support cardiovascular health and that a small loss of renal function may cause a disproportionate amount of cardiovascular damage. For example, the kidney may clear insulin, metabolize vitamin D, or remove a toxin from the blood. Such a function might explain why atherosclerosis and ischemic heart disease are observed so often in those who receive a kidney transplant (and thus are uni-nephric) and in those on dialysis. If the kidney does contribute to cardiovascular health, then one might argue that transplants should contain a larger renal mass, that is, transplants should be of two kidneys, or that the transplants need to include a larger number of a specific cell type. This concept suggests the possibility that transplantation of the kidneys or of a type of renal cell might someday be undertaken to prevent vascular disease in those with minimal decreases in renal function, and that scenario could clearly increase the demand for renal transplantation by yet another order of magnitude.

Clearly, the number of kidneys available for transplantation today is by any measure too small. Hence, one can anticipate a growing interest in seeking alternatives to the use of human organs for renal replacement. This chapter will consider various technologies that might be used to augment renal function and some strategies through which those technologies may some day be applied.

XENOTRANSPLANTATION

The most obvious alternative to the use of human organs and cells for transplantation is xenotransplantation, the transplantation of animal organs, tissues, or cells into humans. Xenotransplantation has been advocated and tried at various times during the past century for replacement of renal function. The experience with clinical xenotransplantation of the kidney is summarized in Table 41–1. The sections that follow will consider the biologic barriers that prevent clinical application of xenotransplantation. The reader is referred to a collection of recent reviews for more detailed consideration.[7] Although kidneys from nonhuman primates have been used in some trials of xenotransplantation,[8–10] and the results in one were quite good,[11] we shall focus on the use of lower animals as a source of kidneys, because among other problems nonhuman primates, such as baboons, are too small and not sufficiently numerous to address the need. Larger mammals, particularly the pig, are suitable in size, available in large numbers, and these animals can be genetically engineered and bred.

Barriers to Xenotransplantation

Three factors pose barriers to clinical xenotransplantation. These factors are the immune response of the recipient against

Table 41–1 Experience with Clinical Xenotransplantation

Year	Recipients (Surgeon)	Source of Kidney	Survival	Ref.
1906	2 (Jaboulay)	pig and goat	3 days	124
1910	1 (Unger)	macaque	<2 days	125
1914	1 (Ullman)		unsuccessful	126
1923	1 (Neuhof)	sheep	9 days	127
1963/64	13 (Reemtsma)	chimpanzee (12), macaque (1)	9 months, 12 days	8,11,128
1964	3 (Traeger)	chimpanzee	49 days	129
1964	1 (Hume)	chimpanzee	1 day	130
1964	6 (Starzl)	baboon	60 days	9
1964	1 (Hitchcock)	baboon	5 days	131
1965	2 (Goldsmith)	chimpanzee	4 months	132
1966	1 (Cortesini)	chimpanzee	31 days	133

the graft, the physiologic limitations of the transplant in the foreign host, and the possibility of transferring infectious agents from the graft to the recipient and potentially to others in society. Because xenotransplantation has been attempted on a number of occasions over the past 100 years, much more is known about these barriers than the barriers to other technologies, such as stem cells and tissue engineering. Because we believe that the immune response to xenotransplantation is the most difficult barrier to overcome, we shall focus especially on this subject.

The immune responses to xenotransplantation are much more severe than the immune responses to allotransplantation.[12] One reason why immune responses to xenografts are severe is that all normal individuals have innate immune reactants—including xenoreactive natural antibodies, complement, and natural killer cells—against xenogeneic cells. Not only can innate immunity destroy a xenograft, but it also amplifies adaptive immune responses. Another reason why immune responses to xenografts are severe is that xenografts carry a diverse set of foreign antigens against which cellular and humoral immune responses can be elicited (in allotransplants, the main foreign antigens are MHC antigens).[13] Finally, immune responses to xenografts may be severe because immune-regulation, which might partially control responses to allografts, may fail to do so in responses to xenografts.

The Barrier to Xenotransplantation of Cells and Tissues

As the preceding discussion suggested, one might seek to replace or amplify some aspect of renal function by a cellular transplant. The main barrier to transplanting xenogeneic cells and tissues is cellular rejection (Figure 41–1). Cell-mediated

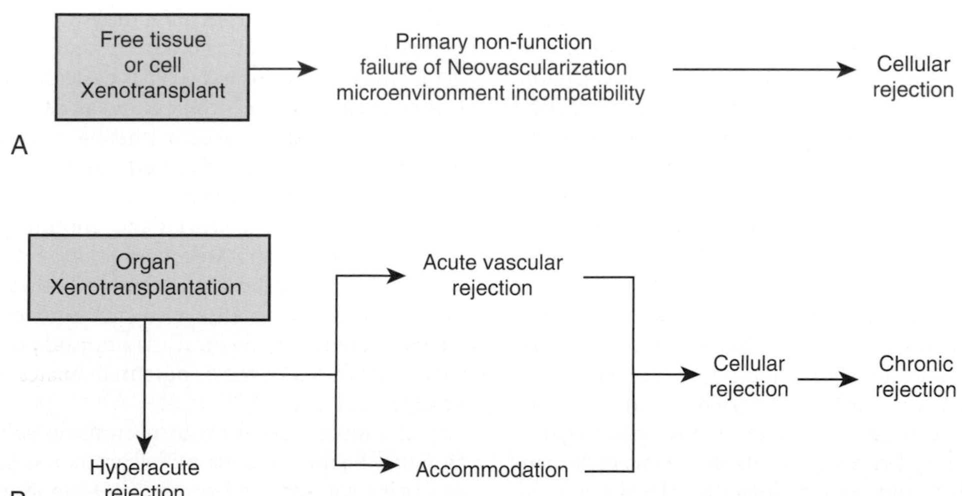

Figure 41–1 Biologic hurdles for xenotransplantation. ***A***, Tissue or cell xenotransplants are subject to failure caused by primary nonfunction that may reflect failure of engraftment or a very rapid immune response. If primary nonfunction is bypassed and the tissue or cells engraft, they are then subject to cellular rejection. Humoral rejection is not usually observed because the blood vessels are of recipient origin. ***B***, Organ transplantation between disparate species can lead to hyperacute rejection. If hyperacute rejection is averted by depletion of xenoreactive natural antibodies or inhibition of the complement system, the xenograft is subject to acute vascular rejection, or "accommodation." If acute vascular rejection is prevented, the graft will be subject to cellular rejection or chronic rejection.

immune responses to xenotransplantation are thought to be especially severe[13–15] and may, in our view, be further amplified by the humoral immune reactions and by failure of immune regulation between species.[12,16] Some fundamental aspects of the cellular immune response to xenotransplantation have been reviewed by us[12,17] and others.[18,19] What is pertinent to mention here is that, despite the severity of cell-mediated rejection of cell and tissue transplants between disparate species, it appears to be subject to control by immunosuppressive agents currently available.[20–23] In fact, under some conditions, xenogeneic cellular grafts survive and function without immunosuppression.[23] Thus, if one were to identify or engineer a xenogeneic cell or cell line that could replace critical metabolic functions of the kidney, that xenograft might be undertaken today without new methods of immune modulation.

The Barriers to Xenotransplantation of Vascularized Organs

The barriers to transplantation of whole organs, such as the kidney, are much higher than the barriers to transplantation of cells or tissues. In kidney transplants, the donor blood vessels are directly exposed to components of the immune system of the recipient, and this interaction gives rise to severe vascular disease in various forms, which has, to this point, prevented clinical xenotransplantation (Figure 41–1). The types of vascular disease observed in xenografted organs are the same as those observed in allografted organs; however, the incidence, severity, and resistance to therapy are greater in xenografts.

Renal xenografts are quite susceptible to hyperacute rejection, which can destroy the graft within minutes to a few hours.[17,20,24] Hyperacute rejection of porcine organs transplanted into primates is triggered by xenoreactive natural antibodies, which are found in all immunocompetent people and higher primates and are specific for Galα1-3Gal, a saccharide expressed by pigs and other lower mammals.[25] The binding of these antibodies activates complement, and complement activation in blood vessels of the graft causes hyperacute rejection.

How complement activation triggers hyperacute rejection has been elucidated largely through the study of experimental xenografts. Hyperacute rejection is caused by the rapid insertion of terminal complement complexes into the cell membranes of the endothelial lining of blood vessels in the donor organ.[20,26] What makes hyperacute rejection of xenografts especially severe is that activation of complement in the graft is poorly controlled by endogenous complement regulators, such as decay accelerating factor, membrane cofactor protein, and CD59.[27,28] These proteins function poorly across species, and, consequently, the complement regulators in a porcine organ would provide only a low level of protection against human complement.[17] Consistent with this concept, organs from transgenic pigs expressing human complement regulatory proteins are protected from hyperacute rejection.[29–32] Today, pigs expressing these proteins have been widely used in experimental studies, and hyperacute rejection is no longer viewed as a substantial barrier to xenotransplantation.

If hyperacute rejection is prevented, a renal xenograft becomes susceptible to a condition we have called acute vascular rejection.[33,34] Acute vascular rejection, sometimes called acute humoral rejection or delayed xenograft rejection, may well be the main hurdle to clinical application of xenotransplantation.[35–37] Acute vascular rejection appears to be caused by xenoreactive antibodies that bind to the xenograft, causing "activation" of endothelium in the graft.[33,38,39] Whereas the endothelium of normal blood vessels promotes blood flow and inhibits thrombosis and inflammation, activated endothelium promotes vasoconstriction, thrombosis and inflammation, giving rise to the picture of ischemia and thrombosis characteristic of acute vascular rejection of xenografts.[34,35,40] These pathophysiologic changes in endothelium are due, at least in part, to coordinated elaboration of tissue factor, plasminogen activator inhibitor type I, E-selectin and thromboxane A2, and other products of genes induced by the action of xenoreactive antibodies, small amounts of complement, or platelets.[17,36,38,40–42] Because acute vascular rejection is thought to be the main biologic obstacle to xenotransplantation of organs, much effort is now directed at developing the means to prevent or treat this disorder. Here we summarize the main approaches.

One way to prevent acute vascular rejection may be to suppress the production of xenoreactive antibodies by drug therapy or through induction of tolerance. However, various regimens of immunosuppressive agents have failed to control the humoral response to xenotransplantation. Another way to prevent acute vascular rejection is to induce immunologic tolerance to xenografts. Various approaches to tolerance have been tried[43]; however, most approaches effective in rodents have not proven applicable in humans. One approach that might be sufficiently effective is the engraftment of hematopoietic cells.[44,45] Unfortunately, the biologic hurdles to engraftment of xenogeneic bone marrow cells, which include the action of antibodies and complement on the cells, the incompatibility of host growth factors,[46,47] and induction of thrombosis,[48,49] have precluded application of this method to the present.

Another way to prevent acute vascular rejection might be to eliminate the antigens targeted by xenoreactive antibodies. Although porcine cells express many antigens potentially recognized by the human immune system, the main antigen target by the earliest observed types of acute vascular rejection is Galα1-3Gal.[50] Recent progress in the cloning of pigs[51–53] and in gene targeting[54] makes it possible to knock out the gene encoding the enzyme (α1,3-galactosyltransferase) responsible for synthesis of this saccharide.[55–57] Pigs lacking this enzyme have been recently produced and are under study. As of this date, it is not clear that this manipulation has solved the problem. Indeed, some have questioned whether knocking out this enzyme would eradicate the sugar.[58] And, even if it is possible to eliminate this antigen, it may not be possible to eliminate many other xenogeneic potential antigens present in the xenogeneic kidney.[59–61]

Still another approach to preventing acute vascular rejection may be the inducing of "accommodation." First described in organs transplanted across ABO-blood group barriers,[62,63] accommodation is an acquired resistance of an organ to immune-mediated injury.[17] Accommodation has been used to prevent acute vascular rejection in rodents and, arguably, in pig-to-primate xenografts.[41,50,64]

How can accommodation be reliably induced and what mechanisms underlie it? Accommodation might reflect a change in xenoreactive antibodies or a change in the antigens in the graft[65]; however, experimental work in xenograft models suggest accommodation results at least in part from an acquired resistance of the graft to humoral injury.[64] Consistent with the later possibility are experiments showing that endothelial cells exposed to xenoreactive antibodies acquire resistance to complement mediated injury, owing to increased expression of CD59[66] and other inhibitors of injury.[67] Studies in rodents have shown that accommodation is associated with expression of genes, such as Bcl-2 that inhibit apoptosis and hemoxygenase-1 (HO-1) that confer protection against toxic injury.[68] Organ grafts deficient in HO-1 or in functional complement-regulatory proteins appear to be subject to severe vascular injury,[69] and current study suggests that the regulatory function of HO-1 is related to carbon monoxides generated by HO-1.[70] However, efforts to prevent vascular injury by expression of these genes may not be sufficient to induce a state of accommodation, because grafts with increased expression of HO-1 and/or CD59 may still undergo acute vascular rejection.[71,72] (unpublished observations). This suggests that accommodation is multifactorial.

When acute vascular rejection is prevented, xenografts are susceptible to cellular rejection, as discussed previously, and presumably to chronic rejection.[73] If chronic rejection is caused by an immune response to the graft, as some experimental evidence suggests,[74] then it should be common and severe in xenotransplants. If chronic rejection is caused by qualities of the graft, such as preservation time, ischemia, and donor age, then it should not be much of a problem. In any case, since xenotransplantation offers an unlimited supply of organs, the impact of chronic rejection may be less serious, because the chronically-rejected organ can be replaced.

Physiologic Hurdles to Xenotransplantation

Studies in which porcine kidneys have been transplanted into nonhuman primates suggest that they function sufficiently in a human to sustain life.[75] In fact, the main functional impairment of these xenogeneic organ grafts is from rejection. However, porcine erythropoietin appears to work poorly on human cells, so supplementation with the human hormone would probably be needed. While other defects might still be discovered, these defects are probably no worse than abnormalities imposed by dialysis.

Infectious Agents

Another barrier to xenotransplantation is infection.[76,77] Infection should be less severe a risk in xenotransplantation than in allotransplantation because the animal source can be raised in an environment free of known pathogens, and the organisms associated with the animal can be fully characterized. However, attention has been focused on endogenous retroviruses of the pig, which cannot be eliminated by breeding or special handling.[78] The porcine endogenous retrovirus or PERV can infect human cells in culture and in *in vivo* model systems,[79] hence there is concern it might be transmitted to a xenograft recipient and possibly more widely in the population. However, studies of human subjects who received experimental xenografts or treatment with porcine cells have failed to reveal even a single instance in which PERV has been transmitted to a human subject.[80] Moreover, a recent study suggests that those viruses known at present could be eradicated from pig herds being bred for xenotransplantation.[81]

Although the question of relevance of PERV to public health cannot be entirely dismissed, the question may now be viewed as one that could be resolved by careful attention to the recipients of xenografts, rather than as a reason for abandoning xenotransplantation.[77,82]

Of all the barriers to xenotransplantation, immune responses against the graft appears to be the most difficult to surmount. Nevertheless, it is reasonable to assume that these responses, or their consequences, will be addressed in the coming years. The main question then will not be whether xenotransplantation is feasible, but rather whether the physiologic "cost" of immunosuppression and immune modulation needed to allow the prolonged survival and function of a xenograft justifies this approach to renal replacement. For the patient with renal failure, this biologic cost may well be justified, and xenotransplantation might be welcomed. On the other hand, the biologic costs of xenotransplantation might not justify application as a preemptive procedure, and, for this purpose, other technologies will probably be needed. One type of xenograft that could achieve widespread use is a cellular xenograft. Recent studies have shown that xenogeneic cells can be successfully engrafted with little[22] or no[23] immunosuppression. If the xenotransplantation of a renal cell or another cell suitably engineered could overcome the vascular disease putatively caused by small decrements in renal function or microalbuminuria, such grafts might be found useful at some point in the future.

Stem Cells for Augmentation and Replacement of Organ Function

Stem cells are cells capable of self-renewal and of generating at least one, and often more than one, differentiated line of cells. Stem cells obtained from the inner cell mass of the blastocysts are called *embryonic* stem cells. Stem cells may also be isolated from mature individuals or generated by transfer of nuclei from mature cells to immature cell bodies, that is, cloning (Figure 41–2). Stem cells are thought to be capable of regenerating diseased or damaged tissues[83] and of being coaxed to generate tissues and organs de novo.[84,85] However, depending

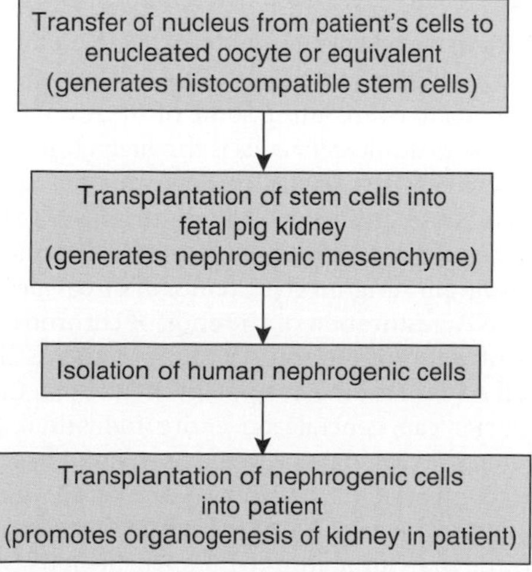

Figure 41–2 A potential approach to replacement of the kidney, using multiple technologies—cloning, stem cells, and organogenesis.

on the type of stem cells used, application may be limited by (1) the proliferative senescence of the cells; (2) constraints on the ability of the cells to differentiate into mature, functional tissues; (3) the possibility that the cells might transform in culture, and (4) immune response against foreign antigens expressed by the cells. A full consideration of these limitations is beyond the scope of this chapter, but some potential applications and limitations will be discussed.

Embryonic stem cells have the capacity to proliferate indefinitely and generate all tissues and organs, including kidney-like tissue.[86] In principle, then, embryonic stem cells might be grown into a kidney. How exactly to coax organ formation, rather than kidney-like tissue, is not known. As discussed later, isolated fetal cells and organ rudiments do have the capacity to form an entire organ, a process known as *organogenesis*, but making less differentiated, less committed cells behave in this way would appear to be a challenge. One application of embryonic stem cells that might be considered is providing whatever metabolic functions are lacking in those with mild renal insufficiency. Given progress in devising methods for coaxing embryonic stem cells to serve endocrine functions,[84] it is reasonable to think the means could be devised to make the cells secrete erythropoietin or carry out needed metabolic functions. Because embryonic stem cells express allogeneic histocompatibility antigens, use of the cells might require immunosuppression. However, some recent work in rodents suggests that embryonic stem cells may not be immunogenic or may even help induce tolerance.[87]

Stem cells can be isolated from adults, and these cells do have the capacity to differentiate into complex structures.[88] The advantage of using "adult" stem cells are that the cells might be isolated from the patient themselves, thus avoiding immune reactions and ethical problems associated with use of totipotent embryonic cells. Adult stem cells can migrate through the blood and take up residence in injured tissues.[82,89] Thus, stem cells regenerate diseased tissues. However, effective application of stem cells for regeneration may require overcoming barriers still unknown that prevented the natural stem cells of the patient from regenerating the diseased kidney in the first place. The generating of a whole organ, such as the kidney, by adult stem cells is less feasible than doing so with embryonic stem cells, because adult stem cells appear to have less ability to proliferate and differentiate. However, adult stem cells might someday be used to provide metabolic functions, as discussed previously.

One approach to overcoming some of the limitations to use of embryonic and adult stem cells is through cloning. Cloning is accomplished by harvesting nuclei from the cells of one individual and implanting the nuclei in primitive cells, such as oocytes or zygotes, that have the capacity to "reprogram" the nuclei. Reprogramming involves removal of covalent modifications of DNA, restoration of the ends of chromosomes, and expression of appropriate transcription elements that allow the new cell to function as totipotent stem cells. Cloning by nuclear transfer can generate an entire individual, a process called *reproductive* cloning, or a tissue or organ, a process called *therapeutic* cloning. One advantage of therapeutic cloning is that it generates cells with the same histocompatibility antigens as the individual from whom the nucleus is obtained (except for mitochondrial antigens, which derive from the oocyte). Another advantage is that the cells, like embryonic stem cells, can develop into any tissue. However, like embryonic stem cells, it is still unknown how to make the cells form an organ ex vivo. However, cloning might be used as a source of cells for bioengineering of tissues and organs. Indeed, one recent report claims to have generated kidney-like devices using cloned cells of cattle.[90] However, the method described used cells actually harvested from a fetus, and thus reproductive rather than therapeutic cloning was performed.

The application of cloning faces ethical hurdles. Use of a zygote or even an oocyte as a "recipient" for the donor nucleus has provoked opposition because it is seen by some as creating life. Similarly, reproductive cloning has been widely seen as unethical to undertake. However, new insights into the mechanisms of nuclear reprogramming may allow reprogramming to be directly undertaken without the use of a primitive human cell. Further, if the cloned cells can be engineered to be of limited potential, it may avert the concern about disrupting human life.

Tissue Engineering

Although embryonic stem cells or cloned cells have the capacity to differentiate any type of cell and contribute to formation of mature tissues and organs, they may not be able to form intact organs, as discussed previously. Organogenesis, as such, requires cues from complex cell–cell and cell–matrix interactions that may not be easily recapitulated outside the embryo. One way to deliver some of these cues is through tissue engineering, the use of scaffolds consisting of synthetic or biologic polymers, to coax growth and development.[91] Tissue engineering has been used to generate blood vessels,[92–95] heart valves,[96–98] cardiac muscle,[99–101] bone,[102] liver,[103–105] nerve,[106] and islets.[107] The most successful applications have been engineered cartilage[108,109] and skin.[110–113] Tissue engineering is not generally thought to be applicable for organ replacement because the matrices in current use do not permit the growth of cells into a sufficient mass or anatomic complexity to yield a whole organ.

Organogenesis

What may be needed to meet the needs for kidneys and to overcome some of the limitations mentioned earlier is a method to grow organs de novo, that is, organogenesis. The growing of organs has been carried out for experimental purposes for many years. Nephrogenic mesenchyme cultured under suitable conditions has been shown to develop into kidney-like structures in vitro.[114] Since human fetal nephrogenic mesenchyme will not be available, what is needed is a way either to use xenogeneic nephrogenic mesenchyme or to drive stem cells to become nephrogenic mesenchyme. Both will be discussed.

Fetal kidney tissues from various sources have been found to mature after implantation into adult animals.[115–118] Organs grown in this way are vascularized by ingrowth of blood vessels of the "recipient." Recently, Rogers[119] showed that fetal porcine kidney tissue can mature in an adult rat and that the tissue exhibits some renal function. Aside from the question of whether full function could be achieved by this approach, there is the concern that the xenogeneic organs would be destroyed by the immune response of the treated individual,[120,121] as described earlier. Although immune-injury is an important concern, the immune response is not as severe a hurdle as it might seem. Since the blood vessels in the organ would derive from the animal host,[115] that is, the treated individual, the graft would not be subject to the various types of vascular rejection described previously, but rather in principle, it would be subject only to cellular rejection. Still, preventing cellular rejection would require treatment with immunosuppressive agents,[119,120] and hence this application would be less appealing for preemptive therapy.

An alternative approach to organogenesis would be to use stem cells originating from the affected individual, perhaps derived by nuclear transfer. As already indicated, these stem cells may lack the ability to grow into an intact organ, but, in a natural environment, the cells are clearly capable of forming nephrogenic mesenchyme.[90] We have proposed that stem cells might be implanted into a fetal animal and there acquire the capacity to form the kidney.[122,123] The human cells might then be harvested and placed into the subject from which they originated, and in that subject organogenesis could proceed further. Under these conditions, the parenchymal cells would be from the clones and thus might express foreign mitochondrial antigens, but blood vessels in the organ would be derived from the human host,[115] and hence severe immune reactions might be avoided. An important limitation to this approach and indeed to application of tissue engineering in general is that it might be too expensive or complex to allow routine application.

Approaches to Augmentation and Replacement of Renal Function: A Synthesis

Given the various technologies that might be applied to replacement or augmentation of renal function, what strategies can be envisioned for application in the future? To address that question, we envision certain strategies to match certain clinical needs.

Those with severe chronic renal failure require immediate replacement of function. They might receive renal allografts as a permanent therapy, as currently practiced. Such individuals might be candidates for an "engineered" organ, as discussed later; however, in this case, temporary renal replacement would be needed, and an allograft, or even a xenograft, might serve that purpose.

For preemptive treatment (e.g., the patient with early diagnosis of renal cancer), the ideal therapy would involve removing the patient's kidneys and replacing them with organs engineered to be genetically similar or identical to the patient. This approach would avoid use of immunosuppression. The sequence of steps that might generate such an organ is shown in Figure 41–2. The steps include therapeutic cloning to generate stem cells that are nearly identical to the patient genetically (only proteins encoded by mitochondrial DNA would differ). The stem cells might be used to fashion a device[90]; however, we believe the better solution might be to generate nephrogenic mesenchyme in a xenogeneic host as described previously and then use it for organogenesis in the patient.[123] Applying this approach of the "engineered kidney" is labor intensive and undoubtedly quite expensive, but it would finally address the hurdle of immune compatibility between the graft and the host.

Another potential solution for full renal replacement would involve the use of a fully implantable device, which might be envisioned in the coming years, together with a cellular implant that would provide the metabolic functions deficient in the device. The cells used to replace renal metabolic functions would ideally be generated by therapeutic cloning to make them nearly compatible or nearly so with the patient.

For those who need a renal metabolic function to forestall vascular disease, one can envision use of cellular transplants. Such transplants might consist of xenogeneic cells, embryonic stem cells, or cells cloned by nuclear transfer. Clearly, the stem cells are preferable to the extent that their use obviates need for immunosuppression. However, if effective treatment were to be widely applied and were to require extensive genetic engineering to confer metabolic function, then xenogeneic cells might be preferred because the engineering could be carried out through germline modifications, yielding a well-characterized line of engineered animals.

CONCLUSION

Any discussion of future therapies, particularly complex therapies that might be applied for the augmentation or replacement of renal function, is fraught with hazard. Some technologies may be blocked by unforeseen barriers, or new technologies may eclipse the usefulness of those discussed earlier. New treatments may eradicate diabetes, hypertension, and glomerulonephritis, which underlie most cases of renal failure in the United States (although, these diseases may soon be replaced by aging). Also, improvements in existing technologies, such as implantable devices, may reduce the need for more complex therapies. However, we believe there is much to be gained by considering what approaches might be applied at a remote time. This consideration helps to determine which technologies need to be improved and which new technologies may be needed. Certainly, there must be an advantage to anticipating such needs well in advance of potential application.

References

1. Evans RW: Coming to terms with reality: Why xenotransplantation is a necessity. *In* JL Platt (ed): Xenotransplantation. Washington, D. C., ASM Press, 2001, pp 29-51.
2. Kasiske BL, Snyder JJ, Matas AJ, et al: Preemptive kidney transplantation: The advantage and the advantaged. J Am Soc Nephrol 2002; 13:1358-1364.
3. Rudin C, Pritchard J, Fernando ON, et al: Renal transplantation in the management of bilateral Wilms' tumour (BWT) and of Denys-Drash syndrome (DDS). Nephrol Dial Transplant 1998; 13:1506-1510.
4. Heathcott RW, Morison IM, Gubler MC, et al: A review of the phenotypic variation due to the Denys-Drash syndrome-associated germline WT1 mutation R362X. Hum Mutat 2002; 19:462.
5. Mann JFE, Gerstein HC, Pogue J, et al: Renal insufficiency as a predictor of cardiovascular outcomes and the impact of Ramipril: The HOPE randomized trial. Ann Intern Med 2001; 134:629-636.
6. Kasiske BL: The kidney in cardiovascular disease. Ann Intern Med 2001; 134:707-709.
7. Platt JL: Xenotransplantation. Washington, D.C., ASM Press, 2001, p 298.
8. Reemtsma K, McCracken BH, Schlegel JU, et al: Heterotransplantation of the kidney: Two clinical experiences. Science 1964; 143:700-702.

9. Starzl TE, Marchioro TL, Peters GN, et al: Renal heterotransplantation from baboon to man: Experience with 6 cases. Transplantation 1964; 2:752-776.
10. Reemtsma K, Benvenisty AI: Experience with clinical kidney xenotransplantation. *In* Cooper DKC, Kemp E, Reemtsma K, White DJG (eds): Xenotransplantation: The Transplantation of Organs and Tissues Between Species. New York, Springer-Verlag, 1991, pp 531-540.
11. Reemtsma K: Renal heterotransplantation from nonhuman primates to man. Ann N Y Acad Sci 1969; 162:412-418.
12. Cascalho M, Platt JL: The immunological barrier to xenotransplantation. Immunity 2001; 14:437-446.
13. Dorling A, Lombardi G, Binns R, et al: Detection of primary direct and indirect human anti-porcine T cell responses using a porcine dendritic cell population. Eur J Immunol 1996; 26: 1378-1387.
14. Murray AG, Khodadoust MM, Pober JS, et al: Porcine aortic endothelial cells activate human T cells: Direct presentation of MHC antigens and costimulation by ligands for human CD2 and CD28. Immunity 1994; 1:57-63.
15. Yamada K, Sachs DH, DerSimonian H: Human anti-porcine xenogeneic T cell response. Evidence for allelic specificity of mixed leukocyte reaction and for both direct and indirect pathways of recognition. J Immunol 1995; 155:5249-5256.
16. Platt JL, Lin SS: The future promises of xenotransplantation. Ann N Y Acad Sci 1998; 862:5-18.
17. Platt JL, Vercellotti GM, Dalmasso AP, et al: Transplantation of discordant xenografts: A review of progress. Immunol Today 1990; 11:450-456.
18. Auchincloss H Jr: Xenogeneic transplantation. Transplantation 1988; 46:1-20.
19. Auchincloss H Jr, Sachs DH: Xenogeneic transplantation. Annu Rev Immunol 1998; 16:433-470.
20. Platt JL: Hyperacute Xenograft Rejection. Austin, TX, R.G. Landes, 1995.
21. Marchetti P, Scharp DW, Finke EH, et al: Prolonged survival of discordant porcine islet xenografts. Transplantation 1996; 61:1100-1102.
22. Gunsalus JR, Brady DA, Coulter SM, et al: Reduction of serum cholesterol in Watanabe rabbits by xenogeneic hepatocellular transplantation. Nat Med 1997; 3:48-53.
23. Nagata H, Ito M, Cai J, et al: Treatment of cirrhosis and liver failure in rats by hepatocyte xenotransplantation. Gastroenterology 2003; 124:422-431.
24. Platt JL, Fischel RJ, Matas AJ, et al: Immunopathology of hyperacute xenograft rejection in a swine-to-primate model. Transplantation 1991; 52:214-220.
25. Galili U, Clark MR, Shohet SB, et al: Evolutionary relationship between the natural anti-Gal antibody and the Gal a1-3Gal epitope in primates. Proc Natl Acad Sci USA 1987; 84:1369-1373.
26. Brauer RB, Baldwin WM III, Daha MR, et al: Use of C6-deficient rats to evaluate the mechanism of hyperacute rejection of discordant cardiac xenografts. J Immunol 1993; 151:7240-7248.
27. Hourcade D, Holers VM, Atkinson JP: The regulators of complement activation (RCA) gene cluster. Adv Immunol 1989; 45: 381-416.
28. Lachmann PJ: The control of homologous lysis. Immunol Today 1991; 12:312-315.
29. McCurry KR, Kooyman DL, Alvarado CG, et al: Human complement regulatory proteins protect swine-to-primate cardiac xenografts from humoral injury. Nat Med 1995; 1:423-427.
30. Cozzi E, Yannoutsos N, Langford GA, et al: Effect of transgenic expression of human decay-accelerating factor on the inhibition of hyperacute rejection of pig organs. *In* Cooper DKC, Kemp E, Platt JL, White DJG (eds): Xenotransplantation: The Transplantation of Organs and Tissues Between Species. Berlin, Springer, 1997, pp 665-682.
31. Cozzi E, Bhatti F, Schmoeckel M, et al: Long-term survival of nonhuman primates receiving life-supporting transgenic porcine kidney xenografts. Transplantation 2000; 70:15-21.
32. Diamond LE, Quinn CM, Martin MJ, et al: A human CD46 transgenic pig model system for the study of discordant xenotransplantation. Transplantation 2001; 71:132-142.
33. Leventhal JR, Matas AJ, Sun LH, et al: The immunopathology of cardiac xenograft rejection in the guinea pig-to-rat model. Transplantation 1993; 56:1-8.
34. Magee JC, Collins BH, Harland RC, et al: Immunoglobulin prevents complement mediated hyperacute rejection in swine-to-primate xenotransplantation. J Clin Invest 1995; 96:2404-2412.
35. Holzknecht ZE, Kuypers KL, Plummer TB, et al: Apoptosis and cellular activation in the pathogenesis of acute vascular rejection. Circ Res 2002; 91:1135-1141.
36. Parker W, Saadi S, Lin SS, et al: Transplantation of discordant xenografts: A challenge revisited. Immunol Today 1996; 17:373-378.
37. Platt JL: New directions for organ transplantation. Nature 1998; 392(suppl):11-17.
38. Blakely ML, Van Der Werf WJ, Berndt MC, et al: Activation of intragraft endothelial and mononuclear cells during discordant xenograft rejection. Transplantation 1994; 58:1059-1066.
39. Lin SS, Weidner BC, Byrne GW, et al: The role of antibodies in acute vascular rejection of pig-to-baboon cardiac transplants. J Clin Invest 1998; 101:1745-1756.
40. Nagayasu T, Saadi S, Holzknecht RA, et al: Expression of tissue factor mRNA in cardiac xenografts: Clues to the pathogenesis of acute vascular rejection. Transplantation 2000; 69:475-482.
41. Bach FH, Winkler H, Ferran C, et al: Delayed xenograft rejection. Immunol Today 1996; 17:379-384.
42. Saadi S, Holzknecht RA, Patte CP, et al: Endothelial cell activation by pore forming structures: Pivotal role for IL-1a. Circulation 2000; 101:1867-1873.
43. Samstein B, Platt JL: Xenotransplantation and tolerance. Philos Trans R Soc Lond 2001; 356:749-758.
44. Sachs DH, Sablinski T: Tolerance across discordant xenogeneic barriers. Xenotransplantation 1995; 2:234-239.
45. Sablinski T, Emery DW, Monroy R, et al: Long-term discordant xenogeneic (porcine-to-primate) bone marrow engraftment in a monkey treated with porcine-specific growth factors. Transplantation 1999; 67:972-977.
46. Gritsch HA, Glaser RM, Emery DW, et al: The importance of nonimmune factors in reconstitution by discordant xenogeneic hematopoietic cells. Transplantation 1994; 57:906-917.
47. Ierino FL, Kozlowski T, Siegel JB, et al: Disseminated intravascular coagulation in association with the delayed rejection of pig-to-baboon renal xenografts. Transplantation 1998; 66:1439-1450.
48. Robson SC, Cooper DKC, d'Apice AJF: Disordered regulation of coagulation and platelet activation in xenotransplantation. Xenotransplantation 2000; 7:166-176.
49. Buhler L, Goepfert C, Kitamura H, et al: Porcine hematopoietic cell xenotransplantation in nonhuman primates is complicated by thrombotic microangiopathy. Bone Marrow Transplant 2001; 27:1227-1236.
50. Lin SS, Hanaway MJ, Gonzalez-Stawinski GV, et al: The role of anti-Gala1-3Gal antibodies in acute vascular rejection and accommodation of xenografts. Transplantation (Rapid Communication) 2000; 70:1667-1674.
51. Betthauser J, Forsberg E, Augenstein M, et al: Production of cloned pigs from in vitro systems. Nat Biotechnol 2000; 18:1055-1059.
52. Onishi A, Iwamoto M, Akita T, et al: Pig cloning by microinjection of fetal fibroblast nuclei. Science 2000; 289:1188-1190.
53. Polejaeva IA, Chen S, Vaught TD, et al: Cloned piglets produced by nuclear transfer from adult somatic cells. Nature 2000; 407:86-90.

54. Denning C, Burl S, Ainslie A, et al: Deletion of the a(1,3) galactosyl transferase (GGTA1) gene and the prion protein (PrP) gene in sheep. Nat Biotechnol 2001; 19:559-562.
55. Dai Y, Vaught TD, Boone J, et al: Targeted disruption of the alpha1,3-galactosyltransferase gene in cloned pigs. Nat Biotechnol 2002; 20:251-255.
56. Lai L, Kolber-Simonds D, Park KW, et al: Production of α-1,3-galactosyltransferase knockout pigs by nuclear transfer cloning. Science 2002; 295:1089-1092.
57. Phelps CJ, Koike C, Vaught TD, et al: Production of alpha 1,3-galactosyltransferase-deficient pigs. Science 2003; 299:411-414.
58. Matthiesen L, Berg G, Ernerudh J, et al: Lymphocyte subsets and mitogen stimulation of blood lymphocytes in normal pregnancy. Am J Reprod Immunol 1996; 35:70-79.
59. McCurry KR, Parker W, Cotterell AH, et al: Humoral responses in pig-to-baboon cardiac transplantation: Implications for the pathogenesis and treatment of acute vascular rejection and for accommodation. Hum Immunol 1997; 58:91-105.
60. Platt JL: Knocking out xenograft rejection. Nat Biotechnol 2002; 20:231-232.
61. Miyata Y, Platt J: Xeno: Still stuck without a-Gal. Nat Biotechnol 2003; 21:359-360.
62. Chopek MW, Simmons RL, Platt JL: ABO-incompatible renal transplantation: Initial immunopathologic evaluation. Transplant Proc 1987; 19:4553-4557.
63. Bannett AD, McAlack RF, Morris M, et al: ABO incompatible renal transplantation: A qualitative analysis of native endothelial tissue ABO antigens after transplant. Transplant Proc 1989; 21:783-785.
64. Lin Y, Vandeputte M, Waer M: Accommodation and T-independent B cell tolerance in rats with long term surviving hamster heart xenografts. J Immunol 1998; 160:369-375.
65. Andres G, Yamaguchi N, Brett J, et al: Cellular mechanisms of adaptation of grafts to antibody. Transpl Immunol 1996; 4:1-17.
66. Dalmasso AP, Benson BA, Johnson JS, et al: Resistance against the membrane attack complex of complement induced in porcine endothelial cells with a Gal alpha(1-3)Gal binding lectin: Up-regulation of CD59 expression. J Immunol 2000; 164:3764-3773.
67. Delikouras A, Hayes M, Malde P, et al: Nitric oxide-mediated expression of Bcl-2 and Bcl-xl and protection from TNFα - mediated apoptosis in porcine endothelial cells after exposure to low concentrations of xenoreactive natural antibody. Transplantation 2001; 71:599-605.
68. Bach FH, Ferran C, Hechenleitner P, et al: Accommodation of vascularized xenografts: Expression of "protective genes" by donor endothelial cells in a host Th2 cytokine environment. Nat Med 1997; 3:196-204.
69. Soares MP, Lin Y, Anrather J, et al: Expression of heme oxygenase-1 can determine cardiac xenograft survival. Nat Med 1998; 4:1073-1077.
70. Sato K, Balla J, Otterbein L, et al: Carbon monoxide generated by heme oxygenase-1 suppresses the rejection of mouse-to-rat cardiac transplants. J Immunol 2001; 166:4185-4194.
71. Diamond LE, McCurry KR, Oldham ER, et al: Characterization of transgenic pigs expressing functionally active human CD59 on cardiac endothelium. Transplantation 1996; 61:1241-1249.
72. Imai T, Morita T, Shindo T, et al: Vascular smooth muscle cell-directed overexpression of heme oxygenase-1 elevates blood pressure through attenuation of nitric oxide-induced vasodilation in mice. Circ Res 2001; 89:55-62.
73. Sebille F, Guillet M, Brouard S, et al: T-cell-mediated rejection of vascularized xenografts in the absence of induced anti-donor antibody response. Am J Transplant 2001; 1:21-28.
74. Hancock WW, Buelow R, Sayegh MH, et al: Antibody-induced transplant arteriosclerosis is prevented by graft expression of anti-oxidant and anti-apoptotic genes. Nat Med 1998; 4:1392-1396.
75. Sablinski T, Lorf T, Monroy R, et al: Absorption of preformed primate anti-swine antibodies by extracorporeal perfusion through galα(1,3)gal columns. 1995; Poster-33 (115):18.
76. Takeuchi Y, Weiss RA: Xenotransplantation: Reappraising the risk of retroviral zoonosis. Curr Opin Immunol 2000; 12:504-507.
77. Boneva R, Folks TM, Chapman LE: Infectious disease issues in xenotransplantation. Clin Microbiol Rev 2001; 14:1-14.
78. Patience C, Takeuchi Y, Weiss RA: Zoonosis in xenotransplantation. Curr Opin Immunol 1998; 10:539-542.
79. Van der Laan LJW, Lockey C, Griffeth BC, et al: Infection by porcine endogenous retrovirus after islet xenotransplantation in SCID mice. Nature 2000; 407:501-504.
80. Paradis K, Langford G, Long Z, et al: Search for cross-species transmission of porcine endogenous retrovirus in patients treated with living pig tissue. Science 1999; 285:1236-1241.
81. Clark DA, Fryer JF, Tucker AW, et al: Porcine cytomegalovirus in pigs being bred for xenograft organs: Progress towards control. Xenotransplantation 2003; 10:142-148.
82. Ogle BM, Butters KA, Cascalho M, et al: Spontaneous fusion of cells between species yields transdifferentiation and retroviral transfer in vivo. FASEB J 2004; 18:548-550.
83. Anversa P, Nadal-Ginard B: Myocyte renewal and ventricular remodelling. Nature 2002; 415:240-243.
84. Lumelsky N, Blondel O, Laeng P, et al: Differentiation of embryonic stem cells to insulin-secreting structures similar to pancreatic islets. Science 2001; 292:1389-1394.
85. Bianco P, Robey PG: Stem cells in tissue engineering. Nature 2001; 414:118-121.
86. Thomson JA, Itskovitz-Eldor J, Shapiro SS, et al: Embryonic stem cell lines derived from human blastocysts. Science 1998; 282:1145-1147.
87. Fandrich F, Lin X, Chai GX, et al: Preimplantation-stage stem cells induce long-term allogeneic graft acceptance without supplementary host conditioning. Nat Med 2002; 8:171-178.
88. Krause DS, Theise ND, Collector MI, et al: Multi-organ, multi-lineage engraftment by a single bone marrow-derived stem cell. Cell 2001; 105:369-377.
89. Quaini F, Urbanek K, Beltrami AP, et al: Chimerism of the transplanted heart. N Engl J Med 2002; 346:5-15.
90. Lanza RP, Chung HY, Yoo JJ, et al: Generation of histocompatible tissues using nuclear transplantation. Nat Biotechnol 2002; 20:689-696.
91. Griffith LG, Naughton G: Tissue engineering: Current challenges and expanding opportunities. Science 2002; 295:1009-1016.
92. Ogle BM, Mooradian DL: The role of vascular smooth muscle cell integrins in the compaction and mechanical strengthening of a tissue-engineered blood vessel. Tissue Eng 1999; 5:387-402.
93. Niklason LE, Gao J, Abbott WM, et al: Functional arteries grown in vitro. Science 1999; 284:489-493.
94. L'Heureux N, Paquet S, Labbe R, et al: A completely biological tissue-engineered human blood vessel. FASEB J 1998; 12:47.
95. Shum-Tim D, Stock U, Hrkach J, et al: Tissue engineering of autologous aorta using a new biodegradable polymer. Ann Thorac Surg 1999; 68:2298-2304.
96. Shin-oka T, Breuer CK, Tanel RE, et al: Tissue engineering heart valves: Valve leaflet replacement study in a lamb model. Ann Thorac Surg 1995; 60:S513-S516.
97. Stock UA, Nagashima M, Khalil PN, et al: Tissue engineered valved conduits in the pulmonary circulation. J Thorac Cardiovasc Surg 2000; 119:732-740.
98. Jockenhoevel S, Zund G, Hoerstrup SP, et al: Fibrin gel: Advantages of a new scaffold in cardiovascular tissue engineering. Eur J Cardiothorac Surg 2001; 19:424-430.
99. Li RK, Yau TM, Weisel RD, et al: Construction of a bioengineered cardiac graft. J Thorac Cardiovasc Surg 2000; 119:368-375.
100. Li RK, Weisel RD, Mickle DA, et al: Autologous porcine heart cell transplantation improved heart function after a myocardial infarction. J Thorac Cardiovasc Surg 2000; 119:62-68.

101. Leor J, Aboulafia-Etzion S, Dar A, et al: Bioengineered cardiac grafts: A new approach to repair the infarcted myocardium. Circulation 2000; 102:III-56-III-61.
102. Yoshikawa T, Ohgushi H, Nakajima H, et al: In vivo osteogenic durability of cultured bone in porous ceramics: A novel method for autologous bone graft substitution. Transplantation 2000; 69:128-134.
103. Kaufmann PM, Sano K, Uyama S, et al: Evaluation of methods of hepatotrophic stimulation in rat heterotropic hepatocyte transplantation using polymers. J Pediatr Surg 1999; 34:1118-1123.
104. Kim SS, Kaihara S, Benvenuto MS, et al: Small intestinal submucosa as a small caliber venous graft: A novel model for hepatocyte transplantation on synthetic biodegradable polymer scaffolds with direct access to the portal venous system. J Pediatr Surg 1999; 34:124-128.
105. Mayer J, Karamuk E, Akaike T, et al: Matrices for tissue engineering-scaffold structure for a bioartificial liver support system. J Control Release 2000; 64:81-90.
106. Chamberlain LF, Yannas IV, Hsu HP, et al: Connective tissue response to tubular implants for peripheral nerve regeneration: The role of myofibroblasts. J Comp Neurol 2000; 417:415-430.
107. Pollok JM, Begemann JF, Jaufmann PM: Long-term insulin-secretory function of islets of Langerhans encapsulated with a layer of confluent chondrocytes for immunoisolation. Pediatr Surg Int 1999; 15:164-167.
108. Vacanti CA, Langer R, Schloo B, et al: Synthetic polymers seeded with chondrocytes provide a template for new cartilage formation. Plast Reconstr Surg 1991; 88:753-759.
109. Vanjak-Novakovic G, Freed L, Biron RJ, et al: Effects of mixing on the composition and morphology of tissue engineered cartilage. AIChE J 1996; 42:850-860.
110. Burke JF, Yannas IV, Quimby WCJ, et al: Successful use of a physiologically acceptable artificial skin in the treatment of extensive burn injury. Ann Surg 1981; 194:413-448.
111. Winfrey ME, Cochran M, Hegarty MT: A new technology in burn therapy: INTEGRA artificial skin. Dimens Crit Care Nurs 1999; 18:14-20.
112. Boyce ST, Supp AP, Wickett RR, et al: Assessment with the dermal torque meter of skin pliability after treatment of burns with cultured skin substitutes. J Burn Care Rehabil 2000; 21:55-63.
113. Waymack P, Duff RG, Sabolinski M, et al: The effect of a tissue engineered bilayered living skin analog, over meshed split-thickness autografts on the healing of excised burn wounds. Burns 2000; 26:609-619.
114. Grobstein C: Inductive epithelio-mesenchymal interaction in cultured organ rudiments of the mouse. Science 1953; 118:52-55.
115. Sariola H: Interspecies chimeras: An experimental approach for studies on embryonic angiogenesis. Med Biol 1985; 63:43-65.
116. Dekel B, Burakova T, Ben-Hur H, et al: Engraftment of human kidney tissue in rat radiation chimera: II. Human fetal kidneys display reduced immunogenicity to adoptively transferred human peripheral blood mononuclear cells and exhibit rapid growth and development. Transplantation 1997; 64:1550-1558.
117. Rogers SA, Lowell JA, Hammerman NA, et al: Transplantation of developing metanephroi into adult rats. Kidney Int 1998; 54:27-37.
118. Rogers SA, Hammerman MR: Transplantation of rat metanephroi into mice. Am J Physiol 2001; 280:R1865-R1869.
119. Hammerman MR: Xenotransplantation of renal primordia. Curr Opin Nephrol Hypertens 2002; 11:11-16.
120. Dekel B, Marcus H, Herzel BH, et al: In vivo modulation of the allogeneic immune response by human fetal kidneys: The role of cytokines, chemokines, and cytolytic effector molecules. Transplantation 2000; 69:1470-1478.
121. Hammerman MR: Transplantation of embryonic organs—kidney and pancreas. Am J Transplant 2004; 4:14-24.
122. Cascalho M, Platt JL: Xenotransplantation and other means of organ replacement. Nat Rev Immunol 2001; 1:154-160.
123. Ogle BM, Cascalho M, Platt JL: Fusion of approaches to the treatment of organ failure. Am J Transplant 2004: 4:74-77.
124. Jaboulay M: De reins au pli du coude par soutures arterielles et veineuses. Lyon Med 1906; 107:575-577.
125. Unger E: Ueber Nierentransplantationen. Berlin, Wehnschr, 1909.
126. Ullman E: Tissue and organ transplantation. Ann Surg 1914; 60:195-219.
127. Neuhof H: The Transplantation of Tissues. New York, D. Appleton, 1923.
128. Reemtsma K, McCracken BH, Schlegel JU, et al: Renal hetero-transplantation in man. Ann Surg 1964; 160:384-410.
129. Traeger J, Gonin A, Delahaye J: Pericardite uremique a evolution constrictive subaigue. A propos d'une observation anatomo-clinique chez un Brightique traite par les epurations extra renale; au long cours. Lyon Med 1964; 211:383-401.
130. Hume DM, Magee JH, Prout GR: Studies of renal homotransplantation in man. Ann N Y Acad Sci 1964; 120:578-606.
131. Hitchcock CR, Kiser JC, Telander RL, et al: Baboon renal grafts. JAMA 1964; 189:934-937.
132. Kauffman HM, Cleveland RJ, Hume DM: Bibliography of kidney transplantation. Transplantation 1965; 3:278-285.
133. Casciani SP, Cortesini R: The renal transplant: Experimental research and first clinical experiences. Minerva Med 1966; 57:2973-298

Chronic Kidney Disease and the Kidney Transplant Recipient

John S. Gill, M.D., M.S.

The premature death of kidney transplant recipients is an important factor that limits the long-term success of kidney transplantation. Early recognition, prevention, and treatment of chronic kidney disease (CKD) related complications prior to transplantation and during the period of allograft function may improve the survival of kidney transplant recipients. Recent investigations indicate that there are important differences in the clinical presentation of CKD between transplant recipients and patients with native kidney disease. This chapter will review how aggressive management of CKD may decrease the incidence of premature death with graft function (DWGF) and thus lead to improvements in long-term graft survival. In addition, the unique aspects of CKD management in kidney transplant recipients will be reviewed. The medical complications of kidney transplantation are also discussed in Chapter 38.

THE IMPACT OF DEATH WITH GRAFT FUNCTION

The two major causes of graft loss after the first year of transplantation are chronic allograft nephropathy and DWGF. Although the risk of DWGF decreased by 67% between 1988 and 1997, patient death still accounted for 43% of all graft loss.[1] The perception that DWGF is an indicator of the success of kidney transplantation is dispelled because most cases of DWGF are premature; the median time to DWGF is only 23 months, and the projected survival of transplant recipients is between 5 and 15 years, lower than that of age-matched individuals in the general population.[1,2]

The impact of DWGF on long-term graft survival is illustrated by the fact that transplant recipients die with a considerable degree of residual transplant kidney function; in an analysis of data from the United States Renal Data System (USRDS), the most recent serum creatinine prior to death was 1.9 ± 0.8 mg/dL, and 60% of patients had serum creatinine less than 2.0 mg/dL.[1] Therefore, when a patient dies with graft function, a significant amount of "potential graft function" is lost. The amount of "potential graft function" that is lost can be estimated by the difference in graft survival when death is both included and excluded as a cause of graft loss. Between 1985 and 1996, the half-life for cadaveric transplant recipients increased by 5.9 years; however, the half-life would have increased by 8.5 years, if death was excluded as a cause of graft loss.[3] Similarly, projected graft half-lives in the absence of DWGF would be 19.5 and 35.9 years for cadaveric and live donor recipients, respectively.[3] Therefore, although some transplant recipients attain a full life, premature death with graft function is an important reason why more marked improvements in long-term graft survival have not been recognized.

PREVALENCE OF CHRONIC KIDNEY DISEASE IN TRANSPLANT RECIPIENTS

Like dialysis, transplantation falls short of replacing normal kidney function. Figure 42–1 shows the prevalence of CKD in 69,394 adults, first kidney transplant recipients between 1987 and 1997 with graft survival of at least 1 year in the United States Renal Data System (USRDS).[4] Glomerular filtration rate (GFR) was estimated at 1, 3, and 5 years after the time of transplantation with an equation derived from the Modification of Diet in Renal Disease (MDRD) Study,[5] and patients were classified by K/DOQI CKD stage.[6] At each time point, the mean GFR was approximately 50 mL/min/1.73 m^2, and the prevalence of K/DOQI CKD Stages 3, 4, or 5 was greater than 70%. This information demonstrates that kidney transplant recipients are rarely cured of their kidney disease and remain at risk for CKD-related complications.

PRESENTATION OF CHRONIC KIDNEY DISEASE IN TRANSPLANT RECIPIENTS

Prior to Transplantation

The clinical manifestations of CKD in a given transplant recipient will primarily depend on the duration and burden of CKD prior to transplantation and the level of kidney function achieved after transplantation. In addition, exposure to immunosuppressive medications after transplantation may exacerbate CKD-related complications, such as hypertension, diabetes, dyslipidemia, and anemia. Early recognition and treatment of CKD-related complications, maximization of allograft function, and minimization of immunosuppressive-related side effects should decrease the impact of CKD in transplant recipients.

Aggressive CKD care should begin prior to transplantation because the preexisting burden of CKD present at the time of transplantation will not be undone by the provision of a functional allograft. In contrast, many of the complications of CKD, such as hypertension, dyslipidemia, anemia, and malnutrition, may be prevented or delayed by early detection and treatment prior to transplantation.[7] Prolonged exposure to

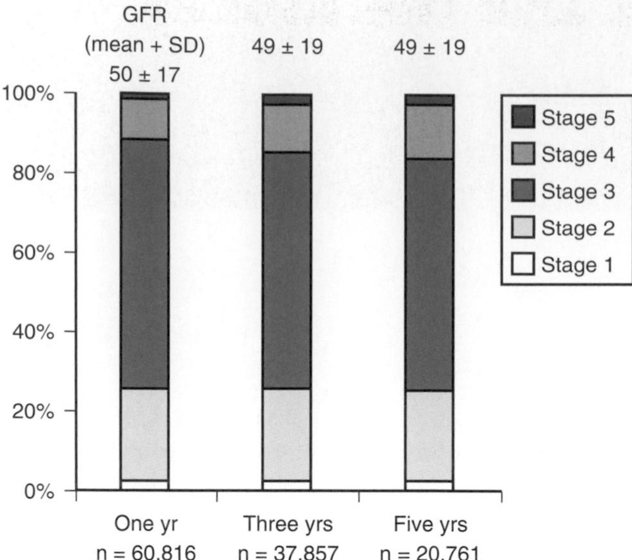

Figure 42–1 Mean ± standard deviation (*SD*) of estimated glomerular filtration rate (GFR) (mL/min/1.73 m^2) and prevalence of K/DOQI chronic kidney disease stages among adult first transplant recipients in the United States between 1987 and 1997 at 1, 3, and 5 years after transplantation.

dialysis prior to transplantation has been associated with reduced allograft survival,[8,9] and preemptive transplant recipients have an allograft survival advantage.[10,11] The reasons underlying these associations are somewhat uncertain; however, a lower burden of CKD in patients with no or limited dialysis exposure is a likely explanation.[12] Reducing dialysis exposure through live donor transplantation and preemptive transplantation should be encouraged.

For patients without the possibility of a live donor transplant, aggressive CKD management prior to transplantation will become increasingly important due to longer transplant waiting times. The United Network of Organ Sharing waiting list for cadaveric kidney transplantation is increasing at a rate of 20% per year and will include an estimated 95,000 patients by 2010.[13] Under current conditions, waiting times of a decade or more are anticipated,[14] and CKD management of wait-listed individuals will be more difficult. Of particular concern is the increased risk of perioperative morbidity and mortality.[15] A detailed perioperative risk assessment and implementation of preventive measures shown to reduce operative risk in non-transplant patient populations should be considered as part of the CKD management of transplant candidates. Appropriate pre-transplant management of CKD-related complications, such as anemia, that are associated with an increased risk of perioperative mortality in non-CKD populations,[16,17] should also be prioritized. In this regard, implementation of an organ allocation strategy that facilitates the optimization of pre-transplant preventive measures may be desirable.

The Peri-Transplant Period

Transplant recipients have an increased risk of mortality in the peri-transplant period compared to wait-listed patients who remain on dialysis. Recently, data from the USRDS and Medicare claims were used to describe the incidence of cardiovascular morbidity and mortality in the peri-transplant period.[18] There was a marked increase in the rate of all cardiovascular events (death, myocardial infarction, congestive heart failure, coronary revascularization, and stroke) during the peri-transplant period. The estimated probability of myocardial infarction, cardiac arrest, and congestive heart failure in cadaveric transplant recipients in the first post-transplant month was 1.2%, 1.1%, and 5.2%, respectively. Approximately 5% of first kidney transplant recipients will die within the first post-transplant year.[19] The majority of deaths are due to cardiac causes, and patients with comorbid disease (diabetes, peripheral vascular disease, angina) and a longer duration of CKD are at increased risk for mortality. These deaths should be regarded as failures of CKD management rather than failures of transplantation because they result from the accumulated burden of CKD prior to transplantation that may have been prevented by the provision of aggressive pre-transplant CKD care. Post-transplant complications, such as acute rejection and delayed graft function, may contribute to the development of acute coronary syndromes in the peri-transplant period. Delayed graft function may be associated with increase cardiac work due to volume expansion. Because delayed graft function is often predictable, it may be preferable to avoid the allocation of organs at high risk for delayed graft function to patients with a high burden of cardiovascular disease.

The Post-Transplant Period

Cardiovascular disease is the most important threat to long-term patient survival after transplantation. The management of cardiovascular disease in transplant recipients will continue to be an important component of post-transplant CKD care because of the increasing age and burden of CKD in these patients. Between 1995 and 2001, the percentage of cadaveric donor transplant recipients older than 50 years increased from 40% to 51%, whereas the percentage of live donor recipients over 50 years increased from 28% to 45%.[18] During this time, the percentage of cadaveric donor recipients with atherosclerotic heart disease or congestive heart failure increased from 40% to 50%, whereas the percentage of live donor recipients with these comorbid conditions increased from 33% to 40%. Comprehensive reviews of post-transplant cardiovascular disease as well as treatment guidelines for cardiovascular risk reduction are available, and therefore a detailed discussion of these issues is not provided here.[20–22]

There is increasing interest in the effect of different immunosuppressive agents on the development and progression of cardiovascular disease. With the increased choice of available maintenance immunosuppressive agents, individualization of immunosuppression, based not only on patient immunologic risk but also on cardiovascular risk, will become more important. Such strategies should be viewed as adjuncts to the early diagnosis and treatment of well-established cardiovascular risk factors. Direct evidence regarding the efficacy of cardiovascular risk reduction in transplant recipients is lacking, and it is unlikely that randomized trials, such as the recently published ALERT study,[23] will become available for all cardiovascular risk factors in the transplant population. Therefore, transplant clinicians must rely on extrapolation of information from non-transplant populations. Currently, it would appear that there is considerable room for improvement in post-transplant cardiovascular disease management. For example, fewer than one-third of transplant recipients have lipid testing performed in the first post-transplant year.[18]

The level of kidney function achieved after transplantation has been associated with both patient and allograft survival and, more recently, with the development of hospitalized heart disease.[24,25] Because of these associations, it is important that an accurate assessment of allograft function be made. A key component of CKD care in transplant recipients is recognition that patients who are typically thought of as having "good graft function" actually have significantly impaired kidney transplant function and are at risk for the complications of CKD. Serum creatinine alone is not an accurate index of kidney function, and an estimate of the GFR is the preferred measure of kidney function. A number of widely used formulas to estimate GFR are available that perform well in the non-transplant population with CKD. Although these prediction equations have not been validated in large samples of transplant recipients, they are still preferred over the use of serum creatinine alone. The K/DOQI work group has recommended equations derived from MDRD study for use in all adult patients with CKD.[6] The most simple of these formulas includes only four variables:

$$\text{Estimated GFR } (\text{mL/min/1.73m}^2) = 186 \times \text{Serum Creatinine}^{-1.154} \times \text{Age}^{-0.203} \times 0.742 \text{ if female} \times 1.210 \text{ if African American}$$ [5]

The level of kidney function achieved after transplantation is largely determined by donor and immunologic factors. Because the mean level of kidney function established after transplantation is only 50 mL/min/1.73 m^2,[26] preservation of kidney function is an important aspect of CKD management in transplant recipients. Recent studies of administrative data sets and from the experience in single centers have described the change in kidney function after transplantation.[26–28] Of importance is the observation that transplant recipients have a mean rate of kidney function decline that is slower than that in patients with native kidney disease with similar levels of kidney function. Further, many transplant recipients have improvement in kidney function over time. These observations highlight the need for further studies to identify the determinants of the change in kidney function after transplantation and suggest that efforts to maximize the baseline level of kidney function may be more important than efforts to slow the progression of kidney decline after transplantation.

Information regarding the determinants of the change in kidney function after transplantation is emerging. It would appear that there are only relatively small differences in the rate of kidney function decline between the most commonly used maintenance immunosuppressive agents.[29] There is preliminary evidence suggesting that kidney function may be optimized with the use of non-nephrotoxic immunosuppressive agents and reduced calcineurin inhibitor exposure.[30] Surprisingly, little direct information about the role of hypertension and proteinuria in kidney function decline in transplant recipients is available. These factors are known to accelerate the progression of kidney function decline in patients with native kidney disease. Evidence regarding the role of anemia in the progression of kidney function decline is emerging.[31] Further studies to determine the optimal blood pressure, the role of proteinuria, and other modifiable CKD factors, such as anemia, on the rate of kidney function decline after transplantation are needed. In the absence of direct evidence in the transplant population, it is reasonable to advocate aggressive treatment of these factors based on their established role in the progression in native kidney disease and because many of these factors also increase the risk of cardiovascular disease.

PATIENTS WITH ALLOGRAFT FAILURE

Despite the improvements in allografts survival, one-third of cadaveric transplant recipients will suffer graft failure within the first 5 years of transplantation.[2] Moreover, many patients will require more than one transplant in their lifetime. As such, it is appropriate for transplant physicians to consider the survival of patients after transplant failure as part of transplant-related outcomes.

A recent study described the prevalence and treatment of CKD-related complications among 4643 patients returning to dialysis after transplant failure in the United States between 1995 and 1998.[32] Despite being known to physicians with knowledge of CKD, failed transplant recipients initiated dialysis with levels of hematocrit, albumin, erythropoietin use, and residual renal function that were suboptimal and similar to those in the general incident dialysis population (Figure 42–2). These findings demonstrate that there are many opportunities to improve the CKD management of transplant recipients and that there is a need for increased awareness of CKD among the medical professionals involved in the care of these patients.

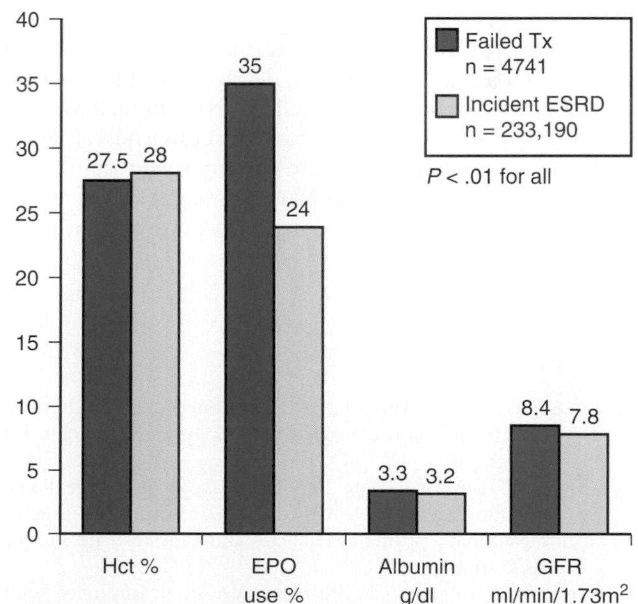

Figure 42–2 Hematocrit (Hct), erythropoietin (EPO) use, albumin, and glomerular filtration rate (GFR) at time of dialysis initiation among failed transplant recipients and general incident dialysis patients.

The survival of patients with transplant failure is known to be poor.[33–35] Between 1995 and 1998, 25% of patients in the United States that remained on dialysis after transplant failure died within 2 years of their return to dialysis date.[33] In a multivariate analysis, the presence of comorbid disease (congestive heart failure, peripheral vascular disease, diabetes) predicted mortality. However, unlike patients with transplant function, immunologic and transplant-related factors (acute rejection, antibody induction, donor source, duration of graft survival, and the maximum attained GFR during transplantation) did not predict mortality.

CONTINUITY OF CARE

Transplant recipients will have multiple care providers before, during, and after transplantation. The overall management of CKD care should be directed by the physician most familiar with CKD. Because aggressive CKD care should begin prior to transplantation and continue after allograft failure, it may be appropriate in some cases for a nontransplant physician to direct the CKD care of transplant recipients. A more realistic and appropriate alternative is that all transplant nephrologists learn and apply the highest standards of CKD care to their transplant patients. Irrespective of who assumes the responsibility for CKD care, communication between the multiple responsible care providers is essential to ensure continuity of care. The inclusion of transplant recipients in the general NKF-K/DOQI classification of CKD should facilitate this process by providing a simple classification system and treatment action plan based on the level of allograft function.[6]

SUMMARY

Most kidney transplant recipients achieve only a modest degree of kidney function and, therefore, are never free of the burden of CKD. Aggressive management of CKD prior to transplantation may attenuate the development of complications after transplantation. Ongoing prevention, diagnosis, and treatment of CKD-related complications and comorbid conditions as patients move from the transplant waiting list through transplantation and back to dialysis after graft failure may be the key to improving long-term outcomes in transplant recipients.

References

1. Ojo AO, Hanson JA, Wolfe RA, et al: Long-term survival in renal transplant recipients with graft function. Kidney Int 2000; 57: 307–313.
2. USRDS 2001 Annual Data Report: Atlas of End-Stage Renal Disease in the United States. Bethseda, MD, National Institutes of Health, National Institute of Diabetes and Digestive and Kidney Diseases, 2001.
3. Hariharan S, Johnson CP, Bresnahan BA, et al: Improved graft survival after renal transplantation in the United States, 1988 to 1996. N Engl J Med 2000; 342:605–612.
4. Gill J, Mix C, Pereira BJG: Glomerular filtration rate and the prevalence of chronic kidney disease in transplant recipients. Am J Transplant 2002; 2:417.
5. Levey A, Greene T, Kusek J, Beck G: A simplified equation to predict glomerular filtration rate from serum creatinine. J Am Soc Nephrol 2000; 11:155A.
6. K/DOQI Clinical Practice Guidelines for Chronic Kidney Disease: Evaluation, classification and stratification. Am J Kidney Dis 2002; 39:S1–S266.
7. Pereira BJG: Optimization of pre-ESRD care: The key to improved dialysis outcomes. Kidney Int 2000; 57:351–365.
8. Meier-Kriesche HU, Port FK, Ojo AO, et al: Effect of waiting time on renal transplant outcome. Kidney Int 2000; 58:1311–1317.
9. Cosio FG, Alamir A, Yim S, et al: Patient survival after renal transplantation: I. The impact of dialysis pre-transplant. Kidney Int 1998; 53:767–772.
10. Mange KC, Joffe MM, Feldman HI: Effect of the use or nonuse of long-term dialysis on the subsequent survival of renal transplants from living donors. N Engl J Med 2001; 344:726–731.
11. Kasiske BL, Snyder JJ, Matas AJ, et al: Preemptive kidney transplantation: The advantage and the advantaged. J Am Soc Nephrol 2002; 13(5):1358–1364.
12. Gill J, Tonelli M, Johnson N, et al: The nature of the benefit of preemptive kidney transplantation. J Am Soc Nephrol 2002; 14: 664.
13. Xue JL, Ma JZ, Louis TA, Collins AJ: Forecast of the number of patients with end-stage renal disease in the United States to the year 2010. J Am Soc Nephrol 2001; 12:2753–2758.
14. Danovitch GM, Hariharan S, Pirsch JD, et al: Management of the waiting list for cadaveric kidney transplants: Report of a survey and recommendations by the Clinical Practice Guidelines Committee of the American Society of Transplantation. J Am Soc Nephrol 2002; 13:528–535.
15. Wolfe R, Ashby V, Milford E, et al: Comparison of mortality in all patients on dialysis, patients on dialysis awaiting transplantation, and recipients of a first cadaveric transplant. NEJM 1999; 341:1725–1730.
16. Dunne JR, Malone D, Tracy JK, et al: Perioperative anemia: An independent risk factor for infection, mortality, and resource utilization in surgery: Effect of anaemia and cardiovascular disease on surgical mortality and morbidity. J Surg Res 2002; 102:237–244.
17. Carson JL, Duff A, Poses RM, et al: Effect of anaemia and cardiovascular disease on surgical mortality and morbidity. Lancet 1996; 348:1055–1060.
18. USRDS 2003 Annual Data Report: Atlas of End-Stage Renal Disease in the United States. Bethesda, MD, National Institues of Health, National Institute of Diabetes and Digestive and Kidney Diseases, 2003.
19. Gill JS, Pereira BJ: Death in the first year after kidney transplantation: Implications for patients on the transplant waiting list. Transplantation 2003; 75:113–117.
20. Kasiske BL, Guijarro C, Massy ZA, et al: Cardiovascular disease after renal transplantation. J Am Soc Nephrol 1996; 7:158–165.
21. Kasiske BL, Vazquez MA, Harmon WE, et al: Recommendations for the outpatient surveillance of renal transplant recipients. American Society of Transplantation. J Am Soc Nephrol 2000; 11(suppl 15):S1–S86.
22. Kasiske BL: Epidemiology of cardiovascular disease after renal transplantation. Transplantation 2001; 72:S5–S8.
23. Holdaas H, Fellstrom B, Jardine AG, et al: Effect of fluvastatin on cardiac outcomes in renal transplant recipients: A multicentre, randomised, placebo-controlled trial. Lancet 2003; 361:2024–2031.
24. Hariharan S, McBride MA, Cherikh WS, et al: Post-transplant renal function in the first year predicts long-term kidney transplant survival: Renal function as a predictor of long-term graft survival in renal transplant patients. Kidney Int 2002; 62: 311–318.
25. Abbott KC, Yuan CM, Taylor AJ, et al: Early renal insufficiency and hospitalized heart disease after renal transplantation in the era of modern immunosuppression. J Am Soc Nephrol 2003; 14:2358–2365.

26. Gill JS, Tonelli M, Mix C, Pereira BJG: The change in allograft function among long term kidney transplant recipients. J Am Soc Nephrol 2003; 16:1636–1642.
27. Djamali A, Kendziorski C, Brazy PC, Becker BN: Disease progression and outcomes in chronic kidney disease and renal transplantation. Kidney Int 2003; 64:1800–1807.
28. Gourishankar S, Hunsicker LG, Jhangri GS, et al: The stability of the glomerular filtration rate after renal transplantation is improving. J Am Soc Nephrol 2003; 14:2387–2394.
29. Gill J, Tonelli M, Johnson N, Pereira BJG: The effect of maintenance immunosuppression on the change in kidney allograft function. Kidney Int 2004; 65(2):692–699.
30. Flechner SM, Goldfarb D, Modlin C, et al: Kidney transplantation without calcineurin inhibitor drugs: A prospective, randomized trial of sirolimus versus cyclosporine. Transplantation 2002; 74:1070–1076.
31. Becker BN, Becker YT, Leverson GE, Heisey DM: Erythropoietin therapy may retard progression in chronic renal transplant dysfunction. Nephrol Dial Transplant 2002; 17:1667–1673.
32. Gill J, Abichandani R, Khan S, et al: Opportunities to improve the care of patients with kidney transplant failure. Kidney Int 2002; 61:2193–2198.
33. Gill JS, Abichandani R, Kausz AT, Pereira BJ: Mortality after kidney transplant failure: The impact of non-immunologic factors. Kidney Int 2002; 62:1875–1883.
34. Ojo A, Wolfe R, Agodoa L, et al: Prognosis after primary renal transplant failure and the beneficial effects of repeat transplantation. Transplantation 1998; 66:1651–1659.
35. Kaplan B, Meier-Kriesche HU: Death after graft loss: An important late study endpoint in kidney transplantation. Am J Transplant 2002; 2:970–974.

SECTION F

Acute Renal Failure

Chapter 43

Acute Renal Failure: Bench to Bedside

Jeremy S. Duffield, M.R.C.P., Ph.D. • Joseph V. Bonventre, M.D., Ph.D.

Acute renal failure (ARF) is a common condition, which carries a high morbidity and mortality.[1] Although many advances have been made over the last 50 years, the management of ARF remains largely supportive. Basic animal and cellular research and human studies have provided limited insight into common disease mechanisms influencing the diverse etiologies of ARF.[2] By pursuing common disease mechanisms at the bench, new insights will hopefully result that will lead to new preventive therapies that could be used in high-risk patients to prevent renal injury or to modify the course of established ARF. In addition, however, fundamental observations will be made at the bedside, which then will be clarified in the laboratory. These clinical insights deriving from the patient will be facilitated by new technologies to probe the disease and by new biomarkers, which will provide better insight into the time-resolved nature of the injury to the kidney. This chapter presents an overview of ARF, including its definition, epidemiology, risk factors and clinical consequences, as well as the complex pathophysiology of this syndrome. To the extent that we have improved our understanding of many of the pathological processes that occur in the injured kidney, these insights have been derived from basic studies *in vitro* using isolated cell systems as well as from animal and human studies *in vivo*. The chapter attempts to summarize how observations at bench have led to modifications of therapeutic approach to humans and may lead to new therapeutic agents in the future.

Definition and Epidemiology

To study ARF, it is necessary to a have clear definition of the disease, for which there is still no clear consensus or standardized approach. Qualitatively, ARF is a clinical syndrome characterized by an acute deterioration of renal function over hours to days, resulting in failure of the kidney to excrete nitrogenous waste and to maintain fluid and electrolyte homeostasis. ARF is a heterogeneous condition with a wide range of etiologies. Unfortunately, there is no unified quantitative definition of the syndrome. There are many different published definitions, ranging from an abrupt (hours or days) rise in serum creatinine of ≥ 0.5 mg/dL (~ 50 μmol/L)[3,4] to an abrupt decline in renal function sufficient for introduction of dialysis. Recent large epidemiological studies have used definitions that vary from a rise in serum creatinine of ≥ 0.5 mg/dL to a rise of normal range serum creatinine to > 2.0 mg/dL.[1] These differences in definition yield markedly different outcomes. In a single-center study of hospital acquired ARF, only 1% of patients had a rise in serum creatinine of ≥ 2.0 mg/dL, whereas 13% had a rise of ≥ 0.5 mg/dL.[5] Depending on the cohort of patients studied, the etiologic spread will be quite different. In a large multicenter study of community- and hospital-acquired ARF, obstructive causes of ARF represented more than 10% of all cases,[6] whereas in a recent hospital-based study, this amounted to only 3% of cases.[5] Thus it is necessary to evaluate studies with full knowledge of the variations in definition of ARF used, the patient population studied, and the breadth of etiologies under investigation.

The necessity for clear definitions of ARF has resulted in the development of new criteria endorsed by the Acute Dialysis Quality Initiative (ADQI). These guidelines recognize definitions based on change in glomerular filtration rate (GFR) from baseline, change in urine output, and duration of these changes. A proposed stratified definition of ARF denoted by the term "RIFLE" divides this syndrome into five groups (Figure 43–1): (1) renal *R*isk (RIFLE-R), (2) renal *I*njury (RIFLE-I), (3) renal *F*ailure (RIFLE-F), (4) renal *L*oss (RIFLE-L), (5) *E*nd stage renal disease (RIFLE-E). This classification incorporates patients with pre-renal ARF who will rapidly restore renal function to baseline if the etiology of the impaired renal parenchymal perfusion is corrected, and such patients will fall into the milder categories. GFR criteria or urine output (oliguria) criteria can also be used in this formulation. When the category is defined by oliguria, a suffix would be used to make the distinction (e.g., RIFLE-Ro). Those patients with chronic kidney disease (CKD) would be distinguished by a suffix (e.g., RIFLE-Fc). The criteria assume patients to be well hydrated and not treated aggressively with diuretic agents. These new criteria have not yet been used in any systematic study of patients with ARF, but offer a standardized approach to acute renal disease both clinically and during investigation. The rationale for the different strata is based on outcome. This new classification has been proposed to allow more consistency across studies and hence greater ability to compare results.[7,8] Future prospective studies validating this new classification and comparing it with more

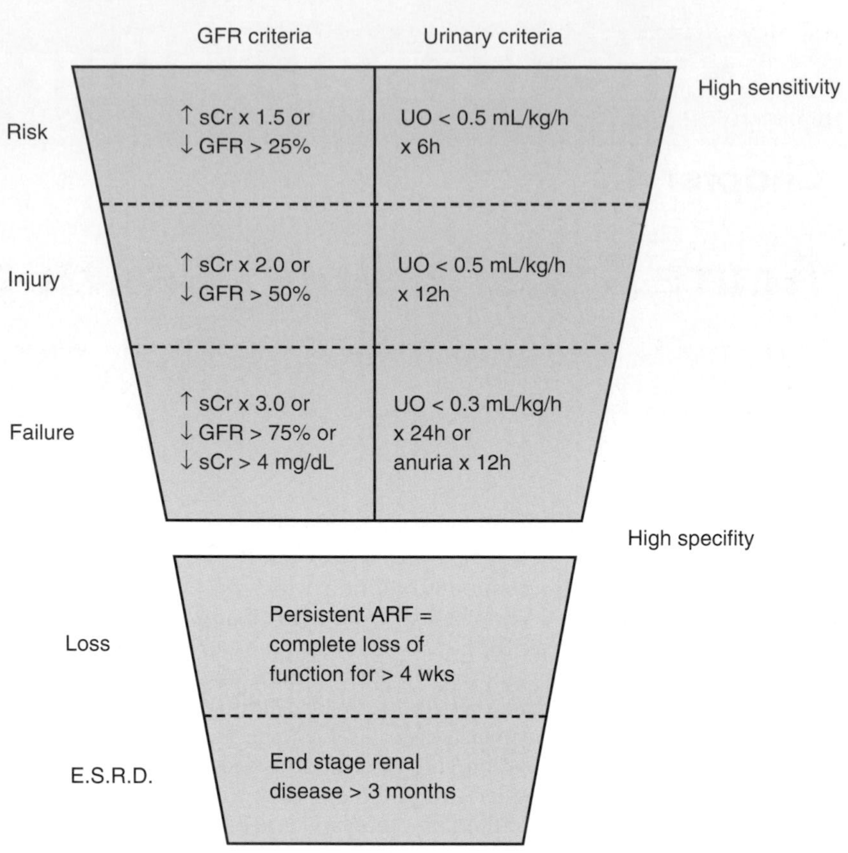

Figure 43–1 RIFLE classification of acute renal failure according to decrease in GFR, urine output and duration of disease. The ARF class (R, I, F, L, or E) is based on the worst criteria following patient assessment. The shape of the figure reflects patient numbers, high for RIFLE-R and low for RIFLE-E. (Taken from ADQI at www.adqi.net.)

traditional definitions of ARF will need to be conducted prior to its more widely accepted use.

Incidence

In the absence of established standardized criteria for ARF, the incidence will vary depending on the definitions used and the patient population studied. In large community-based studies from Europe, the incidence of ARF has been reported as 260 cases per million (0.026%) of total population per year when ARF is defined as a rise of serum creatinine = 2.0 mg/dL,[6] and 140 per million per year (0.014%) when ARF is defined as a rise in serum creatinine > 4.5 mg/dL (>~ 500μmole/L).[9] In the former study from Madrid, more than half of the patients developed ARF in the hospital setting and represented < 0.5% of hospitalized patients. By comparison, a 6-month, U.S. single-center study of in-hospital ARF found an incidence of 13% when defining ARF as a rise of serum creatinine ≥ 0.5mg/dL but only 1% using a rise of serum creatinine ≥ 2.0 mg/dL.[5] These latter data are in broad agreement with large hospital-based studies from the 1980s and 1990s where the incidence of ARF among medical and surgical patients was 5%–8%.[10,11] Thus the in-hospital incidence of ARF is at least 0.5% but may be as high as 13% depending on the definitions used. There are specialized settings in which the incidence of ARF has been reported to be high. For example in the large Madrid study, 7% of patients admitted to the ICU had ARF, and this was replicated in France.[12] The reported incidence of ARF in the ICU varies from 4%-25%.[13,14] ARF has been reported to occur in approximately 7% of patients undergoing cardiac surgery, and more specifically between 15% and 42% of patients undergoing coronary artery bypass graft (CABG) surgery; one small study reported as many as 53% of those requiring cardiac valve replacement developed a 25% rise in serum creatinine.[12,15–19]

The development of ARF is associated with increased hospital length of stay, which further correlates with the severity of the disease. For example, among patients who develop a rise in serum creatinine ≥ 2.0 mg/dL and survive, the length of hospitalization is 9 days longer than patients who do not develop ARF.[5] Development of ARF is associated with more than doubling of the cost of hospital care when compared with patients without the diagnosis of ARF.

Mortality

Many patients with ARF will recover; however, acquisition of the disease is associated with increased mortality. In general, the severity of ARF is correlated with higher mortality. In particular, the requirement for an intensive care facility or renal replacement therapy is associated with increased mortality. Recent data indicate that even small increases in serum creatinine are associated with increased mortality. Using a rise in serum creatinine ≥ 0.5 mg/dL, patients with ARF in the hospital setting are 5.7 times more likely to die than equally sick patients without a rise in creatinine when co-morbidities are accounted for. Mortality increases exponentially with increases in serum creatinine.[5] By comparison, patients admitted with cancer have a 3-fold increased mortality and cardiovascular disease a 1.5-fold increased mortality. Subgroup analysis indicated that even a rise in serum creatinine of 0.3-0.4 mg/dL is associated with a 1.7-fold increase in mortality, although this has not been identified in other studies. Following radiocontrast administration, a 5.5-fold increase in mortality has been reported in those developing ARF when compared with patients without ARF.[20] Of those developing ARF during Amphotericin B administration, a 6.3-fold increase in mortality has been reported.[21] Many studies have looked at mortality and ARF in specific clinical settings (Table 43–1). In summary, ARF is associated strongly with mortality.[12,19,22–25] Patients with ARF who require ICU management have a higher risk of death (e.g., 71% ICU vs. 32% non-ICU)[6] and sepsis is associated with increased mortality in patients with ARF (e.g., 75% sepsis vs. 45% no sepsis).[26]

In many reports it is not possible to dissociate whether the mortality was due to or was simply associated with ARF. However, the study by Liano and colleagues[6] indicates that although 45% of patients with ARF died, only 26% were attributable to ARF as the primary etiology. From a study of 42,000 patients who had cardiac surgery, ARF (defined by a serum creatinine >3 mg/dL) was found to be an independent risk factor for death (7.9 fold), after adjusting for surgical complications and co-morbid conditions.[27] Together with the increased mortality observed after only small rises in serum creatinine,[5] it is fair to conclude that any degree of ARF is an independent risk factor for increased mortality, even if ARF is defined as an increase in serum creatinine of only 0.5 mg/dL.

Etiology

The clinical etiologies of ARF vary widely according to the setting of the study and the cohort of patients. In particular, community-based studies include more patients with prerenal ARF and obstructive ARF than do hospital-based studies. Prostate-related obstructive uropathy accounted for 25% of cases of ARF in one community-based series, and 10% in another.[9] It is likely that many patients with acute obstruction and pre-renal ARF patients are managed in the community without the necessity for hospital admission (Table 43–2). The hospital setting leaves patients at particular risk from low perfusion states; drug toxicities such as aminoglycosides, amphotericin B, and cisplatin; radiocontrast-induced injury; and hemodynamic and septic disturbances associated with major surgery. In one study of all hospital–acquired ARF, these four etiologies accounted for nearly 80% of all cases of ARF.[10]

Within the context of hospital-acquired ARF, certain high-risk groups have been identified. The post-operative period represents greatest risk with 27% of postsurgical patients developing ARF in one study.[6] In addition patients with neoplasia (16%), cardiovascular (30%), respiratory (9%), and gastrointestinal disease (9%), as well as injury/poisoning (14%) and musculoskeletal (5%) disorders, have been shown to be at greater risk of developing ARF in the hospital.[5] In the ICU setting, ARF has been reported to be due to intrinsic renal causes (mainly acute tubular necrosis [ATN]) in 78%, pre-renal in 17%, and post-renal in 5%.[12] In more than 70% of ICU patients with ATN, a combination of hemodynamic instability, nephrotoxins and sepsis can be found reinforcing the view that in most cases of ARF in the ICU there are multiple contributing factors to the etiology (see Table 43–2).[12]

Table 43-1 Mortality of Patients with ARF in Different Clinical Settings*

Author (yr)	Clinical setting	% mortality
Smith (1955)[236]	Trauma patients	68
Kennedy (1973)[22]	Surgical patients	58
Iaina (1975)[237]	Trauma patients	64
Hou (1983)[10]	All hospital patients Cr = 3 mg/dL	60
Berisa (1990)[23]	Aortic aneurysm surgery	61
Frost (1991)[19]	Open heart surgery	63
Spiegel (1991)[24]	ICU patients	88
Groeneveld (1991)[238]	ICU patients	63
Feest (1993)[9]	All patients Cr > 3 mg/dL	46
Brivet (1996)[12]	ICU patients	58
Levy (1996)[20]	Radiocontrast	34
Liano (1996)[6]	All patients Cr >2 mg/dL	45
Liano (1998)[239]	ICU patients	71
Chertow (1998)[27]	Cardiac surgery	63
Metnitz (2002)[14]	ICU patients	63
Nash (2002)[11]	All hospital pts. Cr >3 mg/dL	38

*Note high mortality in all groups, but particularly in ICU and cardiac surgery settings.

Prerenal causes of ARF

When considering the etiologies of ARF, it is useful to categorize according to whether it is due to pre-renal, post-renal or intrinsic renal parenchymal causes (Figure 43–2). Pre-renal kidney dysfunction can return to normal rapidly with correction of the causative insult. It is more common in the community setting, where it is often related to extracellular fluid (ECF) volume losses, associated with gastrointestinal fluid losses. Less often, excessive renal fluid losses or skin losses are implicated (Figure 43–2). In the hospital setting ineffective perfusion of the kidney is often the result of common conditions such as cardiac failure, hemorrhage, sepsis, and liver cirrhosis. In surgical patients—in addition to vasodilatation caused by anesthetic agents, sepsis, or intravascular fluid losses from the surgery—after surgery there are frequently large shifts of intravascular fluid to the extravascular fluid compartment, resulting in effective intravascular fluid depletion. Elderly patients and those with hypertension or diabetes are particularly susceptible to changes in renal perfusion because of preexisting, covert renal vascular disease. Noncompliant intra-renal vasculature from arteriosclerosis disables hemodynamic mechanisms designed to maintain glomerular filtration during variations in renal blood flow.[28,29]

Most cases of ARF are multifactorial in their etiology. In addition to predisposing renal vascular disease, many widely used pharmacological agents alter the response of the vasculature and are frequently implicated in the pathogenesis. Nonsteroidal anti-inflammatory drugs prevent pre-glomerular arteriolar vasodilatation, whereas angiotensin converting enzyme (ACE) inhibitors and angiotensin receptor antagonists prevent post-glomerular arteriolar vasoconstriction.[30,31] Thus in patients at risk for acute deterioration in renal function, these drugs should be temporarily withdrawn or given with caution. There are a number of other drugs that affect the renal vasculature and can potentiate impaired renal perfusion. Calcineurin inhibitors (such as cyclosporine and tacrolimus)

Table 43–2 A Comparison of the Distribution of Etiologies of ARF in Three Different Studies

Author Patient setting	Nash et al (2002) Tertiary referral center	Liano et al (1996) Urban population	Brivet et al (1996) ICU
Number	n=380	n=743	n=350
Definition of ARF	↑Cr > 0.5 mg/dL	Cr > 2.0 mg/dL	Cr > 3.5 mg/dL
Prerenal failure	*	21%	17%
Intrinsic renal	<96%*	63%	65%
ATN	87%	45%	>70%†
Etiologic groups	Renal perfusion 44% Post-operative 18% Radiocontrast 13% Medications 18% Sepsis 7%		Renal perfusion 37% Sepsis 55% Toxic 21%
Glomerulonephritis	1%	3%	
Vasculitis		1%	
Interstitial nephritis	1%	1%	
Acute onset CRF		13%	13%
Vascular	1%	3%	
Unknown	4%		
Multifactorial	6%		
Postrenal	2%	10%	5%

*The proportion of patients with decreased renal perfusion, post operative, and with sepsis who had pre-renal ARF is not defined.
†The proportions of etiologic groups for ARF exceeds 100% since in some patients more than one factor was present.

are used with increasing frequency in transplantation and as therapy for conditions where immunosuppression is required. One side effect of these reagents is intra-renal, pre-glomerular vasoconstriction. In addition, calcineurin inhibitors have a low therapeutic index and are metabolized by liver enzymes. Many drugs that affect liver metabolism can modify plasma levels of calcineurin inhibitors. In high concentrations, radiocontrast agents promote renal vasoconstriction, followed by intratubular contrast precipitation.[32] Cocaine, a widely used recreational drug, promotes cerebral, cardiac, and renal vasoconstriction. Often patients will not report cocaine use, making this diagnosis more challenging.[33]

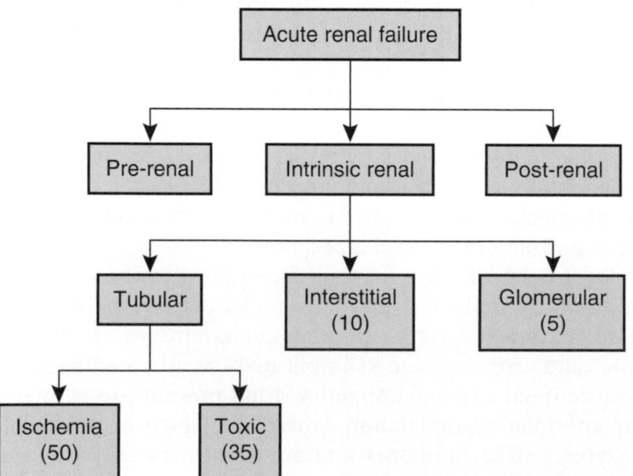

Figure 43–2 Main categories of acute renal failure. Values () indicate approximate percentage of all ARF cases. (Thadhani R, Pascual M, Bonventre JV. Acute renal failure. N Engl J Med 1996; 334:1448-1460. Copyright (C) 1996 Massachusetts Medical Society. All rights reserved.)

Postrenal causes of ARF

Post-renal disease occurs commonly in the community and is frequently due to prostatic disease in men. This condition is readily diagnosed, and therapy to relieve both the obstruction and the ARF is fairly straightforward. One study showed that obstructive causes of ARF occurring in the community had a favorable outcome compared with all other causes of ARF.[9] Similar studies of obstructive disease presenting in the hospital confirm good renal prognosis if the diagnosis is made early.[34] Successful recovery of renal function requires careful attention to fluid balance and electrolytes during the post-obstructive diuretic phase of recovery during which the nephrons are less able to concentrate urine and re-absorb electrolytes.

There are however, many other forms of obstruction that are either silent or intermittent. Unilateral obstruction of the ureter is frequently silent, particularly when caused by neoplastic lesions of the ureteric urothelium, or when caused by external ureteric compression from pelvic neoplasia or inflammation.[35] In one study of bilateral ureteric obstruction, neoplasia accounted for 76% of cases, with prostatic and cervical neoplasia accounting for more than 50%.[36] In such cases of ureteric obstruction, the patient may complain of a change in urinary frequency or vague loin discomfort.[34] When obstruction is unilateral, as is most frequently the case, the GFR in the contralateral kidney can compensate partially so that the net fall in GFR is less than half that of normal and may be reflected only a small rise in serum creatinine. However, if the contralateral kidney does not contribute equally to the overall renal function because of co-existing acute or chronic intrinsic kidney disease, ARF may ensue. In patients with pelvic neoplasia or pelvic inflammation, complicated pathology frequently leads to partial or complete obstruction of both ureters.[36] In these cases, complete understanding of the obstructing lesion requires more detailed anatomical assessment than is afforded by ultrasound scanning alone. Furthermore, the classical features of dilated renal pelvices will not always be present because of encasement of the retroperitoneum.[37,38] Commonly, nephrolithiasis is a cause of unilateral ureteric obstruction. Nephrolithiasis can present with characteristic pain and fever, but like other forms of ureteric obstruction may be silent. In all cases where the normal flow of urine from the pelvis to the urethra is disturbed, the patient is at increased risk of sepsis. Thus frequently obstructive disease presents as part of multifactorial ARF. It is therefore wise to consider an obstructive component to many cases of ARF.

Intrinsic Renal Parenchymal Causes of ARF

Intrinsic renal disease can be subdivided according to the main anatomical site of the injury, including the renal vasculature, the glomeruli, the tubules, and the interstitium (see Figure 43–2). In most clinical settings of ARF, intrinsic causes comprise at least 50% of all ARF with acute interstitial nephritis, glomerulonephritis, and vasculitis making up relatively small proportions of acute renal disease (see Table 43–2). The majority of ARF is exclusively or predominantly as a result of tubular injury, often related to localized or generalized renal ischemia and/or nephrotoxins.

i. Acute Tubular Necrosis (ATN).

ATN is a pathological description and is the most common descriptor used for ARF. Histologically, tubular injury is characterized in the cortex by dilated tubules, and intratubular casts. There is wide variability in the extent of injury to the epithelial cells. With mild injury there is loss of polarity with dislocation of integrins from their usual basal-lateral localization, and loss of the apical brush border. With the change in localization of integrins, some viable cells come off the basement membrane and enter the lumen of the tubule. With more severe injury, tubular cells can undergo apoptosis or necrosis. The glomeruli are usually preserved. A continuum exists between the factors promoting pre-renal disease and ischemic ATN. Renal tubules, in particular the proximal tubules, are susceptible to ischemic injury. This is due to a combination of high metabolic demands, limited anaerobic respiration, and limited blood supply to the straight portion in the outer medulla (see below).[31,39–42] The distribution of tubular injury has been best studied in animals. In humans, where the biopsy data are limited, there may be more distal tubule injury to complement the proximal injury than there is in animals.[43] Those patients experiencing a greater diminution in effective renal perfusion, for a more protracted period, or those patients with predisposing factors affecting the underlying vasculature (diabetes, hypertension, vascular disease, cardiac failure) are more likely to develop ATN. One study of hospital-acquired ARF found sepsis to be the most predisposing factor for the development of ATN.[25] In the ICU setting, 48% of patients with ARF have sepsis as the primary predisposing factor.[12] In addition, a study of community-acquired bacteremia found a doubling of serum creatinine in 24% of patients.[44] Sepsis predisposes to ARF in part by diminished renal perfusion. In addition, however, the circulating toxic milieu of cytokines and chemokines promoting intra-renal local vasospasm and leukocyte activation likely plays an important role.[45–47]

In addition to ischemia and sepsis as contributing factors to ARF, renal tubules are susceptible to many toxins, which often are introduced as therapeutic reagents. Nephrotoxins are implicated in ARF in at least a quarter of all cases.[20,48] Because the nephron functions to filter and then concentrate the filtrate, the concentration of many therapeutic agents often increases along the length of the nephron. Agents commonly associated with ATN include aminoglycosides, amphotericin B, cisplatin, methotrexate, foscarnet, pentamidine, calcineurin inhibitors, and osmotic agents such as mannitol and sucrose (found in intravenous immunoglobulin preparations). In addition, ingestion of heavy metals and organic solvents and excessive ingestion of acetaminophen can induce direct tubular toxicity. Filtration and concentration of free heme pigments by the nephron during rhabdomyolysis or extensive hemolysis, or precipitation of myeloma kappa light chains or uric acid crystals in the tubule leads to direct tubular damage. In the ICU, ATN is associated with multi-organ failure in 90% of cases and is present in as many as 23% of patients at the time of ICU admission. In more than 70% of ICU patients with ATN, a combination of hemodynamic instability, nephrotoxins and sepsis can be implicated as causative.[12] Other patient groups predisposed to ATN include those with hematological malignancies, following cardiac bypass surgery, or with co-existing HIV disease.[19,35,49]

ii. Vascular Disease.

Acute vascular compromise of the large renal vessels is a rare but important cause of ARF. It occurs in patients with critical atherosclerotic vascular disease and is usually accompanied by anuria, and sometimes pain. This is a vascular emergency and requires urgent corrective intervention. Anatomically, this etiology of ARF falls within the category of pre-renal causes. However, it leads to ischemic injury of the parenchyma. On the other hand there are many primary vascular disorders of smaller vessels, which play an important role in ARF and fall under the category of intrinsic renal parenchymal causes. Atheroembolic disease, usually involving cholesterol rich emboli, occurs either spontaneously, especially in patients who are anticoagulated, or following arterial manipulation in those with advanced atherosclerotic vascular disease. In one study, this diagnosis was made in only 5% of those who underwent biopsy with ARF.[6] Although this disease can be characterized by embolic events to the flanks and extremities, presenting as a characteristic rash and the finding of eosinophilia, it is frequently underdiagnosed because it is a relatively silent condition with few diagnostic clues. Therefore a proportion of patients thought to have ATN will have atheroembolic disease as a contributing factor. These vascular diseases compromise blood flow in the kidney and as such will lead to ischemic injury of susceptible components of the nephron. Other vascular conditions such as medium vessel vasculitis as seen in Polyarteritis Nodosa are uncommon and rarely present with ARF. There are a large number of other diseases that primarily affect the vasculature and can present as ARF. These include scleroderma, hypercalcemia, hemolytic-uremic syndrome, malignant hypertension, and pre-eclampsia, to name a few.

iii. Acute Interstitial Nephritis.

Many cases of hospital-acquired ARF have a component of interstitial nephritis, when assessed histologically by biopsy. This is characterized by an excessive interstitial inflammatory infiltrate, often with notable eosinophils amongst the inflammatory cells. The urinary sediment will frequently contain erythrocytes, and leukocytes, less frequently seen in ATN, but this is by no means a reliable finding. There are often relatively few specific diagnostic indicators short of biopsy. In one large study of 748 patients with ARF, 12% had a biopsy, and 10% of those biopsies indicated primary acute interstitial nephritis (AIN) as the cause of ARF.[6]

When presenting as ARF, interstitial nephritis is frequently a response to drug therapy. There are case reports for many and diverse drug therapies that induce interstitial inflammatory response in the kidney. However, β-lactam antibiotics and NSAIDS are implicated in many of these cases.[50–52] Frequently, withdrawal of the drug and supportive management is sufficient to prevent further renal deterioration. In addition, there is an uncommon form of AIN, which is associated with anterior uveitis, known as the tubulo-interstitial nephritis with uveitis syndrome (TINU syndrome). While less common than drug-induced AIN, it can occur in all age groups, and the occurrence of uveitis may be temporally dissociated from the AIN.[53,54] This syndrome is sensitive to glucocorticoid therapy.[54]

iv. Glomerular Diseases.

Glomerular disease can exist as primary glomerular lesions, or alternatively as part of a systemic disorder. Frequently, glomerular disease presents as hypertension, hematuria, proteinuria, nephritic syndrome, or chronic renal dysfunction. There are, however, a proportion of patients who presents with ARF. In one study, 25% of biopsies of patients with ARF had microscopic vasculitis, 25% had primary (idiopathic) glomerulonephritis, and 20% had glomerulonephritis as part of a systemic condition (e.g., systemic lupus erythematosis).[6] A number of these studies point to the importance of the renal biopsy in ARF, even though this important diagnostic tool is used infrequently in these patients.

Diagnosis

History and Physical Examination

Careful assessment of the patient's medical history, current medical condition, recent procedures, medical management, and therapies provides the foundation of a comprehensive assessment of a patient with ARF. A nephrological evaluation will include assessment of risk factors for ARF, underlying CKD, exposure to potential nephrotoxins, and recent disturbance of renal perfusion. The physician should assess the ECF volume status with special attention to the intravascular volume status of the patient. Evidence for focal or systemic infection, focal or systemic injury, or inflammation should be reviewed, and evidence for urinary tract obstruction should be elicited.

Renal Function Tests

One of the major failings of nephrology has been the lack of development of a good marker of acute tubular injury. It is well recognized that an individual can experience an increase of serum creatinine within the normal range, yet lose 75% of GFR.[55] Too often, the diagnosis is delayed by lack of a sensitive marker. In addition to a tubular cell injury marker, it is important to have a sensitive measure of GFR, better than serum creatinine (Figure 43–3). The Cockcroft-Gault (CG) formula is a useful tool in translating the serum creatinine value into an estimate of clearance. It tends to be inaccurate, however, in patients with very high or low GFR, patients who are on drugs that alter renal tubular handling of creatinine, or patients with high body mass.[56] Recently, attempts have been made to introduce new assays to simplify accurate GFR assessment. Cystatin C, a non-glycosylated basic protein, has received significant attention as a more sensitive marker of renal dysfunction. It is synthesized by all nucleated cells and is released into the circulation. Synthesis appears independent of sex, age, and muscle mass. It is freely filtered but totally catabolized by tubules, so that it is neither returned to the circulation nor excreted in the urine.[57] A decline in renal function is associated with a rise in circulating levels. Several studies have compared plasma cystatin C with creatinine concentration and creatinine clearance as estimated by the CG equation, in patients with normal or mild renal dysfunction.[57–61] Overall, the cystatin C assay is

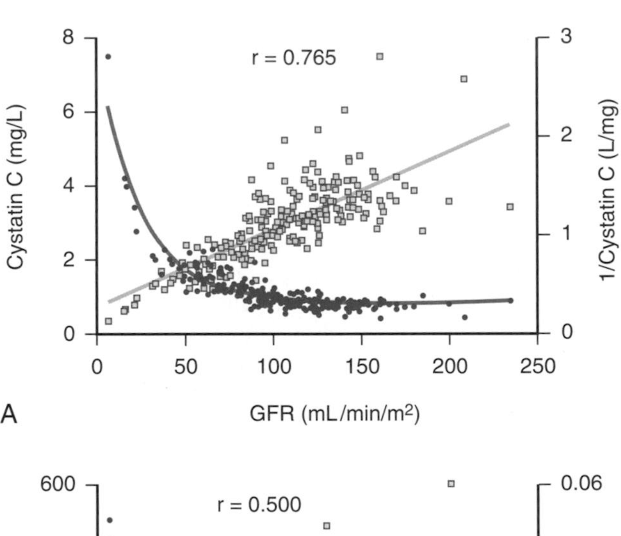

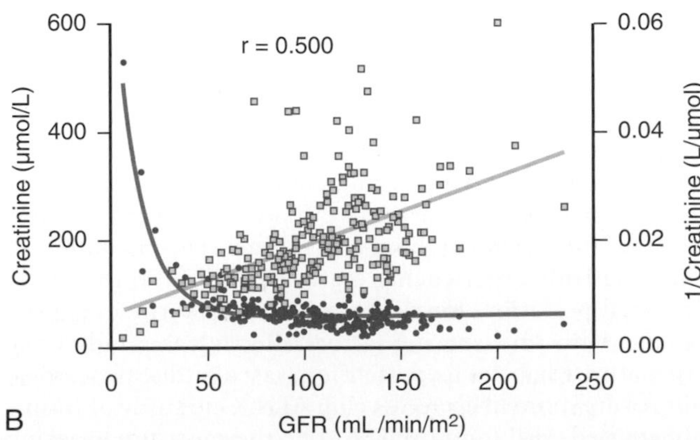

Figure 43–3 Plots of EDTA–measured GFR against ***(A)*** Cystatin C or reciprocal cystatin-C and ***(B)*** creatinine or reciprocal creatinine in the pediatric population. (Taken from Filler G, Priem F, Lepage N, et al. Clin Chem 2002; 48:729-736.) Note the tighter correlation of GFR with 1/cystatin C (r = 0.76 vs. 0.50) and the pronounced rise in Cystatin C at GFR between 50 and 75 mL/min compared with little change to creatinine.

more sensitive than creatinine alone, but comparable with CG creatinine clearance estimates. One advantage of cystatin C over CG equation is that cystatin C clearance declines more than creatinine clearance for mild reductions in GFR. In addition, cystatin C requires only a single measurement, whereas the CG equation requires three variables to be known. Further, several studies have highlighted the utility of cystatin C in specific patient groups, such as the pediatric population or adults with low body mass, whereas low GFR is associated with "deceptively" normal serum creatinine levels (see Figure 43–3).[62–64]

Biomarkers

A novel glycoprotein, KIM-1 is highly upregulated in injured proximal tubular cells, whether that injury is from ischemia or nephrotoxins in both animals and humans.[65–67] The ectodomain of this membrane-associated mucin-rich molecule is shed into the urine of human and rodent kidneys with renal injury, but is not detectable in urine produced by healthy kidneys. Recent evaluation in human disease indicates that it is highly upregulated in ATN, and mildly upregulated in non-ATN ARF and chronic renal failure.[67] Importantly it is not elevated in pre-renal ARF, and increased levels in urine can be detected 12 hours before granular casts in humans and 24 hours before a rise in plasma creatinine in rodents (Figure 43–4).[65,67] Thus assessment of KIM-1 may serve as a useful biomarker to identify tubule injury at an early stage so that aggressive, early, appropriate management can be established. Other biomarkers are being studied. The secreted, cysteine-rich, heparin-binding protein Cyr61 is rapidly induced in proximal straight tubules following renal ischemia, and excreted in the urine where it is detected 3 to 6 hours after the injury in rodents and peaks at 6 to 9 hours after renal injury has occurred, after which it declines rapidly.[68] This marker may serve as an early biomarker of kidney injury. Other studies are ongoing in this area of biomarkers, and the rapid growth of proteomic technologies will likely bring new candidate markers to the forefront of clinical medicine.[69]

Urine Assessment

Patients with ARF often have alterations in urine volume. Oliguria, defined as less than 400 mL/24 hr, is frequently, but not universally seen in patients with ARF. Of all patients developing ARF (defined as a change in serum creatinine of greater than 2.0 mg/dL), nearly 60% have oliguria at first presentation, and this finding tends to be associated with a higher mortality.[10,26,70]

Much information can be determined from careful assessment of dipstick testing and microscopic examination of the urine. Too often, clinicians fail to maintain competence at urine evaluation, yet diagnosis and approach to the care of the patient can often be determined by successful interpretation. The hallmarks of the different diagnoses as determined by assessment of functional analysis of the kidney by composition of the urine are summarized in Table 43–3. There are three considerations: the measurement of urine osmolality, urine sodium excretion, and fractional excretion of sodium. These markers of tubular function help greatly in the assessment and diagnosis of conditions causing ARF (see Table 43–3). Patients with pre-renal ARF, without underlying CKD, who are not taking diuretics, will often retain tubular concentrating capability as well as the ability to absorb sodium from the tubular fluid. Therefore, a concentrated urine specimen with effective resorption of sodium will be present. Similarly a patient with acute glomerulonephritis or obstructive disease will retain tubular function. Patients with ATN and AIN, however, lose tubular function, and will therefore have isotonic urine with high sodium content.

Other Aspects of the Diagnostic Work-Up

In patients in whom the diagnosis is uncertain, early evaluation with a diagnostic ultrasound is essential. Urinary tract obstruction is a common and treatable condition. Although bladder catheterization will expose urethral obstruction such as in prostatic hyperplasia, more proximal obstruction requires visualization. The results of ultrasound must be interpreted with caution, however, since a non-dilated collecting system does not exclude obstruction especially if the assessment is made early in the disease process. Furthermore, encasement of the renal pelvis and ureter may prevent dilatation. In these situations, repeat assessment may be useful or, further, more invasive imaging may be required. In addition to assessment of the collecting system, measurement of renal length with ultrasound may reveal CKD since chronically damaged kidneys are often small.[71–73] In addition to blood tests for evaluating GFR, other serological markers may be useful in diagnosis. Elevated serum calcium or urate may indicate malignancy. Serum or urine electrophoresis may reveal myeloma. Elevated serum creatinine phosphokinase or LDH may reveal rhabdomyolysis or hemolysis, respectively. Elevated neutrophil counts may point to sepsis while eosinophilia and/or eosinophiluria might indicate interstitial nephritis or cholesterol emboli. Where appropriate, tests for systemic immunologic diseases should be performed.

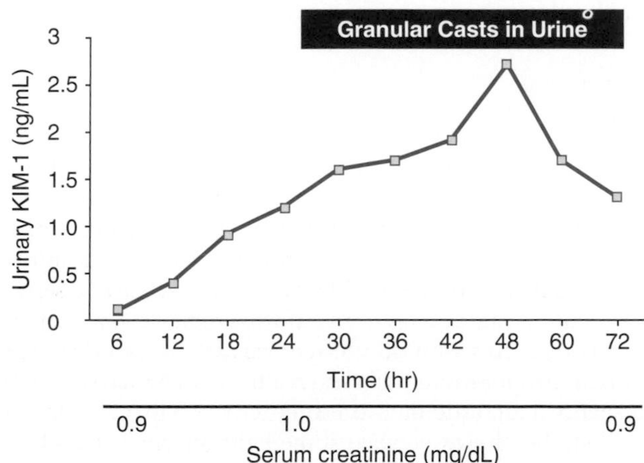

Figure 43–4 The early appearance of Kidney Injury Molecule 1 (KIM-1) in the urine of a patient following abdominal aortic aneurysm repair predates the appearance of granular casts and is seen even without a significant elevation of serum creatinine. (From Han WK, Bailly R, Abichandani R, et al. Kidney Int 2002; 62:237-244.)

Table 43–3 Typical Urinary Findings in Conditions That Cause Acute Renal Failure

Condition	Dipstick Test	Sediment Analysis	urine osmol (mOsm/kg)	fractional excretion of sodium (%)
Prerenal azotemia	Trace or no proteinuria	A few hyaline casts possible	>500	<1
Renal azotemia				
Tubular injury				
Ischemia	Mild-to-moderate proteinuria	Pigmented granular casts	<350	>1
Nephrotoxins	Mild-to-moderate proteinuria	Pigmented granular casts	<350	>1
Acute interstitial nephritis	Mild-to-moderate proteinuria; hemoglobin leukocytes	White blood cells and white blood cell casts; eosinophils and eosinophil casts; red blood cells	<350	>1
Acute glomerulo-nephritis	Moderate to severe proteinuria; hemoglobin	Red blood cells and red blood cell casts; red blood cells can be dysmorphic	>500	<1
Postrenal azotemia*	Trace or no proteinuria; can have hemoglobin, leukocytes	Crystals, red blood cells, and white blood cells possible	<350	>1

* Early in obstruction the urinary indices can mimic those seen in prerenal azotemia.

Kidney Biopsy

One of the great ironies in the field of ARF is that clinicians are still arguing over the pathology of this disease more than 60 years after the disease was first identified. This uncertainty is derived from the reluctance of clinicians to perform biopsies on their patients. Although it is true that it is not necessary for all patients with ARF to be subjected to renal biopsy, in large studies it has been found that it was only by biopsy that the correct diagnosis could be made.[6,10,74,75] Once pre-renal and obstructive causes have been excluded, and assessment suggests in intrinsic renal problem other than ischemic or nephrotoxic ATN, a renal biopsy may establish a diagnosis and direct management. In addition, patients who have protracted ARF despite recovery in other organ systems may benefit from biopsy to exclude occult diagnoses such as cholesterol embolization.[6,74]

Recovery

The normal sequence of events in acute renal injury is recovery of function. Not all patients who survive their illness recover function, however. Some experience partial recovery and a proportion of these later develop progressive kidney failure, as seen following many other forms of kidney injury. The mean duration of ARF (defined as an increase in serum creatinine > 3 mg/dL) has been reported to be 12 days in those surviving patients who do not require dialysis. But dialysis is required, the duration increases to a mean of 17 days.[76] There are surprisingly little data on long-term renal survival. Two recent studies, however, shed some light on this issue. At the more severe end of the spectrum, in those patients discharged from the hospital following ARF requiring renal replacement therapy with at least one other organ failure (e.g., respiratory failure), 10% remained dialysis–dependent, and more than 40% had chronic kidney failure (CKF).[77] This study group was taken from the ICU setting. In this instance, it is reasonable to assume that ATN accounted for most of the causes of ARF. In another recent European study, investigators followed 1100 patients with dialysis-requiring ARF for up to 9 years. Of the survivors, 16% remained dialysis-dependent. A minority (6 patients) who were discharged from the hospital still on dialysis recovered renal function.[78] In a study from Minnesota conducted in the 1980s, among the survivors (31%) of dialysis-requiring ARF, 3% remained dialysis-dependent, 25% had moderate CKD, and a further 10% had severe CKD at 90 days.[79] In a large retrospective study of men with ARF, those with an acute decline in renal function, followed by recovery, had a longer-term (2 to 8 years) outcome that correlate with the severity of the initial insult. Forty percent of patients who had an initial rise in plasma creatinine exceeding three-fold above baseline experienced persistent renal dysfunction. By contrast, fewer than 1% of those whose creatinine increased by less than 50% above baseline developed longer-term renal dysfunction.[80,81]

In studies of mice, 30 minutes of ischemia is followed by return of the serum creatinine to normal within 72 hours; nevertheless, this short ischemic exposure results in progressive interstitial myofibroblast expansion and interstitial fibrosis for at least 12 weeks after reperfusion.[82] These data again point out the insensitivity of the serum creatinine as an indicator of renal parenchymal disease.

Renal Replacement Therapy

Patients with ARF who require renal replacement therapy are at highest risk for death and for developing CKF. Experimental data have been used to justify the approach to the maintenance dialytic therapy of patients with ARF. It has been proposed, but not proven, that in humans who suffer from ARF, the kidney is particularly susceptible to repeated injury because of loss of autoregulatory capacity,[83] persistent inflammation, and intratubular obstruction from tubular cell debris, which are features of the ischemia models of ARF in animals. Thus, while it may be necessary to introduce renal replacement therapies support to help improve survival, there is concern that these therapies not contribute to kidney injury, further delaying recovery of renal function. The loss of autoregulation shown in isolated rodent renal vessel studies (see below) would predict that dialysis therapies that minimize large variations in systemic arterial pressure will benefit renal recovery. The persistence of inflammation in an acutely injured kidney would suggest that dialysis therapies that also minimize systemic inflammation would benefit recovery. Thus, the factors to consider when initiating renal replacement therapy are timing of introduction, choice of modality, choice of dialysis/filtration membrane, adequacy of clearance, potential clearance of inflammatory mediators, and potential loss of anti-inflammatory mediators.

i. Biocompatible Membranes.

The type of membrane used for dialysis or filtration has been shown to affect survival. With the introduction of new biocompatible membrane surfaces, there is less complement activation as a result of interaction of blood with the membrane surface. With greater hydraulic permeability and enhanced adsorptive properties, the biocompatible membranes serve to remove inflammatory mediators from the circulation.[84] Survival of patients dialyzed with biocompatible membranes has been shown in several studies to be enhanced when compared with dialysis using cuprophan membranes.[85] Although there has been controversy in the literature, a recent meta-analysis of survival data from 867 patients confirmed that the synthetic biocompatible membranes do confer substantial survival advantage with an odds ratio of 1.4.[86] Recovery from ARF was not significantly hastened, however.

ii. Dose of Renal Replacement Therapy.

Although it might seem intuitive that since dialysis provides only a small proportion (5%) of the clearance of normally functioning kidneys, more dialysis would be better; however, there are precedents to indicate that such a view might be simplistic. Intermittent hemodialysis (IHD) is not well tolerated in patients with hemodynamic instability and has been considered detrimental in such circumstances. Protracted activation of coagulation and complement cascades clearly could be more detrimental than intermittent activation, and since dialysis or hemofiltration does not selectively remove only harmful substances, the loss of beneficial compounds such as anti-inflammatory cytokines might be deleterious to overall outcome.

When considering the dose of dialysis, many reports indicate that prescribed dose of dialysis overestimates delivered dose in as many as 30% of patients with ARF. The difference between prescribed and delivered dialysis dose appears to be greater when using IHD than continuous venovenous hemofiltration (CVVH).[87,88] Factors such as increased catabolic state, increased total body water, and unusual urea kinetics in patients with ARF may contribute to this phenomenon. In addition, the practicalities of managing dialysis for ARF patients are different from patients with CKF. For example, coagulation of blood in the lines, periods of hemodynamic instability, and procedures requiring disconnection from the dialysis machine are more common in ARF.

Several studies indicate that adjustment of the dialysis dose is important in influencing patient outcome. In a large retrospective study, high Kt/V urea was associated with improved outcome in all patients with moderate disease severity and was subsequently confirmed in a smaller prospective trial (Figure 43–5).[89,90] Recently, Schiffl and colleagues[91] compared daily IHD with thrice-weekly IHD in 160 matched ICU patients. Weekly delivered Kt/V urea was 5.8 and 3.0, respectively. Mortality was 28% and 46%, respectively. There are a number of issues that bring into question the extent to which this study can be generalized.[92] One could look at the study as a comparison of adequate versus inadequate dialysis, since the alternate day group had a substandard (even for patients with CKF) Kt/V urea. Ronco and colleagues,[88] using exclusively CVVH, randomized patients to ultrafiltration rates of 20, 35, or 45 mL/hr/kg (1.3, 2.4, and 2.9 L/hr). Patients treated with the lowest dose had a significantly poorer outcome (41% survival vs. 57% and 58% survival, respectively) at 30 days. In addition the analysis indicated that patients with sepsis had improved outcome on the highest dose compared with the intermediate dose. Furthermore, patients with BUN greater than 60 mg/dL at the onset of CVVH had a worse outcome than those with a BUN less than 60 mg/dL. Thus this study indicates that, using modern dialysis and filtration techniques, more continuous dialysis than has been traditionally used may enhance patient survival (Figure 43–5).

iii. Intermittent Hemodialysis versus Continuous Renal Replacement Therapy.

If it is important to minimize hemodynamic instability to optimize recovery of renal function following the development of ARF, continuous renal replacement therapies (CRRTs), which are associated with less hemodynamic instability, would be superior to intermittent therapies. Consideration of the optimal dialytic modality for patients with ARF is complicated by variability in the delivered dose of dialysis. Several retrospective and three prospective studies have attempted to determine whether continuous dialysis is superior to intermittent therapies. The studies have provided conflicting results.[93–100] Observational retrospective studies have led to findings that patients treated with CRRT had improved survival over IHD patients despite having greater illness severity scores.[101–103] In a relatively small prospective randomized controlled trial of 166 patients, those on CRRT did not have a better outcome than those receiving IHD. This was attributed however, to higher disease severity scores in those on CRRT (despite randomization).[100] The conclusion from two meta-analyses is that there is insufficient evidence to conclude that CRRT is superior to IHD.[104,105] One of the meta-analyses from Kellum and colleagues,[104] however, stratified patients according to disease severity. Their data indicate that in all severity categories, CRRT provided a survival advantage over IHD. In the absence of a clear survival benefit of one modality, and in the absence of a large randomized controlled trial to determine definitively which modality should be used, the choice may rest with local factors such as equipment availability, staffing, and cost, in addition to hemodynamic stability of the patient and disease severity score.

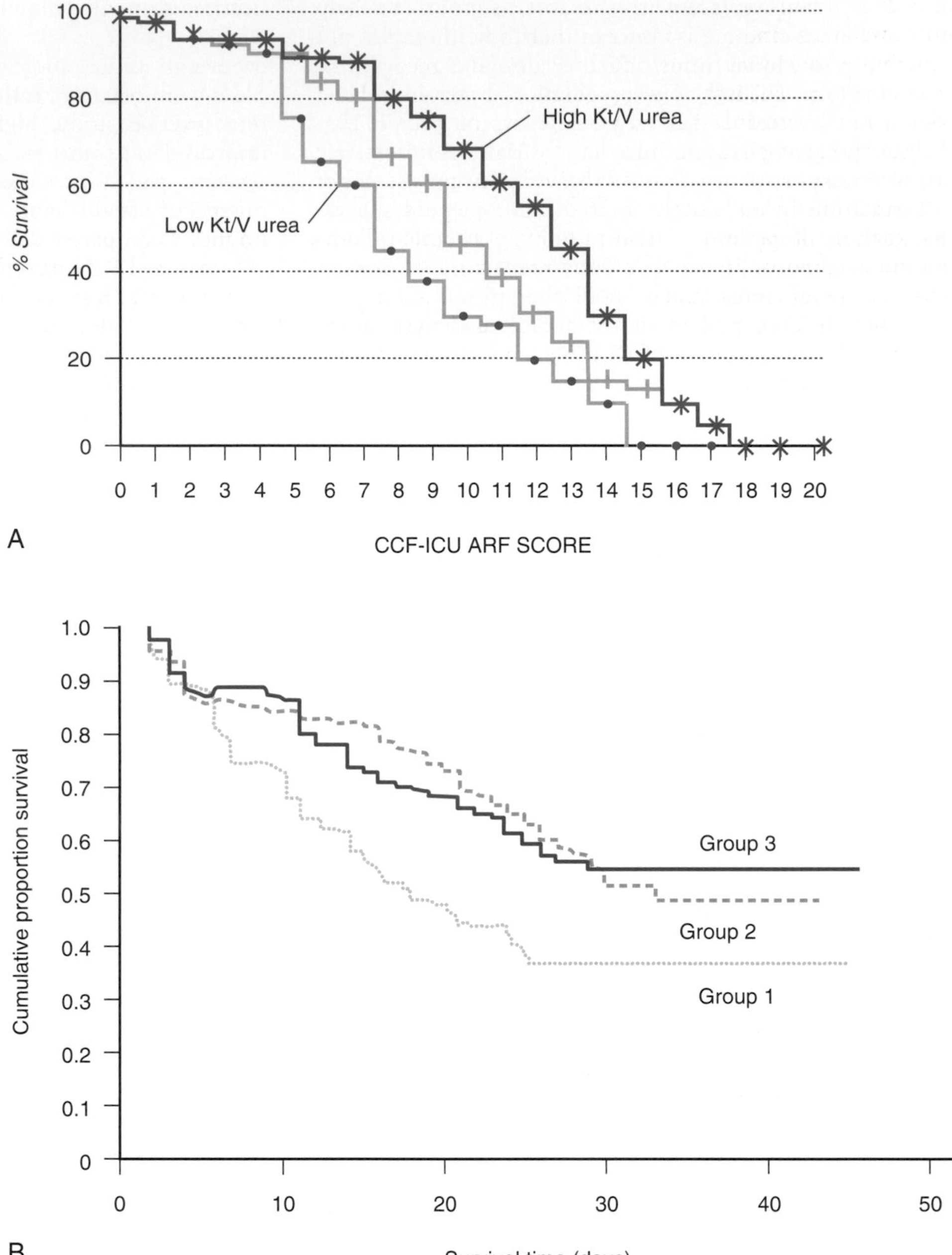

Figure 43-5 (A) The effect of delivered hemodialysis dose as reflected by Kt/V urea, on patient survival according to the Cleveland Clinic Foundation (CCF) acute renal failure ICU severity of illness scores (Adapted from Paganini EP, Halstenberg WK, Goormastic M. *Clin Nephrol* 1996; 46:206-211). **(B)** Kaplan-Meier survival curves for ICU patients receiving CVVH with filtration of 20 mL/kg/hr (Group 1), 35 mL/kg/hr (Group 2), or 45 mL/kg/hr (Group 3). (Adapted from Ronco C, Bellomo R, Homel P, et al. Lancet 2000; 356:26-30.)

Pathophysiology of Acute Renal Failure

i. Intra-Renal Hemodynamic Factors.

Although systemic or localized disturbance of renal blood flow is a major factor in the etiology of ARF, intrinsic renal factors contribute to the pathogenesis of the disease. Two foci of persistent vasoconstriction following injury have been identified. Persistence of pre-glomerular vasoconstriction is proposed to be triggered by a high salt load arriving in the distal tubule as a result of inadequate sodium resorption in the injured, more proximal parts of the tubule. In addition, studies of renal blood flow point to persistent loss of local blood flow to the outer medulla for many hours after renal injury in both experimental models of injury in rodents and in human biopsy specimens.[106–112] Three factors may contribute to a reduction in perfusion in the outer medulla. The medullary blood flow is post capillary, and hence low pressure. Injured endothelial cells swell and, in combination with leukocyte adhesion to the injured endothelium, will impede low-pressure blood flow. In addition, coagulation cascades may become activated. Local production of vasoconstrictor agents is markedly upregulated following ischemic injury. Measurement of renal blood flow in rats 1 week following ischemic injury points to persistent dysregulation of vascular tone at rest and in response to vasodilators and constrictors. In essence, the renal vasculature is tonically more constricted, is hyper-responsive to vasoconstrictors, is hypo-responsive to vasodilators, and responds inappropriately to a fall in perfusion pressure by vasoconstriction (Figure 43–6).[106,107] In the rodent model of ischemia in which the renal artery is clamped, the proximal tubule in the outer medulla is most affected following ischemic injury.[113–114] Even when total perfusion to the kidney is normalized, the outer medulla fails to recover normal blood flow promptly. In the outer medulla, the S3 portion of proximal tubules and the medullary thick ascending limb of Henle (MTAL) dominate. Both nephron segments require substrates for high levels of ATP production. Cell injury is most apparent in the S3 segment of the proximal tubule in most animal models. There is some controversy as to the relative extent of proximal versus distal tubule injury in humans with ARF.[115]

One obvious way to reduce injury and hasten recovery is to reverse inappropriate vascular constriction. Many potent vasoconstrictors have been identified in the ischemic kidney, including endothelin-1, angiotensin II, thromboxane A2, prostaglandin H2, leukotrienes C4, D4, adenosine and sympathetic nerve stimulation.[31,116] A number of studies indicate that blockade of endothelin receptors prior to an ischemic insult protects the rat kidney from injury.[117–120] There are two vascular smooth muscle cell receptors for endothelin, ER-A, and ER-B. The former appears to function primarily in vasoconstriction, and selective blockade in rats has proven beneficial to recovery. Angiotensin receptor blockade, however, is widely implicated in the induction of ischemic injury through paralysis of post glomerular arterioles.[121,122] Successful diminution of post-injury vasoconstriction in animal models with improved functional response has not translated into practical therapies for humans to date.[2] This may relate to the fact that animal studies are performed in a background of normal vasculature, whereas most patients with ARF have at least some degree of underlying vascular disease that could alter the response to vasodilatory drugs. In addition, the agents are given much later in the disease course in humans than they are in animals. These observations, however, suggest the need for directed research into new or combination vasodilators in ischemic injury.

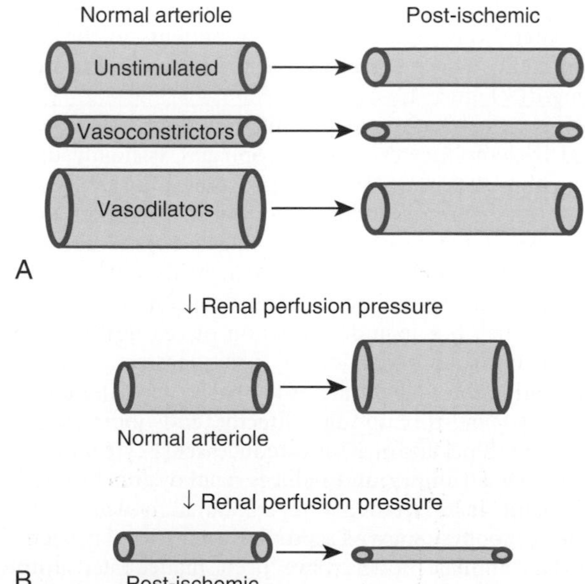

Figure 43–6 ***(A)*** The effect of vasodilators and vasoconstrictors on post-ischemic renal arterioles. ***(B)*** The response to decreased renal perfusion pressure in normal and post-ischemic renal arterioles. (Adapted from studies by J.D. Conger et al.[106–108])

An important finding in animal models of ischemic renal injury is that previous ischemic injury protects from future injury. This "preconditioning" effect lasts for several weeks. These studies indicate that the kidney can activate endogenous protective mechanisms. Endogenous mechanisms appear to protect vessels as well as tubules from injury.[123–125] Exploiting these mechanisms will likely lead to new therapies. Although the deliberate induction of sublethal renal ischemia may appear to have little practical application to patients, studies of pre-conditioning in the myocardium have shown that several pharmacological agents can mediate the same protection as ischemic preconditioning.[126–131] During coronary bypass surgery, ischemic injury sufficient to induce atrial fibrillation (for 5 minutes) protects the myocardium during subsequent surgery. In addition, the use of diazoxide to pharmacologically precondition the myocardium for 5 minutes prior to surgery has also afforded marked benefit to the myocardium during surgery.[132,133] Cardiac studies have highlighted signaling pathways involving protein kinase A, protein kinase D, and mitogen activated kinase pathways in preconditioning. We have found that nitric oxide, a pluripotential molecule derived from inducible nitric oxide synthase (iNOS) contributes to the preconditioning effect in the kidney.[82] Intrinsic cells of the kidney continue to generate NO through increased activation of iNOS for several weeks after injury. NO is the most potent vasodilator yet described. In inflammatory diseases, iNOS-derived NO has been shown to take over the function of eNOS-derived NO in regulating vascular tone.[134] One mechanism by which iNOS-derived NO protects the kidney from injury is by preventing inappropriate vasoconstriction directly as a vasodilator and indirectly by preventing upregulation of vasoconstrictors.[135] In support of this, others have shown that in the preconditioned kidney, production of the vasoconstrictor endothelin-1 is markedly attenuated during ischemia.[136]

ii. Inflammatory Factors.

Injury anywhere in the body promotes an inflammatory response. The kidney is no exception. Intense macrophage accumulation in the outer medulla of postischemic kidneys has been elegantly demonstrated *in vivo* by magnetic resonance imaging and in multiple histological studies (Figure 43–7).[113,137] Injured epithelial and endothelial cells upregulate the production and release of chemokines and cytokines. Although the inflammatory response can be beneficial by promoting repair, increasing evidence is accumulating that in the kidney, the inflammatory response to injury may impede recovery and promote scarring.

Injured endothelial and epithelial cells promote leukocyte adhesion. This combination leads to release of pro-inflammatory cytokines such as TNF-α and IL-1β, and positive feedback in the inflammatory response through generation of chemokines with resultant leukocyte accumulation.[138–141] One of the key molecules involved in leukocyte adhesion is intercellular adhesion molecule-1 (ICAM-1). In addition, other early factors in the inflammatory response, such as complement

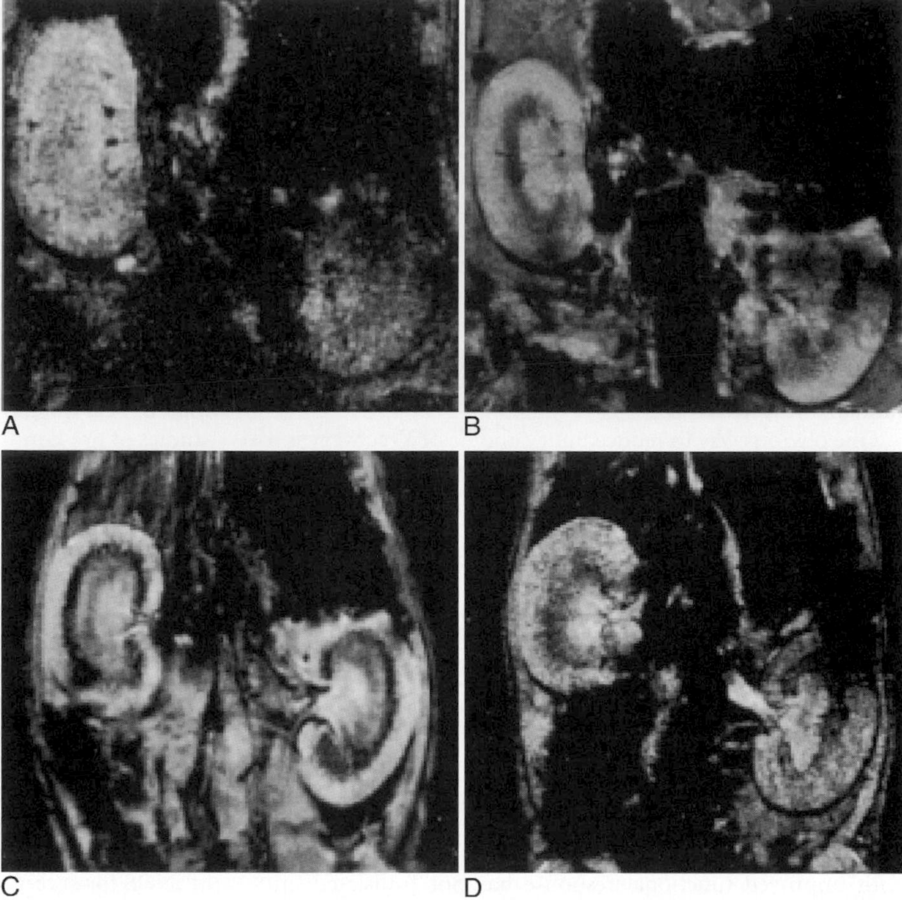

Figure 43–7 Non-invasive evaluation of inflammation in ischemic renal injury. Localization of inflammatory macrophages in the outer medulla captured by MR imaging following administration of ultra-small paramagnetic iron oxide beads to rodents with ischemic injury. Normal kidneys ***(A)***, 48 hr ***(B)***, 72 hr ***(C)***, and 120 hr ***(D)*** following ischemic injury. Note attenuation of signal, a sign of macrophage accumulation, in the outer medullary region only. (Adapted from Jo SK, Hu X, Kobayashi H, et al. Kidney Int 2003; 64:43-51.)

activation and leukotriene generation, are all found in the postischemic kidney.[141] Activated leukocytes release toxic enzymes (elastase) and reactive oxygen intermediates. Blockade of leukocyte adhesion molecules attenuates injury and intravascular accumulation of activated leukocytes with beneficial effects on renal function.[142–145] Blockade of leukocyte adhesion and migration by neutrophil depletion, ICAM-1 antibodies, or antisense oligonucleotides against ICAM-1 mRNA ameliorates ischemia-induced injury in animal models.[146–150] The role of ICAM-1, particularly in renal transplant ischemia-reperfusion injury, has gained significant attention, since ICAM-1 is highly upregulated following revascularization. Recently, a randomized control trial of ICAM-1 blockade was undertaken using humanized anti-ICAM-1 antibodies. There was no significant benefit in reducing delayed graft function, patient survival, graft survival, or acute rejection episodes at 3 months. The study design, however, included delivery of antibody only after reperfusion. Leukocytes accumulate in the kidney very soon after reperfusion. It is possible therefore that the cold-stored kidney has marked upregulation of ICAM-1 and the therapeutic window for ICAM-1 blockade was missed.[151]

Blockade of the effects of toxic products from inflammatory leukocytes and injured parenchymal cells have been proposed as a viable approach to protection of the kidney against ischemic and toxic injury. Targeting reactive oxygen species, such as H_2O_2 and O_2 using scavengers such as *N*-acetylcysteine, or transgenic animals overproducing oxygen radical scavengers, attenuate injury.[46,152–156] The value of such strategies has been suggested for many years, but has only been borne out in humans in a small clinical trial where patients with mild chronic renal failure were given oral *N*-acetylcysteine prior to radiocontrast agent administration. There were significantly more patients in the control group that had an increase in serum creatinine of more than 0.5 mg/dL (Figure 43–8).[4]

TNF-α, the prototypic pro-inflammatory cytokine, produced by lymphocytes and macrophages, is highly upregulated within 30 minutes following ischemic injury.[157] Blockade of TNF-α ameliorates inflammatory disease in other contexts and has led to the creation of blocking agents that are used in human diseases such as rheumatoid arthritis, Crohn's disease, and ankylosing spondylitis.[158] The functions of TNF-α are pluripotential, but include induction of cell death by apoptosis or necrosis, activation of proinflammatory cascades by activating the nuclear factor kappa-B (Nf-κB)–dependent genes, and by functioning directly and indirectly as a chemokine. Blockade of TNF-α reduces leukocyte infiltration, reduces tubular injury, and reduces renal dysfunction following ischemic insult to the kidney in animal models.[159,160]

The pathophysiology of sepsis-induced ARF has been elusive. The animal models have been inadequate, although recently published models capitalizing on increased susceptibility to sepsis-induced ARF in aged animals may change this research platform.[161] In our opinion the systemic inflammatory response syndrome (SIRS), characteristic of sepsis, results in intrarenal inflammation with microvascular and ischemic implications caused by leukocyte activation, pro-coagulant

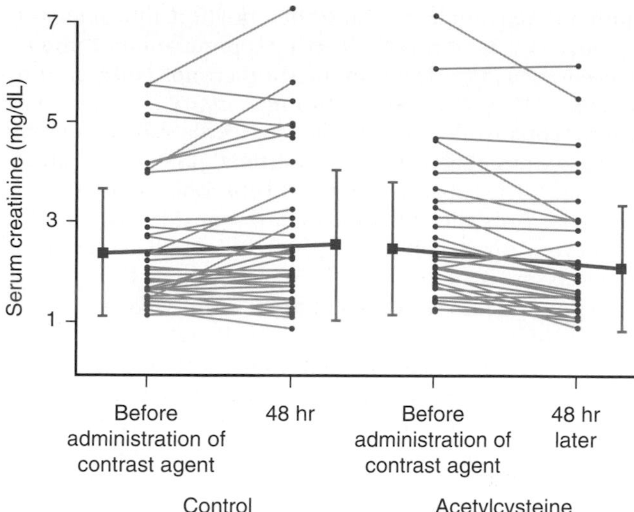

Figure 43–8 *N*-Acetylcysteine protects renal function during radiocontrast-mediated injury. Patients treated with *N*-acetylcysteine 600 mg twice a day for 2 days, in addition to saline hydration (1 ml/kg/hr) for 24 hours, experienced an improvement in renal function compared with a deterioration in renal function in matched controls receiving saline alone ($P < .001$) (Adapted from Tepel M, van der Giet M, Schwarzfeld C, et al. N Engl J Med 2000; 343:180-184.).

effects, and advanced leukocyte-endothelial interactions and adhesion.[162] There is accumulating evidence that genetic predisposition in humans to production of high levels of TNF-α, and low levels of the anti-inflammatory cytokine IL-10, during SIRS associated with organ failure is detrimental to organ and patient survival. This lends further evidence to the view that inflammatory leukocyte-derived cytokines play crucial roles in renal injury during sepsis.[163]

NO may play a critical role in the regulation of the inflammatory response. The importance of NO in protecting the preconditioned kidney has been described previously. The actions of NO in the ischemic kidney are tripartite. NO is involved in maintaining vascular tone. It is known that following injury, endothelial-derived NO is reduced, presumably due to injury to the endothelium.[164,165] Thus generation of iNOS-derived NO by tubular cells and inflammatory cells assists in maintaining some degree of vasodilatation. In addition to a direct role on smooth muscle tone, NO regulates gene expression of endothelin and other vasoconstrictors, directly counteracting the upregulation of this potent vasodilator.[166] It is now widely accepted that a proportion of patients with vascular disease have endothelial dysfunction. In essence, the endothelium does not generate nitric oxide but favors generation of reactive oxygen intermediates (ROI). Thus, upregulation of perivascular NO by interstitial and inflammatory cells may serve to counteract the relative lack of NO generated by the endothelium of patients with endothelial dysfunction.[165] Secondly, NO can counteract the toxic effect of ROI by converting them to harmless nitrites and nitrates as end products. In rare circumstances NO interacts with ROI to generate nitrosyl compounds, which are nitrosylate tyrosine residues, and are very toxic to cells.[167,168] Although this has been observed in the kidney, it remains to be elucidated when NO plays a primarily destructive or primarily beneficial role through interaction with ROI. Finally, NO itself is directly able to induce apoptotic cell death by engaging several mechanisms. It directly disrupts the cell cycle and regulates apoptosis gene expression, including apoptotic death proteases such as Caspase-3. In addition, it interferes with cyclic GMP intracellular signaling, which can also contribute to apoptosis.[169]

Thus in the preconditioned kidney, in addition to its role as a vasodilator, one mechanism by which nitric oxide generation by tubular cells and macrophages might be protective is through reduction of inflammation caused by neutralization of ROI. This protective mechanism has been reported in models of experimental glomerulonephritis in rats.[170] In addition, parenchymal cells generating high levels of NO themselves are resistant to the toxic effects of NO and ROI released from neutrophils and macrophages. Although NO is not currently used as a therapy for renal injury, small human studies of renal injury have confirmed that the use of L-arginine, the substrate for iNOS-dependent NO generation, reduces renal injury.[171]

Complement is deposited specifically on injured endothelial and epithelial cells following ischemic injury. In murine models, C3 is deposited within 2 hours, whereas C6 and C9, which are components of the membrane attack complex (MAC), are deposited later. Specific inhibition of C5 cleavage, which generates C5a, has been reported to inhibit the inflammatory infiltrate, to limit the MAC development, and to limit tubular cell death independently of the inflammatory response.[172,173] These investigations are, however, limited to rodent models.

Later phases of recovery from ischemic injury are characterized by T cell infiltration. CD4/CD8-deficient mice lacking T lymphocytes are protected from ischemia-reperfusion injury,[174] suggesting a causal role for T lymphocytes in mediating injury. In addition, blockade of the interaction of "co-stimulatory" molecules B7-1 and CD28 on antigen presenting cells and T cells, respectively, protects against ischemic injury in rats and significantly inhibits T cell and macrophage infiltration and activation *in situ*.[175,176] These molecular interactions are necessary to trigger an adaptive immune response. However, B7-1 expression by injured endothelium of the vasa recta may have a more general role in leukocyte adhesion, offering an alternative interpretation of these results.[177] Furthermore, mice deficient in both T and B cells are not protected from ARF induced by ischemia. In these experiments, histological assessment of postischemic kidneys found that both tubular necrosis and leukocyte infiltration were comparable with wild-type mice.[178] Thus, the exact role of T cells currently remains unclear.

Inflammatory mediators are generated not only by infiltrating leukocytes, but also by injured proximal tubular cells (PTC). While much of the data concerning inflammatory mediators derived from PTC come from *in vitro* studies, it appears that PTC can generate pro-inflammatory cytokines, including TNF-α, IL-1β, IL-6, growth factors such as M-CSF, and many chemokines including MCP-1, RANTES, IL-8 and fractalkines.[179,180] As indicated above, blockade of the inflammatory response following ischemic injury has been shown to be beneficial in animal models. One of the key functions of the innate inflammatory response is to debride tissue of injured cells, remove debris, destroy invading pathogens, and then promote repair. It is clear that in carrying out these tasks, excessive cellular loss occurs. Tubular cells that could otherwise have recovered may be deleted and removed by the inflammatory response, resulting in an added burden to the repair process. More importantly, however, the inflammatory contribution results in local effects on the peritubular vasculature, causing upregulation of endothelial adhesion molecules and local activation of leukocytes and thus resulting in small vessel occlusion and secondary ischemia.[146]

Factors Affecting Tubular Cell Injury

i. Proximal Tubular Cell Injury.

The S3 segment of the proximal tubule is particularly susceptible to ischemic injury. This is in part due to vascular factors as previously discussed, but in addition, the proximal tubular cells have low glycolytic capacity. Although MTAL cells are subjected to equal hypoxia following ischemic injury, they are resistant to injury. *In vitro*, isolated rat MTAL tubular segments increase lactate generation by 1400% in response to blockage of mitochondrial respiration. Isolated proximal tubules do not generate lactate in identical conditions.[39] Although rat MTAL cells are less vulnerable to ischemia, nevertheless they respond promptly to the stress imposed by ischemia, switching on an array of inflammatory genes that may regulate local inflammatory responses.[181]

ii. Sublethal Injury.

In response to injury, the PTC initially loses polarity. Many molecules, normally polarized to one region or surface of the cell, becoming distributed equally through the cell or to different regions of the cell membrane. The loss of polarity is followed by disruption of the junctions that maintain a barrier between the lumen and the basolateral surface. Key junctions are the tight and adherens junctions.[182,183] Loss of the integrity of these junctions and incorrect targeting of ion transporters results in reduced vectorial transport of NaCl and water, which in turn leads to enhanced sodium delivery to the distal tubule.[184] This might be expected to generate afferent arteriolar vasoconstriction and contribute to post-ischemic vasoconstriction. By definition, this degree of injury is reversible and the altered polarity can ultimately be normalized.

In addition to the functional consequences of the loss of polarity, redistribution of integrins that anchor epithelial cells to the basement membrane allow viable epithelial cells to detach and be shed into the lumen.[185–188] These viable cells undergo a process of dedifferentiation, expressing molecules such as vimentin, NCAM, and the nuclear factor pax-2, normally associated with mesenchymal cells during nephron development and not normally present in epithelial cells.[189–192] Expression of these molecules, normally associated with mesenchymal cells during development, is characteristic of injured epithelial cells that have the potential to migrate to cover areas of denuded basement membrane.

We and others have shown that in animal models of ischemic injury to the kidney, there is expansion of the interstitial myofibroblast population as seen in many forms of renal disease in humans.[82,193] Following injury, there is new evidence that, in addition to acquiring a mesenchymal phenotype within the confines of the tubule, proximal tubular epithelial cells undergo transdifferentiation into interstitial fibroblasts. The normal kidney has a population of interstitial cells, which generate, amongst other molecules, erythropoietin.[194,195] However, during injury, these cells dedifferentiate into myofibroblasts, which produce a number of matrix proteins that, if not resorbed, potentiate scar formation.[196] The expansion of the myofibroblast population is as intrinsic to the inflammatory response as is influx of leukocytes. Renal epithelial cells frequently become myofibroblasts in tissue culture,[197–199] and epithelial cells of the eye, salivary gland, and liver and in tumors have been shown to transdifferentiate *in vivo*.[200–202] Evidence is accumulating from different models of renal injury that injured tubular cells *in vivo* transdifferentiate into myofibroblasts and contribute to the interstitial fibroblast population.[203–205] In a murine model of interstitial fibrosis, most of the interstitial myofibroblasts were derived from the proximal tubule.[203]

Thus it appears that, in addition to epithelial cells mediating repair through migrating to denuded areas of basement membrane, in areas where the basement membrane is damaged, production of extracellular matrix molecules by these cells maintains tissue integrity, preventing secondary damage resulting from tissue collapse (Figure 43–9). In addition to this potentially advantageous effect of enhanced matrix production, however, many studies show that interstitial fibrosis heralds poor outcome in the medium to long term. Repairing tissues, not capable of resorbing matrix, may develop persistent ischemia, progressive cell loss, and loss of function.[206,207] The accumulation of interstitial myofibroblasts appears to be under the regulation of the pluripotential cytokine TGFβ. A natural inhibitor of some of the functions of TGFβ, bone morphogenic protein-7 (BMP-7), is expressed in the developing and injured kidney. BMP-7 *in vitro* is able to counteract the tendency toward epithelial-mesenchymal transdifferentiation and in animal studies of nephritis, BMP-7 has markedly reduced progressive scarring and tubular atrophy.[169,208,209]

iii. Lethal Injury.

While the PTC adapts to injury (noted previously), sufficient injury will result in apoptosis or necrosis. Stimuli that induce necrosis can also induce apoptosis. The more intense the stimuli, the more likely it is that the PTC will not have time to engage the apoptotic death program. Although proximal and distal tubular cells are exposed to similar hypoxic stimuli, it appears that distal tubular cells die predominantly by apoptosis, whereas PTC die predominantly by necrosis.[210,211] The mode of death might be expected to have consequences for the inflammatory response. Removal of apoptotic cells by macrophages is in itself anti-inflammatory whereas removal of necrotic debris is pro-inflammatory.[212,213] Prior treatment with inhibitors of apoptotic and probable necrotic death protects rodent kidneys from functional tubular injury and the inflammatory response following ischemia.[214,215] Given the microvascular blood flow insufficiency, however, it is unclear whether it will be possible to deliver such agents clinically to the tubular structures in the outer medulla of the kidney.

iv. Resistance to Lethal Injury.

While some tubular cells die in response to hypoxia and ATP depletion, many tubular cells come under attack from ROI lib-

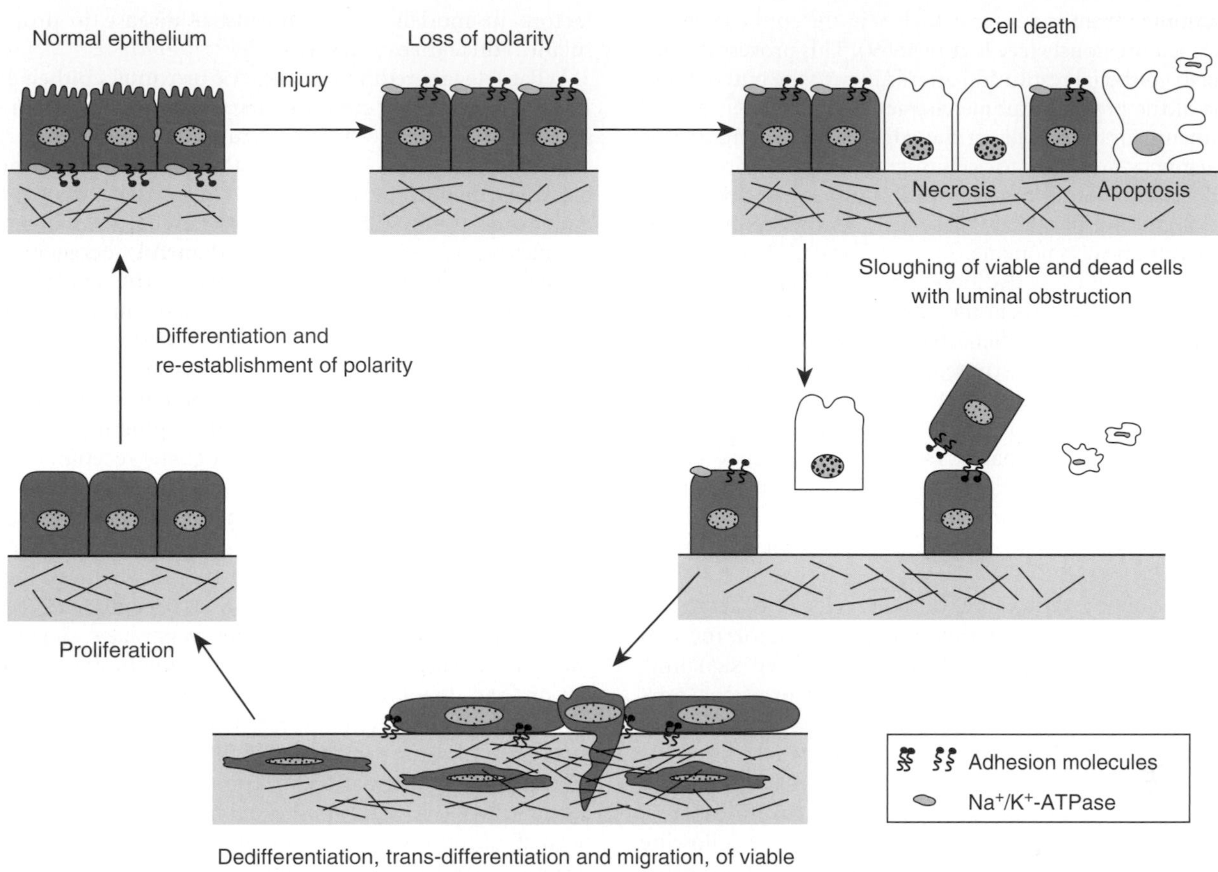

Figure 43–9 Tubular repair following injury. The initial response is loss of cell polarity, histologically and immunohistochemically. Many epithelial cells undergo death by either necrosis or apoptosis. Dead cells and cell debris are sloughed, generating tubular obstruction. Surviving epithelial cells can lift off the basement membrane or remain attached and dedifferentiate, displaying an embryological, mesenchymal phenotype. Some dedifferentiated cells cross the injured basement membrane and transdifferentiating into interstitial fibroblasts, where interstitial matrix is laid down, forming a scaffolding around the injured tubule. Finally, following proliferation of remaining tubular cells, clearance of the lumen and repair of the basement membrane, differentiation to mature epithelial cells can occur.

erated in part by neighboring epithelial cells, and in part by influxing leukocytes. Although cells have intrinsic antioxidant defense in the form of intracellular reducing agents (e.g, glutathione), this defense is frequently overwhelmed during the response to injury. The tubular cells, however, may have the capacity to enhance their ability to deal with the ROI by enhancing the levels of enzymes, which can detoxify these ROI. Following preconditioning of the kidney, one mechanism by which tubular cells resist injury is by generation of iNOS and nitric oxide.[82] It is also apparent that activated tubular cells may have other mechanisms that afford protection from ROI. Many growth factors and cytokines can activate intracellular stress signaling pathways following ligation and activation of specific cell surface receptors on the PTC. In addition, oxidative stress itself can activate the same pathways. These convergent intracellular signaling cascades act on the mitogen-activated protein kinases (MAPK) and involve sequential phosphorylation of proteins in the cascade that results in activation of genes ranging from pro-inflammatory response genes to pro-apoptotic genes. There are essentially three MAPK pathways of parallel signaling into the cell nucleus. It appears that the balance between signaling events in these three stress pathways determines outcome. For example, ROI predominantly activate the Janus kinase (JNK) pathway leading to apoptotic death, whereas growth factors predominantly activate the ERK pathway, which promotes survival. In cultured epithelial cells, inhibition of the JNK pathway prevents ROI-mediated death, whereas overexpression of members of the ERK pathway promotes cell survival in the face of ROI exposure.[123]

KIM-1 is a novel glycoprotein that is highly upregulated in PTC following ischemic injury. It is localized predominantly to the apical membrane and is shed into the urine. Tubular cells *in vitro* that constitutively express this protein are resistant to death induced by ROI.[216] In addition, these cells proliferate more vigorously than control cells. The mechanism by which KIM-1 mediates resistance to a toxic environment is yet to be elucidated.

REGENERATION

Following injury, many tissues engage a program of repair. Proximal tubular cells respond by proliferating and dedifferentiating. These cells alter their shape from cuboidal to fibroblast-like, either prior to or while they spread over the denuded basement membrane to cover breaches in the epithelial lining as described previously (see Figure 43–9). This process is comparable to epithelial restitution after injury to the gut. In those regions of the proximal tubule characterized by extensive cell detachment, surviving cells at the edge of the wound engage the machinery necessary for cell migration.[217,218] The spreading cells also exhibit re-organization of stress fibers that enable migration. It is likely these cells synthesize new basement membrane components.

A proportion of those dedifferentiated epithelial cells leaves the confines of the basement membrane in the form of myofibroblasts.[203] This trans-differentiation may occur where the basement membrane is disrupted, since basement membrane proteins inhibit the process of transdifferentiation into myofibroblasts *in vitro*.[198] A part of the response to injury is the deposit of extracellular matrix (see above). Effective repair, however, leads to resorption of this matrix. It is unclear whether interstitial myofibroblasts redifferentiate or undergo apoptosis followed by phagocytic clearance when repair is effective.[219]

Proliferation of recovering tubular cells is dramatic.[189] This proliferation is under the guidance of autocrine and paracrine growth factors, and integrin-mediated signaling. Epidermal growth factor (EGF), insulin-like growth factors (IGF), hepatocyte growth factor (HGF) and transforming growth factor-β (TGFβ) have all been implicated in governing both proliferation and dedifferentiation. Growth factors are released from tubular cells, interstitial myofibroblasts, and interstitial macrophages. Enhanced recovery following ischemic injury in rodents has been repeatedly demonstrated with IGF-1 therapy. The efficacy of IGF-1 has been shown in tubular repair and proliferation as well as in improving renal blood flow.[220–222] A recent trial of recombinant IGF-1 in moderate human ATN, however, failed to show any benefit.[223]

Although it has been assumed that proliferating tubular cells are derived from remaining tubular cells, it has recently been reported that bone marrow stem cells are recruited to the injured kidney and replace up to 50% of the tubular cells lost to injury.[224,225] Using bone marrow chimeric mice, we have found that bone marrow–derived stem cells make only a minor direct contribution to the repair process.[2] Further work is required to clarify the role of stem cells in human renal repair.

Repair of the endothelium has also become a focus of attention. Without vessels, there cannot be effective repair of the tubules. In experimental models of ischemic injury, clamping of the renal artery for 60 minutes leads to permanent loss of endothelial cells.[193] This degree of ischemia is associated with partial initial recovery followed by progressive interstitial fibrosis, tubular atrophy, and progressive decline in renal function. Following only 30 minutes of arterial clamping we have found that interstitial fibrosis is present at 7 days and persists at 10 weeks.[82] One implication from these studies is that without endothelial repair, resolution of inflammation cannot occur. Further work is required in this area to determine whether there is inadequate or aberrant angiogenesis in the postischemic kidney, and whether this represents a primary mechanism in progressive renal attrition.[226] Work from Johnson and colleagues indicates that microvascular attrition is a central component of interstitial disease in the kidney. Application of pro-angiogenesis factors in models where interstitial disease is prominent might reduce disease severity.[104,227–229]

What triggers redifferentiation of proximal epithelial cells? It is unclear whether cues from the inflammatory response are important or whether the departure of inflammatory cells is necessary. Also, there is evidence that integrity of the normal basement membrane is necessary. During development of the embryonic kidney, it has been proposed that laminin-integrin interactions are likely to be important in mesenchymal to epithelial differentiation. Mesenchymal cell α6β1 integrin interacts with the basement membrane laminin α chain, mediating polarization of the condensed mesenchyme to epithelium.[230] Laminin-5, also known as kalinin, a component of the anchoring filaments of skin basement membrane, is induced in the S3 proximal tubule segment of the post-ischemic kidney, along with its cognate receptor, integrin α3β1. Interactions of laminin-5 with α3β1 are required for epithelialization of skin after wounding, and are necessary for differentiation of enterocytes during migration from the crypt to the villus tip.[231,232] In the S3 segment of the post-ischemic kidney, the induction of laminin-5 and its cognate receptor, α3β1, late after injury during the recovery phase, suggests that this matrix-receptor combination may function in redifferentiation and repolarization critical for restoration of renal function and architecture. A recent study of BMP-7, a natural antagonist of some functions of TGF-β, indicates that it counteracts transdifferentiation of epithelial cells to myofibroblasts.[233] BMP-7 is highly expressed in proximal tubules in the normal kidney. Following ischemic injury in rat models, BMP-7 expression is markedly downregulated. Administration of BMP-7 during acute and chronic disease models promotes recovery and preserves epithelial cell function and morphology.[208,234,235] Thus, rather than promoting redifferentiation to the epithelial phenotype, this endogenous cytokine counteracts the natural tendency of the epithelium to promote interstitial scarring.

CONCLUSIONS

ARF remains a disease with serious consequences for the patient. Although there has been a lack of a unifying diagnosis for ARF, careful analyses of patient groups who acquire ARF indicate that it is a disease syndrome with high mortality, morbidity, and cost to health providers. Increased mortality is apparent even in those with minor increases in serum creatinine. In high-risk groups, such as those undergoing cardiac valvular replacement, patients have as much as a 1 in 2 chance of developing ARF. Trials in the 1990s suggest that, for patients with ARF requiring renal replacement therapy, early introduction of dialysis and achievement of basic lower limits of clearance are necessary to minimize mortality. A better understanding of the inflammatory response and the dysregulation of intra-renal arterioles observed in ARF has informed us that minimizing pro-inflammatory factors and maintaining stable renal blood flow may be applicable that will speed renal recovery.

Fundamental research has revealed that inflammation in the kidney is a hallmark of ARF. Accompanying this is inflammatory damage to intrarenal vessels and tubules. This inflammation adds to the inappropriate intrarenal vasoconstriction, which potentiates damage to susceptible segments of the nephron. Although there are many candidate vasodilators that might counteract this deleterious vasoconstriction, none has emerged from clinical trials as a useful therapy. One aspect of the inflammatory process is that toxic reactive oxygen species play an important role in potentiating damage to injured tubules. Many animal studies indicate that minimizing kidney injury can be afforded by protecting renal cells from these radicals or by neutralizing them at the site of generation. Future management of ARF in humans may derive from modulation of other aspects of the inflammatory response such as leukocyte adhesion and/or generation of inflammatory cytokines by residing cells or transmigrating leukocytes, and such strategies will likely be directed at multiple components of the inflammatory response.

Human studies indicate that many patients with ARF do not recover or only partially recover renal function if they survive their illness. Many of these survivors experience subsequent decline in renal function accompanied by interstitial fibrosis as seen in other forms of renal disease. Animal studies indicate that interstitial fibrosis is a major factor complicating ischemic renal injury. Understanding the processes that lead the injured kidney to initiate and propagate the fibrogenic process is a desirable goal for the design of new therapies that can target this tissue response.

As we develop and evaluate putative therapies for ARF in humans, it becomes clear that we lack useful biomarkers of renal injury. A rise in serum creatinine occurs too late. We need a "troponin"-like biomarker for the kidney so that we can identify tubular epithelial injury early enough in order to intervene therapeutically in a timely fashion.

References

1. Mehta RL, Chertow GM.Acute renal failure definitions and classification: time for change? J Am Soc Nephrol 2003; 14: 2178-2187.
2. Bonventre JV, Weinberg JM. Recent advances in the pathophysiology of ischemic acute renal failure. J Am Soc Nephrol 2003; 14:2199-2210.
3. Solomon R, Werner C, Mann D, et al. Effects of saline, mannitol, and furosemide to prevent acute decreases in renal function induced by radiocontrast agents. N Engl J Med 1994; 331:1416-1420.
4. Tepel M, van der Giet M, Schwarzfeld C, et al. Prevention of radiographic-contrast-agent-induced reductions in renal function by acetylcysteine. N Engl J Med 2000; 343:180-184.
5. Chertow GM, Burdick E, Honour M, et al. Toward and evidence-based definition of hospital-acquired acute renal failure. J Am Soc Nephrol 2003; 8:1042A.
6. Liano F, Pascual J. Epidemiology of acute renal failure: a prospective, multicenter, community-based study. Madrid Acute Renal Failure Study Group. Kidney Int 1996; 50:811-818.
7. Ronco C, Kellum JA, Mehta R. Acute dialysis quality initiative (ADQI). Nephrol Dial Transplant 2001; 16:1555-1558.
8. Kellum JA, Palevsky P, Mehta R, et al. Acute Dialysis Quality Initiative: methodology. Curr Opin Crit Care 2002; 8:500-501.
9. Feest TG, Round A, Hamad S. Incidence of severe acute renal failure in adults: results of a community based study. BMJ 1993; 306:481-483.
10. Hou SH, Bushinsky DA, Wish JB, et al. Hospital-acquired renal insufficiency: a prospective study. Am J Med 1983; 74:243-248.
11. Nash K, Hafeez A, Hou S. Hospital-acquired renal insufficiency. Am J Kidney Dis 2002; 39:930-936.
12. Brivet FG, Kleinknecht DJ, Loirat P, Landais PJ. Acute renal failure in intensive care units–causes, outcome, and prognostic factors of hospital mortality; a prospective, multicenter study. French Study Group on Acute Renal Failure. Crit Care Med 1996; 24:192-198.
13. de Mendonca A, Vincent JL, Suter PM, et al. Acute renal failure in the ICU: risk factors and outcome evaluated by the SOFA score. Intensive Care Med 2000; 26:915-921.
14. Metnitz PG, Krenn CG, Steltzer H, et al. Effect of acute renal failure requiring renal replacement therapy on outcome in critically ill patients. Crit Care Med 2002; 30:2051-2058.
15. Corwin HL, Teplick RS, Schreiber MJ, et al. Prediction of outcome in acute renal failure. Am J Nephrol 1987; 7:8-12.
16. Tuttle KR, Worrall NK, Dahlstrom LR, et al. Predictors of ARF after cardiac surgical procedures. Am J Kidney Dis 2003; 41:76-83.
17. Conlon PJ, Stafford-Smith M, White WD, et al. Acute renal failure following cardiac surgery. Nephrol Dial Transplant 1999; 14:1158-1162.
18. McCullough PA, Wolyn R, Rocher LL, et al. Acute renal failure after coronary intervention: incidence, risk factors, and relationship to mortality. Am J Med 1997; 103:368-375.
19. Frost L, Pedersen RS, Lund O, et al. Prognosis and risk factors in acute, dialysis-requiring renal failure after open-heart surgery. Scand J Thorac Cardiovasc Surg 1991; 25:161-166.
20. Levy EM, Viscoli CM, Horwitz RI. The effect of acute renal failure on mortality. A cohort analysis. JAMA 1996; 275:1489-1494.
21. Bates DW, Su L, Yu DT, et al. Mortality and costs of acute renal failure associated with amphotericin B therapy. Clin Infect Dis 2001; 32:686-693.
22. Kennedy AC, Burton JA, Luke RG, et al. Factors affecting the prognosis in acute renal failure. A survey of 251 cases. Q J Med 1973; 42:73-86.
23. Berisa F, Beaman M, Adu D, et al. Prognostic factors in acute renal failure following aortic aneurysm surgery. Q J Med 1990; 76:689-698.
24. Spiegel DM, Ullian ME, Zerbe GO, Berl T. Determinants of survival and recovery in acute renal failure patients dialyzed in intensive-care units. Am J Nephrol 1991; 11:44-47.
25. Shusterman N, Strom BL, Murray TG, et al. Risk factors and outcome of hospital-acquired acute renal failure. Clinical epidemiologic study. Am J Med 1987; 83:65-71.
26. Neveu H, Kleinknecht D, Brivet F, et al. Prognostic factors in acute renal failure due to sepsis. Results of a prospective multicentre study. The French Study Group on Acute Renal Failure. Nephrol Dial Transplant 1996; 11:293-299.
27. Chertow GM, Levy EM, Hammermeister KE, et al. Independent association between acute renal failure and mortality following cardiac surgery. Am J Med 1998; 104:343-348.
28. Fuiano G, Sund S, Mazza G, et al. Renal hemodynamic response to maximal vasodilating stimulus in healthy older subjects. Kidney Int 2001; 59:1052-1058.
29. Gambaro G, Verlato F, Budakovic A, et al: Renal impairment in chronic cigarette smokers. J Am Soc Nephrol 1998; 9:562-567.
30. Corwin HL, Bonventre JV. Renal insufficiency associated with nonsteroidal anti-inflammatory agents. Am J Kidney Dis 1984; 4:147-152.
31. Conger J. Hemodynamic factors in acute renal failure. Adv Ren Replace Ther 1997; 4:25-37.
32. Lindholt JS. Radiocontrast induced nephropathy. Eur J Vasc Endovasc Surg 2003; 25:296-304.
33. Nzerue CM, Hewan-Lowe K, Riley Jr LJ. Cocaine and the kidney: a synthesis of pathophysiologic and clinical perspectives. Am J Kidney Dis 2000; 35:783-795.
34. Coar D. Obstructive nephropathy. Del Med J 1991. 63:743-749.
35. Harris KP, Hattersley JM, Feehally J, Walls J. Acute renal failure associated with haematological malignancies: a review of 10 years experience. Eur J Haematol 1991; 47:119-122.
36. Norman RW, Mack FG, Awad SA, et al. Acute renal failure secondary to bilateral ureteric obstruction: review of 50 cases. Can Med Assoc J 1982; 127:601-604.

37. Charasse C, Camus C, Darnault P, et al. Acute nondilated anuric obstructive nephropathy on echography: difficult diagnosis in the intensive care unit. Intensive Care Med 1991; 17:387-391.
38. Chong BH, Trew P, Meng L, Pitney WR. Anuric renal failure due to encasement of the ureters by lymphoma–ureteric obstruction without dilatation. Aust N Z J Med 1981; 11:542-544.
39. Bagnasco S, Good D, Balaban R, Burg M. Lactate production in isolated segments of the rat nephron. Am J Physiol 1985; 248:F522-F526.
40. Ruegg CE, Mandel LJ. Bulk isolation of renal PCT and PST. II. Differential responses to anoxia or hypoxia. Am J Physiol 1990; 259:F176-F185.
41. Ruegg CE, Mandel LJ. Bulk isolation of renal PCT and PST. I. Glucose-dependent metabolic differences. Am J Physiol 1990; 259:F164-F175.
42. Torikai S. A bioenergetic explanation for the selective vulnerability of renal medullary tubules to hypoxia. Clin Sci (Lond) 1988; 75:323-330.
43. Bonventre JV, Brezis M, Siegel N, et al. Acute renal failure. I. Relative importance of proximal vs. distal tubular injury. Am. J. Physiol. 1998; 275:F623-F632.
44. Rayner BL, Willcox PA, Pascoe MD. Acute renal failure in community-acquired bacteraemia. Nephron 1990; 54:32-35.
45. Linas SL, Whittenburg D, Parsons PE, Repine JE. Ischemia increases neutrophil retention and worsens acute renal failure: role of oxygen metabolites and ICAM 1. Kidney Int 1995; 48:1584-1591.
46. Ishibashi N, Weisbrot-Lefkowitz M, Reuhl K, et al. Modulation of chemokine expression during ischemia/reperfusion in transgenic mice overproducing human glutathione peroxidases. J Immunol 1999; 163:5666-5677.
47. Lieberthal W, Wolf EF, Rennke HG, et al. Renal ischemia and reperfusion impair endothelium-dependent vascular relaxation. Am J Physiol 1989; 256:F894-F900.
48. Chertow GM, Lazarus JM, Christiansen CL, et al. Preoperative renal risk stratification. Circulation 1997; 95:878-884.
49. Valeri A, Neusy AJ. Acute and chronic renal disease in hospitalized AIDS patients. Clin Nephrol 1991; 35:110-118.
50. Kleinknecht D, Vanhille P, Morel-Maroger L, et al. Acute interstitial nephritis due to drug hypersensitivity. An up-to-date review with a report of 19 cases. Adv Nephrol Necker Hosp 1983; 12:277-308.
51. Ravnskov U. Glomerular, tubular and interstitial nephritis associated with non-steroidal antiinflammatory drugs. Evidence of a common mechanism. Br J Clin Pharmacol 1999; 47: 203-210.
52. Bennett WM, Henrich WL, Stoff JS. The renal effects of nonsteroidal anti-inflammatory drugs: summary and recommendations. Am J Kidney Dis 1996; 28:S56-S62.
53. Sessa A, Meroni M, Battini G, et al. Acute renal failure due to idiopathic tubulo-intestinal nephritis and uveitis: "TINU syndrome." Case report and review of the literature. J Nephrol 2000; 13:377-380.
54. Cacoub P, Deray G, Le Hoang P, et al. Idiopathic acute interstitial nephritis associated with anterior uveitis in adults. Clin Nephrol 1989; 31:307-310.
55. Huang E, Hewitt RG, Shelton M, Morse GD. Comparison of measured and estimated creatinine clearance in patients with advanced HIV disease. Pharmacotherapy 1996; 16:222-229.
56. Rolin HA 3rd, Hall PM, Wei R. Inaccuracy of estimated creatinine clearance for prediction of iothalamate glomerular filtration rate. Am J Kidney Dis 1984; 4:48-54.
57. Coll E, Botey A, Alvarez L, et al. Serum cystatin C as a new marker for noninvasive estimation of glomerular filtration rate and as a marker for early renal impairment. Am J Kidney Dis 2000; 36:29-34.
58. Burkhardt H, Bojarsky G, Gretz N, Gladisch R. Creatinine clearance, Cockcroft-Gault formula and cystatin C: estimators of true glomerular filtration rate in the elderly? Gerontology 2002; 48:140-146.
59. Mussap M, Dalla Vestra M, Fioretto P, et al. Cystatin C is a more sensitive marker than creatinine for the estimation of GFR in type 2 diabetic patients. Kidney Int 2002; 61:1453-1461.
60. Lin J, Knight EL, Hogan ML, Singh AK. A Comparison of Prediction Equations for Estimating Glomerular Filtration Rate in Adults without Kidney Disease. J Am Soc Nephrol 2003; 14:2573-2580.
61. Hoek FJ, Kemperman FA, Krediet RT. A comparison between cystatin C, plasma creatinine and the Cockcroft and Gault formula for the estimation of glomerular filtration rate. Nephrol Dial Transplant 2003; 18:2024-2031.
62. Thomassen SA, Johannesen IL, Erlandsen EJ, et al. Serum cystatin C as a marker of the renal function in patients with spinal cord injury. Spinal Cord 2002; 40:524-528.
63. El Gawad GA, Abrahamsson K, Norten L, Hijalmas. Cystatin C-A superior marker of glomerular filtration rate in cystatin children and adolescents with continent ileal reservoir. Saudi Med J 2003; 24:S46.
64. Filler G, Priem F, Lepage N, et al. Beta-trace protein, cystatin C, beta(2)-microglobulin, and creatinine compared for detecting impaired glomerular filtration rates in children. Clin Chem 2002; 48:729-736.
65. Ichimura T, Bonventre JV, Bailly V, et al. Kidney injury molecule-1 (KIM-1), a putative epithelial cell adhesion molecule containing a novel immunoglobulin domain, is up-regulated in renal cells after injury. J Biol Chem 1998; 273:4135-4142.
66. Ichimura T, Hung CC, Yang SA, et al. Kidney Injury Molecule - 1 (Kim-1): a tissue and urinary biomarker for nephrotoxicant-induced renal injury. Am J Physiol Renal Physiol. 2004 Mar; 286(3):F552-F563.
67. Han WK, Bailly R, Abichandani R, et al. Kidney Injury Molecule-1 (KIM-1): a novel biomarker for human renal proximal tubule injury. Kidney Int 2002; 62:237-244.
68. Muramatsu Y, Tsujie M, Kohda Y, et al. Early detection of cysteine rich protein 61 (CYR61, CCN1) in urine following renal ischemic reperfusion injury. Kidney Int 2002; 62:1601-1610.
69. Bonventre JV. The kidney proteome: a hint of things to come. Kidney Int 2002; 62:1470-1471.
70. Liano F, Pascual J. Outcomes in acute renal failure. Semin Nephrol 1998; 18:541-550.
71. Svarstad E, Ulvik NM, Aslaksen A. [Postrenal acute renal failure with deficient or minimal dilatation of the renal pelvis]. Tidsskr Nor Laegeforen 1992; 112:3194-3196.
72. Somerville CA, Chmiel R, Niall JF, Murphy BF. Non-dilated urinary tract obstruction. Med J Aust 1992; 156:721-723.
73. Thadhani R, Pascual M, Bonventre JV. Acute renal failure. N Engl J Med 1996; 334:1448-1460.
74. Wilson DM, Turner DR, Cameron JS, et al. Value of renal biopsy in acute intrinsic renal failure. Br Med J 1976; 2:459-461.
75. Haas M, Spargo BH, Wit EJ, Meehan SM. Etiologies and outcome of acute renal insufficiency in older adults: a renal biopsy study of 259 cases. Am J Kidney Dis 2000; 35:433-447.
76. Hoste EA, Lameire NH, Vanholder RC, et al. Acute renal failure in patients with sepsis in a surgical ICU: predictive factors, incidence, comorbidity, and outcome. J Am Soc Nephrol 2003; 14:1022-1030.
77. Morgera S, Kraft AK, Siebert G, et al. Long-term outcomes in acute renal failure patients treated with continuous renal replacement therapies. Am J Kidney Dis 2002; 40:275-279.
78. Bhandari S, Turney JH. Survivors of acute renal failure who do not recover renal function. Qjm 1996; 89:415-421.
79. Kjellstrand CM, Ebben J, Davin T. Time of death, recovery of renal function, development of chronic renal failure and need for chronic hemodialysis in patients with acute tubular necrosis. Trans Am Soc Artif Intern Organs 1981; 27:45-50.
80. Salmanullah M, Sawyer R, Hise MK. The effects of acute renal failure on long-term renal function. Ren Fail 2003; 25:267-276.

81. Fink JC, Salmanullah M, Blahut SA, et al.. The inevitability of renal function loss in patients with hypercreatinemia. Am J Nephrol 2001; 21:386-389.
82. Park KM, Byun JY, Kramers C, et al. Inducible nitric-oxide synthase is an important contributor to prolonged protective effects of ischemic preconditioning in the mouse kidney. J Biol Chem 2003; 278:27256-27266.
83. Conger JD, Hammond WS. Renal vasculature and ischemic injury. Ren Fail 1992; 14:307-310.
84. Luyckx VA, Bonventre JV. Dose of dialysis in acute renal failure. Semin Dial 2004; 17:30-36.
85. Pascual M, Swinford RD, Tolkoff-Rubin N. Acute renal failure: role of dialysis membrane biocompatibility. Annu Rev Med 1997; 48:467-476.
86. Subramanian S, Venkataraman R, Kellum JA. Influence of dialysis membranes on outcomes in acute renal failure: a meta-analysis. Kidney Int 2002; 62:1819-1823.
87. Schiffl H. Intermittent hemodialysis and/or continuous renal replacement therapy: are they complementary or alternative therapies? Am J Kidney Dis 2002; 40:1097-1099.
88. Ronco C, Bellomo R, Homel P, et al. Effects of different doses in continuous veno-venous haemofiltration on outcomes of acute renal failure: a prospective randomised trial. Lancet 2000; 356:26-30.
89. Tapolyai M, Fedak S, Chaff C, Paganini E. Delivered dialysis dose may influence acute renal failure outcome in ICU patients. J Am Soc Nephrol 1994; 5:120P.
90. Paganini EP, Halstenberg WK, Goormastic M. Risk modeling in acute renal failure requiring dialysis: the introduction of a new model. Clin Nephrol 1996; 46:206-211.
91. Schiffl H. Biocompatibility and acute renal failure. Lancet 2000; 355:312; author reply 313-314.
92. Bonventre JV. Daily hemodialysis—will treatment each day improve the outcome in patients with acute renal failure? N Engl J Med 2002; 346:362-364.
93. Bellomo R, Mansfield D, Rumble S, et al. Acute renal failure in critical illness. Conventional dialysis versus acute continuous hemodiafiltration. Asaio J 1992; 38:M654-M657.
94. Bellomo R, Farmer M, Boyce N. A prospective study of continuous venovenous hemodiafiltration in critically ill patients with acute renal failure. J Intensive Care Med 1995; 10:187-192.
95. Bellomo R, Ronco C. Acute renal failure in the intensive care unit: adequacy of dialysis and the case for continuous therapies. Nephrol Dial Transplant 1996; 11:424-428.
96. Bellomo R, Boyce N. Continuous venovenous hemodiafiltration compared with conventional dialysis in critically ill patients with acute renal failure. Asaio J 1993; 39:M794-797.
97. John S, Griesbach D, Baumgartel M, et al. Effects of continuous haemofiltration vs intermittent haemodialysis on systemic haemodynamics and splanchnic regional perfusion in septic shock patients: a prospective, randomized clinical trial. Nephrol Dial Transplant 2001; 16:320-327.
98. Kierdorf H. Continuous versus intermittent treatment: clinical results in acute renal failure. Contrib Nephrol 1991; 93:1-12.
99. Mauritz W, Sporn P, Schindler I, et al. [Acute renal failure in abdominal infection. Comparison of hemodialysis and continuous arteriovenous hemofiltration]. Anasth Intensivther Notfallmed 1986; 21:212-217.
100. Mehta RL, McDonald B, Gabbai FB, et al. A randomized clinical trial of continuous versus intermittent dialysis for acute renal failure. Kidney Int 2001; 60:1154-1163.
101. Bellomo R, Farmer M, Parkin G, et al. Severe acute renal failure: a comparison of acute continuous hemodiafiltration and conventional dialytic therapy. Nephron 1995; 71:59-64.
102. McDonald BR, Mehta RL. Decreased mortality in patients with acute renal failure undergoing continuous arteriovenous hemodialysis. Contrib Nephrol 1991; 93:51-56.
103. Kruczynski K, Irvine-Bird K, Toffelmire EB, Morton AR. A comparison of continuous arteriovenous hemofiltration and intermittent hemodialysis in acute renal failure patients in the intensive care unit. Asaio J 1993; 39:M778-M781.
104. Kellum JA, Angus DC, Johnson JP, et al. Continuous versus intermittent renal replacement therapy: a meta-analysis. Intensive Care Med 2002; 28:29-37.
105. Tonelli M, Manns B, Feller-Kopman D. Acute renal failure in the intensive care unit: a systematic review of the impact of dialytic modality on mortality and renal recovery. Am J Kidney Dis 2002; 40:875-885.
106. Conger JD. Vascular abnormalities in the maintenance of acute renal failure. Circ Shock 1983; 11:235-244.
107. Conger JD, Schrier RW. Renal hemodynamics in acute renal failure. Annu Rev Physiol 1980; 42:603-614.
108. Conger J, Robinette J, Villar A, et al. Increased nitric oxide synthase activity despite lack of response to endothelium-dependent vasodilators in postischemic acute renal failure in rats. J Clin Invest 1995; 96:631-638.
109. Vetterlein F, Hoffmann F, Pedina J, et al. Disturbances in renal microcirculation induced by myoglobin and hemorrhagic hypotension in anesthetized rat. Am J Physiol 1995; 268:F839-846.
110. Vetterlein F, Bludau J, Petho-Schramm A, Schmidt G. Reconstruction of blood flow distribution in the rat kidney during postischemic renal failure. Nephron 1994; 66:208-214.
111. Vetterlein F, Petho A, Schmidt G. Distribution of capillary blood flow in rat kidney during postischemic renal failure. Am J Physiol 1986; 251:H510-519.
112. Park KM, Kramers C, Vayssier-Taussat M, et al. Prevention of kidney ischemia/reperfusion-induced functional injury, MAPK and MAPK kinase activation, and inflammation by remote transient ureteral obstruction. J Biol Chem 2002; 277:2040-2049.
113. Jo SK, Hu X, Kobayashi H, et al.. Detection of inflammation following renal ischemia by magnetic resonance imaging. Kidney Int 2003; 64:43-51.
114. Trillaud H, Degreze P, Combe C, et al. USPIO-enhanced MR imaging of glycerol-induced acute renal failure in the rabbit. Magn Reson Imaging 1995; 13:233-240.
115. Zuk A, Bonventre JV, Brown D, Matlin KS. Polarity, integrin, and extracellular matrix dynamics in the postischemic rat kidney. Am J Physiol 1998; 275:C711-731.
116. Brooks DP. Role of endothelin in renal function and dysfunction. Clin Exp Pharmacol Physiol 1996; 23:345-348.
117. Nishida M, Ieshima M, Konishi F, et al. Role of endothelin B receptor in the pathogenesis of ischemic acute renal failure. J Cardiovasc Pharmacol 2002; 40:586-593.
118. Huang C, Hestin D, Dent PC, et al. The effect of endothelin antagonists on renal ischaemia-reperfusion injury and the development of acute renal failure in the rat. Nephrol Dial Transplant 2002; 17:1578-1585.
119. Inman SR, Plott WK, Pomilee RA, et al. Endothelin-receptor blockade mitigates the adverse effect of preretrieval warm ischemia on posttransplantation renal function in rats. Transplantation 2003; 75:1655-1659.
120. Kato A., Hishida A. Amelioration of post-ischaemic renal injury by contralateral uninephrectomy: a role of endothelin-1. Nephrol Dial Transplant 2001; 16:1570-1576.
121. Camaiti A, Del Rosso A, Federighi G. [Acute renal failure caused by treatment with diuretics and ACE inhibitors in the absence of renal artery stenosis]. Minerva Med 1992; 83:371-375.
122. Toto RD. Renal insufficiency due to angiotensin-converting enzyme inhibitors. Miner Electrolyte Metab 1994; 20:193-200.
123. Hung CC, Ichimura, Stevens JL, Bonventre JV. Protection of renal epithelial cells against oxidative injury by endoplasmic reticulum stress preconditioning is mediated by ERK1/2 activation. J Biol Chem 2003; 278:29317-29326.
124. Bonventre JV. Kidney ischemic preconditioning. Curr Opin Nephrol Hypertens 2002; 11:43-48.

125. Ogawa T, Mimura Y, Hiki N, et al. Ischaemic preconditioning ameliorates functional disturbance and impaired renal perfusion in rat ischaemia-reperfused kidneys. Clin Exp Pharmacol Physiol 2000; 27:997-1001.
126. Yellon DM, Downey JM. Preconditioning the myocardium: from cellular physiology to clinical cardiology. Physiol Rev 2003; 83:1113-1151.
127. Vaage J, Valen G. Preconditioning and cardiac surgery. Ann Thorac Surg 2003; 75:S709-714.
128. Asano G, Takashi E, Ishiwata T, et al. Pathogenesis and protection of ischemia and reperfusion injury in myocardium. J Nippon Med Sch 2003; 70:384-392.
129. Nicolini F, Beghi C, Muscari C, et al. Myocardial protection in adult cardiac surgery: current options and future challenges. Eur J Cardiothorac Surg 2003; 24:986-993.
130. Mozzicato S, Joshi BV, Jacobson KA, Liang BT. Role of direct RhoA-phospholipase D1 interaction in mediating adenosine-induced protection from cardiac ischemia. Faseb J 2004; 18:406-408.
131. Loubani M, Hassouna A, Galinanes M. Delayed preconditioning of the human myocardium: signal transduction and clinical implications. Cardiovasc Res 2004; 61:600-609.
132. Ghosh S, Galinanes M. Protection of the human heart with ischemic preconditioning during cardiac surgery: role of cardiopulmonary bypass. J Thorac Cardiovasc Surg 2003; 126:133-142.
133. Wang X, Wei M, Kuukasjarvi P, et al. Novel pharmacological preconditioning with diazoxide attenuates myocardial stunning in coronary artery bypass grafting. Eur J Cardiothorac Surg 2003; 24:967-973.
134. Fagan KA, Tyler RC, Sato K, et al. Relative contributions of endothelial, inducible, and neuronal NOS to tone in the murine pulmonary circulation. Am J Physiol 1999; 277:L472-478.
135. Richard V, Hogie M, Clozel M, et al. In vivo evidence of an endothelin-induced vasopressor tone after inhibition of nitric oxide synthesis in rats. Circulation 1995; 91:771-775.
136. Yamashita J, Ogata M, Itoh M, et al. Role of nitric oxide in the renal protective effects of ischemic preconditioning. J Cardiovasc Pharmacol 2003; 42:419-427.
137. De Greef KE, Ysebaert DK, Persy V, et al. ICAM-1 expression and leukocyte accumulation in inner stripe of outer medulla in early phase of ischemic compared to HgCl2-induced ARF. Kidney Int 2003; 63:1697-1707.
138. Kwon O, Molitoris BA, Pescovitz M, Kelly KJ. Urinary actin, interleukin-6, and interleukin-8 may predict sustained ARF after ischemic injury in renal allografts. Am J Kidney Dis 2003; 41:1074-1087.
139. Rice JC, Spence JS, Yetman DL, Safirstein RL. Monocyte chemoattractant protein-1 expression correlates with monocyte infiltration in the post-ischemic kidney. Ren Fail 2002; 24:703-723.
140. Miura M, Fu X, Zhang QW, et al. Neutralization of Gro alpha and macrophage inflammatory protein-2 attenuates renal ischemia/reperfusion injury. Am J Pathol 2001; 159:2137-2145.
141. Lien YH, Lai LW, Silva AL. Pathogenesis of renal ischemia/reperfusion injury: lessons from knockout mice. Life Sci 2003; 74:543-552.
142. Rabb H, Mendiola CC, Dietz J, et al. Role of CD11a and CD11b in ischemic acute renal failure in rats. Am J Physiol 1994; 267:F1052-1058.
143. Singbartl K, Green SA, Ley K. Blocking P-selectin protects from ischemia/reperfusion-induced acute renal failure. Faseb J 2000;14:48-54.
144. Klausner JM, Paterson I.S, Goldman G, et al. Postischemic renal injury is mediated by neutrophils and leukotrienes. Am J Physiol 1989; 256:F794-802.
145. Hellberg PO, Kallskog TO. Neutrophil-mediated post-ischemic tubular leakage in the rat kidney. Kidney Int 1989; 36:555-561.
146. Kelly KJ, Williams WW Jr., Colvin RB, et al. Intercellular adhesion molecule-1-deficient mice are protected against ischemic renal injury. J Clin Invest 1996; 97:1056-1063.
147. Rabb H, Mendiola CC, Saba SR, et al. Antibodies to ICAM-1 protect kidneys in severe ischemic reperfusion injury. Biochem Biophys Res Commun 1995; 211:67-73.
148. Kelly KJ, Williams WW Jr., Colvin RB, Bonventre JV. Antibody to intercellular adhesion molecule 1 protects the kidney against ischemic injury. Proc Natl Acad Sci U S A 1994; 91:812-816.
149. Dragun D, Tullius SG, Park JK, et al. ICAM-1 antisense oligodesoxynucleotides prevent reperfusion injury and enhance immediate graft function in renal transplantation. Kidney Int 1998; 54:590-602.
150. Dragun D, Lukitsch I., Tullius SG, et al. Inhibition of intercellular adhesion molecule-1 with antisense deoxynucleotides prolongs renal isograft survival in the rat. Kidney Int 1998; 54:2113-2122.
151. Salmela K, Wramner L, Ekberg H, et al. A randomized multicenter trial of the anti-ICAM-1 monoclonal antibody (enlimomab) for the prevention of acute rejection and delayed onset of graft function in cadaveric renal transplantation: a report of the European Anti-ICAM-1 Renal Transplant Study Group. Transplantation 1999; 67:729-736.
152. Yin M, Wheeler MD, Connor HD, et al. Cu/Zn-superoxide dismutase gene attenuates ischemia-reperfusion injury in the rat kidney. J Am Soc Nephrol 2001; 12:2691-2700.
153. DiMari J, Megyesi J, Udvarhelyi N, et al. N-acetyl cysteine ameliorates ischemic renal failure. Am J Physiol 1997; 272:F292-298.
154. Sekhon CS, Sekhon BK, Singh I, et al. Attenuation of renal ischemia/reperfusion injury by a triple drug combination therapy. J Nephrol 2003; 16:63-74.
155. Tepel M. Acetylcysteine for the prevention of radiocontrast-induced nephropathy. Minerva Cardioangiol 2003; 51:525-530.
156. Nakagawa K, Koo DD, Davies DR, et al. Lecithinized superoxide dismutase reduces cold ischemia-induced chronic allograft dysfunction. Kidney Int 2002; 61:1160-1169.
157. Kelly KJ, Meehan SM, Colvin RB, et al. Protection from toxicant-mediated renal injury in the rat with anti-CD54 antibody. Kidney Int 1999; 56:922-931.
158. Reimold AM. TNFalpha as therapeutic target: new drugs, more applications. Curr Drug Targets Inflamm Allergy 2002; 1:377-392.
159. Donnahoo KK, Meng X, Ayala A, et al. Early kidney TNF-alpha expression mediates neutrophil infiltration and injury after renal ischemia-reperfusion. Am J Physiol 1999; 277:R922-929.
160. Donnahoo KK, Meldrum DR, Shenkar R, et al. Early renal ischemia, with or without reperfusion, activates NFkappaB and increases TNF-alpha bioactivity in the kidney. J Urol 2000; 163:1328-1332.
161. Miyaji T, Hu X, Yuen PS, et al. Ethyl pyruvate decreases sepsis-induced acute renal failure and multiple organ damage in aged mice. Kidney Int 2003; 64:1620-1631.
162. Garcia-Fernandez N, Lavilla FJ, Rocha E, Purroy A. Assessment of haemostatic risk factors in patients with acute renal failure associated with severe systemic inflammatory response syndrome. Development of a prognostic index. Nephron 2002; 92:97-104.
163. Jaber BL, Rao M, Guo D, et al. Cytokine promoter gene polymorphisms and mortality in acute renal failure. Cytokine 2004; 25:212-219.
164. Schwartz D, Blum M, Peer G, et al. Role of nitric oxide (EDRF) in radiocontrast acute renal failure in rats. Am J Physiol 1994; 267:F374-379.
165. Brodsky SV, Yamamoto T, Tada T, et al. Endothelial dysfunction in ischemic acute renal failure: rescue by transplanted endothelial cells. Am J Physiol Renal Physiol 2002; 282:F1140-1149.
166. Kourembanas S, McQuillan LP, Leung GK, Faller DV. Nitric oxide regulates the expression of vasoconstrictors and growth

factors by vascular endothelium under both normoxia and hypoxia. J Clin Invest 1993; 92:99-104.

167. Bank N, Kiroycheva M, Singhal PC, et al. Inhibition of nitric oxide synthase ameliorates cellular injury in sickle cell mouse kidneys. Kidney Int 2000; 58:82-89.
168. Bank N, Kiroycheva M, Ahmed F, et al. Peroxynitrite formation and apoptosis in transgenic sickle cell mouse kidneys. Kidney Int 1998; 54:1520-1528.
169. Chung HT, Pae HO, Choi BM, et al. Nitric oxide as a bioregulator of apoptosis. Biochem Biophys Res Commun 2001; 282:1075-1079.
170. Waddington SN, Mosley K, Cattell V. Induced nitric oxide (NO) synthesis in heterologous nephrotoxic nephritis; effects of selective inhibition in neutrophil-dependent glomerulonephritis. Clin Exp Immunol 1999; 118:309-314.
171. Schramm L, La M, Heidbreder E, et al. L-arginine deficiency and supplementation in experimental acute renal failure and in human kidney transplantation. Kidney Int 2002; 61:1423-1432.
172. De Vries B, Matthijsen RA, Wolfs TG, et al. Inhibition of complement factor C5 protects against renal ischemia-reperfusion injury: inhibition of late apoptosis and inflammation. Transplantation 2003; 75:375-382.
173. de Vries B, Kohl J, Leclercq WK, et al. Complement factor C5a mediates renal ischemia-reperfusion injury independent from neutrophils. J Immunol 2003; 170:3883-3889.
174. Rabb H. The T cell as a bridge between innate and adaptive immune systems: implications for the kidney. Kidney Int 2002; 61:1935-1946.
175. Takada M, Chandraker A, Nadeau KC, et al. The role of the B7 costimulatory pathway in experimental cold ischemia/reperfusion injury. J Clin Invest 1997; 100:1199-1203.
176. Takada M, Nadeau KC, Shaw GD, Tilney NL. Prevention of late renal changes after initial ischemia/reperfusion injury by blocking early selectin binding. Transplantation 1997; 64:1520-1525.
177. De Greef KE, Ysebaert DK, Dauwe S, et al. Anti-B7-1 blocks mononuclear cell adherence in vasa recta after ischemia. Kidney Int 2001; 60:1415-1427.
178. Park P, Haas M, Cunningham PN, et al. Injury in renal ischemia-reperfusion is independent from immunoglobulins and T lymphocytes. Am J Physiol Renal Physiol 2002; 282:F352-357.
179. Gerritsma JS, van Kooten C, Gerritsen AF, et al. Production of inflammatory mediators and cytokine responsiveness of an SV40-transformed human proximal tubular epithelial cell line. Exp Nephrol 1998; 6:208-216.
180. Daha MR, van Kooten C. Is the proximal tubular cell a proinflammatory cell? Nephrol Dial Transplant 2000; 15 Suppl 6:41-43.
181. Bonventre JV, Sukhatme VP, Bamberger M, et al. Localization of the protein product of the immediate early growth response gene, Egr-1, in the kidney after ischemia and reperfusion. Cell Regul 1991; 2:251-260.
182. Tsukamoto T, and Nigam SK. Tight junction proteins form large complexes and associate with the cytoskeleton in an ATP depletion model for reversible junction assembly. J Biol Chem 1997; 272:16133-16139.
183. Molitoris BA, Marrs J. The role of cell adhesion molecules in ischemic acute renal failure. Am J Med 1999; 106:583-592.
184. Thurau K, Boylan JW. Acute renal success. The unexpected logic of oliguria in acute renal failure. Am J Med 1976; 61:308-315.
185. Gailit J, Colflesh D, Rabiner I, et al. Redistribution and dysfunction of integrins in cultured renal epithelial cells exposed to oxidative stress. Am J Physiol 1993; 264:F149-157.
186. Goligorsky MS, Lieberthal W, Racusen L, Simon EE. Integrin receptors in renal tubular epithelium: new insights into pathophysiology of acute renal failure. Am J Physiol 1993p; 264:F1-8.
187. Goligorsky MS, Noiri E, Kessler H, Romanov V. Therapeutic effect of arginine-glycine-aspartic acid peptides in acute renal injury. Clin Exp Pharmacol Physiol 1998; 25:276-279.
188. Lieberthal W, McKenney JB, Kiefer CR, et al. Beta1 integrin-mediated adhesion between renal tubular cells after anoxic injury. J Am Soc Nephrol 1997; 8:175-183.
189. Witzgall R, Brown D, Schwarz C, Bonventre JV. Localization of proliferating cell nuclear antigen, vimentin, c-Fos, and clusterin in the postischemic kidney. Evidence for a heterogenous genetic response among nephron segments, and a large pool of mitotically active and dedifferentiated cells. J Clin Invest 1994; 93: 2175-2188.
190. Imgrund M, Grone E, Grone HJ, et al. Re-expression of the developmental gene Pax-2 during experimental acute tubular necrosis in mice 1. Kidney Int 1999; 56:1423-1431.
191. Hay ED, Zuk A. Transformations between epithelium and mesenchyme: normal, pathological, and experimentally induced. Am J Kidney Dis 1995; 26:678-690.
192. Pawar S, Kartha S, Toback FG. Differential gene expression in migrating renal epithelial cells after wounding. J Cell Physiol 1995; 165:556-565.
193. Basile DP, Donohoe D, Roethe K, and Osborn JL. Renal ischemic injury results in permanent damage to peritubular capillaries and influences long-term function. Am J Physiol Renal Physiol 2001; 281:F887-899.
194. Maxwell PH, Osmond MK, Pugh CW, et al. Identification of the renal erythropoietin-producing cells using transgenic mice. Kidney Int 1993; 44:1149-1162.
195. Bachmann S, Le Hir M, Eckardt KU. Co-localization of erythropoietin mRNA and ecto-5'-nucleotidase immunoreactivity in peritubular cells of rat renal cortex indicates that fibroblasts produce erythropoietin. J Histochem Cytochem 1993; 41:335-341.
196. Zhang G, Moorhead PJ, el Nahas AM. Myofibroblasts and the progression of experimental glomerulonephritis. Exp Nephrol 1995; 3:308-318.
197. Stahl PJ, Felsen D. Transforming growth factor-beta, basement membrane, and epithelial-mesenchymal transdifferentiation: implications for fibrosis in kidney disease. Am J Pathol 2001; 159:1187-1192.
198. Zeisberg M, Bonner G, Maeshima Y, et al. Renal fibrosis: collagen composition and assembly regulates epithelial-mesenchymal transdifferentiation. Am J Pathol 2001; 159:1313-1321.
199. Fan JM, Huang XR, Ng YY, et al. Interleukin-1 induces tubular epithelial-myofibroblast transdifferentiation through a transforming growth factor-beta1-dependent mechanism in vitro. Am J Kidney Dis 2001; 37:820-831.
200. Zuk A, Hay ED. Expression of beta 1 integrins changes during transformation of avian lens epithelium to mesenchyme in collagen gels. Dev Dyn 1994; 201:378-393.
201. Aigner T, Neureiter D, Volker U, et al. Epithelial-mesenchymal transdifferentiation and extracellular matrix gene expression in pleomorphic adenomas of the parotid salivary gland. J Pathol 1998; 186:178-185.
202. Lim YS, Kim KA, Jung JO, et al. Modulation of cytokeratin expression during in vitro cultivation of human hepatic stellate cells: evidence of transdifferentiation from epithelial to mesenchymal phenotype. Histochem Cell Biol 2002; 118: 127-136.
203. Iwano M, Plieth D, Danoff TM, et al. Evidence that fibroblasts derive from epithelium during tissue fibrosis. J Clin Invest 2002; 110:341-350.
204. Lan HY. Tubular epithelial-myofibroblast transdifferentiation mechanisms in proximal tubule cells. Curr Opin Nephrol Hypertens 2003; 12:25-29.
205. Jinde K, Nikolic-Paterson DJ, Huang XR, et al. Tubular phenotypic change in progressive tubulointerstitial fibrosis in human glomerulonephritis. Am J Kidney Dis 2001; 38:761-769.
206. Vleming LJ, de Fijter JW, Westendorp RG, et al. Histomorphometric correlates of renal failure in IgA nephropathy. Clin Nephrol 1998; 49:337-344.

207. Howie AJ, Ferreira MA, Adu D. Prognostic value of simple measurement of chronic damage in renal biopsy specimens. Nephrol Dial Transplant 2001; 16:1163-1169.
208. Zeisberg M, Bottiglio C, Kumar N, et al. Bone morphogenic protein-7 inhibits progression of chronic renal fibrosis associated with two genetic mouse models. Am J Physiol Renal Physiol 2003; 285:F1060-1067.
209. Klahr S, Morrissey J. Obstructive nephropathy and renal fibrosis: The role of bone morphogenic protein-7 and hepatocyte growth factor. Kidney Int 2003; Suppl:S105-112.
210. Schume M, Colombel MC, Sawczuk IS, et al. Morphologic, biochemical, and molecular evidence of apoptosis during the reperfusion phase after brief periods of renal ischemia. Am J Pathol 1992; 140:831-838.
211. Oberbauer R, Rohrmoser M, Regele H, et al. Apoptosis of tubular epithelial cells in donor kidney biopsies predicts early renal allograft function. J Am Soc Nephrol 1999; 10:2006-2013.
212. Fadok VA, Bratton DL, Guthrie L, Henson PM. Differential effects of apoptotic versus lysed cells on macrophage production of cytokines: role of proteases. J Immunol 2001; 166:6847-6854.
213. Fadok VA, Bratton DL, Konowal A, et al. Macrophages that have ingested apoptotic cells in vitro inhibit proinflammatory cytokine production through autocrine/paracrine mechanisms involving TGF-beta, PGE2, and PAF. J Clin Invest 1998; 101:890-898.
214. de Vries B, Matthijsen RA, van Bijnen AA, et al. Lysophosphatidic acid prevents renal ischemia-reperfusion injury by inhibition of apoptosis and complement activation. Am J Pathol 2003; 163:47-56.
215. Daemen MA, van't Veer C, Denecker G, et al. Inhibition of apoptosis induced by ischemia-reperfusion prevents inflammation. J Clin Invest 1999; 104:541-549.
216. Ichimura T, Bonventre JV. KIM-1 protects proximal tubualar cells from oxygen radcial mediated death. J Am Soc Nephrol 2003; 9:1569A.
217. Kartha S, Atkin B, Martin TE, Toback FG. Cytokeratin reorganization induced by adenosine diphosphate in kidney epithelial cells. Exp Cell Res 1992; 200:219-226.
218. Kartha S, Toback FG. Adenine nucleotides stimulate migration in wounded cultures of kidney epithelial cells. J Clin Invest 1992; 90:288-292.
219. Rodgers KD, Rao V, Meehan DT, et al. Monocytes may promote myofibroblast accumulation and apoptosis in Alport renal fibrosis. Kidney Int 2003; 63:1338-1355.
220. Noguchi S, Kashihara Y, Ikegami Y, et al. Insulin-like growth factor-I ameliorates transient ischemia-induced acute renal failure in rats. J Pharmacol Exp Ther 1993; 267:919-926.
221. Maestri M, Dafoe DC, Adams GA, et al. Insulin-like growth factor-I ameliorates delayed kidney graft function and the acute nephrotoxic effects of cyclosporine. Transplantation 1997; 64:185-190.
222. Rabkin R. Insulin-like growth factor-I treatment of acute renal failure. J Lab Clin Med 1995; 125:684-685.
223. Hirschberg R, Kopple J, Lipsett P, et al. Multicenter clinical trial of recombinant human insulin-like growth factor I in patients with acute renal failure. Kidney Int 1999; 55:2423-2432.
224. Kale S, Karihaloo A, Clark PR, et al. Bone marrow stem cells contribute to repair of the ischemically injured renal tubule. J Clin Invest 2003; 112:42-49.
225. Poulsom R, Forbes SJ, Hodivala-Dilke K, et al. Bone marrow contributes to renal parenchymal turnover and regeneration. J Pathol 2001; 195:229-235.
226. Nakagawa T, Kang DH, Ohashi R, et al. Tubulointerstitial disease: role of ischemia and microvascular disease. Curr Opin Nephrol Hypertens 2003; 12:233-241.
227. Kang DH, Hughes J, Mazzali M, et al. Impaired angiogenesis in the remnant kidney model: II. Vascular endothelial growth factor administration reduces renal fibrosis and stabilizes renal function. J Am Soc Nephrol 2001; 12:1448-1457.
228. Kang DH, Anderson S, Kim YG, et al. Impaired angiogenesis in the aging kidney: vascular endothelial growth factor and thrombospondin-1 in renal disease. Am J Kidney Dis 2001; 37:601-611.
229. Kim YG, Suga SI, Kang DH, et al. Vascular endothelial growth factor accelerates renal recovery in experimental thrombotic microangiopathy. Kidney Int 2000; 58:2390-2399.
230. Ekblom P. Developmentally regulated conversion of mesenchyme to epithelium. Faseb J 1989; 3:2141-2150.
231. Nguyen BP, Ryan MC, Gil SG, Carter WG. Deposition of laminin 5 in epidermal wounds regulates integrin signaling and adhesion. Curr Opin Cell Biol 2000; 12:554-562.
232. Gout SP, Jacquier-Sarlin MR, Rouard-Talbot L, et al. RhoA-dependent switch between alpha2beta1 and alpha3beta1 integrins is induced by laminin-5 during early stage of HT-29 cell differentiation. Mol Biol Cell 2001; 12:3268-3281.
233. Zeisberg M, Hanai J, Sugimoto H, et al. BMP-7 counteracts TGF-beta1-induced epithelial-to-mesenchymal transition and reverses chronic renal injury. Nat Med 2003; 9:964-968.
234. Simon M, Maresh JG, Harris SE, et al. Expression of bone morphogenetic protein-7 mRNA in normal and ischemic adult rat kidney. Am J Physiol 1999; 276:F382-389.
235. Vukicevic S, Basic V, Rogic D, et al. Osteogenic protein-1 (bone morphogenetic protein-7) reduces severity of injury after ischemic acute renal failure in rat. J Clin Invest 1998; 102: 202-214.
236. Smith LH Jr, Post RS, Teschan PE, et al. Post-traumatic renal insufficiency in military casualties. II. Management, use of an artificial kidney, prognosis. Am J Med 1955; 18:187-198.
237. Iaina A, Reisin E, Eliahou H. Acute renal failure in combat injuries. J Trauma 1975; 15:281-284.
238. Groeneveld AB, Tran DD, van der Meulen J, et al. Acute renal failure in the medical intensive care unit: predisposing, complicating factors and outcome. Nephron 1991; 59:602-610.
239. Liano F, Junco E, Pascual J, et al. The spectrum of acute renal failure in the intensive care unit compared with that seen in other settings. The Madrid Acute Renal Failure Study Group. Kidney Int Suppl 1998; 66:S16-24.
240. Filler G, Pham-Huy A. Cystatin C should be measured in pediatric renal transplant patients! Pediatr Transplant 2002; 6: 357-360.

Pharmacologic Interventions in Acute Renal Failure

Richard Lafayette, M.D.

The incidence rate of acute renal failure (ARF) among patients admitted to the intensive care unit (ICU) has been increasing for several decades and is currently approximately 15%.[1,2] Among subpopulations within the ICU, including those who are aged, those with multiple comorbidities, those with multiple organ failure, and those with septic shock, the incidence rate of ARF can approach 50%.[3,4] Despite substantial advances in techniques of resuscitation and renal replacement therapy, mortality in the critically ill population with ARF remains alarmingly high. Recently, mortality rates in excess of 80% have been reported for ICU patients with multisystem organ failure requiring renal replacement therapy.[5] This scenario is becoming more prevalent as a result of the expansion of invasive medical and surgical procedures and the increasing expectation for aggressive medical management of critically ill patients. The high mortality rate associated with ARF has traditionally been attributed to associated comorbid conditions, but evidence exists to suggest that ARF has an independent negative impact on mortality.[6,7] Presently, there is no specific therapy for established ARF, making the development of agents that can prevent ARF or accelerate recovery from established ARF a priority.

Prerenal azotemia is the most common cause of ARF. When severe or prolonged, renal hypoperfusion is complicated by acute tubular necrosis (ATN). The typical course of ischemic ATN can be conveniently divided into three phases:

1. The *initiation* phase of renal ischemia (usually minutes to hours), during which parenchymal injury occurs
2. The *maintenance* phase (up to 21 days), during which the glomerular filtration rate (GFR) remains compromised and urine output is reduced.
3. The *recovery* phase, characterized by regeneration and repair of tubule epithelial cells and recovery of renal function

Several factors appear to act in concert to depress GFR during the maintenance phase. Studies in animal models of ARF reveal that tubular obstruction by casts is central to the decline in GFR and oliguria.[8,9] Ischemia disrupts osmolar gradients resulting in intracellular Na retention and cellular swelling.[10] If the hypoxic stimulus persists, cellular cytoskeletons are disrupted with the loss of tight junctions, altered epithelial polarity, and accumulation of intracellular Ca.[11,12] Apoptosis ensues with the sloughing of the epithelial brush border, which combines with proteinaceous material in the tubular lumen to form casts.[13] In addition, loss of tight junctions allows for back leak of glomerular filtrate.[14–16] Finally, a tubuloglomerular feedback mechanism may play an important role in the maintenance of prolonged renal insufficiency.[17] It has been postulated that due to tubular obstruction, an excess solute load is delivered to the macula densa resulting in renin release from the juxtaglomerular apparatus. The renin induced release of angiotensin II results in afferent arteriolar vasoconstriction.[18]

A plethora of therapeutic strategies have been tested or are in development directed at these key pathophysiologic events. This chapter critically reviews studies that evaluated the efficacy of low-dose dopamine and fenoldapam as well as atrial natriuretic peptide (ANP) in the treatment of ischemic ATN and discusses the existing evidence for growth factors as agents that promote tubule epithelial cell regeneration and renal recovery.

DOPAMINE

Low-dose dopamine (1–3 μg/kg/min) is prescribed worldwide for the treatment and prevention of ARF, to correct oliguria, and in conjunction with systemic vasopressors to preserve renal perfusion. The animal literature revealed optimistic results for both its use in the prevention and treatment of ARF.[19,20] In healthy persons, low-dose dopamine can cause selective renal vasodilatation and inhibit sodium reabsorption at proximal and distal portions of the nephron. The resulting increases in renal blood flow (RBF), natriuresis, and diuresis form the basis for the use of low-dose dopamine in ARF. Most clinical studies, however, have failed to demonstrate convincingly that low-dose dopamine either prevents ARF in high-risk patients or improves renal function or outcome in patients with established ARF. Further, some editorials have advised against its use, owing to the paucity of supportive scientific evidence and an increasingly recognized side-effect profile.[21,22] In the following section, we hope to clarify this controversial area by reviewing the renal effects of dopamine, discussing the rationale for administering dopamine in ARF, and summarizing the data from the numerous clinical studies in humans.

PHYSIOLOGY

Intrarenal Dopamine

Early studies in humans revealed that urinary dopamine levels exceed filtered dopamine levels and that the quantity of dopamine in the renal vein exceeds that in the renal artery. Furthermore, urinary dopamine levels increase with extracellular fluid volume expansion, and inhibition of renal dopamine synthesis results in an abrogation of the natriuresis induced by sodium loading.[23] It has subsequently been confirmed that the kidney is an important source of dopamine and that intrarenal dopamine is an important paracrine natriuretic agent.[24–26]

Proximal tubule epithelial cells synthesize dopamine from the substrate L-dopa using the enzyme L-amino acid decarboxylase.[27] L-Dopa enters the cell from the tubular fluid by a sodium-coupled cotransport mechanism. Dietary sodium intake is the major factor controlling intrarenal dopamine synthesis, but the mechanism by which increased salt intake leads to increased renal dopamine production is not fully understood.[26] Upon synthesis, intrarenal dopamine may act in an autocrine fashion by binding to dopamine receptors on the proximal tubule cell or may pass along the urinary space to bind to specific receptors in distal portions of the nephron. At the level of the proximal tubule, binding to the dopamine receptors DA_1 and DA_2 mediates inhibition of the basolateral Na^+-K^+-ATPase and luminal Na^+-H^+ exchange transporters, inhibiting sodium reabsorption and inducing natriuresis.[28] Dopamine also inhibits Na^+-K^+-ATPase at the medullary thick ascending limb of the loop of Henle, the distal collecting tubule, and the cortical and medullary collecting ducts. Finally, binding to DA_2 receptors in the inner medullary collecting duct stimulates both the synthesis and release of prostaglandin E_2 (PGE_2).[29] PGE_2 antagonizes the effect of antidiuretic hormone (ADH) on the collecting duct and increases inner medullary blood flow, resulting in medullary urea washout, two mechanisms by which dopamine leads to increased free-water clearance.

The influence of intrarenal dopamine on renal hemodynamics is less clearly defined and is probably species-dependent. Both DA_1 and DA_2 receptors are located on the renal vasculature, albeit at a lower density than that found on tubular cells. DA_1 receptors are localized within the vessel media, whereas DA_2 receptors are present in the adventitia and are probably localized presynaptically on sympathetic nerve terminals.[25] Experimental studies, however, have failed to show that intrarenal dopamine influences renal hemodynamics. Intrarenal infusion of dopamine antagonists abrogates the natriuresis induced by volume expansion without altering renal hemodynamics,[24] suggesting that intrarenal dopamine does not exert a basal influence over glomerular hemodynamics and that the natriuresis induced by intrarenal dopamine is mediated predominantly by its tubular effects. In agreement with these findings, studies have shown preferential release of dopamine from the proximal tubule into the tubular lumen rather than from the renal interstitium.[30]

Exogenous Dopamine

Dopamine can bind to at least three types of receptors: the dopamine receptor, the β-adrenoreceptor, and the α-adrenoreceptor.[31] Differences in these receptor's affinity for dopamine account for its distinct dose-response profile. To define the dose-response relationship for infused dopamine in humans, invasive hemodynamic and renal function tests were performed during graded dopamine infusions in the presence or absence of α- or β-adrenoreceptor blockade.[32] This study showed selective dopamine receptor stimulation within an infusion rate range of 0.5 to 3 μg/kg/min. Further increases in infusion rate between 3 and 10 μg/kg/min resulted in increasing β-adrenoreceptor stimulation, and increased α-adrenoreceptor stimulation occurred at a rate between 5 and 20 μg/kg/min.

Dopamine infusion increases RBF in healthy subjects.[32,33] At so-called renal doses, selective binding to dopamine receptors on the renal vasculature can result in renal vasodilatation and increased RBF, even in the absence of changes in systemic hemodynamics. Renal vasodilatation under these circumstances is mediated by stimulation of DA_1 receptors on both preglomerular and postglomerular vessels, resulting in vascular smooth muscle relaxation.[26] To confirm that low-dose dopamine can increase RBF purely through selective renal vasodilatation and independent of β-adrenoreceptor ligation, the effects of coadministration of the β-adrenoreceptor antagonist metoprolol in healthy adults were examined.[34] Although metoprolol inhibited the chronotropic effect of low-dose dopamine infusion, it did not abrogate the increase in RBF as assessed by para-aminohippuric acid (PAH) clearance, confirming predominant dopamine receptor stimulation at low infusion rates. With higher infusion rates, RBF is increased further by increases in cardiac output, mediated by β-adrenoreceptor stimulation.[34] More evidence for a direct vascular effect of low-dose dopamine is provided by studies comparing the effects of dopamine to dobutamine, a β- and α-receptor agonist deficient of dopamine receptor activity. When dopamine and dobutamine are infused into healthy adults at rates that lead to equivalent increases in cardiac index, dopamine induces a greater increase in RBF, in keeping with a selective effect on the renal vasculature.[35] Finally, dopamine-induced renal vasodilatation has been observed directly with Doppler ultrasound imaging.[36,37]

The effect of low-dose dopamine on the intrarenal distribution of blood flow is less clearly defined. Animal models have shown a preferential increase in cortical flow with dopamine.[26] In humans, preferential increases in cortical flow with dopamine has been confirmed in healthy kidney donors using the xenon washout technique,[38] and, more recently, in healthy volunteers using contrast-enhanced harmonic ultrasonography.[39] Dopamine-induced PGE_2 production by the inner medullary collecting duct results in enhanced inner medullary blood flow.[25] Low-dose dopamine may therefore result in shunting of blood away from the outer medulla, a potentially detrimental effect, given that the outer medulla contains the pars recta of the proximal tubule and the medullary thick ascending limb of the loop of Henle segments, two highly metabolically active portions of the nephron considered vulnerable to hypoxic injury.

Low-dose dopamine has a less dramatic effect on the GFR in healthy subjects. Most studies report only a mild increase in GFR on the order of 10% to 25%, at best.[35,40] Increases in GFR are mediated by preferential afferent arteriolar vasodilatation and an increase in intraglomerular pressure. The ultrafiltration coefficient remains unchanged with dopamine infusion.[26] Natriuresis, on the other hand, is the most consistent renal response to low-dose dopamine infusion. The effect is rapid in onset and may be profound, particularly in healthy persons.[35,40] It is abrogated by extracellular fluid volume depletion[41] and typically wanes after 24 hours of infusion,[42,43] perhaps as a result of counteractive effects of antinatriuretic agents or of dopamine receptor downregulation.

Like endogenous dopamine, inhibition of tubular sodium reabsorption is the predominant mechanism by which dopamine infusion induces a natriuresis. Comparison of sodium and lithium clearance rates in humans demonstrates that dopamine inhibits sodium reabsorption in both the proximal and distal tubule.[35] Low-dose dopamine infusion reduces plasma aldosterone concentrations, which may contribute to its natriuretic effect.[44] Additional effects of low-dose dopamine infusion include phosphaturia and renal tubular acidosis mediated by inhibition of proximal tubule Na^+-phosphate cotransport and proximal tubule Na^+-H^+ exchange, respectively.

The hemodynamic effects of low-dose dopamine infusion differ at the extremes of age, which is likely a result of developmental differences in the maturation of receptor subtypes and differences in the metabolic clearance rates of plasma dopamine.[45] In neonates, activation of the α-adrenoreceptors occurs at a much lower infusion rate.[45] Although dopamine receptor maturation occurs early in life, some studies have demonstrated absence of selective vasodilatory effects of dopamine in children younger than 5 years of age. With increasing age, the effects of dopamine on RBF and GFR are attenuated.[46,47] This attenuated effect may be due to impaired renal prostaglandin production or organic changes in the renal vasculature with increasing age like atherosclerosis.

Whereas low-dose dopamine consistently causes renal vasodilatation in healthy adults, again this effect is often attenuated or absent in ill patients. Several factors may account for this, including hypertensive arteriopathy or counterregulatory effects of other vasoactive hormones, such as activity of the renin-angiotensin-aldosterone system or sympathetic nervous system. Both extracellular volume depletion and hypoxemia have been shown to abrogate the renal effects of dopamine.[42] Table 44–1 lists clinical settings in which studies have reported diminished renal hemodynamic effects of dopamine.

In patients with renal disease, the increase in RBF and GFR observed with low-dose dopamine infusion correlated with the baseline GFR. Patients with a baseline GFR of less than 50 mL/min showed no change in RBF or GFR with dopamine infusion.[48] Low-dose dopamine does not increase RBF in patients with clinical and radiologic heart failure,[40] which may be due to either downregulation of dopamine receptors or the counteractive effects of the sympathetic nervous system and angiotensin II on the renal vasculature in heart failure. In a group of patients who underwent infrarenal aortic surgery, dopamine (4 μg/kg/min) resulted in increased RBF; however, this was entirely due to an increase in cardiac output. No selective renal vasodilatory effect was observed.[44] Furthermore, in a prospective crossover study comparing dobutamine (mean dose, 2.5 μg/kg/min) to dopamine (mean dose, 2.9 μg/kg/min) in critically ill patients, dopamine acted primarily as a diuretic and had no effect on creatinine clearance, whereas dobutamine, which had a greater effect on cardiac index, increased creatinine clearance.[49]

Table 44–1 Effects of Low-Dose Dopamine on Renal Hemodynamics and Na^+ Excretion in Disease States

Disease State	Reference	RBF	GFR	UNa^+
Hypertension	Bughi[225]	↔	NR	↑
Cardiac failure	McDonald[40]	↔	↔	↑
Septic shock on NE	Lherm[93]	NR	↔	↔
After vascular surgery	DeLasson[226]	↑*	↔	↑
After vascular surgery	Girbes[44]	↑*	↔	↑
Critically ill	Duke[49]	NR	↔	↑
Critically ill	Parker[227]	NR	↔	↑
Hypoxemia	Olsen[228]	↔	↔	↑
Renal impairment	Ter Wee[48]	↔	↔	↑

*Increase in renal blood flow mediated by increase in cardiac output, not renal vasodilatation.

RBF, renal blood flow; *GFR*, glomerular filtration rate; *NE*, norepinephrine; *NR*, not recorded; *UNa^+*, urinary sodium excretion; ↔, no change; ↑, increase.

Potentially Deleterious Effects of Dopamine

Table 44–2 outlines common adverse effects of low-dose dopamine. Administration of dopamine requires a central venous catheter, and local extravasation of dopamine adjacent to an artery may provoke distal ischemia and gangrene. Even at low infusion rates all three receptor subtypes may be activated. Even low-dose dopamine can, through β-receptor agonism, increase myocardial oxygen demand and precipitate tachyarrhythmias and myocardial ischemia.[50] In fact, a trial assessing the use of the orally active dopamine agonist ibopamine in patients with chronic heart failure was discontinued early because of the excess mortality in the ibopamine group (25% vs. 20%). This excess mortality was considered to be secondary to ibopamine-induced tachyarrhythmias.[51]

Normally, dopamine is an inhibitory neurotransmitter in the carotid bodies, and dopamine infusion can suppress the respiratory drive induced by hypoxemia. Dopamine can also lower blood PaO_2 by altering ventilation-perfusion matching within the lung, an effect arising from a shunt of blood away from alveolar capillaries.[49] Hypoxemia may worsen myocardial ischemia in susceptible patients and delay recovery from ischemic ATN. The natriuresis and diuresis induced by dopamine may cause severe volume depletion unless close monitoring of the patient permits appropriate fluid replacement. Potassium depletion is also a common result of the increased delivery of sodium to the distal tubule. Hypophosphatemia and hypomagnesemia have also been reported. Low-dose dopamine suppresses pituitary gland function and inhibits prolactin and growth hormone secretion and, hence, may exacerbate the catabolic state in critically ill patients.[52] Hypoprolactinemia suppresses T-cell proliferation.[53]

Table 44–2 Deleterious Effects of Low-Dose Dopamine

Effect	Cause
Distal gangrene	Local extravasation of dopamine
Fluid and electrolyte imbalance	Inhibition of salt and water reabsorption
Tachyarrhythmias and myocardial ischemia	β-Adrenoreceptor stimulation
Hypoxemia	Reduced respiratory drive; pulmonary shunting
Gut ischemia and bacterial translocation	Shunting of blood away from mucosal capillary bed
Catabolic	Inhibition of growth hormone release
Immunosuppression	Inhibition of prolactin release

Although low-dose dopamine increases total splanchnic blood flow, elegant studies in experimental animal models have shown that absolute intestinal mucosal flow is decreased as a result of dopamine-induced shunting of blood away from the mucosa.[54,55] This complication is of extreme concern, particularly in the critically ill patient, in whom critical intestinal mucosal ischemia may lead to bacterial translocation and sepsis. When high-dose dopamine was compared with norepinephrine in patients with septic shock, dopamine was associated with a drop in gastric mucosal pH (an indicator of mucosal ischemia), compared with a rise in pH observed with norepinephrine.[56]

Prevention of Acute Renal Failure in High-Risk Patients

Renal hypoperfusion is the leading cause of ARF in humans. It may be caused by intravascular volume depletion, decreased cardiac output, systemic vasodilatation (e.g., sepsis and liver failure), or conditions that directly promote renal vasoconstriction, including drugs (e.g., cyclosporine), radiocontrast agents, hypercalcemia, liver failure, and sepsis. The renal vasodilatory effect of low-dose dopamine might be expected to be beneficial under these circumstances, particularly when the period of renal hypoperfusion is short-lived, such as during surgery and radiocontrast administration. However, as outlined previously, in a variety of conditions, including renal failure, the selective renal vasodilatory effects of dopamine are frequently absent, placing doubt on the rationale for using this agent in preventing ARF. Table 44–3 summarizes data from prospective, controlled trials performed to determine the value of low-dose dopamine infusion in a variety of high-risk clinical situations.

Numerous studies have compared the effects of perioperative administration of low-dose dopamine to usual care in patients undergoing cardiovascular surgery.[57–62] To date, no study has demonstrated a beneficial effect of low-dose dopamine as assessed by postoperative increase in serum creatinine,[61,62] creatinine clearance,[57–59] or 51Cr-EDTA GFR.[60] Similarly, no benefit in postoperative renal function in patients undergoing abdominal aortic surgery treated with a combination of low-dose dopamine and mannitol[63] or low-dose dopamine infusion alone[64] has been reported. In the first study, RBF assessed during the aortic clamp procedure decreased by 50% in both groups.[63] When low-dose dopamine was compared with intravenous nifedipine in patients undergoing aortic surgery, dopamine was less effective in preserving postoperative GFR.[65]

Five studies have examined the role of perioperative low-dose dopamine infusion during renal transplantation, including four prospective studies[66–69] and a retrospective studies.[70] End points measured included incidence of post-transplantation ARF, delayed graft function, requirements for dialysis, and graft GFR measured at various points after transplantation. Five studies indicated no beneficial effects of perioperative dopamine infusion on graft function. In fact, dopamine-induced natriuresis and diuresis were often associated with fluid and electrolyte management problems in these patients. A single prospective study reported a small but significantly higher GFR at 1 month in the dopamine-treated transplantation group; however, there were no significant differences in the rate of delayed graft function or in the requirement for dialysis between groups in this study. In a recent study that measured renal blood flow velocity and vascular resistance by Doppler ultrasound, transplanted grafts were determined to be insensitive to the vascular effects of dopamine infusion.[71]

Patients undergoing liver transplantation have a high incidence of postoperative ARF precipitated by the major stresses of hepatobiliary surgery superimposed on the chronic renal hypoperfusion that complicates liver failure. In a study of 34 patients undergoing live transplantation, prophylactic dopamine was associated with a lower incidence of renal insufficiency as compared with controls (10% vs. 67%, respectively).[72] However, in a larger, prospective controlled study involving 48 patients, perioperative infusion of dopamine was not associated with lower blood urea nitrogen or creatinine clearance rates measured 24 hours after surgery or GFR measured 1 month later.[73] Similarly, when administered to patients undergoing elective surgery for obstructive jaundice, dopamine was not associated with improved creatinine clearance 5 days after surgery.[74]

Radiocontrast agents can cause potent intrarenal vasoconstriction and may result in transient renal impairment, particularly in patients with diabetic nephropathy and baseline renal impairment. The role of prophylactic dopamine therapy to prevent radiocontrast-induced nephropathy (RCIN) has been assessed in six controlled trials.[75–80] A randomized controlled trial involving 40 diabetic patients, with a mean baseline serum creatinine level of 1.5 mg/dL, showed that low-dose dopamine prevented a 25% increase in serum creatinine levels observed in the control group.[79] Similar results were reported in two other studies.[77,78] In one study, the beneficial effect was more striking in patients with baseline creatinine levels greater than 2 mg/dL.[78] In contrast, no decrease in the rate of RCIN was found with prophylactic dopamine therapy, and unexpectedly, the patients within the dopamine group who subsequently developed RCIN exhibited the greatest increase in RBF.[81] The two most recent trials failed to show a benefit for dopamine infusion.[75,76] In one study, dopamine combined with furosemide and mannitol to achieve a forced diuresis did not reveal a difference in the change in serum creatinine at 48 hours compared to hydration alone.[75] In the second trial, dopamine prolonged the course of renal failure in patients with contrast nephropathy.[76]

Treatment of Established Acute Renal Failure

More severe or prolonged renal hypoperfusion can provoke ischemic renal parenchymal injury. It has been postulated that the renal vasodilatory action of dopamine is beneficial in established ATN, but several issues need to be considered:

1. Dopamine may not induce renal vasodilatation in patients with ARF because of counterregulatory factors causing preglomerular vasoconstriction, such as increased endothelin levels, inhibition of nitric oxide synthesis, and activation of tubuloglomerular feedback.
2. Tubular obstruction and back-leakage are thought to play a more important pathogenic role in maintaining a low GFR in these conditions. Indeed, GFR frequently remains low despite restoration of total RBF.
3. A consistent finding in established ATN is an abnormal distribution of RBF rather than an absolute reduction. This

Table 44–3 Prospective, Controlled Trials on the Value of Low-Dose Dopamine in the Prevention of Acute Renal Failure in High-Risk Patients*

				Renal Function					
				Control		Dopamine			
Study	Clinical Setting	Dopamine Regimen	Parameter	Preop	Postop	Preop	Postop	Significant Difference?	Comments
Myles[57] (N=52)	Elective CABG	3 μg/kg/min presurgery and 24-hr post	BUN	NR	NR	NR	NR	?	CrCl and UO assessed at day 7 postop. SCr assessed at day 7 postop. No ARF in control group
			SCr	1.02 ± 0.05	1.03 ± 0.05	1.05 ± 0.05	1.13 ± 0.14	No	
			CrCl	127 ± 12	107 ± 15	91 ± 16	91 ± 16	No	
Piper[58] (N=40)	Cardiac surgery	2.5 μg/kg/min 24-hr presurgery and 72-hr postop	BUN	NR	NR	NR	NR	?	Parameters assessed at 48 hr postop. Markers of tubular injury (α-GST, α(1)-MG, & NAG) also assessed without significant difference
			SCr	NR	NR	NR	NR	?	
			CrCl	72.0 ± 6.9	76.1 ± 11.6	78.1 ± 8.4	73.9 ± 7.7	No	
Yavuz[59] (N=30)	Elective CABG	2 μg/kg/min 48-hr postop	BUN	NR	NR	NR	NR	?	Parameters assessed at 72 hr postop. No further significant difference in β_2-microglobulin was noted.
			SCr	NR	NR	NR	NR	?	
			CrCl	74.4 ± 9.7	52.7 ± 13.9	67.4 ± 8.7	61.4 ± 7.5	No	
Sumeray[60] (N=36)	Cardiac surgery	2.5 μg/kg/min presurgery and 48-hr postop	BUN	NR	NR	NR	NR	?	GFR was assessed preoperatively and on postop day 5 by 51 Cr EDTA. Urinary markers of tubular injury were significantly lower in the dopamine group
			SCr	103.9 ± 3.5	NR	106.5 ± 2.7	NR	?	
			CrCl	68.2 ± 4.2	70.0 ± 3.8	67.1 ± 5.1	68.4 ± 4.7	No	
			GFR	75.4 ± 3.2	81.4 ± 5.7	74.4 ± 2.8	73.3 ± 4.6	No	
Lassnigg[61] (N=62)	Cardiac surgery	2 μg/kg/min presurgery and 48-hr postop	BUN	17.3 ± 0.94	23.7 ± 1.70	16.2 ± 0.94	25.7 ± 1.25	No	Parameters assessed at 48 hr postop.
			SCr	0.96 ± 0.04	1.10 ± 0.06	0.98 ± 0.04	1.21 ± 0.07	No	
			CrCl	99 ± 7.46	95 ± 8.57	101± 5.38	72 ± 5.38	No	
Tang[62] (N=40)	Cardiac surgery	2-4 μg/kg/min presurgery and 48-hr postop	BUN	5.2 ± 0.09	5.8 ± 0.24	4.5 ± 0.07	6.1 ± 0.4	No	Parameters assessed at 7 days postop.
			SCr	120 ± 1.13	119 ± 1.24	110 ± 1.33	113 ± 2.22	No	
			CrCl	NR	NR	NR	NR	?	
Paul[63] (N=27)	Elective infrarenal aortic clamping	3 μg/kg/min presurgery 40 min post-clamp and mannitol (200 mg/kg/hr)	BUN	NR	NR	NR	NR	?	Parameters assessed at day 1 postop. CrCl decreased in both groups by about 50% during clamp period.
			SCr	NR	NR	NR	NR	?	
			CrCl	96 ± 10	92 ± 7	91 ± 8	92 ± 7	No	
Baldwin[64] (N=37)	Elective abdominal aortic surgery	3 μg/kg/min postsurgery for 24 hr	BUN	6.8	5.8	6.8	5.8	No	Parameters assessed at day 5. No ARF in control group. Trend towards increased UO in dopamine group.
			SCr	1.3	1.2	1.2	1.2	No	
			CrCl	72	83	89	85	No	

Continued

Table 44–3 Prospective, Controlled Trials on the Value of Low-Dose Dopamine in the Prevention of Acute Renal Failure in High-Risk Patients*—cont'd

				Renal Function					
				Control		Dopamine			
Study	Clinical Setting	Dopamine Regimen	Parameter	Preop	Postop	Preop	Postop	Significant Difference?	Comments
Antonucci[65] (N=16)	Elective infrarenal aortic clamping	1.5–2 μg/kg/min during surgery	BUN	NR	NR	NR	NR	?	GFR assessed immediately postop. Control group received nifedipine infusion. Improved renal function postop in nifedipine group.
			SCr	NR	NR	NR	NR	?	
			CrCl	85	110	1-5	70	Yes	
			GFR	62 ± 10	77 ± 25	87 ± 20	65 ± 15	Yes	
Carmellini[66] (N=60)	Renal transplantation	3 μg/kg/min started during and for 48 hr	DGF	NR	33%	NR	20%	No	DGF defined as % pts. requiring dialysis in 1st week. SCr and CrCl assessed at 1 month. No difference in the time of onset of function after DGF.
			SCr	NR	2.2 ± 0.3	NR	1.9 ± 0.2	No	
			CrCl	NR	53.7 ± 5.3	NR	68.1 ± 3.7	Yes	
Donmez[67] (N=40)	Renal transplantation	2 μg/kg/min started during and for 48 hr	BUN	NR	38.80 ± 4.15	NR	43.15 ± 4.10	No	
			SCr	NR	2.69 ± 0.54	NR	3.20 ± 0.51	No	
			CrCl	NR	NR	NR	NR	?	Parameters were assessed on postop day 7.
Grundmann[68] (N=50)	Renal transplantation	2 μg/kg/min post-surgery for 4 days	BUN	NR	NR	NR	NR	?	CrCl assessed at day 4. No difference in requirement of hemodialysis in the 1st postop week between groups (76%).
			SCr	NR	NR	NR	NR	?	
			CrCl	NR	9.0 ± 3.2	NR	7.0 ± 2.2	No	
Kadieva[69] (N=60)	Renal transplantation	3 μg/kg/min started during and for 48 hr	BUN	NR	NR	NR	NR	?	CrCl assessed at day 7. Incidence of ARF in dopamine group 33% vs. 23% in controls.
			SCr	NR	NR	NR	NR	?	
			CrCl	NR	55.2 ± 1.6	NR	57.5 ± 17	No	
Swygert[73] (N=43)	Liver transplantation	3 μg/kg/min pre-surgery and 24 hr post	BUN	14 ± 1.7	33.5 ± 4.5	19.4 ± 3.7	31.6 ± 5.3	No	BUN/SCr assessed at day 7 and GFR (iothalamate) at 1 month postop (after 30 days of cyclosporine). Incidence of postop ARF in both groups was 4%.
			SCr	1.0 ± 0.1	1.4 ± 0.1	1.3 ± 0.2	1.4 ± 0.2	No	
			CrCl	82	58 ± 10	84	59 ± 6	No	
Parks[74] (N=23)	Elective surgery for obstructive	3 μg/kg/min pre-surgery and 24 hr post	NR	5.1 ± 0.6	4.8 ± 0.6	4.9 ± 0.6	6.0 ± 1.0	No	Parameters assessed at day 5. No ARF in control group. All pts. received a bolus of saline and furosemide postop.
			SCr (mmol/L)	72 ± 6	70 ± 7	72 ± 5	68 ± 8	No	
			CrCl	70 ± 17	75 ± 10	90 ± 10	78 ± 12	No	

Hall[77] (N=24)	Peripheral arteriography	3 μg/kg/min 12 hr pre and 24 hr post	BUN	NR	NR	NR	NR	?	SCr assessed at day 3. Subgroup analysis of 22 patients. Control group received mannitol. There was no benefit of dopamine. Infusion in group with SCr <2.0.
			SCr	2.6 ± 0.4	3.9 ± 1.9	3.0 ± 1.5	2.5 ± 1.5	Yes	
			CrCl	NR	NR	NR	NR	?	
Hans[78] (N=60)	Peripheral arteriography	2.5 μg/kg/min during and 12 hr post	BUN	1.75 ± 0.69	NR	NR	NR	?	Parameters assessed at day 3. Small improvement in CrCl in dopamine group not sustained after day 1.
			SCr	50.42 ± 19.36	1.98 ± 0.71	1.93 ± 0.47	1.98 ± 0.43	Yes	
			CrCl		47.16 ± 18.54	49.59 ± 19.36	57.25 ± 27.8	No	
Kapoor[79] (N=40)	Coronary angiography	5 μg/kg/min 30 min pre and 6 hr post	BUN	19.9 ± 13.4	23.25 ± 12.7	16.3 ± 8.05	14.7 ± 5.5	Yes	BUN/SCr assessed 24 hr postop. 50% of patients in control group had a 25% rise in SCr. No patients required dialysis.
			SCr	1.52 ± 0.68	1.96 ± 1.2	1.5 ± 0.32	1.37 ± 0.25	Yes	
			CrC	NR	NR	NR	NR	?	
Weisberg[80] (N=50)	Coronary angiography	2 μg/kg/min during and 2 hr post	RBF	24.7 ± 55	NR	17.1 ± 23	NR	?	RCIN defined as 25% increase in SCr. Dopamine increased RBF, but pts. who developed RCIN had the greatest improvement in RBF.
			SCr	>1.8	NR	>1.8	NR	No	
			CrCl	NR	NR	NR	NR	?	
			RCIN	—	40%	—	30%	No	
Stevens[75] (N=76)	Coronary angiography	3 μg/kg/min during with furosemide and	SCr	2.55 ± 0.91	3.08 ± 1.20	2.20 ± 0.38	2.72 ± 1.19	No	Parameters assayed at 48 hr postop. RCIN defined as 25% increase in SCr.
			CrCl	30.48 ± 12.95	NR	33.73 ± 10.00	NR	?	
			RCIN	—	30.9%	—	31.8%	No	
Abizaid[40] (N=)	Coronary angioplasty	2 μg/kg/min 2 hr prior and during procedure	SCr	2.3 ± 0.18	2.8 ± 0.24	1.9 ± 0.07	2.3 ± 0.16	No	The SCr was expressed as the peak SCr post-procedure. RCIN defined as 25% increase in SCr.
			CrCl	NR	NR	NR	NR	?	
			RCIN	—	30%	—	35%	No	

Yes denotes *P*<.005 when comparing postoperative parameters.

*Data were expressed as means and were estimated from figures where not reported in original text. Standard errors of means are included where reported or derivable from figures.

BUN, blood urea nitrogen (mg/dL); *CABG*, coronary artery bypass grafting; *CrCl*, creatinine clearance (mL/min); *DGF*, delayed graft function; *GFR*, glomerular filtration rate (mL/min); *NR*, not reported; *RBF*, renal blood flow (mL/min); *RCIN*, radiocontrast-induced nephropathy; *SCr*, serum creatinine (mg/dL).

manifests in medullary hypoperfusion and persistent ischemia of the pars recta of the proximal tubule and the medullary thick ascending limb of the loop of Henle. Most studies report a selective increase in cortical rather than medullary perfusion with dopamine.

It has, however, been suggested that low-dose dopamine may improve the course of ARF by other mechanisms:

1. Through inhibition of Na^+-K^+-ATPase, dopamine may favorably alter the oxygen supply/demand ratio of the tubular epithelial cells, rendering them less prone to ischemic injury.
2. By causing natriuresis, dopamine may help to flush out obstructing tubular casts.
3. The frequent use of low-dose dopamine in ARF has evolved from the belief that increasing urine output improves outcome in this condition. This opinion is based on the improved prognosis and lower mortality rates observed in patients with nonoliguric ARF compared with patients who have oliguric ARF. Unfortunately, there is no evidence that converting oliguric ARF to a nonoliguric state improves prognosis.

Low-dose dopamine has been commonly prescribed to critically ill intensive care unit patients with established ARF. Early uncontrolled studies reported variable success with low-dose dopamine in established ARF.[82, 83] Multiple studies have confirmed the natriuretic and diuretic effects of dopamine in this patient population.[82–85] In critically ill oliguric patients, a response of greater than a 50% increase in urine output on low-dose dopamine has been documented.[84] Interpretation of these results, however, requires caution because oliguria is a notoriously poor indicator of ARF, and conversion from an oliguric to a nonoliguric state has not been shown to improve renal prognosis. In addition, such a response is not universal[86] and may wane over time.[87] Eight hemodynamically stable, critically ill patients with mild nonoliguric renal failure defined as a creatinine clearance between 30 and 80 mL/min, received 4-hour infusion periods with placebo alternating with low dose dopamine.[87] Urine flow rate, creatinine clearance, and FENa increased significantly with maximal changes in each parameter noted at 8 hours. However, the improvements waned considerably by 24 hours and were no longer detectable by 48 hours.

In an observational study, a subgroup of patients who received low-dose dopamine within the placebo arm of a multicenter intervention trial were analyzed.[88] All patients within the placebo arm were adults with ARF having a clinical history consistent with ATN. Dopamine had been administered to a portion of these patients at the discretion of the physician. A total of 86 patients received dopamine (<3 μg/kg/min), and 79 patients did not. Despite complex adjustment for treatment bias, low-dose dopamine treatment was not associated with reduced risk of death or with combined risk of death or dialysis in patients with ATN. A meta-analysis including 58 randomized clinical trials revealed that dopamine did not prevent mortality, onset of ARF, or need for dialysis.[89] Finally, a large, multicenter, randomized, controlled, double-blind trial enrolled 328 patients with ATN to either low dose dopamine (2 μ/kg/min) or placebo.[90] No difference in peak serum creatinine concentration, difference from baseline to peak serum creatinine concentration, the number of patients whose serum creatinine exceeded 300 μmol/L, or the number of patients who required renal replacement therapy was detected. In addition, the durations of ICU and hospital stays were similar.

Low-Dose Dopamine in Conjunction with Systemic Vasopressors

Low-dose dopamine is commonly administered to critically ill patients requiring pressor support with systemic vasoconstrictors, with the goal of maximizing renal perfusion. Justification for combination therapy comes from experimental studies in animals. In dogs with septic shock treated with norepinephrine, low-dose dopamine improved RBF.[91] When pressor doses of norepinephrine are administered to healthy humans, RBF falls but can be normalized by coadministration of low-dose dopamine.[92] There is no evidence, however, that low-dose dopamine improves RBF or renal function in patients with septic shock already receiving norepinephrine. Indeed, it has yet to be demonstrated convincingly that therapeutic doses of norepinephrine compromise renal function. No change in GFR was demonstrated when low-dose dopamine was added to norepinephrine-treated patients with septic shock.[93] Norepinephrine has been shown to be more effective than high-dose dopamine in preserving RBF in patients with septic shock.[94] Finally, it has been demonstrated that the addition of norepinephrine alone is sufficient to restore renal perfusion and urine output in patients with septic shock.[95]

FENOLDOPAM

Fenoldopam mesylate is a specific agonist of the DA_1 receptor. Like dopamine, fenoldopam results in peripheral and renal vasodilation as well as diuresis and natriuresis via stimulation of vascular and renal tubular DA_1 receptors.[24,96] Studies in healthy, salt replete subjects have confirmed dose-dependent increases in renal plasma flow, urine flow rate, and urinary sodium excretion without changes in GFR.[24, 97–102] The lack of increase in the GFR is secondary to parallel vasodilation of both afferent and efferent renal arterioles rendering intraglomerular pressure constant.[103] Animal studies have demonstrated fenoldopam to be markedly more potent than dopamine in decreasing renal vascular resistance and augmenting RBF.[96] Its relative potency, in conjunction with the absence of the potentially deleterious cardiac side effects characteristic of dopamine due to β-adrenoreceptor stimulation[50] were the impetus for trials examining its potential to prevent and treat renal ischemia.

Both animal[104] and uncontrolled human observational studies[105–109] indicated that fenoldopam might have a role in the prevention of contrast-induced nephropathy. More recently, however, three double-blind, randomized, placebo controlled trials failed to confirm any benefit for fenoldopam in the prevention of contrast-induced nephropathy.[110–112] Although the smallest of the three trails revealed a statistically significant increase in renal plasma flow in the patients that received fenoldopam (16% above baseline) as compared to the placebo group (33% below baseline), the difference in the incidence of contrast-induced nephropathy was not significant (21% vs. 41%, respectively; $p = .148$).[112] A second trial randomized 123 patients with renal insufficiency (serum creatinine >1.6 mg/dL or creatinine clearance >60 mL/min) to receive either saline, *N*-acetylcysteine or fenoldopam. The incidence of contrast-induced nephropathy defined as an increase in serum creatinine >0.5 mg/dL 48 hours after the procedure was 15%, 18%, and 16% in the saline, N-acetylcysteine fenoldopam groups, respectively ($p = 0.919$).[111] Finally, in the largest trial to date, 315 well-hydrated patients with renal insufficiency (creatinine clearance <60 mL/min) were randomized to fenoldopam (0.1 mcg/kg/min), beginning 1 hour prior and maintained for 12 hours after the procedure or placebo.[110] No difference was detected in the incidence of contrast-induced nephropathy (a 25% increase in serum creatinine within 96 hours of contrast), which was 34% in the fenoldopam group and 30% in the placebo group. In addition, no significant differences were detected in any of the secondary outcome measures, which included the 30-day rate of death, dialysis, or rehospitalization.

In both animals and humans, uncontrolled studies have demonstrated that fenoldopam can prevent and reverse cyclosporin A-induced renal vasoconstriction.[113,114] Similarly, small human trials that initiated fenoldopam prior infrarenal aortic cross-clamping noted rapid recovery to baseline kidney function[115] and less postoperative decrement in creatinine clearance compared to the placebo group.[116] During cardiopulmonary bypass, no patients at risk for developing postoperative renal failure required dialysis in an uncontrolled study of 70 patients.[117] A small, randomized trial of 31 patients revealed a significant decrease in the creatinine clearance after cardiopulmonary bypass in the placebo but not in the fenoldopam group.[118] This renoprotective effect following cardiopulmonary bypass was replicated in a larger prospective randomized controlled trial of 160 patients.[119] However, further studies are required to determine whether fenoldopam alters more clinically meaningful outcomes like allograft survival, need for renal replacement therapy, or mortality.

ATRIAL NATRIURETIC PEPTIDE

The existence of an atrial natriuretic substance was first postulated in 1981 with the discovery that an atrial myocardial extract from rats produced a potent natriuretic response on reinfusion.[120] This substance was originally named *atrial natriuretic factor* and then *peptide* after its characterization as a protein. Subsequent studies defining the physiology and pharmacology of ANP have cast light on its role in the maintenance of circulatory volume in health and disease. The pharmacologic properties of ANP suggested that it has the potential to reverse the impaired glomerular hemodynamics and tubular obstruction that characterize ARF. We now review the structure and physiology of ANP, discuss the rationale for its use in ARF, and describe the results of animal and human trials.

PHYSIOLOGY

ANP is a member of a family of related homologous natriuretic peptides, which includes brain natriuretic peptide, C-type natriuretic peptide, and urodilatin. ANP is released from secretory granules in the atria and, to a lesser extent, the ventricles. It is stored as a 126-amino acid peptide, pro-ANP, and circulates as a 28-amino acid peptide derived from the C-terminal end of pro-ANP. The main stimulus for ANP secretion is an increase in atrial pressure or stretch.[121] ANP is cleared by the kidney and has a short half-life, of the order of 1 to 4 minutes.[122]

The physiologic effects of ANP are mediated through its action on the systemic vasculature as well as on the renal glomerulus and tubules. Systemic effects of ANP include increased vagal tone,[123] inhibition of the renin-angiotensin-aldosterone system,[121] and preferential vasodilatation of the venous circulation with hypotension.[124] ANP can also reverse the vasoconstrictive effect of other peptides, such as endothelin.[125] ANP augments glomerular capillary hydraulic pressure and GFR by triggering afferent arteriolar dilatation.[126] Total RBF remains largely unchanged. The tubular effects of ANP are mediated at several segments. Micropuncture studies have shown that the natriuretic effects of ANP are exerted predominantly at the level of the inner medullary collecting ducts.[127,128] Here, ANP attenuates transport of Na^+ through epithelial luminal Na^+ channels.[121] This action is mediated through engagement of basolateral cell surface receptors, activation of guanylate cyclase resulting in an increase in intracellular cyclic guanosine monophosphate (cGMP) levels, and activation of a cGMP-dependent protein kinase, which closes the Na^+ channel.[129] At the level of the proximal tubule, ANP inhibits the reabsorption of Na^+, Cl^-, and water,[130] possibly through interactions with other modulators of proximal tubular function, such as angiotensin II or dopamine.[131,132] ANP may also modulate Na^+ reabsorption in the loop of Henle and the cortical collecting duct.[133,134] ANP attenuates the collecting tubule responsiveness to ADH, which promotes a diuretic action.[135]

EFFICACY IN EXPERIMENTAL AND HUMAN ACUTE RENAL FAILURE

ANP possesses several bioactivities that may prevent ischemic ARF or accelerate its resolution. Specifically, ANP can raise GFR, enhance urine flow, redistribute RBF to the medulla, inhibit Na^+ transport, and reduce tubular ATP and oxygen requirements. In addition, reversal of endothelin-related vasoconstriction may also improve blood supply to the renal medulla. These observations were the catalyst for numerous studies in animals and humans, which evaluated the efficacy of ANP as a therapeutic agent in ARF.

The initial studies examining the effects of ANP in experimental ischemic ARF were reported in 1986.[136,137] Improvements in GFR, urine volume, and fractional excretion of sodium and potassium were noted after intrarenal infusion of ANP in norepinephrine-induced renal failure in the rat.[137] In addition, pretreatment with ANP prevented norepinephrine-induced renal failure and GFR, urine volume and sodium, and potassium excretion improved with ANP infusion in a dose-dependent fashion.[136] Subsequent studies also demonstrated a beneficial effect of ANP infusion in experimental ischemic ARF due to renal vasoconstriction induced by norepinephrine[138] or arginine vasopressin[139] as well as by renal artery clamping.[140–150] Beneficial effects were also assessed in ARF induced by glycerol,[151,152] uranyl nitrate, gentamicin,[153] and cisplatin.[154,155] In addition to functional improvement, some studies demonstrated significantly less histologic damage in ANP-treated kidneys.[142,149,152] Although the bulk of experimental evidence favored ANP as a potential therapy for

ATN, several studies noted the beneficial effect of ANP to be transient and not sustained beyond its administration.[139,148] The tendency for ANP to result in systemic hypotension prompted investigators to use it in combination with low-dose dopamine.[138,144,150,155] The improvement in MAP due to the addition of dopamine to ANP may have been responsible for the improved, sustained benefit in these studies. Similarly, mannitol has been reported to potentiate the positive effects of ANP.[146]

The encouraging results in experimental ARF prompted evaluation of the efficacy of ANP in human disease (Table 44–4). Urodilatin is a 32–amino acid peptide generated by cleavage of the pro-ANP peptide 4 amino acids upstream from the usual cleavage site. The efficacy of urodilatin has been examined in patients after cardiac or liver transplantation.[156–158] Ninety-six hours of a low-dose urodilatin infusion was initiated in 51 patients after cardiac transplantation.[158] Compared to historical controls, significant reductions in the peak serum creatinine, peak serum urea, and incidence of hemodialysis were noted in the patients who received urodilatin. In a randomized, placebo-controlled trial, 24 patients were randomized to either urodilatin infusion or placebo immediately post cardiac transplantation.[157] Although urodilatin failed to reduce the incidence of ARF, the duration of hemofiltration and/or hemodialysis was reduced. Nine patients with ARF following liver transplantation were randomized in a double-blind, controlled study to receive either urodilatin or placebo.[156] The frequency of dialysis and the serum creatinine levels were significantly reduced in the treatment group compared with those in the placebo group. However, in trials that examined ARF in the ICU setting, urodilatin infusion did not consistently improve renal function.[159–161]

Improvements in urine flow, GFR, and RBF have been reported in patients with ARF and heart failure receiving ANP infusions after cardiac surgery.[162,163] In an open-label study, 53 patients with established intrinsic ARF were randomized to receive ANP infusion in addition to standard diuretic therapy or diuretic therapy alone.[164] A significant increase in creatinine clearance was found with ANP treatment, rising from 9.9 mL/min to 21 mL/min. No corresponding increase was noted in the control group. The need for dialysis was significantly reduced, from 52% in the control group to 23% in the ANP treatment group. A nonsignificant trend toward reduced mortality was noted in the ANP treatment group.

After these initial results, 504 patients with ATN due to ischemic or nephrotoxic insults were enrolled at centers across the United States and Canada in the largest trial to date.[165] Patients were randomized to receive either anaritide, a 25-amino acid synthetic form of ANP (ANP 4-28), or placebo in a double-blind study. No difference was noted between the anaritide-treated and placebo groups for either the primary end point (dialysis-free survival for 21 days after treatment) or any of the secondary end points (need for dialysis, serum creatinine level, and mortality). A subgroup analysis of patients who were oliguric (120 patients) revealed a greater dialysis-free survival in the anaritide group than in the placebo group (27% vs. 8%, respectively; $p = .008$). Conversely, a trend toward a worse outcome existed among the nonoliguric patients as dialysis-free survival was 59% in the placebo group compared to 48% in the ANP group ($p = .03$). These results prompted a follow-up study involving only oliguric patients. In this study, 222 patients were randomized to either ANP infusion versus placebo. However, no benefit in dialysis-free survival was demonstrated.[166] Of note, in the anaritide multicenter study, hypotension was reported in 46% of the anaritide group.[165] Similarly in the follow-up study, which randomized only oliguric patients, 95% versus 55% of the patients had a systolic blood pressure less than 90 mmHg in the anaritide and placebo groups, respectively.[166] The maximal absolute decrease in systolic blood pressure was approximately 10 mmHg.

Similarly, the results of studies assessing the efficacy of ANP for prevention of contrast nephropathy and for the treatment of delayed graft function after cadaveric renal transplantation were equally disappointing. In an effort to prevent contrast nephropathy, 247 patients with stable chronic renal failure (estimated creatinine clearance ≤ 65 mL/min) were randomized to receive one of three doses of ANP infusion or placebo for 30 minutes before and after contrast administration.[167] The incidence of radiocontrast-induced nephropathy did not differ among the groups. ANP was evaluated in prospective, double-blind controlled trials in cadaveric renal transplantation.[168–170] ANP or vehicle was administered intravenously at the time of revascularization of the allograft to 20 recipients of 10 pairs of cadaveric kidneys.[170] No improvement in serum creatinine, GFR, need for dialysis, or allograft function was observed. In a study of 38 recipients of 19 pairs of cadaveric kidneys, escalating doses of atriopeptin III, a synthetic analogue of ANP, was administered over 12 hours in an intravenous infusion commencing at release of the vascular clamps.[169] No improvement was reported in creatinine clearance or sodium excretion compared with placebo. ANP was compared to a maximal hydration regimen as a means of preventing ATN after cadaveric renal transplantation in an open, randomized study involving 40 patients.[168] Although a nonsignificant trend toward a reduced need for dialysis was noted in the ANP group, no difference was detected in the median rate of renal recovery.

GROWTH FACTORS

Growth factors are known to be key players in renal development. To date, three growth factors have received the most attention in the literature for their ability to alter renal function/structure:

- Insulin-like growth factor-1 (IGF-1)
- Epidermal growth factor (EGF)
- Hepatocyte growth factor (HGF)

The kidney is a site of EGF, HGF, and IGF-1 synthesis.[171,172] These growth factors mediate specific growth-promoting, transport, and metabolic functions within the kidney.[173–176] HGF and EGF are mitogenic for cultured tubular cells *in vitro*.[177,178] IGF-1 is required for the development of the metanephric kidney *in vitro*,[177] a process that has many similarities to recovery from ATN in vivo. In addition, expression of some growth factors or their receptors is augmented after renal injury, suggesting that they may have therapeutic potential in ATN.[179,180]

Clinical recovery from ATN correlates temporally with the relief of intratubular obstruction and, more importantly, with the restoration of the continuity and function of the tubular epithelium.[181] Initial studies in experimental animals revealed

Table 44–4 Summary of Evidence of Benefit in Human Trials for Use of Atrial Natriuretic Peptide in Acute Renal Failure

Reference	Study Design	Total Patients	Treatments Compared	Patient Population	Outcome
Kuse[156]	Double-blind	9	Urodilatin, placebo	Liver transplantation	Increased need for dialysis; decreased serum creatinine, stable serum urea; trend towards increased diuresis
Brenner[157]	Double-blind	24	Urodilatin, placebo	Heart transplantation	Half the patients in each group required RRT, but the duration of RRT was significantly less in the urodilatin group
Hummel[158]	Open, nonrandomized	51	Urodilatin, historical controls	Heart transplantation	Urodilatin group significantly lower peak plasma creatinine and lower incidence of RRT
Herbert[159]	Double-blind	12	Urodilatin, placebo	Post major abdominal surgery	No significant difference in peak serum creatinine or need for RRT
Weibe[160]	Double-blind	14	Urodilatin, placebo	Post cardiac surgery	No patients in the urodilatin vs. 6 in placebo group required RRT ($p < .005$)
Meyer[161]	Double-blind	176	Urodilatin, placebo	Oliguric ARF	No significant difference in need for RRT
Sward[162]	Open, nonrandomized	11	Human ANP 1-28	ARF post cardiac surgery	Increased urine flow, GFR, renal blood flow; decreased renal vascular resistance
Valsson[163]	Open, nonrandomized	12	Human ANP 1-28	ARF and heart failure post cardiac surgery	Increased urine flow, GFR, renal blood flow; decreased renal vascular resistance
Rahman[164]	Open, randomized	53	Human ANP 3-28 or human ANP 4-28, diuretic	Intrinsic ARF	Increased GFR; decreased need for dialysis; trend toward decreased mortality
Allgren[165]	Double-blind	504	Anaritide, placebo	Ischemic or nephrotoxic ATN	No improvement in dialysis-free survival, need for dialysis, serum creatinine level, or mortality; increased dialysis-free survival in oliguric subgroup
Lewis[166]	Double-blind	222	Anaritide, placebo	Oliguric ATN	No benefit in dialysis free survival
Kurnik[167]	Double-blind	247	Anaritide, placebo	Contrast nephropathy	No reduction in the incidence of contrast nephropathy in patients with renal insufficiency, with or without diabetes
Gianello[168]	Open, randomized	40	Human ANP 1-28, maximal hydration regime	Renal transplantation	Trend toward decreased need for dialysis; trend toward decreased incidence of ATN
Ratcliffe[169]	Double-blind	38	Atriopeptin III, placebo	Renal transplantation	No difference in creatinine clearance; no difference in sodium excretion
Sands[170]	Open, nonrandomized	20	Human ANP	Renal transplantation	No improvement in serum creatinine or GFR

ANF, atrial natriuretic peptide; *ARF,* acute renal failure; *ATN,* acute tubular necrosis; *GFR,* glomerular filtration rate; *RRT,* renal replacement therapy.

that in either ischemic or nephrotoxic ATN, administration of these agents not only augmented the process of tubular regeneration, promoted earlier recovery of epithelial morphology, improved GFR and anabolism, but also decreased mortality.[182–185] The next section reviews the physiologic and pharmacologic effects of IGF-1, EGF, and HGF and their potential mechanisms of action in experimental and human ARF (Table 44–5).

Insulin-Like Growth Factor-1

Physiology

IGF-1 is a 70-amino acid peptide synthesized primarily in the liver.[186] The kidney is also a source of IGF-1. IGF-1 expression is normally regulated by growth hormone.[187] The cortical collecting duct is the major site of production in adult rats, and renal synthesis is increased in response to both growth hormone and EGF.[176,188] In blood, IGF-1 binds to one of at least six carrier proteins; these IGF-binding proteins modulate its activity.[186] The IGF-binding proteins are derived mainly from the liver but are also produced locally in most organs, where they act in an autocrine or paracrine fashion.[186] IGF-1 mediates its cellular action by binding to one of two membrane-bound receptors that have tyrosine kinase activity and are found throughout the nephron, especially in the inner medulla.[187] The rationale for the use of IGF-1 in the treatment of ATN is based on the following experimental findings[189,190]:

1. Via stimulation of nitric oxide, IGF-1 increases renal plasma flow and GFR in healthy rats and in the ischemic model of ATN.[191,192] Such an effect could be beneficial by increasing urine flow rates and relieving intratubular obstruction.
2. IGF-1 receptor expression and IGF-1 binding are increased in regenerating tubule cells after injury.[193]
3. At high concentrations, IGF-1 is mitogenic for the proximal tubule in vitro and increases incorporation of 5-bromo-2′-deoxyuridine in the nuclei of tubular cells after an ischemic insult in the rat model, reflecting stimulation of DNA synthesis.[194]
4. ARF is characterized by intense protein catabolism and weight loss. IGF-1 has anabolic effects that could ameliorate this detrimental effect.[195]
5. IGF-1 mRNA levels and immunoreactive IGF-1 decrease dramatically within 48 hours of induction of ischemic ATN in rats. Concomitant with this decrease, however, is the striking upregulation of IGF-1 receptor levels and a decrease in the circulating levels of IGF-binding proteins.[190]

In aggregate, these experimental findings suggest increased bioavailability of IGF-1 could contribute to recovery from ATN.

EFFICACY IN EXPERIMENTAL AND HUMAN ACUTE RENAL FAILURE

IGF-1 has been demonstrated to modify the course of the post-clamp model of postischemic ARF in the rat.[183, 195–197] In a series of studies, postischemic injury was induced by transiently clamping both renal arteries for between 35 and 70 minutes, and then commencing 2 to 7 days of IGF-1 treatment in divided doses, beginning 0.5 to 24 hours after clamp release and reperfusion.[183,195-197] Under these conditions IGF-1 therapy uniformly accelerated recovery from the ARF, such that the maintenance stage of ATN was markedly abbreviated. GFR determined on day 2 or 3 post-injury in the IGF-1 treated rats was elevated above corresponding placebo-treated levels by a factor of twofold to fivefold.[195,197,198] As a result, whereas azotemia persisted in placebo-treated animals, it had almost completely resolved within 7 days in animals that received IGF-1. Similarly, in animal models of delayed graft function, IGF-1 accelerates renal recovery and ameliorates cyclosporin nephrotoxicity.[199,200]

It is not clear whether these improved outcomes are due to specific growth-promoting activities of IGF-1 or to its hemodynamic effects, namely increased RBF and GFR. Increased immunostainable IGF-1 has been demonstrated in areas of regeneration after ischemic injury; however, this increase in IGF-1 was noted after the peak in mitogenesis and in noncycling dedifferentiated cells, suggesting that IGF-1 does not initiate renal recovery but may play a role in cellular differentiation after injury.[193]

Given this potential for therapeutic benefit, a randomized, double-blind, placebo-controlled trial of IGF-1 in patients undergoing major abdominal surgery, in whom interruption of RBF was necessary, was completed.[201] Although a statistically significant smaller proportion of patients in the IGF-1

Table 44–5 Renal Actions of Growth Factors

Growth Factor	Renal Effects
Insulin-like growth factor-1 (IGF-1)	Increases glomerular filtration rate and renal blood flow Mitogenic for proximal tubule cells in in vitro Stimulates NA+ transport in renal epithelial cells Accelerates renal recovery in rat models of ATN Accelerates restoration of anatomic integrity after ATN
Epidermal growth factor	Decreases GFR Mitogenic for proximal tubule cells *in vitro* Renal vasoconstriction Natriuresis Augments IGF-1 levels after ATN Accelerates renal recovery and restoration of anatomic integrity after ATN
Hepatocyte growth factor	Accelerates renal recovery and restoration of anatomic integrity after ATN Stimulates DNA synthesis in tubular cells Induces tubulogenesis in renal epithelial cells *in vitro*
Erythropoietin	Cytokine-like effect inducing tubular cell proliferation

ATN, acute tubular necrosis; *GFR*, glomerular filtration rate.

treated group had a postoperative decline in renal function (22%) compared to the placebo group (33%), none of the study patients developed postoperative ARF. In addition, there was no difference between the two groups with respect to length of ICU stay, length of hospital stay, or discharge serum creatinine. A second multicenter, randomized, placebo-controlled trial involving 72 patients with established ATN failed to show any benefit of IGF-1 (100 μg/kg given subcutaneously twice daily for up to 14 days) versus placebo.[202] No differences were detected in GFR measured by iothalamate clearance, need for renal replacement therapy, or mortality. Like human trials in ANP, the primary criticism of this trial was the delay to initiation of therapy, which for some patients was as late as six days after the onset of ARF.

In an effort to circumvent the limitations that plague trials in the ICU setting, including multiple organ failure, recurrent renal injury, and a delay of several days before commencing treatment, a randomized, double-blind, placebo-controlled trial of IGF-1 in renal transplant recipients with delayed graft function was conducted.[203] Patients with a creatinine clearance of less than 20 mL/min immediately post-transplantation were treated with IGF-1 versus placebo for 6 days. As in the post-clamp model of postischemic ARF in the rat, the therapy was initiated within hours of the isolated, ischemic injury (5 hours). However, no statistically significant difference existed in the primary outcome measure, inulin clearance on day 7 post-transplantation, or in the secondary outcome measures, nadir serum creatinine at 6 months post-transplantation and need for renal replacement therapy. The authors proposed that delayed graft function could be used as a "human" model to screen future agents that show potential in animal trials prior to conducting large, expensive trials in the ICU. See Table 44–6 for a summary of these three studies.

Epidermal Growth Factor

Physiology

Epidermal growth factor is a 6-kD peptide. The kidney is a major site of EGF synthesis, and renal urine concentrations are typically higher than circulating serum levels. The main sites of EGF synthesis are the distal tubule and the medullary component of the thick, ascending limb of the loop of Henle. EGF is synthesized as prepro-EGF, which has a hydrophobic domain that anchors it to the apical cell plasma membrane. The extracellular domain contains several EGF-like domains. Cleavage of the extracellular domain by serine proteases releases mature EGF. EGF binds to a 170-kD receptor, which has tyrosine kinase activity. Receptors are found throughout the nephron on the basolateral cell membrane.[204]

EGF can induce renal vasoconstriction as well as cause diuresis and natriuresis when infused.[205] It is a potent mitogen for cultured proximal tubule cells *in vitro*.[174] The EGF-like protein transforming growth factor-α (TGF-α), which also binds to the EGF receptor, is necessary for the growth of the metanephric kidney *in vitro*.[206]

After acute ischemic injury, an increase in the quantity of mature bound EGF is observed.[207] During the same time period, renal levels of prepro-EGF mRNA decrease rapidly and remain depressed. This decrease is accompanied by a marked decrease in the urinary excretion of EGF, which persists for up to 21 days. Together, these observations suggest that the bound EGF found in ischemic kidneys is not of renal origin. Circulating EGF levels originating from nonrenal tissues are not affected by nephrotoxic insults and are therefore presumed to play a more important role than renally derived EGF in functional recovery from renal injury.

Infiltrating inflammatory cells at the time of tubular injury are another potential source of growth factors.[207] Activated macrophages are known to produce TGF-α, which has been demonstrated to accelerate recovery after ischemia. Local release of TGF-α could interact with the EGF receptor, promoting recovery after ischemic or nephrotoxic insult. Concomitant to an increase in the level of bound mature EGF within the kidney and decreased EGF synthesis, there is upregulation of EGF receptor expression.[180, 208] It is unclear how filtered or indeed renally derived EGF could act in an autocrine or paracrine fashion in vivo. Mature EGF is released after cleavage into the tubular lumen and thus cannot bind to receptors expressed on the basolateral membrane. It is possible that damage to the continuity of the tubular epithelium with sloughing of tubular cells into the lumen could permit

Table 44–6 Human Interventional Studies of Insulin-like Growth Factor-1 in Acute Renal Failure

Reference	Patient Population	Trial	Therapeutic Agent	End-Point	Outcome
Franklin[201]	Aortic aneurysm repair Renal revascularization	Randomized Placebo controlled (n=54)	Recombinant IGF-1 100 μg SC × six doses	GFR	GFR statistically better in IGF-1 group; no difference in mortality
Hirschberg[202]	Established acute renal failure	Randomized Placebo controlled (N=72)	Recombinant IGF-1 100 μg SC bid × 2 wk	GFR Mortality	No significant difference in outcome
Hladunewich[203]	Delayed Graft Function	Randomized Placebo controlled (N=72)	Recombinant IGF-1 100 μg SC bid × 6 days	GFR Nadir SCr RRT	No significant difference in outcome

GFR, glomerular filtration rate; *IGF-1*, insulin-like growth factor-1; *SC*, subcutaneous; *SCr*, serum creatinine; *RRT*, renal replacement therapy intraluminal EGF to bind to the normally inaccessible EGF receptors on the basolateral membrane and cause growth promoting activity. Alternatively, superoxide anion and/or hydrogen peroxide generated during ischemia and reperfusion could activate the EGF receptor.[209]

EFFICACY IN EXPERIMENTAL ACUTE RENAL FAILURE

Administration of EGF to animals with ischemic or nephrotoxic ATN results in accelerated DNA synthesis as indicated by an increase in the incorporation of [3H]-thymidine. Several investigators have also noted accelerated histologic and functional recovery and reduced mortality rates after administration of EGF in these settings.[182,185,210] EGF is a regulator of IGF-1 expression and administration of EGF to rats after ischemic injury prevents the decline in IGF-1 levels, otherwise seen in this setting.[211] This potentially explains the mechanism of action of EGF in ATN. Likewise, the administration of thyroxine, which accelerates recovery after experimental ATN, leads to an increase in serine protease activity, resulting in enhanced cleavage of mature EGF from its membrane-bound precursor.[212] Currently, no data from human studies exist to support a potential role for EGF to facilitate recovery from ATN.

Hepatocyte Growth Factor

Physiology

HGF was first identified in the serum of rats after partial hepatectomy. It is a distinct growth factor consisting of a 68-kD α-subunit and a 34-kD β-subunit.[213] Its main renal site of synthesis is thought to be the interstitium.[214] The HGF receptor is a tyrosine kinase transmembrane protein encoded for by the c-met proto-oncogene.[215] This is expressed in the epithelium of the proximal tubule, thick, ascending limb and cortical collecting ducts.[214] Consistent with a paracrine mechanism of action, there is increased expression of mRNA for both HGF and c-met within the kidney after acute renal injury.[178]

EFFICACY IN EXPERIMENTAL ACUTE RENAL FAILURE

The administration of HGF to rats after ischemic renal injury results in lower serum urea and creatinine levels at 7 days, improved histologic outcome, and lower mortality in treated animals.[184] In contrast to IGF-1, HGF exerts no anabolic effect in experimental ARF. Similar findings have been demonstrated in mercuric chloride and glycerol induced renal injury.[216–218] In cell culture, HGF, but not IGF-1 or EGF, decreased death of MDCK cells after ischemic injury by decreasing necrosis and apoptosis.[219] However, no studies to date have evaluated the potential role of HGF in human ARF.

Erythropoietin

Erythropoietin (EPO) is a growth factor synthesized primarily in the renal cortex. Erythropoietin receptors have been found within the kidney, localized to mesangial cells as well as proximal and distal tubular cells.[220] Although the normal kidney appears to be unresponsive to EPO, limited work in animals suggests that following ischemic injury, EPO may induce tubular cell proliferation.[221–223] Depressed plasma EPO levels have been documented in hemodynamically-mediated acute renal failure.[224] In a rat model of ischemic renal failure, EPO treatment has been demonstrated to ameliorate the anemia and decrease mortality.[221] In a rat model of cisplatinum-induced acute renal failure, EPO has been documented to improve GFR and RPF as well as hasten tubular regeneration.[222] These effects were independent of effects on hematocrit values and blood pressure.[223] Further studies will be required to demonstrate benefits in human disease.

CONCLUSION

Due to the significant incidence and consequences of acute renal failure, multiple efforts have been made to demonstrate the efficacy of hormonal therapies in preventing or treating acute tubular necrosis. Although preliminary studies in animals and small populations had suggested promise, large trials have recurrently failed to demonstrate efficacy of hormonal therapies. Additionally, growth factor therapy has failed to demonstrate efficacy in speeding tubular regeneration or recovery. Whether these failures are damning to the conceptual theory of ATN or due to difficulties in protocol (timing, dosing of agents) is difficult to know. Alternative therapeutic targets, such as oxidant stress and inflammation, are presently being studied. Future efforts may be successful in limiting the dramatic sequelae of ARF, but, presently, supportive therapy continues to be the best physicians can offer.

References

1. Chertow GM: On the design and analysis of multicenter trials in acute renal failure. Am J Kidney Dis 1997; 30(5 suppl 4):S96-S101.
2. Clermont G, Acker CG, Angus DC, et al: Renal failure in the ICU: Comparison of the impact of acute renal failure and end-stage renal disease on ICU outcomes. Kidney Int 2002; 62:986-996.
3. Brivet FG, Kleinknecht DJ, Loirat P, Landais PJ: Acute renal failure in intensive care units? causes, outcome, and prognostic factors of hospital mortality; a prospective, multicenter study. French Study Group on Acute Renal Failure. Crit Care Med 1996; 24:192-198.
4. Rangel-Frausto MS, Pittet D, Costigan M, et al: The natural history of the systemic inflammatory response syndrome (SIRS). A prospective study. JAMA 1995; 273:117-123.
5. Chen YC, Fang JT, Tien YC, et al: Organ system failures predict prognosis in critically ill patients with acute renal failure requiring dialysis. Changgeng Yi Xue Za Zhi 2000; 23:8-13.
6. Chertow GM, Levy EM, Hammermeister KE, et al: Independent association between acute renal failure and mortality following cardiac surgery. Am J Med 1998; 104:343-348.
7. Levy EM, Viscoli CM, Horwitz RI, et al: The effect of acute renal failure on mortality. A cohort analysis. JAMA 1996; 275:1489-1494.
8. Arendshorst WJ, Finn WF, Gottschalk CW: Micropuncture study of acute renal failure following temporary renal ischemia in the rat. Kidney Int Suppl 1976; 6:S100-S105.
9. Bayati A, Nygren K, Kallskog O, Wolgast M: The long-term outcome of postischemic acute renal failure in the rat. Ren Fail 1992; 14:333-336.

10. Mason J, Beck F, Dorge A, et al: Intracellular electrolyte composition following renal ischemia. Kidney Int 1981; 20:61-70.
11. Molitoris BA, Falk SA, Dahl RH: Ischemia-induced loss of epithelial polarity. Role of the tight junction. J Clin Invest 1989; 84:1334-1339.
12. Venkatachalam MA, Weinberg JM: Mechanisms of cell injury in ATP-depleted proximal tubules. Role of glycine, calcium, and polyphosphoinositides. Nephrol Dial Transplant 1994; 9:15-21.
13. Lieberthal W, Levine JS: Mechanisms of apoptosis and its potential role in renal tubular epithelial cell injury. Am J Physiol 1996; 271:F477-F488.
14. Myers BD, Carrie BJ, Yee RR, et al: Pathophysiology of hemodynamically mediated acute renal failure in man. Kidney Int 1980; 18:495-504.
15. Myers BD, Chui F, Hilberman M, Michaels AS: Transtubular leakage of glomerular filtrate in human acute renal failure. Am J Physiol 1979; 237:F319-F325.
16. Yagil Y, Myers BD, Jamison RL: Course and pathogenesis of postischemic acute renal failure in the rat. Am J Physiol 1988; 255:F257-F264.
17. Moran SM, Myers BD: Pathophysiology of protracted acute renal failure in man. J Clin Invest 1985; 76:1440-1448.
18. Myers BD, Churchill P: Hemodynamically mediated acute renal failure. N Engl J Med 1986; 314:97-105.
19. Iaina A, Solomon S, Gavendo S, Eliahou HE: Reduction in severity of acute renal failure (ARF) in rats by dopamine. Biomedicine 1977; 27:137-139.
20. Gomez-Garre DN, Lopez-Farre A, Eleno N, Lopez-Novoa JM: Comparative effects of dopexamine and dopamine on glycerol-induced acute renal failure in rats. Ren Fail 1996; 18:59-68.
21. Szerlip HM: Renal-dose dopamine: fact and fiction. Ann Intern Med 1991; 115:153-154.
22. Thompson BT, Cockrill BA: Renal-dose dopamine: A siren song? Lancet 1994; 344:7-8.
23. Sowers JR, Crane PD, Beck FW, et al: Relationship between urinary dopamine production and natriuresis after acute intravascular volume expansion with sodium chloride in dogs. Endocrinology 1984; 115:2085-2090.
24. Carey RM, Siragy HM, Ragsdale NV, et al: Dopamine-1 and dopamine-2 mechanisms in the control of renal function. Am J Hypertens 1990; 3:59S-63S.
25. Hubbard PC, Henderson IW: Renal dopamine and the tubular handling of sodium. J Molec Endocrinol 1995; 14:139-155.
26. Lee MR: Dopamine and the kidney: Ten years on. Clin Sci 1993; 84:357-375.
27. Hayashi M, Yamaji Y, Kitajima W, Saruta T: Aromatic L-amino acid decarboxylase activity along the rat nephron. Am J Physiol 1990; 258:F28-F33.
28. Seri I, Kone BC, Gullans SR, et al: Locally formed dopamine inhibits Na+-K+-ATPase activity in rat renal cortical tubule cells. Am J Physiol 1988; 255:F666-F673.
29. Huo TL, Grenader A, Blandina P, Healy DP: Prostaglandin E2 production in rat IMCD cells. II. Possible role for locally formed dopamine. Am J Physiol 1991; 261:F655-F662.
30. Wang ZQ, Siragy HM, Felder RA, Carey RM: Preferential release of renal dopamine into the tubule lumen: Effect of chronic sodium loading. Clin Exp Hypertens (New York) 1997; 19:107-116.
31. Schwartz LB, Gewertz BL: The renal response to low dose dopamine. J Surg Res 1988; 45:574-588.
32. D'Orio V, el Allaf D, Juchmes J, Marcelle R: The use of low doses of dopamine in intensive care medicine. Arch Int Physiol Biochim 1984; 92:S11-S20.
33. Goldberg LI: Dopamine? clinical uses of an endogenous catecholamine. N Engl J Med 1974; 291:707-710.
34. Olsen NV, Lang-Jensen T, Hansen JM, et al: Effects of acute beta-adrenoceptor blockade with metoprolol on the renal response to dopamine in normal humans. Br J Clin Pharmacol 1994; 37: 347-353.
35. Olsen NV, Lund J, Jensen PF, et al: Dopamine, dobutamine, and dopexamine. A comparison of renal effects in unanesthetized human volunteers. Anesthesiology 1993; 79:685-694.
36. Yura T, Yuasa S, Fukunaga M, et al: Role for Doppler ultrasound in the assessment of renal circulation: Effects of dopamine and dobutamine on renal hemodynamics in humans. Nephron 1995; 71:168-175.
37. Garwood S, Davis E, Harris SN: Intraoperative transesophageal ultrasonography can measure renal blood flow. J Cardiothorac Vasc Anesth 2001; 15:65-71.
38. Hollenberg NK, Adams DF, Mendell P, et al: Renal vascular responses to dopamine: Haemodynamic and angiographic observations in normal man. Clin Sci Mol Med 1973; 45:733-742.
39. Kishimoto N, Mori Y, Nishiue T, et al: Renal blood flow measurement with contrast-enhanced harmonic ultrasonography: Evaluation of dopamine-induced changes in renal cortical perfusion in humans. Clin Nephrol 2003; 59:423-428.
40. McDonald RH Jr, Goldberg Li, Mcnay JL, Tuttle EP Jr: Effects of dopamine in man: Augmentation of sodium excretion, glomerular filtration and renal plasma flow. J Clin Invest 1964; 43:1116.
41. Bryan AG, Bolsin SN, Vianna PT, Haloush H: Modification of the diuretic and natriuretic effects of a dopamine infusion by fluid loading in preoperative cardiac surgical patients. J Cardiothorac Vasc Anesth 1995; 9:158-163.
42. Agnoli GC, Cacciari M, Garutti C, et al: Effects of extracellular fluid volume changes on renal response to low-dose dopamine infusion in normal women. Clin Physiol 1987; 7:465-479.
43. Orme ML, Breckenridge A, Dollery CT: The effects of long term administration of dopamine on renal function in hypertensive patients. Eur J Clin Pharmacol 1973; 6:150-155.
44. Girbes AR, Lieverse AG, Smit AJ, et al: Lack of specific renal haemodynamic effects of different doses of dopamine after infrarenal aortic surgery. Br J Anaesth 1996; 77:753-757.
45. Seri I: Cardiovascular, renal, and endocrine actions of dopamine in neonates and children. J Pediatr 1995; 126:333-344.
46. Mulkerrin E, Epstein FH, Clark BA: Reduced renal response to low-dose dopamine infusion in the elderly. J Gerontol A Biol Sci Med Sci 1995; 50:M271-M275.
47. Fuiano G, Sund S, Mazza G, et al: Renal hemodynamic response to maximal vasodilating stimulus in healthy older subjects. Kidney Int 2001; 59:1052-1058.
48. ter Wee PM, Smit AJ, Rosman JB, et al: Effect of intravenous infusion of low-dose dopamine on renal function in normal individuals and in patients with renal disease. Am J Nephrol 1986; 6:42-46.
49. Duke GJ, Briedis JH, Weaver RA: Renal support in critically ill patients: Low-dose dopamine or low-dose dobutamine? Crit Care Med 1994; 22:1919-1925.
50. Chiolero R, Borgeat A, Fisher A: Postoperative arrhythmias and risk factors after open heart surgery. Thorac Cardiovasc Surg 1991; 39:81-84.
51. Hampton JR, van Veldhuisen DJ, Kleber FX, et al: Randomised study of effect of ibopamine on survival in patients with advanced severe heart failure. Second Prospective Randomised Study of Ibopamine on Mortality and Efficacy (PRIME II) Investigators. Lancet 1997; 349:971-977.
52. Van den Berghe G, de Zegher F: Anterior pituitary function during critical illness and dopamine treatment. Crit Care Med 1996; 24:1580-1590.
53. Devins SS, Miller A, Herndon BL, et al: Effects of dopamine on T-lymphocyte proliferative responses and serum prolactin concentrations in critically ill patients. Crit Care Med 1992; 20:1644-1649.
54. Segal JM, Phang PT, Walley KR: Low-dose dopamine hastens onset of gut ischemia in a porcine model of hemorrhagic shock. J Appl Physiol 1992; 73:1159-1164.
55. Giraud GD, MacCannell KL: Decreased nutrient blood flow during dopamine- and epinephrine-induced intestinal vasodilation. J Pharmacol Exp Ther 1984; 230:214-220.

56. Marik PE, Mohedin M: The contrasting effects of dopamine and norepinephrine on systemic and splanchnic oxygen utilization in hyperdynamic sepsis. JAMA 1994; 272:1354-1357.
57. Myles PS, Buckland MR, Schenk NJ, et al: Effect of "renal-dose" dopamine on renal function following cardiac surgery. Anaesth Intensive Care 1993; 21:56-61.
58. Piper SN, Kumle B, Maleck WH, et al: Diltiazem may preserve renal tubular integrity after cardiac surgery. Can J Anaesth 2003; 50:285-292.
59. Yavuz S, Ayabakan N, Goncu MT, Ozdemir IA: Effect of combined dopamine and diltiazem on renal function after cardiac surgery. Med Sci Mon 2002; 8:PI45-PI50.
60. Sumeray M, Robertson C, Lapsley M, et al: Low dose dopamine infusion reduces renal tubular injury following cardiopulmonary bypass surgery. J Nephrol 2001; 14:397-402.
61. Lassnigg A, Donner E, Grubhofer G, et al: Lack of renoprotective effects of dopamine and furosemide during cardiac surgery. J Am Soc Nephrol 2000; 11:97-104.
62. Tang AT, El-Gamel A, Keevil B, et al: The effect of 'renal-dose' dopamine on renal tubular function following cardiac surgery: Assessed by measuring retinol binding protein (RBP). Eur J Cardiothorac Surg 1999; 15:717-721; discussion 721-722.
63. Paul MD, Mazer CD, Byrick RJ, et al: Influence of mannitol and dopamine on renal function during elective infrarenal aortic clamping in man. Am J Nephrol 1986; 6:427-434.
64. Baldwin L, Henderson A, Hickman P: Effect of postoperative low-dose dopamine on renal function after elective major vascular surgery. Ann Intern Med 1994; 120:744-747.
65. Antonucci F, Calo L, Rizzolo M, et al: Nifedipine can preserve renal function in patients undergoing aortic surgery with infrarenal crossclamping. Nephron 1996; 74:668-673.
66. Carmellini M, Romagnoli J, Giulianotti PC, et al: Dopamine lowers the incidence of delayed graft function in transplanted kidney patients treated with cyclosporine A. Transplant Proc 1994; 26:2626-2629.
67. Donmez A, Karaaslan D, Sekerci S, et al: The effects of diltiazem and dopamine on early graft function in renal transplant recipients. Transplant Proc 1999; 31:3305-3306.
68. Grundmann R, Kindler J, Meider G, et al: Dopamine treatment of human cadaver kidney graft recipients: A prospectively randomized trial. Klin Wochenschr 1982; 60:193-197.
69. Kadieva VS, Friedman L, Margolius LP, et al: The effect of dopamine on graft function in patients undergoing renal transplantation. Anesth Analg 1993; 76:362-365.
70. Sandberg J, Tyden G, Groth CG: Low-dose dopamine infusion following cadaveric renal transplantation: No effect on the incidence of ATN. Transplant Proc 1992; 24:357.
71. Spicer ST, Gruenewald S, O'Connell PJ, et al: Low-dose dopamine after kidney transplantation: Assessment by Doppler ultrasound. Clin Transplant 1999; 13:479-483.
72. Polson RJ, Park GR, Lindop MJ, et al: The prevention of renal impairment in patients undergoing orthotopic liver grafting by infusion of low dose dopamine. Anaesthesia 1987; 42:15-19.
73. Swygert TH, Roberts LC, Valek TR, et al: Effect of intraoperative low-dose dopamine on renal function in liver transplant recipients. Anesthesiology 1991; 75:571-576.
74. Parks RW, Diamond T, McCrory DC, et al: Prospective study of postoperative renal function in obstructive jaundice and the effect of perioperative dopamine. Br J Surg 1994; 81:437-439.
75. Stevens MA, McCullough PA, Tobin KJ, et al: A prospective randomized trial of prevention measures in patients at high risk for contrast nephropathy: Results of the P.R.I.N.C.E. Study. Prevention of Radiocontrast Induced Nephropathy Clinical Evaluation. J Am Coll Cardiol 1999; 33:403-411.
76. Abizaid AS, Clark CE, Mintz GS, et al: Effects of dopamine and aminophylline on contrast-induced acute renal failure after coronary angioplasty in patients with preexisting renal insufficiency. Am J Cardiol 1999; 83:260-263, A265.
77. Hall KA, Wong RW, Hunter GC, et al: Contrast-induced nephrotoxicity: The effects of vasodilator therapy. J Surg Res 1992; 53:317-320.
78. Hans B, Hans SS, Mittal VK, et al: Renal functional response to dopamine during and after arteriography in patients with chronic renal insufficiency. Radiology 1990; 176:651-654.
79. Kapoor A, Sinha N, Sharma RK, et al: Use of dopamine in prevention of contrast induced acute renal failure?a randomised study. Int J Cardiol 1996; 53:233-236.
80. Weisberg LS, Kurnik PB, Kurnik BR: Risk of radiocontrast nephropathy in patients with and without diabetes mellitus. Kidney Int 1994; 45:259-265.
81. Weisberg LS, Kurnik PB, Kurnik BR: Dopamine and renal blood flow in radiocontrast-induced nephropathy in humans. Ren Fail 1993; 15:61-68.
82. Henderson IS, Beattie TJ, Kennedy AC: Dopamine hydrochloride in oliguric states. Lancet 1980; 2:827-828.
83. Graziani G, Cantaluppi A, Casati S, et al: Dopamine and furosemide in oliguric acute renal failure. Nephron 1984; 37: 39-42.
84. Flancbaum L, Choban PS, Dasta JF: Quantitative effects of low-dose dopamine on urine output in oliguric surgical intensive care unit patients. Crit Care Med 1994; 22:61-68.
85. Pavoni V, Verri M, Ferraro L, et al: Plasma dopamine concentration and effects of low dopamine doses on urinary output after major vascular surgery. Kidney Int Suppl 1998; 66:S75-S80.
86. Marik PE: Low-dose dopamine in critically ill oliguric patients: The influence of the renin-angiotensin system. Heart Lung J Acute Crit Care 1993; 22:171-175.
87. Ichai C, Passeron C, Carles M, et al: Prolonged low-dose dopamine infusion induces a transient improvement in renal function in hemodynamically stable, critically ill patients: A single-blind, prospective, controlled study. Crit Care Med 2000; 28:1329-1335.
88. Chertow GM, Sayegh MH, Allgren RL, Lazarus JM: Is the administration of dopamine associated with adverse or favorable outcomes in acute renal failure? Auriculin Anaritide Acute Renal Failure Study Group. Am J Med 1996; 101:49-53.
89. Kellum JA, M Decker J: Use of dopamine in acute renal failure: A meta-analysis. Crit Care Med 2001; 29:1526-1531.
90. Bellomo R, Chapman M, Finfer S, et al: Low-dose dopamine in patients with early renal dysfunction: A placebo-controlled randomised trial. Australian and New Zealand Intensive Care Society (ANZICS) Clinical Trials Group. Lancet 2000; 356:2139-2143.
91. Schaer GL, Fink MP, Parrillo JE: Norepinephrine alone versus norepinephrine plus low-dose dopamine: Enhanced renal blood flow with combination pressor therapy. Crit Care Med 1985; 13:492-496.
92. Richer M, Robert S, Lebel M: Renal hemodynamics during norepinephrine and low-dose dopamine infusions in man. Crit Care Med 1996; 24:1150-1156.
93. Lherm T, Troche G, Rossignol M, et al: Renal effects of low-dose dopamine in patients with sepsis syndrome or septic shock treated with catecholamines. Intensive Care Med 1996; 22: 213-219.
94. Martin C, Papazian L, Perrin G, et al: Norepinephrine or dopamine for the treatment of hyperdynamic septic shock? Chest 1993; 103:1826-1831.
95. Marin C, Eon B, Saux P, et al: Renal effects of norepinephrine used to treat septic shock patients. Crit Care Med 1990; 18: 282-285.
96. Hunter DW, Chamsuddin A, Bjarnason H, Kowalik K: Preventing contrast-induced nephropathy with fenoldopam. Tech Vasc Interv Radiol 2001; 4:53-56.
97. Ragsdale NV, Lynd M, Chevalier RL, et al: Selective peripheral dopamine-1 receptor stimulation. Differential responses to sodium loading and depletion in humans. Hypertension 1990; 15:914-921.

98. Girbes AR, Smit AJ, Meijer S, Reitsma WD: Renal and endocrine effects of fenoldopam and metoclopramide in normal man. Nephron 1990; 56:179-185.
99. Hughes JM, Beck TR, Rose CE Jr, Carey RM: The effect of selective dopamine-1 receptor stimulation on renal and adrenal function in man. J Clin Endocrinol Metab 1988; 66:518-525.
100. Hughes JM, Ragsdale NV, Felder RA, et al: Diuresis and natriuresis during continuous dopamine-1 receptor stimulation. Hypertension 1988; 11:I69-I74.
101. Allison NL, Dubb JW, Ziemniak JA, et al: The effect of fenoldopam, a dopaminergic agonist, on renal hemodynamics. Clin Pharmacol Ther 1987; 41:282-288.
102. Stote RM, Dubb JW, Familiar RG, et al: A new oral renal vasodilator, fenoldopam. Clin Pharmacol Ther 1983; 34:309-315.
103. Pollock DM, Arendshorst WJ: Tubuloglomerular feedback and blood flow autoregulation during DA1-induced renal vasodilation. Am J Physiol 1990; 258:F627-F635.
104. Bakris GL, Lass NA, Glock D: Renal hemodynamics in radiocontrast medium-induced renal dysfunction: A role for dopamine-1 receptors. Kidney Int 1999; 56:206-210.
105. Madyoon H: Clinical experience with the use of fenoldopam for prevention of radiocontrast nephropathy in high-risk patients. Rev Cardiovasc Med 2001; 2(suppl 1):S26-S30.
106. Kini AA, Sharma SK: Managing the high-risk patient: Experience with fenoldopam, a selective dopamine receptor agonist, in prevention of radiocontrast nephropathy during percutaneous coronary intervention. Rev Cardiovasc Med 2001; 2(suppl 1):S19-S25.
107. Chamsuddin AA, Kowalik KJ, Bjarnason H, et al: Using a dopamine type 1A receptor agonist in high-risk patients to ameliorate contrast-associated nephropathy. Am J Roentgenol 2002; 179:591-596.
108. Kini AS, Mitre CA, Kim M, et al: A protocol for prevention of radiographic contrast nephropathy during percutaneous coronary intervention: Effect of selective dopamine receptor agonist fenoldopam. Cathet Cardiovasc Interv 2002; 55:169-173.
109. Madyoon H, Croushore L, Weaver D, Mathur V: Use of fenoldopam to prevent radiocontrast nephropathy in high-risk patients. Cathet Cardiovasc Interv 2001; 53:341-345.
110. Stone GW, McCullough PA, Tumlin JA, et al: Fenoldopam mesylate for the prevention of contrast-induced nephropathy: A randomized controlled trial. JAMA 2003; 290:2284-2291.
111. Allaqaband S, Tumuluri R, Malik AM, et al: Prospective randomized study of N-acetylcysteine, fenoldopam, and saline for prevention of radiocontrast-induced nephropathy. Cathet Cardiovasc Interv 2002; 57:279-283.
112. Tumlin JA, Wang A, Murray PT, Mathur VS: Fenoldopam mesylate blocks reductions in renal plasma flow after radiocontrast dye infusion: A pilot trial in the prevention of contrast nephropathy. Am Heart J 2002; 143:894-903.
113. Brooks DP, Drutz DJ, Ruffolo RR Jr: Prevention and complete reversal of cyclosporine A-induced renal vasoconstriction and nephrotoxicity in the rat by fenoldopam. J Pharmacol Exp Ther 1990; 254:375-379.
114. Jorkasky DK, Audet P, Shusterman N, et al: Fenoldopam reverses cyclosporine-induced renal vasoconstriction in kidney transplant recipients. Am J Kidney Dis 1992; 19:567-572.
115. Gilbert TB, Hasnain JU, Flinn WR, et al: Fenoldopam infusion associated with preserving renal function after aortic cross-clamping for aneurysm repair. J of Cardiovasc Pharmacol Ther 2001; 6:31-36.
116. Halpenny M, Markos F, Snow HM, et al: The effects of fenoldopam on renal blood flow and tubular function during aortic cross-clamping in anaesthetized dogs. Eur J Anaesth 2000; 17:491-498.
117. Garwood S, Swamidoss CP, Davis EA, et al: A case series of low-dose fenoldopam in seventy cardiac surgical patients at increased risk of renal dysfunction. J Cardiothorac Vasc Anesth 2003; 17:17-21.
118. Halpenny M, Lakshmi S, O'Donnell A, et al: Fenoldopam: Renal and splanchnic effects in patients undergoing coronary artery bypass grafting. Anaesthesia 2001; 56:953-960.
119. Caimmi PP, Pagani L, Micalizzi E, et al: Fenoldopam for renal protection in patients undergoing cardiopulmonary bypass. J Cardiothorac Vasc Anesth 2003; 17:491-494.
120. de Bold AJ, Borenstein HB, Veress AT, Sonnenberg H: A rapid and potent natriuretic response to intravenous injection of atrial myocardial extract in rats. Reprinted from Life Sci 1981; 28:89-94. J Am Soc Nephrol 2001; 12:403-409.
121. Vesely DL: Natriuretic peptides and acute renal failure. Am J Physiol Ren Physiol 2003; 285:F167-F177.
122. Yandle TG, Richards AM, Nicholls MG, et al: Metabolic clearance rate and plasma half life of alpha-human atrial natriuretic peptide in man. Life Sci 1986; 38:1827-1833.
123. Thoren P, Mark AL, Morgan DA, et al: Activation of vagal depressor reflexes by atriopeptins inhibits renal sympathetic nerve activity. Am J Physiol 1986; 251:H1252-H1259.
124. Cohen ML, Schenck KW: Atriopeptin II: Differential sensitivity of arteries and veins from the rat. Eur J Pharmacol 1985; 108:103-104.
125. Opgenorth TJ, Novosad EI: Atrial natriuretic factor and endothelin interactions in control of vascular tone. Eur J Pharmacol 1990; 191:351-357.
126. Fried TA, McCoy RN, Osgood RW, Stein JH: Effect of atriopeptin II on determinants of glomerular filtration rate in the in vitro perfused dog glomerulus. Am J Physiol 1986; 250:F1119-F1122.
127. Sonnenberg H, Cupples WA, de Bold AJ, Veress AT: Intrarenal localization of the natriuretic effect of cardiac atrial extract. Can J Physiol Pharmacol 1982; 60:1149-1152.
128. Sonnenberg H, Honrath U, Chong CK, Wilson DR: Atrial natriuretic factor inhibits sodium transport in medullary collecting duct. Am J Physiol 1986; 250:F963-F966.
129. Zeidel ML, Seifter JL, Lear S, et al: Atrial peptides inhibit oxygen consumption in kidney medullary collecting duct cells. Am J Physiol 1986; 251:F379-F383.
130. Roy DR: Effect of synthetic ANP on renal and loop of Henle functions in the young rat. Am J Physiol 1986; 251:F220-F225.
131. Harris PJ, Thomas D, Morgan TO: Atrial natriuretic peptide inhibits angiotensin-stimulated proximal tubular sodium and water reabsorption. Nature 1987; 326:697-698.
132. Ortola FV, Seri I, Downes S, et al: Dopamine1-receptor blockade inhibits ANP-induced phosphaturia and calciuria in rats. Am J Physiol 1990; 259:F138-F146.
133. Nonoguchi H, *et al*: Atrial natriuretic factor inhibits vasopressin-stimulated osmotic water permeability in rat inner medullary collecting duct. J Clin Invest 1988; 82:1383-1390.
134. Nonoguchi H, Sands JM, Knepper MA: ANF inhibits NaCl and fluid absorption in cortical collecting duct of rat kidney. Am J Physiol 1989; 256:F179-F186.
135. Nonoguchi H, Tomita K, Marumo F: Effects of atrial natriuretic peptide and vasopressin on chloride transport in long- and short-looped medullary thick ascending limbs. J Clin Invest 1992; 90:349-357.
136. Schafferhans K, Heidbreder E, Grimm D, Heidland A: Human atrial natriuretic factor prevents against norepinephrine-induced acute renal failure in the rat. Klin Wochenschr 1986; 64:73-77.
137. Schafferhans K, Heidbreder E, Grimm D, Heidland A: Norepinephrine-induced acute renal failure: Beneficial effects of atrial natriuretic factor. Nephron 1986; 44:240-244.
138. Conger JD, Falk SA, Hammond WS: Atrial natriuretic peptide and dopamine in established acute renal failure in the rat. Kidney Int 1991; 40:21-28.
139. Heidbreder E, Zollner T, Schafferhans K, Gotz R: Atrial natriuretic peptide reverses experimental acute renal failure induced

by arginine vasopressin. Miner Electrolyte Metab 1990; 16: 48-53.
140. Mitaka C, Hirata Y, Habuka K, et al: Atrial natriuretic peptide infusion improves ischemic renal failure after suprarenal abdominal aortic cross-clamping in dogs. Crit Care Med 2003; 31:2205-2210.
141. Nakamoto M, Shapiro JI, Shanley PF, et al: In vitro and in vivo protective effect of atriopeptin III on ischemic acute renal failure. J Clin Invest 1987; 80:698-705.
142. Shaw SG, Weidmann P, Hodler J, et al: Atrial natriuretic peptide protects against acute ischemic renal failure in the rat. J Clin Invest 1987; 80:1232-1237.
143. Gianello P, Poelaert D, Ramboux A, et al: Beneficial effect of atrial natriuretic factor on ischemically injured kidneys in rats. Transplant Proc 1988; 20:921-922.
144. Conger JD, Falk SA, Yuan BH, Schrier RW: Atrial natriuretic peptide and dopamine in a rat model of ischemic acute renal failure. Kidney Int 1989; 35:1126-1132.
145. Gianello P, Squifflet JP, Carlier M, et al: Evidence that atrial natriuretic factor is the humoral factor by which volume loading or mannitol infusion produces an improved renal function after acute ischemia. An experimental study in dogs. Transplantation 1989; 48:9-14.
146. Lieberthal W, Sheridan AM, Valeri CR: Protective effect of atrial natriuretic factor and mannitol following renal ischemia. Am J Physiol 1990; 258:F1266-F1272.
147. Neumayer HH, Blossei N, Seherr-Thohs U, Wagner K: Amelioration of postischaemic acute renal failure in conscious dogs by human atrial natriuretic peptide. Nephrol Dial Transplant 1990; 5:32-38.
148. Klein HG, Dimitrov D, Atanasova I, et al: Atrial natriuretic factor infusion following acute renal ischemia in anesthetized dogs. Ren Physiol Biochem 1992; 15:73-82.
149. Haab F, Farge D, Nochy D, et al: [Beneficial effects of perfusion of atrial natriuretic factor in acute post-ischemic renal insufficiency in the rat]. Chirurgie 1992; 118:678-682.
150. Atanasova I, Girchev R, Dimitrov D, et al: Atrial natriuretic peptide and dopamine in a dog model of acute renal ischemia. Acta Physiol Hung 1994; 82:75-85.
151. Heidbreder E, Schafferhans K, Schramm D, et al: Toxic renal failure in the rat: beneficial effects of atrial natriuretic factor. Klin Wochenschr 1986; 64:78-82.
152. Seki G, Suzuki K, Nonaka T, et al: Effects of atrial natriuretic peptide on glycerol induced acute renal failure in the rat. Jpn Heart J 1992; 33:383-393.
153. Schafferhans K, Heidbreder E, Sperber S, et al: Atrial natriuretic peptide in gentamicin-induced acute renal failure. Kidney Int Suppl 1988; 25:S101-S103.
154. Deegan PM, Ryan MP, Basinger MA, et al: Protection from cisplatin nephrotoxicity by A68828, an atrial natriuretic peptide. Ren Fail 1995; 17:117-123.
155. Chen X, Yang H, Mai W: A study on combined treatment with ANP and dopamine in acute renal failure in rats. Chung Hua Nei Ko Tsa Chih 1995; 34:609-611.
156. Kuse ER, Meyer M, Constantin R, et al: [Urodilatin (INN: ularitide). A new peptide in the treatment of acute kidney failure following liver transplantation.] Anaesthesist 1996; 45: 351-358.
157. Brenner P, Meyer M, Reichenspurner H, et al: Significance of prophylactic urodilatin (INN: ularitide) infusion for the prevention of acute renal failure in patients after heart transplantation. Eur J Med Res 1995; 1:137-143.
158. Hummel M, Kuhn M, Bub A, et al: Urodilatin: A new peptide with beneficial effects in the postoperative therapy of cardiac transplant recipients. Clin Investig 1992; 70:674-682.
159. Herbert MK, Ginzel S, Muhlschlegel S, Weis KH: Concomitant treatment with urodilatin (ularitide) does not improve renal function in patients with acute renal failure after major abdominal surgery? a randomized controlled trial. Wien Klin Wochenschr 1999; 111:141-147.
160. Wiebe K, Meyer M, Wahlers T, et al: Acute renal failure following cardiac surgery is reverted by administration of Urodilatin (INN: Ularitide). Eur J Med Res 1996; 1:259-265.
161. Meyer M, Pfarr E, Schirmer G, et al: Therapeutic use of the natriuretic peptide ularitide in acute renal failure. Ren Fail 1999; 21:85-100.
162. Sward K, Valson F, Ricksten SE: Long-term infusion of atrial natriuretic peptide (ANP) improves renal blood flow and glomerular filtration rate in clinical acute renal failure. Acta Anaesthesiol Scand 2001; 45:536-542.
163. Valsson F, Ricksten SE, Hedner T, Lundin S: Effects of atrial natriuretic peptide on acute renal impairment in patients with heart failure after cardiac surgery. Intensive Care Med 1996; 22:230-236.
164. Rahman SN, Kim GE, Mathew AS, et al: Effects of atrial natriuretic peptide in clinical acute renal failure. Kidney Int 1994; 45:1731-1738.
165. Allgren RL, Marbury TC, Rahman SN, et al: Anaritide in acute tubular necrosis. Auriculin Anaritide Acute Renal Failure Study Group. N Engl J Med 1997; 336:828-834.
166. Lewis J, Salem MM, Chertow GM, et al: Atrial natriuretic factor in oliguric acute renal failure. Anaritide Acute Renal Failure Study Group. Am J Kidney Dis 2000; 36:767-774.
167. Kurnik BR, Allgren RL, Genter FC, et al: Prospective study of atrial natriuretic peptide for the prevention of radiocontrast-induced nephropathy. Am J Kidney Dis 1998; 31:674-680.
168. Gianello P, Carlier M, Jamart J, et al: Effect of 1-28 alpha-h atrial natriuretic peptide on acute renal failure in cadaveric renal transplantation. Clin Transplant 1995; 9:481-489.
169. Ratcliffe PJ, Richardson AJ, Kirby JE, et al: Effect of intravenous infusion of atriopeptin 3 on immediate renal allograft function. Kidney Int 1991; 39:164-168.
170. Sands JM, Neylan JF, Olson RA, et al: Atrial natriuretic factor does not improve the outcome of cadaveric renal transplantation. J Am Soc Nephrol 1991; 1:1081-1086.
171. Hammerman MR: New treatments for acute renal failure: Growth factors and beyond. Curr Opin Nephrol Hypertens 1997; 6:7-9.
172. Hammerman MR, Miller SB: Therapeutic use of growth factors in renal failure. J Am Soc Nephrol 1994; 5:1-11.
173. Harris RC, Daniel TO: Epidermal growth factor binding, stimulation of phosphorylation, and inhibition of gluconeogenesis in rat proximal tubule. J Cell Physiol 1989; 139:383-391.
174. Norman J, Badie-Dezfooly B, Nord EP, et al: EGF-induced mitogenesis in proximal tubular cells: potentiation by angiotensin II. Am J Physiol 1987; 253:F299-F309.
175. Quigley R, Baum M: Effects of epidermal growth factor and transforming growth factor-alpha on rabbit proximal tubule solute transport. Am J Physiol 1994; 266:F459-F465.
176. Rogers SA, Karl IE, Hammerman MR: Growth hormone directly stimulates gluconeogenesis in canine renal proximal tubule. Am J Physiol 1989; 257:E751-E756.
177. Rogers SA, Ryan G, Hammerman MR: Insulin-like growth factors I and II are produced in the metanephros and are required for growth and development in vitro. J Cell Biol 1991; 113:1447-1453.
178. Igawa T, Matsumoto K, Kanda S, et al: Hepatocyte growth factor may function as a renotropic factor for regeneration in rats with acute renal injury. Am J Physiol 1993; 265:F61-F69.
179. Safirstein R, Price PM, Saggi SJ, Harris RC: Changes in gene expression after temporary renal ischemia. Kidney Int 1990; 37:1515-1521.
180. Safirstein R: Gene expression in nephrotoxic and ischemic acute renal failure. J Am Soc Nephrol 1994; 4:1387-1395.
181. Toback FG: Regeneration after acute tubular necrosis. Kidney Int 1992; 41:226-246.

182. Humes HD, Cieslinski DA, Coimbra TM, et al: Epidermal growth factor enhances renal tubule cell regeneration and repair and accelerates the recovery of renal function in postischemic acute renal failure. J Clin Invest 1989; 84:1757-1761.
183. Miller SB, Martin DR, Kissane J, Hammerman MR: Insulin-like growth factor I accelerates recovery from ischemic acute tubular necrosis in the rat. Proc Natl Acad Sci U S A 1992; 89:11876-11880.
184. Miller SB, Martin DR, Kissane J, Hammerman MR: Hepatocyte growth factor accelerates recovery from acute ischemic renal injury in rats. Am J Physiol 1994; 266:F129-F134.
185. Norman J, Tsau YK, Bacay A, Fine LG: Epidermal growth factor accelerates functional recovery from ischaemic acute tubular necrosis in the rat: role of the epidermal growth factor receptor. Clin Sci 1990; 78:445-450.
186. Le Roith D: Seminars in medicine of the Beth Israel Deaconess Medical Center. Insulin-like growth factors. N Engl J Med 1997; 336:633-640.
187. Hammerman MR: The growth hormone-insulin-like growth factor axis in kidney. Am J Physiol 1989; 257:F503-F514.
188. Rogers SA, Miller SB, Hammerman MR: Insulin-like growth factor I gene expression in isolated rat renal collecting duct is stimulated by epidermal growth factor. J Clin Invest 1991; 87:347-351.
189. Hirschberg R, Kopple JD: Effects of growth hormone and IGF-I on renal function. Kidney Int Suppl 1989; 27:S20-S26.
190. Tsao T, Wang J, Fervenza FC, et al: Renal growth hormone—insulin-like growth factor-I system in acute renal failure. Kidney Int 1995; 47:1658-1668.
191. Haylor J, Singh I, el Nahas AM: Nitric oxide synthesis inhibitor prevents vasodilation by insulin-like growth factor I. Kidney Int 1991; 39:333-335.
192. Hirschberg R, Kopple JD: Evidence that insulin-like growth factor I increases renal plasma flow and glomerular filtration rate in fasted rats. J Clin Invest 1989; 83:326-330.
193. Matejka GL, Jennische E: IGF-I binding and IGF-I mRNA expression in the post-ischemic regenerating rat kidney. Kidney Int 1992; 42:1113-1123.
194. Humes HD, Beals TF, Cieslinski DA, et al: Effects of transforming growth factor-beta, transforming growth factor-alpha, and other growth factors on renal proximal tubule cells. Lab Invest 1991; 64:538-545.
195. Ding H, Kopple JD, Cohen A, Hirschberg R: Recombinant human insulin-like growth factor-I accelerates recovery and reduces catabolism in rats with ischemic acute renal failure. J Clin Invest 1993; 91:2281-2287.
196. Clark R, Mortensen D, Rabkin R: Recovery from acute ischaemic renal failure is accelerated by des-(1-3)-insulin-like growth factor-1. Clin Sci 1994; 86:709-714.
197. Noguchi S, Kashihara Y, Ikegami Y, et al: Insulin-like growth factor-I ameliorates transient ischemia-induced acute renal failure in rats. J Pharmacol Exp Ther 1993; 267:919-926.
198. Hirschberg R, Ding H: Mechanisms of insulin-like growth factor-I-induced accelerated recovery in experimental ischemic acute renal failure. Miner Electrolyte Metab 1998; 24: 211-219.
199. Maestri M, Dafoe DC, Adams GA, et al: Insulin-like growth factor-I ameliorates delayed kidney graft function and the acute nephrotoxic effects of cyclosporine. Transplantation 1997; 64:185-190.
200. Petrinec D, Reilly JM, Sicard GA, et al: Insulin-like growth factor-I attenuates delayed graft function in a canine renal autotransplantation model. Surgery 1996; 120:221-225; discussion 225-226.
201. Franklin SC, Moulton M, Sicard GA, et al: Insulin-like growth factor I preserves renal function postoperatively. Am J Physiol 1997; 272:F257-F259.
202. Hirschberg R, Kopple J, Lipsett P, et al: Multicenter clinical trial of recombinant human insulin-like growth factor I in patients with acute renal failure. Kidney Int 1999; 55:2423-2432.
203. Hladunewich MA, Corrigan G, Derby GC, et al: A randomized, placebo-controlled trial of IGF-1 for delayed graft function: a human model to study postischemic ARF. Kidney Int 2003; 64:593-602.
204. Carpenter G, Zendegui JG: Epidermal growth factor, its receptor, and related proteins. Exp Cell Res 1986; 164:1-10.
205. Breyer MD, Jacobson HR, Breyer JA: Epidermal growth factor inhibits the hydroosmotic effect of vasopressin in the isolated perfused rabbit cortical collecting tubule. J Clin Invest 1988; 82:1313-1320.
206. Rogers SA, Ryan G, Hammerman MR: Metanephric transforming growth factor-alpha is required for renal organogenesis in vitro. Am J Physiol 1992; 262:F533-F539.
207. Verstrepen WA, Nouwen EJ, De Broe ME: Renal epidermal growth factor and insulin-like growth factor I in acute renal failure. Nephrol Dial Transplant 1994; 9:57-68.
208. Safirstein R, Zelent AZ, Price PM: Reduced renal preproepidermal growth factor mRNA and decreased EGF excretion in ARF. Kidney Int 1989; 36:810-815.
209. Yano T, Yazima S, Hagiwara K, et al: Activation of epidermal growth factor receptor in the early phase after renal ischemia-reperfusion in rat. Nephron 1999; 81:230-233.
210. Coimbra TM, Cieslinski DA, Humes HD: Epidermal growth factor accelerates renal repair in mercuric chloride nephrotoxicity. Am J Physiol 1990; 259:F438-F443.
211. Fervenza FC, Tsao T, Rabkin R: Response of the intrarenal insulin-like growth factor-I axis to acute ischemic injury and treatment with growth hormone and epidermal growth factor. Kidney Int 1996; 49:344-354.
212. Rogers SA, Miller SB, Hammerman MR: Altered EGF expression and thyroxine metabolism in kidneys following acute ischemic injury in rat. Am J Physiol 1996; 270:F21-F30.
213. Nakamura T, Teramoto H, Ichihara A: Purification and characterization of a growth factor from rat platelets for mature parenchymal hepatocytes in primary cultures. Proc Natl Acad Sci U S A 1986; 83:6489-6493.
214. Matsumoto K, Nakamura T: Hepatocyte growth factor: Renotropic role and potential therapeutics for renal diseases. Kidney Int 2001; 59:2023-2038.
215. Liu Y, Tolbert EM, Sun AM, Dworkin LD: Primary structure of rat HGF receptor and induced expression in glomerular mesangial cells. Am J Physiol 1996; 271:F679-F688.
216. Kawaida K, Matsumoto K, Shimazu H, Nakamura T: Hepatocyte growth factor prevents acute renal failure and accelerates renal regeneration in mice. Proc Natl Acad Sci U S A 1994; 91:4357-4361.
217. Nagano T, Mori-Kudo I, Tsuchida A, et al: Ameliorative effect of hepatocyte growth factor on glycerol-induced acute renal failure with acute tubular necrosis. Nephron 2002; 91:730-738.
218. Yamasaki N, Nagano T, Mori-Kudo I, et al: Hepatocyte growth factor protects functional and histological disorders of HgCl(2)-induced acute renal failure mice. Nephron 2002; 90: 195-205.
219. de Souza Durao M Jr, Razvickas CV, Goncalves EA, et al: The role of growth factors on renal tubular cells submitted to hypoxia and deprived of glucose. Ren Fail 2003; 25: 341-353.
220. Westenfelder C: Unexpected renal actions of erythropoietin. Exp Nephrol 2002; 10(5-6):294-298.
221. Nemoto T, Yokota N, Keane WF, Rabb H: Recombinant erythropoietin rapidly treats anemia in ischemic acute renal failure. Kidney Int 2001; 59:246-251.
222. Bagnis C, Beaufils H, Jacquiaud C, et al: Erythropoietin enhances recovery after cisplatin-induced acute renal failure in the rat. Nephrol Dial Transplant 2001; 16:932-938.

223. Vaziri ND, Zhou XJ, Liao SY: Erythropoietin enhances recovery from cisplatin-induced acute renal failure. Am J Physiol 1994; 266:F360-F366.
224. Giglio MJ, Huygens P, Frid A, et al: Depressed plasma erythropoietin levels in rats with hemodynamically-mediated acute renal failure. Acta Physiol Pharmacol Latinoam 1990; 40:299-308.
225. Bughi S, Horton R, Antonipillai I, et al: Comparison of dopamine and fenoldopam effects on renal blood flow and prostacyclin excretion in normal and essential hypertensive subjects. J Clin Endocrinol Metab 1989; 69:1116-1121.
226. de Lasson L, Hansen HE, Juhl B, et al: A randomised, clinical study of the effect of low-dose dopamine on central and renal haemodynamics in infrarenal aortic surgery. Eur J Vasc Endovasc Surg 1995; 10:82-90.
227. Parker S, Carlon GC, Isaacs M, et al: Dopamine administration in oliguria and oliguric renal failure. Crit Care Med 1981; 9:630-632.
228. Olsen NV, Hansen JM, Kanstrup IL, et al: Renal hemodynamics, tubular function, and response to low-dose dopamine during acute hypoxia in humans. J Appl Physiol 1993; 74:2166-2173.

Dialytic Management for Acute Renal Failure

Geoffrey S. Teehan, M.D., M.S. • Ravindra L. Mehta, M.D. • Glenn M. Chertow, M.D., M.P.H.

Over the last 2 decades, significant advances have been made in dialysis methods for replacement of renal function. These range from modifications in intermittent dialysis (e.g., biocompatible membranes, bicarbonate dialysate, dialysis machines with volumetric ultrafiltration controls) to the development of several modalities for continuous renal replacement therapy (CRRT).[1,2] Several of these techniques may be used to treat acute renal failure (ARF) in the intensive care unit (ICU), but little information exists for the most appropriate therapy in a given circumstance. The goals for treatment, indications and timing of dialytic intervention, choice of dialysis modality, and the effect of dialysis on outcomes from ARF need to be considered. This chapter outlines current concepts in the use of dialysis techniques for ARF and suggests an approach for selecting the optimal method of renal replacement therapy.

GOALS FOR RENAL REPLACEMENT FOR ACUTE RENAL FAILURE IN THE INTENSIVE CARE UNIT

The treatment of ARF with renal replacement therapy (RRT) has the following goals: (1) maintain fluid and electrolyte, acid-base, and solute homeostasis, (2) prevent further insults to the kidney, (3) promote healing and renal recovery, and (4) permit other support measures (e.g., provision of nutrition) to proceed without limitation. Ideally, therapeutic interventions should be designed to achieve the above goals, taking into consideration the clinical course. In practice, these issues are based on physician preferences and experience. No evidence-based criteria have been established, thereby making comparisons between any two centers or even two chosen strategies at the same institution difficult. An important consideration in this regard is to recognize that the patient with ARF is somewhat different than the one with ESRD. The rapid decline of renal function associated with multiorgan failure does not permit much of an adaptive response akin to what characterizes the course of the patient with chronic kidney failure. Consequently, the traditional indications for renal replacement (developed in chronic kidney failure, yet applied to ARF) need to be redefined. For instance, excessive volume resuscitation, a common strategy used for multiorgan failure, may be an indication for dialysis even in the absence of significant elevations in blood urea nitrogen (BUN). In this respect it may be more appropriate to consider dialytic intervention in the ICU patient as a form of renal support rather than replacement. This terminology serves to distinguish between the strategy for replacing individual organ function and one to provide support for all organs. Table 45–1 lists some of the revised indications for dialytic intervention using this approach. It is, thus, possible to widen the indications for renal intervention and provide a customized approach for the management of each patient.

MODALITIES FOR RENAL REPLACEMENT THERAPY (RRT)

Several methods of dialysis are available for renal replacement therapy (Table 45–2). Although most of these have been adapted from dialysis procedures developed for chronic kidney failure, several variations are available specifically for ARF patients. A key distinction among the techniques is the duration of application, that is, intermittent versus continuous dialysis.

Intermittent Procedures

Intermittent hemodialysis (IHD) has been used widely for the last four decades to treat chronic kidney failure and ARF. It remains the standard therapy for treating ARF in both the ICU and non-ICU settings. The vast majority of IHD is performed using single-pass systems with countercurrent dialysate flow at a rate greater than blood flow. Several advances have been made in this area, particularly with respect to availability of variable sodium, bicarbonate-based, and volumetrically controlled machines with precise ultrafiltration control.[3] The advantages offered by volumetric controlled ultrafiltration and bicarbonate dialysate are particularly appealing in the ARF setting, given the propensity for hemodynamic instability, although efficacy of these technologies in this population has not been formally tested. In patients with chronic kidney failure, these machine enhancements have led to the development of a wide variety of different therapeutic regimens of IHD, including variations of high flux and high efficiency dialysis with high blood flow and dialysate flow rates.[4] In contrast in most centers, IHD for ARF utilizes a standard approach with moderate blood flow rates (200–250 mL/min) and dialysate flow rates of 500 mL/min. Often this approach is dictated by the lack of a permanent vascular access capable of supplying a high blood flow rate and the absence of any standardized methods of dialysis prescription and dose delivery.

Sorbent system IHD that regenerates small volumes of dialysate with an in-line Sorbent cartridge has not been very

Table 45–1 Potential Indications for Dialysis in Critically Ill Patients

Renal Replacement	Renal Support
Life-threatening indications	Nutrition
Hyperkalemia	Fluid removal in congestive heart failure
Acidemia	Cytokine manipulation in sepsis
Pulmonary edema	Cancer chemotherapy
Uremic complications	Treatment of respiratory acidosis in ARDS
Solute control	Fluid management in multiorgan failure
Fluid removal	
Regulation of acid-base and electrolyte status	

Table 45–2 Dialysis Modalities for ARF

Intermittent Therapies	
	Hemodialysis (HD): single-pass, sorbent-based
	Peritoneal (IPD)
	Hemofiltration (IHF)
	Ultrafiltration (UF)
Continuous Therapies	
	Peritoneal(CAPD, CCPD)
	Ultrafiltration (SCUF)
	Hemofiltration (CAVH, CVVH)
	Hemodialysis (CAVHD, CVVHD)
	Hemodiafiltration (CAVHDF, CVVHDF)

popular, however, it is a useful adjunct if large amounts of water are not available or in disasters.[5] This system depends upon a sorbent cartridge with multiple layers of different chemicals to regenerate dialysate. In addition to the advantage of needing small amounts of water (6 L for a typical run), which does not need to be pretreated, the unique characteristics of the regeneration process allow greater flexibility in customizing the dialysate. For example, urea removed across the dialyzer is converted to ammonium carbonate by a layer containing urease. In a subsequent layer, zirconium phosphate adsorbs the cations, including ammonium, and exchanges these for sodium and hydrogen ions. The hydrogen ions then react with the carbonate ions to generate bicarbonate. Thus, the dialysate can be tailored to treat a wide range of acid-base disorders and is particularly useful in special circumstances (e.g., metabolic alkalosis). Unfortunately, the improved flexibility comes at the expense of a complex process that requires intense monitoring and is less efficient than single-pass IHD. Two factors account for this: the slower flow of dialysate and the adsorptive capacity of the sorbent cartridges. Cartridges of two different sizes are available and can remove between 20 and 30 g of urea. This degree of clearance may be inadequate for the hypercatabolic patient and may obligate the use of more than one cartridge during a single dialysis session. Additionally, Sorbent systems are infrequently utilized in most centers, and as a consequence, many nephrologists and nursing personnel are unfamiliar with them. Presently, this technique appears best reserved for special circumstances and should be utilized only by highly trained personnel.

In contrast to IHD, intermittent hemodiafiltration (IHDF), which uses convective clearance for solute removal, is popular in Europe but has not been used extensively in the United States, mainly because of the high cost of the sterile replacement fluid. Several modifications have been made to this therapy, including the provision of on-line preparation of sterile replacement solutions. Proponents of this modality claim a greater degree of hemodynamic stability and improved clearance of middle molecule (i.e., molecules in the range of 70–100 kD, relatively poorly cleared with diffusive dialysis).

Intermittent ultrafiltration (UF), in contrast to IHDF, utilizes the same machines as IHD but is used specifically for volume removal alone with minimal solute clearance. Most nephrologists use UF as a method of rapid fluid removal when the major indication for renal replacement or support is pulmonary edema or refractory congestive cardiomyopathy. In most instances where clearance is required, UF requires supplementation with IHD. Some centers use a combination of UF and IHD in the same session (sequential dialysis).[7] This strategy offers a greater degree of hemodynamic stability resulting from the dissociation of solute and fluid removal during the dialysis. The improved hemodynamic status may be related to the attenuation of osmotic flux during the UF phase. Although sequential UF–IHD can be easily implemented, a major potential disadvantage of this strategy is the reduction in time for diffusive solute clearance, if the overall treatment time is fixed. Since solute removal during UF alone is minimal, the treatment may be inadequate in some settings.

A newer modality, extended daily dialysis (EDD), is a hybrid therapy between IHD and CRRT and uses standard IHD equipment. In EDD, patients undergo HD for 6 to 8 hours daily, using blood and dialysate flows of 200 mL/min and 300 mL/min, respectively. Anticoagulation requirements tend to exceed those of IHD but are less than those in bicarbonate-based CRRT. Four major advantages of this modality include the ability to provide as good or better hemodynamic and solute control as that in IHD, less intensive monitoring required by dialysis nurses and ICU staff, training of nurses and support staff is minimal, and it allows sufficient time for patient procedures requiring mobility.[8] Results of a 2-year randomized clinical trial comparing CRRT to EDD are forthcoming.

Continuous Techniques

Although the concept of continuous dialysis was advocated as early as 1960 by Scribner and colleagues,[9] peritoneal dialysis (PD) was the first form of continuous renal replacement therapy and became popular largely because of its highly permeable natural membrane. In patients with ARF, two forms of PD have been used. Most commonly, dialysate is infused and drained from the peritoneal cavity by gravity. The procedure can be performed intermittently but is fairly labor intensive and is best done by personnel trained in PD procedures. More commonly, a variation of the procedure for continuous ambulatory PD termed *continuous equilibrated* PD (CEPD) is utilized.[10] Dialysate is instilled and drained manually every 3 to 6 hours continuously, and fluid removal is achieved by varying the concentration of dextrose in the solutions. Alternatively, the process can be less labor intensive with an automated cycler device that is programmed to deliver a fixed volume of dialysate and the peritoneal cavity drained at fixed intervals. However, cyclic PD suffers from two basic problems: (1) the procedure is relatively inefficient, and total solute removal is limited by the amount of peritoneal effluent; and (2) peritoneal transport characteristics may be altered with hypotension and pressor agents. For instance, in the hypercatabolic postoperative patient, PD may not provide the required amount of solute removal for adequate control of azotemia. Intermittent peritoneal dialysis (IPD) continues to occupy a small niche for renal replacement, particularly in the pediatric population. The small body surface area allows for an adequate clearance without a large number of exchanges.[11]

Over the last decade, a variety of continuous renal replacement therapies (CRRT) have evolved. In general, these techniques use highly permeable synthetic membranes, and the modalities differ principally in the driving force for solute removal. When arteriovenous (AV) circuits are employed, the mean arterial pressure provides the pumping mechanism. Alternatively, external pumps utilize a venovenous (VV) circuit and permit precision in blood flow rates and transmembrane pressure. The letters *AAV* or *AVV* in the terminology serve to identify the driving force in the technique. Solute removal with these techniques is achieved either by convection, by diffusion, or by a combination of both. Convective techniques include ultrafiltration (UF) and hemofiltration (HF) and depend on solute removal by solvent drag.[12] Hemofiltration provides more efficient clearance of the so-called middle molecules that are inefficiently cleared with dialysis alone. While UF implies fluid removal only, HF necessitates partial or complete replacement of the fluid removed. The composition of the replacement fluid can be varied, and the solution can be infused pre- or post-filter.

Diffusion-based continuous techniques are based on the principle of a solute gradient between the blood and the dialysate, as with IHD. However, unlike IHD, the dialysate flow rates (typically 0.5 to 2 L/hr, or 8–34 mL/min) in continuous hemodialysis are significantly slower than the blood flow rates (typically 100–200 mL/min), resulting in complete or near complete saturation of the dialysate. Small molecules are preferentially removed by these diffusion-based methods. If both diffusion and convection are used in the same technique, the process is termed *hemodiafiltration* (HDF). With HDF, dialysate and a replacement solution (hemofiltrate) are used, and small and middle molecules can both be efficiently removed. The letters *UF, H, HD,* and *HDF* serve to identify the operational characteristics in the terminology. Once exposed to these principles, the terminology for the continuous dialysis techniques is easier to understand. As shown in Table 45–2, the letter *C* in all terms describes the continuous nature of the methods, the next two letters (*AV* or *VV*) depict the driving force, and the remaining letters *(UF, H, HD, HDF)* represent the operational characteristics. The exception is the acronym *SCUF* (slow continuous ultrafiltration), which remains as a reminder of the history of these therapies as simple techniques harnessing the power of AV circuits.[13]

Conceptually, it is important to recognize that CRRT are operationally very different from intermittent techniques. As shown in Table 45–3, the major difference is that time is no longer a limiting factor for blood purification. Consequently, it is possible to use slower blood and dialysate flow rates and achieve weekly clearances equivalent and often superior to intermittent techniques. Another major distinction is the ability to dissociate solute removal from fluid balance. For example, by varying the composition of the dialysate, hemofiltrate, or both, solute balance can be altered, while fluid balance over time can be kept negative, positive, or even. Although IHD provides efficient small solute clearance, and is often effective at ultrafiltration over the several hour period of therapy, 24 or more hours go by during which major changes in fluid balance may ensue, without the fine-tuning offered by CRRT.[14]

TIMING OF DIALYTIC INTERVENTION

Whether or not to provide dialytic support, and when, are two of the most fundamental questions facing nephrologists and intensivists in most cases of ARF. The optimal timing of dialysis for ARF is unknown. Relatively few studies have carefully examined this question[15–19]; none in the modern dialysis era, and most studies on timing are confounded by differences in intensity as a result of a chosen therapeutic strategy. Moreover, changes in illness severity, especially in later years, make comparisons of studies extremely difficult.

Fischer and colleagues[16] reported 15 years' experience (1950–1964) of ARF from a single institution (N = 235). The mean age was 41 years; 34% were women. Acute renal failure was associated with major surgery in 114 (49%), trauma in 33 (14%), transfusion reactions in 22 (9%), obstetrical complications in 13 (6%), and other conditions in 53 (22%) patients. One hundred and sixty-two (70%) patients underwent HD. Before 1961 (N = 120), dialysis was performed "only rarely" until the BUN exceeded 200 mg/dL, even when clinical deterioration was observed. Hyperkalemia was the most common indication for dialysis in the early years (1950–1956) of the series. From 1961 to 1964 (N = 115), dialysis was performed when clinical deterioration was first observed or before the BUN reached 150 mg/dL ("early dialysis"). The 1961 to 1964 group had a lower overall mortality rate (57% vs. 74%) that was more striking when only patients requiring dialysis were considered (51% vs. 77%).

The largest study in this area was completed by Kleinknecht and colleagues,[17] who described a comparative case series of 500 patients with ARF between 1966 and 1970. In this study, 279 patients were treated before, and 221 were treated after the institution of a "prophylactic hemodialysis" strategy. Prophylactic hemodialysis was defined as early and frequent dialysis to maintain the BUN below 200 mg/dL, while providing calorie and protein intakes of 30 kcal/kg/day and 1.0 g protein/kg/day, respectively. Prior to July 1968, dialysis was performed only if the BUN exceeded 350 mg/dL or if severe electrolyte disturbances were present. Acute renal failure was associated with surgery or trauma in 230 (46%), obstetrical complications in 142 (28%), and medical conditions in 128 (26%) patients. Overall, 358 patients underwent dialysis. Mortality rates were significantly reduced during the latter study period for patients receiving hemodialysis (29% vs. 42%, $P < .05$); the reduction in peritoneal dialysis patients (22% vs. 40%), although similar in magnitude, did not reach statistical significance. Furthermore, the authors noted a marked reduction in deaths due to gastrointestinal hemorrhage (27% vs. 55%, $P < .01$) and septicemia (12% vs. 24%, $P < .02$) in the prophylactic dialysis group, attributing these findings to improved control of uremia.

Table 45–3 Renal Replacement Therapy: Comparison of Techniques

	SCUF	CAVH	CVVH	CAVHD	CAVHDF	CVVHD	CVVHDF	PD	IHD
Access	A-V	A-V	V-V	A-V	A-V	V-V	V-V	Peritoneal catheter	V-V
Pump	No	No	Yes	No	No	Yes	Yes	No†	Yes
Filtrate (mL/hr)	100	600	1000	300	600	300	800	100	1000
Filtrate (L/day)	2.4	14.4	24	7.2	14.4	7.2	19.2	2.4	1-5
Dialysate flow (L/hr)	0	0	0	1.0	1.0	1.0	1.0	0.4	30
Replacement fluid (L/day)	0	12	21.6	4.8	12	4.8	16.8	0	0
Urea clearance (mL/min)	1.7	10	16.7	21.7	26.7	21.7	30	8.5	200
Weekly urea clearance(L)	16.8	100.8	168	218.8	269	218	302	85.7	144-336
Cost*	1	2	4	3	3	4	4	3	2

*1 = least expensive; 4 = most expensive

†Cycler can be used to automate exchanges, but they add to the cost and complexity

Modified from Seminars in Dialysis 1993; 6:253-259.

SCUF, slow continuous ultra-filtration; *CAVH,* continuous arteriovenous hemofiltration; *CVVH,* continuous venovenous hemofiltration; *CAVHD,* continuous arteriovenous hemodialysis; *CVVHD,* continuous venovenous hemodialysis; *CAVHDF,* continuous arteriovenous hemodiafiltration; *CVVHDF,* continuous venovenous hemodiafiltration; *IHD,* intermittent hemodialysis.

In the studies reviewed previously, there were no inter-era comparisons of patient characteristics or nondialytic therapies and no efforts made to adjust for comorbidity or severity of illness. Therefore, it is difficult to ascribe improvement in outcomes to earlier institution of dialysis, in each case administered in the latter years of the study period. Conger[18] and Gillum and colleagues[19] performed prospective studies of the intensity of dialysis, the former showing beneficial trends in improved survival, although neither was well controlled for timing of intervention.

Case mix clearly differs today compared with these studies dating back several decades. A much smaller proportion of patients require dialysis because of obstetric complications, and many more are elderly and suffer from multiorgan failure accompanying ARF. Furthermore, what was considered *early* in the previous studies would not be considered early by most criteria. Currently, most nephrologists intervene when the BUN exceeds 100 mg/dL, for fear of impending uremic complications.

Two factors tend to dissuade nephrologists from initiating dialysis in the ICU. First, there are well-known risks of the dialysis procedure, including hypotension, arrhythmia, and complications of vascular access placement. Second, strong concern exists that some element of the dialysis procedure may slow the recovery of renal function and increase the risk of developing ESRD.[20–22] This contention is supported by experimental data showing renal lesions consistent with fresh ischemia in animals dialyzed without systemic hypotension, long after their initial renal injury. However, it is difficult to document that earlier initiation of dialysis is of harm, because patients with more severe forms of renal injury may (1) develop indications for dialysis earlier in their ICU course and (2) may be more likely to develop irreversible disease independent of therapy.

In current practice, the decision to dialyze is based most often on clinical features of volume overload and biochemical features of solute imbalance (e.g., azotemia, hyperkalemia). Data from a randomized controlled trial comparing IHD to CRRT[23] suggest that the *indication* for dialysis is an important determinant of outcome. In this study, patients dialyzed predominantly for solute control experienced better outcomes than those dialyzed predominantly for volume overload. Patients dialyzed for control of both azotemia and volume overload experienced the worst outcome. Mukau and colleagues[24] found that 95% of their patients with postoperative ARF had fluid excess of more than 10 L at the time of dialysis. The amount of fluid overload was a strong independent determinant of outcome. Volume resuscitation is a common strategy used in the treatment of multiorgan failure, particularly when accompanied by sepsis syndrome and hypotension. It is often applied indiscriminately in the setting of oliguric ARF, where it is assumed that providing additional volume will improve renal perfusion, prompting correction of renal dysfunction. Although this may be of great benefit to patients with prerenal azotemia, excessive volume administration can lead to pulmonary edema, compromising oxygenation and ventilation, hastening the need for dialysis. These factors collectively suggest the need to develop evidence-based, patient-specific, and nonbiased indications for the initiation of dialysis in ARF.

We favor utilizing an approach that recognizes that the strategy in treating ARF is to minimize and avoid uremic complications, whereas in chronic kidney failure the aim is to keep the patient off dialysis as long as possible, commensurate with maintaining good health and quality of life. Thus, it is not necessary to wait for progressive uremia to initiate dialytic support. As discussed earlier, the indications for dialysis should include a consideration of the need for renal support (as well as renal replacement), and the timing of dialysis should be based on the goals to be achieved.

SELECTION OF DIALYSIS MODALITY

Several factors influence the choice of a dialytic therapy in the ICU. The general principle is to provide adequate renal replacement without adversely affecting the patient. Unfortunately, no consensus exists on the timing, dose, frequency, and duration of dialysis in ARF. Therefore, the choice of dialysis modality is often based on experience with the technique most commonly used in one's facility and availability. In a survey of nephrologists in the United States,[25] IHD was the modality most frequently used for treating ARF, followed by CRRT and PD. An informal survey at the Fourth International Conference on CRRT in 1999 suggested a shift toward even more CRRT. According to the survey participants, the major reasons for choosing IHD in preference to CRRT or PD were the efficacy, ease of use, and familiarity with the IHD technique. CRRT techniques were largely reserved for hemodynamically unstable patients or for those judged to be hypercatabolic or needing aggressive nutritional support. The minority of nephrologists who used PD reported that their choice was related to the facts that PD could be performed effectively without anticoagulation needed and tended to cause less hemodynamic compromise. Nevertheless, a randomized controlled trial (RCT) by Phu and colleagues[26] compared mortality rates among patients with infection-associated ARF in Vietnam assigned to PD or CVVH and found significantly lower mortality rates in the CVVH group (15% vs. 47%, $P = .005$), limiting the likelihood of choosing PD initially to treat ARF. Overall, these findings support the statement that as of 1999, no standard methods exist for the dialytic treatment of ARF. Ideally, therapeutic decisions should be based on some or all of the considerations described below, and future prospective evidence gained.

Patient Factors

Indication for Renal Replacement

The primary indication for dialytic intervention can be a major determinant of the modality chosen, because different procedures have varying efficacy for solute and fluid removal. In the ICU, indications for renal replacement are more diverse and more prone to modification based on the clinical situation. For instance, if the indication for dialysis is to facilitate the removal of a drug such as theophylline, or potassium in the case of severe hyperkalemia, IHD is a logical choice given its efficiency for removal of small molecular weight solutes and the rapidity of response. Conversely, if volume overload is the principle indication for dialysis, particularly where there is hemodynamic instability, CRRT is preferable. In most patients, the indication(s) for dialysis are not clear-cut and both solute and fluid removal is desired. In this setting, the time course of the desired response will also influence this decision.

Presence of Other Organ Failure

Although several studies have aimed to determine factors predicting mortality in ARF, none have uniformly identified factors that prove critical in all populations studied to date. Several investigators have developed independent ARF scoring systems.[27–44] Most of these systems were derived from retrospective analysis of data obtained from relatively small series of ICU and non-ICU patients.[30,31] The predictive variables have differed in many of the studies, and the majority of them have not been validated. One study has been prospectively validated at the same hospital and in an external group of 25 patients.[32] Liano and colleagues[37] developed a linear discriminant model, identifying age, gender, nephrotoxic ARF, oliguria, hypotension, jaundice, coma, level of consciousness, and assisted respiration as risk factors. Using this index, the authors derived a discriminant score of 0.9 beyond, which no patient has survived. It is unclear how this model performs outside of their geographic setting. Paganini and colleagues[30] published a severity system derived from ICU patients with ARF requiring dialysis and identified eight risk factors associated with poor outcome. Although three of Paganini's factors were common to the Liano model (gender, bilirubin, assisted respiration), five were unique. When these authors tested other models in their population, discrimination was poor.[37] Poor generalizability is an obvious limitation of existing systems.

Failure of nonrenal organ systems has been the most widely recognized risk factor across studies.[39,40] Data from the European Dialysis and Transplant Association (EDTA) show that patients with isolated ARF (61 of 474) experience a mortality rate of only 8%, lending support to the fact that ARF per se is not the only reason for the exceptionally high mortality seen.[39] Indeed, several investigators[40–43] have shown that mortality is proportional to the number of failing organ systems. Lohr and colleagues[44] derived a clinical index to predict survival in patients with ARF undergoing dialysis, finding that associated organ system failure in the form of respiratory failure, GI dysfunction, CHF, sepsis, and hypotension were significantly associated with mortality.

When ARF complicates the course of a critically ill patient in the ICU, it worsens the prognosis and contributes to increased mortality.[39] In this setting, ARF is usually associated with multiple organ failure (MOF) that can influence the choice of RRT in two ways. First, the presence of MOF may limit the choice of modalities (e.g., patients with abdominal surgery may not be able to receive peritoneal dialysis because it may increase the risk for wound dehiscence and infection.[9] Further, hemodialysis may be impossible in hemodynamically unstable patients.[45] Second, the requirement for anticoagulation is dependent on the presence of coagulation abnormalities. Peritoneal dialysis avoids anticoagulation, and IHD can usually be performed anticoagulant-free, with frequent saline flushes of the hemodialyzer. In contrast, CRRT can only rarely be performed without anticoagulation. In our experience, patients with thrombocytopenia (<50 K) and liver failure may be treated successfully with no heparin or citrate; otherwise, some degree of anticoagulation is usually required.

Furthermore, the anticipated effect of the modality chosen on previously compromised organ systems is an important consideration. Rapid removal of solutes and fluid during IHD can result in a disequilibrium syndrome and worsen neurologic status. Patients with hepatic encephalopathy, underlying neurologic disorders, and preexisting hyponatremia may be at increased risk for this complication. The risk of disequilibrium can be reduced with the use of continuous techniques, either peritoneal dialysis or CRRT. Peritoneal dialysis may be attractive in ARF complicating acute pancreatitis but would contribute to additional protein losses in the hypoalbuminemic patient with liver failure.[46] Continuous therapies afford hemodynamic stability; however, if not monitored carefully, they can lead to significant volume depletion. The effects of these therapies on respiratory status are an additional area of concern. Peritoneal dialysis may compromise respiratory status by limiting diaphragmatic excursion, especially in patients who are kept supine. A final consideration is the influence of these therapies on drug dosing, particularly of antibiotics and inotropes.[47–50]

Access

The availability of appropriate venous angioaccess is crucial for IHD and CRRT (CVVH, D, or HDF); and an intraperitoneal catheter is required for PD. A variety of vascular catheters are now available that obviate the need for surgically placed central venous catheters and can sustain blood flows consistently above 350 L/min. Arteriovenous shunts are still used in the occasional patients with severe peripheral vascular disease.[51,52] If vascular access cannot be obtained, PD may be the only alternative, particularly in the pediatric patient. The type of catheter and the technique of insertion are important to minimize complications. Access related complications depend on the expertise of the operator and are exacerbated by underlying coagulopathy.[53] It may be possible to use a single needle for access,[54] however, this requires pumped equipment that permits single needle methods.

Requirement for Mobility

A major consideration in the choice of modality is the requirement of patient mobility. If patients are to be moved for different investigations—trips to the operating room or in the bed for different procedures—it becomes more difficult to perform continuous therapies. Similarly, the use of an arterial access for CAVH and CAVHD restricts patient ambulation. In pumped CRRT (CVVH, HD, and HDF), most of the pumps currently available are not equipped with battery packs, thereby making transportation difficult. The location of the patient (ICU or non-ICU) is an additional determinant of therapy because CRRT should only be performed where constant monitoring and 1:1 nursing is available. Extended daily dialysis offers time off dialysis to attend to various investigations.[8]

Anticipated Duration of Treatment

Renal replacement for ARF is based on the premise that there will be a return of kidney function allowing discontinuation of dialysis. Although this is the desired outcome, it does not always occur. This is particularly true for the patient with ARF complicating MOF, wherein the ultimate prognosis depends on recovery of other organ systems. Traditional teaching suggests that most patients with ARF will improve within 4 to 6 weeks, and dialysis requirement beyond this period likely represents chronicity. Although this is true in most instances, two important factors need to be considered: (1) some patients with ARF in the ICU setting may require prolonged dialysis support (>8 weeks) before recovering renal function and recovery may be incomplete,[55] and (2) the duration of dialytic support may need to be predefined in some patients with ARF when other organ system failure accompanies ARF. For instance, a patient with respiratory, cardiac, and liver failure secondary to sepsis requiring dialytic support for ARF should have a finite (1–2 weeks) trial period of dialysis and be reassessed for evidence of improvement in all organ systems. Obviously, dialysis cannot improve nonrenal organ function, and withdrawal of dialysis should be considered in selected patients with severe ARF accompanying MOF who are extremely unlikely to recover organ function. The ultimate prognosis depends on recovery of all organ systems, and dialytic support may serve only to prolong the time to death. Woodrow and Turney[56] reviewed the causes of death in all patients with severe ARF seen at a single center over 33 years. They found that the most important factor contributing to death was the underlying cause of ARF, whereas deaths due to secondary complications had declined over time. Interestingly, withdrawal of active therapy accounted for approximately 6% of all deaths before 1970 but was responsible for 13.3% in 1970 to 1979 and 15.4% cases in 1980 to 1989.[56]

Modality-Specific Factors

Components

Choice of Membrane

One of the key components of any dialysis system is the membrane. In addition to the well-recognized effects of each membrane on solute and fluid removal, two additional factors must be considered in the choice of membranes for renal replacement in ARF.

Biocompatibility Membrane interactions leading to complement activation and neutrophil sequestration have been described predominantly for IHD.[57] However, the exposure time to the membrane is considerably greater in continuous therapy, and membrane effects may also influence outcome in CRRT. Although various membranes have been shown to have different intensities of complement activation,[58,59] polysulfone and polyacrylonitrile membranes do not appear to result in this activation.[58] Development of newer membranes with heparin bonding[60–63] is promising, although they have been associated with increased complement activation.[64] An additional area is the finding of cytokine induction by various membranes during dialysis.[65] Some data suggest that this may be related to the passage of endotoxin fragments across the membrane from the dialysate.[66] Use of an ultrapure dialysate has been found to markedly reduce production of tumor necrosis factor (TNF)-α.[67,68] Additionally, the role of various soluble receptors and natural antagonists to cytokines in this setting is still unclear.[69,70]

Two conflicting meta-analyses were published in 2002, looking at trials comparing biocompatible (BCM) and bioincompatible (BICM) membranes and mortality. In the first meta-analysis 722 patients were examined, after selecting the most inclusive and updated trials to maximize the sample size. Overall death rate was not different between BCM and BICM (45% vs. 46%). Using a random effects model, a more conservative model for combining data that incorporates both within and between study variability, the relative risk of death was not significantly lower among patients dialyzed with BCM (RR = 0.92; 95% CI = 0.76, 1.13; P = .44).[71] The second meta-analysis added one study, which markedly affected the overall result.[72] Indeed, this study was an observational study of patients with ARF, where dialysis modality was not limited to IHD, and where dialysis membrane use reflected the practice pattern of the participating centers. Further, it contributed more patients than any other study in the meta-analysis (n = 169).[73] The inclusion of this study carried significant weight in the compiled meta-analysis, resulting in a statistically significant overall lower relative risk of death among patients dialyzed with BCM compared with BICM (RR = 0.73; 95% CI = 0.55, 0.98; P = .03). Neither meta-analysis demonstrated an overall impact of dialysis membranes on recovery of renal function.

Cytokine Modulation An additional area of intense interest is the effect of the dialytic techniques in removing mediators of inflammation, such as TNF-α, interleukin-1, and interleukin-6. Because these cytokines are an integral component of the response to sepsis and may mediate some of the detrimental hemodynamic consequences, it is theoretically possible that their removal might be beneficial. Clearance of molecules in the size range of these inflammatory mediators (10–30,000 Da) is increased in the hemofilters used with CRRT compared with hemodialyzers used with IHD. It has been previously shown that TNF-α and IL-1 are removed from the circulation by CRRT.[74,75] In fact, cytokine extraction may be dependent on the membrane used.[76] In an in-vitro model of CRRT, the AN69 polyacrylonitrile (PAN) membrane was twofold to threefold more efficient at removing TNF compared with polysulphone and polyamide membranes.[76] Hemofiltration was found to be useful in initial studies from animal models of sepsis and in some patients.[77–86] Similar membranes can be used for IHD, however, the potential for cytokine removal will be limited. Any assessment of cytokine removal has to consider the influence of cytokine induction by various membranes and the induction of receptors and receptor antagonists of these mediators. Although complex, and thus far unsuccessful, additional investigation into the use of dialysis for modification of the inflammatory milieu should be pursued. Combination of dialysis techniques, for example, coupled filtration adsorption[87,88] and the bioartificial renal assist device developed by Humes and colleagues[89] may play a role in this area in the near future.

Dose of Dialysis

The ideal dialysis prescription for ARF should incorporate an assessment of the dose of dialysis delivered. Unfortunately, no standard methods for assessing dose of dialysis exist in ARF. In chronic kidney failure, the dose of dialysis prescribed and delivered is usually based on an assessment of the amount of urea removed, using urea kinetic modeling either via direct dialysis quantification or using regression formulas or urea reductions.[90–93] A key feature of these methods is the assumption that patients with chronic kidney failure are in steady state with respect to urea generation, volume status, and renal and extrarenal clearance. However, dialysis dosing in ARF needs to account for highly variable body water volumes and varying urea generation rates, as well as different methods of dialysis and changes in renal and extrarenal clearance. Unfortunately, these issues have not been properly quantified or studied sufficiently to date.

In general the dose of dialysis is based on modality-specific criteria (e.g., membrane choice, operational characteristics, and the duration of each dialysis session). For patients treated with IHD, the frequency of dialysis is another determinant of the overall dose of dialysis delivered. Table 45–4 shows a comparison of the factors affecting dose of dialysis for IHD and CRRT. Several investigators have attempted to quantify the dose of dialysis delivered in ARF using methods used for patients with chronic kidney failure. Clark and colleagues[94] compared IHD to CRRT techniques using a computer model to derive the required IHD frequency (per week) or required CRRT for a given patient weight for desired BUN values of 60, 80, and 100 mg/dL. For the attainment of intensive IHD metabolic control (BUN = 60 mg/dL) at steady state, a required treatment frequency of 4.4 dialyses per week was predicted for a 50-kg patient. However, the model predicted that the same degree of metabolic control could not be achieved even with daily IHD therapy in patients 90 kg or more. On the other hand, for the attainment of intensive CRRT metabolic control (BUN = 60 mg/dL), required urea clearance rates of approximately 900 mL/hr and 1900 mL/hr were predicted for 50 and 100 kg patients, respectively. These data suggest that, for many patients, rigorous control of azotemia equivalent to that readily attainable with most CRRT programs can be achieved with intensive (nearly daily) IHD regimens only. In practice, the frequency of dialysis usually depends on the patient's clinical and biochemical status. It is noteworthy that reimbursement policies currently do not support the practice of daily IHD. In the absence of obvious uremic symptoms, the height of the interdialytic rise in BUN is usually paramount, although there are few data to support this approach (see previous text).

Table 45–4 Factors Affecting Dialysis Dose in CRRT and IHD

	Dialysis Dose Delivered	
	IHD	**CRRT**
Patient Factors		
Hemodynamic stability	+++	+
Recirculation	+++	+
Infusions	++	+
Technical factors		
Blood flow	+++	++
Concentration repolarization	+	+++
Membrane clotting	+	+++
Duration	+++	+
Other Factors		
Nursing errors	+	+++
Interference	+	+++

The role of aggressive dialysis on outcome from ARF has been addressed in previous studies[18,19] A controlled study done several years ago failed to show any difference in outcome (e.g., survival, need for long-term dialysis) in patients dialyzed daily to maintain BUN levels less than 60 mg/dL compared with those dialyzed to BUN levels of greater than 100 mg/dL.[18] Although this study is often cited as evidence against early and intensive dialysis, it has several weaknesses, which should be considered: (1) the study did not evaluate the role of early dialysis as patients were enrolled only after their serum creatinine levels were greater than 8 mg/dL, (2) the aggressively treated patients were treated to levels of only BUN 60 mg/dL, (3) the study compared only a single modality of renal replacement (i.e., IHD) without the option of CRRT, and (4) only cellulosic dialysis membranes were used (see previous text).

Recently, Schiffl and colleagues conducted a randomized clinical trial comparing conventional every other day dialysis to daily dialysis among 160 patients with ARF, assessing 14-day survival. The groups were similar with respect to baseline characteristics and illness severity and were analyzed by intention to treat. In the daily group, the weekly delivered Kt/V was 5.8 ± 0.4, and in the conventional group it was 3.0 ± 0.6. The duration of therapy was 3.3 hours per session in the daily group and 3.4 hours per session in the conventional group. The daily HD group had improved survival (28% vs. 46%, P = .01) and recovered renal function more quickly (9 ± 2 days vs. 16 ± 6 days, P = .001). Factors significantly associated with an increased odds of death included alternate day HD (vs. DHD) (OR 3.92, 95% C.I. 1.68–9.18, P = .002), higher APACHE III scores (OR 1.06, 95% C.I. 1.01–1.12, P = .02), oliguria (OR 3.02, 95% C.I. 1.35–6.77, P = .007), and sepsis (OR 3.27, 95% C.I. 1.43–7.50, P = .005).[95,96]

This was a landmark study. It was as large as any to date, randomized, and showed that patients with ARF benefited from more frequent HD and, consequently, a higher weekly Kt/V. Unfortunately, a formal expression of concern regarding potential scientific misconduct during the trial was published a year later in the same journal, rendering the findings of the trial suspect. A full report is forthcoming.[97]

From another perspective, a retrospective analysis of patients with ARF showed a mortality rate of 75% in patients dialyzed once, 67% and 50% in those dialyzed between 2 to 10 times, and 10 to 20 times, respectively.[98] An additional consideration is that unlike intermittent techniques the dose of dialysis delivered in CRRT is not time dependent.[99] In IHD, hemodynamic instability, shortened dialysis times, and logistic factors often impact adversely on the delivered dose of dialysis.[100] Paganini and colleagues[101] found that in patients with ARF, 65% of all IHD treatments resulted in lower Kt/V than prescribed. In a subsequent study the same group reported that nonsurvivors had significantly lower dose of dialysis delivered.[102]

Intermittent Versus Continuous

The choice of intermittent or continuous therapy is currently largely based on the availability of CRRT and the familiarity of the nephrologist and other personnel, particularly ICU staff, with the procedure. In centers where CRRT is routinely done, this choice is usually based on the experience of the nephrologist. Currently, only limited information exists comparing

CRRT with IHD; however, results with these techniques should be compared to those obtainable with the gold standard, IHD. It is helpful to compare the operating characteristics of the two therapies to recognize the strengths and weaknesses of each modality (Table 45–5). Although difficult, comparisons of solute control, fluid balance, nutritional support, and outcome are relevant for the choice of modality and are discussed briefly in the following text.

The shorter duration of intermittent techniques results in higher levels of solutes and a greater difficulty in achieving fluid and nutritional balance in comparison to continuous techniques.[103,104] These effects are further influenced by differences in the dose prescribed and delivered. In practice this shortcoming goes largely unrecognized and probably contributes to decreased solute clearance. Because continuous therapies provide renal replacement 24 hours a day, they compensate for some of the factors resulting in decreased dose delivery.

Fluid removal is a desirable component of any renal replacement therapy and is a major goal of renal replacement for ARF.[105] There is some evidence that volume overload may be an independent contributor to mortality in ICU patients, even in the absence of uremia. Fluid removal in IHD is easily achieved in many cases, however, because the process has been typically prescribed over 3 to 4 hours, the rate of volume removal has to be high (>1 L/hr). As a consequence, large shifts in fluid balance generally result and contribute to hemodynamic instability.[106–109] Additionally, fluid removal and, hence, fluid balance, is limited to the period of dialysis. If the patient is hemodynamically unstable during this period, it may be difficult to remove any fluid. By contrast, CRRT has the advantage of providing renal replacement continuously and, hence, fluid removal, or replacement can be precisely adjusted for each patient. Ronco and colleagues[110] randomly assigned 425 ICU patients with ARF requiring CVVH to an ultrafiltration rate of 20 (group 1), 35 (group 2) and 45 (group 3) mL/kg/hr, and found higher survival in groups 2 and 3 compared with group 1 (P <.001), leading the authors to conclude that the ultrafiltration rate in ARF should be at least 35 mL/kg/hr. Because the process is gradual, hemodynamic stability is usually maintained, and these therapies allow ongoing modulation of fluid balance. The high efficacy of these therapies in continuous fluid removal lends them for use in situations other than renal failure.[111,112] Pediatric patients are better suited for PD and CRRT, and these modalities have been used successfully in the management of ARF in neonates.[113,114]

Continuous therapies have a major advantage over IHD in permitting optimal nutrition provision because fluid removal is not a limiting factor of therapy. In the overall nutritional balance of the patient, two other factors need to be recognized: the composition of the dialysate and composition of hemofiltrate or replacement fluid. Lactate-based dialysis and hemofiltration solutions can rarely result in hyperlactatemia and worsening of acid-base status. Additionally, the lactate-buffered substitution fluids used in CRRT tend to have higher urea generation rates, as compared to bicarbonate solutions.[115,116] Second, glucose containing dialysate solutions result in glucose absorption during the dialysis procedure, which contributes to the caloric load. This glucose content is also associated with an increase in endogenous insulin secretion in most patients, and some patients may require exogenous insulin.[117] Avoidance of peritoneal dialysate and the use of a lower dextrose concentration-based dialysate in CRRT usually obviates this complication. A second nutritional factor is the dialysance of amino acids, vitamins, and trace elements across the filter. Losses appear to depend more on the serum levels than on the underlying clinical status of the patient.[118–123]

A major question, still unanswered, is the effect of the dialysis modality on outcome. Two issues are pertinent: the outcomes of interest and the causal link of choice of modality to the outcome. Dialysis has been utilized in the management of ARF over the last 3 decades. In spite of improvements in technology and enhanced understanding of the pathobiology of ARF and its treatment, mortality rates remain distressingly high (>60% in series limited to ICU patients). Both IHD and PD were the major therapies until a decade ago. Although continuous therapies appear promising in some regards, the effect of CRRT on overall patient outcome is still unclear.[124,125] The absence of an effect on mortality may represent an initial bias in patient selection because, in general, continuous therapies have until recently been given only to patients who were hemodynamically unstable and "too sick" to receive IHD.[126] In this situation CRRT is likely to be used infrequently and, as a result, there might be an increased risk of failure related to lack of expertise and experience with the procedure. Critical evaluation of CRRT in comparison with IHD is scant. As shown in Table 45–6 only two prospective, randomized controlled trials have evaluated this question, and both failed to show a survival advantage for CRRT.[127,128] It appears that the underlying severity of illness is a more important determinant of outcome than the modality.

Recently, two meta-analyses were published on the available trials comparing IHD and CRRT and led to conflicting results.[129,130] In the first, Kellum and colleagues included 13 publications in the analyses, which consisted of 3 RCTs, 1 non-RCT, and 9 prospective cohort studies. The inclusion criterion was the use of some form of CRRT compared to IHD. Methods and results were appraised with a predefined study instrument and a numeric score assigned to each study. The APACHE II score assessed illness severity. The authors also attempted to deal with modality switches after treatment allocation, a potential source of bias. Using a less conservative estimate (fixed effects model), the unadjusted cumulative relative risk of death among patients receiving CRRT in all 13 studies was not significantly lower than IHD (relative risk = 0.93, 95% confidence interval = 0.79, 1.09; P = .29). However, CRRT was associated with a significantly decreased relative risk of death after adjustment for study quality, baseline severity of illness or both (relative risk = 0.72, 95% confidence interval = 0.60, 0.87; P <.01). Despite this reduced relative risk, the authors cautiously concluded that there were not enough data to answer the question and that more studies were needed.

Table 45–5 Operating Characteristics of IHD and CRRT

Membrane Characteristics	IHD Variable Permeability	CRRT High Permeability
Anticoagulation	Short duration	Prolonged
Blood flow rate	>200 mL/min	<200 mL/min
Dialysate flow	>500 mL/min	17–34 mL/min
Duration	3–4 hr	Days
Clearance	High	Low

Table 45–6 Clinical trials of Intermittent Hemodialysis vs. Continuous Renal Replacement Therapies

		IHD		CRRT		
Investigators	**Type of Study**	**No.**	**Mortality%**	**No.**	**Mortality %**	***P* Value**
Mauritz 1986	Retrospective	31	90	27	70	NS
Alarabi 1989	Retrospective	40	55	40	45	NS
Mehta 1991	Retrospective	24	85	18	72	NS
Kierdorf 1991	Retrospective	73	93	73	77	<.05
Bellomo 1992	Retrospective	167	70	84	59	NS
Bellomo 1993	Retrospective	84	70	76	45	<.01
Kruzinski 1993	Retrospective	23	82	12	33	<.01
Simpson 1993	Retrospective	58	82	65	70	NS
Kierdorf 1994	RCT	47	65	48	60	NS
Mehta 2001	RCT	82	48	84	66	NS

RCT, randomized controlled trial.

Tonelli and colleagues[130] examined the same question but came to a different conclusion. The authors identified six RCTs, of which two were published in abstract form. The selection process was equally systematic, except the appraisal was not conducted with a systematic scoring system, and instead qualitative details of the individual studies were reported. The relative risk for death of CRRT, as assessed with a random effects model, was not significantly different from IHD (relative risk = 1.03, 95% confidence interval = 0.86, 1.22; $P = .74$). Of note, the dialysis modality also had no impact on recovery of renal function. The authors concluded that CRRT does not improve survival if used for unselected patients with ARF.

The results of these two meta-analyses highlight the importance of case definition in the selection criteria of trials comparing treatment effects. Indeed, whereas Tonelli and colleagues restricted their analysis to RCTs, Kellum and colleagues combined RCTs, non-RCTs, and cohort studies, which further compromised the quality of the overall analysis, due to the inevitable introduction of confounders. Of note, Tonelli and colleagues attempted to minimize publication bias by including two non–peer-reviewed publications. In one of the highest quality RCT, at randomization, the sickest patients were by chance assigned to CRRT.[127] Further efforts to determine an *optimal* therapy in ARF will require rigorous evaluation of only the highest quality randomized trials to avoid the pitfalls inherent in nonrandomized studies.[131]

Although mortality is obviously an important end point for consideration, it has become the *only* outcome of interest in most publications. This preoccupation with mortality tends to obscure some other issues pertinent to the patient with ARF, forced to make decisions in the throes of critical illness. It is thus helpful to consider that in ARF, dialysis is offered under the premise that there will likely be a return of renal function. Renal functional recovery, thus, becomes an important proximate outcome of interest. There is some evidence that the choice of modality may influence this outcome. Hemodynamic instability, reflected by hypotension and cardiac arrhythmias, is encountered in approximately 25% to 50% of dialysis patients.[132] A major area of concern is that episodes of hypotension during dialysis can adversely influence renal outcome.[133] Development of oliguria following initiation of dialysis is fairly common and may be more frequent with IHD in comparison with CRRT or PD.[134]

As the modalities differ also in their efficacy of solute and fluid removal, another area for consideration is whether the dialysis dose delivered is an important determinant of mortality and other outcomes. Evidence from the Cleveland Clinic suggests that the dose of dialysis may play an important role in survival following severe ARF. There was a difference in the delivered dose of dialysis in survivors (Kt/V 1.09) and nonsurvivors (Kt/V 0.89) in ARF patients treated with equivalent prescriptions of dialysis (similar membrane, blood flow rate, time).[135]

In ARF there is a marked discrepancy between prescribed and delivered dose of dialysis. Indeed, whereas delivered Kt/V in patients with chronic kidney failure is 10% lower than prescribed,[136] observed Kt/V values in patients with ARF have been shown to be 30% lower than prescribed.[95,137] These differences are thought to be related in part to early discontinuation of dialysis due to hypotension, dialyzer hollow-fiber clotting due to constrained use of anticoagulation, and vascular access blood recirculation, an unavoidable complication of central venous catheters.[138]

Table 45–7[126] summarizes the studies examining the removal of urea by IHD in patients with ARF.[95,137,139–141] In these studies, treatment time ranged from 3 to 4 hours, and venous catheter blood flow rates were limited to less than 300 mL/min. Furthermore, there was wide variability in heparin use, ranging from 15% to 64% of treatment sessions. More importantly, mean URR and mean Kt/V were less than 65% and less than 1.2, respectively. Using the minimally accepted dialysis dose defined by the DOQI guidelines for patients on chronic HD, only 15% to 32% of treatment sessions achieved a Kt/V greater or equal to 1.2.[137,140,141]

A further concern relates to the suitability of BUN as the surrogate marker of dialysis adequacy in ARF. Van Bommel and colleagues[142] found no difference in the BUN amongst deceased and surviving patients with ARF who were treated with dialysis. Other possibilities include the role of removal of middle molecules, including cytokines. Storck and colleagues compared spontaneous hemofiltration (CAVH) to pump-driven hemofiltration (CVVH) and found that both treatments adequately controlled uremia and fluid overload. However, survival was significantly higher with CVVH than with CAVH (29% vs. 13%). Because ultrafiltrate volumes were higher with CVVH as compared to CAVH, the authors postulated that improved middle- and large-molecule clearance may have had a salutary effect on survival.[143] However,

Table 45–7 Summary of Observational Studies Examining Urea Removal by Hemodialysis in Acute Renal Failure

Authors and Colleagues	Year	Treatment Time (min)	Blood Flow Rate (mL/min)	Heparin Use (%)	URR* (%)	Kt/V*
Lo	1997	190	194	NR	NR	0.82
Evanson	1998	233	263	50	55	1.04
Evanson	1999	223	260	64	54	0.96
Jaber	2001	188	291	15	51	0.83
Schiffl	2002	195	243	NR	NR	0.94

NR, not reported; *URR*, urea reduction ratio.
*The minimally accepted dialysis dose defined by the Dialysis Outcomes Quality Initiative (DOQI) guidelines for patients on chronic HD, corresponds to a URR ≥ 65% or Kt/V ≥1.2. (From Mehta RL, McDonald B, Pahl M, et al: ARF Collaborative Study Group: Indications for dialysis influence outcomes from acute renal failure. J Am Soc Nephrol 1997; 8[9].)

Journois and colleagues[144] found no relationship between ultrafiltrate volumes and patient outcome, but they did find a negative correlation between ultrafiltrate volume produced and recovery from oliguria. Still unclear is whether any one of these therapies is superior in terms of outcome.

It is clearly evident that further research is warranted in the area of ARF treatment, including modality, as it relates to dose. Once dose of dialysis can be identified, the ability of a modality to deliver a particular dose (possibly higher than that currently delivered with three to four times per week IHD) may be an important determinant for its choice. It would appear that in this circumstance CRRT would have an edge over IHD. However, it should be emphasized that CRRT provides increased opportunities for complications, and prolonged exposure to the membrane increases the risks of bioincompatibility.[145]

Other Factors

Procedure - Related Complications

Complications associated with continuous therapies are due mostly to the potential for volume depletion, particularly if monitoring is inadequate and calculations are inaccurate, hemostatic alterations related to anticoagulation, and metabolic changes.[120–122] Since large volumes of fluid can be rapidly removed, meticulous monitoring is essential and often requires a nursing to patient ratio of 1:1, if not more.[132] Access-related problems include peripheral embolism and dissection resulting in limb ischemia with arterial catheters. Fortunately, these complications are rare, but it should be emphasized that intra-arterial catheters should be of an appropriate size and be placed by experienced personnel.[133] In addition to the usual luer-lock mechanisms, connections should be reinforced with tape to reduce the risk of accidental disconnection. Other vascular complications can occur with the arteriovenous techniques, including the undesired development of arteriovenous fistulas, and large hematomas, which can become secondarily infected. Bellomo[145] has shown that venovenous techniques offer equivalent, if not slightly enhanced, clearance characteristics compared with arteriovenous techniques and a significantly lower risk of vascular access-related complications.[145]

Complications with IHD (Table 45–8) are usually related to the rapid changes in fluid and solutes resulting in hypotension and rarely, disequilibrium. As blood flow rates and transmembrane pressures are higher, membrane leaks are more common. Because CRRT requires anticoagulation for a longer period of time, the risk for complications related to anticoagulation may be higher; however, this has not been the case in our experience.[146] In EDD, moderate blood flow rates and anticoagulation requirements may limit hypotension relative to IHD and bleeding complications relative to CRRT.[8]

Cost

Information on the costs of the three dialytic techniques for ARF is scanty. Most investigators have found that CRRT costs are somewhat greater than IHD.[147,148] Our experience suggests that to a large extent the major difference pertains to the costs of supplies for CRRT. In most centers the costs for hemofilters, tubing, dialysate, and so forth, for IHD are significantly discounted for bulk buying because the same membranes are used for patients with chronic kidney failure. In contrast, hemofilters for CRRT are usually priced 3 to 4 times higher than comparable IHD filters. This disparity may be greatly reduced if continuous therapy is used more frequently, allowing for further reduction in prices of the filters. It has also been our experience that physician time is greater for CRRT, however, this represents a learning curve with these techniques. In our institution, we have standardized protocols and have found that as physicians become experienced with CRRT the time required is reduced. Whether these techniques are cost-effective still requires further research,[147,148] especially in the cost of ICU nursing labor.

Nursing Expertise and Other Support

IHD, CRRT, and APD are renal nursing procedures, however, CRRT and APD requires a significant effort by ICU nurses in addition to nephrology nursing support.[149,150] It is impossible to institute CRRT without an adequate in-servicing of ICU nurses and their active participation in the procedure. This is usually facilitated by the availability of flow sheets, manuals (for pumped circuits), and backup attending physician support. Additionally, since CRRT requires changes in drug dosing, nutrition pharmacy, and clinical nutrition, personnel should be actively involved.[49,151] If CRRT is performed infrequently, there is a greater chance of problems and the continued need for frequent in-servicing of dialysis and ICU personnel to maintain skills.[149,150]

Table 45–8 Selected Major Complications of Intermittent Hemodialysis and Methods of Prevention

Complication	Preventive Measure(s)
Hypotension	Extend dialysis time Perform sequential ultrafiltration hemodialysis Discontinue antihypertensive (not antianginal) agents Decrease dialysate temperature Increase dialysate calcium concentration Increase hemoglobin concentration Consider administration of colloid Consider change in estimated dry weight
Arrhythmia	Increase dialysate potassium concentration Consider discontinuing digoxin and other antiarrhythmic agents Supplemental oxygen during dialysis
Muscle cramps	Extend dialysis time Consider hypertonic saline Consider vitamin E Consider quinine sulfate
Pyrogen reaction	Culture dialysate Immediate water testing for LPS
Dialysis disequilibrium	Attenuate clearance by limiting time, dialyzer surface area, blood flow, and dialysate flow consider mannitol
Hypoxemia	Use noncellulosic dialyzer Supplemental oxygen during dialysis
Hemolysis	Examine blood lines Immediate water testing for chloramine

Recommendations for Initial Choice of Renal Replacement

Despite the lack of definitive results derived from randomized clinical trials, it is possible to develop a rational approach to the selection of a dialysis modality for the initial treatment of ARF in critically ill patients. A primary consideration is the availability of a technique at the center and familiarity and comfort of personnel with the technique. The latter point is extremely important with respect to continuous techniques as infrequent use may be associated with a higher incidence of iatrogenic complications.[152,153] The next consideration is the complexity of the patient, the location in the hospital, and need for mobility.

Patients with uncomplicated ARF can be treated with IHD or PD, and the choice is based on other patient characteristics (e.g., pregnancy, hemodynamic tolerance, access and urgency for treatment). Patients with multiple organ failure and ARF can be treated with CRRT or IHD. In general, hemodynamically unstable, catabolic, and excessively fluid overloaded patients are ideally treated with CRRT, whereas IHD may be better suited for patients requiring early mobilization and who are more stable.[126] Table 45–9 depicts a potential therapy for several different clinical scenarios. Amongst continuous therapies, those that include hemofiltration (CVVH, CVVHDF) may be superior in sepsis or the systemic inflammatory response syndrome because of the ability to more efficiently remove (or adsorb) larger molecular weight solutes.[154,155] For most clinical scenarios, we favor the use of hemodiafiltration techniques that combine hemodialysis and hemofiltration and are thus providing optimal clearance for both small and large molecules. It is important to stress that one of the key factors in the choice of renal replacement is to tailor the therapy to the patient. This implies an ongoing assessment of the patient and modification of the therapy used based on clinical criteria (e.g., in a hemodynamically unstable patient CRRT may be an initial choice, however, when the patient is more stable and needs to be mobilized IHD may be more appropriate). We would suggest that flexibility in utilizing the entire range of renal replacement therapies is an important overall philosophy in the management of ARF.

Table 45–9 Renal Replacement Therapy for ARF: Initial Choice

Indication	Clinical Setting	Modality
Uncomplicated ARF	Antibiotic nephrotoxicity	IHD, PD
Fluid removal	Cardiogenic shock, CP bypass	SCUF, CVVH
Uremia	Complicated ARF in ICU	CRRT (CVVHD, CVVH, CVVHDF) IHD
Increased intracranial pressure	Subarachnoid hemorrhage, Hepatorenal syndrome	CRRT (CVVH, CVVHDF)
Shock	Sepsis, ARDS	CRRT (CVVH, CVVHDF)
Nutrition	Burns	CRRT (CVVHD, CVVHDF, CVVH)
Poisons	Theophylline, barbiturates	Hemoperfusion, IHD, CVVHD
Electrolyte abnormalities	Marked hyperkalemia	IHD, CVVHD

SUMMARY

Several new methods of dialysis are now available to treat ARF. Rational use of these techniques requires an understanding of factors influencing the choice of a modality and appreciation of the advantages and disadvantages of each technique. Management of ARF is different from that of chronic kidney failure, and the dialysis prescription should incorporate the unique characteristics of each patient. Therapeutic alternatives to traditional IHD now permit nephrologists to match the modality to the patient. This approach (and additional research) will allow better management of patients with ARF and ultimately improve survival and other important outcomes.

References

1. von Albertini B, Bosch JP: Short hemodialysis. Am J Nephrol 1991; 11:169-173.
2. Paganini EP: Slow continuous hemofiltration and slow continuous ultrafiltration. Trans Am Soc Artif Intern Organs 1988; 34: 63-66.
3. de Vries PM, Olthof CG, Solf A, et al: Fluid balance during hemodialysis and hemofiltration: The effect of dialysate sodium and a variable ultrafiltration rate. Nephrol Dial Transplant 1991; 6:257-263.
4. Collins A: *In* Heinrich WL (ed): High-flux, High-Efficiency Procedures in Principles and Practice of Hemodialysis. Baltimore, Williams & Wilkins, 1994, pp 76-88.
5. Shapiro WB: The current status of sorbent hemodialysis. Semin Dial 1990; 3:40-45.
6. Botella J, Ghezzi P, Sanz-Moreno C, et al: Multicentric study on paired filtration dialysis as a short, highly efficient dialysis technique. Nephrol Dial Transplant 1991; 6:715-721.
7. Wehle B, Asaba H, Castenfors J: The influence of dialysis fluid composition on the blood pressure response during dialysis. Clin Nephrol 1978; 10(2):62-66.
8. Kumar VA, Craig M, Depner TA, Yeun JY: Extended daily dialysis: A new approach to renal replacement for acute renal failure in the intensive care unit. Am J Kidney Dis 2000; 36(2):294-300.
9. Scribner BH, Caner JEZ, Butri R, et al: The technique of continuous hemodialysis. Trans Am Soc Artif Intern Organs 1960; 6:88-103.
10. Steiner RW: Continuous equilibration peritoneal dialysis in acute renal failure. Perit Dial Intensive 1989; 9:5-7.
11. Reznick VM, Ferris ME, Mendoza SA: Peritoneal dialysis for acute renal failure in children. Pediatr Nephrol 1991; 5:715-717.
12. Henderson LW: Hemofiltration: From the origin to the new wave. Am J Kidney Dis 1996; 28(5) S3:100-104.
13. Kramer P, Wigger W, Rieger J, et al: Arteriovenous hemofiltration: A new and simple method for treatment of overhydrated patients resistant to diuretics. Klin Nochen 1977; 55:1121-1122.
14. Mehta RL: Fluid management in continuous renal replacement therapy. Semin Dial 1996; 9(2):140-144.
15. Parsons FM, Hobson SM, Blagg CR, McCracken BH: Optimum time for dialysis in acute reversible renal failure. Description and value of an improved dialyzer with large surface area. Lancet 1961; 1:129-134.
16. Fischer RP, Griffen WO, Reiser M, Clark DS: Early dialysis in the treatment of acute renal failure. Surg Gynecol Obstet 1966; 123: 1019-1023.
17. Kleinknecht D, Jungers P, Chanard J, et al: Uremic and non-uremic complications in acute renal failure: Evaluation of early and frequent dialysis on prognosis. Kidney Int 1972; 1:190-196.
18. Conger JD: A controlled evaluation of prophylactic dialysis in post traumatic acute renal failure. J Trauma 1975; 15:1056-1063.
19. Gillum DM, Dixon BS, Yanover MJ, et al: The role of intensive dialysis in acute renal failure. Clin Nephrol 1986; 25:249-255.
20. Adams PL, Adams PF, Bell PD, Navar LG: Impaired renal blood flow autoregulation in ischemic acute renal failure. Kidney Int 1980; 18-22.
21. Conger J: The role of blood flow autoregulation in pathophysiology of acute renal failure. Circ Shock 1983; 11:235-244.
22. Conger JD: Does hemodialysis delay recovery from acute renal failure? Semin Dial 1990; 3:146-147.
23. Mehta RL, McDonald B, Pahl M, et al: ARF Collaborative Study Group: Continuous vs intermittent dialysis for acute renal failure (ARF) in the ICU: Results from a randomized multicenter trial. J Am Soc Nephrol 1996; 7(9):1456.
24. Mukau L, Latimer RG: Acute hemodialysis in the surgical intensive care unit. Am Surg 1988; 54:548-552.
25. Mehta RL, Letteri J: Renal replacement therapy for ARF, current trends: A survey of US nephrologists. Am J Nephrol 1999; 19(3): 377-382.
26. 26. Phu NH, Hien TT, Mai NT, et al: Hemofiltration and peritoneal dialysis in infection-associated acute renal failure in Vietnam. N Engl J Med 2002; 347(12):895-902.
27. Mehta RL, McDonald B, Pahl M, et al: ARF Collaborative Study Group: Indications for dialysis influence outcomes from acute renal failure. J Am Soc Nephrol 1997; 8(9):144A.
28. Barton IK, Hilton PJ, Taub NA, et al: Acute renal failure treated by haemofiltration: Factors affecting outcome. Q J Med 1993; 86: 81-90.
29. Chertow GM, Christiansen CL, Cleary PD, et al: Prognostic stratification in critically ill patients with acute renal failure requiring dialysis. Arch Intern Med 1995; 155:1505-1511.
30. Paganini EP, Halstenberg WK, Goormastic M: Risk modeling in acute renal failure requiring dialysis: The introduction of a new model. Clin Nephrol 1996; 46:206-211.
31. Cioffi WG, Ashikaga T, Gamelli RL: Probability of surviving postoperative acute renal failure. Ann Surg 1984; 200:205-211.
32. Lohr JW, McFarlane MJ, Grantham JJ: A clinical index to predict survival in acute renal failure requiring dialysis. Am J Kidney Dis 1988; 11:254-259.
33. Liano F, Gallego A, Pascual J, et al: Prognosis of acute tubular necrosis: An extended prospectively contrasted study. Nephron 1993; 63:21-31.
34. Bullock ML, Armen AJ, Finkelstein M, Keane WF: The assessment of risk factors in 462 patients with acute renal failure. Am J Kidney Dis 1985; 5:97-103.
35. Routh SG, Briggs JD, Mone JE, Ledingham ImcA: Survival from acute renal failure with and without multiple organ dysfunction. Post Grad Med J 1980; 56:244-247.
36. Biesenbach G, Zazgornik J, Kaiser W, et al: Improvement in prognosis of patients with acute renal failure over a period of 15 years. An analysis of 710 cases in a dialysis center. Am J Nephrol 1992; 12:319-325.
37. Liano F: Severity of acute renal failure: The need of measurement. Nephrol Dial Transplant 1994; 9(suppl 4):229-238.
38. Halstenberg WK, Goormastic M, Paganini EP: Utility of risk models for renal failure and critically ill patients. Semin Nephrol 1994; 14:23-32.
39. Maher ER, Robinson KN, Scoble JE, et al: Prognosis of critically-ill patients with acute renal failure: APACHE II score and other predictive factors. Q J Med 1989; 72:857-866.
40. Schaefer JH, Jochimsen F, Keller F, et al: Outcome prediction of acute renal failure in medical intensive care. Int Care Med 1991; 17:19-24.
41. Wheeler DC, Feehally J, Walls J: High risk acute renal failure. Q J Med 1986; 234:977-984.
42. Cioffi WG, Ashikage T, Gamelli RL: Probability of surviving postoperative acute renal failure: Development of a prognostic index. Ann Surg 1984; 200:205-211.
43. Biesenbach G, Zazgornik J, Kaiser W, et al: Improvement in prognosis of patients with acute renal failure over a period of 15 years. An analysis of 710 cases in a dialysis center. Am J Nephrol 1992; 12:319-325.
44. Lohr JW, McFarlane MJ, Grantham JJ: A clinical index to predict survival in acute renal failure patients requiring dialysis. Am J Kidney Dis 1988; 11:254-259.
45. Ronco C, Brendolan A, Bellomo R: Continuous versus intermittent renal replacement therapy in the treatment of acute renal failure. Nephrol Dial Transplant 1998; 13(suppl 6):79-85.
46. Coles GA, Williams JD: What is the place of peritoneal dialysis in the integrated treatment of renal failure? Kidney Int 1998; 54(6): 2234-2240.
47. Bellomo R, McGrath B, Boyce N: In vivo catecholamine extraction during continuous hemodiafiltration in inotrope dependent patients. Trans Am Soc Artif Intern Organs 1991; 37:M324-M325.
48. Vos MC, Vincent HH, Yzerman EPF: Clearance of imipenem/cilastin in acute renal failure patients treated by continuous hemodiafiltration. Int Care Med 1992; 18:282-285.

49. Keller E: Pharmacokinetics during continuous renal replacement therapy. Int J Artif Organs 1996; 19(2):113-117.
50. Kroh UF: Drug administration in critically ill patients with acute renal failure. New Horizons 1995; 3(4):748-759.
51. Ahmad Z: Introduction of percutaneous arteriovenous femoral shunt: A new access for continuous arteriovenous hemofiltration. Am J Kidney Dis 1990; 16:116-117.
52. Al-Wakeel JS, Milwalli AH, Malik GH, et al: Dual-lumen femoral vein catheterization as vascular access for hemodialysis: A prospective study. Angiology 1998; 49(7):557-562.
53. Canaud B, Leray-Moragues H, Leblanc M, et al: Temporary vascular access for extracorporeal renal replacement therapies in acute renal failure patients. Kidney Int 1998; 66(suppl):S142-S150.
54. Takeda K, Harada A, Kubo M, et al: Successful use of single-lumen, urokinase immobilized femoral catheters as a temporary access for haemodialysis. Nephrol Dial Transplant 1998; 13(1): 130-133.
55. Spurney RF, Fulkerson WJ, Schwab SJ: Acute renal failure in critically ill patients: Prognosis for recovery of kidney function after prolonged dialysis support. Crit Care Med 1991; 19:8-11.
56. Woodrow G, Turney JH: Cause of death in acute renal failure. Nephrol Dial Transplant 1992; 7:230-234.
57. Cheung A: Biocompatibility of hemodialysis membranes. J Am Soc Nephrol 1990; 1:150-161.
58. Horl WH, Riegel W, Schollmeyer P, et al: Different complement and granulocyte activation in patients dialyzed with PMMA dialyzers. Clin Nephrol 1986; 25:3.
59. Bohler J, Kramer P, Gotze O, et al: Leucocyte counts and complement activation during pump driven and arteriovenous hemofiltration. Contrib Nephrol 1983; 36:15.
60. Bohler J, Dressel B, Reetze-Bonorden P, et al: Ca2+ not complement is the key trigger for neutrophil degranulation during hemodialysis. Nephrol Dial Transplant 1992; 7:721.
61. Akizawa T, Sekiguchi T, Nakayama F, et al: Complement activation during hemodialysis: Effects of membrane materials and anticoagulants. *In* Nose Y, Kjellstrand C, Ivanovich P (eds): Progress in Artificial Organs. Cleveland, ISAO Press, 1986, pp 1169-1173.
62. Arakawa M, Nagao M, Gejyo F, et al: Development of a new antithrombogenic continuous ultrafiltration system. Artif Organs 1991; 15:171-179.
63. Tong SD, Hsu LC: Non-thrombogenic hemofiltration system for acute renal failure treatment. Proceedings of 38 Annual Meeting of ASAIO, Nashville, Tennessee, 1992, p 82.
64. Cheung AK, Parker CJ, Janatova J, Brynda E: Modulation of complement activation on hemodialysis membranes by immobilized heparin. J Am Soc Nephrol 1992; 2:1328-1337.
65. Zaoui P, Green W, Hakim RM: Hemodialysis with cuprophane membranes modulates interleukin-2 receptor expression. Kidney Int 1991; 39:1020-1026.
66. Patarca R, Perez G, Gonzalez A, et al: Comprehensive evaluation of acute immunological changes induced by cuprophane and polysulphone membranes in a patient on chronic hemodialysis. Am J Nephrol 1992; 12:274-278.
67. Lonnemann G, Linnenweber S, Burg M, Koch KM: Transfer of endogenous pyrogens across artificial membranes? Kidney Int 1998; 66(suppl):S43-S46.
68. Tetta C, Fidelio T, Licata C, et al: Production of tumor necrosis factor alpha in patients on hemodiafiltration. Nephron 1992; 61: 135-138.
69. Swinford RD, Baid S, Pascual M: Dialysis membrane adsorption during CRRT. Am J Kidney Dis 1997; 30(5 suppl 4):S32-S37.
70. Cheung AK, Leypoldt JK: The hemodialysis membrane: A historical perspective, current state and future prospect. Semin Nephrol 1997; 17(3):196-213.
71. Jaber BL, Lau J, Schmid CH, et al: Effect of biocompatibility of hemodialysis membranes on mortality in acute renal failure: A meta-analysis. Clin Nephrol 2002; 57(4):274-282.
72. Subramanian S, Venkataraman R, Kellum JA: Influence of dialysis membranes on outcomes in acute renal failure: A meta-analysis. Kidney Int 2002; 62(5):1819-1823.
73. Neveu H, Kleinknecht D, Brivet F, et al: French Study Group on Acute Renal Failure: Prognostic factors in acute renal failure due to sepsis: Results of a prospective multicentre study. Nephrol Dial Transplant 1996; 11:293-299.
74. Jacobs C: Membrane biocompatibility in the treatment of acute renal failure: What is the evidence in 1996? Nephrol Dial Transplant 1997; 12(1):38-42.
75. Hakim R, Wingard RL, Lawrence P, et al: Use of biocompatible membranes improves outcome and recovery from acute renal failure. J Am Soc Nephrol 1992; 3:367.
76. Schiffl H, Sitter T, Lang S, et al: Bioincompatible membranes place patients with acute renal failure at increased risk of infection. ASAIO 1995; 41(3):M709-M712.
77. Himmelfarb J, Tolkoff-Rubin N, Chandran P, et al: A multicenter comparison of dialysis membranes in the treatment of acute renal failure requiring dialysis. J Am Soc Nephrol 1998; 9(2):257-266.
78. Schiffl H, Lang SM, Haider M: Bioincompatibility of dialyzer membranes may have a negative impact on outcome of acute renal failure, independent of the dose of dialysis delivered: A retrospective multicenter analysis. ASAIO 1998; 44(5):M418-M422.
79. Brown A, Mehta RL: Effect of CAVH membranes on transmembrane flux of TNF alpha. J Am Soc Nephrol 1991; 2:316.
80. Silvester W: Mediator removal with CRRT: Complement and cytokines. Am J Kidney Dis 1997; 30(suppl 4):S38-S43.
81. Staubach KH, Rau HG, Kooistra A, et al: Can hemofiltration increase survival time in acute endotoxemia: A porcine shock model. Second Vienna Shock Forum, Liss Inc, 1989, pp 821-826.
82. Stein B, Pfenninger E, Grunert A, et al: Influence of continuous hemofiltration on hemodynamics and central blood volume in experimental endotoxic shock. Int Care Med 1990; 16:494-499.
83. Lee PA, Weger GW, Pryor RW, Matson JR: Effects of filter pore size on efficacy of continuous arteriovenous hemofiltration therapy for staphylococcus aureus-induced septicemia in immature swine. Crit Care Med 1998; 26(4):730-737.
84. Kellum JA, Johnson JP, Kramer D, et al: Diffusive vs. convective therapy: Effects on mediators of inflammation in patient with severe systemic inflammatory response syndrome. Crit Care Med 1998; 26(12):1995-2000.
85. Rodby RA: Hemofiltration for SIRS: Bloodletting, twentieth century style? Crit Care Med 1998; 26(12):1940-1942.
86. Grootendorst AF, van Bommel EF, van der Hoven B, et al: High volume hemofiltration improves right ventricular function in endotoxin-induced shock in the pig. Int Care Med 1992; 18:235-240.
87. Jaber BL, Pereira BJ: Extracorporeal adsorbent-based strategies in sepsis. Am J Kidney Dis 1997; 30(suppl 4):S44-S56.
88. Tetta C, Cavaillon JM, Camussi G, et al: Continuous plasma filtration coupled with sorbents. Kidney Int 1998; 66(suppl):S186-S189.
89. Humes HD, Mackay SM, Funke AJ, Buffington DA: The bioartificial renal tubule assist device to enhance CRRT in acute renal failure. Am J Kidney Dis 1997; 30(suppl 4):S28-S30.
90. Garred LJ: Dialysate-based kinetic modeling. Adv Ren Replacement Ther 1995; 2:305-318.
91. Ing TS, Yu AW, Wong FKM: Collection of a representative fraction of total spent dialysate. Am J Kidney Dis 1995; 25:810-812.
92. Keshaviah P, Star RA: A new approach to dialysis quantification: An adequacy index based on solute removal. Semin Dial 1994; 7: 85-90.
93. Gotch FA: Kinetic modeling in hemodialysis. *In* Nissensen AR, Gentile DE, Fine RN (eds): Clinical Dialysis, 2nd ed. Norwalk, CT, Appleton and Lange, 1989, pp 118-146.
94. Clark WR, Mueller BA, Kraus MA, Macias WL: Extracorporeal therapy requirements for patients with acute renal failure. J Am Soc Nephrol 1997; 8(5):804-812.

95. Schiffl H, Lang SM, Fischer R: Daily hemodialysis and the outcome of acute renal failure. N Engl J Med 2002; 346(5):305.
96. Schiffl H, Lang SM, Konig A, Held E: Dose of intermittent hemodialysis and outcome of acute renal failure: A prospective randomized study. J Am Soc Nephrol 1997; 8:290A-292A.
97. Schiffl H, Lang SM, Fischer R: Daily hemodialysis and the outcome of acute renal failure. N Engl J Med 2002; 346:305-310.
98. Jindal KK, Manuel A, Goldstein MB: Percent reduction in blood urea concentration during hemodialysis (PRU). Trans Am Soc Artif Intern Organs 1987; 33:286-288.
99. Daugirdas JT: The post: Pre-dialysis plasma urea nitrogen ratio to estimate Kt/V and NPCR: Mathematical modeling. Int J Artif Organs 1989; 12:411-416.
100. Kindler J, Rensing M, Sieberth HG: Prognosis and mortality of acute renal failure. Continuous Arteriovenous Hemofiltration (CAVH). Int Conf on CAVH, Aachen 1984, HG Sieberth, H Mann (eds); Karger, Basel, 1985, pp 129-142.
101. Paganini EP, Pudelski B, Bednarz D: Dialysis delivery in the ICU: Are patients receiving the prescribed dialysis dose? J Am Soc Nephrol 1992; 3:384.
102. Paganini EP, Tapolyai M, Goormastic M, et al: Establishing a dialysis therapy/patient outcome link in intensive care unit acute dialysis for patients with acute renal failure. Am J Kidney Dis 1996; 28(5)S3:81-90.
103. Mehta RL: Renal replacement therapy for acute renal failure: Matching the method to the patient. Semin Dial 1993; 6:253-259.
104. Bellomo R, Ronco C: Acute renal failure in the intensive care unit: Adequacy of dialysis and the case for continuous therapies. Nephrol Dial Transplant 1996; 11:424.
105. Van Bommel EFH: Are continuous therapies superior to intermittent hemodialysis for acute renal failure on the intensive care unit? Nephrol Dial Transplant 1995; 10:311-314.
106. Lowell JA, Schifferdecker C, Driscoll DF, et al: Postoperative fluid overload: Not a benign problem. Crit Care Med 1990; 18:728-733.
107. Stevens PE, Rainford DJ: Isovolumic hemodialysis combined with hemofiltration in acute renal failure. Ren Fail 1990; 12:205-211.
108. Sivak ED, Tita J, Meden G, et al: Effects of furosemide versus isolated ultrafiltration on extravascular lung water in oleic acid induced pulmonary edema. Crit Care Med 1986; 14:48-51.
109. Mukau L, Latimer RG: Acute hemodialysis in the surgical intensive care unit. Am Surg 1988; 54:548-552.
110. Ronco C, Bellomo R, Homel P, et al: Effects of different doses in continuous veno-venous haemofiltration on outcomes of acute renal failure: A prospective randomised trial. EDTNA ERCA J 2002; suppl 2:7-12.
111. Bagshaw ONT, Anaes FRC, Hutchinson A: Continuous arteriovenous hemofiltration and respiratory function in multiple organ systems failure. Int Care Med 1992; 18:334-338.
112. Bosworth C, Paganini EP, Cosentino F, et al: Long term experience with continuous renal replacement therapy in intensive care unit acute renal failure. Contrib Nephrol 1991; 93:13-16.
113. Heney D, Brocklebank JT, Wilson N: Continuous arteriovenous hemofiltration in the newly born with acute renal failure and congenital heart disease. Nephrol Dial Transplant 1989; 4:870-876.
114. Yorgin PD, Krensky AM, Tune BM: Continuous veno-venous hemofiltration. Pediatr Nephrol 1990; 4:640-642.
115. Davenport A, Will EJ, Davison AM: Hyperlactatemia and metabolic acidosis during hemofiltration using lactate buffered fluids. Nephron 1991; 59:461-465.
116. Olbricht CJ, Huxmann-Nageli D, Koch KM: Anticatabolic effect of bicarbonate substitution solution in patients with acute renal failure on CAVH. Proceedings of 2nd Hospal International Forum on Contemporary Management of Renal Failure, Jomtien, Thailand, 1992, p 64.
117. Bellomo R, Colman PG, Caudwell J, et al: Acute continuous hemofiltration with dialysis: Effect on insulin concentrations and glycemic control in critically ill patients. Crit Care Med 1992; 20:1672-1676.
118. Davenport A, Roberts NB: Amino acid losses during continuous high flux hemofiltration in the critically ill patient. Crit Care Med 1989; 17:1010-1014.
119. Sigler MH, Teehan BP: Solute transport in continuous hemodialysis: A new treatment for acute renal failure. Kidney Int 1987; 32:562-571.
120. Bellomo R, Martin H, Parkin G, et al: Continuous arteriovenous hemodiafiltration in the critically ill: Influence on major nutrient balances. Int Care Med 1991; 17:399-402.
121. Kuttnig M, Zobel G, Ring E, et al: Nitrogen and amino acid balance during total parenteral nutrition and continuous arteriovenous hemofiltration in critically ill anuric children. Child Nephrol Urol 1991; 11:74-78.
122. Frankenfield DC, Badellino MM, Reynolds HN, et al: Amino acid loss and plasma concentration during continuous hemodiafiltration. JPEN 1993; 17:551-560.
123. Story DA, Ronco C, Bellomo R: Trace element and vitamin concentrations and losses in critically ill patients treated with continuous venovenous hemofiltration. Crit Care Med 1999; 27(1):220-223.
124. Bellomo R, Ronco C: Continuous versus intermittent renal replacement therapy in the intensive care unit. Kidney Int 1998; 66(suppl):S125-S128.
125. Manns M, Sigler MH, Teehan BP: Continuous renal replacement therapies: An update. Am J Kidney Dis 1998; 32(2):185-207.
126. Teehan GS, Liangos O, Jaber BL: Update on dialytic management of acute renal failure. J Int Care Med 2003; 18(3):130-138.
127. Mehta RL, McDonald B, Gabbai FB, et al: A randomized clinical trial of continuous versus intermittent dialysis for acute renal failure. Kidney Int 2001; 60(3):1154-1163.
128. Kierdorf H: Acute renal failure in sight of the 21st century. Etiology, prognosis, and extracorporeal treatment modalities (Abstract). Nieren und Hochdruck 1994; 23:614-621.
129. Kellum JA, Angus DC, Johnson JP, et al: Continuous versus intermittent renal replacement therapy: A meta-analysis. Int Care Med 2002; 28(1):29-37.
130. Tonelli M, Manns B, Feller-Kopman D: Acute renal failure in the intensive care unit: A systematic review of the impact of dialytic modality on mortality and renal recovery. Am J Kidney Dis 2002; 40(5):875-885.
131. Teehan GS, Liangos O, Lau J, et al: Dialysis membrane and modality in acute renal failure: Understanding discordant meta-analyses. Semin Dial 2003; 16(5):356-360.
132. Jones CH, Goutcher E, Newstead CG, et al: Hemodynamics and survival of patients with acute renal failure treated by continuous dialysis with two synthetic membranes. Artif Organs 1998; 22(8):638-643.
133. Manns M, Sigler MH, Teehan BP: Intradialytic renal haemodynamics: Potential consequences for the management of the patient with acute renal failure. Nephrol Dial Transplant 1997; 12(5):870-872.
134. Bellomo R, Ronco C: Acute renal failure in the intensive care unit: Adequacy of dialysis and the case for continuous therapies. Nephrol Dial Transplant 1996; 11:424–426.
135. Paganini EP: Slow continuous hemofiltration and slow continuous ultrafiltration. Trans Am Soc Artif Intern Organs 1988; 34: 63-66.
136. United States Renal Data System: 1999 Annual Data Report. Bethesda, MD, National Institutes of Health, Diabetes and Digestive and Kidney Diseases, 1999.
137. Jaber B, King A, Cendoroglo M, et al: Correlates of urea kinetic modeling during hemodialysis in patients with acute renal failure. Blood Purif 2002; 20:154-160.

138. Chertow GM, Lazarus MJ: Intensity of dialysis in established acute renal failure. Semin Dial 1996; 9:476-480.
139. Lo AJ, Depner TA, Chin ES, Craig MA: Urea disequilibrium contributes to underdialysis in the intensive care unit (Abstract). J Am Soc Nephrol 1997; 8:287A.
140. Evanson JA, Himmelfarb J, Wingard R, et al: Prescribed versus delivered dialysis in acute renal failure patients. Am J Kidney Dis 1998; 32:731-738.
141. Evanson JA, Ikizler TA, Wingard R, et al: Measurement of the delivery of dialysis in acute renal failure. Kidney Int 1999; 55:1501-1508.
142. Van Bommel EFH, Bouvy ND, So KL, et al: High-risk surgical acute renal failure treated by continuous arteriovenous hemodiafiltration: Metabolic control and outcome in sixty patients. Nephron 1995; 70:185-192.
143. Storck M, Hartl WH, Zimmerer E, et al: Comparison of pump driven and spontaneous hemofiltration in postoperative acute renal failure. Lancet 1991; 337:452-455.
144. Journois D, Chang D, Safton D: Pump driven hemofiltration. Lancet 1991; 337:985.
145. Bellomo R, Ronco C: Continuous renal replacement therapy: Continuous blood purification in the intensive care unit. Ann Acad Med (Singapore) 1998; 27(3):426-429.
146. Mehta RL, McDonald BR, Aguilar MM, et al: Regional citrate anticoagulation for continuous arteriovenous hemodialysis in critically ill patients. Kidney Int 1990; 38:976-981.
147. Mehta RL, Turner D, Black E: Cost effectiveness of intermittent versus continuous renal replacement therapy in the treatment of acute renal failure: A preliminary report (Abstract). Abstracts Xth Intensivists Cong Nephrol 1989; 325.
148. Moreno L, Heyka RJ, Paganini EP: Continuous renal replacement therapy: Cost considerations and reimbursement. Semin Dial 1996; 9(2):209-214.
149. Martin RK, Jurschak J: Nursing management of continuous renal replacement therapy. Semin Dial 1996; 9:192-199.
150. Politoski G, Mayer B, Davy T, Swartz MD: Continuous renal replacement therapy. A national perspective AACN/NKF. Crit Care Nurs Clin N Am 1998; 10(2):171-177.
151. Joos B, Schmidli M, Keusch G: Pharmacokinetics of antimicrobial agents in anuric patients during continuous venovenous haemofiltration. Nephrol Dial Transplant 1996; 11(8):1582-1585.
152. Meloni C, Morosetti M, Meschini L, et al: Blood purification procedures for acute renal failure: Convenient strategy related to clinical conditions. Blood Purif 1996; 14(3):242-248.
153. Bellomo R, Mehta R: Acute renal replacement in the intensive care unit: Now and tomorrow. New Horizons 1995; 3(4):760-767.
154. Bellomo R: Continuous hemofiltration as blood purification in sepsis. New Horizons 1995; 3(4):732-737.
155. Van Bommel EF: Should continuous renal replacement therapy be used for non-renal indications in critically ill patients with shock? Resuscitation 1997; 33(3):257-270.

Extracorporeal Treatment of Poisoning

Stuart Abramson, M.D., M.P.H.

The 2001 Annual Report of the American Association of Poison Control Centers (AAPCC) Toxic Exposure Surveillance System recorded 2,267,979 human exposure cases reported by 64 poison centers during 2001.[1] This was an increase of 5% compared with 2000. A total of 218.5 million people were served by the participating centers, with an average of eight exposures per 1000 people. Of the exposures, 93% were acute and 92% involved a single poison.[1]

Approximately 22% of recognizably poisoned patients require admission to the hospital, and less than 1% of these patients die.[2] Ten percent of the recognizably poisoned patients require intensive medical care, including hemodynamic and ventilatory support with close monitoring in an intensive care unit.[1] The remainder recover with general support and ward nursing supervision. Fewer than 5% of cases of recognizable poisoning are amenable to techniques that facilitate the elimination of poisons.[3]

Certain types of exposures still carry a high morbidity and mortality secondary to the toxic effect of the poison or its metabolic by-products. For example, conversion of methyl alcohol to formate, and of ethylene glycol to oxalic acid, can lead to severe metabolic abnormalities and end organ damage. Accidental or intentional poison exposure or drug overdose can cause reversible illnesses, such as arrhythmias, congestive heart failure, noncardiogenic pulmonary edema, aspiration pneumonia, brain swelling with subsequent seizures and decreased mentation or psychosis, and hypotension with tissue hypoxia and lactic acidosis or permanent end organ damage (prolonged coma and permanent neurologic deficits, blindness, renal and liver failure, and pancreatitis), and, subsequently, death.

Initial treatment modalities are fairly standardized. The first intervention is decontamination, which consists of the following:

- Dilution or irrigation
- Activated charcoal
- Cathartics
- Gastric lavage
- Syrup of ipecac
- Bowel irrigation

These methods are used in the majority of cases. Of the cases of poisoning reported in 2001, 1,335,900 were treated with one of these therapeutic modalities.[1]

The AAPCC describes the number of patients receiving a specific mode of decontamination or specific antidote. Primarily owing to limitations in reporting and data gathering, the values reported in Tables 46–1 and 46–2 should be interpreted as the minimum frequency with which a particular therapy was administered. Substances of exposure that accounted for the largest number of deaths were analgesics (531 total), sedatives (266 total), and antidepressants (255 total).[1] Tables 46–1 and 46–2 summarize the 2001 data according to the distribution of the exposures and deaths compiled by age, gender, and substance, along with the type of therapy received and the percentages requiring medical intervention.

This chapter reviews the general approach to the poisoned patient, focusing on techniques used to increase removal of drugs and toxins. We begin with a brief discussion of strategies to minimize toxin accumulation, and then focus on the use of extracorporeal therapies to increase elimination of toxins, poisons, or endogenous compounds. We examine the following:

1. Removal of alcohols, lithium, and salicylate with hemodialysis.[2]
2. Use of hemofiltration for the elimination of *N*-acetylprocainamide,[4] methotrexate,[5] lithium,[6] theophylline,[7] and metal-chelator complexes.[8]
3. Use of hemoperfusion for the removal of lipid-soluble drugs, such as barbiturates,[9] digoxin,[10] and theophylline[11,12]; hemoperfusion can also be used to greatly enhance the clearance of salicylates.[13]

We mention briefly other techniques that are more limited in their application, such as peritoneal dialysis, plasmapheresis, and exchange transfusion.

APPROACH TO THE POISONED PATIENT

After supplying supportive measures to maintain airway, breathing, and circulation ("ABCs"), the management for a poisoned patient should be directed toward decreasing or limiting toxin accumulation.[14]

Prevention of Further Absorption

The first therapeutic intervention should be directed at preventing further absorption of the compound in question. Gastrointestinal lavage, with a solution of electrolytes and polyethylene glycol in a dose of 25 mL/kg/hr in children and 1.2–1.8 L/hr in adults, for a total of 4 liters, can be beneficial in the elimination of undissolved tablets or pills. This mode of therapy, also referred to as *whole bowel irrigation*, may be helpful in the management of toxins that are poorly adsorbed by activated charcoal, such as arsenic[15] and lithium. It is time-consuming and contraindicated in patients with an ileus, hemodynamic instability, or a compromised airway.[16] Cleansing of the skin with soap and water helps bind and remove unabsorbed drug or toxin from the surface of the body.

Table 46–1 Exposures and Treatments of Reported Poisonings in the United States for 2001

Exposure	
Number	2,267,979
Age	<6 years of age (52%)
Gender	
Unintentional: male = female	
Intentional: female = 61%	
Treated in health care facility	22%
Treated and released	54.5%
Intensive care unit	14.1%
Noncritical care	7.3%
Treatment	
Decontamination*	1,335,900
Urine alkalinization	6944
Hemodialysis	1280
Hemoperfusion	45
Other extracorporeal therapy	26
Transplant	8
ECMO6	
Antidotes	44,772

*See text for definition.
ECMO, extracorporeal membrane oxygenation. (From Litovitz TL, Klein-Schwartz W, Rogers GC, et al: 2001 Annual Report on the American Association of Poison Control Centers Toxic Exposure Surveillance System. Am J Emerg Med 2002; 20:391-401.)

Table 46–2 Fatalities of Reported Poisonings in the United States for 1995

Number	1074
Age >19 years old (89%)	
Age (intentional) >19 years old (>93%)	
Route	
Ingestion	77%
Inhalation	9.4%
Substances accounting for death	
Analgesics	531
Sedatives	266
Antidepressants	255
Stimulants	207
Cardiovascular drugs	153
Alcohols	108
Chemicals	60

(From Litovitz TL, Klein-Schwartz W, Rogers GC, et al: 2001 Annual Report on the American Association of Poison Control Centers Toxic Exposure Surveillance System. Am J Emerg Med 2002; 20:391-401.)

Oral sorbents (primarily activated charcoal) can bind unabsorbed drug in the gastrointestinal tract and therefore promote its elimination by decreasing its absorption. Activated charcoal is most helpful in the elimination of salicylates,[17] phenobarbital,[18] β-methyl-digoxin,[19] and theophylline.[21] It is administered as an aqueous suspension with a minimum of 8 mL of water to each gram of powder. Commercial premixed formulations are available that may contain activated charcoal with a lubricant (i.e., propylene glycol or carboxymethylcellulose) or a cathartic (i.e., sorbitol). The mean transit time of activated charcoal in fasting subjects is 25 hours; this can be reduced to 1.1 hours with sorbitol.[21] The American Academy of Clinical Toxicology recommends limiting cathartic use to a single dose to lower the risk of adverse effects.[22] Activated charcoal can be administered orally or via nasogastric tube.[23] The recommended dose is 10 times the weight of the ingested chemical or as much as possible, if the dose of poison is unknown up to 1 g/kg. Single-dose activated charcoal has been shown to be most effective if given within 1 hour of ingestion. It should be used only in patients with an intact or protected airway.[24] Multidose activated charcoal has been shown to increase drug elimination significantly, but there have been no studies that show that it decreases morbidity or mortality. The American Academy of Clinical Toxicology recommends that its use be considered only in patients who have ingested a potentially lethal amount of carbamazepine, dapsone, phenobarbital, quinine, or theophylline.[25] The standard regimen is to administer activated charcoal 1 g/kg then 0.5 g/kg at 2- to 6-hour intervals.[25,26]

Gastrointestinal lavage can directly remove ingested chemicals from the gastrointestinal tract and therefore prevent their absorption.[27,28] The efficacy of gastrointestinal lavage decreases as the time increases from ingestion to treatment. The efficacy of gastrointestinal lavage is enhanced, if it is preceded and followed by a dose of activated charcoal.[29] The lavage fluid of choice for patients more than 2 years of age is tap water.[30] Gastrointestinal lavage should be considered only when a patient has ingested a life-threatening amount of a poison and the lavage can be performed within 1 hour of ingestion.[31]

Forced Diuresis

The second step in minimizing toxin accumulation or promoting its removal is to facilitate endogenous excretion through forced diuresis or decreasing tubular reabsorption. Forced diuresis is useful only for compounds and metabolites that are excreted by the kidneys; even then, it is limited to very few poisonings. Alkaline diuresis can be used to enhance the elimination of salicylates[32] and phenobarbital,[33,34] and acidification can be used to enhance the elimination of chloroquine,[35] amphetamine,[36,37] quinine,[38,39] and phencyclidine.[40] If this maneuver decreases the concentration in the "toxic compartment," it may be adequate, but in most instances forced diuresis is not used as the sole method of treatment.

The kidneys are perfused with plasma at a rate of 36 L/hr; only one fifth of the plasma entering the kidney is filtered. Nearly all of the remaining plasma flows past the proximal tubules, where solutes are extracted from the plasma by tubular cells and actively secreted into the urine. Thus, plasma is filtered, then modified by a combination of tubular secretion and reabsorption processes. Even at maximal tubular secretion rates, production of urine volumes of 200 to 300 mL/hr limits tubular reabsorption because a large concentration gradient is prevented by urine dilution.[41–43] If high urine flow rates are applied with either acidification or alkalinization, elimination of certain toxins can be enhanced.

Manipulation of the urine pH can enhance the excretion of acidic or basic chemicals through a mechanism known as *ion trapping.*[44,45] The membranes of the nephron are generally more permeable to nonionized and nonpolar molecules. Compounds are filtered and secreted in a nonionized form of weak acids or bases by nonionic diffusion across cell membranes. They subsequently become ionized in extreme pH conditions and become trapped in urine.

Alkalinization of the urine helps promote elimination of weak acids, such as salicylates[32] and barbiturates[33,34] (phenobarbital and barbital). Acidification techniques help promote elimination of weak bases, such as amphetamine,[36,37] quinine,[38,39] phencyclidine,[40] and fenfluramine.[46,47] This change in the intraluminal pH promotes the formation of a higher intratubular fraction of ionized drug, effectively trapping the ionized moiety in the urinary space secondary to the impermeability of the nephron to charged substances. Thus, reabsorption is decreased and renal elimination enhanced.

Table 46–3 summarizes the methods for alkalinization and acidification of the urine.[48] Intravenous sodium bicarbonate is most commonly used for alkalinization. The carbonic anhydrase inhibitor acetazolamide can be used as well but should be used with caution and only with sodium bicarbonate because of the risk of systemic acidosis. Acidification techniques are no longer recommended because of their questionable effectiveness and the complications of the acid diuresis, which include myoglobinuria, acute renal failure, and hyperkalemia.

The limitation of forced diuresis is that it requires volume expansion with the possible induction of volume overload. Alkalinization or acidification of the urine occurs through systemic loading of the agents listed in Table 46–3 and can lead to systemic acid-base and electrolyte disturbances. Hypokalemia is a common consequence of attempts at forced diuresis or alkalinization of the urine, and addition of potassium chloride to the fluids used is often necessary. These techniques require adequate renal function, and, therefore, their use is limited to only a few poisonings and a few clinical situations.

Antidotes

The third strategy is to convey protection against the toxin by administering specific antidotes, antibodies, or substrate inhibitors. Antidotes and antibodies are available for a limited number of poisonings (Table 46–4). The timing of their administration can be crucial, and most antidotes are only adjunctive therapy to aggressive supportive care.[49] For example, with opiate poisoning, naloxone may reverse or prevent cardiac or respiratory arrest when administered rapidly.[49] This agent can prevent hypoxic brain damage or death when administered early in the course of treatment. As well, flumazenil is very beneficial in benzodiazepine poisoning or overdose. Additional therapy with vasopressors or ventilatory support is occasionally necessary until other means of therapy have been initiated or have taken effect. Ethanol and fomepizole are employed in methanol and ethylene glycol intoxications (see later). Deferoxamine is used for acute iron poisoning.

Digoxin-specific (digoxin immune Fab) antibody is one example of an antidote used in life-threatening *digitalis* intoxication. This antibody should be administered early, if the patient has digitalis-induced ventricular arrhythmias, high-grade atrioventricular block, severe hyperkalemia, or cardiac arrest.[50] There is great variability in the threshold of serum digoxin level at which cardiotoxicity may develop. Therefore, clinical judgment is paramount in the evaluation of

Table 46–3 Urine Alkalinization and Acidification*

To Achieve an Alkaline Diuresis
Sodium bicarbonate, 1–2 mEq/kg every 3–4 hours
Goal: urine pH = 7.5–8.5
For example: 1 amp sodium bicarbonate bolus followed by 3 amps of sodium bicarbonate per liter of 5% dextrose in water to run at 250 mL/hr
To Achieve an Acid Diuresis
10 g arginine or lysine hydrochloride IV over 30 minutes
Then ammonium chloride, 4 g every 2 hours orally
Goal: urine pH = 5.5–6.5

*Both therapies require some degree of volume expansion. (From Mudge GH, Silva P, Stibitz GR: Renal excretion by non-ionic diffusion. Med Clin North Am 1975; 59:681–698.)

Table 46–4 Drugs and Poisons Treated with Specific Antidotes

Poison	Antidote
Acetaminophen	*N*-acetylcysteine
β-Blocking drugs	Glucagon, atropine, isoproterenol
Carbon monoxide	Oxygen (100% or hyperbaric)
Cyanide	Amyl nitrite, sodium nitrite, sodium thiosulfate, oxygen
Digoxin	Digoxin-specific Fab antibody fragment
Ethylene glycol	Fomepizole, ethyl alcohol,
Methanol	Fomepizole, ethyl alcohol
Isoniazid	Pyridoxine
Metallic poisons	
Arsenic	Dimercaprol
Iron	Deferoxamine
Lead	Dimercaprol, edetate disodium calcium, penicillamine
Mercury	Dimercaprol, penicillamine
Nitrates, nitrites, phenacetin	Methylene blue
Opioid drugs (codeine, heroin, meperidine, morphine, propoxyphene)	Naloxone HCl
Organophosphates	Atropine, pralidoxime
Sympathomimetic agents	β-Blockers, phentolamine,
Benzodiazepines	Flumazenil

(From Goldberg MJ, Spector R, Park GD, et al: An approach to the management of the poisoned patient. Arch Intern Med 1986; 16:1381–1385; Mokhlesi B, Leikin JB, Murray P, Corbridge TC: Adult toxicology in critical care: Part I: General approach to the intoxicated patient. Chest 2003; 123:897-922.)

digitalis-intoxicated patients. Loss of digitalis effect after Fab antibody administration may lead to congestive heart failure, increased ventricular rate in the setting of atrial fibrillation, or hypokalemia, especially when there was previous treatment of hyperkalemia.[51] Patients with anuria may have a rebound in the digoxin level because of slow clearance of the digoxin-antibody complex.[52] One vial of Digibind (Burroughs Wellcome), the proprietary formulation of this agent, contains 38 mg of digoxin-specific antibody; each vial neutralizes 0.6 mg of absorbed digoxin. When the ingested dose of digoxin is unknown, 1 to 20 vials (38 to 760 mg) should be administered for acute ingestions and 6 vials for chronic toxicity.[53]

Cyanide poisoning is difficult to diagnose but may be suspected in victims of smoke inhalation, especially those exposed to burning plastic or polyurethane.[54] An elevated anion gap metabolic acidosis secondary to lactic acidosis with an oxygen (O_2) saturation gap[55] (a decreased measured arterial percent O_2 saturation with a normal calculated percent O_2 saturation) may be present. Blood cyanide levels greater than 0.5 mg/L are considered toxic.[56] The treatment includes an amyl nitrite–sodium nitrite–sodium thiosulfate combination, which is marketed as the Lilly Cyanide Antidote Kit (Eli Lilly). Nitrite-induced methemoglobin (Fe^{3+}) has a greater affinity for cyanide than does the ferric iron moiety of cytochrome oxidase and attracts cyanide from the respiratory enzyme. Sodium thiosulfate allows for the formation of thiocyanate, which is renally excreted.[51] Recent work with hydroxycobalamin has shown that it will safely reduce red blood cell and plasma cyanide levels. The currently recommended dose is 5 g IV.[57]

Poisoning due to *anticholinesterase pesticides* (organophosphates, carbamates) and *military nerve agents*[58] can be treated with atropine and pralidoxime. Atropine is a physiologic antidote acting by competitive inhibition of acetylcholine at muscarinic receptor sites, blocking the clinical effect of excessive parasympathetic activity. The dose of atropine is 2 mg by the intravenous route (IV) every 15 minutes, with therapeutic response being judged from drying of excessive secretions.[59] Pralidoxime (Protopam Chloride, 2-PAM) reactivates cholinesterase that has been phosphorylated by the organophosphate. The recommended dose for pralidoxime is 1 to 2 g IV over 10 to 20 minutes.[60] By 24 to 36 hours after exposure, the efficacy of pralidoxime decreases as the cholinesterase is irreversibly bound. However, ongoing release of organophosphate from fat stores may warrant treatment with pralidoxime.[61]

Laboratory Evaluation

A few measurements that are commonly done in the emergency room can give a hint about the nature and amount of the toxin ingested. Three simple calculations are most helpful in determining the type of ingestion: anion gap, osmolar gap, and oxygen saturation gap.

Anion Gap

The calculation of the difference between the measured cations and the measured anions can be used to estimate the difference between the *unmeasured* anions and the *unmeasured* cations. The normal anion gap is 8 to 12 mEq/L, and a value above 12 mEq/L can signify an increase in unmeasured anions. The most common intoxications to cause a high anion gap acidosis are ethylene glycol, methanol, and salicylates. Also, an elevated anion gap from lactic acidosis can signify an intoxication with acetaminophen, carbon monoxide, metformin, phenformin and NSAIDs.[62] It is important to note that a normal anion gap does not rule out an intoxication because many toxins do not cause a gap or there may be a coexisting condition that lowers the gap. The most common condition to lower the gap is hypoalbuminemia: the anion gap falls 2.5 mEq/L for every 1 g/dL drop in serum albumin.[63] A few toxins, such as methanol and ethylene glycol, need to be metabolized before they create an anion gap acidosis. In these cases, intoxication may not be associated with an anion gap early on, especially when there is ethanol coingestion.[64]

Osmolar Gap

Ingestion of low molecular weight toxins will increase the difference between the measured and the calculated plasma osmolarity or osmolar gap. The calculated osmolarity is

$$2 \times \text{Na} + \text{BUN}/2.8 + \text{glucose}/18 + \text{ethanol}/4.6 \quad (1)$$

[65,66]

$$\text{Osmolar gap} = \text{measured Osm} - \text{calculated Osm}$$

An osmolar gap greater than 10 mOsm indicates the presence of osmotically active substances, such as ethanol, methanol, isopropyl alcohol, and ethylene glycol.[67] Hospitalized patients may develop an osmolar gap from glycerol, IV immunoglobulin, propylene glycol, radiocontrast media, and sorbitol.[14] Propylene glycol is a common vehicle for intravenous medications and can cause an osmolar gap, and its metabolite, lactic acid, can contribute to a high anion gap acidosis.[68] Accumulation of propylene glycol in patients receiving high doses of IV medications, such as diazepam, which have propylene glycol as their carrier, may cause severe acidosis with hemodynamic instability and can be treated with hemodialysis.[69] Table 46–5 lists the contribution to the osmolar gap of various drugs and toxins.

A number of toxins, such as ethylene glycol and methanol, will no longer produce an osmolar gap because they are metabolized, and, in these cases, a normal gap does not exclude intoxication—only a late presentation.[70] Another factor that lowers the sensitivity of the osmolar gap is the considerable variation in the normal osmolar gap in the general population. Indeed, patients may have an increased gap that is still below 10 mOsm/kg.[71] Thus, a high osmolar gap is supportive of intoxication, but a normal gap does not rule it out. On the other hand, the osmolar gap can also be falsely elevated. Patients who are critically ill may have an elevated gap because of the presence of endogenous substances, such as amino acids. Patients with hyperlipidemia or hyperproteinemia will have spurious hyponatremia leading to an elevated gap.[71] There is also an accumulation of osmotically active substances in chronic renal failure.[72]

Oxygen Saturation Gap

A saturation gap exists when there is more than a 5% difference in the calculated saturation from the partial pressure of oxygen and the measured saturation with co-oximetry. Co-

Table 46–5 Osmolar Contribution of Various Toxins and Drugs

Alcohol	Osmolar Gap (mOsm/L)	Serum Concentration (mg/dL)
Ethanol	10	46
Methanol	10	32
Ethylene glycol	10	62
Isopropanol	10	60
Acetone	10	58
Propylene glycol	10	76
Mannitol	10	182

Osm, osmolar gap: measured Osm – calculated Osm.

oximetry is often performed on blood gas samples and can measure the levels of four different hemoglobin species: oxyhemoglobin, carboxyhemoglobin, methemoglobin, and reduced hemoglobin.[73] Pulse oximetry will measure carboxyhemoglobin and methemoglobin as oxyhemoglobin and will therefore overestimate the oxygen saturation in cases of carbon monoxide intoxication or methemoglobinemia.[74] This difference between oxygen saturation as measured by co-oximetry and that measured by pulse oximetry is often referred to as the pulse oximetry gap and suggests carbon monoxide poisoning or methemoglobinemia.[73,75]

DRUG OR TOXIN REMOVAL BY EXTRACORPOREAL TECHNIQUES

To determine the ability of a drug or toxin to be removed by a specific extracorporeal technique, one should consider both dialysis-related factors and drug-related factors. The characteristics of a drug that determine whether it can be removed by a specific extracorporeal technique are molecular weight, protein binding, volume of distribution, lipid or water solubility, rebound, charge, and membrane binding. The type of extracorporeal therapy, whether hemodialysis, peritoneal dialysis, or hemofiltration, also influences drug or toxin removal. Some of the important properties of the hemodialysis system that are discussed are properties of the dialysis membrane, blood flow rate (Q_b), dialysate flow rate (Q_d), pH, and temperature.

Drug-Related Factors

Molecular Weight

The molecular weight of a compound is the most reliable predictor of drug removal by a dialysis system.[76,77] The molecular size, which comprises the molecular weight, shape, charge, and steric hindrance of a molecule, is also an important determinant of the molecule's ability to permeate a dialysis membrane pore. *Low-molecular-weight* compounds or small molecules are those classified as being less than 500 D. These molecules cross conventional low-flux (low porosity, low surface area) dialysis membranes readily, with the extent depending more on Q_b, Q_d, and effective membrane surface area. *High-molecular-weight* compounds or "large solutes" are those greater than 5000 D; they diffuse slowly across membranes. *Middle-molecular-weight* compounds are those between 500 and 5000 D. Their removal is intermediate to the other two categories mentioned.

Drugs with molecular weights of more than 1000 D depend more upon convection for dialytic clearance[77] and are substantially removed only with high-flux dialysis because of the higher rate of water movement across the membranes. Common features of high-flux dialysis are (1) Q_b greater than 300 mL/min, (2) urea clearance greater than 200 mL/min, and (3) ultrafiltration coefficients (K_{Uf}) greater than 15 mL/mm Hg/hr for the dialyzers and the dialysis membranes utilized. Removal of large solutes is enhanced by the use of a porous membrane with a large surface area along with high Q_b and Q_d. Over the past 5 years, there has been a trend toward higher flux dialysis membranes. Most membranes in use today have considerably higher ultrafiltration fractions as compared to filters used 5 years ago allowing for greater clearances of *middle-molecular-weight* compounds.

Protein Binding

Protein binding renders the drug or compound pharmacologically inactive; only the unbound fraction of the drug can be readily metabolized and excreted. Unbound drug is the pharmacologically active form because it can be distributed to receptor sites, metabolic inactivating sites, or excretory sites (the kidney or dialyzer). Malnutrition and proteinuria lower serum protein levels and therefore lead to a higher fraction of free drug owing to a reduced number of protein binding sites.[78]

Drug-protein complexes are too large to cross conventional dialysis membranes and are therefore not available for removal by most renal replacement therapies. The accumulation of compounds during uremia decreases the affinity of albumin for drugs, such as penicillin, digitoxin, phenobarbital, phenytoin, warfarin, morphine, primidone, salicylate, theophylline, and sulfonamides.[79,80] If the affinity for albumin is decreased, more free or unbound drug is available for both pharmacologic effect and elimination.

Because of the chronic organic acidosis that accompanies renal failure,[81] acidic drugs have a higher free fraction than basic drugs in patients with renal failure. Examples of acidic drugs are cephalosporins, imipenem, vancomycin, and ciprofloxacin. The free fraction of basic drugs, on the other hand, is often decreased as a result of elevations of the acute-phase reactant α_1-acid glycoprotein, which binds these drugs readily.[81,82]

Free fatty acids can compete with drugs, such as tryptophan, sulfonamides, salicylates, phenylbutazone, phenytoin, thiopentone, and valproic acid for protein-binding sites. Use of heparin during hemodialysis stimulates the activity of lipoprotein lipases, subsequently increasing free fatty acid levels by triglyceride breakdown.[83–85] This increases the free fraction of the previously mentioned drugs during the time that heparin is used. Elevated free fatty acids can displace a drug, such as cefamandole, but may enhance the binding of other cephalosporins, such as cephalothin and cefoxitin.[86]

The molar ratios of drug to protein can also affect protein binding or fraction of free drug. Altered protein binding becomes clinically important in the setting of highly bound drugs with a low therapeutic index.

Volume of Distribution

The *volume of distribution* (Vd) is defined as that volume of water into which a specified amount of an agent would have to be diluted to yield the concentration found in plasma (Cp). Avid tissue binding expands the apparent Vd. The relationship can be defined as:

$$\text{Vd (L)} = \text{dose (mg)} / \text{Cp (mg/L)} \qquad (2)$$

The Vd does not necessarily correspond to a particular anatomic compartment or fluid space but denotes a mathematical relationship that assumes the body is homogenous. Substances, such as alcohols, atenolol, 2,4-dichlorophenoxyacetic acid, paracetamol, phenobarbitone, paraquat, salicylate, sotalol, aminoglycosides, and theophylline, have a relatively small or moderate Vd of less than or equal to 1 L/kg. These compounds are more likely to be removed by extracorporeal techniques.

Compounds with high degrees of tissue binding or protein binding are not substantially removed by hemoperfusion or hemodialysis. For most other β-blockers, calcium channel blockers, chloroquine, colchicine, diazepam, digoxin, flecainide, quinidine, tricyclic antidepressants, organochlorine pesticides, strychnine, quinine, and phenothiazines, the Vd is 2 L/kg or greater. These compounds are ineffectively cleared by any extracorporeal technique because of a low plasma concentration relative to the total body burden.

As discussed by Gibaldi,[87] the fraction of unbound drug in the blood and tissue can influence the Vd. In patients with impaired plasma protein binding, there is an increase in the apparent Vd of the drug. This is seen in patients with renal failure, owing to decreased albumin and impaired binding capacity of albumin. Renal failure decreases the Vd for digoxin but increases the Vd for phenytoin.

Rebound

If the rate of distribution of an agent from the extravascular tissues is slower than the elimination of the substance from the vascular space, the agent is removed from the blood more rapidly than it can be replaced from tissue stores. This is most noticeable with compounds with a large Vd (>1 L/kg) because the largest burden of drug is outside the vascular space.

Rebound refers to the movement of drug or compound from peripheral storage compartments (cells or tissues) to plasma or blood. This is characteristic of lithium, which distributes predominately within cells and exhibits slow diffusion across cell membranes.[88] After a short hemodialysis treatment, lithium plasma levels rebound or rise,[89] and repeated dialysis or continuous therapy may be required to effectively remove a substantial amount of the drug.[90] With middle- and large-molecular-weight solutes, intracellular equilibration with extracellular fluid can be slow.[91] There may be a post-hemodialysis rebound of 10% to 25% with intercompartmental equilibration.[92] The removal of other compounds, such as methotrexate,[93] paraquat,[94] and tricyclic antidepressants,[95] is hindered by slow distribution from peripheral tissues to the blood even after the blood compartment has been depleted.

Dialysis-Related Factors

In addition to drug or toxin characteristics, extracorporeal removal is also determined by the properties of the dialysis system. For hemodialysis, these factors are (1) membrane type, (2) dialyzer size, (3) dialysate composition, (4) blood flow, and (5) dialysate flow. Solute removal during hemodialysis is accomplished primarily by diffusion, with a smaller contribution coming from convection.

The factors in peritoneal dialysis that contribute to drug or toxin removal are (1) transport characteristics of the peritoneal membrane, (2) composition of the dialysate solution, (3) frequency of exchanges, and (4) dwell times. For hemofiltration, the solutes, drug, or toxin is removed primarily by convective mass transfer, meaning that solutes dissolved in plasma water are removed in the filtrate. Thus, toxin removal depends on high rates of ultrafiltration.

Hemodialyzer Properties

Removal of small solutes depends on the concentration gradient between blood and dialysate. Therefore, countercurrent flow combined with increased blood and dialysate flow rates creates a high concentration gradient for maximal solute removal. The gradient can also be maximized by enlarging the surface area of the dialysis membrane, thus exposing more undialyzed blood to areas of fresh dialysate. As the solute increases in molecular size or volume, its removal becomes limited by the pore size of the membrane and is more dependent on the property of *convection*, which is the net flow or ultrafiltration of plasma water from the blood to the dialysate. For larger molecules, diffusion across the membrane is decreased. Drug removal is limited by the membrane area times the permeability. The overall clearance of compounds can be enhanced by an increase in (1) the surface area of the membrane, (2) Q_b, and (3) the ultrafiltration rate.[96] Furthermore, drugs may bind to dialysis membranes and are removed from the circulation by adsorption, as first noted by Rumpf and associates.[97]

Peritoneal Dialysis

Although employed infrequently for toxin removal, peritoneal dialysis can be used for compounds with low molecular weight, low Vd, low protein binding, and high water solubility. Depending on the transport characteristics of the peritoneal membrane (high, average, or low), the composition of the dialysate solution, the frequency of exchanges, and dwell times can be altered to enhance clearance or removal of certain compounds or toxins. For example, the addition of albumin to the dialysate may enhance or promote removal of protein-bound substances, and modification of the pH with alkalinization may promote removal of weak acids.

Exaire and associates[98] have shown that the addition of albumin to peritoneal dialysate solutions can increase the dialytic clearance from 8 to 20 mL/min in barbiturate intoxication. With hypertonic dialysate solutions, such as 4.25% dextrose rather than 1.5% dextrose, water-soluble compound removal should be enhanced owing to higher convective losses.

When hemodynamically unstable patients are being treated with peritoneal dialysis, dopamine would be the pressor agent of choice because, at least in animal studies, it has been shown to increase peritoneal solute transport.[99] Peritoneal dialysis is the least effective method of removing drugs and should be used only if other methods are unavailable.

Hemofiltration

Hemofiltration depends on adequate blood flow (150 to 250 mL/min) to the filter for maximal performance. The removal of drug depends on its delivery to the filter, which, in turn, depends on the Vd of the drug or toxin in question. If a drug is displaced from protein, its pharmacologic effect, metabolism, and removal are enhanced.

As already described, many factors can affect drug-protein binding and Vd. Drug removal may be partially due to drug-membrane binding. Kraft and Lode[100] noted membrane binding of gentamicin to an RP-6 hemofilter, whereas Kronfol and associates[101] described the binding of both tobramycin and amikacin to AN69 filters. The *sieving coefficient* (S) is also an important factor in hemofiltration; it is the permeability of a membrane to a certain solute during ultrafiltration. A sieving coefficient of 1 means the membrane is fully permeable to the compound in question, whereas a value of 0 indicates total impermeability.[102] This relationship can be described as follows:

$$S = C(f)/C(p) \tag{3}$$

where C(f) is concentration in ultrafiltrate and C(p) is concentration in plasma.

In hemofiltration, the clearance rate is proportional to the sieving coefficient and the ultrafiltration rate:

$$\text{Clearance rate} = \text{ultrafiltration rate} \times \text{sieving coefficient}.$$

EXTRACTION RATIO

The extraction ratio (ER) is determined by measuring the concentration of the drug (plasma or blood levels) before it enters (A) the hemoperfusion cartridge or hemodialyzer filter and just after it exits (V). The ER can refer to the removal or the extraction of a drug from whole blood or plasma. It is calculated by the following formula:

$$ER = (A - V)/A \tag{4}$$

A value of 1.0 indicates that the drug was completely removed (extracted) in one pass through the extracorporeal system. The clearance rate can thus be calculated by knowing the flow rate (blood or plasma) through the system:

$$\text{Clearance rate} = \text{flow rate} \times \text{extraction ratio} \tag{5}$$

High ER can be misleading with respect to total body removal of a drug or compound. After absorption, the drug is distributed in various body compartments in different ways according to its (1) molecular weight, (2) ionization at various body fluid pH values, (3) lipid solubility, (4) protein binding, and (5) tissue binding. These factors determine the amount of drug in various body tissues, extracellular fluid, and plasma as well as the ease with which the drug moves between compartments.

Both hemodialysis and hemoperfusion are directed at drug or compound available in plasma or blood. The ease with which a compound moves from the peripheral tissue compartments to the central blood compartment must be considered when determining the practicality of these therapies for removal of the compound in question. In other words, the availability of the drug for removal is important in determining the total body clearance and decreasing toxicity with extracorporeal therapy. High ERs or clearance rates are only prerequisites to suggest the effectiveness of hemoperfusion or hemodialysis; they indicate nothing about the clinical efficacy of the removal technique.[2] They indicate the amount of drug or toxin removed only from the blood compartment not from the total body. Pharmacokinetically, hemodialysis is an appropriate removal technique when the drug or toxin is primarily distributed in extracellular water, is not highly protein bound, and has a small Vd.

Techniques of Extracorporeal Drug Removal

Dialysis to treat poisonings was introduced by Doolan and associates,[103] was championed by Schreiner and associates[104] in the 1950s, and became widely accepted in the 1960s and early 1970s. By 1972, it was believed that dialysis could treat practically all known toxic exposures.[105] The first successful treatment of a poisoned patient was achieved in 1955 by Schreiner and associates[104] for the removal of aspirin.

Anionic exchange resins were first proposed for the removal of uremic toxins in 1948[106] and for the extraction of exogenous poisons in 1958.[107] Hemoperfusion was first applied by Muirhead and Reid[106] in 1948, who used mixed ion exchange resins to remove "uremic toxins" from animals. Coated charcoal for hemoperfusion was introduced in the 1970s.[108]

Hemodialysis, Hemofiltration, and Hemoperfusion

Hemodialysis is most useful for removal of compounds with the following characteristics:

- Vd less than 1 L/kg
- Low molecular weight
- Less than 80% protein bound

These compounds include alcohols, salicylates, theophylline, and lithium.[109]

Lithium can readily be removed by hemodialysis. However, because of its moderate Vd (0.7–0.9 L/kg) and intracellular distribution with slow diffusion across cell membranes,[77] multiple treatments or continuous therapy may be required to effectively decrease the body burden of lithium.

The efficiency of hemodialysis depends not only on drug-related factors or characteristics but also on the extracorporeal system in regard to Q_b, Q_d, and dialysis membrane properties. Increasing Q_b and Q_d helps maintain a large concentration gradient with greater diffusion.

In hemofiltration, convective transport of solutes is affected by the ultrafiltration of plasma water with its dissolved constituents. The clearance of a toxin is proportional to the sieving coefficient for that toxin and the ultrafiltration rate. Therefore, to maximize the clearance in hemofiltration, one must maximize the ultrafiltration rate. In most cases, clearances of small molecules are 2 to 5 times greater with hemodialysis as compared to hemofiltration due to the limit on ultrafiltration.[110] High-volume hemofiltration may be able to overcome this difficulty by allowing for ultrafiltration rates up to 6 to 10 L/hr.[111] Hemofiltration can be employed in the removal of metal-chelator complexes, such as aluminum-deferoxamine and iron-deferoxamine. Aluminum toxicity, although now rare, can be treated with deferoxamine and the aluminum-deferoxamine complex then removed with hemodialysis or hemofiltration. Hemofiltration has been shown to be more efficient than other methods for this therapy.[8]

In hemoperfusion, blood is passed through a cartridge of sorbent material, such as coated charcoal[112] or polystyrene resin.[113] Resins were initially introduced for the removal of lipid-soluble compounds but offered little advantage over charcoal hemoperfusion, and they were withdrawn from the market in the early 1980s. In 1964, Yatzidis[114] demonstrated that a column containing activated charcoal could adsorb from plasma a considerable amount of barbital, phenobarbital, pentobarbital, salicylic acid, and glutethimide. Activated charcoal cartridges now contain charcoal covered with an ultrathin, porous coating (microencapsulation).[115] This coating decreases the direct contact between constituents of blood and charcoal, minimizing trauma to all cellular elements. Platelets are the most vulnerable; the average platelet loss is 30% with conventional hemoperfusion devices using coated charcoal.[116] There are also reductions in serum calcium and glucose levels.[13] Complications of hemoperfusion include thrombocytopenia, hypocalcemia, hypoglycemia, hypothermia, and charcoal embolization. To prevent the latter, the system contains a filter in the venous line to remove loosened charcoal particles prior to returning blood to the patient. It has been shown to be effective in removal of theophylline, phenobarbital, phenytoin, carbamazepine, paraquat, and glutethimide.[117] Hemoperfusion is not beneficial in control of electrolyte disturbances, acid-base disorders, or fluid overload but may be applied concurrently with hemodialysis or hemofiltration to correct these disorders.

Peritoneal Dialysis and Plasma Exchange

Peritoneal dialysis can be used for removal of compounds with low or middle molecular weight, low Vd, low protein binding, and polar substances that readily dissolve in water. They include alcohols, lithium, salicylates, and theophylline. Peritoneal dialysis is less efficient than other extracorporeal techniques because clearances rarely exceed 10 mL/min. In some situations, however, it may be beneficial, especially if it is the only extracorporeal therapy available.

With the use of hypertonic dialysate, convective forces can increase recovery of water-soluble compounds. Other modifications can be made to promote drug removal; for example, adding albumin to the dialysate may help promote removal of protein-bound substances,[118] and modification of the pH through alkalinization of the dialysate may promote the removal of weak acids.[119]

Plasma exchange is most applicable to removal of drugs that have an extremely high affinity for circulating proteins. It has been used rarely in chromic acid and chromate poisonings.[120] It has also been used to remove antibody-digoxin complexes following treatment with digoxin-specific antibody for patients with digoxin toxicity and anuria.[121] Exchange transfusion is not applicable to poisonings. It has been used for treatment of hemolysis and methemoglobinemia secondary to various poisonings.[122]

Continuous hemofiltration techniques are useful for patients in need of renal replacement therapy along with continuous drug removal. These techniques are particularly useful for removal of drugs that have high degrees of tissue binding or intracellular distribution and slow intercompartmental transfer, such as lithium.[88,111]

Indications for Extracorporeal Therapy

Indications for extracorporeal elimination of drugs or toxins depend most strongly on the clinical severity and potential complications of the poisoning. The following issues must be considered:

1. Characteristics of the individual patient (age and other comorbid conditions, such as congestive heart failure, end-stage renal disease, and liver failure).
2. Toxic side effects of the compound ingested, along with dose ingested, potential complications, and impaired pathways of metabolism.
3. Nature, dose, and plasma concentration of the toxic substance.

Appropriate interpretation of the drug concentration must take into account hepatic or renal elimination, delayed gastrointestinal absorption, active metabolites, altered distributional characteristics, and saturable elimination pathways. Extracorporeal elimination that increases the total body clearance by 30% or more is believed to be a worthwhile intervention in the proper clinical setting.[123,124]

Extracorporeal therapy may be considered when all of the following conditions are met:

1. The drug or toxin diffuses readily through the dialysis membrane (e.g., alcohol) or is readily bound by the adsorbent (e.g., barbiturate).[125]
2. A clinically significant proportion of the poison is present in plasma water or is capable of rapid equilibration with plasma water (e.g., alcohols).
3. The pharmacologic effect of the toxin is directly related to its blood concentration (e.g., lithium).
4. Dialysis or hemoperfusion will add significantly to total body elimination (>30%) (e.g., alcohols or procainamide).

Indications for extracorporeal removal of poisons are not universally agreed on, however. Table 46–6 lists characteristics of poisonings for which there is general agreement that extracorporeal therapy should be used.[109,126]

SPECIFIC TOXINS

The rest of the chapter will focus on specific toxins and drugs that are frequent causes of intoxication and whose elimination is significantly enhanced with either hemodialysis or hemoperfusion. They include ethanol, methanol, ethylene glycol, isopropyl alcohol, salicylates, lithium, and theophylline. Table 46–7 shows the number of reported exposures and the mortality rates for these toxins.[1]

Alcohols

Alcohols are readily dialyzed because of their rapid diffusibility, water solubility, poor protein binding, and small Vd.

Ethanol

Ethanol is rapidly metabolized without toxic metabolites. A level greater than 350 mg/dL is dangerous, and a level greater

Table 46–6 Indications for Extracorporeal Therapy

1. A patient whose status is deteriorating despite full supportive care.
2. Normal routes of detoxification and elimination of the toxic agent are impaired.
3. A patient who has ingested a compound that will cause serious morbidity (tissue damage) or death and for which supportive care is ineffective. Examples: (a) Methyl alcohol metabolism to a toxic byproduct: poisoning of concentration >50 mg/dL or >16 mmol/L can lead to blindness; (b) theophylline intoxication can cause seizures with permanent neurologic impairment or death.
4. A patient who is unduly susceptible to the effect of an overdose because of age or comorbid conditions. These patients poorly tolerate prolonged coma and its complications (intubation, respirator support, pneumonia, septicemia, or hemodynamic instability or immobilization).
5. Severe central nervous system depression, primarily of midbrain function, leading to hypoventilation, hypothermia, and hypotension.
6. Patient who presents with overt signs and symptoms of toxicity.

than 500 mg/dL may be fatal.[2] The total body clearance of ethanol is increased by 50% with hemodialysis.[127] There may be circumstances in which hemodialysis is indicated for ethanol intoxication (i.e., pediatric intoxication). However, the relevance of a 50% reduction in ethanol concentration by hemodialysis is better applied when ethanol is used to treat poisonings with other alcohols. Severe acidosis is not usually seen with ethanol intoxication. There is a rise in the osmolar gap of 22 mOsm/kg for every 100 mg/dL rise in serum ethanol concentration.[128] Table 46–5 lists the osmolar contributions of the various alcohols and other low–molecular-weight toxins.

Methanol

Methanol is a highly toxic alcohol that is found in a variety of commercial products, including antifreeze, windshield wiper fluid, paint thinner, and canned solid fuel for keeping food warm.[129] There were 12 reported deaths from methanol exposure in 2001.[1] The estimated minimum lethal dose for adults is approximately 10 mL. There are also reports of patients surviving ingestions greater than 400 mL without sequelae.[130]

Methanol is rapidly absorbed after ingestion. It has a distribution volume of 0.6 L/kg and a molecular weight of 32 g/mol. The metabolism of methanol to its end products is displayed in Figure 46–1. Methanol is oxidized by alcohol dehydrogenase in the presence of NAD to formaldehyde. Formaldehyde is then quickly oxidized to formate. Formate produces much of the toxic effect as well as the high anion gap acidosis. The formation of lactate also contributes to the anion gap acidosis. Pyruvate is metabolized to lactate because of the reduction of NAD to NADH during the oxidation of methanol.[131,132] Ethanol and fomepizole will slow the oxygenation of methanol by inhibiting alcohol dehydrogenase.[133,134]

Most of the clinical effects of methanol intoxication are due to the accumulation of formate. Before it is metabolized, methanol's major effect is to cause central nervous system depression. This is of short duration and is followed by a latent period. The latent period is due to the time it takes for formate to accumulate and lasts 14 to 18 hours or longer with ethanol or fomepizole treatment.[135]

The latent period is followed by a number of systemic findings as formate accumulates. Metabolic acidosis can be severe and a pH less than 7.0 has been found to be the strongest predictor of mortality. Patients with a pH less than 7.0 have 20 times the mortality as compared to patients with pH greater than 7.0.[130] Central nervous system effects in this stage can include headache, lethargy, convulsions, delirium, and coma. Patients who present with seizure or coma have over 10 times the mortality as patients without these symptoms.[136] Serum methanol levels have very little prognostic value for either permanent visual changes or death.[130,136]

Table 46–7 Exposures and Fatalities from Toxins Substantially Removed by Extracorporeal Techniques

Toxin	Exposures (% of total)	Fatalities (% of total)	Mortality (% of exposures)
Methanol	1142 (0.05)	12 (1.1)	1.0
Ethylene glycol	5833 (0.2)	34 (3.1)	0.6
Isopropyl alcohol	9745 (0.4)	0 (0)	0
Salicylates	17,075 (0.7)	66 (6.1)	0.4
Lithium	4607 (0.2)	8 (0.7)	0.2
Theophylline	1146 (0.05)	18 (1.6)	1.5

(From Litovitz TL, Klein-Schwartz W, Rodgers GC Jr, et al: 2001 Annual report of the American Association of Poison Control Centers Toxic Exposure Surveillance System. Am J Emerg Med 2002; 20:391-452.)

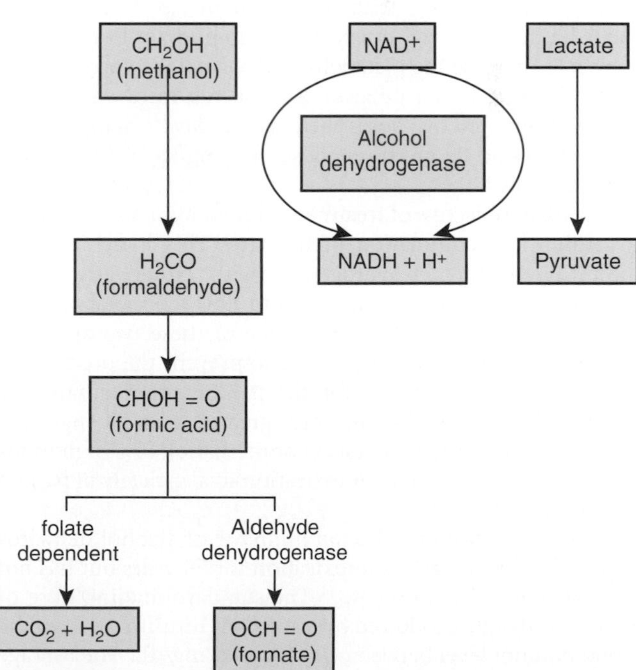

Figure 46–1 Metabolism of methanol to its toxic intermediates. See text for explanation.

Ocular findings can be prominent and may include photophobia, central scotoma, visual field defects, fixed pupils, and difficulty with light adaptation. Pupillary dysfunction has also been shown to be a strong predictor of mortality.[136] Funduscopic signs include hyperemia, disk edema, and possible optic atrophy.[137] The ocular findings are due to the direct cytotoxic effect of formate on the retina. Other systemic findings can include nausea, vomiting, diaphoresis, and abdominal pain. The abdominal pain is often due to pancreatitis.[138]

As already stated, the accumulation of formate produces a high anion gap metabolic acidosis. Some of the anion gap is from the increased lactate production. A patient who presents early after an ingestion or later after a coingestion ethanol, may have little or no acidosis making the diagnosis of methanol intoxication much more difficult. These same patients receive the most benefit from alcohol dehydrogenase inhibition since the ingested methanol still needs to be metabolized to formate to have its toxic effect.[131]

Methanol also produces an osmolar gap. A serum level of 32 mg/dL increases the measured serum osmolarity by 10 mOsm/kg, and the serum methanol level can be estimated by multiplying the osmolar gap by 3.2. A high serum methanol level should therefore cause a gap between the calculated serum osmolarity and the measured osmolarity by freezing point depression.[139] However, patients with methanol intoxication may have a normal gap (<10 mOsm/kg), if they present late after ingestion and the methanol has been converted to formate. Formate does not contribute to the serum osmolarity because it is balanced by sodium, which is included in the calculated osmolarity. For this reason, the osmolarity gap should be used to help support the diagnosis of methanol intoxication, but it is not sensitive enough to rule out intoxication when there is no gap.[64]

Supportive treatment for methanol intoxication includes airway protection, circulatory support, correction of metabolic abnormalities, and control of seizures. Bicarbonate is indicated for patients with pH less than 7.3.[140] The use of folate has not been rigorously studied in humans but has been shown to increase the metabolism of formate to carbon dioxide and water. It can be given as a 50 mg intravenous dose every 4 hours for five doses then once a day.[141] Symptomatic patients should be given one dose of 1 mg/kg of folinic acid intravenously.[140]

The main objective of treatment of methanol intoxication is to limit the accumulation of formate. This is achieved by inhibiting alcohol dehydrogenase with either ethanol or fomepizole. Both have been shown to slow the metabolism of methanol to formate.[130,132,142–144] One of these two antidotes should be used as soon as possible to prevent the production of formate.[140] Indications for the use of either ethanol or fomepizole include a serum level greater than 20 mg/dL, a high osmolar gap after ingestion of methanol, or a high index of suspicion for methanol intoxication in a critically ill patient (Table 46–8).[140]

Ethanol has been used as an inhibitor of alcohol dehydrogenase in ethylene glycol intoxication for 50 years but has not been approved by the FDA.[144] The standard loading dose of ethanol is 0.6 g/kg followed by a constant infusion to keep the blood ethanol level between 100 and 200 mg/dL. The average maintenance dose of ethanol is 100 mg/kg/hr but is significantly higher for alcoholics and for patients on dialysis. Blood ethanol levels should be checked every 1 to 2 hours until a steady state has been reached and then every 2 to 4 hours (Table 46–9). The potential adverse effects of ethanol include central nervous system depression, hypoglycemia, respiratory depression, and aspiration.[67,78,146]

Fomepizole should be given at a loading dose of 15 mg/kg followed by 10 mg/kg every 12 hours for 48 hours. After 48 hours, the dose should be increased to 15 mg/kg every 12 hours.[142] Fomepizole should be continued until the serum methanol level is less than 20 mg/dL and the patient is asymptomatic with a normal pH. Fomepizole is dialyzed and therefore needs to be dosed every 4 hours during dialysis (Table 46–10).[147]

The dose of both inhibitors of alcohol dehydrogenase have to be increased during dialysis.[148,149] Fomepizole may be the preferred antidote in methanol intoxication because levels do

Table 46–8 Indications for Fomepizole or Ethanol Therapy in Methanol or Ethylene Glycol Intoxication

1. Serum level of ethylene glycol or methanol >20 mg/dL
   or
2. History of ingestion of ethylene glycol or methanol and osmolar gap >10 mOsm/L
   or
3. Strong suspicion of ingestion of ethylene glycol or methanol and at least two of the following:
   a. Arterial pH <7.3
   b. Serum bicarbonate <20 mEq/L
   c. Osmolar gap >10 mOsm/L
   d. Calcium oxalate crystals in urine (for suspected ethylene glycol ingestion)

(From Barceloux DG, Bond GR, Krenzelok EP, et al: The American Academy of Clinical Toxicology Ad Hoc Committee on the Treatment Guidelines for Methanol P: American Academy of Clinical Toxicology practice guidelines on the treatment of methanol poisoning. J Toxicol Clin Toxicol 2002; 40:415-446; Barceloux DG, Krenzelok EP, Olson K, Watson W: American Academy of Clinical Toxicology Practice Guidelines on the Treatment of Ethylene Glycol Poisoning. Ad Hoc Committee. J Toxicol Clin Toxicol 1999; 37:537-560.)

Table 46–9 Ethanol Dosing in Methanol and Ethylene Glycol Intoxications

- IV loading dose 0.6–0.7 g/kg
- Followed by 66 mg/kg/hr constant infusion
- Keep serum concentration between 100–150 mg/dL
- Check serum concentration every 1–2 hr
- Increase maintenance dose to 154 mg/kg/hr for chronic drinkers
- Increase maintenance dose to 169 mg/kg/hr during dialysis
- Increase maintenance dose to 257 mg/kg/hr for chronic drinkers during dialysis

(From Barceloux DG, Krenzelok EP, Olson K, Watson W: American Academy of Clinical Toxicology Practice Guidelines on the Treatment of Ethylene Glycol Poisoning. Ad Hoc Committee. J Toxicol Clin Toxicol 1999; 37:537-560.)

Table 46–10 Fomepizole Dosing in Methanol and Ethylene Glycol Intoxications

- IV loading dose 15 mg/kg (1 g/mL, 1.5 mL/vial)
- Followed by 10 mg/kg every 12 hr for 48 hr
- Then 15 mg/kg every 12 hours until ethylene glycol or methanol levels <20 mg/dL
- All doses should be administered over 30 minutes
- Increase the frequency to every 4 hours during hemodialysis

(From Brent J, McMartin K, Phillips S, et al: Fomepizole for the treatment of ethylene glycol poisoning. Methylpyrazole for Toxic Alcohols Study Group [Comment]. N Engl J Med 1999; 340:832-838.)

not need to be followed, it has fewer side effects, does not cause further sedation, and it has a much simpler dosing scheme both with and without concurrent dialysis. Finally, because of the low side effect profile, some patients treated with fomepizole may not need observation in an intensive care unit, if they are otherwise stable.[142] With either antidote, the treatment should be continued until the methanol level is undetectable or both symptoms and acidosis resolve and the level is less than 20 mg/dL.[129]

Hemodialysis will remove both methanol and formic acid efficiently and will help correct the acidosis. It should be considered in any patient with severe acidosis or other refractory metabolic disturbance, high formate levels, seizures, visual changes, funduscopic abnormalities, or mental status changes (Table 46–11).[140,149] Since the serum methanol level has not been linked to permanent visual changes or death and with the availability of fomepizole, a less toxic antidote as compared to ethanol, some authors have argued that a high methanol level is no longer an indication for dialysis, if no other indication for dialysis is present.[151,152] Patients with a high methanol level that are not treated with dialysis should be watched closely for the development of acidosis or vision changes that would indicate the need for urgent dialysis. Clearance constants with high efficiency membranes have been as high as 200 mL/min for both formate and methanol.[148] The dose of both ethanol and fomepizole need to be increased during hemodialysis. Hemodialysis can hinder the maintenance of adequate ethanol levels, and a number of authors have described the use of ethanol enriched dialysate solutions.[153] Hemodialysis should be continued until the serum methanol level is undetectable or the patient is asymptomatic with a normal serum pH and the level is less than 20 mg/dL.[154]

Table 46–11 Indications for Dialysis in Patients with Methanol Intoxication

1. Metabolic acidosis with pH <7.30
2. Vision or funduscopic abnormalities
3. Deteriorating vital signs, seizures or mental status despite supportive care
4. Renal failure
5. Refractory electrolyte imbalance
6. Methanol level >50 mg/dL (controversial if fomepizole is available)

(From Barceloux DG, Bond GR, Krenzelok EP, et al: The American Academy of Clinical Toxicology Ad Hoc Committee on the Treatment Guidelines for Methanol P: American Academy of Clinical Toxicology practice guidelines on the treatment of methanol poisoning. J Toxicol Clin Toxicol 2002; 40:415-446.)

Ethylene Glycol

Ethylene glycol is a sweet-tasting substance that is a common constituent of antifreeze. Because of its sweet taste and its ability to intoxicate, it is sometimes used as a substitute for ethanol. It is also often found as an accidental ingestion in children, or as a suicidal agent, accounting for approximately 0.2% of all exposures and 3.0% of all deaths due to poisonings. In 2001, there were 5833 exposures to ethylene glycol and 34 deaths reported to the Toxic Exposure Surveillance System (TESS) (see Table 46–7).[1] The estimated minimum lethal dose for adults is approximately 100 mL. A number of patients have survived ingestions of over 2000 mL.[155–157] In a case report by Johnson and associates,[155] one patient who underwent rapid treatment with ethanol infusion and hemodialysis in the emergency room survived an ingestion of 3000 mL without sequelae. The ethylene glycol level was found to be 1889 mg/dL.

Ethylene glycol reaches a peak serum level 2 to 4 hours after ingestion. It is water-soluble and has a volume of distribution that is equal to total body water (0.6 L/kg). It has a molecular weight of 62 g/mol. Figure 46–2 displays the metabolism of ethylene glycol to its end products. Ethylene glycol is oxidized by alcohol dehydrogenase in the presence of nicotinamide

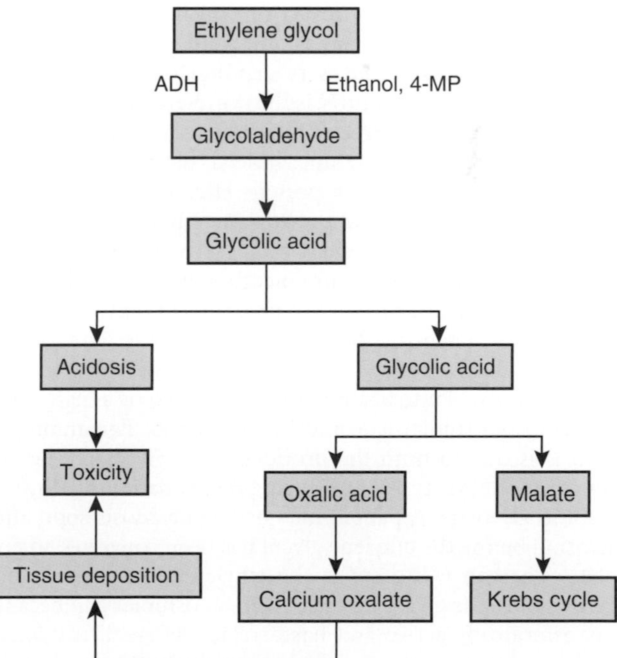

Figure 46–2 Ethylene glycol elimination. The metabolite glycolic acid produces the acidosis, and calcium oxalate damages tissue. Metabolism to these toxic species can be diminished if one saturates alcohol dehydrogenase (ADH) with ethanol. *4-MP,* 4-methylpyrazole.

adenine dinucleotide (NAD) to glycoaldehyde, which is then rapidly oxidized to glycolate.[158] Ethanol and fomepizole slow the metabolism of ethylene glycol by inhibiting the enzyme alcohol dehydrogenase.[144] Glycolate is the toxic metabolite and produces the high anion gap acidosis. Glycolate may be metabolized to oxalate, α-hydroxy-β-ketoadipate, and glycine. Oxalate causes some of the end organ damage as a direct toxin and through calcium oxalate deposition. Some part of the acidosis stems from the production of lactate and is due to the reduction of NAD to NADH, which drives the conversion of pyruvate to lactate (see Figure 46–1).[159] Without treatment, the elimination half-life of ethylene glycol is 3 to 8 hours. Ethanol and fomepizole will prolong the half-life fivefold to 15 to 20 hours.[141,160]

The clinical course of ethylene glycol intoxication can be divided into three phases.[161] The first phase occurs less than an hour after ingestion and is characterized by mental status depression similar to alcohol intoxication. In severe intoxication, coma, seizures, and respiratory depression can complicate this phase. This stage lasts about 12 hours as the ethylene glycol is oxidized to glycoaldehyde and glycolate.[72] In the second phase, glycolate has a toxic effect on the cardiopulmonary system. In severe intoxications, patients can develop acidosis, heart failure, pulmonary edema, or adult respiratory distress syndrome (ARDS).[72] The timing of this stage depends on the metabolism of the ethylene glycol to glycolate and usually starts approximately 12 hours after ingestion but will be delayed by alcohol coingestion. Review of data from TESS suggests that most deaths occur during this stage.[1] The final stage occurs 24 to 72 hours after ingestion and is characterized by flank pain, acute tubular necrosis, hypocalcemia, and renal failure. During this stage, the production of oxalate leads to calcium oxalate precipitation in the kidney and other tissues and hypocalcemia. The renal toxicity is probably due to a combination of hydronephrosis from calcium oxalate crystals and a direct toxic effect from the metabolites of ethylene glycol.[162] Most renal damage is reversible, and renal recovery, which may take a few months, is the norm even after anuria.[163]

There is very little correlation between serum ethylene glycol levels and clinical outcome. Indeed, patients may have a very high mortality, if they present after their serum levels have begun to decrease and the ethylene glycol has been converted to its toxic metabolites.[158] There is better correlation between the arterial pH, serum bicarbonate, or glycolate level and the clinical outcome. A number of studies of patients treated with fomepizole have shown that those who present without acidosis or a high glycolate level do well.[160,164]

Ethylene glycol intoxication is characterized by a high anion gap acidosis, osmolar gap, and hypocalcemia. The anion gap acidosis is due to both the production of glycolate and the reduction of NAD to NADH during the oxidation of ethylene glycol to glycolate. A patient may have no acidosis soon after ingestion before the ethylene glycol has been converted to glycolate. The gap will grow as the ethylene glycol is metabolized.[165] Ethylene glycol will also form an osmolar gap because it is osmotically active and has a relatively small molecular weight. In ethylene glycol intoxication, the serum level of the toxin can be estimated by multiplying the osmolar gap by 6.2.[166] An osmolar gap lacks the sensitivity and specificity to be an ideal screening test for intoxications. Glycolate does not contribute to the osmolar gap so that as the ethylene glycol is metabolized to glycolate, the osmolar gap will, in fact, fall. Therefore, patients who present late after an ingestion, may have a normal osmolar gap.[70]

The urine may contain two forms of calcium oxalate crystals in ethylene glycol intoxication. The dumbbell-shaped monohydrate forms are more common, but the octahedral-shaped dihydrate form is more specific for ethylene glycol intoxication.[156] Individuals who ingest a large amount of vitamin C or urate-containing foods may have monohydrate calcium oxalate crystals in their urine. The dihydrate form requires higher oxalate concentrations for its formation and therefore is more indicative of intoxication with ethylene glycol.[159]

Supportive treatment includes airway protection, circulatory support, correction of metabolic abnormalities, and control of seizures. Bicarbonate is indicated for patients with pH less than 7.3.[158] Asymptomatic hypocalcemia is generally not treated because of the risk of increasing the formation of calcium oxalate crystals. Seizures may be due to hypocalcemia but should be first treated with standard anticonvulsants. There is no role for activated charcoal, cathartics, or gastric lavage in ethylene glycol intoxication.[158] Alcoholics and patients likely to be malnourished should be given thiamine and pyridoxine. The addition of thiamine, 100 mg intramuscularly (IM) or IV, and pyridoxine, 50 mg IV every 6 hours, should shunt the metabolism of ethylene glycol to less toxic metabolites.[67] Thiamine promotes the metabolism of glyoxylate from glycolic acid to a nontoxic metabolite, α-hydroxy-β-ketoadipate, and pyridoxine promotes the metabolism of glyoxylate to glycine.[169]

As with methanol intoxication, fomepizole and ethanol will slow the metabolism of ethylene glycol to its more toxic metabolites. The indications for the use of one of the antidotes have been outlined by the American Academy of Clinical Toxicology.[158] These indications include a plasma ethylene glycol concentration greater than 20 mg/dL, a recent ingestion of ethylene glycol and an osmolar gap greater than 10 mOsm/kg, or a high clinical suspicion and two of the following: pH less than 7.3, serum bicarbonate less than 20 mEq/L, osmolar gap greater than 10 mOsm/kg, or urinary oxalate crystals (see Table 46–8). The dosing schedule of each antidote is the same as that for methanol intoxication and is listed in Tables 46–9 and 46–10.

As with methanol intoxication, fomepizole may be the preferred antidote in ethylene glycol poisoning because of its ease of administration and because it does not cause CNS depression or hypoglycemia. Some patients treated with fomepizole may not need observation in an intensive care unit if they are otherwise stable.[142] Fomepizole is removed with dialysis and therefore needs to be dosed every 4 hours during dialysis.[147]

Hemodialysis is very effective at clearing ethylene glycol and its metabolites. The clearance rate of ethylene glycol ranges between 200 and 250 mL/min, depending on the filter and blood flow. Glycolate, which is the major toxic metabolite, has a half-life of up to 18 hours without hemodialysis, but the half-life is reduced by a factor of 6 with hemodialysis.[159] Patients with acidosis may therefore still benefit from hemodialysis even in the face of a low serum ethylene glycol level.[168]

The indications for hemodialysis include those patients who have or are likely to develop the major sequelae of ethylene glycol ingestion. These include patients with metabolic acidosis (pH <7.3) or deteriorating clinical status with respiratory failure or hypotension. Patients with acute renal failure and a metabolic derangement that is unresponsive to standard therapy should be considered for hemodialysis as well (Table 46–12). In the past, an ethylene glycol level of 50 mg/dL was considered an indication for hemodialysis. Recent experience suggests that patients with normal renal function and no acidosis may be treated with fomepizole without hemodialysis even in the setting of an ethylene glycol level greater than 50 mg/dL.[164] These patients would require close monitoring for the development of renal insufficiency or acidosis.

Both fomepizole and ethanol are cleared during dialysis. The addition of ethanol to the dialysate has been shown to maintain blood ethanol levels during dialysis.[157] The use of fomepizole during hemodialysis is more straightforward and only requires an increase in the frequency of the doses to every 4 hours to maintain adequate levels.[160]

Dialysis should be continued until the ethylene glycol level is less than 20 mg/dL, the acidosis has resolved and there are no signs of systemic toxicity, or until the ethylene glycol level is undetectable. Prolonged dialysis up to 8 to 10 hours may be required for very high ethylene glycol levels and severe acidosis.[155] First-order kinetics can be used to estimate the required dialysis time in both methanol and ethylene glycol intoxication. Using the kinetics equation $C_1/C_0 = e^{-kt/V}$ where C_1 = desired drug level, C_0 = current level, k = clearance constant (~0.2 L/min), and Vd = volume of distribution (0.6 L/kg), and t is time in minutes,[154] the required dialysis time in minutes is therefore:

$$t = -\,Vd/k \times \ln(C_1/C_0) \quad (6)$$

For example, a 100 kg man with an ethylene glycol level of 100 mg/dL will need dialysis for

$$t = -\,(60\ L/0.2\ L/min) \times \ln(20/100) = 483\ \text{minutes} \sim 8\ \text{hours.} \quad (7)$$

Alternatively, dialysis can be continued until the serum osmolar gap and anion gap resolve, suggesting that ethylene glycol and glycolate levels have dropped.

Isopropyl Alcohol

Isopropanol is a colorless liquid with a bitter taste. It is used in the manufacture of acetone and glycerin. It is often used as the solvent in rubbing alcohol. Most rubbing alcohol contains 70% isopropanol.

There were 9745 exposures to isopropanol and 0 deaths reported to TESS in 2001.[1] This represents 0.4% of all exposures reported (see Table 46–7). It has a much smaller percentage of deaths per exposure as compared to either ethylene glycol or methanol. The estimated minimum lethal dose for adults is approximately 100 mL. Patients have survived ingestions of over 1000 mL.

Isopropanol reaches a peak serum level 15 to 30 minutes after ingestion. It is water-soluble and has a volume of distribution that is equal to total body water (0.6 L/kg). It has a molecular weight of 60 g/mol. Isopropanol is oxidized by alcohol dehydrogenase to acetone. The elimination half-life of isopropanol is 3 to 7 hours but is prolonged with ethanol coingestion.[167] The elimination of acetone is much slower and is due to excretion in the breath and urine.[171]

Unlike ethylene glycol and methanol, most of the clinical effects in isopropanol intoxication are due to the parent compound. Acetone causes only mild central nervous system depression.[139] The clinical signs of isopropanol intoxication will occur within an hour of ingestion and include effects on the central nervous system, gastrointestinal, and cardiovascular systems. The CNS effects include ataxia, confusion, stupor, and coma. The GI effects include nausea, vomiting, abdominal pain, and gastritis. Patients with severe intoxication can present with hypotension due to cardiac depression and vasodilatation.[172] Hypotension is the strongest predictor of mortality.[173] Many patients will have fruity breath from the acetone elimination via respiration.

A serum level of isopropanol equal to 60 mg/dL will increase the serum osmolarity by 10 mOsm/kg. A high serum level should therefore produce a gap between the calculated serum osmolarity and that measured by freezing point depression.[174] Acidosis is rare following isopropanol ingestion because neither the parent compound nor its metabolites are organic acids. Therefore, a finding of a high serum or urine acetone level with an osmolar gap but without acidosis is suggestive of a recent isopropanol ingestion.[167] Renal failure can occur in the setting of significant hypotension. Hypoglycemia can result from the interference of gluconeogenesis by isopropanol.[139]

Supportive treatment for isopropyl alcohol intoxication includes circulatory support with fluids or vasoconstrictors in patients with hypotension. Inhibition of alcohol dehydrogenase is not indicated because acetone is less toxic than isopropanol. Hemodialysis is indicated for patients with an isopropanol level greater than 400 mg/dL and significant CNS depression, renal failure, or hypotension.[173] Hemodialysis will remove both isopropanol and acetone effectively.[175] High-efficiency membranes can produce clearance constants greater than 200 mL/min for both acetone and isopropanol.

Table 46–12 Indications for Dialysis in Patients with Ethylene Glycol Intoxication

1. Metabolic acidosis with pH <7.30
2. Deteriorating vital signs or mental status despite supportive care
3. Renal failure
4. Refractory electrolyte imbalance
5. Ethylene glycol >50 mg/dL (controversial if fomepizole is available)

(From Barceloux DG, Krenzelok EP, Olson K, Watson W: American Academy of Clinical Toxicology Practice Guidelines on the Treatment of Ethylene Glycol Poisoning. Ad Hoc Committee. J Toxicol Clin Toxicol 1999; 37:537-560.)

Salicylates

Salicylate intoxication accounted for approximately 0.7% of all exposures and 6.1% of all deaths reported to the TESS (see Table 46–7).[1] Salicylates are found in many commonly used medications. The most common is acetylsalicylic acid or aspirin. Acetylsalicylic acid is converted to salicylic acid in the stomach and is then rapidly absorbed. The symptoms of salicylate intoxication differ according to the age of the patient and whether the intoxication is acute or chronic.[176] Most people will have some clinical effects of intoxication with serum levels greater than 40 mg/dL.[177] In chronic intoxication and in the elderly, symptoms will occur at lower levels.[178]

The common symptoms in all settings are nausea, vomiting, hyperventilation, tinnitus, stupor, coma, and convulsions. The acidosis is due to uncoupling of oxidative phosphorylation in the Krebs cycle and accumulation of lactic acid and ketoacids.[179,180] Hyperventilation occurs from direct stimulation and can lead to a respiratory alkalosis. Children are more likely to demonstrate fever and severe metabolic acidosis,[181–183] whereas adults are more likely to experience noncardiogenic pulmonary edema, especially among those with a history of smoking.[176,184–186]

Activated charcoal is effective in reducing the gut absorption of salicylate in acute intoxication.[187–189] Salicylate undergoes both glomerular filtration and tubular secretion. Renal excretion is very important at toxic and therapeutic serum salicylate levels. Reabsorption of salicylate in the proximal convoluted tubule depends on the urine flow rate and urine pH. In an acid environment, salicylate is nonionized. For this reason, urinary alkalinization can increase the renal clearance significantly through ion trapping.[190] Sodium bicarbonate can be used to increase serum pH and raise urine pH to greater than 7.5.[191] Forced diuresis does not appear to increase clearance and may lead to volume overload. The use of acetazolamide should be avoided because it can increase the risk of systemic acidosis.

Salicylates have a small Vd (0.21 L/kg), a low molecular weight (138 D), and a moderate degree of protein binding (about 50% at toxic levels).[192] All of these characteristics enable salicylates to be removed by hemoperfusion or hemodialysis.[105] Hemodialysis is the preferred method because of the inability of hemoperfusion to correct acid-base and electrolyte disorders and volume disturbances.[193] Hemodialysis should be considered for serum levels greater than 100 mg/dL in acute ingestion and as low as 60 mg/dL in chronic ingestion.[109] Hemodialysis can be advantageous in the patient with a high serum salicylate level, fluid overload, and metabolic acidosis associated with clinical deterioration and coma.[194, 195] The end point of dialysis is considered to consist of:

1. Return to a nontoxic level of the serum salicylate level.
2. Clinical improvement.
3. Correction of acid-base disturbances.[180]

Lithium

Lithium is a commonly used mood stabilizer. It has a low therapeutic index and can therefore cause inadvertent toxicity fairly easily. The risk of toxicity increases when it is used as long-term therapy, both when lithium is ingested in overdose and when a patient's elimination pathways are impaired. Few patients require intervention with extracorporeal therapy, especially if treated promptly. The severity of intoxication is related to the duration of the poisoning, the possibility of delayed absorption, and the actual serum lithium level.[196–198] In 2001, there were 4607 toxic exposures but only 8 deaths reported to TESS (see Table 46–7).[1]

Lithium Absorption and Elimination

An alkali metal, lithium is well absorbed in the stomach and proximal small intestine,[199] with a peak serum concentration in 5 hours for regular-release preparations and 4 to 12 hours for sustained-release preparations. It is not bound to plasma proteins and has a low molecular weight (74 D), but its Vd is moderate (0.7 to 0.9 L/kg), approximately that of total body water.[200] Lithium is predominately intracellular but diffuses across cell membranes slowly,[200] making its removal by extracorporeal techniques a slow process, requiring up to 8 to 10 hours and repeated treatments for thorough removal.[90]

Lithium elimination is almost exclusively renal.[201] This drug is freely filtered and 60% reabsorbed, mostly in the proximal tubule by the same active process that promotes sodium reabsorption.[90,202] Conditions associated with a reduction in either glomerular filtration rate or tubular sodium concentration result in decreased elimination secondary to greater reabsorption. These conditions include sodium and volume depletion, cardiac failure, liver failure, use of thiazide diuretics, nonsteroidal anti-inflammatory drugs, or angiotensin-converting enzyme inhibitors.[196,200,203]

Toxicity

Extracorporeal therapy for lithium intoxication should be based on clinical criteria rather than on serum lithium levels.[196,204–206] Patients with serum lithium levels as high as 8.0 mEq/L have survived lithium intoxication without hemodialysis.[196,207,208] The serum lithium level is a more reliable indicator of intracellular lithium levels in chronic intoxication or acute intoxication superimposed on chronic intoxication.[206,209]

For acute intoxication, the failure of severe or moderate clinical signs or symptoms to improve within 6 hours of supportive therapy is an indication for hemodialysis. The correlation between serum lithium level and clinical presentation is not always close; therefore, clinical symptoms must be the main determinant of the need for dialysis. Hemodialysis is recommended for all patients with severe clinical manifestations. If the clinical condition fails to improve or progresses after 6 hours of corrective or supportive care, or if renal clearance is impaired, dialysis should be considered even in the patient who has moderate clinical manifestations.[206,210–213]

Table 46–13 categorizes the clinical symptoms of lithium intoxication as mild, moderate, or severe, irrespective of whether the intoxication is acute or chronic. The hallmark of the lithium-intoxicated patient is the CNS toxicity. This effect may range from coarse tremor to mental status changes,

Table 46–13 Toxic Manifestations of Lithium

Mild (lithium level <2.5 meq/L)
Tremor, ataxia, photophobia, nystagmus, light-headedness, weakness
Nausea, emesis
Moderate (lithium level 2.5–3.5 mEq/L)
Hyperreflexia, twitching, tinnitus, apathy, drowsiness, confusion
Diarrhea
Bradycardia, hypotension
Severe (lithium level >3.5 mEq/L)
Seizure, clonus, delirium, coma
Severe bradycardia, cardiovascular collapse

(From Timmer RT, Sands JM: Lithium intoxication. J Am Soc Nephrol 1999; 10:666-674.)

ataxia, and subsequent coma. The cardiovascular manifestations range from benign flattening and inversion of the T waves on electrocardiogram to severe hypotension and cardiovascular collapse.[214,215] Lithium-related intraventricular conduction defects are observed only with toxic concentrations of lithium, in patients with established heart disease, or in those taking other cardiotoxic agents.[216,217] Severe ventricular arrhythmias occur almost exclusively with acute intoxications.[218] With severe acute ingestion, vomiting and profuse diarrhea develop soon afterward secondary to the high lithium concentrations in the gastrointestinal tract. If the patient fails to improve or deteriorates after 6 hours of supportive care, the status of the CNS and cardiovascular systems dictates the need for extracorporeal therapy.[196] As an unmeasured cation, severe lithium intoxication will decrease the anion gap.

It is estimated that 75% to 90% of the patients given long-term lithium therapy have some signs of toxicity.[210] Eighty percent report a fine tremor that may resolve spontaneously to a decrease in lithium dose or to administration of a β-blocker. Manifestations of mild chronic lithium toxicity[219,220] include:

- Poor memory
- Loss of concentration
- Fatigue
- Muscle weakness
- Slowed reaction time
- Lack of spontaneity

Long-term lithium use can lead to tubular atrophy, polyuria secondary to decreased urine-concentrating ability, and, ultimately, nephrogenic diabetes insipidus.[221,222] Factors associated with an increased risk of renal damage[223] include:

- A history of lithium intoxication
- Advanced age
- Underlying renal disease
- A multiple-dose regimen
- Duration of therapy

Therapeutic Interventions

The lithium-intoxicated patient should be managed like other intoxicated patients, with supportive care, enhancement of lithium elimination, and prevention of further absorption. Gastrointestinal lavage for pill fragments and whole bowel irrigation with polyethylene glycol can help decrease absorption, especially with ingestion of sustained release tablets or if started within 1 hour of ingestion.[224,225] Sodium polystyrene sulfonate (Kayexalate) administration has been shown to bind lithium and decrease absorption in both healthy volunteers and in toxic ingestions.[226,227] The dehydrated patient should be given crystalloid resuscitation but there are no data to support the use of forced diuresis or large volume saline infusion to increase elimination when the patient is not dehydrated.[224] Both techniques run the risk of causing volume overload and electrolyte disturbances.

Extracorporeal therapy for lithium intoxication should be based more on clinical criteria not on serum lithium levels.[196,204–206] The serum lithium level can be a poor indicator of toxicity in acute ingestion. Patients with serum lithium levels as high as 8.0 mEq/L from an acute ingestion have survived without hemodialysis.[196,207,208] The serum lithium level is a more reliable indication of intracellular lithium levels in chronic intoxication or acute intoxication superimposed on chronic intoxication.[206,209]

Lithium is readily dialyzable because of its low molecular weight, water solubility, and lack of protein binding. It does have a moderate Vd (0.7 to 0.9 L/kg), is predominantly intracellular, and diffuses slowly across cell membranes.[200] For this reason, 8 to 10 hours or more of treatment are needed, to bring the serum level to less than 1 mEq/L.[196,219,228] The serum lithium level should be measured 6 to 8 hours after dialysis is completed to evaluate for rebound.[199,209,229] The indications for hemodialysis are listed in Table 46–14. The correlation between serum lithium level and clinical presentation is not always close; therefore, clinical symptoms must be the main determinant of dialysis. For acute intoxication, the failure of severe or moderate clinical signs or symptoms to improve with 6 hours of supportive therapy is an indication for hemodialysis. Hemodialysis is recommended for all patients with severe clinical manifestations. If the clinical condition fails to improve or progresses after 6 hours of corrective or supportive care, or if renal clearance is impaired, dialysis should be considered even in the patient who has moderate clinical manifestations.[196,206,210–213]

Because of the slow equilibration between intracellular and extracellular lithium stores, continuous renal replacement therapy may be advantageous. Leblanc and associates[6] suggest that continuous renal replacement therapy should be performed instead of conventional intermittent hemodialysis for the treatment of lithium intoxication, particularly in cases of chronic poisoning associated with a large intracellular accumulation of the drug. In these cases, it may be advisable to first start with conventional hemodialysis and then switch to a continuous modality because the initial clearance will be higher with standard hemodialysis.[230]

If the patient's clinical condition (1) has failed to improve or (2) again deteriorates after initial improvement, further dialysis may be needed. Specifically, if the patient continues with moderate or severe clinical toxicity 6 to 8 hours after dialysis is terminated, another dialysis treatment is recommended. Neurologic improvement may lag behind improvement in

Table 46–14 Indications for Dialysis in Patients with Lithium Intoxication

1. Serum lithium >3.5 mEq/L
2. Serum lithium >2.5 mEq/L and
   a. Severe symptoms
   b. Renal insufficiency
   c. Conditions that increase renal sodium reabsorption (heart failure, cirrhosis)
   d. Chronic ingestion and moderate to severe symptoms
3. Any lithium level with one of the following:
   a. Severe symptoms
   b. Moderate symptoms that have failed to improve with 6 hours of support
   c. Large ingestion where rising levels are anticipated

(From Okusa MD, Crystal LJ: Clinical manifestations and management of acute lithium intoxication. Am J Med 1994; 97: 383-389.)

serum lithium levels, cardiac toxicity, or gastrointestinal symptoms because of the slow equilibration of lithium from brain to blood.[198,229,231]

Theophylline

Theophylline is a methylxanthine bronchodilator used for obstructive airway disease. Although the number of patients using it and the number of toxic exposures are declining, toxic exposure to theophylline continues to have a very high morbidity and mortality (see Table 46–7).[1] It is metabolized by the liver, with 10% being recovered unchanged in the urine. Its half-life is prolonged in patients with liver disease[232–234] or congestive heart failure,[232,235,236] with the use of supratherapeutic doses, and if it is ingested with cimetidine[237–239] or erythromycin.[240,241] Raoof and associates[242] observed an average increase in the serum theophylline level of 87% when ciprofloxacin and theophylline were administered concurrently. In addition, 61% of the patients these researchers evaluated had a mean increase in the serum theophylline level of 10.5 mg/L, resulting in toxic concentrations of the drug.[242] The half-life of theophylline is decreased by smoking, phenobarbital,[243] and phenytoin (secondary to hepatic enzyme induction).[244]

Signs of mild theophylline toxicity are nausea, vomiting, abdominal pain, tachycardia, and muscle tremor.[245,246] Severe toxicity consists of cardiac arrhythmias, hypotension, impaired consciousness, seizures, cardiorespiratory arrest, and, ultimately, death.[247–249] The risk of major toxicity is influenced by the method of intoxication. Patients who use theophylline as long-term therapy have a greater risk of major toxicity at lower serum theophylline concentrations than patients with acute intoxication. The serum levels are more predictive of major toxicity with acute theophylline intoxication. Toxicity usually appears when the serum level is around 20 to 25 mg/L and increases with rising serum levels.[250]

Theophylline is 60% protein bound; the free fraction distributes in interstitial fluid and the intracellular space with a Vd equal to 0.4 to 0.6 L/kg. Activated charcoal can bind theophylline in the gastrointestinal tract and should be used initially in intoxication. The dose of activated charcoal is 20 g every 2 hours[251,252] in adults for 6 to 12 hours, depending on the serum theophylline level. Because of its enterohepatic circulation, multidose activated charcoal has a role in increasing the elimination of theophylline.[25]

Conventional hemodialysis using a hollow-fiber filter with a Q_b of 180 to 250 mL/min and a Q_d of 500 mL/min can result in plasma ER of 0.5, a dialysis clearance rate of 75 to 98 mL/min, and the removal of 40% of the administered dose of theophylline in 3 hours.[253] Hemoperfusion is more effective than hemodialysis, achieving an ER of 0.6[254] to 0.9.[255] Extracorporeal therapy should be performed for the patient with:

1. Severe acute theophylline intoxication and whose serum theophylline level is higher than 80 mg/L.
2. Chronic theophylline intoxication and whose serum theophylline level is higher than 60 mg/L.
3. Inability to tolerate oral charcoal and who is either at least 60 years of age or who has underlying liver or heart disease.[256,257]

Hemodialysis should be considered when hemoperfusion is indicated but unavailable. Charcoal hemoperfusion appears to be the most efficacious therapy to treat severe toxicity.[254,258,259] β-Blockade has been used to treat refractory hypotension[260–262] and dysrhythmias.[249,261,262] Hypokalemia may be present secondary to intracellular shift of potassium; one must take care to avoid hyperkalemia[263] when giving supplementary potassium. The end point for dialysis in theophylline intoxication is met when the patient has improved clinically and the serum drug level is well below the upper limit of therapeutic (about 15 mg/L).

OTHER TECHNIQUES FOR DRUG REMOVAL

Additional techniques for removing protein-bound drugs or toxins were introduced by Stange and associates[264] in 1993. The categories of these toxins are quite varied and include:

- Albumin-bound toxins that accumulate in hepatic failure with encephalopathy[265–268]
- Ingested drugs that have high protein binding[269,270]
- Albumin-bound toxins that accumulate in chronic renal failure[264] and sepsis

This system involves an asymmetric, highly permeable dialysis membrane that is albumin-coated before use on both blood and dialysate sides. An albumin dialysate is used in a closed-loop system for regeneration of the albumin.[264] A column of activated charcoal is used to deligandize the albumin in the dialysate for regeneration of free albumin. This arrangement was found to be advantageous over other methods of hemoadsorption because (1) there is no direct contact between cellular components of blood and the charcoal cartridge, and (2) the albumin is cleaned (deligandized and regenerated). The hemocompatibility of this system appears to be better than that of conventional systems because the patient's blood comes in contact with only tubing and a dialysis membrane coated with albumin.

References

1. Litovitz TL, Klein-Schwartz W, Rodgers GC Jr, et al: 2001 Annual report of the American Association of Poison Control Centers Toxic Exposure Surveillance System. Am J Emerg Med 2002; 20: 391-452.
2. Culter RE, Forland SC, Hammond P, et al: Extracorporeal removal of drugs and poisons by hemodialysis and hemoperfusion. Ann Rev Pharmacol Toxicol 1987; 27:169–191.
3. Vale A, Meredith T, Buckley B: ABC of poisoning: Eliminating poisons. Br Med J 1984; 289:366–369.
4. Domoto DT, Brown WW, Bruggensmith P: Removal of toxic levels of N-acetyl-procainamide with continuous arteriovenous hemofiltration or continuous arteriovenous hemodiafiltration. Ann Intern Med 1987; 106:550–552.
5. Montagne N, Milano G, Caldani C, et al: Removal of methotrexate by hemodiafiltration. Cancer Chemother Pharmacol 1989; 24:400–401.
6. Leblanc M, Raymond M, Bonnardeaux A, et al: Lithium poisoning treated by high-performance continuous arteriovenous and venovenous hemodiafiltration. Am J Kidney Dis 1996; 27: 363–372.
7. Horton MW, Godley PJ, Moore ES, et al: Estimation of theophylline clearance during continuous arteriovenous hemodiafiltration. Artif Organs 1990; 14:416–420.

8. Weiss LG, Danielson BG, Fellstroem B, et al: Aluminum removal with hemodialysis, hemofiltration and charcoal hemoperfusion in uremic patients after deferoxamine infusion: A comparison of efficiency. Nephron 1989; 3:325–329.
9. Vale JA, Rees AJ, Widdop B, Goulding R: Use of charcoal haemoperfusion in the management of severely poisoned patients. Br Med J 1975; 1:5–9.
10. Shah G, Nelson HA, Atkinson AJ, et al: Effect of hemoperfusion on the pharmacokinetics of digitoxin in dogs. J Lab Clin Med 1979; 93:370–380.
11. Ehlers SM, Zaske DE, Sawchuck RJ: Massive theophylline overdose—rapid elimination by charcoal hemoperfusion. JAMA 1978; 240:474–475.
12. Muir KT, Pond SM: Removal of theophylline from the body by haemoperfusion. Clin Pharmacokinet 1979; 4:320–321.
13. Gelfand MC, Winchester JF, Knepshield JH, et al: Treatment of severe drug overdose with charcoal hemoperfusion. Trans Am Soc Artif Organs 1977; 23:599–605.
14. Mokhlesi B, Leikin JB, Murray P, Corbridge TC: Adult toxicology in critical care: Part I: General approach to the intoxicated patient. Chest 2003; 123:897-922.
15. Lee DC, Roberts J, Kelly J, et al: Whole-bowel irrigation as an adjunct in the treatment of radiopaque arsenic. Am J Emerg Med 1995; 13:244–245.
16. Tenenbein M: Position statement: Whole bowel irrigation. American Academy of Clinical Toxicology; European Association of Poisons Centres and Clinical Toxicologists. J Toxicol Clin Toxicol 1997; 35:753-762.
17. Hillman RJ, Prescott LF: Treatment of salicylate poisoning with repetitive oral charcoal. Br Med J 1985; 291:1472.
18. Boldy DA, Vale JA, Prescott LF: Treatment of phenobarbitone poisoning with repeated oral administration of activated charcoal. Q J Med 1986; 61:997–1002.
19. Belz GG: Plasma concentrations of intravenous beta-methyldigoxin with and without oral charcoal. Klin Wochenschr 1974; 52:749–750.
20. Sintek C, Hendeles L, Weinberger M: Inhibition of theophylline absorption by activated charcoal. J Pediatr 1979; 94:314–316.
21. Krenzelok EP: Gastrointestinal transit times of cathartics combined with charcoal. Ann Emerg Med 1985; 14:1152–1155.
22. Barceloux D, McGuigan M, Hartigan-Go K: Position statement: Cathartics. American Academy of Clinical Toxicology; European Association of Poisons Centres and Clinical Toxicologists. J Toxicol Clin Toxicol 1997; 35:743-752.
23. Ohning BL, Reed MD, Blumer JL: Continuous nasogastric administration of activated charcoal for the treatment of theophylline intoxication. Pediatr Pharmacol 1986; 5:241–245.
24. Chyka PA, Seger D: Position statement: Single-dose activated charcoal. American Academy of Clinical Toxicology; European Association of Poisons Centres and Clinical Toxicologists. J Toxicol Clin Toxicol 1997; 35:721-741.
25. Anonymous: Position statement and practice guidelines on the use of multi-dose activated charcoal in the treatment of acute poisoning. American Academy of Clinical Toxicology; European Association of Poisons Centres and Clinical Toxicologists. J Toxicol Clin Toxicol 1999; 37:731-751.
26. Ilkhanipour K, Yealy DM, Krenzelok EP: The comparative efficacy of various multiple-dose activated charcoal regimens. Am J Emerg Med 1992; 10:298–300.
27. Easom JM, Lovejoy FH: Efficacy and safety of gastrointestinal lavage in the treatment of oral poisoning. Pediatr Clin North Am 1979; 26:827–836.
28. Cupit GC, Temple AR: Gastrointestinal decontamination in the management of the poisoned patient. Emerg Med Clin North Am 1984; 2:15–28.
29. Burton BT, Bayer MJ, Barron L, et al: Comparison of activated charcoal and gastric lavage in the prevention of aspirin absorption. J Emerg Med 1984; 1:411–416.
30. Rudolph JP: Automated gastric lavage and a comparison of 0.9% normal saline solution and tap water irrigant. Ann Emerg Med 1985; 14:1156–1159.
31. Vale JA: Position statement: Gastric lavage. American Academy of Clinical Toxicology; European Association of Poisons Centres and Clinical Toxicologists. J Toxicol Clin Toxicol 1997; 35: 711-719.
32. Smith PK, Gleason HL, Stoll CG, et al: Studies on the pharmacology of salicylates. J Pharmacol Exp Ther 1946; 87:237–255.
33. Bloomer HA: A critical evaluation of diuresis in the treatment of barbiturate intoxication. J Lab Clin Med 1966; 67:898–905.
34. Linton AL, Luke RG, Speirs I, et al: Forced diuresis and haemodialysis in severe barbiturate intoxication. Lancet 1964; 1:1008.
35. Jailer JW, Rosenfeld M, Shannon JA: The influence of orally administered alkali and acid on the renal excretion of quinacrine, chloroquine and santoquine. J Clin Invest 1947; 26: 1168–1172.
36. Beckett AH, Rowland M, Turner P: Influence of urinary pH on excretion of amphetamine. Lancet 1965; 1:303.
37. Asatoor AM, Galman BR, Johnson JR, Milne JD: The excretion of dexamphetamine and its derivatives. Br J Pharmacol Chemother 1965; 24:293–300.
38. Haag HB, Larson PS, Schwartz JJ: The effect of urinary pH on the elimination of quinine in man. J Pharmacol Exp Ther 1943; 79:136–139.
39. Sabto JK, Pierce RM, West RH, Gurr FW: Hemodialysis, peritoneal dialysis, plasmapheresis and forced diuresis for the treatment of quinine overdose. Clin Nephrol 1981; 16:264–268.
40. Done AK, Aronow R, Micelli JN: The pharmacokinetics of phencyclidine in overdosage and its treatment. Natl Inst Drug Abuse Res Monogr Ser 1978; 21:210–217.
41. Gerdes U, Kristensen J, Moller JV, et al: Renal handling of phenol red: Bidirectional transport. J Physiol 1978; 277:115–129.
42. Mudge GH, Silva P, Stibitz GR: Renal excretion by non-ionic diffusion. Med Clin North Am 1975; 59:681–698.
43. Weiner LM, Blanchard KC, Mudge GH: Factors influencing renal excretion of foreign organic acids. Am J Physiol 1964; 207, 953–963.
44. Garrettson LK, Geller RJ: Acid and alkaline diuresis: When are they of value in the treatment of poisoning? Drug Saf 1990; 5: 220–232.
45. Temple AR: Acute and chronic effects of aspirin toxicity and their management. Arch Intern Med 1981; 141:364–369.
46. Beckett AH, Brookes LG: The absorption and urinary excretion in man of fenfluramine and its main metabolite. J Pharm Pharmacol 1967; 19(suppl 1):505–525.
47. Von Muhlendahl KE, Krienke EG: Fenfluramine poisoning. Clin Toxicol 1979; 14:97–106.
48. Vale A, Meredith T, Buckley B: ABC of poisoning. Br Med J 1984; 289:366–369.
49. Jacobsen D: The relative efficacy of antidotes. Clin Toxicol 1995; 33:705–708.
50. Bayer MJ: Recognition and management of digitalis intoxication: Implications for emergency medicine. Am J Emerg Med 1991; 9(suppl 1):29–32.
51. Bolgiano EB, Barish RA: Use of new and established antidotes. Emerg Med Clin North Am 1994; 12:317–334.
52. Mehta RN, Mehta NJ, Gulati A: Late rebound digoxin toxicity after digoxin-specific antibody Fab fragments therapy in anuric patient. J Emerg Med 2002; 22:203-206.
53. Package insert: Digoxin-immune Fab (ovine), Digibind. Research Triangle Park, NC, Burroughs Wellcome, June 1996.
54. Baud FJ, Barriot P, Toffis V, et al: Elevated blood cyanide concentrations in victims of smoke inhalation. N Engl J Med 1991; 325:1761–1766.
55. Hall AH, Rumack BH: Clinical toxicology of cyanide. Ann Emerg Med 1986; 15:1067–1074.

56. Litovitz T, Larkin R, Myers R: Cyanide poisoning treated with hyperbaric oxygen. Am J Emerg Med 1983; 1:94-101.
57. Sauer S, Keim M: Hydroxocobalamin: Improved public health readiness for cyanide disasters. Ann Emerg Med 2001; 37:635-641.
58. Dunn MA, Sidell FR: Progress in medical defense against nerve agents. JAMA 1989; 262:649–652.
59. Lee P, Tai D: Clinical features of patients with acute organophosphate poisoning requiring intensive care. Intensive Care Med 2001; 27:694-699.
60. Mokhlesi B, Leikin JB, Murray P, Corbridge TC: Adult toxicology in critical care: Part II: Specific poisonings. Chest 2003; 123: 897-922.
61. De Kort WL, Kiestra SH, Sangster B: The use of atropine and oximes in organophosphate intoxications: A modified approach. Clin Toxicol 1988; 26:199–208.
62. Oster JR, Singer I, Contreras GN, et al: Metabolic acidosis with extreme elevation of anion gap: Case report and literature review. Am J Med Sci 1999; 317:38-49.
63. Figge J, Jabor A, Kazda A, Fencl V: Anion gap and hypoalbuminemia. Crit Care Med 1998; 26:1807-1810.
64. Hazouard E, Ferrandiere M, Paintaud G, Perrotin D: Delayed toxicity in acute ethanol-methanol copoisoning in a chronic alcohol abuser: Usefulness of continuous 4-methylpyrazole (fomepizole) infusion. Intensive Care Med 2000; 26:827-828.
65. Glasser L, Sternglanz PD, Combie J, Robinson A: Serum osmolality and its applicability to drug overdose. Am J Clin Pathol 1973; 60:695-699.
66. Geller RJ, Spyker DA, Herold DA, Bruns DE: Serum osmolal gap and ethanol concentration: A simple and accurate formula. J Toxicol Clin Toxicol 1986; 24:77-84.
67. Goldfrank L, Flomenbaum N, Lewin N, et al: The liquid time bomb. Hosp Physician 1982; 2:38–60.
68. Arbour R, Esparis B: Osmolar gap metabolic acidosis in a 60-year-old man treated for hypoxemic respiratory failure. Chest 2000; 118:545-546.
69. Wilson KC, Reardon C, Farber HW: Propylene glycol toxicity in a patient receiving intravenous diazepam. N Engl J Med 2000; 343:815.
70. Darchy B, Abruzzese L, Pitiot O, et al: Delayed admission for ethylene glycol poisoning: Lack of elevated serum osmol gap. Intensive Care Med 1999; 25:859-861.
71. Poulose V: Factors influencing the serum osmolar gap. Chest 2002; 122:381; discussion 381.
72. Piagnerelli M, Lejeune P, Vanhaeverbeek M: Diagnosis and treatment of an unusual cause of metabolic acidosis: Ethylene glycol poisoning. Acta Clin Belg 1999; 54:351-356.
73. Konig MW, Dolinski SY: A 74-year-old woman with desaturation following surgery. Co-oximetry is the first step in making the diagnosis of dyshemoglobinemia. Chest 2003; 123:613-616.
74. Wahr JA, Tremper KK, Diab M: Pulse oximetry. Respir Care Clin N Am 1995; 1:77-105.
75. Bozeman WP, Myers RA, Barish RA: Confirmation of the pulse oximetry gap in carbon monoxide poisoning. Ann Emerg Med 1997; 30:608-611.
76. Vincent HH, Vos MC, Akcahuseyin E, et al: Blood flow, ultrafiltration and solute transport rate in CAVD: The AN69 flat plate haemofilter. Nephrol Dial Transplant 1992; 7:29–34.
77. Keller F, Wilms H, Schultze G, et al: Effect on plasma protein binding, volume of distribution, and molecular weight on the fraction of drugs eliminated by hemodialysis. Clin Nephrol 1983; 19:201–205.
78. Maher JF: Principles of dialysis and dialysis of drugs. Am J Med 1977; 62:475–481.
79. Gulyassy PF, Depner TA: Impaired binding of drugs and endogenous ligands in renal disease. Am J Kidney Dis 1983; 2:578–601.
80. McNamara PJ, Lalka D, Gibaldi M: Endogenous accumulation products and serum protein binding in uremia. J Lab Clin Med 1981; 98:730–740.
81. Vos MC, Vincent HH: Continuous arteriovenous hemodiafiltration predicting the clearance of drugs. Contrib Nephrol 1991; 93:143–145.
82. Piafsky KM: Disease-induced changes in the plasma binding of basic drugs. Clin Pharmacokinet 1980; 5:246–262.
83. Lee CC, Marbury TC: Drug therapy in patients undergoing haemodialysis. Clin Pharmacokinet 1984; 9:42–66.
84. Dromgoole SH: The effect of hemodialysis on the binding capacity of albumin. Clin Chim Acta 1973; 46:469–472.
85. Rutstein DD, Castelli WP, Nickerson RJ: Heparin and human lipid metabolism. Lancet 1969; 2:1003–1008.
86. Suh B, Craig WA, England AC, Elliot RL: Effect of free fatty acids on protein binding of antimicrobial agents. J Infect Dis 1981; 143:609–616.
87. Gibaldi M: Drug distribution in renal failure. Am J Med 1977; 62:471–474.
88. Okusa MD, Crystal LJT: Clinical manifestations and management of acute lithium intoxication. Am J Med 1994; 97:383–389.
89. Jaeger A, Sauder P, Kopferschmitt J, et al: Toxicokinetics of lithium intoxication treated by hemodialysis. Clin Toxicol 1985; 6:501–517.
90. Leblanc M, Raymond M, Bonnardeaux A, et al: Lithium poisoning treated by high-performance continuous arteriovenous and venovenous hemodiafiltration. Am J Kidney Dis 1996; 27: 365–372.
91. Fabris A, La Greca G, Chiaramonte S, et al: Total solute extraction versus clearance in the evaluations of standard and short hemodialysis. ASAIO Trans 1988; 34:627–629.
92. De Bock V, Verbeelen D, Naes V, et al: Pharmacokinetics of vancomycin in patients undergoing hemodialysis and hemofiltration. Nephrol Dial Transplant 1989; 4:635–639.
93. Grimes DJ, Bowles MR, Buttsworth JA, et al: Survival after unexpected high serum methotrexate concentrations in a patient with osteogenic sarcoma. Drug Saf 1990; 5:447–454.
94. Hampson EC, Pond SM: Failure of haemoperfusion and haemodialysis to prevent death in paraquat poisoning: A retrospective review of 42 patients. Med Toxicol 1988; 3:64–71.
95. Pond S, Rosenberg J, Benowitz NL, et al: Pharmacokinetics of haemoperfusion for drug overdose. Clin Pharmacokinet 1979; 4:329–354.
96. Von Albertini B, Miller JH, Gardner PW, et al: Performance characteristics of high-flux haemodiafiltration. Proc Eur Dial Transplant 1985; 21:447–453.
97. Rumpf KW, Rieger J, Ansorg R, et al: Binding of antibiotics by dialysis membranes and its clinical relevance. Proc Eur Dial Transplant 1977; 14:607–609.
98. Exaire E, Trevino-Becerra A, Monteon F: An overview of treatment with peritoneal dialysis in drug poisoning. Contrib Nephrol 1979; 17:39–43.
99. Hirszel P, Lasrich M, Maher JF: Augmentation of peritoneal mass transport by dopamine. J Lab Clin Med 1979; 94:747–754.
100. Kraft D, Lode H: Elimination of ampicillin and gentamicin by hemofiltration. Klin Wochenschr 1979; 57:195–196.
101. Kronfol NO, Lau AH, Barakat MM: Aminoglycoside binding to polyacrylonitrile hemofilter membranes during continuous hemofiltration. ASAIO Trans 1987; 33:300–303.
102. Colton CK, Henderson LW, Ford CA, et al: Kinetics of hemodiafiltration. I: In vitro transport characteristics of a hollow-fiber blood filter. J Lab Clin Med 1975; 85:355–371.
103. Doolan PD, Walsh WP, Kyle LH, et al: Acetylsalicylic acid intoxication: A proposed method of treatment. JAMA 1951; 146: 105–106.
104. Schreiner GE, Berman LB, Griffin J, et al: Specific therapy for salicylism. N Engl J Med 1955; 253:213–217.
105. Winchester JF, Gelfand MC, Knepshield JH, Schreiner GE: Dialysis and hemoperfusion of poisons and drugs-update. Trans ASAIO 1972; 23:762–842.

106. Muirhead EE, Reid AF: Resin artificial kidney. J Lab Clin Med 1948; 33:841–844.
107. Schreiner GE: The role of hemodialysis (artificial kidney) in acute poisoning. Arch Intern Med 1958; 102:896–913.
108. Gelfand WC, Winchester JF: Hemoperfusion in drug overdosage: A technique when conservative management is not sufficient. Clin Toxicol 1980; 17:583–602.
109. Garella S: Extracorporeal techniques in the treatment of exogenous intoxications. Kidney Int 1988; 33:735-754.
110. Golper TA: Drug removal during continuous hemofiltration or hemodialysis. Contrib Nephrol 1991; 93:110-116.
111. van Bommel EF, Kalmeijer MD, Ponssen HH: Treatment of life-threatening lithium toxicity with high-volume continuous venovenous hemofiltration. Am J Nephrol 2000; 20:408-411.
112. Andrade JD, Van Wagenen RA, Chen C, et al: Coated absorbents for direct blood perfusion. Trans ASAIO 1972; 18:473–483.
113. Zmuda MJ: Resin hemoperfusion in dogs intoxicated with ethchlorvynol. Kidney Int 1980; 17:303–311.
114. Yatzidis H: A convenient haemoperfusion microapparatus over charcoal for the treatment of endogenous and exogenous intoxications: Its use as artificial kidney. Proc Eur Dial Transplant Assoc 1964; 1:83–87.
115. Chang TMS: Removal of exogenous and endogenous toxins by microencapsulated adsorbent. Can J Physiol Pharmacol 1969; 47:1043–1045.
116. Koffler A, Bernstein M, Lasette A: Fixed-bed charcoal hemoperfusion treatment of drug overdose. Arch Intern Med 1978; 138:1691–1694.
117. Rommes JH: Haemoperfusion, indications and side-effects. Arch Toxicol 1992; 15:40-49.
118. Berman LB, Vogelsang P: Removal rates for barbiturates using two types of peritoneal dialysis. N Engl J Med 1964; 270:77–80.
119. Nahas GG, Giroux JJ, Gjessing J, et al: The use of THAM in peritoneal dialysis. Trans ASAIO 1964; 10:345–349.
120. Meert KL, Ellis J, Aronow R, et al: Acute ammonium dichromate poisoning. Ann Emerg Med 1994; 24:748–750.
121. Rabetoy GM, Price CA, Findlay JW, Sailstad JM: Treatment of digoxin intoxication in a renal failure patient with digoxin-specific antibody fragments and plasmapheresis. Am J Nephrol 1990; 10:518-521.
122. Harrison MR: Toxic methaemoglobinaemia: A case of acute nitrobenzene and aniline poisoning treated by exchange transfusion. Anaesthesia 1977; 32:270–272.
123. Levy G: Pharmacokinetics in renal disease. Am J Med 1977; 62:461–463.
124. Gibson TP: Problems in designing hemodialysis drug studies. Pharmacotherapy 1985; 5:23–29.
125. Yatzidis H, Voudiclari S, Oreopoulos D, et al: Treatment of severe barbiturate poisoning. Lancet 1965; 2:216–217.
126. Cutler RE, Forland SC, Hammond PG, Evans JR: Extracorporeal removal of drugs and poisons by hemodialysis and hemoperfusion. Ann Rev Pharmacol Toxicol 1987; 27: 169-191.
127. Elliott RW, Hunter PR: Acute ethanol poisoning treated by hemodialysis. Postgrad Med J 1974; 50:515–517.
128. Glasser L, Sternglanz PD, Combie J, et al: Serum osmolality and its applicability to drug overdose. Am J Clin Pathol 1973; 60:695–699.
129. Liu JJ, Daya MR, Mann NC: Methanol-related deaths in Ontario. J Toxicol Clin Toxicol 1999; 37:69-73.
130. Meyer RJ, Beard ME, Ardagh MW, Henderson S: Methanol poisoning. N Z Med J 2000; 113:11-13.
131. Sullivan M, Chen CL, Madden JF: Absence of metabolic acidosis in toxic methanol ingestion: A case report and review. Del Med J 1999; 71:421-426.
132. Kerns W II, Tomaszewski C, McMartin K, et al: META Study Group. Methylpyrazole for Toxic Alcohols: Formate kinetics in methanol poisoning. J Toxicol Clin Toxicol 2002; 40:137-143.
133. Burns MJ, Graudins A, Aaron CK, et al: Treatment of methanol poisoning with intravenous 4-methylpyrazole. Ann Emerg Med 1997; 30:829-832.
134. Pamies RJ, Sugar D, Rives LA, Herold AH: Methanol intoxication. How to help patients who have been exposed to toxic solvents. Postgrad Med 1993; 93:183-184, 189-191, 194.
135. Williams GF, Hatch FJ, Bradley MC: Methanol poisoning: A review and case study of four patients from central Australia. Aust Crit Care 1997; 10:113-118.
136. Liu JJ, Daya MR, Carrasquillo O, Kales SN: Prognostic factors in patients with methanol poisoning. J Toxicol Clin Toxicol 1998; 36:175-181.
137. Sullivan-Mee M, Solis K: Methanol-induced vision loss. J Am Optom Assoc 1998; 69:57-65.
138. Kruse JA: Methanol poisoning. Intensive Care Med 1992; 18: 391-397.
139. Church AS, Witting MD: Laboratory testing in ethanol, methanol, ethylene glycol, and isopropanol toxicities. J Emerg Med 1997; 15:687-692.
140. Barceloux DG, Bond GR, Krenzelok EP, et al: The American Academy of Clinical Toxicology Ad Hoc Committee on the Treatment Guidelines for Methanol P: American Academy of Clinical Toxicology practice guidelines on the treatment of methanol poisoning. J Toxicol Clin Toxicol 2002; 40: 415-446.
141. Abramson S, Singh AK: Treatment of the alcohol intoxications: Ethylene glycol, methanol and isopropanol. Curr Opin Nephrol Hypertens 2000; 9:695-701.
142. Brent J, McMartin K, Phillips S, et al: Methylpyrazole for Toxic Alcohols Study G: Fomepizole for the treatment of methanol poisoning. N Engl J Med 2001; 344:424-429.
143. Casavant MJ: Fomepizole in the treatment of poisoning. Pediatrics 2001; 107:170.
144. Roe O: Methanol poisoning: Its clinical course, pathogenesis and treatment. Acta Med Scand 1946; 126(suppl 182):1–253.
145. Sivilotti ML, Burns MJ, McMartin KE, Brent J: Toxicokinetics of ethylene glycol during fomepizole therapy: Implications for management. For the Methylpyrazole for Toxic Alcohols Study Group. Ann Emerg Med 2000; 36:114-125.
146. King L: Acute methanol poisoning: A case study. Heart Lung 1992; 21:260-264.
147. Jobard E, Harry P, Turcant A, et al: 4-Methylpyrazole and hemodialysis in ethylene glycol poisoning. J Toxicol Clin Toxicol 1996; 34:373-377.
148. Chow MT, Di Silvestro VA, Yung CY, et al: Treatment of acute methanol intoxication with hemodialysis using an ethanol-enriched, bicarbonate-based dialysate. Am J Kidney Dis 1997; 30:568-570.
149. Megarbane B, Borron SW, Trout H, et al: Treatment of acute methanol poisoning with fomepizole. Intensive Care Med 2001; 27:1370-1378.
150. Wadgymar A, Wu GG: Treatment of acute methanol intoxication with hemodialysis. Am J Kidney Dis 1998; 31:897.
151. Bekka R, Borron SW, Astier A, et al: Treatment of methanol and isopropanol poisoning with intravenous fomepizole. J Toxicol Clin Toxicol 2001; 39:59-67.
152. Battistella M: Fomepizole as an antidote for ethylene glycol poisoning. Ann Pharmacother 2002; 36:1085-1089.
153. Dorval M, Pichette V, Cardinal J, et al: The use of an ethanol- and phosphate-enriched dialysate to maintain stable serum ethanol levels during haemodialysis for methanol intoxication. Nephrol Dial Transplant 1999; 14:1774-1777.
154. Hirsch DJ, Jindal KK, Wong P, Fraser AD: A simple method to estimate the required dialysis time for cases of alcohol poisoning. Kidney Int 2001; 60:2021-2024.
155. Johnson B, Meggs WJ, Bentzel CJ: Emergency department hemodialysis in a case of severe ethylene glycol poisoning. Ann Emerg Med 1999; 33:108-110.

156. Davis DP, Bramwell KJ, Hamilton RS, Williams SR: Ethylene glycol poisoning: Case report of a record-high level and a review. J Emerg Med 1997; 15:653-667.
157. Nzerue CM, Harvey P, Volcy J, Berdzenshvili M: Survival after massive ethylene glycol poisoning: Role of an ethanol enriched, bicarbonate-based dialysate. Int J Artif Organs 1999; 22:744-746.
158. Barceloux DG, Krenzelok EP, Olson K, Watson W: American Academy of Clinical Toxicology Practice Guidelines on the Treatment of Ethylene Glycol Poisoning. Ad Hoc Committee. J Toxicol Clin Toxicol 1999; 37:537-560.
159. Moreau CL, Kerns W II, Tomaszewski CA, et al: Glycolate kinetics and hemodialysis clearance in ethylene glycol poisoning. META Study Group. J Toxicol Clin Toxicol 1998; 36:659-666.
160. Brent J, McMartin K, Phillips S, et al: Fomepizole for the treatment of ethylene glycol poisoning. Methylpyrazole for Toxic Alcohols Study Group. N Engl J Med 1999; 340:832-838.
161. Zimmerman HE, Burkhart KK, Donovan JW: Ethylene glycol and methanol poisoning: Diagnosis and treatment. J Emerg Nurs 1999; 25:116-120.
162. Poldelski V, Johnson A, Wright S, et al: Ethylene glycol-mediated tubular injury: Identification of critical metabolites and injury pathways. Am J Kidney Dis 2001; 38:339-348.
163. LaKind JS, McKenna EA, Hubner RP, Tardiff RG: A review of the comparative mammalian toxicity of ethylene glycol and propylene glycol. Crit Rev Toxicol 1999; 29:331-365.
164. Borron SW, Megarbane B, Baud FJ: Fomepizole in treatment of uncomplicated ethylene glycol poisoning. Lancet 1999; 354:831.
165. Scalley RD, Ferguson DR, Piccaro JC, et al: Treatment of ethylene glycol poisoning. Am Fam Physician 2002; 66:807-812.
166. Glaser DS: Utility of the serum osmol gap in the diagnosis of methanol or ethylene glycol ingestion. Ann Emerg Med 1996; 27:343-346.
167. Pappas AA, Ackerman BH, Olsen KM, Taylor EH: Isopropanol ingestion: A report of six episodes with isopropanol and acetone serum concentration time data. J Toxicol Clin Toxicol 1991; 29:11-21.
168. Peterson CD, Collins AJ, Himes JM, et al: Ethylene glycol poisoning: Pharmacokinetics during therapy with ethanol and hemodialysis. N Engl J Med 1981; 304:21–23.
169. Beasley VR, Buck WB: Acute ethylene glycol toxicosis. Vet Hum Toxicol 1980; 22:255–263.
170. Jacobsen D, Hewlett TP, Webb R, et al: Ethylene glycol intoxication: Evaluation of kinetics and crystalluria. Am J Med 1988; 84: 565–574.
171. Jones AW: Elimination half-life of acetone in humans: Case reports and review of the literature. J Anal Toxicol 2000; 24:8-10.
172. Gaudet MP, Fraser GL: Isopropanol ingestion: Case report with pharmacokinetic analysis. Am J Emerg Med 1989; 7:297-299.
173. Lacouture PG, Wason S, Abrams A, Lovejoy FH Jr: Acute isopropyl alcohol intoxication. Diagnosis and management. Am J Med 1983; 75:680-686.
174. Monaghan MS, Ackerman BH, Olsen KM, et al: The use of delta osmolality to predict serum isopropanol and acetone concentrations. Pharmacotherapy 1993; 13:60-63.
175. Rosansky SJ: Isopropyl alcohol poisoning treated with hemodialysis: Kinetics of isopropyl alcohol and acetone removal. J Toxicol Clin Toxicol 1982; 19:265-271.
176. Anderson RJ, Potts DE, Gabow PA, et al: Unrecognized adult salicylate intoxication. Ann Intern Med 1976; 85:745–748.
177. Yip L, Dart RC, Gabow PA: Concepts and controversies in salicylate toxicity. Emerg Med Clin North Am 1994; 12:351-364.
178. Anderson RJ, Potts DE, Gabow PA, et al: Unrecognized adult salicylate intoxication. Ann Intern Med 1976; 85:745-748.
179. Temple AR: Acute and chronic effects of aspirin toxicity and their treatment. Arch Intern Med 1981; 141:364-369.
180. Gabow PA, Anderson RJ, Potts DE, Schrier RW: Acid-base disturbances in the salicylate-intoxicated adult. Arch Intern Med 1978; 138:1481-1484.
181. Winters RW, White J, Hughes M, et al: Disturbances of acid-base equilibrium in salicylate intoxication. Pediatrics 1959; 23: 260–285.
182. Proudfoot AT, Brown SS: Acidaemia and salicylate poisoning in adults. Br Med J 1969; 2:547–550.
183. Gabow PA, Anderson RJ, Potts DE, et al: Acid-base disturbances in the salicylate-intoxicated adult. Arch Intern Med 1978; 138: 1481–1484.
184. Hormaechea E, Carlson RW, Rogove H, et al: Hypovolemia, pulmonary edema and protein changes in severe salicylate poisoning. Am J Med 1979; 66:1046–1050.
185. Heffner JE, Sahn SA: Salicylate-induced pulmonary edema: Clinical features and prognosis. Ann Intern Med 1981; 95: 405–409.
186. Walters JS, Woodring JH, Stelling CB, et al: Salicylate-induced pulmonary edema. Radiology 1983; 146:289–293.
187. Kirshenbaum LA, Mathews SC, Sitar DS, Tenenbein M: Does multiple-dose charcoal therapy enhance salicylate excretion? Arch Intern Med 1990; 150:1281-1283.
188. Levy G, Tsuchiya T: Salicylate accumulation kinetics in man. N Engl J Med 1972; 287:430–432.
189. Filippone GA, Fish SS, Lacoutre PG, et al: Reversible adsorption (desorption) of aspirin from activated charcoal. Arch Intern Med 1987; 147:1390–1392.
190. Prescott LF, Balali-Mood M, Critchley JA, et al: Diuresis or urinary alkalinisation for salicylate poisoning? Br Med J (Clin Res Ed) 1982; 285:1383-1386.
191. Temple AR: Pathophysiology of aspirin overdosage toxicity, with implications for management. Pediatrics 1978; 62: 873-876.
192. Wosilait WD: Theoretical analysis of the binding of salicylate by human serum albumin: The relationship between free and bound drug and therapeutic levels. Eur J Clin Pharmacol 1976; 9:285–290.
193. Winchester JF, Glefand MC, Helliwell M, et al: Extracorporeal treatment of salicylate or acetaminophen poisoning—Is there a role? Arch Intern Med 1971; 141:370–374.
194. Temple AR, George DJ, Done AK, Thompson JA: Salicylate poisoning complicated by fluid retention. Clin Toxicol 1976; 9:61-68.
195. Heffner JE, Sahn SA: Salicylate-induced pulmonary edema. Clinical features and prognosis. Ann Intern Med 1981; 95: 405-409.
196. Hansen HE, Amdisen A: Lithium intoxication. Q J Med 1978; 47:123–144.
197. Tunkel AR, D'Antonio J, Engel-Kominsky S, et al: Predicting the clinical course in intentional drug overdose. Arch Intern Med 1988; 148:253.
198. Lydiard RB, Gelenberg AJ: Hazards and adverse effects of lithium. Ann Rev Med 1983; 33:327–344.
199. Friedberg RC, Spyker DA, Herold DA: Massive overdoses with sustained-release lithium carbonate preparations: Pharmacokinetic model based on two case studies. Clin Chem 1991; 37:1205–1209.
200. Okusa MD, Crystal LJT: Clinical manifestations and management of acute lithium intoxication. Am J Med 1994; 97: 383–389.
201. Krishel S, Jackimczyk K: Cyclic antidepressants, lithium, and neuroleptic agents: Pharmacology and toxicology. Emerg Med Clin North Am 1991; 9:53–86.
202. Thomsen K, Holstein-Rathlou NH, Leyssac PP: Comparison of three measures of proximal tubular reabsorption: Lithium clearance, occlusion time and micropuncture. Am J Physiol 1981; 241:F348–F355.
203. Jaeger A, Sauder P, Kopferschmitt J, et al: When should dialysis be performed in lithium poisoning? A kinetic study in 14 cases of lithium poisoning. Clin Toxicol 1993; 31:429–447.
204. Annitto WJ: Recognizing lithium associated neurotoxicity. Drug Ther 1979; 9:125.

205. El-Mallakh RS: Treatment of acute lithium toxicity. Vet Hum Toxicol 1984; 26:31–35.
206. Gadallah MF, Feinstein EI, Massry SG: Lithium intoxication: Clinical course and therapeutic considerations. Miner Electrolyte Metab 1988; 14:146–149.
207. Horowitz LC, Fisher GU: Acute lithium toxicity. N Engl J Med 1969; 281:1369.
208. Wolpert EA: Nontoxic hyperlithemia in impending mania. Am J Psychiatry 1977; 134:580–582.
209. Singer I, Rotenberg D: Mechanisms of lithium action. N Engl J Med 1973; 289:254–260.
210. Amdisen A: Clinical features and management of lithium poisoning. Med Toxicol 1988; 3:18–32.
211. Hall RCW, Perl M, Pfefferbaum B: Lithium therapy and toxicity. Am Fam Physician 1979; 19:133–139.
212. Hauger RL, O'Conner KA, Yudofsky S, et al: Lithium toxicity: When is hemodialysis necessary? Acta Psychiatr Scand 1990; 81: 515–517.
213. Mateer JR, Clark MR: Lithium toxicity with rarely reported ECG manifestations. Ann Emerg Med 1982; 11:208–211.
214. Guerin JM, Barbotin-Larrieu P, Lustman C: Acute voluntary life-threatening carbonate lithium poisoning. Arch Intern Med 1990; 150:920.
215. Demers RG, Rivenbark JF III: Lithium intoxication and its clinical management. South Med J 1982; 75:738–739.
216. Brady HR, Horgan JH: Lithium and the heart, unanswered questions. Chest 1988; 93:166–169.
217. Ong AC, Handler CE: Sinus arrest and asystole due to severe lithium intoxication. Int J Cardiol 1991; 30:364–366.
218. Perrier A, Martin PY, Favre H, et al: Very severe self-poisoning lithium carbonate intoxication causing a myocardial infarction. Chest 1991; 100:863–865.
219. Goddard J, Bloom SR, Frackowiak RS, et al: Lithium intoxication. Br Med J 1991; 302:1267–1269.
220. Lewis DA: Unrecognized chronic lithium neurotoxic reactions. JAMA 1983; 250:2029–2030.
221. Hansen HE, Pedersen EB, Amdisen A: Renal function and plasma aldosterone during acute lithium intoxication. Acta Med Scand 1979; 205:593–597.
222. Waller DG, Edwards JG: Lithium and the kidney: An update. Psychol Med 1989; 19:825–831.
223. Hetmar O, Povlsen UJ, Ladefoged J, et al: Lithium: Long term effects on the kidney: A prospective follow-up study ten years after kidney biopsy. Br J Psychiatry 1991; 158:53–58.
224. Scharman EJ: Methods used to decrease lithium absorption or enhance elimination. J Toxicol Clin Toxicol 1997; 35:601-608.
225. Smith SW, Ling LJ, Halstenson CE: Whole-bowel irrigation as a treatment for acute lithium overdose. Ann Emerg Med 1991; 20:536-539.
226. Tomaszewski C, Musso C, Pearson JR, et al: Lithium absorption prevented by sodium polystyrene sulfonate in volunteers. Ann Emerg Med 1992; 21:1308-1311.
227. Linakis JG, Lacouture PG, Eisenberg MS, et al: Administration of activated charcoal or sodium polystyrene sulfonate (Kayexalate) as gastric decontamination for lithium intoxication: An animal model. Pharmacol Toxicol 1989; 65:387-389.
228. Cohen WJ, Cohen NH: Lithium carbonate, haloperidol, and irreversible brain damage. JAMA 1974; 230:1283–1287.
229. Clendeninn NJ, Pond SM, Kaysen G, et al: Potential pitfalls in the evaluation of the usefulness of hemodialysis for the removal of lithium. J Toxicol 1982; 19:341–352.
230. Beckmann U, Oakley PW, Dawson AH, Byth PL: Efficacy of continuous venovenous hemodialysis in the treatment of severe lithium toxicity. J Toxicol Clin Toxicol 2001; 39:393-397.
231. Depaulo JR Jr, Folstein MF, Correa EI: The course of delirium due to lithium intoxication. J Clin Psychiatry 1982; 43:447–449.
232. Ogilvie RI: Clinical pharmacokinetics of theophylline. Clin Pharmacokinet 1978; 3:267–293.
233. Piafsky KM, Sitar DS, Rangno RE, et al: Theophylline disposition in patients with hepatic cirrhosis. N Engl J Med 1977; 296: 1495–1497.
234. Mangione A, Imhoff TE, Lee RV, et al: Pharmacokinetics of theophylline in hepatic disease. Chest 1978; 73:616–622.
235. Jusko WJ, Gradner MJ, Mangione A, et al: Factors affecting theophylline clearances: Age, tobacco, marijuana, cirrhosis, congestive heart failure, obesity, oral contraceptives, benzodiazepines, barbiturates, and ethanol. J Pharm Sci 1979; 68: 1358–1366.
236. Powell JR, Vozeh S, Hopewell P, et al: Theophylline disposition in acutely ill hospitalized patients: The effect of smoking, heart failure, severe airway obstruction and pneumonia. Am Rev Respir Dis 1978; 118:229–238.
237. Reitberg DP, Bernhard H, Schentag JJ, et al: Alteration of theophylline clearance and half-life by cimetidine in normal volunteers. Ann Intern Med 1981; 95:582–585.
238. Jackson JE, Powell JR, Wandell M, et al: Cimetidine decreases theophylline clearance. Am Rev Respir Dis 1981; 123:615–617.
239. Powell JR, Rogers JF, Wargin WA, et al: Inhibition of theophylline clearance by cimetidine but not ranitidine. Arch Intern Med 1984; 144:484–486.
240. Zarowitz BJM, Szefler SJ, Lasezkay GM: The effect of erythromycin base on theophylline kinetics. Clin Pharmacol Ther 1981; 29:601–605.
241. Reisz G, Pingleton SK, Melethil S, et al: The effect of erythromycin on theophylline pharmacokinetics in chronic bronchitis. Am Rev Respir Dis 1983; 127:581–584.
242. Raoof MB, Wollschlager C, Khan FA: Ciprofloxacin increases serum levels of theophylline. Am J Med 1987; 82(suppl 4A): 115–118.
243. Landay RA, Gonzalez MA, Taylor JC: Effect of phenobarbital on theophylline disposition. J Allergy Clin Immunol 1978; 62: 27–29.
244. Marquis JF, Carruthers SG, Spence JD, et al: Phenytoin-theophylline interaction. N Engl J Med 1982; 307:1189–1190.
245. Skinner MH: Adverse reactions and interactions with theophylline. Drug Saf 1990; 5:275–285.
246. Tsiu SJ, Self TH, Burns R: Theophylline toxicity: Update. Ann Allergy 1990; 64:241–257.
247. Aitken ML, Martin TR: Life-threatening theophylline toxicity is not predictable by serum levels. Chest 1987; 91:10–14.
248. Zwillich CW, Sutton FD, Neff TA, et al: Theophylline-induced seizures in adults. Correlation with serum concentrations. Ann Intern Med 1975; 82:784–787.
249. Greenberg A, Piraino BH, Kroboth PD, et al: Severe theophylline toxicity: Role of conservative measures, antiarrhythmic agents, and charcoal hemoperfusion. Am J Med 1984; 76:854–860.
250. Jacobs MH, Senior RM, Kessler G: Clinical experience with theophylline: Relationships between dosage, serum concentration, and toxicity. JAMA 1976; 235:1983–1986.
251. Park G, Radomski L, Goldberg M, et al: Effects of size and frequency of oral doses of charcoal on theophylline clearance. Clin Pharmacol Ther 1983; 34:663–666.
252. Park GD, Spector R, Goldberg MJ, et al: Effect of the surface area of activated charcoal on theophylline clearance. J Clin Pharmacol 1984; 24:289–292.
253. Lee CS, Marbury TC, Perrin JH, et al: Hemodialysis of theophylline in uremic patients. J Clin Pharmacol 1979; 19:219–226.
254. Russo ME: Management of theophylline intoxication with charcoal-column hemoperfusion. N Engl J Med 1979; 300:24–26.
255. Van Kesteren RG, Van Dijk A, Klein SW, et al: Massive theophylline intoxication: Effects of charcoal haemoperfusion on plasma and erythrocyte theophylline concentrations. Hum Toxicol 1985; 4:127–134.
256. Park GD, Spector R, Roberts RJ, et al: Use of hemoperfusion for treatment of theophylline intoxication. Am J Med 1983; 74: 961–966.

257. Goldberg MJ, Park GD, Berlinger WG: Treatment of theophylline toxicity. J Allergy Clin Immunol 1986; 78:811–817.
258. Olson KR, Benowitz NL, Woo OF, et al: Theophylline overdose: Acute single ingestion versus chronic repeated overmedication. Am J Emerg Med 1985; 3:386–394.
259. Lynn KL, Buttimore AL, Begg EJ, et al: Treatment of theophylline poisoning with haemoperfusion. N Z Med J 1988; 101:4–5.
260. Kearney TE, Manoguerra AS, Curtis GP, et al: Theophylline toxicity and the beta-adrenergic system. Ann Intern Med 1985; 102:766–769.
261. Biberstein MP, Ziegler MG, Ward DM: Use of beta-blockade and hemoperfusion for acute theophylline poisoning. West J Med 1984; 141:485–490.
262. Amin DN, Henry JA: Propranolol administration in theophylline overdose. Lancet 1985; 1:520–521.
263. Amitai Y, Lovejoy FH: Hypokalemia in acute theophylline poisoning. Am J Emerg Med 1988; 6:214–218.
264. Stange J, Mitzner S: A new procedure for the removal of protein bound drugs and toxins. ASAIO J 1993; 39:M621–M625.
265. Brunner G: What is needed for an artificial liver? *In* Nose Y, Kjellstrand C, Ivanovich P (eds): Artificial Organs. Cleveland, OH, ISAO Press, 1986, pp 715–720.
266. Brunner G, Tegtmeier F: Enzymatic detoxification using lipophilic hollow-fiber membranes. Artif Organs 1984; 8: 161–166.
267. Mitzner SR, Stange J, Klammt S, et al: Extracorporeal detoxification using the molecular adsorbent recirculating system for critically ill patients with liver failure. J Am Soc Nephrol 2001; 12:S75-S82.
268. Di Campli C, Zileri Dal Verme L, Andrisani MC, et al: Advances in extracorporeal detoxification by MARS dialysis in patients with liver failure. Curr Med Chem 2003; 10:341-348.
269. Sen S, Ratnaraj N, Davies NA, et al: Treatment of phenytoin toxicity by the molecular adsorbents recirculating system (MARS). Epilepsia 2003; 44:265-267.
270. Shi Y, He J, Chen S, et al: MARS: Optimistic therapy method in fulminant hepatic failure secondary to cytotoxic mushroom poisoning: A case report. Liver 2002; 22:78-80.

Economic Issues and Drug Dosing

Chapter 47

Chronic Kidney Disease: Cost of Care in this High-Risk Outlier Population

Allan J. Collins, M.D., F.A.C.P.

Amendments passed in 1972 expanded the Medicare program to include end-stage renal disease (ESRD) as a covered condition. The enabling legislation envisioned that the number of ESRD patients to be covered at a given time would be approximately 40,000. It was not anticipated that the program would grow to cover more than 400,000 individuals by the year 2002, a doubling over the previous 10 years and 10 times greater than the estimates made in the early 1970s. Projections suggest that 650,000 individuals will be under treatment in 2010 and that this number may reach 2.2 million by 2030, if the patterns of the previous 30 years continue.[3] The growth of the ESRD patient population is fueled by a reservoir of patients with progressive chronic kidney disease (CKD) in the general population. Until recently, the size of this reservoir was unknown. Coresh and associates[1] investigated the size of the CKD pool in the United States, using data from the Third National Health and Nutrition Examination Survey (NHANES III), taking advantage of the extensive biochemical data collected and applying criteria that reasonably would reflect evidence of kidney damage. Based on these methods, the National Kidney Foundation (NKF) published a classification system for CKD and estimated the total population to be 8 to 20 million individuals, depending on the severity of the kidney damage.[2] Although there has been some debate regarding the precise number of individuals in the general population who show evidence of CKD, there is little doubt that the burden is significant and that the CKD pool is the feeder population for the ESRD program. Although 100,000 individuals begin receiving ESRD care every year, it is clear that others with advancing disease die before ESRD treatment.[3,4]

The CKD population has predominantly been studied in a cross-sectional manner, with researchers investigating reductions in kidney function and identifying associated complicating conditions, biochemical abnormalities, and demographic characteristics of those affected.[1] Little information is available on the cost of CKD. To investigate this important area, one needs a data set containing both clinical and cost information. Unfortunately, large data sets that contain information on both kidney function and cost are not available. Data from the available alternatives are less precise regarding the degree of kidney damage but are drawn from patients with clinically recognized disease. Administrative claims represent the best source of information on kidney disease and cost. The Medicare claims data and information from employer group health plans can be used to study the population of patients who have a diagnosis of CKD, identifying the clinical services rendered to these patients and determining the expenditures paid to providers for the cost of these services. For example, the Medicare+Choice risk adjustment payment system contains data on a variety of patients who have been diagnosed with kidney disease, such as diabetics with nephropathy, patients with hypertensive nephropathy, patients with kidney failure due to other primary causes, and those with combinations of comorbid conditions that are strongly associated with advancing kidney disease. Although the use of this approach identifies patients with more advanced disease, the patients identified are the ones that providers have found to require specific services that generate increased cost.

Using data in the 5% sample of the Medicare population, investigators can identify CKD patients from diagnosis codes recorded on claims for services.[3–5] These codes have allowed United States Renal Data System (USRDS) investigators to determine that 1.1 million elderly individuals (age ≥ 65 years) carry a diagnosis of CKD. This number represents only one fifth of the 5.9 million elderly with an estimated glomerular filtration rate (GFR) of less than 60 mL/min, as determined from the NHANES III cohort.[1,3] With this approach to identifying individuals with CKD, associated expenditures can be identified and categorized into cost groups for sake of comparison. To illustrate this investigative approach, this chapter reports on Medicare patients who advance to ESRD, identifying services rendered and associated costs in a period preceding the start of dialysis. Material presented includes information on the range of clinical conditions associated with advancing kidney disease.

Chronic Kidney Disease and Complicating Conditions

The complicating medical conditions associated with CKD are discussed elsewhere in this book. The reader is referred to other chapters for detailed discussions of cardiovascular disease, peripheral vascular disease, lipid disorders, and bone and mineral diseases that are associated with CKD. Investigators have demonstrated associations between increasing degrees of kidney damage and blood pressure elevations,[6] ischemic heart disease, congestive heart failure, and peripheral vascular disease.[7] The largest population studied is the Medicare population assessed by the USRDS. In diabetic patients, CKD is highly associated with congestive heart failure, ischemic heart disease, and peripheral vascular disease. Proteinuria has been associated with a range of cardiovascular disease in both diabetic and nondiabetic patients.

Cardiovascular disease appears to advance at almost twice the rate in the CKD population than in the non-CKD population, with CHF being the leading complicating condition.[3] Heart failure hospitalization rates are four times higher in CKD patients than in non-CKD patients; infectious complications, almost five times higher. These rates of disease generate large expenditures from services to treat the conditions.

Transitional Comorbidity and Expenditures Associated with CKD Patients Entering ESRD Treatment

Because CKD patients who advance to ESRD appear to have complications that advance at a rate comparable to the rate observed in those who die before reaching ESRD, an assessment of the patients approaching ESRD would provide insight into their services and expenditures. Investigators have reported information on Medicare and non-Medicare patients who advance to ESRD.[8,9] In the elderly population, almost two-thirds of patients who were age 67 years or greater and entered dialysis between 1995 and 1998 carried a diagnosis of congestive heart failure. Sixty percent carried a diagnosis of ischemic heart disease, with almost 20% carrying a diagnosis of acute myocardial infarction. Forty percent carried a diagnosis of cardiac dysrhythmias, and 43% carried a diagnosis of peripheral vascular disease. In addition, almost 60% carried a diagnosis of diabetes (primary or secondary). Therefore, it is clear that patients who finally enter ESRD have significant comorbid conditions. Looking at the period between 24 months before (Month −24) and 6 months after (Month +6) dialysis initiation, average expenditure was $932 per member, per month (PMPM) at Month −24. These costs increased between Month −5 to Month −2 to $1740 PMPM. Between the months just before and after initiation of dialysis, the cost was $8600 PMPM. The cost stabilized at $5490 PMPM between Months +4 and +5. As expected, those who died after initiation of dialysis had costs that were higher, by 20% to 50%.

A similar analysis is shown in Figure 47–1. The changing composition of the primary causes of hospitalization is shown for individuals age 67 years or greater who advanced to ESRD from 1995 to 1997. Congestive heart failure, ischemic heart disease, and other cardiovascular disease accounted for half of the hospitalization events. These events steadily increased as the patients advanced toward ESRD, with vascular access emerging as the dominant cause of hospitalization near dialysis initiation. Figure 47–2 shows that the number of hospital days per month increased with advancing CKD (as patients approached ESRD). Diabetic patients had more hospital days than nondiabetic patients until the last 2 months before ESRD; from Month −2 to Month +2, the nondiabetic patients had more hospital days per month than the diabetic patients. Figures 47–3 and 47–4 show that expenditures escalate (as expected), with the most rapid growth occurring in the final 6 months before dialysis initiation. Peak expenditures occur in the month of dialysis initiation ($14,000 PMPM). These transitional expenses are driven by hospitalization for cardiovascular disease and vascular access. Table 47–1 shows the

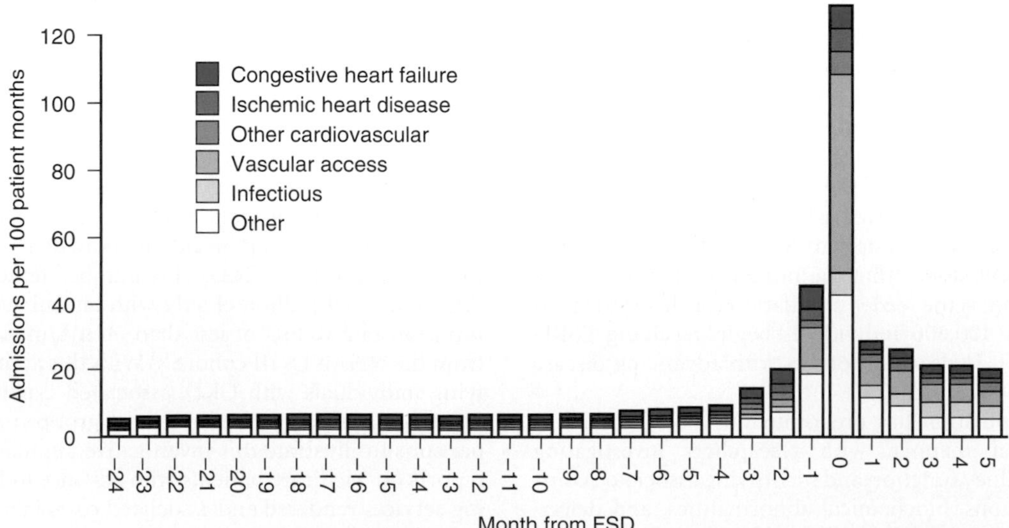

Figure 47–1 1995 to 1997 admission rates by category: 24 months before (Month −24) to 6 months after (Month +6) dialysis initiation. *FSD,* first service date.

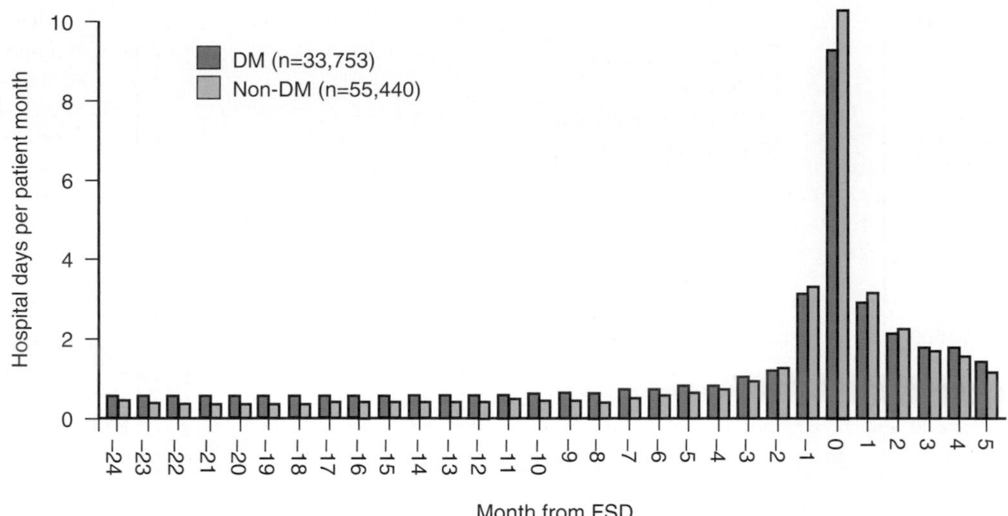

Figure 47–2 Hospital days per month at risk: combined cohorts by diabetic status. *DM,* diabetes mellitus; *FSD,* first service date.

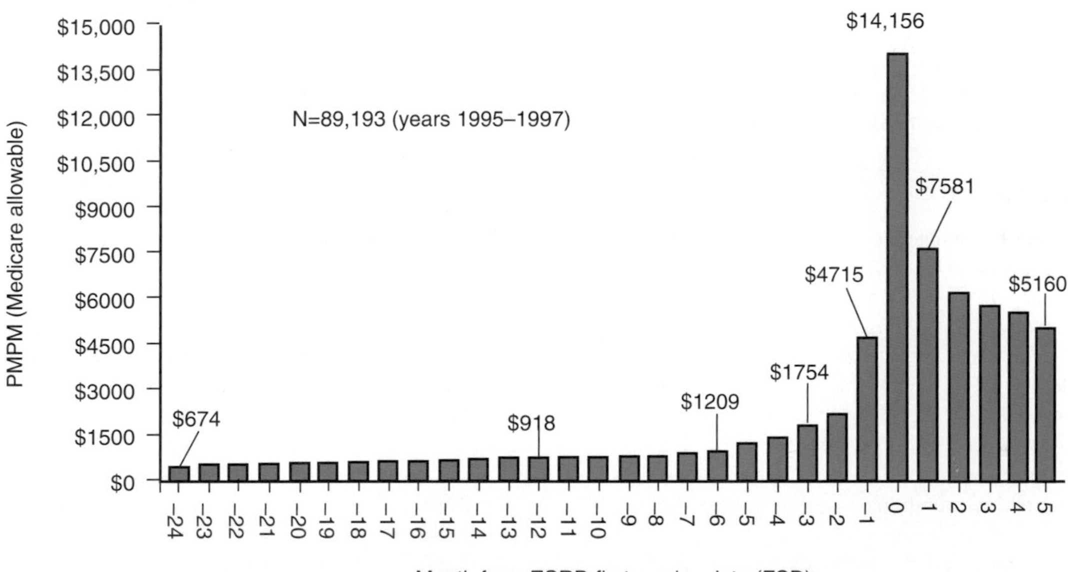

Figure 47–3 1995 to 1997 per-person, per-month (PMPM) total Medicare allowable expenditures, 24 months before (Month −24) to 6 months after (Month +6) dialysis initiation. *ESRD,* end-stage renal disease; *FSD,* first service date.

principal diagnoses related to the hospitalizations before, at, and after the ESRD first service date. Congestive heart failure, ischemic heart disease, renal failure complications, and infections are major sources of complication. As expected, vascular access represents a major cost component near and after initiation of dialysis. These data suggest that efforts to preemptively address the cardiovascular complications, metabolic and electrolyte disturbances, and infectious events may reduce the high cost of care in this population.

Expenditures Associated with the CKD Population

The magnitude of the expenditures associated with the large population of patients with evidence of CKD is undetermined. This is mainly because a lack of information precludes our ability to identify the at-risk group and link the clinical evidence of reduced kidney function to associated expenditures. Two recent attempts to develop information in this area are of note, one by the Centers for Medicare & Medicaid Services (CMS), in its aforementioned risk adjustment payment system and the other by the USRDS. Each of these efforts has yielded convincing evidence that the CKD population is very costly and an important outlier population that consumes considerable resources.

Work by the USRDS investigators was preliminarily presented in 2003 at the annual meeting of the American Society of Nephrology. Drs. Lawrence Hunsicker and John Brooks of the University of Iowa, investigators for the USRDS Economic Special Studies Center, in collaboration with investigators at the

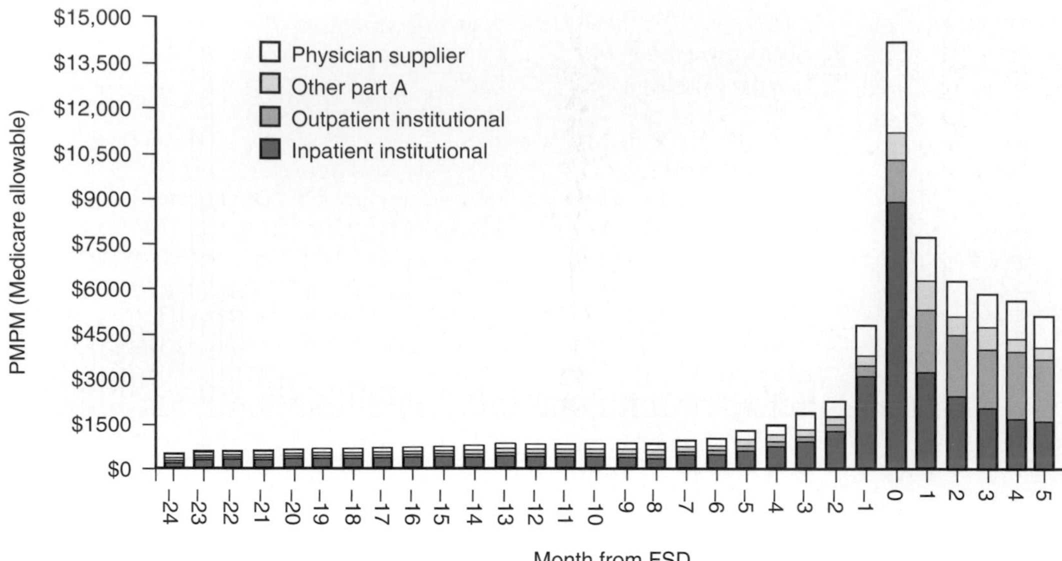

Figure 47–4 Cost breakdown by source of claim.

Table 47–1 Principal Diagnosis Related to Hospitalization in Study Patients, 1995-1997

	Percent of Admissions			
Cause of Admission	**Pre-FSD**	**FSD Mo.**	**Post-FSD**	**Total**
Vascular access (noninfectious)	7.1%	45.8%	22.4%	19.0%
Congestive heart failure	19.1%	5.3%	6.8%	13.2%
Renal failure	12.7%	19.0%	8.3%	12.9%
Ischemic heart disease	9.7%	4.9%	4.9%	7.5%
Other	7.4%	5.1%	8.8%	7.3%
Gastrointestinal	6.7%	2.7%	6.1%	5.7%
Respiratory infection	5.0%	1.9%	4.6%	4.3%
Circulatory system	3.0%	2.1%	4.9%	3.3%
Cerebrovascular disease	3.9%	1.0%	3.1%	3.1%
Metabolic, endocrine, nutrition	3.6%	0.9%	2.9%	2.9%
Septicemia	1.1%	1.5%	4.8%	2.1%
Conduction disorders and dysrhythmias	2.1%	1.2%	2.7%	2.1%
Electrolyte, acid-base	2.3%	0.9%	1.9%	1.9%
Other infection	1.9%	0.7%	2.8%	1.9%
Respiratory	1.7%	1.3%	2.5%	1.8%
Cancer	2.0%	1.1%	1.3%	1.6%
Skin and musculoskeletal	1.8%	0.5%	1.4%	1.4%
Genitourinary and breast	2.0%	0.6%	0.6%	1.4%
Immune and hematologic	1.6%	0.4%	0.8%	1.1%
Surgical complications	0.8%	0.7%	1.9%	1.1%
Urinary tract infection	1.2%	0.3%	1.0%	1.0%
Vascular access infection	0.1%	0.9%	2.6%	0.9%
Mental disorder	0.8%	0.2%	1.0%	0.7%
Central nervous system	0.7%	0.3%	0.8%	0.6%
Other cardiovascular	0.7%	0.4%	0.5%	0.6%
Hypertensive heart and renal disease w/o CHF	0.8%	0.1%	0.1%	0.5%
Osteomyelitis	0.2%	0.0%	0.2%	0.2%
Cardiac infection	0.1%	0.1%	0.1%	0.1%
Human immunodeficiency virus	0.0%	0.0%	0.0%	0.0%
Total Admits	196,449	75,699	88,803	360,921

CHF, congestive heart failure; *FSD,* first service date; *Mo.,* month.

USRDS Coordinating Center in Minneapolis, Minnesota, assessed associations in Medicare patients with a diagnosis of CKD. This study, which evaluated 1997 to 1998 patients in the fee-for-service Medicare system, compared costs between those with CKD diagnosis codes and those who did not have CKD diagnosis codes, and also considered Medicare patients with ESRD. The non-CKD population consisted of 1.07 million individuals; almost 39,000 had a diagnosis of CKD. The dialysis population of comparable age (=67 years) was taken from 1999 and consisted of 62,000 individuals. Inpatient, outpatient, and physician services were assessed on a PMPM basis. Table 47–2 summarizes the age, gender, and race distribution of individuals in the CKD, non-CKD, and dialysis groups. Of note, the CKD patients were older and the dialysis patients were younger than the non-CKD patients. There was also a more equal distribution of males and females who carried a diagnosis of CKD and who were on dialysis, compared to the general Medicare population. This observation suggests that the survival advantage for women in the general population is not present in women who carry a diagnosis of CKD or women who reach dialysis. There was also an increasing representation of black patients who were carrying a diagnosis of CKD or were on dialysis. The follow-up year was 1999; Figure 47–5 shows the distribution of Medicare expenditures for the three groups for the follow-up year in comparison with 1997 to 1998. Whereas the Medicare patients aged 67 years or greater who were on dialysis represented only 0.28% of the Medicare population, they generated almost 10 times the expenditures in the Medicare system. The Medicare patients age 67 years or greater who were carrying a diagnosis of CKD represented 3.5% of the Medicare population, yet they generated 9% of the Medicare expenditures. Together, the dialysis and CKD patients identified by a diagnosis code represented 3.8% of the Medicare population and accounted for 12.5% of the Medicare budget annually. This is an underestimate, because only the dialysis population is known (because of a registration system) and the CKD population is only one-fifth of those with the most advanced disease identified by the providers. A greater accounting of this population is needed.

Figure 47–6 shows the unadjusted average PMPM allowable Medicare expenditures in 1999 by patient group. Table 47–3

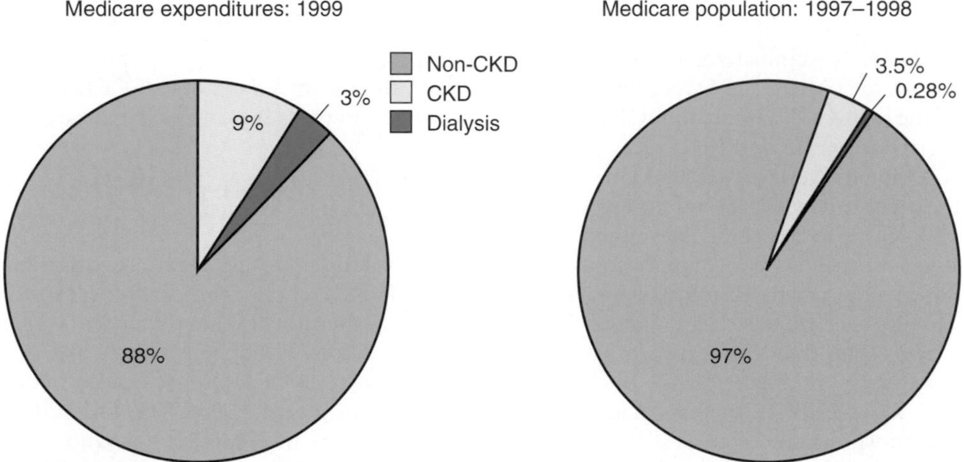

Figure 47–5 Distribution of Medicare expenditures by study group for the study period 1997 to 1998 and for the follow-up year, 1999. *CKD,* chronic kidney disease.

Table 47–2 Distribution of Study Patients by Demographic Characteristics and Study Group

	Non-CKD Patients	CKD Patients	Dialysis Patients
Sample size	1,066,607	38,781	61,697
Age (yr)			
67 to 74	45.1%	34.2%	51.7%
75 to 84	40.5%	44.8%	41.2%
= 85	14.4%	21.1%	7.1%
Gender			
Male	38.8%	47.5%	47.5%
Female	61.2%	52.5%	52.5%
Race			
White	89.3%	83.5%	61.8%
Black	6.9%	11.9%	32.2%
Other	3.8%	4.6%	6.0%

CKD, chronic kidney disease.

Table 47–3 Unadjusted Average Per-Person, Per-Month Allowable Medicare Expenditures in 1999 by Age, Gender, and Race within Patient Group

	Non-CKD Patients	CKD Patients	Dialysis Patients
Sample size	1,066,607	38,781	61,697
Age (yr)			
67 to 74	$405	$1328	$5270
75 to 84	$553	$1402	$5178
= 85	$694	$1385	$5126
Gender			
Male	$533	$1388	$5052
Female	$487	$1359	$5377
Race			
White	$501	$1317	$5092
Black	$559	$1689	$5492
Other	$491	$1576	$5064

CKD, chronic kidney disease.

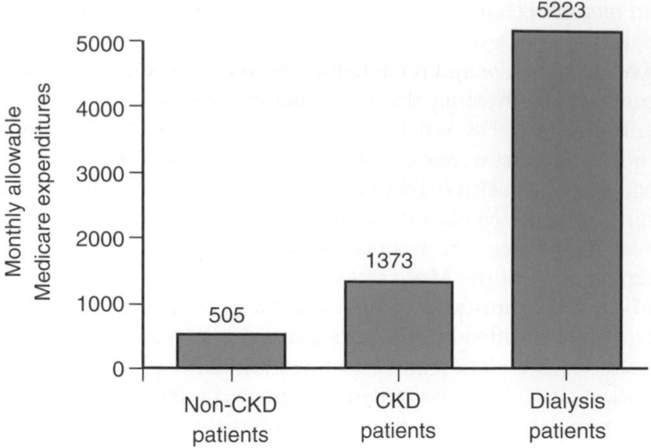

Figure 47–6 Unadjusted average per-person, per-month allowable Medicare expenditures in 1999 by patient group. *CKD*, chronic kidney disease.

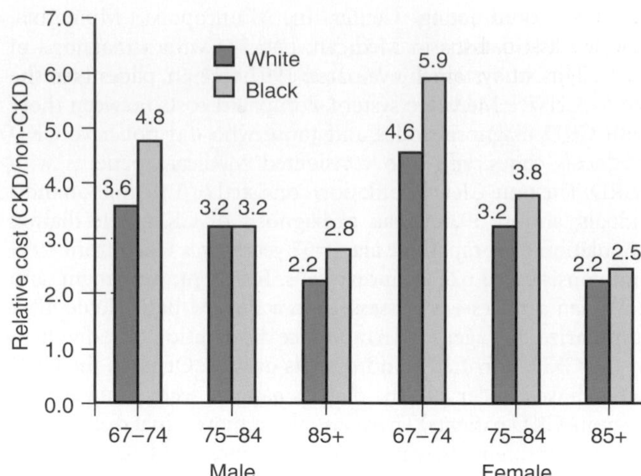

Figure 47–7 Adjusted comparison of CKD and non-CKD costs by age, gender, and race. From log transformed monthly expenditures, regressed by ordinary least squares. *CKD*, chronic kidney disease.

provides detail by age, gender, and race. Given advancing age, the non-CKD patients showed the expected increase in expenditures; however, this was not the case in the CKD and dialysis patients, who had expenditures that were more consistent, regardless of age. Table 47–4 summarizes the results from regression estimates addressing the CKD population as a group, compared to the non-CKD population. Of particular note, after adjustments for age, gender, and race, Medicare expenditures for CKD patients are 467% greater than expenditures for non-CKD patients. These data are very consistent with the reported differences in the event rates noted earlier for cardiovascular disease and infectious complication.[3] These relative costs were not equally distributed across all age groups. The interaction between age, gender, race, and CKD also appeared to be associated with different degrees of comparative expenditures, as shown in Figure 47–7. Interestingly enough, the youngest group (aged 67 to 74 years) had the highest relative costs between women and men as well as between blacks and whites. At older ages, the difference between blacks and whites decreased, and the difference between CKD and non-CKD patients also decreased. Therefore, on a population basis, those with a diagnosis of CKD carry a heavy burden of comorbidity and associated expenditures.

CKD and the New Medicare+Choice Risk Adjustment Payment System

The evolution of the Medicare capitated payment system is beyond the scope of this chapter. However, it is important to note that the effort to identify patients with increased comorbid conditions is not new. Comorbidity profiling methods have been developed to relate disease intensity to cost of care; examples include the Johns Hopkins Adjusted Clinical Groups (ACG) system, the Brandeis risk adjusters, and quality of life adjusters. Such efforts ultimately led to Congressional passage of a Budget Reconciliation Act that included a directive to CMS to develop a more comprehensive risk adjustment

Table 47–4 Predictors of Expenditures from Multiple Linear Regression Estimates on the Allowable Monthly Expenditures in 1999*

Risk Factor	% Effect on PMPM	Coefficient	SE	*P*
Intercept		4193	0.005	<.0001
Age 67 to 74 yr reference				
Age 75 to 84 yr	+80.3%	0.589	0.006	<.0001
Age =85 yr	+160%	0.957	0.008	<.0001
Female reference				
Male	−19.3%	−0.214	0.005	<.0001
White reference				
Black	−38.1%	−0.479	0.010	<.0001
Other race	−35.9%	−0.445	0.014	<.0001
Non-CKD reference				
CKD	+467%	1.74	0.014	<.0001

CKD, chronic kidney disease; *PMPM*, per-member, per-month expenditures; *SE*, standard error.
*Log transformed monthly expenditures, regressed by ordinary least squares.

payment system for the Medicare population. After considerable work and discussion, in May 2003 CMS announced the new payment system for Medicare+Choice enrollees (see the May 12, 2003, announcement of the Medicare+Choice payment rates for calendar year 2004 at *www.cms.hhs.gov/healthplans/rates/2004/cover.pdf*). This payment system is unique in that it is based on the identification of groups of diseases analyzed through standard actuarial regression models to determine their relative costs to the Medicare program, with a resulting hierarchical order of diseases applied to the payment system. Because this model is being implemented in the United States over the next 4 years, it will attract increasing attention, particularly for its handling of chronic diseases, such as CKD.

A full description of the Medicare+Choice hierarchical care model can be viewed at *www.cms.hhs.gov/healthplans/rates/default.asp*. The expenditure models used by CMS created risk adjusters with dollar coefficients, which are then divided by the national average to create a predicted expenditure ratio determined by the fee-for-service beneficiaries. The average dollar expenditures for the base year (2002) were $5129, which were used to establish the 2004 rates. As in most risk adjustment systems for payment of individuals, age and gender were strongly predictive of expenditures in the Medicare system. Not surprisingly, disability or receipt of combinations of Medicare and Medicaid payments were also predictive of high expenditures. For example, higher costs were associated with AIDS, metastatic cancer, and acute leukemia. Of particular note are categories of diseases that were indicated to have renal failure among their major manifestations. The risk-adjusted disease groupings that were identified as significantly associated with renal failure are given in Table 47–5.

Within Table 47–5, the hierarchical condition categories are additive to previous adjustments for age, gender, disability status, and other medical conditions that the patient may have. Within the renal failure categories is that patients undergoing dialysis were the most expensive in the Medicare system, with dialysis alone adding almost three times the cost per year. For patients not on dialysis, a diagnosis of renal failure resulted in an expenditure increase almost twice that of those with diagnoses associated with primary kidney diseases other than from diabetes. The interaction of kidney failure with heart failure and diabetes also significantly increased the costs. On the basis of Medicare's findings, it is clear that renal failure, heart failure, and diabetes, especially in combination, are associated with major increases in expenditures for the disabled and the elderly in the United States. The renal failure categories established in the Medicare+Choice system are well known to medical practitioners: diagnoses associated with hypertension and renal failure or hypertension with congestive heart failure and renal failure, as well as chronic renal failure and cystic kidney disease, to name a few.

The second major category of renal failure diagnoses (beyond diabetes and the renal failure category) is the group of kidney diseases associated with relatively acute onset. Conditions, such as proliferative nephritis, acute nephritis, and rapidly progressive nephritis, as well as nephrotic syndrome, dominate the disease defined as nephritis. The new Medicare+Choice hierarchical payment system is unique in that each individual's associated chronic diseases are additive to the payment system. Because this was the first attempt to identify the various diseases associated with increased expenditures, insight was gained into the additive nature of the costs of treating renal failure in the elderly and/or disabled population. As this new payment system is adopted, it will be evaluated to determine whether it provides a better fit between the complexities of the individual patient and the payments a health plan receives as compensation for care delivered by providers.

CKD and Associated Costs in the Non-Medicare Population

Findings regarding the cost of treating CKD in the elderly Medicare population cannot necessarily be extrapolated to younger populations. Unfortunately, few economic analyses have assessed the cost of caring for younger patients with CKD. Because CKD patients have significant comorbid conditions, it is likely that the younger CKD population has similar differential costs as the older CKD population. To a certain extent, younger CKD patients may have greater proportional costs than their non-CKD counterparts because of the high association between CKD, ischemic cardiovascular disease, heart failure, hypertension, and diabetes. Compared to Medicare patients, younger patients tend to have fewer complicating medical conditions, thereby potentially magnifying the effects of CKD. Economic evaluations are sorely needed to assess the cost of CKD in the non-Medicare population.

Cost-Effectiveness of Screening for CKD

Boulware and associates studied the cost-effectiveness of screening for proteinuria in U.S. adults.[10] These investigators used a Markov decision analytic model to compare annual screening to no screening for proteinuria in patients at age 50 years. For those without a diagnosis of hypertension or diabetes,

Table 47–5 Disease Groups Associated with Renal Failure in the Medicare+Choice Hierarchical Risk-Adjustment Model

Disease Group	Description	Relative (Community) Weight	Institutional Weight
HCC #15	DM with renal failure or peripheral circulatory manifestation	0.764	0.612
HCC #130	Dialysis	3.076	3.112
HCC #131	Renal failure	0.576	0.420
HCC #132	Nephritis	0.273	0.420
Interaction terms	Renal failure + CHF	0.234	
Interaction 6	Renal failure + CHF + DM	0.864	

CHF, congestive heart failure; *DM*, diabetes mellitus; *HCC*, hierarchical condition category.

screening appeared cost-prohibitive, with quality-adjusted life years adding $282,000 for the investment in screening. However, for individuals age 60 years or greater or those with a history of hypertension, the cost per quality-adjusted year of life saved was approximately $20,000. Cost-effectiveness appeared improved with use of angiotensin- converting enzyme inhibitor or an angiotensin II-receptor blocker therapy. The investigators concluded that proteinuria screening efforts were not particularly cost-effective unless directed at high-risk groups, such as individuals with hypertension.

The conclusions reached by Boulware and associates appear to be borne out by the recent reposting of results for the NKF's Kidney Early Evaluation Program (KEEP). The KEEP program is directed at individuals with a family history of diabetes, hypertension, or kidney disease as well as those who currently have a diagnosis of diabetes or hypertension. Started in 2000, this nationwide effort has resulted in the screening of more than 27,000 individuals through December 2003. The first 11,000 individuals screened were reported in October 2003.[6] In this target population, 2% to 3% of screened individuals knew they had evidence of CKD before screening, yet 50% had evidence of albuminuria or an estimated GFR of less than 60 mL/min. Of individuals with stage 3+ kidney disease, 80% had a blood pressure higher than 130/85. These findings in a targeted population are consistent with the high yield needed to be cost-effective. Health plans and providers need to develop methods to more actively identify those at high risk of kidney disease because this population carries a heavy burden of cardiovascular disease and expenditures. On the basis of the emerging evidence, it appears that CKD plays a much greater role in the morbidity, mortality, and cost of care of the general population than previously appreciated.

References

1. Coresh J, Astor BC, Greene T, et al: Prevalence of chronic kidney disease and decreased kidney function in the adult U.S. population: Third National Health and Nutrition Examination Survey. Am J Kidney Dis 2003; 41:1-12.
2. National Kidney Foundation: K/DOQI clinical practice guidelines for chronic kidney disease: Evaluation, classification and stratification. Am J Kidney Dis 2002; 39(suppl 1):S1-S266.
3. U.S. Renal Data System: USRDS 2003 Annual Data Report. Bethesda, MD, National Institutes of Health, National Institute of Diabetes and Digestive and Kidney Diseases, 2003.
4. Collins AJ, Li S, Gilbertson DT, et al: Chronic kidney disease and cardiovascular disease in the Medicare population. Kidney Int 2003; 64(suppl 87):S24-S31.
5. U.S. Renal Data System: USRDS 2002 Annual Data Report. Bethesda, MD, National Institutes of Health, National Institute of Diabetes and Digestive and Kidney Diseases, 2002.
6. National Kidney Foundation: KEEP (Kidney Early Evaluation Program) Annual Data Report. Am J Kidney Dis 2003; 42 (suppl 4): S3-S60.
7. Foley RN, Wang C, Collins AJ: Cardiovascular risk profile and declining kidney function. The NHANES III study (Abstract). J Am Soc Nephrol 2003; 14:678A.
8. London R, Solis A, Goldberg GA, et al: Health care resource utilization and the impact of anemia management in patients with chronic kidney disease. Am J Kidney Dis 2002; 40:539-548.
9. Peter WL, Khan SS, Ebben JP, et al: Chronic kidney disease: The distribution of health care dollars. Kidney Int 2004, 66:313-321.
10. Boulware LE, Jaar BG, Tarver-Carr ME, et al: Screening for proteinuria in U.S. adults: A cost-effectiveness analysis. JAMA 2003; 290:3101-3114.

Drug Dosing in Chronic Kidney Disease

George R. Aronoff, M.D., F.A.C.P.

The number of patients with impaired renal function has increased. Advances in the treatment of chronic diseases have permitted patients to live longer. Many of them develop decreased renal function over time. Kidney function also decreases with age, and older patients make up the most rapidly growing patient group for which special understanding of drug disposition is important. When chronic renal failure occurs, age, diabetes mellitus, and coronary artery disease are no longer barriers to renal replacement strategies.

Because uremia affects every organ system in the body, the physiological changes associated with renal disease profoundly alter the pharmacology of many drugs. Caregivers must consider how decreased renal function changes the bioavailability, distribution, metabolism, and elimination of medications and their active or toxic metabolites. Hypertension, diabetes mellitus, and heart disease compound the management of drugs in patients with renal diseases.

Novel strategies for treating renal failure contribute to the need for understanding drug removal during extracorporeal therapies. New dialysis membranes and devices, acceptance of intermittent and continuous peritoneal dialysis, and the application of continuous extracorporeal renal replacement therapies require that clinicians understand drug transport across biological and artificial membranes. This chapter outlines a rational approach to pharmacotherapy for patients with chronic kidney disease and those requiring renal replacement therapies.

PATIENT ASSESSMENT

Figure 48-1 shows a practical clinical approach to drug prescribing for patients with renal insufficiency. Pharmacotherapy for patients with kidney disease begins with a careful history and physical examination. Previous medications, adverse drug reactions, and concurrent medications influence the choice and dose of drugs in patients with impaired renal function.

On average, dialysis patients routinely receive 11 different medications and have three times the incidence of adverse drug events as patients with normal renal function.[1–3] Limiting the number of different drugs and choosing medications carefully decreases the potential for adverse drug effects, as does establishing a specific diagnosis before beginning treatment. Individualizing treatment can take advantage of using one medication to treat several conditions. For example, a calcium channel antagonist used to lower blood pressure in a hypertensive patient can also decrease angina or prevent certain tachyarrhythmias.

Physical examination to assess hydration status allows an estimate of the volume of distribution of many drugs. Water-soluble drugs are distributed in the extracellular fluid. Dehydrated patients have smaller distribution volumes, whereas patients with edema or ascites demonstrate expanded volumes of distribution.

Appropriate dosing requires measurements of the patient's height and weight. In dosing obese patients, many clinicians use the average of the patient's measured weight and the calculated ideal body weight (IBW) as a guide. For men, IBW is 50 kg plus 2.3 kg for each inch over 5 feet. For women, IBW is 45.5 kg plus 2.3 kg for each inch over 5 feet.[4]

Liver disease alters drug therapy in patients with renal insufficiency by limiting alternative pathways for drug and metabolite elimination. Finding the stigmata of liver failure is a strong indication of the need to further decrease drug doses in patients with decreased kidney function.

Measurement of Renal Function

The rate of elimination of drugs or drug metabolites excreted by the kidneys is proportional to the glomerular filtration rate. The serum creatinine or creatinine clearance is needed to determine renal function before prescribing any drug. The Cockcroft and Gault[5] equation is useful for this purpose as shown in the formula:

$$\text{Clcr} = \frac{(140 - \text{age}) \times (\text{IBW})}{72 \times \text{Scr}} \times (0.85 \text{ if female})$$

where:

Clcr = Creatinine clearance (mL/min)
Scr = Serum creatinine (mg/dL)

IBW (in kg)	= Ideal body weight (men)	=	50 kg + 2.3 kg per inch over 5 feet
	= Ideal body weight (women)	=	45.5 kg + 2.3 kg per inch over 5 feet

For obese men and women, the equation should be modified:

$$\text{Clcr(obese men)} = \frac{(137 - \text{age}) \times [(0.285 \times \text{wgt}) + (12.1 \times \text{hgt}^2)]}{51 \times \text{Scr}}$$

$$\text{Clcr(obese men)} = \frac{(146 - \text{age}) \times [(0.287 \times \text{wgt}) + (9.74 \times \text{hgt}^2)]}{60 \times \text{Scr}}$$

where:
wgt = patient's weight in kg
hgt = patient's height in cm

In cases of changing renal function, the serum creatinine will no longer reflect the true clearance rate. In these cases, a timed urine collection is needed to estimate renal function.

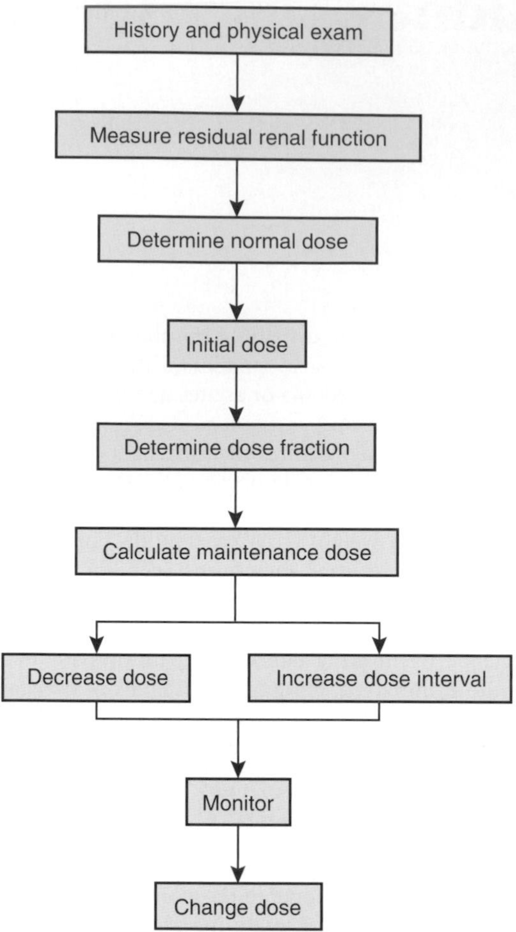

Figure 48–1 A clinical approach to drug dosing in renal failure.

The midpoint serum creatinine is useful to calculate the creatinine clearance for the collection period.

The serum creatinine reflects muscle mass as well as glomerular filtration rate. Serum creatinine measurements within the "normal" range are frequently used to establish "normal" renal function. This erroneous assumption may cause serious overdose and resultant toxic drug accumulation in elderly or debilitated patients with decreased muscle mass. A 72-kg man with a serum creatinine of 1 mg/dL has half the renal function at the age of 80 years as he did with the same body mass and serum creatinine at the age of 20 years. If the same doses of medications are given to the 80-year-old as to the 20-year-old, adverse drug events are likely because of drug and metabolite accumulation.

The serum creatinine measurement alone does not accurately estimate renal function in dialysis patients and should not be used to estimate drug dosing. Some patients may still have substantial renal function when they initiate dialysis therapies. The presence of residual renal function in dialysis patients increases the rate of drug or metabolite elimination. However, residual renal function decreases over time and may be assumed negligible for estimating drug doses in oliguric patients or in those who have required dialysis for longer than a year.

Serum creatinine measurements are a poor measure of intrinsic renal function in dialysis patients. Residual renal function in non-oliguric dialysis patients is difficult to estimate, because the serum creatinine reflects the adequacy of dialysis and muscle mass, as well as residual glomerular filtration. Unfortunately, creatinine clearance measurements do not accurately estimate the glomerular filtration rate in patients with renal failure requiring dialysis. The plasma clearance of radioisotopes or inulin can be a precise measure of renal function, but their use is cumbersome and expensive.

EFFECTS OF UREMIA ON DRUG DISPOSITION

Bioavailability

The bioavailability is the rate and extent to which a drug enters the systemic circulation. The rapid onset of action observed with intravenously administered drugs is the result of entering the central circulation directly. When drugs must cross biological membranes or pass through metabolizing organs, only a fraction of the dose reaches the site of action. Bioavailability is the percentage of the dose that reaches the systemic venous circulation. The rate of drug absorption determines the time required to achieve the maximum concentration of the drug in venous blood.

As oral drugs traverse gastrointestinal membranes, they may be metabolized by enzymes in the intestinal epithelium.[6,7] Once in the portal circulation, they must next pass through the liver, where hepatic biotransformation or excretion into the bile may prevent the drug from reaching the systemic circulation.

Gastrointestinal drug absorption is decreased in patients with renal failure. Nausea, vomiting, and gastroparesis are common in uremia and may discourage patients from taking oral medications. Unfortunately, little is known about bowel function in renal failure, but some drugs are not well absorbed when given orally. For example, ferrous iron salts require acid hydrolysis for absorption. It has been postulated that salivary urea is converted to ammonia in the stomach of uremic patients, buffering gastric acid and causing decreased absorption of drugs requiring acid hydrolysis.[8]

Patients with renal impairment often ingest large quantities of antacids to bind dietary phosphate. Chelation and the formation of non-absorbable complexes with multivalent cations frequently used in antacids decreases the bioavailability of some drugs.[9,10] This effect is particularly important for the absorption of some antibiotics and digoxin.

Gastrointestinal absorptive function is decreased in patients with impaired renal function. Craig and colleagues[11] showed the absorption of D-xylose is diminished in patients with renal failure. Gastroparesis prolongs gastric emptying and delays drug absorption in diabetics with renal impairment. Conversely, diarrhea shortens gut transit time and diminishes drug absorption by the small bowel.

The interaction between absorption and first-pass hepatic metabolism is complex and causes variable drug bioavailability in patients with renal impairment. Decreased hepatic or gastrointestinal biotransformation increases the active drug entering the systemic circulation from the portal system. However, impaired protein binding results in more free drug at the site of hepatic metabolism and more drug removal during the hepatic first pass.

Distribution

At equilibrium, the amount of drug in the body divided by its plasma concentration is the drug's apparent volume of distribution. This mathematical construct is used to estimate the dose of a drug to be given in order to achieve a desired plasma concentration, rather than an actual anatomical space. Highly protein-bound drugs, or those that are water soluble, are restricted to the extracellular fluid space and have small distribution volumes. Lipid-soluble drugs penetrate body tissues and exhibit large volumes of distribution.

A drug's apparent volume of distribution can be altered by factors frequently present in patients with renal insufficiency. Water-soluble drugs demonstrate increased distribution volume in patients with edema or ascites. Drug doses will need to be increased somewhat for edematous patients to avoid ineffectively low plasma levels. Dehydration or muscle wasting decreases the volume of distribution of water soluble and highly protein bound drugs. In these cases, initial drug doses should be decreased to avoid toxic plasma concentrations.

Protein-bound drugs attach reversibly either to albumin or glycoprotein in plasma. Binding to serum proteins may be decreased in uremic patients. This protein-binding defect is believed to be the result of a combination of decreased serum albumin concentration and a reduction in albumin affinity for the drug, but it may be present even when the plasma albumin concentration is normal.[12–14]

The extent of drug binding to serum proteins influences the volume of distribution, the amount of free drug available for action, and the degree to which the drug is eliminated by hepatic or renal excretion. Decreased plasma protein binding in patients with renal insufficiency increases drug action, but may also increase the rate of drug removal because it is the free fraction that is available for hepatic biotransformation.[15]

Impaired plasma protein binding in uremia has important clinical effects. Toxicity can occur if the total plasma concentration of a protein bound drug is pushed into the therapeutic range by increasing the dose. In cases where there is a significant protein-binding defect, the concentration of free drug may be toxic. For highly protein bound drugs, it may be useful to measure total and unbound plasma concentrations. The variable effects of protein binding on elimination and toxicity make predicting the clinical effects of altered protein binding in uremia difficult.

Metabolism

Surprisingly, renal failure slows the rate of non-renal drug elimination. The rate of reduction and hydrolysis reactions can be decreased in patients with renal failure, while glucuronidation and sulfate conjugation usually occur at normal rates.[16] Uremia in rats may decrease the protein expression of CYP450 isoforms up to 50% as well as their mRNA.[17]

The biotransformation of drugs to active or toxic metabolites is important in patients with renal failure, because polar metabolites are frequently eliminated by the kidneys. Metabolite accumulation explains, in part, the increased incidence of adverse drug reactions seen in renal failure.

Drug dosing calculations for dialysis patients are usually derived from studies in patients with stable, chronic renal failure. These recommendations are frequently extrapolated to seriously ill patients with acute renal failure. Although metabolic drug removal is often decreased in patients with chronic renal failure, acute renal failure may spare non-renal drug clearance.[18] Extrapolation of drug dosing recommendations from patients with stable chronic renal failure could result in potentially ineffectively low drug concentrations in patients with acute renal dysfunction.

DRUG DOSING CALCULATIONS

The initial dose of a drug given to patients with renal failure should be the same as that given to a patient with normal renal function, unless there is evidence of edema, ascites, dehydration, or severe muscle wasting. This initial loading dose of any drug can be calculated from the following expression:

$$\text{Loading Dose} = \text{Vd} \times \text{IBW} \times \text{Cp}$$

where Vd is the drug's volume of distribution in liters per kilogram, IBW is the patient's ideal body weight in kilograms, and Cp is the desired steady state plasma drug concentration.

For subsequent drug doses, the fraction of the normal dose recommended for a patient with renal failure can be calculated as follows:

$$\text{Df} = t\tfrac{1}{2}\ \text{normal} \,/\, t\tfrac{1}{2}\ \text{renal failure}$$

where Df is the fraction of the normal dose to be given; $t\frac{1}{2}$ normal is the elimination half-life of the drug in a patient with normal renal function; and $t\frac{1}{2}$ renal failure is the elimination half-life of the drug in a patient with renal failure. To maintain the normal dose interval in patients with renal impairment, the amount of each dose, following the loading dose, can be determined from the following relationship:

$$\text{Dose in Renal Impairment} = \text{Normal Dose} \times \text{DF}$$

The resulting dose is usually given at the same dose interval as that for patients with normal renal function. This method is effective for drugs with a narrow therapeutic range and a short plasma half life. Figure 48–2 illustrates plasma concentrations following an initial loading dose and reduction of the individual doses.

A convenient method for decreasing the amount of drug given to a patient with renal insufficiency is to prolong the dose interval. This method is used for drugs with a wide therapeutic window and long plasma half-life. The dose interval in renal impairment can be estimated from the following expression:

$$\text{Dose interval in renal impairment} = \text{Normal dose interval} \,/\, \text{Df}$$

The resulting plasma concentrations from prolonging the dose interval in an individual with impaired renal function are shown in Figure 48–3. If the range between therapeutic and toxic levels is too narrow, either potentially toxic or subtherapeutic plasma concentrations result.

Combining dose reduction and interval prolongation is a practical and convenient approach to reducing the amount of a medication given to a patient with renal impairment. The daily dose is calculated by multiplying the normal daily dose by the dose fraction. This modified dose can be divided into convenient dosing intervals.

The decision to extend the dosing interval beyond a 24-hour period should be based on the need to maintain therapeutic peak or trough levels. The dosing interval may be prolonged if the peak level is most important. When the minimum trough level must be maintained, it is preferable to modify the individual dose or use a combination of dose and interval methods to determine the correct dosing strategy. Drugs removed by dialysis and given once daily should be given after

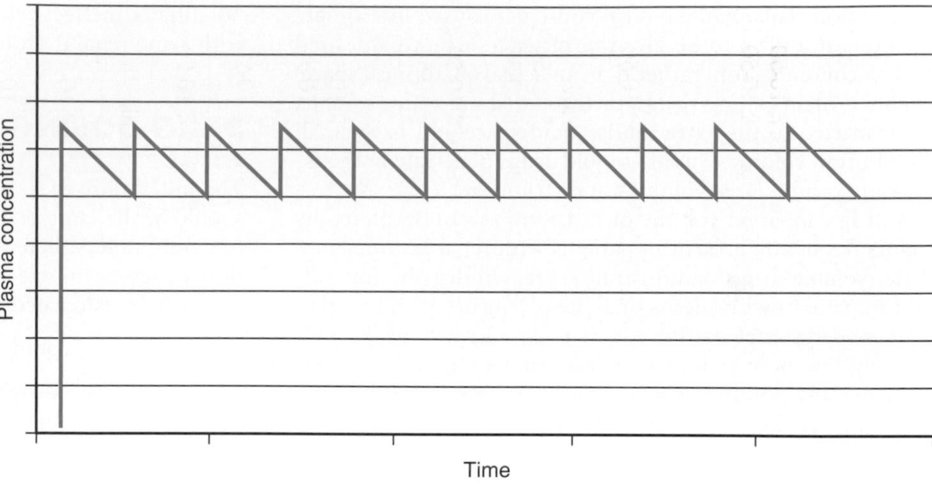

Figure 48–2 A normal loading dose and reduced maintenance doses avoids high peak and low trough concentrations. This approach is best for drugs with a narrow range between the therapeutic and toxic concentrations.

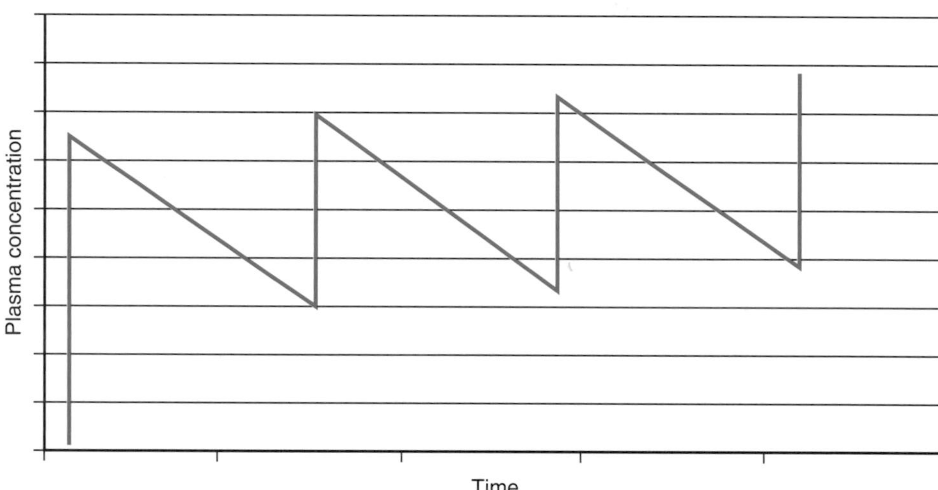

Figure 48–3 A normal loading dose and repeated normal doses at a prolonged dose interval result in higher peak and lower trough concentrations.

the dialysis treatment. Recommendations for drug dosing in patients with renal impairment are given in Table 48–1.[19]

DRUG REMOVAL BY DIALYSIS

Drug removal by hemodialysis occurs primarily by the process of drug diffusion across the dialysis membrane down a concentration gradient from the plasma to the dialysate. It is most effective for drugs that are less than 500 Daltons (Da), are less than 90% protein bound, and have small volumes of distribution. Removal of small molecular weight drugs is enhanced by increasing the blood and dialysate flow rates and by using large surface area dialyzers. Larger molecules require more porous membranes for increased removal. The hemodialysis clearance of a drug can be estimated from the following relationship:

$$Cl_{HD} = Cl_{urea} \times (60/MW_{drug})$$

where Cl_{HD} is the drug's clearance by hemodialysis, Cl_{urea} is the clearance of urea by the dialyzer, and MW_{drug} is the molecular weight of the drug.[20] The urea clearance for most standard dialyzers is about varies between 150 and 200 mL/min.[21]

The use of porous dialysis membranes to perform high flux dialysis decreases the importance of drug molecular mass in determining drug removal during extracorporeal circulation. During high flux dialysis, the volume of distribution and percent protein binding of the drug are more important determinants dialysis drug clearance. The removal of drugs during high-flux dialysis depends more on treatment time, blood and dialysate flow rates, distribution volume, and binding of the drug to serum proteins. Much more drug is removed during high-flux dialysis than previously estimated for conventional hemodialysis.

Peritoneal dialysis is less efficient at removing drugs than is hemodialysis and most effective for smaller molecular weight drugs that are not extensively bound to serum proteins.[22] Larger molecular weight drugs are removed by peritoneal dialysis by secretion into peritoneal lymphatic fluid. Drugs that have small volumes of distribution are more effectively removed than those that are distributed in adipose tissue or have extensive tissue binding. Removal of small molecular weight drugs is dependent on the number of peritoneal dialysis exchanges done daily. Peritoneal drug clearance can be estimated from the relationship:

$$Cl_{PD} = Cl_{urea} \times \frac{\sqrt{60}}{\sqrt{MW_{drug}}}$$

where Cl_{PD} is the peritoneal drug clearance; Cl_{urea} is the peritoneal urea clearance; and MW_d is the molecular weight of the

Continued on page 868

Table 48–1 Recommendations for Drug Dosing in Patients with Renal Impairment

Drug	Dose Method	GFR > 50 (mL/min)	GFR 10-50 (mL/min)	GFR < 10 (mL/min)	Supplemental dose after hemodialysis	CAPD	CRRT
Acarbose	D	50%-100%	Avoid	Avoid	Unknown	Unknown	Avoid
Acebutolol	D	100%	50%	30%-50%	None	None	Dose for GFR 10-50
Acetaminophen	I	q4h	q6h	q8h	None	None	Dose for GFR 10-50
Acetazolamide	I	q6h	q12h	Avoid	No data	No data	Avoid
Acetohexamide	I	Avoid	Avoid	Avoid	Unknown	None	Avoid
Acetohydroxamic acid	D	100%	100%	Avoid	Unknown	Unknown	Unknown
Acetylsalicylic acid	I	q4h	q4-6h	Avoid	Dose after dialysis	None	Dose for GFR 10-50
Acrivastine	D	Unknown	Unknown	Unknown	Unknown	Unknown	Unknown
Acyclovir	D,I	5 mg/kg q8h	5 mg/kg q12-24h	2.5 mg/kg q24h	Dose after dialysis	Dose for GFR <10	3.5 mg/kg/day
Adenosine	D	100%	100%	100%	None	None	Dose for GFR 10-50
Albuterol	D	100%	75%	50%	Unknown	Unknown	Dose for GFR 10-50
Alcuronium	D	Avoid	Avoid	Avoid	Unknown	Unknown	Avoid
Alfentanil	D	100%	100%	100%	Unknown	Unknown	Dose for GFR 10-50
Allopurinol	D	75%	50%	25%	1/2 dose	Unknown	Dose for GFR 10-50
Alprazolam	D	100%	100%	100%	None	Unknown	NA
Altretamine	D	Unknown	Unknown	Unknown	No data	No data	Unknown
Amantadine	I	q24-48h	q48-72h	q7d	None	None	Dose for GFR 10-50
Amikacin	D,I	60%-90% q12h	30%-70% q12-18h	20%-30% q24-48h	2/3 normal dose	15-20 mg/L/day	Dose for GFR 10-50
Amiloride	D	100%	50%	Avoid	Not applicable	Not applicable	Not applicable
Amiodarone	D	100%	100%	100%	None	None	Dose for GFR 10-50
Amitriptyline	D	100%	100%	100%	None	Unknown	NA
Amlodipine	D	100%	100%	100%	None	None	Dose for GFR 10-50
Amoxapine	D	100%	100%	100%	Unknown	Unknown	NA
Amoxicillin	I	q8h	q8-12h	q24h	Dose after dialysis	250 mg q12h	Not applicable
Amphotericin	I	q24h	q24h	q24-36h	None	Dose for GFR <10	Dose for GFR 10-50
Amphotericin B colloidal	I	q24h	q24h	q24-36h	None	Dose for GFR <10	Dose for GFR 10-50
Amphotericin B lipid	I	q24h	q24h	q24-36h	None	Dose for GFR <10	Dose for GFR 10-50
Ampicillin	I	q6h	q6-12h	q12-24h	Dose after dialysis	250 mg q12h	Dose for GFR 10-50
Amrinone	D	100%	100%	50%-75%	No data	No data	Dose for GFR 10-50
Anistreplase	D	100%	100%	100%	Unknown	Unknown	Dose for GFR 10-50
Astemizole	D	100%	100%	100%	Unknown	Unknown	NA
Atenolol	D,I	100% q24h	50% q48h	30%-50% q96h	25-50 mg	None	Dose for GFR 10-50
Atovaquone		100%	100%	100%	None	None	Dose for GFR 10-50
Atracurium	D	100%	100%	100%	Unknown	Unknown	Dose for GFR 10-50
Auranofin	D	50%	Avoid	Avoid	None	None	None
Azathioprine	D	100%	75%	50%	Yes	Unknown	Dose for GFR 10-50
Azithromycin	D	100%	100%	100%	None	None	None
Azlocillin	I	q4-6h	q6-8h	q8h	Dose after dialysis	Dose for GFR <10	Dose for GFR 10-50
Aztreonam	D	100%	50%-75%	25%	0.5 g after dialysis	Dose for GFR <10	Dose for GFR 10-50

(*Continued*)

Table 48–1 Recommendations for drug dosing in patients with renal impairment—cont'd

Drug	Dose Method	GFR > 50 (mL/min)	GFR 10-50 (mL/min)	GFR < 10 (mL/min)	Supplemental dose after hemodialysis	CAPD	CRRT
Benazepril	D	100%	50%-75%	25%-50%	None	None	Dose for GFR 10-50
Bepridil		Unknown	Unknown	Unknown	None	None	No data
Betamethasone	D	100%	100%	100%	Unknown	Unknown	Dose for GFR 10-50
Betaxolol	D	100%	100%	50%	None	None	Dose for GFR 10-50
Bezafibrate	D	70%	50%	25%	Unknown	Unknown	Dose for GFR 10-50
Bisoprolol	D	100%	75%	50%	Unknown	Unknown	Dose for GFR 10-50
Bleomycin	D	100%	75%	50%	None	Unknown	Dose for GFR 10-50
Bopindolol	D	100%	100%	100%	None	None	Dose for GFR 10-50
Bretylium	D	100%	25%-50%	25%	None	None	Dose for GFR 10-50
Bromocriptine	D	100%	100%	100%	Unknown	Unknown	Unknown
Brompheniramine	D	100%	100%	100%	Unknown	Unknown	NA
Budesonide	D	100%	100%	100%	Unknown	Unknown	Dose for GFR 10-50
Bumetanide	D	100%	100%	100%	None	None	Not applicable
Bupropion	D	100%	100%	100%	Unknown	Unknown	NA
Buspirone	D	100%	100%	100%	None	Unknown	NA
Busulfan	D	100%	100%	100%	Unknown	Unknown	Dose for GFR 10-50
Butorphanol	D	100%	75%	50%	Unknown	Unknown	NA
Capreomycin	I	q24h	q24h	q48h	Give dose after HD only	None	Dose for GFR 10-50
Captopril	D,I	100% q8-12h	75% q12-18h	50% q24h	25%-30%	None	Dose for GFR 10-50
Carbamazepine	D	100%	100%	100%	None	None	None
Carbidopa	D	100%	100%	100%	Unknown	Unknown	Unknown
Carboplatin	D	100%	50%	25%	1/2 dose	Unknown	Dose for GFR 10-50
Carmustine	D	Unknown	Unknown	Unknown	Unknown	Unknown	Unknown
Carteolol	D	100%	50%	25%	Unknown	None	Dose for GFR 10-50
Carvedilol	D	100%	100%	100%	None	None	Dose for GFR 10-50
Cefaclor	D	100%	50%-100%	50%	250 mg after dialysis	250 mg q8-12h	Not applicable
Cefadroxil	I	q12h	q12-24h	q24-48h	0.5-1.0 g after dialysis	0.5 g/day	Not applicable
Cefamandole	I	q6h	q6-8h	q12h	0.5-1.0 g after dialysis	0.5-1.0 g q12h	Dose for GFR 10-50
Cefazolin	I	q8h	q12h	q24-48h	0.5-1.0 g after dialysis	0.5 g q12h	Dose for GFR 10-50
Cefepime	I	q12h	q16-24h	q24-48h	1.0 g after dialysis	Dose for GFR <10	Not recommended
Cefixime	D	100%	75%	50%	300 mg after dialysis	200 mg/day	Not recommended
Cefmenoxime	D,I	1.0 g q8h	0.75 g q8h	0.75 g q12h	0.75 g after dialysis	0.75 g q12h	Dose for GFR 10-50
Cefmetazole	I	q16h	q24h	q48h	Dose after dialysis	Dose for GFR <10	Dose for GFR 10-50
Cefonicid	D,I	0.5 g/day	0.1-0.5g/day	0.1 g/day	None	None	None
Cefoperazone	D	100%	100%	100%	1 g after dialysis	None	None
Ceforanide	I	q12h	q12-24h	q24-48h	0.5-1.0 g after dialysis	None	1.0 g/day
Cefotaxime	I	q6h	q8-12h	q24h	1 g after dialysis	1 g/d	1 g q12h
Cefotetan	D	100%	50%	25%	1 g after dialysis	1 g/d	750 mg q12h
Cefoxitin	I	q8h	q8-12h	q24-48h	1 g after dialysis	1 g/d	Dose for GFR 10-50
Cefpodoxime	I	q12h	q16h	q24-48h	200 mg after dialysis	Dose for GFR <10	Not applicable

Cefprozil	D,I	250 mg q12h	250 mg q12-16h	250 mg q24h	250 mg after dialysis	Dose for GFR <10	Dose for GFR <10
Ceftazidime	I	q8-12h	q24-48h	q48h	1 g after dialysis	0.5 g/day	Dose for GFR 10-50
Ceftibutin	D	100%	50%	25%	300 mg after dialysis	Dose for GFR <10	Dose for GFR 10-50
Ceftizoxime	I	q8-12h	q12-24h	q24h	1 g after dialysis	0.5-1.0 g/day	Dose for GFR 10-50
Ceftriaxone	D	100%	100%	100%	Dose after dialysis	750 mg q12h	Dose for GFR 10-50
Cefuroxime axetil	D	100%	100%	100%	Dose after dialysis	Dose for GFR <10	Not applicable
Celiprolol	D	100%	100%	75%	Unknown	None	Dose for GFR 10-50
Cephalexin	I	q8h	q12h	q12h	Dose after dialysis	Dose for GFR <10	Not applicable
Cephalothin	I	q6h	q6-8h	q12h	Dose after dialysis	1 g q12h	1 g q8h
Cephapirin	I	q6h	q6-8h	q12h	Dose after dialysis	1 g q12h	1 g q8h
Cephradine	D	100%	50%	25%	Dose after dialysis	Dose for GFR <10	Not applicable
Cetirizine	D	100%	100%	30%	None	Unknown	NA
Chloral hydrate	D	100%	Avoid	Avoid	None	Unknown	NA
Chlorambucil	D	Unknown	Unknown	Unknown	Unknown	Unknown	Unknown
Chloramphenicol	D	100%	100%	100%	None	None	None
Chlorazepate	D	100%	100%	100%	Unknown	Unknown	NA
Chlordiazepoxide	D	100%	100%	50%	None	Unknown	Dose for GFR 10-50
Chloroquine	D	100%	100%	50%	None	None	None
Chlorpheniramine	D	100%	100%	100%	None	Unknown	NA
Chlorpromazine	D	100%	100%	100%	None	None	Dose for GFR 10-50
Chlorpropamide	D	50%	Avoid	Avoid	Unknown	None	Avoid
Chlorthalidone	I	q24h	q24h	Avoid	Not applicable	Not applicable	Not applicable
Cholestyramine	D	100%	100%	100%	None	None	Dose for GFR 10-50
Cibenzoline	D,I	100% q12h	100% q12h	66% q24h	None	None	Dose for GFR 10-50
Cidofovir	D	50%-100%	avoid	avoid	No data	No data	Avoid
Cilastin	D	100%	50%	Avoid	Avoid	Avoid	Avoid
Cilazapril	D,I	75% q24h	50% q24-48h	10%-25% q72h	None	None	Dose for GFR 10-50
Cimetidine	D	100%	50%	25%	None	None	Dose for GFR 10-50
Cinoxacin	D	100%	50%	Avoid	Avoid	Avoid	Avoid
Ciprofloxacin	D	100%	50%-75%	50%	250 mg q12h	250 mg q8h	200 mg iv q12h
Cisapride	D	100%	100%	50%	Unknown	Unknown	50%-100%
Cisplatin	D	100%	75%	50%	Yes	Unknown	Dose for GFR 10-50
Cladribine	D	Unknown	Unknown	Unknown	Unknown	Unknown	Unknown
Clarithromycin	D	100%	75%	50%-75%	Dose after dialysis	None	None
Clavulanic acid	D	100%	100%	50%-75%	Dose after dialysis	Dose for GFR <10	Dose for GFR 10-50
Clindamycin	D	100%	100%	100%	None	None	None
Clodronate	D	Unknown	Unknown	Avoid	Unknown	Unknown	Unknown
Clofazamine		100%	100%	100%	None	None	No data
Clofibrate	I	q6-12h	q12-18h	Avoid	None	Unknown	Dose for GFR 10-50
Clomipramine	D	Unknown	Unknown	Unknown	Unknown	Unknown	NA
Clonazepam	D	100%	100%	100%	None	Unknown	NA
Clonidine	D	100%	100%	100%	None	None	Dose for GFR 10-50
Codeine	D	100%	75%	50%	Unknown	Unknown	Dose for GFR 10-50
Colchicine	D	100%	100%	50%	None	Unknown	Dose for GFR 10-50

(Continued)

Table 48–1 Recommendations for drug dosing in patients with renal impairment—cont'd

Drug	Dose Method	GFR > 50 (mL/min)	GFR 10-50 (mL/min)	GFR < 10 (mL/min)	Supplemental dose after hemodialysis	CAPD	CRRT
Colestipol	D	100%	100%	100%	None	None	Dose for GFR 10-50
Cortisone	D	100%	100%	100%	None	Unknown	Dose for GFR 10-50
Cyclophosphamide	D	100%	100%	75%	1/2 dose	Unknown	Dose for GFR 10-50
Cycloserine	I	q12h	q12-24h	q24h	None	None	Dose for GFR 10-50
Cyclosporine	D	100%	100%	100%	None	None	100%
Cytarabine	D	100%	100%	100%	Unknown	Unknown	Dose for GFR 10-50
Dapsone		100%	No data	No data	None	Dose for GFR <10	No data
Daunorubicin	D	100%	100%	100%	Unknown	Unknown	Unknown
Delavirdine		100%	100%	100%	None	No data	Dose for GFR 10-50
Desferoxamine	D	100%	100%	100%	Unknown	Unknown	Dose for GFR 10-50
Desipramine	D	100%	100%	100%	None	None	NA
Dexamethasone	D	100%	100%	100%	Unknown	Unknown	Dose for GFR 10-50
Diazepam	D	100%	100%	100%	None	Unknown	100%
Diazoxide	D	100%	100%	100%	None	None	Dose for GFR 10-50
Diclofenac	D	100%	100%	100%	None	None	Dose for GFR 10-50
Dicloxacillin	D	100%	100%	100%	None	None	Not applicable
Didanosine	I	q12h	q24h	q24-48h	Dose after dialysis	Dose for GFR <10	Dose for GFR <10
Diflunisal	D	100%	50%	50%	None	None	Dose for GFR 10-50
Digitoxin	D	100%	100%	50%-75%	None	None	Dose for GFR 10-50
Digoxin	D,I	100% q24h	25%-75% q36h	10%-25% q48h	None	None	Dose for GFR 10-50
Dilevalol	D	100%	100%	100%	None	None	Unknown
Diltiazem	D	100%	100%	100%	None	None	Dose for GFR 10-50
Diphenhydramine	D	100%	100%	100%	None	None	None
Dipyridamole	D	100%	100%	100%	Unknown	Unknown	NA
Dirithromycin		100%	100%	100%	None	None	Dose for GFR 10-50
Disopyramide	I	q8h	q12-24h	q24-40h	None	None	Dose for GFR 10-50
Dobutamine	D	100%	100%	100%	No data	No data	Dose for GFR 10-50
Doxacurium	D	100%	50%	50%	Unknown	Unknown	Dose for GFR 10-50
Doxazosin	D	100%	100%	100%	None	None	Dose for GFR 10-50
Doxepin	D	100%	100%	100%	None	None	Dose for GFR 10-50
Doxorubicin	D	100%	100%	100%	None	Unknown	Dose for GFR 10-50
Doxycycline	D	100%	100%	100%	None	None	Dose for GFR 10-50
Dyphylline	D	75%	50%	25%	1/3 dose	Unknown	Dose for GFR 10-50
Enalapril	D	100%	75%-100%	50%	20%-25%	None	Dose for GFR 10-50
Epirubicin	D	100%	100%	100%	None	Unknown	Dose for GFR 10-50
Erbastine	D	100%	50%	50%	Unknown	Unknown	Dose for GFR 10-50
Erythromycin	D	100%	100%	50%-75%	None	None	None
Estazolam	D	100%	100%	100%	Unknown	Unknown	NA
Ethacrynic acid	I	q8-12h	q8-12h	Avoid	None	None	Not applicable
Ethambutol	I	q24h	q24-36h	q48h	Dose after dialysis	Dose for GFR <10	Dose for GFR 10-50
Ethchlorvynol	D	100%	Avoid	Avoid	None	None	NA

Ethionamide	D	100%	100%	50%	None	None	None
Ethosuximide	D	100%	100%	100%	None	Unknown	Unknown
Etodolac	D	100%	100%	100%	None	None	Dose for GFR 10-50
Etomidate	D	100%	100%	100%	Unknown	Unknown	Dose for GFR 10-50
Etoposide	D	100%	75%	50%	None	Unknown	Dose for GFR 10-50
Famciclovir	I	100%	q 12-48 h	50% q48h	Dose after dialysis	No data	Dose for GFR 10-50
Famotidine	D	50%	25%	10%	None	None	Dose for GFR 10-50
Fazadinium	D	100%	100%	100%	Unknown	Unknown	Dose for GFR 10-50
Felodipine	D	100%	100%	100%	None	None	Dose for GFR 10-50
Fenoprofen	D	100%	100%	100%	None	None	Dose for GFR 10-50
Fentanyl	D	100%	75%	50%	Not applicable	Not applicable	NA
Fexofenadine	I	q12h	q12-24h	q24h	Unknown	Unknown	Dose for GFR 10-50
Flecainide	D	100%	100%	50%-75%	None	None	Dose for GFR 10-50
Fleroxacin	D	100%	50%-75%	50%	400 mg after dialysis	400 mg/day	Not applicable
Fluconazole	D	100%	100%	100%	200 mg after dialysis	Dose for GFR <10	Dose for GFR 10-50
Flucytosine	I	q12h	q16h	q24h	Dose after dialysis	0.5-1.0 g/day	Dose for GFR 10-50
Fludarabine	D	100%	75%	50%	Unknown	Unknown	Dose for GFR 10-50
Flumazenil	D	100%	100%	100%	None	Unknown	NA
Flunarizine	D	100%	100%	100%	None	None	None
Fluorouracil	D	100%	100%	100%	Yes	Unknown	Dose for GFR 10-50
Fluoxetine	D	100%	100%	100%	Unknown	Unknown	NA
Flurazepam	D	100%	100%	100%	None	Unknown	NA
Flurbiprofen	D	100%	100%	100%	None	None	Dose for GFR 10-50
Flutamide	D	100%	100%	100%	Unknown	Unknown	Unknown
Fluvastatin	D	100%	100%	100%	Unknown	Unknown	Dose for GFR 10-50
Fluvoxamine	D	100%	100%	100%	None	Unknown	NA
Foscarnet	D	28 mg/kg	15 mg/kg	6 mg/kg	Dose after dialysis	Dose for GFR <10	Dose for GFR 10-50
Fosinopril	D	100%	100%	75%-100%	None	None	Dose for GFR 10-50
Furosemide	D	100%	100%	100%	None	None	Not applicable
Gabapentin	D,I	400 mg tid	300q 12-24h	300 mg qd	300mg load, then 200-300		Dose for GFR 10-50
Gallamine	D	75%	Avoid	Avoid	Not applicable	Not applicable	Dose for GFR 10-50
Ganciclovir	I	q12h	q24-48h	q48-96h	Dose after dialysis	Dose for GFR <10	2.5 mg/kg day
Gemfibrozil	D	100%	100%	100%	None	Unknown	Dose for GFR 10-50
Gentamicin	D,I	60%-90% q8-12h	30%-70% q12h	20%-30% q24-48h	2/3 normal dose	3-4 mg/L day	Dose for GFR 10-50
Glibornuride	D	Unknown	Unknown	Unknown	Unknown	Unknown	Avoid
Gliclazide	D	Unknown	Unknown	Unknown	Unknown	Unknown	Avoid
Glipizide	D	100%	100%	100%	Unknown	Unknown	Avoid
Glyburide	D	Unknown	Avoid	Avoid	None	None	Avoid
Gold sodium thiomalate	D	50%	Avoid	Avoid	None	None	Avoid
Griseofulvin	D	100%	100%	100%	None	None	None
Guanabenz	D	100%	100%	100%	Unknown	Unknown	Dose for GFR 10-50

(Continued)

Table 48–1 Recommendations for drug dosing in patients with renal impairment—cont'd

Drug	Dose Method	GFR > 50 (mL/min)	GFR 10-50 (mL/min)	GFR < 10 (mL/min)	Supplemental dose after hemodialysis	CAPD	CRRT
Guanadrel	I	q12h	q12-24h	q24-48h	Unknown	Unknown	Dose for GFR 10-50
Guanethidine	I	q24h	q24h	q24-36h	Unknown	Unknown	Avoid
Guanfacine	D	100%	100%	100%	None	None	Dose for GFR 10-50
Haloperidol	D	100%	100%	100%	None	None	Dose for GFR 10-50
Heparin	D	100%	100%	100%	None	None	Dose for GFR 10-50
Hexobarbital	D	100%	100%	100%	None	Unknown	NA
Hydralazine	I	q8h	q8h	q8-16h	None	None	Dose for GFR 10-50
Hydrocortisone	D	100%	100%	100%	Unknown	Unknown	Dose for GFR 10-50
Hydroxyurea	D	100%	50%	20%	Unknown	Unknown	Dose for GFR 10-50
Hydroxyzine	D	100%	Unknown	Unknown	100%	100%	100%
Ibuprofen	D	100%	100%	100%	None	None	Dose for GFR 10-50
Idarubicin		Unknown	Unknown	Unknown	Unknown	Unknown	Unknown
Ifosfamide	D	100%	100%	75%	Unknown	Unknown	Dose for GFR 10-50
Iloprost	D	100%	100%	50%	Unknown	Unknown	Dose for GFR 10-50
Imipenem	D	100%	50%	25%	Dose after dialysis	Dose for GFR<10	Dose for GFR 10-50
Imipramine	D	100%	100%	100%	None	None	NA
Indapamide	D	100%	100%	Avoid	None	None	Not applicable
Indinavir		100%	100%	100%	None	dose for GFR<10	No data
Indobufen	D	100%	50%	25%	Unknown	Unknown	NA
Indomethacin	D	100%	100%	100%	None	None	Dose for GFR 10-50
Insulin	D	100%	75%	50%	None	None	Dose for GFR 10-50
Ipratropium	D	100%	100%	100%	None	None	Dose for GFR 10-50
Isoniazid	D	100%	100%	50%	Dose after dialysis	Dose for GFR <10	Dose for GFR <10
Isosorbide	D	100%	100%	100%	10-20 mg	None	Dose for GFR 10-50
Isradipine	D	100%	100%	100%	None	None	Dose for GFR 10-50
Itraconazole	D	100%	100%	50%	100 mg q12-24h	100 mg q12-24h	100 mg q12-24h
Kanamycin	D,I	60%-90% q8-12h	30%-70% q12h	20%-30% q24-48h	2/3 normal dose	15-20 mg/L day	Dose for GFR 10-50
Ketamine	D	100%	100%	100%	Unknown	Unknown	Dose for GFR 10-50
Ketanserin	D	100%	100%	100%	None	None	Dose for GFR 10-50
Ketoconazole	D	100%	100%	100%	None	None	None
Ketoprofen	D	100%	100%	100%	None	None	Dose for GFR 10-50
Ketorolac	D	100%	50%	50%	None	None	Dose for GFR 10-50
Labetolol	D	100%	100%	100%	None	None	Dose for GFR 10-50
Lamivudine	D,I	100%	50-150 mg qd	25 mg qd	Dose after dialysis	dose for GFR <10	Dose for GFR 10-50
Lamotrigine	D	100%	100%	100%	Unknown	Unknown	Dose for GFR 10-50
Lansoprazole	D	100%	100%	100%	Unknown	Unknown	Unknown
Levodopa	D	100%	100%	100%	Unknown	Unknown	Dose for GFR 10-50
Levofloxacin	D	100%	50%	25%-50%	Dose for GFR <10	Dose for GFR <10	Dose for GFR 10-50
Lidocaine	D	100%	100%	100%	None	None	Dose for GFR 10-50
Lincomycin	I	q6h	q6-12h	q12-24h	None	None	Not applicable

Lisinopril	D	100%	50%-75%	25%-50%	20%	None	Dose for GFR 10-50
Lispro Insulin	D	100%	75%	50%	None	None	None
Lithium carbonate	D	100%	50%-75%	25%-50%	Dose after dialysis	None	Dose for GFR 10-50
Lomefloxacin	D	100%	50%-75%	50%	Dose for GFR <10	Dose for GFR <10	Not applicable
Loracarbef	I	q12h	q24h	q 3-5day	Dose after dialysis	Dose for GFR <10	Dose for GFR 10-50
Lorazepam	D	100%	100%	100%	None	Unknown	Dose for GFR 10-50
Losartan	D	100%	100%	100%	Unknown	Unknown	Dose for GFR 10-50
Lovastatin	D	100%	100%	100%	Unknown	Unknown	Dose for GFR 10-50
Low-molecular-weight heparin	D	100%	100%	50%	Unknown	Unknown	Dose for GFR 10-50
Maprotiline	D	100%	100%	100%	Unknown	Unknown	NA
Meclofenamic acid	D	100%	100%	100%	None	None	Dose for GFR 10-50
Mefenamic acid	D	100%	100%	100%	None	None	Dose for GFR 10-50
Mefloquine		100%	100%	100%	None	None	Dose for GFR 10-50
Melphalan	D	100%	75%	50%	Unknown	Unknown	Dose for GFR 10-50
Meperidine	D	100%	75%	50%	Avoid	None	Avoid
Meprobamate	I	q6h	q9-12h	q12-18h	None	Unknown	NA
Meropenem	D,I	500 mg q6h	250-500 mg q12h	250-500 mg q24h	Dose after dialysis	Dose for GFR <10	Dose for GFR 10-50
Metaproterenol	D	100%	100%	100%	Unknown	Unknown	Dose for GFR 10-50
Metformin	D	50%	25%	Avoid	Unknown	Unknown	Avoid
Methadone	D	100%	100%	50%-75%	None	None	NA
Methenamine mandelate	D	100%	Avoid	Avoid	Not applicable	Not applicable	Not applicable
Methicillin	I	q4-6h	q6-8h	q8-12h	None	None	Dose for GFR 10-50
Methimazole	D	100%	100%	100%	Unknown	Unknown	Dose for GFR 10-50
Methotrexate	D	100%	50%	Avoid	Yes	None	Dose for GFR 10-50
Methyldopa	I	q8h	q8-12h	q12-24h	250 mg	None	Dose for GFR 10-50
Methylprednisolone	D	100%	100%	100%	Yes	Unknown	Dose for GFR 10-50
Metoclopramide	D	100%	75%	50%	None	Unknown	50%-75%
Metocurine	D	75%	50%	50%	Unknown	Unknown	Dose for GFR 10-50
Metolazone	D	100%	100%	100%	None	None	Not applicable
Metoprolol	D	100%	100%	100%	50 mg	None	Dose for GFR 10-50
Metronidazole	D	100%	100%	50%	Dose after dialysis	Dose for GFR <10	Dose for GFR 10-50
Mexiletine	D	100%	100%	50%-75%	None	None	None
Mezlocillin	I	q4-6h	q6-8h	q8h	None	None	Dose for GFR 10-50
Miconazole	D	100%	100%	100%	None	None	None
Midazolam	D	100%	100%	50%	Not applicable	Not applicable	NA
Midodrine		5-10mg q8h	5-10mg q8h	Unknown	5mg q8h	No data	Dose for GFR 10-50
Miglitol	D	50%	Avoid	Avoid	Unknown	Unknown	Avoid
Milrinone	D	100%	100%	50%-75%	No data	No data	Dose for GFR 10-50
Minocycline	D	100%	100%	100%	None	None	Dose for GFR 10-50
Minoxidil	D	100%	100%	100%	None	None	Dose for GFR 10-50
Mitomycin C	D	100%	100%	75%	Unknown	Unknown	Unknown
Mitoxantrone	D	100%	100%	100%	Unknown	Unknown	Dose for GFR 10-50

(Continued)

Table 48–1 Recommendations for drug dosing in patients with renal impairment—cont'd

Drug	Dose Method	GFR > 50 (mL/min)	GFR 10-50 (mL/min)	GFR < 10 (mL/min)	Supplemental dose after hemodialysis	CAPD	CRRT
Mivacurium	D	100%	50%	50%	Unknown	Unknown	Unknown
Moricizine	D	100%	100%	100%	None	None	Dose for GFR 10-50
Morphine	D	100%	75%	50%	None	Unknown	Dose for GFR 10-50
Moxalactam	I	q8-12h	q12-24h	q24-48h	Dose after dialysis	Dose for GFR <10	Dose for GFR 10-50
Nabumetone	D	100%	100%	100%	None	None	Dose for GFR 10-50
N-Acetylcysteine	D	100%	100%	75%	Unknown	Unknown	100%
Nadolol	D	100%	50%	25%	40 mg	None	Dose for GFR 10-50
Nafcillin	D	100%	100%	100%	None	None	Dose for GFR 10-50
Nalidixic acid	D	100%	Avoid	Avoid	Avoid	Avoid	Not applicable
Naloxone	D	100%	100%	100%	Not applicable	Not applicable	Dose for GFR 10-50
Naproxen	D	100%	100%	100%	None	None	Dose for GFR 10-50
Nefazodone	D	100%	100%	100%	Unknown	Unknown	NA
Nelfinavir		No data	No data	No data	No data	No data	No data
Neostigmine	D	100%	50%	25%	Unknown	Unknown	Dose for GFR 10-50
Netlimicin	D,I	50%-90% q8-12h	20%-60% q12h	10%-20% q24-48h	2/3 normal dose	3-4 mg/L day	Dose for GFR 10-50
Nevirapine	D	100%	100%	100%	None	dose for GFR <10	Dose for GFR 10-50
Nicardipine	D	100%	100%	100%	None	None	Dose for GFR 10-50
Nicotinic acid	D	100%	50%	25%	Unknown	Unknown	Dose for GFR 10-50
Nifedipine	D	100%	100%	100%	None	None	Dose for GFR 10-50
Nimodipine	D	100%	100%	100%	None	None	Dose for GFR 10-50
Nisoldipine	D	100%	100%	100%	None	None	Dose for GFR 10-50
Nitrazepam	D	100%	100%	100%	Unknown	Unknown	NA
Nitrofurantoin	D	100%	Avoid	Avoid	Not applicable	Not applicable	Not applicable
Nitroglycerine	D	100%	100%	100%	No data	No data	Dose for GFR 10-50
Nitroprusside	D	100%	100%	100%	None	None	Dose for GFR 10-50
Nitrosoureas	D	100%	75%	25%-50%	None	Unknown	Unknown
Nizatidine	D	75%	50%	25%	Unknown	Unknown	Dose for GFR 10-50
Norfloxacin	I	q12h	q12-24h	Avoid	Not applicable	Not applicable	Not applicable
Nortriptyline	D	100%	100%	100%	None	None	NA
Ofloxacin	D	100%	50%	25%-50%	100 mg bid	Dose for GFR <10	300 mg/day
Omeprazole	D	100%	100%	100%	Unknown	Unknown	Unknown
Ondansetron	D	100%	100%	100%	Unknown	Unknown	Dose for GFR 10-50
Orphenadrine	D	100%	100%	100%	Unknown	Unknown	NA
Ouabain	I	q12-24h	q24-36h	q36-48h	None	None	Dose for GFR 10-50
Oxaproxin	D	100%	100%	100%	None	None	Dose for GFR 10-50
Oxatomide	D	100%	100%	100%	None	None	NA
Oxazepam	D	100%	100%	100%	None	Unknown	Dose for GFR 10-50
Oxcarbazepine	D	100%	100%	100%	Unknown	Unknown	Unknown
Paclitaxel	D	100%	100%	100%	Unknown	Unknown	Dose for GFR 10-50
Pancuronium	D	100%	50%	Avoid	Unknown	Unknown	Dose for GFR 10-50

Paroxetine	D	100%	50%-75%	50%	Unknown	Unknown	NA
PAS	D	100%	50%-75%	50%	Dose after dialysis	Dose for GFR <10	Dose for GFR <10
Penbutolol	D	100%	100%	100%	None	None	Dose for GFR 10-50
Penicillamine	D	100%	Avoid	Avoid	1/3 dose	Unknown	Dose for GFR 10-50
Penicillin G	D	100%	75%	20%-50%	Dose after dialysis	Dose for GFR <10	Dose for GFR 10-50
Penicillin VK	D	100%	100%	100%	Dose after dialysis	Dose for GFR <10	Not applicable
Pentamidine	I	q24h	q24-36h	q48h	None	None	None
Pentazocine	D	100%	75%	50%	None	Unknown	Dose for GFR 10-50
Pentobarbital	D	100%	100%	100%	None	Unknown	Dose for GFR 10-50
Pentopril	D	100%	50%-75%	50%	Unknown	Unknown	Dose for GFR 10-50
Pentoxifylline	D	100%	100%	100%	Unknown	Unknown	100%
Perfloxacin	D	100%	100%	100%	None	None	Dose for GFR 10-50
Perindopril	D	100%	75%	50%	25%-50%	Unknown	Dose for GFR 10-50
Phenelzine	D	100%	100%	100%	Unknown	Unknown	NA
Phenobarbital	I	q8-12h	q8-12h	q12-16h	Dose after dialysis	1/2 normal dose	Dose for GFR 10-50
Phenylbutazone	D	100%	100%	100%	None	None	Dose for GFR 10-50
Phenytoin	D	100%	100%	100%	None	None	None
Pindolol	D	100%	100%	100%	None	None	Dose for GFR 10-50
Pipecuronium	D	100%	50%	25%	Unknown	Unknown	Dose for GFR 10-50
Piperacillin	I	q4-6h	q6-8h	q8h	Dose after dialysis	Dose for GFR <10	Dose for GFR 10-50
Piretanide	D	100%	100%	100%	None	None	Not applicable
Piroxicam	D	100%	100%	100%	None	None	Dose for GFR 10-50
Plicamycin	D	100%	75%	50%	Unknown	Unknown	Unknown
Pravastatin	D	100%	100%	100%	Unknown	Unknown	Dose for GFR 10-50
Prazepam	D	100%	100%	100%	Unknown	Unknown	NA
Prazosin	D	100%	100%	100%	None	None	Dose for GFR 10-50
Prednisolone	D	100%	100%	100%	Yes	Unknown	Dose for GFR 10-50
Prednisone	D	100%	100%	100%	None	Unknown	Dose for GFR 10-50
Primaquine		100%	100%	100%	None	None	Dose for GFR 10-50
Primidone	I	q8h	q8-12h	q12-24h	1/3 dose	Unknown	Unknown
Probenecid	D	100%	Avoid	Avoid	Avoid	Unknown	Avoid
Probucol	D	100%	100%	100%	Unknown	Unknown	Dose for GFR 10-50
Procainamide	I	q4h	q6-12h	q8-24h	200 mg	None	Dose for GFR 10-50
Promethazine	D	100%	100%	100%	Unknown	Unknown	Dose for GFR 10-50
Propafenone	D	100%	100%	100%	None	None	Dose for GFR 10-50
Propofol	D	100%	100%	100%	Unknown	Unknown	Dose for GFR 10-50
Propoxyphene	D	100%	100%	Avoid	None	None	NA
Propranolol	D	100%	100%	100%	None	None	Dose for GFR 10-50
Propylthiouracil	D	100%	100%	100%	Unknown	Unknown	Dose for GFR 10-50
Protryptyline	D	100%	100%	100%	None	None	NA
Pyrazinimide	D	100%	Avoid	Avoid	Avoid	Avoid	Avoid
Pyridostigmine	D	50%	35%	20%	Unknown	Unknown	Dose for GFR 10-50
Pyrimethamine	D	100%	100%	100%	None	None	None

(Continued)

Table 48–1 Recommendations for drug dosing in patients with renal impairment—cont'd

Drug	Dose Method	GFR > 50 (mL/min)	GFR 10-50 (mL/min)	GFR < 10 (mL/min)	Supplemental dose after hemodialysis	CAPD	CRRT
Quazepam	D	Unknown	Unknown	Unknown	Unknown	Unknown	NA
Quinapril	D	100%	75%-100%	75%	25%	None	Dose for GFR 10-50
Quinidine	D	100%	100%	75%	100-200 mg	None	Dose for GFR 10-50
Quinine	I	q8h	q8-12h	q24h	Dose after dialysis	Dose for GFR <10	Dose for GFR 10-50
Ramipril	D	100%	50%-75%	25%-50%	20%	None	Dose for GFR 10-50
Ranitidine	D	75%	50%	25%	1/2 dose	None	Dose for GFR 10-50
Reserpine	D	100%	100%	Avoid	None	None	Dose for GFR 10-50
Ribavirin	D	100%	100%	50%	Dose after dialysis	Dose for GFR <10	Dose for GFR <10
Rifabutin		100%	100%	100%	None	None	Dose for GFR 10-50
Rifampin	D	100%	50%-100%	50%-100%	None	Dose for GFR <10	Dose for GFR <10
Ritonavir		100%	100%	100%	None	Dose for GFR <10	Dose for GFR 10-50
Saquinavir		100%	100%	100%	None	Dose for GFR <10	Dose for GFR 10-50
Secobarbital	D	100%	100%	100%	None	None	NA
Sertraline	D	100%	100%	100%	Unknown	Unknown	NA
Simvastatin	D	100%	100%	100%	Unknown	Unknown	Dose for GFR 10-50
Sodium valproate	D	100%	100%	100%	None	None	None
Sotalol	D	100%	30%	15%-30%	80 mg	None	Dose for GFR 10-50
Sparfloxacin	D,I	100%	50%-75%	50% q48h	dose for GFR <10	No data	Dose for GFR 10-50
Spectinomycin	D	100%	100%	100%	None	None	None
Spironolactone	I	q6-12h	q12-24h	Avoid	Not applicable	Not applicable	Avoid
Stavudine	D,I	100%	50% q12-24h	50% q24h	Dose after dialysis	No data	Dose for GFR 10-50
Streptokinase	D	100%	100%	100%	Not applicable	Not applicable	Dose for GFR 10-50
Streptomycin	I	q24h	q24-72h	q72-96h	1/2 normal dose	20-40 mg/L day	Dose for GFR 10-50
Streptozotocin	D	100%	75%	50%	Unknown	Unknown	Unknown
Succinylcholine	D	100%	100%	100%	Unknown	Unknown	Dose for GFR 10-50
Sufentanil	D	100%	100%	100%	Unknown	Unknown	Dose for GFR 10-50
Sulbactam	I	q6-8h	q12-24h	q24-48h	Dose after dialysis	0.75-1.5 g/day	750 mg q12h
Sulfamethoxazole	I	q12h	q18h	q24h	1 g after dialysis	1 g/d	Dose for GFR 10-50
Sulfinpyrazone	D	100%	100%	Avoid	None	None	Dose for GFR 10-50
Sulfisoxazole	I	q6h	q8-12h	q12-24h	2 g after dialysis	3 g/d	Not applicable
Sulindac	D	100%	100%	100%	None	None	Dose for GFR 10-50
Sulotroban	D	50%	30%	10%	Unknown	Unknown	Unknown
Tamoxifen	D	100%	100%	100%	Unknown	Unknown	Dose for GFR 10-50
Tazobactam	D	100%	75%	50%	1/3 dose	Dose for GFR <10	Dose for GFR 10-50
Teicoplanin	I	q24h	q48h	q72h	Dose for GFR <10	Dose for GFR <10	Dose for GFR 10-50
Temazepam	D	100%	100%	100%	None	None	NA
Teniposide	D	100%	100%	100%	None	None	Dose for GFR 10-50
Terazosin	D	100%	100%	100%	Unknown	Unknown	Dose for GFR 10-50
Terbutaline	D	100%	50%	Avoid	Unknown	Unknown	Dose for GFR 10-50
Terfenadine	D	100%	100%	100%	None	None	NA
Tetracycline	I	q8-12h	q12-24h	q24h	None	None	Dose for GFR 10-50

Theophylline	D	100%	100%	100%	1/2 dose	Unknown	Dose for GFR 10-50
Thiazides	D	100%	100%	Avoid	Not applicable	Not applicable	Not applicable
Thiopental	D	100%	100%	75%	Not applicable	Not applicable	NA
Ticarcillin	D,I	1-2 g q4h	1-2 g q8h	1-2 g q12h	3 g after dialysis	Dose for GFR <10	Dose for GFR 10-50
Ticlopidine	D	100%	100%	100%	Unknown	Unknown	Dose for GFR 10-50
Timolol	D	100%	100%	100%	None	None	Dose for GFR 10-50
Tobramycin	D,I	60%-90% q8-12h	30%-70% q12h	20%-30% q24-48h	2/3 normal dose	3-4 mg/L d	Dose for GFR 10-50
Tocainide	D	100%	100%	50%	200 mg	None	Dose for GFR 10-50
Tolazamide	D	100%	100%	100%	Unknown	Unknown	Avoid
Tolbutamide	D	100%	100%	100%	None	None	Avoid
Tolmetin	D	100%	100%	100%	None	None	Dose for GFR 10-50
Topiramate	D	100%	50%	25%	Unknown	Unknown	Dose for GFR 10-50
Topotecan	D	75%	50%	25%	Unknown	Unknown	Dose for GFR 10-50
Torsemide	D	100%	100%	100%	None	None	NA
Tranexamic acid	D	50%	25%	10%	Unknown	Unknown	Unknown
Tranylcypromine	D	Unknown	Unknown	Unknown	Unknown	Unknown	NA
Trazodone	D	100%	Unknown	Unknown	Unknown	Unknown	NA
Triamcinolone	D	100%	100%	100%	Unknown	Unknown	Dose for GFR 10-50
Triamterene	I	q12h	q12h	Avoid	Not applicable	Not applicable	Avoid
Triazolam	D	100%	100%	100%	None	None	NA
Trihexyphenidyl	D	Unknown	Unknown	Unknown	Unknown	Unknown	Unknown
Trimethadione	I	q8h	q8-12h	q12-24h	Unknown	Unknown	Dose for GFR 10-50
Trimethoprim	I	q12h	q18h	q24h	Dose after dialysis	q24h	q18h
Trimetrexate	D	100%	50%-100%	Avoid	No data	No data	No data
Trimipramine	D	100%	100%	100%	None	None	NA
Tripelennamine	D	Unknown	Unknown	Unknown	Unknown	Unknown	NA
Triprolidine	D	Unknown	Unknown	Unknown	Unknown	Unknown	NA
Tubocurarine	D	75%	50%	Avoid	Unknown	Unknown	Dose for GFR 10-50
Urokinase	D	Unknown	Unknown	Unknown	Unknown	Unknown	Dose for GFR 10-50
Vancomycin	D,I	500 mg q6-12h	500 mg q24-48h	500 mg q48-96h	Dose for GFR <10	Dose for GFR <10	Dose for GFR 10-50
Vecuronium	D	100%	100%	100%	Unknown	Unknown	Dose for GFR 10-50
Venlafaxine	D	75%	50%	50%	None	Unknown	NA
Verapamil	D	100%	100%	100%	None	None	Dose for GFR 10-50
Vidarabine	D	100%	100%	75%	Infuse after dialysis	Dose for GFR <10	Dose for GFR 10-50
Vigabatrin	D	100%	50%	25%	Unknown	Unknown	Dose for GFR 10-50
Vinblastine	D	100%	100%	100%	Unknown	Unknown	Dose for GFR 10-50
Vincristine	D	100%	100%	100%	Unknown	Unknown	Dose for GFR 10-50
Vinorelbine	D	100%	100%	100%	Unknown	Unknown	Dose for GFR 10-50
Warfarin	D	100%	100%	100%	None	None	None
Zafirlukast	D	100%	100%	100%	Unknown	Unknown	Dose for GFR 10-50
Zalcitabine	I	100%	q 12 h	q 24 h	Dose after dialysis	No data	Dose for GFR 10-50
Zidovudine (AZT)	D,I	200 mg q8h	200 mg q8h	100 mg q8h	Dose for GFR <10	Dose for GFR <10	100 mg q8h
Zileuton		100%	100%	100%	None	Unknown	Dose for GFR 10-50

drug. Peritoneal urea clearance is approximately 20 mL/min. In general, if a drug is not removed by hemodialysis, it will not be removed by peritoneal dialysis.

Drug transport by the peritoneal membrane is unidirectional.[23] Although peritoneal dialysis does not rapidly remove drugs, many are well absorbed when placed in peritoneal dialysate.

Molecular weight, membrane characteristics, blood flow rate, and the addition of dialysate determine the rate and extent of drug removal during continuous renal replacement therapies (CRRT). Molecular weight effects drug removal by diffusion during dialysis more than during convection during CRRT because of the large pore size of membranes used for CRRT. Because most drugs are less than 1500 Da, drug removal by CRRT does not depend greatly on molecular weight.

The volume of distribution of a drug is the most important factor determining removal by CRRT. Drugs with a large volume of distribution are highly tissue bound and not accessible to extracorporeal circuit in quantities sufficient to result in substantial removal by CRRT. Even if the extraction across the artificial membrane is 100%, only a small amount of a drug with a large volume of distribution is removed. A volume of distribution greater than 0.7 L/Kg substantially decreases CRRT drug removal.

Drug protein binding also determines how much is removed during CRRT. Only unbound drug is available for elimination by CRRT. Protein binding of more than 80% provides a substantial barrier to drug removal by convection or diffusion. During continuous hemofiltration, an ultrafiltration rate of 10-30 mL/min is achieved. The addition of diffusion by continuous dialysis increases drug clearance, depending on blood and dialysate flow rates. As during high flux dialysis, drug removal parallels the removal of urea and creatinine. The simplest method for estimating drug removal during CRRT is to estimate urea or creatinine clearance during the procedure.[24]

Recommendations for dosing selected drugs in patients with impaired renal function are given in Table 48–1. These recommendations are meant only as a guide and do not imply efficacy or safety of a recommended dose in an individual patient. A loading dose equivalent to the usual dose in patients with normal renal function should be considered for drugs with a particularly long half-life. The table indicates potential methods for adjusting the dose, either by decreasing the individual doses (D) or increasing the dose interval (I). In the table, when the dose method is suggested, the percentage of the dose for normal renal function is given. When the interval method is suggested, the actual dose interval is provided.

Prolonging the dose interval is often more convenient and less expensive. When the dose interval can safely be lengthened beyond 24 hours, extended parenteral therapy may be completed without prolonging hospitalization. In patients requiring chronic hemodialysis, many drugs need to be given only at the end of the dialysis treatment. Further, compliance with any drug regimen may be better when fewer doses can be taken at convenient times. In practice, a combination interval prolongation and dose-size reduction is often effective and convenient.

The effect of the standard clinical treatment on drug removal is shown for hemodialysis, chronic ambulatory peritoneal dialysis, and continuous renal replacement therapy. Most of these recommendations were established before very high efficiency hemodialysis treatments were practical, continuous cycling nocturnal peritoneal dialysis was common, and diffusion was added to hemofiltration in continuous renal replacement therapies. Some drugs that have high dialysis clearance do not require supplemental doses after dialysis, if the amount of the drug removed is not sufficient, as would be the case if the volume of distribution were large. To ensure efficacy when information about dialysis loss is not available and to simplify dosimetry, maintenance doses of most drugs should be given after dialysis.

Peritonitis is a major complication of peritoneal dialysis, and treatment usually involves intraperitoneal administration of antibiotics. For some drugs, sophisticated pharmacokinetic studies are available, whereas for others use is still based on empirical dosage recommendations. In general, there is excellent drug absorption after intraperitoneal administration of common antibiotics. Factors favoring absorption include inflamed membranes and concentration gradients. For many drugs, peritoneal fluid levels after intravenous or oral administration are inconsistent.

DRUG LEVEL MONITORING

If there is a known relationship between drug efficacy or toxicity and plasma drug concentrations, blood levels may serve as a guide to drug therapy. These measurements are most important for drugs with a narrow therapeutic range and they are useful when pharmacological effects are difficult to determine.

To ensure that steady state serum concentrations have been obtained, three or four doses of the drug should be administered before serum levels are measured. Peak levels are most meaningful when measured after rapid drug distribution has occurred. Conversely, minimum concentrations are usually measured just before giving the next scheduled dose.

Patients with renal disease are heterogeneous and their response to drug therapy is variable. Dosage nomograms, drug tables, and computer-assisted dosing recommendations provide guidelines for an initial drug administration in patients with decreased renal function. Individualizing the dose regimen for each patient requires continuing evaluation of the therapeutic response for drug efficacy and toxicity.

References

1. Manley HJ, Bailie GR, Grabe DW. Comparing medication use in two hemodialysis units against national dialysis databases. Am J Health Syst Pharm 2000; 57(9):902-906.
2. Jick H. Adverse drug effects in relation to renal function. Am J Med 1977; 62:514-517.
3. Pearson TF, Pittman DG, Longley JM, et al. Factors associated with preventable adverse drug reactions. Am J Hosp Pharm 1994; 51(18):2268-2272.
4. Aronoff GR, Abel SR. Principles of administering drugs to patients with renal failure. In: Bennett WM, McCarron DA, Brenner BM, Stein JH, eds. Contemporary issues in nephrology. Pharmacotherapy of renal diseases and hypertension. New York: Churchill-Livingston, 1987:1.
5. Cockcroft DW, Gault MH. Prediction of creatinine clearance from serum creatinine. Nephron 1976; 16(1):31-41.
6. Baily DG, Arnold JM, Munoz C, Spence JD. Grapefruit juice - felodipine interaction: mechanism, predictability, and effect of naringin. Clin Pharmacol Ther 1993; 53:637.

7. Min DI, Ku YM, Perry PJ, et al. Effect of grapefruit juice on cyclosporine pharmacokinetics in renal transplant patients. Transplantation. 1996; 62(1):123-125.
8. Anderson RJ, Gambertoglio JG, Schrier RW. Clinical use of drugs in renal failure. Springfield, IL: Charles C. Thomas, 1976.
9. Hurwitz A. Antacid therapy and drug kinetics. Clin Pharmacokin 1977; 2:269-280.
10. Maton PN, Burton ME. Antacids revisited: a review of their clinical pharmacology and recommended therapeutic use. Drugs 1999; 57(6):855-870.
11. Craig RM, Murphy P, Gibson TP, Quintanilla A. Kinetic analysis of D-xylose absorption in normal subjects and in patients with chronic renal failure. J Lab Clin Med 1983; 101:496-506.
12. Dromgoole SH. The binding capacity of albumin and renal disease. J Pharmacol Exp Ther 1974; 191:318-323.
13. Reidenberg MM, Affrime M. Influence of disease on binding of drugs to plasma proteins. Ann NY Acad Sci 1973; 226:115-126.
14. Reidenberg MM, Odar-Cederlof I, Von Bahr C, et al. Protein binding of diphenylhydantoin and desmethylimipramine in plasma from patients with poor renal function. N Engl J Med 1971; 285:264-267.
15. Reidenberg MM. The binding of drugs to plasma proteins and the interpretation of measurements of plasma concentration of drugs in patients with poor renal function. Am J Med 1977; 62: 466-470.
16. Reidenberg MN. The biotransformation of drugs in renal failure. Am J Med 1977; 62:482-485.
17. Leblond F, Guevin C, Demers C, et al. Downregulation of hepatic cytochrome P450 in chronic renal failure. J Amer Soc Neph 2001; 12(2):326-332.
18. Macias WL, Mueller BA, Scarim SK. Vancomycin pharmacokinetics in acute renal failure; preservation of nonrenal clearance. Clin Pharmacol Ther 1991; 50:688-694.
19. Aronoff GR, Berns JS, Brier ME, et al. Drug prescribing in renal failure. dosing guidelines for adults. Philadelphia: American College of Physicians, 1999.
20. Maher JF. Pharmacokinetics in patients with renal failure. Clin Nephrol 1984; 21:39-46.
21. Oosterhuis WP, de Metz M, Wadham A, et al. In Vivo Evaluation of Four Hemodialysis Membranes: Biocompatibility and Clearances. Dialysis & Transpl 1995; 24(8):450-4.
22. Paton TW, Cornish WR, Manuel MA, Hardy BG. Drug therapy in patients undergoing peritoneal dialysis: clinical pharmacokinetic considerations. Clin Pharmacokin 1985; 10:404-426.
23. Bunke CM, Aronoff GR, Brier ME, Sloan RS, Luft FC. Cefazolin and cephalexin kinetics in continuous ambulatory peritoneal dialysis. Clin Pharm Ther 1983; 33:66-72.
24. Keller F, Bohler J, Czock D, et al. Individualized drug dosage in patients treated with continuous hemofiltration.Kidney Int Suppl 1999; 72:S29-S31.

Index

Page numbers followed by f indicate figures; t, tables

D

E

H

J

K

T

W

X

Z